Institute for Safe Medication Practices

ISMP's List of *Error-Prone Abbreviations, Symbols, and Dose Designations* (continued)

Dose Designations and Other Information	Intended Meaning	Misinterpretation	Correction
Drug name and dose run together (especially problematic for drug names that end in "l" such as Inderal40 mg; Tegretol300 mg)	Inderal 40 mg Tegretol 300 mg	Mistaken as Inderal 140 mg Mistaken as Tegretol 1300 mg	Place adequate space between the drug name, dose, and unit of measure
Numerical dose and unit of measure run together (e.g., 10mg, 100mL)	10 mg 100 mL	The "m" is sometimes mistaken as a zero or two zeros, risking a 10- to 100-fold overdose	Place adequate space between the dose and unit of measure
Abbreviations such as mg. or mL. with a period following the abbreviation	mg mL	The period is unnecessary and could be mistaken as the number 1 if written poorly	Use mg, mL, etc. without a terminal period
Large doses without properly placed commas (e.g., 100000 units; 1000000 units)	100,000 units 1,000,000 units	100000 has been mistaken as 10,000 or 1,000,000; 1000000 has been mistaken as 100,000	Use commas for dosing units at or above 1,000, or use words such as 100 "thousand" or 1 "million" to improve readability

Drug Name Abbreviations	Intended Meaning	Misinterpretation	Correction
ARA A	vidarabine	Mistaken as cytarabine (ARA C)	Use complete drug name
AZT	zidovudine (Retrovir)	Mistaken as azathioprine or aztreonam	Use complete drug name
CPZ	Compazine (prochlorperazine)	Mistaken as chlorpromazine	Use complete drug name
DPT	Demerol-Phenergan-Thorazine	Mistaken as diphtheria-pertussis-tetanus (vaccine)	Use complete drug name
DTO	Diluted tincture of opium, or deodorized tincture of opium (Paregoric)	Mistaken as tincture of opium	Use complete drug name
HCl	hydrochloric acid or hydrochloride	Mistaken as potassium chloride (The "H" is misinterpreted as "K")	Use complete drug name unless expressed as a salt of a drug
HCT	hydrocortisone	Mistaken as hydrochlorothiazide	Use complete drug name
HCTZ	hydrochlorothiazide	Mistaken as hydrocortisone (seen as HCT250 mg)	Use complete drug name
MgSO4**	magnesium sulfate	Mistaken as morphine sulfate	Use complete drug name
MS, MSO4**	morphine sulfate	Mistaken as magnesium sulfate	Use complete drug name
MTX	methotrexate	Mistaken as mitoxantrone	Use complete drug name
PCA	procainamide	Mistaken as patient controlled analgesia	Use complete drug name
PTU	propylthiouracil	Mistaken as mercaptopurine	Use complete drug name
T3	Tylenol with codeine No. 3	Mistaken as liothyronine	Use complete drug name
TAC	triamcinolone	Mistaken as tetracaine, Adrenalin, cocaine	Use complete drug name
TNK	TNKase	Mistaken as "TPA"	Use complete drug name
ZnSO4	zinc sulfate	Mistaken as morphine sulfate	Use complete drug name

Stemmed Drug Names	Intended Meaning	Misinterpretation	Correction
"Nitro" drip	nitroglycerin infusion	Mistaken as sodium nitroprusside infusion	Use complete drug name
"Norflox"	norfloxacin	Mistaken as Norflex	Use complete drug name
"IV Vanc"	intravenous vancomycin	Mistaken as Invanz	Use complete drug name

Symbols	Intended Meaning	Misinterpretation	Correction
ℨ	Dram	Symbol for dram mistaken as "3"	Use the metric system
♏	Minim	Symbol for minim mistaken as "mL"	
x3d	For three days	Mistaken as "3 doses"	Use "for three days"
> and <	Greater than and less than	Mistaken as opposite of intended; mistakenly use incorrect symbol; "< 10" mistaken as "40"	Use "greater than" or "less than"
/ (slash mark)	Separates two doses or indicates "per"	Mistaken as the number 1 (e.g., "25 units/10 units" misread as "25 units and 110" units)	Use "per" rather than a slash mark to separate doses
@	At	Mistaken as "2"	Use "at"
&	And	Mistaken as "2"	Use "and"
+	Plus or and	Mistaken as "4"	Use "and"
°	Hour	Mistaken as a zero (e.g., q2° seen as q 20)	Use "hr," "h," or "hour"

© ISMP 2006

**These abbreviations are included on TJC's "minimum list" of dangerous abbreviations, acronyms and symbols that must be included on an organization's "Do Not Use" list, effective January 1, 2004. Visit www.jointcommission.org for more information about this TJC requirement.

Institute for Safe Medication Practices
www.ismp.org

MEDICAL-SURGICAL
NURSING
Clinical Management for Positive Outcomes

MEDICAL-SURGICAL NURSING
Clinical Management for Positive Outcomes

EIGHTH EDITION

Joyce M. Black,
PhD, RN, CPSN, CWCN, FAPWCA
Associate Professor
College of Nursing
University of Nebraska Medical Center
Omaha, Nebraska

Jane Hokanson Hawks,
PhD, RN, BC
Professor of Nursing
Nebraska Methodist College
Omaha, Nebraska

SAUNDERS

ELSEVIER

SAUNDERS
ELSEVIER

11830 Westline Industrial Drive
St. Louis, Missouri 63146

MEDICAL-SURGICAL NURSING   ISBN: 978-1-4160-3641-8 (Single Volume)
Clinical Management for Positive Outcomes   978-4160-4687-5 (Two-Volume Set)

Copyright © 2009 by Saunders, an imprint of Elsevier Inc.

Notice

Knowledge and best practice in this field are constantly changing. As new research and experience broaden our knowledge, changes in practice, treatment and drug therapy may become necessary or appropriate. Readers are advised to check the most current information provided (i) on procedures featured or (ii) by the manufacturer of each product to be administered, to verify the recommended dose or formula, the method and duration of administration, and contraindications. It is the responsibility of the practitioner, relying on their own experience and knowledge of the patient, to make diagnoses, to determine dosages and the best treatment for each individual patient, and to take all appropriate safety precautions. To the fullest extent of the law, neither the Publisher nor the Authors assume any liability for any injury and/or damage to persons or property arising out of or related to any use of the material contained in this book.

The Publisher

Previous editions copyrighted 2005, 2001, 1997, 1993, 1987, 1980, 1974.

Library of Congress Control Numbers: 2008922504 (Single Volume)
2008922503 (Two-Volume Set)

Executive Publisher: Tom Wilhelm
Managing Editor: Maureen Iannuzzi
Senior Developmental Editor: Jennifer Ehlers
Publishing Services Manager: Deborah L. Vogel
Design Direction: Louis Forgione

Printed in China

Last digit is the print number: 9 8 7 6 5 4 3 2

When I walked into the hospital, I used to see a sign that said, "Enter in to learn, go forth to serve." Therefore this book is dedicated to those patients and students who taught me the value of caring and teaching, and I hope they can serve others through my efforts here. I continue to appreciate the quiet contributions and support of my colleagues. And I thank my family—Steve, Jon, Katy, and Tricia, and my newest family members, Katie, Josh, and Elly—for their ongoing understanding of the considerable strain on my time and energy.

— J.M.B.

To the clients, nurses, students, and faculty I learned and continue to learn from; to my parents, Esther and the late Charles Hokanson, who laid the foundation for my role as a nurse, author, editor, speaker, and educator; and to my husband, Edward, and my daughter, Jennifer, whose love, support, and understanding remain constant.

— J.H.H.

About the Authors

Joyce M. Black, PhD, RN, CPSN, CWCN, FAPWCA, is an Associate Professor of Nursing at the University of Nebraska Medical Center, College of Nursing, in Omaha, Nebraska. She teaches medical-surgical nursing to junior- and senior-level nursing students. Dr. Black also teaches advanced pathophysiology to graduate students. Dr. Black received her Doctor of Philosophy degree from the University of Nebraska Medical Center; her Master of Science in Nursing degree and Clinical Nurse Specialist designation from the University of Nebraska Medical Center; her Bachelor of Science in Nursing degree from Winona State University in Winona, Minnesota; and her Associate's degree in Nursing from Rochester Community College in Rochester, Minnesota.

Dr. Black has had several years of clinical experience as a medical-surgical nurse at Saint Mary's Hospital in Rochester, Minnesota, which is affiliated with the Mayo Clinic. Her clinical practice has been in orthopedics, critical care, burn care, respiratory diseases, wound care, and plastic surgery. She is certified by the Wound, Ostomy and Continence Nurses Society and the American Society of Plastic Surgical Nurses. She is also a Fellow in the American Professional Wound Care Association. Dr. Black is the immediate past president of the National Pressure Ulcer Advisory Panel. She was chairperson of the NPUAP task force to update the stages of pressure ulcers and co-chairperson of the deep tissue injury task force. Her primary research expertise is in the area of deep tissue injury, pressure ulcers, and wound healing.

Jane Hokanson Hawks, PhD, RN, BC, is a Professor of Nursing at Nebraska Methodist College in Omaha, Nebraska. She teaches students in the MSN Nurse Executive track. Previously, she taught undergraduate students in medical-surgical nursing, advanced medical-surgical nursing, trends and issues, and nursing management. Dr. Hawks received her Doctor of Philosophy in collegiate nursing education from Widener University in Chester, Pennsylvania; her Master of Science in Nursing degree in medical-surgical nursing and nursing administration from the University of Nebraska Medical Center College of Nursing in Omaha, Nebraska; and her Bachelor of Science in Nursing degree from St. Olaf College in Northfield, Minnesota.

Dr. Hawks has worked in and has taught medical-surgical nursing for more than 30 years. She has practiced in a variety of areas, including critical care, renal transplantation, orthopedics, general surgery, and urology. She serves as the editor of *Urologic Nursing*. Her areas of research include empowerment, mentoring, nursing education, active teaching strategies, and alcoholism. She and her colleagues developed the NANDA nursing diagnosis Altered Family Process: Alcoholism (now known as Dysfunctional Family Processes: Alcoholism). Dr. Hawks co-authored *Mentoring for Mission: Nurturing New Faculty at Church-Related Colleges,* which was funded through a grant from the Lilly Fellows Foundation.

Section Editors

Robert G. Carroll, PhD
Professor
Department of Physiology
Brody School of Medicine
East Carolina University
Greenville, North Carolina

Susanne A. Quallich, BS, BSN, MSN, APRN, BC, NP-C, CUNP
Adjunct Faculty
University of Michigan School of Nursing
Andrology Nurse Practitioner
Division of Andrology and Microsurgery
Department of Urology
University of Michigan Medical Center
Ann Arbor, Michigan

Contributors

Donna M. Barker, MS, APRN, ANP-BC, ONC, RN-C
Pain Management Nurse Practitioner
St. Alexius Medical Center
Hoffman Estates, Illinois

Francie Bernier, PhD(c), RNC
Doctoral Candidate
University of Virginia
School of Nursing
Charlottesville, Virginia;
Principal Clinical Research Scientist
Hollister Incorporated
Libertyville, Illinois

Meg Blair, RN, MSN, CEN, PhD(c)
Associate Professor
Nebraska Methodist College of Nursing and Allied Health
Omaha, Nebraska

Lisa Bowman, MSN, RN, CRNP, CNRN
Nurse Practitioner
Division of Cerebrovascular Disease and Neurological Critical Care
Thomas Jefferson University Hospital
Philadelphia, Pennsylvania

Robert G. Carroll, PhD
Professor
Department of Physiology
Brody School of Medicine
East Carolina University
Greenville, North Carolina

Gretchen J. Carrougher, RN, MN
Research Nurse Supervisor
Department of Surgery
University of Washington Burn Center at Harborview
   Medical Center
Seattle, Washington;
Clinical Instructor
Department of Biobehavioral Nursing and Health Systems
University of Washington School of Nursing
Seattle, Washington

'Lissa D. Clark, BS, BSN, MSN, CNE
Instructor, Adult Health and Illness Department
College of Nursing
University of Nebraska Medical Center
Omaha, Nebraska

Linda Carman Copel, PhD, APRN BC, NCC, DAPA
Associate Professor
Villanova University
Villanova, Pennsylvania

Melissa Craft, RN, PhD, AOCN
Adjunct Clinical Professor
University of Oklahoma
Oklahoma City, Oklahoma;
Oncology Clinical Nurse Specialist
Breast Imaging of Oklahoma
Edmond, Oklahoma

Sherill Nones Cronin, PhD, RN, BC
MSN Program Director and Professor of Nursing
Bellarmine University
Louisville, Kentucky;
Consultant
Baptist Hospital East
Louisville, Kentucky

Beth F. Crowder, BSN, MNSc, PhD, RN, APN
Advanced Practice Nurse
Little Rock Cardiology Clinic
Little Rock, Arkansas

Susan L. Dean-Baar, RN, PhD, CRRN, FAAN
Associate Dean for Academic Affairs
University of Wisconsin–Milwaukee
Milwaukee, Wisconsin

Marie A. DeFrancesco-Loukas, MSN, CRNP
Nurse Practitioner; Clinical Manager
GoodNights Urgent Care
Hershey, Pennsylvania;
Pediatric Inpatient Nurse Practitioner
Harrisburg Hospital
Harrisburg, Pennsylvania

Jean E. DeMartinis, PhD, APRN-BC, FNP
Associate Professor and Director DNP and CNL Graduate
   Programs
School of Nursing
University of Massachusetts–Amherst
Amherst, Massachusetts

Margaret M. Ecklund, RN, MS, CCRN, APRN-BC
Clinician VI/Nurse Practitioner
Rochester General Hospital
Rochester, NY

Charlotte Eliopoulos, PhD, RNC, MPH, ND
Executive Director
American Association for Long Term Care Nursing
Glen Arm, Maryland

James A. Fain, PhD, RN, BC-ADM, FAAN
Dean and Professor, College of Nursing
University of Massachusetts–Dartmouth
North Dartmouth, Massachusetts

Kathryn Fiandt, DNS, FAANP
Professor and Associate Dean for Clinical Affairs
University of Texas Medical Branch
Galveston, Texas

Nancy J. Girard, RN, PhD, FAAN
Associate Professor and Chair
Acute Nursing Care Department
University of Texas Health Science Center–San Antonio
School of Nursing
San Antonio, Texas

Patricia E. Graham, MSN, RN, BC
Assistant Professor
Department of Nursing Education
Morningside College
Sioux City, Iowa

Mikel Gray, PhD, FNP, PNP, CUNP, CCCN, FAAN, FAANP
University of Virginia
Department of Urology and School of Nursing
Charlottesville, Virginia

Sheila A. Haas, PhD, RN, FAAN
Professor
Niehoff School of Nursing
Loyola University Chicago
Chicago, Illinois

Diana P. Hackbarth, RN, PhD, FAAN
Professor
Niehoff School of Nursing
Loyola University Chicago
Chicago, Illinois

Judith S. Halpern, MS, NP, APRN, BC
Lecturer, RN Studies
School of Nursing
University of Michigan
Kalamazoo, Michigan

Allen Hanberg, RN, MSN, PhD(c)
Assistant Professor
Clinical College of Nursing
University of Utah
Salt Lake City, Utah

Karen Hanson, RN, MS, CNP
Gastroenterology Nurse Practitioner
Mayo Clinic
Rochester, Minnesota

Debra E. Heidrich, MSN, RN, ACHPN, AOCN
Palliative Care Clinical Nurse Specialist
Bethesda North Hospital, TriHealth, Inc.
Cincinnati, Ohio

Lianne F. Herbruck, MSN, RN, CNM
Health Care Consultant and Nursing Educator
Chagrin Falls, Ohio

Patricia A. Keresztes, RN, PhD, CCRN
Assistant Professor of Nursing
Saint Mary's College
Notre Dame, Indiana;
Staff Nurse, Cardiovascular Intensive Care Unit
Memorial Hospital
South Bend, Indiana

Helene J. Krouse, PhD, APRN, BC, CORLN, FAAN
Professor of Nursing
Wayne State University
Detroit, Michigan

Judi L. Kuric, PhD, MSN, RN, APRN-BC, CRRN-A, CNRN
Adjunct Assistant Professor
University of Southern Indiana
Acute Care Nurse Practitioner
Tri State Neurosurgical, Inc.
Evansville, Indiana

Sharon Lanzetta, MSN, RN, C
Ambulatory Care Nurse Manager
University of Michigan Health System
Ann Arbor, Michigan

Joan M. Lappe, PhD, RN, FAAN
Criss/Beirne Endowed Chair in Nursing and Professor
  of Medicine
Creighton University
Omaha, Nebraska

Mira Lessick, PhD, RN
Associate Professor
The University of Toledo
College of Nursing
Toledo, Ohio

Patricia A. MacDonald, RN, NP
Senior Clinical Research Specialist
TAP Pharmaceutical Products, Inc.
Lake Forest, Illinois

Patricia A. Manion, RN, MS, CCRN, CEN
Trauma Program Administrator
Genesys Regional Medical Center
Grand Blanc, Michigan

Karen S. Martin, MSN, RN, FAAN
Health Care Consultant
Martin Associates
Omaha, Nebraska

Norma D. McNair, MSN, RN, CCRN, CNRN, APRN-BC
Assistant Clinical Professor
University of California–Los Angeles School of Nursing
Neuroscience Clinical Nurse Specialist
University of California–Los Angeles Medical Center
Los Angeles, California

Anita Meehan, MSN, RN, ONC, CNOR(e)
Clinical Nurse Specialist
Medical/Surgical and Gerontology
Akron General Medical Center
Akron, Ohio;
Clinical Faculty
Kent State University College of Nursing
Kent, Ohio
University of Akron College of Nursing
Akron, Ohio

Lindsay A. Middelton, BSN, CGC
Genetic Counselor and Senior Research Nurse
Urologic Oncology Branch
National Institutes of Health
National Cancer Institute
Bethesda, Maryland

Kim Miracle, MSN, RN, C
Clinical Coordinator
Quality Care and Outcomes Management Department
Jewish Hospital
Louisville, Kentucky

Anita E. Molzahn, PhD, MN, BScN
Professor
School of Nursing
University of Victoria
Victoria, British Columbia
Canada

Diana Moxness, RN, BSN, MSN
Assistant Professor
Department of Nursing
Midland Lutheran College
Fremont, Nebraska

Mark Moyad, MD, MPH
Phil F. Jenkins Director of Complementary Medicine
Urologic Oncology
Clinical Cancer Researcher/Consultant
University of Michigan
Ann Arbor, Michigan

Dawn P. Murphy, MSN, CRNP
Oncology Nurse Practitioner
Abramson Cancer Center
Hospital of The University of Pennsylvania
Philadelphia, Pennsylvania

Louise Nelson LaFramboise, RN, PhD
Director, Undergraduate Program
University of Nebraska Medical Center
Omaha, Nebraska

Susan Newton, RN, MS, AOCN, AOCNS
Oncology Advanced Practice Nurse
Project Leader, Innovex
Dayton, Ohio

Noreen Heer Nicol, MS, RN, FNP
Clinical Senior Instructor
University of Colorado
Denver, Colorado;
Affiliate Assistant Professor
University of Northern Colorado
Greeley, Colorado;
Chief Clinical Officer/Chief Nursing Officer
National Jewish Medical and Research Center
Denver, Colorado

Catherine Nosek, PhD, RN
Associate Professor
Undergraduate Nursing Education
Winona State University
Winona, Minnesota

Barbara B. Ott, RN, PhD
Associate Professor
Villanova University
Villanova, Pennsylvania

Mary Ellen Pike, RN, MSN, MA, PhD(c)
Assistant Professor
Bellarmine University
Louisville, Kentucky

Susanne A. Quallich, BS, BSN, MSN, APRN, BC, NP-C, CUNP
Adjunct Faculty
University of Michigan School of Nursing
Andrology Nurse Practitioner
Division of Andrology and Microsurgery
Department of Urology
University of Michigan Medical Center
Ann Arbor, Michigan

Sharon R. Redding, MN, RN, CNE
Associate Professor of Nursing
College of Saint Mary
Omaha, Nebraska

Dottie Roberts, MSN, MACI, RN, CMSRN, OCNS-C
Clinical Nurse Specialist
Palmetto Health Baptist
Columbia, South Carolina

Vicki M. Ross, RN, PhD
Graduate Faculty/Research Assistant Professor
University of Kansas School of Nursing
Kansas City, Kansas

Charlie Sandidge, RN, BSN, MN, CWCN
Registered Nurse, Burn Center
Harborview Medical Center
University of Washington
Seattle, Washington

Susan A. Sandstrom, MSN, RN, BC, CNE
Associate Professor in Nursing
College of Saint Mary
Omaha, Nebraska

CDR Linda M. Scott, CRNP
Nurse Practitioner
National Institute of Allergy and Infectious Diseases
Laboratory of Allergic Diseases
National Institutes of Health
Bethesda, Maryland

Clare M. Sekerak, MSN, APRN, BC, NP-C, CNRN
Nurse Practitioner
Neurosurgery
Veterans Administration Ann Arbor Healthcare System
Ann Arbor, Michigan

Nancy Christine Shoemaker, APRN-PMH, BC
Nurse Psychotherapist
University of Maryland Fayette Street Clinic;
Associate Faculty
University of Maryland School of Nursing
Baltimore, Maryland

Mary Sieggreen, MSN, APRN, BC, NP, CVN
Associate Clinical Professor
Wayne State University;
Nurse Practitioner, Vascular Surgery
Harper University Hospital
Detroit Medical Center
Detroit, Michigan

Karen A. Sikorski, MS, BSN, APN
Clinical Nurse Specialist, Pain
OSF Saint Anthony Medical Center
Rockford, Illinois

Terran Warren Sims, MSN, ACNP-C, COCN, CNN
Nurse Practitioner, ACNP-C
Genitourinary Oncology
Hematology/Oncology and Urology
University of Virginia Health System;
Course Preceptor/Lecturer
Acute Care Nurse Practitioner
Wound, Ostomy, and Continence Programs
University of Virginia School of Nursing
Charlottesville, Virginia

Sarah C. Smith, RN, MA, CRNO, COA
Medical/Surgical Nursing Division
Department of Ophthalmology
University of Iowa Hospitals & Clinics
Iowa City, Iowa

Dianne M. Smolen, PhD, CNE, RNBC, CNS
Professor
College of Nursing
The University of Toledo
Toledo, Ohio

Christina Stewart-Amidei, MSN, RN, CNRN, CCRN, CS
Instructor
University of Central Florida
Orlando, Florida

Cynthia M. Sublett, DNSc, RN
Adjunct Faculty
Xavier University
Cincinnati, Ohio

Peggy Ward-Smith, RN, PhD
Associate Professor
University of Missouri–Kansas City
School of Nursing
Kansas City, Missouri

Mary Wcisel, RN, MSN
Associate Professor of Nursing
Saint Mary's College
Notre Dame, Indiana

Carol J. Weber, RN, BSN, MSN, PhD
Professor and Chair, Online Nursing Program
Regis University
Denver, Colorado

Bernadette White, RN, MSN, APRNc, CHTP
Assistant Professor
Creighton University School of Nursing
Nurse Practitioner
Creighton University Oncology/Hematology Clinic
Omaha, Nebraska

Lynn White, MSN, CCRN, APRN, BC
Assistant Professor
Augustana College
Sioux Falls, South Dakota;
Clinical Nurse Specialist
Avera McKennan Transplant Institute
Sioux Falls, South Dakota

Connie White-Williams, RN, MSN, FAAN
Cardiothoracic Transplant Coordinator
University of Alabama at Birmingham
Birmingham, Alabama

Linda H. Yoder, RN, MBA, PhD, AOCN, FAAN
Associate Professor
Director, Nursing Systems Graduate Program
Luci Baines Johnson Fellow in Nursing
University of Texas–Austin
School of Nursing
Austin, Texas

Nancy L. York, PhD, RN
Assistant Professor of Nursing
University of Nevada-Las Vegas
Las Vegas, Nevada

Reviewers

Katrina D. Allen, RN, MSN, CCRN
Faulkner State Community College
Bay Minette, Alabama

Daria U. Amato, MSN, RN, CNE
Springfield, Virginia

Rebecca S. Appleton, RN, PhD
Marshall University
Huntington, West Virginia

Susan D. Arbogast, RN, MS
Maricopa Community College
Sun City, Arizona

Meg Blair, RN, MSN, CEN, PhD(c)
Nebraska Methodist College of Nursing and
    Allied Health
Omaha, Nebraska

Therese M. Bower, EdD, RN, MSN, CNS, CNE
Firelands Regional Medical Center School of
    Nursing
Sandusky, Ohio

Donna J. Bowles, EdD, MSN, RN, CNE
Indiana University Southeast
New Albany, Indiana

Lavoy Bray, Jr., RN, Med
Southside Regional Medical Center
    Professional Schools
Petersburg, Virginia

Patricia Louise Brown, RN, MN, PhD
Kansas Wesleyan University
Salina, Kansas

Michele Bunning, RN, MSN
Good Samaritan College of Nursing & Health
    Sciences
Cincinnati, Ohio

Catherine M. Concert, RN, MS, APRN, BC,
    FNP
Wyckoff Heights Medical Center & Long Island
    University
Brooklyn, New York

Claire Cottrell, RN, MSN
Mississippi Gulf Coast Community College
Perkinston, Mississippi

Judy A. Criner, PhD, RN
Germantown, Maryland

Mary F. Crowely, MS, RN
Regis College
Weston, Massachusetts

Sheryl L. Currie, RN, MN
Butler Community College
El Dorado, Kansas

Patricia Delmoe, RN, MN
Boswell/Mesa Nursing Education Program
Sun City, Arizona

R. Eric Doerfler, NP, MSN, AAHIVS
The Pennsylvania State University School of
    Nursing
Harrisburg, Pennsylvania

Sharon Kay Evans-Bernard, APRN-BC
The Hospital of Saint Raphael
New Haven, Connecticut

Kathleen Walsh Free, MSN, RN-C, ARNP-BC
Indiana University Southeast
New Albany, Indiana

Richard Freedberg, RN, MSN, MPA
Lansing Community College
Lansing, Michigan

Toni J. Galvan, RN, MSN, CNS, CCRN, CEN
Texas Tech University Health Sciences Center
    School of Nursing
Lubbock, Texas

Karen Heys, MN, RN
Everett Community College
Everett, Washington

Michelle N. Hough, MS, RN
Massachusetts Bay Community College
Framingham, Massachusetts

Donna Walker Hubbard, MSN, RN, CNN
University Mary Hardin-Baylor
Belton, Texas

Jaclynn A. Johnson, RNC, MSN
Otero Junior College/Arkansas Valley Regional
    Medical Center
La Junta, Colorado

Juanita F. Johnson
Oklahoma Baptist University
School of Nursing
Shawnee, Oklahoma

Leah Kelly
Jackson, New Jersey

Maria Lasater, RN, MSN, CCRN, CNRN
Texas County Technical Institute
Houston, Missouri

Gavin O'Connor, MS
Ozarks Technical Community College
Springfield, Missouri

Cynthia K. Olson, RN, MSN, C-FNP
Riverland Community College
Austin, Minnesota

Shelly Orr, RN, BS, MSN
Southside Regional Medical Center School of
    Nursing
Petersburg, Virginia

Stacey L. Rosenberg
Riverland Community College
Austin, Minnesota

Janet E. Shimek, RN, MSN, MSEd,
    CCRN, CNE
Carroll Community College
Westminster, Maryland

Fernisa Sison, MSN, RN, FNP
San Joaquin Delta College
St. Joseph's Medical Center
Lodi Hospital
Pacific Heart & Vascular
Stockton, California

Preface

In revising this textbook to keep pace with the rapidly evolving field of nursing, a perennial dilemma for us has been deciding which advancements to include in each new edition. As important new evidence-based protocols and guidelines have been issued, new legislation has taken effect, and our knowledge base has expanded in areas such as genetics, pain management, and wound healing, we've broadened our coverage to encompass each major development. Students and instructors alike have told us that even with many excellent resources available online, including those that accompany this book, they still want a reliable, comprehensive print reference. Yet as every experienced nursing instructor knows, students who are struggling to absorb the core concepts underlying this complex field can become overwhelmed by too much detail.

In this eighth edition of *Medical-Surgical Nursing: Clinical Management for Positive Outcomes*, we believe we've achieved just the right balance by offering thorough coverage in all key areas yet maintaining a constant focus on what the student needs to know. Though streamlined in design and content to approximately 2,200 pages, this eighth edition remains the most comprehensive medical-surgical nursing text in the field. It provides a solid foundation in anatomy and physiology, pathophysiology, medical management, and nursing care for the full spectrum of adult health conditions.

A key theme of this edition is evidence-based practice. Throughout the text, an integrated icon system continually highlights evidence-based content and clinical guidelines. These icons, which link in-text citations to research-based references, serve as visual reminders that clinical practice must be based on peer-reviewed research evidence and established clinical guidelines. In addition, *Translating Evidence into Practice* boxes show students that evidence-based practice is not simply an academic exercise—it's a practical way of improving measurable outcomes, such as preventing falls, ventilator-associated pneumonia, and endocarditis. To further underscore the text's evidence-based practice orientation, all Complementary and Alternative Therapy boxes report findings from research studies, many of which are randomized, controlled trials.

Another important strength of the book is its clear delineation of various healthcare professionals' roles in managing each disorder. Within each topic, nursing management is clearly identified and organized by assessment, diagnosis, desired outcome, interventions, and evaluation, allowing students to see how the nurse's actions dovetail with those of the other members of the healthcare team.

Critical thinking skills have been emphasized throughout the eighth edition, including a new chapter in Unit 1 entirely devoted to the topic. Once again, the focus is evidence based and practical. The chapter explains how sharpening their critical thinking skills can help nurses determine the significance of diagnostic findings, for example, or ensure early identification of complications ranging from dehydration to transplant rejection.

PHILOSOPHY AND APPROACH

This textbook grew out of the belief that nurses and physicians do not compete with each other but instead collaborate to reach certain outcomes in cooperation with the client and family. Nonetheless, nursing and medicine are separate disciplines and are not intermingled in this text. However, because it is often difficult for nursing students to understand one without understanding the other, we present thorough coverage of both nursing management and medical management.

With the increased emphasis on outcomes in health care, we have organized client care under the heading of Outcome Management. Several subheadings appear under this heading, including Medical Management, Nursing Management of the Medical Client, Surgical Management, and Nursing Management of the Surgical Client, as appropriate.

In this text, we use the nursing process to describe nursing management, but we do not apply the nursing process to every disorder. Instead, we have designated the nursing process for major or prototypical disorders. Within the presentation of the nursing process for those disorders, we have developed nursing diagnoses and collaborative problems, as appropriate, with their own outcomes and interventions. Collaborative problems are defined as client problems that cannot be resolved through independent nursing actions; they are complications that may develop because of a disorder, surgical procedure, or nonsurgical treatment. Collaborative problems complete the picture of nursing care and eliminate the need to force-fit every client problem into the framework of a nursing diagnosis. We have written Outcomes and Interventions sections for *each* identified nursing diagnosis and collaborative problem because we have found from our teaching experience that students cannot easily pull apart lists of diagnoses followed by lists of outcomes and interventions and then rebuild them into care plans. Each care plan is written with the problems listed in priority order and then proceeding through the trajectory of the illness. As we know from our years of teaching, setting priorities for nursing care is a skill that students struggle to master.

ORGANIZATION

This edition is organized from simple to complex and from common to uncommon disorders. The early portion of the text focuses on the care of clients usually assigned to beginning students. The book then progresses to address the care of clients with more complex disorders, which are more commonly taught in upper-division classes. Within each chapter, we begin with the most important diseases for students to grasp; this organization stems from our belief that students often trim their reading time to prioritize the most essential material. We believe that by placing the most important information first, we encourage students to read it first.

Although the text retains its familiar 18-unit format, the assessment chapters in the disorders units have been streamlined and significantly modified using simple yet innovative visual diagrams to present clinical manifestations, review-of-systems information, and standard diagnostic work-ups for many common problems, such as hematuria, anemia, and dyspnea. These concise algorithms complement the text by offering at-a-glance summaries of practical information, such as what questions to ask the client during a GI assessment and what diagnostic studies may be ordered when kidney stones are suspected. Developed in response to reviewers' suggestions, the diagrams are especially useful as study tools for today's visual learners and as quick refreshers in the clinical setting.

The first five units in the book are devoted to content that is applicable to all medical-surgical clients. The material in this first portion of the book will guide the student in learning to provide comprehensive care regardless of the specific diagnosis or problem. Concepts that span medical-surgical practice, such as health promotion, care delivery settings, physical assessment, complementary and alternative therapies, fluid and electrolyte balance, genetics, infectious diseases, pain, palliative care, perioperative care, and oncology, are found in this portion of the book. The remainder of the text, beginning with Unit 6, is divided into common

responses to health disorders. Each unit begins with a review of anatomy and physiology, followed by a chapter on health and diagnostic assessment; one or more chapters then present the nursing care of clients with specific disorders. A brief description of each unit is given below.

Unit 1 introduces the essential principles of health promotion and disease prevention (Chapter 1), such as wellness, health literacy, self-care, injury prevention, and early detection of illness. A thoroughly updated chapter on health assessment (Chapter 2) focuses on a hospital-based assessment rather than a comprehensive assessment and provides an introduction to the revised assessment format used throughout the text. A new chapter on Critical Thinking (Chapter 3; see "New Features" on p. xxii) provides a solid foundation in the increasingly important skill of thinking critically in order to provide high-level nursing care. We have approached critical thinking as a science and have provided foundational material for students to apply in the clinical setting. Chapter 4 discusses why people choose alternative therapies and considers how to discuss complementary and alternative therapies with clients.

Unit 2 presents an overview of health care delivery systems, allowing students to become oriented to care in various settings. Chapters 5 through 10 address nursing care in ambulatory care, acute care, critical care, home health care, long-term care, and rehabilitation settings.

Unit 3 explores the foundations of care for medical-surgical clients, including separate chapters on fluid and electrolyte imbalances (Chapters 11 and 12), acid-base disorders (Chapter 13), and perioperative care (Chapter 14).

Unit 4 discusses physiologic concepts basic to medical-surgical nursing care. The unit begins with a look at the field of genetics (Chapter 15) and continues with chapters related to cancer (Chapters 16 and 17), wound healing (Chapter 18), and infectious disease, including expanded information about bioterrorism (Chapter 19).

Unit 5 covers psychosocial concepts basic to medical-surgical nursing care. The unit begins with a chapter on pain management (Chapter 20) and continues with chapters on palliative care (Chapter 21), sleep and rest disorders (Chapter 22), psychosocial and mental health concerns (Chapter 23), and substance abuse (Chapter 24).

Units 6 through 17 focus on the management of clients with specific disorders. Each unit begins with an overview of the structure and function of pertinent body systems. These anatomy and physiology reviews are complemented by many new pieces of full-color artwork. Next, the unit progresses to chapters on assessment and nursing care. As mentioned earlier, the assessment chapters in the disorders units now feature concise, innovative diagrams to present clinical manifestations, review-of-systems information, and standard diagnostic work-ups for the most common problems students will encounter in daily practice. These algorithms encapsulate the assessment process and summarize critical diagnostic pathways for conditions such as neurologic pain and sensory impairments, musculoskeletal derangements, and reproductive disorders. This efficient new format puts essential information at students' fingertips for quick reference and study. In Unit 8, for example, new content related to management of chronic kidney disease has been added to Chapter 35, which concerns renal disorders. In Unit 11, author Joyce Black offers her own cutting-edge research on pressure ulcers in a chapter on managing clients with integumentary disorders (Chapter 49). In Unit 13, chronic stable heart failure is explained in Chapter 56, and STEMI versus NSTEMI is addressed in Chapter 58.

In general, the discussion of specific disorders includes section headings for Etiology, Pathophysiology, Clinical Manifestations, and Outcome Management. The etiology topics in the disorders chapters focus on health promotion, maintenance, and restoration. Within the Outcome Management sections, students are linked back to the pathophysiology of the disorder. These linkages help the student to connect the concepts of pathophysiology and the treatments used to reverse or control the pathophysiology.

Unit 18 presents the care of clients with multisystem disorders. Chapter 80 examines organ donation issues, the transplantation process, quality-of-life questions, and specific interventions for clients requiring organ transplantation. Shock and multisystem disorders are discussed in Chapter 81. Chapter 82 introduces the basic concepts of triage, ethical issues, and maintaining the chain of custody of medicolegal evidence. This chapter organizes emergency conditions according to the various nursing diagnoses identified and treated.

HALLMARK FEATURES

A completely new full-color design focuses on guiding the reader to the Evolve website, where a wealth of supplemental content resides. Each chapter opens with a list of web enhancements, which introduces the reader to that chapter's features on the Evolve website. Many of the web features—including those that begin in the text and continue on the Evolve website with interactive exercises and bonus material—contain a reference within the text and are designated with a marginal icon: `evolve`

The following is a list of the book's hallmark features, including a description and the location of the feature:

- **Anatomy and Physiology Reviews** introduce each body system unit and provide a brief review of the relevant anatomy and physiology. Many new full-color illustrations depict anatomic units, such as the cell and the genetic code, and complex physiologic processes, such as the sleep cycle and the body's response to pain.
- **Bridge to Critical Care** boxes highlight major critical care concerns, such as burn injury, defibrillation, and alarm troubleshooting. This feature appears in selected chapters in the text.
- **Bridge to Home Health Care** boxes describe specific applications and strategies for medical-surgical care in the home. Some bridges appear on the Evolve website, and others remain in the text for this edition.
- **Care Plans** use the nursing process format to highlight nursing diagnoses and collaborative problems, expected outcomes, interventions with rationales, and evaluation. These problems are presented in priority order to guide nursing care decisions anywhere along the disease trajectory. For the eighth edition, NIC and NOC designations have been incorporated into the Nursing Care Plans to demonstrate the applicability of these standardized nursing taxonomies to everyday clinical practice. Some care plans appear on the Evolve website, but most remain in the text for this edition.
- **Case Studies** present complex, in-depth client scenarios, most of which feature multiple clinical problems. Each Case Study is introduced in the text, and the body of the Case Study is continued on the Evolve website, along with discussions, multiple-choice questions, and a nursing care plan.
- **Client Education Guides** use client-centered language to help students teach clients how to collaborate in their own care. Some guides appear in the text, while others are found only on the Evolve website. All Client Education Guides in the text have been translated into Spanish and appear on the Evolve website.
- **Complementary and Alternative Therapy** boxes present nontraditional therapies used by clients and health care providers to treat various conditions. They discuss alternative and complementary therapies related to specific diseases or body systems. Some boxes are featured in the text, and others appear on the Evolve website. Each box outlines the findings of specific research studies, many of which are randomized, controlled trials.
- **Concept Maps** are full-color flowcharts linking pathophysiological processes, clinical manifestations, and medical and nursing interventions. This feature appears throughout the text, and new maps are provided for liver failure and heart failure.
- **Critical Monitoring** boxes highlight clinical manifestations that must be reported to the physician without delay and, in some cases, show how critical values are calculated. This feature appears throughout the text. New Critical Monitoring features for this edition include a consensus formula

for fluid resuscitation and an explanation of arterial blood gas analysis.

- **Evolve Web Enhancement** boxes on the first page of each chapter list the supplemental features that appear on the Evolve website.
- **Genetic Links** boxes link a disease, such as breast cancer or polycystic kidney disease, with its corresponding genetics. This feature provides the student with the description, genetics, diagnosis/testing, and management of a specific disease. It appears throughout the text.
- **Integrating Pharmacology** boxes help students understand how medications can be used for disease management and examine iatrogenic complications of certain drugs by exploring common classifications of medications. This feature appears throughout the text and is designed to present material on medications for clinical consideration.
- **Management and Delegation** boxes present the primary concerns nurses need to address when delegating care activities to unlicensed assistive personnel. This feature appears in the text and includes new topics such as infection control precautions.
- **Physical Assessment Findings in the Healthy Adult** serves both to remind students of the relevant normal findings for each body system and to demonstrate how to chart those findings with clinical precision. This feature appears in the text.
- **Terrorism Alert** boxes provide cutting-edge material on bioterrorism preparedness and response. They aid the student in recognizing the clinical manifestations and diseases associated with bioterrorism. This feature appears throughout the text.
- **Thinking Critically Questions** conclude each nursing care chapter. This feature presents short, typical client scenarios and poses questions about what actions to take. Discussions of all the questions, found on the Evolve website, provide insight into the reasoning behind appropriate actions.

NEW TO THIS EDITION

In addition to the hallmark features listed in the previous section, the eighth edition includes new features that underscore the book's commitment to evidence-based practice and critical thinking.

NEW FEATURES

- **Evidence-Based Practice icons** remind students that daily clinical decision making must be based on reliable research evidence.
  - **Red lamp icons** ( ) identify primary research applicable to practice interventions, especially evidence-based recommendations that supersede

previously accepted nursing knowledge (for example, Homans' sign having been proved an unreliable indicator of DVT). Corresponding references in the bibliography are highlighted in red for easy retrieval.
  - **Blue lamp icons** ( ) precede standardized guidelines, protocols, and classification systems that have evolved from evidence-based practice to govern patient care. Corresponding references in the bibliography are highlighted in blue to direct readers to print media and to the web, where they can link to online journals and to resources offered by government agencies and nonprofit health care organizations.
- **Integrating Diagnostic Testing** boxes on topics such as dyspnea and pelvic pain give students examples of the laboratory and imaging studies that may be ordered during the course of a client's illness. These boxes, accompanied by brief explanations in the text, appear in most assessment chapters and in several of the disorders chapters. They help students understand which clinical manifestations prompt specific tests and what the tests identify. However, they do not unnecessarily repeat the nursing implications of each test or the typical pre- and post-testing nursing interventions, since that information is covered in assessment courses and in diagnostic testing handbooks.
- **NIC and NOC designations** have been incorporated into the Nursing Care Plans to demonstrate how these standardized nursing taxonomies are used in everyday clinical practice.
- **Safety Alert** icons identify common hospital emergencies, National Patient Safety Goals established by The Joint Commission (TJC), and TJC sentinel events.
- **Translating Evidence into Practice** boxes present a topic in the form of a clinical question and summarize the conclusions of four to five research articles. This feature shows students that evidence-based practice occurs in the care setting, not in the ivory tower, allowing nurses to improve measurable outcomes in areas such as injury prevention, infection control, and management of chronic conditions.
- **Many new pieces of full-color art** illustrate pathologic processes such as airway obstruction and osteoarthritis, products and equipment such as a voice prosthesis and types of casts, and surgical procedures such as scleral buckling.

EXPANDED AND NEW CHAPTERS

- A **thoroughly updated chapter on Health Assessment** (Chapter 2) provides an introduction to this vital skill set and introduces the assessment format used throughout the text.

- A **new chapter on Critical Thinking** (Chapter 3) provides a solid foundation in the increasingly important skill of thinking critically in order to provide high-level nursing care. The chapter explores the necessity of applying critical thinking skills to evidence-based practice and explains how mastering the principles of critical thinking can help in setting practical priorities. Case studies are used to illustrate critical thinking skills in action in various care settings.
- An **expanded infectious-disease chapter** (Chapter 19: Perspectives on Infectious Disease and Bioterrorism) now includes vital content on bioterrorism.
- A **completely revised and newly illustrated chapter on structural cardiac disorders** (Chapter 55: Management of Clients with Structural Cardiac Disorders) provides the latest information on the expected outcomes of transplantation and the related nursing care.
- An **expanded kidney disorders chapter** (Chapter 35: Management of Clients with Renal Disorders) includes a new section on chronic kidney disease management.
- **All assessment chapters have been streamlined using simple yet innovative diagrams** to summarize clinical manifestations, review-of-systems information, and critical diagnostic pathways.

ANCILLARY PACKAGE

The ancillary package supplies both instructors and students with a variety of additional resources to enhance the utility of the book. Instructors are provided with all of the tools required for a vibrant, media-rich, successful classroom experience: Instructor's Manual, Test Bank, Image Collection, PowerPoint Presentations, and iClicker Question Suite. Students are offered content enhancements such as animations, video and audio clips, and audio pronunciations. They benefit from study and testing aids such as NCLEX® Examination Style Review Questions, Open-Book Quizzes, and Chapter Review Audio Summaries. In addition, students are given the tools to promote a successful clinical experience, such as Client Education Guides.

INSTRUCTOR RESOURCES

All Student Ancillaries, as described below, are available for instructor use. In addition, the **Instructor's Electronic Resource,** available both on **CD-ROM** and on the **Evolve Resources** website at http://evolve.elsevier.com/Black/medsurg, contains an Instructor's Manual, PowerPoint Presentations, a Test Bank, an Image Collection (including all images in the text), and an iClicker Question Suite:

- The **Instructor's Manual** consists of critical points to emphasize, to facilitate student comprehension

in both the classroom and the clinical setting. Classroom exercises include Review Activities, Class Assignments, Lectures and Discussions, suggestions for Guest Speakers, Group Activities, and Concept Map Activities (where applicable). The clinical activities include Skills Laboratories, Clinical Site Activities, and Clinical Conference Activities. For this new edition, the Chapter Objectives in the Instructor's Manual have been coordinated with those in the *Study Guide* (see below) for effective student learning.
- The **PowerPoint Presentations** include more than 2,500 slides and provide instructors with lecture aids for each chapter. Illustrations from the text as well as bonus health assessment images are included in the PowerPoint Presentations.
- The electronic **Test Bank** offers approximately 2,500 questions, including more than 300 questions in multiple-select format. Each test question includes a rationale, nursing process step, cognitive level, NCLEX category of client needs, and text reference.
- The **Image Collection** consists of more than 800 full-color images.
- **NEW!** The iClicker Question Suite contains more than 325 questions, covering topics for every chapter in the book. These questions are designed to elicit curiosity and motivate students for a dynamic classroom experience.

The **Evolve Course Management System** is an interactive learning environment that works in coordination with *Medical-Surgical Nursing: Clinical Management for Positive Outcomes,* eighth edition, to provide Internet-based course management tools you can use to reinforce and expand on the concepts you deliver in class. You can use the Evolve website to do the following:

- Publish your class syllabus, outline, and lecture notes
- Set up "virtual office hours" and e-mail communication
- Share important dates and information through the online class *Calendar*
- Encourage student participation through *Chat Rooms* and *Discussion Boards*

STUDENT RESOURCES
Student CD-ROM
The **Companion CD-ROM** for students includes the following resources:

- **Audio Pronunciations**
- **NEW! 3-D Animations** illustrating pathophysiology, drug actions, and medical treatments
- **Health Assessment Video Clips**
- **Health Assessment Audio Clips**
- **Assessment Finding Photographs**

- **Bonus Features**, including Bridges to Home Health Care; Care Plans; Case Management boxes; Clinical Pathways; discussions of Complementary and Alternative Therapy, Diversity in Health Care, and Ethical Issues; and selected tables and illustrations
- Discussions of the **Thinking Critically** questions in the text, offering students the opportunity to compare their responses to those of the authors

Student Resources on the Evolve Website

The **Evolve Resources** website, available at http://evolve.elsevier.com/Black/medsurg, contains a wealth of student assets. Students are encouraged at both the beginning and the end of each chapter to take advantage of these resources, which include all of the materials on the Companion CD-ROM in addition to the following materials:

Interactive Online Resources

- **NEW! Interactive NCLEX® Examination Style Review Questions** for every chapter, with answers and rationales
- **Interactive Open-Book Quizzes,** consisting of multiple-choice, matching, and fill-in-the-blank questions for each chapter
- **Interactive Case Studies** consisting of 12 exercise sets composed of multiple-choice quizzes and care-planning activities drawn from the Case Study feature boxes in the text
- **Interactive Concept Map Creator,** a one-of-a-kind program that allows students to create customized concept maps. Students are prompted to enter the following client data: medical diagnosis, pathophysiology, risk factors, clinical manifestations, nursing diagnoses, collaborative problems, expected outcomes, and nursing interventions. The program then generates a concept map in two formats: (1) a graphic "map" that clearly illustrates the relationships among various client data and components of the nursing process, and (2) a tabular word-processing file that students can print and use to record client responses/evaluation data, thereby completing the nursing process.

Supplemental Online Resources

- **Appendices** titled "Religious Beliefs and Practices Affecting Health Care" and "A Health History Format That Integrates the Assessment of Functional Health Patterns" supplement information in the printed text.
- **Case Management** boxes, written by a practicing case manager, present key coordination and anticipatory issues under the consistent headings of Assess, Advocate, and Prevent Readmission, thus linking nursing care with client-focused case management.
- **NEW! Chapter Review Audio Summaries** supply the major teaching points of each management chapter in downloadable MP3 files.

- **Client Education Guides,** in Spanish and English, are available for selected chapters.
- **Clinical Pathways** are excerpted from actual pathways used in specific hospitals. They are accompanied by a guide to show what should occur during specific times in the pathway and how to stay on track when caring for the client.
- **Crossword Puzzles** are supplied for each chapter.
- **Diversity in Health Care** boxes are focused discussions of health and illness related to particular populations.
- **Ethical Issues in Nursing** boxes feature an ethical dilemma in the form of a question, with the discussion immediately following.
- **Fluid and Electrolyte Tutorial** is a user-friendly module that helps students master the difficult concepts of fluid and electrolyte balance and imbalance. This self-paced program includes animations to help illustrate important concepts. Its accessible, inviting user interface helps make the program easy to navigate. The program is divided into five sections: an introduction, three sections on fluid and electrolyte balance and imbalance, and a quiz section with approximately 75 questions to test students on information learned throughout the program.
- The complete **NANDA taxonomy,** a complete listing of **NIC labels,** and a complete listing of **NOC labels** have all been updated for the new edition.
- **Spanish Assessment Phrases,** for nurses who work with Spanish-speaking clients, are supplied for selected chapters.
- **WebLinks** are provided for each chapter.

Additional Resources for Students

Other student ancillaries are available separately and include the following texts:

Study Guide for Medical-Surgical Nursing: Clinical Management for Positive Outcomes, **8th edition.** Keyed chapter-by-chapter to the text, this resource provides engaging and challenging exercises in many different formats to clarify and reinforce the textbook content. The *Study Guide* is offered in a traditional print-format text and has been completely revised for this edition, offering students the opportunity to review terminology and best practices, understand theories and trends, keep drug skills sharp, and test and apply their knowledge.

Virtual Clinical Excursions for Medical-Surgical Nursing: Clinical Management for Positive Outcomes, **8th edition.** This workbook/CD-ROM package helps students prepare for the average clinical rotation by immersing them in a realistic, yet safe, virtual hospital. The VCE workbook serves as a map, providing textbook reading assignments that correspond with the software before guiding students through the CD-ROM, where they care for patients in the virtual hospital. It presents significant real-world problems that place the student in nursing situations where they can set priorities for care, collect and analyze data, prepare and administer medications, and reach conclusions about complex and changing problems. Using multiple information sources (such as an Electronic Patient Record, Charts, a Medication Administration Record, and a Drug Guide), students make connections between what they experience in the virtual hospital and what they have learned in the text, creating a true-to-life, hands-on, multimedia learning experience.

ACKNOWLEDGMENTS

To our surprise, the preparation of this text has never become routine from one edition to the next. As medical-surgical nursing has evolved, we've only quickened our own step to see that the text keeps pace with the exciting and often momentous developments in this dynamic field. Many people have walked this path with us. Our contributing authors have led the way by lending broad clinical expertise in their respective areas of specialization. We continue to be impressed by the depth of their knowledge, the scope of their experience, and most of all, their enthusiasm for sharing it with students. Likewise, our reviewers are dedicated scholars and educators whose suggestions and comments have helped us sharpen our focus and present each topic with precision and clarity.

We would also like to thank the publishing professionals who, once again, have turned our extensively revised manuscript into a finished book. Barbara Nelson Cullen, our former Executive Publisher at Elsevier, encouraged us and gave her unflagging support to the project. Maureen Iannuzzi, Managing Editor, brought a keen eye for detail and helped us negotiate every bump in the road. Jennifer Ehlers, Senior Developmental Editor, developed the book's new features, kept the manuscript flowing in on schedule from the contributors, and handled the entire print and online ancillary package with finesse. Kathy Macciocca and Mary Ann Zimmerman, Editorial Assistants, dispatched every administrative task with an efficiency we truly appreciate. Louis Forgione, Design Director, is responsible for the bold new look that makes each page attractive and inviting. Deborah Vogel, Publishing Services Manager, and her team shepherded the manuscript through its complex production phase with an ease that could come only from experience.

Hand in hand with Elsevier, freelance editor Beth Welch overlooked nothing in copyediting the text to make it straightforward and user friendly. Melissa Kinsey and Monica Groth Farrar, of Nicholson & Stillwell Publishing Services, were thorough and responsive in developing the manuscript and the new scientific art for the book. Imagineering Media Services, of Toronto, Canada, provided contemporary, accurate medical illustration work, and Top Graphics, of St. Louis, Missouri, rendered the less complex drawings cleanly and attractively. Our thanks also go to SPi Technologies for handling the mammoth task of typesetting the manuscript.

Finally, we would like to extend our heartfelt gratitude to the educators and students nationwide who allow us to walk by their side as the practice of medical-surgical nursing is passed on to a new generation of nurses.

JOYCE M. BLACK AND JANE HOKANSON HAWKS

Contents

UNIT 2
**Health Care Delivery
Systems,**   57

UNIT 3
Foundations of Medical-Surgical Nursing, 119

UNIT 4

Physiologic Foundations, 229

CHAPTER **19**

Perspectives on Infectious Disease and Bioterrorism, 323

Carol J. Weber

UNIT **5**

Psychosocial Foundations, 343

CHAPTER **20**

Clients with Pain, 351

Karen A. Sikorski and Donna M. Barker

UNIT 6

Musculoskeletal Disorders, 451

UNIT **7**
Nutritional Disorders, 545

UNIT 8
Elimination Disorders, 643

CHAPTER 32
Assessment of Elimination, 653
Karen A. Hanson and Susanne Quallich

CHAPTER 33
Management of Clients with Intestinal Disorders, 678
Dawn P. Murphy and Jane Hokanson Hawks

CHAPTER **34**

Management of Clients with Urinary Disorders, 727
Francie Bernier and Terran Warren Sims

UNIT **9**

Sexuality and Reproductive Disorders, 839

CHAPTER **40**

Management of Clients with Breast Disorders, 940

Melissa Craft

CHAPTER **41**

Management of Clients with Sexually Transmitted Infections, 972

Meg Blair

UNIT 10
Metabolic Disorders,   995

ANATOMY AND PHYSIOLOGY REVIEW: The Metabolic Systems,   996
   Robert G. Carroll

CHAPTER **42**
Assessment of the Endocrine and Metabolic Systems,   1006
Dianne M. Smolen

CHAPTER **43**
Management of Clients with Thyroid and Parathyroid Disorders,   1019
Allen Hanberg

CHAPTER **44**

Management of Clients with Adrenal and Pituitary Disorders, 1040

Allen Hanberg

CHAPTER **45**

Management of Clients with Diabetes Mellitus, 1062

James A. Fain

UNIT 11

Integumentary Disorders, 1179

CHAPTER **48**

Assessment of the Integumentary System, 1186

    Noreen Heer Nicol

CHAPTER **49**

Management of Clients with Integumentary Disorders, 1199

    Noreen Heer Nicol and Joyce M. Black

UNIT **12**
Vascular Disorders,   1271

ANATOMY AND PHYSIOLOGY REVIEW: The Vascular System,   1272
Robert G. Carroll

UNIT 13
Cardiac Disorders, 1341

UNIT **14**
Oxygenation
Disorders, 1513

UNIT **15**
Sensory Disorders,   1667

UNIT **16**

Cognitive and Perceptual Disorders, 1745

UNIT 17
Protective Disorders, 1975

CHAPTER **76**

Management of Clients with Immune Disorders, 2040

Linda M. Scott

CHAPTER **77**

Management of Clients with Rheumatic Disorders, 2053

Patricia A. MacDonald

UNIT 18
Multisystem Disorders, 2135

Special Features

COMMUNITY-BASED PRACTICE

COMPLEMENTARY AND ALTERNATIVE THERAPY

CONCEPT MAP

CRITICAL MONITORING

GENETIC LINKS

INTEGRATING DIAGNOSTIC TESTING

INTEGRATING PHARMACOLOGY

MANAGEMENT AND DELEGATION

Physical Assessment Findings in the Healthy Adult

TERRORISM ALERT

TRANSLATING EVIDENCE INTO PRACTICE

Additional Online Content

THE FOLLOWING LEARNING TOOLS AND KEY REFERENCE CONTENT CAN BE FOUND ON THE EVOLVE WEBSITE AT

http://evolve.elsevier.com/Black/medsurg/

Audio Pronunciations for more than 250 words
Audio Clips, Animations, and Video Clips for physical examination and health assessment
Fluid & Electrolyte Module
Concept Map Creator
List of Nursing Interventions Classification (NIC) Labels
List of Nursing Outcomes Classifications (NOC) Labels
List of NANDA International Approved Nursing Diagnoses

APPENDIX A
Religious Beliefs and Practices Affecting Health Care

APPENDIX B
A Health History Format that Integrates the Assessment of Functional Health Patterns

U N I T 11

INTEGUMENTARY DISORDERS

ANATOMY AND PHYSIOLOGY REVIEW:

The Integumentary System

Robert G. Carroll

The integument, or skin, makes up 15% to 20% of the body's weight. Intact skin is the body's primary defense system. It protects us from invasion by organisms, helps to regulate body temperature, manufactures vitamins, and provides our external appearance. Skin has three primary layers (i.e., *epidermis,* or outer layer; the *dermis,* or inner layer; and the *hypodermis,* or subcutaneous layer) as well as epidermal appendages (i.e., eccrine glands, apocrine glands, sebaceous glands, hair follicles, and nails).

The skin's *epithelium* is composed of cells that provide a continuous barrier between the body contents and the outside environment. Epithelial cells also cover the gastrointestinal (GI) tract, pulmonary airways and alveoli, renal tubules and the urinary system, and the ducts that empty onto the surface of the skin (lumen) of the GI and respiratory systems. Epithelial cells allow the selective transport of ions, nutrients, and metabolic wastes and have a permeability to water that is partially regulated. Epithelial cells are joined to each other through tight junctions and express different populations of protein transporters on the apical side (generally facing a lumen) and the basolateral (facing the blood, or serosal) side. The functional significance of epithelial transport is covered in the GI and renal chapters (see the Anatomy and Physiology Review for Units 7 and 8).

STRUCTURE OF THE INTEGUMENTARY SYSTEM

EPIDERMIS

The epidermis is the thin, stratified outer skin layer that is in direct contact with the external environment (Figure A&P11-1). The thickness of the epidermis ranges from 0.04 mm on the eyelids to 1.6 mm on the palms and soles. *Desmosomes* (points of intercellular attachment that are vital for cell-to-cell adhesion) are found in the epidermis.

Keratinocytes, the principal cells of the epidermis, produce *keratin* in a complex process. The cells begin in the basal cell layer and change constantly, moving upward through the epidermis. On the surface, they are sloughed off or lost by abrasion. Thus the epidermis constantly regenerates itself, providing a tough keratinized barrier.

Skin color reflects both the production of pigment granules *(melanin)* by melanocytes and, in light-skinned people, the presence of blood *(hemoglobin)*. Skin color reflects a combination of four basic colors:

- Exogenously formed carotenoids (yellow)
- Melanin (brown)
- Oxygenated hemoglobin in arterioles and capillaries (red)
- Reduced hemoglobin in venules (blue or purple)

Melanin plays the largest role in skin color; it is produced in the epidermis and in corresponding layers of the hair follicle. Although melanin is not produced in the dermis, it can be deposited in the dermis from the epidermis through various processes (such as inflammation).

Melanosomes are granules in melanocytes that synthesize melanin. Skin color differences result from the size and quantity of melanosomes as well as from the rate of melanin production. In natives of equatorial Africa, there is an increase in the size and number of melanosomes (not melanocytes) as well as increased melanin production. The melanosomes are large, discrete, and dispersed. In natives of northern Europe, the melanosomes are small and aggregated, producing less melanin. Sun exposure initially increases the size and functional activity of both melanocytes and melanosomes. With chronic sun exposure, there is an increase in the concentration of melanocytes as well as in size and functional activity. The presence of melanin limits the penetration of sun rays into the skin and protects against sunburn and the development of ultraviolet light–induced skin carcinomas.

Epidermal Appendages

Epidermal appendages are down-growths of epidermis into the dermis. They consist of eccrine glands, apocrine units, sebaceous glands, hair, and nails.

Glands

Eccrine glands produce sweat and play an important role in thermoregulation. They are found throughout the skin except on the vermilion border (junction of the pink area of the lip with the surrounding skin), the ears, nail bed, glans penis, and labia minora. They are more numerous on the palms, soles, forehead, and

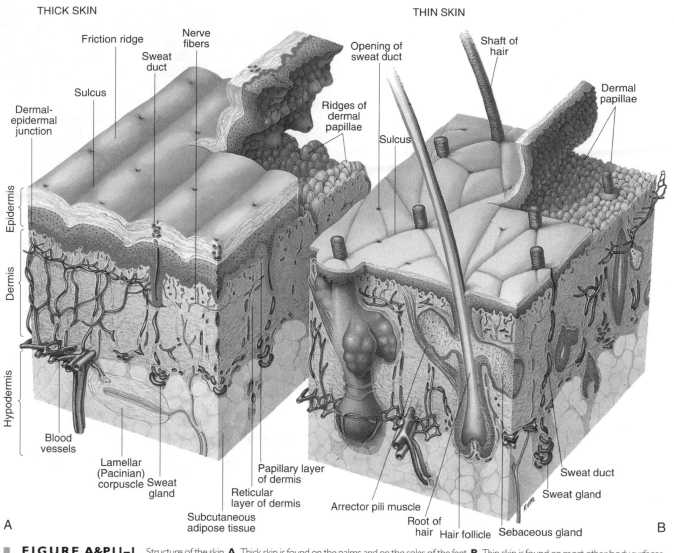

THICK SKIN

THIN SKIN

Labels (Thick skin, A):
- Friction ridge
- Nerve fibers
- Sweat duct
- Sulcus
- Dermal-epidermal junction
- Epidermis
- Dermis
- Hypodermis
- Blood vessels
- Lamellar (Pacinian) corpuscle
- Sweat gland
- Subcutaneous adipose tissue
- Reticular layer of dermis
- Papillary layer of dermis

Labels (Thin skin, B):
- Opening of sweat duct
- Shaft of hair
- Dermal papillae
- Ridges of dermal papillae
- Sulcus
- Arrector pili muscle
- Root of hair
- Hair follicle
- Sebaceous gland
- Sweat gland
- Sweat duct

A   B

■ **FIGURE A&PII–I**   Structure of the skin. **A,** Thick skin is found on the palms and on the soles of the feet. **B,** Thin skin is found on most other body surfaces.

axillae. Sweat is similar to plasma but sweat is more dilute. Eccrine gland secretion is stimulated by heat and emotional stress. Eccrine glands exit the body independently of the hair shaft (see Figure A&P11-1).

Apocrine glands occur primarily in the axillae, breast areolae, anogenital area, ear canals, and eyelids. In lower-order animals, apocrine secretions function as sexual attractants *(pheromones),* and the apocrine secretion musk is used as a perfume base. The role, if any, in humans is not established. Mediated by adrenergic innervation, apocrine glands secrete a milky substance that becomes odoriferous when altered by skin surface bacteria. These glands do not function until puberty, and they require a high output of sex hormone for activity.

Sebaceous glands are found throughout the skin except on the palms and soles and are most abundant on the face, scalp, upper back, and chest. They are associated with hair follicles that open onto the skin surface, where *sebum* (a mixture of sebaceous gland–produced lipids and epidermal cell–derived lipids) is released. Sebum has a lubricating function and bactericidal activity. Androgen is responsible for sebaceous gland development. In utero androgen causes neonatal acne; after puberty sebum production can cause acne in adolescents.

Hair and Nails

Hair is a nonviable protein end product found on all skin surfaces except the palms and soles. Each hair follicle functions as an independent unit and goes through intermittent stages of development. Hair develops from the mitotic activity of the hair bulb. The rate of hair growth varies in different parts of the body. In a typical adult scalp, 85% to 90% of hairs are in an *anagen* (growth) phase. The remainder is in a *telogen* (rest) phase. About 50 to 100 hairs are lost each day. As a rule, the growing phase of hair on the eyebrows, trunk, and extremities does not exceed 6 months. Its resting phase is 3 to 4 months.

Hair form (straight or curly) depends on the shape of the hair in cross-section. Straight hair has a round cross-section; curly hair has an oval or ribbon-like cross-section. Curved follicles also affect the curliness of hair. Melanocytes in the bulb determine hair color. Hair follicles usually occur with sebaceous glands, and together they form a *pilosebaceous unit*. *Arrector pili* muscles of the dermis attach to hair follicles and elevate the hairs when body temperature falls or strong emotions are present, producing "goose bumps."

Nails are horny scales of epidermis. The nail matrix is the source of specialized, nonkeratinized cells. They differentiate into keratinized cells, which make up the nail protein. The matrix for nail formation is located in the proximal nail bed. It grows forward from the nailfold to cover the nail bed. Fingernails grow about 0.1 mm each day; complete reproduction takes 100 to 150 days. Toenails grow one third as fast as fingernails do. A damaged nail matrix, which may result from trauma or aggressive manicuring, produces a distorted nail. Nails are also sensitive to physiologic changes; for instance, they grow more slowly in cold weather and during periods of illness.

Nails and hair consist of keratinized and, therefore, "dead" cells. The ingestion of gelatin has not been shown to increase nail growth or strength.

DERMIS

The dermis, a dense layer of tissue beneath the epidermis, gives the skin most of its substance and structure. It varies from 1 to 4 mm in thickness and is thickest over the back. The dermis contains fibroblasts, macrophages, mast cells, and lymphocytes, which promote wound healing. The skin's lymphatic, vascular, and nerve supplies, which maintain equilibrium in the skin, are in the dermis.

The dermis is divided into two parts: papillary and reticular. The papillary dermis, which contains increased amounts of collagen, blood vessels, sweat glands, and elastin, is in contact with the epidermis. The *reticular* dermis also contains collagen but with increased amounts of mature elastic tissue. The dermis houses many specialized cells, blood vessels, and nerves.

The epidermis and dermis meet at the *dermoepidermal junction*. This area contains wave-like projections from the dermis called *papillae* (or rete pegs), which correspond to reciprocal structures in the epidermis.

These projections increase the area of contact between the layers of skin, and help to prevent the epidermis from being sheared off. They are not present in the skins of unborn babies but rapidly develop after birth, and are very noticeable in a young person's skin when it is examined under the microscope. As skin ages, the papillae get smaller and flatter.

The *subepidermal basement membrane zone* is a semipermeable filter that permits fluid exchange of components such as nutrients, metabolites, and waste products.

HYPODERMIS

The *subcutaneous layer* is a specialized layer of connective tissue. It is sometimes called the *adipose layer* because of its fat content. This layer is absent in some sites, such as the eyelids, scrotum, areola, and tibia. Age, heredity, and many other factors influence the thickness of the subcutaneous layer. Subcutaneous fat is generally thickest on the back and buttocks, giving shape and contour over the bone. This layer functions as insulation from extremes of hot and cold, as a cushion to trauma, and as a source of energy and hormone metabolism.

FUNCTION OF THE INTEGUMENTARY SYSTEM

The skin is a morphologically complex structure that serves several functions essential to life. The skin differs anatomically and physiologically in various areas of the body. Functions of the skin include protection, maintenance of homeostasis, thermoregulation, sensory reception, vitamin synthesis, and processing of antigenic substances.

PROTECTION

The skin protects the body against many forms of trauma (e.g., mechanical, thermal, chemical, radiant). The intact tough epidermal layer is a mechanical barrier. Bacteria, foreign matter, other organisms, and chemicals can penetrate it with difficulty. The oily and slightly acid secretions of its sebaceous glands protect the body further by limiting the growth of many organisms. The thickened skin of the palms and soles provides additional covering to absorb the constant use of or trauma to these areas.

Cells in both the epidermis and the dermis of the skin are important in immune function. Skin is now recognized not only as a physical barrier but also as a participant in immunologically mediated defense against various antigens. *Langerhans cells* are scattered among the keratinocytes located primarily in the epidermis; however, they can also be seen in the dermis. These cells originate in the bone marrow and migrate to the epidermis. Langerhans cells play a role in the cell-mediated immune responses of the skin through antigen presentation. An antigen entering immunologically competent skin is likely to encounter a coordinated response of Langerhans and T cells to neutralize its effect. An antigen entering diseased skin can induce and elicit immune responses. These reactions may be involved in the pathogenesis of many inflammatory skin diseases.

HOMEOSTASIS

Skin forms a barrier that prevents excessive loss of water and electrolytes from the internal environment. Intact skin also prevents the subcutaneous tissues from drying out. The effectiveness of this impermeable membrane is readily recognized when one observes the extreme loss of fluids that occurs with damage to the skin, as with burns and other injuries. Insensible loss of water and electrolytes occurs only through pores in this effective barrier.

THERMOREGULATION

Body temperature represents the balance between heat generation and heat loss processes. The skin, with its ability to alter the rate of heat loss, is the major point of regulation of body temperature. The rate of heat loss depends primarily on the surface temperature of the skin, which is in turn a function of the skin's blood flow. The blood flow of the skin varies in response to changes in the body's core temperature and to changes in temperature of the external environment.

The flow of blood to the skin is derived in two processes. Direct perfusion is from capillary beds entering in lateral directions. Skin is also perfused vertically from vessels that enter from the muscle and fascia supporting it.

In general, the vessels dilate during warm temperatures and constrict in cold temperatures. The hypothalamus is partly responsible for regulating skin blood flow, particularly to the extremities, the face, ears, and the tip of the nose. Maintenance of the thermal balance allows the internal temperature of the body to remain at approximately 37° C (98.6° F).

Under severe heat stress, increased cutaneous blood flow is inadequate to dissipate the thermal load. Eccrine glands produce sweat, and cooling is enhanced by fluid evaporation from the skin. Eccrine gland innervation is unique in that these sympathetic cholinergic nerves use acetylcholine (rather than norepinephrine) as the neurotransmitter. Sweating significantly enhances the body's capacity for thermoregulation.

SENSORY RECEPTION

Apart from sight and hearing, the major human sensory apparatus is in the skin. Sensory fibers responsible for pain, touch, and temperature form a complex network in the dermis. This information is transmitted in compartments to the spinal cord and is relayed to the somatosensory cortex, where the information is integrated into a somatotopic representation of the body.

The skin contains specialized receptors to detect discriminative touch and pressure. *Touch* (flutter) is sensed by Meissner's corpuscles; *pressure,* by Merkel cells and Ruffini endings; *vibration and pressure,* by Pacinian corpuscles; and *hair movement,* by hair follicle endings. Together these receptors communicate information to the somatosensory cortex via the dorsal column spinal pathways.

A second grouping of nerves communicates information about temperature and pain to the somatosensory cortex via the anterolateral spinal pathways. *Temperature* is sensed by specific thermoreceptors in the epidermis, and *pain* is sensed by free nerve endings throughout the epidermal, dermal, and hypodermal layers. The speed of conduction of pain information to the cortex results in a functional division. "Fast" pain is well localized and has a short latency. "Slow" pain is more diffuse, has a longer latency, and is more difficult to endure.

The density of receptors determines the sensitivity of the skin. For example, two-point discrimination is most accurate on the skin of the fingers and face, where the highest density of touch receptors occurs. In contrast, the skin on the back has a low density of touch receptors, and the ability to localize touch is therefore reduced.

VITAMIN D PRODUCTION

The epidermis is involved in synthesis of vitamin D. In the presence of sunlight or ultraviolet radiation, a sterol found on the malpighian cells is converted to form cholecalciferol (vitamin D_3) in the liver to its active form. Vitamin D_3 assists in the absorption of calcium and phosphate from ingested foods.

DERMATOLOGIC CARE

As the largest and most visible organ of the body, the skin plays a major role in our physical and mental health and protects us from an array of natural and man-made attacks. Yet the skin is rarely taken as seriously as other organ systems, such as the heart and the lung. In both outpatient and inpatient practice settings, as a nurse you have a unique opportunity to affect a client's dermatologic care. You can teach clients to appreciate the skin's important role and to recognize that some skin conditions are indeed life-threatening. For example, skin cancers and especially malignant melanoma are rising at rapid rates. Malignant melanoma is an aggressive form of skin cancer, and often fatal. In the United States today, one person dies every hour from skin cancer. Also, burn injuries continue despite advances in fireproofing homes and clothes. Pressure ulcers, a serious alteration in skin integrity, pose a growing concern as the older population increases, and may result in 60,000 deaths per year.

APPEARANCE AND SELF-ESTEEM

Skin is integral to self-image and self-esteem. Each client's unique appearance is established through the skin. The skin was once thought to reflect the normal "aging process" and how that aging process affected the genetic skin types we inherit. We now know that skin type more likely reflects the cumulative amount of sun exposure over a lifetime. It is hoped that with education, people will once again view untanned skin as attractive and healthy. Cosmetic surgery should not be considered a procedure for vanity but a procedure to enhance self-esteem.

Today's society has a long-standing prejudice that needs to be dispelled regarding impaired skin. Historically, skin diseases were perceived as divine punishment for being spiritually and physically "unclean." Subtle punishment for skin diseases still exists because of ignorance. For example, a woman with atopic dermatitis may sit isolated and shunned in a waiting room because others view eczematous lesions as contagious. A server at a restaurant may be encouraged to work in the back of the kitchen so that customers will not notice the healed burn scars on his or her hands and body. Vitiligo, loss of pigment in the skin, is sometimes mislabeled "white leprosy," and so on. Clients who have visible chronic skin problems often withdraw from social situations and have altered interpersonal relationships and increased social isolation. When these clients seek professional care for skin problems, psychosocial as well as physical concerns need to be met.

Another function of skin, hair, and nails is to provide an outward appearance or *cosmetic adornment*. The appearance of our skin, hair, and nails is crucial to our psychosocial well-being and can affect our experiences positively or negatively. Skin disorders are often a major cause of morbidity because we live in a beauty-conscious society. Health care providers must be acutely aware of the role of the skin in a person's self-esteem and ability to function in relationships.

EFFECTS OF AGING

The skin undergoes numerous changes that can be seen and felt throughout the life span. Many of these changes are natural, unchangeable, and harmless. Some may be bothersome or painful and are treated until there is an acceptable resolution or acceptance of the condition. Other skin changes may go unnoticed or might not be bothersome because they are slow growing, such as senile keratosis. Table A&P11-1 lists some age-associated changes.

Adolescence

During puberty, hormone secretion stimulates the maturation of hair follicles, sebaceous glands, and apocrine and eccrine units in certain body areas. Hair follicles on the face (males), pubic region, and axillae activate to produce coarse terminal hairs. Normal changes may bother teenagers, but adolescents must be cautioned about the potential for irritating the skin with excessive use of over-the-counter products.

New nevi can appear after adolescence. At any age, raised, pigmented lesions that bleed or change in color or size should be assessed by a physician to determine whether they require only minor care or removal because of early malignant changes.

Adulthood

Temporary *hormonal changes* account for some adult skin changes. Pregnancy and birth control pills may alter

TABLE A&P11-1	Common Skin Changes Associated with Aging
Skin Change	**Description**
Adolescence	
Folliculitis	Hair follicle inflammation
Acne	Inflammation of pilosebaceous follicle
Increased perspiration	Response to heat, emotional stress, exercise
Apocrine secretion	Related to sex hormone activity
Skin irritation	Often caused by overuse of over-the-counter skin products
Pigmented nevi	Benign cluster melanocyte-like cells
Adulthood	
Melasma	Blotchy hyperpigmentation
Alopecia	Baldness (hormonal and genetic factors)
Excessive facial or body hair	Androgen-related problem in women
Actinic keratosis	Slightly raised, red papules (premalignant)
Sebaceous cyst	Enclosed cyst in dermis (potentially infectious)
Acrochordon	Small, flesh-colored papule
Older Adulthood	
Xerosis	Dry skin (decreased natural oils and sweat)
Wrinkling	Natural change affected by many factors (e.g., loss of elasticity and subcutaneous fat, sun exposure, gravity, cigarette smoking)
Skin tears	Epidermal thinning; seen most in clients using oral corticosteroids
Senile lentigenes	Black or brown flat lesions ("liver spots")
Seborrheic keratosis	Harmless raised black or brown spots or wart-like growths
Cherry angiomas	Dilated blood vessels that form loops

hormonal status and thus change skin structures that are hormonally linked. Pregnancy may cause changes in hair growth patterns and a temporary thinning of hair after pregnancy. Pregnancy also leads to darkening skin of the areola and a linea nigra (dark line on the abdomen).

Heredity and exposure to environmental factors, such as sun, tobacco, alcohol, and chemicals, play a major role in many of the skin changes that occur in adults. Some lesions (i.e., seborrheic keratosis and acrochordons) may be removed for cosmetic reasons, if desired, or if physically irritating. Actinic keratoses (because of their premalignant status) and sebaceous cysts (because of their infectious potential) need to be assessed and may be removed. Basal and squamous cell cancers develop from sunlight exposure.

Older Adulthood

The skin of older people reflects the cumulative influence of environmental insults, decreased circulation, and diminished function of various skin structures. As the stratum corneum becomes thinner, the skin reacts more readily to minor changes in humidity, temperature, and other irritants. The skin also becomes more transparent. Hair loss is often noticeable on the trunk, pubic area, axillae, and limbs. Loss of pigment causes gray hair. Nails become brittle and may yellow or thicken. Skin may be leathery from overexposure to ultraviolet light.

There is no known treatment for past overexposure; protection from ultraviolet light is the only preventive measure. Wrinkles develop because of loss of tensile strength and elasticity in the skin.

CONCLUSIONS

The skin is the largest and most visible organ of the body. Anatomically, the skin is divided into (1) the epidermis (outer layer), (2) the dermis (inner layer), and (3) the hypodermis (subcutaneous layer). The skin serves many functions. It is the first line of defense against many forms of trauma. Skin maintains body temperature, prevents water loss, and provides sensations of touch, temperature, and pain. Skin also produces vitamin D and recognizes antigens. Finally, healthy skin is aesthetically pleasing.

BIBLIOGRAPHY

1. Berne, R., et al. (2004). *Physiology* (5th ed.). St. Louis: Mosby.
2. Carroll, R.G. (2007). *Elsevier's integrated physiology*. Philadelphia: Saunders.
3. Kierszenbaum, A.L. (2007). *Histology and cell biology: An introduction to pathology* (2nd ed.). St. Louis: Mosby.
4. Guyton, A., & Hall, J. (2006). *Textbook of medical physiology* (11th ed.). Philadelphia: Saunders.
5. Silverthorn, D. (2006). *Human physiology* (4th ed.). San Francisco, Calif: Pearson Benjamin Cummings.

CHAPTER 48

Assessment of the Integumentary System

Noreen Heer Nicol

Assessment of skin disorders is a complex process because many skin disorders undergo a characteristic evolution. Observation is often required on more than one occasion for diagnosis. Additionally, diagnosis may require the information provided by a complete history, physical examination, laboratory tests, and histopathologic analysis. A complete health history assists in the diagnosis of integumentary disorders, such as occupationally related contact dermatitis, or in revealing psychosocial aspects of skin disorders. The medication history is important because side effects of certain medications can cause skin changes. The physical examination can confirm integumentary disorders as well as disclose disorders that the client may have omitted during the history.

HISTORY

The history includes questions about the chief complaint and current manifestations, a review of systems, past health history, past surgical history, allergies, medications, psychosocial history, and family health history.

Current Health
Chief Complaint

The most common problems related to the integument are itching (pruritus), dryness, rashes, lesions, ecchymoses (small hemorrhagic patches), lumps, masses, and cosmetic appearance. The onset, duration, and suspected trigger of each manifestation should be discussed. Ask about changes in the skin, hair, and nails that may be related to the chief complaint. Sample questions that elicit pertinent information related to the presenting dermatologic problem are listed in the website table Dermatologic Assessment History: Sample **evolve** Questions.

Clinical Manifestations

Conduct an analysis of clinical manifestations including the questions located in the Dermatology Assessment: Sample Questions located on the website. The sexual history may **evolve** be significant if the differential diagnosis includes a sexually transmitted infection (STI) (see Chapter 41). Figure 48-1 demonstrates assessment information for clinical manifestations specific to skin complaints.

Pruritus. Persistent itching or pruritus is a manifestation that frequently brings clients to a health care provider. Note whether the itching is associated with skin lesions and whether it is localized or generalized. Persistent itching without associated lesions could suggest significant systemic disease such as biliary obstruction, diabetes mellitus, uremia, lymphoma, or hyperthyroidism. If pruritus is associated with skin lesions, consider scabies, many types of dermatitis, psoriasis, xerosis, and dermatophytosis in the diagnostic process.

Lesions. A change or new skin lesion will often prompt a client to seek evaluation. When assessing any lesion, it is important to inquire about the time the lesion has been present, any color changes, any exudate, and any other changes that have occurred. The lesion may have been altered because of scratching, trauma, or infection and scarring. It is also necessary to establish if the

evolve **Web Enhancements**

Appendix B A Health History Format That Integrates the Assessment of Functional Health Patterns

Tables Dermatologic Assessment History: Sample Questions

Glossary of Dermatologic Terms

Be sure to check out the bonus material on the Evolve website and the CD-ROM, including free self-assessment exercises. **http://evolve.elsevier.com/Black/medsurg**

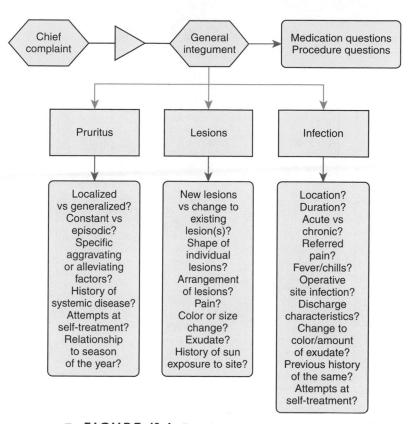

■ FIGURE 48–1 Expanded integumentary assessment.

lesion is in an area of skin that has received significant sun exposure.

Infection. Skin infections will prompt clients to seek further evaluation, especially if there is a history of failure at attempts at self-treatment. As with any infection, establish if there has been fever, chills, the amount and type of exudate, and the presence of pain at the suspected site of infection.

Review of Systems

Obtain a complete history of the skin. Specifically, ask about past problems with unusual itching, dryness, lesions, rashes, lumps, ecchymoses, and masses. Determine if the client has problems with moles or other lesions, especially if they have undergone changes in size, shape, or color. Refer to Figure 48-2 for a guide to compiling an expanded integument history.

Past Medical History

Recent past medical history may be significant. For example, a recent acute or unresolved *Streptococcus* infection might explain diffuse hair loss or an unresolved rash. Ask about childhood diseases, and find out about the vaccination status.

Various systemic diseases are characterized by cutaneous manifestations. Does the client have other systemic disorders relevant to the skin (immunologic, endocrine, collagen, vascular, renal, or hepatic conditions)? Ask about childhood diseases, and find out about the vaccination status.

Surgical History

Evaluating previous trauma, procedure sites, and surgical interventions may explain unusual lesions and/or scars or their location.

Allergies

An *allergy* is an immunologic response that happens consistently with exposure. *Irritation* can occur unpredictably. Inquire about substances that may cause local skin irritation or lesions on direct contact, such as textiles or metals. Wool is irritating to most people. Jewelry that contains nickel can cause skin discoloration, irritation, rash, or other problems in people who are sensitive to this metal.

Ask the client about allergies to medications, foods, inhalants, latex, and other chemicals. Does the ingestion of certain foods cause itching, burning, or eruption of rashes? Does contact with pollens, inhalants, or animals result in hives? A history of past allergic reactions to foods or medications is important for avoiding inadvertent reaction through readministration. A history of contact with and discussion of compounds in the work environment, hobbies, and recent travel is

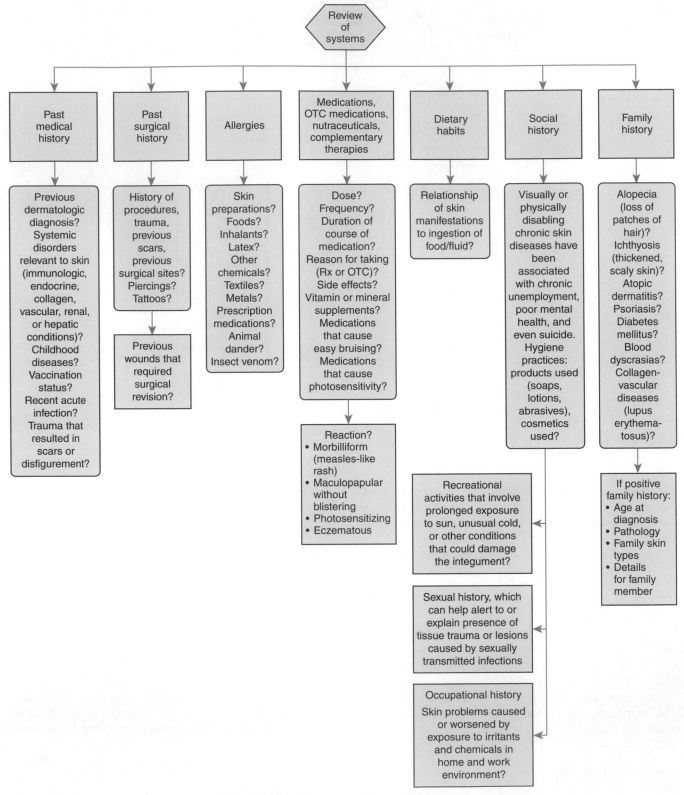

■ **FIGURE 48–2** Expanded integumentary history.

particularly useful when evaluating conditions such as suspected occupational or contact dermatitis or urticaria, which are very common reasons for dermatology consultation.

Medications

Note prescription and over-the-counter medications that the client is currently taking or has recently finished. Complications from these products can range from nuisance skin rashes to rare or life-threatening events. Medication reactions can be limited to the skin or may be part of a systemic process.

The most common type of allergic drug reactions is cutaneous. Most of these skin reactions are *morbilliform* (measles-like rash) or maculopapular without blistering or pustulation. These eruptions can be caused by many drugs, including penicillins, sulfonamides, nevirapine, and antiseizure medications. Sensitivity to antibiotics or other drugs that is manifested in the form of a skin rash may not occur until the end of a routine course of therapy or with subsequent exposures. Photosensitizing drugs (phenothiazines, tetracycline, diuretics, sulfonamides) may cause a sunburn-like rash in areas of sun exposure.[8] Topical preparations may include preservatives or active ingredients that are known sensitizers that frequently produce an eczematous rash. The most commonly encountered are neomycin, benzocaine, and diphenhydramine hydrochloride. Oral corticosteroids (prednisone), if used at high doses or routinely, can cause acne breakouts, thinning of skin, stretch marks, and many other systemic side effects.

Complementary and alternative medicine has grown in the United States, and providers at all levels realize that clients may be anxious to try these products, especially if they suffer from chronic skin disorders such as atopic dermatitis, psoriasis, or wounds. Some components of these medications are beneficial, but for others scientific evidence is lacking and is actually detrimental. When possible, clients need to be educated about these modalities and their possible adverse physiologic and immunologic side effects. Aloe vera *(Aloe barbadensis, Aloe ferox, Aloe africana, Aloe spicata)* is promoted for the relief of eczema and psoriasis and to aid in wound healing. Chamomile *(Matricaria recutita, Chamaemelum nobile),* comfrey *(Symphytum officinale),* evening primrose *(Oenothera biennis),* gotu kola *(Centella asiatica),* and Oregon grape *(Mahonia aquifolium)* have similar uses. Although these products in pure forms or in high quantities may have pharmacologic activities such as antiseptic, diaphoretic, diuretic, or analgesic effects, the effect of diluted topical formulas is not known.[1] Care must also be taken to watch how clients administer products. The answer to future use of these products is the need for more high-quality evidence-based studies.

Dietary Habits

The benefit of balanced nutrition in the areas of wound healing and general skin health continues to be common knowledge. However, discussions of other supplemental nutrition, such as megavitamins taken orally, continue to be causes of concern especially with fat-soluble vitamins. Another myth is the one associated with water and fluid intake for the correlation to xerosis or dry skin conditions. One needs to have almost clinical dehydration before turgor changes become apparent on clinical examination. And while good routine intake of water is a healthy practice for the genitourinary and other systems, there is no scientific evidence that it plays a role in routine hydration of the skin. Suspected food allergy can play a role in specific dermatologic conditions such as atopic dermatitis and urticaria. In these situations, true food allergy needs to be evaluated and established to avoid unnecessary elimination of food types or groups.

Social History

Psychosocial factors that influence dermatologic disorders often play a large role, particularly in long-term and chronic processes. Skin disease can greatly affect lifestyle and self-image. Cultural and familial influences in caring for a particular disorder may conflict with prescribed therapies. Misconceptions about skin problems (e.g., that acne lesions can be scrubbed away) need to be determined and corrected. Visually or physically disabling chronic skin diseases have been associated with chronic unemployment, poor mental health, and even suicide. Assess the client's sexual history, which can help to explain the presence of tissue trauma or lesions caused by STIs (see Chapter 41).

Socioeconomic factors may influence an individual's compliance with outlined therapies and return for follow-up care. When recommending therapies or medications, consider the impact on the client's day-to-day routine as well as the type of prescription insurance plan. Many topical therapies—whether or not they are covered by insurance—are expensive, and expense affects compliance.

Occupational history is important because a large number of skin problems are caused or worsened by exposure to irritants and chemicals in the home and work environment. The travel history can be helpful as well, especially if it includes hiking or exposure to outdoor agents that result in dermatologic disorders, such as poison ivy, poison sumac, poison oak, or Lyme disease. Ask about recent exposure to ticks, other insects, or infections.

Inquire about the client's habits, such as the frequency of hygiene practices, the products used (soaps, lotions, abrasives), and whether cosmetics are used. Record the products used, including brand names. Inquire whether there have been any changes in clothing or bedding, and discuss how these items are cleaned.

Does the client engage in recreational activities that involve prolonged exposure to the sun, unusual cold, or other conditions that could damage the integument? For example, does the client visit tanning salons? Advise clients that exposure to sun and tanning beds leads to premature aging, increased risk of skin cancer, risk of corneal burns if eye guards are not worn, exacerbation of photosensitivity disorders, and increased development of lentigines (age spots) and other types of photodamage.

Family Health History

A personal or family health history helps to determine genetic predisposition to skin disorders as well as a predisposition to parasitic or other conditions related to the family's lifestyle and living environment. Many dermatologic disorders or systemic disorders with a dermatologic presentation have a genetic or familial component. Genetically transmitted dermatologic conditions include *alopecia* (loss of patches of hair), *ichthyosis* (thickened, scaly skin), atopic dermatitis, and psoriasis. Systemic diseases with dermatologic manifestations include diabetes mellitus, blood dyscrasia, and collagen-vascular diseases (lupus erythematosus). Other diseases, such as scabies, are likely to be passed on to family members because of close and frequent exposure.

PHYSICAL EXAMINATION

Examine the skin as thoroughly as any other body organ. This procedure cannot be done properly in the hall or at a quick glance, which the health care provider is often requested to do. Use inspection, palpation, and olfaction to assess hair, nails, and skin. Effective assessment requires knowledge, awareness, and practice in describing the skin of people of all ages, ethnicities, and different lifestyles and in recognizing normal and abnormal skin changes. A description of normal conditions of the integumentary system is given in the Physical Assessment Findings in the Healthy Adult feature above, right.

Terminology

The terms routinely used in dermatology have been referred to as a "foreign language" and have been known to inhibit use of the correct terminology for skin disorders by health care providers. Use of standardized terminology often leads to differential diagnosis. This section clarifies some commonly used dermatologic terms and should assist the reader in recognizing and *evolve* describing skin disorders. See the Glossary of Dermatologic Terms on the website.

Types of Lesions

Examining and making the correct diagnosis of skin disorders depend on identifying skin lesions or changes. Two major types of lesions are distinguished: *primary* and *secondary* lesions.

The primary lesion is the first lesion to appear on the skin and has a visually recognizable structure. Figure 48-3, *A* depicts nine primary lesions: macule, papule, plaque, nodule, wheal, vesicle, bulla, cyst, and

---

Physical Assessment Findings in the Healthy Adult

The Integumentary System

INSPECTION

Skin. Even skin tones, darker on exposed areas of face, neck, arms, and lower legs; lighter on trunk and back. Small tan freckles scattered over face and arms. Scars, striae absent.

Hair and Scalp. Hair evenly distributed over scalp. Clean, without nits or lice. No dandruff, scaling, or scalp lesions. Axillae and legs probably shaved; pubic hair distributed as inverted triangle from symphysis pubis to perineum (female). Pubic hair distributed in diamond pattern from below umbilicus to perineum (male).

Nails. Regular, smooth, oval shape. Pink nail beds. Cuticles manicured, clean. Nail bed angle 160 degrees (no clubbing).

PALPATION

Skin. Warm, well hydrated, smooth, elastic, nontender. No lesions, masses, or lumps.

Hair and Scalp. Hair non-oily, even textured, resilient. Scalp smooth, intact, nontender.

Nails. Firm without tenderness or bogginess. Rapid blanch response.

---

pustule. Frequently, the health care provider does not see a primary lesion but sees only secondary lesions; the health care provider then must depend on the client's description of "how it looked when it first appeared." An in-depth look should be made to find a primary lesion because these are often key to clarifying the diagnosis.

When a primary lesion undergoes changes, it becomes a secondary lesion. These alterations, brought about by the client or by the client's environment, often occur in the epidermal layer. The changes may result from many factors, including scratching, rubbing, medication, natural disease progression over time, or processes of involution and healing. Figure 48-3, *B* presents eight secondary lesions: scale, crust, erosion, deep ulcer, scar, lichenification, excoriation, fissure, and atrophy.

Examination Environment

The best setting for conducting a dermatologic assessment is a well-lighted, private room with moderate temperature and neutral, white, or cream-colored walls. Excessive warmth can produce changes in skin color (redness) by causing vasodilation. Colored walls can affect normal skin hue (color). For a complete examination, ask the client to undress and provide a gown. Explain that all skin surfaces will be examined. Having a second health care provider in the room during a total body examination is frequently recommended. Avoid unnecessary exposure during the examination. Have

MACULE: Skin color change without elevation, i.e., flat (freckles or petechia). Described as a "patch" if greater than 1 cm (vitiligo).

PAPULE: Elevated, solid lesion of less than 1 cm, varying in color (warts or elevated nevus).

PLAQUE: Raised, flat lesion formed from merging papules or nodules.

NODULE: Larger than a papule. Raised solid lesion extending deeper into the dermis. A large nodule is referred to as a tumor.

WHEAL (hive): Fleeting skin elevation that is irregularly shaped because of edema (mosquito bite or urticaria).

VESICLE (blister): Elevated, sharply defined lesion containing serous fluid. Usually less than 1 cm (blister, chickenpo, or herpes simplex).

BULLA (plural, bullae): Large, elevated, fluid-filled lesion greater than 1 cm (partial-thickness burn).

CYST: Elevated, thick-walled lesion containing fluid or semisolid matter.

PUSTULE: Elevated lesion less than 1 cm containing purulent material. Lesions larger than 1 cm are described as boils, abscesses, or furuncles (acne or impetigo).

SCALE: Dried fragments of sloughed epidermal cells, irregular in shape and size and white, tan, yellow, or silver in color (dandruff, dry skin, or psoriasis).

EROSION: A moist, demarcated, depressed area due to loss of partial- or full-thickness epidermis. Basal layer of epidermis remains intact (ruptured chickenpox vesicle).

DEEP ULCER: Irregularly shaped, exudative, depressed lesion in which entire epidermis and all or part of dermis are lost. Results from trauma and tissue destruction (pressure ulcer).

SCAR: Mark left on skin after healing. Replacement of destroyed tissue by scar tissue.

LICHENIFICATION: Epidermal thickening resulting in elevated plaque with accentuated skin markings. Usually results from repeated injury through rubbing or scratching (chronic atopic dermatitis).

EXCORIATION: Superficial, linear abrasion of epidermis. Visible sign of itching caused by rubbing or scratching (atopic dermatitis).

FISSURE: Deep linear split through epidermis into dermis (tinea pedis).

KELOID: Irregularly shaped, elevated, progressively enlarging scar; extends beyond the boundaries of the wound; caused by excessive collagen formation during post-surgical healing.

■ **FIGURE 48–3 A,** Primary lesions: visually recognizable structural changes in the skin that have specific characteristics. **B,** Secondary lesions: primary lesions that have changed because of the natural progression of the lesion or because of physical change (scratching, irritation, or secondary infection).

warm hands to avoid stimulation of the skin and to add to the client's overall comfort.

Depth of Examination

The examination is systematic and as complete as appropriate. A total-body skin examination involves assessment of the hair, scalp, nails, mucous membranes, and skin, including the axillae, areas in skinfolds, external genitalia, webs between toes and fingers, palms of hands, and soles of feet. Begin at the head, and proceed to the toes. General changes can alter total-body skin color (jaundice, cyanosis, pallor), thickness, turgor, temperature, and vascularity (purpura, petechiae). General findings can suggest systemic disease and may require complete physical examination and appropriate evaluation. The diagnosis of skin disorders is accomplished by careful observation and evaluation of individual lesions. This discussion is limited to assessment of hair, scalp, nails, and skin lesions.

Considerations in Ethnic Populations

As the demographics of the United States continue to change, the background and skills of the health care providers must continue to expand. Providers must learn to distinguish between normal and pathologic dermatologic variations in all ethnic populations, including Asians, African Americans, and Hispanics, as well as Caucasians (e.g., recognizing how inflammation, erythema, or follicular reactivity can appear in different skin pigments). Inflammation is underrecognized in dark-skinned people because erythema is difficult to assess. In diseases such as atopic dermatitis, nummular eczema, pityriasis rosea, or sarcoidosis, follicular accentuation is clearly visible in darker-skinned people. Post-inflammatory hyperpigmentation may persist longer after the disease has cleared in dark-pigmented skin than in fair-skinned people. In addition to appreciating physical differences in the skin of various ethnic populations, one must learn to value the social customs, traditional beliefs, mistrust, and fear that may influence adherence to treatment regimens.

Inspection and Palpation
Hair and Scalp

Examine the hair distribution patterns for symmetry and distribution according to the client's age and sexual development. Fine hair covers much of the body and is the same color as scalp hair. Increased distribution occurs normally in the axillae and pubic area. Having excess body hair is known as *hirsutism*.

Inspect the hair and scalp under good light, and always wear protective gloves while examining open lesions or if you suspect infestation with lice. Inspect

and palpate the hair for distribution, thickness, texture, lubrication, and signs of infestation or infection. Because natural hair color varies greatly, ask the client whether hair dye is used because it alters the hair's texture. Hair should be resilient and distributed evenly over the scalp. Texture and lubrication are affected by the type of hair care products used as well as by a protein-deficient diet or severe health problems, which tend to leave hair dry and brittle. Hair loss or thinning *(alopecia)* can result from genetic predisposition to baldness or a health problem, such as recent chemotherapy or a thyroid disorder.

Inspect and palpate the scalp for lesions, excoriations (from scratching), lumps, or bruises, which should be absent. Examine hair shafts for the presence of nits, which are the eggs of the human head louse. Adult lice often bite the scalp behind the ears and along the back of the neck, which results in pustular lesions.

If you see lesions, describe them and ask the client about recent trauma or injury to the head. If the client has not already provided information during the health history interview, conduct an analysis of clinical manifestations.

Nails

Inspect the client's nails for color, shape, texture, integrity, and thickness (Table 48-1). The nails reflect the client's overall health, indicating nutrition and respiratory status.

Color and Shape. The nail plate is usually transparent and colorless and, when viewed from the side, has a convex shape. The vascular bed underlying the nail plate gives the nail its color. The color is pink in white clients and darker in dark-skinned clients. A hemoglobin deficiency is seen in the nail bed as pallor, and decreased arterial circulation appears as cyanosis.

Texture. Texture should be smooth; healthy nails are of uniform thickness with no signs of dryness, softness, brittleness, splitting, peeling, ridges, or pitting. The *angle* formed between the nail plate and the posterior nailfold is about 160 degrees without separation (see Table 48-1). Changes in nail shape and nail bed angle can indicate health problems. Clubbing of the nails refers to an increase of more than 160 degrees in the angle between the nail plate and nail base. The base of a clubbed nail is spongy and soft on palpation. These changes result from hypoxia (diminished tissue oxygenation). Nail clubbing commonly occurs in clients with congenital heart defects or chronic lung disease.

Integrity. The tissue surrounding the nail should appear intact without signs of inflammation, jagged edges

TABLE 48–1 Assessing the Nails	
Assessment Finding	**Description**
Normal nail About 160° 	Nail shape is convex, and nail plate angle is approximately 160°
Beau's line Beau's line 	Horizontal depression in nail plate; depressions can occur singly or in multiples Cause: Nail growth is disturbed temporarily; related to systemic illness (infection) or direct injury to the nail root
Splinter hemorrhages 	Linear (vertical) red or brown streaks in nail bed Cause: Minor trauma to nail bed; subacute bacterial endocarditis; trichinosis
Paronychia 	Inflammation of skinfold at nail margin Cause: Trauma; skin infection at nail base
Spoon shape 	Nail shape is concave as nail curves upward from nail bed Cause: Use of strong detergents; iron deficiency anemia; syphilis
Clubbing 	Increased angle between nail plate and nail base Cause: Long-standing hypoxia

(hangnail), or dryness. Inferior or lateral nailfold inflammation is a sign of paronychia (nailfold infection). If these abnormalities are noted, ask the client about nail care habits such as biting or cutting cuticles.

Thickness. While examining the fingers and toes, you may note common abnormalities such as calluses or corns. A *callus* is a flat, painless thickening of a circumscribed area of skin. Calluses usually occur on the hands and feet. A *corn* is a horny induration and thickening of the skin caused by friction and pressure and is often painful.

Skin
Color. Assess overall skin color during the health history interview. Observe the client's face and visible skin surfaces for color tones, which should be congruent with the stated race. Abnormal findings include pallor

(paleness), a flushed or ruddy complexion, cyanosis (blue cast), jaundice (yellow cast), and areas of irregular pigmentation. Normal variation occurs from one region of the body to another, particularly in areas protected from the sun and exposure by clothing; these areas are lighter. Overall color should be uniform, but may range over a variety of colors.

Examine local areas of color change closely. *Hyperpigmentation* describes areas of increased pigmentation; *hypopigmentation* describes areas of decreased pigmentation. Skin color also results from the circulation; an increased blood supply may lead to the redness of inflammation *(rubor),* whereas extreme pallor may be a result of anemia or impeded arterial circulation to the area. Areas that are less pigmented reveal abnormal findings more readily than more heavily pigmented surfaces. *Pallor* is best seen in the buccal (mouth) mucosa, especially in clients with dark skin. *Cyanosis* is evident more readily in less pigmented areas, such as the nail beds, lips, and palms. *Jaundice* sharply contrasts with the white of the sclera, especially in dark-skinned clients who have more carotene deposits. Jaundice is best assessed in dark-skinned clients by inspecting color changes in the hard palate.

Moisture. Moisture refers to the skin's hydration level. Overall skin moisture in healthy individuals can be described as well hydrated. Skin moisture often reflects ambient temperature and humidity levels. Moistness usually occurs in intertriginous areas (where skin touches skin), such as the axillae and groin. Skin that feels overly moist and cool (clammy) or overly dry, scaling, or cracked is abnormal.

Temperature. Assess temperature with the dorsum of the hand. The skin should feel uniformly warm because it reflects circulation. Compare areas of hypothermia or hyperthermia with the same areas on the opposite side (Figure 48-4).

Texture. Palpate *texture* by stroking the skin lightly with the fingertips. The skin should feel smooth, soft, and resilient. There should be no areas of lumps or unusual thickening or thinning *(atrophy).*

Turgor. Turgor, a reflection of the skin's elasticity and hydration status, is measured by the time needed for the skin and underlying tissue to return to their original contour after being "pinched up." Lightly pinch the skin over the forearm between the thumb and index finger, and then release it. Skin with normal turgor is mobile and elastic and should return to baseline contour within 3 seconds. If the skin remains elevated (tented) for more than 3 seconds, turgor is decreased. Turgor decreases with age as the skin loses elasticity.

■ **FIGURE 48–4** Assessing skin temperature uses the backs of the hands for the most accurate assessment.

Edema. Palpate for *edema* (fluid retention), particularly if areas of taut, shiny skin are noted. Edema refers to a collection of fluid in underlying tissues that separate the skin's surface from pigmented and vascular layers, resulting in a blanched appearance. It is an abnormal finding. Palpate edematous areas for consistency, temperature, shape (extent), tenderness, and mobility. Assess and describe edematous areas using the technique described in Chapter 51. Areas examined for edema include those over the sacrum (especially in bedridden clients), the feet, the ankles, and over the tibia.

Tenderness. Tenderness is an abnormal finding and is elicited with palpation. No areas of tenderness should be found in a healthy, uninjured client.

Odor. The skin should be free of pungent odors. Odors, when noted, are usually present in the axillae and skinfolds or in open wounds and are related to the presence of bacteria on the skin, inadequate hygiene, or infection. Assess odor in open wounds after cleansing the wound because odor can be related to the drainage itself or to the type of dressing used (hydrocolloid).

Lesions. Inspect the skin for detectable lesions. Assess and describe lesions in an orderly fashion: location, distribution, size, arrangement, color, configuration, secondary changes, and presence of drainage. Palpate skin lesions to determine the characteristics of contour (flat, raised, or depressed), size (using a measuring device), consistency (firm, soft), mobility, and tenderness. Lesions can be mobile or immobile (fixed to underlying tissue). Photographing lesions of concern is an excellent way to document changes over time.

Location, Distribution, and Size. Location is described in reference to anatomic landmarks. Measure the lesions for *size* to help classify their type (macule, papule). If multiple lesions are present, the *distribution pattern* can be helpful in determining the diagnosis. Note the extent of the lesions. Lesions can be (1) localized (confined to a specific area), (2) regional, or (3) generalized (present over a large surface). Compare sides bilaterally to determine whether lesions are symmetrical or asymmetrical. Another commonly noted distribution is on sun-exposed areas. Certain diseases feature a classic lesion distribution; for example, lesions of herpes zoster follow along a nerve root dermatome. Table 48-2 presents common configurations and distributions. Figure 48-5 depicts the locations of common skin disorders found during physical examination.

Arrangement. The *arrangement* refers to the pattern of nearby lesions. Two of the typical patterns are *linear* and *satellite,* which can also be helpful in confirming diagnosis. Linear lesions appear in a straight line (scabies). Satellite lesions appear as small peripheral lesions around a central larger lesion (diaper candidiasis).

Color. Skin lesions are found in a wide variety of colors; they may be skin-colored, brown, red, yellow, tan, or blue. Color can be influenced by many factors,

TABLE 48–2 Terminology for Skin Lesion Configuration and Distribution

Configuration*	Description
Annular	Ring-shaped
Iris	Concentric rings, "bull's eyes"
Gyrate	Spiral-shaped
Linear	Forming a line
Nummular	Coin-like
Polymorphous	Occurring in several forms
Punctate	Marked by points or dots
Serpiginous	Snake-like
Distribution†	**Description**
Solitary	Single lesion
Satellite	Single lesion occurring in close proximity to but separate from a large group of lesions
Grouped	Clustered
Confluent	Merged together
Diffuse	Widely distributed
Discrete	Separate from other lesions
Generalized	Diffusely distributed
Localized	Limited, clearly defined
Symmetrical	Bilaterally distributed
Asymmetrical	Unilaterally distributed
Zosteriform	Band-like distribution of lesions along a dermatome

* Position of lesions relative to other lesions.
† Grouping, or pattern, of lesions over entire skin surface.

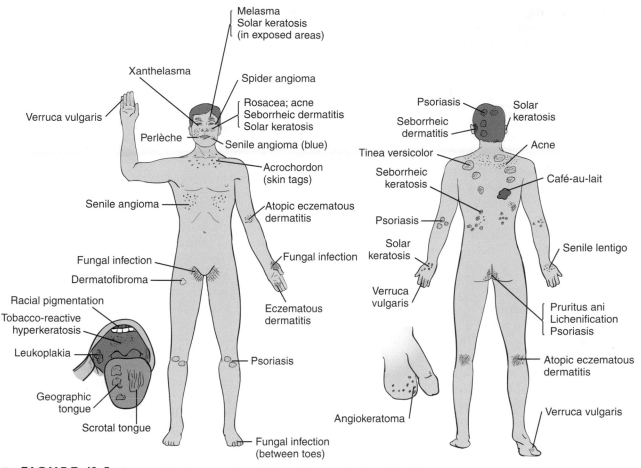

■ **FIGURE 48–5** Common disorders encountered during physical examination of the skin.

including the client's normal skin hue, which may make accurate description difficult. Slight color changes can best be assessed in areas having the least amount of natural pigmentation and those with superficial capillary beds (buccal membrane of the mouth, mucosa, lips, nail beds, ocular conjunctiva, palms, and soles). These areas are especially important in assessing darkly pigmented skin.

Configuration. The term *configuration* refers to the shape or the outline of the lesion. Most lesions are circular. The term *nummular* is used for a circular lesion that is the size of a large coin (nummular eczema). *Annular* describes lesions with an active ring-shaped border and some central clearing (granuloma annulare). Table 48-2 describes other configurations that may be found during assessment.

Skin Self-Examination

Although it is crucial that all health care providers learn to perform an accurate and complete assessment of the skin, it is more important to teach every individual how to perform a skin self-examination. Routine self-examination promotes skin health and awareness and greatly lowers individual risk for severe skin disorders, such as skin cancer. Teach clients to examine their entire bodies to look for any changes in the skin or in their moles or skin lesions. See the Client Education Guide feature on Skin Self-Examination in Chapter 49. Encourage clients to visit their health care provider for further evaluation of any suspicious-looking lesions.

Danger signals to look for are the *ABCDEs* of melanoma:

A, *Asymmetry:* one half is unlike the other half
B, *Border:* irregular, scalloped, or poorly circumscribed border
C, *Color:* varied from one area to another, shades of two colors, or changing colors
D, *Diameter:* larger than 6 mm as a rule (diameter of a Number 2 pencil eraser)
E, *Evolving:* any change (e.g., in size, shape, color, elevation), or another trait, or a new manifestation (such as bleeding, itching, or crusting)

Diagnostic Testing

Before a diagnostic skin procedure (or treatment), perform an assessment and document the findings. Nursing intervention for diagnostic procedures includes explaining the procedure to the client and the client's significant others and allowing them to ask questions and express concerns. Explain appropriate wound care and indications of possible side effects and complications that should be reported, such as prolonged bleeding or infection (indicated by swelling, redness, drainage, increased discomfort, or temperature elevation).

Provide instructions (preferably written) for follow-up care as well as follow-up appointment and telephone number. Documentation of diagnostic procedures (exactly what was done and by whom) and the specific location of the lesion must be completed by appropriate personnel.

Skin Culture and Sensitivity

Bacterial, fungal, and certain viral infections of the skin can be confirmed by culture. Because of the cost and delay in getting results, culture is usually reserved for infections that have been unresponsive to routine care. Clients who have had frequent courses of systemic antibiotics and still experience bacterial skin infections are candidates for a culture and sensitivity test to determine which antibiotic is indicated for treatment.

Potassium Hydroxide Examination and Fungal Culture

Fungal infection of skin, hair, or nails can be confirmed by microscopic identification or culture of scrapings from the area, or both. Any area of scaly dermatitis may be scraped for this test. Typical sites are the scalp, intertriginous areas (between the toes, axillae, groin, under or between the breasts, abdominal folds), and the nailfold.

Fine scales from the edge of the site are scraped with a number 15 scalpel blade or the edge of a glass slide onto a second glass slide. A drop of 10% to 20% potassium hydroxide is added to the scale, and a coverslip is placed over the specimen. Gentle pressure is applied to the coverslip to flatten the scales. The slide may be gently heated to dissolve the keratin or the cells more quickly. The scrapings are examined under the microscope. For a culture, scrapings from a suspicious lesion are implanted in the appropriate culture medium. For a nail culture, an altered, dystrophic nail is snipped and implanted in the medium. Debris from the nail's subungual area is less suitable for culture.

Tzanck's Smear

Tzanck's smear is used for microscopic assessment of fluids and cells from vesicles or bullae. The presence of multinucleated giant cells establishes a diagnosis of viral infection, such as herpes simplex or herpes zoster infection. An intact, recently evolved vesicle top is removed, and its base is scraped with a scalpel or small curette. The debris is smeared onto a labeled slide and sent for cytologic assessment.

Scabies Scraping

The most difficult part of the test for scabies is selecting an unscratched lesion from which to take the specimen. Often several areas need to be prepared. When visible, a linear burrow is sampled to look for the mite, its eggs, or feces. The top of the lesion is shaved off with a number 15 scalpel blade or removed by curette. The specimens are placed on a microscope slide, covered with immersion oil and a coverslip, and examined under low power on the microscope. Local anesthesia is not necessary, and fine bleeding is expected. Some discomfort occurs when the lesion is opened.

Wood's Light Examination

Wood's light ("black light") uses a high-pressure mercury lamp that transmits long-wave ultraviolet light (UVA, or 360-nm light); it has limited diagnostic uses. For example, Wood's light can (1) detect few superficial fungal and bacterial skin infections, (2) delineate pigmentary disorders by highlighting the degree of contrast between lesions and normal skin color, and (3) accentuate the contrast between hypopigmented and totally amelanotic areas. It is important to recognize that the most common types of fungi do not fluoresce, and for years this test has been of questionable use in diagnosing fungus.[11] Wood's light examination is done in a darkened room.

Patch Testing

Patch testing is done to attempt to identify substances that produce allergic skin responses.[4,13] It is a painless procedure, and a skilled evaluator must be on hand to read and interpret the results. Patch testing is often done to differentiate between an *irritant* contact dermatitis and an *allergic* contact dermatitis. Small amounts of various substances or allergens are applied to the skin using a commercially prepared tape containing the allergens, or allergens are placed on aluminum disks on a special tape. The client and the client's significant others need to understand that whereas potential allergic substances (allergens) can produce inflammatory skin reactions, compounds of low concentration are used to prevent possible excessive irritation.

Patch testing should not be performed if acute dermatitis is present or if the client is taking substantial amounts of oral steroids; the potential allergen might worsen the dermatitis.

TABLE 48–3 **Methods of Lesion Biopsy**

Biopsy Type	Details
Punch	Obtains skin specimen with full thickness (epidermal, dermal, and subcutaneous tissue) using circular sharp instrument of varying cutting diameters (2-8 mm) for diagnosis
Shave	Obtains tissue sample of epidermis and generally upper portion of dermis using blade-type instrument to remove lesions/specimen around the plane of surrounding skin for diagnosis or treatment
Snip excision	Used to remove lesion/specimen that can be cut off with blade-type instrument or scissor at base of pedunculated lesion for diagnosis or treatment
Curettage	Used to remove/obtain tissue/specimen using an oval or round scalpel-type instrument for diagnosis or treatment
Excision	Obtains a larger full-thickness specimen than is attainable by punch; usually used on large irregular lesion for diagnosis or treatment of a recurrent or aggressive lesion
Surgical excision	Used (1) when it is necessary to excise lesion completely (when full skin thickness is needed), (2) when lesion's borders are indistinct from surrounding skin, or (3) when there is recurrent or aggressive cancer. Lesion is excised with scalpel by means of a variety of surgical techniques

The tape must be worn for 48 hours without disturbing the patches; then it is removed. Interpretations are made at 48, 72, and 96 hours and sometimes at 1 week. A specific eczematous response at the test site with erythema, papules, or small vesicles indicates a positive reaction and confirms an allergic contact sensitivity to the substance on the disk. Counseling regarding allergen avoidance in a positive test or the meaning of the negative result is a critical part of the test.[4]

Biopsy

Skin biopsy refers to the removal of a skin tissue specimen for histologic (cellular microscopic) assessment and/or immunofluorescence (special media before special microscopic evaluation). In all procedures, local anesthesia is generally used. Small-gauge (26- to 30-gauge) needles are recommended to limit trauma to the skin. Refer to Table 48-3 for specifics regarding the types of biopsy.

Depending on the size and location of the biopsy specimen and the skill of the practitioner, the procedure is usually quick and almost painless. The most common source of pain is the initial administration of local anesthetic. The specimen is placed in a preservative such as formalin solution, properly identified, and sent for pathologic assessment. Clean or sterile technique is used as appropriate to dress or cover the biopsy site.

Preprocedure Care. Depending on the procedure, instruct the client to avoid the use of aspirin and products containing aspirin for 48 hours before the biopsy to avoid a prolonged postprocedure bleeding time. If the client is taking anticoagulants (heparin or warfarin), notify the physician. Review the client's medical history for systemic disorders such as liver malfunction, which affects clotting time. If the client has a history of cardiac valve replacement, be sure that prophylactic antibiotics are prescribed. Obtain an informed consent. The client may eat a light meal before the procedure to avoid syncope (fainting).

Postprocedure Care. After the procedure, cover most biopsy sites with an antibiotic ointment and a clean bandage or dry dressing unless ordered otherwise. Many nonadhesive types of dressings are available and may be preferable for clients who have fragile or sensitive skin. The client should be reminded that a follow-up assessment is necessary, and a follow-up appointment should be scheduled if needed for suture removal. Tell the client how and when biopsy results will be reported; individuals have different levels of anxiety about biopsy results.

CONCLUSIONS

The skin is the largest organ in the body, and it presents many health care challenges. The key to assessment of the skin or to the assessment of a rash or lesion is use of a comprehensive, systematic approach. Remember, the current view does not tell the whole story; multiple assessments over time or anticipating the changes that came before or those that will occur next will be important.

BIBLIOGRAPHY

Citations appearing in red refer to primary research.

Citations appearing in blue refer to evidence-based practice guidelines and protocols.

1. Boguniewicz, M. (2002). *Immunology and allergy clinics of North America: Atopic dermatitis.* Philadelphia: Saunders.
2. Callen, J.P. (2000). *Color atlas of dermatology* (2nd ed.). Philadelphia: Saunders.
3. Deleo, V.A., Elsner, P., & Marks, J.G. (2002). *Contact & occupational dermatology* (3rd ed.). St. Louis: Mosby.
4. Fitzpatrick, T.B., Johnson, R.A., & Wolff, K. (2001). *Color atlas and synopsis of clinical dermatology: Common and serious diseases* (4th ed.). New York: McGraw-Hill.
5. Freedberg, I.M., Eisen, A.Z., Wolff, K., et al (2003). *Fitzpatrick's dermatology in general medicine* (6th ed.). New York: McGraw-Hill.
6. Gilchrest, B.A. (2002). *Geriatric dermatology part II.* Philadelphia: Saunders.
7. Greaves, M.W., & Leung, D.Y.M. (2000). *Allergic skin disease: A multidisciplinary approach.* New York: Marcel Dekker.
8. Hill, M.J. (2003). *Dermatologic nursing essentials: A core curriculum* (2nd ed.). Pitman, NJ: Dermatology Nurses' Association.

9. Huether, S., & McCance, K. (2004). *Understanding pathophysiology* (3rd ed.). St. Louis: Mosby.
10. Lane, A.T., Morelli, J.G., & Weston, W.L. (2002). *Color textbook of pediatric dermatology* (3rd ed.). St. Louis: Mosby.
11. Lookingbill, D.P., & Marks J.G. (2006). *Principles of dermatology* (4th ed.). Philadelphia: Saunders.
12. McCance, K., & Huether, S.E. (2006). *Pathophysiology: The biological basis for disease in adults and children* (5th ed.). St. Louis: Mosby.
13. Williams, J.D., Berger, T.G., & Elston, D.M. (2006). *Andrews' diseases of the skin: Clinical dermatology* (10th ed.). Philadelphia: Saunders.

evolve *Did you remember to check out the bonus material on the Evolve website and the CD-ROM, including NCLEX®-Examination Style Review Questions, Open-Book Quizzes, and Chapter Review Audio Podcasts?*

http://evolve.elsevier.com/Black/medsurg

CHAPTER 49

Management of Clients with Integumentary Disorders

NOREEN HEER NICOL AND JOYCE M. BLACK

The skin is the largest and most visible organ of the body. Disorders of the skin offer the nurse an opportunity to provide care that makes a noticeable difference to clients. Anger, frustration, depression, and anxiety are commonly experienced by clients with skin disorders, particularly those with chronic dermatoses. Clients can become embarrassed about their appearance and shun socializing.

The educational needs of people affected by skin disease are vast. Health care providers need to consistently provide information that includes detailed skin care plans, general disease information, and availability of client-oriented support organizations as well as updates on encouraging research results. It behooves health care providers to stay current with new therapies to assist clients in obtaining information and treatment advances. Clients tend to forget or confuse important skin care treatment programs without written instructions. Clearly outlining the skin care recommendations orally and in writing is essential for increased compliance and good outcomes.

COMMON SKIN DISORDERS

PRURITUS

Pruritus (itching), one of the most common manifestations of skin problems, is a symptom, not a disease. Pruritus can lead to damage if scratching injures the skin, increasing risk for infection and scarring. Pruritus can be seen in conditions ranging from dry skin to severe systemic disease. Systemic diseases that can cause generalized and severe pruritus include chickenpox, liver and renal failure, diabetes mellitus, drug hypersensitivity reaction, immunodeficiency disorders, intestinal parasites, leukemia, and lymphoma. Relieving itching, especially for chronically ill clients, is challenging

because of its common occurrence, detrimental effect on skin health, and the major effect it may have on quality of life.

Itching can begin by irritation from almost any chemical or physical substance, or allergic reaction, especially if skin is damaged. Once the itch sensation starts, the client has an almost uncontrollable urge to scratch; and scratching leads to further skin damage and increased inflammation. Thus the itch-scratch-itch cycle develops. To minimize skin trauma caused by scratching, fingernails should be short, smooth, and clean.

Appropriate management of itching requires a complete assessment that attempts to discover the underlying cause and knowledge of appropriate therapeutic modalities for treatment. Dry skin may be either the source of pruritus or a contributing factor, and good hydration is often helpful (see Xerotic Eczema), in addition to any other topical therapy. The Integrating Pharmacology feature on Common Topical Preparations describes medications used to treat dermatologic conditions (see p. 1200).

One bath or shower per day for 15 to 20 minutes with warm water and a gentle cleanser is recommended, immediately followed by the application of a sealing

---

evolve **Web Enhancements**

Care Plan The Client with Atopic Dermatitis

Case Management The Client with Impaired Skin Integrity

Client Education Guide Skin Self-Examination (Spanish Translation)

Topical Corticosteroids (Spanish Translation)

Simple Guidelines to Help Protect You from the Damaging Rays of the Sun (English Version and Spanish Translation)

Postoperative Care After Rhinoplasty (English Version and Spanish Translation)

Be sure to check out the bonus material on the Evolve website and the CD-ROM, including free self-assessment exercises. **http://evolve.elsevier.com/Black/medsurg**

Common Topical Preparations

The skin's large surface area allows the absorption, penetration, and permeation of topically applied preparations. The factors that determine how well these processes occur in the skin's layers include the client's age, the size of the affected region of skin, the condition of the stratum corneum, the cutaneous blood supply, the molecular weight of the drug, and the medication vehicle (the word *vehicle* is used here to mean the substance containing the medication or the form in which the medication is delivered).

Topical medications are chosen both for the action of the active ingredients (which are delivered directly to the skin surface) and for the vehicle. Topical medications have many different actions and cover a large spectrum of drug categories, including anti-infective, antipruritic, and anti-inflammatory.

Examples of various topical medication vehicles are ointments, creams, gels, lotions, solutions, and powders. Ointments are more occlusive, providing better delivery of the medication by preventing water loss from the skin. Use ointments cautiously with excessive heat or humidity because occlusion may result in increased itching or skin infection. When the weather is hot and humid, creams may be better tolerated. Although creams spread more easily than ointments, they are less occlusive, leading to increased skin drying in some people because of the evaporative property of the water. Creams also can be water based with ethyl alcohol and not be as drying as creams have been in the past. Sprays and lotions are available for use on the scalp and other hairy areas. The various ingredients used to formulate the different bases may be irritating to the skin, and care must be taken when recommending any product.

Both the active ingredient and the vehicle must be appropriate for the condition being treated. For acute dermatoses (i.e., weeping, blistering lesions), an aqueous (water-based) compound provides a drying effect. A greasy vehicle has the opposite effect; it promotes lubrication and occlusion and helps treat the dryness and scaling caused by chronic dermatosis. Differences in skin permeability also influence the effectiveness of topical medications. For example, absorption is increased in inflamed skin. Depending on the medication and the specific condition, topical medication may be applied to localized lesions or to larger skin surfaces. When increased absorption of the medication is needed, topical medication may be prescribed for application under an occlusive dressing. Be aware that some topical medication drug package-insert information states that they should or should *not* be used with or under occlusion. Ointments, creams, and gels have greatly increased absorption if they are applied to skin that is wet.

emollient, with or without other topical medications, to prevent evaporation of water from the hydrated epidermis. Other topical medications often added to emollients to help alleviate itching include menthol (0.25% to 0.5%), camphor (0.25% to 0.5%), urea (10% to 20%), and lactic acid (12%). Camphor and menthol produce a cooling effect. Urea and lactic acid moisturize scaly skin by drawing moisture into the cell structure of the stratum corneum. Topically applied antihistamines and anesthetics are relatively ineffective and are best avoided because they can be potent allergic sensitizers. The sensitizing effect is especially pronounced if these products are used on inflamed skin. Use of topical corticosteroids should be reserved for the treatment of specific steroid-responsive dermatoses, not pruritus of unknown origin. Long-term application of topical steroids, especially on skin not affected with an eczematous condition, may result in thinning of the skin, striae, telangiectases, and easy bruising.

Systemic antihistaminic agents are most helpful in disorders in which histamine is the principal mediator but may be of benefit through a sedative or even placebo effect. A trial of a histamine$_1$ (H$_1$) blocker (hydroxyzine, diphenhydramine, cetirizine) is appropriate either on a regular schedule or as indicated for itching. Tricyclic antidepressants have a high binding capacity for H$_1$ receptors and may be helpful in clients who would benefit from their antidepressant as well as antipruritic effect. Mild analgesia can also be effective.

Older clients may have difficulty applying the needed topical agents properly, and assistive personnel may be required to ensure proper therapy. Oral sedating antihistamines should be administered carefully, with use of small doses initially, because many older people have a very low tolerance of these agents and may experience severe drowsiness, especially at the initiation of therapy.

ECZEMATOUS DISORDERS

Eczema is not a specific disease. *Dermatitis* and *eczema* are terms that may be used interchangeably to describe a group of disorders with a characteristic clinical appearance. Types of dermatitis are listed in Box 49-1.

BOX 49-1   Types of Dermatitis

- *Allergic contact dermatitis:* eruptions from allergy to poison ivy, sumac, or oak or another proven allergen
- *Irritant dermatitis:* eruptions from direct contact with irritating substances, which can be almost anything including cosmetics, chemicals, dyes, or detergents
- *Nummular eczema:* appearance of coin-shaped, oozing, crusting patches
- *Seborrheic dermatitis:* yellowish pink scaling of the scalp, face, and trunk
- *Stasis dermatitis:* eruptions resulting from peripheral venous disorders
- *Atopic dermatitis:* characteristic distribution of eczema in people with a family history of asthma, hay fever, or eczema

Eczema/dermatitis has three primary stages; the condition may be limited to any one of the three stages, or the three stages may coexist.

- *Acute dermatitis* is characterized by extensive erosions with serous exudate or by intensely pruritic, erythematous papules and vesicles on a background of erythema.
- *Subacute dermatitis* is characterized by erythematous, excoriated, scaling papules or plaques that are either grouped or scattered over erythematous skin; the scaling may be so fine and diffuse that the skin acquires a silvery sheen.
- *Chronic dermatitis* is characterized by thickened skin and increased skin marking secondary to rubbing and scratching (lichenification); excoriated papules, fibrotic papules, and nodules (prurigo nodularis); and postinflammatory hyperpigmentation and hypopigmentation.

ATOPIC DERMATITIS

Atopic dermatitis is a common, chronic, relapsing, pruritic type of eczema that begins in childhood. Clients with atopic dermatitis have familial hay fever, asthma, sensitive skin, and/or a history of atopic dermatitis.

Etiology

Atopic dermatitis (AD) is due to a combination of heredity and environmental factors. Genetic aspects are clear; most clients with atopic dermatitis report a family history of atopic diseases. The Genetic Links feature below lists other genetic disorders involving the skin. Atopic dermatitis is becoming increasingly prevalent in northern, industrialized, temperate countries. Many factors have been implicated in the increased prevalence of this disorder. Researchers point to environmental pollutants, food additives, a decrease in breast-feeding, and lifestyles involving primarily indoor dwelling, which increase exposure to house dust mites and indoor air pollution. Some theories suggest that an overly sterile, modern lifestyle, with its lack of exposure to immune-stimulating parasites, infections, and bacteria, creates an imbalance and immaturity of the immune system that predisposes to atopic disorders.

Pathophysiology

The pathophysiology of AD is poorly understood. Atopic dermatitis appears to be caused by dysfunction of skin T cells. A complex chain of events leads to T-cell activation and proliferation, resulting in the release of cytokines and inflammatory mediators, leading to the clinical manifestation of atopic dermatitis. Compared with normal skin, the dry skin of atopic dermatitis has reduced water-binding capacity, higher rate of transepidermal water loss, and decreased water content. Water loss leads to further drying and cracking of the skin, which leads to more itching. Rubbing and scratching of itchy skin are responsible for many of the changes seen in the skin.

GENETIC LINKS

Examples of Genetic Disorders Involving the Skin

Disorder	Skin Features	Inheritance	Metabolic/Gene Defect	Genetic Testing Available
Neurofibromatosis, type 1	Dermal neurofibromas, multiple café-au-lait spots, axillary and inguinal freckling	AD	Mutation in *NF1* gene on chromosome 17	Yes
Tuberous sclerosis	Hypomelanotic macules, facial angiofibromas, shagreen patches, fibrous facial plaques	AD	Mutation in *TSC1* gene on chromosome 9; *TSC2* gene on chromosome 16	Yes
Oculocutaneous albinism, type 1	Hypopigmentation of skin, hair, and eyes	AR	Mutation in tyrosinase gene, *TYR*, on chromosome 11	Yes
Waardenburg's syndrome	Hypopigmentation of skin and hair; white forelock; premature gray hair	AD	Mutation in *PAX3* gene on chromosome 2	Yes
Fabry's disease	Vascular cutaneous lesions (angiokeratomas)	XR	Mutation in *GLA* gene on chromosome X; deficient activity of enzyme alpha-galactosidase (α-Gal A)	Yes
Bloom syndrome	Sun-sensitive, telangiectatic, hypo- and hyperpigmented skin; predisposition to cancer	AR	Mutation in *BLM* gene on chromosome 15	Yes

AD, Autosomal dominant; *AR,* autosomal recessive; *XR,* X-linked recessive.

Clinical Manifestations

Atopic dermatitis begins in many clients during infancy. The dermatitis is usually of acute onset, with a red, oozing, crusting rash. Over time, the skin tends to show the chronic form of dermatitis, with thickened dry texture, brownish-gray color, and scales. The rash tends to become localized to the large folds of the extremities as the client becomes older (Figure 49-1). In older children and adults, it is found mainly on elbow bends, the backs of the knees, the neck, the eyelids, and the backs of the hands and feet. Hand and foot dermatitis becomes a significant problem in some adults.

Pruritus is the major clinical manifestation of atopic dermatitis and causes the greatest morbidity. The condition may be mild and self-limiting, or it may be intense, provoking scratching that results in severely excoriated lesions, infection, and scarring.

Clients with atopic dermatitis tend to experience viral, bacterial, and fungal skin infections. It is not clear whether these cutaneous infections arise secondary to a disruption of normal barrier function or are due to reduced local immunity. Honey-colored crusting, extensive serous weeping, folliculitis, pyoderma, and furunculosis indicate bacterial infection, usually secondary to *Staphylococcus aureus* colonization in clients with atopic dermatitis. Clients with atopic dermatitis are frequently heavily colonized with *S. aureus*. Superficial fungal infections may also appear more frequently. The most common viral infection is herpes simplex, which tends to spread locally or become generalized.

OUTCOME MANAGEMENT

The goal of therapy is to break the inflammatory cycle that causes excess drying and cracking as well as the itching and scratching.

■ **FIGURE 49-1** Atopic dermatitis. Intense pruritus leads to scratching and open lesions.

Medical Management

Hydrate the Skin

Hydration is the key to management but is often difficult to achieve. Management begins with daily skin care that hydrates and lubricates the skin. Soaks followed by application of occlusive substances are usually prescribed.

Remove Allergens

Understanding each client's disease pattern and the discovery and reduction of exacerbating factors are crucial to effective management of this chronic disorder. Allergens, food, aeroallergens, and emotional stresses may be inciting factors. Many of these triggering factors are the same irritants or allergens that contribute to generalized pruritus (see Pruritus). Clients should avoid exposure to substances for which there is a positive result on allergy testing that correlates with history of precipitating dermatitis. Stringent restrictions on lifestyle and activities do not change the outcome.

Dietary management of atopic dermatitis has continued to be controversial. Food allergies in the causation of atopic dermatitis seem to be more significant in certain populations of young children and infants. The most common allergens appear to be eggs, cow's milk, soy, wheat, nuts, and fish. Proven allergens are avoided. People with food allergies must be taught to read labels. Care must be taken to avoid malnutrition when any type of restrictive diet is used.

Reduce Inflammation

Systemic medications may include antibiotics and antihistaminics (see Pruritus). The use of a systemic corticosteroid is rarely warranted in atopic dermatitis. Although systemic steroids can be a "quick and easy cure," they should be avoided in this chronic, non–life-threatening disorder. Although there may be dramatic improvement with their use, the recurrence of dermatitis after their discontinuation is equally dramatic. The side effects of long-term systemic steroid use are both unpleasant (moon face and buffalo hump) and dangerous (adrenal suppression, delayed healing).

Nursing Management of the Medical Client

Assess the client with atopic dermatitis for bathing habits, use of moisturizers, medication regimen, exposure to known allergens, environmental exposure, and history of skin eruptions. The Integrating Pharmacology feature on p. 1203 describes interventions for clients with atopic dermatitis. See also the Care Plan on The Client with Atopic Dermatitis on the website.

Soaks and Wet Wraps

Soaks serve several purposes. Moisture softens dry epidermis, which aids in removal of crusts. Removal of cellular skin debris promotes healing and improves absorption of topical medication. The risk of infection is reduced by removal of necrotic tissue and occlusive crusts. Cooling also results from the gradual evaporation of water and has an anti-inflammatory effect, thus relieving itching (pruritus).

Soaks can be accomplished by either soaking the affected area or bathing for 15 to 20 minutes in warm water. The agent added to the soaks is the least important aspect of this therapy. Addition of substances such as colloidal oatmeal (Aveeno) or starch to the bath water may be soothing for some people but does nothing to increase water absorption. Coal tar preparations (Balnetar, T/Derm) have an anti-inflammatory effect and can be helpful in some eczematous and psoriatic conditions. Aluminum acetate (Burow's solution), aluminum sulfate and calcium acetate (Domeboro), povidone-iodine (Betadine), and diluted bleach in appropriate quantities are also effective antibacterial substances; however, they have drying effects and may cause increased stinging and noncompliance. Bath oils are usually not recommended because they give the client a false sense of lubrication and make the soaking area very slippery.

After soaking, clients should remove excess water by gently patting the skin with a soft towel. Then they should immediately apply the recommended topical substance. Immediate application of this substance to damp skin is the most important detail, because if the occlusive barrier is not provided within 3 to 5 minutes, evaporation begins to occur.

For moisturization and to seal in the water, use occlusives such as white petrolatum (Vaseline) or petrolatum with mineral oil and wool wax alcohol (Aquaphor ointment). Occlusives can be greasy and may be cosmetically unacceptable to some people. Clients may prefer creams or lotions because they are cosmetically pleasing products. Lotions and even creams may be irritating and drying because of the evaporative property of the water and the substances used as preservatives, solubilizers, and fragrances.

Wet wraps used immediately after soaking and occlusion can optimize hydration and topical therapy; this also promotes cooling of the skin. Wet wraps and occlusion can be applied in various ways and should not be confused with wet-to-dry dressings used for debridement. The location and severity of lesions often determine the choices. Total-body wet wraps can be accomplished by putting on wet pajamas or wet long underwear followed by dry pajamas or a dry or plastic sweat suit. The hands and feet can be covered with wet tube socks or wet cotton gloves followed by dry tube socks. Any extremity or the trunk can be covered with wet rolled (e.g., Kerlix) gauze and occluded with elastic bandages or by pieces of tube sock, wet followed by dry. The face can be wrapped with two layers of wet Kerlix gauze, followed by two layers of dry Kerlix gauze held in place with elasticized netting or other tubular dressings; holes are cut out for the eyes, nose, and mouth. If the dressing becomes dry, it should be rewetted before removal because debridement by the wet-to-dry method produces tissue damage and pain. Gentle debridement usually still occurs if dressings are removed when damp.[19]

Modifications for Older Clients

Dermatitis is a common skin disorder in the older population. It may be caused by venous insufficiency, allergens, irritants, or underlying malignancy such as leukemia or lymphoma. Because older adults often take many medications, the potential for dermatitis from drug-drug interactions is increased. The fragility of the skin as a result of the flattened epidermal-dermal junction and loss of dermis should be considered in planning any form of treatment.

XEROTIC ECZEMA

Xerotic (dry) skin lacks moisture in the top layer of the skin. Xerotic eczema may present as erythematous, scaling, and finely cracked skin. Xerosis occurs in patches and may involve any skin surface. It is common in the older population. If xerosis is severe, the skin is tight, itchy, and painful. Water loss causes xerotic chapping and fissures. The problem may be accentuated by use of drying skin cleansers, soaps, disinfectants, and solvents and infrequent use of moisturizers. Environmental factors play a large role, especially those that increase water loss in the stratum corneum. Any factors that decrease the relative humidity exacerbate this condition, such as cold or dry winter air, especially in artificially heated rooms.

Management includes hydration and moisturizing the skin plus avoiding irritating factors. Teaching the client correct daily skin care is essential to treating this condition (see Integrating Pharmacology feature on Soaks and Wet Wraps). Clients known to have xerosis every winter are advised to increase skin moisturizing before severe weather starts.

CONTACT DERMATITIS

Contact dermatitis is an inflammatory response of the skin. There are two types based on the etiology: irritant or allergic. Irritant contact dermatitis (ICD) is most common and is from exposure to anything that produces a chemical or physical irritant response. Allergic contact dermatitis (ACD) is a delayed hypersensitivity reaction resulting from contact with an allergen. This hypersensitivity reaction is an immune-mediated response by previously sensitized lymphocytes to a specific allergen. Common allergens are poison ivy, nickel, bacitracin, and formaldehyde.

The two conditions are difficult to distinguish. Clinical manifestations begin at the site of exposure with itching, stinging, erythema, and edema, which may extend to involve more distant sites. Manifestations may develop within an hour of contact or as late as 7 to 14 days after contact and may range from mild erythema to vesicles to ulceration (Figure 49-2). With even brief contact of the substance with the skin, an allergic response is possible. For example, contact with poison ivy may have happened quickly and the allergen washed off. However, areas of dermatitis may continue to appear for many days following the initial exposure.

Management begins with identification of the causative agent. First, question the client about recent exposure to substances such as plants, chemicals, and metals. Pain and itching may be controlled with topical medication or wet dressings (see Integrating Pharmacology on Soaks and Wet Wraps). Oral antihistaminic agents and topical or systemic steroids may be required. The Client Education Guide at right provides teaching information on topical corticosteroids. Patch testing is a test done to attempt to determine the specific agent. Each patch in a standardized test panel (TRUE test [thin-layer, rapid-use epicutaneous test]) contains a substance that is known to be one of the most common causes of allergic contact dermatitis. When these tests elicit a positive reaction, much can be done to teach the client about what to avoid (see Chapter 48).

INTERTRIGINOUS DERMATITIS

Intertriginous areas are between folds of skin. When the skin lays one fold on top of another, a superficial inflammatory dermatitis occurs. Inadequate ventilation

■ **FIGURE 49–2** Contact dermatitis. Note the distinct line of erythema.

CLIENT EDUCATION GUIDE

Topical Corticosteroids

Corticosteroids are still among the most commonly used medications for treatment of a variety of dermatologic conditions. Corticosteroids can also be injected directly into the lesion, applied topically, or given systemically. Diagnosing the condition before any corticosteroid use is important because the effects of the medication can mask or change the clinical manifestations. Topical corticosteroids work through broad mechanisms, including anti-inflammatory, antimitotic, immunosuppressant, and vasoconstrictive actions. The effectiveness of these agents largely depends on the potency of the agent used and the degree of absorption through the skin. The greater the potency of a steroid, however, the greater the safety concerns. Skin hydration just before application increases absorption and effectiveness.

Topical steroids range in potency from low to high. Low-potency topical steroids are now available in over-the-counter (OTC) formulations (e.g., hydrocortisone, 0.5% or 1%) and in prescription strength (e.g., desonide, alclometasone). Generally, low-potency steroids are safe to use for longer periods of time and even on thin-skinned areas like the face, groin, or axilla. Prolonged use should still be monitored. Medium-potency (e.g., triamcinolone, fluocinolone) to high-potency (e.g., halcinonide, fluocinonide) corticosteroids should be used with caution and for short periods of time and not on the face, groin, or axilla. High-potency or super high-potency (e.g., betamethasone dipropionate, clobetasol) steroids should be reserved for use on acute or resistant dermatoses (e.g., contact dermatitis) or areas with thick plaque such as in psoriasis.

Clients should know the strength of the topical steroid they are using and its potential side effects. The lowest potency corticosteroid that is effective should be used. Side effects are more likely with prolonged use of medium-potency to high-potency topical corticosteroids. The most common side effect is skin atrophy, which presents as thin or shiny skin with increased prominence of blood vessels, telangiectases, and easy bruising. Other possible side effects include acne-like conditions, folliculitis, hypopigmentation, delayed wound healing, and striae.

Clients must clearly understand how, when, and where to use topical steroids. Properly applying the medication evenly and sparingly once or twice daily to the affected areas can eliminate many potential problems. More frequent application increases the chance of side effects, makes the therapy more costly, and does not usually increase effectiveness. The condition can recur if treatment is stopped abruptly. When the skin disease disappears or is under good control, a tar preparation, moisturizer, or other topical preparation may be substituted for the topical steroid.

especially in hot or humid weather, friction, heat, and moisture buildup result in maceration, erosions, fissures, itching, and burning. Skin folds prone to intertrigo are in the neck, axillae, antecubital fossae, the perineum, finger and toe webs, abdomen, and beneath the breasts, particularly in obese clients. One of the most common causes of intertrigo is contamination with body fluids, as occurs in urinary incontinence. Secondary bacterial (*Pseudomonas* or *Staphylococcus*) or *Candida albicans* infection may occur. Whenever candidiasis is present, a careful evaluation is indicated. In an otherwise healthy person, candidiasis is a self-limiting disease that responds well to topical antifungal therapy; however, it can be the presenting manifestation of underlying systemic disease affecting the endocrine system (e.g., diabetes) or the immune system (e.g., immunodeficiency syndromes).

Treatment of intertrigo is to eliminate maceration by promoting drying and to aerate the body skinfolds. For mobile clients, review environmental changes that promote drying of the body folds, such as wearing loose-fitting cotton-blend clothing or periodic removal of clothing to dry off. Instruct clients to avoid tight-fitting clothing such as jeans as well as activities that promote sweating. Care recommendations depend on the degree of involvement and the overall condition of the skin. If the skin is still intact, recommendations include washing the area gently with tap water twice daily and then rinsing and drying the area, followed by sprinkling of a talc-containing powder or a cellulose-containing powder (e.g., Zeasorb) for extra absorption. Avoid using cornstarch in pure form because it encourages *C. albicans* overgrowth. Applying folded gauze or clean cotton handkerchiefs in skinfolds promotes healing by keeping skin surfaces apart. Wash cloths and paper towels should not be used; they do not wick drainage from the skin. Silver-impregnated dressings (e.g., InterDry), have been shown to work well for these skin folds. Apply cool, wet soaks with tap water or Burow's solution (an antiseptic) three to four times daily for removal of exudate if secondary infection is present.

If inflammation is present, a low-potency topical corticosteroid in a nonocclusive vehicle (e.g., hydrocortisone 1.0% or 2.5% cream or lotion) or a combination steroid-antibiotic-antifungal agent (Vytone 1%) may initially be helpful, but long-term use should be avoided (see the Client Education Guide on topical corticosteroids on p. 1204).

STASIS DERMATITIS

Stasis dermatitis is characterized by the development of areas of very dry, dark skin and sometimes shallow ulcers on the lower legs, primarily as a result of venous insufficiency. The dermatitis is treated with moisturizing agents and antihistamines; antifungal preparations may also be helpful. When fragile skin ulcerations are present, the wound is called a *venous stasis ulcer*. The treatment of these wounds is discussed in Chapter 53.

INCONTINENCE ASSOCIATED DERMATITIS

Dermatitis from exposure to urine or stool is called incontinence associated dermatitis (IAD). Risk factors include frequent exposure to urine or diarrheal stool and use of absorptive containment device. Secondary cutaneous infection (usually fungal) is common. When skin is exposed to urine, the urea is absorbed by the keratinocytes and once they are swollen, they cannot provide a barrier. The skin also develops an odor of ammonia. Diarrhea contains digestive enzymes that denude the skin.

These skin ulcers can be confused with pressure ulcers and may coexist with pressure ulcers. IAD ulcers are diffuse, often occurring as multiple areas of open skin in the perineum and perineal skin folds. They are partial thickness ulcers and do not develop necrotic tissue.

Treatment of IAD begins by determining the reason for the incontinence, for example, urinary tract infection. Skin must be kept clean by quickly cleansing incontinent clients. Reduce exposure of the skin to irritants. Keep the skin moisturized and provide a barrier on the skin by using wipes that contain dimethicone. It is most efficient and effective to keep the skin care products at the beside.

PSORIASIS VULGARIS

Psoriasis vulgaris is a chronic, recurrent, erythematous, inflammatory disorder with a worldwide distribution. The prevalence varies according to race and geographic location. Psoriasis occurs equally in both genders, usually starting in the early 20s to 40s. The Latin *vulgaris* (from *vulgus,* or "the public") means "common" and does not refer to "vulgar." Psoriasis is a genetic systemic disease with an immunologic basis that frequently manifests in the skin and joints.

Pathophysiology

T cells are one of the immune cells. In psoriasis, hordes of activated T cells are found in psoriatic skin and almost none in healthy skin. These activated T cells secrete interleukin-6, which has as one of its effects the ability to stimulate skin cell growth. A normal skin cell matures and is shed in 28 to 30 days, but a psoriatic skin cell takes only 3 to 4 days to mature and move to the surface. Instead of shedding, the cells pile up and form lesions.

Clinical Manifestations

The epidermis thickens with extra skin cells, and blood vessels dilate with increased blood supply to nourish those cells. At the surface, skin cells pile up. Dead cells create a white, flaky layer of silvery white scales over the patch of inflamed skin.

The eruptions (usually in a symmetrical distribution) commonly occur on the scalp, elbows, knees, genital,

■ **FIGURE 49–3** Plaque psoriasis of the buttocks.

and sacral regions (Figure 49-3). Lesions may develop at the site of an injury, which is known as *Koebner's phenomenon*. A generalized eruption may occur with severe psoriasis vulgaris. Another type is palmar plantar psoriasis, which can be pustular or of a plaque type and only affects the palms and soles. In a rare form of psoriasis, known as *pustular psoriasis,* generalized, sterile cutaneous pustules are produced. Severe systemic involvement can be fatal. Up to one third of clients with moderate to severe psoriasis have psoriatic arthritis, which primarily affects the distal joints and may be deforming. Nail dystrophies and pitting occur frequently.

OUTCOME MANAGEMENT

The course of psoriasis vulgaris is unpredictable. It can be controlled with aggressive therapies but cannot be cured. Exacerbations and remissions are common. As with other chronic diseases, changes in physical and emotional health can precede flares. The goals of medical management of psoriasis are to decrease the T-cell counts in the epidermis, control the rate of epidermal cell turnover, and monitor for complications of therapy. Some individuals also may have associated psoriatic arthritis. In this group, selecting the appropriate treatment option is necessary to provide adequate pain relief and possibly reduce or prevent joint destruction.

Medical Management

Suppress T-Cell Activation

Steroids can be used to suppress the immune system (see the Client Education Guide Topical Corticosteroids on p. 1204). Injecting small, dilute amounts of corticosteroids (e.g., triamcinolone acetonide) into or just beneath a lesion gives a high drug concentration at the injection site. Systemic steroids are contraindicated in psoriasis. Tazarotene is a retinoid derivative that very commonly causes irritation and as such is typically used in conjunction with a topical steroid. Retinoid derivatives

alter the delayed hypersensitivity response and increase the number of Langerhans cells in the psoriatic lesion. For plaque psoriasis, retinoids can be used in combination with ultraviolet phototherapy to minimize the dose of each. Keratolytic agents (e.g., salicylic acid) may remove scales and allow greater penetration of topical agents. Anthralin reduces mitotic action in the cell and is an effective topical agent for treatment of psoriasis with widespread discrete lesions consisting primarily of thick plaques, but it is rarely used in the United States because of its complicated protocol. Calcipotriene is a synthetic vitamin D_3 analog that regulates skin cell production; however, it is not in widespread use.

Promote Desquamation

Artificial forms of ultraviolet light (UVL) are used therapeutically with topical or systemic photosensitizing drugs to cause desquamation (shedding or peeling of the epidermis). Ultraviolet A (UVA) light and ultraviolet B (UVB) light are used to treat diseases responsive to UVL, such as psoriasis, vitiligo, cutaneous T-cell lymphoma, uremic pruritus, and chronic eczematous eruptions. At present, two treatment modalities involve UVL: (1) broadband and narrowband UVB and (2) photochemotherapy, or PUVA (psoralen plus UVA). Initially, many of these regimens are given two or three times a week with the frequency decreased to two to four times per month for maintenance.

Obtaining a complete history and physical examination in every client before initiation of any UVL therapy is very important. One must take care to include the complete medication history, because the client may be taking one or more of the many photosensitizing drugs (e.g., thiazide diuretics, tetracycline). Ask clients specifically about previous herpes simplex infections, which can be reactivated by UVL. Pretreatment assessment includes identifying solar energy–induced skin malignancies, premalignant lesions, cataracts, or lupus erythematosus and any additional photodamage. Potential benefit must be weighed against potential risk. The skin changes of lupus erythematosus (LE) are worsened by sun exposure, and phototherapy is thus contraindicated. If LE is suspected, an antinuclear antibody (ANA) test should be obtained to rule out this condition before therapy is initiated.

A complete ophthalmologic examination before full body box treatment begins is important and should be performed yearly during long-term treatment. A history of cataract formation is a potential contraindication to PUVA therapy. Clients who exhibit early cataract changes need extra photoprotective measures (e.g., the complete occlusion provided by goggles or PUVA glasses) and more frequent ophthalmologic assessments (every 3 to 6 months).

Because UVL treatments add to the cumulative effects of natural and artificial UVL, minimize exposure by shielding the head, face, and male genitalia to reduce the risk of skin cancers. Periodic assessments must be done throughout the course of therapy for manifestations of actinic damage (e.g., severe wrinkling, "tissue paper" transparency) or cutaneous malignancy. All phototherapy should be administered by qualified and well-trained dermatologic personnel. Use of home UVL equipment and tanning salons should be considered only when the client has no access to qualified dermatologic personnel. Numerous risks and significantly diminished responses are associated with home and salon therapy.

Ultraviolet Light B Therapy

UVB therapy requires no oral medications and is usually the first-line UVL therapy used before progression to PUVA. Types of UVB therapy include (1) broadband or narrowband UVB treatment as monotherapy and (2) broadband or narrowband UVB in combination with topicals (tar, anthralin, calcipotriene, corticosteroids, or tazarotene). Topical anthralin and tar used with UVB are mainly of historical interest because they have generally been replaced by newer developments that are reimbursable and that are not as time-consuming.

Photochemotherapy

Photochemotherapy (PUVA) combines oral or topical 8-methoxypsoralen with UVA. PUVA is used to treat severe, unresponsive forms of psoriasis, atopic dermatitis, cutaneous T-cell lymphoma, graft-versus-host disease, and alopecia areata or vitiligo. The potent systemic photosensitizing medications (psoralens) used in PUVA increase skin sensitivity to long-wave UVL (UVA). In conjunction with exposure to artificially reproduced forms of UVA light, these medications induce repigmentation (melanin production) in vitiligo and have an antimitotic effect and reduce T-cell population in psoriasis and cutaneous T-cell lymphoma.

The skin and eyes must be protected from ambient UVL irradiation from the time psoralens are ingested until 8 hours after taking the photosensitizing medication. The client should (1) wear protective clothing, such as long sleeves, (2) apply sunscreen to exposed skin, (3) minimize natural skin exposure with topical psoralen, and (4) wear both UVA and UVB protective eyewear for 24 hours after taking the medication when outside or in an automobile.

Areas that are difficult to treat, such as the scalp and nails, remain a challenge. Scalp care in psoriasis consists of reducing scales and treating inflammation. Clients are instructed to avoid picking and scratching. Use of steroids and oil vehicles under occlusion is often necessary to enhance percutaneous absorption; on the scalp, a plastic shower cap can be used for this purpose. Other products such as tars, medicated shampoos, and

nonsteroidal treatments also play an important role in scalp care. There is no consistently effective treatment of psoriatic involvement of the nails. Tazarotene is showing promising results in reducing nail dystrophy. However, the scalp and nails do improve with clearing of psoriasis on the body surface.

Systemic treatments are being increasingly prescribed for psoriasis affecting 10% or more of the body surface area. Systemic agents are used to block the activation of T cells and prevent the migration of T cells into the skin. Agents include acitretin, methotrexate, and cyclosporine. Methotrexate and cyclosporine are potentially toxic to the renal, hepatic, and hematopoietic systems. Thus baseline assessment (e.g., blood chemistry, complete blood count, liver biopsy) is important before this medication is started. During treatment, periodic assessments are needed, including biopsy of the liver. If any serious side effects develop, such as bone marrow depression or gastrointestinal tract bleeding, treatment is discontinued. To limit potential liver damage, advise the client not to consume alcohol throughout therapy. Because methotrexate may cause chromosomal abnormalities, effective birth control methods are important for both women and men before and during treatment and for 3 months after completing methotrexate. Nausea, the most common side effect, can be limited by taking methotrexate with food, using prophylactic antiemetics, and adding supplemental folic acid.

Biologic drugs are the newest drugs in managing psoriasis and psoriatic arthritis and include etanercept, alefacept, efalizumab, and infliximab. This class of drugs is injected or infused and require specific monitoring.

Self-Care

Assist the client in coping with an altered self-concept. Psoriatic disease can have enormously negative effect on client quality of life, causing depression, disrupting work, and producing economic hardships. The appearance of skin lesions may make the client feel "dirty" or untouchable. Because open lesions are at high risk for secondary infection, the client should be taught to keep the creams or ointments on and to keep the area clean and dry. To keep psoriasis in remission, the client needs to control the causative factors. Stress should be minimized, and illness and infection should be treated early.

ACNE VULGARIS

Acne vulgaris is a common, multifactorial follicular disorder that affects pilosebaceous follicles, primarily of the face, neck, and upper trunk. It is characterized by both noninflammatory and inflammatory lesions. Acne is the most common chronic skin disease, affecting up to 85% of the population between the ages of 12 and 25. Genetic influences may determine client's susceptibility and severity of disease. Numerous topical and systemic drugs are available for the treatment of acne vulgaris; see a pediatric nursing textbook for further discussion.

ACNE ROSACEA

Acne rosacea is a chronic inflammatory skin eruption characterized by erythema, papules, pustules, and telangiectases. It occurs on the face, especially the cheeks and over the bridge of the nose. The onset is insidious, usually occurring between 30 and 50 years of age, and women are affected more frequently than men. It is more common in fair-skinned people with a history of easy facial flushing. Precipitating factors that appear to make the flushing worse include tea, coffee, alcohol (especially wine), caffeine-containing products, sunlight, extremes of hot and cold, spicy foods, and emotional stress.

Sebaceous hyperplasia of the nose (rhinophyma) often develops after many years of chronic acne rosacea. This condition results from chronic inflammation with an increase in the amount of connective tissue and may be mistaken for an indication of excessive alcohol consumption. Ocular changes such as eyelid inflammation and conjunctivitis may occur.

Avoidance of the stimuli that trigger acne rosacea may be sufficient for management of mild forms of the disorder. Treatment of rosacea is sometimes difficult. The topical agents generally used include antibiotics, metronidazole (MetroGel), and retinoids. Systemic drugs include antibiotics, isotretinoin, and metronidazole, but the pros and cons of using these must be weighed.

SKIN TEARS

Skin tears are wounds resulting from separation of the epidermis from the underlying connective tissue. The most common sites for skin tears, in order of frequency, are the forearm, hand, elbow, and upper arm. Skin tears are most common in older adults as a result of a thinning of the epidermis, a flattening of the dermal-epidermal junction, and a reduced adhesion of the dermis to the epidermis. They are very common in clients who have taken long-term oral steroids for conditions such as emphysema. Skin tears often result from trauma, such as falls and injury from wheelchair handles or brakes or injury that incurred during transfer to a chair. Even though the actual skin damage is minor, families and residents are disturbed by the presence of skin tears, often perceiving the injury as resulting from abuse.

OUTCOME MANAGEMENT

For tears with small to moderate losses of epidermal tissue, irrigate the wound with normal saline to remove blood or debris. Replace any flaps of epidermis and secure with strips of paper tape. Cover the open wound with nonocclusive, moisture-retentive dressing, such as petrolatum-impregnated gauze or opaque foam dressing. Do not use adherent clear dressings; when these dressings are removed, the skin can tear again. Table 49-1 shows how to select an appropriate dressing.

Prevention is important. Use protective gloves on the client's hands and soft armrests on wheelchairs, and train caregivers in proper transfer techniques (e.g., use of transfer belts). Daily assessment by unlicensed assistive personnel is critical to identify lesions early. The Management and Delegation feature on p. 1209 describes reportable skin abnormalities.

PRESSURE ULCERS

A pressure ulcer is localized injury to the skin and/or underlying tissue, usually over a bony prominence, as a result of pressure or pressure in combination with

TABLE 49–1 Choosing a Dressing for a Wound	
Desired Purpose	**Dressing Options**
Prevent contamination of puncture sites	Transparent dressings
Prevent contamination from stool/urine	Skin protection with dimethicone
	Topical pastes and creams (dressings often lift up at the edges)
Prevent injury periulcer skin from frequent dressing changes	Hydrocolloids for window frame around wound
	Tubular gauze to hold dressing in place
Prevent injury to intact skin	Transparent dressings
Prevent injury to intact blisters	Lightly adhesive foams if removed often
Absorb drainage from incisions	Gauze and combination dressings
Absorb exudate from deep wounds	Alginate rope or dressings
	Foams
	Gauze packing
Control infection	Products with silver or iodine
	Dressings soaked with antibiotic solutions
Control odor	Products with iodine, silver, activated charcoal, or diluted Dakin's solution
	Crushed metronidazole
Control pain	Hydrogels
	Adaptic gauze
	Mepitel
Promote tissue hydration	Transparent dressings and films
	Hydrocolloids
	Gels
Promote autolytic debridement	Gels
	Transparent dressings and films
Conform to irregular body areas	Extra thin types of hydrocolloids
	Extra thin layers of foams
	Transparent films
Conform to depth for packing	Gels
	Rope alginate
	Gauze strips (do not pack deep wounds with single dressings)

Skin Inspection

Unlicensed assistive personnel frequently are in the position to observe the skin of clients as they assist with various activities of daily living and provide assistance with personal hygiene. Be sure to fully delineate their role in identifying and reporting skin abnormalities. Reportable findings are listed as follows.

Bruising or a change in skin color. Ecchymosis, erythema, jaundice, and pallor may indicate a serious disease process or acute deep tissue injury. Identification of these changes in skin color by unlicensed assistive personnel should be immediately reported to you for thorough assessment and intervention. Redness overlying bony structures may indicate prolonged or undue pressure. Purple areas over bony prominences or pressure prone areas may indicate deep tissue injury. Unlicensed assistive personnel should ensure pressure relief by assisting the client with frequent position changes.

Lumps. Assess any skin lesion or growth in further detail.

Dry, scaling, or cracked skin. Dry skin may indicate dehydration or other integumentary disorders. You may delegate the application of over-the-counter lotions to unlicensed assistive personnel if the skin is not broken. Some clients may need specific lubricants or medications prescribed by a physician; therefore have any findings of dry skin reported to you.

Skin that feels excessively moist and cool or excessively warm. It is appropriate for unlicensed assistive personnel to cover clients with extra bedding if they feel cool or to offer cool compresses for warm skin (see Chapter 27). Be certain that the client is not febrile. Localized areas of warmth may indicate underlying processes that need prompt attention. Clearly communicate that any of these findings should be immediately reported to you for prompt assessment and intervention.

Any break in the skin with drainage or bleeding. You may delegate the application of sterile gauze to the surface of the skin to unlicensed assistive personnel for the purpose of containing drainage (see Chapter 14). Skin tears should be treated with nonstick dressings. Assess such skin abnormalities promptly after identification by unlicensed assistive personnel.

Taut or shiny skin. This finding may indicate fluid shifting from the intravascular space. Such skin is susceptible to breakdown and infection. Employ proactive measures to prevent any undue pressure or damage to the skin. Assess the area carefully, and report any unknown disorders or significant change to a physician. Elevate the area to decrease swelling if present.

Client complaints of itching or tenderness. Instruct unlicensed assistive personnel identifying such client complaints to communicate these findings to you promptly. Assess the client for potential allergic reaction, an underlying tissue pathologic process, or the need for additional analgesics.

Rashes. New rashes or other skin eruptions sometimes suggest allergic reactions. Instruct that such findings be reported to you promptly.

You are ultimately responsible for thorough, ongoing assessment and evaluation of integument.

shear and/or friction. Although pressure ulcers are most common over bony prominences, they can be located in any area of the body that is subjected to pressure, shear, or friction. Pressure ulcers have also been called "bed sores" and "decubitus ulcers." The word *decubitus* comes from the Latin *decumbere,* which means to lie down. The ulcers were so named because they are common in bedridden clients.

Etiology and Risk Factors

Classically, pressure ulcers develop when soft tissues (skin, subcutaneous tissue, and muscle) are compressed between a bony prominence and a firm surface for a prolonged period. Recently, deep tissue injury pressure ulcers have been identified. These pressure ulcers develop during shorter periods of intense pressure, with the major site of injury initially being in the muscle. Therefore immobility and inactivity are major risk factors. In bedridden clients, infrequent turning and repositioning or lack of padding between surfaces that touch (e.g., knees) may lead to tissue damage. In addition, clients in bed are often positioned in semi-Fowler position to facilitate breathing or eating. This position increases the risk of ulcers on the sacrum and heels. The ischia are common sites of pressure ulcers in chairbound clients, especially if they sit erect in the chair. The length of time of exposure to pressure before skin breakdown varies among clients; in very debilitated clients, permanent tissue damage can result in less than 2 hours. Cognitive or sensory impairments also increase risk because the client cannot recognize the need to turn or move.

Protein-calorie malnutrition is another major risk factor. Malnourished clients have poor skin integrity, and their skin is damaged easily. In addition, incontinence, friction, and skin shearing can also lead to breakdown. These factors reduce the tolerance the skin has for pressure.

The reported incidence (number of new cases per year) of pressure ulcers in acute care facilities ranges from 2.7% to 29.5%. The prevalence (number of cases at one point in time) in acute care settings ranges from 3.5% to 29.5%. Several populations are at increased risk. Quadriplegic clients, older adults with femoral fractures, and clients in critical care units have the highest risk. Prevention of pressure ulcers begins with identifying the client at risk. Risk factors can be determined by assessing sensory perception, moisture, activity, mobility, nutrition, friction, and shear. Risk for pressure ulcers can be expressed numerically by using an instrument to appraise risk such as the Braden or Norton tool (see later discussion).

Pathophysiology

Pressure on soft tissues between bony prominences and external surfaces (mattress, chair) compresses capillaries and occludes blood flow. If the pressure is relieved, a brief period of rebound capillary dilation (called *reactive hyperemia*) occurs, and there is no tissue damage. If pressure is not relieved, microthrombi form in capillaries and completely occlude blood flow. A blister may form initially. When the blister breaks, an open wound is present. The open wound is rapidly colonized with surface bacteria. These bacteria can proliferate and cause a biofilm to develop. Today, slough in the wound is known to be a biofilm of bacteria covered by a surface that is not easily penetrated by antibiotics.

During periods of intense pressure it is hypothesized that the muscle becomes ischemic, resulting in necrosis of the injured muscle. The leakage of old blood causes the overlying skin to become purple. The necrotic tissue develops into eschar.

Healing occurs through secondary intention. Granulation tissue fills the base of full-thickness ulcers. Contraction of the ulcer edges closes the wound. Eventually, epithelial cells cover the wound. Stage III and IV pressure ulcers often require debridement and surgery to close the wound. Scar tissue predominates in ulcers that close without surgery.

Clinical Manifestations

The clinical manifestations of pressure ulcers have been described in four stages (Figure 49-4). Stage I is characterized by intact skin with nonblanchable redness of a localized area, usually over a bony prominence. Darkly pigmented skin may not have visible blanching, but its color may differ from the surrounding area. The area may be painful, firm or soft, and warmer or cooler compared with adjacent tissue. Stage I may be difficult to detect in clients with dark skin tones. This stage, considered a heralding sign, may indicate the client is at risk for pressure ulcers.

A stage II pressure ulcer is characterized by partial-thickness loss of dermis presenting as a shallow, open ulcer with a reddish-pink wound bed without slough. An ulcer at this stage may also present as an intact (serum-filled) or open (ruptured) blister. The wound is shiny or dry and shallow, without slough or bruising. (Bruising suggests a likelihood of deep tissue injury.) This stage should not be used to describe skin tears, tape burns, perineal dermatitis, maceration, or excoriation.

Ulcers classified as stage III are wounds that have full-thickness tissue loss. Subcutaneous fat may be visible, but bone, tendon, and muscle are not exposed. Slough may be present but does not obscure the depth of tissue loss. These ulcers may include undermining and tunneling. The depth of a stage III pressure ulcer varies by anatomic location. Ulcers most commonly occur on the sacrum, heel, greater trochanter, and ischial tuberosities. The bridge of the nose, ear, occiput, and malleolus do not have subcutaneous tissue, so stage III ulcers can be shallow. In contrast, areas of significant adiposity can

Stage I

Intact skin with non-blanchable redness of a localized area usually over a bony prominence. Darkly pigmented skin may not have visible blanching; its color may differ from the surrounding area

The area may be painful, firm, soft, warmer, or cooler as compared to adjacent tissue. Stage I may be difficult to detect in individuals with dark skin. May indicate "at risk" persons (a heralding sign of risk)

Stage II

Partial-thickness loss of dermis presenting as a shallow open ulcer with a red pink wound bed, without slough. May also present as an intact or open/ruptured serum-filled blister

Presents as a shiny or dry shallow ulcer without slough or bruising.* This stage should not be used to describe skin tears, tape burns, perineal dermatitis, maceration, or excoriation

*Bruising indicates suspected deep-tissue injury

Stage III

Full-thickness tissue loss. Subcutaneous fat may be visible, but bone, tendon, or muscle are not exposed. Slough may be present but does not obscure the depth of tissue loss. May include undermining and tunneling

The depth of a stage III pressure ulcer varies by anatomical location. The bridge of the nose, ear, occiput, and malleolus do not have subcutaneous tissue, and stage III ulcers can be shallow. In contrast, areas of significant adiposity can develop extremely deep stage III pressure ulcers. Bone/tendon is not visible or directly palpable

Stage IV

Full-thickness tissue loss with exposed bone, tendon, or muscle. Slough or eschar may be present on some parts of the wound bed. Often includes undermining and tunneling

The depth of a stage IV pressure ulcer varies by anatomical location. The bridge of the nose, ear, occiput, and malleolus do not have subcutaneous tissue and these ulcers can be shallow. Stage IV ulcers can extend into muscle and/or supporting structures (e.g., fascia, tendon, or joint capsule), making osteomyelitis possible. Exposed bone/tendon is visible or directly palpable

Unstageable

Full-thickness tissue loss in which the base of the ulcer is covered by slough (yellow, tan, gray, green, or brown) and/or eschar (tan, brown, or black) in the wound bed

Until enough slough and/or eschar is removed to expose the base of the wound, the true depth, and therefore stage, cannot be determined. Stable (dry, adherent, intact without erythema or fluctuance) eschar on the heels serves as the body's natural (biological) cover and should not be removed

Deep tissue injury

Purple or maroon localized area of discolored intact skin or blood-filled blister due to damage of underlying soft tissue from pressure and/or shear. The area may be preceded by tissue that is painful, firm, mushy, boggy, warmer, or cooler as compared to adjacent tissue

Deep-tissue injury may be difficult to detect in individuals with dark skin. Evolution may include a thin blister over a dark wound bed. The wound may further evolve and become covered by thin eschar. Evolution may be rapid, exposing additional layers of tissue even with optimal treatment

■ **FIGURE 49-4** Stages of pressure ulcers.

develop extremely deep stage III pressure ulcers. Bone and tendon are neither visible nor directly palpable.

Stage IV ulcers show full-thickness tissue loss with exposed bone, tendon, or muscle. Slough or eschar may be present on some parts of the wound bed, and undermining and tunneling are often evident. The depth of a stage IV pressure ulcer varies by anatomic location. The bridge of the nose, ear, occiput, and malleolus do not have subcutaneous tissue, so these ulcers can be shallow. Stage IV ulcers can extend into muscle or supporting structures, such as fascia, tendon, and joint capsules, making osteomyelitis possible. Exposed bone or tendon is visible or directly palpable.

Some pressure ulcers cannot be staged because the bottom of the ulcer cannot be seen. These unstageable ulcers are characterized by full-thickness tissue loss in which the base of the ulcer is covered by slough (yellow, tan, gray, green, or brown) and/or eschar (tan, brown, or black) in the wound bed. Until enough slough or eschar is removed to expose the base of the wound, the true depth, and therefore the stage, cannot be determined. Some pressure ulcers will be "unstageable" for a long time, because the eschar provides a "biologic dressing." This is seen in stable (dry, adherent, and intact, without erythema or fluctuation ("buoyant") eschar on the heels, which serves as the body's natural (biological) cover and should not be removed.

Deep tissue injury is a new stage of pressure ulcers. Deep tissue injury is a purple or maroon localized area of discolored intact skin or blood-filled blister due to damage of underlying soft tissue from pressure and/or shear. This ulcer may be preceded by tissue that is painful, firm, mushy, boggy, and warmer or cooler as compared with adjacent tissue. Deep tissue injury may be difficult to detect in individuals with dark skin tones. Evolution may include a thin blister over a dark wound bed. The wound may further evolve and become covered by thin eschar. Evolution may be rapid, exposing additional layers of tissue even with optimal treatment.

Terminal ulcers, sometimes referred to as "Kennedy terminal ulcers," are pressure ulcers seen near the time of death. They are due to pressure in very poorly perfused skin and may represent "skin failure," especially because they are noted in conjunction with failure of other organs, such as the heart and lungs.

With pressure ulcers, few additional diagnostic assessments are required. Nurses can stage pressure ulcers based on their appearance. Sometimes osteomyelitis is present in deep wounds. Bone scans are used for confirming this problem. If malnutrition is suspected as a cause, serum protein, albumin, or prealbumin levels may be monitored. It is important to distinguish pressure ulcers from other wounds, such as arterial or venous ulcers. See Chapter 53 for a discussion of these wounds.

Medical Management

Management of the client with a pressure ulcer begins with a complete history and physical examination. There are many causes of delayed wound healing, and delayed healing of pressure ulcers may be the result of other health problems. The goal of medical management is to heal the ulcer by redistributing pressure over the ulcer (sometimes called decreasing tissue load), cleaning and dressing the wound, and improving nutrition. In addition, the ulcer is monitored for healing, and the client is monitored for complications.

Decrease Tissue Load

The term *tissue load* refers to the distribution of pressure, friction, and shear on the tissues. Interventions are designed to decrease tissue load and thereby decrease pressure. Increasing the frequency of turning helps disperse pressure over time. Clients should not lie on a pressure ulcer. Restricting blood flow to the ulcer delays healing. If the ulcer is on the sacrum, sitting should be reduced to 1 to 2 hours at a time and only for meals. If the client can turn or be repositioned so as not to lie on a pressure ulcer, a pressure-redistributing overlay may be placed on the mattress. However, these overlay devices can be compressed by the client's weight, and rendered ineffective. Check for bottoming out when using overlay mattresses (Figure 49-5). Special low-pressure beds may be required for clients with pressure ulcers on two or more turning surfaces (Figure 49-6). Heels should be floated from the bed by placing pillows under the calf or using pressure reduction boots. Chair cushions should be used if the client is sitting in a chair or getting up to a chair; 4 inches of foam is effective. In addition, clients who sit in chairs need to be repositioned hourly. Specialty cushions also exist for wheelchair-dependent clients.

Provide Ulcer Care

Moist, devitalized tissue supports bacterial growth. Therefore devitalized tissue must be removed from the ulcer. Several forms of debridement can be used depending on the client's goals and the type of wound. *Sharp debridement* is the use of a scalpel to excise devitalized thick, adherent eschar; this form of debridement is completed in the operating room by the physician. *Conservative sharp* debridement is carried out at the bedside using a scalpel and forceps to remove loose necrotic tissue. This form of debridement is done by trained personnel. *Mechanical debridement* is the use of wet-to-dry dressings, hydrotherapy, and high-pressure

At least 1 inch of support surface

■ **FIGURE 49–5** Assessment of pressure relief ("bottoming out"). Slide your hand (palm up and fingers flat) under the support surface, just under the pressure point. Do not flex your fingers. With adequate support, there will be at least 1 inch of uncompressed support surface between your hand and the client's body. *(Modified from Gaymar Industries, Inc., Orchard Park, NY.)*

wound irrigation to soften and remove devitalized tissues. *Enzymatic debridement* is the use of topical debriding agents to dissolve the collagen anchors that hold the necrotic slough tissue to the wound bed. *Biodebridement* is the use of sterile larvae (maggots), which secrete enzymes that digest wound tissue. Honey may also be used as a biodebriding agent. Finally, *autolytic debridement* involves the use of synthetic dressings to cover an ulcer, allowing enzymes in the wound bed to digest the devitalized tissues. This form of debridement is the slowest and is usually reserved for clients who cannot tolerate the other forms. Some ulcers should not be debrided, for example, ulcers on limbs where perfusion is insufficient to support healing and dry, stable eschar on heels. Stable eschar is hard and intact. If the eschar becomes soft, cracks, or exposes underlying open skin, it should be removed. Sharp, conservative debridement is painful; the client should be given analgesics before debridement begins. Some clients report burning pain with the enzymatic debriding agents.

Improve Nutrition

The association of malnutrition with pressure ulcer formation and delayed healing is clear. In fact, many clinicians believe that pressure ulcers are a specific indicator of malnutrition. If the client's serum albumin or prealbumin concentration is low, if the client is not eating, or if the client's body weight is less than 80% of ideal, consider nutritional supplementation. If the client has no gastrointestinal disorders and can swallow, provide oral supplements. Some clinicians use the phrase "if the gut works, use it" to summarize this recommendation. If the client cannot swallow without aspiration, tube-feeding may be required. If the client has digestive problems, consider total parenteral nutrition. These more aggressive forms of feeding must be compatible with the client's wishes, but in many cases a few weeks

A

B

■ **FIGURE 49–6** Pressure redistribution surfaces. **A,** KinAir beds provide controlled air suspension to redistribute body weight away from bony prominences. **B,** FluidAir beds use air flow and bead fluidization. Both of these beds are covered with Gore-Tex fabric, which resists tearing. This fabric is also waterproof and acts as a barrier against bacteria. *(Courtesy KCI Licensing, Inc., 2008.)*

of improved nutrition can "jump start" healing. Monitor nutritional status with repeated measurement of prealbumin, weight monitoring, or calorie counts. If tube-feeding must be stopped several times a day for medications or treatments, consider increasing the rate during the nighttime.

Monitor Healing

If the ulcer does not heal within 2 weeks despite adequate nutrition, pressure redistribution, daily cleaning, and use of appropriate dressings, the ulcer may be infected. An infected pressure ulcer looks like any other infected wound, with foul-smelling drainage, increasing size, increasing pain in the wound, and fever or elevation in white blood cell count. Older clients do not invariably demonstrate all of the manifestations of infection and are at risk for development of confusion; therefore vigilance in assessing the ulcer for changes is critical. If infection is suspected, a 2-week trial of topical antibiotics is considered. Swab cultures are not appropriate for diagnosis of infection in the ulcer, but can be used to diagnose heavy colonization or the presence of antibiotic resistance bacteria. Use a quantitative culture for suspected infection. Systemic antibiotics are used when the infection cannot be controlled locally or for systemic infection (manifested by fever or positive blood cultures).

Many conditions are associated with delays in healing. Diabetes, paralysis, and arterial diseases require close assessment because of increased risk of infection as a result of reduced blood flow to the wound. Urine and bowel incontinence lead to dermatitis and can contaminate open wounds.

Monitor for Complications

Many complications have been associated with pressure ulcers, including osteomyelitis, bacteremia and sepsis, and cellulitis. Wounds with osteomyelitis usually do not heal; if they do heal, they soon open again. The wound may become increasingly painful and drainage may be foul, often infected with *S. aureus, Enterobacter* species, and *Pseudomonas* species. Sepsis can follow osteomyelitis; confusion, reduced levels of consciousness, fever, hypotension, elevated white blood cell count, and other manifestations of septic shock may develop. The word *cellulitis* literally means "inflammation of the cells." It generally indicates an acute spreading infection of the dermis and subcutaneous tissues, resulting in pain, erythema, edema, and warmth. Associated red streaking visible in skin proximal to the area of cellulitis is characteristic of ascending lymphangitis. Cellulitis characterized by violaceous color and bullae suggests infection with *Streptococcus pneumoniae* (pneumococcus).

Nursing Management of the Medical Client

Assessment. All clients should be assessed for risk of pressure ulcers on admission and then daily, depending upon the client's condition. Less frequent assessment may be done if the client's condition is stable. The assessment of the client at high risk for development of pressure ulcers should identify any specific risk factors. The Braden scale (Figure 49-7) is an assessment tool that assists the nurse in predicting which clients are at greatest risk. Assess laboratory values on hemoglobin, hematocrit, albumin, prealbumin, total protein, and lymphocytes to further identify risks related to protein calorie malnutrition.

Skin should be fully assessed on admission and on each shift. To fully assess skin, look between folds of skin, remove anti-embolic stockings or devices, and use a mirror to see the heels. Also assess under oxygen tubing, especially on the ears and the cheeks, beneath splints and other medical devices. Pressure ulcers beneath medical devices are commonly overlooked! If the bath has been delegated to an unlicensed assistive person, arrange a time when the skin can be fully assessed. Sometimes helping with the bath is a convenient means to do a full skin assessment.

If the client has a pressure ulcer on admission to the facility, it must be recorded. Note objective data about the pressure ulcer (i.e., stage, length, width, depth, wound bed appearance, drainage, and condition of periulcer tissue). Reassessment of the ulcer is completed each time dressings are changed or sooner if the ulcer shows manifestations of deterioration. Analyses of the trends in healing are an important step in assessment. Consider whether the ulcer is increasing in size or depth or is developing more purulent drainage or odor, or whether the periulcer tissue is showing manifestations of deterioration. These changes in the pressure ulcer indicate that it is deteriorating and a change in treatment is needed. The physician or wound nurse should be notified, unless the agency protocol allows independent changes in treatment.

Diagnosis, Outcomes, Intervention

Diagnosis: Risk for Impaired Skin Integrity. Traditionally, clients who score between 12 and 16 on the Braden risk assessment scale are considered at risk for pressure ulcers. Scores below 12 indicate a high risk. A newer approach to reduce risk is to examine each risk factor independently and not rely on the total risk score, but rather the subscale score. This nursing diagnosis is written as *Risk for Impaired Skin Integrity related to malnutrition, unrelieved pressure, and/or incontinence as evidenced by Braden total risk score or subscale score.*

Outcomes. The client will have reduced risk of impairment of skin integrity, as evidenced by no actual tissue breakdown and no persistent reddened areas.

RISK PREDICTORS FOR SKIN BREAKDOWN

Patient's Name _____

Evaluator's Name _____

	1	2	3	4
SENSORY PERCEPTION ability to respond to discomfort	**1. Completely limited:** Unresponsive to painful stimuli, either because of state of unconsciousness or severe sensory impairment, which limits ability to feel pain over most of body surface	**2. Very limited:** Responds only to painful stimuli (but not verbal commands) by opening eyes or flexing extremities. Cannot communicate discomfort verbally, OR has a sensory impairment which limits the ability to feel pain or discomfort over one half of body surface	**3. Slightly limited:** Responds to verbal commands by opening eyes and obeying some commands, but cannot always communicate discomfort or need to be turned, OR has some sensory impairment which limits ability to feel pain or discomfort in one or two extremities.	**4. No impairment:** Responds to verbal commands by obeying. Can communicate needs accurately. Has no sensory deficit which would limit ability to feel pain or discomfort
MOISTURE degree to which skin is exposed to moisture	**1. Very Moist:** Skin is kept moist almost constantly by perspiration and urine. Dampness is detected every time patient is moved or turned. Linen must be changed more than one time each shift	**2. Occasionally Moist:** Skin is frequently, but not always kept moist, linen must be changed two to three times every 24 hours	**3. Rarely Moist:** Skin is rarely moist more than three to four times a week, but linen does require changing at that time	**4. Never Moist:** Perspiration and incontinence are never a problem; linen changed at routine intervals only
ACTIVITY degree of physical activity	**1. Bedfast:** Confined to bed	**2. Chairfast:** Ability to walk severely impaired or nonexistent and must be assisted into chair or wheelchair. Is confined to chair or wheelchair when not in bed	**3. Walks occasionally:** Walks occasionally during day, but for very short distances, with or without assistance. Spends majority of each shift in bed or chair	**4. Walks frequently:** Walks a moderate distance at least once every 1 to 2 hours during waking hours
MOBILITY ability to change and control body position	**1. Completely Immobile:** Unable to make even slight changes in position without assistance	**2. Very limited:** Makes occasional slight changes in position without help but unable to make frequent or significant changes in position independently	**3. Slightly limited:** Makes frequent though slight changes in position without assistance but unable to make or maintain major changes in position independently	**4. No limitations:** Makes major and frequent changes in position without assistance
NUTRITION usual food intake pattern	**1. Very Poor:** Never eats a complete meal. Rarely eats more than 1/3 of any food offered. Intake of protein is negligible. Takes even fluids poorly. Does not take a liquid dietary supplement, OR is NPO and/or maintained on clear liquids or IV for more than 5 days	**2. Probably Inadequate:** Rarely eats a complete meal and generally eats only about one half of any food offered. Protein intake is poor. Occasionally will take a liquid dietary supplement, OR receiving less than optimum amount of liquid diet or tube feeding	**3. Adequate:** Eats over half of most meals. Eats moderate amount of protein source one to two times daily. Occasionally will refuse a meal. Will usually take a dietary supplement if offered OR is on a tube feeding or TPN regimen which probably meets most of nutritional needs	**4. Excellent:** Eats most of every meal. Never refuses a meal. Frequently eats between meals. Does not require a dietary supplementation
FRICTION AND SHEAR	**1. Problem:** Requires moderate to maximum assistance in moving. Complete lifting without sliding against sheets is impossible. Frequently slides down in bed or chair, requiring frequent repositioning with maximum assistance. Either spasticity, contractures or agitation leads to almost constant friction	**2. Potential Problem:** Moves feebly independently or requires minimum assistance. Skin probably slides against bedsheets or chair to some extent when movement occurs. Maintains relatively good position in chair or bed most of time but occasionally slides down	**3. No Apparent Problem:** Moves in bed and in chair independently and has sufficient muscle strength to lift up completely during move. Maintains good position in bed or chair at all times	

Key: 16, minimum risk; 13–14, moderate risk; 12 or less, high risk; NPO, nothing by mouth; IV, intravenously; TPN, total parenteral nutrition.

■ **FIGURE 49–7** The Braden Scale for evaluation of risk of pressure ulcers. *(Courtesy Barbara Braden and Nancy Bergstrom. © 1988.)*

Interventions. Preventive measures to reduce the risk of pressure ulcers cannot be overemphasized (Box 49-2). Interventions are chosen to match the specific risk factors present (Table 49-2). Shearing injury can happen quickly in clients who are in semi-Fowler position. These clients should be repositioned often to reduce the risk of shear injury to the sacral area. Flexing the knee gatch of the bed will also prevent shearing when the head is elevated. It is also important to float heels from the bed by placing pillows under the calves.

Clients who have been placed on pressure-redistribution surfaces cannot be considered to be free from pressure ulcer risk. These clients must still be turned side to side and the skin inspected during turning. If the skin manifests stage I pressure ulcers, the turning frequency must be increased. If the client has been turned every 2 hours and is still showing stage I pressure ulcers, a higher level of pressure-redistribution device (e.g., mattress replacement) should be applied to the bed or a bed replacement should be used (e.g., low-air-loss bed).

Adequate hydration and nutrition are also important aspects of pressure ulcer prevention. Ask the unlicensed assistive personnel to offer food and fluids often and to accurately record what food and fluids are consumed. Skin should be lubricated when dry, and skin vulnerable to damage from incontinence should be protected with skin barriers. Indwelling catheters are commonly used in acute care settings; however, the continued use of catheters increases the risk of urinary tract infection.

Evaluation. Outcomes should be met in 24 to 48 hours. Recall that skin integrity can be impaired in just 2 hours. Therefore several hours are needed to determine whether skin injury occurred before risk reduction measures are implemented. If so, a more aggressive prevention plan is needed.

Diagnosis: Impaired Skin Integrity. If the client has a pressure ulcer, state the nursing diagnosis as *Impaired Skin Integrity related to pressure ulcer secondary to prolonged immobility, malnutrition, and unrelieved pressure as evidenced by (add description of the ulcer).*

BOX 49-2   Interventions for Treatment of Pressure Ulcers

- Continue to reduce risk of pressure ulcers using appropriate interventions.
- Assess and manage pain associated with the ulcer and its care. Even though clients cannot report pain, they still may be able to feel pain.
- Position the client to stay off the ulcer. If there is no turning surface without a pressure ulcer, use a pressure-redistribution bed and continue to turn the client. Do not rely on the bed exclusively to move the client. The client still needs to be repositioned and turned. Establish a written turning schedule.
- Elevate heels off the bed by using pillows or heel elevation boots. Fleece heel covers do not relieve pressure, but they can reduce friction.
- Maintain the head of the bed at the lowest elevation consistent with the client's medical condition. If the client must have the head elevated to prevent aspiration, reposition into a 30-degree lateral position. Use a seat cushion in the chair, and assess for sacral ulcers daily. For dyspneic clients, position erect and assess for sacral and ischial ulcers daily.
- Use support cushions (4 inches of foam, gels, flotation cushions) for the wheelchair-bound client or for any client who prefers to sit. Teach wheelchair-bound clients to reposition themselves every 15 minutes.
- Use support surfaces for clients with multiple ulcers or when there is no position for the client that does not place the client on an ulcer. Consider upgrading the support surface for those who are not able to keep off the ulcer surface. Begin with a reactive or active surface or mattress overlay. Progress to low-air-loss beds or air-fluidized beds if the ulcer does not heal. Check for bottoming out beneath the mattress. Place your hand between the mattress and the bed. If you feel less than an inch between the client's body and the mattress surface, the support is not adequate.

- Ensure adequate dietary intake to prevent malnutrition and delayed healing. Review the dietitian's recommendations for caloric and protein needs. Communicate these recommendations to the physician as needed.
- Provide oral supplementation, tube-feeding, or hyperalimentation to achieve positive nitrogen balance. For many clients, the decision not to eat is an important one that can give a sense of control over some aspect of existence. However, pressure ulcers cannot heal in clients with severe malnutrition.
- Supplement the diet with vitamins and minerals. Vitamin C and zinc are commonly prescribed to support wound healing in clients who are not consuming adequate calories.
- Remove devitalized tissue from the wound bed, except in avascular tissue or on the heels. Begin by cleansing the ulcer bed with normal saline; then use the appropriate technique for debridement. Once the ulcer is free of devitalized tissue, apply dressings that keep the wound bed moist and the surrounding skin dry. Do not use occlusive dressings on ulcers that may be infected.
- Prevent the ulcer from being exposed to urine and feces. Use indwelling catheters, bowel containment systems, and topical creams or dressings to prevent contamination.
- Follow body substance isolation precautions; use clean gloves and clean dressings for wound care.
- Monitor healing.

If the ulcer does not show signs of healing in 2 weeks or if manifestations of infection develop, the treatments must change to reduce the risk of sepsis and osteomyelitis.

SAFETY
ALERT

TABLE 49–2   Interventions to Reduce Pressure Ulcer Risk Based on Braden Subscale Scores

	Score 3	Score 2	Score 1
Sensory perceptual	Remind client to turn self and remain in off-loaded positions. Examine position of paralyzed limbs to be certain they are not trapped or pinned and do not rest on each other. Float heels from bed.	Inspect skin every shift. Protect client from self-injury on side rails, opposite limb, tubing, devices/monitors.	Assess all bony prominences (occiput, scapulae, elbows, heels). If positioned with head of bed elevated for tube-feeding, position in 30-degree lateral position rather than always supine. Examine skin beneath medical devices every shift
Activity	Place bed setting on prevention mode. Consider physical therapy consult.	Use padding of at least 4 inches of foam or a wheelchair cushion in wheelchair. Reposition wheelchair-bound clients every hour. Teach clients who are able to shift their weight every 15 min.	Depending on other factors (e.g., whether this client can turn at all), consider an upscaled bed. Float heels from bed.
Mobility	Use side rails and trapeze to facilitate self-movement.	Turn every 2 hr or more often and inspect bony prominences for skin breakdown. Do not massage red areas. Use pillows to keep bony prominences apart.	Turn every 2 hr using a written schedule for consistency. Consider an upscaled bed if other risk factors are present.
Moisture	Keep clean and dry between episodes of incontinence. Use skin protectant sprays, wipes, or lotions to protect skin. Treat dry skin with moisturizers. Keep skin care products at the bedside	Consider urinary tract infection as cause of incontinence. Consider infectious forms of diarrhea. Consider side effects of medications or tube-feeding as cause of diarrhea. Obtain order for antifungal powder or dressings if rash between skinfolds appears fungal.	Consider placing an indwelling catheter if denudement is severe. Consider a rectal bag if fecal incontinence is frequent. Monitor for dehydration from fluid loss. Avoid using plastic incontinence pads on specialty beds.
Nutrition	Offer oral supplements to diet. Monitor weight weekly.	Provide dietary consultation. Assess condition of mouth and ability to swallow. Monitor oral intake; consider calorie count.	Offer tube-feeding or hyperalimentation if within the goals of client or family.
Friction/shear	N/A	Apply lotions and creams to abraded areas. Apply cotton sleeves, socks, or heel and elbow protectors. Consider treatment for agitation or spasms.	Keep head of bed as low as possible. Use a lifting device to move client in bed. Apply adhesive dressings to abraded areas. If head of bed is elevated, monitor sacrum and heels closely for shear injury. Treat early manifestations of shear with protective dressings.

Outcomes. The client will experience healing of the ulcer, as evidenced by development of granulation tissue and decreasing ulcer size. Do not use lower stages of pressure ulcers to describe healing. For example, do not state a stage IV will heal to a stage III. The body does not heal by regeneration of tissue but, rather, by scar tissue. For clients who are terminally ill, outcomes such as healing may not be appropriate. For these clients, outcomes of pain management, comfort, or reducing risk of infection may be more appropriate.

Interventions. Consistency in the nursing care provided is an important aspect of interventions directed at achieving wound healing. It is important to develop scientific protocols in ulcer care and to use them consistently. It is also important to give one protocol time to work before changing to another. See Box 49-2 and Chapter 18 for information on wound healing.

Reducing the risk of pressure ulcer development and identifying early manifestations of pressure ulcers are frequently delegated to unlicensed assistive personnel. The Management and Delegation feature on p. 1217 highlights important nursing instructions to give to unlicensed personnel caring for clients with pressure ulcers. Case managers often assist in managing care between facilities. When preparing for discharge to home, case managers assist with advocating and preventing readmission (see the Case Management feature on The Client with Impaired Skin Integrity on the website).

evolve

MANAGEMENT AND DELEGATION

Care of Clients with Pressure Ulcers

When working with unlicensed assistive personnel (UAP) in the care of clients with pressure ulcers, help them to keep the following points in mind:

- Report any areas of skin redness that do not disappear after pressure relief.
- Report any new areas of purple or bruised skin.
- Report any development of foul odor or drainage from pressure ulcers.
- Reposition the client *at least* every 2 hours. Sometimes small shifts in the client's body weight may be sufficient, but the client must not be consistently positioned on the same tissue
- *Do not position the client on the ulcer.* If an ulcer is on the client's trunk, use a reactive mattress or an overlay mattress. However, the use of these support surfaces does not eliminate the need for turning.
- If the client is wheelchair-bound, instruct the UAP to reposition the client hourly. Ensure that the padding provides adequate pressure relief by checking for "bottoming out."
- Keep all pressure off the client's heels. Instruct the UAP how to float the heels using pillows for short term leg immobility. Be certain that any boots are applied properly. Instruct UAPs to remove boots and other devices on the legs to inspect the skin every shift.
- Keep the head of the bed at the lowest elevation to reduce shear and friction on the skin of the client's lower back.
- Keep the client's skin dry; clean any episodes of incontinence immediately.

Even though you have delegated the skin care of these clients, you are still accountable for their skin condition. Assess the entire skin surface every day. Ask for help in turning the client so that you can see the client's heels and sacrum. Use an assessment guide such as the Braden scale to determine the risk of further ulceration.

Evaluation. As the ulcer heals, assess the degree of outcome attainment every 3 to 4 days. Allow 2 weeks before changing the plan of care, unless the ulcer is deteriorating.

Self-Care

Clients at high risk for development of pressure ulcers who are going home should be referred to a home health agency before discharge from the acute care facility so that devices to reduce pressure can be obtained for home use. The family and the client need to understand the importance of frequent turning. A client who is wheelchair-bound and has arm function should be taught to lift the body, using the arms, off the chair twice every hour for repositioning. "Tilt in space" wheel chairs can be used for long-term wheelchair-dependent clients to assist with pressure redistribution. A client who is incontinent needs to wear protective pads to absorb the urine or stool and should be assessed often.

If the client is going home with an unhealed ulcer, the client and one or more family members must be taught wound care, wound assessment, and in some cases the administration of intravenous (IV) antibiotics. Teach these interventions before the day of discharge, so that return demonstrations can be used to evaluate learning. In addition, procurement of equipment is often necessary, which takes time. Community nurses need to be involved early in the planning for the discharge of the client with an ulcer. The Bridge to Home Health Care feature on p. 1218 describes ways to help the client and family manage pressure ulcers.

Surgical Management

Surgical repair is frequently performed on stage III and stage IV ulcers, on ulcers greater than 2 cm in diameter, and in clients who can tolerate surgery. In stage III ulcers, undamaged tissue near the wound is rotated to cover the ulcer. In stage IV ulcers, musculocutaneous flaps are often used (see later discussion).

PRECANCEROUS CHANGES IN THE SKIN

Precursors to cancer of the skin include damage from recurrent skin trauma and various skin lesions. To understand the role of prevention of skin cancer, these precursor conditions are discussed first. *Photodamage* refers to a spectrum of medical conditions caused by the sun. The spectrum includes sunburn; spider veins (telangiectasias); rough, thick skin; fine and deep wrinkling; actinic keratoses; and carcinomas. Sun protection at every age is the key to preventing short-term damage (sunburn and acute events), as well as the long-term damaging effects of sunlight such as photodamage and skin cancer. Tips for sun protection include daily use of sunscreen with SPF 15 or higher with broad-spectrum protection, wearing a T-shirt, broad-brimmed hat, and sunglasses, and staying out of the sun in the middle of the day. Use extra caution near water, snow, and sand because they reflect the damaging rays of the sun. Tanning beds should be avoided, and clients should be taught to check their skin regularly and consult a health-care provider if they see any skin lesions that are changing. Recall that "a change in a wart or mole" is one of the signs of cancer.

BRIDGE TO HOME HEALTH CARE

Managing Pressure Ulcers

For the client with pressure ulcers, a smooth transition from hospital to home care requires planning, preparation, and communication. For example, it may take a home health nurse several days to obtain special wound care supplies or pressure redistribution devices not ordinarily stocked by the home health agency. If a pressure redistribution bed or mattress overlay is required, the agency then contacts a durable medical equipment company and arranges delivery at a predetermined time. To facilitate the transition from hospital care, the home health agency should be notified of the referral before the client's discharge from the hospital and should receive specific instructions per physician orders for wound cleansing, dressing materials, and frequency of dressing changes. In addition, sending a day's supply home with the client minimizes disruption in the wound treatment regimen.

Clients who have stage IV or draining, infected pressure ulcers may initially require daily skilled nursing visits. However, as the infection is treated and drainage subsides, the frequency of skilled nursing visits is usually decreased and the family member or informal caregiver is taught to perform the dressing change. Caregivers should participate in or at least observe dressing change procedures in the hospital, and should receive information about turning and other aspects of care. The earlier the caregiver is introduced to prevention and treatment goals, the faster the client can reach the desired clinical outcome. Hospital nurses can significantly enhance the continuity of care by coordinating educational efforts with the home health agency. The home health nurse should obtain copies of any teaching materials distributed in the hospital. Older adults are often fearful of leaving the security of an inpatient setting; therefore

reinforcing familiar teaching materials and wound care procedures helps to ensure a more seamless transition from inpatient to outpatient management.

Maintaining equipment and supplies is more difficult in the home than in inpatient settings. Estimate the needed amount of skin and wound care supplies, and arrange for delivery in a timely manner. Establish an intercommunication sheet in the home that flags a change in wound care orders for other members of the health care team. Leave specific directions for product use, especially when more than one product is being used. *Normal saline* can be made by using the following recipe: mix 8 teaspoons of salt in 1 gallon of bottled or boiled water. Do not use water from an outdoor well or an unknown water source.

Adapting the home environment to meet the needs of the client and family members or other caregivers requires creativity and skill. Note the conditions under which the client spends prolonged periods of time. Any firm, unyielding surface can contribute to development of a pressure ulcer in unusual body areas. Sitting on ridged, corded edges of chairs or stools or a firm toilet seat for extended periods can restrict blood flow, leading to pressure ulcer development.

The limitations of older clients and their older caregivers pose additional changes. For example, it may not be possible for a debilitated client to be turned as often as needed during the night to relieve pressure over bony prominences. Frequent turning schedules usually result in increased anxiety and sleep deprivation for older caregivers. Accurately assessing the client's risk category and using an effective pressure-relieving mattress overlay can help to reduce the physical demands for caregivers and increase the possibility that the client can receive needed care and remain at home.

SUNBURN

Sunburn is an acute inflammatory skin response that occurs as a reaction to excessive exposure to sunlight. Pathologic changes in the skin include the production of epidermal cells that exhibit cytoplasmic and nuclear changes. These changes are cumulative over the life span and lead to an increased incidence of skin cancer with aging.

A first-degree sunburn produces mild, tender erythema followed by desquamation (peeling), which heals without scarring. Second-degree sunburn causes more extreme erythema and edema, and blistering results from damage to the epidermal cells. Deep sunburn is uncommon unless it is induced by artificial sources such as tanning lamps or booths. Deep sunburn produces burns (see Chapter 50).

Prevention is the best approach to management of sunburn. Client teaching emphasizing sun protection should never be omitted when caring for the sunburned client. For a list of specific precautions, see the Client Education Guide feature on Simple Guidelines to Help Protect You from the Damaging Rays of the Sun on the website.

Treating sunburn involves decreasing inflammation and rehydrating the damaged skin. For localized, *superficial, partial-thickness* sunburn, use cool tap water soaks for 20 minutes or until the skin is cool. This measure limits skin destruction, prevents edema, and potentially reduces blisters. Tepid tap water baths are indicated for large sunburned areas. After a bath or soak, apply water-based emollients, lotions, foams, gels, or sprays, preferably refrigerated for an additional cooling effect. Emollients should also be applied throughout the day to soothe the skin and relieve dryness. Lotions, foams, or sprays containing camphor and menthol (e.g., Sarna) can also be beneficial. Avoid the use of OTC remedies containing local anesthetics—such as benzocaine, dibucaine (Nupercaine), or lidocaine (Xylocaine)—because they are rarely effective and have the potential to induce contact sensitivity.

For *partial-thickness* sunburn, apply continuous cool, normal saline soaks or soaking baths to reduce oozing and edema. Very large blisters may be aspirated and dressed with sterile dressings. Avoid debridement unless there is evidence of secondary bacterial infection. Silver sulfadiazine may be prescribed.

Prostaglandin inhibitors (nonsteroidal anti-inflammatory drugs [NSAIDs]) may be used to reduce erythema and inflammation in adults. Topical corticosteroids may be prescribed to be used sparingly in nonocclusive vehicles (lotion, spray, gel) for their vasoconstrictive effects. Systemic corticosteroids are prescribed only for clients with extensive, painful burns, but their use has declined because they seem to offer little efficacy when given in a reasonable dose range.

ACTINIC KERATOSIS

Actinic keratosis, the most common epithelial precancerous lesion in Caucasians, is primarily caused by sun exposure. It affects nearly 100% of older Caucasian adults. There is a small but definite risk of malignant degeneration and subsequent metastatic potential in neglected lesions.

Actinic keratosis most frequently occurs in areas of chronic, usually high-intensity sun exposure, including the face, the tops of the ears, the back of the neck, the forearms, the backs of the hands, and the chest. The clinical appearance of actinic keratoses is varied. The typical lesion is an irregularly shaped, flat, slightly erythematous macule or papule with indistinct borders and an overlying hard keratotic scale or horn that feels rough or sharp to palpation. In some cases, the erythema or the horn may be absent. This scale can be periodically shed or peeled off, but then it regrows. The lesion varies in size from the size of a pinhead to several centimeters across and is often more easily palpated than observed. Single lesions may be seen, but more often they appear in groups on a background of sun-damaged skin.

OUTCOME MANAGEMENT

Medical Management

Topical application of fluorouracil (Carac, Efudex, and Fluoroplex), a topical antineoplastic, is currently one of the best approaches to treatment of widespread actinic damage with multiple lesions. The advantage is that large areas of widespread disease can be treated at the same time. Use not only removes the majority of premalignant and superficial malignant lesions that can be seen but also uncovers and destroys clinically undetectable lesions of this type. However, the major disadvantage is the inflammatory response that often accompanies successful treatment. This response sequence is erythema usually followed by vesiculation, erosion, ulcerations, necrosis, and epithelialization.

The medication should be applied twice daily with a gloved hand, carefully avoiding the eyes, folds around the nose, the mouth, and the scrotum. Medication should be continued until the inflammatory response reaches the erosion, necrosis, and ulceration stage, at which time the medication should be stopped. The usual duration of therapy is 2 to 4 weeks; by then, the client may experience extreme discomfort requiring pain medication. At the time these products are stopped, topical corticosteroid creams may be applied to reduce inflammation and provide the client with additional pain reduction. Complete healing of the lesions may not be evident for 1 to 2 months after cessation of therapy.

Surgical Management

Cryotherapy

Cryotherapy using liquid nitrogen is a common treatment for single lesions or for small numbers of actinic keratoses. Liquid nitrogen is usually applied with a cotton-tipped applicator or spraying device. No local anesthetic is required but the freezing process is associated with a small amount of discomfort, which may linger afterward. Intermittent application of a warm, damp wash cloth to the site may bring relief. Freezing frequently results in inflammation with blister formation, and blister care should be reviewed with the client.

Electrodesiccation and Curettage

Electrodesiccation produces superficial destruction. The procedure may be done using local anesthetics. The tissue is destroyed by mechanical disruption of cells and heat. The tissue is removed by scraping or scooping with a loop-shaped instrument called a curet. This method can provide tissue for histologic diagnosis if needed. The curetted areas usually heal quickly, with adequate wound care resulting in a small white permanent scar. The wound site should be kept moist with a less sensitizing topical antibiotic ointment such as bacitracin.

Laser Excision

Laser uses light energy to vaporize lesions. Depending upon the wavelength of the light, various portions of the cell are heated. Tissue is not available for histologic examination. Local anesthesia is used.

Punch or Excisional Biopsy

Punch or excisional biopsy is indicated for lesions that are large or have other characteristics of cancer. It is often difficult to distinguish a large actinic keratosis from a squamous cell carcinoma without histologic diagnosis. Biopsy should also be done on lesions that persist after adequate treatment. Local anesthesia is used for the biopsy procedure and allows electrodesiccation to be done painlessly after biopsy. Excisional biopsy requires primary closure of the site and may be a more extensive procedure than the lesion warrants; however, it ensures more complete removal of the growth (see Chapter 48).

SKIN CANCER

Skin cancer is the most common cancer in the United States, and the number of new skin cancers and the number of skin cancer deaths are increasing at alarming rates. Skin cancer is a malignant condition caused by uncontrolled growth and spread of abnormal cells in a specific layer of the skin. The several different kinds of skin cancer are distinguished by the types of cells involved. The three most common types are (1) basal cell carcinoma, (2) squamous cell carcinoma, and (3) malignant melanoma. More than 90% of all skin cancers fall into the first two classifications. Both basal cell carcinoma and squamous cell carcinoma are slow-growing tumors with a cure rate of 95% or greater after early treatment

Etiology and Risk Factors

The cause of skin cancer is well known. Prolonged or intermittent, repeated exposure to UVL radiation from the sun, especially when it results in sunburn and blistering, plays a key role in the induction of skin cancer, especially malignant melanoma. Most non-melanoma skin cancers occur on parts of the body unprotected by clothing (face, neck, forearms, and backs of hands) and in people who have received considerable exposure to sunlight. All people are at risk of skin cancer regardless of skin tone and hair color, although some are at much greater risk than others. In general, people with red, blond, or light brown hair with light complexions or freckles, many of Celtic or Scandinavian origin, are most susceptible; blacks and Asians are least susceptible. The Genetic Links feature at right describes skin care for clients with reduced melanin synthesis.

Due to the rising numbers of skin cancers, all clients should be encouraged to use sunscreen. Clients should be taught to examine their own skin regularly and have someone examine their back looking for new moles or lesions. Danger signals in moles (pigmented nevi) are presented in Box 49-3. Suspicious lesions should be examined by a physician.

The pattern of reaction to acute sun exposure can be correlated with the development of actinic keratosis and skin cancer. People who never tan and always burn after 1 to 2 hours of midday summer sun are most susceptible. People who burn once or twice at the beginning of

summer and then tan are somewhat less susceptible. Those who never burn and always tan are the least susceptible. The most severely affected people usually have a history of long-term occupational (farmers, construction workers, surveyors, sailors) or recreational (swimmers, skiers, surfers, sunbathers) sun exposure. It is imperative that all people at risk of skin cancer examine their skin systematically. The Client Education Guide on p. 1222 summarizes teaching instructions recommended by The Skin Cancer Foundation.

GENETIC LINKS

Oculocutaneous Albinism Type I (OCA1)

DESCRIPTION

OCA1 is an autosomal recessive disorder characterized by reduced synthesis of melanin in the skin, hair, and eyes, and associated characteristic ocular findings. Ocular findings include nystagmus, reduced iris and retinal pigment, foveal hypoplasia with reduced visual acuity, and misrouting of the optic nerves, producing alternating strabismus and reduced stereoscopic vision. There are two categories of OCA1: OCA1A (most common), associated with absent melanin synthesis in all tissue; and OCA1B, associated with varying amounts of melanin synthesis in the skin, hair, and eyes. Clients with OCA1A have white hair, white skin that does not tan, and blue, fully translucent irises. Clients with OCA1B have white or light yellow hair that darkens with age, white skin that gradually develops some generalized pigment, and blue irises that may change color with age to green/hazel or brown/tan.

GENETICS

OCA1 is caused by mutations in the tyrosinase gene, *TYR*, located on chromosome 11. Molecular genetic testing of the *TYR* gene is clinically available. The carrier rate for OCA1 is approximately 1 in 100 in most populations throughout the world. OCA1 is an autosomal recessive disorder, and offspring of carrier parents have a 25% chance of being affected with OCA1, a 50% chance of being a carrier, and a 25% chance of being unaffected and not a carrier.

DIAGNOSIS AND TESTING

Diagnosis of OCA1 is established by clinical features of hypopigmentation of the skin and hair and eye findings. Genetic testing is rarely used in diagnosis and is most commonly used for carrier detection in genetic counseling.

MANAGEMENT

A critical aspect of the ongoing care of clients with OCA1 is ophthalmologic care, including, for example, correction of refractive errors (e.g., myopia, hyperopia, astigmatism) to improve visual acuity and annual eye examination. Skin care is dictated by the amount of skin pigment and cutaneous response to sunlight. Clients with OCA1A need to be protected from sun exposure with clothing and sunscreens.

BASAL CELL CARCINOMA

Basal cell carcinoma (BCC), the most common form of skin cancer, is a malignant epithelial tumor of the skin that arises from the basal cells in the epidermis. The tumor is usually painless and slow growing, generally appearing on sun-exposed skin of the face, ears, head, neck, or hands. Occasionally, basal cell carcinoma may appear on the trunk, especially the upper back and chest. The majority of cases are caused by chronic over-exposure to UVL radiation, and only a few cases can be linked to arsenic, burns, scars, exposure to radiation, or genetic predisposition. Clinical and histologic findings are used to identify the tumor.

The most common clinical presentation of basal cell carcinoma is the nodular lesion (Figure 49-8, *A*). This is a dome-shaped papule with a well-defined border having a classic "pearly" texture. Basal cell carcinoma has this flesh-colored "pearly" or shiny appearance because it does not keratinize. Telangiectatic (small spider-like) vessels frequently overlie the lesion. As the lesion enlarges, the center may flatten or ulcerate, but the border is still raised, giving a "rolled-edge" appearance.

Although basal cell carcinomas almost never metastasize, they can be locally destructive and invasive through tissue. This is particularly true on the face, where a lesion can invade deep structures with resultant loss of an eye or ear or the nose. If untreated, the tumor can invade bone and brain. If the tumor is identified and treated early, local excision or even nonexcisional destruction is usually curative.

Clients who have had one basal cell carcinoma are at risk for development of another. Recurrences of previously treated basal cell carcinomas are also possible but more unusual; recurrence is generally noted within the first 2 years after removal or therapy.

SQUAMOUS CELL CARCINOMA

Squamous cell carcinoma (SCC) (Figure 49-8, *B*) is the second most common skin cancer in Caucasians. It is a tumor of the epidermal keratinocytes and rarely occurs in dark-skinned people. It is found on areas often exposed to the sun, typically the rim of the ear, the face, the lips and mouth, and the backs of the hands.

Squamous cell carcinoma is more difficult to characterize than basal cell carcinoma. The tumor is poorly marginated; the edge often blends into surrounding sun-damaged skin. Squamous cell carcinoma may present as an ulcer, a flat red area, a cutaneous horn, an indurated plaque, or a hyperkeratotic papule or nodule. Often it presents as a red- to skin-colored papule surmounted by varying amounts of scale.

The lesions grow more rapidly than does basal cell carcinoma. These tumors are potentially dangerous because they may infiltrate surrounding structures and metastasize to lymph nodes, with a fatal outcome.

MALIGNANT MELANOMA

Malignant melanoma (Figure 49-8, *C* and *D*) is a cancer of melanocytes; it is the deadliest form of skin cancer. The incidence of melanoma is increasing, such that currently about 1 in 100 people in the United States can expect to develop this cancer in a lifetime. The incidence of and death rate from melanoma are increasing worldwide. In countries populated with fair-skinned Caucasian people, the incidence of melanoma and the death rate have increased 7% to 15% per year, more than doubling during the 1990s.

Exposure to UVL continues to be one of the most important causes of malignant melanoma. What causes melanocytes to transform to melanoma cells is poorly understood. Primary cutaneous melanoma may develop in precursor melanocytic nevi (common acquired, congenital, and atypical or dysplastic types), although more than 50% of cases are believed to arise without a pre-existing pigmented lesion. Melanoma is multifactorial and appears to be related to multiple risk factors including (1) fair complexion, (2) excessive childhood sun exposure and blistering childhood sunburns, (3) increased number of common and dysplastic moles, (4) family history of melanoma, and (5) presence of a changing mole on the skin. The suspicion of melanoma is based on history as well as the clinical appearance.

Clinical Manifestations

The cardinal clinical manifestation of melanoma is a change in a skin lesion observed over a period of months. If a lesion grows so fast that it doubles in size in 10 days, it is usually an inflammation. If a lesion changes so slowly that neither the client nor the family

CLIENT EDUCATION GUIDE

Skin Self-Examination

You will need a bright light, a full-length mirror, a hand mirror, two chairs or stools, a blow dryer, body maps, and a pencil.

A. Examine your face—especially the nose, lips, mouth, and ears—front and back. Use one or both mirrors to get a clear view.

B. Thoroughly inspect your scalp, using a blow dryer and mirror to expose each section to view. Get a friend or family member to help, if you can.

C. Check your hands carefully: palms and backs, between the fingers, and under the fingernails. Continue up the wrists to examine both the front and back of your forearms.

D. Standing in front of the full-length mirror, begin at the elbows and scan all sides of your upper arms. Do not forget the underarms.

E. Next, focus on the neck, chest, and torso. Women should lift breasts to view the underside.

F. With your back to the full-length mirror, use the hand mirror to inspect the back of your neck, shoulders, upper back, and any part of the back of your upper arms you could not view previously.

G. Still using both mirrors, scan your lower back, buttocks, and backs of both legs.

H. Sit down; prop each leg in turn on the other stool or chair. Use the hand mirror to examine the genitals. Check front and sides of both legs, thigh to shin; ankles; and tops of feet, between toes, and under toenails. Examine soles of the feet and the heels.

From The Skin Cancer Foundation (1992). *Skin cancer. If you can spot it, you can stop it.* New York: Author.

is sure of a change, it is usually benign. Changes that may signal melanoma are called the *A, B, C, D* changes in moles:

- Asymmetry
- Border notching
- Color variegation with black, brown, red, or white hue
- Diameter greater than 6 mm

Other changes include doubling size in 3 to 8 months, bleeding, itching, ulceration, a change in color, or development of a palpable lymph node. Four types of melanoma are presented in Table 49-3. The tumor can metastasize, usually to the brain, lungs, bones, liver, and skin, and is ultimately fatal.

OUTCOME MANAGEMENT

Management is directed at removing the tumor, if possible. Survival is directly related to the depth of tumor invasion: 10-year survival is greater than 90% if the tumor is less than 1 mm in depth, but if the tumor is larger than 4 mm in depth, 10-year survival decreases to only 40%. Microscopic ulceration is the next most

■ **FIGURE 49–8 A,** Basal cell carcinoma characterized by rolled edges and a crater in the center of the lesion. Scars are from previous destruction of skin cancers. **B,** Squamous cell carcinoma on the hand. **C,** Superficial spreading melanoma. **D,** Nodular melanoma with satellite lesions.

important adverse prognostic pathologic feature. Metastatic melanoma is universally fatal. It is therefore extremely important for a malignant melanoma to be diagnosed early according to the ABCD rules.

Medical Management

Medical management begins with a high level of suspicion for any type of skin cancer but specifically for melanoma. The need for early detection cannot be overemphasized. Any indication, whether it is a confirmed risk factor or a suspicious lesion, is adequate reason for referral. Clients with localized cutaneous disease have been treated with adjuvant chemotherapy, nonspecific passive immunotherapy, radiation therapy, and biologic therapy. No increase in survival has been reported with these adjunctive therapies. Adjuvant interferon (IFN) alfa-2b and various experimental melanoma vaccines show promise in individuals with high-risk primary cutaneous melanoma and those with regional nodal disease. Melanoma vaccines are being investigated for therapeutic use. A variety of vaccines targeting melanoma cell antigens are in the clinical trial phase. The Complementary and Alternative Therapy feature on p. 1224 lists interventions that could reduce the risk or recurrence of melanoma.

Surgical Management

Treatment of all skin cancers requires removal of the lesion. The margins of the resected specimen must be free of tumor to a specified distance (depending on the type of skin cancer) to guarantee full removal.

A special surgical technique primarily used for the removal of skin malignancies such as basal cell carcinoma and squamous cell carcinoma is *Mohs' surgery,* which is also indicated for primary lesions in areas in which preservation of normal skin is necessary (e.g., eyelids, pinna, nasolabial folds). The technique involves a series of excisions with careful microscopic tissue assessment to "map" the presence or absence of malignant cells within each specimen. The procedure may be lengthy. After all tumor tissue is removed, the wound is closed with sutures or a flap, or is allowed to close by secondary intention.

Basal cell carcinomas and squamous cell carcinomas can also be excised and the surgical wound closed primarily (with skin edges sewn together) or with a skin flap. The advantage of this technique is that it requires much less time, and a fine line scar is produced. The tumor is completely excised with adequate margins of tumor-free tissue. If there is doubt about adequacy of margins, the specimen is sent for pathologic diagnosis (by permanent section technique).

TABLE 49–3 Types of Melanoma

Tumor Type	General Information	Clinical Manifestations
Superficial spreading melanoma (SSM)	Most common form of melanoma; slowly changing lesion with more rapid growth just before diagnosis	Deeply pigmented area contained within a brown nevus (freckle); usually flat and asymmetrical; as lesion grows, color changes may occur, ranging from jet black to dark blue to pale gray or white; looks lacy; lesions may have areas of no color; usually 2 cm wide
Nodular melanoma (NM)	Second most common form of melanoma; more aggressive tumor than SSM, with shorter clinical onset time	Common on trunk, head, and neck; usually 1-2 cm in diameter; often begins in normal skin, rather than in a pre-existing lesion; dark and more uniform in color; may resemble a blood blister or hemangioma; dome-shaped with sharp borders
Lentigo maligna melanoma (LMM)	Fairly uncommon tumor; typically appears on face of Caucasian women; usually has been present for long time (5-15 yr)	Generally a large, flat lesion that looks like a stain on the skin; typically tan with various shades of brown; metastasis less common
Acral-lentiginous melanoma (ALM)	Commonly occurs on palms and soles; more common in dark-skinned people; usually occurs in older adults; may evolve over a few months to years	Large lesion, about 3 cm in diameter; resembles LMM (a tan or brown flat lesion on palm or sole); can be misdiagnosed as a corn; ulceration is common; likely to metastasize

The treatment of malignant melanoma is wide local excision. Surgical excision begins with biopsy to determine the stage of the cancer. Excisional biopsy is the removal of the lesion and a narrow margin of normal-appearing tissue. The tumor is excised with a 1- to 2-cm margin of normal-appearing tissue. The margin width is based on the type of melanoma. The surgical wound is closed either primarily or with grafts or flaps.

Surgeons differ on the timing of the definitive surgery. Some surgeons excise the lesion after frozen section examination while the client is still on the operating table. Other surgeons wait for the results of permanent section pathologic diagnosis and then proceed with definitive treatment. The final excision is usually completed within 1 week of biopsy. Although there is a theoretical risk of tumor spread during biopsy, there is no convincing evidence that waiting 1 to even 6 weeks after biopsy jeopardizes the outcome. In fact, sometimes the delay gives the client time to prepare for surgery, both physically and psychologically.

Most clients with metastatic melanoma live less than 1 year. Currently, there is no cure for metastatic melanoma, but some of the new developments in clinical trials may change currently accepted treatments. A treatment plan is formulated on the basis of several factors: site of the tumor, number of metastases, rate of tumor growth, previous treatments, response to treatment, and the age, general health, and desires of the client. Some treatments include surgery to remove metastatic lesions, radiation therapy, chemotherapy, and local hyperthermia. Alternatively, the client can opt for no further treatment.

COMPLEMENTARY AND ALTERNATIVE THERAPY

Chemoprevention of Melanoma

A recent review of chemoprevention studies for melanoma found that several interventions could reduce the risk or the recurrence of melanoma. These include higher intakes of polyunsaturated fatty acids (such as fish oil), vitamin E from food, normal levels of selenium, green tea, soy, and nonsteroidal anti-inflammatory drugs (NSAIDs). More research is needed, but these are interesting initial data.

REFERENCE
Demierre M.-F., Nathanson L. (2003) Chemoprevention of melanoma: An unexplored strategy. *Journal of Clinical Oncology,* 21:158-165.

CUTANEOUS T-CELL LYMPHOMA (MYCOSIS FUNGOIDES)

Cutaneous T-cell lymphoma (CTCL), or mycosis fungoides, is a malignant disease involving the T helper cells. Malignant T cells in the blood migrate to the skin, where they have an affinity for the epidermis. The malignant cells continue to grow and change, eventually moving into the dermis. The cause is not known, and the course is unpredictable, varying with the type of presentation.

The three distinct clinical presentations are patch, plaque, and tumor. Clinical manifestations include eversion of the eyelids and hyperkeratosis of the palms and soles, often with fissuring. Finally, the plaques form tumors that ultimately ulcerate. Tumors can also develop spontaneously in previously unaffected areas, and eventual visceral or organ involvement ensues. This disease is often described as a slow-growing but highly disfiguring debilitating cancer. Clients often feel desperate by the time diagnosis is confirmed, which adds to the psychological difficulties. The tumor presentation carries the worst prognosis, with a survival period of 3 years or less.

CTCL is extremely difficult to diagnose and is often misdiagnosed. In its early stages, CTCL can clinically mimic eczematous processes. The initial erythematous papules resemble those in other eczematous conditions, including psoriasis and atopic dermatitis. The original eruptions of CTCL may be either transitory or of prolonged duration and sometimes are pruritic.

OUTCOME MANAGEMENT

Control of pruritus is essential at all stages and is accomplished by rehydration of the skin, various dry skin therapies (see Xerotic Eczema), topical corticosteroids, and PUVA therapy (see Ultraviolet Light B Therapy). Prevention of secondary infections is important. Nitrogen mustard and other chemotherapy agents are administered topically. Daily application of chemotherapeutic agents often constitutes the initial treatment. Photophoresis, a treatment involving the removal of small amounts of blood that is irradiated and then returned to the body, is used frequently in more advanced stages. Total-body electron beam therapy with or without adjuvant chemotherapy is an aggressive approach often used.

The primary systemic drug used for treatment of CTCL was formerly intravenous methotrexate. With advances in treatment, newer drugs have replaced methotrexate: one is denileukin diftitox (Ontak), used primarily in the treatment of persistent or recurrent CTCL. This agent has produced sustained regression of the tumors, in some cases for longer than 2 years. Fatalities remain extremely high in this disease as a result of progression to systemic involvement.

BULLOUS DISORDERS: PEMPHIGUS

Pemphigus is a chronic disorder that results in the development of blisters (*bullae*). It is fairly uncommon in the general population, but the incidence is increased in Jewish and Mediterranean people. There are several types: pemphigus vulgaris, pemphigus foliaceus, and pemphigus erythematosus. This discussion focuses on pemphigus vulgaris, the most common type.

Pemphigus is an autoimmune disease caused by circulating immunoglobulin G (IgG) autoantibodies. These autoantibodies react with the intracellular cement—the substance that holds epidermal cells together. The reaction causes intraepidermal bulla (blister) formation and acantholysis (loss of cohesion between epidermal cells).

Clinical manifestations include flaccid bullae that rupture easily, emitting a foul-smelling drainage and leaving crusted, denuded skin. Nikolsky's sign is the result when the epidermis can be rubbed off by slight friction or injury; this sign is a hallmark of pemphigus. Even slight pressure on an intact blister may cause it to spread to adjacent skin. The lesions are common on the face, back, chest, groin, and umbilicus.

OUTCOME MANAGEMENT

Management includes large doses of steroids and immunosuppressives. Plasmapheresis has been of some benefit in the treatment of pemphigus. If a large proportion of the skin is denuded, management is similar to that for a burn-injured client. The client is at increased risk for infection, fluid and electrolyte imbalance, and stress response complications (i.e., stress ulcers, body system failure). In addition, nursing management focuses on self-concept and pain management. Potassium permanganate baths may be used to reduce the risk of infection, control the odor of the drainage, and ease the pain.

INFECTIOUS DISORDERS

Several organisms lead to skin infections and infestations. Common skin infections are described in Table 49-4. The Terrorism Alert feature on p. 1227 describes smallpox, a serious viral infection. A few others are discussed in detail here.

ERYSIPELAS AND CELLULITIS

Cellulitis is a skin infection that extends into the deeper dermis and subcutaneous tissues and causes deep, red erythema without sharp borders that spreads widely through tissue spaces (Figure 49-9 on p. 1228). The skin is erythematous, edematous, tender, and sometimes nodular. *Streptococcus pyogenes* is the usual cause of this infection, although other pathogens may be responsible. Lymphangitis may occur; if cellulitis is untreated, gangrene, metastatic abscesses, and sepsis result.

Older clients are at increased risk for cellulitis due to lowered resistance from diabetes, malnutrition, steroid therapy, or the presence of wounds or ulcers. Other predisposing factors include the presence of edema and other cutaneous inflammation or wounds (e.g., tinea, eczema, burns, trauma). There is a tendency for recurrence, especially at sites of lymphatic obstruction.

Oral or IV antibiotics are used that are effective against both streptococci and *S. aureus*. Before antibiotics are administered, a wound specimen for culture and sensitivity testing should be obtained, although culture rarely yields the causative organism. Soaks may reduce edema and inflammation. The enzymes that facilitate a rapid spread of infection also seem to produce other significant manifestations such as high fever, tachycardia, confusion, and hypotension; appropriate interventions should be undertaken if these occur. Monitor

TABLE 49–4 Common Skin Infections and Infestations

Disease with Causative Organism	Clinical Manifestations	Management
Parasitic		
Scabies: *Sarcoptes scabiei*	Multiple straight or wavy thread-like lines beneath skin, itching	Application of a scabicide with retreatment in 1 wk to kill residual eggs. All clothing and linen should be washed and dried in hot cycles or dry-cleaned.
Lice: *Pediculus humanus, Phthirus pubis*	Intense itching; scratch marks may be evident	Application of pediculicides. For *head lice,* shampoo should be worked into dry hair until it is saturated. A fine-toothed comb should be used to remove dead lice and nits. Brushes and combs should be washed in pediculicide also. For *body lice,* pediculicide lotion is applied to involved body areas. Clothing should be washed and dried in hot cycles or dry-cleaned. Other items can be stored in plastic bags for 30-35 days. Family members, close contacts, and sexual partners should also be treated.
Bacterial		
Impetigo: group A streptococci, staphylococci	Pruritic vesicle or pustule that breaks and leaves a thick honey-colored crust	Antibiotics given until culture results available include erythromycin or dicloxacillin. Mupirocin is preferable to oral antibiotics when lesions are limited to small, localized area. **Teach control of contagion; infection is contagious as long as skin lesions are present. Use thorough hand-washing, separate laundry for client's linens, and separate washing of client's dishes.**
Folliculitis, furuncles, carbuncles: *Staphylococcus aureus*	White pustules on forehead, chest, upper back, neck, thighs, groin, and axillae; furuncles are deeper inflamed nodules; carbuncles are interconnected furuncles and often rupture, expelling purulent, foul-smelling thick drainage	Localized folliculitis is treated with warm compresses, gentle washing, and topical antibiotics. Furuncles are treated as for folliculitis with incision and drainage (I&D) to avoid rupture. Carbuncles are treated with systemic antibiotics and I&D. Instruct client to use disposable razors to avoid reinfection. **Reduce spread of infection by careful hand-washing and separate laundry of linens.**
Fungal		
Candidiasis: *Candida albicans*	Appearance depends on location; in *mouth,* infection is called thrush and appears as white plaques with an underlying red base with fissures on corners of mouth; *skin* lesions are pruritic, red, and moist with eroded scales, commonly found in axilla and gluteal, perianal, and interdigital folds; *vaginal* thrush causes intense itching and cheesy drainage	Eliminate or control predisposing factors such as antibiotics (which alter flora), malnutrition, diabetes, immunosuppression, pregnancy, or birth control pills. Use topical antifungal powders and creams. Keep skin dry and environment cool.
Tinea: variety of dermatophytes (tinea corporis, on body; tinea capitis, on scalp; tinea cruris, jock itch; tinea pedis, athlete's foot)	*Tinea corporis:* round red macules and papules with scales—lesions have advancing borders and healing centers; *tinea capitis:* patchy hair loss, inflammation, scales, and folliculitis; *tinea cruris:* red lesions with raised borders; *tinea pedis:* scaling, maceration, pain, and vesicles	Infection is controlled with antifungal solutions and creams. Acute lesions may require wet dressings, keratolytic agents, or both to remove scales. Client is taught to reduce risk by thoroughly drying after a bath or shower, wearing absorbent underwear and socks, applying talc to intertriginous areas, and wearing open shoes during warm weather.
Viral		
Herpes simplex: herpes simplex virus	Vesicles preceded by sensation of itching or burning; clear exudate from vesicles, followed by crusting; common to nose, lips, cheeks, ears, and genitalia	No cure is available. Treatment includes pain relief and topical anesthetics. Acyclovir, an antiviral drug, may decrease viral shedding and hasten healing. Avoiding sun and using sunscreens reduce recurrent lesions on lips. Reduce contagiousness by using frequent hand-washing, not picking at lesions, avoiding sexual intercourse and kissing while lesions are active, and not sharing lipsticks. Try to identify (and avoid or control) personal triggers for lesions.
Warts: human papillomavirus	Rough, fresh, or gray-colored skin protrusion	Numerous therapies, some with over-the-counter medication. May require electrodesiccation or cryosurgery. Intralesional injections of cytotoxic drugs may also be used. No treatment is also an acceptable option.

SAFETY
⚠
ALERT

SAFETY
⚠
ALERT

TERRORISM ALERT

Smallpox

Smallpox is a serious, contagious, and sometimes fatal infectious disease caused by the variola virus. Smallpox outbreaks have occurred from time to time for thousands of years, but the disease has been eradicated after a successful worldwide vaccination program. The last case of smallpox in the United States was in 1949 and the last naturally occurring case in the world was in Somalia in 1977. After the disease was eliminated from the world, routine vaccination against smallpox among the general public was stopped because it was no longer necessary for prevention. Except for laboratory stockpiles, the variola virus has been eliminated. However, there is heightened concern that the variola virus might be used as an agent of bioterrorism.

Smallpox normally spreads from contact with infected people. Generally, direct and fairly prolonged face-to-face contact is required to spread smallpox from one person to another. Smallpox also can be spread through direct contact with infected body fluids or contaminated objects such as bedding or clothing. Indirect spread is less common. Rarely, smallpox has been spread by virus carried in the air in enclosed settings such as buildings, buses, and trains. Smallpox is not known to be transmitted by insects or animals.

There are two clinical forms of smallpox. *Variola major* is the severe and most common form of smallpox, with a more extensive rash and higher fever. *Variola minor* is a less common presentation of smallpox, and a much less severe disease, with death rates historically of 1% or less. There is no specific treatment for smallpox disease, although some medications are in laboratory trials; currently, the only prevention is vaccination.

The first phase of smallpox is an incubation period of 7 to 17 days after exposure to the virus. The person is not contagious and does not feel ill. The first manifestations of smallpox include fever, headache, muscle pain, and malaise (weakness, tiredness) over a 2- to 4-day time frame. A person with smallpox becomes most contagious with the onset of rash on the tongue and mouth. As the lesions open, the virus enters the mouth and airway, and the person is highly contagious. The rash spreads throughout the body over the next 2 to 3 days. The pox areas become pustular,

eventually form a crust, and then a scab. A person is contagious until the last smallpox scab falls off.

It is important to distinguish smallpox from other diseases that have skin eruptions, such as chickenpox. People with smallpox report a fever 1 to 4 days before the skin eruptions, all skin eruptions are at the small stage of development, and the skin lesions are deep-seated, round, and pustular that may be draining purulent, thick fluid. The person may recall that the first lesions were in the mouth and that they evolved over 2 to 3 days. Suspicious cases should be isolated and reported to the Centers for Disease Control and Prevention (CDC).

There is a detailed nationwide smallpox preparedness program to protect Americans against smallpox used as a biologic weapon. This program includes the creation of preparedness teams that are ready to respond to a smallpox attack on the United States. Members of these teams—health care and public health workers—are being vaccinated so that they might safely protect others in the event of a smallpox outbreak.

Data from Henderson, D.A. (1999). Smallpox as a biological weapon: Medical and public health management. *Journal of the American Medical Association, 281,* 2127-2137.

the client's temperature and administer prescribed antipyretic medication. Prevent cross-contamination by teaching the client proper hand-washing technique and careful handling of soiled linen, clothing, and dressings. Standard precautions should be used as appropriate. Close follow-up evaluation is necessary.

HERPES ZOSTER (SHINGLES)

Herpes zoster, or shingles, is an infection caused by the reactivation of the varicella zoster virus in clients who

have had chickenpox. Although zoster is much less communicable than varicella, people who have not had chickenpox are at risk after exposure to a person with herpes zoster. An increased incidence of herpes zoster is seen in clients with lymphoma, leukemia, or acquired immunodeficiency syndrome, probably because of their decreased immunologic response. Diagnostic tests may not be necessary because of the specific characteristics of herpes zoster; however, a Tzanck test demonstrates multinucleated giant cells (see Chapter 48), and a viral culture is also helpful.

■ **FIGURE 49–9** Cellulitis in a client with long-standing diabetes and stasis dermatitis.

The primary lesion of zoster is a vesicle. The classic presentation is grouped vesicles on an erythematous base along a dermatome. The vesicles appear 1 to 2 days after onset of pain and itching at the site. Occasionally, only papules appear and not vesicles. Because they follow nerve pathways, the lesions do not cross the body's midline; however, rarely, the nerves of both sides may be involved. Herpes zoster lesions evolve into ulcers on the superficial mucous membrane.

The eruption generally clears in about 2 weeks, unless the period between the pain and the eruption is longer than 2 days. In such cases, a prolonged convalescence may be expected. Residual pain, called *postherpetic neuralgia,* and itching are the major complications with herpes zoster. The pain may be constant or intermittent and may range from light burning to a deep visceral sensation. The duration of the pain can be weeks or months to years. In older clients, the pain generally lasts months to years. Another potential complication is loss of sight when herpes zoster involves the facial or acoustic nerve. Involvement of the ophthalmic branch of the facial nerve requires close medical attention to avoid ocular damage.

OUTCOME MANAGEMENT

The primary goals of therapy are to limit extent, duration, and severity of pain and rash in the primary dermatome, prevent spread of the disease, and prevent postherpetic neuralgia. Treatment for herpes zoster is administration of antiviral medications. Antivirals, when started early in the course of the disease, reduce acute pain and accelerate healing of the lesions. Studies suggest that early oral antiviral therapy may assist in reducing postherpetic neuralgia. Analgesics and sedatives are prescribed for pain reduction.

Topical therapy is primarily symptomatic: applications of cool compresses; use of cooling antipruritic preparations, cornstarch, or baking soda; and measures to prevent secondary infection. If pain is present, the client's normal pain tolerance and current pain level must be assessed. Systemic analgesics are usually required, and occasionally opioids; however, in chronic pain, use of these agents raises the possibility of addiction. Assess the effectiveness and side effects of prescribed analgesics. Because postherpetic neuralgia can last a long time, the client and significant others need continued intervention and support. Chronic pain management may include the use of tricyclic antidepressants, phenothiazines, and other local physical modalities such as electrical stimulating units.

PLASTIC SURGERY AND OTHER COSMETIC/ RESTORATIVE PROCEDURES

Plastic surgery is the surgical subspecialty that concentrates on the restoration of function and form to body structures damaged by trauma, transformed by the aging process, changed by disease processes (such as skin cancer), or malformed as a result of congenital defects. Plastic surgery can be divided into two major areas: (1) aesthetic (cosmetic) and (2) reconstructive.

Aesthetic plastic surgery improves physical features that are already within "normal" range. It is performed for changes that result from aging, to alter inherited features, or because of a client's personal desire. Because aesthetic surgery is considered "cosmetic," it is not covered by insurance; clients pay out of pocket. Most clients are enthusiastic and happy because the surgery is a culmination of a personal desire that they may have held for a long time. In contrast, other clients may or may not have social support for their decision. The client may feel vain, embarrassed, or guilty about taking health care away from "people who really need it." Become sensitive to these feelings in the client, and be comfortable with a person's normal desires to feel good about the way he or she looks.

Reconstructive surgery attempts to restore a more normal appearance or function in a person who has an abnormal body part or in whom a body part is missing. The abnormality may be a result of injury or disease, it may be congenital, or it may be the cause of other medical problems. People undergoing reconstructive surgery are typically motivated to try to gain increased function of body parts and to improve their appearance. Although they may hope that plastic surgery will make them "normal," they usually know this may be unrealistic. Such clients are often struggling with diverse emotions: hope for a future without disease recurrence, eagerness to see final surgical results, anxiety over the surgery itself and impending postoperative pain, and weariness of the illness. The client having reconstructive surgery does have the advantage of social approval. Inasmuch as such a client is seen as a victim, society, as represented by either individuals or institutions, often provides treatment or makes appeals for payment of the operations.

Because of the significant impact of plastic surgery procedures on body image and self-esteem, psychological care is imperative. Plastic surgery not only is an operation on the skin but also reaches into the psyche of the person undergoing the surgery.

Minimal postoperative scarring is the hallmark of successful plastic surgery. It is important to understand that no surgery can be done without creating a scar. Plastic surgery is conducted to minimize scars, so at times it seems that surgery can be done without scars. The quality of scarring is affected by many variables, such as the client's age, general health, skin type, and healing ability. Surgical technique and the quality of wound care also affect the healing process.

Blacks, people of Mediterranean origin, and other people with dark skin tend to have more noticeable scars. Wounds located in areas in which the tissue moves as it heals (e.g., over joints) are also more susceptible to scarring. The skin of malnourished clients heals slowly, and those wounds may also develop more obvious scars.

BODY IMAGE AND SURGERY

The desire to be attractive or beautiful is present in people of all cultures, but the perception of what is attractive varies. The importance of physical appearance varies from person to person; however, it is an integral part of the sense of self. The desire to want to physically resemble one's peers reasonably closely—for instance, to have acceptably "normal" facial features—is a normal desire. A significant portion of any deformity rests in the client's perception of the abnormality. Perceptions develop in part from body image. Body image describes a person's perception of his or her body—how the person *thinks* he or she looks, rather than an objective assessment of the person's characteristics. Body image is a factor in determining self-image, self-concept, and self-esteem. People with a positive body image display more confidence and interact more easily with others. Body image changes continually, depending on individual expectations and feedback from others.

A person with a physical deformity, real or perceived, can have a severely damaged body image. Even the usual processes of aging can be detrimental to body image. A self-perception of "getting old" can impair self-confidence, affect behavior, and interfere with interactions in society. Body image is an important factor in the nursing assessment of the client having plastic surgery.

The client's ability to cope with a temporary or permanent or a perceived or actual disfigurement is also assessed. Assess the client's coping mechanisms. Some coping mechanisms may be effective; others may be ineffective. Men may have more difficulty expressing their feelings about their appearance than that typically noted in women. Listen to the client, be alert for positive and negative self-statements, and note the degree of anxiety and fear. Evaluate the client's willingness or unwillingness to touch or look at involved body areas and the client's comfort with being near other people.

Techniques for working with clients who have alterations in body image are presented in Box 49-4.

FACIAL REJUVENATING PROCEDURES

In childhood, skin is very elastic and is fully supported by adipose tissue ("baby fat"). During aging, the skin loses elasticity and the subcutaneous fat diminishes and changes character. Skinfolds and wrinkles become increasingly noticeable. Tissue around the eyes and jaw line sags, producing a drooping, tired, weary, or worried expression. The rate of skin change varies among people. Weight loss, habitual sun exposure, genetic tendencies, and alcohol and tobacco use affect the speed and character of the changes.

Facial Resurfacing
Skin Peels
Various products (alpha-hydroxy acid, glycolic acid, trichloroacetic acid) can be used to lift superficial layers of skin and remove fine wrinkles from the skin. These products are usually applied in an office setting with the client awake. The best candidates are those clients with fair skin and fine wrinkles. Trained nurses perform the peel procedure. Most skin peel procedures require a regimen of skin care before treatment. Care after the peel includes application of skin moisturizers, use of hydrocortisone to reduce edema and erythema, gentle cleansing, and use of sunscreen. The client often resumes the pre-peel skin regimen after the peel. Hyperpigmentation is the most common complication.

Laser Resurfacing
Laser treatment creates a shallow burn injury to the skin. Dormant herpes can be reactivated; therefore antiviral agents are used before treatments. Clients are sedated, or topical anesthetics such as eutectic mixture of local anesthetic (EMLA) are used. Postoperative edema can be reduced somewhat with ice packs and oral corticosteroids for 48 hours. Some clients also experience a burning sensation for 12 to 18 hours after treatment. The skin reepithelializes in about 5 to 10 days, depending on the depth of the injury. Sun-blocking agents are a must, in that hyperpigmentation can develop.

BOX 49-4 Supporting the Client Who Has a Changed Body Image

Many clients undergoing plastic surgery experience some form of body image alteration. Clients may experience body image changes before surgery because of disease or injury. They may also have problems after surgery from edema, bruising, or less than desired results. Try to anticipate these problems and work with the client as soon as possible to facilitate needed adjustments. You may want to work with the nursing diagnosis of *Risk for Disturbed Body Image* or *Situational Low Self-Esteem related to perceived or actual disfigurement and changes in self-concept*. The expected outcome must be tailored to the client but may include improved self-image with incorporation of the changed body part into the body image, as evidenced by effective coping and appropriate use of defense mechanisms; verbalizing feelings comfortably and appropriately; expressing satisfaction with the changed body image; having the ability to openly verbalize feelings; making positive statements about self; having a normal level of anxiety and normal fears; comfortably looking at self in mirror and/or touching the deformed body area, healed surgical site, or other scars; being able to be with others comfortably; and having no indications of depression.

Some interventions that you may find effective with clients who are experiencing body image disturbances include the following:

■ Continue to assess apparent self-concept, coping methods, defense mechanisms, degree of anxiety, and fears frequently.

■ Assist the client to explore and express feelings; do not use phrases such as "I know how you feel." These empty phrases create barriers to communication, whereas

statements such as "you are angry" or "you seem depressed," for example, identify the feeling.

■ Be sensitive to and acknowledge the client's feelings and needs.

■ Present reality; building false hope is detrimental (reality need not be brutal, however).

■ Healing is unpredictable; refer questions about healing to the surgeon.

■ Do not force the client to view or touch himself or herself; gently assist the client to look at and touch the deformity or healed surgical site (help incorporate it into the client's self-concept and body image).

■ Encourage the client to begin meeting in public to begin desensitization to the reactions of others, such as by taking walks in halls; desensitization begins in safe environments and proceeds to new situations; prepare the client for stares and remarks.

■ Discuss others' reaction to the client; support grief reactions.

■ If the client has a facial deformity, prepare visitors and family members before they see the client.

■ Look for vocal expressions or hand gestures in cases of facial disfigurement; facial expression may be limited in clients with extensive facial scars or skin grafts.

■ Refer the client and family to local support groups, such as About Face.

■ Assist the client with techniques to camouflage scars; licensed aestheticians can assist with make-up choices and techniques.

Dermabrasion

Dermabrasion is a process of sanding the surface layers of skin on cheeks and forehead with an electric rotating brush to smooth out pitting and surface blemishes. This operation is the preferred treatment for depressed acne scars and other deep scars. Local anesthesia with sedation is used. The abraded surfaces are covered with antibiotic ointment and gauze. After removal of the gauze, the facial skin weeps serous fluid for 5 to 7 days. Once the weeping stops and new skin has appeared, the client can apply make-up to camouflage the redness. The redness fades over the following 6 weeks.

Dermal Fillers

Soft tissue augmentation has become a popular means of addressing contour defects that result from aging, photodamage, trauma or scarification, or disease. Several products can be used (e.g., autologous fat, collagen, hyaluronic acid, Hylaform, Restylane to fill in small wrinkles or depressed blemishes in the skin. The client's reaction to collagen is tested before treatment, because some people experience induration (hard, raised area) and swelling at the injection site. Clients with autoimmune disorders

are not candidates for collagen injection. Restylane can also be used to fill medium to deep creases and folds.

Botulinum Injections

Botulinum toxin type A (Botox) can be injected to temporarily improve the appearance of moderate to severe frown lines between the eyebrows (glabellar lines). Botox is a protein produced by the bacterium *Clostridium botulinum*. Small doses of the toxin are injected into the affected muscles and block the release of the chemical acetylcholine that would otherwise signal the muscle to contract. The toxin thus paralyzes or weakens the injected muscle for up to 120 days. Following injection, some clients report headache, respiratory tract infection, flu syndrome, blepharoptosis (droopy eyelids), and nausea. Less frequent adverse reactions include pain in the face, redness at the injection site, and muscle weakness.

Rhytidectomy (Face Lift)

A rhytidectomy (*face lift*) may restore a more youthful appearance to the face (perhaps from 5 to 10 years younger) by removing wrinkled skin from the forehead and around the eyes and mouth (Figure 49-10).

■ FIGURE 49–10 Face lift (rhytidectomy) and blepharoplasty. Face lifts enable removal of large wrinkles and folds of skin from the face and neck. **A,** Area in pink shows amount of tissue that is undermined (lifted from the fascial connection) and moved during a face lift. For the face lift, the incision lines go around the ear and into the hair-bearing scalp; other incisions may also be used. Note also the incision line beneath the eyelid for the blepharoplasty, which enables removal of excess eyelid tissue. **B,** The postoperative near-final result, with tightened facial skin and neck folds.

A Before face lift and blepharoplasty

B After face lift and blepharoplasty

Rhytidectomy is usually performed on an outpatient basis with the client under general anesthesia, or using local anesthesia with IV sedation. Incisions are made from the temple along the ear and out into the hair-bearing scalp behind the ear. Through the incisions, excess facial skin is undermined and pulled back toward the ear. *Undermining* is a surgical technique in which the skin is separated from underlying structures.

Postoperatively, the client is placed in the Fowler position to reduce the risk of edema. Cold compresses can also be used to reduce swelling and bleeding. Suction drains are used to eliminate dead space and remove wound drainage. Drains are removed in 24 to 48 hours, when drainage has subsided. Facial movement (talking and chewing) should be limited. Increases in blood pressure should be avoided by keeping the head elevated; any prescribed antihypertensive medications should also be resumed. Coughing also increases blood pressure and should be avoided (by not operating on clients with colds) or treated if it manifests after surgery.

Complications include hematomas, which can cause tissue necrosis and must be surgically removed. Hematoma formation occurs most often in people who smoke or have pre-existing hypertension. Postoperative nausea and vomiting can also increase bleeding and hematoma formation. Hematoma development is first noted as increasing facial asymmetry associated with pain or tightness on one side of the face. Increasing drainage and changes in facial sensation should also be reported.

Blepharoplasty

Blepharoplasty is the surgical removal of excess skin and periorbital fat from the upper or lower eyelid.

Blepharoplasty is usually performed on an outpatient basis. General or local anesthesia with sedation can be used. Wide elliptical incisions are made on the upper eyelids. The excised wedge of excess tissue is lifted off, and herniated fat is removed. A lower-lid blepharoplasty incision is placed ⅛ inch below the edge of the eyelid.

Assess preoperative near and distant vision in each eye by asking the client to read from a book and from something in the distance while one eye is covered. These baseline data are crucial to assess postoperative visual changes. An ophthalmologic examination is indicated before surgery if vision problems are noted.

After blepharoplasty, the head is elevated to reduce edema. Iced normal saline compresses or patches are applied to the eyes as prescribed. Activity is limited for 1 week to reduce blood pressure elevations that often lead to increased edema and ecchymosis (bruising). Normally, severe pain is not experienced after blepharoplasty. An itching sensation, similar to that associated with dry eyes, is usually experienced as a result of slight corneal swelling. This can be prevented with cold wet dressings.

Rhinoplasty

Rhinoplasty is the surgical correction of nasal deformities. This procedure is frequently performed as an outpatient procedure using either local anesthesia and sedation or general anesthesia. Incisions are made inside the nose to reshape the dorsum, ala, or internal cartilage. After surgery, the inside of the nose may be packed and an external splint applied.

Preoperative nursing care focuses on teaching the client to breathe through the mouth after surgery and to not touch the nose. Postoperatively, assess for bleeding.

While the client is sleepy from the anesthesia, excessive swallowing may be the only manifestation of bleeding. Examine the back of the throat with a flashlight to look for blood. Some bleeding is normal down the back of the throat and on the nasal packs and dressings. The nurse promptly reports excessive bleeding to the surgeon. The head of the bed is kept elevated to control postoperative edema. Nasal packing can be very uncomfortable. Pain management is important and can usually be achieved with oral analgesics (e.g., codeine, acetaminophen). Aspirin is avoided for 1 week before and 3 weeks after surgery. (See the Client Education Guide feature on Postoperative Care After Rhinoplasty on the evolve website.)

BODY-CONTOURING SURGERY (LIPECTOMY)

Body-contouring surgical procedures (lipectomy) remove excess fatty tissue, skinfolds, or subcutaneous fat from various body parts, including the abdomen, thighs, arms, and buttocks.

Liposuction

Liposuction is a technique used (1) to aspirate fatty tissue from areas of the body resistant to diet and exercise (lipodystrophy), (2) to contour flaps, and (3) to remove lipomas (benign fatty tumors). A blunt, hollow cannula is inserted through very small incisions and then attached to a powerful suction machine that vacuums out adipose tissue. After surgery, compression garments are used to prevent fluid collection (hematoma and seroma), to maintain the desired body contour, and to promote healing. Tumescent technique involves the additional use of large volumes of dilute lidocaine and epinephrine. These medications promote vasoconstriction to minimize bleeding and provide postoperative analgesia. Ultrasonic lipectomy is the use of ultrasound to ease the removal of fat.

Complications of liposuction include hematoma, skin necrosis, infection, and undesirable scars or skin dimpling. If large volumes of fat are removed, hypovolemia may develop. Pulmonary embolism has also been reported.

After liposuction, assess the client for hypovolemia and electrolyte imbalance (manifested by syncope, dizziness, and abnormal blood values). If drains are used, monitor the quantity and quality of drainage. Ice and oral analgesics are effective in managing postoperative pain. Dressings usually remain in place for at least 24 hours. Nurses must ensure that dressings remain smooth and uniform; otherwise, contour irregularities can result. Sometimes the client wears a compression garment for several weeks postoperatively.

Clients may gradually resume normal activity except for strenuous exercise. It may be 4 to 6 weeks before the client works up to the preoperative level of exercise.

Resuming activity too rapidly may result in soreness and swelling. Bruising is common after liposuction and may take weeks to disappear completely.

Many clients expect the results of liposuction to be immediate. Usually up to 6 months is required for final results to be apparent after edema subsides and subcutaneous tissue heals. Reinforce that results may not be apparent for 6 months following surgery. This period of time is required for complete resolution of edema and reconnection of soft tissues.

Abdominoplasty

Abdominoplasty is the removal of excess abdominal skin and fat and the repair and tightening of separated abdominal muscles. An incision is made across the lower abdomen, and tissue is undermined to the costal margin. The excess skin and fatty tissue are excised and recontoured. The umbilical stalk is detached and reattached once the overlying skin is in its proper position.

After surgery, inspect the incision line for manifestations of pallor or lack of capillary refill. The operative site can swell, with resulting impairment of capillary blood supply. Smoking is prohibited, because nicotine further restricts blood flow to the skin. Tension on the suture line must be minimized; therefore the client must lie in semi-Fowler position with the knees flexed (a contouring position). The client also needs to walk in a "hunched-over" position until the swelling decreases and abdominal skin relaxes. Teach the client postoperative pain management techniques. Abdominoplasty is an abdominal operation and produces significant postoperative discomfort. Adequate analgesia and other pain-relieving measures are essential. As suggested in the Management and Delegation feature below, reinforce to unlicensed personnel that these plastic surgery clients require usual postoperative care.

MANAGEMENT AND DELEGATION

Care of Clients Recovering from Plastic Surgery

When unlicensed assistive personnel are caring for clients after plastic surgery, reinforce the need for adequate pain management and routine postoperative care. It is not uncommon for these clients to feel uncomfortable about asking for pain medications and for nursing assistance. Some people have the notion that surgery "for vanity" should hurt a little. This is a dangerous philosophy and should not be condoned. Any incision hurts, and these clients do not differ in their need for pain control. Likewise, measuring routine vital signs, providing pulmonary care, monitoring intake and output, and encouraging ambulation are routine aspects of postoperative nursing care. Withholding care is not acceptable.

Panniculectomy

In people who have experienced major weight loss, excess loose skin and subcutaneous tissue may remain over the abdomen, thighs, and arms, hanging in large folds. The folds of tissue are called *pannus,* and panniculectomy is the surgical removal of these tissue folds. As much as 10 pounds of redundant tissue has been surgically removed during one of these operations. Clearly, this operation is not for the cure of the client's obesity, but it can offer some positive gains in self-esteem and reduction in health-related problems.

Postoperative care is usually focused on reducing stress on the long suture lines. For example, place the client in the Fowler position after abdominal panniculectomy. Monitor the suture lines closely for manifestations of nonhealing. Fatty tissue is poorly perfused, and the client may have pre-existing diet-induced malnutrition. During the healing phase, the client needs to consume adequate amounts of protein and carbohydrate to heal. Other tissue folds must be treated for intertriginous dermatitis (see earlier discussion on intertrigo).

RECONSTRUCTIVE PLASTIC SURGERY

One of the greatest challenges in plastic surgery is the reconstruction of deformities. Skin grafting is discussed in Chapter 50. This section discusses flap surgery.

Flaps are areas of tissue raised from one area of the body without being completely detached, so that the blood supply is intact; the flap is transferred (e.g., by rotation) to adjacent areas. Flaps of tissue can also be transferred to distant areas, where a blood supply is reestablished; these are called *free flaps* and are discussed later. Local flaps are rotated or advanced to reconstruct an adjacent defect (Figure 49-11).

Preservation of the nutrient blood vessels is paramount to flap survival. The tissue attachment containing these vessels is sometimes called the *pedicle,* because in the past flaps were moved from site to site with a visible portion of tissue that "carried" the flap to the recipient site. This style of flap can be seen in the deltopectoral flaps used to repair neck resection tissue loss. Flaps are also used to cover extensive wounds from pressure ulcers and long-standing defects from osteomyelitis.

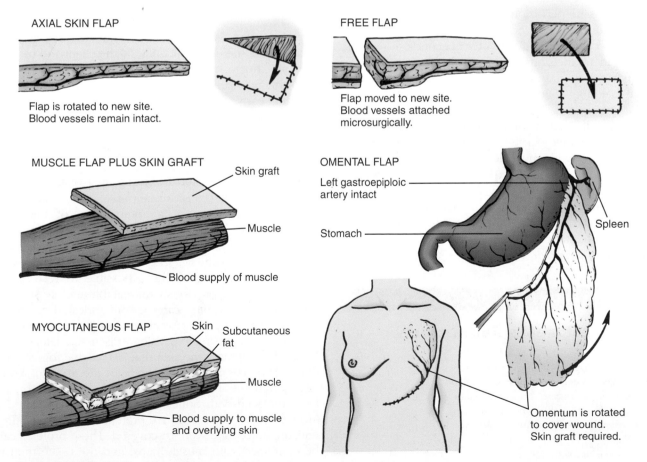

AXIAL SKIN FLAP

Flap is rotated to new site.
Blood vessels remain intact.

FREE FLAP

Flap moved to new site.
Blood vessels attached microsurgically.

MUSCLE FLAP PLUS SKIN GRAFT
Skin graft
Muscle
Blood supply of muscle

MYOCUTANEOUS FLAP
Skin
Subcutaneous fat
Muscle
Blood supply to muscle and overlying skin

OMENTAL FLAP
Left gastroepiploic artery intact
Stomach
Spleen
Omentum is rotated to cover wound. Skin graft required.

■ **FIGURE 49-11** Common flaps.

Skin Flaps

Skin flaps are sections of skin rotated from their origin to cover a defect. Common uses of skin flaps are to reconstruct a neck after excision of cancer (deltopectoral flap) or the face (rotation flap). Occasionally skin flaps are used to close pressure ulcers on the pelvis. Blood flow to the flap must be protected. Avoid securing dressings or tracheotomy ties across the flap.

Musculocutaneous Flaps

Flaps comprising both muscle and skin are called *musculocutaneous flaps*. They are commonly used to fill in defects where muscle is missing or where muscle can provide ample blood flow to heal osteomyelitis. These flaps are named by the muscle of origin. For example, large trochanteric pressure ulcers can be repaired with tensor fasciae latae flaps, named for the tensor fasciae latae muscle of the lateral thigh. Intrathoracic muscle flaps used for chest wall reconstruction include serratus anterior, latissimus dorsi, and pectoralis muscles.

Nursing care centers on maintaining perfusion and reducing tissue injury to the flap. You may choose to design your nursing care under the nursing diagnosis of *Risk for Ineffective Tissue Perfusion related to tissue transfer*.

The outcome is that the client will maintain effective peripheral tissue perfusion, as evidenced by usual color of skin, no pallor or cyanosis, warm and dry skin, blanching (capillary refill) in 3 to 5 seconds, no edema or blebs, intact incisions, and controllable pain.

The flap is monitored for color, capillary refill, and dermal bleeding. Look for pallor, coolness, decreased capillary refill, or dark dermal blood on lancing (lancing may not be allowed in some settings). The Critical Monitoring feature below lists findings to report immediately in clients with musculocutaneous reconstruction. It takes a fair amount of experience in clinical assessment of flaps to predict early flap demise using these subjective methods. Findings can vary because of oxygen content of the blood, capillary dilation, blood flow, and skin pigmentation. Therefore in complex flaps, temperature and Doppler monitors are used to monitor

---

CRITICAL MONITORING

Musculocutaneous Reconstruction

Report the following findings immediately:
- Development of coolness in the flap
- Development of duskiness or pallor in the flap
- Slowing of capillary refill in the flap
- Loss of pulses (palpable or detected by Doppler) in the flap
- Increasing pain in the flap

---

circulation. The extremity is usually elevated to improve venous return as long as elevation does not interfere with arterial flow.

Protecting the blood supply to a flap is a primary nursing responsibility. Nursing interventions are designed to avoid factors that can jeopardize blood flow. Position the client so that the flap is relaxed and elevated. Gravity promotes edema and venous congestion, both of which impede blood flow. Interventions to increase venous return include elevating the involved body part and applying elastic stockings or wraps as prescribed. Tension on the flap can stretch or kink the feeding blood vessels, reducing the flow of blood to the tissues. A blood clot can restrict blood flow. The first manifestation of compromised blood flow is pallor.

Know the location of the pedicle that carries blood vessels to the flap. Most of the time the pedicle is buried, and little can be done to harm it. Some exceptions exist, though. When skin flaps are used, such as the deltopectoral flap, the pedicle is visible. Tracheostomy ties should not be tied tightly around the flap; otherwise, circulation to the distal portions will be compromised. When the breast is reconstructed after mastectomy with a latissimus dorsi flap, the pedicle is located in the ipsilateral axilla. The client cannot lie on the ipsilateral side or blood flow to the flap will be impaired.

Hydrate the client well, if prescribed, to help perfuse the flap. Maintain any postoperative splints to prevent tension on vessels. Limit the use of caffeine by the client and prohibit the use of nicotine by the client and by visitors once home.

Problems resulting from impaired arterial supply are apparent early after surgery. Altered perfusion caused by venous obstruction may not be evident for a few hours.

Free Flaps

Free flaps are harvested from one area of the body to reconstruct a defect in a distant area. The donor tissue (skin, muscle, bone, or a combination of these) is detached from its blood supply at the donor site and reattached by microvascular anastomosis to arteries and veins at the recipient site. The development of microvascular techniques has made it possible to reconstruct defects that were previously untreatable. Before surgical reconstruction, a flap can be prefabricated to build exactly what is needed for repair. Supplemental techniques, such as tissue expansion (discussed later), may be used to augment the skin that is available for closure. Other advances have been made in the areas of bone and soft tissue reconstruction. Bone has traditionally been replaced with bone grafts or alloplastic materials. More recently, osteoinductive proteins capable of differentiating into bone were discovered. These proteins can be combined with muscle flaps, and the tissue then is transformed into useful bone.

Preoperative client characteristics to consider include health status and condition of potential donor tissue. Diabetes and cardiovascular, renal, and pulmonary disease do not present absolute contraindications, but these diseases do increase risk of flap failure. The vessels used for a flap must not be in proximity to sites of previous trauma or irradiation. After trauma, widespread changes occur in the walls and perivascular tissues of the major vascular bundles. These changes have been labeled as *post-traumatic vessel disease* (PTVD). Vessels with PTVD are more difficult to dissect, are easily damaged, and have little resistance against clots. Donor sites are chosen according to guidelines presented previously. The donor site pedicle is deliberately planned so that the flap can comfortably reach the recipient site.

Free Flap Failure

When all goes well, the advantages of free flaps are obvious. Nevertheless, the phantom called *free flap failure* looms large, limiting use of the procedure. Thrombosis is the most common cause of failure. After surgery, the free flap site is seldom dressed, so that clinical assessments can be performed. Several techniques have been developed in large clinical trials, but no consensus exists as to which is the best technique. The ideal monitoring system would provide a continuous recording of flap perfusion or flap metabolism. It should monitor both visible and buried tissues. Finally, the data should be easily interpreted by nursing personnel and junior medical staff.

Assess for trends in color, texture, and temperature of the flap, as well as Doppler pulses and drainage from wound drains. Other postoperative care includes maintaining adequate hydration, keeping the client warm, managing pain, and allowing only appropriate activities. Clients may express some concern with the decision to salvage a body part or may fear that the flap will fail

and amputation will be required. The nurse needs to be supportive of the decision for surgery and allow time for expression of fears.

SKIN EXPANSION

Skin expansion is a technique used to increase the amount of local tissue available to reconstruct a defect. An inflatable silicone balloon is placed under the skin or muscle flap adjacent to a defect. The expander is inflated sequentially over several weeks or months to stretch the overlying tissue. When tissue is sufficient to resurface the adjacent defect, the balloon is removed and the flap is contoured (shaped) and advanced to cover the defect.

REPAIR OF TRAUMATIC INJURIES

Facial Fractures

Fractures can occur in the individual bones of the face: the nasal bones, orbit, malar prominence, mandible, or maxilla (Figure 49-12). The client with facial fractures has often been involved in an automobile accident or an assault or has suffered a sports injury. Pain, improper bite (malocclusion), swelling, bruising, diplopia (double vision), facial asymmetry, enophthalmos (sunken eye), and exophthalmos (bulging eye) are clinical manifestations of facial fractures. Diagnostic assessment includes x-ray studies.

Life-threatening problems (e.g., airway obstruction, hemorrhage, or cervical spine injury) that may accompany facial trauma must be managed immediately. Because of the proximity of the injury to the airway, assess airway patency and breath sounds every 2 hours (more often if bleeding is present). Place suction equipment at the bedside. Teach the client to breathe through the nose. Trying to open the mouth may dislocate the fracture.

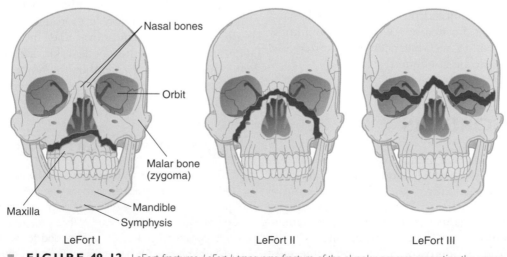

■ **FIGURE 49–12** LeFort fractures. *LeFort I:* transverse fracture of the alveolar process separating the upper dental arch from the maxilla; *LeFort II:* fracture of the mid face, maxilla, and orbits; *LeFort III:* fracture of the orbit that creates craniofacial dissociation.

Repair of facial fractures can be delayed for up to 3 weeks and still achieve good results. Like all fractures, facial fractures must be reduced, stabilized, and immobilized to ensure proper healing. Methods vary according to the location of the fractures.

When the client has intermaxillary wiring, wire cutters should be in the client's possession at all times. If airway problems develop that cannot be managed with suction, the wires that secure the upper and lower jaws should be cut. The nurse and the client need to be informed about which wires should be cut. These are the only wires that attach the top and bottom teeth. Do not try to cut off the bands attached to the teeth.

A liquefied diet is used until the wires are removed. Without adequate nutrition, clients can lose 10 to 20 pounds during convalescence. Instruct the client how to "blenderize" food and to maintain an adequate balance of carbohydrates, fat, protein, and calories. Milkshakes can be made with a wide variety of foods. High-calorie food supplements can augment the regular diet, and liquid multivitamins may be useful. Alcoholic and carbonated beverages can cause nausea and can fizz and foam in the back of the throat, leading to airway problems; they are to be avoided.

Oral hygiene aids in healing of oral wounds, prevents infection and destruction of teeth and gums, increases comfort, and enhances self-esteem. Rinsing the mouth with water or a mouthwash followed by use of an oral irrigation device on low pressure removes particles from the front of the mouth while the tissues are still tender. Once the initial swelling and tenderness subside, the teeth must be brushed and the mouth rinsed after every meal and at bedtime. Pieces of dental wax can be placed on the open ends of the wires if they irritate buccal surfaces.

Before discharge, the client and family members need to be taught about the wires, diet, and oral care. Once the incisions have healed, the client can resume normal activities. However, as noted previously, while the jaws are wired, the client must carry a wire cutter and know which wires to cut. A well-balanced blenderized diet and oral care should be continued.

NAIL DISORDERS

Disorders of the nail can indicate any of several dermatologic processes. Potential causes include an infection of the nail (e.g., paronychia), a fungal infection of the nail (e.g., onychomycosis), a dermatologic disease with prominent nail changes (e.g., psoriasis), or pigmentary abnormalities of the nail (as in melanoma).

Unguis incarnatus (ingrown nail) is one of the most common nail conditions and is caused by improper nail trimming and by wearing tight or ill-fitting shoes. It primarily involves the nail of the great toe that acts as a foreign body, leading to inflammation. A painful, warm inflammatory reaction results from excessive lateral growth of the nail into the nailfold. Decrease inflammation with warm soaks for 20 minutes several times a day. If the problem is minor, lifting the lateral portion of the nail by inserting a cotton wick prevents contact with the nailfold. Sometimes, the involved segment of the nailfold needs to be excised.

Paronychia, or infection around the nail, is characterized by red, shiny skin often associated with painful swelling. These infections frequently result from trauma, picking at the nail, or disorders such as dermatitis. Often these sites become secondarily infected with bacteria or fungi, which later involve the nail. As with ingrown toenail, warm soaks three or more times a day may reduce pressure and pain; however, incision and drainage of inflamed sites is frequently required. Samples for appropriate cultures of the purulent material and the nail should be obtained.

Onychomycosis refers to any fungal infection of the nail, whether caused by dermatophytes or candidiasis. Topical or systemic antibiotic or antifungal therapy is prescribed, with emphasis on medication regimen compliance. Unfortunately, even with good compliance, recurrence of fungal infections in nails is frequent.

Clients should understand the importance of reducing trauma and irritation to involved nails by (1) trimming nails straight across to reduce further trauma, (2) avoiding overmanicuring or self-induced trauma, (3) limiting harsh chemical irritants such as abrasive cleansers and drying nail products, and (4) keeping the nails dry.

CONCLUSIONS

Skin disorders range from those that are a mere nuisance (such as dry skin) to life-threatening disorders (such as melanoma). Nurses frequently manage skin disorders independently; therefore a thorough knowledge of the use of topical medications and therapies is crucial. Because much of the needed skin care is provided by the client or a family member, the nurse must use excellent teaching skills to convey the necessary self-care information.

THINKING CRITICALLY

1. You are caring for an older woman who has had a stroke that left her with residual paralysis on the left side. She also has a pressure ulcer on the left trochanter, in part because she lies on her left side all the time. While caring for her on Monday, you convince her to sit in a chair and to lie on her right side. When you care for her again on Thursday, the ulcer is twice as large and deeper. She refuses to turn to the right and says "I like lying on my left side." What can you do to help this client?

Factors to Consider. What pressure-redistribution methods should be instituted? Is there any harm in lying on a pressure ulcer? Why might she be at increased risk because of malnutrition?

2. The client is a 72-year-old Caucasian man who had undergone a wide excisional biopsy on his forearm to rule out squamous cell carcinoma. The next day the client calls the office complaining of pain at the surgery site. What additional questions need to be asked? What potential interventions might be necessary?

Factors to Consider. What clinical manifestations would indicate an infection is present? Is age a factor in wound healing?

3. The client is an otherwise healthy 41-year-old woman who presented to the clinic with a week-long history of intensely itchy, erythematous red lesions under her breasts. The rash appears to be spreading, and the centers of some of the lesions are seen to contain tiny pustules. In addition, the woman complains of a 12-pound weight loss over the past 6 months despite always feeling hungry and thirsty. She denies any medical problems and reports that she does not currently take systemic or topical medications.

Factors to Consider. What is the common cause of intertriginous dermatitis? What diagnostic study can determine the cause of the problem? What endocrine disorder is suggested by the history of skin rash, thirst, and weight loss?

Discussions for these questions can be found on the website.

BIBLIOGRAPHY

Citations appearing in red refer to primary research.

Citations appearing in blue refer to evidence-based practice guidelines and protocols.

1. Aly, R., Bayles, C., & Forney, R. (2001). Treatments for common superficial fungal infections. *Dermatology Nursing, 13*(2), 91-101.
2. American Society of Plastic Surgical Nurses. (2007). *Core curriculum for plastic and reconstructive surgical nurses* (3rd ed.). Pensacola, Fla: Author.
3. Ankrom, M., Bennett, R., Sprigle, S., & the National Pressure Ulcer Advisory Panel. (2005). Pressure-related deep tissue injury under intact skin and the current pressure ulcer staging systems. *Advances in Skin and Wound Care, 18*(1), 35-42.
4. Ayello, E.A., & Franz, R.A. (2003). Pressure ulcer prevention and treatment: Competency-based nursing curricula. *Dermatology Nursing, 15*(1), 44-55.
5. Berger, T.G., James, W.D., & Odom, R.B. (2000). *Andrews' diseases of the skin: Clinical dermatology* (9th ed.). Philadelphia: Saunders.
6. Bergstrom, N., & Braden, B. (1987). The Braden Scale for predicting pressure sore risk. *Nursing Research, 36*(4), 205-210.
7. Bergstrom, N., et al. (1994). *Treatment of pressure ulcers: Clinical practice guideline No. 15* (AHCPR Pub No. 95-0652). Rockville, Md: U.S. Department of Health and Human Services, Public Health Service, Agency for Health Care Policy and Research.
8. Bergstrom, N., et al. (1992). *Pressure ulcers in adults: Prediction and prevention* (AHCPR Pub No. 95-0050). Rockville, Md: U.S. Department of Health and Human Services, Public Health Service, Agency for Health Care Policy and Research.
9. Bielory, L., & Kanuga, M. (2002). Complementary and alternative interventions in atopic dermatitis. In M. Boguniewicz (Ed.), *Immunology and Allergy Clinics of North America: Atopic Dermatitis, 22* (1), 153-173.

10. Black, J., Baharestani, M., Cuddigan, J., et al. (2007). National Pressure Ulcer Advisory Panel's updated pressure ulcer staging system. *Advances in Skin and Wound Care, 20*(5), 269-274.
11. Black, J. (2006). Saving the skin during kinetic bed therapy. *Nursing 2006, 36,* 17.
12. Black, J., & National Pressure Ulcer Advisory Panel. (2005). Moving toward consensus on deep tissue injury and pressure ulcer staging. *Advances in Skin and Wound Care, 18*(8), 415-421.
13. Black, J. (2005). Treating heel pressure ulcers. *Nursing 2005, 35*(1), 68.
14. Black, J. (2004). Preventing heel pressure ulcers. *Nursing 2004, 34* (11), 17.
15. Black, J., & Black, S. (2003). Deep tissue injury. *Wounds: A Compendium of Clinical Research and Practice, 16*(11), 380.
16. Black, J. (2000). Improving outcomes in the elderly after pressure ulcer repair. *Plastic Surgical Nursing, 20*(3), 139-143, 170.
17. Boguniewicz, M., et al. (2003). Evolution in the treatment of atopic dermatitis: New approaches to managing a chronic skin disease. *Dermatology Nursing* (Suppl), *15*(4), 3-19.
18. Boguniewicz, M., & Leung, D.Y.M. (2001). Pathophysiologic mechanisms in atopic dermatitis. *Seminars in Cutaneous Medicine and Surgery, 20*(4), 217-225.
19. Boguniewicz, M., & Nicol, N.H. (2002). Conventional therapy for atopic dermatitis. In M. Boguniewicz (Ed.), *Immunology and allergy clinics of North America, atopic dermatitis* (pp. 107-124). Philadelphia: Saunders.
20. Bratcher, C., & Stover, B. (2001). Varicella-zoster virus: Infection, control, and prevention. *American Journal of Infection Control, 26*(3), 369-381.
21. Callen, J.P. (2000). *Color atlas of dermatology* (2nd ed.). Philadelphia: Saunders.
22. Camisa, C., & Warner, M. (1998). Treatment of pemphigus. *Dermatology Nursing, 10*(2), 115-118, 123-131.
23. Cohen, P.R., Schulze, K.E., Tolz, R., et al. (2006). Allergic contact dermatitis. *Dermatology Nursing, 18*(1), 48-49.
24. Christos, P.J., Oliveria, S.A., Masse, L.C., et al. (2004). Skin cancer prevention and detection by nurses: Attitudes, perceptions and barriers. *Journal of Cancer Education, 19*(1), 50-57.
25. Coolum, N., McInnes, E., Bell-Syer, S.E., et al. (2004). Support surfaces for pressure ulcer prevention. *Cochrane Database of Systematic Reviews* (electronic resource), CD001735.
26. Cullum, N., Deeks, J., Sheldon, T., et al. (2002). Beds, mattresses and cushions for pressure sore prevention and treatment. *The Cochrane Library, 1.*
27. DeLeo, V.A., Elsner, P., & Marks, J.G., Jr. (2002). *Contact & occupational dermatology* (3rd ed.). St. Louis: Mosby.
28. Duvic, M., et al. (2003). Analysis of long-term outcomes of combined modality therapy for cutaneous T-cell lymphoma. *Journal of the American Academy of Dermatology, 51*(1), 35-54.
29. Freedberg, I.M., Eisen, A.Z., & Wolff, K. (2003). *Fitzpatrick's dermatology in general medicine* (6th ed.). New York: McGraw-Hill, Health Professions Division.
30. Gilchrest, B.A. (2002). *Geriatric dermatology part II.* Philadelphia: Saunders.
31. Greaves, M.W., & Leung, D.Y.M. (2000). *Allergic skin disease: A multidisciplinary approach.* New York: Marcel Dekker.
32. Guile, K., & Nicholson, S. (2004). Does knowledge influence melanoma-prone behavior? Awareness, exposure, and sun protection among five social groups. *Oncology Nursing Forum, 31*(3), 641-646.
33. Heddens, C. (2001). Belt lipectomy: Procedure and outcomes. *Plastic Surgical Nursing, 21*(4), 185-189, 199.
34. Hill, M.J. (2003). *Dermatology nursing essentials: A core curriculum—Dermatology Nurses' Association* (2nd ed.). Pitman, NJ: Anthony J. Jannetti.
35. Kanzler, M.H., & Swetter, S.M. (2003). Malignant melanoma. *Journal of the American Academy of Dermatology, 48*(5), 781-783.
36. Leone, G., Rolston, K., & Spaulding, G. (2003). Alefacept for chronic plaque psoriasis: A selective therapy with long-lasting disease remissions and an encouraging safety profile. *Dermatology Nursing, 15*(3), 216-220.
37. Madison, L.K. (2001). Shingles update: Common questions in caring for a patient with shingles. *Dermatology Nursing, 13*(1), 51-55.
38. Memierre, M.F., Allten, S., & Brown, R. (2005). New treatments for melanoma. *Dermatology Nursing, 17*(4), 287-295.

39. Menter, M.A. (Ed.) (2003). Psoriasis for the clinician: A new therapeutics era ("the biologics") beckons. *Journal of the American Academy of Dermatology, 51*(Suppl), 39-142.

40. Naeyaert, J.M., & Brochez, L. (2003). Dysplastic nevi. *New England Journal of Medicine, 349*(23), 2233-2240.

41. Nicol, N.H. (2003). Dermatitis/eczemas. In M.J. Hill (Ed.), *Dermatologic nursing essentials: A core curriculum* (2nd ed., pp. 103-116). Pitman, NJ: Anthony J. Jannetti.

42. Nicol, N.H. (2000). Managing atopic dermatitis in children and adults. *Nurse Practitioner, 25*, 58-79.

43. Nicol, N.H., & Baumeister, L. (1997). Topical corticosteroid therapy: Considerations for prescribing and use. *Lippincott's Primary Care Practice, 1*(1), 62-69.

44. Nicol, N.H., & Boguniewicz, M. (1999). Understanding and treating atopic dermatitis. *Nurse Practitioner Forum, 10*(2), 48-55.

45. Noel, S., & Strohl, R. (2002). The management of high-risk melanoma: Staging, treatment, and nursing issues. *Dermatology Nursing, 14*(6), 363-371.

46. Nunley, J.R. (2000). Cutaneous manifestations of HIV and HCV. *Dermatology Nursing, 12*(3), 163-173.

47. Oliveria, S.A., Dusza, S.W., Phelan, S.L., et al. (2004). Patient adherence to skin self-examination. Effect of nurse intervention with photographs. *American Journal of Preventive Medicine, 26*(2), 152-155.

48. Pinnell, S.R. (2003). Cutaneous photodamage, oxidative stress, and topical antioxidant protection. *Journal of the American Academy of Dermatology, 48*(1), 1-22.

49. Smith, P., Black, J., & Black, S. (1999). Infected pressure ulcers in the long-term care facility. *Infection Control and Hospital Epidemiology, 20*(5), 358-361.

50. Spilsbury, K., Nelson, A., Cullum, N., et al. (2007). Pressure ulcers and their treatment and effects on quality of life: Hospital inpatient perspectives. *Journal of Advanced Nursing, 57*(5), 494-504.

51. Stulberg, D.L., Penrod, M.A., & Blatny, R.A. (2002). Common bacterial skin infections. *American Family Physician, 66*(1), 119-124.

52. Trioa, C. (2002). Promoting positive outcomes in obese patients. *Plastic Surgical Nursing, 22*(1), 10-17, 28.

53. Wheeler, T. (2006). Psychological consequences of malignant melanoma: Patients' experiences and preferences. *Nursing Standard, 21*(10), 42-46.

54. Wound Ostomy and Continence Nurses Society. (2003). *Guideline for prevention and management of pressure ulcers.* Glenview, Ill: Author.

55. Wound Ostomy and Continence Nurses Society. (2003). *Guideline for prevention and management of incontinence.* Glenview, Ill: Author.

evolve *Did you remember to check out the bonus material on the Evolve website and the CD-ROM, including NCLEX®-Examination Style Review Questions, Open-Book Quizzes, and Chapter Review Audio Podcasts?*

http://evolve.elsevier.com/Black/medsurg

CHAPTER 50

Management of Clients with Burn Injury

GRETCHEN J. CARROUGHER AND CHARLES SANDIDGE

Injuries that result from direct contact with or exposure to any thermal, chemical, electrical, or radiation source are termed *burns*. Burn injuries occur when energy from a heat source is transferred to the tissues of the body. The depth of injury is related to the temperature and the duration of exposure or contact.

Burn care has improved in recent decades, resulting in a lower mortality for victims of burn injuries. Dedicated burn centers have been established in which multidisciplinary burn team members work together to care for the burn client and family. Advances in pre-hospital and inpatient care have contributed to survival. However, despite these advances, many people are still injured and die each year from burns. In the United States, it is estimated that 500,000 people are treated every year for a burn injury. Of these, approximately 40,000 will require hospitalization.[2]

Etiology

Burns can be caused from a number of substances or items that come into direct contact with the skin or lungs. To facilitate treatment, burn injuries are categorized according to the mechanism of injury.

Thermal Burns

Thermal burns are caused by exposure to or contact with flame, hot liquids, semiliquids (e.g., steam), semisolids (e.g., tar), or hot objects. Specific examples of thermal burns are those sustained in residential fires, explosive automobile accidents, cooking accidents, or with ignition of poorly stored flammable liquids.

Chemical Burns

Chemical burns are caused by contact with strong acids, alkalis, or organic compounds. The concentration, volume, and type of chemical, as well as the duration of contact, determine the severity of a chemical injury. Chemical burns can result from contact with certain household cleaning agents and various chemicals used in industry, agriculture, and the military. Chemical injuries to the eyes and inhalation of chemical fumes can be very serious.

Electrical Burns

Electrical burn injuries are caused by heat that is generated by the electrical energy as it passes through the body. Electrical injuries can result from contact with exposed or faulty electrical wiring or high-voltage power lines. People struck by lightning also sustain electrical injury.

The extent of injury is influenced by the duration of contact, the intensity of the current (voltage), the type of current (direct or alternating), the pathway of the current, and the resistance of the tissues as the electrical current passes through the body. Contact with electrical current greater than 40 volts (V) is potentially dangerous because of cardiac dysrhythmias; current greater than 1000 V is considered to be high-voltage current and is associated with extensive tissue damage.

Radiation Burns

Radiation burns are the least common type of burn injury and are caused by exposure to a radioactive source. These types of injuries have been associated with nuclear radiation accidents, the use of ionizing radiation in industry, and therapeutic irradiation. Sunburn, from prolonged exposure to ultraviolet rays (solar radiation), is also considered to be a radiation burn.

The amount of radioactive energy received after exposure depends on the distance the person is from the source of the radiation, the strength of the radiation source, the duration of exposure, the extent of body surface area exposed, and the amount of shielding between the source and the person. An acute, localized radiation injury appears similar to a cutaneous thermal injury. The injury is characterized by skin erythema, edema, and pain. In contrast, whole-body radiation exposure manifestations may begin with nausea, vomiting, diarrhea, and fatigue, continuing with a headache and fever within hours of exposure. As time proceeds, hematopoietic and gastrointestinal complications are seen. The severity of manifestations is dose-dependent.

Inhalation Injury

Exposure to asphyxiants (e.g., carbon monoxide) and smoke commonly occurs with flame injuries, particularly if the victim was trapped in an enclosed, smoke-filled space (e.g., in a residential fire). Victims who die at the scene of a fire usually do so as a result of hypoxia and carbon monoxide poisoning. The pulmonary pathophysiologic changes that occur with inhalation injury are multifactorial and relate to the severity and type of smoke or gases inhaled. Exposure to asphyxiants, smoke poisoning, and direct thermal (heat) injury to lung tissue constitute the three facets of an inhalation injury. However, not all of these injury components may be present in the client suffering from an inhalation injury. An inhalation injury increases the risk of mortality 7 times after controlling for the size of the cutaneous burn injury and other clinical and demographic factors.

Risk Factors and Injury Prevention

Adults with burn injuries are more likely to be male and in the 20 to 40 age group. Contact with fire/flame occurs in more than 60% of injuries. Structural fires account for approximately 5% of burn-related hospital admissions; however, they are responsible for the greatest number of burn-related deaths. Approximately 30% of all burn-related deaths are a result of structural fires, seemingly from the associated smoke inhalation. Ignition from cigarettes is the nation's largest single cause of all fire deaths. Alcohol and drug intoxication, which contributes to careless smoking, has been reported as a factor in 40% of residential fire deaths. In approximately 10% of cases of residential fire deaths, the fires were caused by children playing with matches or other ignition sources. Additionally, faulty chimneys, flue vents, fixed heating units, fireplaces, central heating systems, wood-burning stoves, ignition of wood-shingled roofs, as well as human error have all been implicated as causes of residential fires that have resulted in deaths.

Clothing ignition during routine meal preparation has been cited as a leading cause of burn injury, particularly in the older population. Synthetic fabrics are especially dangerous, because they melt and adhere to the skin, causing prolonged contact with heat. Another age group at risk for clothing ignition is the pediatric population. During the early 1970s, the fatality rate among young children burned from ignition of sleepwear was significant. In 1975 it was mandated that children's sleepwear, sizes 0 to 6X, pass a standard flame test. This action significantly lowered mortality associated with children's clothing ignition. The mandate for sleepwear to pass a flame test has since been repealed, and testing is no longer required. Since the repeal, some have reported an increase in clothing-related flame burns occurring in 2- to 11-year-old girls.[19]

Scald burns occur in approximately 10% of adults, but 30% in children. Toddlers (children 2 to 4 years of age) suffer more scald injuries than people in any other age group. Scald injuries are frequently the result of mishaps in the performance of everyday tasks such as bathing and cooking. Overturned coffeepots, cooking pans spilling hot liquid and grease, overheated foods, liquids cooked in microwave ovens, and hot tap water have been identified as specific causes.

Of primary importance in reducing injuries and deaths from residential fires is the presence of a working smoke detector and fire extinguisher. It has been estimated that the risk of dying in a residential fire is reduced 50% when an operating smoke detector is in place.[5] One national burn prevention activity is the "Change Your Clock, Change Your Battery" campaign. This program is designed to remind people in the United States that when they set their clocks back in the fall, they should change the batteries in their smoke detector as well. Prevention efforts have also focused on passing legislation mandating the commercial production and sale of fire-safe cigarettes that are designed with a reduced propensity for ignition. To date, these efforts have been unsuccessful in achieving legislation in all states.

To reduce the incidence of scald injuries, the Consumer Products Safety Commission and Underwriters Laboratory has recommended that the maximum temperature on the thermostats of hot water heaters be lowered and that a warning label identifying the potential for injury be affixed to hot water heaters. Legislation requiring public buildings to lower water temperature to 120° F (48.8° C) has been successful in reducing scald injuries. In addition, a thermostatic control system (anti-scald device) has been developed that, when installed at the faucet or shower head, shuts off the flow of water when the temperature rises above a predetermined temperature, typically 119° F (48.3° C). Box 50-1 summarizes burn injury prevention recommendations.

BOX 50-1 Burn Injury Prevention Recommendations

In the kitchen:

- Turn pot handles toward the back of the stove.
- Purchase a stove with controls on the front or side to reduce the likelihood of clothing ignition as one reaches across hot elements.
- Use a cooking timer with an audible alarm.
- The use of turkey fryers to prepare holiday meals carries a high risk of severe injury and fire—consumers are encouraged to seek out commercial professionals to prepare the turkey or order the turkey from a supermarket or restaurant.

In the home:

- Store all matches and lighters securely so they are inaccessible to children.
- Infants and young children should wear flame-resistant sleepwear and costumes.
- Teach children to STOP, DROP, and ROLL on the ground if their clothing were to catch fire.
- Install smoke detectors on each level of the house and outside all sleeping areas. Test the batteries once a month and change the batteries twice a year.
- Install carbon monoxide detectors on each level of the house.
- Check the temperature on the hot water heater; the recommended setting is 120° F (48.8° C).
- Install water temperature-regulating valves (anti-scald device) that obstruct the flow of water when the water temperature exceeds a preset level.

In the community:

- Attend public fireworks displays conducted by professionals.
- Support fire-safe cigarette legislation in your state.

Pathophysiology

The pathophysiologic changes that occur following a cutaneous burn injury depend on the extent or size of the burn. For smaller burns, the body's response to injury is localized to the burned area. However, with more extensive burns (i.e., involving 25% or more of the total body surface area [TBSA]), the body's response to injury is systemic and proportional to the extent of the injury. The clinical manifestations of an extensive burn injury evolve in dramatic fashion over the post-injury clinical course. Extensive burn injuries affect all major systems of the body. The systemic response to burn injury is typically biphasic, characterized by early hypofunction followed later by hyperfunction of each of the organ systems.

Direct Injury to the Skin

With direct injury to the skin, heat from an external source is conducted to the skin, where it destroys tissue. The amount of damage depends on the length of exposure to the heat and the temperature. At sustained temperatures of 40° to 44° C (104° to 111.2° F), various cellular enzyme systems and cellular systems fail. The sodium-potassium pump fails, which leads to cellular edema. As the temperature rises to 44° C, cell necrosis occurs. In addition, free radicals are produced, which leads to further cellular damage. These destructive processes continue until the heat source is withdrawn and the mechanisms for cooling return the cell temperature to a tolerable range.

Some types of burn create unique patterns of injury. In electrical injuries, heat is generated by electricity as it travels through the body, resulting in internal tissue damage. The concept of the "tip of the iceberg," where the true extent of the injury is not visually apparent, is helpful to understand these injuries. For instance, the cutaneous burn injury may appear negligible in size, but underlying muscle and soft tissue damage may be extensive, particularly with high-voltage electrical injuries. The voltage, type of current (direct or alternating), moisture content at the contact site, composition of the skin at the contact site, and duration of contact are important considerations affecting mortality and morbidity. Once the electrical current enters the body, it seeks to go to ground; en route, it creates heat and may damage vital organs as it passes through them. Alternating current (AC) is more dangerous than direct current (DC). AC produces more heat-related injury and, related to its rapid intermittent flow of electricity, is often associated with cardiopulmonary arrest, ventricular fibrillation, tetanic muscle contractions, and long bone or vertebral compression fractures. The risk of acute renal failure is noteworthy in clients following an electrical injury. Hemoglobin (released from heat-damaged erythrocytes) and myoglobin (the protein that supplies muscles with oxygen) are released in significant quantities into the bloodstream after deep burn injuries involving muscle damage. These substances pass through the glomeruli and are excreted in the urine. However, released in larger than normal quantities as a result of the muscle damage, they may precipitate and obstruct the renal tubules, causing renal damage. This damage can be minimized with the maintenance of a brisk urine output. In addition, victims of electrical injuries may have fallen from the point of electrical contact and sustained associated trauma-related injuries. Cataract formation is also associated with high-voltage electrical injury, especially when contact points are on the head or neck.

In chemical burns, systemic toxic effects may result from cutaneous absorption of the offending agent. Organ failure and even death have resulted from prolonged contact with and absorption of different chemicals.

Fluid Shifts

Immediately following a burn injury, vasoactive substances (catecholamines, histamine, serotonin, leukotrienes, kinins, and prostaglandins) are released from the injured tissues. These substances initiate changes in capillary integrity, allowing plasma to seep into surrounding tissues (Figure 50-1). Direct damage to vessels from heat further increases capillary permeability, which permits sodium ions to enter the cell and potassium ions to exit. The overall effect of these changes is creation of an osmotic gradient, which leads to increases in intercellular and interstitial fluid that further deplete intravascular fluid volumes. These vasoactive substances exert their effects both locally (in the area of injury) and systemically (throughout the body) with extensive injuries. The burn-injured client's hemodynamic balance, metabolism, and immune status are altered.

The body responds initially by shunting blood toward the brain and heart and away from all other body organs. Prolonged lack of blood flow to these other organs is detrimental. The resulting damage depends on the basal needs of the body organ. Some organs can survive for only a few hours without nutrient blood supply. For example, the lack of renal blood flow decreases

Fluid and electrolyte shift during burn shock

Fluid and electrolyte shift after burn shock

■ **FIGURE 50–1** Changes in capillary permeability allow plasma to seep into interstitial spaces. In addition, the sodium pump fails and sodium remains in the cell. There is a corresponding increase in serum potassium concentration.

glomerular filtration rate, leading to oliguria (low urine output). If fluid resuscitation is delayed or inadequate, hypovolemia progresses, and acute renal failure may occur. However, with adequate fluid resuscitation and an increase in cardiac output, renal blood flow returns to normal. After resuscitation, the body begins to reabsorb the edema fluid and eliminate it through diuresis.

Blood flow to the mesenteric bed is also diminished initially, leading to the development of intestinal ileus and gastrointestinal dysfunction in clients with burns greater than 25% TBSA. With the reduction in blood flow to the gastric mucosa, ischemic changes to the upper gastrointestinal tract occur, which slows production of the protective mucous lining, resulting in small, superficial erosions to the stomach and duodenum. If the gastrointestinal tract is left untreated and unprotected by antacids or histamine H_2-receptor antagonists, the erosions can progress to ulcerations—called *Curling's ulcers* in burn-injured clients—and gastrointestinal bleeding.

Pulmonary System

Minute ventilation is often normal or slightly decreased early after an extensive burn injury. Following fluid resuscitation, an increase in minute ventilation—manifested by hyperventilation—may occur, especially if the client is fearful, anxious, or in pain. This hyperventilation is the result of an increase in both respiratory rate and tidal volume and appears to be the result of the hypermetabolism that is seen after burn injury. It typically peaks in the second post-injury week and then gradually returns to normal as the burn wound heals or is closed by grafting.

Pulmonary vascular resistance may increase slightly, and lung compliance may decrease. The changes in lung compliance cause a proportionate increase in the work of breathing. However, these changes are typically small, and in the absence of any pulmonary parenchymal (tissue) damage, they require no specialized treatment.

Inhalation Injury. Exposure to asphyxiants is the most common cause of early mortality from inhalation injury. Carbon monoxide (CO), a common asphyxiant, is produced when organic substances (e.g., wood or coal) burn. It is a colorless, odorless, and tasteless gas that has an affinity for the body's hemoglobin that is 200 times greater than that of oxygen. With inhalation of CO, the oxygen molecules are displaced, and CO binds to hemoglobin to form carboxyhemoglobin (COHb). Tissue hypoxia occurs from an overall decrease in the blood's oxygen-delivering capability.

Direct heat injury to the upper airway results from inhalation of the air heated by fire. The heat immediately produces injury to the airway, which results in edema, erythema, and ulceration. Thermal burns to the lower airways of the pulmonary system are rare because of the protective reflex closure of the glottis and the ability of the respiratory tract to exchange heat effectively. However, thermal burns to the lower airways can occur with the inhalation of steam or explosive gases or with aspiration of scalding liquids, especially in the unconscious victim.

Smoke poisoning results from the inhalation of the by-products of combustion: noxious chemicals (e.g., carbon monoxide, hydrogen cyanide, acrolein, ammonia) and particulate matter. The pulmonary response includes a localized inflammatory reaction, a decrease in bronchial ciliary action, and a decrease in alveolar surfactant. Mucosal edema occurs in the smaller airways. After several hours, sloughing of the tracheobronchial epithelium may occur, and hemorrhagic tracheobronchitis may develop. Adult (acute) respiratory distress syndrome may follow.

Myocardial Depression

Some research investigators have suggested that a myocardial depressant factor exists with more extensive injuries and circulates in the early post-injury period. A significant and immediate depression in cardiac output (CO) occurs, even before circulating plasma volumes decrease, suggesting a neurogenic response to some circulating agent. This depression in CO often continues for several days even after plasma volumes have been restored and urinary output normalizes. More recently, a combination of inflammatory mediators and hormones has been suggested as the cause of myocardial depression occurring after the injury.

Altered Skin Integrity

The burn wound itself exhibits pathophysiologic changes caused by disruption of the skin and alterations to the tissue beneath the surface. The skin, nerve endings, sweat glands, and hair follicles injured by the burn lose normal functioning. Most important, the skin's barrier function is lost. Intact skin normally keeps bacteria from entering the body and body fluids from seeping out, controls evaporation, and maintains body warmth. With destruction of the skin, mechanisms for maintaining normal body temperature can be altered, the risk of infection from invasion of bacteria increases, and evaporative water loss increases. Depending on the depth of the injury, nerve endings either become exposed, resulting in pain and discomfort until wound closure, or are damaged, leaving the innervated area insensate, with potential for permanent impairment of the ability to sense touch, pressure, and pain.

Individuals with severe burn injuries are at risk for developing hypertrophic scarring. This type of scar is best described as reddened, raised (above adjacent uninjured skin), rigid, and uncomfortable. Clients often suffer from pruritus (itch) and increased sensitivity. Hypertrophic scars can result in skin and tissue contractures, especially when the scar crosses over a joint The incidence of hypertrophic scarring varies; however, it is thought that the depth of burn and age and ethnic background of the survivor are key factors in whether or not this type of scar develops.

Immunosuppression

Immune system function is depressed following burn injury. Depression of lymphocyte activity, a decrease in immunoglobulin production, suppression of complement activity, and an alteration in neutrophil and macrophage functioning are evident following extensive burn injuries. In addition, the burn injury disrupts the body's primary barrier to infection—the skin. Together these changes result in an increased risk of infection and life-threatening sepsis.

Psychological Response

Numerous psychological and emotional responses to burn injuries have been identified, ranging from fear to psychosis. A victim's response is influenced by age, personality, cultural and ethnic background, the extent and location of the injury, impact on body image, and pre-injury coping abilities. In addition, separation from family and friends during hospitalization and the change in the client's normal role and responsibilities affect the reaction to burn trauma.[1]

Clinical Manifestations
Degree of Injury

Depending on the skin layers damaged, burn wounds are termed either *partial-thickness* burns or *full-thickness* burns. Burn wounds are also classified as first-, second-, third-, or fourth-degree burns. Partial-thickness burns involve injury to the epidermis and portions of the dermis. *First-degree* partial-thickness burns are superficial and painful and appear red. They heal on their own by epidermal cell regeneration within about 3 to 7 days. Sunburn is a good example of a first-degree partial-thickness burn. *Second-degree* partial-thickness burns appear wet or blistered and are extremely painful. They heal on their own (that is, without skin grafting) as long as they are fairly small and they do not become infected (Figure 50-2).

Third-degree full-thickness burns are characterized by damage through the entire epidermis and dermis (Figure 50-3). A full-thickness burn appears dry and may be mottled and colored black, brown, white, or red. The denatured skin is called *eschar* (pronounced "ES-car"). The burned tissue is most often painless as a result of damage to the nerve endings; however, the surrounding skin may be painful. Upon palpation, individuals with a full-thickness burn may feel pressure. Full-thickness injuries heal by formation of granulation tissue to fill the wound defect and contracture of the epithelium, also known as scarring, to close the wound. Unless the area is very small (the size of a half-dollar or less), the full-thickness burn will not heal adequately and must be skin-grafted to close the wound. *Fourth-degree* full-thickness burns involve skin, subcutaneous (fat) tissue, muscle, and sometimes bone. The skin appears charred or may be completely burned away. Fourth-degree burns require extensive surgical debridement and skin grafting. Amputations are common in these extensive injuries (Figure 50-4). The appearance of the burn relative to the depth of injury is described in Figure 50-5.

Hypothermia

In addition to altered physical appearance, the loss of skin leads to other problems. Hypothermia results from loss of body heat through the burn wound and is characterized by a core body temperature below 98.6° F (37° C). Hypothermia is extremely harmful because it leads to shivering, which in turn increases oxygen consumption and caloric demands as well as vasoconstriction in the periphery. Hypothermia is most common in extensive injuries during the early hours following injury, evacuation, and transport to a burn facility.

Fluid and Electrolyte Imbalance

The evaporative water loss through the burn contributes to the client's diminished fluid volume and compromised hydration status. Evaporative losses not compensated for by fluid replacement are evidenced by a low blood pressure, decreased urine output, dry mucous membranes, and poor skin turgor.

Hyponatremia, hypernatremia, and hyperkalemia are common electrolyte abnormalities that affect the burn-injured client at different points in the recovery process. Extensive burns (greater than 25% TBSA) result in generalized body edema affecting both burned and non-burned tissues and in a decrease in circulating intravascular blood volume. Hematocrit levels are elevated in the first 24 hours after injury, demonstrating hemoconcentration from the loss of intravascular fluid. In addition, evaporative fluid losses through the burn wound are 4 to 20 times greater than normal and remain elevated until complete wound closure is obtained. The result is a decrease in organ perfusion. If the intravascular space is not replenished with intravenous (IV) fluids, hypovolemic (burn) shock and, ultimately, death ensue for the victim of an extensive burn.

Urine output for the adult client receiving insufficient fluid replacement following a major burn injury diminishes to less than 30 ml/hour. Physical findings of the urine sample demonstrate dehydration, characterized by dark amber, concentrated urine and elevated specific gravity. Laboratory tests reveal elevated blood urea nitrogen (BUN) levels until the client is adequately hydrated.

■ **FIGURE 50–2** Partial-thickness burn injury (second-degree burn).

■ **FIGURE 50–3** Full-thickness burn injury (third-degree burn).

■ **FIGURE 50–4** Full-thickness burn injury of the forearm and hand caused by high-voltage electrical current. Injury extends into the muscle and bone of the hand and forearm (fourth-degree burn).

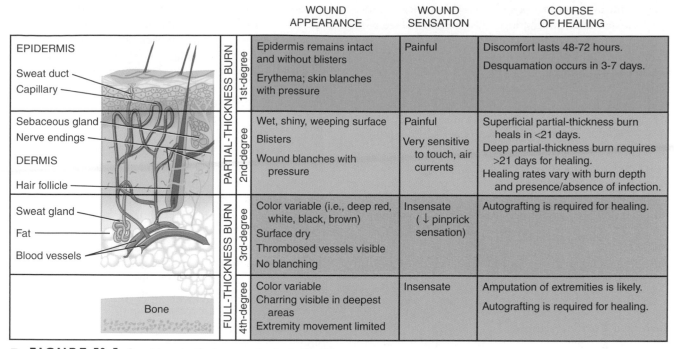

		WOUND APPEARANCE	WOUND SENSATION	COURSE OF HEALING
EPIDERMIS Sweat duct Capillary	**PARTIAL-THICKNESS BURN** 1st-degree	Epidermis remains intact and without blisters Erythema; skin blanches with pressure	Painful	Discomfort lasts 48-72 hours. Desquamation occurs in 3-7 days.
Sebaceous gland Nerve endings **DERMIS** Hair follicle	2nd-degree	Wet, shiny, weeping surface Blisters Wound blanches with pressure	Painful Very sensitive to touch, air currents	Superficial partial-thickness burn heals in <21 days. Deep partial-thickness burn requires >21 days for healing. Healing rates vary with burn depth and presence/absence of infection.
Sweat gland Fat Blood vessels	**FULL-THICKNESS BURN** 3rd-degree	Color variable (i.e., deep red, white, black, brown) Surface dry Thrombosed vessels visible No blanching	Insensate (↓ pinprick sensation)	Autografting is required for healing.
Bone	4th-degree	Color variable Charring visible in deepest areas Extremity movement limited	Insensate	Amputation of extremities is likely. Autografting is required for healing.

■ **FIGURE 50–5** Burn injury classification according to depth of injury.

Manifestations of decreased gastrointestinal motility following major burn injuries include the absence of bowel sounds, stool, or flatus; nausea and vomiting; and abdominal distention. After adequate fluid resuscitation, gastrointestinal motility returns, signaled by a return of hunger and appetite, bowel sounds, flatus, and stool production.

At approximately 18 to 36 hours after burn injury, capillary membrane integrity begins to be restored. The initial increase in hematocrit, seen early after injury, falls to below normal by the third or fourth day after injury. The fall in hematocrit occurs as a result of red blood cell loss and damage incurred at the time of injury. Over the ensuing days and weeks, the body begins to reabsorb the edema fluid, and the excess fluid is excreted via diuresis.

Alterations in Respiration

Initially, the client may exhibit tachypnea following the burn injury. Arterial blood gas analysis may demonstrate a relatively normal arterial partial pressure of oxygen (Pao_2), with oxygen saturation lower than expected relative to the Po_2. In those with an inhalation injury, respiratory insufficiency may develop during the resuscitative phase when fluid shifts are greatest and the injured lung parenchyma is particularly susceptible to edema formation. Later on in the course of recovery, respiratory failure may occur because of infection (often 10 days to 2 weeks following injury).

Diagnosis of CO poisoning is made by measuring the COHb level in the blood. The clinical manifestations of acute CO poisoning, shown in the Bridge to Critical Care

feature below, are directly related to the level of COHb saturation and relative degree of tissue hypoxia. The onset of clinical manifestations typically does not occur until COHb levels reach 15%. Initial manifestations are related to decreased cerebral tissue oxygenation and are neurologic in nature. The neurologic problems caused by CO exposure can lead to progressive and permanent cerebral dysfunction.

Thermal burns to the upper airways (mouth, nasopharynx, and larynx) characteristically appear erythematous and edematous, with mucosal blisters or ulcerations. Increasing mucosal edema can lead to upper airway obstruction, typically within the first 24 to 48 hours after

▢ BRIDGE TO CRITICAL CARE

Clinical Manifestations of Carbon Monoxide (CO) Poisoning

CO Level (%)	Clinical Manifestations
5-10	Impaired visual acuity
11-20	Flushing, headache
21-30	Nausea, impaired dexterity
31-40	Vomiting, dizziness, syncope
41-50	Tachypnea, tachycardia
>50	Coma, death

From Cioffi, W.G. (1998). Inhalation injury. In G.J. Carrougher (Ed.), *Burn care and therapy* (p. 42). St. Louis: Mosby.

injury. Clinical manifestations observed in critical narrowing of the airway include stridor, dyspnea, increased work of breathing, use of respiratory accessory muscles, and eventually cyanosis.

Admission physical findings indicative of smoke exposure include soot on the face and nares, facial burns, soot in the sputum, coughing, and wheezing. The manifestations of tracheobronchitis typically do not present until 24 to 48 hours after injury. Early manifestations consist of bronchospasm evidenced as wheezing and bronchorrhea. Lung compliance is decreased, causing an increased work of breathing. Impaired clearance of secretions accentuates the problem. Normally, ventilation and perfusion are matched by equal volumes of air and blood at the alveolar-capillary level. The client with smoke inhalation exhibits pathophysiologic changes that reduce alveolar ventilation, causing a ventilation-perfusion ($\dot{V}/\dot{Q}$) mismatch, which impairs gas exchange.[8]

Decreased Cardiac Output

Following an extensive burn injury, heart rate and peripheral vascular resistance increase in response to the release of catecholamines and to the relative hypovolemia, but initial cardiac output decreases (hypofunction). At approximately 24 hours after burn injury in clients receiving adequate fluid resuscitation, cardiac output returns to normal and then increases (2 to 2.5 times normal) to meet the hypermetabolic needs of the body (hyperfunction). This change in cardiac output occurs even before circulating intravascular volume levels are restored to normal. Arterial blood pressure is normal or slightly elevated unless severe hypovolemia exists. The decreased cardiac output seen initially after burn injury is evidenced by decreased blood pressure, decreased urine output, weak peripheral pulses, and, if monitored via a pulmonary artery catheter, a cardiac output of less than 4 L/min, cardiac index of less than 2.5 L/min, and systemic vascular resistance of less than 900 dynes.

Pain Responses

The client experiences substantial pain as a result of the burn wound and exposed nerve endings from lack of skin integrity. Burn survivors typically describe three types of pain resulting from their injury: background, breakthrough, and procedural pain. Background pain is experienced when the client is at rest or engages in non–procedure-related activities, such as shifting position in bed, or with chest or abdominal wall movements that occur with deep breathing or coughing. Background pain is described as continuous in nature and low in intensity, typically lasting the duration of recovery. Management of background pain is often with the use of long-acting analgesic agents using such modalities as patient-controlled analgesia (PCA), continuous infusion, or sustained-release oral agents. Breakthrough pain is an increase in the pain experienced that exceeds the low intensity level of background pain. Like background pain, it is experienced when the client is at rest or engages in activities of daily living or other minor activities that require movement of injured areas. Breakthrough pain occurs intermittently throughout the day. The intensity and frequency of breakthrough pain lessen as the burn heals. Management of breakthrough pain is often with the use of short-acting agents. Procedural pain is experienced during the performance of therapeutic measures commonly used in burn care, such as wound cleansing, dressing changes, and physical/occupational therapy. Procedural pain is described as acute and high in intensity. Management depends on the phase of recovery and includes short-acting opioids (e.g., morphine sulfate, fentanyl, hydromorphone, oxycodone, ketamine). Inhaled agents, such as nitrous oxide, may also be used to treat procedural pain.[11]

Clinical responses to pain may include an increase in blood pressure, heart rate, and respiratory rate with dilated pupils, rigid muscle tone, and guarded positioning. To assess pain, several different pain measurement tools are available for use in adults; they include numerical scales (e.g., 1 to 5, or 1 to 10), verbal descriptive scales (e.g., none, mild, moderate, or severe), and visual analog scales (e.g., 0 to 10 rating scale with verbal descriptors of none at the 0 mark to worst pain possible at the 10 mark).[16]

Altered Level of Consciousness

Rarely do burn-injured clients suffer neurologic damage unless prolonged exposure to smoke has occurred. The client with a major burn injury is most often awake and alert on admission to the hospital. If agitation develops in the immediate post-injury period, the client may be suffering from hypoxemia or hypovolemia and needs further assessment for identifying the origin of these changes. When an alteration in level of consciousness is present on admission to the hospital, it is most often related to neurologic trauma (e.g., fall, motor vehicle accident), impaired perfusion to the brain, hypoxemia (as from a closed-space fire), inhalation injury (as from exposure to asphyxiates or other toxic materials from the fire), electrical burn injury, or the effects of drugs present in the body at the time of injury.

Clients with associated head trauma may have scalp lacerations, swelling, tenderness, or ecchymosis. Level of consciousness may fluctuate between intervals of lucidity followed by rapid deterioration. Pupils may be of unequal size. Neurologic manifestations may include headache, dizziness, memory loss, confusion or loss of consciousness, disorientation, visual changes, hallucinations, combativeness, and coma.

Psychological Alterations

Immediately after injury, those with a major injury may respond with psychological shock, disbelief, anxiety, and feelings of being overwhelmed. The client and family members may be aware of what is happening but may be coping with the situation poorly. Because the client will have a limited ability to process new information, the familiar presence of family and friends can help alleviate anxiety. Simple preparatory instructions and information, especially before procedures, is important. Families of critically ill clients have a need for assurance, proximity to the injured person, and information. Specifically, families want to know how the client is being treated, specific facts about the client's progress, and why certain procedures are being done.

Once stabilized, the client may cope psychologically in many ways. The most common problems during the acute phase of recovery include grief, depression, anxiety, and acute stress disorder (i.e., persistent re-experiencing of the trauma, avoidance of stimuli associated with the trauma, and manifestations of increased arousal). Clients may experience nightmares or flashbacks of the injury, sleep problems, and behavioral regression. A combination of pharmacologic and psychological treatments is often used during this phase. Brief supportive therapy and behavior modification are psychological treatments often used, as is group therapy (e.g., inpatient support groups for burn survivors).

Following hospital discharge, clients may continue to suffer from anxiety and depression. They may report difficulties as they relate to vocational and emotional adjustment. However, the intensity of emotional difficulties often decreases significantly after a year post-burn.[1]

OUTCOME MANAGEMENT

The burn client undergoes a wide range of physiologic and metabolic changes in response to the burn injury. To accomplish the best outcomes, it is essential to have a clear understanding of the pathophysiologic process and the necessary treatment modifications needed over the entire recovery continuum. Three distinct periods or phases of treatment can be defined in the care of clients with major burns: the resuscitative, the acute, and the rehabilitation phases of recovery.

Resuscitative Phase

The resuscitative phase of burn injury consists of the time between the initial injury and 36 to 48 hours after injury. This phase ends when fluid resuscitation is complete. During this phase, life-threatening airway and breathing problems are of major concern. It is also characterized by the development of hypovolemia, which results as

capillaries leak fluid from the intravascular spaces into the interstitial spaces, causing edema. Although the fluid remains in the body, it is unable to contribute to maintaining adequate circulation, because it is no longer in the vascular space. The burn itself, except for initial assessment of severity and depth, is of less immediate concern; in certain cases, however, escharotomy may be performed to restore perfusion to areas exhibiting circulatory compromise. The adequacy of initial treatment of pulmonary and circulatory abnormalities sets the stage for subsequent management. Management of the burn client begins at the scene of the accident. The first step should be to remove the victim from the area of immediate danger, followed by stopping the burning process. Basic life support measures should be implemented during transport of the client to the hospital.

Medical Management in the Resuscitative Phase of Burn Injury

Assess Burn Severity

The American Burn Association has published a severity classification schedule for burn injuries, shown in the Bridge to Critical Care feature on p. 1248.[3] These guidelines are intended to assist the clinician in determining injury severity for the burn client. This classification schedule separates injuries into major, moderate, and minor categories. Clients with major burns are usually transferred to a specialized burn care facility after local emergency treatment has been provided. Clients with moderate burns can usually be managed on an inpatient basis at the receiving hospital. Clients with minor burns usually receive initial care in the emergency department and are then discharged for follow-up care on an outpatient basis.

The severity of a burn injury is classified according to the risk of mortality and the risk of cosmetic or functional disability. Several factors influence injury severity.

Burn Depth.   The deeper the burn wound, the more serious the injury. Deep partial-thickness and full-thickness burns are more likely to become infected, have more profound systemic effects, and are more frequently associated with scarring and development of skin contractures.

Burn Size.   The size of a burn (percentage of injured skin, excluding first-degree burns) is determined by one of three techniques: (1) the rule of nines; (2) the palm method; and (3) an age-specific burn diagram or chart. Burn size is expressed as a percentage of TBSA. The *rule of nines* was introduced in the late 1940s as a quick assessment tool for estimating burn size in the adult. The basis of the rule is that the body is divided into

American Burn Association Severity Classification for Burn Injuries

MAJOR BURN INJURY

■ 25% TBSA* burn in adults <40 yr of age
■ 20% TBSA burn in adults >40 yr of age
■ 20% TBSA burn in children <10 yr of age

or

Burns involving the face, eyes, ears, hands, feet, and perineum likely to result in functional or cosmetic disability

or

High-voltage electrical burn injury

or

All burn injuries with concomitant inhalation injury or major trauma

MODERATE BURN INJURY

■ 15-25% TBSA burn in adults <40 yr of age
■ 10-20% TBSA burn in adults >40 yr of age
■ 10-20% TBSA burn in children <10 yr of age

with

Less than 10% TBSA full-thickness burn without cosmetic or functional risk to the face, eyes, ears, hands, feet, or perineum

MINOR BURN INJURY

■ <15% TBSA burn in adults <40 yr of age
■ <10% TBSA burn in adults >40 yr of age
■ <10% TBSA burn in children <10 yr of age

with

<2% TBSA full-thickness burn and no cosmetic or functional risk to the face, eyes, ears, hands, feet, or perineum

TBSA, Total body surface area.
Modified from American Burn Association. (1984). Guidelines for service standards and severity classification in the treatment of burn injury. *American College of Surgeons Bulletin, 69*(10), 24-28.

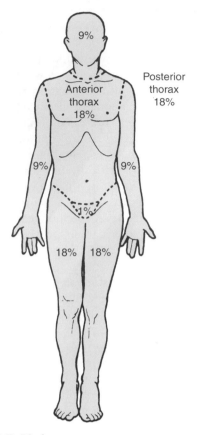

■ **FIGURE 50–6** The rule of nines provides a quick method for estimating the extent of a burn injury in the adult.

anatomic sections, each of which represents 9%, or a multiple of 9%, of the TBSA (Figure 50-6). This method is easy and requires no diagrams to determine the percentage of TBSA injured. Therefore it is frequently used in emergency departments, where initial triage occurs. A second method for estimating the size of a burn is the *palm method.* The client's palm and digits make up approximately 1% of the total body surface area. The percent burn is derived by visualizing the number of client hands it would take to cover the burn area. This method is useful when the burned area or areas is small, less than 5%. Lastly, a *burn diagram* charts the percentages for body segments according to age and provides a more accurate estimate of burn size (Figure 50-7). It should be noted that the extent of burn injury is most accurate after initial debridement and should therefore be verified again at that time.

Burn Location. The location of injury on the body can affect outcome. Pulmonary complications are frequent with burns of the head, neck, and chest. When burns involve the face, associated injuries often include corneal abrasions. Burns of the ears are susceptible to auricular chondritis, infection, and further loss of tissue. Management of burns of the hands and joints often requires intense physical and occupational therapy, with the potential for major loss of work time and for permanent physical and vocational disability. Burns involving the perineal area are susceptible to infection because of auto-contamination by urine and feces. Circumferential burns of extremities may produce a tourniquet-like effect, leading to distal vascular compromise. Circumferential thorax burns may lead to inadequate chest wall expansion and pulmonary insufficiency.

Age. The client's age affects the severity and outcome of the burn. Death rates are higher for children younger than 4 years, particularly in newborns and infants up to 1 year of age, and for clients older than 65 years. High mortality and morbidity rates in the older burn-injured client are from the combination of age-related functional impairments (slower reaction time, impaired judgment, and decreased mobility), living alone, environmental

Area	1 Year	1 to 4 Years	5 to 9 Years	10 to 14 Years	> 15 Years	Adult	Shallow	Indeterminate or deep
Head	19	17	13	11	9	7		
Neck	2	2	2	2	2	2		
Ant. Trunk	13	13	13	13	13	13		
Post. Trunk	13	13	13	13	13	13		
R. Buttock	2½	2½	2½	2½	2½	2½		
L. Buttock	2½	2½	2½	2½	2½	2½		
Genitalia	1	1	1	1	1	1		
R. U. Arm	4	4	4	4	4	4		
L. U. Arm	4	4	4	4	4	4		
R. L. Arm	3	3	3	3	3	3		
L. L. Arm	3	3	3	3	3	3		
R. Hand	2½	2½	2½	2½	2½	2½		
L. Hand	2½	2½	2½	2½	2½	2½		
R. Thigh	5½	6½	8	8½	9	9½		
L. Thigh	5½	6½	8	8½	9	9½		
R. Leg	5	5	5½	6	6½	7		
L. Leg	5	5	5½	6	6½	7		
R. Foot	3½	3½	3½	3½	3½	3½		
L. Foot	3½	3½	3½	3½	3½	3½		
Total								

■ **FIGURE 50–7** A sample chart for recording the extent and depth of a burn injury using the Berkow formula. To estimate burn extent using this chart, the nurse outlines the injured areas, excluding first-degree burns. Shallow (second-degree) burns are designated by parallel lines, and deeper (third-degree and fourth-degree) burns are designated by shading in the appropriate areas. The percentage of each injured anatomic area is then estimated using the age-specific table. Total body surface area (TBSA) burn is then calculated.

hazards, and significant pre-injury morbidity. Compounding this vulnerability to burn injury is the thinning of the skin and atrophy of skin appendages that occur with aging.

General Health. Debilitating cardiac, pulmonary, endocrine, and renal disease—specifically, cardiopulmonary insufficiency, diabetes, alcoholism-related disease, and renal failure—can influence the client's response to injury and treatment. The death rate for clients with pre-existing cardiac disorders is 3.5 to 4 times higher than that for burn-injured clients without cardiac disorders. Clients suffering from alcoholism and a significant burn injury have a three-fold increase in mortality over that of clients with only a burn injury. In addition, those clients with alcoholism who survive their burn injury have longer hospital stays and more complications. The increased morbidity may be related to impaired immune function. Obese clients with burn injury are at increased risk because of cardiopulmonary complications.

Mechanism of Injury. The mechanism of injury is another factor used to determine the severity of injury. In general, special attention to this aspect of the injury is required for any electrical or chemical burn injury or any burn associated with inhalation injury. The client, people at the scene of the injury, and emergency medical personnel may have important information that could help in determining the severity of the burn. Useful information includes the time of injury, the level of the client's consciousness at the scene, whether the injury occurred in an enclosed or open space, the presence of associated trauma, and the specific mechanism of injury. If the victim has suffered a chemical burn, knowledge of the offending agent, its concentration, the duration of exposure, and whether irrigation was initiated at the scene is useful. For victims of electrical injuries, knowledge of the electrical source, type of current, and the current voltage is useful in determining the extent of the injury. Information concerning the client's past medical history as well as general health should be obtained. Specifically, information regarding cardiac, pulmonary, endocrine, or renal disease may have implications for treatment. Also, it is important to identify known allergies and current medication regimen, including herbal remedies.

Treat Minor Burns

Care of the client with only minor burn injuries is usually provided on an ambulatory or outpatient basis. In making the decision about whether to manage a client as an outpatient, the seriousness of the injury must first be assessed. As outlined in the Bridge to Critical Care feature on p. 1248, a minor burn injury in the adult is generally considered to be less than 15% TBSA in clients younger than 40 years or 10% TBSA in clients older than 40 years, without a risk of cosmetic or functional impairment or disability. In addition, the client or caregiver's ability to perform wound care in the home environment must be considered. Medical care of the minor burn includes wound evaluation and initial care, tetanus immunization, and pain management. While providing initial wound care, the nurse is responsible for teaching home wound care and the clinical manifestations of infection that necessitate further medical care. Other teaching needs

include the need to perform active range-of-motion (ROM) exercises to maintain normal joint function and to decrease edema formation. The need for any follow-up evaluations or treatments should be confirmed with the client at this time.

Major Burns

The medical goals for burn care depend on the phase of care. Initial goals are saving life, maintaining and protecting the airway, and restoring hemodynamic stability. Later goals focus on promoting healing, and assessing and correcting complications.

Monitor Airway and Breathing

The adequacy of the airway and breathing should take prime importance during the resuscitative phase. The oropharynx should be inspected for evidence of erythema, blisters, or ulcerations, and the need for endotracheal intubation should be considered.

SAFETY ALERT

If inhalation injury is suspected, administration of 100% oxygen via a tight-fitting non-rebreathing face mask continues until COHb levels fall below 15%. Hyperbaric oxygen may be considered with any exposure to CO. However, depending on the location of the hyperbaric chamber and transport time, this treatment option may carry additional risk. If breathing appears to be compromised by tight circumferential trunk burns, bilateral escharotomies of the trunk may be necessary to relieve ventilatory compromise.

Prevent Burn (Hypovolemic) Shock

In adults with burn injuries affecting more than 15% TBSA, intravenous (IV) fluid resuscitation is generally required. Two peripheral large-bore IV lines placed through nonburned skin, proximal to any extremity burns, are recommended. IV lines may be placed through burned skin if necessary; however, these lines should be secured with a suture. For clients with extensive burns or limited peripheral IV access sites, cannulation of a central vein (subclavian, internal or external jugular, or femoral) by a physician may be necessary.

Fluid resuscitation is used to minimize the deleterious effects of the fluid shifts. The goal of fluid resuscitation is to maintain vital organ perfusion while avoiding the complications related to either inadequate or excessive fluid administration. Several different formulas exist that are used to calculate fluid requirements. The formula currently recommended by the American Burn Life Support (ABLS) course, outlined in the Critical Monitoring feature on p. 1251, is 2 to 4 ml/kg/24 hours of lactated Ringer's solution. In the calculation of fluid infusion rates, the time of injury, not the time at which fluid resuscitation was initiated, serves as time zero. Thus if a burned client is

Consensus Formula for Fluid Resuscitation

Adults: Ringer's lactate solution 2 to 4 ml × kg body weight × percent burn

The infusion rate is adjusted so that half of the estimated volume is administered in the first 8 hours post-burn. The remaining half of the estimated resuscitation volume is administered over the subsequent 16 hours.

delayed 2 hours in reaching an emergency department, those 2 hours must be considered in any calculation of needed fluid. However, adjustment to the fluid infusion rate is based on the client's physiologic response (e.g., urine production, vital signs, and lung sounds) and not missed resuscitation fluid.

SAFETY

⚠

ALERT

It is important to remember that this resuscitation formula is only a guide and that fluid resuscitation volumes should be adjusted according to the client's physiologic response. Adequacy of fluid resuscitation is based on urine output and hemodynamic monitoring (if necessary and available). An indwelling urethral catheter connected to a closed drainage system should be placed to measure hourly urine production in order to guide IV fluid replacement in those with extensive or major burn injuries.

The exact amount of fluid is based on the client's weight and the extent of injury. Other factors to be considered include the presence of an inhalation injury or a high-voltage electrical injury, delay in initiation of resuscitation, history of excessive alcohol intake, associated trauma, and deep tissue damage. These factors tend to increase the amount of IV fluid required for adequate resuscitation above the calculated amount. Colloid-containing solutions are not given during this period because of the changes in capillary integrity that allow leakage of protein-rich fluid (e.g., albumin) into the interstitial space, resulting in the formation of additional edematous fluid. During the second 24 hours after burn injury, colloid-containing solutions may be administered, along with 5% dextrose and water in varying amounts.

Vital signs are used to provide a baseline of information as well as additional data for determining the adequacy of fluid resuscitation. Baseline laboratory studies should include blood glucose, BUN, serum creatinine, serum electrolytes, and hematocrit levels. Arterial blood gas and COHb levels should be obtained, particularly if an inhalation injury is suspected. A chest x-ray film should be obtained for all clients with extensive burns

or inhalation injury. Other laboratory tests in addition to the radiographic study should be performed in all clients with associated trauma, as indicated. Depending on the circumstance of the injury, an alcohol or drug screen may be appropriate. Continuous electrocardiographic (ECG) monitoring should be initiated in all clients with major burn injuries, particularly those who have suffered a high-voltage electrical injury or who have a history of cardiac ischemia. ECG leads should be placed on nonburned skin, therefore interpretation of the rhythm must be interpreted in light of where the leads are placed.

Prevent Aspiration

Many burn centers advocate the placement of a nasogastric tube for management of unresponsive clients and clients with burns of 20% to 25% TBSA or more, to prevent emesis and reduce the risk of aspiration. Gastrointestinal dysfunction results from the intestinal ileus that develops almost universally in clients during the early post–burn injury period. All oral fluids should be restricted at this time.

Minimize Pain and Anxiety

During the resuscitative phase, pain management for the client with a major burn is achieved through the administration of IV opioids, typically morphine sulfate or fentanyl. In the adult, small doses are given and repeated in 5- to 10-minute intervals until pain is under control.

The intramuscular and subcutaneous routes are *not* used during the resuscitative phase because absorption from the soft tissues is unreliable when peripheral perfusion is sporadic. The oral route for pain medication administration is not used because of the likelihood of gastrointestinal dysfunction.

SAFETY

⚠

ALERT

Clients presenting to emergency departments with minor or moderate burn injuries often are initially given small doses of IV opioids (e.g., morphine sulfate). Oral analgesic agents are then prescribed.

To minimize anxiety, simple explanations concerning the hospital environment (e.g., cardiac monitoring devices, pumps used to administer intravenous fluids) and preparatory information before all procedures should be provided.[6,16]

Wound Care

Stop the Burning Process. All burn wound care begins at the scene of the injury. Clothing that continues to smolder should be carefully removed. In the case of a scald injury, all hot, wet clothing (includes diapers) should be removed immediately. Once the clothing is removed, the client should be covered with a dry sheet and blanket to preserve body heat.

Treatment of chemical burn injuries also begins at the scene of the injury. All clothing should be promptly removed, and any chemical powder brushed off the skin. Chemical burns should be irrigated continuously with copious amounts of water for at least 20 minutes and until the burning sensation stops. Neutralizing agents are not recommended because the neutralizing reaction causes heat, which results in further tissue damage.

For chemical eye injuries, irrigate the eyes with a gentle stream of normal saline, flushing both the injured eye and the conjunctiva. The recommended method is to irrigate the eyes from the inner canthus outward, to avoid washing any chemicals down the tear duct or toward the other eye.

Electrical burn care includes stopping the burning process.

SAFETY ALERT

It is important to remember, for your safety and the client's, to shut off any power source before approaching the victim.

Early care is directed at assessment of the entire person, because of the potential path of the electricity through the body (e.g., dysrhythmias, fractures).

Immediate Care. When transfer to a burn center will be accomplished within 12 hours of injury, wound care should consist of covering the wound with sterile towels and placing clean, dry sheets and blankets over the client. Initiation of debridement and application of topical antimicrobial agents are unnecessary. Definitive wound care begins following inpatient admission to the hospital.

Definitive wound care for burns consists of cleansing, debridement of devitalized tissue, removal of any damaging agents (e.g., chemicals, tar), and application of an appropriate topical agent and a dressing. Burn wounds should be washed with a mild soap and rinsed thoroughly with warm water. Loose, devitalized tissue should be carefully trimmed away, and any hair should be shaved to within a 1-inch margin around the burn wound (exception: do not shave eyebrows or eyelashes as they may not grow back in a normal pattern) to minimize surface organisms.

The removal of tar or asphalt is more easily accomplished with the use of a citrus-petroleum product such as Medisol (Orange-Sol, Inc., Chandler, Ariz) or with mineral oil and a petroleum-based antibiotic ointment such as bacitracin or polymyxin-neomycin-bacitracin (Neosporin ointment, Pfizer Inc., New York, NY).

Clients with minor burns are generally taught wound care and discharged home with instructions to continue wound care once to twice daily and return to the outpatient clinic or their private physician for follow-up assessment and care.

Prevent Tetanus. Burns, even minor ones, are susceptible to tetanus. The current protocol for tetanus immunization in clients with any burn injury is the same as those with other types of trauma. Clients who have not received immunization against tetanus within the past 5 years should receive a tetanus toxoid booster. For clients who have not been immunized, tetanus immunoglobulin (a passive immunizing agent) and the first of a series of active immunizations with tetanus toxoid should be administered.[4]

Prevent Tissue Ischemia. Circumferential burns of the extremities may compromise circulation in the affected limb. Elevating injured extremities 15 degrees above the level of the heart and performing active exercises help to reduce dependent edema formation. However, circulatory compromise may still occur. Therefore frequent assessment of distal extremity perfusion is necessary. Doppler flowmeter assessment of the palmar arch vessels (for the upper extremity) and the posterior tibial artery (for the lower extremity) provides the most precise indication of peripheral perfusion and should be performed regularly during the resuscitation period. The absence of flow or the progressive diminution of the Doppler flowmeter signal intensity is an indication that perfusion is impaired.

An escharotomy is the appropriate treatment for circulatory compromise caused by constricting, circumferential burns (Figure 50-8). A midlateral or midmedial incision of the involved extremity is made from the most proximal to the most distal extent of the full-thickness burn. The depth of the incision is limited to the eschar. It is generally performed at the bedside without local or general anesthesia, because full-thickness burns are insensate. However, viable tissue beneath the escharotomy may bleed if cut, and then the client may feel pain. Bleeding can be controlled with pressure, a topical clotting agent, suture ligation, or electrocautery. Pain control is achieved with IV opioid administration. After escharotomy, the burn wound can be dressed with topical antimicrobial creams and gauze dressings.

■ **FIGURE 50–8** Escharotomy. Incision is made through the constricting burn eschar to permit expansion of the underlying subcutaneous tissues as edema forms. *(Courtesy University of Washington Burn Center at Harborview Medical Center, Seattle, Wash).*

If adequate tissue perfusion does not return following escharotomy, a fasciotomy may be necessary. This procedure, in which the fascia is incised, is performed in the operating room with the client under general anesthesia. A fasciotomy is usually necessary only in injuries caused by high-voltage electricity or those with concomitant crush injury.

Transport to a Burn Facility. Consideration of transfer to a specialized burn care facility is appropriate for all clients with major burn injuries (see the Bridge to Critical Care feature on p. 1248 for burn classifications). Prompt contact with the receiving burn center is important to facilitate a smooth transfer. All copies of medical records, including administered fluids and medications, hourly urine output values, and vital signs, must accompany the client. The client's burn wounds should simply be covered with a dry sheet and blankets. Burn center personnel will perform a complete assessment of the wound; therefore it is best if topical wound care has not been initiated.

Nursing Management of the Medical Client in the Resuscitative Phase of Burn Care

Assessment. Because the body's immediate physiologic responses to burn injury can either be life-threatening or lead to significant morbidity, prudent nursing assessment during the resuscitative phase of burn injury is crucial.

Diagnosis, Outcomes, Interventions
Diagnosis: Impaired Gas Exchange. Effective gas exchange may become impaired when clients have experienced smoke inhalation because of tracheobronchial swelling, the presence of carbonaceous debris in the airway, or CO poisoning.

Outcomes. The client will have adequate gas exchange evidenced by a Pao_2 greater than 90 mm Hg, oxygen saturation (Sao_2) greater than 95%, arterial partial pressure of carbon dioxide ($Paco_2$) 35 to 45 mm Hg, respiratory rate 16 to 24 breaths/min with a normal pattern and depth, and clear bilateral breath sounds.

Interventions. The client must be frequently assessed for manifestations of respiratory distress such as restlessness, confusion, labored breathing, tachypnea, dyspnea, diminished or adventitious breath sounds, tachycardia, decrease in Pao_2 and Sao_2, and cyanosis. Monitor Sao_2 continuously in clients with major burns during the resuscitative phase of burn injury. Monitor arterial blood gas and COHb levels per physician order. Report changes in the client's condition immediately.

Instruct the client on the use of the incentive spirometer to encourage deep breathing every 2 hours. Elevate the head of the bed to facilitate lung expansion and to reduce facial and neck edema.

Diagnosis: Ineffective Airway Clearance. Because of the occurrence of airway epidermal sloughing, increase in secretions, inflammation and swelling of the nasopharyngeal mucous membranes from smoke irritation, and depressed ciliary action from inhalation injury, the client becomes at risk for *Ineffective Airway Clearance.*

Outcomes. Clients will have an effective airway clearance, as evidenced by clear bilateral breath sounds, clear to white pulmonary secretions, effective mobilization of pulmonary secretions, and unlabored respiration with a respiratory rate of 16 to 24 breaths/min.

Interventions. A thorough pulmonary assessment should be performed every 1 to 2 hours during the first 24 hours after injury, and every 2 to 4 hours the second 24 hours after injury, evaluating breath sounds, rate and depth of respirations, and level of consciousness.

> **Be alert to a declining respiratory status as evidenced by crackles, rhonchi, stridor, labored breathing, dyspnea, tachypnea, restlessness, or a decreasing level of consciousness. Report significant findings promptly.**
> SAFETY ⚠ ALERT

Have the client turn, cough, and deep breathe every 1 to 2 hours for 24 hours and then every 2 to 4 hours. Place an oral suctioning device within the client's reach for independent use. Perform endotracheal or nasotracheal suction as needed. Assess and document the character and amount of secretions.

Diagnosis: Deficient Fluid Volume. The client with an extensive burn injury is at risk for hypovolemia, most significantly during the first 36 hours after burn injury. The *Deficient Fluid Volume* is directly related to the increased capillary leakage and fluid shift from the intravascular to the interstitial space after the burn insult.

Outcomes. The client will have improved fluid balance, as evidenced by a urine output of 30 ml/hour, clear sensorium, pulse rate less than 120 beats/min, absence of dysrhythmias, adequate amplitude of peripheral pulses (2+ or better), and blood pressure within the expected range for age and medical history.

Interventions. Assess the client for manifestations of hypovolemia every hour for 36 hours, including tachycardia, decreased blood pressure, decreased amplitude of peripheral pulses, urine output of less than 30 ml/hour, thirst, and dry mucous membranes. Report significant findings.

> **Carefully monitor and document intake and output, administering fluid therapy as prescribed; titrate the infusion to maintain a urine output of 30 ml/hour. Early in the resuscitative phase, nurses should not wait for the full hour to adjust infusion of fluids; if little to no urine is present, fluid rates should be adjusted.**
> SAFETY ⚠ ALERT

Monitor serum electrolyte and hematocrit values. Hyponatremia, hyperkalemia, and elevated hematocrit levels are common findings during the resuscitative phase. As the circulation is restored, levels should return to normal values.

Diagnosis: Ineffective Tissue Perfusion: Renal. Clients who have suffered deep burn tissue injury, such as in electrical injury or crush injuries, and those in who adequate fluid resuscitation has not been achieved are at risk for renal failure. Myoglobin and hemoglobin are released from the damaged muscles and red blood cells and precipitate in the renal tubules, where they can create acute tubular necrosis.

Outcomes. The client with evidence of deep burn tissue injury will maintain a urine output of 75 to 100 ml/hour until the pigment load has decreased.

Interventions. Monitor and document hourly output and urine color. A dark brown or red color is indicative of the presence of hemochromogens. Send urine samples for myoglobin or hemoglobin assay per physician order to provide quantitative information for documentation of the client's condition. Ensure that the catheter is patent, because the tubing may become plugged with hemochromogens. Administer IV fluids per physician orders. Hemochromogens must be flushed from the body; therefore the rate of fluid administration is based on maintaining an hourly urine output of 75 to 100 ml/hour.

Diagnosis: Ineffective Tissue Perfusion: Peripheral. The client may exhibit *Ineffective Peripheral Tissue Perfusion* as a result of constricting circumferential burns and/or edema of peripheral tissues.

Outcomes. The client will have adequate peripheral perfusion, as evidenced by the presence of pulses on palpation or Doppler flowmeter assessment, capillary refill time for unburned skin of less than 2 seconds, absence of numbness or tingling, and absence of increased pain with active range-of-motion (ROM) exercises.

Interventions. Remove all constricting jewelry and clothing as early as possible, because constricting items may compromise circulation as edema formation ensues. Limit the use of the blood pressure cuff on the affected extremity, because the cuff can reduce arterial inflow and venous return. Elevate the burned extremity above the level of the heart to promote venous return and to prevent excessive dependent edema formation.

Monitor arterial pulses by palpation or with the use of an ultrasonic flow detector (Doppler flowmeter) hourly for up to 72 hours after burn injury. Pulses will diminish with circulation impairment. Assess capillary refill of unburned skin on the affected extremity; capillary refill will be prolonged with impaired circulation. Encourage ROM exercises, and assess the level of pain associated with efforts. Increasing pain with movement is a result of tissue ischemia. When pain is not present, increased movement of the affected area will promote venous return and assist in decreasing edema.

If tissue perfusion is threatened, anticipate and prepare the client for an escharotomy. Once the underlying tissue edema has exceeded the expansion ability of the burned skin, an escharotomy will be needed to restore perfusion. After the procedure is complete, recheck for restoration of circulation by assessing pulses, color, movement, and sensation of the affected extremity. Anticipate some bleeding after escharotomy, because the tissue beneath the eschar may bleed. Bleeding can be controlled by pressure, electrocautery, or suturing by the physician. Continue to observe and assess the extremity after the procedure.

Diagnosis: Acute Pain. The client can be expected to experience a significant amount of pain during the resuscitative phase of recovery. The pain experienced is associated with the burn wound and wound-related procedures.

Outcomes. The client will verbalize a level of acceptable pain control.

Interventions. Assess for pain, and administer appropriate opioids. Time the administration of medications so that the client receives the benefit of the drug's peak performance during painful procedures, and evaluate the effectiveness of interventions. Explain all procedures and allow adequate time for preparation. Assess the need for an anxiolytic medication, as anxiety can be a major contributor to pain. Document findings, including the client's response to pain interventions.

Diagnosis: Anxiety. The client can be expected to experience a significant amount of anxiety. The anxiety experienced is associated with the critical nature of the injury, wound- and care-related procedures, and pain.

Outcomes. The client will verbalize a level of acceptable anxiety control.

Interventions. Assess for anxiety. Explain all procedures and allow adequate time for preparation. Provide adequate pain medications to reduce pain-related anxiety. Assess the need for anxiolytic agents. Document findings.

Diagnosis: Risk for Infection. The burn-injured client faces an increased *Risk for Infection* related to inadequate primary and secondary defenses resulting from traumatized tissue, bacterial proliferation in burn wounds, and an immunocompromised status.

Outcomes. The client will remain free from significant burn wound microbial invasion, as evidenced by quantitative wound cultures containing less than 100,000 colony-forming units (CFUs)/g. In addition, core body temperature will be maintained between 99.6° and 101°F (37.5° C to 38.3° C); there will be no swelling, redness, or purulence present at IV line insertion sites; and results of blood, urine, and sputum cultures will be negative.

Interventions. Tetanus prophylaxis should be administered per physician order because the anaerobic environment beneath eschar is ideal for tetanus organism growth. Topical antimicrobial agents are used to deter the growth of bacteria on the surface of the wound.

SAFETY ALERT

It is essential to maintain infection control techniques at all times during the client's hospitalization to prevent cross-contamination. Ensure aseptic technique when administering care to burned areas and performing invasive techniques. Enforce strict hand-washing, and instruct family members or significant others on infection control measures.

When wound care is performed, it is important to debride the wound of loose, devitalized tissue, which serves as a medium for bacterial growth. Hair within and around a wound should be shaved (with the exception of eyebrows and eyelashes), because hair is contaminated and prevents adherence of the burn cream. Apply a topical antimicrobial agent or skin substitute per physician order.

Diagnosis: Impaired Physical Mobility. The client's mobility during the resuscitative phase of burn injury is impaired by tissue edema, pain, and dressings.

Outcomes. The outcomes related to physical mobility are measured throughout the hospitalization and recovery process. The long-term outcome goal is return of the client to maximum independence in performance of activities of daily living (ADL) with minimum disability and disfigurement. Although this outcome is demonstrated long after the resuscitative phase, it is important to initiate care on the day of admission and to follow through continually throughout hospitalization.

Interventions. Encourage the client to participate in self-care and ROM exercises at the earliest time possible. During the early postinjury fluid shifts, physical movement helps to improve circulation and decrease edema. Consult with occupational and physical therapists for initial assessment and follow-up care throughout the hospitalization.

Diagnosis: Disabled Family Coping. Because of the urgent and critical nature of the injury, the client and family are at risk for ineffective coping skills.

Outcomes. Family members and significant others will have accurate information about the immediate status of the client, as evidenced by their ability to verbalize an understanding of the client's injury and treatment goals. Support services will be provided as needed.

Interventions. It is important to prepare family members or significant others for their first visit with the client after injury. Provide a simple explanation of procedures and equipment, communicate the extent of the burn, and describe changes in the client's appearance. When client transfer is impending, provide family members or significant others with support services to assist with

travel arrangements. Providing support at this time will help to reduce their anxiety during the client's transfer. Families of clients remaining in the facility should be provided with information that meets their basic needs (e.g., information about lodging, location of cafeteria, parking).

Acute Phase

The acute phase of recovery following a major burn begins when the client is hemodynamically stable, capillary integrity is restored, and diuresis has begun. This time-point begins at approximately 48 to 72 hours after the time of injury. Many of the same principles of care outlined for the resuscitative phase apply to the acute phase; however, more emphasis is placed on restorative therapies. For clients with either a minor or a moderate burn, the acute phase essentially begins at the time of injury. The acute phase continues until wound closure is achieved.

Medical Management in the Acute Phase of Burn Injury

Prevent Infection

SAFETY ALERT

Infection control is a major component of burn management. An infection control policy is necessary for managing burn-injured clients to control the transmission of microorganisms that can lead to infection. Standard precautions should be followed in caring for all clients with burn injuries; however, specific infection control practices and isolation techniques exist for all burn centers. These practices include the use of gloves, caps, masks, shoe covers, scrub clothes, and plastic aprons. Strict hand-washing is stressed to reduce the incidence of cross-contamination between clients and is the single most important means of preventing the spread of infection. Staff and visitors are generally prevented from client contact if they have any skin, gastrointestinal, or respiratory tract infections. See Box 50-2 for basic infection control strategies. All visitors as well as health care providers from other departments should be educated concerning established infection control practices before their first contact with the burn-injured client. Some burn centers limit the number of visitors in burn units.

Provide Metabolic Support

Maintenance of adequate nutrition during the acute phase of burn care is essential in promoting wound healing and preventing infection. Basal metabolic rates may be 40% to 100% higher than normal levels, depending on the extent of the burn. This response is thought to be the result of a resetting of the homeostatic "thermostat" of the hypothalamic-pituitary-adrenal axis, leading

BOX 50-2 Basic Requirements of Infection Control

1. Hands should be washed before and after each client contact with antimicrobial agent and water or an alcohol hand rinse.
2. Appropriate garb, including clean aprons or gowns and clean gloves, should be donned before each client contact and discarded immediately after leaving the bedside or room.
3. Gloves should be changed when contaminated with secretions or excretions from one body site before contact with another site on the client.
4. Sterile gloves, hats, and masks should be worn when caring for an open burn wound and when preparing for and performing other sterile procedures.
5. Equipment, materials, and surfaces should be considered contaminated with organisms from the client and should be appropriately decontaminated before use on other clients.
6. Appropriate garb should be worn when handling or touching equipment, materials, and surfaces contaminated by clients.

Personal communication with Joan M. Weber, RN, BSN, CIC, Infection Control Coordinator, Shriners Burn Hospital, 51 Blossom St., Boston, Mass.

to an increase in heat production. Metabolic rates decrease as wound coverage and healing are achieved.

Aggressive nutritional support is required to meet the increased energy requirements necessary to promote healing and to prevent the untoward effects of catabolism. Several different formulas, shown in the Critical Monitoring feature below, are currently used to estimate energy requirements by factoring different indices: weight, gender, age, extent of burn, and amount of activity. Additional support is generally indicated for the burn-injured client with any of the following: 30% or greater TBSA burn, clinical course requiring multiple

CRITICAL MONITORING

Energy Calculation Formulas Used for the Adult with a Burn Injury

Formula/Author Name	Formula for Daily Caloric Expenditure Estimate
Curreri	(25 kcal/kg body weight) + (40 kcal × % TBSA burn)
Modified Harris-Benedict	RMR × Activity factor × Injury factor
U.S. Army Institute of Surgical Research	(Age- and gender-specific BMR) × (0.89142 + 0.01335 × % TBSA burn) × (m² × 24 × Activity factor)

BMR, Basal metabolic rate; *RMR,* resting metabolic rate; *TBSA,* total body surface area.
From Weber, J.M., & Tompkins, D.M. (1993). Improving survival: Infection control and burns. *AACN Clinical Issues in Critical Care Nursing, 4*(2), 418-419.

operations, need for mechanical ventilatory support, compromised mental status, and poor pre-injury nutritional state. Methods for delivering nutritional support include oral intake, enteral tube feedings, peripheral parenteral nutrition, and total parenteral nutrition, which may be used alone or in combination. The preferred feeding route is oral or enteral; however, the decision of how to best meet the client's nutritional needs should be individualized. Typically, parenteral nutrition is reserved for clients with a prolonged ileus or for those in whom enteral feedings fail to meet nutritional needs.

Minimize Pain

Procedural, background, and breakthrough pain continue to be important issues during this part of the recovery. During the acute phase of injury, an attempt is made to find the right combination of medications and interventions to minimize the discomfort and pain.

As in the resuscitative phase, the most common approach to pain control is with the use of pharmacologic agents. However, in addition to the opioids used during the resuscitative phase, other modalities may be used during the acute phase of burn injury to help alleviate the client's pain. Patient-controlled analgesia devices, inhalation analgesics such as nitrous oxide, oral analgesic "pain cocktails," and opioid agonist-antagonist agents may be beneficial during the acute phase of burn injury. Nonsteroidal anti-inflammatory drugs (NSAIDs) can be prescribed for the treatment of mild to moderate pain. When NSAIDs are used, extra precautions must be taken to prevent gastric ulceration.[11]

Nonpharmacologic modalities used to treat burn-related pain include hypnosis, guided imagery, art and play therapy, relaxation techniques, distraction, biofeedback, and music therapy. These modalities have been found to be effective in decreasing anxiety, thereby decreasing the perception of pain. They are often used as adjunctive therapies to the pharmacologic treatment of burn pain.[9]

Provide Wound Care

Care of the burn wound is ultimately aimed at promoting wound healing. Daily wound care involves cleansing, debridement of devitalized tissue, and dressing of the wound.

Wound Cleansing. The practice of hydrotherapy remains a mainstay of burn treatment plans for cleansing the wounds. This is accomplished by immersion, showering, or spraying (Figure 50-9). A hydrotherapy session of 30 minutes or less is optimal for clients with acute burns. Longer time periods may increase sodium loss (water is hypotonic) through the burn wound and may promote heat loss, pain, and stress. During hydrotherapy, the wounds are gently washed using any one of a variety of solutions.

■ FIGURE 50–9 A low-boy whirlpool tank is used for immersion hydrotherapy treatment of burn wounds. *(Courtesy of Shriners Hospitals for Children of Northern California.)*

Care should be taken to minimize bleeding and to maintain body temperature during this procedure. To prevent cross-contamination, single-use plastic hydrotherapy tub liners are available, with tub cleansing performed between clients. Clients excluded from hydrotherapy are generally those who are hemodynamically unstable and those with new skin grafts. If hydrotherapy is not used, wounds are washed and rinsed while the client is in bed, before the application of topical antimicrobial agents.

Debridement. Burn wound debridement involves the removal of eschar, exudate, and crusts. This promotes wound healing by preventing bacterial proliferation in and under the devitalized tissue. Debridement of the burn wound is accomplished through mechanical, enzymatic, or surgical means.

Mechanical debridement can be accomplished with careful use of scissors and forceps to lift and trim away loose devitalized tissue. Hydrotherapy softens and loosens devitalized tissue so that it is more easily removed. Wet-to-dry dressing changes are another effective means of mechanical debridement. Coarse gauze dressings are saturated with a prescribed solution, wrung out until the dressing is slightly moist, and applied to the wound. The dressing is left in place to dry. Typically 6 to 8 hours later the gauze is carefully removed from the wound, mechanically lifting drainage, exudate, and loose necrotic tissue that have dried onto the gauze. However, this method of wound debridement must be used cautiously, as it will also debride viable tissue. Mechanical debridement of the burn wound can be extremely painful; therefore effective pain management is paramount.

Enzymatic debridement involves the application of commercially prepared proteolytic and fibrinolytic topical enzymes (Accuzyme, Healthpoint Ltd., Ft. Worth, Tex;

Santyl, Abbott Laboratories, Columbus, Ohio) to the burn wound, which facilitates devitalized tissue removal. These agents require a moist environment to be effective and are applied directly to the burn wound.

Caution must be used when enzymes are used as pain and bleeding are common side effects. As the enzyme digests necrotic tissue, it may open up thrombosed blood vessels. This causes some oozing of blood from the vessels and creates a site for bacteria to enter the bloodstream. Bacteremia, pain, and bleeding can occur; therefore if enzymatic debridement is used, the client should be assessed for complications continuously throughout the course of treatment. The use of enzymatic debridement agents is contraindicated for wounds communicating with major body cavities and for wounds with exposed nerves or nervous tissue.

SAFETY

⚠

ALERT

Surgical debridement of the burn wound involves excision of the devitalized tissue and coverage of the wound. Early surgical excision begins during the first week after injury, once the client is hemodynamically stable. Advantages of early excision include early mobilization, early wound closure (which reduces the potential for wound infection), and reduced length of hospitalization. A disadvantage of early excision is the risk of excising viable tissue that may heal with time.

Two techniques of surgical debridement are currently used. In *tangential* excision, very thin layers of devitalized tissue are sequentially shaved until viable tissue is reached. *Fascial* excision involves removing the burn tissue and underlying fat down to fascia. This technique is frequently used for debridement of very deep burns.

Topical Antimicrobial Treatment. Deep partial-thickness or full-thickness burn wounds are treated initially with topical antimicrobial agents. These agents are applied once or twice daily following cleansing, debridement, and inspection of the wound. The nurse assesses for separation of devitalized tissue, the presence of granulation tissue or reepithelialization, and manifestations of infection. The most commonly used topical antimicrobial agents are listed in Table 50-1. Although no single agent is used universally, many burn centers choose silver sulfadiazine cream as the initial topical agent.[7,14]

Burn wounds are treated using either an open or a closed dressing technique. For the *open method,* the antimicrobial cream is applied with a gloved hand and the wound is left open to the air without gauze dressings. The cream is reapplied as needed, although formal reapplication is common every 12 to 24 hours. The advantages of the open method include increased visualization of the wound, greater freedom for mobility and joint motion, and simplicity in wound care. The disadvantages include an increased chance of hypothermia and pain from exposure.

TABLE 50–1   Topical Antimicrobial Agents Used in Burn Care

Agent	Antimicrobial Spectrum	Application	Side Effects	Nursing Considerations
Water-Based Creams				
1% Silver sulfadiazine	Broad spectrum; effective against some fungi and yeast	1-2 times daily, $\frac{1}{16}$-inch thickness	Transient leukopenia typically appearing after 2 or 3 days of treatment Macular rash	Do not store in warm environment (e.g., warm client room)
Mafenide acetate	Broad spectrum; little antifungal activity	Gauze dressing not required	Hyperchloremic metabolic acidosis from bicarbonate diuresis because of inhibition of carbonic anhydrase Pain/burning sensation on application to superficial burns Maculopapular rash	Assess for side effects Assess adequacy of pain management; if pain and discomfort continue, consider other topical treatments Use cautiously in clients with acute renal failure
Solutions				
5% Mafenide acetate	Broad spectrum	2 times daily, $\frac{1}{16}$-inch thickness	Pain on application Pruritus Rash Fungal colonization	Assess for side effects Assess adequacy of pain management
0.5% Silver nitrate	Broad spectrum; effective against *Candida* species	Gauze dressing not required	Hyponatremia Hypochloremia Hypokalemia Hypocalcemia	Check serum electrolyte levels daily Penetrates eschar poorly Remoisten dressings every 2 hr to avoid wound desiccation Protect environment; stains everything blackish-brown color
Petroleum-Based Ointments				
Polymyxin B	Gram-negative organisms	Gauze dressing required, moistened with solution for application to wound	Hypersensitivity (rash)	Assess for side effects
Neomycin sulfate	Predominantly gram-negative organisms	Multiple layers of gauze dressing required, moistened with solution for application to wound	Overgrowth of nonsusceptible organisms including fungi	
Bacitracin	Predominantly gram-positive organisms	Apply as needed in a thin layer; gauze dressing not used unless clothing protection is needed		

In the *closed method* of wound care, gauze dressing is impregnated with antimicrobial cream and applied to the wound. To prevent circulatory compromise in extremity burns, the gauze should be wrapped from the most distal portion of the extremity in a proximal direction. The advantages of the closed method are decreases in evaporative fluid and heat loss from the wound surface. In addition, gauze dressings may aid in debridement. The disadvantages of gauze dressings are mobility limitations and a potential decrease in effectiveness of range-of-motion (ROM) exercises. Wound assessment is also limited to the times at which dressing changes are performed.

Temporary wound coverings (skin substitutes) are frequently used as a kind of wound "dressing." Table 50-2 outlines the most common biologic, biosynthetic, and synthetic wound coverings available. These products are temporary wound coverings, and each has specific indications. The character of the wound (depth of injury, amount of exudate, location of the wound on the body, and phase of recovery) and treatment goals are considered in choosing the most appropriate wound covering.

🪔 Maximize Function

Maintenance of optimal physical functioning in the client with a burn injury is a challenge for the entire team. Nurses work closely with occupational and physical therapists to identify the rehabilitative needs of the burn-injured client. An individualized program of splinting, positioning, exercise, ambulation, performance of ADL, and pressure therapy should be implemented in the acute phase of recovery to maximize functional recovery and cosmetic outcome. Therapeutic goals at

TABLE 50-2 Wound Coverings Used in Burn Care

Category/Examples	Description/Indications	Nursing Considerations
Biologic		
Allograft (homograft/cadaver)	Donated human cadaver skin used to: Debride exudative wounds Protect excised wounds and test for receptivity before autograft placement Cover and protect meshed autografts	Gauze cover dressing is applied over allograft to protect from shearing forces and, with meshed allograft, used to absorb drainage. Staples may be used to hold allograft in place. Staples are placed intraoperatively. Negative pressure therapy may be used over allograft to increase vascularization of wound bed.
Xenograft (heterograft/pigskin)	Harvested porcine (pig) skin used to: Promote healing of clean, superficial partial-thickness burn wounds Debride exudative wounds	Gauze cover dressing applied over xenograft for first 24 hr until adhered (for clean partial-thickness wounds). Once xenograft is adhered, it may be left open to air. Gauze cover dressing applied over xenograft to protect from shearing forces and, with meshed xenograft, to absorb wound drainage. Xenograft is changed daily when used to promote debridement.
Biosynthetic		
Biobrane (Bertek Pharmaceuticals, Morgantown, WV)	Nylon fabric bonded to a silicone membrane containing collagenous porcine peptides used to: Cover donor sites Protect and facilitate healing of clean, superficial partial-thickness burn wounds	Secure to surrounding intact skin with tape, skin closure strips, or staples. Wrap Biobrane with coarse mesh roller gauze dressing. For donor sites, gauze wrap is secured with an outer dressing. Once Biobrane is adhered (usually at 48 hr postoperative), outer dressings can be removed and Biobrane left exposed to air. New and healing donor sites of legs require support during ambulation; figure-eight elastic (Ace) bandage wrapping technique is recommended to minimize trauma to newly formed capillaries. For superficial partial-thickness wounds, Biobrane is applied and secured with tape or skin closure strips. Assess for purulent drainage beneath fabric and at wound periphery (indicative of infection).
Integra (Integra Life Sciences, Plainsboro, NJ)	Bilayer matrix of bovine collagen and glycosaminoglycan covered by silicone layer used to: Provide a dermal layer to excised burn wounds	Applied in OR to excised wounds and secured with staples or securing devices. Silastic (outer) layer is removed approximately 2 weeks following application and covered with very thin split-thickness skin graft. Assess for infection; may appear as pockets of purulent fluid beneath Integra. If indicated, these areas may require debridement and topical antimicrobial coverage. Protect from shearing forces.
Calcium alginate (Kaltostat, ConvaTec/Bristol-Myers & Squibb Co., New York, NY; SeaSorb Ag, Coloplast Corp, Marietta, Ga; Silver Cel, Johnson & Johnson/Ethicon, Inc., Somerville, NJ) Hydrofiber (Aquacel/Aquacel Ag—ConvaTec/Bristol-Myers & Squibb Co., New York, NY)	Dressing produced from alginates found in brown seaweed or synthetically produced to create hydrofibers that are used to: Absorb exudate from moderate to heavily draining wounds Cover donor sites Reduce wound bioburden (those with silver (Ag) added to them)	Applied to wounds and donor sites following irrigation with physiologic solution, such as saline. Absorptive dressing covers calcium alginate or Hydrofiber dressing. Entire dressing should be changed when outer dressing is saturated with drainage.
Non-adhering fine mesh gauze (Aquaphor gauze, Beiersdorf Inc., Norwalk, Conn; Adaptic, Johnson & Johnson/Ethicon, Inc., Somerville, NJ; Xeroform gauze, Sherwood Medical, St. Louis, Mo)	Gauze impregnated with ointment used to: Cover meshed autograft Cover donor sites Cover and protect fragile, newly healed skin	Gauze dressing over healing autograft is often changed daily. Gauze dressing over donor sites should remain in place until healed (10-14 days; may be longer in older adults). Healing donor sites on legs require vascular support when out of bed; figure-eight (Ace) wrapping technique is recommended to minimize trauma to newly formed capillaries.

this stage in recovery are to prevent early contracture formation and to maintain soft tissue length.

Wound contracture and hypertrophic scarring are two major problems for the burn-injured client. Wound contractures are typically more severe with extensive burns. Areas seemingly predisposed to contracture are the hands, head and neck, and axilla. Measures used to prevent and treat wound contractures include therapeutic positioning, ROM exercises, splinting, and client and family education.

Table 50-3 lists corrective and therapeutic techniques for positioning clients with specific areas of burn injury during periods of inactivity or immobilization. Allowing the burn-injured client to assume a position of comfort most often contributes to contracture formation. Therefore proper positioning, both in and out of bed, should be maintained for the burn-injured client. These techniques place affected body parts in positions that are in opposition to positions of potential contracture or deformity. The natural tendency with healing and immobility is for muscles and joints to contract into a shortened, flexed position. For example, to reduce the risk of neck contractures, the use of pillows—which place the neck in flexion—is not allowed.

Active ROM exercises are prescribed early in the acute phase of recovery to promote resolution of edema and to maintain strength and joint function. In addition, ADL can be effective in maintaining function and ROM. Ambulation maintains strength and ROM of the lower extremities. They should begin as soon as the client is physiologically stable. Passive ROM and stretching exercises should be included as part of the daily treatment plan when the client is unable to perform active ROM exercises.

Splints are used to maintain proper joint position and to prevent or correct contractures. Two types of splints are frequently used. A *static splint* immobilizes the joint. Static splints do not replace exercise and are frequently applied for periods of immobilization or during sleeping hours or are used for clients who cannot maintain proper positioning. In contrast, *dynamic splints* exercise the affected joint. Care must be taken to ensure that all splints fit properly and do not apply excessive pressure, which may lead to further tissue or nerve damage.

Provide Psychological Support

The longest period of adjustment occurs during the acute phase. The burn-injured adult may demonstrate a variety of emotional and psychological responses. Anxiety and fearfulness related to potential disfigurement and perceived changes in role and identity plague the client during this time period. Depression, withdrawal, and regression may result.

The client may begin discussing the burn injury or accident, recounting significant events and searching for the meaning of what has happened. Allowing the

expression of these worries and validating that they are "normal" are essential in providing support. Staff members need to actively listen and to allow the client to talk about the accident. Detailed and repetitious recounting of the injury is useful in desensitizing clients to the horror of what has happened and in decreasing nightmares.

Clients who have little information about specific treatment procedures, potential associated discomfort or pain, and available resources or options for pain management typically react with anxiety and a heightened pain response. Providing the client with information about what will occur during a particular procedure or what is expected over the course of recovery is a concept known as *providing preparatory information*. This technique is a psychologically based method that has proved successful in reducing pain and anxiety during certain procedures. To enhance the client's sense of personal control, teaching should include education about various coping mechanisms and the use of nonpharmacologic methods for pain control.

Involving clients in their own care helps them to feel some control over the situation at hand. Clients can be encouraged to participate in wound care (e.g., bathing, simple debridement, dressing application) and physical therapy (e.g., active versus passive ROM exercises, application of splints and pressure garments). These interventions have been found to be effective in supporting the client's psychological needs.

Nursing Management of the Medical Client in the Acute Phase of Burn Injury

Assessment. Once fluid balance is achieved, the client moves into the acute phase of burn care. During this phase, closure of the wounds is a major focus of care. Wounds are assessed daily with every dressing change for evidence of healing and infection. Other areas of assessment include respiratory condition; pain control; nutritional status, and stress ulceration; mobility and contractures; and psychological adjustments by both the client and the family.

Diagnosis, Outcomes, Interventions

Diagnosis: Impaired Gas Exchange. Note that the consequences of smoke inhalation may not be fully appreciated until the acute phase of burn care. The decreased ciliary action in the airways leads to a high risk for pulmonary infection (which usually is not manifested until day 3 or 4 after the burn injury), which is demonstrated first by tracheobronchitis and is followed by bronchopneumonia.

Outcomes. The client will have improved gas exchange, as evidenced by unlabored respirations, a respiratory rate

TABLE 50–3   Anticontracture Positioning for the Client with a Burn Injury

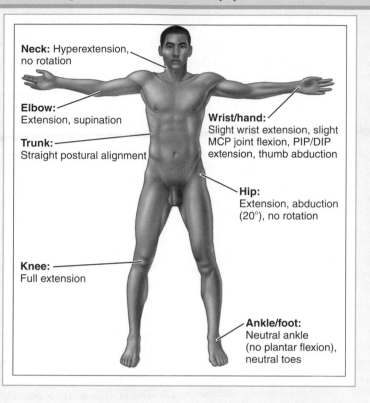

Neck: Hyperextension, no rotation

Elbow: Extension, supination

Trunk: Straight postural alignment

Wrist/hand: Slight wrist extension, slight MCP joint flexion, PIP/DIP extension, thumb abduction

Hip: Extension, abduction (20°), no rotation

Knee: Full extension

Ankle/foot: Neutral ankle (no plantar flexion), neutral toes

Burned Area	Therapeutic Position	Positioning Techniques
Neck		
Anterior	Extension	No pillow
		Small towel roll beneath shoulders to promote neck extension
Circumferential	Neutral toward extension	No pillow
Posterior or asymmetrical	Neutral	No pillow
Shoulder/axilla	Arm abduction to 90-110 degrees	Splinting
		Arms positioned away from body and supported on arm troughs
Elbow	Arm extension	Elbow splint
		Elbows positioned in extension with slight bend at elbow (no more than 10 degrees of elbow flexion)
		Arms supported on arm troughs with forearm in slight pronation
Hand		
Wrist	Wrist extension	Hand splint
MCP	MCP flexion at 90 degrees	Hand splint
PIP/DIP	PIP/DIP extension	Hand splint
Thumb	Thumb abduction	Hand splint with thumb abduction
Finger web spaces	Finger abduction	Web spacers of foam, silicone products, or custom-fitted pressure garments to decrease webbing formation
Hip	Hip extension	Supine with head of bed flat and legs extended
		Trochanter roll to maintain neutral hip rotation (toes should be pointing toward ceiling)
		Prone positioning
Knee	Knee extension	Supine with knees extended (toes should be pointing toward the ceiling)
		Prone positioning with feet extended over end of mattress
		Sitting in chair with legs extended and elevated
		Knee splint
Ankle	Neutral	Padded footboard
		Ankle positioning devices (avoid heel cord tightening)— provide heel protection to prevent pressure sore development

MCP, Metacarpal interphalangeal joint(s); *PIP/DIP,* proximal/distal interphalangeal joint(s).

of 16 to 24 breaths/min, Pao_2 greater than 90 mm Hg, $Paco_2$ of 35 to 45 mm Hg, Sao_2 greater than 95%, and clear bilateral breath sounds.

Interventions. Interventions continue unchanged from the resuscitative phase of injury. Comprehensive respiratory assessment and preventive pulmonary toilet should be performed every 2 hours while the client is awake.

Diagnosis: Ineffective Airway Clearance. Upper airway and facial edema caused by heat-induced tissue and mucosal damage begins to resolve between 2 and 4 days after injury with superficial burns. Full-thickness injuries, however, resolve more slowly, making *Ineffective Airway Clearance* a problem that may last well into the acute phase of treatment.

Outcomes. The client will have effective airway clearance, as evidenced by clear bilateral breath sounds, clear to white pulmonary secretions, effective mobilization of pulmonary secretions, and unlabored breathing.

Interventions. Continue interventions begun in the resuscitative phase of treatment. Pulmonary toilet including turning, coughing, and deep breathing; use of an incentive spirometer every 2 to 4 hours while the client is awake; and endotracheal suctioning as needed facilitates clearance of secretions and sputum. Leave an oral suctioning device within the client's reach for independent use.

Diagnosis: Hypothermia. Clients remain at risk for loss of body heat through burn injuries until wound closure is complete. During hydrotherapy, dressing changes, and lengthy operative procedures, clients are at increased risk for hypothermia.

Outcomes. The client will maintain a core body temperature between 99.6° and 101° F (between 37.5° and 38.3° C).

Interventions. To help prevent the loss of heat from open wounds that occurs as a result of evaporation, limit hydrotherapy treatment sessions to 30 minutes or less with water temperatures of 98° to 102° F (36.6° to 38.8° C). Cover the client with warm blankets after the hydrotherapy session, exposing only limited areas of body surface during topical agent and dressing application. Provide heat lamps or heat shields and increase the ambient temperature in the treatment room or in the client's room if the client exhibits subnormal temperatures. Intravenous fluids and warming blankets may be used in the operating room to maintain body temperature.

Diagnosis: Risk for Infection. During the acute phase of injury, infection remains an ongoing risk because of inadequate primary and secondary defenses resulting from traumatized tissue, bacterial proliferation in the burn wound, presence of invasive lines or urinary catheters, and an immunocompromised status.

Outcomes. The client will have no significant burn wound microbial invasion, as evidenced by quantitative wound cultures containing less than 100,000 CFUs/g. In addition, the client will maintain core body temperature at 99.6° to 101° F; will demonstrate evidence of no swelling, redness, or purulence at invasive line insertion sites; and will have negative results on blood, urine, and sputum cultures.

Interventions

Continue to follow infection control policy for burn-injured clients in an effort to prevent cross-contamination. Assess for clinical manifestations of infection in the burn wound: discoloration of wounds (e.g., brown, black, or hemorrhagic), drainage, odor, delayed healing, or spongy eschar. As in the resuscitative phase, provide meticulous wound care in an aseptic fashion, cleaning and rinsing the wound, and debriding loose devitalized tissue to discourage bacterial growth. Apply a topical antimicrobial agent to the wound to decrease the risk for local wound infection. Continue to shave or cut body hair around wound margins until complete wound closure (exception: do not shave eyebrows or eyelashes).

SAFETY ALERT

Observe for clinical indicators of sepsis: headache, chills, anorexia, nausea, changes in vital signs, hyperglycemia and glycosuria, paralytic ileus, and confusion, restlessness, or hallucinations. Assess for manifestations of infection at catheter insertion sites and wounds. Obtain cultures per physician order, and administer antibiotics and antipyretics as prescribed.

Collaborative Problem: Risk for Stress Ulceration. Stress ulcers can occur at any time after a burn injury. The assessment and preventive treatment started in the resuscitative phase of injury should continue until wound coverage is complete.

Outcomes. The nurse will monitor for manifestations of gastrointestinal bleeding and will maintain gastric pH greater than 5.

Interventions. Monitor and document gastric pH values and heme content every 2 hours while the client's nasogastric tube is in place. Administer antacids, H_2 blockers, or proton pump inhibitors per physician order to reduce the gastric acid content, because high acid levels may lead to bleeding. Monitor stools for occult blood.

Diagnosis: Imbalanced Nutrition: Less Than Body Requirements. The burn-injured client must maintain adequate protein and caloric intake to meet metabolic demands for wound healing.

Outcomes. The client will have adequate nutrition, as evidenced by maintenance of 85% to 90% of pre-burn weight and healing of burn wounds, donor sites, and skin grafts.

Interventions. Caloric needs are based on pre-injury weight. For clients with a major burn, obtain a daily weight to assess whether caloric needs are being met and to provide documentation for staff to follow trends. Weekly weight assessments are adequate for the client who is stable and has less than 25% TBSA burn wound. Assess eating habits and patterns, and identify food preferences and food allergies. Order meals high in calories and proteins. Encourage family members or significant others to bring favorite nutritional foods from home. Provide supplements between meals.

Document daily caloric intake, and consult with the dietitian to perform a nutritional assessment. Consider other methods to meet caloric needs such as tube-feeding or total parenteral feeding, because oral feeding may not provide adequate calories for healing.

Performing oral hygiene during each nursing shift and as needed helps to prevent stomatitis and enhance appetite. Provide an aesthetically pleasing environment that is conducive to eating. Treatments are scheduled to provide for uninterrupted meal times. Allow a period of rest before meal times if the client has endured a painful procedure or treatment, because pain will decrease appetite.

Diagnosis: Acute Pain. The client can be expected to experience a significant amount of pain during the acute burn phase. The pain experienced during this phase of recovery is associated with the burn wound, donor sites, wound care procedures, and ROM exercises.

Outcomes. The client will verbalize a level of acceptable pain control.

Interventions. Continue to assess for pain frequently, and administer appropriate opioids. Time the administration of medications so that the client receives the benefit of the drug's peak performance during painful procedures, and evaluate the effectiveness of interventions.

During the acute phase, nonpharmacologic interventions should be initiated to enhance medication effects and to assist in controlling pain. Explore the benefits of relaxation techniques, guided imagery, music therapy, distraction, and biofeedback. Explain all procedures and allow adequate time for preparation. Assess the need for anxiolytic agents, as anxiety can be a major contributor to pain. Document findings including response to pain interventions.

Diagnosis: Anxiety. The client can be expected to experience a significant amount of anxiety. The anxiety experienced is associated with wound- and care-related procedures, and pain.

Outcomes. The client will verbalize a level of acceptable anxiety control.

Interventions. Assess for anxiety. Explain all procedures and allow adequate time for preparation. Provide adequate pain medications to reduce pain-related anxiety. Provide a consistent treatment schedule (e.g., wound care and physical therapy times are prescheduled with the client on a daily basis). Assess the need for anxiolytic agents. Document findings.

Diagnosis: Impaired Physical Mobility. *Impaired Physical Mobility* during the acute phase of burn treatment is related to pain, the presence of dressings and splints, surgical procedures, and wound contractures.

Outcomes. The client will maintain soft tissue length, as evidenced by maintaining ROM without manifestations of early contracture formation.

Interventions. The main interventions during the acute phase of injury are splinting, positioning, and ROM exercises. Collaboration with physical and occupational therapists is essential for guidance in an individualized program for each client.

Optimal positioning of the client involves continuing use of anticontracture positions. Maintaining burned areas in a position of physiologic function by either splinting or positioning will help to prevent or reduce contracture development.

Encourage the client to participate in ADL, to ambulate, and to spend time sitting up in a chair. These activities will not only improve mobility but also assist in moving the client toward independence.

Diagnosis: Disturbed Personal Identity. During the acute burn phase, the client recognizes the extent of injury and realizes that his or her body is changed. Depression, grief, fear, and anxiety confront the client.

Outcomes. The client will acknowledge body changes and demonstrate movement toward incorporating these changes into the self-concept. The client will not exhibit maladaptive responses such as severe depression.

Interventions. The client can be expected to experience emotional lability while progressing through recovery. Staff members should provide an accepting atmosphere for the client, although the client should be assisted to exercise control over any destructive behaviors. Family members or significant others should be involved in care as much as possible to demonstrate continued support for the client. Staff members should be available to provide information about the appearance of burns and grafts and to explain changes that can be expected over time (healed burn wounds, graft sites, and donor sites may change in appearance for up to 1 year after injury). Providing information helps to reduce misconceptions and can give hope that the painful procedures can produce good cosmetic results.

Diagnosis: Disabled Family Coping. Recognize that families often imagine that the survival of the family unit is threatened following a member's injury. Normal coping mechanisms become overwhelmed.

Outcomes. Family members will demonstrate coping strategies, as evidenced by verbalizing realistic expectations for client outcomes, expressing knowledge of the goals of the treatment regimen, interacting appropriately with the client, and demonstrating decreased emotional stress.

Interventions. Once beyond the resuscitative phase, it is important to provide the family members or significant others with information about what to expect for the burn-injured client in the future. It is helpful to provide families with daily updates regarding changes in the client's condition. This assists in maintaining realistic perceptions of the client's progress. Assist the family in finding ways to nurture the client and to participate in some aspects of care. These measures not only assure the client of the family's love and acceptance but also allow family members or significant others to regain some feelings of control. It may also be useful to introduce the family members to the local burn support group. Burn survivors and their families can provide emotional support and validation and can reinforce the concept that it is possible to survive and live happily and productively after a burn injury.

Surgical Management in the Acute Phase of Burn Injury

Definitive wound care for full-thickness burns is accomplished by *autografting,* the surgical removal of a superficial layer of the client's own unburned skin, which is subsequently grafted to the excised or granulating burn wound. Because the epidermis is split (in layers) rather than taken in full, these grafts are referred to as *split-thickness grafts.* This procedure is performed in the operating room while the client is under general anesthesia. Autografts can be applied either as a sheet *(sheet graft)* or in a meshed form *(meshed graft).*

A sheet autograft is applied to the excised wound bed without alteration in its integrity (Figure 50-10). Sheet autografts are frequently used to graft burns in visible areas (e.g., face, neck, hands).

In contrast, a meshed autograft contains many little slits that allow for expansion of the donor skin (Figure 50-11). Meshing permits coverage of larger areas of irregularly shaped wounds and allows for drainage from a bleeding wound bed. When healed, the meshed pattern of the autograft remains visible. Therefore meshed grafts are often used on hidden body areas. When a thicker layer of skin is removed, consisting of the epidermis and the dermis, this is referred to as a *full-thickness graft.* For all autografts, the area of the body from which the skin was removed is referred to as the *donor site* (Figure 50-12).

■ **FIGURE 50–10** Split-thickness sheet autograft of the hand on postoperative day 3. Note the use of medical adhesive tape (white coloring) that has been used at the junctions between grafts and graft and intact skin to help affix the graft to the wound bed. Tape is removed at postoperative day 7-10.

■ **FIGURE 50–11** Split-thickness meshed autograft of the foot on postoperative day 5. Note the thin layer of dressing material covering the meshed graft. This dressing provides protection while not preventing wound drainage.

■ **FIGURE 50–12** Harvesting donor skin from the lateral portion of the client's thigh.

Graft adherence is dependent on the formation of a fibrin bond between the recipient bed and the graft. There are no vascular connections between the graft and the wound bed immediately after surgery. The graft is held in place only by weak fibrin bonds and is nourished by the diffusion of serum from the wound bed. The graft begins to stabilize after 3 days as a fibrovascular and collagen network form and provide durability to the graft.

SAFETY ALERT

A bleeding wound bed, hematoma formation, or shearing of the graft disrupts formation of this bond between graft and bed. Care must be taken during the postoperative period to assess for bleeding, remove accumulated serum beneath sheet grafts (as described next in the discussion on nursing management of the surgical client), and prevent unwanted movement and shearing of autografts.

Various types of dressings are used to cover donor sites, depending on the size, location, and condition of adjacent skin or tissue (see Table 50-2).

SAFETY ALERT

However, despite the differences in dressings, the donor site wound requires the same meticulous care as for other partial-thickness wounds, to expedite healing and prevent infection. If the donor site becomes infected, the dressing should be gently removed or soaked off. The wound can then be thoroughly cleansed and an antimicrobial agent applied.

Once the donor site has healed, lubricating lotions can be applied to soften the area and reduce itching. Donor sites can be reused after they are healed.

Cultured *epithelial autografting* is a technique for closure of massive burn wounds. The process of autologous epithelial cell growth begins with taking a full-thickness skin specimen from an uninjured body site. This specimen is sent to a specialized laboratory for culture and growth. Typically, in 3 to 4 weeks, several sheets of cultured epithelial autografts are ready for application. In the operating room, the cultured epithelial autograft sheets are carefully applied to an excised and nonbleeding wound bed and are secured in place with staples. Dressings are applied and moistened with an antibiotic solution shown to be nontoxic to the cultured epithelial autografts.

Reports demonstrating the success of cultured epithelial autografts in the treatment of massive burn wounds have been limited. Both early and late cultured epithelial autograft loss resulting from mechanical shearing, nutritional imbalance, infection, or an autoimmune response has been reported.

Nursing Management of the Surgical Client in the Acute Phase of Burn Injury

Preoperative Care

Routine care of clients undergoing surgery is discussed in Chapter 14. Specific preoperative care of the client scheduled for burn surgery includes providing information about areas to be excised and plans for pain control. Specific orders for medications to be given or withheld and the time to begin *nil per os* (NPO) (i.e., nothing by month) status should be obtained.

Before skin grafting, clients need information on the type of skin graft to be placed (e.g., sheet graft, meshed graft, cultured epithelial autografts), the location of the donor site, the postoperative plans for pain control, and the need for immobility and elevation of the graft site postoperatively. Fears over scarring should be addressed; in general, scarring cannot be predicted because scar tissue requires a full year to mature. Both debridement and grafting can require multiple procedures, and clients may become anxious over repeated surgical procedures. Severe anxiety should be communicated to the surgeon and anesthesia personnel.

Postoperative Care

Routine postoperative care is discussed in Chapter 14. Care specific to excised wounds includes assessment of bleeding and pain control. Many clients report more pain in donor sites (because of exposed nerve endings) than in recipient sites. Donor sites are dressed with occlusive dressings. Skin-grafted sites must be immobilized to promote adherence of the graft to the wound bed. Various techniques are used, including suture, staples, tape, splints and dressings. Because blebs (pockets) of serum or hematomas may develop beneath the sheet graft, postoperative dressings are often removed within 24 hours for an assessment. If blebs or hematomas are evident, they must be removed or the risk of graft loss is high. A small needle (e.g., 25 gauge) is used to aspirate fluid beneath the graft, or a small slit in the graft is made with a scalpel and the fluid is rolled out with a cotton-tipped applicator. Skin-grafted sites are elevated to prevent edema. Swelling of edematous tissue can lift the graft off of the wound bed. Bed rest may be prescribed. When the graft is on the lower legs, the client should typically not walk until postoperative day 3 to 7 to be certain the graft has appropriately adhered.

Rehabilitation Phase

The rehabilitation phase of recovery represents the final phase of burn recovery and encompasses the time from wound closure to discharge and beyond. In order for the best outcomes to be achieved, caregivers must understand the consequences of burn injury, and treatment for rehabilitation must begin from the day of injury. Rehabilitation should overlap the acute care phase and last well beyond the acute inpatient hospitalization. Ultimately, a burn rehabilitation program is designed for maximal functional and emotional recovery. Measures to promote wound healing, to prevent or minimize deformities and hypertrophic scarring, to increase physical strength and function, to promote emotional support, and to provide education are a part of the ongoing rehabilitation phase.

The Bridge to Home Health Care feature below describes rehabilitative care for the client after discharge from the hospital.

Medical Management in the Rehabilitation Phase of Burn Injury

Minimize Functional Loss

Early wound excision helps minimize short-term and long-term functional loss by closing the wound, minimizing infection, and eliminating wound pain. A skin graft, although more elastic than eschar, still does not have normal elasticity. The resultant wound stiffness must be counterbalanced with aggressive therapy and splinting.

Exercise, splinting, and positioning continue through all phases of burn injury; however, it is during this phase that the importance of these efforts becomes paramount. These measures are crucial to the client's progression to optimal functional independence.

Hypertrophic scarring, which results from an overabundant deposition of collagen in the healed burn wound, can be minimized with the use of massage and pressure therapy. Constant pressure applied to healing burn wounds through the use of custom-fit pressure garments has been found to reduce scarring in some individuals. Several commercially available products provide the constant, even pressure that is required. Although hypertrophic scarring usually does not peak until several months after the injury, it is important to plan ahead before the onset of loss of function. If custom-fit pressure garments are to be prescribed, the client should have been measured for the garments by the time of hospital discharge or by their first outpatient visit (Figure 50-13). It is important that these garments fit properly and are checked often during the early post-discharge phase of recovery.

Provide Psychosocial Support

In this last phase of recovery, during which the wounds are almost healed and specific plans are made for hospital discharge, the client will face numerous issues and concerns. Self-image issues, pain, physical limitations,

BRIDGE TO HOME HEALTH CARE

Managing After Burns

When admitting the burn-injured client to home health services, remember that each client is unique and involves detailed treatment instructions. In the nursing assessment, include the responses of both the client and the family members to hospital discharge and return home. If clients require assistance with wound care and activities of daily living (ADL), they will need a primary caregiver to provide both emotional support and direct care. This person is a critical member of the home health care delivery team.

Work with the client and the primary caregiver to set up a place in the home for dressing changes and storage of needed dressing materials. This area should be clean, comfortable, relaxing, and off-limits to family pets. If possible, select a room that clients do not use for other activities, especially sleeping, so that they do not associate these activities with painful dressing changes. The dressing materials and a current wound care plan can be neatly organized and stored in a sealed plastic box or plastic bag. Dressing supplies should be ordered in quantities that allow for single dressing changes, thus reducing wastage. In some agencies, prepackaged wound care kits provide an excellent method of infection control and significantly reduce the amount of waste.

Although dressing changes and physical therapy can be painful experiences for the client, both are essential for recovery. Identify ways to decrease the pain or the length of time during which pain is experienced. Work with the physical therapist, the client, and the family to determine the best schedule for these activities. Consider scheduling joint visits if this would improve

the care given to the client. Instruct a family member on when to give prescribed pain medications in order to provide the best relief for the client. Timing of medication administration depends on the dose and route of pain medication. Typically, at this stage in the recovery, the client is receiving only oral medications. While changing dressings, consider the use of music or relaxation techniques, and involve the client and family as much as possible. These strategies offer a sense of control and can decrease anxiety and the perception of pain.

Unless mechanical debridement of the wound is necessary, the dressings should not stick to the wound bed. Avoid removing dried-on, adhered dressings because they cause unnecessary pain. If the dressings are adhered to the wound, soak them off with normal saline or water. Collaborate with the primary physician or a wound care nurse to obtain an appropriate moisture-retentive dressing to reduce or eliminate pain with dressing changes.

Rehabilitation of clients who have suffered burn injury involves more than dressing changes and physical therapy. It is also important to consider the psychological stress of the initial injury, scarring, and surgical procedures and other treatments as well as the financial burden from loss of work time and the lengthy recovery period.[12] Evaluate the need of the client and family members for referrals to local agencies that offer social, counseling, financial, and spiritual services as well as support groups. Such services may be essential in order for clients and their families to cope with the traumatic life event that a major burn injury with its sequelae represents.

■ **FIGURE 50–13** Custom-fit pressure garments. Pressure therapy helps to minimize the development of hypertrophic (raised, reddened) scars.

reintegration into society, and fear of rejection represent only a few of the issues the client must handle as discharge nears. During this time, it is important to maintain good communication with the client. It is beneficial to the client for the staff to encourage independence and convey the message that survivors can find ways to achieve whatever goals they set for themselves. Pain control and anxiety prevention continue to require assessment and medical management as needed. Psychosocial assistance for the client and family members or significant others should carry through to hospital discharge. Providing information on local community resources that will be of assistance after hospital discharge is important for continued support and assistance. Additionally, national survivor organizations such as the Phoenix Society for Burn Survivors (www.phoenix-society.org) can be of great benefit and support. Providing clients with the names and telephone numbers of burn clinic staff and rehabilitation staff for urgent questions has also been found to be helpful during this transition period from hospital to home. Vocational rehabilitation may also be required if the burns involved the hands and arms.

Nursing Management of the Medical Client in the Rehabilitation Phase of Burn Injury

Assessment. Once the client and family are able to manage the care of the client, the focus becomes preparing them for discharge to a home setting (for some clients, other settings will be necessary). Nurses will assess the client and family's comprehension of teaching and ability to perform needed care. Nurses will also determine the best methods to teach the client and family. The client's psychological status and need for vocational rehabilitation will be addressed during this final phase.

Diagnosis, Outcomes, Interventions
Diagnosis: Impaired Physical Mobility. During the rehabilitation phase of burn injury, the client's physical mobility and ability to provide self-care are impaired by the presence of dressings, pain, scarring, contracture, and muscle atrophy.

Outcomes. The client will have improved physical mobility, as evidenced by maximum independence in performance of ADL, with minimum disability and disfigurement.

Interventions. The physical and occupational therapy consultations initiated in the early phases of burn injury are especially important for continued treatment in the rehabilitation phase as the client works toward functional independence. Typically, the therapist provides an individualized rehabilitation schedule as well as needed assistive devices for the client.

Motivate the client to participate in self-care activities such as brushing teeth and self-feeding, because this increased activity will not only improve mobility but also lessen dependence. Provide assistive devices furnished by therapy consultants to assist the client with any limitations. Expect tasks to take longer when the client works independently. Allow adequate time for the client to complete the undertaking. Self-confidence will be gained with independent functioning regardless of the time spent.

Encourage active ROM every 2 to 4 hours while the client is awake unless contraindicated because of a recent grafting procedure. Increased activity prevents muscle atrophy, tendon adherence, joint stiffness, and capsular tightness. Help the client to ambulate to promote muscle strength and cardiopulmonary reserve. Provide passive exercise and stretching if the client is unable to actively participate.

Wrap donor sites on both burned and unburned legs with elastic bandage wraps (Ace bandages), using a figure-eight technique at the feet and a spiral up the legs, before placing the limbs in a dependent position. The support will decrease capillary venous stasis, which impairs wound healing.

Explain the rationale for activities to the client and family members, because understanding improves compliance. Avoid the position of comfort, and maintain burned areas in the position of physiologic function, within the client's limit of endurance. Continue to follow the splinting and positioning regimen recommended in the therapy consultation.

Diagnosis: Acute Pain and Chronic Pain. Pain experienced during the rehabilitation phase of burn injury is typically associated with wound care and therapeutic activity, particularly ROM exercises.

Outcomes. The client will have an acceptable level of comfort, as evidenced by verbalizing relief or control of pain or discomfort and actively participating in care.

Interventions. Formulate a plan for controlling the client's pain based on an assessment of the client's response to pain and documentation of previous successful treatment regimens. As in the earlier phases of injury, allow adequate time for the onset of the medication for maximum benefits of the medication. Nonpharmacologic methods of pain control, such as relaxation techniques, music therapy, guided imagery, distraction, and hypnosis, may improve the client's comfort, even if such methods were not successful in the earlier phases of injury. In preparation for impending discharge, the client should at some point during the rehabilitation phase progress to analgesia given only by the oral route. Again, document pain scores before and after analgesia.

Diagnosis: Disturbed Personal Identity. The client is at risk for self-esteem disturbances related to threatened or actual change in body image, physical loss, and loss of role responsibilities.

Outcomes. The client will develop improved self-esteem, as evidenced by making social contact with others outside the immediate family, developing effective coping mechanisms throughout the stages of recovery, and verbalizing feelings about self-concept.

Interventions. Allowing time for two-way communication with the client is especially important during this phase of injury. Provide an atmosphere of acceptance as the client tries various coping strategies to deal with the injury. Provide honest and accurate information about the client's projected appearance to reduce misconceptions that he or she may have.

Assess the need for limit setting for maladaptive behavior. Consult with burn team members to establish such limits and to formulate a treatment plan for such behaviors; explain limit setting to family members or significant others and assist them to maintain the same limits. Promote the client's self-confidence by providing information about the progress made, and support the client's role in care and treatment, providing encouragement and positive reinforcement.

Encourage family members to interact with the client, because this encouragement facilitates societal reintegration. During this phase of recovery, encourage the client to interact with others outside the facility. Use of a family day pass during this time is useful. Help to prepare the client for social interaction after discharge by discussing potential situations and how the client might deal with them. Such preparation provides rehearsal of events and reduces anxiety.

Diagnosis: Impaired Skin Integrity. The expectation is that by the time the client reaches the rehabilitation phase of burn injury, the majority of wounds will be healed (either by reepithelialization or autograft). The new skin over areas of donor site, graft, and healed burn is characteristically very thin, with disrupted oil glands. The healed skin is fragile; it can be very dry and shears or cracks easily.

Outcomes. The client will have intact skin with no evidence of infection, breakdown, or blistering.

Interventions. Daily wound and skin care should continue throughout hospitalization. Clean burned areas, grafts, and donor sites daily with a mild soap (without fragrance) and water. Rinse thoroughly to remove the soap. After cleaning, the healed skin should be lubricated with a nonirritating, alcohol-free moisturizer. Itching associated with dry skin can be minimized with application of the moisturizer at least three times a day. Avoid any shearing of skin with dressings, clothing, or splints.

Diagnosis: Deficient Knowledge. The burn-injured client or a family member or significant other must have knowledge of important treatment modalities that need continuation after discharge from the hospital.

Outcomes. The client or a family member or significant other will verbalize knowledge and demonstrate techniques that facilitate continued wound healing and limb mobility.

Interventions. Demonstrate and discuss the following skin care interventions with the client and appropriate family member or significant other: daily skin and wound care and dressing instructions if any; lubrication of grafts, donor sites, and healed burn wounds using an alcohol-free skin moisturizer; wearing pressure dressings or garments for 23 hours daily; and avoidance of direct sunlight for 1 year after injury because of increased sensitivity to ultraviolet rays.

Review current medications and the dosage, precautions, and potential side effects. Discuss nutritional needs and the benefits of diets with adequate protein and calories.

Provide information on support groups of peers and/or counseling as needed for adjustment to life outside the hospital setting. Stress the need for follow-up care, and provide appointment dates and times if these have been established.

CONCLUSIONS

Nursing care of the burn-injured client is both complex and challenging. The psychological and physical trauma sustained following a burn injury can be devastating for both the survivor and the family members or significant others. Having a thorough understanding of the pathophysiologic changes that occur after a burn, knowing what to expect clinically as a result of the injury, and becoming familiar with the standards of care will guide nursing care. As a key member of the burn team, you are responsible for an individualized plan of care that reflects the client's changing needs during progression through the different phases of recovery. Priority issues and care change as the client moves from the critical resuscitative phase into and, ultimately, through the rehabilitation period.

THINKING CRITICALLY

1. You are working on the night shift in your hospital's burn center and receive a call that a client is in transport via ambulance to your unit. He will be a direct admission and bypass the emergency department. The telephone report describes that the client was found unconscious on the floor of the bedroom. He is covered with soot and has obvious burns on his face, arms, and torso. An intravenous line of lactated Ringer's solution is started and is running wide open. Oxygen is being administered via face mask. On admission, the client is received lying in the supine position on a gurney. He is restless, confused, and combative. He appears anxious and in pain. The eyebrows, eyelashes, and hair are singed. There is soot in the nares and mouth and on the tongue. His voice is raspy, and he is coughing up thick black sputum. Breath sounds are scattered crackles; oxygen saturation is 75%. A face mask is in place but was disconnected from the oxygen tank while the client was being moved onto the burn center gurney.

Heart rate is 142 beats/min, with sinus tachycardia. Respiratory rate is 40 breaths/min and labored. Blood pressure is 144/88 mm Hg; temperature is 35° C. Bowel sounds are absent. There is thick, white leathery eschar on the chest, neck, left and right arms, and hands. The skin of the face and back are pink, moist, and blistered. The body from the waist to the feet is unburned. An IV line is infusing lactated Ringer's solution through the right antecubital vein. Weight is 85 kg. What priorities should be set for the client's care? What interventions should be undertaken?

Factors to Consider. What is the client's respiratory status? Do the physical examination and history provided by the ambulance crew give any clues to his respiratory status? What should you consider when administering analgesia or anxiolytics to this client? What is the client's fluid volume status? How will you monitor fluid resuscitation?

2. It is now 7 days after the injury and the client has just returned to the burn intensive care unit after receiving autografts on his chest, neck, bilateral arms, hands, and axillae. Donor skin was taken circumferentially from both thighs. What assessments should you perform? What interventions should be undertaken?

Factors to Consider. What factors disrupt graft adherence? What can you do to help prevent contracture formation?

3. It is now 2 months since the client was injured and discharge plans are being finalized. The client tells you that he is concerned about his ability to manage at home. What can you do to help the client?

Factors to Consider. What concerns might a burn survivor face upon discharge from the hospital? What professional resources might be helpful? What lay resources might be helpful?

Discussions for these questions can be found on the website.

BIBLIOGRAPHY

Citations appearing in red refer to primary research.

Citations appearing in blue refer to evidence-based practice guidelines and protocols.

1. Adcock, R., Boeve, S., & Patterson, D. (1998). Psychological and emotional recovery. In G.J. Carrougher (Ed.), *Burn care and therapy* (pp. 329-347). St. Louis: Mosby.
2. American Burn Association. (2006). *Burn incidence and treatment in the US: 2007 fact sheet* [online]. Available at www.ameriburn.org/resources_factsheetphp.
3. American Burn Association. (1984). Guidelines for service standards and severity classification in the treatment of burn injuries. *Bulletin of the American College of Surgeons, 69*, 24-28.
4. American College of Surgeons: Committee on Trauma. (1987). *A guide to prophylaxis against tetanus in wound management.* Chicago: American College of Surgeons.
5. Barillo, D.J., & Goode, R. (1996). Fire fatality study: Demographics of fire victims. *Burns, 22*, 85-88.
6. Carrougher, G.J., Ptacek, J.T., Honari, S., et al. (2006). Self-reports of anxiety in burn injured hospitalized adults during routine wound care. *Journal of Burn Care and Research, 27*, 676-681.
7. Carrougher, G.J. (1998). Burn wound assessment and topical treatment. In G.J. Carrougher (Ed.), *Burn care and therapy* (pp. 133-159). St. Louis: Mosby.
8. Cioffi, W.G. (1998). Inhalation injury. In G.J. Carrougher (Ed.), *Burn care and therapy* (pp. 35-59). St. Louis: Mosby.
9. deJong, A.E.E., Middelkoop, E., Faber, A.W., VanLoey, N.E.E. (2007). Non-pharmacological nursing interventions for procedural pain relief in adults with burns: A systematic literature review. *Burns, 33*, 811-827.
10. Esselman, P.C., Thombs, B.D., Magyar-Russell, G., et al. (2006). Burn rehabilitation: State of the science. *American Journal of Physical Medicine and Rehabilitation, 85*, 383-413.
11. Faucher, L., & Furukawa, K. (2006). Practice guidelines for the management of pain. *Journal of Burn Care and Research, 27*, 659-668.
12. Fauerbach, J.A., Engrav, L., & Kowalske, K. (2001). Barriers to employment among working-aged patients with major burn injury. *Journal of Burn Care and Rehabilitation, 22*, 26-34.
13. Hall, B. (2005). Wound care for burn patients in acute rehabilitation settings. *Rehabilitation Nursing, 30*, 114-119.
14. Honari, S. (2004). Topical therapies and antimicrobials in the management of burn wounds. *Critical Care Nursing Clinics of North America, 16*, 1-11.
15. Kramer, G., Lund, T., & Herndon, D.N. (2002). Pathophysiology of burn shock and burn edema. In D.N. Herndon (Ed.), *Total burn care* (pp. 78-87). London: Saunders.
16. Marvin, J.A. (1998). Management of pain and anxiety. In G.J. Carrougher (Ed.), *Burn care and therapy* (pp. 167-183). St. Louis: Mosby.
17. Pruitt, B., Goodwin, C., & Mason, A. (2002). Epidemiological, demographic and outcome characteristics of burn injury. In D.N. Herndon (Ed.), *Total burn care* (pp. 16-20). London: Saunders.
18. Runyon, C.W., Bangdiwala, S.I., & Linzar, M.A. (1992). Risk factors for fatal residential fires. *New England Journal of Medicine, 327*, 859-863.
19. Wilson, D., & Bailie, F. (1999). Night attire burns in young girls: The return of an old adversary. *Burns, 25*, 269-271.

evolve *Did you remember to check out the bonus material on the Evolve website and the CD-ROM, including NCLEX®-Examination Style Review Questions, Open-Book Quizzes, and Chapter Review Audio Podcasts?*

http://evolve.elsevier.com/Black/medsurg

UNIT 12

VASCULAR DISORDERS

ANATOMY AND PHYSIOLOGY REVIEW:

The Vascular System

Robert G. Carroll

The vascular system is a vast network of vessels through which blood circulates in the body. The major functions of the cardiovascular system—delivery of nutrients to tissues and removal of metabolic wastes—are accomplished in the capillaries. Blood leaving the ventricles is distributed through arteries and arterioles, in progressively smaller branches to the capillaries (a *divergent* pattern, like a river to a delta). Blood leaving the capillaries follows progressively larger venules and veins on its way back to the atria (a *convergent* pattern, like tributaries flowing into a river).

The anatomic arrangement of blood vessels allows regulation of blood flow at the individual tissue level so that blood flow delivery can be proportional to the tissue's metabolic needs. Because the volume of blood flowing from the arteries to the capillaries is a major determinant of blood pressure, the blood pressure control systems also include control of arteriolar diameter by the sympathetic nervous system and circulating hormones.

STRUCTURES OF THE VASCULAR SYSTEM

Two series of blood vessels—the systemic and the pulmonary circulations—distribute blood to the capillaries and return blood to the heart. Blood exiting the left ventricle enters the *systemic circulation,* passing progressively through the aorta, arteries, arterioles, capillaries, venules, veins, and finally the vena cava before entering the right atrium (Figure A&P12-1). For the *pulmonary circulation,* blood flows from the right ventricle into the pulmonary artery, and then passes through arterioles, pulmonary capillaries, and venules before returning to the pulmonary vein and the left atrium.

GENERAL BLOOD VESSEL STRUCTURE

The anatomic division of blood vessels into arteries, arterioles, capillaries, venules, and veins is based on the presence of up to three histologic layers (Figure A&P12-2):

1. The *tunica intima* (innermost layer) consists of endothelial cells that separate the blood from the extravascular spaces. The tightness of the junctions

between the endothelial cells varies among tissues. For example, the very tight junctions of cerebral capillaries restrict movement of some drugs to brain cells (the blood-brain barrier). In contrast, the endothelial cell holes and relatively loose junctions in the liver and spleen allow easy transit between the blood and tissue spaces in those organs. The endothelium has surface proteins, or *adhesion molecules,* that facilitate the attachment of white blood cells and their movement from the circulation to the tissues. The endothelium generates substances such as endothelial-derived relaxing factor (EDRF, or nitric oxide), allowing nitroglycerin, friction, and stress to cause vasodilation. Damage to the endothelium may allow blood to enter the middle layer of a blood vessel, creating an aneurysm.

2. The *tunica media* (middle layer) consists of elastic connective tissue and smooth muscle cells. Particularly in the aorta and large arteries, the elastic tissue contributes to the shape of the arterial pressure pulse. Smooth muscle contraction regulates the diameter of the vessel and causes a change in blood flow and blood pressure. Smooth muscle is normally partially contracted because of sympathetic nerve activity (also known as sympathetic tone). Smooth muscle contraction can also be regulated by circulating hormones and (in the smaller vessels) by tissue metabolic factors.

3. The *tunica adventitia* (outermost layer) consists of a relatively thin layer of connective tissue that provides shape for the blood vessels. This layer also houses the *vasa vasorum,* the small arteries and veins that provide nutrients to the cells of the blood vessel.

VASCULAR SEGMENTS

Arteries and Arterioles

Arteries, particularly the aorta, have an extensive elastic tissue layer that accounts for the difference between arterial pressure (120/80 mm Hg) and left ventricular pressure (120/10 mm Hg). The elastic tissue stretches during ventricular ejection, storing energy. When the aortic valve closes and ventricular ejection stops, recoil of the elastic tissue slows the fall of arterial pressure during the interval until the next period of ventricular ejection. The efficiency of the elastic tissue decreases with age and with

Right and left common carotid arteries
Right subclavian a.
Axillary a.
Ascending aorta
Brachial a.
Diaphragm
Hepatic a.
Superior mesenteric a.
Ulnar a.
Radial a.
Inguinal ligament
Deep palmar arch
Superficial palmar arch
Digital a.
Descending branch of lateral circumflex a.
Peroneal a.
Posterior tibial a.
Anterior tibial a.
Dorsalis pedis a.
Digital a.

Brachiocephalic a.
Left subclavian a.
Aortic arch
Thoracic aorta
Splenic a.
Renal a.
Abdominal aorta
Inferior mesenteric a.
Common iliac a.
External iliac a.
Obturator and gluteal a.
Internal iliac a.
Femoral a.
Deep femoral a.

ARTERIES

Brachiocephalic vein
Cephalic v.
Brachial v.
Basilic v.
Hepatic v.
Median cubital v.
Median antebrachial v.
Superficial palmar network
Digital v.
Great saphenous v.
Small saphenous v.
Tibial v.
Dorsal venous arch
Digital v.

Internal jugular v.
External jugular v.
Superior vena cava
Renal v.
Inferior vena cava
Common iliac v.
External iliac v.
Internal iliac v.
Femoral v.

VEINS

From heart
Arteriole
Endothelium
Smooth muscle fiber
Metarteriole
Precapillary sphincters (relaxed)
True capillary
Capillary bed
Smooth muscle fiber
Throroughfare channel
Endothelium
Venule
To heart

■ **FIGURE A&P12–1** Major systemic arteries and veins. *Inset,* Capillary network.

■ **FIGURE A&P12–2** Structure of blood vessels.

atherosclerosis, contributing to the rise in systolic arterial blood pressure usually seen in older adults.

Arterioles (5 to 100 μm in diameter) contain a high proportion of vascular smooth muscle. The degree of contraction of this muscle is regulated by background activity of the autonomic nervous system, primarily the sympathetic nerves. In addition, circulating hormones such as epinephrine, norepinephrine, and angiotensin II can cause smooth muscle contraction. These substances are produced as metabolic by-products, so they allow the individual tissue beds to receive the blood they need.

Microcirculation

The microcirculation consists of the small arterioles, the capillary beds, and the small venules (see Figure A&P12-1, *inset*). Blood flows freely between an arteriole and a venule through a vessel channel called a thoroughfare channel. Capillaries extend from this channel, and structures called precapillary sphincters control the flow of blood between the arteriole and capillaries. The precapillary sphincters contain muscle fibers that allow them to control blood flow.

The smooth muscle of the small arterioles is contracted by sympathetic nerves, but local factors become increasingly important as the diameter of the vessel decreases. The *precapillary sphincters* (the last band of smooth muscle before the capillaries) respond only to local factors. Blood passes from the arterioles into capillaries (5 to 10 μm in diameter). The capillary diameter approaches that of the red blood cell (7 μm). Capillaries have only a tunica intima (see Figure A&P12-2), and the small wall thickness facilitates exchange by diffusion. In tissues such as the skin, blood also passes through *metarterioles* (10 to 100 μm in diameter). Metarterioles are not exchange vessels but serve a separate role. Decreased blood flow through cutaneous metarterioles helps the body conserve heat; increased flow enhances heat loss.

Venules and Veins

Venules (10 to 100 μm in diameter) collect drainage from the capillaries in a convergent flow pattern. Venule smooth muscle is innervated by sympathetic nerves. Along with the veins, venules serve as capacitance (volume storage) areas, containing up to 75% of the circulating blood volume as a result of their ability to expand. Permeability of the postcapillary venules is regulated by hormones such as histamine and bradykinin. Note that angiogenesis is initiated in the postcapillary venules.

Veins are characterized by high volume and low pressure. Sympathetic nerve activity constricts the smooth muscle of the veins and helps move blood toward the heart. Blood flow toward the heart is also assisted by gravity (for veins in the head) and valves that ensure a unidirectional flow along with surrounding muscle contraction. Damage to venous valves can cause swellings, such as varicose veins, and lack of leg muscle movement can lead to venous stasis and clotting.

Lymphatics

Lymph is excess fluid in the interstitial space not removed by the venous system. Lymphatics are a network of endothelial tubes that merge to form two large ducts that enter the vena cava. Terminal lymphatics lack tight junctions, allowing large proteins (and metastasizing cancer cells) to enter the circulatory system through the lymphatic system. In the gastrointestinal tract, lymphatics allow digested fats to enter the circulation. Lymph is propelled by (1) massaging from adjacent muscle, (2) tissue pressure, and (3) contraction of the lymph vessels. Valves ensure that the flow of lymph, which over 24 hours is a volume equal to the total blood volume, is toward the vena cava. Lymph is filtered in lymph nodes before progressing back to the circulation (Figure A&P12-3).

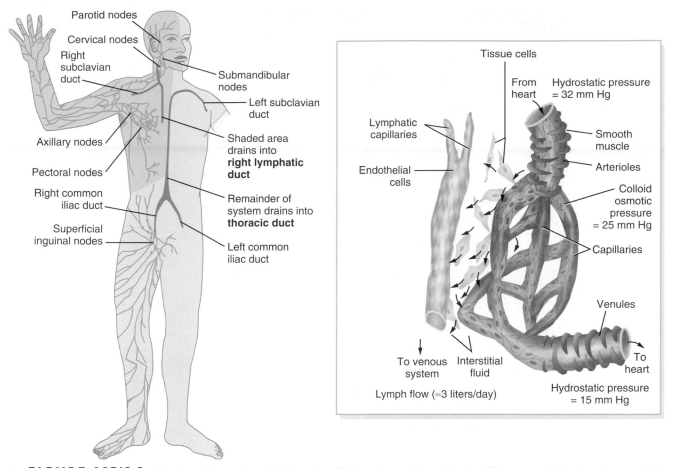

■ **FIGURE A&PI2–3** Major lymphatic vessels and drainage. *Inset,* Fluid exchange at the capillary bed. The primary driving force to move fluids from the capillary is *hydrostatic pressure.* The primary pulling force to bring fluids back into the vessel is *colloid osmotic pressure* from the proteins in the capillary fluids (e.g., albumin). The hydrostatic pressure at the arterial end of the capillary is 32 mm Hg. As the fluid moves through the capillary, the pressure falls. Because proteins do not move across the capillary endothelium, colloid osmotic pressure is constant at 25 mm Hg. Thus at the arterial end the hydrostatic pressure is greater than the colloid osmotic pressure, and fluids then move into interstitial spaces. The opposite is true at the venous end where pressure falls to 15 mm Hg. The hydrostatic pressure is lower than the colloid osmotic pressure, and fluids thus return to the capillary. There is a net loss of fluids out of the capillary (approximately 3 L/day). This fluid is absorbed by the lymphatic system and is returned to circulation at the lymphatic duct.

FUNCTION OF THE VASCULAR SYSTEM

PRESSURE, FLOW, AND RESISTANCE

The relationship of arterial pressure, cardiac output, and total peripheral resistance is shown by the following equation:

$$Q = \frac{\Delta P}{R}$$

Or

$$\text{Flow} = \frac{\text{Pressure Gradient}}{\text{Resistance}}$$

Resistance

In the body, arterial *pressure* is regulated. A decrease in arterial pressure is corrected by a reflex increase in cardiac output and an increase in total peripheral resistance, both mediated by an increase in sympathetic nervous system activity. For a capillary bed, however, *flow* is regulated. If flow is too low, the arteriole dilates and the decrease in resistance allows flow to increase.

Resistance affects blood flow according to the (1) radius of the vessel, (2) fluid viscosity, and (3) length of the vessel. Of these factors, vessel radius is the most powerful mechanism for controlling resistance and the one that is physiologically most important. If the radius of the vessel decreases to one half the starting value, resistance to flow increases 16-fold. The body utilizes vascular smooth muscle to alter the diameter of arteries and arterioles and therefore to regulate both pressure and flow. Occasionally, changes in blood viscosity can alter resistance, particularly when the hematocrit is increased (*polycythemia*) or decreased (*anemia*). Resistance increases as viscosity increases and decreases as viscosity decreases.

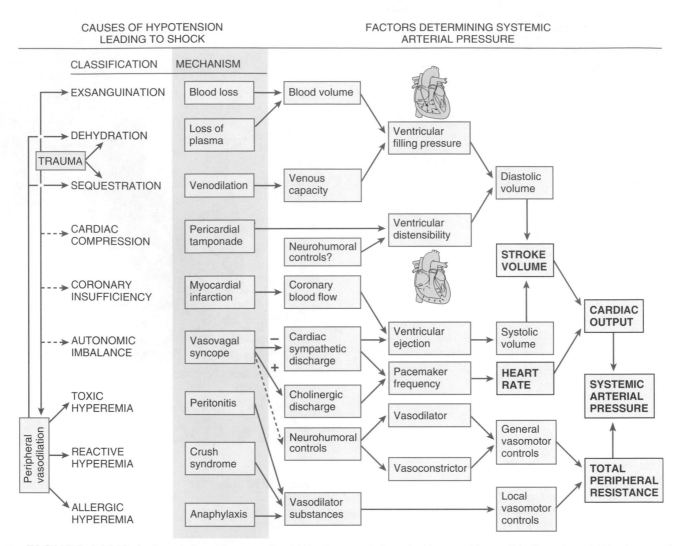

FIGURE A&P12–4 Control of arterial pressure. Arterial blood pressure is determined by several factors. *Right,* Systemic arterial blood pressure is controlled by two major factors: cardiac output and total peripheral vascular resistance. Cardiac output is also a function of two factors: stroke volume and heart rate. Reading the diagram from the right, you will find the factors that govern each step. Each bifurcation represents possible compensatory mechanisms. *Far left,* Disorders that can lead to shock. *(Modified from Rushmer, R.F. [1976]. Cardiovascular dynamics [p. 207]. Philadelphia: Saunders.)*

CAPILLARY EXCHANGE

Exchange of nutrients and wastes between the blood and the tissues is the primary purpose of the cardiovascular system. The movement of nutrients from the blood to the tissue and removal of metabolic wastes are driven by diffusion, filtration, and pinocytosis.

Diffusion

Diffusion is quantitatively the most important process. The rate of diffusion is enhanced by (1) increasing the surface area available for exchange, (2) increasing the concentration gradient, and (3) decreasing the distance that a substance must travel. In tissues such as exercising skeletal muscle, an increase in the number of perfused capillaries enhances the delivery of nutrients to the tissues. Altering arteriole flow to individual tissue beds is used to meet metabolic need.

Filtration

Fluid movement across the capillary depends on the balance of the hydrostatic pressure gradient (which favors filtration) and the oncotic pressure gradient from plasma proteins (which favors reabsorption) (Figure A&P12-4). In normal situations, the net force favors filtration at the arteriolar end of the capillary bed, and reabsorption at the venular end of the capillary bed. In most capillary beds, the volume filtered is slightly greater than the volume absorbed, and the excess fluid is removed from the tissue spaces by the lymph vessels. *Edema* (accumulation of fluid in the tissue spaces) occurs because of (1) increased filtration, (2) decreased reabsorption, or (3) impaired lymph drainage.

Pinocytosis

Pinocytosis is the movement of vesicles, especially from outside the cell to inside the cell. Pinocytosis is thought to be important only as a route for large proteins to cross the capillary wall.

CARDIOVASCULAR CONTROL

Much like the power and water supply systems in a city, the distribution of blood flow in the body depends on a sufficient driving pressure (arterial pressure), allowing the end users (capillary beds) to determine how much of the resource to utilize. Cardiovascular control is best described in terms of (1) regulation of arterial pressure and (2) local regulation of tissue blood flow.

Regulation of Arterial Pressure

The normal arterial pressure is maintained by a negative feedback mechanism called the *baroreceptor reflex* (Figure A&P12-5). A decrease in blood pressure immediately activates the sympathetic nervous system, increasing cardiac output (heart rate, venoconstriction for venous return, and cardiac contractility) and increasing peripheral resistance to trap blood within the arteries, and restores arterial blood pressure.

Longer term management of blood pressure is through baroreceptor control by volume-sensitive receptors in the low-pressure atria and veins. The volume of circulating blood is controlled by renal fluid balance and by endocrine vasoconstrictor agents such as angiotensin II, antidiuretic hormone (ADH), and norepinephrine. Chronic regulation of blood pressure depends on the volume of blood in the system and, ultimately, is tied to renal regulation of body fluid balance.

Chemoreceptors in the carotid body and aortic body are associated primarily with respiratory control but can elicit cardiovascular responses. A decrease in arterial O_2 concentration, an increase in arterial CO_2 concentration, or a drop in arterial pH can elicit a sympathetic response similar to that caused by a drop in arterial blood pressure.

Local Regulation of Blood Flow

If arterial pressure is sufficient, tissues can regulate their blood flow to match their metabolic needs. If blood flow is inadequate, metabolites such as carbon dioxide, adenosine, potassium, and acids accumulate, acting as vasodilators of the arteriolar smooth muscle to promote blood flow only in that local area. The resulting increase in blood flow washes out the metabolites and diminishes the vasodilator stimulus. This control system allows tissue blood flow to increase as tissue metabolic activity

Legend:
- Stimulus
- Receptor
- Integrating center
- Efferent pathway
- Effector
- Tissue response
- Systemic response

■ **FIGURE A&P12–5** Baroreceptor control of blood pressure. When baroreceptors sense a drop in blood pressure, they elicit an increase in sympathetic nervous system activity and a decrease in parasympathetic activity. The resultant vasoconstriction, increase in heart rate, and increase in ventricular contractility help to restore blood pressure to the starting point. *SA*, Sinoatrial. *(Modified from Silverthorn, D. [2001]. Human physiology [2nd ed.]. Upper Saddle River, NJ: Prentice Hall.)*

increases and accounts for the period of increased blood flow that follows a period of occlusion (called reactive hyperemia). In the long term, inadequate blood flow to a tissue can cause the growth of new capillaries (called collateral circulation), again matching blood flow to the tissue's metabolic needs. Blood flow to tissues such as the brain and myocardium is dominated by local control. The brain is exceptional at altering local flow, and in brain edema the systolic pressure rises in an attempt to provide the edematous brain with blood.

At the other extreme of regulation, cutaneous blood flow responds primarily to neural control. Because skin blood flow is tied to thermoregulation rather than nutrition, metabolic control is poorly developed. Other vascular beds, such as the kidney and the splanchnic circulation, respond both to sympathetic control and to local control. During increased sympathetic activity, blood flow to these tissues is decreased and is shunted to the brain and the myocardium.

CARDIOVASCULAR ADJUSTMENT TO EXERCISE

Cardiovascular control must balance the need for a steady arterial blood pressure against the ability to respond to a physiologic challenge. Exercise, which increases skeletal muscle consumption of oxygen and other nutrients, requires a marked increase in both cardiac output and skeletal muscle blood flow. The increase in cardiac output results from a cerebral cortical stimulation of the medullary cardiovascular center and activation of the sympathetic nervous system. The increased cardiac output requires an increased venous return, accomplished both by the arteriolar dilation of the skeletal muscle beds and by a sympathetic-mediated venous constriction. In rhythmic activity such as running, compression of the veins by the contracting skeletal muscle along with the negative intra-thoracic pressure from breathing assists the flow of venous blood toward the heart. In low cardiac output states, the brain and heart preferentially receive blood flow.

The increased cardiac output is preferentially directed to the exercising muscles (including the heart). Local factors in the exercising muscles cause a vasodilation of those vascular beds. The sympathetic activity constricts the arteriolar smooth muscle of the nonexercising vascular beds, such as the gastrointestinal tract, the kidney, and the nonworking muscles. Cerebral blood flow remains unchanged because that vascular bed is regulated primarily by local control. Cutaneous blood flow may be diminished initially but increases as the heat generated by the exercising muscles raises body core temperature, and cutaneous vasodilation helps to cool the body.

CONCLUSIONS

The vascular system is a series of vessels that transport blood to the capillary exchange vessels. In the capillaries, nutrients pass to the tissues and wastes pass into the blood for transport to excretory organs. Blood pressure regulation by the baroreceptor reflex ensures that arterial pressure remains sufficient to propel blood toward the tissues. Tissue blood flow is controlled by the metabolic needs of the tissues, and it increases when tissue metabolism increases.

BIBLIOGRAPHY

1. Berne, R., et al. (2004). *Physiology* (5th ed.). St. Louis: Mosby.
2. Carroll, R.G. (2007). *Elsevier's integrated physiology*. Philadelphia: Saunders.
3. Kierszenbaum, A.L. (2007). *Histology and cell biology: An introduction to pathology* (2nd ed.). St. Louis: Mosby.
4. Guyton, A., & Hall, J. (2006). *Textbook of medical physiology* (11th ed.). Philadelphia: Saunders.
5. Silverthorn, D. (2006). *Human physiology* (4th ed). San Francisco, Calif: Pearson Benjamin Cummings.

CHAPTER 51

Assessment of the Vascular System

MARY SIEGGREEN AND SUSANNE A. QUALLICH

There are several well-established risk factors for the development of atherosclerosis, including smoking, hyperlipidemia, hypertension, and diabetes. Several other conditions are contributors as well, such as obesity, a sedentary lifestyle, stress, hypertriglyceridemia, and family history.

Peripheral vascular disease is common among older clients and diabetic clients. It is characterized by disturbances of blood flow through the peripheral vessels. These disturbances eventually damage tissues as a result of ischemia, excessive accumulation of waste and fluid, or both. Damage can be a result of any disorder that narrows, obstructs, or injures blood vessels, thus impeding blood flow. Without intervention, damage may progress to the point of tissue or organ death.

HISTORY

When assessing the client, note risk factors for atherosclerosis and vascular disease (see Chapter 53), hypertension (see Chapter 52), diabetes mellitus (see Chapter 45), and cardiac (see Chapters 55 to 58) as well as lymphatic disorders. Some clients are reluctant to mention what they believe to be minor manifestations (swelling, intermittent discomfort). Consequently, perform a careful assessment, ask specific questions skillfully, and be alert for information that may indicate early manifestations of insidious conditions.

Studies have found that the effects of peripheral arterial disease (PAD) have significant psychosocial and emotional consequences. Assessment of quality of life as well as functional changes and symptom manifestations is needed to establish effective interventions. Seven themes emerged from one study[8] designed to evaluate the effects of PAD from clients' perspectives. The themes are (1) PAD diagnosis and management, (2) clinical manifestation (symptom) experience, (3) limitations in physical functioning, (4) limitations in social functioning, (5) compromise

of self, (6) uncertainty and fear, and (7) adaptation (see the website for a table with more information on these themes—Themes, Definitions, and Characteristics of Peripheral Arterial Disease).

Biographical and Demographic Data

Biographical data that are particularly relevant to the vascular system include the client's age. Atherosclerosis (hardening of the arteries) is more prevalent in older people. Venous disease, although also more prevalent in older clients, may be identified in younger people. Ask about occupation, and clarify whether the occupation increases the risk for vascular disease.

Current Health

Ask about the onset, precipitating factors, frequency, duration, and persistence of clinical manifestations that may indicate a vascular disorder. The following section describes the typical complaints of clients who have arterial and venous disorders.

Chief Complaint

Arterial Disorders. Arterial manifestations may occur in the head, upper extremities, abdomen, chest, or lower

---

evolve Web Enhancements

Assessment Terms English and Spanish

Appendix B A Health History Format That Integrates the Assessment of Functional Health Patterns

Figure Head-to-Toe Bilateral Pulse Assessment

Table Themes, Definitions, and Characteristics of Peripheral Arterial Disease

Be sure to check out the bonus material on the Evolve website and the CD-ROM, including free self-assessment exercises. **http://evolve.elsevier. com/Black/medsurg**

extremities. Clinical manifestations related to the head include visual disturbances, orientation, movement of extremities, facial symmetry, speech, and swallowing. These manifestations may be found in neurologic disorders as well as vascular disorders. Document the activity required to cause pain when it is present. In lower extremity arterial disorders the extent of disease involvement can be gauged by the distance the client is able to walk without pain, or claudication distance.

Venous Disorders. Chronic venous disease has an insidious onset. Many clients do not recall a precipitating event. A positive family history, a job history involving standing in one place, multiple pregnancies, varicose veins, or a history of phlebitis or obesity may be factors. Acute venous disorders usually present as sudden swelling in a localized area. Upper extremity superficial venous occlusion causes discomfort along the course of the affected vein. Suspect deep vein thrombosis in the upper extremity if there is significant edema in the affected arm. Pain in chronic venous disease has a slow onset. Heaviness in the legs or nighttime cramping may be reported. Exercise and elevation improve venous return to the heart and generally relieve the discomfort and swelling.

Clinical Manifestations

Vascular disease may be arterial, venous, or lymphatic, but there are also neurologic conditions that cause similar manifestations. Table 51-1 compares arterial and venous clinical manifestations in the lower extremities. Figure 51-1 provides a guide for the evaluation of clinical manifestations related to vascular disease.

Pain. In arterial insufficiency of the lower extremities, the client may complain of cramping leg pain in the calf muscles that occurs during ambulation but disappears with 1 to 2 minutes of rest. The pain is called intermittent claudication. The pain occurs in the muscle group distal to the diseased artery and is a pathologic process similar to angina pectoris (chest pain). As an artery becomes more stenosed, the pain may become more severe. The Integrating Diagnostic Testing feature on p. 1283 demonstrates the evaluation of a claudication complaint.

Pain in chronic venous disease has a slow onset and is not associated with exercise or rest. The client who has venous disease may report chronic aching pain in the legs when they are in a dependent position.

Skin Changes. Skin changes noted with chronic venous disorders may include erythema (redness), followed in the late stages by lipodermatosclerosis (brawny, thick, darkly pigmented skin). The skin becomes dry and flaky, which leads to itching and scratching. With chronic

arterial insufficiency, the skin is pale when the legs are elevated above heart level and dusky red after they are placed in a dependent position.

Sensory Changes. Clients may report distal forefoot burning, numbness or tingling, pain at rest, or pain that awakens them during the night (rest pain). These complaints may indicate that urgent attention is needed. This pain is related to arterial disease and exacerbated by decreased cardiac output during sleep.

Edema. In more severe forms of chronic venous disorders, lower extremity edema may be the initial complaint. Edema worsens toward the end of the day and diminishes after nighttime leg elevation. Skin temperature remains normal or slightly elevated and pulses are present, although they may be difficult to palpate through the edema. Pitting edema (see later discussion of edema) may be seen at first, but as the edema becomes more chronic, tissue sclerosis develops and the tissue becomes more difficult to compress. Lymphatic disorders also lead to edema. If the lymphatic obstruction is prolonged, edematous tissue becomes fibrotic and almost impossible to compress.

Lower Extremity Ulcers. With chronic venous disorders, the continued fluid leakage results in stasis dermatitis and the skin eventually ulcerates. Ulcers develop in the lower third of the leg, most commonly above the medial malleolus, where venous pressure is highest and there are more perforator veins than elsewhere in the leg.

Review of Systems

Review each body system as it relates to peripheral vascular disorders. Inquire about headaches, dizziness, pulmonary emboli, phlebitis, and leg or foot ulcers. Refer to Figure 51-2 on p. 1284 for vascular system-specific information to gather for the health history and review of systems.

Past Medical History

Note any history of vascular impairment. Inquire about changes that indicate vasospastic disorders, such as changes in color or temperature of digits. Ask specifically whether the client has a history of hypertension, diabetes, stroke, transient ischemic attacks (TIAs), changes in vision, pain in legs during activity, leg cramps, phlebitis, venous or arterial blood clots, pulmonary emboli, edema, varicose veins, or extremities that are cold, pale, or blue. Question any previous history of frostbite, which increases risk of vasospasm. Visual changes and TIAs may indicate carotid artery disease. Ask about previous treatment for diabetes mellitus, collagen disorders, or hypertension.

TABLE 51–1 Manifestations of Lower Extremity Arterial and Venous Disorders

	Arterial	Venous	Differentiating Neuropathic Disorder (Spinal Stenosis or Disc Disease)
Location of manifestation	Distal to arterial stenosis, buttocks, thigh, calf muscles, feet	Around ankle, over course of veins, often on medial side, may be entire leg	May radiate down lower back, legs, and buttocks after ambulation
Pain	Claudication, cramping pain occurs predictable distance Rest pain Continuous pain worsens with elevation	Aching, throbbing, burning, heaviness at end of day, nocturnal cramping	Burning, sharp, or aching pain
Relief of manifestation	Claudication—cessation of muscle use Rest pain—dependent position	Leg elevation	Must sit or flex lower back for relief May be able to walk only if bent over
Infection	May be present if open ulcer Thick toenails often indicate fungal infection but may also indicate arterial insufficiency	May be present if open ulcer	No
Skin	Pale Cooler than other skin areas In long-standing disease, skin is thin with absence of hair	Darkened brown color in gaiter area (area above the ankle to the knee) Dependent cyanosis Temperature may be higher than other skin areas Brawny edema Skin also may be thick and fibrotic (woody) May be oozing and crusted	No change
Sensation	Decreased Tingling, numbness may be present	Pruritus may be present	Numbness, tingling, or other paresthesias in affected limb
Edema	Minimal unless leg kept dependent	May be severe	Not present
Pulses	Absent or diminished Often disappears with exercise	Usually present with only venous etiology but may be difficult to palpate if edema is present	Present
Muscle mass	Reduced in chronic disease	Unaffected in pure venous disease	Muscle wasting possible with long-term disease
Ankle-brachial index (ABI)	Decreased, 0.50 to 0.75	Not affected	Normal, 1.0 or greater
Ulcer description	Dry, pale gray or yellow May be necrotic Small, painful ulcers on pressure points, points of trauma, between toes, or distal points, especially lateral malleolus and toes	Broad, shallow, but may be deep pink or beefy red base with granulation tissue Ulcer bed moist; may have copious drainage Surrounding skin is brown, fibrotic	No ulcer
Operative procedures	Arterial bypass Angioplasty Stent placement	Vein ligation/stripping Valve grafts Sclerotherapy Laser or radiofrequency ablation	May require nerve decompression

Past Surgical History

Detail any previous operations that the client has endured, particularly vascular bypass surgery. Note if there has been any previous angiography, endovascular graft or stent placement, or harvesting of arteries or veins from the lower extremities. These are discussed in more detail in the following chapters on vascular and cardiac disorders.

Allergies

Note allergies, especially to iodine. Iodine is found in contrast agents used in diagnostic testing for vascular disorders.

Medications

Note specific medications that the client takes, including over-the-counter drugs and herbal remedies. Some

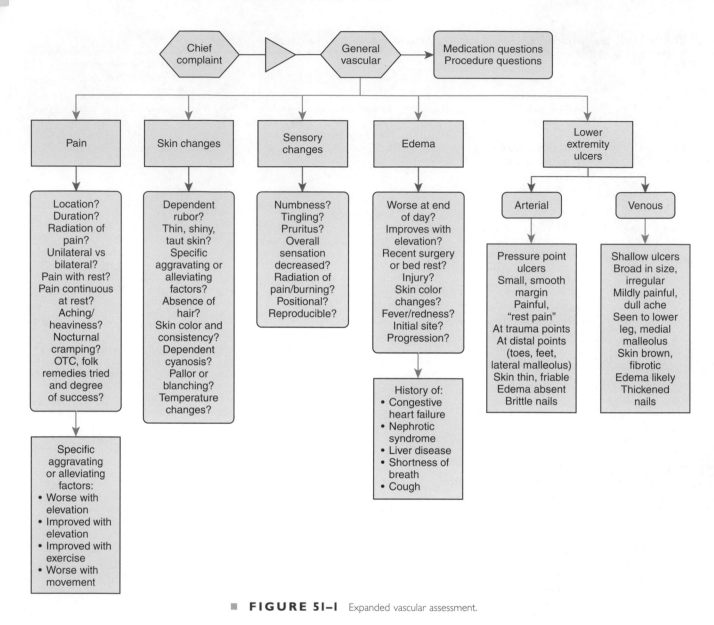

FIGURE 51–1 Expanded vascular assessment.

medications increase the risk for vascular disorders (such as birth control pills). Ask specifically about the use of prescription and over-the-counter nicotine products. Ask about use of illegal or street drugs.

Herbal remedies used to self-treat peripheral vascular disorders include those for hypertension, varicose veins, atherosclerosis, and vascular spasm. Herbs with antihypertensive action include garlic *(Allium sativum),* hawthorn *(Crataegus oxyacantha),* kudzu *(Pueraria lobata),* nettle *(Urtica dioica),* onion *(Allium cepa),* purslane *(Portulaca oleracea),* reishi mushroom *(Ganoderma lucidum),* and valerian *(Valeriana officinalis).* Garlic is thought to be preventive for atherosclerosis. Ginkgo biloba is used for varicose veins, obliterative arterial disease of the lower extremities, and intermittent claudication. Horse chestnut

(Aesculus hippocastanum) and butcher's broom *(Ruscus aculeatus)* are used for varicose veins and phlebitis, and valerian is used as an antispasmodic. Spices with possible antihypertensive effects include basil, black pepper, fennel, and tarragon.

Dietary Habits

Determine the client's nutrient and fluid intake (see Chapter 28). Ask about the usual intake of protein and calories. Also ask about sodium, cholesterol, and fat intake. The client who is underweight or overweight can be at risk for compromised healing and progression of vascular ulcers. Does the client report shortness of breath or fatigue when eating? Overall dietary intake

INTEGRATING DIAGNOSTIC TESTING

Claudication Pain

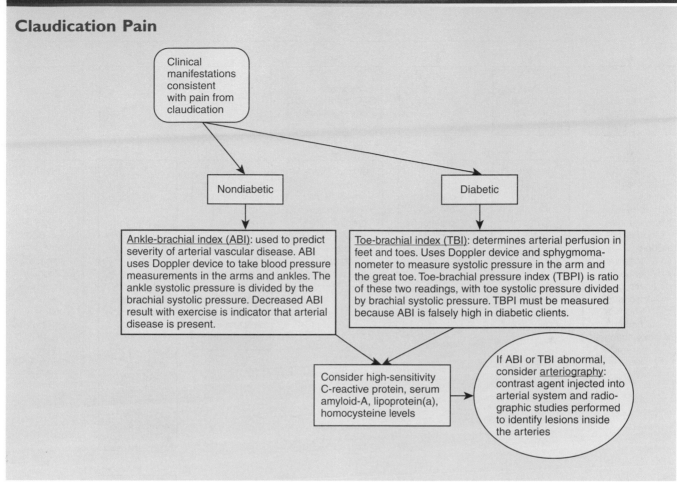

---

should support maintenance of ideal body weight. Ask about recent weight loss or pain in the abdomen within 20 minutes of eating. This may indicate mesenteric artery ischemia.

Social History

Record the occupational history, including the number of hours spent in various positions or activities (standing, prolonged sitting, walking, using vibrating machinery). Some occupations involve contact with chemicals or are associated with cold or wet environments; these should be noted as well.

Nicotine in any form is a potent vasoconstrictor. A complete smoking history is necessary as part of the vascular assessment. Discuss previous and current use of chewing tobacco, cigarettes, cigars, and pipe tobacco.

Assess the client's activity, rest, and sleep habits. Assess the extent to which the clinical manifestations illustrated in Figure 51-1 interfere with activities of daily living. Obtaining information about the frequency and

duration of manifestations, precipitating activities, and their influence on daily life enables determination of disease severity.

Disorders of the aorta and iliac vessels can lead to impotence. If a male client has aortoiliac disease, ask about problems with erectile function. Assessment of the client's stress level, emotional state, and coping mechanisms is important. Remain sensitive to the emotional effect of peripheral vascular disorders. Clients who have visible lesions may be embarrassed. Clients may have concern about the inability to perform self-care and about changes in role and sexual performance. Fear of amputation or functional loss may be significant.[2]

Family History

The family health history helps determine risk factors and provides clues about reported and observed manifestations. Note any family history of diabetes, hypertension, coronary artery disease, collagen diseases, and peripheral vascular disease.

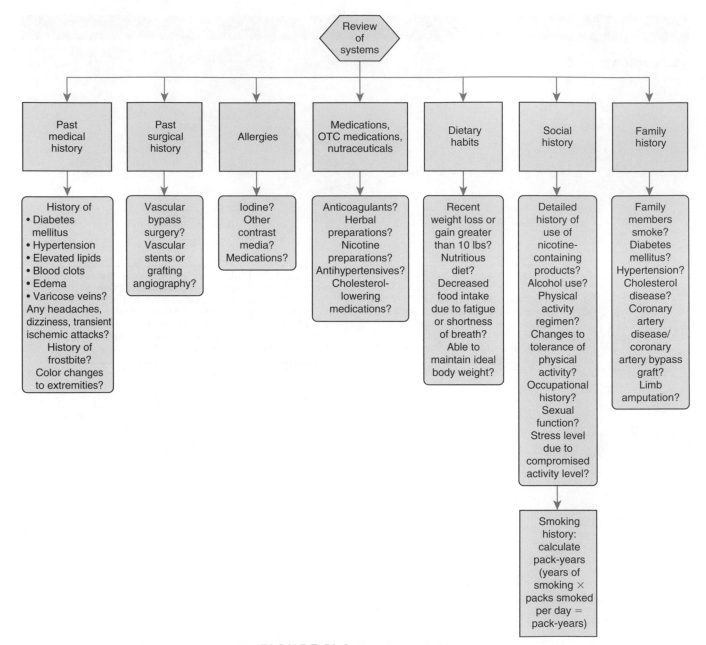

■ **FIGURE 51–2** Expanded vascular history.

PHYSICAL EXAMINATION

Assessment of the vascular system allows for the comparison of one side to the other. Blood pressure, pulse examination, color, and temperature assessment are bilateral. Differences between bilateral measurements may signify vascular disorders. Refer to the normal findings described in the Physical Assessment Findings in the Healthy Adult feature on p. 1285.

Inspection

Observe the extremities, noting skin color, hair distribution, nail beds and capillary refill time, presence of muscle atrophy or edema, venous pattern, and ulcers. Compare one side with the other. Begin with the head and upper extremities, and proceed toward the legs and feet.

Skin Color

There is a range of normal skin color. Localized areas of cyanosis, rubor, or pallor are easily noticed in a person with fair skin (Figure 51-3) but are more difficult to see in a person with darker skin tones (Figure 51-4). For all clients, changes in skin color are best assessed by comparison with the contralateral limb. Ischemic pallor may be detected by comparing the palms of the hands, the soles of the feet, or the nail beds. Clients with

The Peripheral Vascular System

INSPECTION

Extremities of even contour, without edema. Even hair distribution; symmetrical venous pattern. Varicosities, skin lesions, and ulcers absent. Capillaries refill in less than 3 seconds on blanching.

PALPATION

Extremities warm and dry without areas of localized heat or tenderness. Pulses (temporal, carotid, brachial, radial, ulnar, femoral, popliteal, posterior tibial, dorsalis pedis) are bilaterally equal and regular. No aneurysmal dilation of aorta.

AUSCULTATION

Blood pressures equal in contralateral extremities. Orthostatic hypotension absent. No bruits.

arterial disorders may have pale extremities and cyanotic (blue-tinged) or red extremities with venous disorders.

Hair Distribution

Lack of hair growth may indicate chronically inadequate circulation to an area. It is not a valid indicator of acute arterial insufficiency.

Capillary Refill Time

Capillary refill time is an evaluation of peripheral perfusion and cardiac output. This assessment is usually completed while pulses are assessed. Depress the nail bed or the pad of the toe or finger until it blanches or becomes pale. Release pressure on the blanched area, and note the length of time for usual skin color to return. Capillaries usually refill in a fraction of a second, but "normal" times range up to 3 seconds for color return.

Muscle Atrophy

There can be many reasons for muscle atrophy in an extremity. If atrophy is suspected, compare it with the muscle on the opposite side.

Edema

To assess edema of the leg, push with your thumb on the skin over the client's foot or tibia for 5 seconds. If the skin is edematous, an indentation or pit will remain (thus the term *pitting edema*) (Figure 51-5). Edema is often graded; however, scales used to grade edema are not universal. Clinicians should use their institution's approved scale. This may include documentation as basic as noting if edema is present or absent and, if present, whether it is pitting or non-pitting.

Edema resulting from cardiac disease is bilateral and occurs in dependent areas (in the legs of a client who is ambulatory and the sacrum of a client who is bedridden). Unilateral edema indicates venous or lymphatic obstruction. Long-standing edema destroys the structure of the skin and the subcutaneous tissue and is easily recognized from its fibrotic appearance and firm texture.

■ **FIGURE 51–3** Dependent rubor is noted as a ruddy color in severe arterial insufficiency in this white client's left leg just minutes before amputation. (Note area of ulceration and necrosis on the third toe.)

■ **FIGURE 51–4** Dependent rubor in dark skin (which can be difficult to see) in the client's left foot has a reddish hue when compared with the unaffected right foot.

No edema

A barely detectable
depression accompanied
by normal foot and leg contours

A deeper depression
(less than 5 mm) accompanied
by normal foot and leg contours

A deep depression
(5 to 10 mm) accompanied
by foot and leg swelling

An even deeper depression
(more than 1 cm) accompanied by
severe foot and leg swelling

■ **FIGURE 51–5** To assess peripheral edema, press a finger into the skin over the client's tibia. Note the presence, depth, and persistence of any resulting depression. Use descriptive terms to record your findings.

Ulcers

Note the presence of skin lesions or scar tissue (indicating healed ulcers); fissures of the feet and ulcers of the ankles and heels may be signs of arterial insufficiency. Tissue necrosis (see Figure 51-4) and gangrene may be present with severe arterial disease. Examine between the toes for moist ulcers penetrating into the web spaces.

Palpation
Temperature

Palpate the arms and legs with the dorsal surface of your hand, and note the temperature (see Chapter 48). Temperature should be similar in contralateral limbs. Vasoconstriction produces cold, pale skin. Bilateral vasoconstriction may be caused by smoking, environmental temperature, anxiety, or generalized arterial disease. Unilateral or localized arterial vasoconstriction indicates arterial disease. Venous disorders may cause an increase in local skin temperature.

Pulses

Palpate pulses by placing the first three fingers of your dominant hand along the length of the selected artery. Apply gentle pressure against the artery, followed by a gradual release. Palpate temporal, carotid, brachial, radial, and ulnar pulses (upper extremities), and femoral, popliteal, posterior tibial, and dorsalis pedis pulses (lower extremities), as shown in the website figure Head-to-Toe Bilateral Pulse Assessment. Palpate

pulses bilaterally and simultaneously, except for the carotid pulse. Palpate carotid pulses separately to avoid stimulation of the carotid sinus, which may produce bradycardia or sinus arrest. Assess the ulnar pulse during Allen's test (Box 51-1). Homans' test, which was used in the past to assess for deep venous thrombosis, is no longer used because the test itself

BOX 51-1

ALLEN'S TEST

Blood flow to the hand is supplied by both the ulnar and the radial arteries, which join at the volar arch in the palm. Allen's test is used to assess the patency of the radial and ulnar arteries distal to the wrist. It is commonly performed before arterial blood samples are drawn for analysis or before an arterial line is inserted. Perform Allen's test as follows:

1. Ask the client to make a tight fist while you compress the radial and ulnar arteries.
2. Have the client open the hand, which should be pale and mottled.
3. Release the pressure on the radial artery while continuing to compress the ulnar artery. If the client's hand regains full color within about 6 seconds, the radial artery has normal patency.
4. Repeat steps 1 to 3, this time releasing the pressure on the ulnar artery to assess its patency.

If the client's hand remains pale during either portion of the test, the artery being tested may be occluded. Allen's test is shown in Figure 59-13 on p. 1539.

may cause a clot to dislodge and become an embolus (Box 51-2).

Always note the rhythm, amplitude, and symmetry of pulses. Compare peripheral pulses on both sides for rate, rhythm, and quality. There are no standard numerical grades or rating scales for pulses although some systems use a numerical scale. It is most accurate to describe the pulse as palpable (or present), diminished (weak), absent, or aneurysmal (easily palpable, bounding).

Note whether a pulse feels unequal bilaterally. The dorsalis pedis pulse is congenitally absent in approximately 10% to 17% of the normal adult population.[1] The posterior tibial pulse is absent congenitally in 9% of the black adult population of the United States.[1] In older clients, dorsalis pedis and posterior tibial pulses may be more difficult to palpate. If they are found, mark the site with a pen to facilitate later examinations. Clients who have arterial grafts may have palpable pulses along the length of the graft. The aorta can easily be palpated on a thin person by placing the hand on the upper abdomen just below the xyphoid process.

Auscultation
Limb Blood Pressure
The measurement of arterial blood pressure is the most commonly performed noninvasive test of cardiac and vascular function. It may be the best single indicator of arterial perfusion. Arterial stenosis or occlusion produces regional hypotension. Auscultate the blood pressure in both arms. 🪔 A difference of 20 mm Hg between extremity readings may indicate aortic dissection or subclavian artery stenosis. Document asymmetrical readings. All subsequent blood pressure measurements should be performed on the arm with the higher reading. Measure blood pressure with the client in supine, sitting, and standing positions on the first assessment, and document the position of the client and the site used for each reading. Note orthostatic (positional) changes in blood pressure.

Auscultate over the carotid artery, the aorta, and the renal, femoral, and popliteal arteries to assess for the presence of bruits. A bruit is a "whooshing" sound that may be soft or loud; it results from turbulent blood flow from vessel wall irregularities. The presence of a bruit indicates arterial narrowing. These arterial sounds are best heard with the bell of the stethoscope.

DIAGNOSTIC TESTING
The following is a summary of tests used to assess the extent of a client's vascular disease. For specifics on the nursing role with and pre- and postprocedure care with each test, consult a diagnostic testing textbook.

Noninvasive Tests
Noninvasive diagnostic techniques have assumed an increasingly important role in the management of vascular disorders. Noninvasive diagnostic tests provide reliable, objective data that can be used to evaluate the extent of vascular disease. Variables include blood flow velocity, blood flow abnormality, and some measure of functional limitations.

Ankle-Brachial Index
The ankle-brachial index (ABI) is a commonly used parameter for overall evaluation of extremity status. This test measures blood pressure at the ankle and in the arm while a person is at rest. Measurements are repeated at both sites after 5 minutes of walking on a treadmill. This ABI result is used to document the severity of lower extremity arterial disease. A decrease in the ABI measurement with exercise is an indicator that arterial disease is present.

Doppler Ultrasonography
Hand-held Doppler ultrasonographic instruments permit assessment of arterial disease through evaluation of audible arterial signals or measurement of limb blood pressures. Doppler ultrasonography is simple and inexpensive, but the technique may not detect minor disease, and it is less accurate than duplex scanning (see later discussion).

Brightness-mode (B-mode) ultrasound refers to the creation of a two-dimensional image from ultrasound waves. It can be used to assess the size and compressibility of a vessel, flow patterns, the presence or absence of thrombus, and valve function.

Ultrasonic Duplex Scan
Ultrasonic duplex scanners are used to localize vascular obstruction, evaluate the degree of stenosis, and determine the presence or absence of vascular reflux (backward flow). This anatomic and physiologic test evaluates the hemodynamic effects of arterial lesions. 🪔 It is also the most sensitive and specific noninvasive modality for detecting DVT. Both an ultrasound image of the vessel and a Doppler audible signal and waveform are provided. The visual ultrasound data allow more specific localization of

stenosis than simple pressure or waveform techniques. No special client preparation is required.

Air Plethysmography

Air plethysmography (APG) uses a pneumatic plethysmograph to measure volume changes in the legs. Venous reflux, venous obstruction, calf muscle pump function, and venous volume can be measured. A large cuff is applied to the client's calf, and a known volume of air is instilled to calibrate the cuff. Venous volume, ejection fraction, and residual volume fractions are then measured.

Impedance Plethysmography

Impedance plethysmography (IPG) and photoplethysmography (PPG) are also used to measure venous blood volume changes in the extremities. During the procedure, electrodes from a plethysmograph are applied to a limb along with a pressure cuff. As pressure is increased, electrical resistance is increased; thus the quality of venous blood flow is demonstrated.

Exercise Testing

Exercise or stress testing provides an objective measurement of the severity of intermittent claudication. The most commonly used 🔦 method for stress testing is the treadmill exercise test. This test is similar to that used for clients who have cardiac stress testing, except that walking speed is usually 1.5 to 2 miles per hour (mph) with a grade elevation of 10% to 20% and a time limit of 5 minutes. A client who can walk 5 minutes is considered mildly symptomatic; a walking time of 1 minute represents severe disease.

Performance on the treadmill test is also gauged by measurement of ankle systolic pressure. In asymptomatic clients, the time required for return to pre-exercise ankle pressure is usually less than 3 minutes with a decline from baseline of 20% or less. In clients with intermittent claudication, recovery time is longer; ankle pressure is usually less than 50 mm Hg and may be unrecordable during recovery.

Computed Tomography

Computed tomography (CT) provides a cross-section of vessel walls and other structures. CT scans can be used to diagnose abdominal aortic aneurysms and postoperative complications, such as graft infection, graft occlusion, hemorrhage, and abscess.

Magnetic Resonance Imaging

Magnetic resonance imaging (MRI) is used to detect tissue changes, such as tumors, aneurysms, and DVT, in the pelvic iliac veins and leg veins. Blood flow in an extremity is evaluated, with the limb to be examined placed in a cradle-like support in a flow cylinder.

In the future, MRI techniques likely will supply much of the information that currently is available only with invasive angiography. Although MRI does not require ionizing radiation or injection into the arterial system, the expense and time necessary limit its use for routine screening and follow-up.

Invasive Tests

Arteriography

Contrast arteriography is performed if the client is willing to undergo a surgical or percutaneous intervention. It is used to identify lesions inside the arteries and intraoperatively to evaluate the results of an operation. The procedure involves injecting a contrast agent into the arterial system and performing radiographic studies.

Venography

Venography, performed in a manner similar to that for arteriography, is used to examine the venous system. Venograms can be used to detect DVT and other abnormalities, such as incompetent valves. This diagnostic test is performed less frequently than in the past. Newer, noninvasive vascular laboratory studies pose less risk, are more accurate, and provide functional information as well.

Magnetic Resonance Angiography

Magnetic resonance angiography (MRA) uses magnetic imaging techniques to access blood vessels. The advantage of this technique is that the images are not obscured by bone, bowel gas, fat, or vascular calcification. The vessel anatomy is displayed as a three-dimensional angiogram. MRA can be used to measure blood flow volume and blood viscosity. It is a noninvasive modality. The disadvantages are its limited availability, its cost, and the need for the client to hold still during the procedure. MRA cannot be used for people who have cardiac pacemakers or intracranial aneurysm clips.

Vascular Endoscopy (Angioscopy)

Vascular endoscopy permits imaging of intra-arterial disease with the use of fiberoptic technology. Images are in color and in three dimensions. The major advantage of angioscopy is the internal visualization of the vessel lumen. This enables identification of thrombus (blood clot), plaque, hemorrhage, ulceration, or embolus (clot that has broken off from a thrombus and lodged in a more distal artery). Angioscopes can be used to remove debris from vessels and to check the integrity of an anastomosis (suture line that connects a vessel grafted to a native vessel) from within a vessel. They may also be used to remove venous valves in preparation for use of the vein as a bypass graft.

Complications of vascular endoscopy are rare but may include intimal damage, vessel spasm, thrombosis or embolism, perforation, fluid overload, and infection. Postprocedure care is similar to that for clients who have undergone angiography.

Intravascular Ultrasonography

Intravascular ultrasonography provides information about the atherosclerotic intima beneath the luminal surface. It can thus determine the thickness of the arterial wall and can distinguish thrombus and calcified vessel walls from vascular tissue, allowing more exact removal of lesions. Specialized interpretation of the scan is necessary.

Laboratory Tests

Elevations in the total lipid profile, or specific portions of it, are a major risk factor in the development of atherosclerosis, and measures of the coagulation properties of a client's blood are part of the evaluation of the severity of cardiovascular disease. Refer to the discussion of the relevance of these laboratory values in the chapter about vascular disorders (Chapter 53) and functional cardiac disorders (Chapter 56).

CONCLUSIONS

Vascular assessment requires inspection, palpation, and auscultation skills. Knowledge of anatomy is critical for correct performance of assessments. Diagnostic modalities can range from simple, noninvasive tests to complex, sophisticated, invasive technology. A clear understanding of the indications for diagnostic tests and interpretation of the findings assists the clinical decision making.

BIBLIOGRAPHY

Citations appearing in red refer to primary research.

Citations appearing in blue refer to evidence-based practice guidelines and protocols.

1. Fahey, V. (2004). Clinical assessment of the vascular system. In V.A. Fahey (Ed.), *Vascular nursing* (4th ed.). Philadelphia: Elsevier Saunders.
2. Hirsch, A., Haskal, Z., Hertzer, N., et al. (2006). ACC/AHA guidelines for the management of patients with peripheral arterial disease (lower extremity, renal, mesenteric, and abdominal aortic). *Journal of the American College of Cardiology, 147*, 1239-1312.
3. Hirsch, A.T. (Ed.) (2001). Primary care series: Peripheral arterial disease and intermittent claudication: A compilation of the American Journal of Medicine Continuing Education Series. An office based approach to the diagnosis and treatment of peripheral arterial disease. *Excerpta Medica*. Philadelphia: Elsevier.
4. Hirsch, A.T., et al. (2001). Peripheral arterial disease detection, awareness, and treatment in primary care. *Journal of the American Medical Association, 11*(286), 1317-1324.
5. Jaff, M.R., & Hiatt, W.R. (2001). Clinical and vascular laboratory evaluation of peripheral arterial disease. In W.R. Hiatt, A.T. Hirsch, & J.G. Regensteiner (Eds.), *Peripheral arterial disease handbook* (pp. 81-94). Boca Raton, Fla: CRC Press.
6. Moore, W.S. (Ed.) (2005). *Vascular and endovascular surgery: A comprehensive review* (7th ed.). Philadelphia: Saunders.
7. Negus, D. (2005). Diagnosis: History and examination. In D. Negus, P. Coleridge Smith, & J. Bergan (Eds.), *Leg ulcers: Diagnosis and management* (3rd ed., pp. 75-83). London: Hodder Arnold.
8. Treat-Jacobson, D., et al. (2002). A patient-derived perspective of health-related quality of life with peripheral arterial disease. *Journal of Nursing Scholarship, 34*(1), 55-60.

evolve *Did you remember to check out the bonus material on the Evolve website and the CD-ROM, including NCLEX®-Examination Style Review Questions, Open-Book Quizzes, and Chapter Review Audio Podcasts?*

http://evolve.elsevier.com/Black/medsurg

CHAPTER 52

Management of Clients with Hypertensive Disorders

JEAN ELIZABETH DEMARTINIS

HYPERTENSION

Arterial hypertension, simply stated, is high blood pressure. It is defined as a persistent elevation of the systolic blood pressure (SBP) at a level of 140 mm Hg or higher and diastolic blood pressure (DBP) at a level of 90 mm Hg or higher. The National Institutes of Health's report titled *The Seventh Report of the Joint National Committee on Detection, Evaluation, and Treatment of High Blood Pressure (JNC VII)* and the Centers for Disease Control and Prevention (CDC) publications *Healthy People 2000* and *2010* have documented the advances made over the last few decades in the prevention, detection, and treatment of hypertension. Members of the public have become more knowledgeable about high blood pressure, are more likely to visit a health care provider for hypertension, and are more likely to comply with medical advice. The use of increasingly effective antihypertensive agents has also dramatically reduced the death rate associated with hypertension. The percentage of people has increased significantly who receive treatment for hypertension and keep their blood pressure controlled. The combined effects from increased access to treatment and better control of existing hypertension have contributed to a greater than 60% decline in stroke and greater than 50% decline in the death rate from coronary artery disease. These impressive gains have been seen across all age groups, in both men and women, and in special populations.

The *JNC VII* and *Healthy People 2010*, however, also document some disturbing current trends. After years of decline, the death rates for coronary heart disease and stroke leveled off and have begun to rise again. The prevalence of hypertension is on the rise, and control rates are variable, with the majority of people with hypertension undercontrolled. Arterial hypertension affects more than 50 million people—1 in 4—in the United States, with the highest rates of occurrence among older adults, blacks, less educated people, and lower socioeconomic groups. Estimates are that only about 25% of all people with hypertension have blood pressure controlled at a target level. Lack of client compliance and providers' continued ignorance of the need to prescribe and manage complex holistic treatment protocols are cited as the two major factors that have contributed to this abysmal decline in improved client outcomes.

Acute coronary syndrome events such as a "heart attack" are still the most common result of hypertension. Hypertension is also related to increased severity of atherosclerosis, stroke, nephropathy, peripheral vascular disease, aortic aneurysms, and heart failure. Nearly all people with heart failure have antecedent hypertension. If hypertension is left untreated, nearly half of hypertensive clients will die of heart disease, one third will die of stroke, and the remaining 10% to 15% will die of renal failure. Hypertension is also a "silent factor" leading to many deaths attributed to stroke or heart attacks.

These disturbing trends indicate the need for increased vigilance in the battle against hypertension. Hypertension-related morbidity and mortality rates will not significantly decrease until providers appreciate the need for adjustments or refinements in their existing treatment protocols that are based on current practice guidelines that suggest options for evidence-based practice that produce

---

evolve Web Enhancements

Client Education Guide Low-Sodium Diet (English Version and Spanish Translation)

Low-Fat, Low-Cholesterol Diet (English Version and Spanish Translation)

Calorie-Restriction Diet (English Version and Spanish Translation)

Concept Map Understanding Hypertension and Its Treatment

Be sure to check out the bonus material on the Evolve website and the CD-ROM, including free self-assessment exercises. **http://evolve.elsevier.com/Black/medsurg**

quantifiable client outcomes. For example, there are readily available non-invasive assessment devices that indirectly measure a client's internal hemodynamics; these measurements can be used to guide a provider's choices for appropriate medications and dosages for each individual client.

The *Healthy People 2010* guidelines are prevention focused, and the *JNC VII* guidelines are also now primarily prevention focused and strongly recommend the use of nonpharmaceutical as well as pharmaceutical measures to prevent and treat hypertension. The Translating Evidence into Practice feature at right examines new guidelines for preventing and managing hypertension. Nurses are faced with a profound urgency to enhance public and professional education toward this end and to translate the results of research into improved practice. An ambitious, but nevertheless feasible, goal is the diagnosis and treatment of hypertension in all affected people in the United States.

Types of Hypertensive Disease, Etiology, and Severity

Hypertension is characterized by type, cause, and severity. Most clients with a combination of systolic and diastolic blood pressure elevation are diagnosed with *primary hypertension,* also known as *essential* or idiopathic hypertension. The etiology is multifactoral, with no identifiable cause, but several interacting homeostatic forces are generally involved. The blood pressure remains elevated and continues to rise over time because of a persistent, progressive increase in peripheral arterial resistance. The persistent rise in arterial resistance is due to inappropriate renal retention of salt and water or abnormalities of or within the vessel wall. The severity of the condition directly relates to the number and magnitude of risk factors present, the length of time for which these risk factors have been present, and the presence of accompanying disease states. The severity of complications from hypertension increase as the blood pressure, both systolic and diastolic, increases.

Clients who develop hypertension from an identifiable cause—a specific disease state or problem—are diagnosed with *secondary hypertension,* and in many cases the underlying cause is correctable (Box 52-1 on p. 1294). Therefore it is important to isolate the root of the problem so that the most appropriate treatment regimen can be prescribed. Severity depends on underlying causes, personal and environmental factors, and duration of concurrent disease states.

When the systolic blood pressure is 140 mm Hg or higher but the diastolic blood pressure remains less than 90 mm Hg, the client is diagnosed with *isolated systolic hypertension* (ISH). ISH can result from increased cardiac output or atherosclerosis-induced changes in blood vessel compliance or both. Regardless of cause, this form of hypertension is treated in the same manner as

⊶ TRANSLATING EVIDENCE INTO PRACTICE

Guidelines for Hypertension Prevention and Management

The Seventh Report of the Joint National Committee on Prevention, Detection, Evaluation, and Treatment of High Blood Pressure provides a new guideline for hypertension prevention and management. The following are the report's key messages:

- In people older than 50 years, systolic blood pressure greater than 140 mm Hg is a much more important cardiovascular disease (CVD) risk factor than diastolic blood pressure.
- The risk of CVD beginning at 115/75 mm Hg doubles with each increment of 20/10 mm Hg; individuals who are normotensive at age 55 have a 90% lifetime risk for developing hypertension.
- Individuals with a systolic blood pressure of 120 to 139 mm Hg or a diastolic blood pressure of 80 to 89 mm Hg should be considered as prehypertensive and require health-promoting lifestyle modifications to prevent CVD.
- Thiazide-type diuretics should be used in drug treatment for most clients with uncomplicated hypertension, either alone or combined with drugs from other classes. Certain high-risk conditions are compelling indications for the initial use of other antihypertensive drug classes (such as angiotensin-converting enzyme inhibitors, angiotensin receptor blockers, beta-blockers, calcium channel blockers).
- Most clients with hypertension will require two or more antihypertensive medications to achieve goal blood pressure (<140/90 mm Hg, or <130/80 mm Hg for clients with diabetes or chronic kidney disease).
- If blood pressure is >20/10 mm Hg above goal blood pressure, consideration should be given to initiating therapy with two agents, one of which usually should be a thiazide-type diuretic.
- The most effective therapy prescribed by the most careful clinician will control hypertension only if clients are motivated. Motivation improves when clients have positive experiences with, and trust in, the clinician. Empathy builds trust and is a potent motivator.
- In presenting these guidelines, the committee recognizes that the responsible physician's judgment remains paramount.

From National High Blood Pressure Education Program, National Institutes of Health, National Heart, Lung and Blood Institute. (2003). *The Seventh Report of the Joint National Committee on Detection, Evaluation, and Treatment of High Blood Pressure.* Bethesda, Md: U.S. Government Printing Office.

primary hypertension. The likelihood of the development of ISH increases with advancing age, as does the severity of ISH.

Clients who develop refractory hypertension with persistent systolic or diastolic elevation and/or if diastolic blood pressure is protracted above 110 to 120 mm Hg are diagnosed with *resistant hypertension.* It results when hypertension is left untreated or is unresponsive to treatment and becomes a truly severe emergency condition as the pressure continues to rise unchecked. The unrelenting rise in arterial resistance is due to inappropriate renal retention of salt and water or abnormalities of or within the vessel wall. The severity of the condition directly relates to the number and magnitude of risk factors present, the length of time for which these risk factors have been present, and the presence of accompanying disease states.

Epidemiology and Risk Factors

Primary hypertension constitutes more than 90% of all cases of hypertension. Fewer than 5% to 8% of adult hypertensive clients have secondary hypertension; however, hypertension, regardless of type, results from an array of genetic and environmental factors. These risk factors are grouped into those that are modifiable and those which are not. Education for lifestyle change is directed at the modifiable risk factors.

Nonmodifiable Risk Factors

Family History

Hypertension is thought to be polygenic and multifactorial—that is, in any person with a family history of hypertension, several genes may interact with each other and the environment to cause the blood pressure to elevate over time. The genetic predisposition that makes certain families more susceptible to hypertension may be related to an elevation in intracellular sodium levels and to lowered potassium-to-sodium ratios, which are found more often in blacks than in other groups. Clients with parents who have hypertension are at greater risk for hypertension at a younger age.

Age

Primary hypertension typically appears between the ages of 30 and 50 years. The incidence of hypertension increases with age; 50% to 60% of clients older than 60 years have a blood pressure over 140/90 mm Hg. Epidemiologic studies, however, have shown a poorer prognosis in clients whose hypertension began at a young age. Isolated systolic hypertension occurs primarily in people older than 50 years, with almost 24% of all people affected by age 80 years. Among older adults, SBP readings are a better predictor of possible future events such as coronary heart disease, stroke, heart failure, and renal disease than are DBP readings.

Gender

The overall incidence of hypertension is higher in men than in women until about age 55 years. Between the ages of 55 and 74 years, the risk in men and that in women are almost equal; then, after age 74 years, women are at greater risk.

Ethnicity

Mortality statistics indicate that the death rate for adults with hypertension is lowest for white women at 4.7%; white men have the next lowest rate at 6.3%, and black men have the next lowest at 22.5%; the death rate is highest for black women at 29.3%. The reason for the increased prevalence of hypertension among blacks is unclear, but the increase has been attributed to lower renin levels, greater sensitivity to vasopressin, higher salt intake, and greater environmental stress.

Modifiable Risk Factors

Diabetes

Hypertension has been shown to be more than twice as prevalent in diabetic clients according to several recent research studies. Diabetes accelerates atherosclerosis and leads to hypertension from damage to the large vessels. Therefore hypertension *will* become a prevalent diagnosis in diabetics, even if diabetes is well controlled. When a diabetic client is diagnosed with hypertension, treatment decisions and follow-up care must be totally individualized and aggressive.

Stress

Stress increases peripheral vascular resistance and cardiac output and stimulates sympathetic nervous system activity. Over time hypertension can develop. Stressors can be many things, and noise, infection, inflammation, pain, decreased oxygen supply, heat, cold, trauma, prolonged exertion, responses to life events, obesity, old age, drugs, disease, surgery, and medical treatment can elicit the stress response. These noxious stimuli are perceived by a person as a threat or as capable of causing harm; subsequently, a psychophysiologic "fight-or-flight" response is initiated in the body. If stress responses become excessive or prolonged, target organ dysfunction or disease will result. A report from the American Institute of Stress estimates that 60% to 90% of all primary care visits involve stress-related complaints. Because stress is a matter of perception, people's interpretations of events are what create most stressors and stress responses.

Obesity

Obesity, especially in the upper body (giving an "apple" shape), with increased amounts of fat about the midriff, waist, and abdomen, is associated with subsequent development of hypertension. People who are overweight but carry most of the excess weight in the buttocks, hips, and thighs (giving them a "pear" shape) are at far less risk for development of hypertension secondary to increased weight alone. The combination of obesity with other factors can be labeled as metabolic syndrome, which also increases the risk of hypertension.

Nutrients

Sodium consumption can be an important factor in the development of essential hypertension. At least 40% of clients who eventually develop hypertension are salt-sensitive and the excess salt may be the precipitating cause of the hypertension in these individuals. A high-salt diet may induce excessive release of natriuretic hormone, which may indirectly increase blood pressure. Sodium loading also stimulates vasopressor mechanisms within the central nervous system (CNS). Studies also show that low dietary intake of calcium, potassium, and magnesium can contribute to the development of hypertension.

Substance Abuse

Cigarette smoking, heavy alcohol consumption, and some illicit drug use all are risk factors for hypertension. The nicotine in cigarette smoke and drugs such as cocaine cause an immediate rise in blood pressure that is dose dependent; however, *habitual* use of these substances has been implicated in an increased incidence of hypertension over time. The incidence of hypertension is also higher among people who drink more than 3 ounces of ethanol per day. The impact of caffeine is controversial. Caffeine raises blood pressure acutely but does not produce sustained effects.

Pathophysiology
Primary (Essential) Hypertension

The exact pathologic underpinnings of primary hypertension remain to be established. Any factor that produces an alteration in peripheral vascular resistance, heart rate, or stroke volume affects systemic arterial blood pressure (see Figure A&P12-4 in the Anatomy and Physiology Review on p. 1276). Four control systems play a major role in maintaining blood pressure: (1) the arterial baroreceptor and chemoreceptors' system; (2) regulation of body fluid volume; (3) the renin-angiotensin system; and (4) vascular autoregulation. Primary hypertension most likely occurs from a defect or malfunction in some or all of these systems. Probably no single defect causes essential hypertension in all affected people.

Arterial baroreceptors and chemoreceptors work reflexively to control blood pressure (see Figure A&P12-5 in Anatomy and Physiology Review on p. 1277). Baroreceptors, major stretch receptors, are found in the carotid sinus, aorta, and wall of the left ventricle. They monitor the level of arterial pressure and counteract increases through vasodilation and slowing of the heart rate via the vagus nerve. Chemoreceptors, located in the medulla and carotid and aortic bodies, are sensitive to changes in concentrations of oxygen, carbon dioxide, and hydrogen ions (pH) in the blood. A decrease in arterial oxygen concentration or pH causes a reflexive rise in pressure, whereas an increase in carbon dioxide concentration causes a decrease in blood pressure. Changes in fluid volume affect systemic arterial pressure. Thus an abnormality in the transport of sodium in the renal tubules may cause essential hypertension. When sodium and water levels are excessive, total blood volume increases, thereby increasing blood pressure. Pathologic changes that alter the pressure threshold at which kidneys excrete salt and water alter systemic blood pressure. In addition, the overproduction of sodium-retaining hormones has been implicated in hypertension.

Renin and angiotensin play a role in blood pressure regulation. *Renin* is an enzyme produced by the kidney that catalyzes a plasma protein substrate to split off angiotensin I, which is removed by a converting enzyme to the lung to form angiotensin II and then angiotensin III. Angiotensins II and III act as vasoconstrictors and also stimulate aldosterone release. With increased sympathetic nervous system activity, angiotensins II and III also seem to inhibit sodium excretion, which results in elevated blood pressure. Increased renin secretion has been investigated as a cause of increased peripheral vascular resistance in primary hypertension.

Vascular endothelial cells are being shown to be important in hypertension. The cells of the endothelium produce nitric oxide that dilates the arteriole and endothelium that constricts it. Dysfunction of the endothelium has been implicated in human essential hypertension.

Secondary Hypertension

Many renal, vascular, neurologic, endocrine, and drug- and food-induced problems that directly or indirectly negatively affect the kidneys can result in serious insult to these organs that interferes with sodium excretion, renal perfusion, or the renin-angiotensin-aldosterone mechanism, leading to an elevation in blood pressure over time (Box 52-1).

Chronic glomerulonephritis and renal artery stenosis are the most common cause of secondary hypertension. Also, the adrenal glands can cause secondary hypertension if they produce excessive aldosterone, cortisol, and catecholamines. Excess aldosterone causes renal retention of sodium and water, expands blood volume, and elevates blood pressure. *Pheochromocytoma*, a small tumor of the adrenal medulla, can cause dramatic hypertension because of the release of excessive amounts of epinephrine and norepinephrine (called catecholamines). Other adrenocortical problems can result in excess production of cortisol (Cushing's syndrome). Clients with Cushing's syndrome have an 80% risk for development of hypertension. Cortisol increases blood pressure by increasing renal sodium retention, angiotensin II levels, and vascular reactivity to norepinephrine. Chronic stress elevates blood levels of catecholamines, aldosterone, and cortisol.

BOX 52-1   Causes of Secondary Hypertension

ACUTE STRESS
- Alcoholism
- Acute alcohol withdrawal
- Burns
- Chronic intermittent vasovagal response
- Hyperventilation
- Hypoglycemia
- Psychogenic

VASCULAR DISORDERS
- Arteriosclerosis
- Coarctation of the aorta
- Increased intravascular volume
- Sickle cell crisis
- Dissecting aortic aneurysm

ENDOCRINE DISORDERS
- Acromegaly
- Adrenal disorders
  - Cortical
    - Cushing's syndrome
    - Primary aldosteronism
  - Medullary
    - Pancreatitis
    - Pheochromocytoma
- Hypothyroidism
- Hyperthyroidism

NEUROLOGIC DISORDERS
- Autonomic dysreflexia
- Increased intracranial pressure
  - Brain tumor
  - Encephalitis
  - Respiratory acidosis
- Sleep apnea

MEDICATIONS
- Abrupt medication withdrawal
- Amphetamine use
- Anabolic and adrenogenic steroids
- Antihistamines/decongestants
- Cocaine use
- Cyclosporine
- Ergot alkaloids
- Erythropoietin
- Glucocorticoids
- Heavy metal poisons (lead, arsenic)
- Mineralocorticoids
- Monoamine oxidase inhibitors
- NSAIDs
- Oral contraceptives
- Sympathomimetics
  - Ephedrine
  - Phenylephrine
- Tricyclic antidepressants

PROBLEMS WITH PREGNANCY
- Pregnancy-induced hypertension
- Eclampsia

RENAL DISORDERS
- Renal artery stenosis
- Renal parenchymal disease
  - Acute glomerulonephritis
  - Chronic pyelonephritis
  - Connective tissue diseases
  - Diabetic nephropathy
  - Hydronephrosis
  - Polycystic disease
- Renin-producing tumors
- Renovascular diseases
- Atherosclerosis
- Vasculitis

SEVERE ANEMIA

TYRAMINE-CONTAINING FOODS
- Aged cheeses (especially cheddar)
- Beer, wine
- Chicken liver
- Yeast extract

From National High Blood Pressure Education Program, National Institutes of Health, and National Heart, Lung and Blood Institute. (2003). *The Seventh Report of the Joint National Committee on Detection, Evaluation, and Treatment of High Blood Pressure.* Bethesda, MD: U.S. Government Printing Office.

Vessel Changes

Early in the course of development of hypertension, no obvious pathologic changes in the blood vessels and organs may be seen other than intermittent elevations of blood pressure *(labile hypertension)*. Slowly, widespread pathologic changes take place both in the large and small blood vessels and in the heart, kidneys, and brain.

The large vessels, such as the aorta, coronary arteries, basilar artery to the brain, and peripheral vessels in the limbs, become sclerotic, tortuous, and weak. Their lumina narrow, with resultant decreased blood flow to the heart, brain, and lower extremities. As the damage continues, large vessels may become occluded or may hemorrhage, causing infarction of the tissue supplied by the vessel that has suddenly been robbed of its blood supply.

Small vessel damage, equally dangerous, causes structural changes in the heart, kidneys, and brain. Elevated DBP damages the intimal lining of the small vessels. Because of intimal damage, fibrin accumulates in the vessels, local edema develops, and intravascular clotting may occur. The net results of these changes are (1) a decreased blood supply to the tissues of the heart, brain, kidneys, and retina; (2) progressive functional impairment of these organs; and (3) finally, as a consequence of the chronic ischemia, infarction of the tissue

supplied by these vessels, originating in much the same way as with occlusion of the large vessels.

Clinical Manifestations

In the early stages of development of hypertension, no clinical manifestations are noted by clients or practitioners. Eventually the blood pressure will rise, and if it is not "found" during routine screening, clients will remain unaware that their blood pressure is elevated. If the condition is left undiagnosed, the blood pressure will continue to rise, clinical manifestations will become apparent, and clients will eventually report to a provider's office with complaints of persistent headaches, fatigue, dizziness, palpitations, flushing, blurred or double vision, or epistaxis.

Assessment of the client with hypertension involves the following three main objectives:

- To assess lifestyle and determine the presence of other cardiovascular risk factors or concomitant disorders that can affect prognosis and guide treatment
- To identify the type of hypertension (primary or secondary) and identifiable causes
- To verify the presence or absence of target organ involvement

Clinicians can obtain information relevant to these areas from the history, physical examination, and laboratory studies (Box 52-2). The diagnosis of hypertension is made after the seated client has been allowed to rest for at least 5 minutes and the average of two or more readings separated by at least 2 minutes is 140 mm Hg or higher for the SBP and 90 mm Hg or higher for the DBP. Follow-up examinations are scheduled to diagnose or rule out the presence of hypertension, unless first-visit measurement averages fall into either stage 2 or stage 3. In such cases, the client is diagnosed with hypertension on the basis of the first-visit measurements, and a temporary management plan is implemented to bring the blood pressure down quickly (see Hypertensive Crises: Urgency Versus Emergency later in this chapter). Careful differentiation of primary from secondary causes of the high blood pressure must precede any long-term management plan.

Hypertension is classified into a prehypertension category and two stages according to blood pressure readings (Table 52-1). It is important to identify "prehypertensive" values because this range of blood pressures is associated with twice the risk of developing hypertension. Clients who are classified as prehypertensive,

---

BOX 52-2 Assessment of the Client with Hypertension

HISTORY

Note the following points when interviewing the hypertensive client:

- Family history of hypertension, diabetes mellitus, cardiovascular disease, hyperlipidemia, or renal disease; smoking; stress; obesity; or sedentary lifestyle.
- Previous documentation of high blood pressure, including age at onset, level of elevation, and currently prescribed medical regimen.
- History of all prescribed and over-the-counter medications and the client's exact compliance with taking the medications. **Note:** Medications that may either raise blood pressure or interfere with the effectiveness of antihypertensive medications include oral contraceptives, steroids, nonsteroidal anti-inflammatory drugs, nasal decongestants, appetite suppressants, cyclosporine, tricyclic antidepressants, monoamine oxidase inhibitors, and erythropoietin.
- History of any disease or trauma to target organs.
- Results and side effects of previous antihypertensive therapy.
- Clinical manifestations of cardiovascular disorders, such as angina, dyspnea, or claudication.
- History of or recent weight gain, exercise activities, sodium intake, fat intake, alcohol use, and smoking.
- Psychosocial and environmental factors (e.g., emotional stress, cultural food practices, economic status) that may influence blood pressure control.

PHYSICAL EXAMINATION

Physical assessment should include an accurate determination of blood pressure as well as an evaluation of target organs:

- Vital signs and weight.
- Blood pressure—because blood pressure is variable and can be affected by multiple factors, it should be measured so that readings are representative of the client's usual level; the following techniques are strongly recommended:
  - The client should be seated with the arm bare, supported, and positioned at heart level. The client should not have smoked tobacco or ingested caffeine within the previous 30 minutes.
  - Measurement should begin after at least 5 minutes of quiet rest. The client's back should be supported, and both feet should be flat on the floor with the legs uncrossed. The client should not speak while the blood pressure is being monitored.
  - Use of the appropriate cuff size will ensure an accurate measurement. The rubber bladder should encircle at least 80% of the limb being measured. The bladder's width should be one third to one half the circumference of the limb. Several sizes of cuffs (e.g., child, adult, large adult) should be available.
- Measurements should be taken with a mercury sphygmomanometer, a recently calibrated aneroid manometer, or a validated electronic device.
- Postural blood pressures should be measured and recorded according to position and arm used, including lying, sitting, and standing measurements from both arms.
  - Both systolic and diastolic blood pressures should be recorded. The disappearance of sound (phase V) should be used for the diastolic reading.
  - Two or more readings should be averaged. If the first two readings differ by more than 5 mm Hg, additional readings should be obtained.
- Funduscopic examination for retinal arteriolar narrowing, hemorrhages, exudates, and papilledema.
- Examination of the neck for distended veins, carotid bruits, and enlarged thyroid.
- Auscultation of the heart for increased heart rate, dysrhythmias, enlargement, precordial impulses, murmurs, and S_3 and S_4 heart sounds.
- Examination of the abdomen for bruits, aortic dilation, and enlarged kidneys.
- Examination of extremities for diminished or absent peripheral pulses, edema, and bilateral inequality of pulses.
- Neurologic evaluation for signs of cerebral thrombosis or hemorrhage.

LABORATORY STUDIES

Studies used in the routine evaluation of hypertension include a complete blood cell count, urinalysis, determinations of serum potassium and sodium levels, fasting blood glucose level, serum cholesterol level, blood urea nitrogen and serum creatinine levels, electrocardiogram, and chest radiography. These tests provide useful information in determining the severity of vascular disease, the extent of target organ damage, and the possible causes of hypertension. Clients with the potential for secondary hypertension may need more extensive studies.

TABLE 52–1   Classification and Management of Blood Pressure for Adults*

BP Classification	SBP* (mm Hg)	DBP* (mm Hg)	Lifestyle Modification	Initial Drug Therapy Without Compelling Indication	With Compelling Indications
Normal	<120	and <80	Encourage		
Prehypertension	120-139	or 80-89	Yes	No antihypertensive drug indicated	Drug(s) for compelling indications‡
Stage 1 hypertension	140-159	or 90-99	Yes	Thiazide-type diuretics for most May consider ACEI, ARB, BB, CCB, or combination§	Drug(s) for compelling indications‡
Stage 2 hypertension	≥160	or ≥100	Yes	Two-drug combination for most† (usually thiazide-type diuretic and ACEI or ARB or BB or CCB)	Other antihypertensive drugs (diuretics, ACEI, ARB, BB, CCB) as needed

*Treatment determined by highest BP category.
†Initial combined therapy should be used cautiously in those at risk for orthostatic hypotension.
‡Treat clients with chronic kidney disease or diabetes to BP goal of <130/80 mm Hg.
§ACEI, Angiotensin-converting enzyme inhibitor; ARB, angiotensin receptor blocker; BB, beta-blocker; CCB, calcium channel blocker; DBP, diastolic blood pressure; SBP, systolic blood pressure.
From National High Blood Pressure Education Program, National Institutes of Health, National Heart, Lung and Blood Institute. (2003). *The Seventh Report of the Joint National Committee on Detection, Evaluation, and Treatment of High Blood Pressure.* Bethesda, Md: U.S. Government Printing Office.

particularly those who have additional risk factors, should be informed that they are at risk of developing hypertension and that they should institute appropriate lifestyle modifications.

Risk Stratification

Risk stratification (Box 52-3) of clients with hypertension is accomplished after assessing each individual for the type and number of major risk factors and the presence or absence of target organ damage (TOD) or clinical cardiovascular disease (CCD). Target organs, sometimes called *end organs,* are the body organs likely to be damaged by untreated disease (e.g., brain, eyes, kidneys).

OUTCOME MANAGEMENT

The goal of management is to normalize blood pressure and reduce risk factors in order to control the progression of the hypertension. The goal is to lower SBP below 140 mm Hg (goal of ≤120 mm Hg) and DBP below 90 mm Hg (goal of ≤80 mm Hg) while modifying and controlling risk factors. For clients with diabetes or progressive renal disease, the goal is <130/80 mm Hg (or 125/75 mm Hg for clients with renal disease and proteinuria >1 g/24 hour).

Long-term compliance and adherence has emerged as the most essential element in reducing morbidity and mortality rates associated with hypertension. The most pronounced positive client outcomes have resulted from a systematic, multifactorial, multidisciplinary team approach for primary and secondary prevention and management of hypertension using diverse qualified health care professionals. Multidisciplinary teams can provide the most comprehensive, cost-effective care of clients with a multitude of prevention and management

needs, including those related to the prevention, diagnosis, and management of hypertension.

Unfortunately, poor compliance with or adherence to antihypertensive therapy persists as one of the most frustrating blocks to effective therapeutic management

BOX 52-3   Cardiovascular Risk Stratification

MAJOR RISK FACTORS

- Hypertension*
- Smoking
- Age (>55 for men; >65 for women)
- Diabetes mellitus*
- Physical inactivity
- Dyslipidemia*
- Gender (men and postmenopausal women)
- Obesity (BMI ≥30)*
- Family history of cardiovascular disease: women <65 years or men <55 years
- Microalbuminuria or estimated GFR <60 ml/min

TARGET ORGAN DAMAGE/CLINICAL CARDIOVASCULAR DISEASE (TOD/CCD)

- Heart diseases
  - Left ventricular hypertrophy
  - Angina/prior myocardial infarction
  - Prior coronary revascularization
  - Heart failure
- Stroke or transient ischemic attack
- Nephropathy
- Peripheral arterial disease
- Retinopathy

*Components of metabolic syndrome.
Modified from National High Blood Pressure Education Program, National Institutes of Health, National Heart, Lung and Blood Institute. (2003). *The Seventh Report of the Joint National Committee on Detection, Evaluation, and Treatment of High Blood Pressure.* Bethesda, Md: U.S. Government Printing Office.

and is often due to clients' belief systems and values. Poor compliance or adherence is the reason that more than two thirds of clients with hypertension do not have adequate control of their blood pressure. For example, clients may choose not to have the initial prescription filled; successfully initiate therapy only to abandon it after a few weeks or months; or comply with only part of the regimen, thus failing to achieve optimal control.

Normalizing Arterial Pressure
The ultimate factors in evaluating whether the correct choice of treatment regimen has been made are as follows: the desired "control" blood pressure is reached, treatment choices are tolerated and safe, and the client is willing to *commit* to the regimen over the long term.

Lifestyle Modifications
Strong research evidence has illustrated conclusively that lifestyle modifications are effective in lowering blood pressure and reducing cardiovascular risk factors at little overall cost and with minimal risk. According to the *JNC VII* (Figure 52-1), lifestyle modifications are suggested as definitive first-line therapy for some clients, at least for the first 6 to 12 months after the initial diagnosis.

Lifestyle modification is also strongly encouraged as adjunctive therapy for all clients with hypertension who are receiving pharmacologic therapy. Continued healthy lifestyle practices, along with pharmacologic therapy, can reduce the number and dosage of antihypertensive medications needed to manage the condition.

Weight Reduction
Excess body weight, exhibited by a body mass index (BMI)—weight in kilograms divided by height in meters squared—of 27 or greater, correlates closely with elevated blood pressure. Also, excess body fat accumulated in the torso with a waist circumference of 35 inches or greater for women and 40 inches or greater for men has been associated with an increased risk for hypertension (waist/hip ratio). For many people with hypertension whose body weight is more than 10% greater than ideal, weight reduction of as little as 10 pounds can lower blood pressure up to 10 mm Hg. Weight reduction also enhances the effectiveness of antihypertensive medications. Therefore reassess the client's blood pressure during weight loss, and make appropriate changes in pharmacologic interventions as needed.

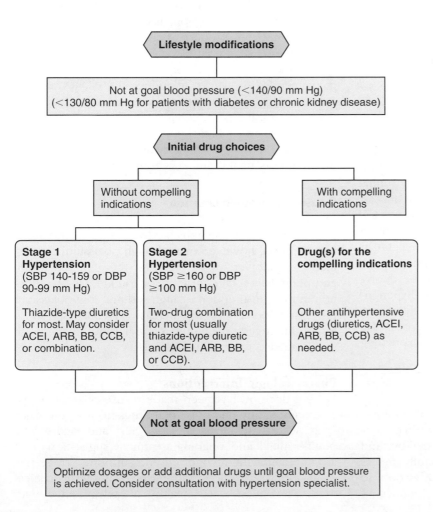

■ **FIGURE 52–1** Algorithm for treatment of hypertension. *ACEI,* Angiotensin-converting enzyme inhibitor; *ARB,* angiotensin receptor blocker; *BB,* beta-blocker; *CCB,* calcium channel blocker; *DBP,* diastolic blood pressure; *SBP,* systolic blood pressure. *(From National High Blood Pressure Education Program, National Institutes of Health, National Heart, Lung and Blood Institute. [2003]. The Seventh Report of the Joint National Committee on Detection, Evaluation, and Treatment of High Blood Pressure. Bethesda, Md: U.S. Government Printing Office.)*

Sodium Restriction

Most hypertensive people are sensitive to sodium, showing rises in BP after sodium intake. Therefore, a moderate restriction of sodium intake to 2 or 3 g of sodium can be used to lower blood pressure. The amount of medication otherwise needed may be decreased if sodium intake is lowered. In addition, this moderate sodium restriction may reduce the degree of potassium depletion that often accompanies diuretic therapy.

Dietary Fat Modification

Modification of dietary intake of fat by decreasing the fraction of saturated fat and increasing that of polyunsaturated fat has little, if any, effect on decreasing blood pressure but can decrease the cholesterol level significantly. Because dyslipidemia is a major risk factor in the development of atherosclerosis, diet therapy aimed at reducing lipids is an important adjunct to any total dietary regimen. In addition to the usual recommendations for sensible eating following the food pyramid (see Chapter 1), the Dietary Approaches to Stop Hypertension (DASH) diet (Table 52-2), which is rich in fruits, vegetables, nuts, and low-fat dairy foods with reduced saturated and total fats, should be recommended for clients who need a more structured, fat-limited dietary intervention.

Exercise

A regular program of aerobic exercise adequate to achieve at least a moderate level of physical fitness facilitates cardiovascular conditioning and can aid the obese hypertensive client in weight reduction and reduce the risk for cardiovascular disease and all-cause mortality. Blood pressure can be reduced with moderate-intensity (as low as 40% to 60% of maximum oxygen consumption) physical activity, such as a brisk walk (about 2.5 to 3 mph) for 30 to 45 minutes most days of the week.

Weight training using *light* weights is a positive addition to any exercise regimen; however, lifting *heavy* weights can be harmful because blood pressure rises, sometimes to high levels, with the vasovagal response that occurs during an intense isometric muscle contraction. Advise hypertensive clients to initiate exercise programs gradually, slowly increasing the intensity and the duration of activity as the body adjusts and becomes more conditioned with ongoing professional surveillance.

Alcohol Restriction

The consumption of more than 1 ounce of alcohol per day is associated with a higher prevalence of hypertension, poor adherence to antihypertensive therapy, and occasionally refractory hypertension. Carefully assess alcohol intake. Advise clients who do drink alcohol to do so in moderation (i.e., no more than 1 ounce of ethanol per day for men and 0.5 ounce for women). There is 1 ounce (30 ml) of ethanol in 2 ounces (60 ml) of 100-proof whiskey, in 10 ounces (300 ml) of wine, or in 24 ounces (720 ml) of beer.

Caffeine Restriction

Although acute ingestion of caffeine may raise blood pressure, chronic moderate caffeine ingestion appears to have no significant effect on blood pressure. Therefore caffeine restriction is not necessary unless cardiac response or other excessive sensitivity to caffeine is present.

Relaxation Techniques

A variety of relaxation therapies, including transcendental meditation, yoga, biofeedback, progressive muscle relaxation, and psychotherapy, can reduce blood pressure in hypertensive clients, at least transiently. Although each modality has its advocates, none has been conclusively shown to be either practical for the majority of hypertensive clients or effective in maintaining a significant long-term effect.

Smoking Cessation

Although smoking has not been statistically linked to the development of hypertension, nicotine definitely increases the heart rate and produces peripheral vasoconstriction, which does raise arterial blood pressure for a short time during and after smoking. Smoking cessation is strongly recommended, however, to reduce the client's risk for cancer, pulmonary disease, and cardiovascular disease. Smokers appear to have a higher frequency of malignant hypertension and subarachnoid hemorrhage. In addition, risk reduction brought about by antihypertensive therapy may not be as great in smokers as in nonsmokers.

Potassium Supplementation

The high ratio of sodium to potassium in the modern diet has been held responsible for the development of hypertension; however, even though potassium supplements may lower blood pressure, they are too costly and potentially too hazardous for routine use. A reduction in the consumption of high-sodium, low-potassium processed foods with an increase in consumption of low-sodium, high-potassium natural foods may be all that is needed for maximum benefits.

Pharmacologic Interventions

Once a decision has been made to use pharmacologic intervention, any one of several drugs from seven major drug classes can be used. Table 52-1 and Figure 52-1 outline initial and ongoing treatment suggestions that are internationally recognized and supported by results of major worldwide, randomized, long-term clinical trials. Prevention-based healthy lifestyle change with

TABLE 52–2   Dietary Approaches to Stop Hypertension (DASH) Diet

The DASH eating plan shown below is based on 2000 calories per day. Depending on your caloric needs, your number of daily servings in a food group may vary from those listed. This eating plan is from the Dietary Approaches to Stop Hypertension (DASH) clinical study supported by the National Institutes of Health. The DASH combination diet lowered blood pressure and so may help prevent and control high blood pressure.

Food Group	Daily Servings (Number)	Serving Size	Examples	Significance of Each Food Group to DASH Diet Pattern
Grains and grain products	7-8	1 slice bread; ½ cup dry cereal; ½ cup cooked rice, pasta, or cereal*	Whole wheat breads, English muffin, pita bread, bagel, cereals and fiber, grits, oatmeal	Major source of energy and fiber
Vegetables	4-5	1 cup raw, leafy vegetable; ½ cup cooked vegetable; 6 oz vegetable juice	Tomatoes, potatoes, carrots, peas, squash, broccoli, turnip greens, collards, kale, spinach, artichokes, beans, sweet potatoes	Rich sources of potassium, magnesium, and fiber
Fruits	4-5	6 oz fruit juice; 1 medium fruit; ¼ cup dried fruit; ½ cup fresh, frozen, or canned fruit	Apricots, bananas, dates, grapes, oranges, orange juice, grapefruit, grapefruit juice, mangoes, melons, peaches, pineapples, prunes, raisins, strawberries, tangerines	Important sources of potassium, magnesium, and fiber
Low-fat or nonfat dairy foods	2-3	8 oz milk; 1 cup yogurt; 1.5 oz cheese	Fat-free or 1% milk, skim or low-fat buttermilk, nonfat or low-fat yogurt, part skim mozzarella cheese, nonfat cheese	Major sources of calcium and protein
Meats, poultry, fish	2 or less	3 oz cooked meats, poultry, or fish	Select only lean; trim away visible fats; broil, roast, or boil, instead of frying; remove skin from poultry	Rich sources of protein and magnesium
Nuts, seeds, and legumes	4-5/wk	1.5 oz or ⅓ cup nuts; ½ oz or 2 tbsp seeds; ½ cup cooked dry beans	Almonds, filberts, mixed nuts, peanuts, walnuts, sunflower seeds, kidney beans, lentils, and peas	Rich sources of energy, magnesium, potassium, protein, and fiber
Fats and oils†	2-3	1 tsp soft margarine; 1 tbsp low-fat mayonnaise; 2 tbsp light salad dressing; 1 tsp vegetable oil	Soft margarine, low-fat mayonnaise, light salad dressing Vegetable oil (such as olive, corn, canola, or safflower)	Besides considering the fats added to foods, choose foods that contain less fat
Sweets	5/wk	1 tbsp sugar; 1 tbsp jelly or jam; ½ oz jelly beans; 8 oz lemonade	Maple syrup, sugar, jelly, jam, fruit-flavored gelatin, jelly beans, hard candy, fruit punch, sorbet ices	Sweets should be low in fat

*Serving sizes vary between ½ and 1½ cups. Check the nutrition label.
†Fat content changes per serving size of fats and oil. For example, 1 tbsp regular salad dressing equals 1 serving, 1 tbsp low-fat dressing equals ½ serving, and 1 tbsp fat-free dressing equals zero servings.
Modified from Kolasa, K.M. (1999). Dietary Approaches to Stop Hypertension (DASH) in clinical practice: A primary care experience. *Clinical Cardiology, 22*(7 Suppl), III-16-22.

the addition of pharmacologic therapy as indicated is the preferred treatment regimen for those clients in stages 1 and 2. If therapy is chosen carefully, more than half of mild hypertension cases can be controlled with one or two drugs. Most clients, however, will require two or more drugs to achieve goal blood pressure.

Antihypertensive medications can be classified into the following categories: diuretics, alpha- and beta-adrenergic antagonists [beta-blocker (BB)], vasodilators, calcium antagonists [calcium channel blocker (CCB)], angiotensin-converting enzyme (ACE) inhibitors, and angiotensin receptor blockers (ARBs). Diuretics, particularly thiazide-type diuretics, will continue to be the first line drug of choice for newly diagnosed, low level, uncomplicated hypertension, and BBs will continue to be first-line choices in other selected cases. However, there are compelling and specific indications for two- and three-drug initial and/or subsequent treatment regimes for various conditions.

Provider Responsibilities

The goal of antihypertensive therapy is to control blood pressure with a minimum of side effects (see the Integrating Pharmacology feature on Antihypertensive Medications at right). Clinicians must be currently knowledgeable regarding drug choices and must be able to extrapolate potential side effects or negative effects quickly and effectively to manage clients' blood pressures most successfully, especially if concomitant conditions exist. See a pharmacologic text for detailed descriptions of each drug or drug combination and its actions and side effects. See the Client Education Guide at right and the Concept Map feature on p. 1301.

If more than one drug is necessary, several combination therapies have proved effective. For example, the combination of a diuretic with a beta-adrenergic blocker or other adrenergic inhibitor has been effective in both blacks and whites, in contrast to the responses to the individual drugs, whereas blacks respond less well to beta-adrenergic blockers alone or as first-line treatment. The combination of a diuretic with an ACE inhibitor or a CCB has additive effects on blood pressure. Finally, combination drugs can be less expensive than the individual drugs, and the need for only one drug may improve compliance in a client who does not like "taking so many pills."

Reducing the number and amounts of antihypertensive medications should be considered once a client's blood pressure has been controlled effectively for at least 1 year. Medication dosages must be decreased slowly and progressively until the lowest effective dosages are reached and maintained. Regular follow-up evaluation is essential if drug therapy has been completely stopped secondary to success of weight loss or other lifestyle change practices because blood pressure can rise again over time.

INTEGRATING PHARMACOLOGY

Antihypertensive Medications

It is common to administer more than one antihypertensive along with diuretics for blood pressure control. Usually the use of more than one medication is designed to lower the dose of any single medication and reduce the side effects. However, when administering these medications, it is important to consider their synergistic effects.

Before administering antihypertensives, be certain that you are aware of the most recent blood pressure (BP). Many events during a hospitalization can lower BP, such as blood loss with surgery and pain control with analgesics. Conversely, fluid overload and stress or anxiety can raise BP. It is common to withhold antihypertensives following surgery during times when BP is low. If the BP is high, administer the antihypertensive medications ahead of schedule (e.g., at 0800 rather than waiting until 0900). Also note the pulse rate; beta-adrenergic blockers can lead to bradycardia.

Also make note of the most recent potassium level. Loop diuretics quickly reduce potassium levels, and potassium-sparing diuretics can lead to elevations in potassium levels. Further, aldosterone blocking agents, such as ACE inhibitors and angiotensin receptor blockers, can also lead to hyperkalemia. ACE inhibitors and calcium channel blockers can lead to orthostatic hypotension, and positional BP measurement may be warranted to reduce the risk of falls.

Recent data have shown that the use of beta-adrenergic blockers before surgery has reduced mortality. Therefore you may be asked to administer these medications before surgery even in clients with no history of hypertension or who do not routinely take beta blockers.

CLIENT EDUCATION GUIDE

Ten Ways to Control Your High Blood Pressure

- Know your blood pressure. Have it checked regularly.
- Know what your weight should be. Keep it at that level or below.
- Do not use too much salt in cooking or at meals. Avoid salty foods.
- Eat a low-fat diet according to American Heart Association recommendations.
- Do not smoke cigarettes or use tobacco products.
- Take your medicine exactly as prescribed. Do not run out of pills even for a single day.
- Keep appointments with the doctor.
- Follow your doctor's advice about exercise.
- Make certain that your parents, brothers, sisters, and children have their blood pressure checked regularly.
- Live a normal life in every other way.

From the American Heart Association. (2004). Retrieved 03/18/04 from http://americanheart.org/presenter.jhtml?identifier=578.

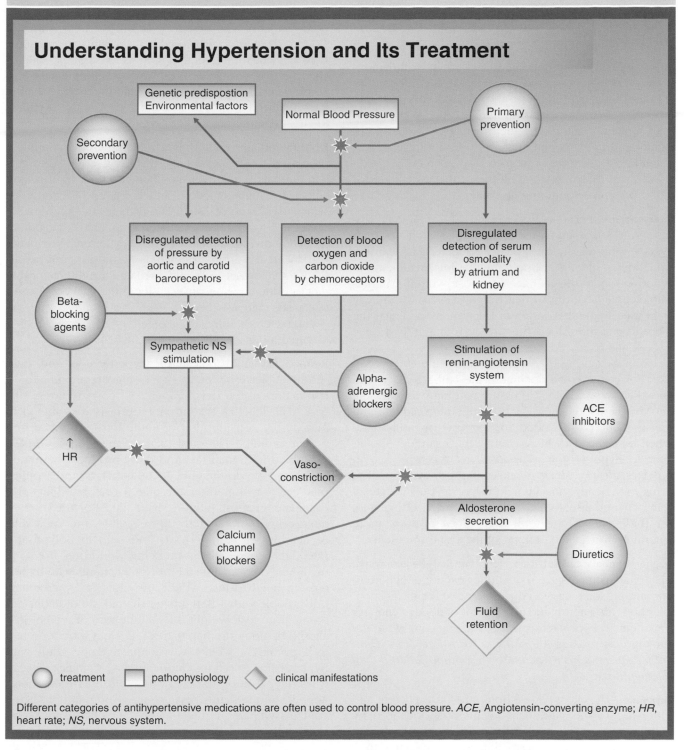

Understanding Hypertension and Its Treatment

Different categories of antihypertensive medications are often used to control blood pressure. *ACE*, Angiotensin-converting enzyme; *HR*, heart rate; *NS,* nervous system.

Nursing Management

Assessment. The many sequelae of untreated hypertension can be prevented, or the severity of such problems reduced, if hypertension is well managed. Client education and understanding are crucial to successful management.

Diagnosis, Outcomes, and Interventions

Diagnosis: Ineffective Therapeutic Regimen Management (Individual). Use the nursing diagnosis *Ineffective Therapeutic Regimen Management (Individual)* to identify the learning needs of the newly diagnosed hypertensive client. The nursing diagnosis can be written *Risk for*

Ineffective Therapeutic Regimen Management (Individual) related to a new diagnosis, no previous learning about the disease process, potential consequences, the rationale for life-long intervention and follow-up, and proper administration of prescribed medications.

Outcomes. The client and significant others will demonstrate knowledge required for self-care as evidenced by (1) describing hypertension and its associated risk factors; (2) discussing the importance of lifelong medical follow-up; (3) listing the prescribed medications, including drug name, rationale for use, dose, frequency, potential side effects, and measures to minimize side effects; and (4) demonstrating the proper technique for blood pressure monitoring at home.

Interventions. Because hypertension is a lifelong disease and has dangerous complications, clients with hypertension need clear, practical, and realistic learning guidelines. Guidelines should include information about hypertension and its management. Use written materials with clear illustrations for teaching the client with newly diagnosed hypertension about the condition. Teach the client to measure blood pressure at home at least once a week and to record the findings in a diary.

When measuring blood pressure, use the correct cuff size. For consistency, document the cuff size used and on which arm the blood pressure reading was assessed. Inform clients of their blood pressure reading, and advise them of the need for periodic measurement. When working with most clients, the examiner should refer to hypertension as *high blood pressure* to help avoid confusion. Many clients unfamiliar with medical terms may believe that hypertension denotes a state of being "hypertense"—that is, being worried or agitated. For these clients, the term *high blood pressure* more accurately conveys the nature of the health problem.

Diagnosis: Imbalanced Nutrition: More Than Body Requirements. Dietary adjustments can reduce the severity of hypertension and in some cases reduce the need for medication. Client teaching about and assessment of needed changes constitute an important aspect of nursing care. Write the nursing diagnosis as *Imbalanced Nutrition: More Than Body Requirements related to high sodium, fat, and total calorie intake.*

Outcomes. The client will demonstrate knowledge of and adherence to the nutritional regimen as evidenced by describing specific dietary modifications (including sodium, fat, and calorie restrictions) and explaining their rationales (reduction in levels of urine sodium and blood cholesterol, weight loss). (See the Client Education Guide features on Low-Sodium Diet, on Low-Fat, Low-Cholesterol Diet, and on Calorie-Restriction Diet on the website.)

Interventions. The two most important aspects of dietary intervention for hypertension are weight reduction (for overweight clients) and mild to moderate sodium restriction. Therefore advise the client with hypertension to eat a diet low in salt, calories, cholesterol, and saturated fat. Discuss the prescribed diet with the household members who prepare food. If possible, enlist the aid of a dietitian to provide detailed dietary instructions. Before dietary intervention begins, assess the client's patterns of food intake; lifestyle; food preferences; and ethnic, social, cultural, and financial influences. A highly individualized approach to dietary counseling is crucial to client compliance and adherence.

Restrict Sodium. Sodium is a hidden ingredient in many processed foods, beverages (including water from certain sources), and over-the-counter drugs (particularly antacids, cough remedies, and laxatives). It cannot be seen and often is not tasted. The average adult daily intake of salt is 5 to 15 g, but the therapeutic effects of sodium reduction on blood pressure do not occur until salt intake is reduced to 6 g/day or lower. Low-salt diets can be difficult to follow, at least initially. Reassure the client that dietary adherence becomes easier as the palate adjusts to decreased salt over several weeks to months. After the client becomes fully accustomed to the low-salt diet, unsalted foods usually cease to taste bland.

Reduce Fat and Cholesterol. Hypertension and high serum cholesterol levels (>250 mg/dl) are linked as risk factors in the development of coronary artery disease. The level of serum cholesterol is determined in part by the consumption of cholesterol, saturated and polyunsaturated fats, and total calories. Cholesterol is contained in animal fats and dairy products. Saturated fats occur predominantly in animal fats and tropical oils (e.g., coconut and palm oils). Unsaturated fats predominate in most plant-derived fats. Polyunsaturated fats occur predominantly in vegetable and seed oils. A diet low in saturated fats and high in polyunsaturated fats is beneficial in reducing blood pressure. (See the DASH diet in Table 52-2.) Not all clients with hypertension need to lose weight. As discussed previously, only people with a BMI greater than 27 should consider the need to lose weight. Ideally the rate of weight loss should be no more than 0.25 kg -0.5 kg (about one-half to 1 pound) a week. Advise the average adult with hypertension to reduce caloric intake by at least 250 calories/day. Caution the client to avoid over-the-counter appetite suppressants because these preparations often contain sympathomimetic agents, which elevate blood pressure.

Diagnosis: Ineffective Health Maintenance. Exercise is like dietary management: A regular exercise program can lower blood pressure in hypertensive clients. This nursing diagnosis can be written as *Ineffective Health Maintenance related to a lack of regular exercise regimen.*

Outcomes. The client will begin and maintain an appropriate exercise program as evidenced by self-report, demonstration of the ability to monitor heart rate during exercise, sensation of reduced physical and emotional stress, and reduced blood pressure.

Interventions. Exercise programs can heighten the client's sense of well-being, provide an outlet for emotional tension, produce relaxation of blood vessels, and raise the levels of high-density lipoproteins (HDLs) relative to total blood cholesterol. Elevated HDL levels are associated with a decreased risk of cardiovascular morbidity and mortality. Instruct the client, however, to avoid heavy weight-lifting, isometric exercises, and other activities inappropriate to the client's physical limitations. A modest but consistent exercise program provides greater benefits than those obtainable with spurts of strenuous activity mixed with periods of inactivity. A gradually increasing program of aerobic activity such as walking, jogging, or swimming can thus be recommended.

Maximum heart rate is calculated by subtracting the client's age from 220. Most clients without diagnosed heart disease or other concomitant conditions can safely exercise to 75% to 85% of the maximal heart rate. Clients with known cardiopulmonary disease and hypertension must be prescreened; a cardio-respiratory exercise stress test is most predictive of cardiopulmonary and exercise functional capacity. An *individualized* target heart rate can be designated from objective data obtained from this test that will allow the client to maximize his or her aerobic exercise. Ultimately, before an exercise prescription is advised and initiated for a hypertensive client, a qualified specialist must conduct a careful performance evaluation.

Diagnosis: Risk for Nonadherence. The greatest problem in the management of chronic hypertension involves the client's lack of adherence to nonpharmacologic and pharmacologic interventions. An estimated 40% to 60% of clients with hypertension fail to comply with prescribed therapy. There are several reasons why hypertensive clients do not follow prescribed regimens:

- The asymptomatic nature of the disease tends to minimize the perceived seriousness of the problem and importance of intervention.
- Therapeutic regimens often demand difficult lifestyle changes, such as low-sodium diets, weight loss, and smoking cessation.
- Many hypertensive agents produce annoying side effects, and clients who require antihypertensive medication may consider the intervention worse than the disease.
- The high cost of medications and the inconvenience of obtaining health care also contribute to noncompliance.

Assess the reasons for possible nonadherence, and then state the nursing diagnosis as *Risk for Nonadherence related to a lack of understanding about the seriousness of high blood pressure, cost of therapy, side effects of*

medications, complexity of management, or *multiple changes in lifestyle.*

Outcomes. The client will actively participate in creating a treatment plan, describing the underlying causes of hypertension and self-care strategies, adhering to scheduled follow-up appointments, describing the actions and side effects of current medications, and expressing commitment to and self-responsibility for controlling hypertension.

Interventions. Nursing interventions for promoting adherence to the antihypertensive treatment regimen include individualizing care, ensuring adequate follow-up, communicating often with the client, and teaching the client and the client's family. Adherence usually improves dramatically when the client understands the causative factors underlying hypertension as well as the consequences of inadequate intervention and health maintenance.

Evaluation. Medications can lower blood pressure quickly. The remainder of the interventions, such as stress management, exercise, and smoking cessation, are more difficult to implement and maintain. Expect the client to struggle with compliance with any and all of the necessary changes in medications and/or lifestyle. Ask specific questions in a nonjudgmental manner. As needed, recommend involvement in various self-help groups, such as smoking cessation groups.

Modifications for Older Clients

Hypertension is one of the most prevalent cardiovascular diseases among older adults, and because of their advanced age, these clients are more likely to suffer from end-organ damage secondary to chronically elevated pressure.[7,14] Blood pressure readings in older adults show greater variability from one measurement to the next compared to younger clients; therefore the diagnosis is made after several readings. Recent research findings indicate a need to treat hypertension in older people, regardless of whether both the SBP *and* DBP are involved or there is evidence of only isolated systolic hypertension. Older adults are more likely to experience adverse reactions to antihypertensive drugs and are monitored closely for evidence of such reactions; they are given detailed advice on the specifics of their medication regimens; and the clinical course of the disease is carefully followed.

The ultimate goal of antihypertensive therapy in older adults is not to try to lower the pressure to "normal" values immediately but rather to lower the pressure gradually to a level sufficient to eliminate target organ damage and to minimize the risk of hypoperfusion. "Start low and go slow" is the principle followed for prescribing medications to the older adult. Too rapid a reduction in blood pressure in older clients, particularly those with chronic hypertension, may produce cerebral hypoperfusion that manifests by decreased mental status, weakness, and dizziness.

HYPERTENSIVE CRISES: URGENCY VERSUS EMERGENCY

Elevated blood pressure alone, in the absence of clinical manifestations or new or progressive target organ damage, rarely requires *emergency* therapy. In most cases the hypertensive crisis really constitutes a hypertensive *urgency* in which a severe elevation in blood pressure has been reached but there is mild or no acute target organ damage. Hypertensive urgencies include cases in which it is desirable to reduce blood pressure within a few hours to 24 hours. Clinicians treat urgent situations primarily with oral medications in an outpatient setting with close follow-up.

Because many clients have chronically elevated blood pressure that has not been diagnosed, the seriousness of any crisis correlates not so much with the level of blood pressure elevation as with the extent of target organ damage secondary to length of time the blood pressure has remained significantly high. Clients who qualify for emergent care are hospitalized, given intravenous medications, and monitored closely for at least 12 to 24 hours.

Without treatment persistent severe hypertension results in a 90% death rate within 1 year secondary to renal or heart failure, stroke, myocardial infarction, or aortic dissection. The most common cause of persistent severe hypertension is untreated hypertension. Other causes include eclampsia, dissecting aortic aneurysm, pyelonephritis, sudden catecholamine release (as from a pheochromocytoma), drug or toxic substance ingestion or exposure, and food and drug interactions (e.g., between a monoamine oxidase inhibitor [MAO] and aged cheese).

Clinical manifestations include those of hypertensive encephalopathy evidenced by restlessness, changes in level of consciousness (e.g., confusion, somnolence, lethargy, memory defects, coma), seizures, blurred vision, dizziness, headache, nausea, and vomiting. Assessment may also reveal renal insufficiency, proteinuria, hematuria, urinary sediment casts, hemolytic anemia, left ventricular failure, and pulmonary edema. Severe headache may be occipital or anterior in location, is steady and throbbing, and is often worse in the morning. Visual blurring, reduced visual acuity, and even blindness can occur. Acute renal failure, rapid vascular deterioration, and stroke can also develop.

OUTCOME MANAGEMENT

The initial goal of therapy in hypertensive crisis is to reduce mean arterial pressure by no more than 25% within the first minutes to 2 hours. Then a reduction in blood pressure toward 160/100 mm Hg is accomplished over the next 2 to 6 hours.

SAFETY

ALERT

Blood pressure is monitored frequently (every 5 to 15 minutes, depending on the drug and the route of administration used), and medications are titrated to manage the course of blood pressure reduction. It is essential to avoid excessive falls in blood pressure, which can precipitate renal, cerebral, or coronary ischemia.

Consequently restoration of normal blood pressure must be done slowly and with care. Once the client is out of immediate danger, oral medications are adjusted while vital signs are monitored continuously, and changes in drug therapy regimens are made if necessary. NOTE: Although sublingual administration of nifedipine had been widely used to reduce blood pressure in an urgent situation, it is no longer considered appropriate therapy because of several reports of severe adverse effects from its use.

COMMUNITY SCREENING AND SELF-CARE

Public Health Initiative

Research showing the importance of normalized blood pressure for clients' optimum health led to the introduction by the National Heart, Lung and Blood Institute (NHLBI) of the National High Blood Pressure Education Program (NHBPEP) in 1972. The NHBPEP is the first large-scale public outreach and education campaign to reduce high blood pressure. Its promotion of the detection, treatment, and control of high blood pressure has been credited with influencing the dramatic increase in the public's understanding of hypertension and its role in heart attacks and strokes.

The prevention and treatment of hypertension continue to be a major public health concern in the United States. Prevention of hypertension and early discovery of new cases depend on a broader national public health effort. With guidance from the *Healthy People/2010* initiatives, this national effort has begun. In addition to the diligent work of the NHBPEP, government support is increasing, and nationwide attention and assistance from business and industry, labor organizations, health care institutions, voluntary associations, and local communities are also on the rise. For example, the *JNC VII* guideline endorses the American Public Health Association (APHA) resolution challenging food manufacturers and restaurants to reduce sodium in foods by 50% over the next decade.

The following are the revised goals of the national public health plan:

- To prevent the rise of blood pressure with age
- To decrease the existing prevalence of hypertension
- To increase hypertension awareness and detection
- To improve control of hypertension
- To reduce cardiovascular risks
- To increase recognition of the importance of controlled isolated systolic hypertension
- To improve recognition of the importance of the persistence and damage from high-normal blood pressures
- To reduce ethnic, socioeconomic, and regional variations in hypertension
- To improve opportunities for treatment
- To enhance community programs

Managed Care and Community Screening

Because high blood pressure is so common, its management requires a major commitment from clinicians and managed care organizations. Managed care programs offer the opportunity for a coordinated systematic, multifactorial, multidisciplinary approach to care. Nurse-managed clinics offer attractive opportunities to improve adherence and outcomes.

Hypertensive clients usually learn of their condition through incidental screening in health care facilities or through organized community screening in public settings (e.g., shopping malls, schools, and the workplace). Nurses are actively involved in both approaches. About 80% of Americans come into contact with some aspect of the health care system at least once a year (e.g., in a health care provider's office, clinic, or hospital). Each encounter with the health care system presents an opportunity for incidental blood pressure screening. Blood pressure measurement should be a routine procedure at every initial encounter with a health care practitioner and annually thereafter.

Organized community screening programs help to assess the remaining 20% of Americans not in contact with any part of the health care system. Such programs identify not only clients with untreated hypertension but also those who have discontinued intervention or whose hypertension is not adequately controlled by current intervention. In addition, screening programs provide an opportunity to educate the public. It is particularly important to screen members of high-risk "target groups," such as black and older populations. Community services need to keep target groups in mind when choosing the setting for blood pressure screenings. Practitioners who take blood pressure readings need to inform clients in writing of their blood pressure and its significance and, if necessary, the importance of follow-up evaluation. Culturally and linguistically appropriate counseling by health care providers is important to those efforts.

Self-Measurement of Blood Pressure

Measurement of blood pressure outside a health care provider's office can provide valuable information for initial evaluation and subsequent follow-up of people with hypertension. Most drug, medical supply, and grocery stores provide standardized blood pressure monitors that their customers can use at no cost. These monitoring stations are generally located near the pharmacy or medical supplies department. Such stores also usually carry a variety of self-measurement blood pressure devices for home use. Choosing a monitoring device may be confusing for some people; however, several models of accurate and appropriate electronic or aneroid-type sphygmomanometers are available. Most insurance packages cover the cost of a home blood pressure unit, and these devices are generally easy to use.

Manual and electronic arm cuffs are the most accurate. Finger and wrist monitors are available but have proved inaccurate in standardized testing. Periodically, the accuracy of the instrument used in the home should be checked by comparing home readings with those obtained in the health care provider's office, at a "health fair," or in a community nursing clinic. It is helpful if the client keeps a record of BP values; these findings will help with follow-up care.

SYNCOPE

Syncope (fainting) is defined as generalized muscle weakness and an inability to stand erect accompanied by loss of consciousness. It is a good measure of cardiovascular status because it may indicate decreased cardiac output, fluid volume deficits, or defects in cerebral tissue perfusion.

Syncope is a common occurrence when a person tries to stand after being bedridden for a while. This form of syncope, called *postural hypotension,* can be seen in clients attempting to ambulate the first few times after surgery, in clients who have been on prolonged bed rest, and in clients who have dysrhythmias. When a person moves quickly to a standing position, blood normally pools in the lower legs. The arterial pressure receptors in the aortic arch detect the fall in cardiac output that occurs with the lack of venous return, and they increase sympathetic tone to compress arterioles to improve venous return. If the sympathetic response is not adequate or is blocked by medication, the person becomes dizzy because of the decreased cerebral perfusion. All medications taken to reduce blood pressure have the potential to cause orthostatic hypotension or postural hypotension—some more than others, such as potent diuretics, alpha$_1$-receptor blockers, and vasodilators.

> **When a client reports dizziness or is at risk of syncope because of medication use or prolonged bed rest, assess fluid volume status and check the pulse for irregularities.**   SAFETY ALERT

If syncope develops, it usually can be managed by having the client move slowly to a sitting position and rest a moment before standing. If the client becomes dizzy, instruct the client to breathe deeply and to keep both eyes open. Syncope should resolve within moments. If it is prolonged, place the client supine, use leg exercises to improve venous return, and wait until the blood pressure returns to a normotensive state.

> **Confused clients who do not wait for syncope to resolve before walking are at risk for falls. Bed alarms may be needed.**   SAFETY ALERT

CONCLUSIONS

New coalitions between health care providers and individual communities are forming to focus on the prevention and management of hypertension throughout all stages of life. Support from the community and greater use of technology such as the Internet will play an increasingly greater role in promoting long-term adherence to lifestyle and pharmacologic regimens. Achieving long-term control of blood pressure risk factors requires that the same interest and attention given to initial evaluation and treatment decisions also be given to long-term lifestyle management issues. In addition, *JNC VII* has taken a strong stance toward mandating better pharmacologic control of high blood pressure. In their report, *JNC VII* stated that clinicians' failure to titrate or combine medications, despite knowing that a client's blood pressure is not at goal, represents clinical inertia and must be overcome.

THINKING CRITICALLY

1. A 50-year-old obese black man arrives at your clinic with persistent elevated blood pressure. He has had hypertension for 7 months. Despite attempts at lifestyle management, his blood pressure has continued to rise. He was started on a regimen of antihypertensive medication 1 month ago and has returned to the clinic today for a follow-up visit. His blood pressure is higher than it was initially. What might explain his continued elevated blood pressure?

Factors to Consider. What other history and physical examination data should you obtain to analyze this case more effectively? When and how long should lifestyle modifications alone be encouraged? How long does it take for various medications to be effective? What diseases worsen hypertension? What psychosocial factors affect compliance with or adherence to a treatment regimen? What modifications in the pharmacologic treatment plan, if any, would be most appropriate at this time?

evolve *Discussions for these questions can be found on the website.*

BIBLIOGRAPHY

Citations appearing in red refer to primary research.

Citations appearing in blue refer to evidence-based practice guidelines and protocols.

1. Ades, P.A. (2001). Cardiac rehabilitation and secondary prevention of coronary heart disease. *New England Journal of Medicine, 345,* 892-902.
2. Agodoa, L.Y., et al. (2001). Effect of ramipril vs amlodipine on renal outcomes in hypertensive nephrosclerosis: A randomized control trial (AASK). *Journal of the American Medical Association, 285,* 2719-2728.
2a. American Heart Association. (2006, December). *Controlling blood pressure: Hypertension among United States adults 1999-2004.* Retrieved November 19, 2007, from www.heart.org/print_presen ter.jhtml?identifier=3044518.
2b. Barlow, C.E., LaMonte, M.J., FitzGerald, S.J., et al. (2006). Cardiorespiratory fitness is an independent predictor of hypertension incidence among initially normotensive healthy women. *American Journal of Epidemiology, 163*(2),142-150.
3. Brenner, B.M., et al. (2001). Effects of losartan on renal and cardiovascular outcomes in patients with type 2 diabetes and nephropathy. *New England Journal of Medicine, 345,* 861-869.
4. Cardiac Rehabilitation Guideline Panel. (1995). *Cardiac rehabilitation* (AHCPR Pub. No. 96-0672). Rockville, Md: Agency for Health Care Policy and Research, Public Health Services, U.S. Department of Health and Human Services.
5. Davidson, M.H. (2002). Strategies to improve adult treatment panel III guideline adherence and patient compliance. *The American Journal of Cardiology* 89(Suppl), 8C-22C.
6. DeMartinis, J. (2001). Relaxation and stress management. In D. Robinson & C.P. Kish (Eds.), *Core concepts in advanced practice nursing.* St. Louis: Mosby.
7. DeMartinis, J. (2003). Principles and methods of the basic physical examination. In R. Jones & R. Rospond (Eds.), *Patient assessment in pharmacy practice.* Baltimore, Md: Lippincott Williams & Wilkins.
8. DeMartinis, J.E., Uphold, C.R., & Graham, M.V. (2003). Cardiovascular problems. In C.R. Uphold & M.V. Graham (Eds.), *Clinical guidelines in adult health* (3rd ed.). Gainesville, Fla: Barmarrae Books.
8a. Dengel, D.R., Brown, M.D., Reynolds, T.H. IV, Supiano, M.A. (2006). Effect of aerobic exercise training on renal responses to sodium in hypertensives. *American College of Sports Medicine, 217-222.* Retrieved November 19, 2007, from www.acsm-msse.org.
9. Epperly, T.D., & Fogarty, J.P. (2001). Syncope. In M.B. Mengel & L.P. Schwiebert (Eds.), *Ambulatory medicine: The primary care of families* (3rd ed.). New York: Lange Medical Books/McGraw-Hill.
10. Furberg, C.D., et al. (2001). Clinical implications of recent findings from the Antihypertensive and Lipid-Lowering Treatment to Prevent Heart Attack Trial (ALLHAT) and other studies of hypertension. *Annals of Internal Medicine, 135,* 1074-1078.
11. Isaacsohn, J., et al. (2002). The impact of the national cholesterol education program adult treatment panel III guidelines on drug development. *The American Journal of Cardiology, 89*(Suppl), 45C-49C.
11a. Margolis, K.L., Piller, L.B., Ford, C.E., et al. (2007). Blood pressure control in Hispanics in the Antihypertensive and Lipid-Lowering Treatment to Prevent Heart Attack Trial. *American Heart Association, 50,* 854-861.
12. McGowan, M.P. (2002). Lipid-lowering therapy in women: New treatment options. *Cardiology Review, December,* 1-12.
13. National Cholesterol Education Program (NCEP), National Institutes of Health, National Heart, Lung and Blood Institute. (2001). *Executive summary of the third report of the National Cholesterol Education Program (NCEP) Expert Panel on detection, evaluation, and treatment of high blood cholesterol in adults (Adult Treatment Panel III)* (NIH Publ. No. 01-3305). Bethesda, Md: U.S. Government Printing Office.
14. National High Blood Pressure Education Program, National Institutes of Health, National Heart, Lung and Blood Institute. (2003). *The Seventh Report of the Joint National Committee on Detection, Evaluation, and Treatment of High Blood Pressure.* Bethesda, Md: U.S. Government Printing Office.
15. Nutrition Committee of the AHA. (2000). AHA dietary guidelines: Revision 2000: A statement for healthcare professionals from the nutrition committee of the American Heart Association. *Circulation, 102,* 2284-2299.
15a. Ong, K.L., Cheung, B.M., Man, Y.B., et al. (2007). Prevalence, awareness, treatment, and control of hypertension among United States adults 1999-2004. *American Heart Association, 49,* 69-75.
16. Opie, L. (1991). *Drugs for the heart* (3rd ed.). Philadelphia, Saunders.
17. Pasternak, R. (2002). Adult treatment panel II versus adult treatment panel III: What has changed and why? *American Journal of Cardiology, 89*(Suppl), 3C-7C.
18. Rader, D. (2002). Lipid disorders. In E.J. Topol (Ed.), *Textbook of cardiovascular medicine* (2nd ed.). Philadelphia: Lippincott Williams & Wilkins.
19. U.S. Department of Health and Human Services. (2000). *Healthy People 2010: National health promotion and disease prevention objectives.* Washington, DC: U.S. Public Health Service.

evolve **Did you remember to check out the bonus material on the Evolve website and the CD-ROM, including NCLEX®-Examination Style Review Questions, Open-Book Quizzes, and Chapter Review Audio Podcasts?**

http://evolve.elsevier.com/Black/medsurg

CHAPTER 53

Management of Clients with Vascular Disorders

JOYCE M. BLACK

PERIPHERAL ARTERY DISORDERS

Peripheral vascular disease (PVD) includes disorders of the arterial, venous, and lymphatic systems. In clinical settings, the term *PVD* is usually used to describe peripheral arterial disease. PVD is increasingly common and has the potential to cause loss of limb or, occasionally, life.

Etiology and Risk Factors

Peripheral arterial occlusive diseases are primarily caused by atherosclerosis, a complex and chronic inflammatory process that slowly occludes the elastic and muscular arteries. The atherosclerotic process gradually may progress to complete occlusion of medium and large arteries.

Primary risk factors for atherosclerosis include diabetes, smoking, hypertension, obesity, and elevated blood lipid levels. Phlebitis, surgery, and autoimmune disease are other risk factors. Clients with PVD often have other forms of atherosclerosis, such as coronary artery disease, myocardial infarction, atrial fibrillation, carotid stenosis, stroke, or renal disease.

Arteries can be occluded acutely from embolism, thrombosis, trauma, vasospasm, or edema. Multiple factors increase risk of thromboses including obesity, sepsis, hypotension, low cardiac output, aneurysms, aortic dissection, bypass grafts, and underlying atherosclerotic narrowing of the arterial lumen. Emboli, the most common cause of sudden ischemia, usually are of cardiac origin during periods of atrial fibrillation, but they also can originate from proximal atheroma, tumor, or foreign objects. Emboli tend to lodge at artery bifurcations or in areas where vessels abruptly narrow such as the femoral artery bifurcation.

Pathophysiology

The progressive nature of atherosclerosis slowly starves the tissues of oxygenated blood. Collateral arterioles develop to attempt to compensate for the occluded arterial supply. However, collateral vessels develop slowly. During the interim, vasodilation and anaerobic pathways are used to meet oxygen and nutrient demands. Vasodilation has a limited effect because arteries that become oxygen-deprived quickly become maximally dilated. Cellular anaerobic metabolism tries to meet the basic requirements, but the waste products of lactic acid and pyruvic acid build up quickly, are extremely toxic, and are excreted slowly.

Stenosis, the narrowing of a vessel, is progressive. The physiologic effect of any given stenosis is variable because it is determined not only by the degree of narrowing but also by the amount of collateral vessels that have developed. However, continued lack of arterial flow eventually results in pain. The pain is called *intermittent claudication* and is analogous to anginal pain. Intermittent claudication occurs when a muscle is forced to work without an adequate blood supply to meet its metabolic demands. Remember, muscles are metabolically active and use aerobic metabolism; therefore without blood they resort to anaerobic metabolism.

Clinical Manifestations

The process of atherosclerosis is insidious and the clinical manifestations of chronic arterial occlusion may not appear for 20 to 40 years.

---

evolve **Web Enhancements**

Client Education Guide Foot Care (Spanish Translation)

Stump and Prosthesis Care (Spanish Translation)

Be sure to check out the bonus material on the Evolve website and the CD-ROM, including free self-assessment exercises. **http://evolve.elsevier. com/Black/medsurg**

Intermittent Claudication

The most important subjective manifestations of chronic arterial occlusive disease are *intermittent claudication* and *rest pain*. The client typically reports pain described as tightening pressure in the calves or buttocks or a sharp cramp or burning sensation that occurs during walking and disappears with rest. Claudication also may present as the hip or leg "giving out" after a certain period of exertion. The pain of claudication usually does not occur with sitting or standing. Claudication generally occurs in men, although there is an increased incidence in women after menopause. Usually, claudication strikes men in their sixth or seventh decade. Nearly half of clients who experience claudication also have associated severe coronary artery disease (Table 53-1).

Intermittent claudication is worsened by the speed or incline of the walk, conditions that increase the demand for oxygen by muscles of the legs. The more rapid the speed or the greater the incline, the faster claudication occurs. The client's exercise tolerance generally decreases over time; episodes of claudication occur with less exertion. Claudication response is constant, reproducible, and not positional. Reproducible means that the client who walks the same distance at the same speed and incline has manifestations at the same distance each time. The client who cannot walk the length of a house because of leg pain one day but can walk indefinitely the next day does not have intermittent claudication.

PVD can occur along any portion of the arterial system. Aortoiliac stenosis and occlusion result in hip, thigh, and buttock claudication with absent or diminished femoral and distal pulses (Figure 53-1). In males, impotence is also part of the syndrome, known as *Leriche syndrome*. A superficial femoral artery and popliteal occlusion leads to calf claudication, which may improve, stay the same, or potentially progress to rest pain. Popliteal artery disease and stenosis in the anterior or posterior tibial artery result in claudication in the distal leg and foot.

Rest Pain

As the disease progresses, clinical manifestations become more severe. The development of pain at rest, usually occurring at night when the client lies supine, indicates limb-threatening disease. Usually described as a dull, deep pain in the toes or forefoot, this sensation awakens the client from sleep and may cause the client to hang the foot over the side of the bed or get up and walk around for relief. The client may start to sleep in a chair with legs dependent. Placing the leg in a dependent position provides increased gravitational supply of blood. This often results in a moderate degree of lower extremity edema. The affected foot usually demonstrates dependent rubor. Ischemic rest pain often is exacerbated by poor cardiac output. PVD may also be acutely compounded by either emboli or thrombi. Many people live daily with PVD; however, in situations such as acute limb ischemia, the disease can be life-threatening and can require emergency intervention to minimize morbidity and mortality.

Lower extremity pain may also occur in several other disorders unrelated to arterial disease. Other conditions that cause a similar type of pain include arthritis, lumbar disk protrusion, neuritis, and muscle cramps. However, the pain of other conditions is not consistent, reproducible, or positional.

Paresthesias with exertion indicate ischemia of the peripheral nerves because of the phenomenon of *arterial steal*. This phenomenon occurs as arterioles of the muscles are maximally dilated because of hypoxia. To meet muscular metabolic needs, these arterioles steal from cutaneous and peripheral nerve vessels, which results in coldness and a "pins and needles" sensation.

Decreased Pulses

Objective data associated with arterial insufficiency include weak or absent peripheral pulses, low ankle-brachial index (ABI) scores (see p. 1287), dependent rubor and pallor with elevation, hypertrophied toenails, coolness of the skin, hairlessness of the extremity, tissue atrophy, ulceration, and gangrene (Figure 53-2). Dependent rubor is a dusky, purplish discoloration of the foot and leg when the foot is placed in a dependent position. This *dependent rubor* changes to white pallor when the leg is elevated. Dependent rubor is common when aortoiliac and femoropopliteal disorders are combined. Mottling, paralysis, and paresthesias tend to occur in limb-threatening conditions and prompt care to restore blood flow is required.

TABLE 53–1	Manifestations of Arterial Insufficiency
Type of Data	**Manifestations**
Subjective	Exertional pain
	Nocturnal pain
	Ischemic rest pain
	Claudication manifestations
	Foot, calf, thigh, or buttock pain
	Pain worse with exertion
	Pain relieved with several minutes rest
	Pain relieved with dependent position
Objective	Decreased skin temperature
	Shiny skin
	Skin hairless over lower extremity (e.g., shin)
	Dystrophic toenails
	Distal extremity color change with position
	Skin pallor when leg elevated
	Skin rubor when leg dependent
	Bilateral leg diminished pulses throughout
	Slow wound healing in legs
	Impotence

ARTERIAL OCCLUSION SITES

☐ Aortic/iliac occlusion

☐ Femoral occlusion

☐ Popliteal/tibial occlusion

RELATED CLAUDICATION AREAS

☐ Gluteal and thigh claudication

☐ Calf claudication

☐ Calf claudication or foot pain

■ **FIGURE 53-1 A,** Major sites of peripheral atherosclerotic occlusive disease. **B,** Specific patterns of claudication in distal tissues.

■ **FIGURE 53-2** Arterial ulcers of the foot. Note the pale, hairless appearance of the leg and the smooth, round shape of the ulcers.

Delayed Wound Healing

Even small or shallow wounds do not heal because of the lack of arterial blood flow. The physician should be made aware of the presence of wounds.

Laboratory findings may reveal abnormal lipid profiles. If the renal arteries are involved, elevated levels of urea nitrogen and creatinine may be noted. An elevated level of total homocysteine (tHcy) in blood is emerging as a prevalent and strong risk factor for atherosclerotic vascular disease in the coronary, cerebral, and peripheral vessels, and for arterial and venous thromboembolism.

Diagnostic Evaluation

Diagnostic evaluation of the lower extremity includes both noninvasive and invasive techniques. ABI can be measured at the bedside. Using Doppler ultrasonography, the systolic pressure both at the brachial artery and at the posterior tibialis artery is measured. The ankle systolic pressure is divided by the brachial pressure, with both measured in the supine position. Normally, the ratio is more than 1. Comparison with ABI in the opposite extremity is helpful to determine the degree of ischemia. ABI is not accurate in diabetic clients using the ankle pulsation; pulsation in the great toe can be used instead.

Doppler ultrasound studies can determine the quality of blood flow (Figure 53-3). The femoral, popliteal, dorsalis pedis, and posterior tibial arteries are evaluated in the lower extremities. The axillary, brachial, ulnar, and radial arteries are evaluated in the arms. The shape of the waveform (i.e., monophasic, biphasic, triphasic) provides data on the presence of disease. A monophasic waveform can indicate proximal stenosis or occlusion in the iliac vessels. The biphasic or triphasic waveform is normal and occurs when the main blood vessels in the leg are elastic and dilated by the increased pressure during systole.

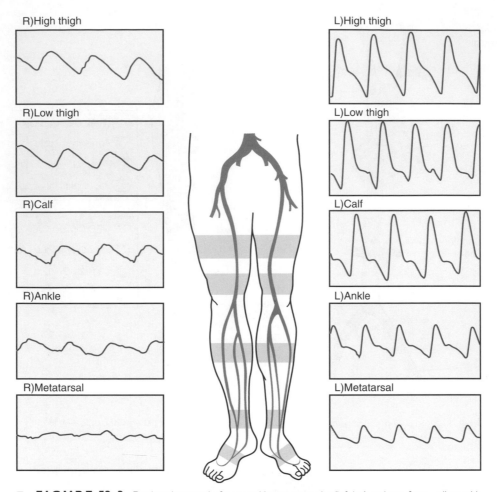

R)High thigh

R)Low thigh

R)Calf

R)Ankle

R)Metatarsal

L)High thigh

L)Low thigh

L)Calf

L)Ankle

L)Metatarsal

■ **FIGURE 53–3** Duplex ultrasound of a normal lower extremity (left leg) and one from a client with rest pain (right leg). *(From Townsend, C.M., Jr., Beauchamp, R.D., Evers, B.M., Mattox, K.L. [2004]. Sabiston textbook of surgery [17th ed.]. Philadelphia: Saunders.)*

Transcutaneous oximetry measures tissue levels of oxygen and carbon dioxide, providing data on impairments of flow in both large and small vessels.

Treadmill examination, a form of lower extremity stress testing, measures the decrease of arterial pressure with ambulation and the rapidity with which it returns to baseline. Color flow imaging visualizes the blood flow in the vessels and records pressures within the vessel.

Arteriography is the definitive examination when surgery is being considered. Arteriography shows the lumen of the blood vessels. It is not a measurement of actual blood flow like the noninvasive assessment, but instead shows the outline of the contrast media within the lumen. Use of contrast media, however, contributes to risk of many potential complications especially renal insufficiency.

OUTCOME MANAGEMENT

Medical Management

The goals of medical management are to reduce the risk of progressive arterial disease, to promote arterial flow, and to save the limb for clients with intermittent claudication and non–limb-threatening ischemia. Additionally, medical management may be the only course of action in the client with multiple morbidities and who is a poor surgical risk.

Promote Arterial Flow

Pentoxifylline (Trental) has been reported to decrease blood viscosity and increase red cell flexibility, thereby increasing peripheral blood flow. Several studies have shown that pentoxifylline increases the duration of exercise in clients with claudication. Cilostazol has also been shown to increase walking distance. It works as a vasodilator and has antiplatelet properties. Platelet inhibitors, such as aspirin and clopidogrel, are used to reduce the risk of embolism in clients with PVD. New medications including L-arginine, which is the precursor of the endothelium-dependent vasodilator nitric oxide, and vasodilator prostaglandins are being studied.

In severe cases of arterial insufficiency, the physician may order reverse Trendelenburg position; this can be achieved by placing the head of the client's bed on 6-inch blocks (or heavy books such as encyclopedias) so that blood from the heart flows more easily to the extremities whenever the client sleeps or rests. Fleece boots may also be used to keep the feet warm and protected from injury. Float the heels from the bed to prevent pressure ulcers.

Reduce Risk

Because of the chronic nature of PAD, all clients are provided with information to reduce their risk of continued ischemia and injury to the peripheral leg and foot.

Smoking Cessation

The importance of stopping cigarette smoking cannot be overemphasized. Cigarette smoke is a potent vasoconstrictor, further impairing blood flow to the extremities. Clients who are able to stop smoking successfully improve their treadmill walking distance. Smoking cessation is extremely difficult, because nicotine is a highly addictive chemical. Social support, especially of friends and family members, seems to be an important factor in assisting smokers to quit their habit. Pharmacologic measures may be instituted by the primary care provider, if necessary. Educate clients about the dangers of cigarette smoke, encourage them to stop smoking, act as role models for nonsmoking, and support policies to prohibit smoking in the workplace. Primary care providers should question clients each time they visit about their desire to quit and the need to quit. (See Chapter 62 for techniques to help with smoking cessation.)

Control of Comorbid Diseases

Diabetes, obesity, hypertension, and lipid abnormalities should all be well controlled to slow the progression of the disease. Clients are advised and counseled to reduce body weight by following a low-fat, low-cholesterol diet containing more fruits and vegetables. Interventions for lowering blood lipid levels are recommended for clients with hyperlipidemia. The initial step for lowering cholesterol level is to reduce calorie intake to achieve ideal body weight. If weight loss is seen as improbable, the client should try to maintain current weight.

The next major step is to reduce the total fat intake in the diet to 30% or less of total calories. Saturated fat intake should be reduced. The most common sources of saturated fat in the American diet are red meat, fried foods, and dairy products, especially whole milk and cheese. Increasing the quantity of fish and poultry and changing to skim milk and nonfat cheese may be sufficient to meet saturated fat recommendations.

The third major goal is to reduce intake of cholesterol, which is found in egg yolks, organ meats, shellfish, and animal meats. Increasing dietary fiber, especially soluble fiber, such as that found in oats, lentils, and beans, has a beneficial effect on lipid levels. Fast foods, snack foods, and restaurant dining account for a large amount of the

increased fat intake in the United States. Dietary counseling by a registered dietitian is a helpful intervention for clients and families who are attempting to change eating habits. See other chapters for treatment of diabetes (Chapter 45) and hypertension (Chapter 52).

Exercise

A prescribed moderate program of exercise and rest reduces claudication. Supervised exercise for 30 to 45 minutes 3 times a week for 12 weeks on a treadmill or track improves claudication by changing the metabolism in muscles, altering the endothelium of the vessels, and improving the gait. Improvements are not due to increased collateral circulation as once thought. The exercise program should begin slowly with the client stopping at the onset of pain and progress gradually until the client has substantially lengthened walking distances. For obese and chronically ill clients, it is important that an exercise program (1) be individually tailored to the client's abilities, goals, interests, and resources and (2) be written with specific instructions. Most clients can significantly increase their walking distance, and many can avoid surgery if they exercise regularly and stop smoking.

Prevention of Injury

As a result of poor blood flow to the feet, supportive measures include meticulous care of the skin. Feet should be kept clean and protected against excessive drying with moisturizing creams. Well-fitting and protective shoes are advised to reduce trauma. Sandals and shoes made of synthetic materials that do not "breathe" should be avoided. Elastic support hose should be avoided, because they reduce blood flow to the skin. In clients with ischemia at rest, "shock blocks" under the head of the bed together with a canopy over the feet may improve perfusion pressure and ameliorate some of the rest pain.

Nursing Management of the Medical Client

Assessment. The history should include questions regarding arterial disease, surgery, medications, and ulcerations. Some clients are not aware of chest pain, shortness of breath, or fatigue because their attention is focused on leg discomfort. Question them carefully about these discomforts. Because of the chronic nature of the problem, perform a psychosocial assessment. Clients may have feelings of powerlessness.

The physical examination should include peripheral pulses (begin with dorsalis pedis, then proceed proximally to the posterior tibial, popliteal, and femoral until a pulse is found); ABI; quality of arterial flow assessed with a hand-held Doppler instrument; notations of skin color, skin temperature, and level of hair on the leg; and assessment of skin integrity (including the presence of ulcers, darkened areas of skin, tinea pedis, or thickened nails), capillary refill time, and the presence of venous filling when the foot is dependent.

The Management and Delegation feature below provides additional information for ongoing assessment of clients with vascular disorders.

Diagnosis, Outcomes, Interventions

Diagnosis: Ineffective Peripheral Tissue Perfusion. The ideal nursing diagnosis for clients with arterial disorders is *Ineffective Peripheral Tissue Perfusion*. Write the diagnosis as *Ineffective Tissue Perfusion related to interruption of blood flow secondary to arterial occlusion*.

Outcomes. The client will maintain adequate peripheral tissue perfusion to affected extremities as evidenced by improvement from baseline of skin color, skin temperature, pulse rate measurements, and level of pain.

Interventions

Promote Arterial Flow. Position clients with arterial disease so that blood flows toward the legs and feet.

MANAGEMENT AND DELEGATION

Management of Clients with Vascular Disorders

Clients with peripheral vascular disorders require frequent monitoring and observation of the neurovascular status (NV) of their affected extremities. Likewise, you will implement interventions to minimize pressure and swelling to the affected extremity. Following your initial assessment and implementation of protective measures in an affected extremity, you may deem it appropriate to delegate the routine monitoring and recording of NV status to an unlicensed assistant.

Your baseline assessment establishes the NV status, including skin temperature, skin color, presence and location of pulses, sensation, and skin integrity. Skin integrity, especially overlying bony prominences like the heels, ankles, and elbows, is at especially high risk for compromise and breakdown and deserves close assessment. Pulses are best noted by marking their location with a waterproof marker, noting whether they are palpable or audible by Doppler.

Inform your assistants of the initial findings and instruct them to notify you of any changes in skin color or temperature, quality or detection of pulses, altered sensation (e.g., "pins and needles"), or client report of pain in the extremity. Assistants can help ensure protective measures are maintained by providing heel protectors, using pillows to elevate the heels from the bed, and implementing other pressure-reducing devices.

Perform ongoing assessment of your client as your institution and the client's clinical condition dictates. Changes in assessment may necessitate a change in delegation considerations. Vascular clients may have postoperative dressings on their affected extremities. Delegation considerations in the care of postoperative clients are described in Chapter 14 and apply in this population as well.

In milder cases, clients can benefit from simply sitting for periods of time with their feet flat on the floor. If reverse Trendelenburg position is used, assess for dependent edema. Remind clients with arterial insufficiency to avoid raising their feet above heart level unless the physician has specifically prescribed this as an exercise.

Explain the dangers of smoking to the client who uses tobacco. Encourage the client to stop smoking completely. The client who realizes that smoking literally threatens life and limbs may develop sufficient motivation to abstain permanently. Help the client locate therapy groups or biofeedback training. Do not advise the use of nicotine patches. Patches provide continuous administration of nicotine and thereby can cause continuous vasospasm.

Encourage the client to avoid stressful situations and to relax, both mentally and physically. Counseling services may be indicated for nervous, "high-strung" clients. Offer information regarding stress reduction classes. Involve significant others.

Prevent the client from becoming chilled. Stockings should be worn to keep the legs warm. Clients should wear protective clothing in layers during cold weather, warm their cars before entering them, and follow winter driving precautions (e.g., not running out of gas).

Be certain that the client understands how to take antiplatelet medications. The effect of these drugs is augmented by other anticoagulants including self-prescribed medications. Side effects often include gastrointestinal upset or bleeding when using aspirin.

Reduce Risk. Nurses should encourage the client to follow all risk reduction programs. These changes are prescribed for life and should be incorporated into daily living. This amount of change can be stressful and clients should be allowed to express their frustration at the changes prescribed, but also strongly encouraged to continue with them.

Diagnosis: Acute Pain. Intermittent claudication is caused by ischemia. The nursing diagnosis can be written *Acute Pain related to inadequate arterial blood supply to the legs*.

Outcomes. The client will experience increased comfort, as evidenced by self-report and demonstrated knowledge of pain reduction measures, both pharmacologic and nonpharmacologic.

Interventions. The pain of ischemia is usually chronic, continuous, and difficult to relieve. Arterial leg ulcers are exquisitely painful. Because of pain, clients with arterial disorders are often depressed and irritable. Pain limits their activities, disturbs their sleep, saps their energy, and has a demoralizing emotional effect. Thus pain must be reduced if the client is to rest and improve.

Help clients assess and plan ways of correcting the position of their beds at home. The head of the bed can be elevated to promote blood flow to the legs. Remind the client with arterial insufficiency of the following points:

- Avoid standing in one position for more than a few minutes.
- Avoid crossing the legs at the knees.
- In general, seek the most comfortable position.
- Watch for and report edema.

Any measure that increases circulation to the extremities helps alleviate ischemic pain. Although pain also can be subdued by analgesics, interventions that augment circulation are best. When strong analgesics, such as morphine, are necessary around the clock, the client may require amputation. Amputation can improve the quality of life by diminishing pain and improving mobility with a prosthesis.

Diagnosis: Risk for Impaired Skin Integrity. Because of altered peripheral tissue perfusion, the client is at risk of arterial ulceration and skin infection. Write the diagnosis as *Risk for Impaired Skin Integrity related to decreased peripheral circulation*. If the client has an arterial ulcer, this diagnosis can still be used for the remaining intact skin.

Outcomes. The client will reduce risk of skin impairment as evidenced by maintaining soft skin, protecting skin from trauma, and showing no signs of skin injury. If the client has an open wound, see later information in this chapter.

Interventions. Prevent injury to the extremities, particularly the feet. Excellent foot care should be an integral part of the daily routine of clients with peripheral vascular disorders, because prevention is easier to initiate and maintain than is correction. For bedridden clients, use fleece leg wraps or cotton stockings to keep the feet warm and reduce friction injury. The Client Education Guide below summarizes client instructions.

CLIENT EDUCATION GUIDE

Foot Care

CLIENT INSTRUCTIONS

Daily Hygiene
- Do not soak your feet; use mild soap and a washcloth to clean them.
- Dry well between your toes.
- Check water temperature with a bath thermometer or your elbow, not your toes, to prevent burns; 32.2° to 35° C (90° to 95° F) is safe.
- Gently rub corns or calluses. Avoid cutting, digging, or using harsh commercial products.

Daily Inspection and Lubrication
- Use good lighting.
- Put on your glasses or contacts, if you wear them.
- Promptly report ulcerations, redness, calluses, blisters, or cracking of the skin on the feet or thickening of the nails to the physician.
- Rub soothing lotions or lanolin on your hands, feet, legs, and arms to prevent dryness.
- Do not use lotion on sores or between your toes.
- Do not use perfumed lotions.
- Dust your feet lightly with cornstarch if they sweat.

Care of Toenails
- Use clippers, not scissors or razor blades.
- Cut straight across the nail.
- Do not perform "bathroom surgery."
- If your eyesight is poor or if you are unable to reach your toes, find qualified assistance.
- Place lamb's wool between overlapping toes.

Proper Footwear
- Never go barefoot, not even at the beach or at home.
- Avoid high heels and shoes with pointed toes.
- Make sure nothing is in your shoes before putting them on your feet.
- Avoid tight socks and shoes.
- Wear cotton socks for absorbency. Change your socks daily.
- Alternate several pairs of comfortable, firm, well-made shoes during the week.
- Avoid shoes that cause your feet to perspire (for example, canvas shoes and rubber boots).
- Make sure that your shoes and slippers fit well and are sturdy enough to prevent foot injury.

Safety
- Avoid sunburn.
- Avoid scratching insect bites on your legs to prevent creating open lesions.
- Do not use heating pads.
- Wear adequate foot protection on cold days.
- Turn on the lights before entering a dark hallway or room.
- Avoid sitting with your legs crossed.
- Use a cane or walker, if indicated.
- When in doubt, ask for help. Have telephone numbers of people who can assist you at hand.

Activity
- Walking is good, but get your physician's permission before beginning a regular program.
- Do not walk if you have open ulcerations.
- Walk until pain begins, stop and rest, and then begin again.
- Elevate your feet if they swell.
- Find a nurse and a physician who will get to know you and your foot problems and will take the time to talk with you when you need help.

Diagnosis: Risk for Activity Intolerance. Intermittent claudication may greatly deter activity. This common nursing diagnosis is written as *Risk for Activity Intolerance related to leg pain after walking.*

Outcomes. The client will develop appropriate levels of activity free from pain and excess fatigue, as evidenced by normal vital signs, absence of pain, and verbalized understanding of the benefits of gradual increase in activity and exercise.

Interventions. When assisting the client with a walking program, assert that *pain* should be the guide to the amount of activity to be undertaken. Intermittent claudication signals that the muscles and tissues of the legs are not receiving enough oxygen.

SAFETY ALERT

Before the client begins a walking program, take a careful history and perform a physical assessment. Establish a cardiopulmonary profile and carefully examine the client's feet and legs to locate open ulcerations or anatomic deformities. The client should have sturdy shoes to prevent foot trauma.

Although exercise helps most clients with vascular disorders, some clients must not exercise. These clients have leg ulcers, pain at rest, cellulitis, deep vein thrombosis, or gangrene. Exercise and activity increase the metabolic needs of tissues and, consequently, tissue requirements for oxygenated blood. Thus clients with tissue breakdown or necrosis must remain for a period of time on complete bed rest. Even minimal activity raises the oxygen requirements of the tissues above that which damaged arteries can provide.

Diagnosis: Deficient Knowledge. The nursing diagnosis *Deficient Knowledge* can be used as a guide to teaching the client about a walking program. State the nursing diagnosis as *Deficient Knowledge related to walking program as evidenced by no previous experience.*

Outcomes. The client will develop and follow a progressive walking program.

Interventions. Remind clients that at first it may be painful to walk any distance and that they may need to stop frequently to rest. Walking on a track or treadmill is the best way to start exercising. Encourage them to walk in enclosed shopping malls in the winter for safety from falls on icy pavement and to avoid vasoconstriction from the environment. In the summer, walking in the malls helps avoid heat exhaustion or stress on other conditions such as heart disease. Clients should walk through the pain as much as possible without causing undue distress. It is important to stress that small increments of exercise increase are not dramatic, but rather are evidence of improvement. Even improvement to the point of being able to shop in the grocery store is a cause for celebration.

Diagnosis: Health-Seeking Behaviors. Health-conscious clients may request information about self-improvement and interventions to reduce the severity of manifestations. Write the nursing diagnosis as *Health-Seeking Behaviors related to lack of knowledge about the role of exercise, weight reduction, and smoking cessation in management of arterial disease.*

Outcomes. The client will begin and maintain the chosen health promotion program, as evidenced by demonstrated knowledge of the specific activities of the program, regular evaluation of goals against performance, and verbalized feelings of increased well-being.

Interventions. Instruct the client in areas of concern or interest. Refer to the nonpharmacologic intervention methods described earlier. Also refer to the Complementary and Alternative Therapy features below and on p. 1315. Refer the client to groups in the community if available. The client with intermittent claudication caused by arterial disease should be routinely reexamined at least every 3 months for progression of disease.

Evaluation. Arterial disorders are chronic, so do not expect to see reversal of the problems. Write outcomes that allow for time and client adjustments.

Modifications for Older Clients

Age-related changes and impairments of physiologic function along with arterial disease affect the nursing diagnoses of *Activity Intolerance* (possibly increased), *Altered Peripheral Tissue Perfusion* (possibly reduced),

COMPLEMENTARY AND ALTERNATIVE THERAPY

Vitamin E Supplements and Peripheral Vascular Disease

Recent data on the ability of vitamin E supplements to reduce the risk of cardiovascular disease have not shown a positive effect. For example, the Heart Outcomes Prevention Evaluation (HOPE) trial was a 4.5-year randomized controlled clinical trial of vitamin E or placebo in 9541 clients ages 55 years or older with a history of coronary artery disease (CAD), stroke, peripheral vascular disease, or diabetes and other cardiovascular disease risk factors. No difference was noted between vitamin E (400 international units/day) and placebo for the outcomes of stroke, death, or other cardiac outcomes for these high-risk clients.

REFERENCE

Yusuf, S., et al. (2000). Vitamin E supplementation and cardiovascular events in high-risk patients. The Heart Outcomes Prevention Evaluation (HOPE) study investigators. *New England Journal of Medicine, 342,* 154-160.

and *Pain* (acute or chronic). Recognition of pain may be complicated by physical or cognitive impairments, ongoing drug therapy, and psychosocial factors (e.g., depression or social isolation). Additionally, sight reduction and flexibility limitations may prevent or decrease self-care. Sight reduction may increase risk for falls or other injury, which may be disastrous in the client with impaired circulation.

Surgical Management

Surgical management of PAD is called *revascularization* and is reserved for clients with progressive, severe, or disabling manifestations, including ischemia at rest. Angiography is commonly used before surgery to mark the level of inflow or areas of obstruction. Revascularization can be done through endovascular techniques or surgical reconstruction with grafting.

Endovascular Interventions

Endovascular procedures include angioplasty, atherectomy, and stent placement. The goal is to operate from within the artery to remove partial or total blockages. Most of the procedures can be done in the radiology department or in cardiac catheterization laboratories. Using local anesthetics for sedation, many of these procedures can be performed through small puncture wounds. The client recovers quickly and costs are reduced. Preprocedural and postprocedural care is discussed in Chapter 51.

Arterial Bypass

Arterial bypass operations are used to revascularize limbs. Selecting the client for surgery begins with a careful history and physical and diagnostic assessments, including arteriography. Arteriography provides a necessary road map to indicate the level of obstruction, because it is essential to reconstruct the arterial inflow to the legs before correcting the outflow. This process prevents newly placed bypass grafts from thrombosing because of inadequate blood supply to the graft. During the operation, the surgeon assesses inflow, and after it is ascertained that inflow to the femoral system is adequate, a distal site is chosen for outflow.

Improvements in vascular surgery have provided outstanding examples of long-term limb salvage in clients who in the past would have required amputation. Current data indicate that revascularization should be the first option considered in clients with critical limb ischemia. This recommendation is based on the following observations: (1) previous revascularization does not raise the level of amputation, (2) mortality rates for amputation are at least as high as for arterial bypass, and (3) there is no difference in cost between amputation and successful bypass.

Various locations along the arterial system can be reconstructed. The femoral artery can be bypassed with grafts anastomosed (surgically connected) to any one of three lower leg arteries (posterior tibial, anterior tibial, or peroneal artery) (Figure 53-4). The success of bypass grafts of the legs depends largely on what material is used for grafting. The client's own saphenous vein is the most successful grafting material. Up to 80% of saphenous vein grafts are patent after 5 years; in contrast, only 30% of synthetic material (polytetrafluoroethylene [PTFE]) is patent after the same length of time. (Gore-Tex is a common brand name for PTFE.) The client's own saphenous vein is not always large enough or long enough for the surgery, however, or it may have been removed during another operation. In these cases, PTFE is used. In situ grafts can also be used for reconstruction. In situ grafting uses the client's own vein for a bypass of the artery. A section of vein is anastomosed proximally and distally and then the valves are disabled. The vein then acts as an artery.

Axillofemoral grafting is reserved for clients who have increased operative risk, usually because of their cardiopulmonary status or the presence of intra-abdominal infection. The graft begins at the axillary artery and travels subcutaneously along the lateral chest wall to the femoral artery. It may then be combined with a femorofemoral graft to revascularize both extremities. Axillofemoral grafts have a higher incidence of occlusion than aortofemoral grafts. The patency rates are 60% to 70%

Superficial
femoral
artery

Popliteal
artery

Superficial
femoral
artery

Popliteal
artery

Anterior
tibial artery

Peroneal
artery

Posterior
tibial artery

Anterior
tibial
artery

Peroneal
artery

Posterior
tibial artery

■ **FIGURE 53–4** The occluded femoral artery can be bypassed into the arteries supplying the lower leg.

at 5 years, in part because thrombi are easily removed from axillofemoral grafts.

Clots in the graft are a major complication after surgery. Clots cause immediate impairment in blood flow and the limb becomes cool, pale, painful, and pulseless. Anticoagulant medications (e.g., low-molecular-weight heparin, heparin sodium) or antiplatelet aggregates (e.g., aspirin and Plavix) can be used prophylactically. If the graft becomes occluded, fibrinolytics may be used depending on the amount of time that has lapsed since surgery (because of marked risk of bleeding) (see Chapter 56).

When an ischemic leg is revascularized and the ischemic muscle is reperfused, a variety of ions, structural proteins, and enzymes that accumulated in the ischemic tissue return to central circulation. This process is called reperfusion syndrome and can lead to renal failure when the myoglobin is trapped in the renal tubules. Lactic acid can lead to myocardial depression, and debris can impair blood flow in the limb as it enters smaller blood vessels. Edema can develop and create compartment syndrome.

Nursing Management of the Surgical Client

Preoperative Care

Preoperatively, obtain baseline vital signs and document the character of peripheral pulses, comparing one side to the other. Know exactly which pulses are

palpable and which pulses can be assessed only with the Doppler. To assist with postoperative assessment, mark with ink the sites where peripheral pulses can be palpated. A lack of pulses postoperatively can be considered an occlusion if the quality of the pulses before surgery was not recorded.

SAFETY

⚠

ALERT

As with any preoperative assessment, perform careful cardiac and pulmonary evaluation. Even though the incision for a femoral artery bypass is peripheral and major complications are infrequent, the client probably has other manifestations of atherosclerosis (such as heart and kidney disease) that may complicate the surgery. If the operation is not an emergency, malnutrition can be reversed and open wounds cleaned. The client should have a complete medical evaluation and hypertension should be controlled. Report to the surgeon or anesthesia department any blood pressure reading outside of normal parameters or well above the client's normal. All infections (e.g., tooth abscesses, urinary tract infections, respiratory tract infections) must be resolved, especially if the synthetic graft is planned.

Before the client goes to surgery, it is common to begin administration of intravenous fluids, insert a urinary catheter, and weigh the client. In addition, broad-spectrum antibiotics normally are administered.

The client and family are taught the various procedures involved and are offered psychological support. First assess the client's readiness and desire to learn about the surgery. The importance of maintaining the medication routine is to be stressed with appropriate guidance from the physician or anesthesia department.

Postoperative Care

The client is placed on bed rest for the evening after surgery, with the leg flat in bed. The leg is wrapped with light dressings or a fleece vascular boot. The Care Plan feature on Postoperative Care of the Client Who Has Had Arterial Bypass Surgery of the Lower Extremity on pp. 1318-1319 describes additional nursing care of the client.

Complications

Bleeding may develop along the suture line and can indicate a disruption in the suture line, pseudoaneurysm formation, or a slipped ligature (suture). These problems require additional surgery. Reclotting of the graft is also possible. Peripheral tissue perfusion is monitored and non-invasive follow-up studies are performed to assess patency.

Infection is not a common complication after bypass surgery, but it can occur, especially when synthetic grafting material is used. Because infection in a synthetic graft necessitates its removal, infection often results in the loss of a limb. Poorly nourished clients appear to be at highest risk of infection and delayed healing.

Reperfusion syndrome can lead to several problems. Compartment syndrome may also develop from swelling around the fascial compartments of the leg. The manifestations of compartment syndrome include pain out of proportion to the surgery, a tense swollen leg and pain with muscle stretching, and decreased sensation. In addition to loss of sensation and function, muscle cells can die and release myoglobin, which can cause acute tubular necrosis in the kidney. A change involving any of these manifestations or a change in the color of the urine to rusty brown should be reported immediately.

Self-Care

Most clients are discharged to home. Because activity was limited by claudication before surgery, the client needs to begin regular permissible exercise, including climbing stairs and going out of doors. The client is taught that swelling of the operative leg is normal and can last for 2 to 3 months. Elastic wraps can be used when the client is ambulating, but they should not be worn continuously. Smoking must stop; it can jeopardize the results of the operation.

CRITICAL LIMB ISCHEMIA

Critical limb ischemia differs from claudication. These clients have rest pain in the forefoot and toes that interferes with sleep as well as ischemic ulcers or gangrene of the forefoot or toes. There may be calf muscle atrophy, loss of hair on the dorsum or the foot, and shiny, scaly skin attributable to loss of subcutaneous tissues. Treatment includes antiplatelet medications and revascularization. The outcomes may not be as predictable, however.

AMPUTATION

Amputation is the oldest operation known to man, existing before recorded history. Early amputations were done as punishment for crime. Today's amputations are used to treat injuries, cancers, overwhelming limb gangrene, and limb-threatening arterial disease or rest pain. Amputation is common; nearly 2 million people in the United States have undergone amputations. Even though prosthetic devices can restore a reasonable degree of function after amputation, the visible loss engenders an additional emotional component that may not occur with other surgeries.

For many years, amputation was performed with an apology and often a sense of failure. Recently there has been increasing media publicity featuring amputees who have "overcome their handicap" and returned to mainstream society. There are organizations of amputee skiers, golfers, and runners. Publicity has removed much of the old stigma.

Clients with peripheral vascular disease are the most frequent candidates for amputation of the lower extremities. Diabetes mellitus is a major cause of arterial

occlusion and has been associated with more than 55% of major amputations in clients with lower extremity occlusive disease. Traumatic injuries are also a common cause of amputation.

Preoperative Assessment

Usual preoperative assessment is performed (see Chapter 14). In addition, a rehabilitation team designs an individualized care plan focusing on the whole client rather than on a diseased or missing limb. Before amputation, the surgeon and rehabilitative team consider the following:

- *The client's physical condition.* The following physical conditions may predicate the rehabilitation potential: the age of the client, the ability to become ambulatory or remain ambulatory, the comprehension level of the client, the willingness of the client to participate in a rehabilitation program, and the condition of pre-existing conditions (e.g., chronic and progressive mental deterioration, advancing neurologic problems, chronic obstructive pulmonary disease, or cardiac disease with heart failure or angina). Ideally, clients should attain independent function with the use of a prosthesis.
- *The type of amputation to be performed.* There are two types of amputation procedures: the open, or guillotine, amputation and the closed, or "flap," amputation. The major indication for guillotine amputation is infection. In open amputation, the surgeon does not close the stump with a skin flap immediately but leaves the end open, allowing the wound to drain freely. Antibiotics are used. Once the infection is completely eradicated, the client undergoes another operation for stump closure.
- During a "flap" amputation, the surgeon closes or covers the stump with a flap of skin sutured over the end of the stump. This type of amputation is the most common and performed when there is no evidence of infection and, consequently, no need for open drainage. However, the surgeon may insert small drains to promote wound healing.
- *The level of amputation required.* The level of amputation for any extremity should be as distal as possible (Figure 53-5 on p. 1320). Arteriography is used to guide the decision about the level of amputation. Clients with below-knee amputations (even bilateral) more successfully achieve independent function with a prosthesis than do those with above-knee amputations (see Figure 53-5).
- *The client's general attitude toward amputation.* Attitude toward amputation depends to a large degree on the client's age and maturity. Young clients may resist amputation even though it would greatly improve their function. For some, the thought of amputation dramatically conflicts with their ideal

Postoperative Care of the Client Who Has Had Arterial Bypass Surgery of the Lower Extremity

Nursing Diagnosis: *Risk for Deficient Fluid Volume related to hemorrhage, hematoma, third-spacing of fluid, or diuresis from contrast given during angiography.*

| NOC OUTCOMES | Fluid Balance, Hydration, Kidney Function, Bleeding Reduction (NOC). |

Interventions	NIC INTERVENTIONS	Rationales
1. Observe the client for an increase in pulse rate, decrease in blood pressure, anxiety, restlessness, pallor, cyanosis, thirst, oliguria, clammy skin, venous collapse, and decreasing level of consciousness.	Bleeding Reduction	1. Hemorrhagic shock can develop from surgical or postoperative blood loss. Blood is shunted from peripheral stores because of the effect of sympathetic nervous system stimulation.
2. Check the client's dressings for excessive drainage. Also check under the leg.	Bleeding Reduction	2. Bleeding may appear on dressings and may also be found beneath the leg because of gravity.
3. Assess the client's pulmonary artery pressures and cardiac output if parameters are available.	Hemodynamic Regulation Invasive Hemodynamic Monitoring	3. Pulmonary artery pressures and cardiac output parameters are reliable indicators of hemodynamic stability.
4. Check the client's daily weights; monitor intake and output closely.	Fluid Monitoring	4. Intake should equal output. Weight is a reliable indicator of fluid balance.
5. Check hematocrit and hemoglobin values and notify the physician if they are abnormal.	Hypovolemia Management	5. Hematocrit and hemoglobin levels normally fall slightly because of surgical blood loss. Transfusion may be required.
6. Check the client's creatinine level after angiography.	Risk Identification	6. Contrast is excreted by the kidneys.

Evaluation: This outcome should be attainable within 24 hours. Bleeding usually occurs within the first few hours after the operation, and if bleeding develops it is usually visible on the dressings. Intravenous fluids are required until the client is drinking without nausea and producing adequate urine volumes.

Nursing Diagnosis: *Acute Pain related to surgical incision.*

| NOC OUTCOMES | Pain Level, Pain Control, Comfort Level. |

Interventions	NIC INTERVENTIONS	Rationales
1. Assess the client's level of pain: type, duration, and location.	Pain Management	1. Baseline data are used to evaluate the effectiveness of treatment and act as a guide to determine type of analgesia needed.
2. Medicate with prescribed analgesics based on current level of pain and prior effectiveness.	Medication Administration: IV, Oral Analgesic Administration	2. Analgesia is provided to obtain comfort, using the previous pain response to analgesia and current level of pain to guide the decision.
3. Evaluate the effectiveness of pain medication after each administration.	Pain Management	3. This helps determine the adequacy of analgesia.
4. Teach the client how pain will be controlled.	Patient-Controlled Analgesia Assistance	4. Clients can participate in pain management by notifying the nurse before intense pain and by using patient-controlled analgesia (PCA) devices.
5. Position the leg to promote blood flow and keep the leg warm.	Circulatory Care: Arterial Insufficiency	5. Arterial inflow and warmth are aided by supine position.

Evaluation: Acute pain should subside over 48 to 72 hours. The client should report less severe pain on a 1 to 10 scale, use less analgesia, and ambulate increasing distances. The client will likely require intravenous opioids for the first 24 hours and then should be able to remain comfortable on oral opioids, tapering to nonsteroidal medications in a few days. Pain that does not follow such a pattern should be investigated.

Nursing Diagnosis: *Impaired Physical Mobility related to a surgical procedure, pain, preoperative deconditioning, or nerve injury secondary to ischemia.*

| NOC OUTCOMES | Ambulation, Balance, Coordinated Movement, Mobility. |

Interventions	NIC INTERVENTIONS	Rationales
1. Assess the causative factors for immobility and the client's range of motion and ability to ambulate.	Exercise Promotion: Ambulation Exercise Promotion: Strength Training	1. Mobility can be facilitated once the cause of immobility is known.
2. Encourage range of motion while the client is in bed.	Exercise Promotion: Strength Training Body Mechanics Promotion	2. These activities promote venous return and muscle strength.

Interventions	NIC Interventions	Rationales
3. Ambulate increasing distances daily. Monitor tolerance of ambulation. Monitor for balance, stamina, and unsteady gait if muscle atrophy is present.	Exercise Promotion: Strength Training Exercise Promotion: Balance Fall Prevention Exercise Therapy: Muscle Control	3. Ambulation increases muscle strength and endurance. Clients who have not ambulated for some time need to be monitored for safety (balance and gait) and stamina.
4. Request a physical therapy consult when appropriate.	Exercise Promotion: Strength Training Body Mechanics Promotion	4. Assistive devices may be necessary for ambulation.
5. Encourage independence in the client's activities of daily living.	Exercise Promotion: Strength Training	5. Independence improves both physical and psychological recovery.

Evaluation: Outcomes related to mobility may require several days, depending on initial physical status. Begin transferring to the bedside chair as soon as possible and proceed with ambulation as tolerated.

Nursing Diagnosis: *Risk for Impaired Skin Integrity related to altered circulation, altered nutritional state, infection, and surgical procedures.*

NOC OUTCOMES Immobility Consequences: Physiologic, Wound Healing: Primary Intention.

Interventions	NIC INTERVENTIONS	Rationales
1. Inspect the client's lower extremities on a daily basis, including footdrop.	Skin Surveillance	1. Early detection of ulceration will allow early treatment of lesions.
2. Monitor the client for low-grade fever, elevated white blood cell count, any drainage from the wound, and graft exposure at each shift.	Incision Site Care	2. These are clinical manifestations of wound infection.
3. Monitor the client's nutritional status, oral intake, weight, and prealbumin and albumin levels. Obtain a dietitian's consultation, if necessary.	Nutritional Therapy	3. Malnutrition is the most common cause of delayed healing.
4. Provide proper skin care using lanolin-based creams.	Skin Care: Topical Treatments	4. Soft skin does not excoriate.
5. Protect the client's lower extremities from trauma.	Pressure Management	5. Tissue perfusion is decreased and injured sites heal poorly.
6. Use fleece vascular boots when appropriate.	Circulatory Precautions	6. Boots protect the skin from breakdown and keep the legs warm.
7. Elevate heels from the bed.	Pressure Ulcer Prevention	7. Pressure ulcers on the heels may be slow to heal because of poor circulation.
8. Avoid using tape on the skin below the client's knee.	Skin Care; Topical Treatments	8. Tape burns from tape removal may be slow to heal.
9. Observe strict aseptic technique during dressing changes.	Infection Control	9. Aseptic technique reduces the risk of infection.
10. Instruct the client to inspect feet and incisions daily. (See Client Education Guide on Foot Care.)	Teaching: Disease Process	10. Circulation to the legs and feet is impaired from arteriosclerosis. Daily assessment and proper care can lead to early intervention.

Evaluation: Expect the wound to heal slowly over 10 days if arteriosclerosis is extensive. Because of delays in wound healing, the client will remain at risk of infection.

Nursing Diagnosis: *Risk for Ineffective Tissue Perfusion related to graft thrombosis, compartment syndrome, progressive arterial disease, or inadequate anticoagulation.*

NOC OUTCOMES Circulation Status, Tissue Perfusion; Peripheral, Kidney Function.

Interventions	NIC INTERVENTIONS	Rationales
1. Assess the client's pedal pulses every hour for 24 hours, then every shift, unless otherwise ordered. Obtain Doppler pressures per doctor's orders. Compare to baseline values.	Lower Extremity Monitoring	1. Pedal pulses indicate graft patency.
2. Assess the sensory and motor function of the client's extremities.	Neurologic Monitoring	2. Compartment syndrome may develop because of bleeding.
3. Assess the client's leg for hematoma or severe swelling.	Circulatory Precautions	3. Severe swelling may impede the flow through the graft.
4. Monitor creatine phosphokinase levels when appropriate.	Laboratory Value Interpretation	4. Enzymes are released from ischemic muscle.
5. Report dark red or brown urine and the presence of red blood cells in the client's urine.	Emergency Management	5. These manifestations may be caused by a release of myoglobin secondary to muscle ischemia.
6. Report any unexpected deviation in perfusion to the physician.	Circulatory Precautions	6. Early reporting allows early intervention.
7. Avoid raising the knee section of the Gatch bed and placing pillows under the client's knees.	Positioning	7. Pressure may increase the risk of thrombosis.

Evaluation: Outcomes related to tissue perfusion should be met within 48 hours. Preoperative decreases in pedal pulse measurements should be restored when the client returns from surgery. Some edema is common but should not become so severe that it impairs blood flow or nerve conduction.

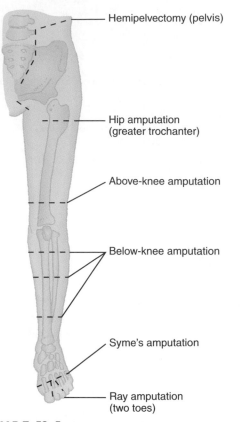

- Hemipelvectomy (pelvis)

- Hip amputation (greater trochanter)

- Above-knee amputation

- Below-knee amputation

- Syme's amputation

- Ray amputation (two toes)

■ **FIGURE 53–5** Common sites of lower extremity amputation.

self-image. Conversely, some clients who suffer from the pain of chronic ischemia may welcome amputation. These clients are often more concerned with removing the source of their pain than they are with altering their body image or function.

Diagnostic assessments include the usual preoperative blood studies and radiographs. In addition, the client may have arteriography to determine the level of blood flow in the extremity. Doppler studies are used to measure blood flow velocity, and transcutaneous tissue oxygen levels may also be measured (see Chapter 51). These studies assist with determining the level of amputation that is most likely to heal.

Phantom Limb Sensation

Phantom sensations are feelings that the amputated part is still present. Although these sensations are often referred to as phantom pain, not all of the sensations are painful. The client may describe sensations of warmth, cold, itching, or pain, especially in amputated fingers or toes. *Phantom sensations* are caused by intact peripheral nerves proximal to the amputation site that carried messages between the brain and the now amputated part. These sensations are normal, and the client should be prepared for them. Phantom sensations often are felt immediately after surgery and their frequency gradually decreases over the next 2 years.

Another condition called *phantom pain* is a form of central pain. The client reports actual pain. The pain is usually burning, cramping, squeezing, or shooting in nature. Phantom pain is less well understood and may occur in a large percentage of clients. It is thought to be caused by a combination of physiologic and psychological components. However, no research has identified a link between phantom pain and any clinical psychological disorder. Phantom pain occurs most often in clients who had pain in the limb before the amputation. Interventions that may reduce phantom pain include range-of-motion exercises, visual imaging, nerve-stabilizing medications, and other interventions for chronic pain (see Chapter 20).

Preoperative Care

Nursing Assessment of the Surgical Client

Assessment. Perform the usual preoperative assessments (see Chapter 14). In addition, support the client and family through their pain, suffering, and decision making as the client is prepared physically and psychologically for amputation. If the amputation is being done for an infectious process, administer antibiotics and monitor for sepsis (changes in mental status, fever and chills, increasing pain or odor from the wound, elevated white blood cell count). If the client has an infection in the leg to be amputated, it is important that the remaining leg is not wounded and also infected. Ulcers on the heel are hazardous, and the legs should be elevated to remove all pressure from the heel. Diabetic clients need close monitoring of blood glucose levels because infection makes blood glucose regulation erratic. Maintaining or promoting strength in the upper arms facilitates rehabilitation. Teach the client to use the trapeze and side rails for independent movement in bed. Maintain or promote nutrition to aid in healing. Older adults may have several problems that can lead to malnutrition. Ask the dietitian to evaluate the nutrient intake and offer suggestions to meet caloric and protein needs.

Diagnosis, Outcomes, Interventions

Diagnosis: Risk for Delayed Surgical Recovery. Some clients require amputation on an emergent basis; for those clients the usual preoperative care to stabilize health conditions cannot occur. The need for emergent surgery can create a risk for delayed recovery. State this nursing diagnosis as *Risk for Delayed Surgical Recovery related to pre-existing health conditions.*

Outcomes. The risk for delayed surgical recovery will be minimized.

Interventions. Clients with diabetes mellitus are a high-risk surgical group and require frequent assessment of their blood glucose level. Blood glucose level is normalized using frequent (e.g., four times daily) blood testing and sliding scale insulin. Clients with ulcerated legs or osteomyelitis may be treated with wound packing, antibiotics, and leg elevation with bed rest. Malnourished clients are nourished with foods high in protein or are administered tube feedings. They also may benefit from vitamin and mineral supplements. Severely anemic clients may require iron preparations and blood transfusions. Dehydrated clients should receive preoperative intravenous fluids to restore fluid balance.

Diagnosis: Anxiety. Clients may fear amputation because it destroys a familiar body image, imposes physical and social limitations, and temporarily upsets personal lifestyle. Such fears and anxiety must be resolved during the preoperative period to ensure successful postoperative recovery. Depending on the reason for the amputation, fear may lead the client to experience anticipatory grief. State this nursing diagnosis as *Anxiety related to impending loss of limb, change in mobility, loss of independence, pain, changes in body image, fear about feelings after amputation.* Other nursing diagnoses may also be appropriate, such as ineffective individual coping, self-esteem disturbance, or body image disturbance.

Outcomes. The client will have reduced anxiety as evidenced by openly discussing feelings and expressing reduced anxiety before surgery.

Interventions. Establish open, honest communication. Allow free expression of fears and negative feelings about the loss of a limb. Ask significant others how they feel about the amputation and how they perceive the client to be responding. The social worker or psychologist may need to be involved if the client is responding poorly.

The client may also be anxious about unknown consequences and sensations after the amputation. Provide and reinforce information. Most clients feel less anxious when they know what to expect on awakening from surgery. Prepare the client for *phantom limb sensation.* Most clients with new amputations experience the peculiar sensation that their missing limb is still present. This phantom limb sensation may or may not be painful. Also, it may either disappear within hours after surgery or persist for years. To avoid misunderstandings, inform clients that phantom limb sensations occur and are normal.

Diagnosis: Acute Pain. The client may experience severe to moderate pain before surgery. The nursing diagnosis of *Acute Pain related to ischemia of the limb* is used.

Outcomes. The client will have improved comfort as evidenced by statements of reduced pain, use of reduced doses of opioids (e.g., pain is controlled without increasing dosage), ability to move about comfortably, and ability to sleep or rest.

Interventions. Administer prescribed analgesics as necessary to reduce pain. Intervene with supportive measures. For example, use footboards and cradles to avoid pressure on injured or ischemic limbs. Keep ischemic limbs warm with wraps or fleece vascular boots.

Diagnosis: Deficient Knowledge. A common nursing diagnosis for clients having surgery is *Deficient Knowledge related to expectations after surgery.*

Outcomes. The client will express an understanding of the usual postoperative regimens.

Interventions. Clients want to know what to expect after surgery and what will be expected of them by health care professionals. Emphasize that the client is the most important member of the rehabilitation team. To achieve independence, teach the client about the following:

- Exercising legs and arms several times a day
- Strictly limiting weight-bearing (for leg amputations) until instructed otherwise
- Learning the intricacies of stump and prosthesis care
- Mastering the use of the prosthesis

Postoperative Care

After the operation is completed, the surgeon applies a small amount of fluffed gauze over the end of the stump. A rigid dressing (usually a cast) is applied, distributing pressure evenly over the end of the stump. The cast protects the stump from injury and reduces swelling by gently compressing the tissues. The socket of the distal end of the cast connects to a pylon. A pylon is an adjustable rigid support, the proximal end of which attaches to the below-knee socket or to the knee unit of an above-knee prosthesis. The distal end connects to a foot-ankle assembly. The rigid dressing is usually changed three to four times before application of a permanent prosthesis. Cast changes are necessary because the stump tends to shrink as it heals and, consequently, is no longer adequately compressed by the original cast.

Edema is controlled by elevating the stump for the first 24 hours after surgery. Then, the stump is placed flat on the bed to reduce hip contracture. Edema is also controlled by stump wrapping techniques. In below-knee amputations, the knee is immobilized to eliminate joint flexion. A trapeze is attached to the bed to assist the client to develop upper arm and shoulder strength.

Nursing Assessment of the Surgical Client

Assessment. Following an amputation, the usual postoperative care is given. Look for bleeding or oozing. If present, outline the drainage, including the time on the temporary prosthesis or soft dressing. If drains were placed in the wound, carefully monitor the amount and type of drainage.

Postoperative management of acute pain is essential. Acute surgical pain assessment and management is like those techniques used for other postoperative clients. To prevent increased pain, the nurse handles the stump carefully when assessing the site or drainage beneath the stump or dressings.

Because of pre-existent conditions such as diabetes, open infected wounds, and decreased perfusion, the client remains at high risk for infection. The nurse monitors the client and the wound for manifestations of wound infection, which usually develops about 72 hours after surgery. Broad-spectrum antibiotics are usually prescribed for several days after surgery, until there is indication that the wound is healing.

Diagnosis, Outcomes, Interventions

Diagnosis: Acute Pain. Following amputation, acute pain from the operation is present and phantom limb sensation can also be present. State this nursing diagnosis as either *Acute Pain related to traumatized tissues and phantom sensation in amputated limb* or *Anxiety related to phantom sensation in amputated limb.*

Outcomes. The client will have comfort and express an understanding of the sensations present and will recognize that they are normal and usually diminish in time.

Interventions. Provide pain control with ordered analgesics. Ischemia in the limb before surgery can sensitize the nerves, making pain somewhat more difficult to control after the amputation. If phantom sensations are present, empathetically reinforce the idea that this sensation is usual and, more importantly, subsides in time. It is not helpful to correct the client, telling the client that the limb cannot be hurting because it is absent.

Diagnosis: Ineffective Coping. For clients with some chronic disorders, such as diabetes, the amputation may signal further losses in their battle. These clients may express anger openly or covertly. Many clients express depression after amputation. The client may cry easily, eat little, sleep poorly or sleep more, or avoid interactions with others. Many times depression is a reaction to the fear of never walking again, and therefore early ambulation is therapeutic. State the nursing diagnosis as *Ineffective Coping related to reaction/response to change in body image, fear over loss of independence.*

Outcomes. The client will openly verbalize fears about changes in body image and loss of independence, and will begin to speak optimistically and realistically about the future.

Interventions. The nurse listens to the client and confronts misconceptions about the rehabilitation. If it is possible, the nurse arranges for the client to meet with another amputee. The client may express concerns that it will be impossible to return to a previous lifestyle, including job, leisure activities, or intimate relationships. With advancements in prosthetic devices, many clients can have both functional and aesthetic prosthetic devices.

Some clients feel the use of the word "stump" to be distasteful and report feeling like they are part of a tree. Use of other terms may be controversial, however, if they encourage or support denial of the problem. Some rehabilitation specialists use the phrase "residual limb" instead.

Diagnosis: Deficient Knowledge. Clients require information and time to learn all the new information about the care of the stump and the prosthesis. Use the nursing diagnosis *Deficient Knowledge related to gait training, care of the stump, care of the prosthesis.*

Outcomes. The client will express an understanding of stump and prosthesis care.

Interventions. *The Prosthesis.* The most common prosthesis for clients with a below-the-knee amputation is a patellar tendon–bearing limb prosthesis. The interior of the prosthesis contacts all surfaces of the stump and weight-bearing is on several areas. Clients with above-the-knee amputation are fitted with either a quadrilateral socket or an ischial containment prosthesis. Weight is borne on the ischial tuberosity or the soft tissues of the proximal stump, respectively.

Prostheses for the upper extremity consist of a hook or hand device, a harness to supply force to the hand, and a socket for attachment. The client coping with an upper extremity amputation must be highly motivated to master the prosthesis and achieve independence. For successful rehabilitation, the client must integrate the prosthetic arm and hand into the total body image.

Cosmetic prostheses are primarily used to enhance self-esteem and make reentry into society minus a limb more tolerable for clients who are not candidates for a functioning prosthesis. Because the construction of cosmetic prostheses does not allow weight-bearing, caution the client never to attempt transfers or ambulation with a cosmetic prosthesis.

Immediate prosthetic fitting is not always possible. However, anyone with a new amputation who is capable of ambulating should receive a temporary prosthesis as soon as possible after surgery. When a conventional delayed prosthesis fitting is anticipated, the client returns from surgery with the stump dressed and covered with elastic bandages or stump socks. (See a fundamentals of nursing text on how to wrap these stumps.) When the sutures are removed 2 to 3 weeks after surgery, the surgeon or prosthetist fits the client with a provisional temporary prosthesis made of plaster of paris or plastic.

A permanent prosthesis is fitted once the stump is healed and molded (Figure 53-6).

Gait Training. Physical mobility will be compromised for the client who has just experienced an amputation. Amputating a limb displaces the center of gravity, normally located just below the umbilicus. A client coping with an amputation must relearn balance because the prosthesis, however similar, will not be an exact replica in weight and movement of the lost limb. Adapting to a change in the center of gravity occurs slowly but progressively until the conscious effort of maintaining balance comes under unconscious control. Physically, the client increases strength and endurance with regularly scheduled exercise, controls weight-bearing until the wound completely heals, and practices ambulating with the new prosthesis until a skillful, automatic gait is developed. Physical therapists usually work with the client twice daily for strengthening and gait training.

When the prosthesis is not worn (e.g., during the night), turning also requires a readaptation in body balance. Consequently, the client may need assistance while turning until awareness of the new center of gravity is present.

Self-Care

When making discharge plans for the client with a new amputation (and probably a prosthesis), consider the client's ambulatory level and the tasks with which the client may need help. Frequently, by the time amputees are aware of their changed circumstances, they are at home, alone, and without the informed and professional advice that can prepare them for their altered lives. Schedule home visits from community health care nurses until such clients have adjusted to their new situation and feel reasonably comfortable and confident in their ability to provide self-care.

The Client Education Guide feature below offers suggestions for care in the health care facility or at home for clients who have had lower limb amputation.

TRAUMATIC AMPUTATION

Not all amputations are planned. Some clients suffer traumatic loss of limb as a result of farm machinery

■ **FIGURE 53–6** Permanent lower-extremity prosthesis. *(Courtesy Otto Bock Health Care, Minneapolis, Minn.)*

CLIENT EDUCATION GUIDE 🄴

Stump and Prosthesis Care

STUMP CARE

- Inspect the stump daily for redness, blistering, or abrasions.
- Use a mirror to examine all sides and aspects of the stump. Skin breakdown on the stump is extremely serious because it interferes with prosthesis training and may prolong hospitalization and recovery. If you have diabetes mellitus, you are particularly susceptible to skin complications, because changes in sensation may obliterate your awareness of stump pain.
- Perform meticulous daily hygiene. Wash the stump with a mild soap, and then carefully rinse and dry it. Apply nothing to the stump after it is bathed. Alcohol dries and cracks the skin, whereas oils and creams soften the skin too much for safe prosthesis use.
- Wear woolen stump socks over the stump for cleanliness and comfort. Wash woolen socks in cool water and mild soap to prevent shrinkage. To prevent stretching, wash socks gently. Dry stump socks flat on a towel. Replace torn socks; mending creates wrinkles that irritate the skin.
- Put on the prosthesis immediately when arising and keep it on all day (once the wound has healed completely) to reduce stump swelling.
- Continue prescribed exercises to prevent weakness.

PROSTHESIS CARE

- Remove sweat and dirt from the prosthesis socket daily by wiping the inside of the socket with a damp soapy cloth. To remove the soap, use a clean damp cloth. Dry the prosthesis socket thoroughly.
- Never attempt to adjust or mechanically alter the prosthesis. If problems develop, consult the prosthetist.
- Schedule a yearly appointment with the prosthetist.

accidents, chain saw accidents, or automobile accidents. Sometimes the amputated limb can be replanted because usually both the client and the limb were healthy up to the time of injury. It is important to properly store and transport the amputated limb before replantation. The limb should be wrapped in a cloth, placed in a plastic bag, and then placed on ice. The limb or digit itself should not come in contact with ice or water to prevent direct tissue damage. No promises should be made to the client about the ability to successfully replant an amputated limb before evaluation by the replantation surgery team. Individuals whose limbs were amputated because of trauma have had no time before surgery to grieve the loss or adjust to their perceived alterations in body image. They may express sadness or anger, or they may show a strong determination not to let the amputation alter their ability to function. Outcomes after replantation vary with the complexity of repair required and the amount of tissue replanted. Months of rehabilitation are required; the peripheral nerve repairs itself very slowly.

ACUTE ARTERIAL OCCLUSION

Acute occlusion of an artery may be caused by trauma, embolism, or thrombosis and may occur in a healthy or diseased artery. About 90% of acute occlusion occurs in the lower limbs. In arterial embolism, the wall of the artery is often healthy; the obstruction in the artery arises most frequently from a thrombus within the heart. Etiologies include atrial fibrillation, myocardial infarction, prosthetic heart valves, and rheumatic heart disease. Sometimes, portions of a blood clot, such as platelet emboli, which form at points of turbulence and then lodge at a bifurcation, can initiate a thrombus. Other noncardiac sources of emboli are clot in an abdominal aortic aneurysm or peripheral aneurysm, and up to 20% are from an unidentified source. Arterial thrombosis is usually superimposed on atherosclerosis and consequently develops in a damaged vessel; however, coagulopathy from heparin-induced thrombocytopenia, inherited coagulation disorders, disseminated intravascular coagulation, or polycythemia vera may also occur.

The circulatory changes that follow arterial occlusion and that predict the outcome are complex and depend on a variety of factors. Acute occlusion produces a decrease in mean and pulse pressures in the distal arteries and a decrease in tissue perfusion and oxygenation. In a normal artery, blood flow is restored by collateral channels, but with acute emboli, collateral vessels have not had time to develop.

It is important to differentiate between arterial thrombosis and arterial embolism. Acute arterial thrombosis is usually caused by arterial obstruction from a blood clot

that forms in an artery that has been damaged by atherosclerosis. Arterial thrombosis may also develop in an arterial aneurysm, especially aneurysms that form in the popliteal artery. Arterial emboli form in the terminal end of an artery and lead to distinct areas of necrotic tissue (Figure 53-7).

The classic manifestations of acute ischemia caused by peripheral thrombus or embolism, which are known as the *six P's,* are shown in Box 53-1. Muscle necrosis may start as early as 2 to 3 hours after occlusion. Paresthesias indicate advanced damage. Complete paralysis with stiffness of muscles and joints (rigor mortis) indicates irreversible damage. The leg must be amputated to prevent systemic reaction to the products of massive muscle destruction and systemic sepsis.

FIGURE 53–7 Distal necrosis of toes from arterial embolization.

BOX 53-1 Clinical Manifestations of Acute Arterial Occlusion: The Six Ps

1. *Pain* or loss of sensory nerves secondary to ischemia
2. *Pulselessness*
3. *Poikilothermia* (coldness)
4. *Pallor* caused by empty superficial veins and no capillary filling; pallor can progress to a mottled, cyanotic, cadaverous, cold leg
5. *Paresthesias* and loss of position sense; the client cannot detect pressure or sense a pinprick; the client cannot tell whether toes are flexed or extended
6. *Paralysis*

Surgery is required to correct arterial embolism. Arterial emboli can be removed by an embolectomy. Surgery for thrombosis usually involves an arterial reconstructive procedure for revascularization of the leg. If the decision is made to remove the occluding embolus or thrombus, surgery should be performed as quickly as possible, generally using local anesthetics. If hours have elapsed since the occlusion occurred, the viability of the limb determines whether embolectomy should be attempted.

If surgery is not performed immediately, anticoagulants are used to reduce the risk of further occlusion. Heparin is usually continued for a minimum of 2 to 7 days, after which a change to an oral anticoagulant may be made. The prevailing practice is to treat all clients who have a definite source of embolism and who have satisfactorily recovered from the acute episode of occlusion with long-term anticoagulant therapy. Fibrinolytic agents may also be used to dissolve a thrombus or embolus (see Chapter 56 for discussion of their use).

While decisions about surgery are being made, put the client to bed in a comfortable, warm room. Protect the limb from pressure and other trauma and keep it at room temperature, neither warm nor chilled. The best position for the limb is level or slightly dependent.

ARTERIAL ULCERS

Areas of an ischemic foot or leg subjected to pressure or minor trauma may have skin breakdown. The usual sites of arterial ulcers are the medial and lateral metatarsal heads and the tip of the toes. The ulcers are painful, which distinguishes them from the achy or "heavy" sensation of venous stasis ulcers. Arterial ulcers also have a sharp edge and pale base, and often are surrounded by atrophic tissue (see Figure 53-2). In contrast, venous stasis ulcers are irregular and have a red healthy base (see later discussion).

Once an ulcer develops, it tends to heal poorly, if at all (especially in diabetic clients). Without adequate blood flow, the damaged tissues fail to receive needed oxygen, nutrients, antibodies, and protective leukocytes, and the process of tissue damage continues. Eventually, the client may be forced to undergo limb amputation.

Although skin grafting may ultimately be required to cover the site of arterial ischemic leg ulcers (once the ulcerated area is free from infection and granulation tissue is evident), intervention for the skin lesion does not cure the underlying disease. Most ulcers require revascularization to heal. Arterial bypass surgery improves circulation when the client has an aortoiliac or femoral-popliteal occlusion. For this surgery to be successful, however, the arteries in the leg must be healthy enough to carry sufficient blood to the foot once the block has been removed or bypassed.

General intervention involves keeping the area of ulceration clean and free from pressure and irritation. Bed rest reduces the oxygen needs of the impaired tissues. Debridement is performed only when the client has reasonable blood flow to heal the wound. Dry, intact eschar should be left in place, that is not softened or removed. If surgical debridement is necessary, a qualified health care provider should perform this procedure. After revascularization, if the ulcer bed is clean and granulating, healing is enhanced with moist dressings.

ANEURYSMS

An aneurysm is a permanent localized dilation, stretching, or ballooning of an artery to around 50% increase in the size (Figure 53-8). The exact cause is unknown, but recent evidence includes atherosclerosis and hypertension. Abdominal aortic aneurysm may be caused by damage to the artery wall by metalloproteinase, infection, congenital weakening of the connective tissue component of the artery wall (e.g., Marfan syndrome or Ehlers-Danlos syndrome), mycotic (fungal) infections, or rarely by trauma. The most common locations for arteriosclerotic aneurysms are the thoracic and abdominal aorta, the iliac arteries, and the femoral and popliteal arteries.

Aneurysms are designated as being either *venous* or *arterial.* They are also described according to the specific vessel they affect (e.g., abdominal aortic aneurysm). Aneurysms are also labeled by their shape and size (see Figure 53-9). True aneurysms contain all three layers of the arterial wall (intima, media, and adventitia); saccular aneurysms have a neck or mouth. Fusiform aneurysms involve the entire circumference of the vessel. A dissecting aneurysm is not a true aneurysm, but rather is a hematoma in the arterial wall that separates the layers of the arterial wall. A *pseudoaneurysm,* or false aneurysm, results from the development of a sac around a hematoma that

■ **FIGURE 53–8** Classification of aneurysms. In a true aneurysm, layers of the vessel wall dilate in one of the following ways: *saccular,* a unilateral outpouching; *fusiform,* a bilateral outpouching; or *dissecting,* a bilateral outpouching in which layers of the vessel wall separate, creating a cavity. In a false aneurysm, the wall ruptures, and a blood clot is retained in an outpouching of tissue, or there is a connection between a vein and an artery that does not close.

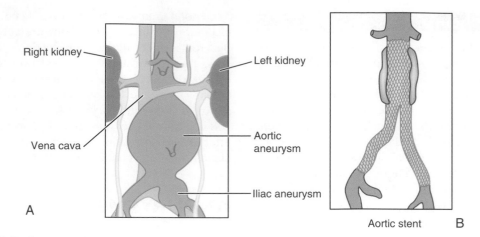

Right kidney

Left kidney

Vena cava

Aortic aneurysm

Iliac aneurysm

Aortic stent

A

B

■ **FIGURE 53–9 A,** An abdominal aortic aneurysm. **B,** A bifurcated synthetic graft in place.

maintains a communication with the lumen of an artery whose wall has been ruptured or penetrated.

ABDOMINAL AORTIC ANEURYSMS

Abdominal aortic aneurysms (Figure 53-9, *A*) are the most common type of aneurysm. They are seen most often in men 40 to 70 years of age. Most abdominal aneurysms are asymptomatic; discovery is usually made on physical or x-ray examination of the abdomen or lower spine for other reasons. When the aneurysm reaches about 5 cm in diameter, it can usually be palpated, except in obese clients. Smaller aneurysms and aneurysms in obese clients may be more difficult to confirm. The most common clinical manifestation is the client's awareness of a pulsating mass in the abdomen, with or without pain, followed by abdominal pain and back pain. Groin pain and flank pain may be experienced because of increasing pressure on other structures. Bruits can be heard over the aneurysm. Sometimes mottling of the extremities or distal emboli in the feet alert the clinician to a source in the abdomen. Ultrasonography and computed tomography (CT) scan are the most accurate diagnostic tools.

OUTCOME MANAGEMENT

Medical Management

Surgery is usually not performed on clients with an asymptomatic abdominal aortic aneurysm smaller than 4 to 5 cm. Every 6 months, an ultrasonographic examination is indicated to determine whether any change in the size has occurred. Antihypertensive medications are usually prescribed if indicated.

Surgical Management

Surgical resection of the aneurysm and creation of a new artery are the definitive treatments for aneurysm. There

are two types of surgery: endovascular surgery and traditional surgery through an abdominal incision.

Endovascular Procedures

Endovascular procedures are a newer method for non-emergency treatment to repair abdominal aortic aneurysm. Two small incisions are made in the groin, and a vascular graft is guided into the aorta (see Figure 53-9, *B*). At the tip of the catheter are a deflated balloon and a tightly wrapped polyester cloth graft. When properly positioned, the graft is secured in place by inflating the balloon and opening the graft to the diameter needed to prevent blood flow into the aneurysm. The balloon is then deflated and removed along with the catheter. At each end of the graft are hooks that help secure it to the inner walls of the aorta. The graft allows blood flow to continue through the aorta to the arteries in the pelvis and legs, without filling the aneurysm.

Postprocedure Care. The usual postoperative care is provided. Assess the surgical sites for swelling and pain (hematoma) and bleeding. Monitor peripheral perfusion closely, comparing findings to baseline. Ambulation is allowed the day after surgery. Clients may ask if they can "feel" the hooks in the aorta. They should be told that they will not be able to feel the hooks because the aorta cannot sense the hooks. Before dismissal, the location of the graft may be confirmed with CT scan, ultrasound, or x-ray study.

Aneurysm Repair

Surgical repair is usually recommended for all aneurysms greater than 6 cm wide. Elective repair is also generally recommended for aneurysms between 4 and 6 cm in clients who are good surgical risks. The more traditional surgical technique for aneurysm repair is done through a midline incision that extends from the xiphoid process to the symphysis pubis. The aneurysm is exposed, the aorta is clamped just above and below the aneurysm to stop the flow of blood, the aneurysm is opened, and a Dacron graft is placed within the aneurysm. The aneurysm sac is then wrapped around the graft to protect it (see Figure 53-9, *B*).

Complications. Abdominal aortic aneurysm repair is considered a major operation, and many specific postoperative complications can develop. Complications after abdominal aortic aneurysm repair are generally caused by underlying coronary artery disease and chronic obstructive pulmonary disease. These conditions decrease excretion of anesthetic, increase the risk of postoperative atelectasis, and decrease the client's tolerance of hemodynamic changes from blood loss and fluid shifts. To reduce the risk of acute myocardial infarction, one of the most serious complications, clients may undergo coronary artery bypass before aneurysm repair.

Prerenal failure can develop for several reasons. The kidney can sustain ischemia from decreased aortic blood flow, decreased cardiac output, emboli, inadequate hydration, or the need for clamps on the aorta above the renal arteries during surgery.

Emboli can also develop and lodge in the arteries of the lower extremities or mesentery. Clinical manifestations include those of acute occlusion in the leg. Bowel necrosis is exhibited as fever, leukocytosis, ileus, diarrhea, and abdominal pain.

The spinal cord can also become ischemic, resulting in paraplegia, rectal and urinary incontinence, or loss of pain and temperature sensation. Spinal cord ischemia tends to occur more commonly when an abdominal aortic aneurysm has ruptured.

Changes in sexual function may also develop following repair of an abdominal aortic aneurysm. Retrograde ejaculation occurs in about two thirds of male clients, and loss of potency occurs in one third of males who have undergone repair of abdominal aortic aneurysm.

Nursing Management of the Surgical Client

Preoperative Care

Abdominal aortic surgery is major surgery; it lasts approximately 4 hours. During the hours under anesthesia, the client faces a great risk of pulmonary and cardiac complications developing. Preoperative assessment must include detection of concurrent coronary artery disease and cerebrovascular disease. Also assess all peripheral pulses for baseline comparison postoperatively. For endovascular repair, the procedure is much shorter. Standard evaluation must occur because the potential for an open repair of the aneurysm still exists.

Postoperative Care

Assessment. Following surgery, clients usually return to an intensive care unit. A comprehensive postoperative assessment of the client after open surgical repair for abdominal aortic aneurysm repair is essential. Potential complications are many, because of the seriousness of the problem and the complexity of the repair. Even though extracorporeal perfusion (cardiopulmonary bypass) is not needed for the surgery, arterial flow to tissues distal to the aneurysm is reduced during the time required to perform the surgery because the aorta is clamped.

Diagnosis, Outcomes, Interventions

Collaborative Problem: Risk for Hemorrhage. Because of the risk of bleeding at the graft site, the client is at risk for hemorrhage. Use the collaborative problem *Risk for Hemorrhage.* You can also use the nursing diagnosis *Risk for Deficient Fluid Volume,* but recognize that the "fluid" that can be lost is blood.

Outcomes. The nurse will monitor for manifestations of hemorrhage and notify the physician if any manifestations occur.

Interventions. Assess for changes indicating hypovolemia.

> **Monitor the client for increase in pulse rate, decrease in blood pressure, clammy skin, anxiety, restlessness, decreasing levels of consciousness, pallor, cyanosis, thirst, oliguria (urine output less than 0.5 ml/kg/hour), increase in abdominal girth, increased chest tube output greater than 100 ml/hour for 3 hours, and back pain (from retroperitoneal bleeding). Monitor central venous pressure, left atrial pressure, pulmonary artery pressure, and pulmonary capillary wedge pressure continuously. Report any of these manifestations immediately.**

SAFETY ⚠ ALERT

Diagnosis: Risk for Impaired Gas Exchange. The large abdominal incision impairs deep inspiration and usually reduced effective coughing. Write the nursing diagnosis as *Risk for Impaired Gas Exchange related to ineffective cough secondary to pain from large incision.*

Outcomes. The client will have improved gas exchange as evidenced by oxygen saturation or Pao_2 greater than 95%, increasing effectiveness in coughing, and clearing of lung sounds.

Interventions. Monitor settings on the ventilator to ensure that the client is adequately oxygenated. Assess lung sounds every 1 to 2 hours. Report any adventitious sounds. Monitor oxygen saturation continuously. Report any desaturation. After extubation, assist with coughing by using incentive spirometry, provide splinting pillows before coughing, encouraging ambulation, and providing adequate analgesia.

Diagnosis: Risk for Ineffective Tissue Perfusion. During the operation, the aorta is clamped to stop bleeding while the graft is placed. During that time, distal peripheral tissues are not perfused. The graft site can also become occluded with thrombus. In addition, the client often has pre-existing arterial disease. Write the nursing diagnosis as *Risk for Ineffective Tissue Perfusion related to temporary decrease in blood supply.*

Outcomes. The client will maintain adequate tissue perfusion as evidenced by pedal pulses, warm feet, capillary refill of less than 5 seconds, absence of numbness or tingling, and ability to dorsiflex and plantiflex both feet equally.

Interventions. Assess dorsalis pedis and posterior tibial pulses every hour for 24 hours. Report changes in pulse quality or absent pulses (assess with Doppler if needed). Assess dorsiflexion and plantiflexion and sensation ("pins and needles" sensation) every hour for 24 hours. Inspect lower extremities for mottling, cyanosis, coolness, or numbness every 4 hours.

Diagnosis: Acute Pain. Abdominal aortic aneurysm repair necessitates a long incision. Write this common postoperative diagnosis as *Acute Pain related to surgical incision.*

Outcomes. The client will have increased comfort as evidenced by self-report of decreasing levels of pain, use of decreasing amounts of opioid analgesics for pain control, and ambulating or coughing without extreme pain.

Interventions. Opioids are usually provided via a patient-controlled analgesia system or through an epidural catheter. Assess the degree of pain often, and record the baseline level of pain and the degree to which pain is reduced by medications or other interventions. When changing to an oral route for pain management, plan to pretreat the pain with oral medications 30 minutes or more before discontinuing the infusion.

Collaborative Problem: Risk for Ischemia of the Bowel. If the client undergoes extensive aortic procedures that involve clamping the mesenteric vessels, ischemic colitis can develop. In addition, the inferior mesenteric artery can embolize. The lack of blood supply can lead to ischemia and ileus.

Outcomes. The nurse will monitor the client for abdominal distention, diarrhea, severe abdominal pain, sudden elevations in white blood cell count, and bowel sounds.

Interventions. Assess bowel sounds every 4 hours. Keep the client nothing by mouth (NPO) and provide oral care every 2 to 4 hours. Provide routine nasogastric (NG) tube care and assess nares for tissue impairment. Perform guaiac tests of NG drainage every 4 hours or if bleeding is suspected (i.e., drainage has dark, coffee-ground appearance or is bright red).

Collaborative Problem: Risk for Spinal Cord Ischemia. A rare but devastating effect of aortic abdominal aneurysm repair is spinal cord ischemia leading to paralysis, with or without bowel and bladder involvement. It appears to be most common in clients who have suprarenal aortic reconstruction.

Outcomes. The nurse will monitor for manifestations of spinal cord damage and report any abnormal data.

Interventions

> **Monitor ability to move lower extremities (dorsiflexion and plantar flexion) and sensation in both legs every 1 to 2 hours. Report any changes from baseline.**   SAFETY ⚠ ALERT

Self-Care

Most clients who require abdominal aortic aneurysm repair have significant degrees of arterial disease. Many of the postoperative instructions should address care of clients with arterial disorders, which is discussed earlier. Review all medications to be used by the client to be certain that the purpose, schedule, and side effects are understood.

> **Instruct the client about incision care and manifestations of infection.**   SAFETY ⚠ ALERT

The client should ambulate as tolerated, including climbing stairs and walking outdoors. If leg swelling develops, the leg should be wrapped in elastic bandages or support stockings should be used. Activities that involve lifting heavy objects, usually more than 15 to 20 pounds, are not permitted for 6 to 12 weeks postoperatively. Activities that involve pushing, pulling, or straining may also be restricted. Driving may also be restricted because of postoperative weakness and decreased response time.

The client can resume sexual activity in about 4 to 6 weeks, when the client is able to walk without shortness of breath (e.g., two flights of stairs). The risk of impotence in male clients should be discussed before discharge. Causes vary from pre-existing aortoiliac disease or diabetes to side effects from aortic cross-clamping. Referral may be appropriate if the client is amenable.

RUPTURE OF AN ABDOMINAL AORTIC ANEURYSM

Rupture of an abdominal aortic aneurysm (AAA) is a catastrophe. Rupture occurs most often in aneurysms

5 cm or more in diameter; an abdominal aneurysm measuring 6 cm or more in diameter has a 20% chance of rupturing in 1 year. Less than 50% of people with a ruptured abdominal aortic aneurysm survive. Abdominal, back, or flank pain of sudden onset is characteristic of a rapidly expanding or ruptured AAA. The diagnosis should be entertained whenever a client older than 50 years presents with abdominal pain, particularly when pain is associated with syncope or signs of hemorrhagic shock.

The Critical Monitoring feature below lists clinical manifestations associated with ruptured abdominal aortic aneurysm.

Surgery is the only intervention for clients with ruptured abdominal aortic aneurysm. New surgical and grafting techniques and faster methods for transport (e.g., helicopters) permit rapid resection of ruptured abdominal aortic aneurysm. However, even with advances in surgery, the operative mortality rate for repair of ruptured abdominal aneurysm may be as high as 50%. Manage hemorrhagic shock with fluid resuscitation, and blood transfusion. If the client is hypertensive before surgery, there is greater risk of rupture. Treat the blood pressure to maintain a systolic pressure between 100 and 120 mm Hg. Care of the client following emergency repair of a ruptured AAA is the same as elective repair, except that the client has more hemodynamic instability because of preoperative blood loss and ischemic organ disease.

AORTIC DISSECTION

Aortic dissection is the longitudinal splitting of the medial (muscular) layer of the aorta by blood flowing through it. It is the most common catastrophe involving the aorta. Dissection occurs following a tear in the intima, or inner lining, of the aorta, which allows blood to dissect between it and the medial layer. As the dissection progresses, blood flow through the arterial branches of the aorta becomes blocked, and blood flow to the organs that are served by these branches is reduced. Aortic dissections occur more often in men between 50 and 70 years of age, most of whom are hypertensive. Aortic dissections differ from aneurysms in that a false lumen is formed by separation of the intima from the medial layers of the aorta. An aneurysm is a dilation of the entire aortic wall.

Etiology and Classification

The exact cause of dissection is not known. The medial layer of the aorta can become necrotic and thereby lose strength. Clients with Marfan syndrome (a hereditary condition of connective tissue that predisposes it to aneurysm formation) have a high incidence of dissection. Blunt trauma to the chest wall, such as impact on the steering wheel during a car accident, can also lead to tearing of the aorta.

Dissections are classified by the anatomic location using the Stanford classification system. There are two types of dissections: type A and type B. Type A involves the ascending aorta; type B does not. This system also helps delineate treatment. Usually, type A dissections require surgery, whereas type B dissections may be managed medically under most conditions.

Clinical Manifestations

Abrupt, excruciating pain is the most common presenting manifestation in clients with aortic dissection. Clients describe the pain as ripping or knife-like tearing sensations that radiate to the back, abdomen, extremities, or anterior part of the chest. Hypertension is a common finding, although the client looks "shocky," is sweating profusely, is severely apprehensive, and has diminished peripheral pulses. Other manifestations from decreased perfusion include unequal pulses, different blood pressures in the arms, paraplegia or hemiplegia, decreased urine output or hematuria, mental status changes, and chest pain. A murmur of aortic regurgitation can be heard if the dissection proceeds proximally.

Chest radiograph reveals a widened mediastinum and may show fractured ribs. Transesophageal echocardiogram can be used to determine the size, shape, and location of the tear. Laboratory tests during emergency settings are usually not helpful, except for hemoglobin and hematocrit assays to calculate blood loss and transfusion needs. If the client's condition is stable, helical CT or magnetic resonance imaging can be used to determine the extent of the dissection.

CRITICAL MONITORING

Ruptured Abdominal Aortic Aneurysm

- Pulsating sensation in the abdomen
- Severe, sudden, persistent or constant pain in the abdomen
  - Pain is not colicky or spasmodic
  - Pain radiates to groin, lower back, buttocks, or legs
- Abdominal rigidity
- Manifestations of shock
  - Pallor
  - Tachycardia with hypotension
  - Dry skin and mouth
  - Excessive thirst
  - Anxiety

Complications

Cardiac tamponade can develop when the client has dissection of the ascending aortic arch. This life-threatening complication occurs when blood escapes from the area of dissection into the pericardial sac. Clients have pulsus paradoxus, muffled heart sounds, narrowed pulse pressure, and distended neck veins. Pulsus paradoxus occurs when beats are weaker in amplitude during inspiration and stronger with expiration. Blood pressure readings decrease more than 10 mm Hg during inspiration and increase with expiration.

Because the dissection decreases blood supply to many vital organs, ischemic changes in many organs can develop. The spinal cord, kidneys, and abdominal organs are most commonly affected. Ischemia of the spinal cord can lead to manifestations ranging from weakness to paralysis. Renal ischemia can lead to oliguria. Ileus is the most common manifestation of decreased bowel perfusion.

OUTCOME MANAGEMENT

Emergency management is directed at lowering the blood pressure to decrease the force of the blood tearing the aorta. Potent vasodilators, such as nitroprusside, are used to quickly reduce blood pressure. Beta-blockers can also be used to decrease myocardial contractility.

If the client's condition is stable, management is directed at pain reduction, blood transfusion (as needed), and management of heart failure (as needed). Pain levels are used as a guide for needed treatment. Pain subsides when the dissection stabilizes.

Surgery is used for clients whose condition is unstable, in whom severe heart failure develops, who have leaking blood, or who have occlusion of arteries to major organs. During surgery, the torn area is resected and repaired with synthetic graft materials. The operation is similar to that for repair of AAA.

Nursing care is directed at reducing blood pressure. The client is maintained on bed rest in a semi-Fowler position. Unnecessary environmental stresses (e.g., noise) should be minimized. Use opioids to reduce pain; tranquilizers may also be needed. If the client is receiving potent antihypertensive agents, blood pressure should be monitored continuously with an arterial line. Usually the desired parameters for blood pressure are maintained by titrating the vasodilators. Observe the client often for manifestations of further tearing or rupture. Monitor peripheral pulses, level of anxiety, level of pain, and pulse pressure and check for pulsus paradoxus.

If the client is being managed medically, teach the client about the need for antihypertensive agents and beta-blocker drugs.

SAFETY

⚠️

ALERT

The client and family should understand that if pain returns they should immediately return to the emergency department.

RAYNAUD'S SYNDROME

Raynaud's syndrome is a condition in which the small arteries and arterioles constrict in response to various stimuli. It is classified as either vasospastic or obstructive. Manifestations of vasospastic Raynaud's syndrome can be induced by cold, nicotine, caffeine, and stress. Obstructive Raynaud's syndrome is often found in association with autoimmune disorders such as systemic lupus erythematosus, scleroderma, or rheumatoid arthritis.

Raynaud's syndrome may be a benign primary disorder (previously called *Raynaud's disease*) or secondary to another disease or underlying cause (previously called *Raynaud's phenomenon*). Manifestations of both types are the same.

Clinical Manifestations

Raynaud's syndrome causes classic color changes in the hands. Exposure to causative stimuli leads to spasm of the digital arteries, which results in pallor. The resulting tissue hypoxia causes the arteries to dilate slightly. Because they carry mainly deoxygenated hemoglobin, the fingers look cyanotic. Finally, rubor develops when arterial spasms stop completely. Criteria for diagnosing primary Raynaud's disease include (1) manifestations for at least 2 years, (2) intermittent attacks of pallor or cyanosis of the digits by exposure to cold or from emotional stimuli, (3) bilateral or symmetrical involvement, (4) no evidence of occlusive disease in the digital arteries or of any systemic disease that might be the cause of the changes, and (5) gangrene, which (when it occurs) is limited to the skin of the tips of the digits.

Noninvasive blood flow studies to determine finger pressures both before and after cold challenge may be necessary. Occasionally, the presence of vasospasm during examination makes the use of cold challenge unnecessary.

OUTCOME MANAGEMENT

Conservative measures are essential. These measures include keeping hands and feet warm and dry, protecting all parts of the body from cold exposure to prevent reflex sympathetic vasoconstriction of the digits, and terminating tobacco use. Biofeedback has been of help to some clients.

Medication is used when the vasospastic attacks interfere with the client's ability to work or to perform activities of daily living. Medications are used to induce smooth muscle relaxation, to relieve spasm, and to increase arterial flow. Calcium antagonists, such as nifedipine, are the drugs of first choice because they have been shown to decrease the frequency, duration, and intensity of vasospastic attacks. Medications may be necessary only during the winter months. Individuals who rarely go out in the cold weather may take medications prophylactically 1 to 2 hours before exposure to the cold.

The manifestations of Raynaud's syndrome may be alarming, so reassure the client that the condition is not likely to lead to a serious disability. Advise the client to stay warm by wearing wool gloves and turtleneck sweaters, turning up the thermostat at home if necessary, and staying out of drafts. Teach the client to warm up a cold car before driving. Body core heating is important to prevent chilling and the shunting of blood from the extremities to the trunk. Encourage clients to limit their intake of caffeine or chocolate. They must stop smoking to control the disease. Stress can also trigger vasospasm, so stress management workshops and biofeedback programs may be beneficial. Also, teach the client about any prescribed medications.

BUERGER'S DISEASE (THROMBOANGIITIS OBLITERANS)

Buerger's disease (thromboangiitis obliterans) is an inflammatory disease of the small and medium-sized arteries and veins of the extremities. It is often seen in men and appears to be directly related to smoking. Many clients have a hypersensitivity reaction to intradermal injection of tobacco products, so there may also be an autoimmune element as well. Raynaud's phenomenon, ulcers, and pain are typically seen.

Pain is the outstanding clinical manifestation. Clients have digital ulcerations and pain from ischemia. The pain may be accompanied by manifestations of ischemia, such as color or temperature changes in the fingers. Cold sensitivity, with color changes and pain, may be another early manifestation. Various types of lower extremity paresthesias may occur. Claudication type pain is common, with pain in the arch of the foot. Pulsations in the posterior tibial and dorsalis pedis arteries are weak or absent. In advanced cases, the extremities may be abnormally red or cyanotic, particularly when dependent.

Ulceration and gangrene are frequent complications and may occur early in the course of the disease. These lesions can appear spontaneously from migratory superficial thrombophlebitis but can also follow trauma. Gangrene usually occurs in one extremity at a time. Edema of the legs is fairly common in advanced cases. Changes in the nails and skin appear, and segmental thrombophlebitis affects the smaller veins in about 40% of clients. The primary diagnostic study is leg arteriography. Biopsy may also be used; inflammatory lesions are usually noted.

OUTCOME MANAGEMENT

The goals for management include arresting progress of the disease, producing vasodilation, relieving pain, and providing emotional support. The need for smoking cessation must be clearly and unequivocally conveyed to the client and family. Information about programs to promote abstinence from tobacco should be provided. Because of vasoconstriction, the client should be taught to avoid exposure to cold. Work-related exposure to cold should be considered.

For clients with rest pain and ischemic lesions, adequate pain control is essential. Vasodilation by calcium-channel blockers may be used. Ulcerations need wound care to facilitate healing. Amputation should be deferred until conservative interventions have failed. Thromboangiitis is usually not life-threatening. It does, however, result in disability from pain and amputation.

VENOUS DISORDERS

Venous disorders can be separated into acute and chronic conditions. Chronic venous disorders can be further separated into varicose vein formation and chronic venous insufficiency. Acute venous disorders include thromboembolism. Acute venous disorders are discussed first.

ACUTE VENOUS DISORDERS

Acute venous disorders are caused by thrombus (clot) formation that obstructs venous flow. Blockage may occur in either the superficial or the deep veins.

THROMBOPHLEBITIS

Superficial thrombophlebitis is usually an easily diagnosed condition; it may iatrogenic, resulting from intravenous catheters or infusion of caustic solutions. Deep vein thrombosis (DVT) is thrombophlebitis of the deep veins. DVT is a common disorder, more so in women than in men, and among hospitalized clients. DVT develops in approximately one third of clients older than 40 years who have had major surgery, orthopedic surgery, or an acute myocardial infarction. In addition, clients with cancer or a family history of clotting disorders are at high risk.

Etiology and Risk Factors

There are many risk factors for the development of venous thrombosis (Box 53-2). Thrombus formation is usually attributed to Virchow's triad: (1) venous stasis, (2) hypercoagulability, and (3) injury to the venous wall. At least two of the three conditions must be present for thrombi to form.

Venous stasis is usually caused by immobilization or lack of use of the calf muscle pump. Other conditions that may cause stasis are age older than 40 years, surgery, immobility, prolonged travel, stroke, obesity, pregnancy, paralysis, and heart disease such as heart failure, myocardial infarction, and cardiomyopathy. Some of the highest risk clients are those having orthopedic surgery.

BOX 53-2 Common Conditions Associated with Venous Thrombosis and Thromboembolism

- Age >40 years
- Surgery requiring more than 30 minutes of general, spinal, or epidural anesthesia
- Postoperative edema in the pelvis
- Prolonged position of hip flexion
- Venous stasis (bed rest, prolonged travel, stroke)
- Previous deep vein thrombosis
- Cardiac disease (heart failure, myocardial infarction, cardiomyopathy)
- Pregnancy
- Trauma, especially of the lower extremities
- Estrogen therapy or oral contraceptives
- Malignancy
- Obesity
- Family history of clotting disorders

Hypercoagulability often accompanies malignant cancers (especially visceral and ovarian tumors). Dehydration and blood dyscrasias may raise the platelet count, decrease fibrinolysis, increase the clotting factors, or increase the viscosity of the blood. Oral contraceptives and hematologic disorders may also increase the coagulability of the blood.

SAFETY ALERT

Conditions that may cause vein wall trauma are intravenous injections; fractures and dislocations; severe blows to an area; chemical injury from sclerosing agents, contrast x-ray studies, or certain antibiotics (such as chlortetracycline); and thromboangiitis obliterans (Buerger's disease). The resulting damage to the vein wall attracts platelets, and blood debris accumulates. Platelets do not stick to an intact endothelium. This injury, in combination with low blood flow and a hypercoagulable state, results in thrombus formation.

Pathophysiology

Usually, venous return is aided by the calf muscle pump. When the legs are inactive or the pump is ineffective, blood pools by gravity in the veins (Figure 53-10). Thrombus development is a local process. It begins by platelet adherence to the endothelium. Several factors promote platelet aggregation, including thrombin, fibrin, activated factor X, and catecholamines. In addition, where the platelets adhere to collagen, adenosine diphosphate (ADP) is released. ADP is also released from the damaged tissues and disrupted platelets. ADP produces platelet aggregation that results in a platelet plug. Approximately 24 to 48 hours after formation, thrombi undergo lysis or become organized and adhere to the vessel wall, a process that diminishes the risk of embolization.

Deep vein thrombi vary from 1 mm in diameter to long tubular masses filling main veins. Small thrombi are found commonly in the pocket of deep vein valves. As thrombi become larger in diameter and length, they obstruct the

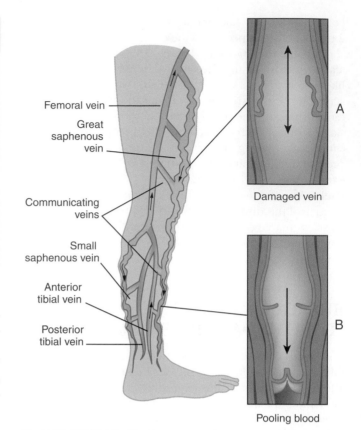

FIGURE 53-10 Venous return from the legs. **A,** Normal flow. **B,** Varicosities and retrograde venous flow.

veins. If a thrombus occludes a major vein (e.g., femoral, vena cava, axillary), the venous pressure and volume increase distally. Conversely, if a thrombus occludes a deep small vein (e.g., tibial, popliteal), collateral venous channels usually relieve the increased venous pressure and volume. The resulting inflammatory process can destroy the valves of the veins; thus venous insufficiency and postphlebitic syndrome are initiated.

Newly formed thrombi may embolize and travel. Pulmonary emboli, most of which start as thrombi in the large deep veins of the legs, are an acute and potentially lethal complication of DVT. Pulmonary embolism (PE) is discussed in Chapter 61.

Prevention

Because of the frequency of DVT and the risk of PE, prevention is imperative. Prevention is geared toward reversing the three risk factors by promoting venous return, treating hypercoagulability, and reducing risk of injury to the venous wall.

Venous stasis is improved by any activity that causes the leg muscles to contract; passive or active contraction promotes venous return. Leg exercises and ambulation promote venous return. Passive leg muscle contraction occurs by using intermittent sequential compression devices (SCDs) (Figure 53-11). These devices are applied

■ **FIGURE 53–11** Pneumatic compression devices, such as the Kendall sequential compression device, are commonly used to prevent deep vein thrombosis in high-risk clients. *(Courtesy Kendall Company, Mansfield, Mass.)*

after surgery and carefully used until the client is ambulatory. Research has shown that SCDs are clinically effective in reducing the incidence of DVT. It is also a good alternative for clients who cannot tolerate anticoagulation. These devices should *not* be used in clients with known DVT. Other methods of promoting venous return include elevating the foot of the bed, applying compression stockings, using motorized foot compressive devices, and providing passive range-of-motion exercises. Encouraging postoperative deep-breathing exercises promotes thoracic pull as a result of the negative thoracic pressure on venous stores in the legs.

Pharmacologic prevention directed at reducing the hypercoagulability includes warfarin, platelet antiaggregation agents (aspirin being the most common), heparin, and low-molecular-weight heparin. Other methods to reduce coagulation include preventing the venous blood from pooling.

SAFETY ALERT

Avoid using pillows under the client's knees postoperatively. Teach the client to avoid sitting or standing in one position for prolonged periods.

Measures to prevent injury to the vein wall include avoidance of (1) infiltration during intravenous therapy, (2) pressure on the calf veins during prolonged surgery, and (3) trauma to veins in procedures requiring prolonged positioning (e.g., childbirth, colonoscopy). In addition, access ports should be used in clients requiring multiple intravenous punctures.

Clinical Manifestations and Diagnostic Findings

Clinical manifestations of superficial thrombophlebitis include redness (rubor), induration, warmth (calor), and tenderness (dolor) along a vein. Discomfort may be relieved by applying heat. Activity should be encouraged, and a supportive wrap or stocking should be applied.

The clinical manifestations of DVT are less distinctive; about half of clients are asymptomatic. The most common clinical manifestation is unilateral leg swelling. Other clinical manifestations include pain, redness or warmth of the leg, dilated veins, and low-grade fever. The first clinical manifestation may be PE. Clients may have thrombi in both legs even though the manifestations are unilateral, but this is more common in the client with malignancy.

Homans' sign—discomfort in the upper calf during forced dorsiflexion of the foot—is commonly assessed during physical examination, but findings are insensitive and nonspecific. Homans' sign is present in less than one third of clients with documented DVT. In addition, more than 50% of clients with a positive Homans' sign do not have venous thrombosis. For example, shin splints from running create a positive Homans' sign without DVT.

Venous duplex scanning has become the primary diagnostic test for DVT because it allows visualization of the vein, which provides a reliable diagnosis of venous thrombus. Venography, the previous gold standard of diagnosis, results in exposure to contrast medium and is seldom used. The D-dimer blood test is being used more frequently in evaluation of DVT. The D-dimer is a product of fibrin degradation and is indicative of fibrinolysis, which occurs with thrombosis. Recent studies seem to indicate that the use of the D-dimer test, a risk assessment score, and duplex imaging are excellent at predicting and diagnosing DVT in an asymptomatic population. Plethysmographic examination of the venous system is seldom used, although results of these studies may be found in client records.

OUTCOME MANAGEMENT

Medical Management

The goals of medical management are to reduce risk of DVT, detect the thrombus early, prevent extension or embolization of the thrombus, and prevent further thrombus formation.

Superficial thrombophlebitis can be managed with local measures, such as warm packs and elevation of the extremity. Ambulation is encouraged. Sometimes anti-inflammatory medications are required. Clients are encouraged to be seen in follow-up, because an extension of a superficial phlebitis can result in a DVT.

Anticoagulation

Anticoagulant therapy is designed to prevent initiation or extension of thrombi by inhibiting the synthesis of clotting factors or by accelerating their inactivation. Anticoagulant agents do not break up or dissolve clots; they prevent new clots from forming. Various agents that can be used for anticoagulation are discussed in the Integrating Pharmacology feature on p. 1334.

Nursing Management of the Medical Client

Goals of nursing management are to prevent DVT in high-risk clients, prevent existing thrombi from becoming emboli, and prevent new thrombi from forming. Nurses also closely monitor the effect of anticoagulant medications.

Prevent DVT

All clients prescribed bed rest should be encouraged to move their legs because blood stasis leads to clotting. Sequential compression devices (SCDs) should be used for those clients expected to be prescribed bed rest for longer than 24 hours. SCDs are removed twice daily to inspect the skin and allow perspiration to evaporate. High-risk clients may also be prescribed anticoagulants.

Promote Venous Return

Elevation of the legs above the level of the heart facilitates blood flow by the force of gravity. The increase of blood flow prevents venous stasis and the formation of new thrombi. Elevation of the legs also decreases venous pressure, which in turn reduces edema and pain. Elevate the foot of the bed 6 inches (Trendelenburg's position), with a slight knee bend to prevent popliteal pressure. The veins of the legs should be level with the right atrium. The head of the bed may be raised to facilitate eating and bathing. Various forms of elastic support are used to promote venous return. Elastic bandages are advantageous for

---

INTEGRATING PHARMACOLOGY

Anticoagulant Therapy for the Prevention and Treatment of Deep Vein Thrombosis

Anticoagulation prevents the extension of the original thrombus and the development of new thrombi while the existing thrombus is lysed naturally by fibrinolysis. Oral warfarin (Coumadin) and parenterally administered heparin have been the mainstays of anticoagulant therapy since the 1940s. Even though it is well-known that these medications are effective, they have several undesirable characteristics, such as unpredictability in dosage required for therapeutic effect, the need for careful laboratory monitoring, and the potential for life-threatening toxicity.

Acute deep vein thrombosis (DVT) is treated with continuous intravenous heparin or injected low-molecular-weight heparin (LMWH). Heparin is normally administered according to the client's weight and blood levels of activated partial thromboplastin time (aPPT or PTT), which is maintained either at more than 60 seconds or at a level 1.5 to 2.5 times a baseline established before the beginning of therapy. Heparin is usually infused in the range of 700 to 1400 units/hour. When the client has marked elevated PTT levels, frequent assessment of bleeding or bruising and institution of bleeding precautions are important. Bleeding precautions include avoidance of injections, brushing teeth with a soft sponge device, supervision with ambulation to prevent falls, and increasing intake of fiber and fluids to prevent straining and constipation. Heparin has a short half-life of 4 hours and can be quickly reversed with protamine. Heparin has increased effects when simultaneously administered with other anticoagulants. Therefore a full list of prescribed and over-the-counter medications must be reviewed for potential drug-drug interactions.

LMWH has been available for the past decade. LMWHs are longer acting, homogeneous molecules, with a reliable dose-response curve requiring little or no monitoring, but they are much more expensive than heparin. The actions of heparin and LMWHs are similar. Both bind to antithrombin III, increasing its activity and inhibiting thrombin and other factors. Whereas the anticoagulant function of heparin can be measured through PTT, no such blood test is available for LMWH. This may seem like a drawback for LMWHs, but the reason that standard heparin therapy must be monitored is because heparin has an unpredictable bioavailability and pharmacokinetics, particularly when administered subcutaneously. LMWHs, however, have extremely high bioavailability. The same bleeding precautions and drug-drug interactions apply with LMWH.

Coumadin (warfarin or coumarin) is an oral anticoagulant. It is often used as a long-term anticoagulant after the acute DVT has been treated with injectable forms of heparin. Coumadin has a long half-life (3 to 5 days). Therefore the drug must be stopped for 3 days before any invasive procedure is done. Coumadin is prescribed based on International Normalized Ratio (INR) levels; the recommended therapeutic range is 2 to 3.5. Coumadin can also be prescribed based on prothrombin (ProTime) levels, but there is variation from one laboratory to another, so INR levels are becoming more common, especially with long-term use of warfarin (Coumadin). For hospitalized clients, warfarin (Coumadin) is administered in the afternoon or early evening. This schedule allows for dose adjustments based on daily INR or ProTime results. Warfarin (Coumadin) can be reversed with injections of vitamin K (phytonadione). The therapeutic effect of warfarin (Coumadin) is altered by a host of medications and foods, and in clients with liver disease. Potential drug-drug and drug-food interactions should be reviewed by a pharmacist if the intended response (e.g., changes in INR) is not seen as predicted.

PREVENTION OF DEEP VEIN THROMBOSIS

Several medications can be used to prevent DVT. Standard heparin is increased by adjusting the dose to maintain the aPTT ratio in the upper normal range. An average dose is 5000 units given subcutaneously in the abdomen twice daily. LMWH is also given subcutaneously. Subcutaneous injection of anticoagulants can lead to bruising at the injection sites. Clients and families should be taught that this is an expected response and does not indicate active bleeding. The development of painful masses in the abdomen should be reported and may indicate more active bleeding.

The use of antiplatelet drugs, aspirin, and nonsteroidal anti-inflammatory drugs may have a place in the prevention of DVT postoperatively or once conventional anticoagulant therapy for DVT has been concluded, although there is still debate on this topic.

clients with large or misshapen legs. Apply elastic wraps snugly from toe to groin. Use a narrower elastic wrap for the foot and a wider one for the leg. Rewrap them every 4 to 8 hours. If compression stockings are prescribed, they must be fitted correctly and removed for a short time every day. Bathe the legs and inspect them closely for manifestations of skin breakdown while the stockings are off.

Reduce Discomfort

Elevation of the extremity and application of warm packs usually reduce discomfort. Some clients need a mild analgesic.

Monitor Anticoagulant Therapy

Most physicians use an algorithm to adjust the dose of heparin based on the client's body weight and partial thromboplastin time (PTT) results. Blood is sampled every 4 to 8 hours for measurement of PTT or International Normalized Ratio (INR), and the dose is adjusted accordingly. Warfarin therapy requires the prothrombin time (PT) or INR be determined on a regular basis. Low-molecular-weight heparin requires no testing.

SAFETY
⚠
ALERT

Bleeding can occur in any client receiving anticoagulation. The client should also be observed for frank bleeding in the urine, tarry or frank blood in the stool, bleeding with brushing the teeth, easy subcutaneous bruising, and flank pain. When invasive studies are necessary (e.g., arterial blood gas analyses), apply pressure for 30 minutes to the puncture site.

Monitor for Pulmonary Embolism

PE is an acute and potentially lethal complication of DVT. Tachypnea and anxiety are the most common manifestations of PE. Pleuritic chest pain can also occur. It is often sudden and aggravated by breathing. Pleuritic pain is caused by an inflammatory reaction of the lung parenchyma or by pulmonary infarction or ischemia caused by obstruction of small pulmonary arterial branches.

Other clinical manifestations may include cough without hemoptysis, diaphoresis, dyspnea, crackles, and wheezing. Hemoptysis can occur as a result of pulmonary infarction, or atelectasis may produce alveolar hemorrhage. Because of the seriousness of PE, promptly notify the physician of these clinical manifestations. Document the lack of manifestations or PE in clients with DVT to provide evidence of monitoring for the condition. PE is fully discussed in Chapter 61.

Surgical Management

Surgical treatment of thrombophlebitis is aimed at reducing PE by inserting a filter into the vena cava to filter the blood before it reaches the lungs (see Chapter 61).

Thrombectomy can also be performed, but it is not common.

Self-Care

Prevention is the key to managing DVT. Therefore teach the client about risk factors of DVT and how to avoid them. Continue teaching with explanations of medications being taken, actions, doses, timing, adverse effects, and importance of monitoring coagulation status. Begin teaching on the first day of heparinization, discussing reasons for anticoagulants. Clients need to know who to contact and how to reach a health care provider in case problems develop. Inform the client about the monitoring required while receiving anticoagulation therapy.

After thrombosis of a deep calf vein, clients should wear elastic support for at least 3 to 6 months and probably for life. Elastic support compresses the superficial veins when the client walks, and blood flow in the larger veins is increased while venous pressure is kept to a minimum. Standing and sitting are not allowed for long periods during the acute phase so as not to increase the hydrostatic pressure in the capillaries, which promotes edema. Encourage walking and exercises in bed to decrease venous pressure and promote blood flow.

CHRONIC VENOUS DISORDERS

VARICOSE VEINS

Varicose veins are permanently distended veins that develop from the loss of valvular competence. Faulty valves elevate venous pressure, causing distention and tortuosity of the superficial veins. The greater and lesser saphenous veins and perforator veins in the ankle are common sites of varicosities.

Varicose veins may be either primary or secondary. Primary varicose veins often result from a congenital or familial predisposition that leads to loss of elasticity of the vein wall. Secondary varicosities occur when trauma, obstruction, DVT, or inflammation causes damage to valves.

Varicose veins affect a large percentage of the adult population. An estimated 24 million Americans have varicose veins. The prevalence increases with age and peaks between the fifth and sixth decades of life. Varicose veins are more common in women; however, the gender ratio decreases with advancing age and almost disappears in clients older than 70 years. Prolonged standing has been implicated as a cause of varicose veins, but epidemiologic studies have not demonstrated an association between standing at work and an increased incidence of varicose veins.

Clients with varicose veins often complain of aching, a feeling of heaviness in the legs, itching, moderate swelling, and, frequently, the unsightly appearance of their legs. Severity of discomfort is difficult to assess and does not seem related to the size of varicosities. A superficial inflammation may occasionally develop along the path of the varicose vein. To assess for varicose veins, carefully examine both of the client's legs in good lighting. Varicosities appear as dilated, tortuous skin veins (Figure 53-12).

■ **FIGURE 53-12** Varicose veins on the surface of the leg *(arrow)*. Note the tortuous pattern.

OUTCOME MANAGEMENT

Medical Management

In early stages of varicose veins, the goal is to reduce venous pooling, prevent complications, and improve comfort levels. The simplest form of treatment is the application of below-the-knee compression stockings or elastic wraps. These stockings are designed to apply the greatest amount of pressure over the ankle.

Nursing Management of the Medical Client

The client should be taught that varicose veins are a chronic problem. Even though they do not subside, various activities can help prevent ulceration or new varicosities. The client should avoid standing still in one position for extended periods of time. Legs should be elevated when seated and, if swelling is present, legs should be elevated higher than the heart. Elastic stockings or support hose should be worn to help with venous blood return. Fit of elastic stockings is important. Many clients with venous disease have misshapen legs and standard stockings do not fit them well, being too tight in the ankle. Custom stockings may be needed. Elastic wraps need to be wrapped twice daily so that that greatest pressure is at the ankle, with lesser pressure gradually applied to the level of the knee.

Surgical Management

Sclerotherapy

Sclerotherapy is the injection of a sclerosing agent into varicose veins. The agent damages the vein and endothelium,

causing an aseptic thrombosis that closes the vein. Application of pressure causes the vein walls to grow together. Sclerotherapy is usually performed for cosmetic reasons, but it may relieve the discomfort of both short segments of varicosities and spider veins. It is most effective in closing small, residual varicosities after surgical intervention for varicose veins. (Sclerotherapy is contraindicated before such surgery, because it makes vein stripping more difficult.) Within minutes after injection of the sclerosing agent, elastic compression and active walking should commence. Elastic bandages are worn for 1 to 3 weeks, from morning to night (but not 24 hours a day).

Vein Ligation and Stripping

Surgical management of varicose veins consists of ligation (tying off) of the greater saphenous vein with its tributaries at the saphenofemoral junction, combined with removal of the saphenous vein (stripping) and ligation of incompetent perforator veins. Removal of the vein is performed through multiple, short incisions. An incision is made at the ankle over the saphenous vein and a nylon wire is threaded up the vein to the groin. The wire is brought out through the groin, capped, and then the wire and vein are pulled out through the ankle incision. If the perforator veins alone are ligated, it may be done through multiple small endoscopic incisions.

Elastic compression bandages are applied from foot to groin. The client is rarely hospitalized overnight. Complications are infrequent and include bleeding, infection, and nerve damage. Hemorrhage most commonly occurs at the surgical wound site in the groin. Bleeding comes primarily from the stripped canal. The risk of serious bleeding can be decreased by carefully wrapping the leg from foot to groin and by applying compression, especially to the upper thigh and groin. Some discoloration and bruising along the stripped tract are normal.

Saphenous nerve damage may occur with surgery. In the distal third of the leg, the saphenous nerve runs close to the saphenous vein. Thus risk of nerve injury increases when the distal part of the vein is involved. DVT, embolism, and infection are rare following varicose vein surgery, especially if postoperative precautions (e.g., bandaging, movement, exercise) are taken.

Saphenofemoral Ligation

Some clients require only tying off of the junction of the saphenous and the femoral vein at the groin. This involves one short incision, often local anesthesia, and no hospital stay. Postoperative care is the same.

Nursing Management of the Surgical Client

Routine postoperative assessment and care are provided. Specific care includes maintaining firm elastic pressure over the whole limb, reducing the risk of thrombophlebitis by promoting regular movement and exercise of the legs, and improving venous return by elevating the foot of the bed 6 to 9 inches so that the legs are above the heart level when the client is in bed. The client ambulates for short periods, starting immediately after surgery. Clients should walk rather than stand or sit. After ambulation, elevate the client's legs again.

CHRONIC VENOUS INSUFFICIENCY

Chronic venous insufficiency is also known as *postphlebitic syndrome* and follows most severe cases of DVT. Chronic venous insufficiency results from dysfunctional valves that reduce venous return, which thus increases venous pressure and causes venous stasis. Because existing valves are destroyed, venous blood flow is bidirectional, resulting in inefficient venous outflow. The net effect of this change is that the weight of the venous blood column from the right atrium is transmitted along the full length of the veins. Very high venous pressure is exerted at the ankle and the venules become the final pathway for the highest venous pressure. The current theory is that the abnormal capillaries lead to extravasation of red blood cells, activation of endothelial cells, and trapping of white blood cells. The end result is capillary thrombosis. Skin ulcerations also occur.

Chronic venous insufficiency is marked by the following characteristics:

- Chronically swollen legs
- Thick, coarse, brownish skin around the ankles (referred to as the "gaiter" area)
- Venous stasis ulceration (Figure 53-13)
- Itchy, scaly skin

■ **FIGURE 53–13** Venous stasis ulcers usually develop in the lower outer leg, appear irregular, and have a beefy red base. Note the dark-stained skin from venous disease.

OUTCOME MANAGEMENT

Goals of management are to increase venous blood return and to decrease venous pressure. Antigravity measures increase blood return to the heart. They include elevating the client's legs above the heart level and avoiding prolonged standing or sitting. Encourage the client to sleep with the foot of the bed elevated 6 inches. At least one third of every 24 hours should be spent with the feet and legs elevated above the heart. The client should also be taught *not* to cross the legs, sit in chairs that are too high to allow the feet to touch the floor or that are too deep (and press on the popliteal area), or wear garters, rolled stockings or tight girdles.

The Bridge to Home Health Care feature on p. 1338 describes how increased venous pressure on the tissues of the leg can be counteracted by the compression of elastic support hose. Ideally, this support should just balance the increased venous pressure. Thus hose should be fitted individually to the client's legs. Measurements of the ankle and calf circumference and from 1 inch below the knee or 1 inch below the groin to the bottom of the foot are usually taken. Measure after the client has been recumbent and leg edema is minimal. Stockings that extend above the knee often bind the popliteal space and act as a tourniquet, especially when the knee is bent. Knee-length elastic stockings are preferable. Elastic wraps are often preferable for clients who have periods of leg swelling. Apply the elastic wrap using a graded technique, placing more tension on the lower leg. The problem with elastic wraps is that they only maintain their elastic properties for a few washings (with a few exceptions), and clients tend to use them long past their effective compression. Additionally, wraps often are not used properly and do not exert adequate compression.

VENOUS STASIS ULCERATION

Venous stasis ulceration is the end stage of chronic venous insufficiency. Prolonged venous pressure slows nutrient blood flow, which deprives cells of needed oxygen, glucose, and other substances. Skin of the lower legs ulcerates, causing a stasis ulcer, which occurs as a result of stasis of blood. It is characteristically located in the malleolar or gaiter (lower third of the leg) area (see Figure 53-13). It is important to determine the cause of the ulcer before beginning treatment. Determining whether arterial disease is present is imperative; compression devices are contraindicated in arterial disease because they can restrict arterial inflow of blood.

Management of venous stasis ulceration includes leg elevation, wound care, moist dressings, and support stockings. Gravity is the major enemy of venous stasis disease. The client should rest with his or her legs elevated 6 inches. Regular walking is encouraged.

When ulcers are present, cultures are often obtained of painful, odorous, or weeping wounds to rule out infection.

Managing Peripheral Vascular Disease

Many clients who are referred to home health agencies or clinics that serve older people have peripheral vascular disease. Consider what you can do to help clients prevent further complications through assessment and evaluation, blood pressure monitoring, health education, and reporting changes in your clients' status to their physicians.

ASSESSMENT

Inspect clients for temperature variations; color changes in the skin; dorsal and ankle foot pulses; extremity size comparisons; shiny, taunt, hairless, or blistered skin; diminished toenail growth and color change; pain with palpation, dependent position, or weight-bearing; and skin breakdown and ulcerations. As part of the assessment, measure the calves, ankles, and feet correctly, as the involved areas of edema indicate. Use a monofilament (thin plastic filament) test for sensation and dorsiflexion and plantar flexion of the great toe (proprioception), especially for diabetic clients. The loss of touch sensation may require special foot protection. The loss of proprioception of the foot (position perception) indicates the need to discourage or stop driving. For many clients, this news is very traumatic. You may want to discuss this safety recommendation with a family member or significant other. Be prepared to problem-solve transportation alternatives.

EDUCATION

Health education is an essential component of the care you provide. It is important for clients to avoid smoking, wearing constrictive clothing, and applying excessive heat to their extremities. Clients need information about elevating their legs and performing daily foot hygiene. They may be able to reduce lower extremity edema by wearing properly fitted anti-embolic hose or compression socks (Sigvaris or TEDS); home health clients need physicians' orders. Before ready-made compression socks are bought, measure the heel to knee or the heel to thigh distance and the largest calf circumference; the cost ranges from $8 to $15. Before purchasing custom-ordered anti-embolic socks, clients need a prescription and are measured by a supply company; these socks cost up to several hundred dollars. Clients need to exercise caution when using compression socks. Most ready-made ones lose significant compression after 6 to 12 months and need to be replaced. When possible, use the "open toe" design to prevent excess pressure on the toes, especially with diabetic clients. The nylon content in these socks causes moisture retention and leads to skin maceration in clients who have poor circulation. The socks should not be worn around-the-clock.

Antibiotics may be required to treat infection or cellulitis. Local wound care is essential and should be provided by a health care provider familiar with the disease process. Some ulcers require debridement of eschar (see Chapter 14).

To clean the ulcer, use normal saline. Clean the dry, scaly skin around the ulcer and on the leg with saline or mild soaps. Gently clean the area and apply a lanolin-containing lotion every day to keep skin moist and supple. Avoid lotions containing alcohol and perfumes because they dry and irritate the skin. Protect granulation tissue with saline gel dressings or antibiotic ointments. Cover with a nonadherent dressing that does not accumulate heat or humidity at the wound bed. Monitor for sensitivity to topical agents, seen as blistering, itching, and erythema on the treated areas. If the ulcer is large and heavily exuding, more frequent dressing changes, with absorptive dressings, are required.

No topical treatment is adequate without compression. Graduated compression systems, with adequate padding capable of sustaining compression for at least a week, should be the first line of treatment for uncomplicated venous leg ulcers with an ABI ≥0.8. Stockings are the easiest to apply, although soiling may be a problem. In addition, stockings do not fit abnormally shaped legs or those clients with dressings over the ulcer. Elastic wraps can be adjusted for size. Elastic wraps must be wrapped with the most tension at the foot and ankle and rewrapped twice daily.

An Unna boot is a popular form of bandage impregnated with calamine, zinc oxide, and glycerin. When wrapped snugly around the leg, it provides excellent compression during ambulation and applies minimal pressure during limb elevation. An Unna boot is a permeable dressing that can be applied directly over skin ulcers, thereby allowing drainage of exudate. It creates a moist and warm interface between the ulcerated skin and the bandage. It can be changed on a weekly or biweekly basis; the client wears the boot without interruption and thereby improves compliance. Disadvantages of the Unna boot include allergy, skin irritation, discomfort, difficulty in bathing, and pain while changing the boot. The Unna boot has been shown to achieve healing rates of 70%.

Skin grafting is rarely necessary to achieve healing. Surgery to remove incompetent varicose veins or incompetent perforator veins may also be necessary.

LYMPHATIC DISORDERS

LYMPHEDEMA

Lymphedema is an accumulation of lymphatic fluid in the interstitial tissue that causes swelling, most often in the arms or legs, and occasionally in other parts of the body. Lymphedema can develop when lymphatic vessels are missing or impaired (primary), or when lymph vessels are damaged or lymph nodes removed (secondary). Lymphedema should not be confused with edema resulting from venous insufficiency, which is not lymphedema.

When the impairment becomes so great that the lymphatic fluid exceeds the lymphatic transport capacity, an abnormal amount of protein-rich fluid collects in the tissues of the affected area. Left untreated, this stagnant, protein-rich fluid not only causes tissue channels to increase in size and number, but also reduces oxygen availability in the transport system, interferes with wound healing, and provides a culture medium for bacteria that can result in lymphangitis (infection).

Primary lymphedema may be classified according to age at onset: congenital (present at birth), praecox (before age 35 years), or tarda (after age 35 years). Congenital and familial lymphedema is also called *Milroy disease*. It is inherited as an autosomal dominant trait. The edema usually appears spontaneously and without known cause.

Secondary lymphedema occurs because of some damage or obstruction to the lymph system by another disease process or by a procedure: trauma, cancers (primary or metastatic), filariasis, inflammation, surgical excision, or high doses of radiation. Postoperative lymphedema is usually seen after surgical excision of axillary, inguinal, or iliac nodes. These operations are usually performed as a prophylactic or therapeutic treatment for metastatic tumor. For example, lymphedema of the arm is encountered after mastectomy (Figure 53-14, *A*). Radiation in moderate amounts does not appear to damage the lymph vessels. However, heavy radiation for a particularly resistant tumor usually leads to lymphatic obstruction.

Filariasis, caused by the filarial nematode *Wuchereria bancrofti* (and others), is one of the most common diseases in undeveloped nations; it is transmitted by mosquitoes from human to human. The living embryos (microfilariae) of the adult worms are found in the bloodstream. The larvae migrate to the lymphatics, where they mature into adult worms. Adult worms in the lymph nodes and lymphatics lead to obstruction, lymphedema, and elephantiasis.

Lymphedema secondary to cancer in the lymph nodes is common. The malignant disease may be primary (lymphoma or Hodgkin's disease) or metastatic from another site.

Clinical Manifestations

Primary lymphedema presents as bilateral mild edema of ankles and legs in women at puberty or shortly after puberty, unilateral edema of the entire leg in men and women, or bilateral edema present at birth or early age. The skin of clients with congenital lymphedema contains vesicles (blisters) filled with lymph. A dull, heavy sensation is present, but actual pain is absent. Elevation of the limb and rest in bed cause a reduction but not disappearance of the sensation. Smooth skin becomes roughened; the edema is nonpitting. Acute lymphangitis and cellulitis are infrequent. Ulceration of the skin does not occur. However, the limb becomes greatly enlarged, uncomfortable, and unsightly (see Figure 53-14, *B*). Lymphedema can be diagnosed with isotopic lymphography, lymphangiography, and phlebography.

OUTCOME MANAGEMENT

There is no known cure for lymphedema once the swelling appears. The goal of treatment is to remove as much fluid as possible from the affected extremity and to maintain as normal-appearing an extremity as possible.

Physical therapy for arm or leg lymphedema involves mechanical or manual squeezing of the tissue in order to

■ **FIGURE 53–14** Types of lymphedema. **A,** Secondary lymphedema of the arm following mastectomy. **B,** Severe lymphedema. The client's feet were bandaged so that shoes could be worn.

press the stagnant lymphatic fluid to the proximal part of the limb. This is followed by specific active and passive exercises to transport the lymph farther into the lymphatic system and finally into the bloodstream. Many pneumatic pumping devices for intermittent compression are available. Diuretics may also be prescribed. Elastic stockings or sleeves are used to maintain the effects of the pneumatic pump.

To reduce the swelling, the extremity is elevated above the right atrium. Pneumatic pumps may be used to reduce the extremity size. If pumps are used, teach the client how to apply the device, the frequency of application, and the reasons for its use. When stockings or sleeves are used, ascertain that they fit and do not gather at the knee or elbow. Activity such as walking, rather than sitting or standing, should be promoted. For bedridden clients, teach bed exercises to promote venous and lymphatic return and to maintain muscle strength.

The client with lymphedema is at high risk for infection. The affected extremity is monitored for clinical manifestations of infection such as redness, warmth, and pain. Meticulous skin care is given to the extremity using mild soaps and lotions. Skin should be gently dried, especially between creases of skin. Nails are kept trimmed. Skin should be lubricated to maintain its suppleness; avoid using products with alcohol, dyes, lanolin, mineral oil, petroleum products, talc, or perfumes. Chemical hair removers and regular razors are not used. If shaving is desired, a well-maintained electric razor should be used. Hot water should be avoided.

SAFETY
⚠
ALERT

Clients with lymphedema may suffer from disturbances in self-concept because of the visibility of their deformity. Encourage the client to discuss these feelings and help the client understand that such feelings are normal. Variations in clothing style may be suggested to disguise the deformity. When caring for clients with lymph disorders, remember that these clients must cope with difficult, chronic diseases. Take time to give emotional support to the client and the family. Emphasize the possible need for lifelong follow-up.

CONCLUSIONS

Clients with vascular diseases can challenge a broad range of the nurse's capability and skill, from monitoring a client with rupture of an abdominal aortic aneurysm in an intensive care unit, to performing and teaching meticulous foot care, to educating and counseling a client to make significant lifestyle changes. Vascular diseases involve a broad spectrum of arterial, venous, and lymphatic problems. Nursing care for clients with arterial disorders centers on promoting circulation and adequate tissue perfusion, protecting against skin breakdown and injury, managing pain, and encouraging positive lifestyle changes. Limb amputation requires particularly sensitive assessment, teaching, and counseling skills. Nursing care for clients with venous disorders focuses on monitoring therapeutic regimens such as thrombolytic therapy, controlling and preventing thrombus formation, and promoting circulation by increasing venous blood return and decreasing venous pressure. Nursing care for lymphedema is palliative.

THINKING CRITICALLY

1. The client is admitted to the hospital for the care of leg ulcers. He is homeless and usually wanders the streets, sleeping on external heating grates in the sidewalk. He has large, irregularly shaped ulcers covered with thick, yellow, devitalized tissue. The ulcers are weeping and his stockings have adhered to the ulcers. What types of ulcers are present? What type of wound care will he need? How can he continue to do wound care after discharge?

Factors to Consider. How are arterial and venous ulcers distinguished? Is it important to remove the devitalized tissue? If so, how? How does his lifestyle influence his recovery?

2. A middle-age man enters the emergency department with complaints of a painful leg. The pain began about 3 hours before he noted a very rapid heartbeat. You note that his leg and foot are cold and white. What may have happened? What other factors need to be addressed in relation to his leg? What are the possible treatments available? What might his post-hospital instructions include?

Factors to Consider. How do you determine the acuteness of the tissue insult? What are the potential outcomes if you delay treatment? What might be the source of emboli, and how can this be assessed?

evolve *Discussions for these questions can be found on the website.*

BIBLIOGRAPHY

Citations appearing in red refer to primary research.

1. Aquila, A.M. (2001). Deep venous thrombosis. *Journal of Cardiovascular Nursing, 15*(4), 25-44.
2. Belkin, M., et al. (2004). Peripheral arterial occlusive disease In C.M. Townsend, et al. (Eds.), *Sabiston textbook of surgery* (17th ed.). Philadelphia: Saunders.
3. Bryant, C., et al. (2002). Abdominal aortic aneurysm repair: A look at the first 24 hours. *Journal of Perianesthesia Nursing, 17*(3), 164-169.
4. Cosmi, B., Conti, E., & Coccheri, S. (2001). Anticoagulants (heparin, low molecular weight heparin, and oral anticoagulants) for intermittent claudication. *Cochrane Database of Systematic Reviews*, Issue 2, Article CD001999, DOI 10.1002/14651858.CD001999.
5. Cumming, J.C.O., Barr, S., & Howe, T.E. (2006). Prosthetic rehabilitation for older dysvascular people following a unilateral transfemoral amputation. *Cochrane Database of Systematic Reviews*, Issue 4, Article CD005260, DOI 10.1002/14651858.CD005260.pub2.
6. Dörffler-Melly, J., Koopman, M.M.W., Prins, M.H., et al. (2005). Antiplatelet and anticoagulant drugs for prevention of restenosis/reocclusion following peripheral endovascular treatment. *Cochrane Database of Systematic Reviews*, Issue 1, Article CD002071, DOI 10.1002/14651858.CD002071.pub2.
7. Doughty, D., & Holbrook, R. (2006). Lower extremity ulcers of vascular etiology. In R. Bryant & D. Nix (Eds.), *Acute and chronic wounds* (3rd ed., pp. 258-306). St. Louis: Mosby.
8. Ennis, W.J., & Meneses, P. (2003). Standard, appropriate and advanced care and medical-legal considerations: Venous ulcerations. *Wounds, 15*(4), 107-122.
9. Eskandari, M., Matsumura, J., & Anderson, L. (2004). Surgery on the aorta. In V. Fahey (Ed.), *Vascular nursing* (4th ed., pp. 215-236). Philadelphia: Saunders.
10. Frost-Rude, J.A., et al. (2000). Buerger's disease. *Journal of Vascular Nursing, 18*(4), 128-130.
11. Hafner, J., et al. (2000). Leg ulcers in peripheral arterial disease: Impaired wound healing above the threshold of chronic critical limb ischemia. *Journal of the American Academy of Dermatology, 43*(6), 1001-1008.
12. Hayes, J.M. (2002). Graduated compression stockings: Updating practice, improving compliance. *MEDSURG Nursing, 11*(4), 163-166.
13. Keeling, W.B., et al. (2007). Plaque excision with the Silverhawk catheter: Early results in patients with claudication or critical limb ischemia. *Journal of Vascular Surgery, 45*(1),25-31.
14. Juynh, T., et al. (2004). Thoracic vasculature. In C.M. Townsend, et al. (Eds.), *Sabiston textbook of surgery* (17th ed.). Philadelphia: Saunders.
15. Leng, G.C., Davis, M., & Baker, D. (2000). Bypass surgery for chronic lower limb ischemia. *Cochrane Database of Systematic Reviews*, Issue 3, Article CD002000, DOI 10.1002/14651858.CD002000.
16. Lewis, C.D. (2001). Peripheral arterial disease of the lower extremity. *Journal of Cardiovascular Nursing, 15*(4), 45-63.
17. Jones, M.A., et al. (2000). Endovascular grafting for repair of abdominal aortic aneurysm. *Critical Care Nurse, 20*(4), 38-48.
18. Nelson, E.A., et al. (2003). Compression for preventing recurrence of venous ulcers. *Cochrane Review The Cochrane Library*, (2). Oxford: Update Software.
19. Rudolph, D. (2001). Standards of care for venous leg ulcers: Compression therapy and moist wound healing. *Journal of Vascular Nursing, 19*(1), 20-27.
20. Treat-Jacobson, D. (2003). Treating patients with peripheral arterial disease and claudication. *Journal of Vascular Nursing, 21*(1), 5-14.

evolve **Did you remember to check out the bonus material on the Evolve website and the CD-ROM, including NCLEX®-Examination Style Review Questions, Open-Book Quizzes, and Chapter Review Audio Podcasts?**

http://evolve.elsevier.com/Black/medsurg

UNIT 13

CARDIAC DISORDERS

ANATOMY AND PHYSIOLOGY REVIEW:

The Heart

Robert G. Carroll

The human heart, through rhythmic contraction, provides the pressure necessary to propel blood through the body. Blood flow is essential to deliver nutrients to the tissues of the body and to transport metabolic wastes, including heat, to removal sites. The presence of an arterial pulse, caused by the beating of the heart, is appropriately designated as a vital sign.

The heart weighs about 300 g and is located within the mediastinum; it is cone-shaped and tilted forward and to the left. Because of a rotation in orientation during fetal development, the apex of the heart (tip of the cone) is at its bottom and lies left of the midline. The base is at the top, where the great vessels enter the heart, and lies posterior to the sternum. The heart consists of four chambers: two smaller atria at the top (the base) of the heart and two larger ventricles at the apex. A band of fibrous tissue separates the atria from the ventricles and seats the four cardiac valves. A muscular septum separates the right from the left atrium and the right from the left ventricle. Table A&P13-1 describes the basic structures and their functions.

Functionally, the heart is actually two pumps working simultaneously (Figure A&P13-1). The right atrium and right ventricle generate the pressure to propel the oxygen-poor blood through the pulmonic circulation; the left atrium and left ventricle propel oxygen-rich blood to the remainder of the body through the systemic circulation. At rest, each side of the heart pumps approximately 5000 ml (5 L) of blood per minute (cardiac output). This is accomplished by a contraction frequency (heart rate) of 72 beats/min, with each contraction ejecting a volume of 70 ml (stroke volume) into the arterial system. Cardiac output can increase five-fold during exercise as a result of increases in both heart rate and stroke volume.

STRUCTURE OF THE HEART

LAYERS OF THE HEART

The heart consists of three distinct layers of tissue: endocardium, myocardium, and epicardium (Figure A&P13-2, inset). The endocardium (innermost layer) consists of thin endothelial tissue lining the inner chambers and the heart valves. The myocardium (middle layer) consists of striated muscle fibers forming interlaced bundles and is the actual contracting muscle of the heart. The epicardium or visceral pericardium covers the outer surface of the heart. It closely adheres to the heart and to the first several centimeters of the pulmonary artery and aorta.

The visceral pericardium is encased by the parietal pericardium, a tough, loose-fitting, fibrous outer membrane that is attached anteriorly to the lower half of the sternum, posteriorly to the thoracic vertebrae, and inferiorly to the diaphragm. Between the visceral pericardium and the parietal pericardium is the pericardial space, which holds 5 to 20 ml of pericardial fluid. This fluid lubricates the pericardial surfaces as they slide over each other when the heart beats. Excessive fluid accumulation in the pericardial space can diminish the filling of the ventricles (cardiac tamponade).

CHAMBERS OF THE HEART

The heart consists of four chambers: two upper collecting chambers (atria) and two lower pumping chambers (ventricles) (see Figure A&P13-2). A muscular wall (septum) separates the chambers of the right side from those of the left side. The right atrium receives deoxygenated blood from the body. The blood moves to the right ventricle, which pumps it to the lungs against low resistance. The left atrium receives oxygenated blood from the lungs. The blood flows into the left ventricle (the heart's largest, most muscular chamber), which pumps it against high resistance into the systemic circulation.

CARDIAC VALVES

The cardiac valves are delicate, flexible structures that consist of fibrous tissue covered by endothelium. They permit only unidirectional blood flow through the heart. The valves open and close passively, determined by pressure gradients between the cardiac chambers (Figure A&P13-3). "Leaky" valves that do not seal when closed are called regurgitant or insufficient. "Stiff" valves that cannot open completely are called stenotic.

Cardiac valves are of two types: (1) atrioventricular (AV) and (2) semilunar (see Table A&P13-1). Atrioventricular valves lie between the atria and ventricles. The tricuspid valve, on the right side, is composed of three leaflets. The mitral (bicuspid) valve, on the left, is composed of two. Attached to the edges of the AV valves are strong, fibrous filaments called chordae

TABLE A&P13–1   The Heart: *Its Structure and Functions*

Structure	Function
Pericardium	Two-layered case that encases and protects heart
Atrium	Upper, receiving chambers of heart
Right atrium	Receives deoxygenated systemic blood via superior and inferior vena cava; blood passes to right ventricle
Left atrium	Receives oxygenated blood from lungs; blood passes to left ventricle
Ventricles	Lower, pumping chambers of heart
Right ventricle	Receives blood from atrium via tricuspid valve; pumps it to pulmonary circulation
Left ventricle	Receives blood from atrium via tricuspid (mitral) valve; pumps it to systemic circulation
Cardiac valves	Prevent backflow of blood
Tricuspid and bicuspid (mitral) valves	Prevent backflow from right ventricle to right atrium and from left ventricle to left atrium, respectively
Semilunar valves	Prevent backflow from pulmonary artery to right ventricle *(pulmonary semilunar)* and from aorta to left ventricle *(aortic semilunar)*
Coronary arteries (common pattern)	Supply blood to heart
Right coronary artery	Perfuses right atrium, right ventricle, inferior portion of left ventricle and posterior septal wall, SA node, and AV node
Left coronary artery	Supplies blood to anterior wall of left ventricle, anterior ventricular septum, and apex of left ventricle
Left anterior descending artery	Supplies blood to left atrium, lateral and posterior surfaces of left ventricle, occasionally posterior interventricular septum; sometimes supplies SA and AV nodes
Circumflex artery	
SA node	"Pacemaker" node; initiates heartbeat by generating an electrical impulse
AV node	Normal pathway for impulses originating in atria to be conducted to ventricles; can be a secondary pacemaker
Bundle of His, bundle branches, Purkinje's fibers	Rapidly transmit cardiac action potentials to enable synchronous contraction of ventricles

tendineae, which arise from papillary muscles on the ventricular walls. The papillary muscles and chordae tendineae work together to prevent the AV valves from bulging back into the atria during ventricular contraction *(systole).*

The *semilunar valves* consist of three cup-like cusps that open during ventricular contraction and close to prevent backflow of blood into the ventricles during relaxation *(diastole).* Unlike the AV valves, the semilunar valves open during ventricular contraction. The *pulmonic semilunar valve* (right ventricle to pulmonary artery) and the *aortic semilunar valve* (left ventricle to aorta) do not have papillary muscles.

CARDIAC BLOOD SUPPLY

The heart muscle requires a rich oxygen supply to meet its own metabolic needs. The *coronary arteries* (right and left) branch off the aorta just above the aortic valve, encircle the heart, and penetrate the myocardium (Figure A&P13-4). Coronary vessel distribution can vary greatly, but the pattern described in Table A&P13-1 is the most common.

Contraction of the muscle of the left ventricle generates enough extravascular pressure to occlude the coronary blood vessels and prevent blood flow to the muscle of the heart during ventricular systole. Thus 75% of the coronary artery blood flow occurs during diastole, when the heart is relaxed and resistance is low. For adequate blood flow through the coronary arteries, the diastolic blood pressure must be at least 60 mm Hg. Coronary blood flow increases with increased heart workload (e.g., exercise). The coronary veins return blood from most of the myocardium to the coronary sinus of the right atrium. Some areas, particularly on the right side of the heart, drain directly into the cardiac chambers.

FUNCTIONS OF THE HEART

ELECTROPHYSIOLOGIC PROPERTIES

The electrophysiologic properties of cardiac muscle regulate the heart rate and rhythm. These properties include excitability, automaticity, contractility, refractoriness, and conductivity.

Excitability

The ability of cardiac muscle cells to depolarize in response to a stimulus—*excitability*—is influenced by hormones, electrolytes, nutrition, oxygen supply, medications, infection, and autonomic nerve activity.

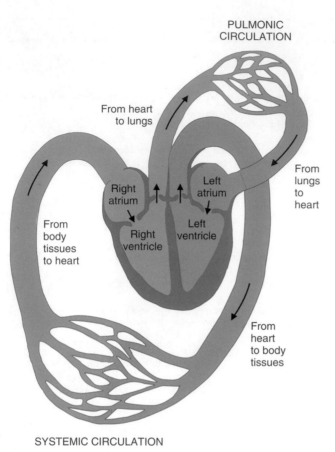

PULMONIC
CIRCULATION

From heart
to lungs

From
lungs
to
heart

Right
atrium

Left
atrium

From
body
tissues
to heart

Right
ventricle

Left
ventricle

From
heart
to body
tissues

SYSTEMIC CIRCULATION

■ **FIGURE A&P13–1** Functions of the heart. In the peripheral capillaries in systemic circulation, blood oxygen is exchanged for carbon dioxide. The oxygen-poor blood returns to the right atrium and right ventricle to be pumped into the lungs, where carbon dioxide is exchanged for oxygen. Oxygen-rich blood from the lungs enters the left atrium and left ventricle of the heart to be pumped once again into the systemic circulation.

In myocardial cells, as in other types of muscle and neurons, differences in intracellular and extracellular ion concentrations create electrical and concentration gradients for ionic movement across the semipermeable cell membrane. At rest, the inside of a myocardial cell is more negative than the outside. This *resting membrane potential* results primarily from the differences in concentrations of potassium (K^+) and sodium (Na^+) ions. Although both ions are present on either side of the cell membrane, potassium has a greater intracellular concentration and sodium has a greater extracellular concentration. Selective channels can increase membrane permeability for specific ions, allowing the ion to move down the electrochemical gradient and to alter the resting membrane potential.

When the cardiac cell is stimulated to a certain threshold, a sequence of ion permeability changes cause a dramatic change in the transmembrane potential; this is known as an *action potential* (Figure A&P13-5, *A*). The action potential consists of depolarization and repolarization phases. The electrocardiogram (ECG) reflects currents generated during the depolarization and repolarization of regions of the heart.

Depolarization is caused by an increase in cell membrane permeability to sodium. The cell returns to its resting (relaxed) state during *repolarization*. Sodium permeability drops sharply, and potassium permeability increases, returning the membrane to the negative resting potential. In the process of depolarization and repolarization, small amounts of sodium leak into the cell and potassium leaks outward. The cell compensates for this by actively pumping sodium back out and potassium inward (using the enzyme Na, K-ATPase).

Other ions, such as calcium and chloride, also play a role in the action potential and the contraction it causes. For the heart, calcium is especially important because it initiates contraction. During depolarization, myocardial cell membrane permeability to calcium increases and calcium moves into the cell. This inward Ca^{++} flux triggers the release of more calcium stored in the sarcoplasmic reticulum (see Contractility). As the intracellular concentration of calcium increases, calcium reacts with contractile proteins and myocardial muscle fibers contract.

Automaticity (Rhythmicity)

The ability of cardiac pacemaker cells to initiate an impulse spontaneously and repetitively, without external neurohormonal control, is known as *automaticity,* or *rhythmicity.* Given the proper conditions, the heart can continue to beat outside the body. In contrast, skeletal muscle must be stimulated by a nerve to depolarize and contract. The sinoatrial (SA) node pacemaker cells have the highest rate of automaticity of all cardiac cells, and thus govern the heart rate. The conduction tissue area with the highest automaticity, or rate of spontaneous depolarization, assumes the role of pacemaker (see Chapter 57). SA node cell automaticity is due to changes in ionic permeability of the membrane. Even at rest, a decreasing potassium permeability and increasing slow channel permeability (for Na^+ and Ca^{++} ions) move the cell membrane potential more positively toward threshold voltage. When threshold is reached, the cell initiates an "all-or-none" action potential. Norepinephrine and acetylcholine cause heart rate to increase and decrease, respectively (Figure A&P13-5, *B*). The rate of spontaneous depolarization can also be affected by other hormones, body temperature, drugs, and disease.

Contractility

The heart muscle is composed of long, narrow cells or fibers. Cardiac muscle fibers, like striated skeletal muscle, contain myofibrils, Z bands, sarcomeres, sarcolemmas, sarcoplasm, and sarcoplasmic reticulum. Contraction results from the same sliding filament mechanism

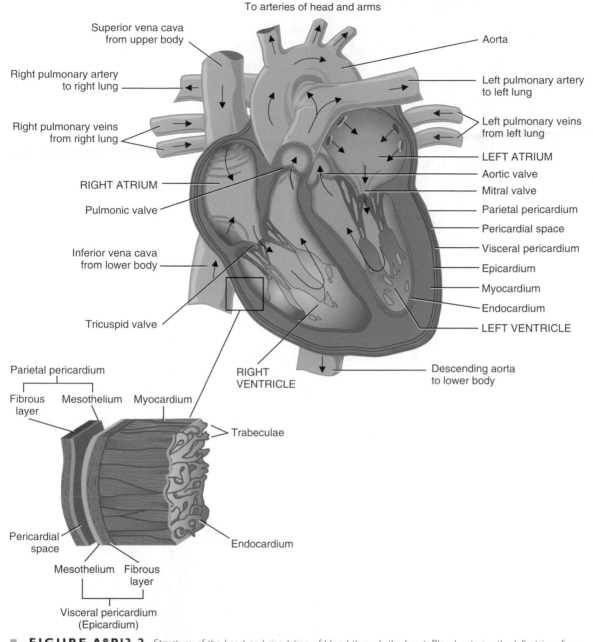

To arteries of head and arms

Superior vena cava
from upper body

Right pulmonary artery
to right lung

Right pulmonary veins
from right lung

RIGHT ATRIUM

Pulmonic valve

Inferior vena cava
from lower body

Tricuspid valve

Aorta

Left pulmonary artery
to left lung

Left pulmonary veins
from left lung

LEFT ATRIUM

Aortic valve

Mitral valve

Parietal pericardium

Pericardial space

Visceral pericardium

Epicardium

Myocardium

Endocardium

LEFT VENTRICLE

RIGHT
VENTRICLE

Descending aorta
to lower body

Parietal pericardium

Fibrous
layer

Mesothelium

Myocardium

Trabeculae

Pericardial
space

Endocardium

Mesothelium

Fibrous
layer

Visceral pericardium
(Epicardium)

■ **FIGURE A&PI3–2** Structure of the heart and circulation of blood through the heart. Blood entering the left atrium from the right and left pulmonary veins flows into the left ventricle. The left ventricle pumps blood into the systemic circulation through the aorta. From the systemic circulation, blood returns to the right atrium through the superior and inferior venae cavae. From there, the right ventricle pumps blood into the lungs through the right and left pulmonary arteries. *Inset,* The pericardium and layers of the heart.

described for skeletal muscle (see the Unit 6 Anatomy and Physiology Review).

The action potential initiates the muscle contraction by releasing calcium through the T tubules of the cell membrane. The calcium reaches the sarcoplasmic reticulum, causing additional calcium release. The intracellular calcium diffuses to myofibrils, where it binds with troponin. When the actin filaments become activated by calcium, the heads of the cross-bridges from the myosin filaments immediately become attracted to the active sites of the actin. Contraction then occurs by power stroke repetition. After contraction, free calcium ions are actively pumped back into the sarcoplasmic reticulum, and muscle relaxation begins.

One important difference between cardiac and skeletal muscle is that cardiac muscle needs extracellular calcium. All the calcium involved in skeletal muscle comes from the sarcoplasmic reticulum. In cardiac muscle, however, extracellular calcium enters through the T tubules and triggers the release of more calcium from

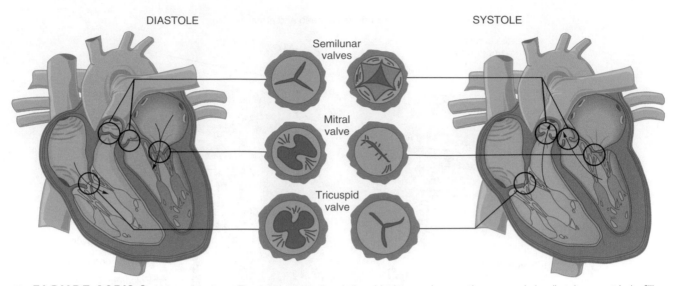

DIASTOLE   SYSTOLE

Semilunar
valves

Mitral
valve

Tricuspid
valve

■ **FIGURE A&P13–3** Valves of the heart. The semilunar, mitral, and tricuspid valves are shown as they appear during diastole, or ventricular filling *(left)*, and during systole, or ventricular emptying *(right)*.

the sarcoplasmic reticulum. Because of this, calcium-channel blockers can alter contraction of the heart, but not the contraction of skeletal muscle.

Refractoriness

Refractoriness is the heart's inability to respond to a new stimulus while still in a state of depolarization from an earlier stimulus. Refractoriness develops when the

sodium channels of the cardiac cell membrane become inactivated and unexcitable during an action potential. Thus the heart muscle does not respond to restimulation, preventing the possibility of tetanic contractions that are seen in skeletal muscle.

Refractoriness occurs in two periods (see Figure A&P13-5, *A*). The *absolute refractory period* occurs during depolarization and the first part of repolarization. During

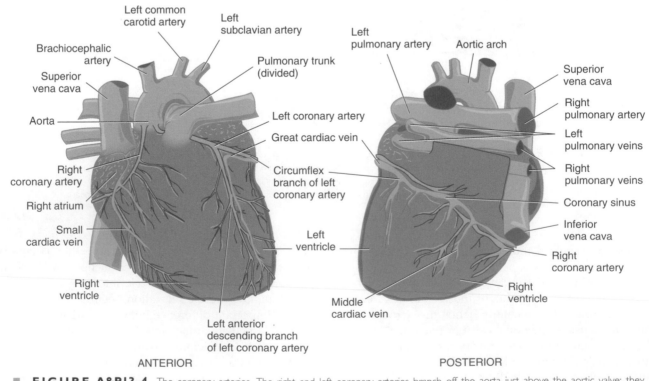

ANTERIOR   POSTERIOR

■ **FIGURE A&P13–4** The coronary arteries. The right and left coronary arteries branch off the aorta just above the aortic valve; they normally supply the myocardium with oxygenated blood.

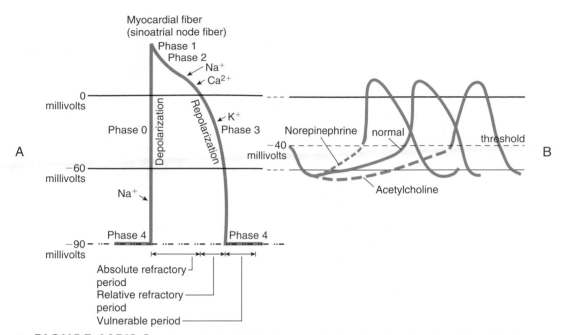

■ **FIGURE A&P13-5** Action potential. **A,** The action potential of cardiac cells has five phases: *Phase 0:* Sodium permeability increases through fast sodium channels, and cell depolarization (contraction) begins. *Phase 1:* The fast sodium channels close. *Phase 2:* Some sodium and calcium permeability remains through slow Na⁺/Ca⁺⁺ channels. *Phase 3:* Potassium permeability increases in the cell. *Phase 4:* The cell returns to its resting potential, sodium is pumped out of the cell, and potassium is pumped into the cell through the cell's sodium-potassium pump. In all cardiac cells, a period occurs during which the cells cannot be stimulated to fire another action potential. During the end of the action potential, the membrane is relatively refractory and can be reexcited only by a larger than usual stimulus. Immediately after the action potential, the membrane has transitory hyperexcitability and is said to be in a vulnerable state. **B,** The sympathetic neurotransmitter norepinephrine increases slow channel activity, allowing cells to reach threshold more rapidly (increased heart rate). Conversely, the parasympathetic neurotransmitter acetylcholine *(dashed line)* increases potassium permeability, moving the cell membrane potential away from threshold, and causes the cell to reach threshold more slowly (decreased heart rate). Calcium-channel blockers slow the heart rate by decreasing slow channel activity.

this period, cardiac cells do not respond to any stimuli, however strong. The *relative refractory period* occurs in the final stages of repolarization; refractoriness diminishes and a stronger-than-normal stimulus can excite the heart muscle to contract. At the end of the refractory period, there is a transient hyperexcitability *(vulnerable period)*. The sodium channels are reset and the cardiac cells can again conduct action potentials. The refractory period is the time when the heart chambers are filling with blood for the next beat.

Normally, the ventricles have an absolute refractory period of 0.25 to 0.3 second, which approximates the duration of the action potential. The relative refractory period for the ventricles lasts about 0.05 second. The atria have a refractory period of about 0.15 second, and they can therefore contract rhythmically much more quickly than the ventricles. The durations of the action potential and the refractory period are not fixed, however; both can shorten as heart rate increases.

Conductivity

Conductivity is the ability of heart muscle fibers to propagate electrical impulses along and across cell membranes.

The heart muscle must conduct the action potential from its origin throughout the heart both rapidly and smoothly so that the atria and ventricles contract as a unit. Intercalated disks join adjacent myocardial cells, allowing the action potential to travel over the entire muscle mass (Figure A&P13-6) through gap junctions. The fibrous band of tissue that separates the atria and ventricles lacks intercalated disks. Therefore the atria are isolated electrically from the ventricles except for the only normal conduction pathway, including the atrioventricular node. Cardiac conduction is a sequential depolarization of the following:

- Sinoatrial (SA) node
- AV node
- Bundle of His and bundle branches
- Purkinje fibers
- Ventricular myocardium

The *SA node,* or *pacemaker,* is located at the junction of the superior vena cava and right atrium. Under normal circumstances, the SA node initiates electrical impulses (heartbeats) approximately 60 to 100 times per minute, but it can adjust its rate. Three internodal and one interatrial tract carry the wave of depolarization through the right atrium to the AV node and to the left

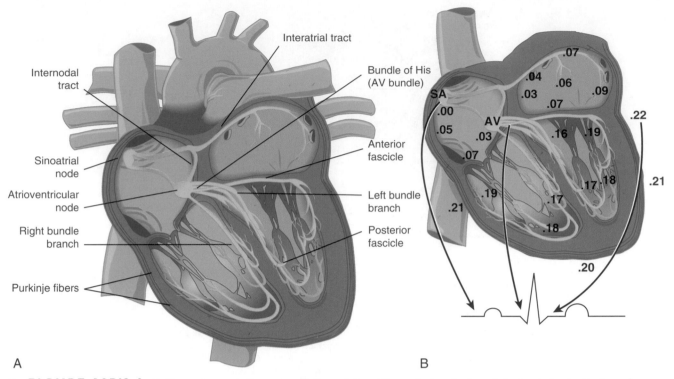

Internodal
tract

Interatrial tract

Sinoatrial
node

Atrioventricular
node

Right bundle
branch

Purkinje fibers

Bundle of His
(AV bundle)

Anterior
fascicle

Left bundle
branch

Posterior
fascicle

SA
AV

A

B

■ **FIGURE A&P13–6 A,** The cardiac conduction system. **B,** Transmission of the cardiac impulse through the heart, showing the time of appearance (in fractions of a second) of the impulse in different parts of the heart. (**B,** *Modified from Guyton, A.C., & Hall, J.E. [2001]. Textbook of medical physiology [10th ed.]. Philadelphia: Saunders.*)

atrium, respectively. The sympathetic and parasympathetic nervous systems regulate the SA node. Any myocardial tissue that generates impulses at a higher rate than the SA node can become an abnormal, or *ectopic,* pacemaker.

The (AV) node, or *AV junction,* is located in the lower aspect of the atrial septum. The AV node can be a secondary cardiac pacemaker, but it normally receives electrical impulses from the SA node and is the only pathway for conducting impulses from the atria to the ventricles. Within the AV node, the impulse is delayed 0.07 second while the atria contract. This delay enables atrial contraction to be completed before the ventricles contract.

The common *bundle of His* in the interventricular septum is relatively short, branching into right and left segments. The *right bundle branch* (RBB) courses down the right side of the interventricular septum. The *left bundle branch* (LBB) bifurcates into anterior and posterior fascicles, both of which extend into the left ventricle. The right and left bundle branches terminate in Purkinje fibers.

Purkinje fibers are a diffuse network of conducting strands beneath the ventricular endocardium; they rapidly spread the wave of depolarization through the ventricles. Activation of the ventricles begins in the septum and then moves from the apex of the heart upward. Within the ventricular walls, depolarization proceeds from endocardium to epicardium. Repolarization occurs in each cell and does not involve the conduction system. Repolarization occurs in reverse order, so that the last cells to depolarize are the first to repolarize. The action potentials of Purkinje fibers have the longest duration, and their repolarization is occasionally seen as a U wave of the electrocardiogram (ECG).

CARDIAC CYCLE

One cardiac cycle (Figure A&P13-7) is equivalent to one complete heartbeat. The sequence of events in the cardiac cycle is divided into two parts: ventricular *systole* (contraction) and ventricular *diastole* (relaxation). The cardiac cycle normally begins with the spontaneous depolarization of the pacemaker cells of the SA node and ends following the filling of the relaxed ventricles.

Atrial Systole

Depolarization of the SA node spreads through the atria, both in a cell-to-cell manner and by using the internodal and interatrial pathways. Depolarization of the atrial cells (P wave of the ECG) allows calcium entry, followed by contraction and pressure generation (a wave of the venous pressure tracing). Contraction of the atria propels a small amount of blood into the ventricles, called the "atrial kick."

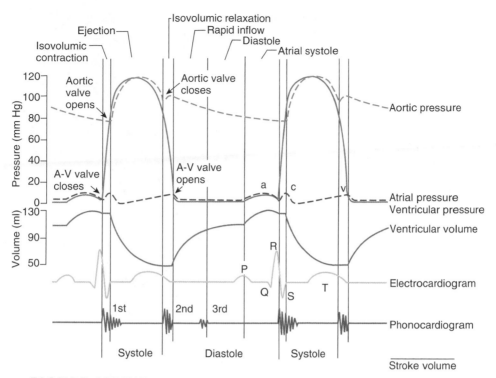

■ FIGURE A&P13–7 Changes that occur during the cardiac cycle in left atrial pressure, left ventricular pressure, aortic pressure, ventricular volume, the electrocardiogram, and the phonocardiogram. *(From Guyton, A.C., & Hall, J.E. [2001]. Textbook of medical physiology [10th ed.]. Philadelphia: Saunders.)*

Ventricular Systole

Following a delay at the AV node, the wave of depolarization enters the ventricles, where it is spread rapidly by the bundle branches and Purkinje fibers (QRS complex of the ECG). Following depolarization, calcium enters, initiating contraction of the ventricle. In the *isovolumic contraction phase,* the ventricles begin to contract, closing the AV valves and building up pressure within the ventricles. As the AV valves close, the first heart sound (S_1) is heard. Because the aortic and pulmonic valves remain closed at this point, no blood leaves the ventricle. The *ejection phase* begins when pressure in the ventricles exceeds the aortic and pulmonic pressures. The semilunar valves open, and the ventricles pump blood into the systemic and pulmonary circulations.

Ventricular Diastole

In early diastole, as the ventricles begin to relax, aortic and pulmonary artery pressures exceed ventricular pressures, and the semilunar valves close. The valve closure causes the second heart sound (S_2). The AV valves remain closed, and no blood moves in or out of the ventricles. This is called *isovolumic relaxation.* As the ventricles continue to relax, pressure in the ventricles falls below that of the atria, and the AV valves open, allowing blood that has been pooling in the atria to flow into the ventricles *(ventricular filling).* When the ventricles have filled passively, the cardiac cycle is ready to begin again.

Extra Heart Sounds

The ventricular wall must expand to accommodate rapid ventricular filling. If ventricular wall compliance is decreased (as in heart failure or valvular regurgitation), blood and structures within the ventricular wall vibrate and a third heart sound (S_3) may be heard. Because of increased filling, an S_3 heart sound may be a normal finding in people younger than age 30 years. During the last phase of ventricular diastole, atrial contraction (atrial systole or atrial kick) occurs, contributing 5% to 30% more blood volume to the ventricles.

A fourth heart sound (S_4) may be heard on atrial systole if resistance to active ventricular filling is present. This is not a normal finding and is commonly caused by a stiff ventricle from hypertrophy, disease, or injury of the ventricular wall.

CARDIAC OUTPUT AND CARDIAC INDEX

Cardiac output (CO) is the volume of blood ejected per minute by rhythmic ventricular contraction. At the end of ventricular diastole, each ventricle contains approximately 140 ml of blood (end-diastolic volume [EDV]). Normally, during systole, the heart ejects approximately half of this volume. The volume ejected with each contraction (heartbeat) of the ventricle is the stroke volume and ejection fraction. Cardiac output can be calculated as follows:

$$CO = [EDV - ESV] \times HR$$

where ESV is the end-systolic volume and HR is the heart rate.

Cardiac output averages between 4 and 8 L/min in adults. For a normal 150-pound (70-kg) adult at rest, cardiac output is 5 to 6 L/min. Adjustments in either stroke volume or heart rate can compensate for fluctuations in the other, or both can rise or fall to maintain cardiac output.

Cardiac output is commonly measured by thermodilution with the use of a pulmonary artery (Swan-Ganz) catheter. Several other approaches can also be used, such as obtaining heart rate from an ECG and stroke volume through ventricular imaging techniques.

Clinicians compute the *cardiac index* (CI) from the cardiac output to compensate for individual differences in body size:

$$CI = \frac{\text{Cardiac output}}{\text{Body surface area}}$$

The normal cardiac index is 2.5 to 4 L/min/m^2.

Stroke volume has a major influence on cardiac output and is determined by (1) preload, (2) afterload, and (3) the contractile state of the heart (reviewed in Figure A&P12-4).

Preload

Preload is the myocardial fiber length of the left ventricle at end diastole. It is determined by the EDV. The Frank-Starling law of the heart states that the greater the resting myocardial fiber length, or stretch, the greater its force of contraction. Preload therefore increases when increased EDV (e.g., from increased venous return) subjects myocardial fibers to greater stretch. The ventricles respond with a greater force of contraction, producing a larger stroke volume and increased cardiac output. This phenomenon, however, has limits (Figure A&P13-8), such as the greatly distended ventricles characteristic of heart failure.

Afterload

Afterload is the resistance to left ventricular ejection. More specifically, it is the amount of pressure required by the left ventricle to open the aortic valve during systole and to eject blood. Afterload directly relates to arterial blood pressure and the characteristics of the valve. If arterial blood pressure is high, the heart must work harder to pump blood into the circulation. Stroke volume is inversely related to afterload. For example, if afterload increases because of peripheral vasoconstriction (which increases arterial blood pressure), myocardial fiber shortening is reduced and ejections are less effective. Then the ventricles cannot eject a normal stroke volume.

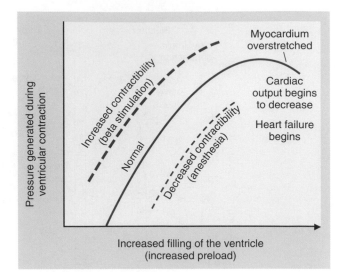

■ **FIGURE A&P13–8** According to the Frank-Starling law, the more the left ventricle fills with blood (preload), the greater the quantity of blood ejected into the aorta. If the left ventricle fills to such an extent that it overdistends the myocardium *(arrow)*, however, cardiac output begins to decrease and the heart begins to fail. Agents that change contractility can shift this relationship. Norepinephrine increases contractility (positive inotrope) and improves cardiac performance; anesthesia decreases contractility (negative inotrope) and impairs cardiac performance.

Contractile State

The contractile *(inotropic)* state refers to the vigor of contraction generated by the myocardium regardless of its blood volume (preload). Unlike skeletal muscle, the myocardium can alter contractile velocity and therefore force. The rate of cross-bridge cycling in the myocardium is calcium dependent, and agents that increase intracellular calcium level thus increase contractile force. For example, sympathetic stimulation increases myocardial contractility and ventricular pressure, thereby ejecting blood more rapidly and increasing stroke volume. Metabolic abnormalities (e.g., hypoxemia) and metabolic acidosis decrease myocardial contractility, therefore reducing stroke volume (see Figure A&P13-8).

Cardiac Pressures

With the use of a pulmonary artery pressure (Swan-Ganz) catheter, pressures in the right atrium, right ventricle, and pulmonary artery can be measured. Inflation of a balloon at the catheter tip allows measurement of pulmonary capillary wedge pressure (PCWP), an estimate of left atrial pressure. Assuming normal aortic valve function, arterial systolic pressure reflects left ventricular systolic pressure. These pressures are useful in determining factors that characterize cardiac performance, such as preload, afterload, volume, filling pressures, and resistance. Normal cardiac pressures are shown in Figure A&P13-9.

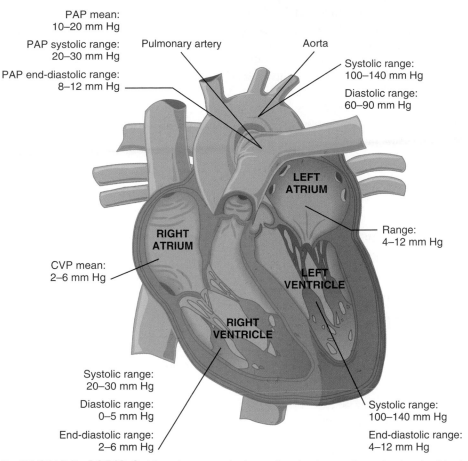

PAP mean:
10–20 mm Hg

PAP systolic range:
20–30 mm Hg

PAP end-diastolic range:
8–12 mm Hg

Pulmonary artery

Aorta

Systolic range:
100–140 mm Hg

Diastolic range:
60–90 mm Hg

LEFT ATRIUM

RIGHT ATRIUM

Range:
4–12 mm Hg

CVP mean:
2–6 mm Hg

LEFT VENTRICLE

RIGHT VENTRICLE

Systolic range:
20–30 mm Hg

Diastolic range:
0–5 mm Hg

End-diastolic range:
2–6 mm Hg

Systolic range:
100–140 mm Hg

End-diastolic range:
4–12 mm Hg

■ **FIGURE A&P13–9** Normal pressures in the cardiac chambers and associated major blood vessels. *CVP,* Central venous pressure; *PAP,* pulmonary artery pressure.

HEART RATE

The normal heart rate is 60 to 100 beats/min. *Sinus tachycardia* is a rate of more than 100 beats/min; *sinus bradycardia* is a rate of fewer than 60 beats/min. (The *sinus* in these terms indicates that the impulse arose in the sinoatrial node, the normal pacemaker region of the heart.) The intrinsic heart rate is 90 beats/min. At rest, the heart rate of 70 beats/min reflects the dominant control by the parasympathetic nervous system. Variations in heartbeat can be caused by exercise, the size of the client, age, hormones, temperature, blood pressure, anxiety, stress, and pain.

ARTERIAL PRESSURE

Arterial pressure (see the Unit 12 Anatomy and Physiology Review) is the pressure of blood against arterial walls. *Systolic pressure* is the maximum pressure of the blood exerted against the artery walls when the heart contracts (normally 100 to 140 mm Hg). *Diastolic pressure* is the force of blood exerted against the artery walls during the heart's relaxation (or filling) phase (normally 60 to 90 mm Hg). *Blood pressure* is expressed as systolic pressure/diastolic pressure (e.g., 120/80 mm Hg). Cardiac output is a key determinant of arterial pressure (see Figure A&P12-4).

Baroreceptors, Stretch Receptors, and Chemoreceptors

Changes in sympathetic and parasympathetic activity occur in response to messages sent from sensory receptors in various parts of the body. Important receptors in cardiovascular reflexes include (1) arterial baroreceptors, (2) stretch-sensitive cardiopulmonary receptors of the atria and veins, and (3) chemoreceptors.

Baroreceptors (pressoreceptors) are stretch-sensitive nerve endings affected by changes in arterial blood pressure. They are located in the walls of the aortic arch and carotid sinuses. Increases in arterial pressure stimulate baroreceptors, which send impulses to the medulla, resulting in heart rate and arterial pressure decreases (the *vagal response*). When arterial pressure decreases, baroreceptors receive less stretch and thus send fewer impulses to the medulla (see Figure A&P12-5). Then sympathetic-mediated increase in heart rate and vasoconstriction occurs.

Cardiopulmonary stretch receptors are located in terminal sections of the vena cava and the atria. These receptors respond to length changes, which reflect circulatory volume status. When blood pressure decreases in the vena cava and the right atrium (e.g., hypovolemia), stretch receptors send fewer impulses than usual to the central nervous system (CNS). This process results in a sympathetic response, particularly to the kidney, to enhance salt and water retention over hours to days. These changes also stimulate release of antidiuretic hormone (ADH) from the posterior pituitary. Hypervolemia produces the opposite effects.

Chemoreceptors, found in the aortic arch and carotid bodies, are primarily sensitive to increased carbon dioxide levels and decreased arterial pH (acidemia) and secondarily sensitive to hypoxemia. When these changes occur, chemoreceptors transmit impulses to the CNS to increase heart rate.

THE AUTONOMIC NERVOUS SYSTEM AND THE HEART

The autonomic nervous system (ANS) is the effector limb of the baroreceptor reflex and plays an important role in regulating the following:

- Heart rate (chronotropic effect)
- Myocardial contractility (inotropic effect)
- AV node conduction velocity (dromotropic effect)
- Peripheral vascular resistance (arteriole constriction and dilation)
- Venous return (venule and vein constriction and dilation)

The two subdivisions of the ANS (sympathetic and parasympathetic) generally exert opposing influences and balance their activities to promote cardiovascular adaptation to internal and external demands. ANS responses are involuntary.

Parasympathetic nerves arise from the dorsal motor nucleus of the vagus nerve, located in the medulla oblongata. They innervate the SA node atria, AV node, and to a lesser extent the ventricles and Purkinje system. When stimulated, parasympathetic nerve endings release the neurotransmitter acetylcholine, which produces inhibitory effects by binding to muscarinic receptors. Parasympathetic stimulation decreases the rate of SA node firing, thus lowering heart rate; atrial conductivity lessens as well.

Sympathetic nerve fibers originate between the first and fifth thoracic vertebrae and terminate in all areas of the heart. With stimulation, the nerve endings release the neurotransmitter norepinephrine and produce the following effects: (1) increased heart rate, (2) increased conduction speed through the AV node, (3) increased atrial and ventricular contractility, and (4) peripheral vasoconstriction, by binding to adrenergic receptors, activating G proteins, and opening ionic channels.

The sympathetic nervous system influences adrenal activity. The adrenal medulla responds to stimulation by secreting catecholamines (norepinephrine and epinephrine) into the circulation. Norepinephrine and epinephrine interact with adrenergic receptors found within cell membranes of the heart and blood vessels. The response to stimulation depends on the type and location of adrenergic receptors involved. The five types of receptors follow:

1. *Alpha$_1$-adrenergic* receptors are located in peripheral arteries and veins. When stimulated, alpha receptors produce a dramatic vasoconstrictive response.
2. *Alpha$_2$-adrenergic* receptors are located in several tissues. Their actions include contraction of some vascular smooth muscle, inhibition of lipolysis, inhibition of neurotransmission, and promotion of platelet aggregation.
3. *Beta$_1$-adrenergic* receptors are predominantly located in the heart. When stimulated, beta$_1$ receptors cause an increase in heart rate, AV node conduction, and myocardial contractility. This may result in increased cardiac output and blood pressure.
4. *Beta$_2$-adrenergic* receptors are found in the smooth muscle of arteriolar and bronchial walls. Stimulation of beta$_2$ receptors causes smooth muscles to dilate, producing vasodilation of arterial vessels and bronchodilation.
5. *Beta$_3$-adrenergic* receptors are found in adipose tissue, where they promote lipolysis. Indirectly, this may assist cardiac performance because the myocardium can utilize fatty acids as metabolic fuels. Currently, no direct cardiac role for beta$_3$ adrenoreceptors has been identified.

Hormonal and Other Influences

In addition to epinephrine and norepinephrine from the adrenal medulla, several other hormones regulate cardiac output indirectly by controlling body fluid volume (and thus venous pressure and venous return). The most important hormones include ADH and the renin-angiotensin-aldosterone mechanism.

Other factors also influence cardiac activity and blood pressure. For example, cerebral cortical input from anger, fear, pain, or excitement can augment the effects of the sympathetic nervous system.

EFFECTS OF AGING

At birth, the neonate ventricles are of equal size; however, the vascular changes associated with birth lead to a decrease in pulmonary vascular resistance and pressure and an increase in systemic vascular resistance and pressure. During childhood, the greater work of the left ventricle to eject its cardiac output into the high-pressure systemic circulation causes a hypertrophy of the left ventricular muscle, which is characteristic of the adult heart. The heart muscle also undergoes changes with further aging that lead to dilation of the cardiac chambers and lessening of contractility. This has little effect on stroke volume, but it reduces cardiac reserve. Coronary arteries become thickened and rigid. These changes decrease the ability of the heart to respond to additional demands and increase the likelihood of coronary artery disease. Heart valves may thicken and become incompetent, resulting in a systolic ejection murmur.

CONCLUSIONS

Although the heart can be viewed simply as a pump, this remarkable, durable organ is much more than that. The heart is a continuously beating organ that never rests. It moves blood throughout the body to oxygenate cells for energy. It propels blood through its four chambers in one direction, from right to left. Left ventricular contraction moves blood into the arteries under high pressure. This pressure propels blood through the systemic circulation.

Heart disease remains the major cause of death and involves disorders both of structure and of function of the heart. These disorders are studied in the following chapters.

BIBLIOGRAPHY

1. Berne, R., et al. (2004). *Physiology* (5th ed.). St. Louis: Mosby.
2. Carroll, R.G. (2007). *Elsevier's integrated physiology.* Philadelphia: Saunders.
3. Kierszenbaum, A.L. (2007). *Histology and cell biology: An introduction to pathology* (2nd ed.). St. Louis: Mosby.
4. Guyton, A., & Hall, J. (2006). *Textbook of medical physiology* (11th ed.). Philadelphia: Saunders.
5. Silverthorn, D. (2006). *Human physiology* (4th ed.). San Francisco, Calif: Pearson Benjamin Cummings.

CHAPTER 54

Assessment of the Cardiac System

BETH F. CROWDER

Since 1918 cardiovascular disease (CVD) has been the number one cause of death in the United States. In 2003 CVD accounted for 37.3% of all deaths, or 1 in every 2.7 deaths, in the United States. In fact, CVD claimed more lives than the next four leading causes of death combined (cancer, chronic lower respiratory tract diseases, accidents, and diabetes mellitus).[3] The 2006 estimated direct and indirect cost of CVD is $403.1 billion. According to the Social Security Administration, CVD is the leading cause of premature, permanent disability in the U.S. labor force today.[3] For those age 60 years and older, CVD is the number one killer worldwide. Of those who die from CVD, 80% to 90% have one or more risk factors. The worldwide incidence and prevalence of CVD are on the rise and CVD is a pandemic that knows no boundaries.[32]

According to World Health Organization estimates for 2003, deaths from CVD totaled 16.7 million. Approximately 80% of CVD deaths occurred in countries with low- and middle-income populations. By 2010 CVD is estimated to be the leading cause of death in developing countries.[32] Heart disease has no geographical, gender, or socioeconomic boundaries; at least 20 million people survive CVD attacks every year. Cardiovascular disease affects individuals in their peak midlife years, disrupting the future of the families dependent on them and undermining the development of nations by depriving them of workers in their most productive years.[32]

It is estimated that more than 50% of CVD deaths and disability can be eliminated by a combination of cost-effective national and individual efforts to reduce risk factors.[3] The goal of *Healthy People 2010* is to improve overall cardiovascular health and quality of life through prevention, assessment, detection, risk factor management, and early diagnosis and treatment.[7,24] The prevalence and complications of CVD have significant implications for nurses, requiring them to use holistic assessment and treatment skills. Assessment of the cardiovascular system involves incorporating data from history-taking, relating the information to the physical examination and diagnostic tests, and correlating the data with the underlying pathophysiology to institute a plan of care.

HISTORY

The history encompasses all of the subjective information gathered from the client and his/her present family members and/or friends. If the client is stable, a detailed history can and should be obtained. A careful history allows a care provider to evaluate the impact the presenting illness has on the client's personal and social life, personality, occupation, and responsibilities.[6]

Biographical and Demographic Data

Biographical and demographic data include name, age, gender, place of birth, race, marital status, occupation, and ethnic background. Alterations in health may have caused changes in the main provider's occupation and

---

evolve Web Enhancements

Client Education Guide Stress Testing (English and Spanish)

Assessment Terms Assessment Terms (English and Spanish)

Appendix A Religious Beliefs and Practices Affecting Health Care

Appendix B Health History Format That Integrates the Assessment of Functional Health Patterns

Tables Common Electrocardiographic Tests

Common Radiographic Cardiac Tests

Common Cardiac Ultrasonographic Tests

Common Cardiac Invasive Procedures

Common Cardiac Laboratory Tests

Be sure to check out the bonus material on the Evolve website and the CD-ROM, including free self-assessment exercises. **http://evolve.elsevier.com/Black/medsurg**

status within the family. There are known transcultural considerations regarding heart disease and stroke among culturally diverse individuals. Economic transition, urbanization, industrialization, and globalization bring about lifestyle changes that promote heart disease.

Prevalence, incidence, and mortality of CVD vary among differing races and by gender. The average incidence of a first major cardiovascular event rises from 7/1000 men ages 35 to 44 to 68/1000 at ages 85 to 94.[3] For women, comparable rates occur a decade later in life. The prevalence of CVD is highest among native Hawaiians (16.6%) followed by American Indians (13.8%), whites (11.4%), and blacks (9.9%).[3] Black and Hispanic women have a higher prevalence of CVD risk factors than white women of comparable socioeconomic status. The age-adjusted death rates for CVD are 17% for Hispanics, 15% for whites, 14% for Asians, 11% for blacks, and 8% for American Indians.[3] The death rates for CVD in men and women were higher compared to the death rates from cancer in the two groups. Among minority women, the CVD death rate is higher in black women compared to white women. For many unaware women, CVD caused greater mortality than the next five leading causes of death combined (cancer, chronic obstructive pulmonary disease [COPD], Alzheimer's disease, diabetes mellitus, and accidents), resulting in about one death every minute.[3]

Current Health

Documenting the progression of the first manifestation to the current complaints or problems helps organize the history and reveals the sequence of events that led the client to seek help.

Chief Complaint

There can be a tendency to rely on objective testing (laboratory values, x-rays, scans, angiography) to diagnose a client's illness. However, the client's history remains the richest source of information concerning the presenting illness or chief complaint.[28] Eliciting a client's history not only assists with individualizing the plan of care but also helps to establish a bond with that client.[6] The history begins with an open-ended question that allows the client to provide his/her own account of clinical manifestations leading up to the illness presentation. Upon completion of the client's clinical manifestations, "probe" questions are asked in order to analyze the manifestations and gather specific information regarding the *o*nset, *l*ocation, *d*uration, *c*haracteristics, *a*ssociated manifestations, *a*ggravating factors, and *r*elieving factors. The mnemonic "OLD CAAR" can help you remember what to ask each client.[11] There are many common cardiac manifestations, however; many disorders can cause chest pain. Table 54-1 differentiates between the various chest pain conditions and clinical manifestations.

Table 54-1 will aid in comparing and contrasting conditions as the mnemonic OLD CAAR assessment skills are reinforced. Some conditions are life-threatening that require immediate attention. As a medical-surgical nurse standing at that client's bedside, you may be the first one to (1) see the client and obtain the history, (2) witness the sudden development of clinical manifestations, or (3) alert the attending health care provider of important information you obtained during assessment of the client. In caring for adults (or children, as they may have congenital anomalies) you will encounter a client with a history of CVD or clinical manifestations that could be due to CVD. What you learn in this chapter may help you diagnose, treat, and save your client's life.

Clinical Manifestations

Conduct an analysis of the client's clinical manifestations to evaluate and clarify the chief complaint. This will help you deduce, or narrow, the possible cause of the presenting illness. While evaluating and caring for any client, keep these three rules foremost in mind: (1) the initial or admitting diagnosis may be incorrect or inconclusive; (2) do not bias the severity of the client's presenting illness based on the client's bed/unit assignment; and (3) keep an open mind to alternative diagnoses.[11] Figure 54-1 on p. 1358 provides questions and manifestations to guide your assessment for cardiac clinical manifestations. The cardinal manifestations of CVD are located in Box 54-1. There may be more than one major manifestation. When this occurs, assess them in the order of importance.

Chest pain. Chest pain is one of the most common manifestations of cardiac disease; however, almost 30% of clients with confirmed myocardial infarction (MI) may not report chest pain at all.[11] Many women and long-standing diabetic clients with neuropathy do not experience chest pain resulting in undiagnosed or unknown cardiac ischemia and a silent MI. Chest pain may also result from pulmonary, gastrointestinal, musculoskeletal, neurologic, and anxiety-related conditions. *Angina pectoris* is the true manifestation, or typical chest pain, of coronary artery disease (CAD). Angina is caused by myocardial ischemia (hypoxia), an imbalance of oxygen supply and demand as the coronary arteries support myocardial tissue. Because chest pain is caused by a number of conditions, it is highly variable.

Chest pain not caused by myocardial ischemia is termed atypical chest pain. Evaluate chest pain and its cause with careful analysis. Table 54-1 compares selected cardiac, pulmonary, gastrointestinal, musculoskeletal, neurologic, and anxiety-related conditions in relation to chest pain. Chest pain manifestations may appear to overlap with the various body systems. A thorough analysis of clinical manifestations will assist in

TABLE 54–1 Differential Assessment of Chest Pain

Conditions	Location	Characteristics	Quantity	Onset/Duration	Aggravating and Relieving Factors	Associated Manifestations
Angina pectoris	Substernal or retrosternal region; radiates to neck, jaw, epigastrium, shoulders, arms (especially left)	Pressure, burning, squeezing, tight heaviness, indigestion	Moderate to severe	<10 min	Aggravated by exertion, cold, stress, or after meals; relieved by rest or nitroglycerin; atypical (Prinzmetal's) angina may be unrelated to activity and caused by coronary artery spasm	Sinus tachycardia, bradycardia, S₄ paradoxical split S₂ during pain episode
Coronary insufficiency	Same as angina	Same as angina	Increasingly severe	>10 min	Same as angina, with gradually decreasing tolerance for exertion	Same as angina
Myocardial infarction	Precordial, substernal; may radiate like angina	Heaviness, crushing pressure, burning, constriction	Severe, sometimes mild (in 30% of clients)	Sudden onset; lasts longer than 15 min	Unrelieved	Dyspnea, sweating, weakness, nausea, vomiting, severe anxiety
Pericarditis	Usually begins over sternum and may radiate to neck and down left upper extremity	Sharp, stabbing, knife-like	Moderate to severe	Lasts many hours to days	Aggravated by deep breathing, rotating chest or supine position; relieved by sitting up and leaning forward	Fever, infection, pericardial friction rub, syncope, dyspnea, orthopnea
Dissecting aortic aneurysm	Anterior chest; radiates to thoracic area of back; may be abdominal; pain shifts in chest	Tearing	Excruciating, tearing, knife-like	Sudden onset, lasts for hours	Unrelated to anything	Lower blood pressure in one arm, absent pulses, stroke, dyspnea, murmur of aortic insufficiency, pulsus paradoxus, stridor; myocardial infarction can occur
Mitral valve prolapse syndrome	Usually not substernal; sometimes radiates to left arm, back, jaw	Stabbing, sharp, sticky quality, "kick"	Variable; generally mild but can become severe	Sudden, recurrent	Not related to exertion, not relieved by nitroglycerin or rest	Variable palpitations, dysrhythmias, dizziness, syncope, dyspnea, late systolic or pansystolic murmur

Condition	Location	Quality	Severity	Timing	Aggravating Factors	Associated Findings
Pulmonary embolism (many pulmonary emboli do not produce chest pain)	Substernal, "anginal"	Deep, crushing; if pulmonary infection, may be pleuritic	Can be absent, mild, or severe	Sudden onset; lasts minutes to <1 hr	May be aggravated by breathing	Fever, tachypnea, tachycardia, hypotension, elevated jugular venous pressure, right ventricular lift, accentuated pulmonary valve (P_2) sound during S_2, occasional murmur of tricuspid insufficiency and right ventricular S_4; with infarction usually in presence of heart failure; crackles, pleural rub, hemoptysis, clinical phlebitis present in minority of cases
Spontaneous pneumothorax	Unilateral	Sharp, well localized, stabbing	Moderate, severe	Sudden onset; lasts many hours	Painful breathing	Dyspnea, shock, tension pneumothorax
Pneumonia with pleurisy	Localized over area of consolidation	Sharp, grabbing, aching	Variable	Sudden	Painful breathing	Dyspnea, cough, fever, hemoptysis, crackles, occasional pleural rub
Gastrointestinal disorders (esophageal reflux)	Lower substernal area, epigastric, right or left upper quadrant	Burning, colic-like aching, tightness, pressure	Moderate to severe	Waves, continuous radiation	Precipitated by recumbency, large meals, alcohol ingestion	Nausea, regurgitation, food intolerance, melena, hematemesis, jaundice
Musculoskeletal disorders	Variable	Aching	Variable	Short or long duration	History of muscle exertion, viral illness	Tender to pressure or movement
Neurologic disorders (herpes zoster)	Dermatomal in distribution	Aching, constant burning, pins and needles, sharp	Moderate, severe	Prolonged period of time	Aggravated by systemic stress	Pain before rash, vesicles
Psychogenic states (depression, self-gain, or attention-seeking)	Usually localized to a point	Vague, burning, diffuse	Mild to moderate, disabling	Unassociated with external events	Situational anger, depression, anxiety	Sighing, chest wall tenderness, fatigue, dyspnea, anorexia

CVA, Cerebrovascular accident; P_2, pulmonic second sound; S_2, second heart sound; S_4, fourth heart sound.
Modified from Andreoli, K., et al. (1987). *Comprehensive cardiac care* (6th ed., pp. 54-55). St. Louis: Mosby; Seller, R.H. (1996). *Differential diagnosis of common complaints* (3rd ed., pp. 57-68). Philadelphia: Saunders; and Hill, B., & Geraci, S.A. (1998). A diagnostic approach to chest pain based on history and ancillary evaluation. *Nurse Practitioner, 23*(2), 20-45.

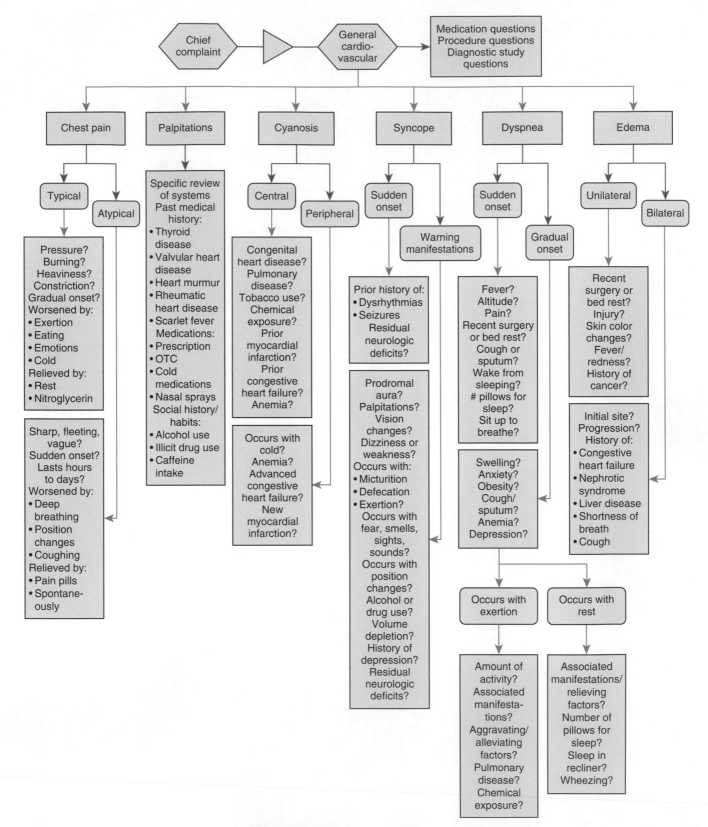

■ **FIGURE 54–1** Expanded cardiac assessment.

BOX 54-1 Common Clinical Manifestations of CVD

- Chest pain
- Dyspnea
- Cyanosis
- Syncope
- Palpitations
- Edema
- Epigastric discomfort
- Fatigue*

*Women often have several weeks of fatigue before a myocardial infarction, so this is often a warning sign for women.

prioritizing treatment and testing strategies.[6,11,16,30] Gender-specific knowledge of CVD is also needed, as research indicates women present with differing (frequently termed "atypical") manifestations, such as fatigue, caused by CVD.[19,20] Although some women may experience chest pain, many women present with dyspnea, nausea, vomiting, fatigue, neck pain, jaw pain, back pain, dizziness, palpitations.[19]

Onset. The onset of chest pain provides not only the time line between when the manifestations began and when the client presented for further evaluation, but also a description of the beginning of pain. Angina pain has a gradual onset that intensifies, especially with continued activities. Pain described as sudden in its onset is atypical for angina.

Location. The site of discomfort provides additional information for determining its cause. Angina pain is ordinarily retrosternal, felt slightly to the left of the midline or partly under the sternum. Angina pain tends to radiate bilaterally across the chest into the arms, left greater than right, and into the neck and lower jaw. Occasionally, radiation to the back or occiput is noted. Chest pain may be diffuse, localized, or so minor that clients dismiss true ischemic pain or possible infarction. Painless or atypical presentation of myocardial infarction occurs in up to 30% of clients, particularly in diabetic and older clients. Diabetic clients in particular have a two-fold to four-fold increase in developing CVD.*

Duration. Note the time the pain begins and ends to determine the duration of discomfort. Several intermittent small episodes of chest pain are not considered as one long period of pain. Generally, angina pain has an increasing pattern that reaches maximum intensity after several minutes and is usually relieved within 10 minutes by rest, with or without the use of vasodilator drugs such as nitroglycerin. Angina pectoris rarely lasts less than 1 minute or longer than 15 minutes. Unstable angina usually lasts less than 20 minutes, and pain from myocardial infarction usually lasts 30 minutes or longer. Pain that is "constant" or "prolonged" is atypical for angina.[‡]

Characteristics. Angina pain may be described as a "strange feeling" in the chest, a "dull heavy pressure, burning, crushing, constricting, squeezing, aching, or tightness." Some clients present with complaints of "gas" or "indigestion" that is caused by angina. Angina pectoris characteristically has a crescendo (gradually increasing) pattern at onset. Pain described as "shooting, stabbing, sudden onset, pleuritic, sharp, or fleeting" is often caused by pulmonary, gastrointestinal, musculoskeletal, neurologic, and anxiety-related conditions.**

To better quantify chest pain, ask the client to use a scale of 1 (least severe) to 10 (most severe). This recorded scale can then be used to compare future episodes of chest pain. For example, the client may report 10/10 for pain on admission and then report 3/10 for pain after administration of a vasodilating medication. Please refer to Chapter 20 for a further discussion of pain and its assessment.

Associated Manifestations. Radiation of pain to the arms (especially the left), throat, jaw, ear, shoulders, or back is typical of angina. Epigastric, unilateral, or right upper quadrant is atypical for angina. Clinical manifestations of dyspnea, nausea, vomiting, diaphoresis, palpitations, or syncope are commonly associated with angina. Fatigue for several weeks before a cardiac episode is common in women and is becoming a well-known warning sign. Tachycardia, coughing, or an associated rash is atypical for angina.[‡]

Aggravating Factors. Angina pain may be associated with certain factors or conditions. Chest pain resulting from stable angina pectoris develops after exertion, eating a heavy meal, or emotional excitement (the three Es), but may also occur with sexual excitement, temperature extremes, or straining to have a bowel movement. Rest or sublingual nitroglycerin will relieve the pain promptly. Chest pain caused by acute coronary syndrome or myocardial infarction occurs at rest or awakens the client from sleep, requiring sublingual nitroglycerin or medical attention for relief. Pain that worsens with position changes, palpation, coughing, deep breathing, or eating is atypical for angina.[6,11,16,17,30]

Relieving Factors. Angina pain is usually relieved by rest, vasodilator drugs such as nitroglycerin, oxygen, and relaxation. Chest pain that is not reduced by these interventions and lasts 20 minutes or longer is suggestive

---

*References 2,6,11,16,17,30.

** References 2,6,8,11,14,16,17,28,30.

‡ References 2, 6, 11, 16, 17, 30.

of an acute coronary syndrome (ACS). Chest pain that is relieved with position changes, eating, antacids, or movement is atypical for angina.[6,11,16,30] The Integrating Diagnostic Testing feature below outlines the steps necessary to integrate the chief complaint of chest pain with clinical manifestations and appropriate tests in order to diagnose the presenting illness.

Palpitations. The word *palpitation* is derived from the Latin *palpitare,* which means "to throb." *Palpitations* are uncomfortable sensations in the chest associated with a wide range of dysrhythmias.[6] Box 54-2 provides common causes of palpitations. Palpitations are commonly caused by extra atrial or ventricular systoles and do not necessarily indicate serious heart disease. The Integrating Diagnostic Testing feature on p. 1361 outlines

the assessment of palpitations and the steps necessary to integrate the chief complaint of palpitations with other clinical manifestations and appropriate tests in order to diagnose the presenting illness.

A palpitation is a sensation of rapid heartbeats, skipping, irregularity, thumping, or pounding and may be accompanied by anxiousness. The onset and termination of palpitations are often abrupt. Some also report manifestations similar to syncopal episodes (vision changes, weakness, dizziness, nausea, or diaphoresis) with the aura they thought they were going to pass out, but do not lose consciousness. This is known as presyncope. Presyncope with palpitations is a more serious occurrence and warrants evaluation consistent with a syncopal evaluation.[6,11,16]

Ask the client about (1) medications, especially the use of over-the-counter cold medications or nasal sprays

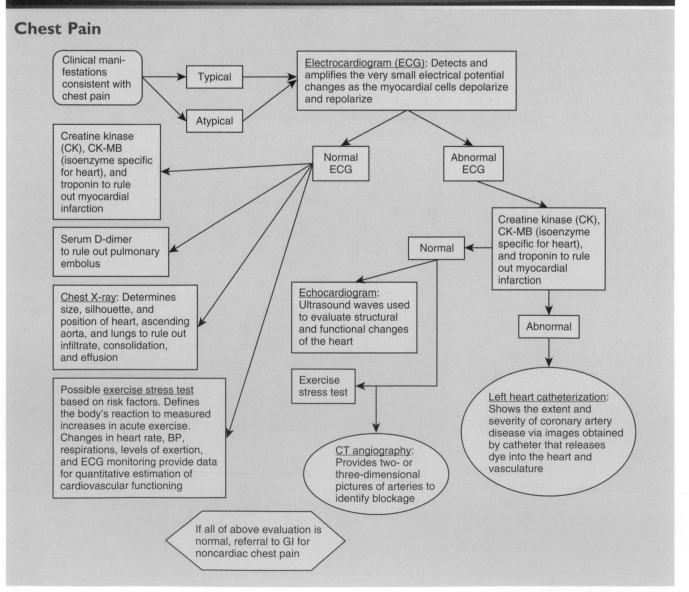

INTEGRATING DIAGNOSTIC TESTING

Chest Pain

BOX 54-2   Common Causes of Palpitations

DYSRHYTHMIAS

1. Bradydysrhythmias
   a. Heart block
   b. Sinus arrest
2. Extrasystoles
   a. Premature atrial contractions (PACs)
   b. Premature nodal contractions
   c. Premature ventricular contractions (PVCs)
3. Tachydysrhythmias
   a. Atrial fibrillation
   b. Atrial flutter
   c. Multifocal atrial tachycardia
   d. Paroxysmal supraventricular tachycardia
   e. Ventricular tachycardia

OTHER

1. Anemia
2. Anxiety states
3. Caffeine
4. Drugs
   a. Antidepressants
   b. Bronchodilators
   c. Digitalis
5. Fever
6. Hyperthyroidism
7. Hypoglycemia
8. Perimenopausal
9. Pheochromocytoma
10. Smoking
11. Thyrotoxicosis

---

with decongestants; (2) caffeine intake; (3) history of thyroid disease; (4) the frequency or pattern (if any) of palpitations; (5) the duration of the palpitations; and (6) any manifestations such as dizziness, shortness of breath, or chest pain associated with the onset of the palpitations. Is there a family history of dysrhythmia or pacemakers?

Cyanosis. Cyanosis is a bluish discoloration of the mucous membranes or skin caused by decreased hemoglobin level or decreased blood perfusion. The two forms of cyanosis are central and peripheral. *Central cyanosis* is a result of decreased arterial oxygen saturation caused by impaired pulmonary function (either a reduced inspired oxygen concentration or an inability to oxygenate blood in the lungs). Causes include advanced pulmonary disease, right-to-left shunting within the heart, or pulmonary edema. Central cyanosis does not occur early in the disease process; it is often a later sign that may indicate advanced disease. *Peripheral cyanosis* is a result of decreased blood flow to the extremities caused by cutaneous vasoconstriction (from exposure to the cold) or low cardiac output (from shock or heart failure).[6,11,16]

Ask clients about any congenital heart disease or history of blood disorder. Inquire about underlying lung or heart disease including chronic obstructive pulmonary disease, emphysema, tobacco use, chemical or asbestos exposure, prior myocardial infarction, or congestive heart failure.

Syncope. Syncope, or fainting, is a transient loss of consciousness related to inadequate cerebral perfusion. The

---

INTEGRATING DIAGNOSTIC TESTING

Heart Palpitations

Clinical manifestations consistent with palpitations → Check serum electrolytes, thyroid function tests

Electrocardiogram (ECG): Detects and amplifies the very small electrical potential changes as the myocardial cells depolarize and repolarize. Will rule out dysrhythmia or prior myocardial infarction

Echocardiogram: Ultrasound waves used to evaluate structural and functional changes of the heart. Will evaluate left ventricular function and rule out structural abnormalities

Exercise stress test: Defines body's reaction to measured increases in acute exercise. Changes in heart rate, BP, respirations, levels of exertion, and ECG monitoring provide data for quantitative estimation of cardiovascular functioning. Will rule out coronary ischemia

24-hour Holter monitor: Detects dysrhythmias that may not appear on routine ECG, but occurs throughout 24-hour period when client is going through normal activity pattern most important tool in the evaluation of syncope is the medical history, which usually uncovers the likely cause. If the syncopal episode was witnessed, it is essential to speak directly to those witnesses in order to obtain a complete history.

Most syncopal episodes have a cardiac origin including either dysrhythmias, vasovagal, or neurocardiogenic syncope. Many syncopal episodes are preceded by warning manifestations such as rapid heart action, vision changes, weakness, dizziness, nausea, or diaphoresis. However, cardiac dysrhythmias (irregular heart rhythms) can precipitate a sudden decrease in cardiac output, causing syncope without warning. Certain medications (antidysrhythmics, antibiotics) can prolong the QT interval in the cardiac cycle, resulting in syncope. Valvular disorders, especially aortic stenosis, may also lead to an adverse change in circulatory hemodynamics precipitated by exertion and cause syncope or vertigo. Micturition, defecation, transient ischemic attacks, or volume depletion (from diuretics, nausea, vomiting, diarrhea, severe anemia) can cause syncope. Seizures often have a prodromal aura (warning manifestations) preceding the seizure, as well as urinary incontinence and a postictal state of confusion.

Vasovagal syncope (caused by heightened vagus nerve tone) occurs after sudden or unexpected pain, fear, or unpleasant sight, smell, or sound. Neurocardiogenic syncope is often preceded by position changes from lying or sitting to standing, or by prolonged standing. Psychiatric disorders (anxiety or major depression), pain disorder, or alcohol or drug dependence can also cause syncope.[6,10,11,16] Ask the client if anyone was with him/her when the episode occurred. Have there been previous episodes of syncope? Were any preceding manifestations noted? Was the syncopal episode preceded by a change in position? Is there a family history of syncope or dysrhythmia?[16]

Dyspnea. Dyspnea is defined as shortness of breath or labored breathing. Like chest pain, this common manifestation affects clients with cardiac and pulmonary disorders, and can also be associated with chest wall, respiratory muscle, and anxiety disorders. *Sudden-onset dyspnea* may occur with a fever, exposure to high altitude, acute pulmonary edema, hyperventilation, anemia, pneumonia, pneumothorax, pulmonary emboli, or airway obstruction. *Chronic dyspnea* also may occur in clients experiencing anxiety, depression, left ventricular heart failure, pulmonary disease, pleural effusion, asthma, obesity, poor physical fitness, or various psychosomatic conditions. Dyspnea accompanied by wheezing is secondary to left ventricular failure (cardiac asthma) or bronchial constriction (bronchial asthma).[6,11,16] Identification and treatment of obstructive sleep apnea (OSA) are additional risk factors for CVD. There are several forms of dyspnea: exertional dyspnea, orthopnea, and paroxysmal nocturnal dyspnea.

Exertional Dyspnea. This is the most common form of cardiac-related dyspnea. Also known as *dyspnea on exertion,* or dyspnea of angina equivalent, this occurs during mild to moderate exercise or activity and disappears with rest. If severe, exertional dyspnea can greatly limit activity tolerance. Ask the client to describe the degree of activity that typically precipitates the onset of dyspnea, for example, walking up one flight of stairs, or walking to the mailbox. How long does the shortness of breath last? Are there any accompanying manifestations with the shortness of breath? What relieves the shortness of breath? Noncardiac conditions such as obesity, poor physical conditioning, anemia, asthma, and obstructions of the nasal passages may also lead to dyspnea after mild exercise.

Orthopnea. Orthopnea (difficult breathing except when sitting erect or standing) results from an increase in pulmonary venous and capillary pressure in the lungs when the person is lying flat, and is relieved when the person sits upright or in a semivertical position. It consists of a cough and dyspnea in clients with left ventricular failure or mitral valve disease, and may also occur with severe chronic obstructive lung disease or asthma. Clients with orthopnea have learned to use two or more pillows when lying down in order to avoid dyspnea.

Ask clients what actions they take to facilitate breathing. In what position do they sleep? On how many pillows do they sleep? Do they sit up in a chair, dangle their feet at the bedside? Record the degree of head elevation required to breathe. Orthopnea usually indicates a more serious compromise of the cardiopulmonary system than does exertional dyspnea.[5,7,8]

Paroxysmal Nocturnal Dyspnea. Paroxysmal nocturnal dyspnea (PND) is dyspnea during sleep that suddenly awakens the sleeper with a "terrifying breathing attack." It is caused by left ventricular failure and commonly occurs 2 to 4 hours after the person goes to bed. It is relieved within 15 to 30 minutes by sitting on the bedside or getting out of bed. The dyspnea usually does not recur after the client goes back to sleep. Episodes can be mild, or they can be severe with wheezing, coughing, gasping, diaphoresis, and apprehension. Some episodes associated with severe left ventricular failure progress to pulmonary edema.[6,11,16] Coughing, either productive or nonproductive, usually occurs after PND as the sleeper tries to expectorate pulmonary secretions. *Hemoptysis* refers to coughing up of blood, including clots of blood as well as blood-tinged sputum. Recurrent episodes of hemoptysis may result from mitral stenosis, pulmonary edema, or pulmonary causes.[6,11,16] Ask clients about their pattern of PND (e.g., nightly, weekly). Are they able to sleep in the bed or do they sleep in a recliner? Also note if they have been diagnosed and treated for OSA.

Fatigue. Fatigue can accompany complaints of dyspnea. Fatigue is weariness or exhaustion with exertion. Women may report experiencing fatigue (rather than chest pain) for several weeks before or during a cardiac episode. Complaints of fatigue in women should be considered a warning sign of an impending cardiac event. Easy fatigability on mild exertion is a frequent problem for clients experiencing cardiac disease; it is a common manifestation of decreased cardiac output. Progressive deterioration of activity tolerance results from the heart's inability to pump an effective volume of blood to meet the varying metabolic demands of the body. Fatigue, however, is not specific for cardiac problems. Other causes of fatigue include anemia, anxiety, chronic diseases, depression, and thyroid dysfunction.[6,11,16]

Edema. Edema, or swelling, is an excess accumulation of fluid in the tissues. The location of the edema aids in clarifying the cause of the edema. For instance, unilateral edema is most commonly caused by deep vein thrombosis, cellulitis, or lymphatic blockage of that extremity. Cardiac edema is generally symmetrical and progresses. It will often start in the feet or ankles and ascend to the thighs, genitalia, and abdomen. In those clients confined to bed, fluid also accumulates in the sacral area. Edema that is diffuse or generalized (anasarca) is usually associated with nephrotic syndrome, severe heart failure, or hepatic cirrhosis. Edema that is localized around the eyes and face is characteristic of nephrotic syndrome, myxedema, angioneurotic edema, acute glomerulonephritis, or hypoproteinemia. Edema evident in the evening that is not present in the mornings is generally caused by heart failure or venous insufficiency.[6,11,16]

Along with locating the edematous area(s), ask the client if there are any associated manifestations such as dyspnea, orthopnea, PND, pain, color changes of the skin, or jaundice. Daily weight measurement is important for clients with cardiac problems. Changes in weight should be reported to the health care provider.[16]

Review of Systems

Following the history of the presenting illness and clinical manifestations, a detailed past medical history follows, including CVD risk factor analysis, past health history and hospitalizations, surgical history, allergies, medications, dietary habits, social habits (tobacco, alcohol, street drugs, exercise), and family history. After all subjective information has been obtained from the client, the physical examination (which began through observation when you walked into the client's room) is completed. Figure 54-2 provides questions to aid with completing an expanded cardiac history.

Past Medical History and Hospitalizations

Ask the client about the following areas: childhood and infectious diseases, immunizations, hospitalizations, obstetric history, major illnesses and hospitalizations. Has CVD been a recurrent or pre-existing illness? Has the client been denied admittance into the armed services or sports, failed an insurance examination, or received a high rating on an insurance examination? Specifically ask about prior history, including rheumatic fever, scarlet fever, severe streptococcal infections, or enlarged heart or heart murmur. These conditions are associated with structural mitral valve disease. Investigate known or corrected congenital anomalies (atrial or ventricular septal defect, persistent patent ductus arteriosus, tetralogy of Fallot, Eisenmenger's syndrome).[6,11,16] Clients with chronic conditions, such as cardiovascular disorders, should be vaccinated yearly against influenza and at least once against pneumococcal pneumonia with additional immunizations every 5 years for high-risk clients. Cardiovascular problems also affect the renal and neurologic systems. Ask about decreased urination, dark or concentrated urine, edema of the legs, dizzy spells, and memory loss.[6,11,16]

Risk Factor Analysis. The Framingham Heart Study of 1961 provided us with today's "risk factor" term. This benchmark cohort study described the natural history and epidemiology of CVD, outlining certain factors that increase the risk of developing CVD.[15] A risk factor assessment not only identifies clients at risk for having manifestations caused by CVD, but also identifies areas to target for nursing intervention. Risk factors are divided into four categories, which are outlined and defined in Table 54-2.[6] Risk factor modification in those with known CVD is referred to as secondary prevention. Risk factor modification in those without CVD is primary prevention.[6] Because of the CVD epidemic, INTERHEART, a worldwide case-control study on acute myocardial infarctions, was conducted to assess the modifiable CVD risk factors.[25] Results revealed that nine modifiable risk factors accounted for greater than 90% of acute myocardial infarction risk in both males and females: smoking, abnormal lipid levels, hypertension, diabetes mellitus, abdominal obesity, psychosocial factors, poor fruit and vegetable consumption, alcohol consumption, and physical activity level. Obstructive sleep apnea (OSA) is also a risk factor for development of CVD and stroke.[1,4]

According to the American Heart Association, for people who are free of CVD at age 50 years, more than 50% of men and 40% of women will develop CVD during their remaining years. The more risk factors that are present, the greater the lifetime risk. Those with known vascular disease in one part of the body, either coronary, cerebrovascular, or peripheral arteries (which includes erectile dysfunction in men), are at higher risk of having

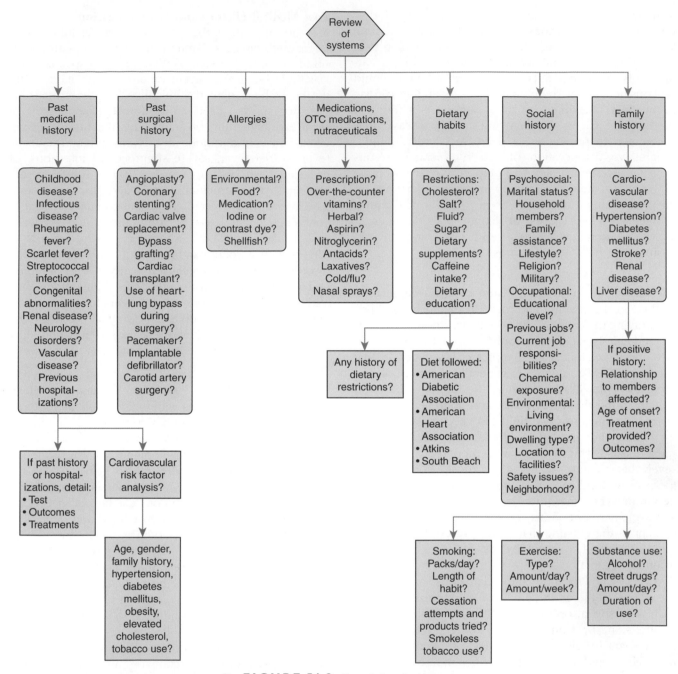

■ **FIGURE 54–2** Expanded cardiac history.

TABLE 54–2 Four Categories of Risk Factors

Category	Risk Factor
Predisposing factors	Age, gender, family history
Modifiable risk factors	Smoking, diet, alcohol intake, inactivity, obstructive sleep apnea
Metabolic risk factors	Dyslipidemia, hypertension, obesity, diabetes mellitus, metabolic syndrome
Identified disease markers	Abnormalities on CT scanning, cardiac catheterization, stress testing, echocardiography, and laboratory results

vascular disease in other areas.[6] Ask if the client experiences muscle cramping in the leg(s) with walking, called claudication, occurring because of arterial blockage supplying blood to those muscles. Ask the client about sleepiness during the day, wakefulness during the night, a dry throat in the morning, and other manifestations of OSA. Table 54-3 summarizes common risk factors for CVD.

Hypertension (defined as systolic pressure of 140 mm Hg or higher, or diastolic pressure of 90 mm Hg or higher) is an important independent risk factor for CVD and requires both primary and secondary prevention.

TABLE 54–3   Risk Factor Analysis for Cardiovascular Disease

Risk Factor	High Risk	Highest Risk
Gender and age	Women after menopause	Men older than 60
Family history of high blood pressure	Two blood relatives	Three or more blood relatives
Family history of heart attack	One relative, before age 60	Two relatives, before age 60
Family history of diabetes mellitus	One or more relatives with type 1 diabetes mellitus	One or more relatives with type 2 diabetes mellitus
Blood pressure[†] (degree of control somewhat modifiable)	Systolic: 160-200 mm Hg	Systolic: >200 mm Hg
	Diastolic: 90-110 mm Hg	Diastolic: >110 mm Hg
Diabetes mellitus[†] (degree of control somewhat modifiable), HbA_{1C} <7%	Type 1 diabetes mellitus uncontrolled or type 2 diabetes mellitus controlled	Type 2 diabetes mellitus uncontrolled
Weight*	30%-40% overweight	50% or more overweight
BMI 18.5-24.9 kg/m^2	Overweight = BMI 25-29.9	Obesity = BMI of 30 or greater
Normal weight		
Waist circumference		
<40 inches (no increased risk for men)	>40 inches (men)	
<35 inches (no increased risk for women)	>35 inches (women)	
Cholesterol level[†]	240-280 mg/dl	>280 mg/dl
HDL-C >40 mg/dl		
LDL-C <100 mg/dl	100-129 mg/dl	130 mg/dl
Serum triglycerides, fasting[†] <150 mg/dl	200-499 mg/dl	>500 mg/dl
Percentage of fat in diet[†]	30%-50%	>50%
Frequency of recreational exercise*	Minimal	No activity
Frequency of occupational exercise*	Minimal	Sedentary occupation
Cigarette smoking*	20-40 per day	>40 per day
Stress at home*	High	Extremely high
Stress at work[†]	High	Extremely high
Behavior pattern (especially men)[†]	Type A	Type A
Use of oral contraceptives (women)[†]	Younger than 40 and use oral contraceptives	Older than 40 and use oral contraceptives
Air pollution[†]	Moderate	High
Sleep patterns*	More than 8 hr sleep a night	4-6 hr sleep a night
		Sleep disrupted by obstructive sleep apnea (OSA)

* Modifable risk factors.
[†] Possibly modifiable risk factors.

According to the American Heart Association, blood pressure (BP) levels to prevent heart attack and/or stroke are as follows: BP maintained below 140/90 mm Hg; below 130/85 mm Hg for people with kidney damage or heart failure; or below 130/80 mm Hg for people with diabetes mellitus.[4] More recent data recommend lower BP values as treatment goals because the risk of CVD, beginning at 115/75 mm Hg, doubles with each increment of 20/10 mm Hg.[23] The report concluded that a systolic BP of more than 140 mm Hg in persons older than 50 years is a much more important CVD risk factor than elevated diastolic BP and that individuals with a systolic BP of 120 to 139 mm Hg or a diastolic BP of 80 to 89 mm Hg should be considered prehypertensive and require health-promoting lifestyle modifications to prevent CVD.[23]

Diabetes mellitus is another important independent risk factor for CVD. The total number of people with diabetes mellitus is projected to increase from 171 million in 2000 to 366 million in 2030.[31] It is estimated that at least 65% of people with diabetes mellitus will die of some form of heart or blood vessel disease, making heart disease the leading cause of diabetes-related death. With the prevalence of obesity, metabolic syndrome and diabetes mellitus have escalated.[3,22,23] See Chapter 45 for information related to diabetes mellitus and metabolic syndrome and their role for development of CVD.

The National Center for Health Statistics began tracking obesity in 1960 through the National Health and Nutrition Examination Survey (NHANES). This continued survey revealed an unanticipated jump in the prevalence of obesity. Obesity is becoming a global epidemic and is now an independent risk factor for CVD. Weight loss therapies (dietary intervention, physical activity, pharmacotherapy, and surgery) can improve or prevent many of the CVD risk factors caused by obesity.[3,22,23] For adults, overweight is a body mass index (BMI) of 25.0 to 29.9 kg/m^2; while obesity is defined as a BMI greater than 30.0 kg/m.[23]

The 2001 National Cholesterol Education Program Adult Treatment Panel III (ATP III) guidelines highlighted several modifiable and nonmodifiable major risk factors for CVD. Serum lipid levels are among the most important modifiable risk factors, and the cardiovascular benefit of lowering lipid levels is well-defined.[13,16,33]

The recently published Multi-Ethnic Study of Atherosclerosis (MESA) findings reveal that ATP III guidelines are not being fully implemented.[5] This coupled with increasing worldwide obesity is increasing the prevalence not only of CVD but also of other co-morbidities such as type 2 diabetes mellitus, hypertension, certain cancers, and sleep apnea.[4]

Those with known CVD or who have two or more risk factors are considered high risk, while those without a CVD history or who have only one risk factor are considered low risk.[6] Data from the Behavioral Risk Factor Surveillance System revealed the reporting of two or more risk factors for CVD increased among successive age groups. The prevalence of having two or more risk factors was highest among blacks (48.7%) and American Indians (46.7%), and lowest among Asians (25.9%). The prevalence of two or more risk factors was similar in men (37.8%) and women (36.4%).[6,7]

The American Heart Association recommends that health care providers routinely assess a client's general risk of CVD beginning at age 20. The AHA guidelines also recommend that providers calculate the risk of developing CVD in the next 10 years for people age 40 and older or for anyone who has multiple risk factors. Risk factor screening includes measuring blood pressure, body mass index, waist circumference, and pulse rate at least every 2 years; obtaining a cholesterol profile and performing glucose testing at least every 5 years beginning at age 20; and obtaining a smoking history.[1]

Past Surgical History

Explore previous cardiac-related outpatient procedures, interventions, or surgery. This includes relatively minor procedures such as a diagnostic cardiac catheterization to major surgery such as a heart transplant. Inquire about the details of each procedure, including any adverse events or prolonged recovery.

Allergies

Note and describe any environmental, food, or drug allergies. Particularly inquire about allergies to Betadine, iodine, shrimp, shellfish, contrast, or dye (in case CT scanning or angiography is warranted). Clearly document the manifestations of an allergic reaction, such as rashes, itching, or anaphylaxis (a sudden severe allergic reaction).[6,16]

Medications

Evaluate the use of prescription medications, over-the-counter medications, herbals, and recreational drugs. Whenever possible, use brand names or simple descriptors

instead of generic names. For example, ask clients whether they are currently taking "water pills," "heart pills," or "blood pressure" medications.[6,16]

Numerous medications can affect the cardiovascular system. Ask specifically about the use of anti-hypertensives, diuretics, vasodilators (nitroglycerin), cardiotonic drugs (digoxin), anticoagulants, bronchodilators, contraceptives, hormones, and steroids. Noncardiac medications can have profound secondary effects on cardiovascular performance. For example, tricyclic antidepressants and other psychotropic medications can potentiate dysrhythmias. Oral contraceptives increase the incidence of thrombophlebitis.[6,27] Steroid use increases fluid retention and may cause hypertension. Various antineoplastic agents may be cardiotoxic, causing dysrhythmias and cardiomyopathy. Elevated levels of thyroid hormones can result in thyrotoxicosis and a resultant hyperdynamic cardiovascular state (bounding pulses, palpitations, tachycardia). Decreased levels of thyroid hormone (hypothyroidism) may explain a client's dyspnea on exertion, fatigue, decreased cardiac output, and heart failure.[6,16,27]

Finally, discuss the use of over-the-counter drugs such as aspirin, cold remedies, and vitamins. Note the dose and times of administration. Inquire about the use of antioxidants (folic acid, vitamin B_6 or B_{12}, nuts, ginger, purslane, or rosemary) or cholesterol-lowering agents (omega 3 fatty acids, niacin, pigweed). Ask about use of herbal remedies. Herbs are used for cardiac disorders such as angina, dysrhythmias, and heart disease and for related disorders such as high blood pressure (BP) and peripheral vascular disease.[27] See Box 54-3 for a list of commonly used antianginal herbs and Box 54-4 for antidysrhythmic herbs.

In addition to the types and names of the medications the client takes, ask how many pills and how often they are taken. Is the client currently taking these medications as prescribed? Clients with cardiac disease occasionally stop taking prescribed medications because they (1) are taking too many pills, (2) are experiencing unwanted

---

BOX 54-3 Antianginal Herbs

- Angelica (*Angelica archangelica*)
- Bilberry (*Vaccinium myrtillus*)
- Evening primrose (*Oenothera biennis*)
- Flaxseed (*Linum usitatissimum*)
- Garlic (*Allium sativum*)
- Ginger (*Zingiber officinale*)
- Hawthorn (*Crataegus laevigata*)
- Khella (*Ammi majus*)
- Kudzu (*Pueraria lobata*)
- Onion (*Allium cepa*)
- Purslane (*Portulaca oleracea*)
- Sichuan lovage (*Ligusticum chuanxiong*)
- Willow (*Salix*)

BOX 54-4   Antidysrhythmic Herbs

- Angelica
- Astragalus (*Astragalus*)
- Barberry (*Berberis vulgaris*)
- Canola (*Brassica*)
- Cinchona (*Cinchona*)
- Gingko (*Gingko biloba*)
- Hawthorn
- Horehound (*Marrubium vulgare*)
- Khella
- Motherwort (*Leonurus cardiaca*)
- Purslane
- Reishi (*Ganoderma lucidum*)
- Scotch broom (*Cytisus scoparius*)
- Valerian (*Valeriana officinalis*)

side effects, (3) believe that the problem has resolved, (4) worry about the cost, or (5) some combination of these factors. A client may neglect to take prescribed diuretics because "it makes me go to the bathroom all the time." Clients who take antihypertensives or lipid-lowering medications may stop taking them when their BP or cholesterol level reaches a normal range because they perceive that the problem has resolved. Careful questioning can identify areas for client teaching.

Dietary Habits

Assess excess or deficit caloric intake and the client's approximate intake of foods high in sodium, cholesterol, saturated fat, and caffeine. Although these are common components of the average American diet, they have been linked to the development of atherosclerosis and hypertensive disease. Elevated serum cholesterol levels are associated with coronary artery disease. The Translating Evidence into Practice feature below details how nurses can help clients make the connection between diet and cardiovascular health.

Caffeine is a stimulant that, in excessive amounts, can increase heart rate and provoke palpitations. For clients with tachycardia or palpitations, caution regarding more than two 8-ounce cups of a caffeinated beverage is

---

TRANSLATING EVIDENCE INTO PRACTICE

Diet and Heart Disease

Being in the medical field, we all know the importance of dieting. Diets have been studied for decades and the choice of diets plans spans from A to Z. In spite of this vast knowledge, disease mortality and morbidity are escalating as a result of both national and international obesity, which not only is a risk factor for CVD but also is now considered a worldwide pandemic.[1]

The importance of dieting, from a medical standpoint, focuses on risk factor modification for disease prevention or control. The DASH (Dietary Approaches to Stop Hypertension) diet showed reduced weight and improved physical fitness with a decreased prevalence of hypertension at 6 months after implementation of the diet.[7] Diabetes mellitus has also been positively impacted through dietary restriction and statin therapy.[2,7]

IMPLICATIONS

Although outcomes are positive regarding dietary restrictions, many people either have not read or do not understand the literature. Implications for nurses include ensuring that every client is made aware of these research findings and is encouraged to follow a heart-healthy diet. Nutrition counseling is recommended, including written literature providing examples of heart-healthy foods. Too often clients have heard of a low-fat or low-cholesterol diet, but do not fully understand their benefits regarding risk factor modification.

For those clients who will not adhere to dietary restrictions, multiple trials using statin medications have replicated previous findings that statin therapy helps to lower LDL-C levels and may actually decrease some of the plaque burden in the artery lumen, thereby decreasing CVD morbidity and mortality.[3-6] Future research is needed to evaluate effective methods for providing dietary information to clients, follow-up on those methods, and client responses to those methods in hopes of better understanding the dietary actions and views of the client.

REFERENCES

1. American Heart Association. (2006). Obesity and cardiovascular disease: Pathophysiology, evaluation, and effect of weight loss: An update of the 1997 American Heart Association Scientific Statement on Obesity and Heart Disease from the Obesity Committee of the Council on Nutrition, Physical Activity, and Metabolism. *Circulation, 113*(6), 898-918.
2. Davidson, M.H. (2006). Statin/fibrate combination in patients with metabolic syndrome or diabetes: Evaluating the risks of pharmacokinetic drug interactions. *Expert Opinions on Drug Safety, 5*, 145-156.
3. Diabetes Prevention Program Research Group. (2002). Reduction in the incidence of type 2 diabetes with lifestyle intervention or metformin. *New England Journal of Medicine, 346*, 393-403.
4. Dierkes, J., Westphal, S., & Luley, C. (2004). The effect of fibrates and other lipid-lowering drugs on plasma homocysteine levels. *Expert Opinions on Drug Safety, 3*, 101-111.
5. Nissen, S.E., Tuzcu, E.M., Schoenhagen, P., et al. (2004). Effect of intensive compared with moderate lipid-lowering on progression of coronary atherosclerosis: A randomized controlled trial. *JAMA, 291*, 1071-1080.
6. Taylor, A.J., Sullenberger, L.E., Lee, H.J., et al. (2004). Arterial Biology for the Investigation of the Treatment Effects or Reducing Cholesterol (ARBITER) 2: A double-blind, placebo-controlled study of extended-release niacin on atherosclerosis progression in secondary prevention patients treated with statins. *Circulation, 110*, 3512-3517.
7. Writing group of the PREMIER Collaborative Research Group. (2003). Effects of comprehensive lifestyle modification on blood pressure control. Main results of the PREMIER clinical trial. *JAMA, 289*, 2083-2093.

recommended. 🪔 Regarding caffeine and blood pressure or coronary artery disease, restriction of caffeine is no longer indicated.[23,29]

Examine not only daily food habits but also attitudes toward food and resistance to therapeutic alterations in diet. Cultural beliefs and economic status greatly affect food choices. Consider these factors before recommending dietary changes. Identify and include the primary food purchaser and preparer in dietary instruction.

Social History/Social Habits

Psychosocial History. The psychosocial history includes data on lifestyle, household members, marital status, children, relationships with significant others, military service, religious beliefs (in relation to perceptions of health and treatment), and hobbies. Note data that help identify support systems and coping mechanisms. Psychosocial data provide information about risk factors for the development of CVD. Background information can be used to formulate a plan to assist the client in making necessary lifestyle adaptations to promote health and lessen disease.

Occupation. Inquire about the client's educational level and all occupations of the client as well as the duration of each job. The present occupation may be relevant to the significance of the disease; that is, coronary artery disease or dysrhythmias may be incompatible with continuing a career as an airline pilot or truck driver. The amount of perceived job-related stress may need to be evaluated; stress is a modifiable risk factor for CVD. Ask about possible occupational exposure to agents or chemicals (asbestos).

Environment.

SAFETY ⚠ ALERT

After a stroke or with deteriorating cardiac function and output, a client may need assistance or environmental adjustments to live safely and fully and meet daily needs. Inquire about the following: (1) the home, such as safety issues, type of dwelling (number of steps), state of repair, exits for fire, heating and cooling adequacy; (2) mode of transportation; (3) the neighborhood, in regard to noise, pollution, and violence; and (4) access to family and friends, grocery store, a pharmacy, laundry, church, and health care facilities.

Smoking. If the client smokes, inquire about the duration of the smoking habit and the number of cigarettes smoked daily. If the client is not smoking currently, does the client use a nicotine inhalation system or a nicotine transdermal product or chew nicotine gum or smokeless tobacco? Determine the pack-year history (number of cigarette packs smoked per day multiplied by the number of years smoked). All nicotine products have a vasoconstrictive effect on the heart and vessels. 🪔 Cigarette smoking increases the risk of coronary artery disease and worsens hypertension. Nicotine, a major ingredient in cigarettes, causes peripheral vasoconstriction, increasing resistance to left ventricular emptying and thus increasing the myocardial workload. 🪔 Cigarette smokers are three to four times more likely to develop CVD than nonsmokers, smoking doubles the risk for stroke, and smokers are 10 times more likely to develop peripheral vascular disease.[3] At 5 to 15 years after tobacco cessation, clients have a death rate from CVD similar to that of nonsmokers.[7]

Substance Abuse. Review for daily substance abuse, including alcohol or street drugs along with the amount(s) ingested. Evidence that alcohol ingestion increases the risk of atherosclerosis is inconclusive. Researchers state that only excessive alcohol intake has deleterious effects on the cardiovascular system and its performance. 🪔 An intake of 100 g of pure (100%) alcohol may slightly increase BP and heart rate; this amount is approximately equal to three beers or one mixed drink. Alcoholism, in contrast, has been associated with the development of hypertension and damage to the heart muscle, leading to cardiomyopathy.[6] Ask about the client's approximate daily and weekly alcohol consumption. Keep in mind that the alcoholic client may lie about the type and amount consumed.

Discuss the use of recreational drugs. Cocaine toxicity is a major threat to the cardiovascular system. The systemic sympathomimetic effects of cocaine result in a "fight-or-flight" reaction that increases heart rate, contractility, blood glucose levels, and peripheral vasoconstriction. 🪔 Cocaine can potentiate the effects of circulating catecholamines (epinephrine and norepinephrine), resulting in sudden death.[6,27]

Exercise. Ask about the type and amount of exercise routinely engaged in during an average week before and after the onset of current manifestations. 🪔 Research confirms that a sedentary lifestyle potentiates the lethality of myocardial infarction or stroke, and it is considered a significant risk factor in the development of coronary artery disease. 🪔 Effective, routine aerobic exercise is thought to lower the likelihood of a coronary event. Aerobic exercise includes such activities as swimming, jogging, brisk walking, bicycling, and rowing.[3,4,6]

🪔 To be beneficial, aerobic exercise should raise the heart rate from 50% to 100% of baseline (depending on age and prior physical conditioning) for at least 30 minutes three to five times a week. Along with general body conditioning, this form of exercise increases the heart's efficiency in using oxygen. Advise clients who are older than 40 years or who have a history of CVD to consult their physician before beginning an exercise program.[1,4]

Ask about current activities and limitations. Do any activities trigger the clinical manifestations discussed in Figure 54-1? How far can the client walk, run, or climb steps? Can the client complete housework, mow the lawn, participate in sports, shop, do a full day's work, or have sexual intercourse?

Family History

Ask about prolonged contact with a communicable disease or the effect of a family member's illness on the client. Specifically, inquire about a family history of heart disease, high BP, stroke, diabetes mellitus, or kidney disease. A detailed health history of the client's family can provide insight into possible genetic, environmental, and lifestyle conditions contributing to a cardiac condition.

PHYSICAL EXAMINATION

The cardiac physical examination begins with a general inspection, followed by assessment of the vital signs, palpation, auscultation, and percussion. The examination logically proceeds from head to toe with the client in supine position (the head of the bed or examination table may be elevated for comfort). Stand at the client's right side. Cardiac examination abnormalities are noted in Table 54-4. Necessary equipment includes a stethoscope with diaphragm and bell, a ruler, and a sphygmomanometer.[6] Please refer to the normal cardiovascular findings described in the Physical Assessment Findings in the Healthy Adult feature on p. 1371.

General Appearance and Level of Consciousness

Begin with inspection. Assessment of *general appearance* and *level of consciousness* provides an initial composite picture of the client and indicates the level of comfort and distress. Look at the client and consider the following: (1) Does the client lie quietly, or is there restlessness or continual moving about? (2) Can the client lie flat, or is only an upright, erect position tolerated? (3) Does the facial expression reflect pain or obvious manifestations of respiratory distress? (4) Are there manifestations of significant cyanosis or pallor? (5) Can the client answer questions without dyspnea during the interview?

Note the client's general *level of consciousness* (LOC). The LOC reflects the adequacy of cerebral perfusion and oxygenation. Also assess whether the client manifests appropriate behavior for the surroundings: (1) What is the client's affect? (2) Are there obvious manifestations of anxiety, fear, depression, or anger? (3) How does the client react to those in the immediate vicinity, including significant others?

Vital Signs

Vital signs include bilateral arm blood pressures, heart and respiratory rates, and temperature. A weight should also be obtained to aid in body mass index calculation and risk factor assessment.

Blood Pressure

Blood pressure measurements should be made with the appropriate cuff size and with the client lying, sitting, and standing, as shown in Figure 54-3. Blood pressure readings normally may vary 5 to 15 mm Hg with postural changes. *Orthostatic hypotension* is a blood pressure drop of more than 15 mm Hg with position changes. Blood pressure readings may also vary with inspiration from 5 to 10 mm Hg. *Pulsus paradoxus* is an abnormal decrease in systolic BP of more than 10 mm Hg during inspiration. If the arms are inaccessible, obtain pressures from the thighs and popliteal arteries or the calves and posterior tibial arteries. When pressures are difficult to auscultate, systolic pressures can be determined through palpation or by Doppler ultrasonography.[6,16]

Pulse

Pulse characteristics can vary. If the pulse is irregular, assess for a pulse deficit by taking apical and radial pulses simultaneously, noting differences in rate. Pulse volume can be described as bounding, thready, or absent. Peripheral pulse assessment is discussed in Chapter 51.

Respiratory Rate

Note the rate, rhythm, depth, and quality of the breathing pattern. Look for accessory muscle use. Does the client have to sit up to breathe easily, or is the client able to lie flat comfortably? (See Chapter 59 for respiratory assessment information.)

Head and Neck

When examining the head, pay particular attention to the eyes, ear lobes, lips, and buccal mucosa. Examine the eyes for *arcus senilis* (a light gray ring around the iris, possibly caused by cholesterol deposits) and *xanthelasma* (yellow raised plaques around the eyelids resulting from lipid deposits).[6,16]

Neck Vein Assessment

Neck vein distention can be used to estimate *central venous pressure* (CVP). The amount of distention reflects pressure and volume changes in the right atrium. The internal jugular veins, although more difficult to detect than the external jugular veins, are more reliable indicators of CVP. The external jugular vein engorges easily with only slight provocation, for example, by holding

TABLE 54–4 Cardiac Examination Abnormalities

Findings	Possible Etiology
Vital Signs	
Unequal arm blood pressures	Aortic dissection, coarctation of the aorta, vascular obstruction, vascular outlet syndrome, measurement error
Pulsus paradoxus	Cardiac tamponade, pericarditis
Tachycardia (>100 beats/min)	Anxiety, hypovolemia, shock, hyperthyroidism
Bradycardia (<60 beats/min)	Medication side effect, SA or AV node abnormality, physical conditioning, hypothyroidism
Irregular pulse	Dysrhythmia, myocardial ischemia, medication side effect
Bounding pulse	Bradycardia, anemia, aortic valve insufficiency
Thready pulse	Hypovolemia, mitral valve stenosis
Absent pulse	Atherosclerosis, embolus, thrombus, trauma
Tachypnea	Anxiety, pain, pulmonary edema, COPD exacerbation
Head	
Arcus senilis	Hyperlipidemia, atherosclerosis
Xanthelasma	Hyperlipidemia, atherosclerosis
Neck	
Neck vein distention	Right ventricular failure, tricuspid failure, cardiac tamponade
Flat jugular veins	Extracellular volume depletion
Carotid bruit	Atherosclerosis, aortic stenosis
Thorax	
Displaced PMI	Left ventricular enlargement, left ventricular aneurysm
Heaves	Valvular heart disease, pulmonary hypertension
Thrills	Valvular heart disease, partially obstructed blood vessels
Crackles	Pulmonary edema
Heart Sounds	
S_3 gallop	Pulmonary edema, myocardial infarction, valvular insufficiency
S_4 gallop	Ventricular hypertrophy, hypertension, cardiomyopathy, cor pulmonale, aortic stenosis, pulmonic stenosis, pulmonary fibrosis
Pericardial rub	Pericarditis
Systolic murmur	Aortic or pulmonic stenosis, anemia, tachycardia
Diastolic murmur	Mitral or tricuspid stenosis, aortic or pulmonic insufficiency
Abdomen	
Ascites	Chronic right ventricular failure; liver failure
Hyperactive bowel sounds	Laxative use, antidysrhythmic medication side effect
Hypoactive bowel sounds	Hyperkalemia
Bruits	Atherosclerosis
Pronounced and widened aortic pulsation	Abdominal aortic aneurysm
Skin	
Central cyanosis	Advanced pulmonary disease, right-to-left shunting within heart, pulmonary edema
Peripheral cyanosis	Cutaneous vasoconstriction, exposure to cold, shock, heart failure
Decreased turgor	Dehydration, volume depletion, rapid weight loss, advanced age
Warm to touch	Thyrotoxicosis
Cool to touch	Vascular disease
Edema	Right ventricular failure, venous insufficiency, medication side effect
Nail	
Clubbing	Advanced pulmonary or cardiovascular disease
Splinter hemorrhages	Subacute bacterial endocarditis

the breath, twisting the neck, and being constricted by clothing (except in weight lifters, football players, and professional speakers and singers, who have overdeveloped neck muscle tendons). The vessels are prominent and visible but soft and compressible.[6,16]

A relaxed supine position with the head of the bed inclined between 15 and 30 degrees maximizes jugular vein prominence. Clients who have greatly increased right atrial pressure may require head elevation from 45 to 90 degrees. Support the client's head with a small

The Cardiovascular System

INSPECTION

Skin color even; capillary refill less than 3 seconds. Thorax symmetrical, without visible lifts or point of maximal impulse (PMI). Jugular venous distention absent with client at 45-degree angle. Lower extremity superficial vessels without tortuosity upon standing.

PALPATION

Skin warm. PMI palpable in fifth intercostal space at left midclavicular line, approximately 1 cm in diameter. Forceful thrusts, heaves, and pulsations absent. No palpable thrills. Abdominal aorta pulsations slightly palpable over epigastrium without lateral radiation. Carotid and peripheral pulses equal and readily palpable bilaterally. Evidence of unimpeded arterial flow and venous return to upper and lower extremities. No edema evident.

PERCUSSION

Right heart border not discerned.

AUSCULTATION

S_1 and S_2 heard without splitting. Apical rate, 72 beats/min, regular. Murmurs and extra heart sounds absent.

pillow and avoid sharp neck flexion. Turn the client's head slightly away from you and loosen or remove clothing that compresses the neck or upper thorax. Tangential (oblique) lighting enhances the appearance of the vein. Observe both sides of the neck. The internal jugular vein lies deep to the sternocleidomastoid muscle and runs parallel along its length to the jaw and ear lobe. Identify the pulsations of the internal jugular. Use the external jugular vein if the internal jugular is not visible.[6]

Note the highest point at which the internal jugular pulses can be seen (the *meniscus*). The *sternal angle* (manubrial joint) is a reference point to measure the height of venous pulsation, approximately 4 to 5 cm above the center of the right atrium. Use a centimeter ruler to measure the vertical distance between the sternal angle and the point of highest venous pulsations (Figure 54-4). The value is usually less than 3 or 4 cm above the sternal angle when the head of the bed is elevated 30 to 40 degrees.[6,16]

Carotid Artery Assessment

Carotid artery examination indicates the adequacy of stroke volume and the patency of the arteries. Using your finger tips, gently palpate the carotid arteries one side at a time in order to avoid vagal stimulation. Check and compare the rate, rhythm, and amplitude of the pulses. Note whether a *bruit* (a blowing sound) is present by listening with the diaphragm of a stethoscope over the arteries while the client holds the breath. Tracheal breath sounds are heard while respiration is ongoing.[6,16]

Thorax
Inspection

Perform inspection and palpation of the precordium together to determine the presence of normal and abnormal pulsations. Ideally, the client should be supine with the chest exposed. The left lateral position allows the heart to move closer to the chest wall, accentuating precordial movements and certain heart sounds. Good lighting and a warm, quiet environment are essential. Stand at the client's right side and observe the anterior chest for size, shape, symmetry of movement, and any evident pulsations. Record the location of pulsation in relation to the intercostal space and the midclavicular line. Confirm your observation with palpation.

STANDING

SITTING

SUPINE

BP = 140/80
P = 80

BP = 124/76
P = 86

BP = 104/68
P = 98

■ **FIGURE 54–3** Recording postural blood pressure (BP). After measuring the client's BP and pulse in the supine position, leave the BP cuff in place and help the client sit. Then measure the BP within 15 to 30 seconds. Help the client stand, and measure again. Postural hypotension is indicated by a BP decrease of more than 10 to 15 mm Hg systolic pressure and more than 10 mm Hg diastolic pressure. Postural hypotension is typically accompanied by a 10% to 20% increase in heart rate (pulse rate).

Centimeter rule

4 cm

Sternal angle

Meniscus:
Highest level
at which pulse
is visible

Right atrium

■ **FIGURE 54–4** Estimation of jugular vein measurement to assess central venous pressure.

Palpation

When palpating, use the fingers and palm of the hand. The *point of maximum intensity* (PMI), or apical impulse, is usually seen at the fifth intercostal space medial to the left midclavicular line. It may be prominent in thin people and obscured in those who are obese or have large breasts. When palpated, the PMI is a single, faint, instantaneous tap beneath the fingers, no more than 2 cm in diameter. The left lateral recumbent position may enhance locating the PMI, but its position is displaced. With left ventricular enlargement and aneurysm, the PMI is more diffuse, sustained, and displaced downward and to the left of the midclavicular line.[6,11]

Right ventricular enlargement can produce an abnormal pulsation, called *"heaves"* or *"lifts,"* that may be seen as a sustained thrust along the left sternal border. *Thrills* represent turbulent blood flow through the heart, especially across abnormal heart valves. Use the heel or ulnar surface of the hand to palpate over each of the five cardiac landmarks (Figure 54-5). Thrills are perceived as a rushing vibration, much like feeling the throat of a purring cat.[6,11,16]

Auscultation of the Posterior Chest

With the client sitting forward, auscultate both sides of the lungs. Crackles (high-pitched, noncontinuous sounds) frequently signal left ventricular failure. As the left ventricle fails, crackles occur because of increasing pulmonary capillary pressure that forces fluid to shift into the intra-alveolar spaces. Crackles are best heard at the lung bases (because of gravitational effects on the fluid) during late inspiration.[6,11,16]

Auscultation of the Precordium

With the client in a supine position, auscultation of the precordium yields valuable information about normal or abnormal heart rate and rhythm, ventricular filling, and blood flow across heart valves. Use the bell to hear low-pitched sounds and the diaphragm to hear high-pitched sounds. Always warm the chestpiece before placing it on the client's skin. A quiet environment is key to successful auscultation. The left lateral position may facilitate auscultation. An upright position, leaning forward and holding the breath after exhalation, helps when assessing early diastolic murmurs and pericardial friction rubs.

Examine heart sounds from the base (right second intercostal space) of the heart to the apex (left fifth intercostal space). Figure 54-5 diagrams specific cardiac areas to auscultate. Use the mnemonic "APE To Man" to remember the areas (aortic, pulmonic, Erb's point, tricuspid, and mitral). Each area corresponds to a specific valvular outflow tract. Concentrate on one component of the cardiac cycle at a time, that is, the first heart sound (S_1), then the second heart sound (S_2), and so on. Listen to several complete cardiac cycles at each of the five precordial areas. Listen carefully, noting the quality (crisp or muffled), intensity (loud or soft), rhythm (irregular or regular), and presence of extra sounds (murmurs, gallops, rubs, or clicks). Repeat this process using the bell over each of the precordial areas.[6,11,16]

Normal Heart Sounds

The *first heart sound* (S_1) is linked to closure of the mitral and tricuspid valves (atrioventricular [AV] valves). It marks the onset of systole (ventricular contraction). It is heard best with the diaphragm at the apex (the mitral valve area) and left lower sternal border (the tricuspid valve area). S_1 results from abrupt closure of the AV valves, which causes some blood turbulence and vibration of structures within the ventricles. This vibration is transmitted across the chest wall as a heart sound. Phonetically, if both heart sounds are appreciated as "lub-dub," S_1 is "lub." Although closure of both mitral and tricuspid valves is heard as a single sound, the mitral valve closes a fraction of a second earlier.[6] If you are not sure which sound is S_1, check the carotid artery for a pulsation (which occurs with S_1 or systole), as outlined in Figure 54-6.

The *second heart sound* (S_2) is related to closure of the pulmonic and aortic (semilunar) valves and is heard best with the diaphragm at the aortic area. Phonetically, it is the "dub" of the heart sounds. It signifies the end of systole and the onset of diastole (ventricular filling). At the base of the heart, normal S_2 is always louder than S_1, whereas both sounds are usually of nearly equal

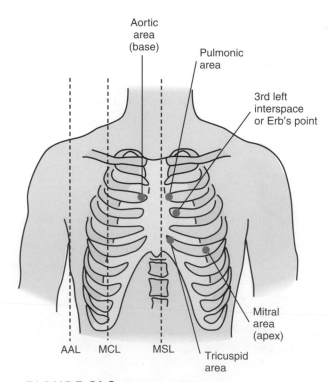

Aortic area (base)

Pulmonic area

3rd left interspace or Erb's point

Mitral area (apex)

AAL   MCL   MSL   Tricuspid area

■ **FIGURE 54–5** Cardiac auscultatory sites. S_1 is heard loudest at mitral and tricuspid areas. S_2 is heard loudest at aortic and pulmonic areas. S_3 and S_4 are heard best at the mitral area. *AAL,* Anterior axillary line; *MCL,* midclavicular line; *MSL,* midsternal line.

intensity at the left sternal border over Erb's point. Usually, S_1 is the louder of the two sounds at the apex and occurs just after or along with the carotid pulse.[6] Figure 54-6 shows the relationship of heart sounds to events during the cardiac cycle.

Abnormal Heart Sounds

Many abnormal heart sounds may indicate a serious heart disorder or change in cardiac function. You may not be able to label each abnormality, but with a thorough understanding of the normal sounds, you should be able to recognize various abnormal sounds and refer the problem to the physician or primary health care provider.

Gallops. Diastolic filling sounds or *gallops* (S_3 and S_4) occur during the two phases of ventricular filling. Sudden changes of inflow volume cause vibrations of the valves and ventricular supporting structures, producing low-pitched sounds that occur either early (S_3) or late (S_4) in diastole. Such sounds can originate in either side of the heart. These extra heart sounds create a triplet rhythm, acoustically mimicking a horse's gallop. For that reason, the term "gallop" is often used to denote these heart sounds. Figure 54-6 shows the timing of S_3 and S_4 during the cardiac cycle.[6,11,16]

A gallop sound that occurs in early diastole, during passive, rapid filling of the ventricles, is known as the *third heart sound* (S_3). It is heard best with the bell at the apex and with the client in the left lateral recumbent position. An S_3 immediately follows S_2 and is a dull, low-pitched sound. An S_3 gallop is considered a normal finding in children and young adults. In adults older than 30 years of age, an S_3 is considered characteristic of left ventricular dysfunction.[6,11,16]

A *fourth heart sound,* or S_4 gallop, occurs in the later stage of diastole, during atrial contraction and active filling of the ventricles. This soft, low-pitched sound is heard immediately before S_1 and is also referred to as an *atrial gallop.* S_4 is heard best with the bell of the stethoscope at the apex, with the client in the supine, left lateral position.[6,11,16] An atrial gallop is found most commonly in disorders involving increased stiffness of the ventricle. The ventricles become resistant to filling, and the structures within the ventricles vibrate in response to the added blood input during the "atrial kick." S_4 is never heard in the absence of atrial contraction (atrial fibrillation).

Pericardial Friction Rub. A pericardial friction rub is produced by inflammation of the pericardial sac. The roughened parietal and visceral layers of the pericardium rub

■ **FIGURE 54–6** Relationship of heart sounds to events during the cardiac cycle. Understanding heart sounds is facilitated when they are correlated with cardiac cycle events and valvular movements. *EC,* Ejection click; *MVc,* mitral valve closing; *MVo,* mitral valve opening; *OS,* opening snap; *PVc,* pulmonic valve closing; *TVc,* tricuspid valve closing; *TVo,* tricuspid valve opening.

against each other during cardiac motion. A pericardial friction rub is best detected with the diaphragm at the apex and along the left sternal border. It may be accentuated when a person leans forward or lies prone and exhales. Friction rubs produce a sound that is described as "to and fro," scratchy, and much like the sound made when rubbing your hair between your thumb and forefinger. Friction rubs may be present during the first week after myocardial infarction or after open heart surgery. Differentiate a pericardial friction rub from a pleural friction rub by noting the timing of the rub in relation to breathing. Pleural friction rubs are heard during inspiration; pericardial friction rubs are heard throughout the respiratory cycle.[6,16]

Murmurs. Murmurs are heard as a consequence of turbulent blood flow through the heart and large vessels. Turbulent blood flow produces vibrations in the heart and great vessels that can be detected as a blowing or swooshing sound. Murmurs are caused by (1) increased rate or velocity of blood flow, (2) abnormal forward or backward flow across stenosed or incompetent valves, (3) flow into a dilated chamber, or (4) flow through an abnormal passage between heart chambers. Murmurs are best heard with the bell of the stethoscope when the client is in the left lateral recumbent position. Certain maneuvers (Valsalva, deep inspiration, sudden postural changes, squatting, isometric exercise) can change the murmur's qualities.[6,11,16] Table 54-5 describes the characteristics of murmurs. Box 54-5 gives the scale for grading the loudness of murmurs.

Systolic murmurs, also called "benign" murmurs, are often caused by vigorous myocardial contraction or strong blood flow. Systolic murmurs begin with or after S_1 and end before S_2. They are common in children, adults younger than 50 years of age, and pregnant women. *Diastolic* murmurs begin with or after S_2 and end before S_1. All diastolic murmurs are pathologic. *Holosystolic* or *continuous* murmurs are present throughout S_1 and S_2.[6,11,16] Table 54-6 presents a comparison of selected heart murmurs.

BOX 54-5	Grading of Heart Murmurs*
Grade I	Faint; heard after listener has "tuned in"
Grade II	Faint murmur heard immediately
Grade III	Moderately loud, with accompanying thrill
Grade IV	Loud
Grade V	Very loud; heard only with the stethoscope
Grade VI	Very loud; heard without the stethoscope

*Heart murmurs are graded on a scale of 1 to 6 (I to VI).

Abdomen
Inspection
Examination of the abdomen provides information regarding cardiac competence. Abdominal assessment is described in Chapter 28, 32 and 42. Inspection may reveal abdominal distention.

Auscultation
Auscultation can yield clues about cardiovascular function including electrolyte imbalance, or atherosclerosis. Aortic bruits are heart just over or above the umbilicus. Renal bruits are heard over the upper midclavicular line laterally from the umbilicus.[6]

Palpitation
Palpation may confirm the presence of *ascites* (fluid accumulation in the peritoneal cavity) and an enlarged liver. In addition, you may elicit a hepatojugular reflex in the client with right ventricular distention. To do this, assess for jugular vein distention. Next, apply mild pressure with one hand over the liver for 1 minute. An increase in jugular vein distention during and immediately after liver compression indicates chronically elevated right ventricular pressure. Also palpate over the abdominal aorta located at midline, superior and inferior to the umbilicus. Assess the pulsation intensity and width.[6,11,16]

TABLE 54–5 Characteristics of Murmurs

Characteristic	Description
Location	Area where murmur is best heard
Loudness	Graded on a 6-point scale from I (barely audible) to VI (audible without stethoscope)
Pitch	Classified as either high or low; describe quality as musical, harsh, blowing, or buzzing
Place and duration	When murmur occurs during cardiac cycle: early, middle, or late; holosystolic or pansystolic murmurs are heard during entire systolic phase; ejection murmur is best heard during midsystole
Quality	A murmur's sound pattern; a *crescendo* starts low and grows louder; a *decrescendo* starts loud and gets softer; a *crescendo-decrescendo* starts softly, becomes loud, and then becomes soft again; a *plateau* is a consistent sound
Radiation	Sound migration to other parts of body; for example, aortic murmurs often radiate to carotid arteries, and mitral murmurs radiate to axillae
Timing	Refers to whether murmur occurs in systole or diastole; systolic murmurs, unlike diastolic murmurs, are harmless
Variations	Changes that occur with movement or interruption of normal respirations

Modified from Alexander, R.W., et al. (Eds.) (1998). *Hurst's the heart* (9th ed.). New York: McGraw-Hill; and O'Hanlon-Nickols, T. (1997). The adult cardiovascular system. *American Journal of Nursing, 97*(12), 34-40.

TABLE 54-6 Heart Murmurs

Type of Heart Sound	Origin	Preferred Method of Auscultation
Systolic Murmurs		
Ejection type	Systolic ejection murmurs are associated with forward blood flow during ventricular contraction across stenotic aortic or pulmonic valves.	Use the stethoscope diaphragm. Ejection murmurs are typically of medium pitch and harsh quality and may be associated with early ejection click. Aortic ejection murmurs are best heard over aortic valve and radiate into neck, down left sternal border, and occasionally to apex. May be accompanied by decreased S_2. Pulmonic ejection murmurs are heard best over pulmonic valve, and they radiate toward left shoulder and left neck vessels. May be accompanied by a wide split S_2.
Pansystolic regurgitant murmurs	Pansystolic murmurs occur when blood regurgitates through incompetent mitral and tricuspid valves (AV valves) or ventricular septal defect as pressures rise during systole and blood seeks chambers of lower pressure. Damage to valve leaflets, papillary muscles, and chordae tendineae results in mitral valve insufficiency (blood regurgitates from left ventricle to left atrium) and tricuspid valve insufficiency (blood regurgitates from right ventricle to right atrium). Ventricular septal defect results in blood regurgitation from left ventricle to right ventricle.	All regurgitant murmurs are high-pitched, and those of AV valve incompetence have blowing quality. Mitral regurgitant murmurs are heard at apex, radiate into left axilla, and may be accompanied by ejection click and signs of left ventricular failure. Tricuspid regurgitant murmurs are heard loudest over tricuspid area and radiate into sternum. Ventricular septal defects are usually loud, harsh, and heard best over left sternal border in fourth, fifth, and sixth intercostal spaces and radiate over precordium but not axilla.
Early systolic murmurs	Early systolic (innocent) murmurs are associated with high cardiac outputs, as blood flow velocity is increased across normal semilunar valves. Causes include anemia, tachycardia, thyrotoxicosis, and fever. Murmur disappears with correction of underlying condition. Normal variant in children.	These are best heard with bell over base of heart or along lower left sternal border. Are usually no greater than grade II, are of medium pitch, and have a blowing quality. Intensity may increase during inspiration with client in left recumbent position or with increased heart rates.
Late systolic murmurs	These imply mild mitral regurgitation as mitral valve balloons into left atrium late in ventricular systole.	Best heard with diaphragm of stethoscope over apex and are often preceded by midsystolic or late systolic ejection click.
Diastolic Murmurs		
Early diastolic murmur	These (decrescendo murmurs) are usually caused by semilunar valve insufficiency, with regurgitation resulting from valvular deformity or dilation of valvular ring. Are heard immediately after S_2 and then diminish in intensity as pressure in aorta or pulmonary artery falls and ventricles fill.	Heard best with diaphragm at base of heart while client leans forward in deep expiration. Are high-pitched and blowing and radiate down left sternal border, perhaps to apex or down right sternal border. Accompanying signs of heart failure may be present.
Diastolic filling rumbles	Caused by blood flow across stenotic AV valves (more often mitral). May also occur during augmented blood flow across normal AV valves. Murmur has two phases, becoming louder as blood flows from atrium to ventricle and increases with passive ventricular filling just after AV valve opening and again during atrial contraction (presystole).	Using bell, this murmur is heard over only a small area at and just medial to apex. Exercise and a left lateral position of the client increase intensity of sound. It is a low-pitched, rumbling sound often accompanied by an augmented S_1 and an opening snap.

AV, Atrioventricular.
Modified from Huang, S.L., et al. (1989). *Coronary care nursing* (2nd ed., p. 19). Philadelphia: Saunders; and Alexander, R.W., et al. (Eds.) (1998). *Hurst's the heart* (9th ed.). New York: McGraw-Hill.

Extremities
Skin
Observe the skin and mucous membranes for abnormalities such as central or peripheral *cyanosis*. The presence of a bluish tinge or duskiness is indicative of central cyanosis. Peripheral cyanosis is seen in lips, ear lobes, and nail beds.[6] Assess *capillary refill* (circulation) by putting slight pressure on a nail bed until it blanches (see

Chapter 51). Quickly release the pressure. When circulation is adequate, nail color returns to baseline in less than 3 seconds. Always check capillary refill before using pulse oximetry; if capillary refill is abnormal, pulse oximetry findings are inaccurate.

Skin Turgor

Assess skin turgor (elasticity) by lifting a fold of skin over the sternum or lower arms and releasing it (see Chapter 48). Normal skin immediately returns to the baseline position, but skin with decreased turgor stays pinched (tenting) for up to 30 seconds. Decreased skin turgor occurs with dehydration, volume depletion, rapid weight loss, and advanced age.

Temperature

The temperature of the skin may reflect cardiac disease. Along with the locations of warm or cold skin areas, the location of temperature changes assists in differentiating underlying pathology.[6,11,16]

Clubbing

Check fingers for clubbing, in which the distal tips of the fingers become bulbous and the angle between the base of the nail and the skin next to the cuticle increases from the normal 160 to 180 degrees or more (see Chapter 48). Also look for splinter hemorrhages of the nails.

Edema

Inspect dependent areas for edema. In the mobile client, edema is best seen in the feet, ankles, and lower legs. In the chair-ridden or bedridden client, edema may be palpated over the sacrum, abdomen, or scapula. Assess the severity of edema by pressing a thumb or finger carefully into the area. A depression that does not rapidly resume its original contour is noted as orthostatic, or pitting, edema.[6,11,16] Record whether edema is present or absent, and, if present, whether it is pitting or non-pitting.

DIAGNOSTIC TESTING

Diagnostic tests add objective findings that when added to the client's subjective information help to diagnose the presenting illness. Cardiac diagnostic procedures are both noninvasive (laboratory, electrocardiograms, Holter monitors, ultrasounds, x-rays, CT scans, stress tests, MRIs, tilt-table tests) and invasive (arteriography, hemodynamic studies, electrophysiologic studies). Nursing responsibilities for these various tests include (1) scheduling the procedure, (2) explaining the purpose and the procedure and answering any questions, (3) witnessing signing of the consent form, (4) providing any necessary preliminary care (adjustments in medications and special diets), (5) promoting maximal emotional and physical comfort, and (6) providing postprocedure care and instructions for home care, returning to work, and general

aftercare.[6,11,16,21] Please refer to a diagnostic and laboratory testing textbook for more specific information for the tests described in the following paragraphs.

Noninvasive Tests
Electrocardiographic Tests

Electrocardiographic tests are noninvasive tests in which patches are placed on the chest wall to obtain the electrical activity of the heart. The table Common Electrocardiographic Tests on the website describes the common electrographic tests and the clinical manifestations that may indicate the need for these tests.

Electrocardiogram. The electrocardiogram (ECG) is an essential tool in evaluating the heart's rhythm and signs of ischemia. The impulse waves, recorded by the ECG machine on graph paper, are designated by the letters P, QRS, and T. Figure 54-7 below depicts the typical ECG pattern formed by these waves. The P wave represents depolarization of the atria. The QRS complex represents depolarization of the ventricles. The T wave represents repolarization of the ventricles.[6]

An ECG tracing also shows the voltage of the waves and the duration of both the waves and the intervals. ECG graph paper is divided into horizontal lines and vertical lines, large squares and small squares. Voltage is represented on the vertical axis of the ECG paper. Each small square is 1 mm in height. Five small squares are equivalent to 5 mm, which is equivalent to 0.5 mV. Voltage yields information about the presence and degree of atrial or ventricular hypertrophy. Time is measured on the horizontal axis. Each small square signifies the passage of 0.04 second. Each large square indicates the passage of 0.20 second. By studying the

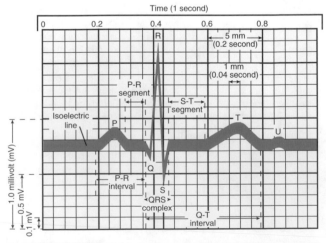

■ **FIGURE 54–7** Normal electrocardiographic (ECG) patterns. The P wave represents depolarization of the atria to the ventricles. The QRS complex represents depolarization of the ventricles, and the T wave represents repolarization of the ventricles. The small U wave is sometimes seen following the T wave. Time and voltage lines of ECG paper: *vertically,* 1 mm = 0.1 mV; 5 mm = 0.5 mV; 10 mm = 1 mV; *horizontally,* one small box = 0.04 second; five small boxes = 0.20 second; 25 small boxes = 1 second.

duration of the waves and intervals, the examiner can diagnose abnormal impulse formation and conduction.[6]

Normal time durations for waves and intervals are as follows:

- *P wave:* less than 0.11 second
- *PR interval:* 0.12 to 0.20 second
- *QRS complex:* 0.04 to 0.11 second
- *QT interval:* in women, up to 0.43 second; in men, up to 0.42 second

The standard ECG has a 12-lead system, offering 12 points of reference for recording the electrical activity of the heart, looking in both horizontal and vertical planes. The placement of 12-lead electrodes is shown in Figure 54-8. The standard 12-lead ECG has 6 *limb* leads (used to view the heart in a frontal or vertical plane) and 6 *precordial* leads (used to view the heart in a horizontal plane). Together, the 12 leads permit multidirectional examination of the electrical events in the heart. The location of pathologic change within the heart, which alters electrical activity (usually ST-segment elevation or depression), can be pinpointed.[6] Table 54-7 correlates the area of infarct with expected ECG changes and coronary artery lesion location.

Holter Monitoring. When the client wears a portable Holter monitor, an ECG tracing is recorded continuously, usually for 24 hours, on an outpatient basis. The Holter monitor may be used to detect dysrhythmias that may not appear on a routine ECG or evaluate the effectiveness of antidysrhythmics or pacemaker therapy. Clients may be asked to record manifestations that develop during the time they are wearing the monitor. A standard ECG records only seconds of cardiac activity.[6]

TABLE 54–7 Coronary Artery Lesion Location, Area of Infarct, and Electrocardiographic Changes

Coronary Artery	Area of Infarct	ECG Leads	Dysrhythmias
LAD	Anterior	V_{2-4}	RBBB, LAH, Mobitz type II, CHB
	Septal	V_{1-2}	
	Anteroseptal	V_{1-4}	
Circumflex	Lateral	I, aV_L	Ventricular and possibly SA and AV node conduction disturbances
	Anterolateral	I, aV_L, V_{5-6}	
	Inferolateral	aV_F, II, III, V_{5-6}	
	Posterior	Reciprocal, V_{1-3}	
RCA	Inferior	II, III, aV_F	SA node, AV node, and His bundle conduction disturbances
	Right ventricle	II, III, aV_R, V_{4-6R}	

AV, Atrioventricular; *CHB,* complete heart block; *LAD,* left anterior descending; *LAH,* left anterior hemiblock; *RBBB,* right bundle branch block; *RCA,* right coronary artery; *SA,* sinoatrial.
From Alspach, J.G. (Ed.) (1992). *Instructor's resource manual for the AACN core curriculum for critical care nursing.* Philadelphia: Saunders.

Exercise Tests

Exercise testing provides physiologic information regarding the heart's functional capacity to meet the metabolic demands caused by increasing exertion. Exercise testing is most often used in conjunction with nuclear scanning, and sometimes echocardiography, using a radionuclide tracer (thallium, dipyridamole, Cardiolite) to provide additional information regarding left ventricular wall motion

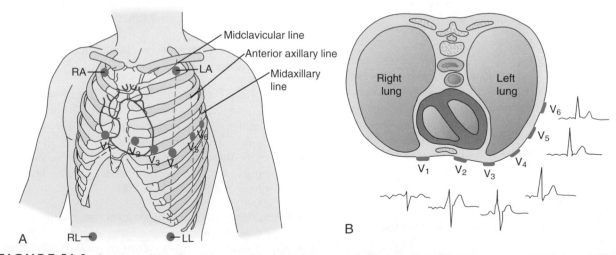

■ **FIGURE 54–8** Common positions for continuous monitoring lead placement. **A,** Five-lead system: RA electrode, below right clavicle at MCL; LA electrode, below left clavicle at MCL; RL electrode, right abdomen at MCL; LL electrode, left abdomen at MCL. V_1 to V_6 are the precordial or chest leads: V_1, fourth ICS at right sternal border; V_2, fourth ICS at left sternal border; V_3, fourth ICS, midway between left sternal border and MCL; V_4, fifth ICS at left MCL; V_5, fifth ICS, midway between left MCL and AAL; V_6, fifth ICS at left AAL. **B,** Normal electrocardiographic findings with corresponding chest leads to cross-section at the fourth rib level. *AAL,* Anterior axillary line; *ICS,* intercostal space; *LA,* left arm; *LL,* left leg; *MAL,* midaxillary line; *MCL,* midclavicular line; *RA,* right arm; *RL,* right leg.

during stress. Echocardiography also aids in revealing any wall motion abnormalities post stress. The perfusion scanning is performed with a special camera that is capable of showing the source of emitted low-energy photons on a screen. Each photon detected by the camera is recorded on film and a computer screen. The computer refines and enhances the images and then provides quantitative perfusion information about the myocardial walls.[21]

Exercise testing helps evaluate the presence, absence, or severity of coronary artery disease, both in clients with known CVD and in those initially seen with chest pain of unknown origin.[6,21] Exercise testing is usually indicated in low-risk clients only but may be indicated in post–open heart clients before beginning cardiac rehabilitation. Box 54-6 lists contraindications to exercise testing. Clients are instructed not to eat or smoke for 2 to 3 hours before the test and to dress appropriately for exercise. Most clients are allowed to take their usual medications unless the clinician orders otherwise.

Exercise testing may include bicycle ergometry or treadmill testing. Clients are exercised in stages in order to increase their heart rates to a value based on their age. Achieving their age-adjusted heart rate increases the reliability of test results. For those who cannot walk on the treadmill, or have underlying left bundle branch block on ECG (which may alter test results), nuclear scanning with intravenous Persantine provides reliable results. Persantine dilates coronary arteries to increase blood flow; however, arteries with plaque and blockage are unable to significantly dilate to allow increased perfusion. Intravenous dobutamine is an option for clients who cannot exercise.

BOX 54-6 Contraindications to Exercise Testing

ACUTE CARDIOVASCULAR DISEASE
- Acute myocardial infarction (usually avoided in clients less than 2 weeks after infarction)
- Unstable angina pectoris
- Heart failure
- Pericarditis
- Myocarditis
- Endocarditis
- Life-threatening dysrhythmias
- Thrombophlebitis
- Recent systemic embolism
- Dissecting or enlarging aneurysm

OTHERS
- Severe diseases restricting mobility
- Renal failure
- Severe pulmonary disruptions
- Orthopedic disorders affecting the spine or lower extremities
- Neurologic impairment (stroke or paralysis)
- Systemic infection
- Left ventricular outflow obstruction (aortic stenosis, hypertension, or hypertrophic cardiomyopathy)

A positive exercise test is indicated by one of the following results: (a) It must be terminated before the predicted maximal (or submaximal) limits have been achieved because of manifestations of cardiovascular intolerance. (b) ST-segment changes have occurred (horizontal ST-segment depression, ST-segment downsloping, or ST-segment upsloping is indicative of abnormal tracings). (c) Echocardiography or nuclear scanning will reveal wall motion abnormalities or reversible perfusion defects. In some people, ST-segment alterations may occur during exercise even though coronary artery disease is not present. Hyperventilation, certain drugs, and electrolyte imbalances can produce false-positive readings. On the other hand, false-negative findings also occur, although with less frequency. Medications such as beta-blocking agents and nitrates can produce false-negative results.[6,21] These medications may be held before the stress test to avoid inaccurate results.

Upright Tilt-Table Tests
Clients are tilted upright to a maximum of 60 to 80 degrees for 20 to 45 minutes while their heart rate and blood pressure are continuously monitored. Tests are positive for vasopressor syncope if both the heart rate and the blood pressure fall in unison. This procedure, when positive, reproduces the client's presenting manifestations.[6] Three to five electrodes are placed on the chest and connected to a monitor (with rhythm recording capabilities) at the client's side.

Radiographic Cardiac Tests
Renal functioning must be obtained before CT scanning or CT angiography because of contrast use. Because of the tracer used with MRI or MRA (which is not cleared through the kidneys), renal function is not a contraindication. This makes these tests especially useful for those clients with renal impairment.[34] Research reassessing the effect of tracer on impaired renal function continues. The table on Common Radiographic Cardiac Tests on the website *evolve* describes these tests and the clinical manifestations indicating the need for these tests.

Chest X-Ray. Posteroanterior, lateral, and oblique chest x-ray films assist in assessing the heart, lungs, and aorta. For the acutely ill client, a portable anteroposterior x-ray study is performed at the bedside. Specific pathologic changes of the heart are difficult to determine with x-ray examination, but anatomic changes, and line or tube placements can be assessed.[6,16]

CT Angiography. Computerized tomography (CT) angiography most commonly includes electron beam tomography (EBT) or modern multivector computerized tomography (MVCT). This scan allows a noninvasive way to evaluate the coronary arteries, great vessels, aorta, renal arteries, and lower extremity arteries through two- or three-dimensional images.[6,16]

CT Scan per Pulmonary Embolus Protocol. In a CT scan with pulmonary embolus protocol, extra contrast is used to enhance the pulmonary arteries. This is an alternative to ventilation-perfusion lung scans, and is now used as the principal diagnostic test to rule out pulmonary emboli.[6,16]

Magnetic Resonance Imaging. Although MRI is one of the most expensive noninvasive diagnostic options, a variety of data may be obtained in a single image. MRI can show the heart beating and the blood flowing in any direction. All standard quantitative functional indices, except transstenotic gradients, can be obtained from an MRI study.[6,16]

Magnetic Resonance Angiography. MRA is similar to MRI, but it uses gadolinium as intravenous contrast medium to evaluate arterial disease. Gadolinium differs from other contrast media because it is not nephrotoxic; thus clients with renal insufficiency can safely undergo this procedure. Research regarding the safety of Gadolinium on impaired renal function is in progress. Along with coronary MRA, pulmonary, renal, and peripheral arteries can also be studied.[6,16]

Viability Scan. Positron emission tomography (PET) allows visualization of regional physiologic function and biochemical changes that often separate normal from diseased myocardium. Cellular metabolic information is obtained by mapping regional myocardial glucose metabolism while a tracer is used to obtain left ventricular perfusion. Combining information from the perfusion and metabolism images provides a thorough assessment of regional cardiac viability. Clients with decreased perfusion but preserved glucose uptake have viable, or hibernating, myocardium. This information is critical regarding the need for coronary artery revascularization, which is indicated if viable myocardium is detected.[21]

Echocardiogram

Echocardiography, a noninvasive diagnostic procedure based on the principles of ultrasonography, provides another way to look at the heart's structure. An echocardiogram is obtained by placing a transducer on several areas of the chest wall. Bursts of ultrasound waves are directed at the part of the heart under investigation. The echocardiogram records the structure, and motion of that area in relation to its distance from the anterior chest wall. An ECG is recorded simultaneously on the graph. Two-dimensional echocardiography generates a continuous picture of the beating heart. The images are recorded on videotape for analysis.[6] The table Common Cardiac Ultrasonographic Tests on the website describes these tests and the clinical manifestations that may indicate the need for these tests.

Invasive Cardiac Tests
Transesophageal Echocardiography

Transesophageal echocardiography (TEE) yields a higher quality picture of the heart than does regular echocardiography. It is especially useful for clients who have thickened lung tissue or thick chest walls or who are obese. Transesophageal echocardiography eliminates the interference of the thoracic structures and provides an excellent image of the heart and great vessels from a posterior view. Because the probe is placed behind the heart, it allows the left atrium to be viewed easily. The procedure may also be used intraoperatively, where conventional echocardiography is ineffective.[6]

Cardiac Catheterization

This complex procedure involves insertion of a catheter into the heart, coronary arteries, and surrounding vessels to obtain detailed information about the structure and performance of the heart, the valves, and the circulatory system. Cardiac catheterization includes both left and right heart catheterization and is performed in a special cardiac catheterization laboratory.[6] Please refer to a diagnostic procedures handbook for discussion of the preprocedure and postprocedure nursing care and possible complications after cardiac catheterization. The table Common Cardiac Invasive Procedures on the website describes the common invasive cardiac procedures and the clinical manifestations that may indicate the need for these tests.

Left Heart Catheterization. Catheters are inserted through the femoral artery or radial artery leading to the aorta and coronary arteries. Each coronary artery is selectively cannulated and contrast is injected into the artery as cineangiography is obtained. Cineangiography provides moving pictures of contrast flow through the coronary arteries or as the left ventricle contracts. These pictures can be viewed at both rapid and slow speeds, permitting detailed and unlimited review of the study. Plaque, or blockage, manifests itself by narrowing of the artery lumen. This information is critical to optimize treatment of atherosclerotic heart disease. There is less that 1% risk of major complication and less than 0.08% mortality risk with this procedure.[6]

Right Heart Catheterization. Although right heart catheterization is conducted in the cardiac catheterization laboratory, hemodynamic monitoring can be conducted at the bedside. A Swan-Ganz catheter is inserted via the brachial vein or femoral vein and progressed through the vena cava into the right atrium, right ventricle, and finally the pulmonary artery. The catheter has several end or side holes that allow blood withdrawal for oxygen analysis from the various cardiac chambers. Hemodynamic pressure monitoring provides information about blood volume, fluid balance, how well the heart is pumping, valvular structures, or shunting.

Current technology allows measurement of right atrial pressure or central venous pressure (CVP); pulmonary artery (PA) pressures during systole and diastole, which reflects right and left ventricular pressures; and pulmonary capillary wedge pressure (PCWP), which is an indirect indicator of left ventricular pressure and cardiac output (CO), reflecting the heart's output in liters per minute, cardiac index (CI), systemic vascular resistance (SVR), pulmonary vascular resistances (PVR) and various stroke volumes. These pressures are obtained by attaching the catheter to a transducer with its connecting amplifier and recording device. Critical care nurses perform all of these studies routinely at the bedside. Hemodynamic studies provide a wealth of information reflecting the earliest changes in the circulatory system that are not yet clinically detectable.[6,11,16] The Bridge to Critical Care feature below and on p. 1381 illustrates Swan-Ganz monitoring.

BRIDGE TO CRITICAL CARE

Swan-Ganz Monitoring (PA Catheter)

POSITIONING THE SWAN-GANZ CATHETER

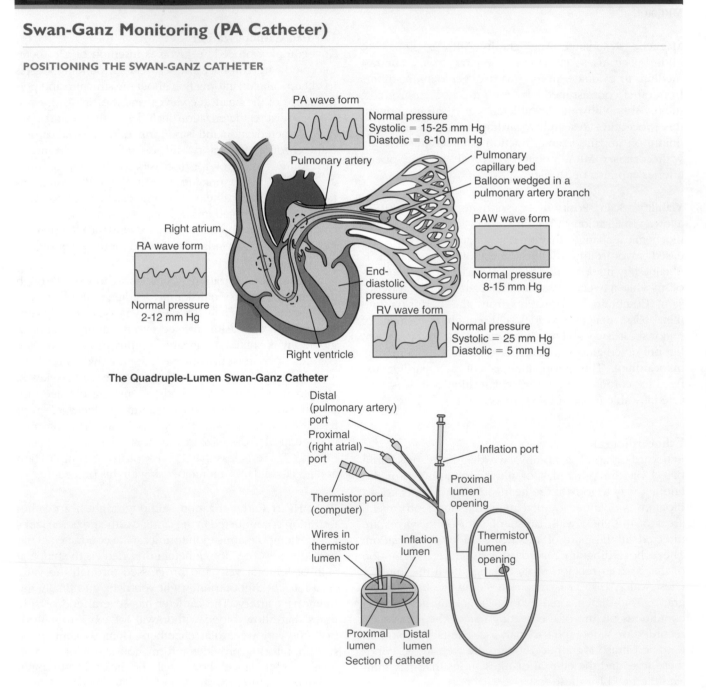

The Quadruple-Lumen Swan-Ganz Catheter

Electrophysiologic Studies

The electrophysiologic study is an invasive method of recording intracardiac electrical activity. It is used to (1) shed light on the mechanisms of dysrhythmias, (2) differentiate between supraventricular and ventricular dysrhythmias, (3) evaluate sinoatrial (SA) or AV node dysfunction, (4) determine the need for a pacemaker, and (5) evaluate the effect of antidysrhythmic agents used to prevent the occurrence of tachycardias. These studies, like cardiac catheterization, are conducted in a specialized laboratory where equipment and monitors are readily available.[6]

The purpose of the procedure is to reproduce any dysrhythmia so that its origin may be isolated. If a dysrhythmia is induced, the client's BP and hemodynamic responses are observed. It is possible to record simultaneously arterial pressure, surface ECGs, and ECGs from intracavitary catheters. The morphology and rate of any induced dysrhythmias are compared with those of the client's spontaneous dysrhythmia.

BRIDGE TO CRITICAL CARE

Swan-Ganz Monitoring (PA Catheter)—Cont'd

MEASURING CARDIAC OUTPUT BY THERMODILUTION

Conditions with Expected Pressure Changes

Condition	Pressure Changes			
	RAP	**RVP**	**PAP**	**PAWP**
Heart failure (volume overload)	↑	↑	↑	↑
Hypovolemia	↓	↓	↓	↓
Cardiogenic shock*	none or ↑	none or ↑	none or ↑	none or ↑ (diastolic)
Pulmonary hypertension	↑	↑	↑	none or ↑
Cardiac tamponade	↑	↑	↑	↑ (diastolic)
Pulmonary emboli	↑	↑	↑	↑ (systolic)
Mitral valve stenosis/insufficiency†	↑	↑	↑	↑

PAP, Pulmonary artery pressure; *PAWP*, pulmonary artery wedge pressure; *RAP*, right atrial pressure; *RVP*, right ventricular pressure.
*Pressure readings depend on the heart's ability to handle circulating volume. Chronic lung disease elevates all readings.
†Mitral valve disease produces unreliable pressure readings.

Laboratory Tests

Laboratory test data are used to (1) diagnose a variety of cardiovascular ailments (myocardial infarction), (2) screen people considered at risk for CVD, (3) determine baseline values, (4) identify concurrent disorders (anemia, diabetes mellitus, electrolyte imbalance, renal or liver abnormalities) that may affect treatment, and (5) evaluate the effectiveness of intervention. Tests that are more commonly used to determine cardiovascular function and disease are discussed here. The table Common Cardiac Laboratory Tests on the website provides a description of the tests and possible etiologies for abnormal findings. Please refer to a laboratory tests textbook for the specifics of collecting and handling these blood samples.

Complete Blood Cell Count

Measuring the packed cell volume, or *hematocrit,* is the easiest way to ascertain the concentration of red blood cells in the blood. Clients with anemia have a significant reduction in red blood cell mass and a decrease in oxygen-carrying capacity. Anemia can be manifested as angina or it can exacerbate heart failure and produce heart murmurs.[6,12]

The *white blood cell (WBC) count* is elevated in infectious and inflammatory diseases of the heart. It is commonly seen after myocardial infarction because large numbers of WBCs are necessary to dispose of the necrotic tissue resulting from the infarction.[6,12]

Cardiac Enzymes

Enzymes are special proteins that catalyze chemical reactions in living cells. Cardiac enzymes are present in high concentrations in myocardial tissue. Tissue damage causes release of enzymes from their intracellular storage areas. For example, myocardial infarction causes cellular anoxia, which alters membrane permeability and causes spillage of enzymes into the surrounding tissue. This leakage of enzymes can be detected by rising plasma levels. Cardiac enzyme levels reflect myocardial infarction (cellular death).[6,12]

Myoglobin is a useful marker of myocardial necrosis; it is rapidly released from the circulation within 1 to 2 hours of infarction. Its release allows very early detection of myocardial infarction, but its short half-life makes it less useful in clients who present several hours after onset. This enzyme is not cardiac specific and although it increases early, it is not the most reliable indicator of an MI. Measurement of myoglobin levels is not recommended if there is evidence of muscle damage, trauma, or renal failure because of the greater potential for false-positive test results in these circumstances.[6,12]

The enzymes most commonly used to detect myocardial infarction because of their excellent sensitivity are *creatine kinase* (CK) and *troponin.* There are three CK isoenzymes: CK-MM (skeletal muscle), CK-MB (myocardial muscle), and CK-BB (brain). Troponin has three components: I, C, and T. Troponin I modulates the contractile state, troponin C binds calcium, and troponin T binds troponins I and C. Although troponin is present in all striated muscle, troponin components in cardiac muscle have different amino acid sequences. Therefore antibodies against cardiac troponins I and T are very specific. Elevated levels of troponin I are as sensitive as CK-MB for the detection of myocardial injury. Because of their higher specificity for myocardial injury, troponins can be used to exclude myocardial infarction when CK-MB may be falsely positive.[6,12,16] Troponin I is the definitive laboratory test for diagnosis of an MI.

Plasma CK-MB can be initially seen within 2 hours of symptom onset, is significantly elevated within 6 to 8 hours of symptom onset, and returns to normal after 48 to 72 hours. Troponin can also be seen in 2 hours after symptom onset, peaks within 6 to 10 hours of symptom onset, and persists for 4 to 7 days. Therefore blood samples should be taken immediately on admission and every 6 to 8 hours for the first 24 hours. Diagnosis of injury requires no fewer than two samples separated by at least 4 hours.[6,10,12,16]

Blood Coagulation Tests

Evaluate coagulation tests such as *prothrombin time* and *partial thromboplastin time* in people with a greater tendency to form thrombi. Research has shown an increase in coagulation factors during and after a myocardial infarction.[6] Therefore the client is at greater risk for thrombophlebitis and extension of clots in the coronary artery. Coagulation studies are ordered to guide dosage of antithrombotic drugs. Chapter 74 discusses coagulation tests in detail.

Serum Lipids

Coronary heart disease is secondary to atherosclerosis and accumulation of lipids within the arterial wall, which is associated with inflammation and vascular remodeling. The cholesterol-containing lipid fraction most closely associated with atherogenesis is low-density-lipoprotein cholesterol (LDL-C). Coronary heart disease risk increases as blood levels of LDL-C increase. The recommended goal for LDL-C is <100 mg/dL, but when the client's risk is very high as with a previous event, the LDL-C goal is <70 mg/dL.[13] A second lipid fraction that plays a major role in determining CVD risk is high-density-lipoprotein cholesterol (HDL-C). Coronary heart disease risk decreases as blood levels of HDL-C increase. These lipids are composed of fatty substances that are insoluble in water. They are derived from fats in the diet or synthesized in the liver.[3,5,12] Serum lipids are discussed in Chapter 56.

C-Reactive Protein

Atherosclerosis is in part a chronic low-grade inflammatory condition. Elevation of levels of C-reactive protein (CRP), an acute-phase protein that measures the presence and degree of inflammation within the arterial walls, has been linked to future cardiovascular risks, including stroke, myocardial infarction, and cardiovascular death.[6,12]

D-Dimer

Plasma D-dimer level is determined by enzyme-linked immunosorbent assay; levels reflect plasmin's breakdown of fibrin (indicating thrombolysis). D-dimer levels are elevated in greater than 90% of clients with pulmonary embolus. If positive, and pulmonary embolus is a suspicion, lung scanning or ventilation-perfusion scanning is recommended.[6,12]

Serum Electrolytes

Fluid and electrolyte regulation may be affected by cardiovascular disorders or medications. In addition, electrolyte levels can alter cardiac muscle contraction.[6,12] Chapters 11 and 12 describe fluids and electrolytes in more detail.

Potassium. *Hypokalemia* (abnormally low potassium level) increases cardiac electrical instability, the occurrence of ventricular dysrhythmias, and the risk of digitalis toxicity. A characteristic change on the ECG is a U wave but this finding alone is not considered diagnostic for hypokalemia. *Hyperkalemia* (elevated potassium level) can lead to a tall T wave on the ECG, asystole, and ventricular dysrhythmias.[6,11,12,16]

Sodium. The serum sodium level reflects water balance. Hyponatremia indicates water excess. Hypernatremia indicates sodium excess.[12]

Calcium. Calcium is considered an important mediator of many cardiovascular functions because of its effect on cardiac excitability, contractility, and vascular tone. Hypocalcemia (low calcium level) can lead to serious ventricular dysrhythmias, a prolonged QT interval, and cardiac arrest. Hypercalcemia (elevated calcium level) shortens the QT interval and causes AV block, tachycardia, bradycardia, digitalis hypersensitivity, and cardiac arrest.[6,12]

Magnesium. Magnesium helps regulate intracellular metabolism, activates essential enzymes, and aids transport of sodium and potassium across the cell membrane. It plays a vital role in neuromuscular excitability. Low magnesium levels (hypomagnesemia) may cause mental apathy, facial tics, leg cramps, respiratory depression, and severe cardiac dysrhythmias, including ventricular tachycardia and fibrillation. Elevated magnesium levels (hypermagnesemia) may cause profound muscle weakness, hyporeflexia, hypotension, and bradycardia with a prolonged PR interval and wide QRS complex.[6,12]

Phosphorus. Most extracellular phosphorus is present in the bone with calcium (85% of the body's total phosphorus). A small amount of phosphorus is found in intracellular fluid. There, it helps regulate energy formation (adenosine triphosphate [ATP]) and maintain acid-base balance and neuromuscular excitability. Phosphate levels are inversely related to calcium levels as the kidneys retain or excrete one or the other. Interpret the two levels together. Low phosphorus levels (hypophosphatemia) may cause bleeding, decreased WBC levels, muscular weakness (including respiratory muscles), and nausea and vomiting. Elevated levels (hyperphosphatemia) may cause manifestations similar to those of hypocalcemia, with muscle tetany being the most common finding.[6,12]

Urea Nitrogen, Creatinine, and GFR. Urea nitrogen, also known as blood urea nitrogen (BUN), serum creatinine, and glomerular filtration rate (GFR) are indicators of renal function, specifically the ability of the kidney to excrete urea and protein. Renal function must be assessed before any procedures using contrast (CT scans, angiography, or angiograms). Contrast is cleared through the kidneys and clients may be at risk for acute renal failure when undergoing those procedures.[6,12]

Serum Glucose. Diabetes mellitus is a major risk factor for the development of atherosclerosis. In addition, the stress of an acute cardiac event can greatly elevate blood glucose level, causing unstable hyperglycemia in clients with latent diabetes mellitus. For these reasons, blood glucose level is routinely assessed in all clients with acute cardiovascular disorders.[6,12,16]

CONCLUSIONS

With the rising incidence and prevalence of CVD, the role of nurses is more important than ever regarding client assessment, treatment, and education. Especially important is education regarding risk factor modification, as it is estimated that more than 50% of CVD deaths and disability can be eliminated by a combination of cost-effective national and individual efforts to reduce risk factors.[3] Learning to obtain a thorough history and conduct a comprehensive physical examination requires repetition and perseverance. These data are just as important as the results of noninvasive and invasive studies if the nurse is to continue to assess the client effectively, provide primary preventive care, and monitor treatment. Assessment skills and nursing interventions can make a significant difference in the client's quality of life by preventing complications and improving outcomes. By helping the client you also impact that client's family and support system, who in turn may by compelled to modify risk factors and seek preventive care. Through these efforts, the goal of *Healthy People 2010* (to improve overall cardiovascular health and quality of life through prevention, assessment, detection, risk factor management, and early diagnosis and treatment) may be attained.

BIBLIOGRAPHY

Citations appearing in red refer to primary research.

Citations appearing in blue refer to evidence-based practice guidelines and protocols.

1. American Heart Association. (2005). *American Heart Association guidelines for primary prevention of cardiovascular disease and stroke.* Accessed 03/28/06 at www.americanheart.org/presenter. jhtml?identifier=4704.
2. American Heart Association. (2003). Case definitions for acute coronary heart disease in epidemiology and clinical research studies: A statement from the AHA Council on Epidemiology and Prevention; AHA Statistics Committee; World Heart Federation Council on Epidemiology and Prevention; the European Society of Cardiology Working Group on National Heart, Lung, and Blood Institute. *Circulation, 108*(20), 2543-2549.
3. American Heart Association. (2006). Heart disease and stroke statistics—2006 update: A report from the American Heart Association Statistics Committee and Stroke Statistics Subcommittee. *Circulation, 113*(6), 85-151.
4. American Heart Association. (2006). Obesity and cardiovascular disease: Pathophysiology, evaluation, and effect of weight loss: An update of the 1997 American Heart Association Scientific Statement on Obesity and Heart Disease from the Obesity Committee of the Council on Nutrition, Physical Activity, and Metabolism. *Circulation, 113*(6), 898-918.
5. American Heart Association. (2006). Prevention of coronary heart disease and the National Cholesterol Education Program. *Circulation, 113*(5), 598-600.
6. Braunwald, E., Zipes, D.P., Libby, P., et al. (2005). *Braunwald's heart disease: A textbook of cardiovascular medicine* (7th ed.). Philadelphia: Saunders.
7. Centers for Disease Control and Prevention. (2004). *Smoking among adults: Coronary heart disease and stroke.* Accessed 8/6/06 at www.cdc.gov.tobacco/sgr/sgr_2004/Factsheets/3.htm.
7a. Centers for Disease Control and Prevention. (2008). Healthy People 2010. Accessed 1/2/08 at www.cdc.gov/nchs/hphome.htm#Healthy%20People%202010.
8. Chahal, P.S., & Rao, S.S. (2005). Functional chest pain: Nociception and visceral hyperalgesia. *Journal of Clinical Gastroenterology, 39*(4, Suppl 3), 204-209.
9. Chen, W., Woods, S.L., & Puntillo, K.A. (2005). Gender differences in symptoms associated with acute myocardial infarction: A review of the research. *Heart & Lung, 34*(4), 240-247.
10. Ferri, F.F. (2006). *Ferri's clinical advisor: Instant diagnosis and treatment.* Philadelphia: Mosby.
11. Fink, M.P., Abraham, E., Vincent, J., et al. (2005). *Textbook of critical care* (5th ed.). Philadelphia: Saunders.
12. Fishbach, F.T. (2004). *A manual of laboratory & diagnostic tests* (7th ed.). Philadelphia: Lippincott.
13. Grundy, S.M., Cleeman, J.L., & Merz, C.N., et al. (2004). Implications of recent clinical trials for the National Cholesterol Education Program Adult Treatment Panel III Guidelines. *Circulation, 110*, 227-239.
14. Habib, P.A., Huang, G., Mendiola, J.A., et al. (2004). Anterior chest pain: Musculoskeletal considerations. *Emergency Radiology, 11*, 37-45.
15. Kannel, W.B. (1961). The Framingham study. *Annals of Internal Medicine, 55*, 33-50.
16. Kasper, D.L., Braunwald, E., Fauci, A.S., et al. (2005). *Harrison's principles of internal medicine* (16th ed.). New York: McGraw-Hill.
17. Kris-Etherton, P.M. (1999). American Heart Association Science Advisory: Monounsaturated fatty acids and risk of cardiovascular disease. American Heart Association Nutrition Committee. *Circulation, 100*, 1253-1258.
18. Kuczmarski, R.J., Flegal, K.M., Campbell, S.M., et al. (1994). Increasing prevalence of overweight among United States adults: The National Health and Nutrition Examination Surveys, 1960 to 1991. *Journal of the American Medical Association, 272*, 205-211.
19. McSweeney, J.C., Cody, M., O'Sullivan, P., et al. (2003). Women's early warning symptoms of acute myocardial infarction. *Circulation, 108*, 2619-2623.
20. McSweeney, J.C., Lefler, L.L., & Crowder, B.F. (2005). What's wrong with me? Women's coronary heart disease diagnostic experiences. *Progress in Cardiovascular Nursing, 20*(2), 48-57.
21. Meltler, F.A., & Guiberteau, M.J. (2006). *Essentials of nuclear medicine imaging* (5th ed.). Philadelphia: Saunders.
22. Mokdad, A.H., Serdula, M.K., Dietz, W.H., et al. (1999). The spread of the obesity epidemic in the United States, 1991-1998. *Journal of the American Medical Association, 282*, 1519-1522.
23. National Heart, Lung, and Blood Institute Joint National Committee on Prevention, Detection, Evaluation, and Treatment of High Blood Pressure. (2003). The seventh report of the Joint National Committee on Prevention, Detection, Evaluation, and Treatment of High Blood Pressure: The JNC-7 report. *Journal of the American Medical Association, 289*(19), 2560-2572.
24. National Institutes of Health. (2005). *Heart and circulation.* Accessed 03/28/06 at www.nih.gov.
25. Ounpuus, S., Negassa, A., & Yusuf, S. (2001). INTER-HEART: A global study of risk factors for acute myocardial infarction. *American Heart Journal, 141*, 711-721.
26. Postgraduate Institute for Medicine. (2006). *New insights in efficacy and safety of combination therapy with statins and fibrates.* [Brochure]. New York: Jobson Publishing Group.
27. *Remington: The science and practice of pharmacy* (21st ed.). (2005). Philadelphia: Lippincott Wilkins & Wilkins.
28. Sapira, J.D. (1990). *Science of bedside diagnosis.* Baltimore: Urban & Schwatzneberg.
29. Sudano, I., Binggeli, C., Spieker, L., et al. (2005). Cardiovascular effects of coffee: Is it a risk factor? *PCVN, 20*(2), 65-69.
30. Swap, C.J., & Nagurney, J.T. (2005). Value and limitations of chest pain history in the evaluation of patients with suspected acute coronary syndromes. *Journal of the American Medical Association, 294*(20), 2623-2630.
31. Wild, S., Roglic, G., Sicree, et al. (2004). Global prevalence of diabetes: Estimates for the year 2000 and projections for 2030. *Diabetes Care, 27*, 1047-1053.
32. World Health Organization. (2005). *Cardiovascular disease.* Accessed 03/28/06 at www.who.int/.
33. World Health Organization Expert Panel on Detection, Evaluation, and Treatment of High Blood Cholesterol in Adults. (May 2001). *Third report of the National Cholesterol Education Program (NCEP)* (NIH Pub No. 01-3670.) Washington, DC: National Heart, Lung, and Blood Institute.

CHAPTER 55

Management of Clients with Structural Cardiac Disorders

BARBARA B. OTT AND MARIE A. DEFRANCESCO-LOUKAS

The movement of blood through the heart is crucial for human life. But in addition to perfusion, blood must flow through the heart in an efficient and orderly manner. This chapter focuses on the cardiac disorders that affect the structure of the heart and impair the efficiency of the heart as a pump.

VALVULAR HEART DISEASE

When heart valves that normally move blood efficiently through the heart chambers cannot fully open or fully close, perfusion of the heart and distal tissues is impaired and the heart muscle is strained. A stenosed valve may impede the flow of blood from one chamber to the next; an insufficient (incompetent) valve may allow blood to regurgitate (flow backward) (Table 55-1). The aortic and mitral valves become dysfunctional more often than do the pulmonary and tricuspid valves. This change occurs because the left side of the heart is a system of higher pressures compared with the lower pressures in the pulmonary circulation.

Valvular heart disease remains fairly common in the United States even though the incidence is steadily decreasing as the incidence of rheumatic fever decreases. Mitral valve prolapse syndrome is one of the most common cardiac abnormalities; as much as 5% of the population is affected, and women are affected more often than men.

MITRAL VALVE DISEASE

The mitral valve separates the left atrium from the left ventricle. Therefore problems with blood flow through the mitral valve affect left ventricular output and hence activity tolerance.

Etiology and Risk Factors

The predominant cause of mitral valve disease is rheumatic fever. Acute rheumatic fever leads to inflammation of the endocardium. The inflammation causes the valve leaflets and chordae tendineae to become fibrous. The chordae tendineae shorten, which narrows the outflow tract (see Table 55-1).

Mitral regurgitation develops from problems with the leaflets, chordae tendineae, papillary muscles, or mitral opening. The major causes of mitral regurgitation are mitral valve prolapse, myocardial ischemia, rheumatic heart disease, cardiomyopathy, and calcification of the opening. Rheumatic heart disease is preventable with early detection of beta-hemolytic streptococcal infections (the precursor to rheumatic heart disease).

Myocardial ischemia from coronary artery disease affects the mitral valve in many ways. Ischemia leads to loss of contractility, which affects mitral valve performance. Portions of the papillary muscle are fed by the coronary vessels, and when the vessels cannot provide blood flow to the myocardium, the leaflets may also not be supplied.

Mitral valve prolapse is the bulging of one or both of the valve leaflets into the left atrium during ventricular systole. Usually it occurs as a primary condition that is not associated with other diseases. However, it can occur in genetic diseases of connective tissues—such as

---

evolve **Web Enhancements**

Care Plan   The Client with Dilated Cardiomyopathy

Client Education Guide   Infective Endocarditis (English Version and Spanish Translation)

Be sure to check out the bonus material on the Evolve website and the CD-ROM, including free self-assessment exercises. **http://evolve.elsevier.com/Black/medsurg**

TABLE 55-1 Mitral and Aortic Valve Stenosis and Regurgitation

Pathophysiology

Mitral stenosis (MS) is a narrowing of the inlet valve into the left ventricle that prevents proper opening during diastolic filling. Clients with mitral stenosis typically have mitral valve leaflets that are thickened, openings that are fused, and/or chordae tendineae that are thickened and shortened. As the opening gets smaller, the left atrial pressure (LAP) rises to maintain a normal cardiac output. The increase in LAP also enlarges the left atrium and raises pulmonary venous and capillary pressures. The resulting pulmonary congestion and reduced cardiac output can mimic primary left ventricular failure, but left ventricular contractility is normal in most cases of mitral stenosis. As the disease evolves, chronic elevation of LAP

Marfan syndrome and osteogenesis imperfecta—and after the ingestion of appetite suppressant drugs.

eventually leads to pulmonary hypertension, tricuspid and pulmonary valve incompetence, and secondary right heart failure. Eventually, there is loss of blood flow into the left ventricle and cardiac output falls.

Mitral insufficiency and regurgitation is due to scarring and retraction of the valve leaflets, resulting in incomplete closure. Mitral regurgitation occurs during systole, when much pressure is generated within the left ventricle to eject it forward into the aorta. When the mitral valve does not close, blood flows backward into the left atrium. The backward flow of blood causes left atrial and left ventricular enlargement. The left atrium dilates and hypertrophies in response to the large volume of blood it is receiving during systole. In response to the large amount of blood lost to the left atrium, the left ventricle must pump harder to preserve cardiac output and also hypertrophies. This hypertrophy of the left ventricle eventually leads to left ventricular failure (see Table 55-1). Over time the increase in blood flow to the left atrium causes a rise in left atrial pressure. This pressure is reflected backward into the pulmonary venous and arterial system. With continued high pressures, right-sided heart failure can develop.

Mitral valve prolapse occurs when the anterior and posterior cusps of the mitral valve billow upward into the atrium during systolic contraction. The chordae tendineae lengthen, allowing the valve cusps to stretch upward. The cusps may be enlarged and thickened. Mitral valve prolapse is often accompanied by mitral regurgitation, causing backward flow of blood into the atrium during systole.

Clinical Manifestations

The clinical manifestations of mitral valvular heart disease may appear gradually or suddenly. Auscultation will reveal a typical pattern of murmur. It is important to note where on the chest wall the murmur is heard best and during what phase of the cardiac cycle it occurs. Asking the client to hold his or her breath may help to distinguish the murmur from respiratory sounds.

Mitral Stenosis

Manifestations of mitral stenosis are usually insidious, occurring over several years after the infection. Clients often report decreased exercise tolerance, dyspnea, orthopnea, and paroxysmal nocturnal dyspnea. On auscultation a loud first heart sound is heard and then an opening "snap" that ushers in a low-pitched, rumbling diastolic murmur. The opening snap is best heard at the apex with the diaphragm of the stethoscope. The diastolic murmur is best heard at the apex using the bell of the stethoscope while the client is in a left lateral recumbent position. Manifestations of right-sided heart failure may also be present.

Atrial fibrillation is a common finding in clients with mitral stenosis. During episodes of atrial fibrillation, the pulse becomes irregular and faint and the blood pressure often drops. Hemoptysis is also seen frequently. Ineffective atrial contractions allow some stagnation of blood in the left atrium and encourage the formation of mural thrombi. These thrombi easily break away and travel as emboli throughout the arterial system, causing tissue infarction. These areas appear as dark areas or areas of necrotic tissue, especially on the toes, where vessels are small.

Mitral Regurgitation

Clients with mitral regurgitation may be asymptomatic until cardiac output falls. Reduced cardiac output first leads to fatigue and dyspnea. Clinical manifestations gradually increase to include orthopnea, paroxysmal nocturnal dyspnea, and peripheral edema. Pulmonary manifestations are less severe than in mitral stenosis because changes in the mean pulmonary capillary pressure are less exaggerated. When the right side of the heart is affected, the manifestations are the same as in mitral stenosis.

Auscultation reveals a blowing, high-pitched systolic murmur with radiation to the left axilla, heard best at the apex. The first heart sound may be diminished, and often a splitting of the second sound is heard. Severe regurgitation is associated with a third heart sound (S_3). Vital signs are usually normal unless mitral regurgitation is severe. Atrial fibrillation is common in clients with this condition; however, emboli and hemoptysis occur far less often than in mitral stenosis.

Mitral Valve Prolapse

It is not uncommon for clients with mitral valve prolapse to be completely asymptomatic. In a healthy client, physical examination may disclose a regurgitant murmur or a midsystolic click on auscultation. Manifestations may be vague; if present, they include tachycardia, lightheadedness, syncope, fatigue, weakness, dyspnea, chest discomfort, anxiety, and palpitations related to dysrhythmias. Minimal morbidity and mortality are associated with mitral valve prolapse, and clinically clients have no physical limitations.

Various diagnostic assessments are used to detect valvular lesions or structural heart changes. These studies include echocardiography, chest radiography, stress tests, and cardiac catheterization.

OUTCOME MANAGEMENT

The goals of treatment for the asymptomatic client are to prevent beta-hemolytic streptococcal infection, which could lead to infective endocarditis, as discussed in the Translating Evidence into Practice feature on p. 1388. The prognosis is good for this group of clients. The goals of medical management of the symptomatic clients are to maintain cardiac output and activity tolerance. When cardiac output falls or the client is unable to tolerate simple activities, the valve can be surgically replaced.

Mitral Stenosis

Clients with mitral stenosis resulting from rheumatic heart disease should receive penicillin prophylaxis for beta-hemolytic streptococcal infections as well as for infective endocarditis. Prompt aggressive treatment of anemia and infections is also warranted. Adolescents and young adults with severe mitral stenosis should avoid entering professions and occupations that may require strenuous physical exertion. For clients that have experienced one or more previous pulmonary embolic episodes, anticoagulant therapy is helpful in preventing venous thrombosis and pulmonary embolism.

TRANSLATING EVIDENCE INTO PRACTICE

Preventing Infective Endocarditis

The number of cases of infective endocarditis is rising and the types of clients are changing. It remains a life-threatening infection responsible for substantial morbidity and mortality. The American Heart Association (AHA) has established guidelines for antibiotic prophylaxis to prevent bacterial endocarditis in high-risk clients.[1,2] Prophylactic antibiotics are administered according to the risk associated with various procedures. Risk for bacteremia is highest with dental extractions and oral surgical procedures, moderate for procedures affecting the genitourinary tract, and lowest for gastrointestinal diagnostic procedures.

Successful prophylaxis depends on client adherence. If clients do not understand the reason for prophylaxis and implications for their health, they may not adhere to the regimen. Nurses can play a key role in preventing bacterial endocarditis in high-risk clients by teaching them and their families the significance of prophylactic antibiotic treatment. Stucki and colleagues found that even after an educational program on the need for prophylaxis, 15% did not remember receiving such education and only 21% had not informed their dentist of their risk for IE.[6] Lynch states that these findings are not surprising considering the volume of information given when a heart lesion is diagnosed.[5] It is understandable that clients' recall of bacterial endocarditis prophylaxis might be poor.

Nurses are often in the ideal position to convey appropriate information to clients about their disease process and available prevention measures. Lynch and Estlow offer examples of teaching modules for promoting awareness of effective bacterial endocarditis prophylaxis in children.[4,5] The teaching package must be understandable, concise, and logical. Nurses possess the education necessary to provide teaching in the most effective manner with content based on the most current medical recommendations. This intervention can result in favorable outcomes such as decreased incidence of bacterial endocarditis, decreased cost for treatment through disease prevention, and decreased morbidity and mortality associated with the disease.

Further research is needed to compare client outcomes and prophylaxis compliance in clients who have received intense nursing instruction compared to those clients who have not had the benefit of such intervention. With the present cost constraints on health care services, research is also needed to quantify the cost-benefit for improved outcomes in preventing bacterial endocarditis when extensive teaching is provided to clients and their families.

Implications for nursing practice include the need to develop a structured program for education. Strong client teaching skills, allocation of adequate nursing hours to provide client teaching, and evaluation methods to measure client outcomes will validate the need for client education provided by qualified nurses.

REFERENCES

1. Taubert, K.A., & Dajani, A.S. (1998). Preventing bacterial endocarditis: American Heart Association guidelines. *American Family Physician, 57*(3), 457-469.
2. Dajani, A.S., et al. (1997). Prevention of bacterial endocarditis: Recommendations by the American Heart Association. *Journal of the American Medical Association, 277*(22), 1794-1801.
3. Durack, D.T. (1995). Prevention of infective endocarditis. *New England Journal of Medicine, 332*(1), 38-44.
4. Estlow, M.M. (1998). Prevention of infective endocarditis in the pediatric congenital heart population. *Pediatric Nursing, 24*(3), 205-212.
5. Lynch, L.I. (1999). A teaching module: Promoting awareness of effective bacterial endocarditis prophylaxis in children. *Pediatric Nursing, 25*(6), 621-626.
6. Stucki, C., Mury, R., & Bertel, O. (2003). Insufficient awareness of endocarditis prophylaxis in clients at risk. *Swiss Medicine Weekly, 133*(9-10), 155-159.
7. Moons, P., De Volder, E., Budts, W., et al. (2001). What do adult patients with congenital heart disease know about their disease, treatment and prevention of complications? A call for structured patient education. *Heart, 86*(1), 74-80.

Heart failure is treated with oral diuretics and a sodium-restricted diet. Digitalis is useful in clients with atrial fibrillation for slowing the ventricular heart rate. Beta-blockers may also decrease the heart rate and therefore increase exercise tolerance. Clients with premature atrial contractions (PACs) should be treated because PACs often precede atrial fibrillation. A client with untreated mitral stenosis can progress from having mild disability to severe disability in less than 10 years.

Mitral Regurgitation

The client should restrict physical activities that produce fatigue and dyspnea. Reducing sodium intake and promoting sodium excretion with diuretics can lessen the work of the heart. Nitrates, digitalis, and angiotensin-converting enzyme (ACE) inhibitors have brought about hemodynamic improvement and symptomatic relief in clients with chronic mitral regurgitation.

Mitral Valve Prolapse

Treatment of mitral valve prolapse depends on the manifestations. Beta-blockers are helpful in relieving syncope, palpitations, and chest pain. Aspirin can also help to prevent transient ischemic attacks. For preventing infective endocarditis, the client may receive antibiotics prophylactically before any invasive procedures are performed.

AORTIC VALVE DISEASE

The aortic valve is the last valve through which blood flows before entering systemic circulation. In aortic stenosis the orifice of the aortic valve becomes narrowed, which causes a decrease in the blood flow from the left ventricle into the aorta and systemic circulation. This obstruction to flow creates a resistance to ejection and increased pressure in the left ventricle. Aortic regurgitation (aortic insufficiency) allows blood to leak back from the aorta into the left ventricle. During systole blood that is ejected into the aorta reenters the left ventricle. To maintain normal pressures, the left ventricle hypertrophies. Both aortic stenosis and aortic regurgitation overwork the left ventricle. Aortic valve disease is far less common than mitral valve disease but often occurs in conjunction with mitral valve disease. A dilation of the ascending aorta, or aortic root disease, is also quite common.

Etiology and Risk Factors

Aortic stenosis can be caused by several congenital defects of the aortic valve and by two degenerative processes: (1) calcification of the valve in older adults and (2) retraction and stiffening of the valve from rheumatic fever. As the population in the United States ages, the incidence of aortic stenosis from calcification has been rising.

Aortic regurgitation is most often a result of infectious disorders such as rheumatic fever, syphilis, and infective endocarditis. Connective tissue disorders can also lead to aortic regurgitation. Acute aortic regurgitation is usually due to aortic dissection, bacterial endocarditis, or trauma, which may be either penetrating or blunt.

Pathophysiology

When aortic stenosis is present, the pressure within the left ventricle rises as the blood is ejected through the narrowed opening. A pressure gradient develops between the left ventricle and the aorta. The elevated pressure in the left ventricle during systole causes the ventricle to hypertrophy. Dilation of the left ventricle occurs over time when the contractility of the hypertrophied muscle deteriorates. Eventually dilation and hypertrophy of the left ventricle are unable to maintain adequate cardiac output, resulting in elevated left ventricular end-diastolic pressure, decreased cardiac output, and increased pulmonary hypertension (see Table 55-1).

Aortic regurgitation is a diastolic event in which blood that is propelled forward into the aorta regurgitates back into the left ventricle through an incompetent valve. The backward flow of blood causes abnormal filling and a volume overload of the left ventricle. The magnitude of the overload depends on the severity of the incompetence; however, a small incompetent area can result in significant aortic regurgitation over time.

Because the left ventricle receives blood from both the atrium and the systemic circulation, aortic regurgitation gradually increases left ventricular end-diastolic volume. Left ventricular stroke volume is increased to produce an effective forward-moving volume into the systemic circulation. Compensatory dilation of the left ventricle occurs, but the increase in left ventricular end-diastolic pressure is minimal.[1] The compensatory mechanisms of dilation and hypertrophy help to maintain an adequate cardiac output. As the condition progresses and the contractile state of the myocardium declines, however, cardiac output declines (see Table 55-1).

Clinical Manifestations

Aortic Stenosis

Clinical manifestations of aortic stenosis tend to occur gradually and late in the course of the disease. Usually a long latent period in which the client is asymptomatic occurs. Manifestations begin to appear as the obstruction and ventricular pressure increase to critical levels. Angina pectoris (chest pain) is a frequent finding in about 66% of clients. The character of the angina is similar to that in clients with coronary artery disease, and pain is commonly brought on by exertion and relieved by rest. Myocardial oxygen consumption is higher in clients with aortic stenosis because of the hypertrophy of the left ventricle, and this probably accounts for the angina.

Syncope, another common clinical manifestation, also occurs during exertion because of a fixed cardiac output during a period of increased demand. Syncope at rest may be due to dysrhythmias. Exertional dyspnea, paroxysmal nocturnal dyspnea, and pulmonary edema occur with increasing pulmonary venous hypertension attributable to left ventricular failure. In severe aortic stenosis, additional manifestations may include palpitations, fatigue, and visual disturbances. On auscultation the systolic murmur may be associated with a diminished second heart sound and an early ejection click. A systolic thrill is present over the aortic areas.

Aortic Regurgitation

Clients with chronic severe aortic regurgitation may be asymptomatic for a long time. During this time the left ventricle gradually enlarges. Clients may complain of an uncomfortable awareness of the heartbeat and palpitations because of the large left ventricular stroke volume with rapid diastolic runoff. Clients may also have prominent pulsations in the neck and even head-bobbing with each heartbeat. Sinus tachycardia or premature ventricular contractions may make palpitations more pronounced.

On physical examination, low systolic blood pressure may be due to the large stroke volume and a decreased diastolic blood pressure resulting from the regurgitation and distal runoff. Carotid artery pulsations may be exaggerated. The arterial pulse pressure widens, and palpable pulse amplitude increases, often noted as a sudden sharp pulse, followed by a swift collapse of the diastolic pulse (Corrigan's or water-hammer pulse). Auscultation reveals a soft, high-pitched, blowing decrescendo diastolic murmur heard best at the second right intercostal space and radiating to the left sternal border. Noninvasive assessment of clients with Doppler echocardiography should be performed at intervals.[1]

OUTCOME MANAGEMENT

Medical Management

The goals of medical management are to maintain or improve cardiac function and activity tolerance. When the client reaches the maximum benefit from medications, surgery may be warranted. Aortic valve surgery may be necessary if angina or heart failure develops even though the client has been on medications.

Aortic Stenosis

Prophylactic antibiotics may be given on an individual basis for invasive medical or dental procedures for the prevention of infective endocarditis (see the Translating Evidence into Practice feature on Preventing Infective Endocarditis on p. 1388). Digitalis and diuretics usually used for ventricular failure must be used with caution because dehydration can reduce the cardiac output. Beta-blockers are not usually ordered because they can depress myocardial function and induce left ventricular failure. Cardiac dysrhythmias should be treated pharmacologically. With aortic stenosis, there is an associated gradual increase in the severity of obstruction that should be monitored with Doppler echocardiography. Advise clients with known or suspected critical obstruction of the aortic valve to avoid vigorous physical activity. Clients with mild obstruction may continue exercise if it is tolerated. For symptomatic clients, it is recommended that exercise stress-testing be avoided. The prognosis for clients with symptomatic aortic stenosis is poor without surgical intervention. The incidence of sudden death rises once myocardial failure develops.

Aortic Regurgitation

Medical intervention for aortic regurgitation is the same as that for aortic stenosis: relief of manifestations of heart failure and prevention of infection in the already deformed aortic cusps. Prompt surgical treatment is indicated when there is left ventricular failure. Death from pulmonary edema, ventricular dysrhythmias, electromechanical dissociation, or circulatory collapse is common in acute severe AR, even with intensive medical management. Early surgical intervention is recommended. Nitroprusside and possibly inotropic agents such as dopamine or dobutamine to augment forward flow and reduce LV end-diastolic pressure may be used temporarily before surgery. Intra-aortic balloon counterpulsation is contraindicated.

TRICUSPID AND PULMONIC VALVE DISEASE

Tricuspid stenosis, or regurgitation, usually develops from rheumatic fever or in combination with other structural disorders of the heart. Because the tricuspid valve is on the right side of the heart, the major hemodynamic alterations are decreased cardiac output and increased right atrial pressure. The inability of the right atrium to propel blood across the stenosed valve may account for these changes. With tricuspid regurgitation, the pressure in the right atrium is also elevated because of regurgitation of the blood volume in the right ventricle back into the right atrium during systole.

Clinical manifestations of tricuspid stenosis are dyspnea and fatigue, pulsations in the neck, and peripheral edema and weight loss. Physical assessment reveals prominent waves in the neck veins as the atrium vigorously contracts against the stenotic valve. A diastolic murmur is heard best along the left lower sternal border. The murmur increases with inspiration. The ECG reveals tall, tented P waves. Tricuspid insufficiency causes hepatic congestion and peripheral edema. Often atrial fibrillation is present, and jugular waves are evident. The murmur is holosystolic along the left sternal border.

Tricuspid stenosis usually responds well to diuretics and digitalis therapy. If the leaflets are severely stenotic, surgery may be required. Surgery for tricuspid regurgitation, however, may not be necessary unless pulmonary hypertension is present.

Abnormalities of the pulmonic valve are usually congenital defects. Few lesions develop after birth. Pulmonary hypertension, caused by mitral stenosis, pulmonary emboli, or chronic lung disease, can precipitate functional pulmonary regurgitation. Pulmonic stenosis and regurgitation lead to a decrease in cardiac output because blood does not reach the left side of the heart in adequate supply for metabolic demands. Pulmonic regurgitation may lead to dyspnea and fatigue. The murmur is a high-pitched diastolic blow along the left sternal border. No significant changes in the ECG are noted. Pulmonic stenosis causes similar clinical manifestations, but the murmur is often a crescendo-decrescendo type. Right-sided heart failure can also develop. Intervention focuses on treating the underlying cause and treating right-sided heart failure.

OUTCOME MANAGEMENT

Nursing Management of the Medical Client

Nursing assessment should address the type, severity, and progress of the valvular disorder; the presence of fatigue; clinical manifestations of heart failure; heart rhythm (including ECG); vital signs; auscultation and palpation of the heart; the client's support systems; and the degree of knowledge that the client and the client's family have concerning the nature of and intervention in the disorder.

The main focus of nursing intervention in valvular heart disease is to help the client maintain a normal cardiac output, thereby preventing manifestations of heart failure, venous or pulmonary congestion, and inadequate tissue perfusion. To evaluate the effectiveness of therapeutic interventions, perform ongoing hemodynamic assessment. Monitor vital signs closely every 1 to 4 hours. A decrease in cardiac output is manifested in a compensatory rise in the heart rate, a drop in blood pressure, and/or a decrease in urine output. Carefully auscultate the chest every 4 hours to identify the presence of abnormal breath sounds (crackles, rhonchi), heart gallops (S_3, S_4) or new heart murmurs.

Self-Care

Clients with valvular heart disease require lifelong management. With a sincere desire to understand and accept each client's response to chronic illness, you can help these clients adapt to difficult lifestyle changes and achieve a positive sense of well-being.

Clients may find it difficult to cope physically and psychosocially after hospital discharge. The chronicity of valvular heart disease and its potential complications can create an atmosphere of uncertainty, fear, and frustration. Take time to help the client identify support people, personal strengths, and coping strategies. Assess how the client handles frustration or anger and which activities are particularly relaxing. Address the client's fears and misconceptions. In some cases counseling referrals may help. Stress the importance of follow-up physical examinations and intervention.

Before discharge prepare detailed teaching materials for the client and family concerning the therapeutic regimen, the disease process, factors contributing to manifestations, and the rationale for intervention. Give information about the prescribed medications. Frequently prescribed medications include digoxin, diuretics, beta-blockers, potassium supplements, anticoagulants, and sometimes prophylactic antibiotics. Explain their rationale, dosages, side effects, and special considerations in their use.

Review the exercise prescriptions with the client. Clients with aortic stenosis often require activity restrictions. The client should demonstrate ability to pace activity, verbalize improvement in fatigue, and accept activity restrictions.

Address dietary restrictions, and plan interdisciplinary follow-up. Make sure the client knows whom to call when questions arise.

Surgical Management

Valves can be reconstructed or replaced. Valve reconstruction can be accomplished if the preoperative assessment indicates that the valve is pliable. If the valve is not pliable, valve replacement is necessary. Indications for valve replacement include the following symptomatic clients:

1. Clients with progressive impairment of cardiac function caused by scarring and thickening of the valve with either impaired narrowing of the valvular opening (stenosis) or incomplete closure (insufficiency, regurgitation)
2. Clients with gradual enlargement of the heart with manifestations of decreased activity, shortness of breath, and heart failure.

Valve Repair Procedures

In clients with mitral regurgitation, valve reconstruction or annuloplasty may be done, which may include the use of a flexible ring that is sewn into the valve for stabilization. Aortic stenosis may be surgically treated with valve replacement or balloon aortic valvuloplasty. In the valvuloplasty procedure, a catheter with a balloon is used to dilate the valve orifice. Commissurotomy is used to repair the leaflets of a valve that have become fused at the base (or annulus).

Balloon Valvuloplasty

Sometimes it is possible to open the valves without resorting to open heart surgery. Balloon valvuloplasty is a procedure in which a narrowed heart valve is stretched open (Figure 55-1). The procedure is performed in a cardiac catheterization laboratory. The client is usually awake but given local anesthesia and sedation. A catheter is placed in the groin and threaded into the heart to measure pressures in the chambers and to gauge the disease in the valve. The first catheter is then withdrawn, and a second catheter which contains a guidewire is threaded into one of the branch pulmonary arteries.

Balloon on catheter (inflated)

■ **FIGURE 55–1** Balloon valvuloplasty is a procedure used to stretch stenotic valves.

The purpose of the wire is to steady the catheter. The balloon catheter is then advanced into the heart and across the narrowed valve. The deflated balloon is positioned in the valve opening and then is inflated repeatedly. The inflated balloon widens the valve's opening by splitting the valve leaflets apart.

The main risk of stretching a mitral valve is for the valve to become severely leaky. A mild increase in the amount of leakage *(regurgitation)* is common with the procedure. In about 5% of clients, however, the valve becomes significantly leaky and will require replacement in 6 months. In about 2% of clients this is necessary as an emergency procedure during the valvuloplasty procedure.

Valve Replacement

Artificial heart valves are continuing to show improvements in design, safety, function, and durability. Mechanical and tissue prosthetic valves are available. The overall advantages and disadvantages of tissue and mechanical valves are almost equal. Mechanical valves are durable, but blood tends to clot on them, and anticoagulant therapy is therefore necessary. Fortunately, some of the newer artificial valves have reduced rates of thrombus formation. Some physicians recommend mechanical valves in clients younger than 65 or 70 years of age and tissue valves in clients 70 years or older. An artificial valve is shown in Figure 55-2. The type of valve prosthesis used is based on a number of considerations. The surgeon primarily considers (1) the durability of the valve and (2) the client's tolerance of anticoagulation. Therefore if the client has a preoperative history of bleeding or noncompliance with pharmacologic regimens, a tissue valve may be preferable.

Tissue valves are commonly from porcine (pig) or bovine (cow) and occasionally from human tissue. These valves do not require anticoagulation therapy, which makes them valuable for older clients, for women of childbearing age, and for clients who live in areas where anticoagulation monitoring is difficult. However, they are less durable. Tissue valves may degenerate or calcify or develop structural abnormalities. The rate of the tissue valve failure is 30% in 10 years, with the rate accelerating over the following 10 years.

Techniques for valve replacement can include the usual sternotomy approach. Advances in valvular surgery include the use of robotic techniques and minimally invasive surgery. Aortic valve replacement incisions are performed through a mini-sternotomy, in which an incision is made from the sternal notch to the third intercostal space. Mitral valve replacement/repair incisions are performed through a right parasternal incision in which small portions of the third and fourth costal cartilages are excised, a limited thoracotomy, or a partial sternotomy. These techniques reduce the size of the incisions and length of recovery. Nursing management of the client after heart surgery is discussed in Chapter 56.

CARDIOMYOPATHY

Cardiomyopathy is a broad term that includes subacute or chronic disorders of the myocardium. It is also used to refer to a group of systemic diseases and processes that are toxic to or alter the myocardium. There are three major types: dilated (congestive), hypertrophic, and restrictive (Figure 55-3). Although there have been several attempts to standardize the classification of the cardiomyopathies,

■ **FIGURE 55–2** Some heart valves are replaced with prosthetic ones. This is a St. Jude bileaflet mechanical valve. *(Courtesy St. Jude Medical, Inc., St. Paul, Minn.)*

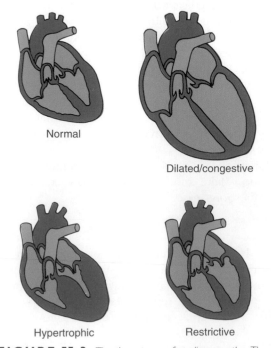

Normal

Dilated/congestive

Hypertrophic

Restrictive

■ **FIGURE 55–3** The three types of cardiomyopathy. The ventricle is enlarged and significantly reduces cardiac output.

the most widely recognized method was devised through a joint effort by the World Health Organization (WHO) and the International Society and Federation of Cardiology. Early research in animal models is being conducted in cardiac stem cell therapy for these clients.

The risk of cardiomyopathy increases in clients who chronically ingest excessive amounts of alcohol, are pregnant, have systemic hypertension, and have had some forms of infections. Table 55-2 compares the diagnostic data for the three types of cardiomyopathy. These forms of cardiomyopathy are described separately.

DILATED CARDIOMYOPATHY

Dilated cardiomyopathy is characterized by ventricular dilation, contractile dysfunction, and heart failure. It is the most common form, seen in about 60% of all cases. This form of cardiomyopathy has also been called hypertrophic subaortic stenosis, idiopathic hypertrophic subaortic stenosis, and asymmetrical septal hypertrophy. Some forms of dilated cardiomyopathy are idiopathic. Other causes include viral myocarditis, infections, metabolic problems, toxins, pregnancy, neuromuscular disorders, connective tissue disorders, and genetic predisposition (20% of cases).

In dilated cardiomyopathy usually both the left and right ventricles dilate, the myocardial fibers degenerate, and fibrotic tissue replaces viable tissue. Fibrotic tissue is not pliable, which leads to reduced contractility and decreased stroke volume and low cardiac output, with

a compensatory increase in heart rate. These changes eventually lead to heart failure accompanied by lethal ventricular dysrhythmias. The combination of ventricular dilation and ineffective myocardial contractility also increases the risk of blood pooling within the heart and subsequent clot formation. Many clients (75%) with idiopathic dilated cardiomyopathy die within 5 years after the onset of manifestations. Spontaneous rapid improvement occurs in some women and early fatality in others. The clinical manifestations of dilated cardiomyopathy are presented in Table 55-2.

OUTCOME MANAGEMENT

Treatment is similar to that for heart failure, including diuretics and sodium-restricted diets, angiotensin-converting enzyme inhibition, and beta-adrenergic blocking agents. Digoxin is also used and because of its narrow window of therapeutic index, the serum level must be closely monitored, keeping the range between 0.5 and 0.8 ng/ml. Inotropic agents are used to enhance myocardial contractility and to unload the heart. Nitroglycerin as a vasodilator can be used to decrease preload and afterload. Anticoagulants may help to prevent clots and emboli. Antidysrhythmic agents may help suppress ventricular irritability. In appropriate candidates implantation of the automatic internal cardiac defibrillator may be used to prevent sudden cardiac death.

Rest improves cardiac function. During the early stages, most clients find it difficult to accept rigidly imposed restrictions on activity. Clients should avoid poorly

TABLE 55–2 Findings in the Three Types of Cardiomyopathy

Dilated	Restrictive	Hypertrophic
Manifestations		
Heart failure, particularly left sided	Dyspnea, fatigue	Dyspnea, angina pectoris
Fatigue and weakness	Right-sided heart failure manifestations of	Fatigue, syncope, palpitations
Systemic or pulmonary emboli	systemic disease (e.g., amyloidosis, iron storage disease)	
Physical Examination		
Moderate to severe cardiomegaly: S_3 and S_4	Mild to moderate cardiomegaly: S_3 or S_4	Mild cardiomegaly
Atrioventricular valve regurgitation, especially mitral	Atrioventricular valve regurgitation; inspiratory increase in venous pressure (Kussmaul's sign)	Apical systolic thrill and heave; brisk carotid upstroke; S_4 common
		Systolic murmur that increases with Valsalva maneuver
Chest X-ray Study		
Moderate to marked cardiac enlargement, especially left ventricle	Mild cardiac enlargement	Mild to moderate cardiac enlargement
Pulmonary venous hypertension	Pulmonary venous hypertension	Paroxysmal nocturnal dyspnea
		Left atrial enlargement
Electrocardiogram		
Sinus tachycardia	Low voltage	Left ventricular hypertrophy
Atrial and ventricular dysrhythmias	Intraventricular conduction defects	ST-segment and T-wave abnormalities
ST-segment and T-wave abnormalities	Atrioventricular conduction defects	Abnormal Q waves
Intraventricular conduction defects		Atrial and ventricular dysrhythmias

Modified from Zipes, D. (2005). *Braunwald's heart disease: A textbook of cardiovascular medicine* (7th ed.). Philadelphia: Saunders.

tolerated activities. Advise clients that physical and emotional stress exacerbate the disease. Most clients experience severe activity intolerance during the later stages of the disease, which automatically limits their activities. Because alcohol depresses myocardial contractility, the client should abstain from drinking alcoholic beverages.

Only transplantation and specific vasodilator therapy (hydralazine plus nitrates) have resulted in prolonged life. Heart transplantation shows a 5-year survival of greater than 70% in appropriately selected clients.

HYPERTROPHIC CARDIOMYOPATHY

The disproportionate thickening of the interventricular septum in hypertrophic cardiomyopathy leads to wall rigidity and thereby increases resistance to blood flow from the left atrium. There is also obstruction of left ventricular outflow. In its severest form, the left ventricular wall reaches tremendous dimensions and encroaches on the left ventricular chamber, which becomes small and elongated. Septal hypertrophy may obstruct the left ventricular outflow tract during systole. Frequently diastolic dysfunction in the form of stiffness of the left ventricle occurs during diastolic filling. This stiffness raises left ventricular end-diastolic pressure, which eventually results in elevation of left atrial, pulmonary venous, and pulmonary capillary pressures.

Hypertrophic cardiomyopathy appears to be a genetically transmitted disease (approximately 50% of cases).[10] It can also be idiopathic, caused by hypertension or hypoparathyroidism. It appears most often in young adults, both men and women.

The clinical manifestations most commonly manifest in late adolescence or early adulthood but may appear at any age. Many clients with hypertrophic cardiomyopathy are asymptomatic and can lead long lives. They often have relatives with incapacitating manifestations of the disease. Sadly, sudden death is frequently the first clinical manifestation of the disease in asymptomatic clients. Sudden death appears more often in younger clients (i.e., less than 30 years of age, family history of sudden death, genetic abnormalities, and syncope, especially in children) and, if the presence of the disease is known, may be avoided by elimination of strenuous exercise. Clients who carry a high risk for sudden death should be considered and evaluated to receive an implantable cardioverter defibrillator (ICD).

The most common manifestation is dyspnea, which occurs in up to 90% of clients.[8] Dyspnea is due to the high pulmonary pressures produced by the elevated left ventricular end-diastolic pressure. Table 55-1 presents the remainder of clinical manifestations.

OUTCOME MANAGEMENT

The goals of intervention for hypertrophic cardiomyopathy are to alleviate manifestations, prevent complications, and reduce the risk of sudden death. Clients with hypertrophic cardiomyopathy should be evaluated using a full history and physical examination, a two-dimensional echocardiography, a 24- to 48-hour ambulatory Holter monitor evaluation, and treadmill or bicycle exercise testing.[11] These goals can be accomplished by reducing ventricular contractility and relieving left ventricular outflow obstruction. Beta-adrenergic blocking agents and calcium channel blocking medications reduce the heart rate, which lowers the myocardial contractility and oxygen consumption and prevents dysrhythmias. With decreased vigor of ventricular contraction, outflow obstruction diminishes. Beta-adrenergic blockade also reduces the heart rate (which further reduces myocardial workload) and prevents dysrhythmias.

Medications that decrease preload (e.g., nitrates, diuretics, morphine) and that increase contractility (e.g., isoproterenol, dopamine, digitalis) should be avoided. Currently, it has not been established whether asymptomatic clients should receive drug therapy because adequate controlled studies are not available.[12-14] Anticoagulants are used if the client is in atrial fibrillation. The client is at risk for endocarditis and should follow the prophylactic care for that condition. Alcohol should be avoided because its vasodilation properties can exacerbate an outflow problem.

RESTRICTIVE CARDIOMYOPATHY

Restrictive cardiomyopathy is the least common of the three clinically recognized and described cardiomyopathies. Its principal abnormality is diastolic dysfunction. Differentiation from constrictive pericarditis, a clinically similar entity, is difficult but important because the treatment options and prognosis differ drastically. Any infiltrative process of the heart that results in fibrosis and thickening can cause restrictive cardiomyopathy. The most frequently associated disease is amyloidosis (deposition of eosinophilic fibrous protein in the heart). Other disorders include glycogen storage disease, hemochromatosis, and sarcoidosis. Fibrotic infiltrations into the myocardium, endocardium, and subendocardium cause the ventricles to lose their ability to stretch. The excessively rigid ventricular walls impair filling during diastole; however, contractility with systole is usually normal. Filling pressures increase, and cardiac output falls. Eventually cardiac failure and mild ventricular hypertrophy occur. As cardiac output falls and intraventricular pressures rise, manifestations of heart failure appear. Table 55-1 presents the clinical manifestations. In severe or end-stage restrictive cardiomyopathy, the clinical manifestations are almost indistinguishable from those for chronic constrictive pericarditis. It is important to distinguish between the two problems because surgery can be used to treat cardiomyopathy.

OUTCOME MANAGEMENT

At present no specific interventions have been established for restrictive cardiomyopathy. Intervention aims at diminishing heart failure using pacemakers, diuretics, vasodilators, and salt restrictions to accomplish this goal. Digitalis may also help in some forms of restrictive cardiomyopathy. Clients with restrictive cardiomyopathy often have dysrhythmias that are refractory to antidysrhythmic drugs. These clients may benefit from a permanent pacemaker. Clients who carry a high risk for sudden death should be considered and evaluated to receive an implantable cardioverter defibrillator (ICD). Death attributable to dysrhythmia may occur suddenly, or a more progressive course may be followed by eventual, intractable heart failure. Candidates with intractable heart failure have been selected to undergo heart or heart-lung transplantation; unfortunately, however, recurrent sarcoid involvement can occur in the transplanted heart. The prognosis depends largely on the underlying cause. Unfortunately, intervention rarely results in long-term improvement.

Nursing management of the client with dilated cardiomyopathy is outlined in the Care Plan feature on The Client with Dilated Cardiomyopathy on the website. In addition, clients who are acutely or chronically ill with cardiomyopathy require strong psychosocial support. The uncertain and serious consequences of the disease create fear and anxiety. The chronic nature of the disorder can deplete coping resources, leaving clients with feelings of helplessness and hopelessness. As physical capabilities diminish, feelings of inadequacy, frustration, and poor self-esteem grow. Clients may become irritable, angry, withdrawn, or dependent.

Even though the prognosis is often poor, you can help clients who suffer from this debilitating disorder to maintain hope and dignity. Encouragement, a caring touch, a listening ear, and attainable goals can promote a high quality of life. Create an environment in which clients can openly express concerns and acknowledge fears. Acceptance, empathy, and kindness can help clients with cardiomyopathies to adopt more successful coping strategies.

Self-Care

SAFETY ALERT

With hypertrophic cardiomyopathy, syncope or sudden death may follow physical exertion. Therefore warn the client with hypertrophic cardiomyopathy to avoid strenuous physical exercise such as running or active competitive sports. In addition, encourage household members to learn cardiopulmonary resuscitation (CPR). Although chest pain often accompanies this disease, nitroglycerin can worsen the obstruction; clinicians can therefore treat chest pain with reduced activity and beta-blocking agents.

Hypertrophic cardiomyopathy predisposes the client to the risk of infective endocarditis. Advise clients

with this cardiomyopathy to check with their physician about taking prophylactic antibiotics before and after dental and surgical procedures because American Heart Association guidelines have changed.[19]

All clients with cardiomyopathy need clear, honest education concerning the disease and its cause and intervention. Both you and the client must be watchful for adverse effects of therapy. Clients with restrictive cardiomyopathy are especially vulnerable to the toxic effects of digitalis (see Chapter 56).

Surgical Management

Surgical procedures have been developed for hypertrophic cardiomyopathy procedures to reduce the outflow gradient. Myotomy is the surgical incision into or resection of a portion of the ventricular septum. The excision of fibrotic endocardium is successful in a limited number of clients with restrictive cardiomyopathy. Surgical ablation can reduce some dysrhythmias.

Heart Transplantation

Cardiac transplantation is now a standard and effective treatment for clients with end-stage cardiac disease.
In 2005, 2125 hearts were transplanted in the United States. About 80% of clients with heart transplants are still living 2 years after the operation. While the benefits are obvious to the recipient, finding a donor can be difficult because the healthy heart must come from a fresh cadaver. Outcomes of heart transplantation depend on how quickly the transplant can be performed once a donor is found. There is a 10% to 20% death rate for clients on the waiting list. As of 2006, 84% to 86% of heart transplant clients survived 1 year and 74% to 78% survived 3 years. (Survival differs by gender; woman have lower survival rates.) Heart transplant recipients who die after the procedure usually do so within the first 30 days postoperatively.

Potential candidates must be evaluated and screened. Their cardiac status is evaluated to determine the need for the heart transplant. The candidates are also evaluated for underlying conditions that predispose to an unfavorable outcome. Box 55-1 shows the selection criteria for heart transplantation

The current orthotopic technique retains a large portion of the right and left atrium in the recipient and implants the donor heart to the atria (Figure 55-4). Cardiopulmonary bypass is used during the operation (see Chapter 56). Temporary pacemaker wires and chest drainage catheters are inserted.

SAFETY ALERT

The newly transplanted heart does not have a vagus nerve or sympathetic nerve fibers. Increases or decreases in cardiac output are due to changes in the venous return causing changes in the stretch of the heart muscle. Therefore the client has a subnormal capacity for exercise. The clients can usually perform

---

BOX 55-1   Indications and Contraindications for Heart Transplant

INDICATIONS

- New York Heart Association (NYHA) class III or IV symptoms
- Dilated cardiomyopathy
- Ischemic cardiomyopathy
- Ejection fraction of less than 25%
- Intractable angina or malignant cardiac dysrhythmias for which conventional therapy has been exhausted
- Age younger than 65 years
- Pulmonary vascular resistance less than 2 Wood's units
- Ability to comply with medical follow-up care

CONTRAINDICATIONS

- Lack of indications
- Active systemic infection
- Active systemic disease such as collagen vascular disease or sickle cell disease
- Active malignancies; clients with malignancies who have been tumor free for 3 to 5 years may be considered depending upon the type of cancer
- An ongoing history of substance abuse (e.g., alcohol, drugs, tobacco)
- Psychosocial instability

---

activities of daily living and at least moderate exercise and probably most importantly enjoy an excellent quality of life. Without nerves, the client cannot experience angina in response to cardiac ischemia or infarction. Instead they will experience dyspnea or dysrhythmias. Treatment of dysrhythmias does not include medications in these clients.

Assisted Circulation and Mechanical Hearts

About 2600 clients in the United States are waiting to receive a heart transplant, but only about 2100 donated hearts are received each year. Clients who are waiting for a heart donor and transplant are at great risk of dying before a heart becomes available. During this waiting period, a ventricular assist device (VAD) may be inserted to keep these clients alive, as explained in the Bridge to Critical Care feature on p. 1397. These high-tech machines help the failing heart to pump blood throughout the body, bridging the time until a donor heart becomes available. In some cases the machine allows the heart to rest and recover so that the VAD can be removed and the client no longer needs a transplant.

Recipient superior vena cava

Recipient aorta

Recipient pulmonary artery

Donor aorta

Pulmonary artery

Donor heart

Small cuff of native left atrial tissue with native pulmonary veins

■ **FIGURE 55–4** During heart transplantation, all but the posterior walls of the atrium are removed. The donor heart is sewn into place.

Management of the Surgical Client

Management of the postoperative client is discussed in Chapter 56. The client will receive immunosuppressant medications, commonly cyclosporine, prednisone, and tacrolimus. Drug therapy is adjusted to give the maximum amount of immunosuppression with the minimum amount of side effects using an individualistic regimen. The risk of acute rejection is highest soon after transplantation and decreases dramatically after 3 months. Even with this intensive regimen, almost all heart transplant recipients experience some acute rejection during the first postoperative year. The most reliable technique for assessing organ rejection is the endomyocardial biopsy, which enables identification of the diffuse interstitial infiltrate associated with rejection.

INFECTIOUS DISORDERS

Bacteria and other microbes are found in abundance in our environment. Because the heart valves do not actually receive any blood supply of their own, which may be surprising given their location, defense mechanisms (such as leukocytes) cannot enter. Therefore if an organism infiltrates the valves, the body cannot combat it. Normally, blood flows smoothly through these valves but if they have been damaged, bacteria have a chance to thrive.

RHEUMATIC FEVER

Rheumatic fever (RF) is a diffuse inflammatory disease characterized by a delayed response to an infection by group A beta-hemolytic streptococci (GAS) in the tonsillopharyngeal area. RF is classified as a collagen-vascular disease or connective tissue disease. Many organs are involved through these rheumatic processes, including the heart, the joints, and the central nervous system. This process is caused by an inflammatory reaction. Although

BRIDGE TO CRITICAL CARE

Left Ventricular Assist Devices

INDICATIONS
- Transplant-ready clients who are in danger of dying before a donor heart is available
- Heart failure not responsive to standard cardiac treatments
- Heart failure following various forms of heart surgery

DEVICES
Consist of a pump, which is implanted in the abdominal wall and connected to the left ventricle of the heart. Although the ventricle may be too weak to pump blood to the entire body, the pump draws blood from the ventricle and, in turn, propels it out to the rest of the body.

Pneumatic: External pulsatile pump that propels blood.

Electric: An electrical line attached to the device connects to a portable, external controller, which fits onto the client's belt and operates and monitors the pump. Clients carry reserve battery packs on their belt or shoulder bag so they can change the batteries every 3 to 4 hours, a procedure like changing the batteries in a cell phone.

PLACEMENT
The surgeon connects the VAD to the bottom of the heart and the main heart artery (aorta). Blood then flows into the heart and out of the aorta by means of a small electrically or pneumatically driven motor that is part of the VAD. A tube is passed through the client's skin. The tube connects to a controller and a battery pack that the client wears or carries. This allows the client to be fully mobile with the device in place.

COMPLICATIONS
- Infection, especially pneumonia related to immobility
- Bleeding from anticoagulant use
- Right-sided heart failure
- Thromboembolism
- Device malfunction

NURSING PRECAUTIONS
- Monitor cardiac output and hemodynamic status.
- Perform range-of-motion exercises to maintain muscle strength and joint flexibility.
- Monitor lung sounds; suction secretions from airway or assist client to deep breathe and cough.
- Monitor level of anticoagulation, especially during weaning.
- Monitor for specific device-related problems.
- Educate about how to change batteries, reportable problems if client is ambulatory.

AbioCor pump.

HeartMate left ventricular assist device.

Data from Mahmood, A.K., et al. (2000). Critical review of current left ventricular assist devices. *Perfusion, 15*(399), 420-432.

this infection remains common, the incidence of RF has declined dramatically to about 2 per 100,000 people in the United States. This decline is due to an emphasis on prevention. The incidence in developing countries is about 100 per 100,000 people.

Etiology and Risk Factors
Rheumatic fever develops in only a relatively small percentage of people (3%), even after a virulent bout of streptococcal infection; there is therefore some evidence of host predisposition. There is also a familial

predisposition to the disease. Once RF is acquired, the client becomes more susceptible than the general population to recurrent infection. Poor hygiene, crowding, and poverty are risk factors for acute RF. If appropriate antibiotic therapy for group A beta-hemolytic streptococcal infection is given within the first 9 days, RF can usually be prevented. The most common age for an initial attack of RF is between 6 and 15 years.

Prevention is the best treatment. The most effective measures against RF are probably socioeconomic. In the affluent neighborhoods of Western cities, where there is spacious housing with no crowding, the incidence of RF is low. Certain populations are at a higher risk for developing streptococcal pharyngitis. These groups include military recruits, people living in crowded conditions, and people in close contact with school-age children. Both males and females have the same incidence for acquiring RF. Identification of high-risk people is also important. Nurses can help to identify mitral valve prolapse (see earlier discussion) early to prevent valvular disease. Nurses in community settings can identify those with beta-hemolytic streptococcal infections and refer clients for appropriate diagnosis and medical management.

Pathophysiology

Rheumatic fever initiates a diffuse, proliferative, and exudative inflammatory process involving all layers of the heart, joints, subcutaneous tissue, central nervous system (CNS), and skin. Although the cellular disease process is not clear, the mechanism is probably an abnormal humoral and cell-mediated response to streptococcal cell membrane antigens. There is a positive correlation that links group A streptococci as the causative agent for initial and recurrent attacks of RF. These antigens bind to receptors on the heart, other tissues, and joints, which begins the autoimmune response. The inflammatory process often produces permanent and severe heart damage. Complications of RF include valvular disorders, cardiomegaly, and heart failure.

All layers of the heart swell, a condition called carditis. Necrosis develops in areas of inflamed myocardium, called Aschoff's bodies. These areas are minuscule nodules with localized fibrin deposits surrounded by areas of necrosis in the myocardium. Endocardial inflammation causes swelling of the valve leaflets, which leads to valve dysfunction and murmurs. Small bacterial vegetations form on the valve tissues. Rough eroded areas of the valves attract platelets, which adhere and form platelet-fibrin clumps that eventually scar and shorten the valve. The valves lose their elasticity, and cardiac function is impaired. After a latent period of about 3 weeks following a group A streptococcal infection, the clinical manifestations of acute rheumatic fever are evident.

First, the damaged valve may become scarred and stenosed, increasing the cardiac workload because higher pressure must be generated to propel blood through the narrow valve. Second, the valve leaflets may become so short that they cannot close securely. As a result blood regurgitates backwards from the damaged valve. Both valvular stenosis and regurgitation eventually cause heart failure from the high workload.

Clinical Manifestations

The clinical manifestations of rheumatic fever are related to the inflammatory response and can last about 3 months.

Major manifestations include the following:

- Carditis is the most destructive consequence of RF. It is present in at least 50% of clients with acute RF and is the most specific manifestation of RF. Characteristics include a significant murmur, cardiomegaly, pericarditis that produces a significant friction rub, and heart failure. Chest pain resulting from pericardial inflammation may be present. Sometimes myocardial involvement produces atrioventricular (AV) conduction defects (first-degree AV block) or atrial fibrillation.
- Arthritis, the most common finding of RF, is painful and migratory. It most often affects the larger joints, such as the ankles, knees, elbows, shoulders, and wrists. The arthritis may or may not be symmetrical. If the client takes aspirin early in the course of the disease, arthritis manifestations may not be as apparent. Joint manifestations may last hours or days. Arthritis that is not treated usually lasts 2 to 3 weeks. RF-associated arthritis has a good response to salicylates.
- Chorea, a disorder of the basal ganglia and caudate nuclei, is a late manifestation of RF, usually appearing 3 months or longer after the streptococcal infection. Chorea, which is from the Greek word for movement and the origin of the word choreography, is manifested by sudden, irregular, aimless involuntary movements. The client may also have emotional lability. Chorea disappears without treatment and produces no permanent sequelae. Chorea may disappear during sleep and be more prevalent when the client is awake and/or under stress.
- Erythema marginatum is an unusual rash that is seen primarily on the trunk. The application of heat may induce this rash. The lesions are crescent-shaped and have clear centers. The rash is transitory and its appearance may change in minutes or hours. This rash is a distinctive feature of RF; however, it is rare.
- Subcutaneous nodules are small, painless, firm yet freely mobile nodules that adhere loosely to the tendon sheaths, especially in knees, knuckles, and elbows. They are usually evident only during the first week or two and generally only in children.

Minor manifestations include the following:

- Fever, with a temperature of 38° C (100.4° F) or higher, alternates with normal temperature. Weakness, malaise, weight loss, and anorexia probably develop as a result of fever, pain, and the general debilitation associated with serious illness. When only a single major manifestation is present, fever is used to support the diagnosis of RF. There is no distinguishing pattern to these fevers in the acute phase of RF.

- A positive throat culture for group A beta-hemolytic streptococci can help to confirm the diagnosis. An elevated white blood cell (WBC) count, erythrocyte sedimentation rate (ESR), and C-reactive protein level may indicate inflammation. An ECG or echocardiogram can help to confirm rhythm problems and structural changes.

The diagnosis is made by the presence of major manifestations; the Jones criteria (Box 55-2) and abnormal laboratory findings are used to make the diagnosis. Not many clients with acute RF have a positive throat culture for group A streptococci. Therefore anti-streptococcal antibody titers are drawn to determine if a recent streptococcal infection has been present.

OUTCOME MANAGEMENT

Medical Management

The goals of medical management include (1) eradicating infection, (2) maximizing cardiac output, and (3) promoting comfort.

BOX 55-2   Jones' Criteria for the Diagnosis of Rheumatic Fever*

MAJOR MANIFESTATIONS
1. Carditis
2. Polyarthritis
3. Chorea
4. Erythema marginatum
5. Subcutaneous nodules

MINOR MANIFESTATIONS
1. Clinical findings
   a. Previous rheumatic fever or rheumatic heart disease
   b. Arthralgia
   c. Fever
2. Laboratory findings
   a. Elevated acute phase reactants
      (1) Erythrocyte sedimentation rate
      (2) C-reactive protein
      (3) Leukocytosis
   b. Prolonged P-R interval

EVIDENCE OF GROUP A STREPTOCOCCAL INFECTION
1. Positive throat culture for Strep A
2. Elevated or rising anti-streptococcal antibody titer
3. Recent scarlet fever

*In some instances, rheumatic fever can be diagnosed without fulfillment of Jones' criteria.
Modified from Special Writing Group of the American Heart Association. (1992). Guidelines for the diagnosis of rheumatic fever: Jones criteria. 1992 update. *Journal of the American Heart Association, 268*(15), 2069-2072.

Eradicate Infection

The first priority is to eradicate the streptococcal infection. At the time of diagnosis of RF, only a few clients will still have throat cultures positive for streptococcal infection. This is because of the elimination of the organism by the host before manifestations of RF appear. Penicillin or erythromycin is usually prescribed for 10 days even if the cultures are negative. The client typically takes prophylactic agents for rheumatic fever for 5 years after the initial attack. After 5 years, recurrences are rare and prophylaxis continues only in high-risk clients. Clients who have had rheumatic fever remain vulnerable to bacterial endocarditis. Therefore in addition to the antibiotics they take to prevent rheumatic fever recurrence, they must be referred for evaluation for possible prophylactic medications before and after any surgical procedure or dental work. Specific evaluation for prophylaxis medication must be individualized according to recommendations by the American Heart Association. (See the Translating Evidence into Practice feature on Preventing Infective Endocarditis on p. 1388.)

Maximize Cardiac Output

Corticosteroids are used to treat carditis, especially if heart failure is evident. If heart failure develops, treatment, including ACE inhibitors, beta blockers, and diuretics, is effective.

Promote Comfort

Clients with arthritic manifestations obtain clinical relief with salicylates; however, because these drugs can result in a misdiagnosis, a firm diagnosis should be in place before salicylates are given. Bed rest is usually prescribed to reduce cardiac effort until evidence of inflammation has subsided. For clients with rheumatic valvular heart disease, bacterial endocarditis prophylaxis may be necessary (see Infective Endocarditis).

Nursing Management of the Medical Client

Assessment. Nursing assessment involves gathering baseline and ongoing subjective and objective data. Obtain baseline vital signs, assess the heart for a friction rub and the lungs for crackles, and palpate peripheral pulses. A baseline ECG is used to determine whether heart block is present. Assess baseline nutritional and hydration data. Continue to reassess vital signs to determine the patterns of fever and the stability of blood pressure. Vital signs are also used as a measure of activity tolerance.

Assess psychosocial data about the client's feelings regarding restrictions of activity, support systems, coping strategies, level of discomfort, and knowledge (both the client and the client's family) concerning the nature of, and intervention for, rheumatic fever.

Diagnosis, Outcomes, Interventions

Diagnosis: Activity Intolerance. A reduced cardiac reserve and enforced bed rest can quickly lead to activity intolerance. The nursing diagnosis statement would be *Activity Intolerance related to reduced cardiac reserve and enforced bed rest.*

Outcomes. The client will have improved tolerance of activity and progress toward an optimal level of physical activity tolerance based on underlying cardiovascular status and psychosocial readiness as evidenced by the ability to (1) steadily increase activity level to include climbing one flight of stairs without chest pain or without ECG changes, while the heart rate remains under 90 beats/min; (2) verbalize improvement in fatigue; (3) express acceptance of any imposed activity restrictions; and (4) pace activities.

Interventions. Bed rest is important in the acute phase because it reduces myocardial oxygen demand and usually continues until the following criteria are met:

- Temperature remains normal without use of salicylates.
- Resting pulse rate remains less than 100 beats/min.
- ECG tracings show no manifestations of myocardial damage.
- ESR returns to normal.
- Pericardial friction rub is not present.

Once ambulatory, the client must still refrain from overexertion. Assess the client's stamina and response to exercise to gauge the degree of gradual activity progression.

SAFETY ⚠ ALERT

Assess vital signs before and after exercise. After 3 to 5 minutes of rest, reassess vital signs. They should have returned to baseline within 3 minutes of cessation of exercise. The client should reduce or discontinue activity if chest pain, vertigo, dyspnea, confusion, a drop in blood pressure, an irregular pulse or abnormal heart rate develops.

The length of activity restriction depends on whether carditis develops and on the extent of permanent heart damage. Restrictions may extend for months. In severe cases of rheumatic carditis, clients may be forced to undergo restrictions on a permanent basis. Encourage a gradual increase in activity within the limits of the client's condition.

The client experiencing chorea requires sedatives, bed rest, and protection from self-injury. A carefully planned and supervised activity schedule should be maintained and evaluated.

Diagnosis: Chronic Pain. The inflammatory response in the joints can lead to pain. The nursing diagnosis statement would be *Chronic Pain related to the inflammatory response in the joints.*

Outcomes. The client will experience increased comfort as evidenced by (1) reports of reduced discomfort, (2) expression of joint pain reduction, (3) reduced use of pain medications, (4) a relaxed body posture and a calm facial expression, and (5) ability to sleep.

Interventions. Obtain a clear description of the pain or discomfort. Identify the source of greatest discomfort as a focus for intervention. Administer analgesics as needed and use salicylates around the clock. Balance rest and activity according to the degree of pain and activity tolerance. Other pain interventions are discussed in Chapter 20.

Diagnosis: Imbalanced Nutrition: Less Than Body Requirements. Hypermetabolism seen with fever and inflammation and other factors in rheumatic fever can lead to protein-calorie malnutrition. This nursing diagnosis is stated as *Imbalanced Nutrition: Less Than Body Requirements, related to fever, inflammation, anorexia, and fatigue.*

Outcomes. The client will maintain or restore adequate nutritional balance as evidenced by (1) the resumption of pre-illness body weight or no further weight loss, (2) consumption of 75% or more of each meal served, (3) normal serum albumin or prealbumin levels, and (4) increasing energy and stamina.

Interventions. A high-protein, high-carbohydrate diet helps maintain adequate nutrition in the presence of fever and infection. Hypermetabolic states (fever and infection) can induce a catabolic state, thus delaying healing. Vitamin and mineral supplements may also benefit the client. Oral hygiene every 4 hours; small, attractive meal servings; and foods that are not overly rich, sweet, or greasy stimulate the appetite. Adequate fluid intake prevents dehydration resulting from fever. If the client shows manifestations of severe carditis or heart failure, sodium and fluids must be restricted. Daily weights can serve as an indication of nutritional and fluid status.

Diagnosis: Risk for Ineffective Therapeutic Regimen Management (Individuals). Following rheumatic fever, the client must follow a lifelong regimen to reduce the risk of rheumatic heart disease. This nursing diagnosis is stated as *Risk for Ineffective Therapeutic Regimen Management (Individuals) related to a need for lifelong therapy.*

Outcomes. The client and the client's family will demonstrate adequate knowledge of rheumatic fever and its ability to lead to rheumatic heart disease including the need to complete the entire course of antibiotics; consuming adequate calories, protein, and fluids; and the rationale for lifelong prevention.

Interventions. Today streptococcal infections do not have to develop into rheumatic fever if the client seeks immediate assessment and begins antibiotics. Clients who have recovered from an episode of rheumatic fever can avoid subsequent attacks by taking prophylactic doses of antibiotics and observing good health practices. Because repeated attacks may lead to serious heart disease and permanent cardiac disability, it is important to emphasize means of avoiding subsequent attacks.

Instruct the client about how to reduce exposure to streptococcal infection as follows:

1. Take good care of the teeth and gums, and obtain prompt dental care for cavities and gingivitis. Prophylactic medication may be needed before invasive dental procedures, and individualized evaluation for prophylaxis medication is needed.
2. Avoid people who have an upper respiratory tract infection or who have had a recent streptococcal infection.
3. Notify the physician if any manifestations of streptococcal sore throat *(pharyngitis)* develop. It is extremely important to begin antibiotic therapy promptly for any infection. The clinical manifestations include fever (102° to 104° F, 38.8° to 40° C), chills, sore throat, and enlarged, painful lymph nodes. Advise clients who have had rheumatic fever that they must guard against infections for the rest of their lives to avoid development of heart disease.

Evaluation. Rheumatic fever is treated over 10 days. Expect activity tolerance to improve once fever and pain are controlled. Altered nutrition may require more than 2 weeks to show improvement, depending on the severity of anorexia and fever.

INFECTIVE ENDOCARDITIS

Endocarditis is an inflammatory process of the endocardium, especially the valves. This disorder carries high morbidity and death rates, but outcomes can be improved greatly with rapid diagnosis and effective treatment.

Many different terms and classifications are used to describe infective endocarditis. Some are defined in the following list:

- Subacute bacterial endocarditis (SBE): develops gradually over several weeks or months; usually caused by organisms of low virulence, such as *Streptococcus viridans,* which has a limited ability to infect other tissues
- Acute bacterial endocarditis: develops over days or weeks with an erratic course and earlier development of complications; commonly caused by *Staphylococcus aureus,* which is capable of infecting other body tissues
- Native valve endocarditis: an infection of a previously normal or damaged valve
- Prosthetic valve endocarditis: an infection of a prosthetic valve
- Nonbacterial thrombotic endocarditis: caused by sterile thrombotic lesions (often aggregates of platelets) that may develop in people with cancer or other chronic diseases

Changes in the population at risk are altering the classic picture of infective endocarditis (IE). The incidence is continuing to rise. Each year 15,000 to 20,000 new cases are diagnosed and IE is now the fourth leading cause of life-threatening infectious disease syndromes. The changes are traced to several notable alterations in the population. The increased incidence of endocarditis caused by yeasts and fungi is attributable to the increased number of people with valve prostheses, to the increased number of people using intravenous (IV) drugs, and to the rising use of long-term antimicrobial therapy or immunosuppression. Nosocomial infections are now the cause of up to 29% of all cases.

The decreased incidence of rheumatic fever results in a lower incidence of endocarditis, whereas the number of children surviving congenital heart disease results in an increased incidence. The growing population of older adults also leads to an increase in the number of endocarditis episodes.

Etiology and Risk Factors

Common infecting organisms include staphylococci *(S. aureus, S. faecalis, S. epidermidis),* streptococci, *Escherichia coli,* gram-negative organisms *(Klebsiella, Pseudomonas, Serratia marcescens),* fungi *(Candida, Aspergillus),* and HACEK organisms *(Haemophilus parainfluenzae, Haemophilus aphrophilus, Actinobacillus actinomycetemcomitans, Cardiobacterium hominis, Eikenella* species, and *Kingella* species). These organisms enter the body through the oral cavity after dental procedures, mouth or tooth abscesses, oral irrigations, or oral irritations from dental floss or bridgework. The upper respiratory tract is another port of entry following surgery, intubations, or infections. Direct exposure of the bloodstream to organisms can occur with prolonged IV catheters, hemodialysis catheters, and IV drug use. Procedures involving the gastrointestinal and genitourinary tracts (e.g., barium enemas, sigmoidoscopy, colonoscopy, percutaneous liver biopsy, catheterization, urethrotomy, prostatectomy, cystoscopy) have been associated with infective endocarditis.

Reproductive conditions have also been linked (e.g., delivery of a newborn, abortion, intrauterine devices, pelvic inflammatory diseases). Defective heart valves causing changes in blood flow and pressures encourage the proliferation of vegetations. Open heart surgery to replace damaged valves increases the risk of endocarditis. Fortunately, coronary artery bypass grafting (CABG), one of the most frequently performed surgical procedures in the United States, carries a low risk of infective endocarditis because the endocardium is not invaded during the operation.

Circulating microorganisms in the bloodstream attach to the endocardial surface and multiply. Usually multiplication of these organisms requires a rough or abnormal endocardium. IV drug abusers may be injecting particulate matter into the bloodstream, causing damage to the previously normal right heart endocardium that allows the organism to adhere, thereby initiating acute bacterial endocarditis.

Pathophysiology

Microorganisms enter the bloodstream in many ways. Once the colonization process begins on the endothelium, replication occurs and bacterial colonies form within layers of platelets and fibrin. As the colonies become entangled within the tight layers of fibrin and platelets, the colony becomes less and less vulnerable to the body's defense mechanisms. The bacteria stimulate the humoral immune system to produce nonspecific antibodies, but the bacteria are protected by the fibrin-platelet aggregation. It is not uncommon for these vegetations to form clots that travel to other organs, forming abscesses. The vegetations can severely damage heart valves by perforating and deforming the valve leaflets (Figure 55-5). Extensions of the bacteria may invade the aorta or pericardium. The amount of damage depends on the type and virulence of the organisms causing the infection.

Many complications are possible. Heart failure may develop as a result of structural valvular damage. Arterial emboli can occur from the vegetation. Systemic embolization occurs in 30% to 40% of clients with left-sided infective endocarditis. Common infarction sites are the kidney, spleen, and brain. Pulmonary embolus is associated with right-sided infective endocarditis. Emboli can also travel to the brain and produce a myriad of manifestations. Occasionally immune complex glomerulonephritis will develop. Renal function usually returns to normal after the infection has been controlled.

Clinical Manifestations

Clinical manifestations of infective endocarditis include those related to the infectious process, heart murmurs, embolization, and the immune response.

■ **FIGURE 55–5** Vegetations of the heart valves resulting from infective endocarditis. *(From Kumar, V.A., Abbas, A.K., & Fausto, N. [2004]. Robbins and Cotran pathologic basis of disease [7th ed.]. Philadelphia: Saunders.)*

Clinical manifestations related to the infection include fever, chills alternating with sweats, malaise, weakness, anorexia, weight loss, pallor, backache, and splenomegaly. Clients may report feeling as though they have the flu, with headaches and musculoskeletal aching. In acute infection, clients appear very ill. Fever, chills, and prostration are so severe that hospital admission is usually necessary within a few days.

Cardiac murmurs eventually develop, but they may be absent in the early stages of infection. In clients with pre-existing valvular disease, new murmurs may be heard. Heart failure may develop suddenly in either acute or subacute endocarditis. Mechanical complications include perforation of a valve leaflet, rupture of one of the chordae tendineae, or development of a functional stenosis from the obstruction of blood flow by large vegetations.

Clinical manifestations related to embolization can occur in any part of the body. They are presented in the following list in order from head to toe:

- Stroke, transient ischemic attacks, aphasia, or ataxia
- Loss of vision from embolization to the brain or retinal artery
- Petechiae on the neck, conjunctiva, chest, abdomen, and mouth
- Roth's spots—a white or yellow center surrounded by a bright red, irregular halo seen by ophthalmoscope
- Myocardial infarction, which may develop as a result of coronary artery embolism
- Pulmonary embolus
- Splinter hemorrhages, which look like tiny splinters under the nail
- Osler's nodes—painful, erythematous, pea-sized nodules on tips of the fingers and toes resulting from inflammation around a small, infected embolus
- Finger clubbing, although less common today, may occur in clients with long-standing infective endocarditis; pathogenesis remains unclear
- Janeway's lesions—flat, small, nontender red spots on the palms of the hands and the soles of the feet
- Evidence of an immunologic reaction to infection, including arthralgia, proteinuria, hematuria, casts, and acidosis

Because the clinical manifestations of endocarditis are numerous and often nonspecific, several modalities are used for the differential medical diagnosis. Blood cultures for bacteria, fungus, and yeast are the most important diagnostic tests. Blood cultures should be obtained for all clients with both fever and heart murmur. ECGs and echocardiograms should be done on admission to the hospital and repeated during the hospital stay.[25] A chest x-ray study is useful in identifying early heart failure. A complete blood count (CBC) and other routine diagnostic procedures are also helpful. Diagnosis is confirmed by clinical manifestations, blood cultures, and echocardiography.

OUTCOME MANAGEMENT

Medical Management

The chief goals of management are to eradicate the infecting organism in the vegetation and to treat the complications. Because the bacteria reside inside the vegetation, getting antibiotics to them is difficult. Antibiotics cannot reach the organism directly, because the valves do not receive a blood supply; therefore antibiotics have to reach the vegetation passively. Penicillin plus ceftriaxone and gentamicin or vancomycin is commonly used. Because of resistive strains of bacteria, other antibiotics might be needed. Therapy is usually administered by the IV route and continued for 4 to 6 weeks. Antibiotics are usually begun in the hospital and continued as an outpatient at the client's home if the living situation is appropriate. Risk for IE will continue for the client's lifetime and prophylaxis against infection will remain important.

IE can lead to valve disease, and surgery may be required once the infection is under control (negative blood cultures, absence of fever, and normal WBC count). Severe valve disease with heart failure can require surgical eradication of the infection.

Nursing Management of the Medical Client

Nursing assessment focuses on gathering data about the client's hemodynamic stability (particularly the presence of a new heart murmur and embolic complications), level of comfort, coping ability, support from significant others, and potential for self-care. Auscultate the heart every 8 hours for murmurs. Assess for rapid pulse rate, easy fatigability, dyspnea, restlessness, manifestations of heart failure, and embolic manifestations. Document these manifestations if they occur, and report them to the physician.

Administer IV antibiotics as prescribed. Antibiotics relieve much discomfort within a few days. Treat fever, when present, with rest, cooling measures, forced fluids, and sometimes salicylates. As with most infectious processes, encourage the client to eat a nutritious diet, drink sufficient fluids, and rest mentally and physically.

The client may need to be hospitalized or transferred to a setting that can provide IV medications for 2 to 6 weeks if home care is not an option. Do not enforce complete bed rest unless fever or manifestations of heart damage develop.

When the client's condition improves, plan and implement a progressive activity schedule and a teaching plan (see the Client Education Guide feature on Infective Endocarditis on the website). As activity increases, monitor the client's physical response to exercise. For example, assess blood pressure, heart rate, diaphoresis, vertigo, and weakness.

Self-Care

The trend toward early hospital discharge has changed the course of treatment for clients with infective endocarditis. IV therapy may now be routinely given in the home. Clients who are alert, cooperative, and reasonably stable and who want to return home may be allowed to do so. Typically the nurse, pharmacist, and physician teach the techniques of self-administered IV antibiotics. Before discharge, the client must demonstrate the knowledge and technique required. The physician's office or home health care nurses often monitor the client's progress.

Home IV antibiotic therapy offers many benefits. It is less costly than hospital care, motivates clients to become active participants in their own care, reestablishes a more normal lifestyle, and promotes a sense of control that aids in psychosocial and physiologic recovery. To be effective, this program calls for exceptional communication and cooperation between members of the health care team and the client.

Invasive procedures, especially dental work, increase the risk of endocarditis. Oral antibiotics are advised before most dental procedures are performed (Box 55-3). Other invasive diagnostic and surgical procedures also require antibiotics.

MYOCARDITIS

Myocarditis is an inflammation of the myocardial wall. Frequently, the inflammation is not limited to the myocardium but extends to the pericardium, with production of an associated pericarditis.

In the United States, most cases of myocarditis are due to viral infections, Coxsackie virus being the most common. Other viral causes include mumps, influenza, rubella, measles, adenoviruses, echoviruses, cytomegalovirus, and Epstein-Barr virus. Bacterial, fungal, rickettsial, spirochetal, helminthic, and protozoal infections can also cause myocarditis. Hypersensitivity immune reactions seen with acute rheumatic fever and postcardiotomy syndrome, toxins and chemicals such as alcohol, and large doses of radiation therapy to the chest for the treatment of malignancy are other causes.

Most viral pathogens enter the body through the upper respiratory or gastrointestinal tract. The virus enters the myocyte, replicates, and destroys the cell. The body's immune system responds. Over the next days to weeks, the cells that survive do not appear normal and are also destroyed by the immune system. If myocardial contractility is impaired, ventricular diastolic pressures and volumes may be elevated to maintain stroke volume. Disruptions leading to cardiac dysrhythmias can decrease cardiac output. Unfortunately, the outcome is commonly dilated cardiomyopathy and heart failure.

BOX 55-3   Dental Procedures and Endocarditis Prophylaxis in Adults

ENDOCARDITIS PROPHYLAXIS RECOMMENDED*

- Dental extractions
- Periodontal procedures, including surgery, scaling and root planing, probing, and recall maintenance
- Dental implant placement and reimplantation of avulsed teeth
- Endodontic (root canal) instrumentation or surgery only beyond the apex
- Subgingival placement of antibiotic fibers or strips
- Initial placement of orthodontic bands but not brackets
- Intraligamentary local anesthetic injections
- Prophylactic cleaning of teeth or implants where bleeding is anticipated
- Restoration of decayed teeth (filling cavities) and replacement of missing teeth
- Selected circumstances that may create significant bleeding

ENDOCARDITIS PROPHYLAXIS NOT RECOMMENDED

- Restorative dentistry (operative and prosthodontic) with or without retraction cord
- Local anesthetic injections (non-intraligamentary)
- Intracanal endodontic treatment; post placement and buildup
- Placement of rubber dams
- Postoperative suture removal
- Placement of removable prosthodontic or orthodontic appliances
- Taking of oral impressions
- Fluoride treatments
- Taking of oral radiographs
- Orthodontic appliance adjustment
- Shedding of primary teeth

*Standard general prophylaxis for adults is amoxicillin 3 g orally 1 hour before procedure, half the dose 6 hours later. If client is allergic to penicillin, erythromycin 800 mg or clindamycin 300 mg 1 hour before procedure, then half the dose 6 hours later.

From Dajani, A.S., et al. (1997). Prevention of bacterial endocarditis. *Journal of the American Medical Association, 277*, 1794-1801.

Clinical Manifestations

Clients who have viral myocarditis will present with a history of recent upper respiratory or gastrointestinal tract infection. After the viral illness is over, there is a delay of days to weeks before cardiac manifestations appear. Cardiac problems include heart failure, lethal dysrhythmias, and embolic problems. The most frequent manifestations are fatigue, dyspnea, palpitations, and chest pain. The client often experiences chest pain as a sharp, stabbing precordial pain, which can then be distinguished from the pressure sensation of angina pectoris. The client also has sinus tachycardia and abnormal heart sounds of murmurs, gallops, and rarely a pericardial friction rub.

ECG abnormalities and elevated serum levels of cardiac enzymes are helpful in the diagnosis. The ECG may show a bundle branch block or complete AV heart block, ST-segment elevation, or T-wave flattening. The chest x-ray may show an enlarged cardiac silhouette resulting from ventricular enlargement or pericardial effusion. Blood tests may show a moderate leukocytosis and elevated cardiac enzymes. Echocardiograms show impairments in the left ventricle and heart wall abnormalities. Ventricular thrombus is not uncommon. Cardiac MRI can reveal abnormal signal intensity in the heart muscle. Endomyocardial biopsies are used in diagnosis of the viral infection.

OUTCOME MANAGEMENT

Clients with acute myocarditis are usually admitted to the hospital for observation. Clients with pericardial effusion, dysrhythmias, heart failure, or hypotension are usually admitted to the intensive care unit (ICU) and may be in cardiogenic shock. Medical management begins with specific therapy for the underlying infection. Bed rest is suggested to decrease cardiac workload. Supplemental oxygen may be prescribed for clients with low cardiac output or dysrhythmias. Immunosuppressive therapy is being investigated. Antipyretic agents are helpful for the fever and its hemodynamic effects, which result in increased myocardial workload. Clients who remain at home may use Holter monitoring, which provides continuous surveillance of the client's heart rhythm. In most cases myocarditis is self-limiting and uncomplicated. Although most clients recover rapidly, some have recurrent or chronic myocarditis and some become very ill and die.

Nursing management for the client experiencing myocarditis is essentially the same as that provided to clients with infective endocarditis and rheumatic fever. Review those sections in this chapter.

Teaching begins when acute manifestations have subsided and the client has demonstrated physical and emotional readiness. Teach clients how to monitor their pulse rate and rhythm. Instruct them to report any sudden changes in heart rate, rhythm, or palpitations immediately. Encourage family members to take CPR training, which can be obtained from such groups as the local fire department, the American Red Cross, or the American Heart Association. Educating family members about CPR can enhance their sense of preparedness for an emergency.

Because the myocardial infectious process resolves slowly and late complications can occur, advise clients to continue self-monitoring and to schedule clinical follow-up appointments, even after apparent recovery.

The potential of lethal dysrhythmias may frighten the client and the client's significant others. The client who is experiencing extreme anxiety, fear, and ineffective coping may manifest insomnia, tearfulness, somatic complaints, an inability to problem-solve, and agitation. Determine with the client (and family) the specific focus of anxiety. Clarify any misconceptions. Speak slowly and calmly, and focus on the present situation, giving feedback about current reality. Encourage the use of relaxation techniques to help allay stress. Schedule activities around periods of undisturbed sleep.

PERICARDITIS

Pericarditis is inflammation of the pericardium and it may be either acute or chronic (recurrent). It is not known why pericarditis may be an acute illness in some clients and recurrent in others.

ACUTE PERICARDITIS

Acute pericarditis is a syndrome resulting from inflammation of the parietal and visceral pericardium. Because of the proximity of the pericardium to the pleura, lungs, sternum, diaphragm, and myocardium, pericarditis may be a consequence of a number of inflammatory or infectious processes (Box 55-4). Acute pericarditis is usually viral (idiopathic) in origin.

Agents or processes causing pericardial inflammation create an exudate of fibrin, WBCs, and endothelial cells. The exudate covers the pericardium and causes further inflammation of the surrounding pleura and tissues. The fibrinous exudate may localize to one region of the heart, or it may be generalized. Acute pericarditis may be either

---

BOX 55-4   Causes of Pericarditis

INFECTIONS
- Viral: Coxsackie, influenza
- Bacterial: tuberculosis, staphylococcus, streptococcus, meningococcus, pneumococcus
- Parasitic
- Fungal

MYOCARDIAL INJURY
- Myocardial infarction (Dressler's syndrome)
- Cardiac trauma: blunt or penetrating
- Post cardiac surgery
- Hypersensitivity

COLLAGEN DISEASES
- Rheumatic fever
- Scleroderma
- Systemic lupus erythematosus
- Rheumatoid arthritis

DRUG REACTION
- Procainamide
- Methysergide
- Hydralazine

RADIATION THERAPY

COBALT THERAPY

METABOLIC DISORDERS
- Uremia
- Myxedema

CHRONIC ANEMIA

NEOPLASM: LYMPHOMA

AORTIC DISSECTION

---

dry (fibrinous) or exudative. Under normal conditions the pericardial sac contains about 50 ml of clear, serous-like fluid. Volumes from 100 to 3000 ml of serofibrinous exudate can accumulate with pericarditis. The exudate accumulates in the pericardial sac, causing cardiac tamponade that restricts cardiac filling and emptying (see below). Without prompt treatment, shock and death can result from decreased cardiac output.

Dry pericarditis can occur after a common viral infection, myocardial infarction, tuberculosis, bacteremia, or renal failure. Delicate adhesions form within the pericardial space along with serous fibrin deposition, hemorrhage, and calcification. Adhesions may eventually obliterate the pericardial sac. Inflammation of the pericardium frequently penetrates the myocardium to some degree, which produces myopericarditis.

Although chest pain is common, the nature of this pain varies. Sometimes the pain is similar to that of myocardial infarction; at other times it mimics the pain of pleurisy. The pain is exacerbated with respiration and rotating the trunk but usually does not radiate to the arms. Sitting up and bending forward often relieves the pain.

Pericardial friction rub is a classic objective manifestation of acute pericarditis. The rub is produced by inflamed, roughened pericardial layers that create friction as their surfaces rub together during heart movement. Auscultation over the precordium reveals a scratchy, leathery, or creaky sound that is heard anywhere over the precordium but most frequently at the third intercostal space left of the sternal border. The rub is best heard with the diaphragm of the stethoscope and with the client holding his or her breath (to eliminate the breath sounds). In some clients the sound is best heard with the client sitting up. Pericardial friction rubs vary in intensity from hour to hour and from day to day.

Fever is another common finding in clients with pericarditis. The temperature may rise to 39.4° C (103° F). Chills, malaise, joint pain, anorexia, nausea, and weight loss accompany the fever. Dyspnea and chest pain can potentiate anxiety. An increase in heart rate usually corresponds to the degree of fever and anxiety.

The ECG may indicate tachycardia, but with underlying heart disease or uremia, bradycardia can occur. Laboratory studies show an elevated ESR and may show an elevated WBC count. Cardiac enzymes are usually normal but may be elevated.

OUTCOME MANAGEMENT

When the cause of acute pericarditis is known, treatment of the cause can be planned accordingly. If no causal agent is known, symptomatic intervention for acute dry pericarditis is provided. Clients may be hospitalized for diagnosis and for the treatment of complications. Pain and fever, usually self-limited, may be eased by aspirin given in the maximally tolerated doses.

Nonsteroidal anti-inflammatory drugs (NSAIDs) may also be prescribed. Stronger analgesia, such as morphine sulfate, may be necessary if chest pain becomes severe.

If acute pericarditis is present after a myocardial infarction (called Dressler's syndrome), reassure the client that the pain experienced with pericarditis does not mean that another infarction is occurring. If the client becomes anxious, worrying about the cause of the pain, oxygen demand increases and myocardial ischemia may develop.

The focus of nursing care related to pericarditis is the same as that described for the other inflammatory cardiac diseases discussed in this chapter. Nursing assessment of the client with pericarditis also includes scrutiny for the presence of pericardial tamponade (pulsus paradoxus, distended neck veins). Vigilant assessment is necessary. Provide reassurance about the temporary nature of the disease.

ACUTE PERICARDITIS WITH EFFUSION

Acute pericarditis with effusion results when fluid accumulates rapidly within the pericardial sac. The fluid may compress the heart and reduce ventricular filling and cardiac output. When fluid accumulates slowly, the fibrous pericardium is better able to stretch and accommodate its presence. Clients can tolerate 1 to 2 L of fluid without an increase in intrapericardial pressure if accumulation is slow and may show no manifestations. The heart sounds are often distant or muffled. The friction rub may disappear. Fever may develop.

Rapid accumulation of only 80 to 200 ml of fluid in the pericardial space can create a decrease in cardiac output. The client usually appears uncomfortable, with varying degrees of reduced cardiac output or even obvious shock. The client may have tachycardia, diaphoresis, cool or cyanotic extremities, and anxiety or confusion. A paradoxical pulse is often present. Carefully assess for an exaggeration of the normal variation in the pulse or a change in blood pressure by 10 mm Hg during the inspiratory phase of respiration, in which the pulse becomes weaker as one inhales and stronger as the client exhales. Echocardiography is the most accurate technique for evaluating pericardial effusion and pericardiocentesis. The fluid withdrawn is sent for analysis. Care of the client with pericardial effusion is similar to the plan of intervention for dry pericarditis. Bed rest, analgesia, and proper positioning can help to alleviate manifestations. Psychological support is important.

CHRONIC CONSTRICTIVE PERICARDITIS

Chronic constrictive pericarditis is a chronic inflammatory condition in which the pericardium changes into a thick,

fibrous band of tissue. This tissue encircles, encases, and compresses the heart, preventing proper ventricular filling and emptying. Cardiac failure eventually results from this slow compression. This condition usually begins with an episode of acute pericarditis characterized by fibrin deposition, often with pericardial effusion. In most cases the visceral and parietal layers become completely fused.

Clinical manifestations include right ventricular failure first, followed by decreased cardiac output manifesting as fatigue on exertion, dyspnea, leg edema, ascites, low pulse pressure, distended neck veins, and delayed capillary refill time. Constrictive pericarditis is a progressive disease without spontaneous reversal of manifestations.

Medical treatment includes digitalis, diuretics, and sodium restriction to relieve manifestations of right ventricular failure. Excision of the damaged pericardium (pericardiectomy) may be required.

CARDIAC TAMPONADE

Cardiac tamponade is a life-threatening complication caused by accumulation of fluid in the pericardium. This fluid, which can be blood, pus, or air in the pericardial sac, accumulates fast enough and in sufficient quantity to compress the heart and restrict blood flow in and out of the ventricles. This is a cardiac emergency.

Large or rapidly accumulating effusions raise the intrapericardial pressure to a point at which venous blood cannot flow into the heart, which decreases ventricular filling. As a result, venous pressure rises and cardiac output and arterial blood pressure fall. A narrowing pulse pressure signals cardiac tamponade. The heart attempts to compensate by beating rapidly (tachycardia), but tachycardia cannot sustain cardiac output for long. Prompt intervention is necessary to prevent shock and death.

Hypotension, tachycardia, jugular venous distention, cyanosis of lips and nails, dyspnea, muffled heart sounds, diaphoresis, and paradoxical pulse (a decrease in systolic arterial pulsation exceeding 10 mm Hg, during inspiration) are present. The client may be comfortable and quiet one minute and then restless with a feeling of impending doom. Clients may panic when fluid accumulates rapidly as a result of seriously reduced cardiac output. Slowly developing tamponade is characterized by manifestations that resemble those of heart failure: nonspecific ECG changes, decreased voltage, and visualization of fluid in the pericardial sac on echocardiogram. These clinical manifestations and related interventions are outlined in the Critical Monitoring feature on p. 1407.

Immediate intervention is required. The emergency intervention of choice is pericardiocentesis, a procedure in which fluid or air is aspirated from the pericardial sac (Figure 55-6). This procedure relieves pressure on the heart, thereby improving cardiac function and perhaps saving the client's life. Pericardiocentesis is performed with a soft catheter to reduce the risk of cardiac lacerations.

CRITICAL MONITORING

Cardiac Tamponade

Report the following manifestations of cardiac tamponade immediately!

- Elevated venous pressure (increased central venous pressure)
- Distended neck veins
- Kussmaul's sign (distended neck veins on inspiration)
- Hypotension
- Narrowed pulse pressure
- Tachycardia
- Dyspnea
- Restlessness, anxiety
- Cyanosis of lips and nails
- Diaphoresis
- Muffled heart sounds
- Pulsus paradoxus
- Decreased friction rub
- Decreased QRS voltage and electrical alternans

CONGENITAL DISORDERS

Congenital heart disorders result from faulty development of cardiac structures in utero. With today's available treatments, about 85% of children with congenital heart disease will survive to adulthood. Therefore we can expect to see more adults with congenital defects in the future. Many people with a congenital heart defect have remained asymptomatic; others have had varying levels of functional ability. Clients may have both residual problems and sequelae. Common lifelong problems include the risk of infective endocarditis in clients with artificial valves or with suture repair of an atrial septal defect. It is not uncommon for a client with a repaired coarctation of the aorta to find that the aorta has gradually become narrowed again. In such cases hypertension may develop. Clients who as children underwent repair for cyanotic defects tend to experience sequelae and complications in adulthood. Some degree of exercise intolerance may be present that can be better managed after proper stress testing.

Dysrhythmias frequently present a lifelong complication. Clients who have had intraventricular repairs may present with ventricular dysrhythmias or complete heart block. A 24-hour Holter monitor and stress testing may help to evaluate the client's tolerance for activity.

Many people who have had surgical procedures as infants and children had to have repeated operations as they "outgrew" their repairs or prosthetic devices. Our growing geriatric population also may be experiencing unknown late consequences of congenital heart disease or surgical repair. It is important to encourage these people to participate in long-term follow-up.

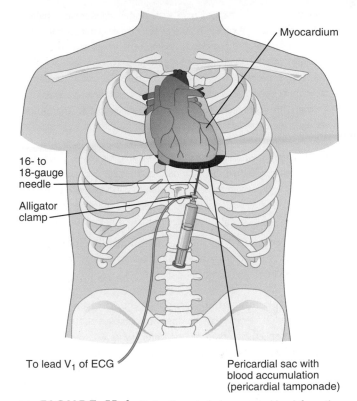

■ **FIGURE 55–6** Pericardiocentesis to remove blood from the pericardial sac during tamponade. *ECG,* Electrocardiogram.

Your role as a nurse who is caring for the adult with congenital heart disease varies with the setting; however, you play an integral role in helping these clients to achieve optimal health and functioning. Nursing assessment, intervention, education, and follow-up are directed toward improving functional levels, managing medications, assisting in psychosocial adjustment, and preventing complications.

CONCLUSIONS

The client with a cardiac disorder frequently has activity intolerance, decreased cardiac output, and ineffective coping because of the seriousness of the disorder. Nurses must be skilled in the physical and psychosocial aspects of disease when providing care.

THINKING CRITICALLY

1. A 52-year-old man with a lengthy history of mitral valve prolapse is recovering from kidney transplantation surgery. This is his fourth postoperative day, and he and his spouse are asking questions about care at home. What priorities for client education should be established?

Factors to Consider. What complication is associated with mitral valve prolapse? How does the medication regimen following transplantation surgery further place the client at risk?

2. The client is a 60-year-old man with dilated cardiomyopathy. His prognosis is very poor. He is able to tolerate only minimal amounts of activity—using the bedside commode, feeding himself, and shaving himself in bed. Today he continues to be short of breath but seems particularly withdrawn. Repeated physical assessment to identify cardiovascular status shows no change in assessment findings. He continues to take his medications at the proper dosages. His physician thinks these medications are at their maximal levels. Repeated psychosocial assessment would show that the client is withdrawn because he is anxious that his physical condition will worsen and that he will be hospitalized and placed on a ventilator again, which he does not wish to happen. He was terrified the last time this was done, and he sees no purpose in just prolonging his dying. What nursing actions might help your client?

Factors to Consider. What are the clinical manifestations of cardiomyopathy? What are the psychological considerations for the client's care?

3. A 45-year-old man arrives in the emergency department after an automobile accident. Initially he does not complain about himself; he is more concerned about his daughter, who was injured in the accident. Neither the child nor the client was wearing a seat belt when their car was struck from behind. While sitting at his daughter's bedside in the emergency department, the client becomes increasingly anxious; his respiratory rate increases, and he becomes restless. The vital signs show a blood pressure of 88/72 mm Hg, pulse rate of 118 beats/min, and respirations of 28 breaths/min. What other assessments are needed to rule out cardiac tamponade? What intervention will relieve pressure on the heart and improve cardiac function?

Factors to Consider. What are the clinical manifestations of cardiac tamponade? How is cardiac output affected by cardiac tamponade?

Discussions for these questions can be found on the website.

BIBLIOGRAPHY

Citations appearing in red refer to primary research.

Citations appearing in blue refer to evidence-based practice guidelines and protocols.

1. American Health Association. (2002). *2002 Heart and stroke statistical update.* Dallas, Tex: American Heart Association.
2. Autore, C., Conte, M.R., Piccininno, M., et al. (2002). Risk associated with pregnancy in hypertrophic cardiomyopathy. *Journal of the American College of Cardiology, 40*(10), 1864-1869.
3. Baddour, L., Wilson, W., Bayer, A., et al. (2005). Infective Endocarditis: American Heart Association Scientific Statement. *Circulation 111,* 3167-3184.
4. Baughman, K.L., & Braunwald, E. (2005). Myocarditis. In E. Braunwald (Ed.), *Heart disease* (7th ed., pp. 1697-1717). Philadelphia: Saunders.
5. Bayer, A.S., et al. (1998). AHA Scientific statement: Diagnosis and management of infective endocarditis and its complications. *Circulation, 98,* 2936-2948.
6. Bond, A.E., Bolton, B., & Nelson, K. (2004). Nursing education and implications for left ventricular assist device destination therapy. *Progress in Cardiovascular Nursing, 19*(3), 85-91.
7. Bonow, R.O., & Braunwald, E. (2005). Valvular heart disease. In E. Braunwald (Ed.), *Heart disease* (7th ed., pp. 1553-1632). Philadelphia: Saunders.
8. Bonow, R.O., Carabello, B., Chatterjee, K., et al. (2006). ACC/AHA 2006 practice guidelines for the management of patients with valvular heart disease: Executive summary: A report of the American College of Cardiology/American Heart Association Task Force on Practice Guidelines. *Journal of American College of Cardiology, 48*(3), 598-675.
9. Bonow, R.O., Carabello, B.A., Chatterjee, K., et al. (2006). ACC/AHA 2006 guidelines for the management of patients with valvular heart disease: A report of the American College of Cardiology/American Heart Association Task force on Practice Guidelines. *Journal of American College of Cardiology, 48*(3), e1-148.
10. Dajani, A.S. (2005). Rheumatic fever. In E. Braunwald (Ed.), *Heart disease* (7th ed., pp. 2093-2099). Philadelphia: Saunders.
11. Dajani, A.S., et al. (1997). Prevention of bacterial endocarditis: Recommendations by the American Heart Association. *Journal of the American Medical Association, 277*(22), 1794-1801.
12. Durack, D.T. (1995). Prevention of infective endocarditis. *New England Journal of Medicine, 332*(1), 38-44.
13. Greffe, G., Chalabreysse, L., Mouly-Bertin, C., et al. (2007). Valvular heart disease associated with fenfluramine detected 7 years after discontinuation of treatment. *Annals of Thoracic Surgery, 83*(4), 1541-1543.
14. Karchmer, A.W. (2005). Infective endocarditis. In E. Braunwald (Ed.), *Heart disease* (7th ed., pp. 1633-1658). Philadelphia: Saunders.
15. LeWinter, M.M., & Kabbani, S. (2005). Pericardial diseases. In E. Braunwald (Ed.), *Heart disease* (7th ed., pp. 1757-1780). Philadelphia: Saunders.
16. Maron, B.J. (2002). Hypertrophic cardiomyopathy: A systematic review. *Journal of the American Medical Association, 287*(10), 1308-1320.
17. McRae, M.E. (2005). Repaired tetralogy of Fallot in the adult. *Progress in Cardiovascular Nursing, 20*(3), 104-110.
18. Mogensen, J., Klausen, I.C., Pedersen, K., et al. (1999). Alpha-cardiac actin is a novel disease gene in familial hypertrophic cardiomyopathy. *The Journal of Clinical Investigation, 103*(10), R39-43.
19. Myers, R.B., & Spodick, D.H. (1999). Constrictive pericarditis: Clinical and pathophysiologic characteristics. *American Heart Journal, 138,* 219-232.
20. Otto, C.M., Burwash, I.G., Legget, M.E., et al. (1997). A prospective study of asymptomatic valvular aortic stenosis: Clinical, echocardiographic, and exercise predictors of outcome. *Circulation, 95*(9), 2262-2270.
21. Rahimtoola, S.H., Durairaj, A., Mehra, A., et al. (2002). Current evaluation and management of patients with mitral stenosis. *Circulation, 106*(10), 1183-1188.
22. Rathore, S.S., Curtis, J.P., Wang, Y., et al. (2003). Association of serum digoxin concentration and outcomes in patients with heart failure. *Journal of the American Medical Association, 289*(7), 871-878.
23. Richardson, P., McKenna, W., Bristow, M., et al. (1996). Report of the 1995 World Health Organization/International Society and Federation of Cardiology Task Force on the Definition and Classification of Cardiomyopathies. *Circulation, 93*(5), 841-842.
24. Shabetai, R. (2000). Sarcoidosis and the heart. *Current Treatment Options in Cardiovascular Medicine, 2*(5), 385-398.
25. Shepler, S.A., & Patel, A.N. (2007). Cardiac cell therapy: A treatment option for cardiomyopathy. *Critical Care Nursing Quarterly, 30*(1), 74-80.
26. Shimada, T., Shimada, K., Sakane, T., et al. (2001). Diagnosis of cardiac sarcoidosis and evaluation of the effects of steroid therapy by gadolinium-DTPA-enhanced magnetic resonance imaging. *American Journal of Medicine, 110*(7), 520-527.
27. Spirito, P., Seidman, C.E., McKenna, W.J., et al. (1997). The management of hypertrophic cardiomyopathy. *New England Journal of Medicine, 336*(11), 775-785.
28. Supino, P.G., Borer, J.S., Preibisz, J., et al. (2006). The epidemiology of valvular heart disease: A growing public health problem. *Heart Failure Clinics, 2*(4), 379-393.

29. Wang, A., Athan, E., Pappas, P., et al. (2007). Contemporary clinical profile and outcome of prosthetic valve endocarditis. *Journal of the American Medical Association, 297,* 1354-1361.

30. Winters, M., & Obriot, P. (2007). Mitral valve repair. *AORN Journal, 85*(1), 152-170.

31. Wynne, J., & Braunwald, E. (2005). The cardiomyopathies. In E. Braunwald (Ed.), *Heart disease* (7th ed., pp. 1659-1696). Philadelphia: Saunders.

32. Yazaki, Y., Isobe, M., Hiroe, M., et al. (2001). Prognostic determinants of long-term survival in Japanese patients with cardiac sarcoidosis treated with prednisone. *American Journal of Cardiology, 88*(9), 1006-1010.

evolve *Did you remember to check out the bonus material on the Evolve website and the CD-ROM, including NCLEX®-Examination Style Review Questions, Open-Book Quizzes, and Chapter Review Audio Podcasts?*

http://evolve.elsevier.com/Black/medsurg

CHAPTER 56

Management of Clients with Functional Cardiac Disorders

PATRICIA A. KERESZTES AND MARY WCISEL

Normal functioning of the heart is based on a balance between oxygen supply and oxygen demand. To function as an effective pump, the heart muscle must be adequately supplied with blood from the coronary arteries. In *coronary heart disease* (CHD), atherosclerosis develops in the coronary arteries, causing them to become narrowed or blocked. When a coronary artery is narrowed or blocked, blood flow to the area of the heart supplied by that artery is reduced. If the remaining blood flow is inadequate to meet the oxygen demands of the heart, the area may become ischemic and injured and myocardial infarction (MI) may result. In addition, the heart may fail to pump sufficient blood supply to the other organs and tissues in the body. Over time, changes resulting from CHD may lead to the development of chronic heart failure.

The terms *coronary heart disease, coronary artery disease,* and *ischemic heart disease* all refer to diseases of the heart that result from a decrease in blood supply to the heart muscle. This chapter reviews the risk factors, etiology, pathophysiology, clinical manifestations, and medical and nursing interventions for two major disorders of cardiac function: CHD and heart failure. The related conditions of angina pectoris and myocardial infarction (MI) are discussed in Chapter 58.

CORONARY HEART DISEASE

CHD is the single largest killer of both men and women in the United States, with nearly 2500 deaths per day. Although these numbers seem high, the death rate from CHD decreased by 30% from 1993 to 2003. Contributing to this decline in the death rate are factors such as improved technology for diagnosis and treatment, the use of thrombolytic drugs in acute MI, improved interventional therapies and surgical techniques, and modification of risk factors in populations at risk.

Etiology and Risk Factors

Although several mechanisms and many risk factors for CHD are present, it appears that the primary cause of CAD is inflammation and lipid deposition in the wall of the artery. Risk factors that precipitate CHD can be presented in two categories: modifiable and nonmodifiable risk factors (Box 56-1). The more risk factors a person has, the greater the risk of CHD. Although risk factors influence the development of CHD in all people, the importance of selected risk factors may vary by gender and race. African-American and Mexican-American women have a higher prevalence of CHD risk factors than white women. The prevalence of having two or more risk factors for CHD has been shown to be higher in African Americans and American Indians/Alaska Natives. There is a lower prevalence of risk factors seen in Asians. Reduction of risk is based on control of the modifiable risk factors.

Nonmodifiable Risk Factors

Heredity (Including Race)

Children whose parents had heart disease are at higher risk for CHD. This increased risk is related to genetic

---

evolve Web Enhancements

Case Management   Heart Failure

Clinical Pathway   Coronary Bypass Grafting

Complementary and Alternative Therapy   Aspirin to Reduce the Risk of Coronary Artery Disease

Eggs and Heart Disease

Do All Fish Products Prevent Heart Disease?

Nuts and the Risk of Sudden Cardiac Death

Be sure to check out the bonus material on the Evolve website and the CD-ROM, including free self-assessment exercises. **http://evolve.elsevier. com/Black/medsurg**

BOX 56–1	Risk Factors for Coronary Heart Disease

NONMODIFIABLE MAJOR RISK FACTORS
- Heredity, including race
- Age
- Gender

MODIFIABLE MAJOR RISK FACTORS
- Cigarette smoking
- Hypertension
- Elevated serum cholesterol level
- Diabetes mellitus
- Physical inactivity
- Obesity

CONTRIBUTING RISK FACTORS
- Stress
- Homocysteine level

predisposition to hypertension, elevated lipid levels, diabetes, and obesity, all of which increase the risk of CHD.

For people 35 to 74 years of age, the age-adjusted death rate from CHD for African-American women is 72% higher than that for white women and Native Americans. The prevalence of CHD is lowest among Mexican Americans.

Increasing Age

Age influences both the risk and the severity of CHD. Symptomatic CHD appears predominantly in people older than 40 years of age, and 4 of 5 people who die of CHD are age 65 years or older. Angina and MI, however, can occur in a person's 30s and even in one's 20s. At older ages, women who have heart attacks are twice as likely as men to die from the heart attack.

Gender

Coronary heart disease is the number one killer of both men and women. In 1999 mortality from CHD was almost equal for men and women. Although men are at higher risk for heart attacks at younger ages, the risk for women increases significantly at menopause, so that CHD rates in women after menopause are two to three times that of women the same age before menopause. Women who take oral contraceptives and who smoke or have high blood pressure are at greater risk for CHD. Women with an early menopause are also at higher risk than are women with a normal or late menopause.

Two lifestyle changes during the past 2 decades may be responsible for the increased incidence of CHD among women. More women (many with full responsibility for the household and children) have entered the work force, and more women have begun to smoke tobacco at an earlier age.

✦ Modifiable Risk Factors

Smoking, hypertension, elevated serum cholesterol levels, physical inactivity, obesity, and diabetes mellitus constitute the modifiable risk factors for CHD. These factors can be modified or reduced by lifestyle changes and treatment.

Smoking

Both active smoking and passive smoking have been strongly implicated as a risk factor in the development of CHD. Currently 23% of men and 18% of women are smokers. The prevalence of smoking is higher in people with 11 years of education or less. Smoking triples the risk of heart attack in women and doubles the risk of heart attack in men. It also doubles the risk of dying from a heart attack and may quadruple the risk of sudden death. Nonsmokers who are exposed to second-hand tobacco smoke at home or work may also have a higher death rate from CHD. The risk of CHD is decreased by 50% 1 year after smokers quit. The risk is further reduced to that of nonsmokers within 5 to 10 years after smoking cessation.

Tar, nicotine, and carbon monoxide contribute to the damage. Tar contains hydrocarbons and other carcinogenic substances. Nicotine increases the release of epinephrine and norepinephrine, which results in peripheral vasoconstriction, elevated blood pressure and heart rate, greater oxygen consumption, and increased likelihood of dysrhythmias. In addition, nicotine activates platelets and stimulates smooth muscle cell proliferation in the arterial walls. Carbon monoxide reduces the amount of blood available to the intima of the vessel wall and increases the permeability of the endothelium.

Hypertension

High blood pressure afflicts nearly 1 in 3 adults in the United States. It increases the workload of the heart by increasing afterload, enlarging and weakening the left ventricle over time. As blood pressure increases, the risk of a serious cardiovascular event also escalates. When clients have hypertension, obesity, tobacco use, high cholesterol levels, and diabetes, the risk of heart attack increases significantly.

More men than women have hypertension until the age of 45, when it is more prevalent in women. The prevalence of hypertension in African Americans is among the highest in the world. In addition, African Americans have hypertension at an earlier age and it is more severe at any age. Consequently, the rate of heart disease in African Americans is 1.5 times greater than that of white Americans. Although hypertension cannot always be prevented, it should be treated to lower the risk of CHD and premature death.

Elevated Serum Cholesterol Levels

The risk of CHD increases as blood cholesterol levels increase. This risk increases further when other risk factors are present. In adults total cholesterol levels of 240 mg/dl are classified as "high" and levels ranging from 200 to 239 mg/dl are classified as "borderline high." At young and middle ages, men have higher cholesterol levels. In women cholesterol levels continue to increase up to about age 70.

Cholesterol circulates in the blood in combination with triglycerides and protein-bound phospholipids. This complex is called a *lipoprotein*. There are four basic groups of lipoproteins, all produced in the intestinal wall. Elevation of lipoproteins is called *hyperlipoprotein-emia*. Elevation of lipids, a component of lipoproteins, is called *hyperlipidemia*. Lipoproteins and their functions are as follows:

- Chylomicrons primarily transport dietary triglycerides and cholesterol.
- Very-low-density lipoproteins (VLDLs) mainly transport triglycerides synthesized by the liver.
- Low-density lipoproteins (LDLs) have the highest concentration of cholesterol and transport endogenous cholesterol to body cells.
- High-density lipoproteins (HDLs) have the lowest concentration of cholesterol and transport endogenous cholesterol to body cells.

People with high levels of HDL in proportion to LDL are at lower risk for CHD than people with a low HDL-LDL ratio. High concentrations of HDL seem to protect against the development of CHD. Experts believe that the cholesterol in HDL, in contrast to that in LDL, does not become incorporated into the fatty plaques that develop in the lining of the artery wall. The ratio of total cholesterol to HDL or of LDL to HDL is the best test for predicting the risk of CHD. Exercise and low-fat, low-cholesterol diets increase the amount of HDL in the blood. The following are the current recommendations for cholesterol and lipoproteins:

- Total blood cholesterol <200 mg/dl
- LDL <160 mg/dl if fewer than two other risk factors (<130 mg/dl if two or more risk factors)
- HDL >40 mg/dl

Triglycerides are not an independent risk factor in men, but their significance in women is unknown; however, the combination of a high triglyceride level and a low HDL level seems to be a more important predictor of CHD in women than in men. The Consensus Panel Statement from the American Heart Association (AHA) recommends that triglyceride levels be below 150 mg/dl.

In the average American diet, about 45% of the total calories come from fat. This level exceeds that recommended in the AHA Step 1 Diet. Dietary fat comes in many forms and "disguises." A high intake of cholesterol and saturated fats is associated with the development of CHD, whereas a proportional intake of polyunsaturated and monounsaturated fats is linked with lower risk. Following a Mediterranean diet, described in the Complementary and Alternative Therapy feature below, may lower the risk of CHD. The AHA Step 1 Diet contains no more than 30% of calories from fat, 55% from carbohydrate (at least half of which should be complex), and 15% from protein. When fat intake does not exceed 30% of total calories, the expected rise in triglyceride levels from a high-carbohydrate diet is minimal. Saturated fats should account for no more than 10% of caloric intake.

COMPLEMENTARY AND ALTERNATIVE THERAPY

Mediterranean Diets and Cardiovascular Disease

A traditional Mediterranean diet may reduce the risk of dying from cardiovascular disease and cancer. Researchers evaluated more than 22,000 apparently healthy individuals ages 22 to 86 in Greece. Participants were rated on how closely they followed a Mediterranean diet. This type of diet is traditionally high in fruits and vegetables, legumes, nuts, cereal grains, and olive oil (monounsaturated fat); contains moderate amounts of fish, dairy (mostly cheese and yogurt), and alcohol; and is low in saturated fat. Adherence to the diet was measured on a scale of 0 (did not follow the diet closely) to 9 (strictly followed the diet). After about 4 years of follow-up, the researchers found that the more closely individuals adhered to the diet, the lower their risk of death, including death from cardiovascular disease and cancer (about a 25% decrease for every 2-point increase on the scale). Thus a greater adherence to the traditional Mediterranean diet was associated with a significant reduction in total mortality.[2]

The first clinical-trial evidence in support of the health benefits of the Mediterranean diet came from the Lyon Diet Heart Study, in which 605 clients with a previous MI were randomly assigned to a Mediterranean diet or a control diet similar to the AHA Step 1 Diet. Clients in the Mediterranean diet arm were encouraged to eat more fruits, vegetables, and fish; to eat less red meat; and to replace butter and cream with margarine high in alpha-linolenic acid (canola oil based margarine). After a mean follow-up of 27 months, the trial was stopped because of a 73% reduction in coronary events and a 70% reduction in all-cause or total mortality in the Mediterranean diet arm of the study.[1]

REFERENCES

1. de Lorgeril, M., et al. (1994). Mediterranean alpha-linolenic acid-rich diet in secondary prevention of coronary heart disease. *Lancet, 343*, 1454-1459.
2. Trichopoulou, A., et al. (2003). Adherence to a Mediterranean diet and survival in a Greek population. *New England Journal of Medicine, 348*, 2599-2608.

See the Complementary and Alternative Therapy features Eggs and Heart Disease, Do All Fish Products Prevent Heart Disease?, and Nuts and the Risk of Sudden Cardiac Death on the website.

Physical Inactivity
In the United States about 25% of adults report no leisure-time physical activity, even though regular aerobic exercise is important in preventing heart and blood vessel disease. There is an inverse relationship between exercise and the risk of CHD. Those who exercise reduce their risk of CHD because they have (1) higher HDL levels; (2) lower LDL cholesterol, triglyceride, and blood glucose levels; (3) greater insulin sensitivity; (4) lower blood pressure; and (5) lower body mass index. The AHA recommends 30 to 60 minutes of physical activity on most days of the week.

Obesity
Obesity places an extra burden on the heart, requiring the muscle to work harder to pump enough blood to support added tissue mass. In addition obesity increases the risk for CHD because it is often associated with elevated serum cholesterol and triglyceride levels, high blood pressure, and diabetes. The prevalence of obesity has increased to 30% in the years 1999 to 2002 compared to 22% from 1988 to 1994. Since 1993 the prevalence of those who are obese increased to 61%.

Distribution of body fat is also important. A waist measurement is a way to estimate fat. For men a high-risk waistline measurement is more than 40 inches, and for women a high-risk waist measurement is more than 35 inches. Body mass index (BMI) is another measure to estimate body fat. A BMI from 18.5 to 24.9 is considered healthy. Extreme obesity, or a BMI greater than 40, is estimated to occur in 4.9% of the population. People can lower their heart disease risk by losing as little as 10 to 20 pounds. An alternating pattern of weight gain and weight loss, however, is associated with an increased risk for CHD.

Diabetes
Since 1990 the prevalence of people diagnosed with diabetes increased by 61%. In addition, the prevalence of diabetes has increased by 8% since 2000 to 2001. Contributing to these statistics is the increased frequency of obesity and sedentary lifestyles. A fasting blood glucose level of more than 126 mg/dl or a routine blood glucose level of 180 mg/dl and glucosuria signals the presence of diabetes and represents an increased risk for CHD. Clients with diabetes have a two- to four-fold higher prevalence, incidence, and mortality from all forms of CHD.

Contributing Risk Factors

Response to Stress
A person's response to stress may contribute to the development of CHD. Some researchers have reported a relationship between CHD risk and stress levels, health behaviors, and socioeconomic status. Stress response appears to increase CHD risk through its effect on major risk factors. For example, some people respond to stress by overeating or by starting or increasing smoking. Stress is also associated with elevated blood pressure. Although stress is unavoidable in modern life, an excessive response to stress can be a health hazard. Significant stressors include major changes in residence, occupation, or socioeconomic status.

Homocysteine Levels
Researchers have reported that elevated levels of plasma homocysteine (an amino acid produced by the body) are associated with an increased risk of CHD (see the Complementary and Alternative Therapy feature on Elevated Homocysteine Levels and Heart Disease on the website). Scientists do not know whether homocysteine directly or indirectly increases CHD risk, however, because homocysteine levels are related to renal function, smoking, fibrinogen, and C-reactive protein (CRP). Elevated homocysteine levels can be reduced by treatment with folic acid, vitamin B_6, and vitamin B_{12}. Experts currently recommend that homocysteine levels be measured in people with a history of premature CHD, stroke, or both in the absence of other risk factors.

Inflammatory Responses
A newly identified risk factor currently being researched is the presence of any chronic inflammatory state that leads to an increase in the body's production of C-reactive protein (CRP). Too much CRP tends to destabilize plaque inside artery walls. When plaque lesions crack or break, a clot is formed and this may lead to a heart attack. Researchers have discovered that a high CRP level is a marker for coronary disease. This means that clients with chronic inflammatory diseases, such as arthritis, lupus, and autoimmune deficiency, may be at higher risk for heart attack.

Menopause
The incidence of CHD markedly increases among women after menopause. Before menopause estrogen is thought to protect against CHD risk by raising HDL and lowering LDL levels. Epidemiologic studies have shown that the loss of natural estrogen as women age may be associated with increases in total and LDL cholesterol and a gradually increasing CHD risk. If menopause is caused by surgical removal of the uterus and ovaries, the risks of CHD and MI increase.

Multiple research studies on the potential benefits of estrogen replacement therapy (ERT) and hormone replacement therapy (HRT) have yielded inconsistent results. Recent recommendations by the AHA outline the potential benefits and risks associated with HRT.

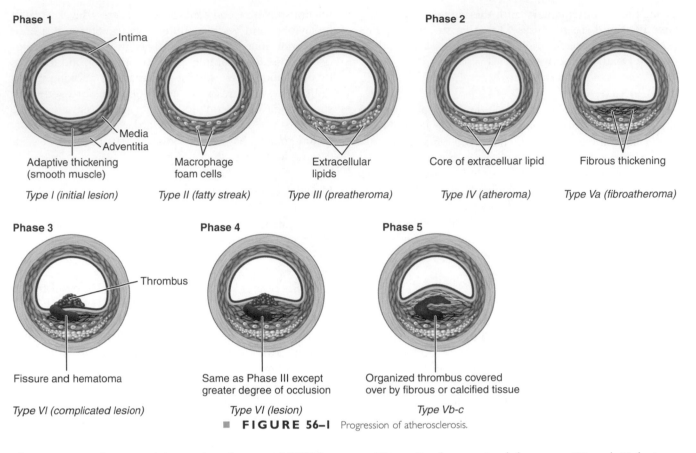

Phase 1

Intima

Media
Adventitia

Adaptive thickening (smooth muscle)

Macrophage foam cells

Extracellular lipids

Type I (initial lesion)   *Type II (fatty streak)*   *Type III (preatheroma)*

Phase 2

Core of extracelluar lipid

Fibrous thickening

Type IV (atheroma)   *Type Va (fibroatheroma)*

Phase 3

Thrombus

Fissure and hematoma

Type VI (complicated lesion)

Phase 4

Same as Phase III except greater degree of occlusion

Type VI (lesion)

Phase 5

Organized thrombus covered over by fibrous or calcified tissue

Type Vb-c

■ **FIGURE 56–1** Progression of atherosclerosis.

The recommendations advise against the use of HRT for the secondary prevention of CHD. There continues to be research to investigate the use of HRT for the primary prevention of CHD.

Pathophysiology

Coronary artery atherosclerosis is a progressive disease that begins early in life. Although several risk factors are present, endothelial injury is caused by an inflammatory response in the intimal layer of the wall and the deposition of lipids into the wall. This process has been shown to occur in five phases that include six progressive types of lesions (Figure 56-1).

Phase 1 is present in most people 30 years of age and younger and is characterized by clinically silent lesions of types I through III that do not appreciably thicken the arterial wall or narrow the arterial lumen. *Type I* lesions are microscopic adaptations of smooth muscle and occur most often near branches in the arteries. Type I lesions progress and mature into *type II* lesions. *Type III* lesions, known as *intermediate* lesions, develop during one's 20s. These lesions surround the smooth muscle cells. Type III lesions are also referred to as *pre-atheromas* because they form the bridge between early and advanced lesions. In phase 1, the progression of lesions is predictable, characteristic, and uniform.

Phase 2, characterized by type IV and V lesions, represents the development of vulnerable plaques. The *type IV* lesion, also called an *atheroma,* is characterized by further changes in the intimal structure caused by the accumulation of large amounts of extracellular lipids and fibrous tissue localized into a lipid core. The lipid core thickens the artery wall but often does not narrow the lumen of the artery. The periphery of type IV lesions is vulnerable to rupture, which may lead to rapid progression to more severe lesions.

When new fibrous connective tissue forms a thin protective cap over the atheroma, the lesion is classified as *type V.* These lesions are further subdivided into types Va, Vb, and Vc. *Type Va* lesions contain irregularly stacked multiple layers of lipid cores separated by thick layers of fibrous connective tissue. These lesions may rapidly progress to a *type VI* lesion or continue to develop into stenotic plaques that eventually occlude the entire lumen of the artery. A type V lesion that contains calcium in the lipid core and other parts of the lesion is referred to as *type Vb.* The absence of a lipid core, with minimal lipid deposition in other parts of the lesion, is characteristic of a *type Vc* lesion. *Type Vc* lesions are often seen in arteries in the legs.

Phase 3 is marked by the acute disruption of type IV and V lesions that causes thrombus formation and the development of a type VI lesion *(complicated).* If thrombus formation during phase 3 does not limit the flow of blood through the artery, these events are often asymptomatic. The net result of phase 3 is a rapid increase in plaque size that may result in stable angina. If the thrombus reduces or significantly blocks flow through the artery *(phase IV),* an acute coronary syndrome such as unstable angina, MI, or sudden cardiac death often results (see Chapter 58). Type VI lesions are characterized by a core that contains extracellular lipids, tissue factor, collagen, platelets, thrombin, and fibrin. These lesions may also be associated with disruption of the plaque surface, hematoma or hemorrhage into the plaque, and thrombosis.

Phase 5 follows a phase 3 or 4 event and occurs when the thrombus over the disrupted plaque begins to calcify (type Vb lesion) or fibrose (type Vc lesion), forming a chronic stenotic lesion. The phase 5 lesion often contains organizing thrombi from several earlier episodes of plaque disruption, ulceration, hemorrhage, and organization. As the phase 5 lesion progresses, it occludes a greater portion of the arterial lumen and eventually may lead to total occlusion. Phase 5 lesions are associated with chronic stable angina and are often accompanied by the development of collateral circulation.

Collateral circulation is the presence of more than one artery supplying a muscle (Figure 56-2). Normally some collateral circulation is present in the coronary arteries, especially in older people. Collateral vessels develop when the blood flow through an artery progressively decreases and causes ischemia to the muscle. Extra blood vessels develop to meet the metabolic demands of the muscle. The development of collateral circulation takes time. Therefore an occlusion of a coronary artery in a younger person is more likely to be lethal because there are no collateral arteries present to supply the myocardium with blood.

■ **FIGURE 56–2** Collateral circulation develops when new vessels form during ischemic periods.

For many years researchers thought that the more obstructive lesions (types Vb and Vc) were responsible for most occlusions of the coronary arteries and acute coronary events. In contrast, more recent studies suggest that lesions that produce mild stenosis (types IV and Va) are more frequently associated with rapid progression to coronary occlusion. In fact nearly 60% to 70% of all acute coronary syndromes occur in arteries with mild (<50% stenosis) or moderate (50% to 70% stenosis) occlusion. It is thought that this occurs because less occlusive lesions are more vulnerable to plaque rupture and thrombosis. Plaque disruption is thought to result from external stresses on the vessel and internal changes that increase plaque fragility. Physical forces that exert external pressure on the atherosclerotic plaques, such as blood and pulse pressures, heart contraction, vasospasm, and shear stress, may trigger plaque rupture. Internal factors, such as inflammation, may increase plaque vulnerability.

Clinical Manifestations

Atherosclerosis by itself does not necessarily produce subjective clinical manifestations. For manifestations to develop, there must be a critical deficit in the blood supply to the heart in proportion to the demands for oxygen and nutrients; in other words, a supply-and-demand imbalance must exist. When atherosclerosis progresses slowly, the collateral circulation that develops generally can meet the heart's demands. Thus whether manifestations of CHD develop depends on the total blood supply to the myocardium (by way of the coronary arteries and collateral circulation) and not solely on the condition of the coronary arteries.

Rapid progression of atherosclerotic lesions (type VI) may cause ischemia and may result in the development of acute coronary syndromes of unstable angina, MI, and sudden cardiac death. Slow progression of atherosclerotic lesions (types Vb and Vc) is associated with stable coronary artery disease and the clinical manifestation of chronic stable angina. These lesions usually cause ischemia during periods when myocardial oxygen demand increases. Angina, MI, and sudden cardiac death are discussed in Chapter 58.

Techniques to determine the extent of CHD and identify the affected vessels include the electrocardiogram (ECG); B-mode ultrasonography; Doppler flow studies; intravascular ultrasound; electron-beam computed tomography; and thallium, sestamibi, or echocardiographic stress tests (see Chapter 58).

OUTCOME MANAGEMENT

Medical Management

The primary goals that guide the medical management of a client with CHD are reducing and controlling risk factors and restoring blood supply to the myocardium.

Reduce Risk Factors

Prevention, rather than treatment, is the goal with regard to CHD. Modification of risk factors can significantly improve prognosis even after an acute coronary event. Recent findings indicate reducing risk factors may limit and even prevent the progression of CHD by increasing the stability of atherosclerotic plaques, decreasing thrombogenicity, and limiting external stress on the vessel. For people without diagnosed CHD, the goal of medical treatment is to prevent the development of risk factors and clinical disease. Cessation of cigarette smoking; participating in regular exercise; and controlling blood pressure, diabetes, cholesterol levels, and weight can reduce the risk of CHD.

Primary and secondary prevention goals are in place for all the major risk factors. Ideally primary prevention should begin with promoting healthy lifestyles in children. Primary care should include family-oriented education about the risk factors, review of the family history, and modification of risk factors. For clients with diagnosed CHD, the goals of prevention are to (1) reduce the incidence of subsequent coronary events, (2) decrease the need for treatments such as angioplasty and coronary artery bypass graft (CABG) surgery, (3) extend overall survival, and (4) improve the quality of life.

Blood pressure should be measured at least every 2 years in adults, and clients should be encouraged to control blood pressure by maintaining ideal weight, exercising regularly, moderating alcohol intake, and following a moderately low sodium diet (alcohol intake is discussed in the Complementary and Alternative Therapy feature at right). Blood pressure should be below 140/90 mm Hg (<130/85 mm Hg for those with heart failure, diabetes, or renal insufficiency). Antihypertensive therapy should begin if blood pressure exceeds 140/90 mm Hg after 6 months of lifestyle modification or if the initial blood pressure exceeds 160/100 mm Hg (130/85 mm Hg for those with heart failure, diabetes, or renal insufficiency). Clients should stop smoking and avoid contact with secondary smoke. Health professionals should provide counseling, nicotine replacement, and referrals to smoking-cessation programs for clients who smoke.

Total, LDL, and HDL cholesterol should be measured annually for adults older than 20 years. The following are the primary prevention goals for cholesterol management:

- LDL <160 mg/dl if no risk factors or only one risk factor
- LDL <130 mg/dl if two or more risk factors
- HDL >40 mg/dl
- Triglycerides <150 mg/dl

The following are the secondary prevention goals for cholesterol management:

- LDL <100 mg/dl
- HDL >40 mg/dl
- Triglycerides <150 mg/dl

COMPLEMENTARY AND ALTERNATIVE THERAPY

Which Type of Alcohol Reduces the Risk of Heart Disease?

Researchers studied the association of alcohol ingestion with the risk of MI among more than 38,000 male health professionals who were free of cardiovascular disease and cancer at baseline. Alcohol consumption and type of alcohol were documented every 4 years using a food-frequency questionnaire. After 12 years of follow-up, the total number of MIs was 1418. Compared with men who consumed alcohol less than once a week, men who consumed alcohol 3 or 4 or 5-7 days per week had a 32% and 37% reduction of MI, respectively. The risk was similar in men who consumed less than 10 g of alcohol per drinking day and those who consumed 30 g or more (a single alcoholic drink contains 11 to 14 g of alcohol). No single type of alcoholic beverage provided an additional benefit. In other words, red wine, white wine, beer, and liquor were similar in their effect. Therefore moderate drinking was associated with a reduced risk of MI. The problem with this large study is that although alcohol in moderation seems to reduce the risk of dying from a MI, researchers are not sure whether or not it reduces the risk of all-cause mortality (this needs to be studied). Regardless, for now moderate consumption reduces the risk of death from cardiovascular disease.

REFERENCE

Mukamal, K., et al. (2003). Roles of drinking pattern and type of alcohol consumed in coronary heart disease in men. *New England Journal of Medicine, 348*, 109-118.

The AHA Step 1 Diet should be recommended for clients who are unable to meet the primary prevention goals, and the Step 2 Diet should be recommended for those with CHD who do not meet the recommended goals. Red-yeast rice supplements may also reduce cholesterol level. This supplement is discussed in the Complementary and Alternative Therapy feature on p. 1417. In addition, drug therapy is recommended for clients who do not meet the recommended goals for cholesterol management. The Complementary and Alternative Therapy features on p. 1417 consider the interplay of statin drugs, diet, and dietary supplements.

During routine physical examinations, health professionals should determine the client's activity level and participation in exercise. Clients should be encouraged to exercise at least five times weekly for 30 minutes and to increase their physical activity in daily life. The Complementary and Alternative Therapy feature on p. 1417 considers the benefits of strength training in men with CHD. An exercise test may be needed to guide an exercise prescription for clients with confirmed CHD.

Clients should be encouraged to maintain ideal body weight as indicated by a BMI between 18.5 and

Red Yeast Rice Supplements to Reduce Cholesterol

Chinese red yeast rice supplements have been available on the U.S. market for several years, and currently they have been involved in litigation because some companies argue that this natural supplement has a similar structure to cholesterol-lowering drugs (statins). This supplement was tested against a placebo in 83 individuals (46 men, 37 women). A total of 2.4 g of red yeast rice or placebo was given daily for 3 months. Levels of total cholesterol, LDL, and triglycerides decreased compared with the placebo arm of the study. Total cholesterol level had the largest reduction, with an average decrease of 45 mg/dl. This supplement showed no effect on HDL (good cholesterol) levels. No apparent adverse effects were seen with this supplement, but this study was of short duration.

REFERENCE

Ashley, J., et al. (1999). Cholesterol-lowering effects of a proprietary Chinese red-yeast-rice dietary supplement. *American Journal of Clinical Nutrition, 69,*231-236.

Statin Drugs and Dietary Supplements

The largest randomized trial of statin drugs in combination with supplements included 160 individuals studied over 3 years. The supplement combination included 800 international units of vitamin E plus 100 mcg of selenium plus 1000 mg of vitamin C and 25 mg of beta-carotene with or without a statin drug plus niacin. Simvastatin plus niacin provided a marked clinical angiographically measurable benefit in clients with coronary disease and low HDL levels. The group taking the supplement combination plus the statin drug experienced a significant reduction in HDL (or "good cholesterol") compared with the group that took the statin drug alone. Further study is needed to determine whether the desired effects of statin drugs are diminished when taken in combination with antioxidant vitamin supplements.

REFERENCE

Brown, B.G., et al. (2001). Simvastatin and niacin, antioxidant vitamins, or the combination for the prevention of coronary disease. *New England Journal of Medicine, 345,*1583-1592.

Diet Versus Statin Therapy for High Cholesterol

A preliminary recent study randomly assigned 55 healthy hyperlipidemic men and women to receive 1 of 3 treatments: a very low saturated fat diet based on low-fat dairy foods and whole-grain cereals (control arm); the same diet plus 20 mg daily of lovastatin (statin group); or a diet with a high intake of plant sterols, soy protein, soluble fibers, and almonds (dietary portfolio group). The data were based on 46 clients who completed the 4-week study. The researchers reported that the statin and dietary portfolio treatment arms had about a 30% decrease in LDL ("bad cholesterol") versus an 8% reduction in the control group. Although a longer and larger trial is needed, this unique study suggests that over a short period, individuals willing to try a more directed dietary change could potentially reduce their cholesterol as much as some cholesterol-lowering drugs; however, cholesterol-lowering drugs are still the treatment of choice for clients who cannot significantly reduce their cholesterol levels with diet and physical activity over a period of 3 to 6 months.

REFERENCE

Jenkins, D., et al. (2003). Effects of a dietary portfolio of cholesterol-lowering foods vs lovastatin on serum lipids and C-reactive protein. *Journal of the American Medical Association, 290,* 502-510.

Lifting Weights and Coronary Heart Disease in Men

A cohort of 44,452 men enrolled in the Health Professionals' Follow-up Study were followed up at 2-year intervals from 1986 to 1998. Men who trained with weights for 30 minutes or more per week had a 23% risk reduction in coronary heart disease compared with men who did not train with weights ($P = 0.03$ for trend). In summary, researchers found that total physical activity, running, weight training, and walking were each associated with a reduced risk of coronary heart disease.

REFERENCE

Tanasescu, M., et al. (2002). Exercise type and intensity in relation to coronary heart disease in men. *Journal of the American Medical Association, 288,* 1994-2000.

24.9 kg/m^2 and a waist circumference less than 40 inches in men and 35 inches in women. Height, weight, BMI, and waist-to-hip ratio should be measured at each visit. People with BMI and waist circumferences higher than those recommended should be counseled regarding weight management and physical activity.

Fasting blood glucose concentration should be maintained near normal levels in clients with diabetes mellitus. Hypoglycemic therapy should be used to achieve normal fasting blood glucose as indicated by hemoglobin A_{1C} (HbA$_{1C}$) value. The recommended goal for HbA$_{1C}$ is <7%. Other risk factors should be treated aggressively.

Hormone replacement therapy should be considered for all postmenopausal women without diagnosed CHD, particularly if they have multiple risk factors. The decision about HRT, however, should be made by considering the risks for breast cancer, gallbladder disease, thromboembolic disease, and endometrial cancer. Estrogen-progesterone therapy reportedly increases cardiovascular events in women with diagnosed CHD during the first year of treatment but decreases events in the fourth and fifth years. Consequently, initiating estrogen-progesterone therapy for women with confirmed CHD is not recommended. For women with CHD who have already been receiving HRT for more than 1 year, continuing therapy is recommended until the results of additional research are known.

Additional management strategies are recommended for clients with diagnosed CHD. These include the use of antiplatelet therapies such as acetylsalicylic acid (aspirin), heparin, and low-molecular-weight heparin if it is not contraindicated. Aspirin reduces the risk of fatal or nonfatal MI by 71% during the acute phase, by 60% at 3 months, and by 52% at 2 years[14] (see the website Complementary and Alternative Therapy feature Aspirin to Reduce the Risk of Coronary Artery Disease). Adjunctive therapies, such as angiotensin-converting enzyme (ACE) inhibitors, beta-blockers, and nitrates, are also recommended.

Glycoprotein IIb/IIIa (GPIIb/IIIa) receptor antagonists are the most recent pharmacologic treatment for secondary prevention of CHD. These drugs prevent platelet aggregation in acute coronary syndromes, and when combined with aspirin they decrease the incidence of recurrent cardiac events. The therapeutic effects, adverse responses, and nursing implications of pharmacologic agents used in the primary prevention of CHD are outlined in the Integrating Pharmacology feature below.

Restore Blood Supply

For some clients even aggressive management of risk factors fails to prevent coronary occlusion. Various techniques have been developed to open the vessels and restore blood flow through the coronary arteries. Percutaneous coronary intervention (PCI) includes percutaneous luminal coronary angioplasty, rotational atherectomy, directional atherectomy, laser angioplasty, and implantation of intracoronary stents. The American College of Cardiology, along with the AHA, issues guidelines for the use of PCI and reports on all procedures collectively. More than 500,000 PCI procedures are performed yearly. The use of percutaneous transluminal coronary angioplasty (PTCA) alone has decreased dramatically, whereas the use of PCTA with placement of intracoronary stents has dramatically increased. Stents have been shown to reduce late restenosis in coronary arteries. The use of GPIIb/IIIa platelet receptor antagonists has also improved outcomes of PCI. PCI is recommended for clients with mild angina, single or multivessel coronary artery disease, unstable angina, and acute MI and following thrombolytic therapy. These procedures are performed in a "catheterization laboratory," which is outfitted with high-resolution fluoroscopy and x-ray.

INTEGRATING PHARMACOLOGY

Preventive Pharmacology for Coronary Heart Disease

Several medications can be prescribed to prevent the development or progression of coronary heart disease. They include statins to reduce elevated LDL levels and antiplatelet aggregates to reduce the risk of clotting in narrowed vessels.

STATINS

A reduction in elevated LDL levels can significantly reduce coronary events in individuals without CHD. Lipid-lowering drug therapy for primary CHD prevention is most clearly indicated when two or more CHD risk factors are present and the LDL level remains higher than 160 mg/dl after an adequate dietary trial. In addition, clients with LDL levels higher than 160 mg/dl and with one other strong risk factor (diabetes, smoking, or a family history of early CHD) may also be candidates for drug therapy. For clients with elevated risk attributable to sudden cardiac death in family members and elevated LDL levels, drug treatment may be beneficial.

Educating the client about the need to take this medication for a lifetime is important. Noticeable effects will not be seen and may lead clients to discontinue the medication without informing their care provider. If cost is an issue, consider prescribing half-pill doses or recommending ingestion of grapefruit juice when the drug is taken to increase drug absorption. Follow-up assessment of serum lipid levels is important to monitor progress.

Clients should be taught that the medication must be taken every day indefinitely to maximize benefit, noting that the LDL level returns to the pretreatment level soon after the medication is discontinued. Dietary adjustments must also be continued.

ANTIPLATELET AGGREGATING AGENTS

Aspirin in low doses is the best known agent for the prevention of coronary heart disease. Aspirin's benefits include reducing the coagulability of blood so that it can flow more freely through tight, narrow vessels. Aspirin is also an anti-inflammatory agent and can reduce the inflammatory process, which destabilizes plaque inside artery walls. A risk factor with the consumption of aspirin is that clients may take the medication because it is readily available without prescription believing it could not harm them. Aspirin should not be used by clients with allergy to aspirin or other salicylates, asthma, uncontrolled high blood pressure, severe liver or kidney disease, excess alcohol consumption, or bleeding disorders. Clients taking other medications that affect bleeding or clotting also should not take aspirin.

Percutaneous Transluminal Coronary Angioplasty. Percutaneous transluminal coronary angioplasty (PTCA) is a technique in which a balloon-tipped catheter is usually inserted into the femoral artery (although the brachial or radial artery can be used) and threaded under x-ray guidance into a blocked coronary artery. The balloon is inflated several times to reshape the lumen by stretching it and flattening the atherosclerotic plaque against the arterial wall (analogous to making footprints in the snow), thus opening the artery (Figure 56-3). PTCA is less invasive and less expensive than open heart surgery and therefore is an attractive alternative.

Directional Coronary Atherectomy. Directional coronary atherectomy (DCA) reduces coronary stenosis by excising and removing atheromatous plaque. The DCA cutter consists of a catheter that contains a rigid cylindrical housing with a central rotating blade (Figure 56-3, *E*). The blade shaves off the atherosclerotic material and deposits it in the nose cone of the housing for later histopathologic study. DCA is appropriate for lesions in medium to large coronary arteries located in the

proximal or middle portions of the vessel. It is not recommended for use with tortuous vessels, distal lesions, or heavily calcified lesions.

Intracoronary Stents. Intracoronary stents were originally designed to reduce restenosis and abrupt closure of coronary vessels resulting from complications of coronary angioplasty. They are now used instead of PTCA to eliminate the risk of acute closure and to improve long-term patency. Several different stent designs are available, but most are balloon-expandable or self-expandable tubes that, when placed in a coronary artery, act as a mechanical scaffold to reopen the blocked artery (Figure 56-3, *C*). Coronary stents are made of numerous materials, ranging from stainless steel to bioabsorbable compounds. The procedure for placing a stent is similar to that for PTCA. Once the coronary lesion is identified by angiography, the balloon catheter bearing the stent is inserted into the coronary artery and the stent is positioned at the site of the occlusion. A major concern related to stent placement is the prevention of acute thrombosis, especially during the first several weeks after the procedure. The use of

Catheter threaded into subclavian artery

Balloon in position in left coronary artery

A

B

C

D

E

■ **FIGURE 56–3** Interventional cardiology can be performed to open occluded coronary arteries. **A,** Percutaneous transluminal coronary angioplasty (PTCA). **B,** The balloon-tipped catheter is centered in the lesion and expanded to compress the blockage. **C,** The artery is restored to its original diameter. **D,** Placement of a coronary artery stent at the site of the lesion. **E,** Atherectomy. If the plaque has hardened and become calcified, atherectomy can be used to pulverize the material. Some catheters are fitted with a laser that dissolves the lesions.

GPIIb/IIIa platelet receptor antagonists has decreased the risk of thrombus formation following stent placement. New technology, including the use of intracoronary gamma and beta radiation with stent placement, has reduced restenosis rates by 3% to 50%. The use of stents coated with antiplatelet drugs has been shown to decrease rates of restenosis.

Laser Ablation. Lasers are used with balloon angioplasty to vaporize atherosclerotic plaque. After the initial balloon angioplasty, a brief burst of laser radiation is administered and additional remaining plaque is removed. Results of clinical trials indicate that laser ablation combined with balloon angioplasty is more effective in treating lesions that typically respond poorly to angioplasty alone. Complications include coronary dissection, acute occlusion, perforation, and embolism.

Transmyocardial Revascularization. A new type of laser catheter, used in a procedure called transmyocardial revascularization (TMR), may be able to help clients who are not candidates for surgery or angioplasty because of ill health or degree of disease. The high-powered laser is guided into the left ventricle between heartbeats when the ventricle is filling with blood. The laser creates from 15 to 40 1-mm channels through the myocardium. The exact mechanism by which TMR works has not been established; however, scientists believe that the "controlled trauma" caused by creating the channels may promote the growth of small new blood vessels, a process called *angiogenesis*. TMR is estimated to cost only slightly more than PTCA, and sustained improvement has been seen up to 27 months following the operation.

Nursing Management of the Medical Client

Reduce Risk Factors

Nursing management for CHD focuses on risk factor modification through risk assessment, screening, and education. The client's level of motivation to reduce cardiovascular risk factors is the primary predictor of success. Nursing researchers are studying methods to improve motivation.

Primary prevention efforts include providing health education about reducing the risk factors for CHD. Encourage clients to reduce their risk by lowering dietary intake of fats and cholesterol, exercising, controlling diabetes and hypertension, keeping body weight near ideal levels, and ceasing smoking (see the Complementary and Alternative Therapy feature on Moderate Lifestyle Change and Coronary Artery Disease on the *evolve* website). The risk and incidence of CHD are so high that many clients are doing these activities on an ongoing basis. Reinforce these behaviors. Participate in risk factor screening for both children and adults, and maintain a high index of suspicion for clients at increased risk for

CHD. Teach stress-reduction techniques, such as progressive muscle relaxation and guided imagery. Instruct postmenopausal women to discuss the need for estrogen HRT with their physician. Monitor blood pressure control in clients with diagnosed hypertension, and monitor HbA_{1C} levels in diabetic clients.

Nursing interventions for clients with diagnosed CHD include assessing their CHD risk and explaining diagnostic tests, when to seek treatment, clinical manifestations of complications, and the actions, dosages, and side effects of prescribed medications. Assess cardiovascular risk factors, and provide individualized education on risk reduction. Emphasize the importance of adopting risk-reduction behaviors and participating in cardiac rehabilitation to prevent recurrence or progression of CHD. Teach clients the clinical manifestations of angina and MI. Monitor therapeutic drug levels as appropriate. Emphasize the importance of keeping follow-up appointments with health care practitioners. Most important, instruct clients to seek prompt medical attention if manifestations of CHD return.

Many clients use forms of alternative therapies for self-treatment of heart disease. The Complementary and Alternative Therapy feature below examines one commonly used therapy.

Restore Blood Supply

Before interventional procedures, the client is usually given an antiplatelet medication, such as aspirin. The client is also given an anticoagulant (heparin) to prevent occlusion and calcium-channel blockers or nitrates to

---

COMPLEMENTARY AND ALTERNATIVE THERAPY

Omega-3 Fatty Acids to Reduce the Risk of Early Mortality

A meta-analysis of omega-3 fatty acids to reduce the risk of death was conducted. A total of 11 randomized trials were included ($n = 15,806$; mean age range, 49-66 years; mean follow-up, 20 months). Of the 11 trials, 2 were dietary, and 9 trials involved supplements of omega-3 fatty acids. The meta-analyses found that in clients with coronary artery disease, dietary or supplemental intake (1 g of fish oil/day) of omega-3 fatty acids reduced fatal MI (27% reduction), sudden death (31% reduction), and overall mortality (19% reduction) greater than a control diet or placebo. The groups did not differ statistically in nonfatal MI, but a nonsignificant 20% reduction was noted. Therefore diets high in omega-3 fatty acids (fish) or fish oil supplements continue to look promising for clients with a history of heart disease.

REFERENCE

Bucher, H., et al. (2002). N-3 polyunsaturated fatty acids in coronary heart disease: A meta-analysis of randomized controlled trials. *American Journal of Medicine, 112,* 298-304.

reduce coronary spasm during the procedure. After the procedure, the client may continue with this drug regimen to prevent reocclusion or arterial spasms.

The client's blood is also typed and crossmatched in the event emergency CABG surgery is needed. A consent form is signed for the interventional procedure and surgery, if required, for spasm, perforation of the artery, or acute occlusion. Following interventional procedures, monitor the vital signs for changes, especially the quality and rhythm of the pulse and in the ECG. Report any indication of coronary ischemia to the physician. ST-segment monitoring is frequently used to detect ischemia.

SAFETY

⚠

ALERT

Complications include bleeding and hematoma formation at the puncture site, acute MI resulting from perforation of an artery, refractory spasm, or occlusion. If the client complains of chest pain, obtain a 12-lead ECG immediately. Force fluids, orally or intravenously, to assist the body in excreting contrast medium, which causes diuresis and may cause acute renal tubular necrosis. Monitor the puncture site for hematoma, and palpate pulses to assess peripheral perfusion.

The physician may order bed rest for longer periods for clients undergoing stent placement and DCA because of the larger sheaths used to dilate the vessels in these procedures.

Nursing considerations specific to the care of the client with a coronary stent include close monitoring of anticoagulation status and ongoing assessment for bleeding. Until the sheath is removed, instruct the client to limit movement of the sheathed leg and keep the head of the bed below 30 degrees to prevent bleeding and hematoma formation at the site. Clients with coronary stents usually have longer hospital stays than clients undergoing other interventional procedures because their antithrombin therapy must be monitored closely.

Surgical Management

Cardiac Surgery

There are three types of cardiac surgery:

1. *Reparative* procedures are likely to produce a cure or excellent and prolonged improvement. Examples are closure of a patent ductus arteriosus, atrial septal defect, and ventricular septal defect; repair of mitral stenosis; and simple repair of tetralogy of Fallot.
2. *Reconstructive* procedures are more complex. They are not always curative, and reoperation may be needed. Examples are CABG and reconstruction of an incompetent mitral, tricuspid, or aortic valve.
3. *Substitutional* procedures are not usually curative because of the preoperative condition of the client. Examples are valve replacement, cardiac replacement by transplantation, ventricular replacement or assistance, and cardiac replacement by mechanical devices.

Open Heart Surgery

Cardiopulmonary bypass is used during cardiac surgery to divert the client's unoxygenated blood to a machine in which oxygenation and circulation occur. Reoxygenated blood is then returned to the client's circulation. This technique, called extracorporeal circulation (ECC, also called the heart-lung machine), allows the surgeon to stop the heart during the time of surgery. The heart-lung machine does the following:

- Diverts circulation from the heart and lungs, providing the surgeon with a bloodless operative field
- Performs all gas exchange functions
- Filters, rewarms, or cools the blood
- Circulates oxygenated, filtered blood back into the arterial system

The three components of cardiopulmonary bypass are hemodilution, hypothermia, and anticoagulation. Hemodilution occurs as the client's blood becomes diluted with the isotonic crystalloid solution used to prime the bypass machine. Hypothermia (28° to 36° C) is used to reduce tissue oxygen requirements by approximately 50% to protect the organs from ischemic injury. Anticoagulation is necessary to prevent coagulation in the bypass machine once the client's blood comes into contact with the surfaces in the machine. These three components contribute to the clinical sequelae and the complications associated with cardiopulmonary bypass, including coagulopathies. Excessive bleeding after cardiac surgery is related to the hemodilution and excessive activation of the hemostatic system because blood cells are injured as they contact the bypass machine. The risk of complications is high when the duration of cardiopulmonary bypass exceeds 2 hours and dramatically increases whenever bypass persists beyond 3 to 4 hours. This proportional increase in complications is attributed to the increase in blood trauma, altered capillary membrane permeability, and subsequent tissue hypoxia.

Coronary Artery Bypass Graft

Coronary artery bypass graft (CABG) surgery involves the bypass of a blockage in one or more of the coronary arteries using the saphenous veins, mammary artery, or radial artery as conduits or replacement vessels. Before surgery, coronary angiography precisely locates lesions and points of narrowing within the coronary arteries.

During traditional CABG surgery, a median sternotomy incision is made so that the heart and aorta can be seen. The client is placed on cardiopulmonary bypass (CPB) and the heart is stopped *(cardioplegia)* using a solution of iced saline containing potassium. After the bypasses have been performed, the client is taken off of the machine, and the heart takes over again. Three different types of "less invasive" CABG surgery are also performed: (1) off-bypass CABG performed through a median sternotomy with a smaller incision; (2) minimally

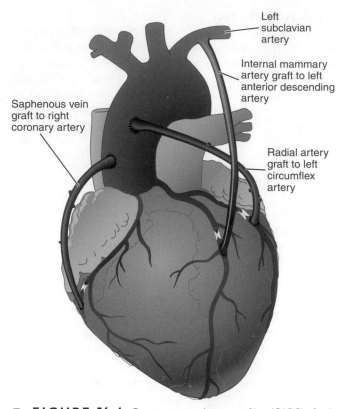

Left subclavian artery

Internal mammary artery graft to left anterior descending artery

Saphenous vein graft to right coronary artery

Radial artery graft to left circumflex artery

■ **FIGURE 56–4** Coronary artery bypass grafting (CABG). **A,** A section of saphenous vein is harvested from the leg and anastomosed (upside down, because of its directional valves) to a coronary artery to bypass an area of occlusion on the right coronary artery. **B,** Bypass of the left coronary artery with the internal mammary artery.

invasive direct CABG (MIDCABG) performed through a left anterior thoracotomy without cardiopulmonary bypass; and port-access CABG with femoral-to-femoral bypass and cardioplegia with a limited incision. Many institutions are performing MIDCABG surgery. In off-bypass CABG, the surgery is performed on a beating heart after a reduction in cardiac motion with several different medications and devices. The benefit of this type of CABG surgery is the avoidance of the use of CPB because of the many potential complications of CPB.

Saphenous veins can be used as the new coronary artery. The distal end of the vein is sutured to the aorta, and the proximal end is sewn to the coronary vessel distal to the blockage (Figure 56-4). The veins are reversed so that their valves do not interfere with blood flow. The internal mammary artery (IMA) can also be grafted to a coronary artery. It is more routinely used to revascularize the portion of the myocardium supplied by the left anterior descending (LAD) artery. The disadvantage of the IMA is that more time is required to remove it and the mammary artery is shorter. An advantage is that IMA grafts have a greater chance of remaining patent. Radial arteries have also been used in repeat CABG and when radiation therapy to the chest makes it impossible to use the IMA. The radial artery has had excellent patency rates.

For clients who need revascularization of the anterior coronary arteries, MIDCABG is a less invasive approach. The IMAs are used as conduits, and the client does not need to be placed on CPB. MIDCABG surgery is less costly than traditional CABG surgery and is associated with fewer postoperative complications. A small study comparing outcomes in CABG to minimally invasive bypass procedures found that fewer cardiac and pulmonary complications were reported in the minimally invasive group.

🪔 **Outcomes.** The use of calcium-channel blockers, PTCA, atherectomy, and stents has reduced the number of CABG surgical procedures being performed. Survival rates using CABG have not been significantly better than those of medically treated clients. CABG nevertheless remains a common procedure; and, because it can reduce angina in 80% to 90% of clients who do not respond to medical management, it will continue to be an important intervention in the management of CHD. Benefits from CABG surgery also include prolongation of life, increased exercise tolerance, reduced need for medication, and ability to resume former activities.

In studies comparing CABG with and without CPB, the advantages of surgery on a beating heart have been documented. These advantages include a decrease in mortality, in postoperative need for mechanical ventilation, in pulmonary complications, and in the incidence of stroke and atrial fibrillation. Clients who benefit from this type of CABG include those who refuse transfusions of blood and blood products and those with advanced respiratory disease, impaired renal function, and heavily calcified aortas.

Regardless of the type of operation, surgical methods only ease the manifestations. Surgery cannot halt the process of atherosclerosis, although it may prolong life in some cases. Recent studies documented an improvement in perceived quality of life following CABG, including improvements in physical functioning, social functioning, and mood states. Data on the outcomes of surgery for CHD in women continue to have conflicting results. Smaller body size in women along with smaller coronary arteries seems to be a consistent finding to explain poorer outcomes for women following CABG. Scientists are continuing to conduct research in this area.

🪔 **Complications.** Possible complications of CABG surgery occur in 6 areas:

Cardiovascular complications include dysrhythmias, decreased cardiac output, and persistent hypotension. While the heart's metabolic demands are reduced during surgery, the myocardium still needs nutrient blood and oxygen supply. Following surgery, the heart can be ischemic and not fully contracting. Dysrhythmias may develop from electrolyte imbalances, surgery near the conduction system, and ischemia. Inotropic medications are used to maintain cardiac output, and antidysrhythmics are used to control dysrhythmias.

When cardiac output is low, other organs can become impaired, including the brain and kidneys. In the absence of treatment, shock can develop. To improve cardiac output, the surgeon may use a mechanical device to support the failing heart if inotropic medications are unsuccessful.

The intra-aortic balloon pump (IABP) is a counterpulsation device that supports the failing heart by increasing coronary artery perfusion during diastole and reducing afterload. It consists of a sausage-shaped balloon catheter that is passed through the femoral artery and positioned in the descending thoracic aorta just distal to the subclavian artery. The catheter is attached to a power console that inflates and deflates the balloon in time with the heart.

The balloon is inflated during diastole; blood is pushed back into the aorta, and coronary artery perfusion is improved. The balloon is deflated during systole; resistance is decreased, and the workload of the heart is thus reduced. This procedure is described in the Bridge to Critical Care feature below. The timing of the balloon inflations and deflations is critical. A nurse educated in the use of the balloon pump is assigned to care for the client. Monitoring the effects of the pumping on the client's vital signs requires special skills.

Hematologic complications include bleeding and clotting. The bypass machine leads to clot formation, so the blood is anticoagulated, but this can lead to persistent

BRIDGE TO CRITICAL CARE

Intra-Aortic Balloon Pumping— Counterpulsation Device

Red line represents an actual pressure tracing. An initial systolic waveform is followed by a pump-generated waveform. Then the systolic waveform is seen following a balloon waveform when systolic pressure is reduced.

When the left ventricle fails to support adequate circulation and perfusion, an intra-aortic balloon pumping (IABP) device can be used to augment coronary artery filling and decrease left ventricular workload. A polyethylene balloon is inserted via the femoral artery into the descending thoracic aorta distal to the left subclavian artery and connected to an external pneumatic pumping system. The pump inflates the balloon with helium or carbon dioxide during diastole and deflates it during systole. The inflation-deflation cycle is triggered by the client's ECG, specifically by the R wave, which signals the beginning of systole. Balloon inflation during diastole augments coronary artery filling. Systolic balloon deflation decreases afterload.

The IABP device is used in clients with cardiogenic shock, septic shock, acute anterior myocardial infarction (MI), complications following MI, angioplasty with MI, ventricular dysrhythmias with ischemia, left ventricular failure, unstable angina refractory to medications, and low cardiac output after surgery.

GUIDELINES FOR MANAGEMENT

1. Select an ECG lead that optimizes the R wave.
2. Time the IABP device using an arterial waveform.
3. Monitor perfusion in the extremity with IABP.
4. Monitor perfusion in arms (catheter can occlude subclavian artery).

5. Monitor arterial pressures (which should improve).
6. Monitor urine output (the catheter can occlude the renal artery).
7. Keep the affected limb straight to prevent dislodgment of the catheter.
8. Monitor for balloon rupture and misplacement (loss of augmentation, wrinkled appearance in safety chamber, blood in tubing).
9. Monitor for bleeding resulting from anticoagulant use.
10. Monitor for aortic dissection (acute back, retroperitoneal, testicular, or chest pain; decreased pulses; variations in blood pressure between arms; decreased cardiac output; tachycardia; decreased filling pressures; decreased hemoglobin and hematocrit levels).
11. Monitor skin integrity on the sacrum, the coccyx, and the heels.
12. Do not elevate the head of the bed above 15 degrees.
13. Clarify or reinforce the client's and family's understanding of the IABP device.

COMPLICATIONS

- Dissection of the femoral or iliac artery or aorta
- Bleeding
- Plaque dislodgment, which can cause embolization
- Balloon rupture
- Arterial occlusion with limb ischemia or neuropathy
- Mechanical destruction of red blood cells
- Inability to wean from the IABP device
- Hematoma at the insertion site
- Mesenteric/renal ischemia (catheter too low)
- Arm ischemia (catheter too high)

WEANING

The ratio of IABP-assisted beats to unassisted beats is decreased from 1:1 to 1:2 based on the following parameters:

- Heart rate <110 beats/min
- No dysrhythmias
- Mean arterial pressure >70 mm Hg without vasopressors
- Pulmonary arterial wedge pressure <18 mm Hg
- Cardiac index >2.5 L/min/m^2
- Capillary refill >3 sec
- Urine output >0.5 ml/kg/min
- SVo_2 between 70% and 80%

bleeding. In addition, the inflammatory response is triggered and leads to edema from increased capillary permeability. Edema is common after surgery; some clients gain 10 kg of fluid.

Renal complications including renal failure can develop if cardiac output is low. Prerenal renal failure can be prevented by managing fluids closely and avoiding medications that further impair renal blood flow, such as nonsteroidal anti-inflammatory drugs.

Pulmonary complications include atelectasis. Because the lungs are not ventilated during bypass surgery, the alveoli collapse. In addition, surfactant may not be produced normally. Both changes make ventilation more difficult, because each breath has to open collapsed lung tissue. Clients also have incisional pain with deep breathing and coughing and guard the chest wall to prevent pain. Early extubation and ambulation have reduced pulmonary complications.

Neurologic complications can be devastating and include stroke and encephalopathy. Stroke can be embolic or thrombotic; embolic from disrupted plaques or air in the bypass machinery. Thrombotic stroke is usually from the walls of the atria or the carotid arteries. Encephalopathy can develop from mild stroke, cerebral edema, or cerebral ischemia.

SAFETY

⚠

ALERT

Wound infection and sternal dehiscence can occur following surgery. Mupirocin nasal ointment has been shown to reduce the risk of mediastinitis. Sternal dehiscence risk can be reduced by preventing strain on the incision line, for example by placing a bra on large-breasted women.

Nursing Management Before Cardiac Surgery

Clients may have experienced cardiopulmonary clinical manifestations for varying amounts of time. Some clients will have had cardiac disease for months or years. Others may have had their first manifestations of heart disease today and already be on their way to surgery.

Note the client's psychological readiness for surgery and his or her reaction to the need for heart surgery. The client may initially experience shock and grief over the impending surgery. Chief concerns may be helplessness and fear of disability or death.

The psychological preparation of the cardiac surgery client is very important. Many hospitals throughout the United States have extensive preoperative education programs that greatly reduce client and family anxiety. Such a program should include a thorough explanation of the preoperative, intraoperative, and postoperative procedures. Also helpful is the introduction of the client to involved health care team members and the health care facility environment. Box 56-2 provides a list of topics for education. Your institution probably has written material for you to use.

Allow clients to tell you in their own words about their heart problem and the surgery. Correct any misconceptions, using pictures and a model of the heart. Clients tend to ask the greatest number of questions about what will happen to them in the recovery room and intensive care unit (ICU).

Explain that they will awaken from the anesthetic with a chest tube in place. Discuss the ventilator that will assist the client's breathing for the first few to 24 hours. Remind clients that during this time they will be unable to talk. Explain that an IV line for fluid or blood will be inserted in an arm, chest and/or neck and that various equipment needed to continuously monitor vital signs will be attached to their skin.

Answer questions concerning the necessity of using blood products. Use these facts to respond to concerns about transfusion. Postoperative blood transfusions are used only as needed; blood is screened carefully, and there is little risk of contracting blood-borne illnesses.

BOX 56–2 Guidelines to Prepare the Client Undergoing Cardiac Surgery

Plan teaching well in advance of the surgical date, if possible. By the time of surgery, the client should be prepared to do the following:

1. Describe the surgical procedure:
   a. All steps, including heart-lung machine
   b. Review of anatomy and physiology of heart and valves
   c. Brief definition of unfamiliar technical terms
   d. Length of time in surgery and approximate time of first visit by family
   e. Give the client pictures of the heart and involved valve for future reference
2. Describe the intensive care unit (ICU) environment and monitoring equipment:
   a. Cardiac monitor and alarm
   b. Endotracheal (ET) tube and projected length of time with ET tube in place
   c. Mechanical ventilator and alarm
   d. Suctioning procedure
   e. Arterial line and automatic blood pressure cuff
   f. Any limitation on visits from family
   g. Chest tubes or mediastinal tubes
   h. Nasogastric tube and length of NPO (nothing by mouth) status
   i. Urinary catheter
   j. High noise level in ICU
   k. Multiple intravenous lines and fluids
3. Describe preoperative preparation:
   a. Showering with antimicrobial soap
   b. Shaving of chest, abdomen, neck, and groin
   c. Special cardiac studies: echocardiogram, electrocardiogram, cardiac catheterization
4. Describe comfort measures:
   a. Pain reduction
   b. Turning, range-of-motion exercises
   c. Out of bed next morning
   d. Medication for sleep, if needed

Emphasize that although the client will experience pain, the pain will be swiftly reduced by medication and comfort measures.

Finally, explain that the client will be awakened frequently following surgery for vital nursing assessments and interventions. Give examples of scheduled activities: vital signs every 15 minutes; temperature every 2 hours; frequent turning, coughing, and deep breathing; blood drawn for tests every morning.

Clients also need information concerning discharge from the ICU and health care facility. Explain the average length of stay in the ICU, the room to which the client will return from the ICU, the average length of stay in the health care facility, and the diet and activities permitted once the client returns home. Be general in the discussion. Remember, many unforeseen events can arise and greatly alter the postoperative course.

Give verbal and written information concerning health care facility services, rules, and regulations; visiting hours; the chaplain's name and visiting hours (if appropriate); and the names of the clinical nurse specialists and other health care professionals who can be contacted for information. Most clients benefit from a tour of the recovery room and ICU. If they are not physically able to participate in a tour, audiovisual material is helpful.

Familiarize the client with the equipment that will be used in the ICU (e.g., chest drainage tubes, oxygen apparatus, ventilators, cardiac monitors, IV setups). Reassure the client that lights and alarm noises are part of the critical care environment and are not indicators that something is wrong.

Nursing Management of the Surgical Client

Clients are usually initially cared for in the intensive care unit (ICU). Initial assessment is focused on the level of consciousness, lung sounds, peripheral pulses and vital signs including heart rhythm, cardiac output/index, and temperature. Clients have continuous blood pressure readings via an arterial line, central venous pressure lines, and occasionally monitors for cardiac output and pulmonary artery pressures. The clients remain intubated and ventilated via a respirator. Mediastinal tube drainage should be measured hourly; surgeons differ on their orders about milking the tubes, but blood should not be allowed to clot in the tube because it would prohibit drainage and lead to tamponade. Urine output is also measured hourly. Laboratory studies are drawn including hemoglobin, hematocrit, platelet count, blood glucose, electrolytes, blood urea nitrogen, creatinine, prothrombin time, partial thromboplastin time, and arterial blood gases. A chest x-ray is taken to verify placement of the endotracheal tube and identify any chest abnormalities (e.g., pneumothorax). Within 4 to 8 hours, if the client is hemodynamically stable, as they awaken and are able to sustain breathing independently, they may be extubated

according to physician's orders. Oxygen will need to be used to maintain desired oxygen saturations.

The goals for the first 24 hours after surgery are to maintain adequate blood pressure and cardiac output, to correct problems with coagulation and calcium levels, and to stabilize intravascular volume. Medications to maintain cardiac output include inotropic agents, calcium, and vasoconstrictors. Vasodilators may also be used to improve flow through the coronary arteries and reduce peripheral vascular resistance and preload.

> **It is imperative that the target parameters (e.g., cardiac output, cardiac index, blood pressure, heart rate) be known and which medications are titrated to achieve these goals. The increments of titration should also be known, along with the side effects and ceiling limits for each drug.**

SAFETY
⚠
ALERT

Many hospitals have initiated rapid recovery programs for cardiac surgery clients that reduce the hospital stay to 4 days. With rapid recovery programs, most of the client's recovery takes place in the home, with the client and family assuming primary responsibility for many aspects of care. Discharge planning begins at the time of admission, activity progression in the postoperative period is accelerated, and client and family education continues on a daily basis throughout hospitalization.

Many hospitals have developed clinical pathways for CABG. See the Clinical Pathway feature on Coronary Bypass Grafting on the website. Immediate care of the client after CABG is shown in the Care Plan on pp. 1426 to 1429. In addition, a three-phase program of activity is implemented.

Phase 1 (In-Hospital) Rehabilitation Programs

Most CABG clients participate in cardiac rehabilitation following surgery. Phase 1 begins immediately after the client returns from surgery. The following are the goals of phase 1 inpatient rehabilitation:

- To prevent the negative effects of prolonged bed rest
- To assess the client's physiologic response to exercise
- To manage the psychosocial issues related to recovery from CABG surgery
- To educate the client and family concerning recovery and the adoption of risk reduction behaviors

While in ICU the client is turned every 2 hours during the first several hours after surgery. Once extubated, the client gets up in a chair and ambulates in the room. After transfer to the intermediate care unit, the client continues to walk three or four times a day, increasing the distance walked each time.

Assess the client's blood pressure, heart rate, ECG, and oxygen saturation before, during, and after activity. Systolic blood pressure should not increase more than 20 mm Hg or decrease more than 10 to 15 mm Hg after exercise. Heart rate should not increase more than 20 beats/min

C A R E P L A N *evolve*

Coronary Bypass Surgical Clients

Nursing Diagnosis: Decreased Cardiac Output related to alterations in preload/afterload/contractility/heart rate.
Outcomes: The client will have improved cardiac output as evidenced by stable blood pressure (and/or cardiac output/
cardiac index) with decreasing need for vasoactive medications, normal sinus rhythm without pacing, clear lung sounds,
warm and dry skin, preoperative mental status, urine output greater than 0.5 ml/kg without diuretics, and palpable pedal
pulses.

NOC OUTCOMES	Cardiac Pump Effectiveness (NOC)

Interventions	NIC INTERVENTIONS	Rationales
1. Monitor cardiac output and/or cardiac index, SVR, PAP, CVP, PCWP as appropriate or according to protocol.	Hemodynamic Regulation	1. Monitoring allows for early intervention.
2. Monitor heart rhythm continuously. Treat dysrhythmias per protocol	Dysrhythmia Management	2. Dysrhythmias can include atrial fibrillation or ventricular dysrhythmias. They must be identified and treated early.
3. Monitor weight daily and compare to previous weights	Fluid Management	3. Body weight is a reliable indicator of fluid volume.
4. Monitor for peripheral edema every 4 hours.	Hemodynamic Regulation	4. Peripheral edema may develop with dilutional hypoproteinemia or heart failure.
5. Auscultate heart sounds every 4 hours.	Hemodynamic Regulation	5. A ventricular gallop (S_3) is an early sign of heart failure. S_4 may indicate decreased ventricular compliance.
6. Auscultate lung sounds for crackles every 4 hours.	Fluid Management	6. Crackles may indicate left ventricular failure.
7. Monitor intake/output, urine output hourly.	Fluid Management	7. Hourly assessment allows for rapid adjustments in fluids to prevent hypotension and maintain renal perfusion.
8. Monitor potassium and calcium levels	Electrolyte Management	8. Hypokalemia and hypocalcemia can lead to ventricular dysrhythmias.
9. Maintain fluid balance by administering IV fluids, packed red blood cells, or colloids.	Shock Management: Cardiac	9. Hypovolemia is a common cause of low cardiac output.
10. Administer prescribed vasodilators (specify).	Cardiac Care: Acute	10. Reducing afterload reduces stress on the left ventricle.
11. Administer positive inotropic/contractility medications as prescribed (specify).	Cardiac Care: Acute	11. Inotropic medications enhance myocardial contractility, leading to improved cardiac output by more complete emptying of the ventricles.
12. Monitor the ECG and arterial blood pressure to verify timing and effect of balloon counterpulsations (IABP). (See also the Bridge to Critical Care feature on IABP.)	Circulatory Care: Mechanical Assist Device	12. IABP must receive a signal to identify the beginning of a new cardiac cycle. Dysrhythmias may affect the timing of balloon deflation and inflation. MAP should remain approximately 80 mm Hg on IABP.
13. Protect external pacemaker wires from water and accidental exposure to electricity by placing them in a rubber glove.	Injury Prevention	13. Static electricity and water can cause the pacer wires to conduct electricity.

Evaluation: The goal for this diagnosis can be written for 24 hours; most clients who were fairly healthy before surgery usually
are awake and up in a chair by the day after surgery.

Nursing Diagnosis: Impaired Gas Exchange related to ventilation/perfusion mismatch or intrapulmonary shunting.
Outcomes: The client will have adequate gas exchange as evidence by Pao_2 >90 mm Hg, $Paco_2$ <35 mm Hg, pH between
7.35 and 7.45, and oxygen saturation >90%.

NOC OUTCOMES	Respiratory Status: Gas Exchange

Interventions	NIC INTERVENTIONS	Rationales
1. Monitor oxygen saturation continuously. If the levels fall below 90%, either encourage the client to deep breathe, or consider if the endotracheal tube needs suctioning.	Mechanical Ventilation	1. Continuous monitoring allows for early intervention

2. Monitor results of ABGs; report abnormal or unexpected findings to the surgeon.	Mechanical Ventilation	2. Hypoxemia or acidosis may require modification in ventilation parameters.
3. Monitor settings on ventilator, position of ET tube, lung sounds, and response to mechanical ventilation.	Artificial Airway Management Mechanical Ventilation	3. Mechanical ventilation is used with positive pressure to facilitate alveolar ventilation. The ET tube must remain at the carina; its position within the airway is monitored by confirming placement. Lung sounds should be present in each lung.
4. Securely tape or hold the ET tube in place; move the tube in the mouth every 12 hours.	Mechanical Ventilation	4. Securing the ET tube allows the client to be moved in bed without dislodgement. Moving the tube prevents pressure ulcers on the lips.
5. Use an oral bite block prn.	Mechanical Ventilation	5. Bite blocks prevent obstruction of the tube from biting.
6. Collaborate with respiratory therapists to assess weaning parameters per protocol.	Mechanical Ventilation	6. Weaning parameters help determine if the client is ready for extubation.

Evaluation: The goal for this care plan can be fairly short term; early extubation (within 4-8 hours after surgery) is becoming more common in clients undergoing elective CABG.

Nursing Diagnosis: Ineffective Airway Clearance related to retained secretions and excess secretions.
Outcomes: The client will have improved airway clearance as evidenced by deep breathing and coughing productively.

NOC OUTCOMES   Respiratory Status: Ventilation

Interventions	NIC INTERVENTIONS	Rationales
1. Monitor lung sounds q 2 hr.	Respiratory Monitoring	1. Fluids in the alveoli accumulate as a result of atelectasis and dilutional hypoproteinemia.
2. Monitor coughing effort.	Respiratory Monitoring	2. After extubation, coughing is used to clear the airways. Because of incisional pain, many clients cough poorly.
3. Administer supplemental oxygen to maintain oxygen saturation levels >93%.	Oxygen Therapy	3. Oxygen saturation levels >93% equate to 90% arterial blood saturation, which is adequate in most clients.
4. Maintain comfort using prescribed opioids.	Cough Enhancement	4. Pain control can facilitate adequate coughing.
5. Splint the incision with "heart pillows" or pillows.	Cough Enhancement	5. Splinting the incision before coughing promotes more intense coughing efforts.
6. Ambulate when tolerated.	Ventilation Assistance	6. Respiratory effort is increased with ambulation; therefore deep breathing occurs.
7. Teach proper use of the incentive spirometer (ICS) once extubated. Demonstrate as needed.	Cough Enhancement	7. Correct use of ICS encourages sustained inspiration to open alveoli.

Evaluation: Expect this outcome to be met after 4 to 5 days; clearing the chest of secretions requires time and client effort.

Collaborative Problem: Risk of Hemorrhage related to inadequate hemostasis, disruption of suture lines, or coagulopathy.
Outcomes: The nurse will monitor for bleeding in excess of expectations (should be less than 70 ml/hr), visible blood loss, decreased blood pressure, and increased heart rate.

NOC OUTCOMES   Blood Loss Severity

Interventions	NIC INTERVENTIONS	Rationales
1. Monitor mediastinal chest tubes for output hourly.	Bleeding Reduction	1. Hourly assessment of output and total output is analyzed. Clients with IMA grafts are at increased risk of bleeding because of the surgical resection needed.
2. Report excess volumes and/or institute prescribed treatments for blood loss.	Bleeding Reduction	2. Agents such as protamine (to reverse heparin), aminocaproic acid (inhibits lysis of clots by blocking the conversion of plasminogen to plasmin), fresh-frozen plasma, platelets, and fluids may be used to restore volume.
3. Retransfuse blood from mediastinum as ordered.	Blood Products Administration	3. Autotransfusion is one mechanism of using the client's own blood for transfusion.

(Continued)

CARE PLAN ~~evolve~~

Coronary Bypass Surgical Clients—Cont'd

Interventions	NIC Interventions	Rationales
4. Keep chest tubes positioned without kinks and/or strip them (per agency or physician protocol).	Tube Care: Chest	4. Maintain patency of the tube. Aggressive chest tube stripping can lead to bleeding by dislodging small clots.
5. Monitor for manifestations of cardiac tamponade: Elevated CVP, PADP, PAP Decreased CO, BP Pulsus paradoxus Muffled heart sounds Sudden cessation of chest tube drainage	Cardiac Care: Acute	5. Cardiac tamponade, which is the collection of blood/fluid in the pericardial sac, can severely restrict ventricular filling.

Evaluation: The risk of bleeding is highest in the first 24 hours after surgery.

Nursing Diagnosis: Acute Pain related to tissue trauma secondary to sternotomy and leg incision.
Outcomes: The client will have improved comfort as evidenced by reporting pain at tolerable levels, using less potent analgesia.

| NOC OUTCOMES | Pain Level, Analgesic Administration |

Interventions	NIC INTERVENTIONS	Rationales
1. Monitor reported level of pain.	Pain Management	1. Reported pain levels are the most accurate method of describing the intensity of pain.
2. Assess the nature of the pain.	Pain Management	2. Angina must be differentiated from incisional pain. Clients with IMA grafts will often have chest wall pain. Saphenous vein graft harvest incisions are often quite painful.
3. Administer ordered opioids for surgical pain by prescribed route management to meet client goal.	Analgesic Administration	3. Treatment of acute pain reduces sympathetic stimulation and thereby cardiac workload. Pain control also enhances recovery.
4. Premedicate before activities such as ambulation and coughing.	Medication Management	4. Premedication assists the client to fully participate.

Evaluation: Expect pain levels to be highest for the first 48 hours after surgery. Clients often require IV analgesia for 24-48 hours, and then the pain should be controllable with oral analgesia.

Collaborative Problem: Risk of Postcardiotomy Delirium or Stroke.
Outcomes: The nurse will monitor for the return to baseline levels of consciousness and mental acuity.

| NOC OUTCOMES | Cognitive Ability: Cranial Sensory/Motor Function |

Interventions	NIC INTERVENTIONS	Rationales
1. Monitor for return of consciousness when off of sedating medications.	Neurologic Monitoring	1. Neurologic examination is accurate only if the client is awake and able to participate.
2. Assess neurologic status every shift. Compare current level of mental acuity to baseline levels. Report any deviations to surgeon.	Neurologic Monitoring	2. Baseline levels of mental acuity provide a comparison. Early intervention for stroke may limit permanent damage.
3. Reorient frequently to setting, timing, and procedures being performed.	Reality Orientation	3. Delirium is short-term, and reorientation is helpful to assist the client in restructuring thoughts.
4. Explain all procedures, using a calm and clear voice.	Reality Orientation	4. The environment of an ICU may threaten the confused client. Explanations also build trust and gain cooperation.
5. Secure all invasive lines and tubes.	Environmental Management: Safety	5. Disoriented clients may accidentally pull or remove lines. Accidental dislodgement may injure the client and/or require replacement of the device.
6. Administer sedative medications cautiously.	Medication Management	6. Mild sedation may help prevent injury. However, the use of sedation in older adults may increase agitation.
7. Avoid restraints in lieu of other methods to prevent self-injury.	Physical Restraint	7. Physical restraints may increase agitation.

8. Explain that changes in mental acuity, agitation, confusion, and/or hallucinations are temporary (as applies).

Reality Orientation

8. Transient changes in acuity are usually caused by decreased cerebral perfusion and microemboli during the cardiac bypass pump run. Discussion of permanent changes is left to the neurologist.

9. Organize nursing care to provide time for sleep. Limit environmental noise as much as possible.

Sleep Enhancement

9. Sleep deprivation may increase confusion.

10. Liberalize visitation time with family.

Reality Orientation

10. Familiar voices and faces will help with reorientation.

Evaluation: Once the sedative effects of the medications and anesthetics wear off, mental acuity of baseline levels should return.

Nursing Diagnosis: Risk for Infection related to sternotomy incision, diabetes, and obesity.
Outcomes: The client will have decreased risk of infection as evidenced by primary healing of the sternotomy and leg incisions.

| NOC OUTCOMES | Wound Healing: Primary Intention

Interventions	NIC INTERVENTIONS	Rationales
1. Initially monitor temperature every hour, and every 4 hr once stable.	Incision Site Care	1. Temperature >38.3° C (101° F) may indicate atelectasis early in recovery. Later fever may indicate sternal wound infection or infective endocarditis.
2. Monitor incision for signs of delayed primary healing.	Incision Site Care	2. Erythema, pain, drainage, or opening of the sternal margin are signs of delayed healing.
3. Administer insulin drip as ordered to control blood glucose levels to desired values as ordered.	Infection Protection	3. Blood glucose levels >200 mg/dl create ineffective phagocytosis and increase the risk of infection.
4. Apply a front-closing brassiere or other supportive dressings for obese female clients.	Incision Site Care	4. Pendulous breasts can create tension on the suture lines and impair sternotomy healing.
5. Collaborate with the dietitian to ensure that a diet of adequate calories and protein is delivered.	Infection Protection	5. Protein and calorie needs increase after major stress and are needed for wound healing.
6. Administer antibiotics as prescribed (specify), including nasal ointments.	Infection Protection	6. Antibiotics reduce the risk of surgical site infection. Nasal application of mupirocin has been shown to reduce the risk of MRSA infections in the sternal incision.

Evaluation: Incisions should heal by primary intention in 7 to 10 days.

BP, Blood pressure; *CI*, cardiac index; *CO*, cardiac output; *CVP*, central venous pressure; *IABP*, intra-aortic balloon pump; *MAP*, mean arterial pressure; *PADP*, pulmonary artery diastolic pressure; *PAP*, pulmonary artery pressure; *PAWP*, pulmonary artery wedge pressure; *PCWP*, pulmonary capillary wedge pressure; *RAP*, right atrial pressure; *SVR*, systemic vascular resistance.

above resting, and no significant dysrhythmias should occur. Activity levels will be reduced if clients have adverse physiologic responses (e.g., tachycardia, dysrhythmias, pain) to exercise. Clients are seated for all meals. Research has demonstrated that early mobilization improves cardiac function and benefits the client psychologically.

Education for a healthier lifestyle is an important part of each phase of cardiac rehabilitation. The emphasis in phase 1 is on the identification and modification of reversible risk factors to prevent further deleterious cardiac events.

Deep breathing and coughing must continue to reduce the risk of pneumonia. The client is taught and encouraged to cough, not just clear the throat, using a pillow to splint the sternum.

Self-Care

Before hospital discharge, instruct the client and family (or significant other) about medication actions and side effects, dietary restrictions, physical activity restrictions and progression, and incisional care. Because it is not always possible to anticipate all the problems clients may encounter the first few days at home, instruct the client whom to call when there is an emergency or when there are questions or concerns. If possible, introduce the client to the home health nurse who will be supervising home care. Following discharge, the home health care nurse provides additional education and counseling and assesses the client for complications.[36] In addition, instruct the client on how to assess response to exercise and activity.[5]

Before discharge, a low-level symptom-limited exercise test may be performed to evaluate the client's ability to perform activities of daily living (ADL) and exercise. The test results are used to prescribe a safe and effective exercise program for the first few weeks at home and serve as a basis for the initial exercise prescription in phase 2.

Phase 2 (Outpatient Exercise Training) Rehabilitation Programs

Outpatient (phase 2) exercise training usually takes place in a facility that provides continuous ECG monitoring, emergency equipment, and medically supervised exercise. Outpatient treatment usually begins 10 to 14 days after discharge and requires physician referral. The following are the goals of phase 2:

- To restore clients to a desirable exercise capacity appropriate to their health status, lifestyle, and occupation
- To provide additional education and support to the client and family for adoption of risk-reduction behaviors
- To meet the psychosocial needs of clients and families, restore confidence, and minimize anxiety and depression
- To promote early identification of medical problems through close observation and monitoring of clients during exercise
- To assist clients in returning to occupational and leisure activities

Exercise therapy is conducted three times weekly for 2 to 3 months. The duration of the aerobic exercise session ranges from 20 to 40 minutes at an intensity of 70% to 85% of the baseline exercise heart rate. During each exercise session, blood pressure, heart rate, respiratory rate, and ECG are monitored before, during, and after exercise. Activity levels are increased gradually, based on the client's response. A nutritionist may counsel clients about proper diet, and a psychologist or social worker may counsel clients about stress management and adoption of other risk prevention behaviors.

At the end of the program, clients are given a symptom-limited exercise test and are reevaluated. Decisions regarding progression to a phase 3 or home program are based on the client's results of the stress test, the client's ability to self-monitor the response to exercise, the client's stability, and the client's psychological or emotional status. Periodic evaluations are scheduled so that activity progression and cardiopulmonary function can be assessed.[5]

Phase 3 (Community) Rehabilitation Programs

Phase 3 programs are conducted in community settings, such as a "Y" or a health club. The following are the goals of phase 3:

- To maintain and, if possible, increase exercise capacity
- To institute long-term follow-up of risk-reduction behavior change
- To encourage clients to take responsibility for continuing lifestyle changes

Exercise consists of walking, jogging, weight training, and recreational games. Clients are usually not monitored while exercising, although some facilities obtain exercise ECGs on a monthly basis. Clients are responsible for monitoring their own heart rate response to exercise, although blood pressure can be taken by program personnel if indicated.[5]

Home Exercise Rehabilitation Programs

For CABG clients, a home exercise program is usually prescribed in conjunction with or in place of the outpatient program. Clients are given detailed exercise instructions and are told to keep a log of heart rates, perceived exertion rates, exercise parameters, and any problems that occur during the home program. Cardiac rehabilitation staff members or the client's physician should analyze the data and adjust the home exercise program if necessary. Once clients reach their optimal level of functional capacity, they are instructed to continue to exercise at least three times weekly so that cardiopulmonary exercise capacity can be maintained.

Modifications for Older Clients

More than half of all CABG procedures are performed on people older than 65 years, and 71% of them are performed on men. Older clients have a postoperative recovery similar to that for younger clients, but the pace is slower and they typically remain hospitalized an average of 2 to 4 days longer. They also have a higher death rate.

Postoperative complications that are more prevalent in older clients include dysrhythmias related to aged sinoatrial node cells, drug toxicity associated with impaired hepatic and renal perfusion, multiple drug interactions, and decreased physical stamina. These complications contribute to a 15-day mean length of hospital stay for clients older than 80 years.

During the first and second weeks after discharge, depression, fatigue, incisional chest discomfort, dyspnea, and anorexia are common. By the fourth to fifth weeks, older clients report improved mood, comfort, and appetite. At 1 year, almost all (93%) clients are pleased with the outcome and improved quality of life.

HEART FAILURE

Despite aggressive medical and surgical treatment, CHD may eventually lead to the development of heart failure. Heart failure is a physiologic state in which the heart cannot pump enough blood to meet the metabolic needs of the body (determined as oxygen consumption). Heart failure results from changes in systolic or diastolic function of the left ventricle. The heart fails when, because of intrinsic disease or structural defects, it cannot handle a normal blood volume or, in the absence of disease, cannot tolerate a sudden expansion in blood volume (e.g., during exercise). Heart failure is not a disease itself; instead, the term refers to a clinical syndrome characterized by manifestations of volume overload, inadequate tissue perfusion, and poor exercise tolerance. Whatever the cause, pump failure results in hypoperfusion of tissue, followed by pulmonary and systemic venous congestion. Because heart failure causes vascular congestion, it is often called *congestive heart failure,* although most cardiac specialists no longer use this term. Other terms used to denote heart failure include *chronic heart failure, cardiac decompensation, cardiac insufficiency,* and *ventricular failure.*

Heart failure affects about 5 million people in the United States, with 500,000 new cases diagnosed each year. In contrast to decreases in mortality associated with other cardiovascular diseases, the incidence of heart failure and the mortality associated with it have increased steadily since 1975. Annually about 300,000 clients die from direct or indirect consequences of heart failure, and the number of deaths attributed to heart failure has increased six-fold over the past 40 years.

Heart failure can affect both women and men, although the mortality is higher among women. There are also racial differences; at all ages death rates are higher in African Americans than in non-Hispanic whites. Heart failure is primarily a disease of older adults, affecting 6% to 10% of those older than 65. It is also the leading cause of hospitalization in older people.

Etiology and Risk Factors

Heart failure is caused by conditions that weaken or damage the myocardium. Heart failure can be caused by factors originating from the heart (i.e., intrinsic disease or pathology) or from external factors that place excessive demands upon the heart. Etiologies of heart failure are shown in Table 56-1.

Intrinsic Factors

The most common cause of heart failure is coronary artery disease. CAD reduces blood flow through the coronary arteries and therefore reduces oxygen delivery to the myocardium. Without oxygen, the muscle cells cannot function. Another common cause of heart failure is myocardial infarction (MI). During MI, myocardium is starved of blood, and the tissue dies and therefore cannot contract. The remaining myocardium must compensate for the loss of tissue. Other intrinsic causes of heart failure include valve disease, cardiomyopathy, and dysrhythmias.

Certain conditions externally compress the heart, thereby limiting ventricular filling and myocardial contractility. Disorders that greatly restrict cardiac chamber filling and myocardial fiber stretch include *constrictive pericarditis,* an inflammatory and fibrotic process of the pericardial sac; and *cardiac tamponade,* which involves the accumulation of fluid or blood within the pericardial sac. Because the pericardium encloses all four heart chambers, compression of the heart both decreases diastolic relaxation, thereby elevating diastolic pressure, and hampers forward blood flow through the heart.

Extrinsic Factors

Factors external to the heart include increased afterload (e.g., hypertension), increased stroke volume from hypervolemia or increased preload, and increased body demands (high output failure; e.g., thyrotoxicosis, pregnancy). The weakened myocardium cannot tolerate the usual changes in the volume of blood entering the left ventricle. These conditions include abnormal volumes of blood reaching the left ventricle (called a load), abnormal muscle in the ventricle from scarring after injury, and problems that reduce the contractility of the heart muscle. They will be examined in more detail.

Abnormal loading occurs when either the pressure or the volume of blood in the ventricle increases. The effect of increasing volume on the ventricle can be explained by the analogy that the heart muscle is like a stretched rubber band. When the rubber band is stretched, it contracts with more force. The heart muscle does the same. Venous return stretches the heart and improves contractility. When the rubber band is overstretched, however, it becomes limp and cannot contract. Likewise, when the heart is overloaded with blood, excessive stretch and decreased contraction occur. Overload develops because blood does not leave the ventricles during contraction. Therefore the workload on the heart increases in an effort to move blood. Loading, called preload and afterload, can occur in normal or abnormal conditions.

TABLE 56–1 Etiology of Heart Failure		
Abnormal Loading Conditions	**Abnormal Muscle Function**	**Limited Ventricular Filling**
Conditions That Increase Preload		
Regurgitation of mitral or tricuspid valve	Myocardial infarction	Mitral or tricuspid stenosis
Hypervolemia	Myocarditis	Cardiac tamponade
Congenital defects (left-to-right shunts)	Cardiomyopathy	Constrictive pericarditis
Ventricular septal defect	Ventricular aneurysm	Hypertrophic obstructive cardiomyopathy
Atrial septal defect	Long-term alcohol consumption	
Patent ductus arteriosus	Coronary heart disease	
	Metabolic heart disease	
	Endocrine heart disease	
Conditions That Increase Afterload		
Hypertension, pulmonary or systemic		
Aortic or pulmonic stenosis		
High peripheral vascular resistance		

Preload can be defined as the initial stretching of the cardiac muscle fiber length before contraction. Changes in ventricular preload dramatically affect ventricular stroke volume by what is called the Frank-Starling mechanism. Increased preload increases stroke volume, whereas decreased preload decreases stroke volume by altering the force of contraction of the cardiac muscle. Preload, therefore, is related to the sarcomere length, but since sarcomere length cannot be determined in the intact heart, other indices of preload are used such as ventricular end-diastolic volume or pressure. For example, when venous return is increased, the end-diastolic pressure and volume of the ventricle are increased, which stretches the sarcomeres (increases their preload). As another example, hypovolemia resulting from a loss of blood by hemorrhage leads to less ventricular filling and therefore shorter sarcomere lengths (reduced preload). Increased pressure load in the ventricle is related to *afterload,* the amount of tension the heart must generate to overcome systemic pressure and to allow adequate ventricular emptying. Thus afterload indicates how hard the heart must pump to force blood into circulation. The tone of systemic arterioles, the elasticity of the aorta and large arteries, the size and thickness of the ventricle, the presence of aortic stenosis, and the viscosity of the blood all determine afterload. High peripheral vascular resistance and high blood pressure force the ventricle to work harder to eject blood. Subjected to prolonged high pressures, the ventricle eventually fails.

Pathophysiology

The healthy heart can meet the demands for oxygen delivery through the use of cardiac reserve. *Cardiac reserve* is the heart's ability to increase output in response to stress. The normal heart can increase its output up to five times the resting level. The failing heart, even at rest, however, is pumping near its capacity and thus has lost much of its reserve. The compromised heart has a limited ability to respond to the body's needs for increased output in situations of stress.

When cardiac output is not sufficient to meet the metabolic needs of the body, compensatory mechanisms, including neurohormonal responses, become activated. These mechanisms initially help to improve contraction and maintain integrity of the circulation, but if continued lead to abnormal cardiac muscle growth and reconfiguration (remodeling) of the heart. The compensatory responses to a decrease in cardiac output are ventricular dilation, increased sympathetic nervous system stimulation, and activation of the renin-angiotensin system. Figure 56-5 depicts the pathophysiology of heart failure in an algorithm.

Ventricular Dilation

Ventricular dilation refers to lengthening of the muscle fibers that increases the volume in the heart chambers. Dilation causes an increase in preload, and thus cardiac output, because a stretched muscle contracts more forcefully (Starling's law); however, dilation has limits as a compensatory mechanism. Muscle fibers, if stretched beyond a certain point, become ineffective. Second, a dilated heart requires more oxygen. Thus the dilated heart with a normal coronary blood flow can suffer from a lack of oxygen. Hypoxia of the heart further decreases the muscle's ability to contract.

Increased Sympathetic Nervous System Stimulation

Sympathetic adrenergic stimulation produces arteriolar constriction, tachycardia, and increased myocardial contractility, all of which work to increase cardiac output and improve delivery of oxygen and nutrients to tissues. Arterial baroreceptors are important components of this response. This compensatory effect occurs at the cost of increasing peripheral vascular resistance (afterload) and myocardial workload, however. In addition, sympathetic stimulation reduces renal blood flow and stimulates the renin-angiotensin system.

Stimulation of the Renin-Angiotensin System

When blood flow through the renal artery is decreased, the baroreceptor reflex is stimulated and renin is released into the bloodstream. Renin interacts with angiotensinogen to produce angiotensin I. When angiotensin I contacts ACE, it is converted to angiotensin II, a potent vasoconstrictor. Angiotensin II increases arterial vasoconstriction, promotes the release of norepinephrine from sympathetic nerve endings, and stimulates the adrenal medulla to secrete aldosterone, which enhances sodium and water absorption. Stimulation of the renin-angiotensin system causes plasma volume to expand and preload to increase.

Cardiac compensation exists when the initial compensatory mechanisms of ventricular dilation, sympathetic nervous system stimulation, and renin-angiotensin system stimulation succeed in maintaining an adequate cardiac output and oxygen delivery to the tissues in the presence of pathologic changes. Once cardiac output is restored, the body produces counter-regulatory substances that restore cardiovascular homeostasis. If underlying pathologic changes are not corrected, prolonged activation of the compensatory mechanisms eventually leads to changes in the function of the myocardial cell and excess production of the neurohormones. These processes are responsible for the transition from compensated to decompensated heart failure. At this point manifestations of heart failure develop because the heart cannot maintain adequate circulation.

When compensatory mechanisms fail, the amount of blood remaining in the left ventricle at the end of diastole increases. This increase in residual blood in turn decreases the ventricle's capacity to receive blood from the left atrium.

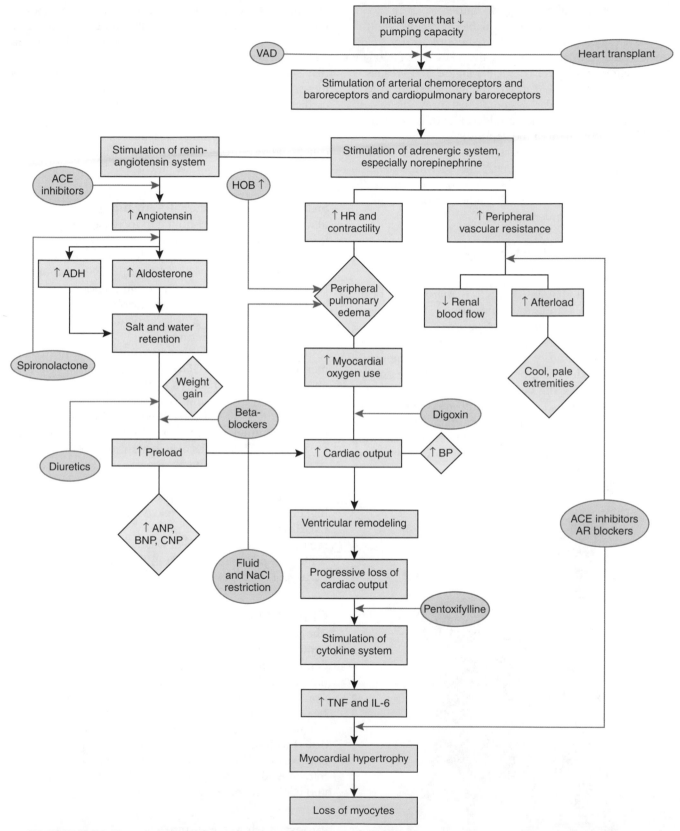

■ **FIGURE 56–5** Pathophysiology of heart failure. *ACE*, Angiotensin-converting enzyme; *ADH*, antidiuretic hormone; *ANP*, atrial natriuretic peptide; *AR*, aldosterone receptor; *BNP*, brain natriuretic peptide; *BP*, blood pressure; *BUN*, blood urea nitrogen; *CNP*, C-natriuretic peptide; *HOB*, head of bed; *HR*, heart rate; *VAD*, ventricular assist device.

The left atrium, having to work harder to eject blood, dilates and hypertrophies. It is unable to receive the full amount of incoming blood from the pulmonary veins, and left atrial pressure increases; this leads to pulmonary edema (Figure 56-6). Left ventricular failure (LVF) results.

The right ventricle, because of the increased pressure in the pulmonary vascular system, must now dilate and hypertrophy to meet its increased workload. It too eventually fails. Engorgement of the venous system then extends backward to produce congestion in the gastrointestinal tract, liver, viscera, kidneys, legs, and sacrum; edema is the main manifestation. Right ventricular failure (RVF) results. RVF usually follows LVF, although occasionally it may develop independently.

Decompensated Heart Failure

Remodeling
Several structural changes, known as *remodeling,* occur in the ventricle during decompensated heart failure. Remodeling is thought to result from hypertrophy of the myocardial cells and sustained activation of the neurohormonal compensatory systems. Recall that one of the initial compensatory responses to a decrease in cardiac output is dilation of the ventricle. This dilation increases cardiac output but also increases wall stress in the ventricle. To reduce wall stress, the myocardial cells hypertrophy, resulting in a thickening of the ventricular wall. According to Laplace's law, an increase in wall thickness reduces wall stress.

■ **FIGURE 56–6** Appearance of a client with both right-sided and left-sided heart failure.

When used over time, these compensatory responses produce changes in the structure, function, and gene expression of the myocardial cell. Changes in the myocardial cells eventually increase failure by reducing myocardial contractility, increasing ventricular wall stress, and increasing oxygen demand. In addition to increasing myocardial dysfunction, the genetically abnormal myocytes die prematurely and at an accelerated rate through the process of *apoptosis* (programmed cell death). Apoptosis affects cells scattered throughout the myocardium and causes a further reduction in cardiac function.

Sustained Neurohormonal Activation
Remodeling changes continue to increase wall stress and further stimulate neurohormonal activity. Long-term sympathetic activation exerts a direct toxic effect on the heart that promotes myocyte hypertrophy and apoptosis. Prolonged activation of the renin-angiotensin system also stimulates myocyte hypertrophy and myocardial fibrosis. This creates a self-perpetuating cycle of cell death and further hypertrophy.

In addition, if renal artery pressure falls, a lowered glomerular filtration rate (GFR) increases retention of sodium and water. In response to a continued reduction in renal blood flow, the renin-angiotensin-aldosterone mechanism is activated. Aldosterone, released from the adrenal cortex, promotes further retention of sodium and water by the renal tubule. This results in an expansion in blood volume of up to 30% and edema. As the sodium concentration in the extracellular fluid increases, so does the osmotic pressure of the plasma. The hypothalamus responds to the higher osmotic pressure by releasing antidiuretic hormone (ADH) from the posterior pituitary. This in turn promotes renal tubular reabsorption of water. Aldosterone, however, is more important than ADH in the production of edema because it promotes sodium retention.

Clinical Manifestations
The manifestations of heart failure depend on the specific ventricle involved, the precipitating causes of failure, the degree of impairment, the rate of progression, the duration of the failure, and the client's underlying condition. Conditions that precipitate heart failure are listed in Box 56-3. Manifestations of pulmonary congestion and edema dominate the clinical picture of LVF; RVF is associated with manifestations of abdominal organ distention and peripheral edema. Heart failure has been classified into several stages based on a client's functional ability and clinical manifestations (Table 56-2).

Types of Heart Failure
Heart failure may be categorized as (1) LVF versus RVF, (2) backward versus forward, and (3) high output versus low output.

BOX 56-3	Conditions That Precipitate Heart Failure

- Dysrhythmias, especially tachycardia
- Systemic infections (sepsis)
- Anemia
- Thyroid disorders
- Pulmonary embolism
- Thiamine deficiency
- Chronic pulmonary diseases
- Medication dose changes
- Physical or emotional stress
- Endocarditis, myocarditis, or pericarditis
- Fluid retention from medication or salt intake
- A new cardiac condition

Left Ventricular Versus Right Ventricular Failure

The theory of LVF versus RVF is based on the fact that fluid accumulates behind the chamber that fails first. Because the circulatory system is a closed circuit, however, impairments of one ventricle commonly progress to failure of the other. This is referred to as *ventricular interdependence*. Figure 56-7 depicts clinical manifestations that differentiate LVF from RVF.

Left Ventricular Failure. Left ventricular failure causes either pulmonary congestion or a disturbance in the respiratory control mechanisms. These problems in turn precipitate respiratory distress. The degree of distress varies with the client's position, activity, and level of stress.

Dyspnea (difficult breathing) is a subjective problem, and it does not always correlate with the extent of heart failure. Because breathing is usually effortless at rest, the feeling of breathlessness can mean anything from an awareness of breathing to extreme distress. An apprehensive client with only moderate ventricular failure may be more aware of dyspnea than a client with advanced disease. To some degree, exertional dyspnea occurs in all clients. Therefore elicit from the client a description of the degree of exertion that results in the sensation of breathlessness. The mechanism of dyspnea may be related to the decrease in the lung's air volume *(vital capacity)* as air is displaced by blood or interstitial fluid. Pulmonary congestion can eventually reduce the vital capacity of the lungs to 1500 ml or less.

Orthopnea is a more advanced stage of dyspnea. The client often assumes a "three-point position," sitting up with both hands on the knees and leaning forward. Orthopnea develops because the supine position increases the amount of blood returning from the lower extremities to the heart and lungs (preload). The client learns to avoid respiratory distress at night by supporting the head and thorax on pillows. In severe heart failure, the client may resort to sleeping upright in a chair.

Paroxysmal nocturnal dyspnea (PND) resembles the frightening sensation of suffocation. The client suddenly awakens with the feeling of severe suffocation and seeks relief by sitting upright or opening a window for a "breath of fresh air." Respirations may be labored and wheezing *(cardiac asthma)*. PND represents an acute exacerbation of pulmonary congestion. It stems from a combination of increased venous return to the lungs during recumbency and suppression of the respiratory center to sensory input from the lungs during sleep. Once the client is upright, relief from the attack of PND may not occur for 30 minutes or longer.

Cheyne-Stokes respirations sometimes occur in clients with severe forms of heart failure. Cheyne-Stokes respirations probably result from the prolonged circulation time between the pulmonary circulation and the central nervous system (CNS).

Cough is a common manifestation of LVF. The cough, often hacking, may produce large amounts of frothy, blood-tinged sputum. The client coughs because a large amount of fluid is trapped in the pulmonary tree,

TABLE 56–2 Stages of Heart Failure and Treatments

Stage	Extent of Disease	NYHA Class	Outcomes and Goals in Order of Importance	Treatments
1	Asymptomatic myocardial dysfunction with mild heart failure	I/II	Reverse or prevent remodeling Prevent overt heart failure	ACE inhibitors or ARBs Beta-adrenergic blockers
2	Mild to moderate heart failure	II/III	Reverse or prevent remodeling Improve symptoms and functional capacity Reduce disability and hospitalizations Reduce mortality	ACE inhibitors or ARBs/beta-adrenergic blockers Diuretics, digoxin
3	Advanced heart failure	III/IV	Reduce mortality Reduce disability and hospitalizations Improve symptoms and functional capacity	ACE inhibitors, spironolactone, beta-adrenergic blockers Positive inotropic agents, including digoxin
4	Severe heart failure with frequent or sustained decompensation	III/IV	Reduce disability and hospitalizations Improve symptoms and functional capacity Reduce mortality	Diuretics, ACE inhibitors Positive inotropic agents for periods of decompensation Beta-adrenergic blockers

ACE, Angiotensin-converting enzyme; *ARB,* angiotensin receptor blocker; *NYHA,* New York Heart Association.

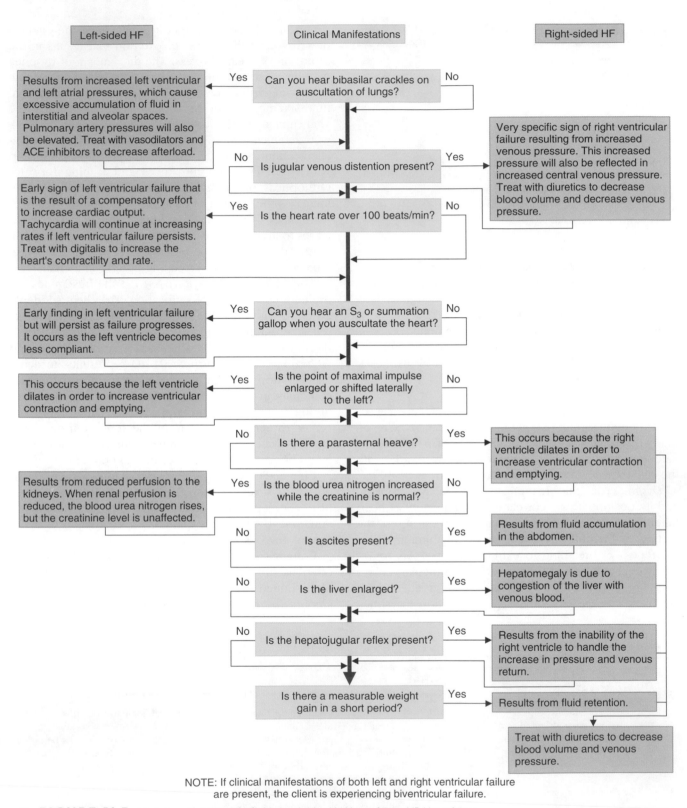

NOTE: If clinical manifestations of both left and right ventricular failure
are present, the client is experiencing biventricular failure.

■ FIGURE 56–7   Clinical manifestations of left-sided and right-sided heart failure. *HF,* Heart failure.

irritating the lung mucosa. On auscultation bilateral crackles may be heard.

Cardiovascular manifestations also denote LVF. Inspecting and palpating the precordium may reveal an enlarged or left laterally displaced apical pulse. This occurs because the left ventricle dilates in an effort to supplement ventricular contraction and emptying. Heart gallop (S₃ or S₄) sounds may be an early finding in heart failure as the left ventricle becomes less compliant and its walls vibrate in response to filling during diastole. The appearance of pulsus alternans (alternating strong and weak heartbeats) may also herald the onset of LVF.

Cerebral hypoxia may occur as a result of a decrease in cardiac output, causing inadequate brain perfusion. Depressed cerebral function can cause anxiety, irritability, restlessness, confusion, impaired memory, bad dreams, and insomnia. Impaired ventilation with resultant hypercapnia may also be a precipitant.

Fatigue and muscular weakness are often associated with LVF. Inadequate cardiac output leads to hypoxic tissue and slowed removal of metabolic wastes, which in turn cause the client to tire easily. Disturbances in sleep and rest patterns may worsen fatigue.

Renal changes can occur in both RVF and LVF but are more striking in LVF. Nocturia occurs early in heart failure. During the day the client is upright, blood flow is away from the kidneys, and the formation of urine is reduced. At night urine formation increases as blood flow to the kidneys improves. Nocturia may interfere with effective sleep patterns, which may contribute to fatigue. As cardiac output declines, decreased renal blood flow may result in oliguria, a late manifestation of heart failure.

Complications of Left Ventricular Failure. Acute pulmonary edema, a medical emergency, usually results from LVF. In clients with severe cardiac decompensation, the capillary pressure within the lungs becomes so elevated that fluid is pushed from the circulating blood into the interstitium and then into the alveoli, bronchioles, and bronchi. The resulting pulmonary edema, if untreated, may cause death from suffocation. Clients with pulmonary edema literally drown in their own fluids. The dramatic manifestations of acute pulmonary edema, listed in the Critical Monitoring feature above, right, terrify the client and the client's significant others.

Right Ventricular Failure. When right ventricle functioning decreases, peripheral edema and venous congestion of the organs develop. Liver enlargement (*hepatomegaly*) and abdominal pain occur as the liver becomes congested with venous blood. If this occurs rapidly, stretching of the capsule surrounding the liver causes severe discomfort. The client may notice either a constant aching or a sharp pain in the right upper quadrant. In chronic heart failure, abdominal tenderness generally disappears.

In severe RVF, the lobules of the liver may become so congested with venous blood that they become anoxic. Anoxia leads to necrosis of the lobules. In long-standing heart failure, these necrotic areas may become fibrotic and then sclerotic. As a result, a condition called *cardiac cirrhosis* develops, manifested by ascites and jaundice.

In chronic heart failure, the increased workload of the heart and the extreme work of breathing increase the metabolic demands of the body. Anorexia, nausea, and

---

CRITICAL MONITORING

Acute Pulmonary Edema

- Severe dyspnea
- Orthopnea
- Pallor
- Tachycardia
- Expectoration of large amounts of frothy, blood-tinged sputum
- Fear
- Wheezing
- Sweating
- Bubbling respirations
- Cyanosis
- Nasal flaring
- Use of accessory breathing muscles
- Tachypnea
- Vasoconstriction
- Hypoxia in ABG findings

---

bloating develop secondary to venous congestion of the gastrointestinal tract. The combination of increased metabolic needs and decreased caloric intake results in a marked wasting of tissue mass, called *cardiac cachexia*. Anorexia and nausea may also result from digitalis toxicity.

Dependent edema is one of the early manifestations of RVF. Venous congestion in the peripheral vascular beds causes increased hydrostatic capillary pressure. Capillary hydrostatic pressure overwhelms the opposing pressure of plasma proteins, and fluid shifts out of the capillary beds and into the interstitial spaces, with resultant pitting edema. Edema is usually symmetrical and occurs in the dependent parts of the body, where venous pressure is highest. In ambulatory clients edema begins in the feet and ankles and moves up the lower legs. It is most noticeable at the end of the day and often subsides after a night's rest. In the recumbent client, pitting edema may develop in the presacral area and, as it worsens, progress to the genital region and medial thighs. Concurrent jugular vein distention differentiates the edema of heart failure from that of lymphatic obstruction, cirrhosis, and hypoproteinemia.

Anasarca, a late manifestation in heart failure, is substantial and generalized edema. It can involve the upper extremities, genital area, and thoracic and abdominal walls. Cyanosis of the nail beds appears as venous congestion reduces peripheral blood flow.

Clients with heart failure often feel anxious, frightened, and depressed. Almost all clients realize that the heart is a vital organ and that when the heart begins to fail, health also fails. As the course of the disease progresses and manifestations worsen, the client may have an overwhelming fear of permanent disability and death. Clients express their fears in varying ways: nightmares, insomnia, acute anxiety, depression, or withdrawal from reality.

Backward Versus Forward Failure

The clinical presentation of heart failure arises from inadequate cardiac output, the pooling of blood behind the failing chamber, or both. *Backward* failure focuses on the ventricle's inability to eject completely, which increases ventricular filling pressures, causing venous and pulmonary congestion. *Forward* failure is a problem of inadequate perfusion. It results when reduced contractility produces a decrease in stroke volume and cardiac output. As cardiac output falls, blood flow to vital organs and peripheral tissues diminishes. This causes mental confusion, muscular weakness, and renal retention of sodium and water. Each of these types of failure is usually present to some degree in the client with heart failure.

High-Output Versus Low-Output Failure

High-output failure occurs when the heart, despite normal-output to high-output levels, is simply not able to meet the accelerated needs of the body. Causes include sepsis, Paget's disease, beriberi, anemia, thyrotoxicosis, arteriovenous fistula, and pregnancy.

Low-output failure occurs in most forms of heart disease, resulting in hypoperfusion of tissue cells. The underlying disorder is related not to increased metabolic needs of the tissues but to poor ventricular pumping action and a low cardiac output.

Decompensated Versus Chronic Heart Failure

The onset of heart failure may be *acute,* leading to decompensation, or stable, called *chronic* heart failure.

Diagnostic Findings

The diagnosis of heart failure rests primarily on presenting manifestations and pertinent data from the client's health history. Diagnostic studies assist in determining the underlying cause and the degree of heart failure. B-type natriuretic peptide (BNP) is a protein secreted from the ventricles in response to overload, such as occurs in heart failure. As the degree of heart failure worsens, the level of BNP secreted into the blood increases. Liver enzymes may reflect the degree of liver failure. Elevated blood urea nitrogen (BUN) and creatinine levels reflect decreased renal perfusion.

Additional studies include an echocardiogram, chest x-ray, and ECG. A two-dimensional (2-D) echocardiogram, coupled with Doppler flow studies, provides information about cardiac chamber size and ventricular function. These tests aid in assessing myocardial, valvular, congenital, endocardial, and pericardial heart disease, allowing the clinician to determine whether the dysfunction is systolic or diastolic. In LVF, chest x-ray often depicts an enlarged cardiac silhouette, pulmonary and venous congestion, and interstitial edema. On x-ray interstitial edema produces images called Kerley's B lines. Pleural effusions may develop and generally reflect biventricular failure. An ECG may give clues to the cause of LVF. Abnormalities in the ECG arise from the underlying cardiac disorder and from therapeutic agents. It may demonstrate evidence of a prior MI, dysrhythmias, or left ventricular dysfunction.

Arterial blood gas analysis may be performed. Early heart failure with pulmonary edema may lead to respiratory alkalosis that is due to hyperventilation. As the disorder progresses and oxygenation becomes more impaired, acidosis develops. Pulse oximetry values show decreased oxygen levels.

OUTCOME MANAGEMENT OF DECOMPENSATED HEART FAILURE

Medical Management

The management of heart failure is divided into two situations: the treatment of decompensated heart failure and the treatment of stable chronic heart failure. Diuretics, nitrates, analgesics, and inotropic agents are indicated for the treatment of decompensated heart failure and pulmonary edema. The goals of the management are to reduce myocardial workload, improve ventricular pump performance, perfuse essential organs, and prevent further heart failure by affecting the process of cardiac remodeling.

Reduce Myocardial Workload

Diuretics are an important aspect of treatment because of the central role of the kidney as the target organ of many of the neurohormonal changes in response to the failing heart. First-line therapy generally includes a loop diuretic such as furosemide, which will inhibit sodium chloride reabsorption in the ascending loop of Henle. Diuretics reduce circulating blood volume, diminish preload, and lessen systemic and pulmonary congestion. Loop diuretics can also produce mild to severe electrolyte imbalance. Hypokalemia, a particularly dangerous side effect, can cause myocardial weakness and cardiac dysrhythmias. Hypokalemia also potentiates digitalis toxicity. Moreover, vigorous diuresis may produce hypovolemia and hypotension, jeopardizing cardiac output.

Vasodilators also reduce myocardial workload by reducing both preload and afterload. Nitroglycerin reduces myocardial oxygen demand by lowering preload and afterload. It is often given intravenously. Morphine IV is often used for clients with acute heart failure. In addition to being both an anxiolytic and an analgesic, its most important effect is venodilation, which reduces preload. Morphine also causes arterial dilation, which reduces systemic vascular resistance (SVR) and increases cardiac output. Medications can be direct vasodilators acting through nitric oxide on the vessel walls. Nesiritide is a newer medication and also works by dilating arteries and veins.

Beta-adrenergic antagonists (beta-blockers) are used to inhibit the effects of the sympathetic nervous system and reduce the oxygen needs of the myocardium. They increase clinical improvement and decrease mortality. These findings are apparent when clients are concurrently receiving ACE inhibitory therapy, suggesting that the combination of two agents that have inhibitory effects on two neurohormonal systems may have an additive effect. Beta-blockers, possibly by restoring beta$_1$-receptor activity or via prevention of catecholamine activity, appear to be cardioprotective in clients with depressed left ventricular function.

Elevate the Client's Head

The client is placed in a high Fowler position or chair to reduce pulmonary venous congestion and to relieve the dyspnea. The legs are maintained in a dependent position as much as possible. Even though the legs are edematous, they should not be elevated. Elevating the legs rapidly increases venous return.

Reduce Fluid Retention

Controlling sodium and water retention improves cardiac performance. Sodium restrictions are placed on the diet to prevent, control, or eliminate edema. Diets with 2 to 4 g of sodium are usually prescribed (Table 56-3).

From the use of some loop diuretics, potassium is lost via the kidneys, which can lead to dysrhythmias and electrolyte imbalances. Hypokalemia sensitizes the myocardium to digitalis and therefore predisposes the client to digitalis toxicity. Potassium supplements and adequate dietary potassium are important.

It is usually not necessary to restrict fluid intake in clients with mild or moderate heart failure. In more advanced cases, however, it is beneficial to limit water to 1000 ml/day (1 L/day). The reason is that excessive water intake tends to dilute the amount of sodium in body fluids and may produce a low-salt syndrome *(hyponatremia)*. Hyponatremia is characterized by lethargy and weakness; it results more often from the combination of a restricted sodium diet, increased sodium loss during diuresis, and excessive water intake.

Improve Ventricular Pump Performance

The most powerful way to increase contractility of the heart is to use adrenergic agonist, or inotropic medications. Angiotensin-converting enzyme (ACE) inhibitors also commonly yield pronounced improvement in hemodynamics, and are discussed below.

Inotropes. Principal inotropic agents include dobutamine, milrinone, dopexamine, and digoxin. In the hypotensive client with heart failure, dopamine and

TABLE 56–3 Sodium Content of Selected Foods	
Foods Low in Sodium	
Dairy products	Skim milk, eggs, cottage cheese, cream cheese, ice cream
Meats*	Turkey, chicken, veal, lamb, liver, fresh fish, tuna packed in water (meats should be unprocessed)
Fruits and vegetables*	Any fresh or frozen food in this group
Beverages	Any juice (except tomato or V8 brand vegetable), coffee, tea, bottled water
Breads	Some breads and cereals
Seasonings	Garlic, onion, bay leaf, pepper, dill, nutmeg, rosemary, allspice, thyme, sage, caraway, cinnamon, almond and vanilla extract, fresh dried herbs
Fats	Margarine, oils, shortening, unsalted salad dressings
Desserts	Sherbet, fruit ice, gelatin, fruit drinks
Miscellaneous	Unbuttered, unsalted popcorn; unsalted nuts; vinegar
Foods High in Sodium	
Milk and dairy products	Aged, hard cheese; pasteurized, processed cheese; buttermilk
Meats	Sausage, frankfurters, ham, bacon, corned beef; all smoked, pickled, or cured meats; canned meats, salami, most luncheon meats, beef jerky; frozen dinners
Fruits and vegetables	Pickled or canned fruits and vegetables, olives, sauerkraut, pickles
Breads and cereals	Salted crackers, macaroni and cheese, pretzels, rye rolls, pizza, commercial pancake mixes
Beverages	Tomato juice, V8 vegetable juice, beef broth, bouillon
Fats	Commercial salad dressings, dips and party spreads, peanut butter
Seasonings	Garlic, celery, or onion salt; Accent, monosodium glutamate (MSG), meat tenderizer, soy sauce, ketchup, steak sauce, mustard, canned soup
Desserts	Fruit pies, doughnuts, cakes, commercial puddings
Miscellaneous	Baking soda, baking powder, salted popcorn, salted nuts, potato chips

*Food sources high in potassium.

dobutamine are agents usually used. These medications facilitate myocardial contractility and enhance stroke volume. They also can lead to dysrhythmias.

Dobutamine is a very useful medication for heart failure because it produces strong beta-stimulatory effects within the myocardium; it increases heart rate, atrioventricular (AV) conduction, and myocardial contractility. Dobutamine is capable of increasing cardiac output without increasing myocardial oxygen demands or reducing coronary blood flow.

Dopamine is a naturally occurring catecholamine with alpha-adrenergic, beta-adrenergic, and dopaminergic activity. Dopamine, given in small doses

(<4 mcg/kg/min), opens the kidney's vascular beds. Vasodilation in the kidney is especially advantageous, leading to improved GFR, urine output, and excretion of sodium. When dopamine is given in higher doses it produces tachycardia and dysrhythmias; therefore it is not commonly used in decompensated heart failure.

Milrinone is another inotropic medication and also dilates the pulmonary vascular beds. Amrinone, the first of the phosphodiesterase inhibitors, is seldom used because it leads to thrombocytopenia. Dopexamine has been used in some clients, and is still being investigated. Digoxin is used less and less in the emergency management of heart failure. Digoxin is discussed with chronic heart failure; it has little to no role in the treatment of decompensated heart failure.

Supplement Oxygen

High concentrations of oxygen by mask or cannula are provided to relieve hypoxia and dyspnea and to improve oxygen–carbon dioxide exchange. For hypoxemia, partial rebreather masks with a flow rate of 8 to 10 L/min can be used to deliver oxygen concentrations of 40% to 70%. A non-rebreathing mask can achieve even higher oxygen concentrations. If these methods do not raise the arterial oxygen tension (Pao_2) above 60 mm Hg, the client may need intubation and ventilatory management. Intubation also provides a route for removing secretions from the bronchi. If severe bronchospasm or bronchoconstriction occurs, bronchodilators are given. The heart rhythm is monitored because some bronchodilators may lead to dysrhythmias.

Control Dysrhythmias

Atrial fibrillation with a rapid ventricular response is the most common dysrhythmia seen in heart failure clients. Atrial fibrillation can lead to embolic stroke, so clients are given anticoagulants. The rhythm is often controlled with medications such as amiodarone.

Reduce Myocardial Remodeling

Angiotensin-converting enzyme inhibitors are now considered first-choice treatment and are the cornerstone of heart failure drug therapy. ACE inhibitors have proved to slow the progression of heart failure by reducing remodeling changes in the heart. ACE inhibitors reduce afterload by blocking the production of angiotensin, a potent vasoconstrictor. They also increase renal blood flow and decrease renal vascular resistance, which enhances diuresis. Side effects include orthostatic hypotension, persistent hacky cough and kidney problems, skin rashes, an altered sense of taste, and hyperkalemia. Potassium levels should be monitored, especially if diuretics or potassium supplements are being used.

Reduce Stress and Risk of Injury

In addition to improving ventricular pump performance and reducing myocardial workload, the client also needs to reduce physical and emotional stress. Sometimes clinicians overlook rest as an intervention to diminish the workload of the heart. The proper use of rest as the initial step in management offers many benefits. Rest can promote diuresis, slow the heart rate, and relieve dyspnea, all of which allow more conservative use of pharmacologic agents (e.g., ACE inhibitors, diuretics, beta-blockers).

Whether the physician prescribes complete, modified bed rest depends on the seriousness of the client's condition. The physician may prescribe a mild sedative or small doses of barbiturates and tranquilizers to promote rest and overcome problems of restlessness, insomnia, and anxiety.

The client may also be at risk for injury because of immobility. The client should be confined to bed only long enough to regain cardiac reserve but not so long as to promote complications of immobility. Give the client confined to bed rest specific guidelines to prevent the harmful effects of immobility. Clients should perform passive leg exercises several times daily to prevent venous stasis, which may lead to the formation of venous thrombi and pulmonary emboli. Anticoagulant therapy prevents these potentially deadly complications.

SAFETY
⚠
ALERT

Nursing Management of the Medical Client

The following are the goals of nursing management for the client with heart failure:

- To monitor for reduced cardiac output
- To maintain adequate fluid balance
- To reduce myocardial workload
- To monitor for pulmonary edema
- To assess response to medical therapies

Consider the psychosocial effect of heart failure on the client and family. Nursing diagnoses that may apply to the client with heart failure are discussed in the Care Plan on pp. 1441-1445.

Surgical Management for Heart Failure

Ventricular Assist Devices

Advances continue to be made in perfecting methods of mechanical ventricular support. The goal of mechanical circulatory support is to decompress the hypokinetic ventricle, decrease myocardial workload, reduce oxygen demands, and maintain adequate systemic perfusion to sustain end-organ function. In the client with heart failure, the two most common options are ventricular assist

C A R E   P L A N   *evolve*

The Client with Decompensated Heart Failure

Nursing Diagnosis: Decreased Cardiac Output related to heart failure or dysrhythmias or both.

Outcomes: The client will have an increase in cardiac output as evidenced by regular cardiac rhythm, heart rate, blood pressure, respirations, and urine output within normal limits.

NOC OUTCOMES   Cardiac Pump Effectiveness

Interventions	NIC INTERVENTIONS	Rationale
1. Assess blood pressure for hypotension or hypertension and respiratory rate for tachypnea q 1 hr (more or less frequently, depending on the client's stability).	Vital Signs Monitoring	1. Hypotension may indicate decreased cardiac output and may lead to a decrease in coronary artery perfusion. Hypertension may be caused by chronic vasoconstriction or may indicate fear or anxiety, and increased respiratory rate may indicate fatigue or increased pulmonary congestion.
2. Assess heart rate and rhythm q 1 hr for tachycardia. Continuously monitor for dysrhythmias.	Vital Signs Monitoring	2. Tachycardia can increase myocardial and oxygen demands and may be a compensatory mechanism related to the decreased cardiac output (increased heart rate to compensate for decrease in stroke volume). Ventricular enlargement decreases conduction of cardiac impulses and may lead to dysrhythmias. Dysrhythmias further compromise cardiac output by reducing ventricular filling time and myocardial contractility and by increasing myocardial oxygen demands.
3. Document rhythm strips q 8 hr and if dysrhythmias occur. Measure and note rate; QRS, PR, and QT intervals; and ST segment with each strip and note any deviations from baseline.	Acute Cardiac Care	3. Common dysrhythmias include premature atrial contractions (PACs), premature ventricular contractions (PVCs), and paroxysmal atrial tachycardia (PAT). Changes in the ST segment may indicate myocardial ischemia, which may be present because of decreased coronary artery perfusion.
4. Report dysrhythmias to the physician, or follow protocol for emergency treatment.	Acute Cardiac Care	4. Dysrhythmias can decrease cardiac output. Particular attention must be paid to ventricular dysrhythmias because they can increase the chance of sudden death.
5. Monitor lab values for isoenzymes, atrial peptide, CK, LDH, AST, BUN, creatinine, liver function tests, CBC, electrolytes, glucose, thyroid function, blood lipids.	Acute Cardiac Care	5. These lab values may indicate myocardial infarction, severe heart failure, renal failure, or liver failure. Thyroid disease can precipitate heart failure.
6. Auscultate heart rate q 2 hr for changes in heart sounds such as murmurs, S_3, or S_4.	Vital Signs Monitoring	6. Delayed filling time, incomplete ejection, and structural changes within the heart and fluid overload may cause abnormal heart sounds detected by auscultation. S_3 may indicate a noncompliant or stiff ventricle, and S_4 may indicate a weak, overdistended ventricle.
7. Monitor lung sounds q 2 hr for adventitious sounds such as crackles and for the presence of coughing.	Vital Signs Monitoring	7. Increased ventricular pressures are transmitted back to the pulmonary circulation, increasing pulmonary capillary hydrostatic pressure and exceeding oncotic pressure fluid moving within the alveolar septum; evidenced by auscultation of crackles, increased shortness of breath, and sputum production. This indicates a further decrease in cardiac output and the possibility of the development of pulmonary edema. Coughing can be caused by the increased fluid in the lungs or by angiotensin-converting enzyme (ACE) inhibitors.

(Continued)

C A R E   P L A N   *evolve*

The Client with Decompensated Heart Failure—Cont'd

8. Monitor intake and output (I&O) and analyze findings q 8 hr and as required (prn). Note color and amount of urine q 2 hr and prn.	Acute Cardiac Care	8. If intake exceeds output, the client is at risk for fluid overload and may not be excreting fluids because of a decompensating heart. Dark, concentrated urine and oliguria may reflect a decrease in renal perfusion. Diuresis is expected in clients receiving diuretic therapy.
9. Assess for changes in mental status.	Acute Cardiac Care	9. Change in mental status may indicate decreased cerebral perfusion or hypoxia.
10. Assess peripheral pulses for strength and quality and for pulsus alternans.	Acute Cardiac Care	10. Decreased strength of peripheral pulses is often found in clients with decreased cardiac output, and a further decrease in pulses from baseline may indicate further cardiac failure. Pulsus alternans may be detected and indicates severe heart failure.
11. Administer prescribed medications and evaluate responses by the client for the intended effect (specify).	Acute Cardiac Care	11. Prescribed medications are used to increase contractility responses and decrease preload or afterload, and their effects must be evaluated. Therapeutic levels and side effects must be monitored.
12. Encourage physical and psychological rest.	Cardiac Precautions	12. Increased physical or mental strain can increase myocardial oxygen demands.
13. Avoid rectal temperatures, rectal meds, enemas, and rectal examinations.	Cardiac Precautions	13. Stimulation of the rectum causes a Valsalva response, which can trigger bradycardia.
14. Encourage clients to eat small meals and rest afterward.	Cardiac Precautions	14. Larger meals increase myocardial workload and may cause vagal stimulation, which may lead to bradycardia.

Evaluation: Following the administration of ACE inhibitors and diuretics, dyspnea should improve. Heart failure is a chronic disorder and complete resolution is not possible; expect small gains in cardiac output in the days that follow.

Nursing Diagnosis: Excess Fluid Volume related to reduced glomerular filtration, decreased cardiac output, increased antidiuretic hormone (ADH) and aldosterone production, and sodium and water retention.

Outcomes: The client will demonstrate adequate fluid balance as evidenced by output equal to or exceeding intake, clearing breath sounds, and decreasing edema.

NOC OUTCOMES Fluid Balance		
Interventions	**NIC INTERVENTIONS**	**Rationales**
1. Monitor I&O q 4 hr (more or less frequently).	Fluid Monitoring	1. I&O balance reflects fluid status (depending on client's status).
2. Weigh clients daily and compare to previous weights.	Fluid Monitoring	2. Body weight is a sensitive indicator of fluid balance and an increase indicates fluid volume excess.
3. Auscultate breath sounds q 2 hr and prn for the presence of crackles and monitor for frothy sputum production.	Fluid Monitoring	3. When increased pulmonary capillary hydrostatic pressure exceeds oncotic pressure, fluid moves within the alveolar septum and is evidenced by the auscultation of crackles. Frothy, pink-tinged sputum is an indicator that the client is developing pulmonary edema.
4. Assess for presence of peripheral edema. Do not elevate the legs if the client is dyspneic.	Fluid Monitoring	4. Heart failure causes venous congestion, resulting in increased capillary pressure. When hydrostatic pressure exceeds interstitial pressure, fluids leak out of the capillaries and present as edema in the legs, sacrum, and scrotum. Elevation of the legs increases venous return to the heart.
5. Assess for jugular vein distention, hepatomegaly, and abdominal pain.	Fluid Monitoring	5. Elevated volumes in the venae cavae occur from inadequate emptying of the right atrium. The excess fluid is transmitted to the jugular vein, liver, and abdomen and manifests as distention.

6. Follow low-sodium diet and/or fluid restriction.	Hypervolemia Management	6. Decreased systemic blood pressure can lead to stimulation of aldosterone, which causes increased renal tubular absorption of sodium. Low-sodium diet helps prevent increased sodium retention, which decreases water retention. Fluid restriction may be used to decrease fluid intake, hence decreasing fluid volume excess.
7. Administer diuretic therapy as ordered and evaluate effectiveness of therapy. Empty indwelling catheter bags before administration of diuretics to record volume diuresed.	Hypervolemia Management	7. Diuretics are commonly prescribed to promote the diuresis of accumulated fluid. The nurse should expect an increase in urine output, improved breathing, and weight loss after the client receives diuretic therapy.
8. Encourage or provide oral care q 2 hr.	Oral Health Maintenance	8. The client senses thirst because the body senses dehydration. Oral care can alleviate the sensation without an increase in fluid intake.

Evaluation: After administration of diuretics, expect profound urine output if the client has reasonable cardiac output. Weight loss and output should stabilize in 2 to 3 days. Expect fairly rapid improvement in peripheral edema.

Nursing Diagnosis: Impaired Gas Exchange related to fluid in alveoli.
Outcomes: The client will have improved gas exchange as evidenced by decreased dyspnea, no cyanosis, normal arterial blood gases, and a decrease in pulmonary congestion on auscultation.

NOC OUTCOMES   Respiratory Status: Gas Exchange

Interventions	NIC INTERVENTIONS	Rationales
1. Auscultate breath sounds q 2 hr.	Vital Sign Monitoring	1. Auscultation of crackles may indicate pulmonary congestion.
2. Encourage the client to turn, cough, and deep breathe and use the incentive spirometer q 2 hr.	Cough Enhancement	2. This will help facilitate oxygen delivery and clear the airways.
3. Administer oxygen as ordered. Monitor for the development of dry nasal mucous membranes and skin injury from the oxygen tubing.	Oxygen Therapy	3. Oxygen therapy will improve oxygenation by increasing the amount of oxygen available for delivery. Administration of nonhumidified oxygen can dry and injure nasal membranes. Tubing pulled tightly can lead to pressure ulcers on the face and ears.
4. Assess respiratory rate and rhythm q 2 hr and prn.	Vital Sign Monitoring	4. Increased respiratory rate indicates difficulty with oxygenation, and a decreased respiratory rate may indicate impending respiratory failure.
5. Assess for cyanosis q 4 hr and prn.	Respiratory Monitoring	5. Circumoral cyanosis or cyanosis to the finger tips or end of nose indicates hypoxia from lack of oxygen in peripheral tissues. Cyanosis is a late sign of poor oxygenation.
6. Position the client to facilitate breathing and observe for paroxysmal nocturnal dyspnea.	Airway Management	6. Fowler position and orthopneic positioning facilitate diaphragmatic excursion. Paroxysmal nocturnal dyspnea may occur because as the client assumes a supine position, venous return to the heart is increased. This increase in return increases preload and will increase pulmonary capillary hydrostatic pressure and lead to pulmonary edema.
7. Monitor pulse oximetry. Move the probe to ensure good contact with the skin or ear.	Vital Sign Monitoring	7. A low SaO_2 reflects hypoxia.
8. Obtain arterial blood gases if ordered.	Acid-Base Management	8. Arterial blood gases indicate whether the client has hypoxia, acidosis, or both.
9. Administer diuretic therapy as ordered, and monitor for effectiveness.	Hypervolemia Management	9. Diuretics promote fluid loss in the alveoli as well as systemically.

Evaluation: Expect dyspnea to improve rapidly once the diuresis has occurred unless the client has significant lung disease from other problems. Because the lung is a low-pressure area, the redevelopment of edema in the lung can occur quickly and continued monitoring is important.

(Continued)

C A R E   P L A N   *evolve*

The Client with Decompensated Heart Failure—Cont'd

Nursing Diagnosis: Ineffective Tissue Perfusion related to decreased cardiac output.
Outcomes: The client will have adequate tissue perfusion as evidenced by warm, dry skin, peripheral pulses, and adequate urine output.

NOC OUTCOMES Tissue Perfusion

Interventions	NIC INTERVENTIONS	Rationales
1. Note color and temperature of the skin q 4 hr.	Acute Cardiac Care	1. Cool, pale skin is indicative of decreased peripheral tissue perfusion.
2. Monitor peripheral pulses q 4 hr.	Acute Cardiac Care	2. Decreased pulses are indicative of decreased tissue perfusion from vasoconstriction of the vessels.
3. Provide a warm environment.	Temperature Regulation	3. A warm environment promotes vasodilation, which decreases preload and promotes tissue perfusion.
4. Encourage active range of motion.	Circulatory Precautions	4. Range of motion helps decrease venous pooling and promotes tissue perfusion.
5. Monitor urine output q 4 hr.	Fluid Monitoring	5. Decreased perfusion to the kidneys may result in oliguria.
6. Protect the skin from trauma by applying cotton socks or fleece boots.	Circulatory Precautions	6. Poorly perfused skin heals slowly, if at all, once injured.

Evaluation: Once cardiac output is improved, expect peripheral blood flow to improve slightly. Pre-existing atherosclerosis will prevent the skin from making dramatic improvement, but the client should return to baseline condition.

Nursing Diagnosis: Risk for Activity Intolerance related to decreased cardiac output.
Outcomes: The client will have improved levels of activity without dyspnea.

NOC OUTCOMES Activity Tolerance

Interventions	NIC INTERVENTIONS	Rationales
1. Space nursing activities.	Energy Management	1. Clustering activities increases myocardial demand and may cause extreme fatigue.
2. Schedule rest periods.	Energy Management	2. Rest periods help alleviate fatigue and decrease myocardial workload.
3. Monitor the client's response to activities. Assess vital signs before and after an activity.	Vital Sign Monitoring	3. Dyspnea, tachycardia, angina, diaphoresis, dysrhythmias, and hypotension are all indicative that the activity required more myocardial demand than the heart was able to supply. The time it requires for the vital signs to return to baseline indicates the degree of cardiac deconditioning.
4. Increase activity as ordered or according to the rehabilitation nurse's directions.	Exercise Promotion: Ambulation	4. Gradually and appropriately increasing physical activity may help the client gain cardiac conditioning and improve activity tolerance.
5. Instruct the client to avoid activities that increase cardiac workload.	Counseling	5. Activities such as stair climbing, working with arms above the head, or sustained arm movement may cause extreme fatigue and demand more cardiac output than the body can supply.

Evaluation: The client will perform spaced activities without dyspnea and will gradually increase activity tolerance. This goal will require time; deconditioning caused by marked dyspnea often prevents rapid improvement.

Nursing Diagnosis: Risk for Impaired Skin Integrity related to decreased tissue perfusion and activities.
Outcomes: The client will have reduced risk of skin impairment.

NOC OUTCOMES Tissue Integrity: Skin

Interventions	NIC INTERVENTIONS	Rationales
1. Reposition the client q 2 hr if client moving self. Turn side to side q 2 hr if client unable to turn self.	Pressure Ulcer Prevention	1. Changing position frequently deters the formation of pressure ulcers by decreasing the amount of time there is pressure on any given area.
2. Provide a therapeutic mattress or bed while the client is in bed.	Pressure Ulcer Prevention	2. Pressure-redistribution mattresses and beds are available to decrease the pressure on the sacrum when the client is sitting up in bed.

3. Assess the skin, especially bony prominences, for redness each shift and as needed. Use protective devices if redness is noted. Inspect between skinfolds in obese clients.	Skin Surveillance	3. Redness is indicative of increased pressure to an area and is the first sign of breakdown. Risk areas include the sacrum, coccyx, heels, elbows, and back of the head.
4. Float the heels from the bed if the client has little spontaneous leg movement.	Pressure Ulcer Prevention	4. The posterior prominence of the heels makes them high risk for breakdown in clients in Fowler position.
5. Assist the client with morning care and lubricate the skin.	Pressure Ulcer Prevention	5. Clients may have difficulty providing themselves with adequate skin care, and the nurse must ensure the skin is clean and has proper moisture to prevent cracking.

Evaluation: Intact skin should remain intact.

Nursing Diagnosis: Risk for Anxiety related to decreased cardiac output, hypoxia, diagnosis of heart failure, and fear of death or debilitation.

Outcomes: The client will not exhibit manifestations of anxiety and will be able to express concerns.

| NOC OUTCOMES | Anxiety Control |

Interventions	NIC INTERVENTIONS	Rationales
1. Provide a calm environment.	Anxiety Reduction	1. A calm environment decreases additional anxiety.
2. Explain in advance all procedures and routine regimens.	Anticipatory Guidance	2. By providing information in advance, the client should not feel anxious about the routine care being provided.
3. Encourage the client to ask questions.	Anxiety Reduction	3. By encouraging the client to ask questions, the nurse is providing an open forum for discussion with the client.
4. Provide emotional support to clients and their significant others.	Anxiety Reduction	4. By allowing clients and their support systems to vent fears and anxiety, the nurse assists them in decreasing anxiety.
5. Encourage the client to use additional support systems.	Coping Enhancement	5. Additional support people such as religious leaders, social workers, counselors, and clinical nurse specialists may increase the client's support system and decrease anxiety.

Evaluation: Anxiety should improve once dyspnea improves. Concerns over deteriorations in health will require additional time for discussion and may require changes in living arrangements.

---

devices (VADs) as a bridge to transplantation and as permanent support.[28] VADs have the capability to support circulation, either partially or totally, until the heart recovers or is replaced. Devices may be right ventricular, left ventricular, or biventricular VADs. Complications of any VAD include bleeding, hemolysis, thromboembolism, infection, and multiorgan failure. Intra-aortic balloon pumping as a treatment for VAD is discussed in the Bridge to Critical Care feature on p. 1423.

Traditionally nonpulsatile pumps have been used as VADs. Difficulties with these devices include end-organ dysfunction, thromboembolic complications, and the need for full anticoagulation. Their use in clients with heart failure is diminishing because better technology has become available. These pumps can be used for a relatively short period of about 10 days.

Total artificial hearts provide complete control of the cardiovascular system and allow total mobility. Their use is limited in smaller people because the device may not fit the client's small body. Complications include infection, thromboembolism, and the possibility of mechanical failure. Initially, total artificial hearts were limited to people awaiting transplantation. Currently, these devices are being used when there are contraindications to transplantation, such as advanced age.

Extracorporeal membrane oxygenation (ECMO) systems are widely used for short-term hemodynamic stabilization. These devices remove blood from the inferior vena cava to a centrifugal pump that pumps the blood to an oxygenator. The oxygenated blood is returned to the client via the femoral artery. Long-term use (<48 hours) does not promote recovery. In addition, bleeding is a concern because anticoagulation therapy is needed.

Heart Transplantation

When the heart is irreversibly damaged and no longer functions adequately and when the client is at risk of dying, cardiac transplantation and the use of an artificial heart to assist or replace the failing heart are measures of last resort. With the development of cyclosporine, and more recently FK-506 and mycophenolate mofetil, and with improvements in the procurement and preservation of donor hearts, cardiac transplantation has become an accepted therapeutic procedure. One-year survival rates after transplantation are greater than 85%. Although transplantation may not be appropriate for all clients, it may be the only option available to some. Heart transplantation is discussed in Chapter 55.

Cardiomyoplasty

For clients with low cardiac output who are not candidates for cardiac transplantation, a procedure called *cardiomyoplasty* may support the failing heart. This procedure involves wrapping the latissimus dorsi muscle around the heart and electrostimulating it in synchrony with ventricular systole.

Immediate postoperative care is similar to that of any cardiac surgery client. Continuous cardiac and hemodynamic monitoring is initiated. Inotropic and vasopressor agents are administered to maintain cardiac output until the pulse generator is activated (within 2 to 3 weeks). Because the muscle flap obliterates the left upper lobe of the lung and can reduce vital capacity by as much as 20%, aggressive pulmonary hygiene and judicious pain management are essential to prevent atelectasis or pneumonia. In addition an upper-extremity exercise regimen is prescribed.

OUTCOME MANAGEMENT OF CHRONIC HEART FAILURE

Chronic heart failure has been classified according to severity (see Table 56-2). Outcome management for clients with chronic heart failure usually follows guidelines based on the degree of severity. This form of heart failure is treated by the client at home, as described in the Bridge to Home Health Care feature below. Interventions must be tailored to the client and taught to improve adherence. Specific instructions should include the following guidelines:

- Adhere to dietary restrictions. Sodium in the diet should be limited to 4 g per day initially until fluid and weight gain are controlled. Fluid restrictions may also be needed. Clients should be shown how to weigh themselves daily and how to adjust sodium and fluid intake if their weight fluctuates from day to day.
- Monitor blood pressure. Clients or family members should be taught how to measure BP daily, especially if the client has diastolic heart failure.
- Modify activity. During severe stages of heart failure, the client should remain on bed rest with the head

---

BRIDGE TO HOME HEALTH CARE

Managing Heart Failure

One third of all clients hospitalized for heart failure are readmitted within 90 days of discharge. Problems with self-monitoring techniques, medication, and diet are the primary reasons. Home health and outpatient care nurses can make a positive difference in readmission rates through nursing interventions.

Review clients' cardiovascular history, disease etiology, and medical management plan to guide your assessment. Auscultate the heart and lungs during each visit, and look for manifestations of fluid accumulation. Measure blood pressure with the client both sitting and standing. If blood pressure decreases significantly and the client experiences lightheadedness or dizziness upon standing, it may be necessary to adjust diuretic or vasoactive medications. Worsening cardiac status or drug toxicities can cause changes in pulse rate or rhythm.

Clients may experience unique manifestations such as fullness in their ears, increased urination at night, and chest heaviness. The client, family members, and informal caregivers need to be educated about the correlation between manifestations and clinical status. Evaluate changes in the prevalence and severity of manifestations. The assessment can include measuring food and fluid intake, abdominal girth and lower extremities, and weight. Instruct clients to call you or their physicians if they lose or gain 2 to 3 pounds in 1 day or 5 to 7 pounds in 1 week. When manifestations are noted and cardiac decompensation is detected early, heart failure can be managed successfully in non-institutional outpatient settings.

Use various techniques to help clients manage their medications. Write the medication schedule clearly, and suggest reminder systems such as pill boxes. Examine all pill bottles for the

drug name, strength, expiration date, and available refills. Review brand versus generic labeling to minimize confusion and prevent drug administration errors. Simplify dosing frequencies; by limiting doses to twice a day (bid), three times a day (tid), or four times a day (qid), medication administration can be associated with daily routines such as meals and bedtime. Flexible dose times can promote drug tolerance and increase accurate administration. Discourage the use of over-the-counter medications because of the potential for drug interactions.

Limiting sodium intake to 2000 mg a day can help prevent fluid retention. Rarely do clients need to restrict fluid intake to less than 2000 ml/day. Evaluate the client's appetite, meal frequency, portion sizes, and food preferences, and provide appropriate health education. If possible, open cupboards and the refrigerator to gain insight into the client's eating patterns. Suggest a food diary to assess intake accurately. Teach clients, family members, and informal caregivers how to distinguish the sodium content of foods by reading food labels.

Because a client's functional status is often severely impaired, explain energy-conservation techniques before initiating limited mobility and aerobic routines. Even the most severely affected client may benefit from chair exercises done in a sitting position. Instruct clients to keep an activity log to demonstrate their progress toward activity goals. Clients should perceive their activities as only somewhat hard to do and should not participate in activities that worsen their manifestations or produce fatigue.

Clients who have chronic illnesses, including heart failure, often have feelings of depression. Consider whether clients need psychosocial and financial assistance. Antidepressant medications benefit some clients and improve their sense of well-being.

of the bed elevated and elastic stockings or wraps worn to mobilize edema. Once the client can breathe comfortably during activity, activity should be increased gradually to help increase strength.

- Adhere to medications. The multiple medications will require some type of system to prevent missed or duplicate doses. Be certain that the client knows how to monitor for side effects. Many people find it best to take diuretics in the morning so that trips to the bathroom to urinate happen during the day. Taking diuretics in the evening or at night often results in interrupted sleep because the urge to empty the bladder continues for hours.

Digoxin

Digoxin is often added to the medication regimen in chronic heart failure. Digoxin is a positive inotrope, often taught to clients as a medication that "slows and strengthens the heart beat." Improved cardiac output enhances kidney perfusion, which may create a mild diuresis of sodium and water. Digoxin does not appear to have an effect on long-term mortality in clients with heart failure. Digoxin therapy may also be initiated to control the ventricular response in atrial fibrillation, the most common dysrhythmia in heart failure.

Digoxin has a narrow therapeutic index, and toxicity occurs in about one in five clients. Clients at risk for the toxic effects of digoxin are older adults; those with advanced heart disease, severe dysrhythmias, or acute MI; and those concurrently using quinidine, verapamil, and amiodarone. Digoxin dosage may need to be reduced if the client is taking any of these medications. Digoxin toxicity is more prevalent when the serum concentration is equal to or greater than 2 mcg/L, serum potassium level is less than 3 mEq/L, or serum magnesium level is low. Digoxin toxicity, described in the Critical Monitoring feature below, may be a life-threatening condition.

CRITICAL MONITORING

Digoxin Toxicity

Digoxin remains a common medication for clients in heart failure because it increases ventricular contractility and emptying by slowing the heart rate, which promotes ventricular filling. Digoxin preparations, however, have a narrow window of therapeutic efficacy, and toxicity from digitalis is not uncommon. Nurses play a significant role in early detection of the subtle manifestations of digoxin toxicity. The diagnosis of digoxin toxicity remains a clinical challenge, in part because therapeutic and toxic digoxin concentrations overlap from one individual to another.

Several causes are known:
- Deteriorating renal function, especially in clients with hyperthyroid conditions
- Dehydration
- Electrolyte imbalances, especially potassium and magnesium imbalances
- Myocardial ischemia
- Acidosis
- Medication interactions:
  - Amiloride
  - Amiodarone
  - Calcium-channel blockers
  - Hydrochlorothiazide and other loop diuretics
  - Indomethacin
  - Propafenone
  - Quinidine
  - Quinine
  - Spironolactone
  - Triamterene

CLINICAL MANIFESTATIONS
- Nausea, vomiting, diarrhea
- Anorexia
- Palpitations
- Irregular heart block, bradycardia and junctional tachycardia

- Confusion
- Lethargy, ataxia
- Visual changes (unusual)
  - Halos or rings of light around objects
  - Seeing lights or bright spots
  - Changes in color perception, especially yellow-green
  - Blind spots in vision
  - Diagnosis

Serum levels of digoxin are used to determine whether toxicity is present. A key factor in determining digoxin toxicity is whether or not blood is drawn at least 6 hours after the last digoxin dose, which ensures that adequate distribution of the drug has been achieved before blood sampling. Blood levels would not be elevated in acute forms of toxicity, such as overdose. Toxic plasma levels are greater than 2.4 ng/ml.

TREATMENT
Because of its long half-life of 38 to 48 hours, treatment is directed at removing the drug. Acute toxicity can be treated with gastric lavage, activated charcoal to limit absorption, or digoxin-Fab fragments (Digibind), which is an antidote. Digibind is composed of digoxin-specific antibody fragments prepared from the immunoglobulin G (IgG) of sheep immunized with digoxin. The smaller Fab fragment avidly binds digoxin but is minimally immunogenic in humans and is excreted renally. Clients are admitted for cardiac monitoring. Factors that led to the toxicity are addressed.

PREVENTION
- Assess potential drug-drug interactions.
- Assess for manifestations of toxicity.
- Assess electrolyte levels (potassium, magnesium).
- Hold the medication if the heart rate is below 60 beats/min or if a new dysrhythmia has developed.
- Push IV digoxin slowly over 5 minutes.
- Schedule serum digoxin levels to be drawn at least 4 hours after an intravenous (IV) dose and 6 hours after an oral dose.

Modifications for Older Clients

Heart failure is becoming increasingly a disorder of the very old. Decompensated heart failure can be triggered by seemingly minor illnesses and dietary indiscretions. Medications commonly used by older people may have an impact on heart performance even though they pose little risk of interaction with cardiovascular medications. Nonsteroidal anti-inflammatory drugs (NSAIDs) tend to worsen heart disease because they promote sodium retention; tricyclic antidepressants (TCAs) and neuroleptic agents lead to orthostatic hypotension. Conversely, cardiac performance can affect the medication's action. The development of RVF can markedly increase the prothrombin time and thereby increase the action of anticoagulants. See the Case Management feature on Heart Failure on the website. Continuous monitoring of homebound clients with heart failure can be facilitated by computer-assisted programs. Nurse researchers are studying the effect of daily interaction via the computer with heart failure clients.

CONCLUSIONS

Disorders of cardiac function are the leading causes of death in the industrialized world. It is imperative that you fully understand the care of clients with heart disease to improve the outcomes and quality of life and to reduce morbidity and mortality. CHD is the precursor to several problems. Your role is to educate the client about risk reduction. Heart failure is a frequent endpoint of cardiac disease. It is important to maximize cardiac output and reduce system demands on the heart.

THINKING CRITICALLY

1. Your client is a 67-year-old man with newly diagnosed insulin-dependent diabetes in end-stage heart failure. The client was recently released from the hospital. You are to begin intravenous dobutamine therapy during this initial home visit. What assessment should be made before initiating dobutamine therapy? What other assessment interventions might be done?

Factors to Consider. How does heart failure respond to the administration of dobutamine? What teaching or learning needs might be assessed in the client?

2. A 70-year-old man is scheduled for a coronary artery bypass graft. What postoperative complications are most prevalent in older adults?

Factors to Consider. How is CABG surgery accomplished? Why is the CABG surgery a popular option?

Discussions for these questions can be found on the website.

BIBLIOGRAPHY

Citations appearing in red refer to primary research.

Citations appearing in blue refer to evidence-based practice guidelines and protocols.

1. Ades, P. (2001). Cardiac rehabilitation and secondary prevention of coronary heart disease. *New England Journal of Medicine, 345*(12), 892-900.
2. Albert, N. (1999). Heart failure: The physiologic basis for current therapeutic concepts. *Critical Care Nurse, 19*(Suppl 6), 2-13.
3. Allen, B., et al. (1999). Comparison of transmyocardial revascularization with medical therapy in patients with refractory angina. *New England Journal of Medicine, 341,* 1029-1036.
4. American Heart Association. (2002). *2002 Heart and stroke facts statistical update.* Dallas: Author.
5. Baig, M.K., et al. (1998). The pathophysiology of advanced heart failure. *Heart and Lung, 28,* 87-97.
6. Balady, G., et al. (2000). Core components of cardiac rehabilitation/secondary prevention programs. *Circulation, 102,* 1069-1073.
7. Chen-Scarabelli, C. (2002). Beating heart coronary artery bypass graft surgery: Indications, advantages, and limitations. *Critical Care Nurse, 22*(5), 44-58.
8. Coffey, M., Crowder, G., & Cheek, D. (2003). Reducing coronary artery disease by decreasing homocysteine levels. *Critical Care Nursing, 23*(1), 25-30.
9. Colbert, K., & Greene, M. (2003). Nesiritide (Natrecor): A new treatment for acutely decompensated congestive heart failure. *Critical Care Nursing Quarterly, 26*(1), 40-44.
10. Collins, A. (2001). More than a pump: The endocrine functions of the heart. *American Journal of Critical Care, 10*(2), 94-96.
11. Cosgrove, J., et al. (2006). Drug-eluting stent restenosis. *Journal of the American College of Cardiology, 47,* 2399-2409.
12. Doering, L.V. (1999). Pathophysiology of acute coronary syndromes leading to acute myocardial infarction. *Journal of Cardiovascular Nursing, 13*(3), 1-20.
13. Eagle, K., et al. (2004). ACC/AHA 2004 guideline update for coronary artery bypass graft surgery. Available at www.acc.org.
14. Epstein, F. (1999). Hormones and hemodynamics in heart failure. *New England Journal of Medicine, 341*(8), 577-585.
15. Fischer, A., et al. (1999). Thrombosis and coagulation abnormalities in the acute coronary syndromes. *Cardiology Clinics, 17,* 283-294.
16. Hunt, S., et al. (2005). ACC/AHA 2005 guideline update for the diagnosis and management of chronic heart failure in the adult: Summary article. *Circulation, 112,* 1825-1852.
17. Kherea, A., et al. (2006). Relationship between C-reactive protein and subclinical atherosclerosis. *Circulation, 113,* 38-43.
18. Kim, W., et al. (2006). The clinical results of a platelet glycoprotein IIb/IIIa receptor blocker (abciximab-ReoPro)-coated stent in acute myocardial infarction. *Journal of the American College of Cardiology, 47,* 933-938.
19. LaFramboise, L., et al. (2003). Comparison of health buddy with traditional approaches to heart failure management. *Family and Community Health, 26*(4), 275-288.
20. Lorenz, B., & Coyle, K. (2002). Coronary artery bypass graft surgery without cardiopulmonary bypass: A review and nursing implications. *Critical Care Nurse, 22*(1), 51-60.
21. MacKlin, M. (2001). Managing heart failure: A case study approach. *Critical Care Nurse, 21*(2), 36-51.
22. Maglish, B.L., et al. (1999). Outcomes improvement following minimally invasive direct coronary artery bypass surgery. *Critical Care Nursing Clinics of North America, 11*(2), 177-208.
23. Mosca, L., et al. (2001). Hormone replacement therapy and cardiovascular diseases. *Circulation, 104,* 499-503.
24. National Institutes of Health. (2001). *Detection, evaluation, and treatment of high blood cholesterol in adults (Adult Treatment Panel III)* (NIH Pub No. 01-3670). Bethesda, Md: NIH.
25. Packer, M., & Cohn, J.N. (1999). Consensus recommendation for the management of chronic heart failure. *American Journal of Cardiology, 83,* 1A-38A.

26. Parson, C. (1999). Evidence based clinical outcome management in interventional cardiology. *Critical Care Nursing Clinics of North America*, 11(2), 143-157.
27. Pasternak, R., et al. (2002). ACC/HA/NHLBI clinical advisory on the use and safety of statins. *Circulation, 106*, 1024-1028.
28. Piano, M., Bondmass, M., & Schwertz, D. (1998). The molecular and cellular pathophysiology of heart failure. *Heart and Lung, 27*, 3-19.
29. Poirier, V. (1997). The HeartMate left ventricular assist system: Worldwide clinical results. *European Journal of Cardio-Thoracic Surgery, 11*, 539-544.
30. Puskas, J. (2004). Off-pump versus conventional coronary artery bypass grafting. Early and 1-year graft patency, cost and quality of life outcomes. *Journal of the American Medical Association, 291*, 1841-1849.
31. Reger, T., & Vargas, G. (1999). The return of the radial artery in CABG. *American Journal of Nursing, 99*(9), 26-32.
32. Ross, A., & Ostrow, L. (2001). Subjectively perceived quality of life after coronary artery bypass surgery. *American Journal of Critical Care, 10*(1), 11-16.
33. Scherr, K., Jensen, L., & Koshal, A. (1999). Mechanical circulation as a bridge to cardiac transplantation: Toward the 21st century. *American Journal of Critical Care, 8*, 324-335.
34. Shah, P.K. (1996). Pathophysiology of plaque rupture and the concept of plaque stabilization. *Cardiology Clinics, 14*(1), 17-28.
35. Shekar, P. (2006). On-pump and off-pump coronary artery bypass grafting. *Circulation, 113*, e51-e52.
36. Smith, A., & Brown, C. (2003). New advances and novel treatments in heart failure. *Critical Care Nurse Supplement*, 11-20.
37. Smith, S., et al. (2001). ACC-AHA guidelines for percutaneous coronary intervention (revision of the 1993 PTCA guidelines)—Executive summary. *Circulation, 103*, 3019-3041.
38. Smith, S., et al. (2006). AHA/ACC guidelines for secondary prevention for patients with coronary and other atherosclerotic vascular disease—2006 update. *Journal of the American College of Cardiology, 47*, 2130-2139.
39. St. Joer, S., et al. (2001). Dietary protein and weight reduction: A statement for healthcare professionals from the nutrition committee on nutrition, physical activity, and metabolism of the American Heart Association. *Circulation, 104*, 1869-1874.
40. Stary, H.C., et al. (1995). A definition of advanced types of atherosclerotic lesions and a histological classification of atherosclerosis. *Circulation, 92*, 1355-1374.
41. Stevenson, L., & Kormos, R. (2001). Mechanical Cardiac Support 2000: Current applications and future trial design. *Journal of Thoracic and Cardiovascular Surgery.* 121(3),418-24.
42. Taccetta-Chapnick, M. (2002). Using carvedilol to treat heart failure. *Critical Care Nurse, 22*(2), 36-58.
43. Teirsteine, P., et al. (2000). Three-year clinical and angiographic follow-up after intracoronary radiation. *Circulation, 101*, 360-370.
44. Wenger, N.K. (1999). Women, myocardial infarction, and coronary revascularization. *Cardiology in Review, 7*, 117-120.
45. Zhou, J., et al. (1999). Plaque pathology and coronary thrombosis in the pathogenesis of acute coronary syndromes. *Scandinavian Journal of Clinical and Laboratory Investigation, 59*(Suppl 230), 3-11.
46. Zimmerman, L., et al. (2002). Comparison of recovery patterns for patients undergoing coronary artery bypass grafting and minimally invasive direct coronary artery bypass in the early discharge period. *Progress in Cardiovascular Nursing, 17*(3), 132-141.

evolve *Did you remember to check out the bonus material on the Evolve website and the CD-ROM, including NCLEX®-Examination Style Review Questions, Open-Book Quizzes, and Chapter Review Audio Podcasts?*

http://evolve.elsevier.com/Black/medsurg

CHAPTER 57

Management of Clients with Dysrhythmias

BETH F. CROWDER*

The heart is endowed with a specialized conduction system for generating rhythmic electrical impulses and for moving these impulses rapidly throughout the heart to cause coordinated contraction of the myocardium. When this system functions normally, the atria contract about one sixth of a second ahead of the ventricles. This orderly electrical activity must precede contraction to provide adequate cardiac output for perfusion of all body organs and tissues.

The rhythmic and conduction systems of the heart are susceptible to damage by heart disease, especially by ischemia of the heart tissues resulting from decreased coronary artery blood flow. The consequence is often a bizarre heart rhythm or abnormal sequence of contraction through the heart chambers. The abnormal rhythms, called dysrhythmias (or arrhythmias), can severely decrease the heart's ability to pump effectively, even causing death.

In 2003 dysrhythmias caused or contributed to 479,000 of more than 2,400,000 deaths in the United States.[1] Dysrhythmias are historically linked to human awareness of the strength and rhythm of the palpable pulse.[14] As early as the 6th century BC, the irregularity of the pulse was observed in China, and then later by the Greeks. Many irregularities were discovered before the availability of electrocardiography. In 1895 Willem Einthoven published a paper on the electrical system of the heart noting five distinct electrical patterns, labeled P, Q, R, S, and T. In 1903 Einthoven modified his string galvanometer, enabling him to record more extensive electrocardiograms (ECGs). In 1912 Einthoven and Thomas Lewis separately published works representing decades of research, observations, and findings regarding cardiac dysrhythmias. Through their discoveries and publications of the heart's electrical system and irregularities, Einthoven and Lewis are considered the pioneers of electrocardiography.[14] Before reading about dysrhythmias, you may want to review the electrical conduction system of the heart in the Unit 13 Anatomy and Physiology Review and the electrocardiogram (ECG) in Chapter 54.

NORMAL SINUS RHYTHM

A normal sinus rhythm is the usual heart rhythm that begins in the sinoatrial (SA) node, is between 60 and 100 beats/min, and has normal intervals and no aberrant or ectopic beats (Figure 57-1). Characteristics of normal sinus rhythm are shown in Table 57-1 and discussed in Chapter 54.

DYSRHYTHMIAS

Dysrhythmias are disorders of the heart rhythm. Dysrhythmias are common in people with cardiac disorders but also occur in people with normal hearts. Dysrhythmias are often detected because of associated manifestations of dizziness, palpitations, and syncope. Abnormalities in conduction are dangerous because of reduced cardiac output, which can lead to impaired cerebral perfusion. The most serious complication of a dysrhythmia is sudden death.[5] Because seconds can literally make the difference between life and death for the person who is experiencing

*The author would like to thank Andrea R. Cain and Sheila Melander for their contribution to this chapter in the seventh edition of Medical-Surgical Nursing.

evolve Web Enhancements

Client Education Guide The Client with a Permanent Pacemaker (Spanish Translation)

Ethical Issues in Nursing What Is Your Role in a "Do Not Resuscitate" Decision?

Be sure to check out the bonus material on the Evolve website and the CD-ROM, including free self-assessment exercises. **http://evolve.elsevier.com/Black/medsurg**

■ **FIGURE 57–1** Normal sinus rhythm as seen on an electrocardiogram (ECG) strip. Note the regular R-R interval, a rate of 80 beats/min, and a P-R interval of 0.16 second.

a serious dysrhythmia, evaluating responsiveness, quickly activating the emergency medical service (EMS), and initiating cardiopulmonary resuscitation (CPR) can determine the outcome.[2]

Etiology and Risk Factors

Dysrhythmias result from disturbances in three major mechanisms: (1) automaticity, (2) conduction, and (3) reentry of impulses.[3,6]

Disturbances in Automaticity

Automaticity is used here to describe the normal processes of generating a heart rhythm. This process of automatically initiating an impulse can be altered if the normal pacemaker cells are firing too rapidly or if an impulse is generated by a cell that normally does not initiate heartbeats, called an ectopic pacemaker. Enhanced normal automaticity occurs when cells conduct an impulse because they were not suppressed. An ectopic pacemaker occurs when cardiac muscle cells that normally do not exhibit pacemaker potential or activity (latent cells) fire to originate an impulse.

Recall that the SA node is the pacemaker of the heart because it possesses the highest level of automaticity. It normally produces a rhythm of 60 to 100 beats every minute. The SA node is regulated by the nervous system through the vagus nerve. Sympathetic stimulation increases the rate of firing, while lack of sympathetic stimulation or vagal stimulation (which is parasympathetic) decreases the rate. If the SA node fails to fire, other latent sites in the atria can fire (60 to 100 beats/min). If the atria

do not initiate a beat, it can begin in the atrioventricular (AV) node; if the AV node does not initiate a beat, one can start in the ventricles. This fail-safe mechanism is crucial during heart disease. Latent pacemaker cells in the AV junction usually assume the role of pacemaker of the heart but at a slower rate (40 to 60 beats/min). Such a pacemaker is called an *escape* pacemaker. If the AV junction cannot take over as the pacemaker because of disease, an escape pacemaker in the electrical conduction system below the AV junction (i.e., in the bundle branches or Purkinje fibers) can take over, but at a still lower rate (less than 40 beats/min). In general, the further the escape pacemaker is from the SA node, the slower the impulse rate generated.

Risk Factors. Abnormal automaticity is commonly caused by myocardial ischemia, decreased left ventricular function, valvular heart disease, electrolyte imbalance, hypoxia, adrenergic (sympathetic nervous system) stimulation, impaired cellular metabolism, use of antidysrhythmic medications, digitalis toxicity, and administration of atropine (which blocks vagal stimulation).

Disturbances in Conduction

Conduction is the speed the impulse travels through the sinus node, AV node, and Purkinje fibers. Latent pacemaker cells can also fire at rates above or below their inherent rate. A rhythm slower than the intrinsic rate is called *bradycardia*. A rhythm faster than the intrinsic rate is called *accelerated* or *tachycardia*. For example, sinus bradycardia is identified as a heart rate below 60 beats/min and sinus tachycardia is defined as a heart rate above 100 beats/min. An accelerated junctional tachycardia can develop with a rate higher than 60 beats/min (the inherent AV node rate).

Impulses can also occur prematurely or may be blocked anywhere between the SA node and the Purkinje fibers. Premature beats are ones that occur before the expected impulse. Premature beats can develop from any of the latent pacemaker cells. Blocks are impulses that are generated normally, but do not reach their destination. Blocks need more time to travel to their destination; the ECG wave is wider than normal. Disturbances in conduction can also lead to decreased cardiac output and life-threatening dysrhythmias.

Risk Factors. Conduction disturbances can result from myocardial ischemia, scarring and compression of conduction pathways, valvular heart disease or valvular surgery, inflammation of the AV node, extreme vagal stimulation of the heart, electrolyte imbalances, increased atrial preload, digitalis toxicity, beta-blocking agents, non-dihydropyridine calcium-channel blockers, impaired cellular metabolism, and myocardial infarction (MI) (especially inferior).

TABLE 57–1	Characteristics of Normal Sinus Rhythms
Rhythm	Regular, P-P intervals and R-R intervals may vary as much as 3 mm and still be considered regular
Rate	60-100 beats/min
P waves	One P wave preceding each QRS complex
P-R interval	0.12-0.20 sec, consistent with each complex
QRS complex	0.04-0.10 sec, consistent with each complex
Q-T interval	<0.40 sec

Reentry of Impulses

Reentry of impulses occurs when cardiac tissue is depolarized multiple times by the same impulse. Normally the impulse enters into the tissue, excites the tissue (causing depolarization), and leaves the tissue after the refractory period is over (repolarization). It occurs along one pathway with a constant conduction velocity. Reentry of impulses occurs when two pathways are present (a "slow" pathway and a "fast" pathway). Two pathways can develop from anatomic abnormalities (accessory pathway, fibrosis) or functional defects (ischemia, drug interactions). The two pathways are separated by an area of unexcitable tissue. As the impulse enters both pathways, the "fast" pathway exhibits a resistance that will not allow the impulse to travel forward but the impulse is able to travel down the slow pathway. When the impulse reaches the distal end of the slow pathway, it travels backwards into the fast pathway, causing the impulse to repeat itself.[3] Reentry of impulses creates problems because some cells have been repolarized sufficiently so that they can prematurely depolarize again, producing ectopic beats and rhythm disturbances.

Risk Factors. Reentry can result from myocardial ischemia, the action of antidysrhythmic medications, myocardial fibrosis, existence of an accessory pathway, or bundle-branch block.

Pathophysiology

The significance of all dysrhythmias is their effect on cardiac output and therefore cerebral and vascular perfusion. Recall that cardiac output is the result of stroke volume times the heart rate. During normal sinus rhythm, the atria contract to fill and stretch the ventricles with about 30% more blood. This process, called the *atrial kick,* increases the amount of blood (stroke volume) in the ventricles before contractility, thereby increasing cardiac output by 30%. When the impulse originates below the SA node, or more than one area fires in the atria to originate a beat (such as with atrial fibrillation or atrial flutter), the atrial kick is lost and cardiac output falls that 30%.[3]

Clinical Manifestations

The reduced cardiac output leads to clinical manifestations of palpitations, dizziness, presyncope or syncope, pallor, diaphoresis, altered mentation (restlessness and agitation to lethargy and coma), shortness of breath, chest pain, orthopnea, paroxysmal nocturnal dyspnea, hypotension, sluggish capillary refill, swelling of the extremities, and decreased urine output.

The initial assessment includes a careful history regarding the onset, duration, associated manifestations, aggravating factors, and relieving factors. Following the history and symptom analysis, a detailed past medical history follows including cardiovascular disease (CVD) risk factor analysis, past health history and hospitalizations, surgical history, allergies, medications, dietary habits, social habits (tobacco, alcohol, street drugs, exercise), and family history. Complete your review of systems and proceed to the physical examination with emphasis on the auscultation of the heart for abnormal heart tones, slow or fast rate, irregularity, murmur(s), or displaced point of maximum intensity.

Diagnostic Assessment
Noninvasive Recording

Electrocardiography. Electrocardiography remains the most important and definitive noninvasive diagnostic test for dysrhythmias. Each rhythm strip or ECG must be approached in a systematic manner for analysis (Box 57-1). The key to dysrhythmia interpretation is the analysis of the form and interrelations of the P wave, the P-R interval, and the QRS complex. Are P waves present? Is there a P wave preceding every QRS complex? What is the duration of the P-R interval? Is the P-R interval constant? What is the duration of the QRS complex? What are the atrial and ventricular rates? Are the P-P and R-R intervals regular? Are all P waves and QRS complexes identical? The ECG should also be analyzed with respect to its rate, rhythm, and site of the dominant pacemaker as well as the configuration of the P and QRS waves (Table 57-2). Remember, any ECG findings should be correlated with clinical observations of the client; that is, treat the client, not the monitor.

Holter Monitors. Holter monitors continuously record the cardiac rhythm for 24 hours. This method of prolonged ECG monitoring, with clients engaged in their usual daily activities, is one of the most useful noninvasive methods for capturing and documenting the type, frequency, and complexity of the dysrhythmia. Holter monitors also allow correlation between the dysrhythmia and the client's manifestations. The Holter tape is timed and clients keep a diary noting the clinical manifestation and the time the manifestation was noted.

Event Monitors. For those clients who do not experience dysrhythmia within that 24-hour period of recording, event monitors are available. This monitor is smaller with fewer electrodes placed on the client. Unlike the 24-hour Holter monitor (which records continuously), the event monitor is client activated. When a dysrhythmia is noted, the client pushes a small button to activate the recorder. Multiple episodes can be recorded and downloaded over the telephone. Clients usually keep event monitors for 2 weeks (or longer) in order to capture their dysrhythmia.

Invasive Electrophysiologic Studies

An electrophysiologic (EP) study involves the positioning of a multipolar catheter electrode into the venous

BOX 57-1 Electrocardiographic Interpretation of Dysrhythmias

There are seven basic steps to assist you in the identification of dysrhythmias. The electrocardiogram (ECG) should be studied in an *orderly* fashion as follows:

Step 1. Calculate the heart rate. The simplest method for obtaining the rate is to count the number of R waves in a 6-inch strip of the ECG tracing (which equals 6 seconds). Multiply this sum by 10 to get the rate per minute (beats/min). Because the ECG paper is marked into 3-inch intervals (at the top margin), the approximate heart rate can be rapidly calculated.

Another method is to count the number of large squares between R waves. Find an R wave crossing a large square. Count the number of large squares until the next R wave. The approximate heart rate is as follows:

- 1 large square = 300 beats/min
- 2 large squares = 150 beats/min
- 3 large squares = 100 beats/min
- 4 large squares = 75 beats/min
- 5 large squares = 60 beats/min
- 6 large squares = 50 beats/min
- 7 large squares = 43 beats/min
- 8 large squares = 37 beats/min
- 9 large squares = 33 beats/min
- 10 large squares = 30 beats/min

Step 2. Measure the regularity (rhythm) of the R waves (ventricular rhythm). This can be done by gross observation or actual measurement of the intervals (R-R).

If the R waves occur at regular intervals (variance <0.12 second between beats), the ventricular rhythm is normal. When there are differences in R-R intervals (>0.12 second), the ventricular rhythm is said to be irregular. The division of

ventricular rhythm into regular and irregular categories assists in identifying the mechanism of many dysrhythmias.

Note atrial regularity and measure the atrial rate. Measure the regularity (rhythm) of the P waves (P-P). Use the previously described method, but calculate the distance between the same point on two consecutive P waves.

Step 3. Examine the P waves. If P waves are present and precede each QRS complex, the heartbeat originates in the sinus node and a sinus rhythm exists. The absence of P waves or an abnormality in their position with respect to the QRS complex indicates that the impulse started outside the sinoatrial node and that an ectopic pacemaker is in command.

Step 4. Measure the P-R interval. Normally this interval should be between 0.12 and 0.20 second. Prolongation or reduction of this interval beyond these limits indicates a defect in the conduction system between the atria and the ventricles.

Step 5. Measure the duration of the QRS complex. If the width between the onset of the Q wave and the completion of the S wave is greater than 0.12 second (three fine lines on the paper), an intraventricular conduction defect exists.

Step 6. Examine the ST segment. Normally this segment is isoelectric, meaning it is neither elevated nor depressed because the positive and negative forces are equally balanced during this period. Elevation or depression of the ST segment indicates an abnormality in the onset of recovery of the ventricular muscle, usually because of injury (e.g., acute myocardial infarction).

Step 7. Examine the T wave. Normally the T wave is upright and one third the height of the QRS complex. Any condition that interferes with normal repolarization (e.g., myocardial ischemia) may cause the T waves to invert. An abnormally high serum potassium level causes the T wave to become very tall, sometimes the height of the QRS complex.

---

system, placing the electrode at various sites along the atria, ventricles, His bundle, bundle branches, accessory pathways, and other structures to record electrical activity. These areas can also be stimulated through the catheter tip to assess for function or rhythm disturbances. Electrophysiologic studies are performed for three primary reasons:

(1) diagnostically (to provide information on the dysrhythmia type and its origin), (2) therapeutically (to evaluate the effects of antidysrhythmic drugs or function of an automatic internal cardioverter-defibrillator), and (3) prognostically (to identify clients at risk for sudden death).[3]

TABLE 57-2 Cardiac Dysrhythmia Characteristics

Type of Dysrhythmia	Atrial Rate (beats/min)	P-Wave Rhythm/Contour	Ventricular Rate (beats/min)	QRS Complex Rhythm/Contour
Sinus rhythm	60-100	Regular/normal	60-100	Regular/normal
Sinus tachycardia	>100	Regular/normal	>100	Regular/normal
Sinus bradycardia	<60	Regular/normal	<60	Regular/normal
Atrial fibrillation	350-600	Irregular/undulations	100-180	Irregular/normal
Atrial flutter	220-350	Regular/sawtooth	75-175	Regular/normal
1° AV block	60-100	Regular/normal	60-100	Regular/normal
2° AV block type I	60-100	Regular/normal	30-100	Regular/normal
2° AV block type II	60-100	Regular/normal	30-100	Regular/normal
3° (complete) AV block	60-100	Regular/normal	40-60	Regular/normal
Ventricular tachycardia	Cannot calculate	Absent	70-250	Fairly regular to irregular/wide
Ventricular fibrillation	Cannot calculate	Absent	150-300	Grossly irregular/wide

OUTCOME MANAGEMENT

The goal of management is to control or ablate the dysrhythmia and reduce potential complications. The specific management of dysrhythmias depends on the type and on the client's response to the dysrhythmia. All dysrhythmias can reduce cardiac output, which can cause a client to have no manifestations or to have many. Rhythm disturbances resulting in syncope, near-syncope, or near sudden death warrant further evaluation. Ventricular dysrhythmias can be life-threatening, demanding immediate treatment. This chapter reviews dysrhythmias and their management, including rhythm disturbances arising (1) in the sinoatrial node, (2) in the atria, (3) in the AV junction, (4) in an accessory pathway, (5) in the ventricles, and (6) with impulse conduction.

SINOATRIAL NODE DYSRHYTHMIAS

DISTURBANCES IN AUTOMATICITY

Sinus Tachycardia

Sinus tachycardia in an adult is defined as a heart rate faster than 100 beats/min. Sinus tachycardia begins in the sinus node, with a regular rhythm between 100 and 180 beats/min. The P wave and QRS complex are normal duration (Figure 57-2, *A*). It often occurs in response to an increase in sympathetic stimulation or decreased vagal (parasympathetic) stimulation.

Causes include the following:

- Fever
- Emotional and physical stress
- Heart failure
- Fluid volume loss
- Hyperthyroidism
- Hypercalcemia
- Medications, including atropine, nitrates, epinephrine, isoproterenol, and over-the-counter cold medications containing decongestants (pseudoephedrine, dextromethorphan)
- Caffeine
- Nicotine
- Exercise

Sinus tachycardia usually does not produce noticeable clinical manifestations except for occasional palpitations; however, if the heart rate is very rapid it will reduce cardiac output. Between these quick beats, there is little time for atrial contraction and ventricular filling. Clients with underlying heart disease may not tolerate the increased myocardial workload and reduced coronary artery filling time that accompany the increased heart rate. These clients may experience hypotension and *angina pectoris* (chest pain).

Management

Management focuses on alleviating the underlying cause and reducing further demands on the heart. Medications such as digitalis, beta-blocking agents (e.g., propranolol), and calcium-channel blockers (e.g., verapamil) may be prescribed, or intravenous fluids may be given

■ **FIGURE 57–2**   Atrial dysrhythmias. **A,** Sinus tachycardia—regular R-R interval, rate 125 beats/min; P-R interval, 0.16 second. **B,** Sinus bradycardia—regular R-R interval, rate 40 beats/min; P-R interval, 0.16. **C,** Premature atrial contractions. The second and fifth beats are premature atrial contractions (PACs). Note the difference in the appearance of the P wave and the shortened R-R interval.

if hypovolemia is suspected.[5,6] Bed rest or decreased physical activity reduces metabolic demand. Oxygen may be prescribed to supply the myocardium adequately. Elimination of tobacco, alcohol, caffeine, and other stimulants is recommended.

Sinus Bradycardia

Sinus bradycardia in an adult occurs when the SA node fires at a rate of less than 60 beats/min. The P wave and QRS complex are normal (Figure 57-2, *B*). Sinus bradycardia may result from the following:

- Increased vagal (parasympathetic) tone, as with vomiting or Valsalva's maneuver (straining with bowel movements)
- Drugs (especially digitalis, propranolol, or verapamil)
- MI (most often inferior MI)
- Hyperkalemia
- Various diseases, such as hypothyroidism, myxedema, and obstructive jaundice
- Severe hypoxia
- Increased intracranial pressure

Asymptomatic sinus bradycardia frequently occurs in young, healthy adults or athletes because of conditioning and a greater than normal stroke volume. In adolescents and young adults during sleep, the normal heart rate may fall to 40 beats/min.

Manifestations develop when cardiac output is decreased and can include fatigue, hypotension, lightheadedness, dizziness, presyncope, syncope, shortness of breath, decreased level of consciousness, pulmonary congestion, or heart failure. The slowed rate of SA discharge may allow junctional or ventricular pacemakers to take over, thereby producing ectopic beats sensed as palpitations.

Management

The goal of management is to correct the underlying cause of sinus bradycardia, and the goal of intervention is to increase the heart rate just enough to relieve manifestations but not enough to cause tachycardia. The intervention sequence for treating hospitalized symptomatic bradycardia is atropine; transcutaneous pacing if available; dopamine, epinephrine, and isoproterenol; or insertion of a temporary transvenous pacemaker.[5,6] Permanent transvenous pacemakers can also be inserted if warranted. Medications to increase the heart rate safely and reliably over long periods without side effects are not available.

Sinus Dysrhythmia

Sinus dysrhythmia is characterized by phasic changes in the automaticity of the SA node, causing it to fire at varying speeds. The heart rate generally ranges between 60 and 100 beats/min. The ECG shows a normal P wave, P-R interval, and QRS complex, with the only abnormality being an irregular P-P interval. Sinus dysrhythmia may develop from alterations in vagal tone and in response to delayed atrial filling with inspiration. During inspiration, venous return to the right atrium is delayed because of increased intrathoracic pressure. In quiet respiration, the heart rate can decrease about 5%; with deep inspiration, the rate can decrease up to 30%.[3] Clients with sinus dysrhythmia do not usually require intervention unless blood pressure is affected, particularly with orthostatic position changes. If dizziness, presyncope, or syncope occur, elastic support stockings and/or sodium-retaining drugs (to expand the vascular volume) are helpful.

Sick Sinus Syndrome

Sick sinus syndrome encompasses different abnormalities of the sinus node including (1) persistent sinus bradycardia (not caused by medications or physiologic disturbances), (2) sinus arrest or pauses, (3) combinations of SA and AV nodal conduction disturbances, and (4) alternating paroxysms of rapid atrial tachycardias. Manifestations are intermittent and unpredictable, and affect client lifestyles. Causes are also similar to those for tachycardia and bradycardia.[3]

Management

Often, clients are found to have tachycardia and are prescribed digitalis, propranolol, verapamil, or other medications that slow the SA node impulse. The drugs then affect the impulse conduction and can lead to bradycardia. Decreasing the drug dose usually leads to recurrence of tachycardia. For clients with sick sinus syndrome, treatment is two-fold including drugs to slow the automaticity and heart rate, along with insertion of a permanent transvenous pacemaker to prevent symptomatic bradycardia.

DISTURBANCES IN CONDUCTION

SINOATRIAL NODE CONDUCTION DISTURBANCES

Under certain circumstances, the impulse from the SA node is either (1) not generated in the SA node (*SA arrest*) or (2) not conducted from the SA node (*sinus exit block*). Causes of SA node conduction abnormalities include the following:

- Conditions that increase vagal tone
- Coronary artery disease
- MI
- Digitalis and calcium-channel blocker toxicity
- Hypertensive disease
- Tissue hypoxia
- Scarring of intra-atrial pathways
- Electrolyte imbalances

SA Arrest

During *SA arrest,* neither the atria nor the ventricles are stimulated, resulting in a pause in the rhythm. An entire

PQRST complex will be missing for one or more cycles. After the pause of sinus arrest, a new pacemaker focus assumes the pacing responsibility. The new pacemaker paces the heart at its inherent rate, which is usually slower than the original SA node rate. The new pacemaker site is often another atrial focus, but the AV junction or ventricle can also assume pacing responsibility.

Management

Intervention may include administration of a vagolytic (atropine) or a sympathomimetic (isoproterenol) agent to increase the rate of SA node firing. If pharmacologic measures fail, a temporary transvenous pacemaker may be required. A permanent transvenous pacemaker may also be warranted depending on the underlying cause of the dysrhythmia.[3,5]

Sinus Exit Block

During *sinus exit block,* a conduction delay occurs between the sinus node and the atrial muscle. Unlike the rhythm in SA arrest, the rhythm of SA node discharge in sinus exit block remains constant and uninterrupted. The ECG characteristically displays a normal sinus rhythm interrupted intermittently by pauses. This creates a pattern of pauses that, when measured, comprises multiples of the underlying P-P interval. Sinus arrest differs from SA exit block in that the SA node at times does not fire at all. The result is the occurrence of pauses that are longer and not a multiple of the underlying P-P interval. These pauses are also frequently terminated by escape ectopic beats. Sinus arrest often is associated with a more serious prognosis.[3] The client usually remains asymptomatic, depending on the duration and frequency of the pauses; however, lengthy pauses can cause lightheadedness, dizziness, presyncope, or syncope. Intervention is unnecessary unless the client becomes symptomatic and exhibits manifestations of decreased cardiac output.

Management

Management is similar to SA arrest and is based on symptoms or alterations in vital signs.

ATRIAL DYSRHYTHMIAS

DISTURBANCES IN AUTOMATICITY

Premature Atrial Contractions

Premature atrial contractions (PACs) are early beats arising from ectopic atrial foci, interrupting the normal rhythm. They commonly result from enhanced automaticity of the atrial muscle and can occur in both normal and diseased hearts. PACs are associated with valvular disease and atrial chamber enlargement; they may also be seen with stress, fatigue, alcohol or caffeine ingestion, smoking, coronary artery disease (CAD), cardiac ischemia, heart failure, cardioactive medications (digitalis, quinidine, procainamide), pulmonary congestion, and pulmonary hypertension. Frequent PACs may mark the onset of atrial fibrillation or heart failure or may reflect electrolyte imbalances.[3]

In clients with PACs, P waves are premature and often differ from the normal sinus P wave in appearance, size, or shape (Figure 57-2, *C*). When a PAC occurs, conduction may not be normal as the AV node may still be refractory from the preceding beat. Thus the impulse may be blocked or slowed, prolonging the P-R interval. Premature beats from any ectopic focus can be palpated as skipped or irregular beats. The client who experiences numerous PACs may note palpitations, or "missed beats." PACs are usually benign; however, if the client has increasing numbers of "skipped beats" or feels palpitations often, the problem should be evaluated.

Management

PACs generally do not require treatment. Intervention usually focuses on correcting the underlying cause and may include administration of digitalis, a beta-blocker, or a calcium-channel blocker.

REENTRY OF IMPULSES

Paroxysmal Atrial Tachycardia

Paroxysmal atrial tachycardia (PAT) is the sudden onset and sudden termination of a rapid firing from an ectopic atrial pacemaker (Figure 57-3, *A*). Atrial tachycardias are referred to as *supraventricular* because the dysrhythmia source is above the ventricles and often P waves are difficult to detect, which leads to difficulty in trying to name the dysrhythmia. The atrial rate is 150 to 200 beats/min with change in P-wave contour from the sinus P wave. At faster atrial rates, the P waves may become lost in the preceding T wave. Rapid atrial rates may overcome the conduction limits of the AV node, causing varying degrees of AV block [2:1 block (i.e., two P waves for every QRS complex)]. If the atrial rate is not excessive, then conduction through the AV node is usually 1:1. If the atrial rate is excessive, the AV node blocks some of the impulses from further conduction. The QRS complexes are usually normal, although aberrant ventricular conduction may occur at very rapid atrial rates or when a conduction defect exists within the ventricle.[3]

Occasionally PAT appears in clients with a normal heart but most commonly develops in clients with cardiac disease. Common cardiac problems precipitating PAT include the following:

- Coronary artery disease
- MI
- Cardiomyopathy
- Extreme emotions
- Caffeine ingestion

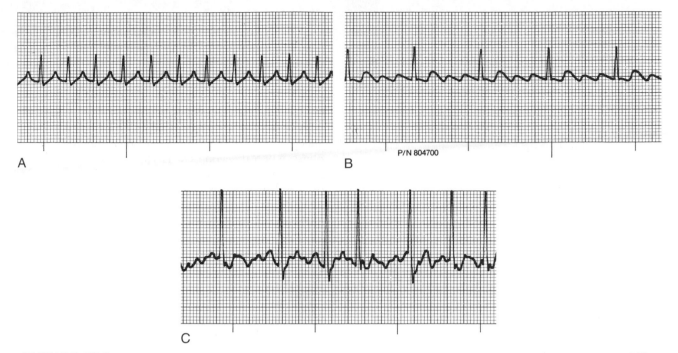

P/N 804700

■ **FIGURE 57–3 A,** Paroxysmal atrial tachycardia (PAT). The rate is rapid, about 175 beats/min. The P wave is not distinguishable, but the QRS complex is narrow, indicating that the impulse began above the atrioventricular node. **B,** Atrial flutter. Note the saw-toothed appearance of the P waves. There are three P waves for every QRS complex, indicating a 3:1 block. Atrial rate is 75 beats/min. **C,** Atrial fibrillation is identifiable by a chaotic P wave, not one clear P wave, and an irregular R-R interval.

- ■ Cor pulmonale (heart failure from lung disease)
- ■ Digitalis toxicity
- ■ Hypokalemia

Less common causes include rheumatic heart disease, valvular disease, pulmonary emboli, thyrotoxicosis, and cardiac surgery. Paroxysmal atrial tachycardia decreases ventricular filling time and mean arterial pressure and also increases myocardial oxygen demand. Clients may report palpitations, heart racing, dizziness, and lightheadedness.

Management

🪔 Management varies with the severity of manifestations. Clients with extremely rapid heart rates or significant underlying cardiovascular disease may experience syncope and heart failure. In such instances, heart rate must be immediately slowed. Any maneuver that stimulates the vagus nerve can successfully terminate PAT or increase AV block. The vagus nerve can be stimulated by carotid sinus massage and/or Valsalva's maneuver. Useful pharmacologic agents include adenosine, verapamil, and beta-blockers. Sedatives may also be used to reduce sympathetic stimulation. If medications and vagal stimulation are not effective, cardioversion (discussed later in this chapter) is an effective means of terminating PAT. Ablation procedures that block a part of the reentrant path are being more widely used (discussed later in this chapter). Such procedures can result in a long-term cure in selected clients.[3–11]

ATRIAL FIBRILLATION

Atrial fibrillation (A Fib) is the most common supraventricular dysrhythmia encountered in the emergency department, affecting 1% to 2% of the general population, especially older adults.[3,6] Atrial fibrillation is characterized by rapid, chaotic atrial depolarization from a reentrant pathway. Ectopic atrial foci produce impulses between 350 and 600 beats/min. At extremely rapid rates, however, the entire atrium may not be able to recover from one depolarization wave before the next begins, resulting in mechanical and electrical disorganization of the atria without effective atrial contraction. Small irregular baseline undulations that vary in size and shape, called f waves, are identified, which differ from the formed "saw-toothed" waves of atrial flutter. Similar to atrial flutter, the AV node is bombarded with more impulses than it can conduct so a rapid ventricular response comparable to the atrial rate cannot occur. Most of these impulses are blocked; however, as a result of the erratic atrial impulses, the ventricular rhythm is very irregular. The ventricular rate ranges from 100 to 180 beats/min.

Examination of the ECG reveals erratic unidentifiable P waves and underlying ventricular rhythm that appears to be irregular (Figure 57-3, *C*). Because of atrial disorganization, "atrial kick" is lost, thereby decreasing cardiac output by as much as 30%. With increasing ventricular rates allowing less filling time, cardiac output declines even further and may result in dyspnea, angina pectoris, heart failure, and shock. The client may have a pulse deficit between apical and radial pulses.

Atrial fibrillation most commonly occurs because of the following:

- Coronary artery disease
- Congestive heart failure
- Valvular heart disease (particularly mitral and aortic)
- Sick sinus syndrome
- Advanced age
- Longstanding hypertension
- Pericarditis

During atrial fibrillation, blood pools in the "quivering" atria because of lack of adequate contraction of atrial appendages. Pooling blood is prone to clot, forming a mural thrombus, which increases the risk of cerebral and peripheral vascular emboli. Most clients with sudden onset of atrial fibrillation are given anticoagulants to reduce risk of thrombus formation and embolic events. Approximately 20% to 25% of cerebral vascular accidents are due to cardiogenic emboli.[11]

OUTCOME MANAGEMENT

The initial treatment goal is to reduce the risk of thromboembolism and to convert the rhythm to sinus rhythm or control the ventricular response. Anticoagulation in the form of heparin or a low-molecular-weight heparin is started. Oral anticoagulation in the form of Coumadin or warfarin should be started on any reliable client. The dose of Coumadin or warfarin should achieve an international normalized ratio (INR) of 2.0 to 3.0 for stroke prevention. Clients with contraindications to anticoagulation (previous cerebral hemorrhage, history of hemorrhage or gastrointestinal bleeding while taking Coumadin, prone to falls, or cannot reliably follow dosing regimen) can be treated with aspirin therapy. Anticoagulation therapy is 50% more effective than aspirin for stroke prevention.[3,11] Conversion of the atrial fibrillation back to sinus rhythm can be accomplished with medications or cardioversion. Diltiazem, verapamil, beta-blockers, or digoxin is used to control the ventricular heart rate. Chemical cardioversion, usually after 4- to 6-week period of anticoagulation therapy, can then be attempted with procainamide, quinidine, sotalol, propafenone, amiodarone, or other antidysrhythmic agent. Electrical cardioversion is another therapeutic option. The risk of stroke following cardioversion, whether chemical or electrical, in clients not treated with anticoagulation is up to 7%. An alternative option to 4 to 6 weeks of anticoagulation therapy, especially in symptomatic clients, is transesophageal echocardiogram to exclude the presence of atrial thrombus. Please see Chapter 54 for a review of transesophageal echocardiography. After return to sinus rhythm, anticoagulation therapy is continued for an additional 4 to 6 weeks.[3]

Electrical Cardioversion

Cardioversion, most often an elective procedure for dysrhythmias caused by reentry, involves the use of a synchronized biphasic direct current (DC) electrical countershock that depolarizes all the myocardial cells simultaneously, allowing the SA node to resume the pacemaker role. The electrical discharge is synchronized with or triggered by the client's QRS complex for avoidance of accidental discharge during the repolarization phase when the ventricle is vulnerable to the development of ventricular fibrillation. A QRS complex must be present for successful conversion of the dysrhythmia.

Biphasic defibrillators have replaced monophasic defibrillators because biphasic energy requires about half the joules for successful cardioversion. Low voltages (50 to 100 J) are tried initially. If the attempt is unsuccessful, cardioversion using larger voltages can be repeated. Only specially trained physicians can perform this procedure.[3]

Cardioversion is used to treat atrial fibrillation, atrial flutter, and supraventricular tachycardia (see later discussion) that is resistant to medication, and is also used in ventricular tachycardia in an unstable client. The unstable client may be hypotensive or dyspneic, may be experiencing chest pain, or may have evidence of heart failure, MI, or ischemia. Analgesia or sedation may be provided before the electrical shock.[11]

Care Before Cardioversion

The physician evaluates the ECG to identify the type of dysrhythmia present. The client must sign an informed consent, after which the intervention is scheduled. The client and family must receive a full explanation of the cardioversion procedure. The client should be in a fasting state with normal electrolyte balance. For those clients receiving digoxin, a therapeutic drug level must be present. Digitalis toxicity may predispose the client to ventricular dysrhythmias during cardioversion. An INR should between 2.0 and 3.0 after 4 to 6 weeks of receiving anticoagulation therapy (or may be normal if transesophageal echocardiography precedes the cardioversion).[3]

Cardioversion is typically performed at the client's bedside in the critical care unit, or similar specialized area, along with the physician, nurses, and respiratory therapist. If a life-threatening dysrhythmia develops after cardioversion, emergency equipment and trained clinicians are immediately at hand. Start an intravenous (IV) line for medication delivery. Self-adhesive pads (instead of paddles) are used and placed in the standard apex-anterior or apex-posterior positions.

The client is premedicated with a rapid, short-acting sedative. Anesthesia personnel may be present to sedate the client. Oxygen is administered before cardioversion, and discontinued if oxygenation saturation is within normal limits.

Care During Cardioversion

The physician performs the following steps and they are repeated with each increase in joules:

1. Sets the biphasic machine within a range of 50 to 200 joules (more or less, depending on the underlying impedances)
2. Turns the synchronizer switch to "on" to deliver the shock during the QRS complex, not on the downslope of the T wave
3. Calls for all health care personnel to stand back from the bed
4. While standing back from the bed, depresses and holds the buttons on the paddles until the shock is delivered
5. Reassess the cardiac rhythm, rate, blood pressure, and pulse oximetry and client's airway after every shock delivered.

Care After Cardioversion

Clinicians immediately assess the ECG, pulse, blood pressure, and respiratory status after the procedure. In some cases ventricular fibrillation or ventricular tachycardia occurs, demanding emergency action. Monitor the client's ECG rhythm and vital signs continuously for at least 2 hours, and carefully assess for rhythm changes and complications. A successful response to cardioversion resolves the dysrhythmia and restores normal sinus rhythm. The client's airway is protected until sedation lightens. With a good response and no complications, the client may be discharged later that day when fully awake and able to eat.

Surgical Management

The Cox-Maze procedure (typically called the MAZE procedure) is an open heart operation for clients with lone atrial fibrillation and no other structural heart disease. The operation involves making a series of incisions that encircle abnormal foci usually near the pulmonary veins. The client requires the usual care of anyone having open-heart surgery (see Chapter 54).

ATRIAL FLUTTER

Atrial flutter is a dysrhythmia from an ectopic pacemaker or the site of a rapid reentry circuit in the atria, characterized by rapid "saw-toothed" atrial wave formations that are usually followed by a slower, regular ventricular response. Atrial flutter differs from PAT in that it produces a much more rapid atrial rate. The P waves are actually inverted or bidirectional because of the clockwise or counterclockwise reentrant pathway, producing a "saw-toothed" pattern of "flutter waves" (Figure 57-3, *B*). The atrial rate generally ranges from 220 to 350 beats/min. The AV node cannot conduct all the atrial impulses that bombard it; therefore the ventricular rate is

always slower than the atrial rate. Thus the pulse, which reflects the ventricular rate, may be normal even though the atrial rate may be quite rapid. The ratio of atrial to ventricular beats may be constant (2:1, 3:1, 4:1, and 5:1, for example), or it may vary. A variable degree of block produces an irregular ventricular rhythm.[3,6]

Atrial flutter most commonly occurs in association with the following:

- Coronary artery disease
- Mitral valve disease
- Atrial enlargement caused by septal defects
- Pulmonary embolus
- Thyrotoxicosis
- Alcoholism
- Pericarditis

In addition, it may occur after cardiac surgery. The client may sense palpitations, shortness of breath, and chest pain, especially when rapid ventricular rates exist. The use of carotid massage helps to slow the ventricular response temporarily so that flutter waves can be identified.

Medical Management

Intervention is based on manifestations and aims at controlling rapid ventricular rates. Anticoagulation is imperative, initially with heparin or a low-molecular-weight heparin, followed by Coumadin or warfarin therapy with an international normalized ratio (INR) of 2.0 to 3.0. Intravenous ibutilide, a short-acting antidysrhythmic medication, has a 60% to 90% success rate for converting atrial flutter. Cardioversion also promptly restores sinus rhythm, usually at energy levels as low as 25 to 100 J. Other medications used include digitalis, diltiazem, flecainide, propafenone, amiodarone, procainamide, and sotalol. Clients with atrial flutter should be referred for electrophysiologic evaluation/study in hopes of dysrhythmia ablation.[3,5,6]

ATRIOVENTRICULAR JUNCTIONAL DYSRHYTHMIAS

If the SA node fails to fire and an impulse is not initiated in other ectopic sites in the atria, the AV junction is the next pacemaker for the heart. An impulse begins in the AV junction and simultaneously spreads up to the atria and down into the ventricles. During junctional rhythms, cardiac output decreases because there is no atrial kick to the ventricles. A junctional rhythm is not dependable as the long-term cardiac pacemaker because its intrinsic rate is slow and more irritable ectopic foci may fire, such as from the ventricles. Consider junctional rhythms to be a warning or forerunner of more serious dysrhythmias.[6]

Two major types of dysrhythmias arise in the AV junction:

- Disturbances in automaticity, with the AV junctional tissue assuming the role of the pacemaker
- Disturbances in conduction, with the AV junction blocking impulses journeying from the atria to the ventricles

Both types of dysrhythmias can result from ischemia, MI, congenital heart disease, valvular heart disease, hyperkalemia, thyrotoxicosis, infectious or inflammatory diseases, or with the use of digoxin, beta-blockers, certain calcium-channel blockers, or certain antidysrhythmics.

Junctional rhythms produce abnormal upward direction of impulse (e.g., in lead II the P waves are inverted) because the impulse is traveling through the atria in a direction opposite that found in normal sinus rhythm. Also, the P-R interval shortens to less than 0.12 second. The impulse may spread through the atria at the same time that the ventricles are being activated by the AV junction. In this instance, the P wave would be buried in the QRS complex and not observed on the ECG. Also, the atria may contract after the ventricles. In this case the P wave would follow the QRS complex. The QRS complex is normal if ventricular conduction is normal.

DISTURBANCES IN AUTOMATICITY

The major junctional dysrhythmias caused by changes in automaticity are (1) premature junctional contractions (PJCs), (2) junctional escape rhythm, and (3) junctional tachycardias. As with PACs, an ectopic focus in the AV junctional tissue may develop increased automaticity and discharge prematurely, initiating depolarization of the heart.[3]

Premature Junctional Contractions

A PJC is the single, early firing of a junctional ectopic focus (Figure 57-4). PJCs are slower as a result of lower intrinsic rates. Usually clients can tolerate junctional rhythms without significant loss of cardiac output; however, clients with underlying cardiac disease may become symptomatic depending upon the amount and frequency

■ **FIGURE 57–4** A premature junctional contraction. The beats marked with *arrows* are premature junctional contractions. Note the absence of a P wave but otherwise normal deflection, indicating that the impulse was initiated above the ventricles.

of ectopic beats. Clients are usually asymptomatic and no interventions are warranted.

Paroxysmal Junctional Tachycardia

A junctional rhythm with a rate that exceeds 60 beats/min is termed a *junctional tachycardia*. It usually stops and starts abruptly, thereby acquiring the name *paroxysmal junctional tachycardia,* or PJT. The usual rate is 140 to 220 beats/min. Causes of PJT include metabolic imbalances and increased sympathetic stimulation. Rapid ventricular rates can lead to left ventricular failure resulting from increased myocardial oxygen demand and decreased myocardial blood supply. PJT that cannot be distinguished from PAT on the ECG is called *supraventricular tachycardia* (SVT).

Medical Management

Management of rapid junctional rhythms begins with vagal stimulation, such as carotid sinus massage. If clinical manifestations develop, treatment consists of pharmacologic agents and cardioversion. Common medications include propranolol, quinidine, and digitalis. Assessment of serum electrolytes and digitalis levels is indicated.[3,6]

DISTURBANCES IN IMPULSE CONDUCTION

The second group of dysrhythmias arising in the area of the AV junction is the AV block. Impulses passing through the AV junction are blocked to varying degrees. Therefore the conduction of impulses from the atria to the ventricles slows or stops entirely, depending on the degree of the AV block. Normally the impulse coming from the SA node is delayed at the AV junction for less than 0.20 second before traveling on to the bundle of His. If the AV junction has been damaged (by one or more of the above etiologies), impulses are delayed or completely blocked at the AV junction for abnormally long periods. Impulse conduction disturbances are classified by the severity of block: first-degree, second-degree, or third-degree AV block.

FIRST-DEGREE ATRIOVENTRICULAR BLOCK

First-degree AV block is a delay in passage of the impulse from atria to ventricles creating a prolonged P-R interval that is greater than the normal 0.20 second. This delay usually occurs at the level of the AV node. Although conduction time is prolonged, all impulses are conducted. The rhythm is regular and each P wave is followed by a QRS complex. The P-R interval usually remains constant (Figure 57-5, *A*). This characteristic is an important differentiation between first-degree AV block and other AV blocks. This block is often associated with structural abnormalities, such as right atrial enlargement or atrial septal defect.

■ **FIGURE 57–5** Junctional dysrhythmias. **A,** First-degree atrioventricular (AV) block. **B,** Second-degree AV block (Mobitz type I, Wenckebach phenomenon; note the regularly occurring P waves and the increasing P-R intervals). **C,** Second-degree AV block (Mobitz type II). **D,** Third-degree AV block (note variable P-R interval and lack of association of the P wave with the QRS complex).

It occurs in 0.5% of young adults without heart disease; however, in the older population it is often seen with idiopathic degenerative disease of the conduction system.[3,6]

Management

First-degree AV block, existing alone as the only abnormal feature of a client's ECG, produces no clinical manifestations and requires no intervention. If the block is a result of digitalis, the medication may be discontinued. Because first-degree AV block can progress to a higher-degree AV block, the client requires routine evaluation including ECG monitoring.[3]

SECOND-DEGREE ATRIOVENTRICULAR BLOCK

Second-degree AV block is a more serious form of conduction delay in the heart; some impulses are conducted and others are blocked. Second-degree block results in intermittently dropped QRS complexes. Atrial depolarization continues producing normal-appearing P waves at regular intervals. Second-degree AV block does not usually affect conduction through the ventricles, and QRS complexes appear normal in configuration. Second-degree AV block develops from coronary artery disease (CAD), digitalis toxicity, rheumatic fever, viral infections, and inferior wall MI.[3,6]

Second-degree AV block is subdivided into two additional types: Mobitz type I (Wenckebach phenomenon) and Mobitz type II.

Mobitz Type I Block (Wenckebach Phenomenon)

The Mobitz type I form of second-degree block is an abnormally long refractory period at the AV node. This delay causes the P-R interval to progressively lengthen until the P wave fails to conduct to the ventricles and a QRS complex is dropped (Figure 57-5, *B*). As the P-R interval lengthens, the R-R interval becomes shorter. With Wenckebach phenomenon, the QRS complexes are typically "grouped" into twos, threes, fours, and so on. Because of this characteristic grouping, the rhythm is described by recording the number of P waves compared to the number of QRS complexes (e.g., 3:2 or 4:3).[3,6]

Mobitz type I is the mildest form of second-degree heart block and carries a better prognosis compared to type II. The etiology is similar to first-degree AV block, except that Mobitz type I is caused by a block in the AV node. Mobitz type I is a stable rhythm that usually does not result in clinical manifestations because the ventricular rate is adequate; however, the client may have an irregular pulse rate. Vertigo, weakness, or other manifestations of low cardiac output may be experienced if the ventricular rate drops precipitously.

Management

Intervention is not required as long as the ventricular rate remains adequate for perfusion. The client is assessed for progression to a higher (more serious) degree of block. Clinicians focus primarily on managing the underlying cause. Intervention, if needed, is similar to that described for Mobitz type II block.[3]

Mobitz Type II Block

Mobitz type II block occurs when a P wave is not conducted, resulting in a dropped QRS complex. Although a QRS complex is dropped in type I, in type II the P-R interval remains constant without prolongation. In type II the P waves are normal and are followed by normal QRS complexes at regular intervals until suddenly a QRS complex is dropped (Figure 57-5, *C*). The block is described by the ratio of the number of P waves to QRS complexes (e.g., 2:1, 3:1, 4:1). This is considered an unstable rhythm that is usually caused by an infranodal conduction disturbance. Mobitz type II blocks result from ischemia, MI, drug toxicity, idiopathic fibrosis of the conduction system, congenital or valvular heart disease, or hyperkalemia.[3,6]

Mobitz type II is a more serious condition than Mobitz type I because it may progress to third-degree AV block, especially in clients with an anterior wall MI. Clients with second-degree AV block require close ECG monitoring for possible progression to complete heart block.

Management

Interventions include (1) administration of atropine or isoproterenol (which speed the rate of impulse conduction), (2) insertion of a temporary or permanent pacemaker, and (3) withholding cardiac depressant drugs (e.g., digitalis, beta-blockers, certain calcium-channel blockers). Second-degree block, which occurs after MI, particularly an inferior MI, may be reversible as the ischemic myocardium heals.[3]

THIRD-DEGREE ATRIOVENTRICULAR BLOCK

Third-degree AV block is the complete dissociation of the impulse between the atria and ventricles. The atria are regularly paced by the SA node, but because the message is completely blocked, the ventricles are being regularly paced by a ventricular ectopic pacemaker (Figure 57-5, *D*). Third-degree heart block is sometimes called *AV dissociation* or complete heart block because upper and lower chambers of the heart are working independently of each other. The atrial rate is always equal to or faster than the ventricular rate in complete heart block. The ventricular rate is typically 40 to 60 beats/min.[3,6]

Other features of the ECG in third-degree heart block include (1) regular P-P intervals, (2) regular R-R intervals, (3) an absence of meaningful or consistent P-R intervals, and (4) normal-appearing P waves. The greatest danger inherent in third-degree AV block is ventricular standstill or asystole. If an ectopic focus in the ventricles does not initiate a heartbeat, asystole will lead to immediate loss of consciousness and in some cases even death.

Third-degree AV block results from a variety of causes, including the following:

- Fibrotic or degenerative changes in the conduction system
- MI (especially inferior wall MI)
- Congenital anomalies
- Cardiac surgery
- Myocarditis
- Viral infections of the conduction system
- Drug toxicity (digitalis, beta-blockers, calcium-channel blockers)
- Trauma
- Cardiomyopathy
- Lyme disease

The slow ventricular rate leads to decreased cardiac output and circulatory impairment. Clients may experience hypotension, angina pectoris, heart failure, dyspnea, dizziness, presyncope, or syncope.

Management

The major interventions for complete heart block are atropine, transcutaneous pacing, catecholamine infusions (dopamine or epinephrine), and transvenous pacemaker. If asystole develops, CPR is used until a transvenous pacemaker can be inserted. Isoproterenol is rarely indicated. Long-term management for irreversible causes includes permanent pacemaker implantation.[3,5]

INTRAVENTRICULAR IMPULSE CONDUCTION ABNORMALITIES

Bundle-Branch Block

Bundle-branch block indicates that conduction is impaired in one of the bundle branches (distal to the bundle of His), and thus the ventricles do not depolarize simultaneously. The abnormal conduction pathway through the ventricles is causing a wide (greater than 0.20 second) or notched QRS complex.

The defect may result from the following:

- Myocardial fibrosis
- Chronic CAD
- MI
- Cardiomyopathy
- Inflammation
- Pulmonary embolism
- Severe left ventricular hypertrophy
- Congenital anomalies

These disturbances of conduction through the ventricles result in either a right bundle-branch block (RBBB) or a left bundle-branch block (LBBB). A 12-lead electrocardiogram is needed to distinguish left and right BBB. In LBBB the QRS complex in V_1 is described as rS or QS (Figure 57-6, *B*). In RBBB the QRS complex in V_1 is described as rsR (Figure 57-6, *C*). Because of its association with left ventricular disease, LBBB carries a worse prognosis. The left bundle branch is composed of anterior and posterior fascicles (small bundles), and one or both fascicles may be involved. No specific intervention for this conduction defect has been established; however, if RBBB exists along with block in one of the fascicles of the left bundle, the one remaining fascicle represents the only conduction pathway to the ventricles. Therefore in this situation, a pacemaker is required.[3]

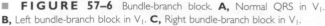

■ **FIGURE 57–6** Bundle-branch block. **A,** Normal QRS in V_1. **B,** Left bundle-branch block in V_1. **C,** Right bundle-branch block in V_1.

VENTRICULAR DYSRHYTHMIAS

Ventricular dysrhythmias arise below the level of the AV junction. Like dysrhythmias in the atria or junction, dysrhythmias in the ventricles are caused by abnormalities of automaticity or conduction. Ventricular dysrhythmias are generally more serious and life-threatening than atrial or junctional dysrhythmias because ventricular dysrhythmias more commonly develop in association with intrinsic heart disease. Also, ventricular dysrhythmias usually cause greater hemodynamic compromise (e.g., hypotension, heart failure, shock). The independent contraction of the ventricles results in a reduced stroke volume and therefore a reduced cardiac output. Rapid ventricular rates prevent optimal filling of the ventricular chambers and reduce stroke volume even further. At rates of less than 40 contractions per minute, cardiac output is simply not sufficient to support the body's vital functions.[13]

The ECG tracing of a client with ventricular dysrhythmias reveals wide and bizarre QRS complexes. Normally impulses traverse the ventricles via the shortest, most efficient route. This normal pathway results in a narrow QRS complex. When an impulse originates in the ventricles, however, the impulse follows an abnormal pathway through the ventricular muscle tissue. This abnormality appears as a wide (greater than 0.12 second) complex on the ECG.

DISTURBANCES IN AUTOMATICITY

Dysrhythmias resulting from problems in automaticity are characterized by ectopic impulses, which result from either myocardial irritability or the phenomenon of reentry. Ventricular dysrhythmias caused by problems with automaticity are premature ventricular contractions (PVCs), ventricular tachycardia (VT), and torsades de pointes.

Premature Ventricular Contractions

Premature ventricular contractions are the most common of all dysrhythmias other than those of the sinus node. They are usually caused by firing of an irritable pacemaker in the ventricle and result from enhanced ventricular automaticity or reentry. Factors promoting PVCs are listed in Box 57-2.[3,6] Premature ventricular contractions

BOX 57-2 **Causes of Premature Ventricular Contractions**	
■ Myocardial hypoxia	■ Heart failure
■ Hypokalemia	■ Toxic agents (e.g.,
■ Hypocalcemia	digitalis, tricyclic
■ Acidosis	antidepressants)
■ Alcohol	■ Exercise
■ Caffeine	■ Hypermetabolic states
■ Nicotine	■ Intracardiac catheters
■ Coronary artery disease	

produce easily recognized ECG changes. They occur earlier than the expected beat of the underlying rhythm and are not preceded by a P wave. The QRS complex is wide (greater than 0.12 second) and bizarre. The T wave is commonly large and in the opposite direction of the QRS deflection (Figure 57-7, *A*).

■ **FIGURE 57-7** Ventricular dysrhythmias. **A,** Beats 2 and 4 are unifocal premature ventricular contractions (PVCs). **B,** Multifocal PVCs. **C,** Paired PVCs. **D,** R-on-T phenomenon, leading to ventricular fibrillation. **E,** Ventricular tachycardia. **F,** Polymorphic ventricular tachycardia.

In the following situations PVCs are considered dangerous:

- Frequent (greater than 6 per minute)
- Coupled with normal beats (bigeminy)
- Multiform (Figure 57-7, *B*)
- In pairs after every third beat (trigeminy) (Figure 57-7, *C*)
- A result of acute MI
- On the T wave (Figure 57-7, *D*)

Clinicians refer to "falling on the T wave" as the R-on-T phenomenon. The downward slope of the T wave is the most vulnerable period of the cardiac cycle. If the heart is stimulated at this time, it often cannot respond to the stimulus in an organized fashion because the muscle fibers are in various stages of repolarization. Therefore PVCs that occur during this vulnerable period can precipitate the more life-threatening dysrhythmias of VT (Figure 57-7, *E*) and ventricular fibrillation.

Management

Isolated PVCs are usually not treated. If the client becomes symptomatic because of decreased cardiac output, lidocaine or any of the other class I, II, or III antidysrhythmics can be given to treat PVCs. Intravenous magnesium may also be useful. In clients with acute MI, the development of PVCs indicates that the myocardium is ischemic and irritated. Treatment with beta-blockers can help to suppress PVCs along with restoring myocardial blood flow. In the ischemic setting, PVCs can progress to VT or ventricular fibrillation quickly, so prompt attention and treatment is warranted.[3,6]

OUTCOME MANAGEMENT OF NONTHREATENING DYSRHYTHMIAS

Medical Management

Suppress Irritable Foci
Management of dangerous PVCs involves the administration of antidysrhythmic agents that have myocardial depressant actions. In acute situations the clinician may administer class I and class II antidysrhythmic agents intravenously (IV), followed by a continuous IV drip. The Integrating Pharmacology feature on Toxicity and Antidysrhythmic Agents on p. 1465 describes a variety of antidysrhythmic agents.[3]

Improve Myocardial Oxygen
Oxygen is an essential component of dysrhythmia management, especially for dysrhythmias that result from irritable foci in an ischemic myocardium. These include PVCs and other ventricular dysrhythmias. Oxygen should be given to all clients at risk of ventricular dysrhythmias, such as those with chest pain or hypoxemia or during cardiac arrest.

Nursing Management of the Medical Client

Assessment. Assess the client for clinical manifestations of decreased cardiac output. Monitor the ECG continuously for patterns of dysrhythmias that indicate further deterioration (e.g., sudden onset of atrial fibrillation, PVCs increasing in number; PVCs from different foci, moving closer to the preceding T wave).

Diagnosis, Outcomes, Interventions
Diagnosis: Decreased Cardiac Output. Dysrhythmias often lead to decreased ventricular filling as a result of the rapid rate or from not being coordinated to allow for atrial kick. Express this common nursing diagnosis as *Decreased Cardiac Output related to decreased ventricular filling time secondary to (name the rhythm)*.

Outcomes. The client will have an adequate cardiac output as evidenced by (1) return of normal heart rate, rhythm, palpable pulse, and blood pressure to baseline levels; (2) return of level of consciousness to baseline value; (3) warm, dry skin; (4) clear lung sounds; (5) the absence of S_3 or S_4; (6) the absence of dysrhythmias; and (7) adequate urine output.

Interventions. Monitor heart rate and rhythm and vital signs continuously, aided by the computer as needed. Assess skin temperature, lung sounds, heart sounds, and peripheral pulses every 2 to 4 hours. Monitor laboratory studies, especially if a myocardial infarction is suspected. Give antidysrhythmic medications according to orders. Use blood levels as a guide to dosage. Many medications, especially antidysrhythmics, can rise to toxic levels, especially if the client has a pre-existing liver, renal, or electrolyte disorder. Do not attempt to memorize the Integrating Pharmacology box; rather, commit a few drugs to memory (amiodarone, lidocaine, verapamil, and sotalol). Some of these medications can be administered orally or by continuous IV infusion. You must be diligent in monitoring for the intended effect and side effects of the medication.

> **Assess for manifestations of stroke in clients with atrial fibrillation or flutter. Teach the client to report to the nursing staff any unusual manifestations, especially changes in speech or ability to move.** SAFETY ALERT

Administer anticoagulant medications to maintain target partial thromboplastin time (PTT) or INR. If the client is discharged on Coumadin, be certain that the need for follow-up monitoring of INR and the effect of diet on anticoagulation are understood.

Maintain a quiet atmosphere, and administer analgesics to control pain. Stimulation can lead to increased levels of catecholamine release and may trigger tachycardias and

Toxicity and Antidysrhythmic Agents

Numerous antidysrhythmic agents are used to treat and prevent disturbances in cardiac rhythms. Antidysrhythmic drugs have and will continue to have a significant role in decreasing the incidence of sudden cardiac death. Unfortunately, antidysrhythmic drugs also can lead to dysrhythmias at both therapeutic and toxic drug concentrations. See Chapter 56 for a discussion of digoxin toxicity.

CLASS I: SODIUM CHANNEL BLOCKERS

All class I agents block fast sodium channels and reduce the rate of increase of the action potential (phase 0) in certain cells. They inhibit depolarization of neuronal cells, thereby producing local anesthesia. They inhibit depolarization in atrial, ventricular, and Purkinje myocytes, thereby decreasing conduction velocity and automaticity. Class I agents are further categorized as A, B, or C subclasses based on the degree of sodium channel blockade and effects on repolarization. Class IA agents prolong action potential duration and produce moderate slowing of cardiac conduction; prolongation of action potential duration occurs from blockade of outward-rectifying potassium channels. Class IB agents shorten the duration of action potentials and selectively depress cardiac conduction in ischemic cells. Class IC agents have little effect on the potential duration of action potentials but markedly depress cardiac conduction (potent sodium channel blockers).

Procainamide is a commonly used class IA medication used to treat sustained ventricular dysrhythmias. At toxic levels it leads to prolongation of the Q-T interval and QRS complex. Other toxic manifestations include gastrointestinal disturbances, headache, mild hypotension, rash, insomnia, dizziness, ataxia, hallucinations, and weakness.

Lidocaine is a class IB agent used for suppression of VTach or dysrhythmias associated with cardiac surgery. Evidence supporting the efficacy of lidocaine is lacking at this time. ACLS protocol recommends other antidysrhythmics, such as amiodarone, as a better choice. Lidocaine blocks sodium channels and shortens the action potential. Side effects are blurred vision, tinnitus, drowsiness, nausea or vomiting, lightheadedness, confusion, hypotension, and atrioventricular block.

CLASS II: BETA-ADRENERGIC BLOCKERS

Class II beta-adrenergic blockers indirectly block calcium-channel opening and block the ability of catecholamines to cause dysrhythmias. Beta-blockers are used to treat hypertension and myocardial infarction. They are also used to treat migraine headaches, essential tremors, thyrotoxicosis, glaucoma, anxiety, and various other disorders. As a result of their expanded use, the incidence of overdose with these agents has also increased. Manifestations of beta-blocker overdose are related to blocking sympathetic beta-adrenergic receptors. Seizures have been reported.

CLASS III: POTASSIUM CHANNEL BLOCKERS

Class III potassium channel blockers prolong refractoriness and delay repolarization by blocking potassium channels; they have little direct effect on sodium channels. Amiodarone is commonly used to suppress dysrhythmias. Toxic effects include photosensitivity, neurotoxicity, hyperthyroidism, heart failure, complete heart block, pulmonary fibrosis, skin pigmentation (blue nail coloration), and corneal deposits. It may induce Q-T prolongation.

CLASS IV: CALCIUM-CHANNEL BLOCKERS

Class IV calcium-channel blockers slow sinoatrial node pacemaker cell and atrioventricular conduction by direct blockade of L-type voltage-gated calcium channels. Calcium-channel blocker overdose is rapidly emerging as the most lethal prescription drug ingestion. Overdose by short-acting agents is characterized by rapid progression to cardiac arrest. Overdose by extended-relief formulations results in delayed onset of dysrhythmias, shock, sudden cardiac collapse, and bowel ischemia.

As in the case of any client with suspected or known acute poisoning, attempt to obtain the original medication containers, pill counts, the quantity that may have been ingested, approximate time of ingestion, and a report of any potential co-ingestants. To clarify the role of the antidysrhythmic agent, ask the client the following:

- What were the indications for starting the drug?
- How long has the client used this medication?
- How do the manifestations correlate with the initiation of drug therapy?
- Is the client compliant with the drug regimen? Does the client take any extra doses?
- What other medications has the client begun recently? Include nonprescription and herbal medications as well.

From Cummings, R. (2001). *ACLS provider manual.* Dallas, Tex: American Heart Association; Asselin, M.E., & Cullen, H.A. (2002). A new beat for BLS and ACLS guidelines. *Nursing Management, 33*(2), 31-38; Ophie, L.H., & Marcus, F.I. (2001). Antiarrhythmic drugs. In L.H. Ophie (Ed.), *Drugs for the heart* (5th ed.). Philadelphia: Saunders; and Miller, J.M., & Zipes, D.P. (2001). Management of the patient with cardiac arrhythmias. In E. Braunwald (Ed.), *Heart disease* (6th ed.). Philadelphia: Saunders.

increased oxygen demand. Apply oxygen with nasal prongs to supplement serum levels. Hypoxia can lead to further myocardial ischemia and dysrhythmias.

If life-threatening dysrhythmias develop, many nurses are trained to use defibrillation for the client. Other emergency interventions include CPR, various medications, and preparation of the client for a transcutaneous or permanent pacemaker (see the Bridge to Critical Care feature on Defibrillation on p. 1466).

Diagnosis: Anxiety. The risk of death from sudden onset of life-threatening dysrhythmias, fear of the unknown, or fear of defibrillation weighs heavily on most clients.

Outcomes. The client will experience a reduced level of anxiety as evidenced by (1) reporting less anxiety or fewer feelings of helplessness or hopelessness, (2) an increased ability to sleep and rest, (3) a return of the heart rate to baseline level, and (4) a reduction of dyspnea.

BRIDGE TO CRITICAL CARE

Defibrillation

When a client is in ventricular fibrillation or pulseless ventricular tachycardia, the nurse must be able to safely and effectively use an automatic external defibrillator (AED) or conventional (manual) defibrillator (monophasic or biphasic).

GUIDELINES FOR USE OF AN AUTOMATIC EXTERNAL DEFIBRILLATOR (AED)

1. Turn the power on the AED device.
2. Attach cables to the adhesive defibrillator pads.
3. Peel paper from pads and attach pads to the client's chest at the upper right sternal border and the cardiac apex.
4. Place the AED in analyze mode.
5. Announce loudly, "Analyzing rhythm, stand clear!"
6. If VF/VT is present, the AED will charge to the appropriate joules and signal that a shock is indicated.
7. Announce, "Shock is indicated, stand clear!"
8. Confirm that no one is touching the client.
9. Press the shock button when indicated.
10. Repeat the analyze and shock steps until VF/VT is no longer present. The device will signal "No shock indicated."
11. For each set of three shocks, provide 1 minute of CPR.

GUIDELINES FOR THE USE OF CONVENTIONAL DEFIBRILLATORS (MONOPHASIC AND BIPHASIC)

1. Turn on the defibrillator.
2. Select energy level at 200 J for monophasic defibrillation.
3. Set the lead switch to paddles.
4. Apply gel on the paddles or use conductor pads, and place on the client's chest (at second right intercostal space and at the anterior axillary line in fifth left intercostal space).
5. Look at the monitor display, and assess the cardiac rhythm. If VF/VT is present, proceed to the next step.
6. Press the charge button on the apex paddle (the right hand).
7. When the defibrillator is fully charged, state loudly, "Shocking on three, all clear!"
8. Chant "Shocking on three. One, I'm clear. Two, you're clear. Three, all clear!"
9. Apply 25 pounds of pressure with both paddles, and press the discharge button on both paddles simultaneously.
10. Look at the monitor display. If VF/VT is still present, immediately recharge the defibrillator.
11. Shock at 200 to 300 J, then at 360 J. Always remember to make sure the client's surroundings are clear, repeating the chant and assessing for safety each time before shocking.

From Cummings, R. (2001). *ACLS provider manual.* Dallas, Tex: American Heart Association.

Interventions. Identify the client's anxiety and assist the client in discussing sources of fear. Clarify misconceptions. Commonly the client or a member of the family has had a heart condition, and the client's ability to cope may be directly influenced by that experience.

Explain the equipment present in the room. Most rooms are stocked with several types of equipment, and its presence does not always indicate the severity of the client's condition. Remain with the client, and tell the client and family what is happening now and what will be happening (e.g., blood will be drawn soon, an ECG will be obtained).

Finally, explore the usual coping methods with the client. Positive coping methods are usually supported; discuss maladaptive coping mechanisms, and suggest substitutions. For example, smoking may be a common coping mechanism, but it is not permitted in hospitals. Therefore if smoking is the client's coping mechanism when stressed, a substitute would need to be found, such as nicotine patches or chewing gum. Be aware that these patches can lead to chest pain because of vasoconstriction from the nicotine. Adjust the dose of the patch appropriately, beginning with the lowest levels.

Ventricular Tachycardia

Ventricular tachycardia is a life-threatening dysrhythmia that occurs when an irritable ectopic focus in the ventricles takes over as the pacemaker. It occurs in the presence of significant cardiac disease, such as in clients with CAD,

cardiomyopathy, mitral valve prolapse, heart failure, acute MI with hypoxia and acidosis, and digitalis toxicity.[13]

Ventricular tachycardia is characterized by a rapidly occurring series of PVCs (three or more) with no normal beats in between (Figure 57-7, *E*). P waves are absent, and the P-R interval is absent. The QRS complex is wide (greater than 0.12 second) and bizarre. The ventricular rate ranges between 70 and 250 beats/min, usually 130 to 170 beats/min. The ventricular rhythm is slightly irregular. VT produces a very low cardiac output that can quickly lead to cerebral and myocardial ischemia. At any time, VT can develop into ventricular fibrillation. Clients with VT commonly express feelings of impending death.[3,6]

Ventricular tachycardia can be described as monomorphic or polymorphic. Monomorphic VT originates from one focal site in the ventricle, producing VT that has a similar contour throughout the run. Polymorphic VT, on the other hand, results from discharges from multiple foci in the ventricle, producing differing contours throughout the run (Figure 57-7, *E*). Polymorphic VT usually occurs because of a prolonged Q-T interval (similar to torsades de pointes discussed later in this section) or as a result of underlying cardiac ischemia.[3]

Management

Manifestations of VT depend on underlying structural cardiac disease, the ventricular rate, and the duration of the VT. Sustained but hemodynamically stable VT is initially treated with antidysrhythmics (i.e., lidocaine, procainamide, or amiodarone). If the dysrhythmia does not respond to antidysrhythmics, cardioversion may be required for conversion to sinus rhythm (see earlier discussion). When the client is in VT and unconscious, defibrillation is indicated. Striking the client's sternum, called a precordial thump or thumpversion, may interrupt the dysrhythmia. The physician may also order IV antidysrhythmic agents, usually lidocaine or amiodarone. Another drug gaining favor is magnesium sulfate, particularly if the client has low magnesium levels.[3,5,9] The goal of long-term therapy includes class IC antidysrhythmics or implantation of an automatic internal cardiodefibrillator by an electrophysiologist.

Differentiating VT from SVT
It can be difficult to differentiate VT from SVT when ventricular rates are rapid and the QRS complex is not wide. Some clues to help distinguish SVT follow: (1) onset of dysrhythmia included a premature P wave, (2) slowing of the ventricular rate or termination of the dysrhythmia by vagal stimulation, (3) a very short R to P interval (less than 100 milliseconds or 0.1 second), (4) a QRS configuration similar to previously documented supraventricular ectopy, and (5) a noted P wave or notch before every QRS complex signaling that ventricular activation is linked to atrial activity.[3]

Torsades de Pointes
Torsades de pointes is a form of VT in which the QRS complexes appear to be constantly changing or twisting around an isoelectric line. Delayed repolarization of the ventricle is revealed as a prolonged Q-T interval and a broad flat T wave in the preceding sinus rhythm. The rhythm is regular or irregular with a ventricular rate of 150 to 250 beats/min (Figure 57-8, *A*). The QRS complex is wide and bizarre.[3,6]

Torsades de pointes is usually a result of drug toxicity (procainamide, quinidine, disopyramide) or electrolyte imbalances (hypokalemia or hypomagnesemia), which can lengthen the Q-T interval (see the Genetic Links feature on Long Q-T Syndrome, p. 1468). Clinical manifestations begin with palpitations and syncope. This rhythm often precedes ventricular fibrillation and sudden death.[13]

Management
Torsades de pointes is treated only if the Q-T interval is prolonged. Intravenous magnesium is the initial treatment of choice, along with intravenous potassium if indicated, followed by temporary ventricular or atrial pacing. Discontinuation of offending agents is also crucial.[3,6,9]

REENTRY OF IMPULSES
Two rhythms occur in the ventricles as a result of the reentry phenomenon: ventricular fibrillation and preexcitation syndromes. The usual pathway through the ventricles is not used and the wave of depolarization must spread from cell to cell. As a result the complex is wide and prolonged.

Ventricular Fibrillation
Ventricular fibrillation (VF) is a life-threatening dysrhythmia characterized by extremely rapid, erratic impulse formation and conduction (Figure 57-8, *B*). Ventricular fibrillation (VF) leads to inadequate myocardial contractions. The heart consequently immediately loses its ability to function as a pump. As the initial reentry pattern of excitation breaks up into multiple smaller wavelets, the level of disorganization increases. Sudden loss of cardiac output with subsequent tissue hypoperfusion creates global tissue ischemia; brain and myocardium are most susceptible. VF is the primary cause of sudden cardiac death (SCD).

This lethal dysrhythmia usually results from severe myocardial damage (such as MI), hypothermia, R-on-T phenomenon, hypoxia, contact with high-voltage electricity,

■ **FIGURE 57–8 A,** Torsades de pointes. **B,** Coarse ventricular fibrillation. **C,** Ventricular asystole in a dying heart. (**B** from Phillips, R.E., Feeney, M.K. [1990]. *The cardiac rhythms: A systematic approach to interpretation* [3rd ed., p. 393]. Philadelphia: Saunders.)

GENETIC LINKS

Long Q-T Syndrome*

DESCRIPTION

Long Q-T syndrome (LQT) produces episodic tachydysrhythmias including *torsades de pointes* (TdP), which may eventually lead to ventricular fibrillation. The most common manifestation of LQT is syncope typically occurring without warning. Undetected or untreated ventricular fibrillation may result in premature sudden death.

GENETICS

LQT is inherited in an autosomal-dominant pattern of inheritance with most individuals (90%) inheriting the gene from an affected parent. Offspring of an affected parent have a 50% chance of inheriting the disease-causing mutation. LQT is caused by mutations in one of five known genes associated with this disorder: *KCNQ1, KCNH2, SCN5A, KCNE1,*

and *KCNE2.* A family history of syncope, sudden death, or successful reversal of cardiac arrest may be suspicious of LQT syndrome.

DIAGNOSIS/GENETIC TESTING

LQT syndrome produces a prolongation of the Q-T interval and T-wave abnormalities, which can be determined clinically by electrocardiography. Clinical molecular genetic testing of the five genes associated with LQT may also make the diagnosis of LQT. About 30% of clinically affected families do not have a detectable mutation in one of these five genes. It is thought that one or more genes not yet identified may be responsible.

MANAGEMENT

Most affected individuals live normal lifestyles. Management is focused on client education, avoidance of triggering events, administration of beta-blockers, insertion of pacemakers, and ready availability of external defibrillators.

*Also known as Romano-Ward syndrome (RWS).

---

electrolyte imbalance, antidysrhythmic drug side effect, or toxicity from quinidine, procainamide, or digitalis.[13]

The ECG tracing displays bizarre fibrillatory wave patterns, and it is impossible to identify P waves, QRS complexes, or T waves (Figure 57-9, *A*). VF may be either coarse or fine with ventricular rates between 150 and 300 beats/min. Untreated, the deflections become smaller, and eventually all ventricular activity ceases. Death results within minutes without immediate intervention (i.e., CPR, defibrillation, and medications).[3,6]

Management

When VF appears, the clinician must immediately initiate CPR until the defibrillator is engaged. Defibrillate up to three times if needed. Defibrillation can be performed by nurses who have advanced training (see Defibrillation). A standard monophasic pattern of energy and current can be used. Defibrillation begins with 200 joules (J); if not successful, it is advanced to 300 J, and then to 360 J. With persistent VF, epinephrine is given and the clinician defibrillates at 360 J. Most defibrillators now are biphasic and each manufacturer has it's own recommendations, but the energy used is significantly less than with an old monophasic defibrillator. Other medications are alternated with defibrillation (lidocaine, magnesium sulfate, sodium bicarbonate), depending on the client's cardiac rhythm and electrolyte and acid-base balance.[3,5,6]

Pre-Excitation Syndromes

Accessory connections between the atrium and ventricle are the result of anomalous embryonic development of myocardial tissue bridging the fibrous tissues that separate the two chambers. This tissue allows for electrical conduction between the atria and ventricles at sites other than the atrioventricular node (AVN). Passage through this accessory pathway circumvents the usual conduction delay between the atria and ventricles, which normally occurs at the AVN and predisposes the client to develop tachydysrhythmias. Although dozens of locations for bypass tracts can exist in pre-excitation, including atriofascicular, fasciculoventricular, intranodal, or nodoventricular, the

A

B

■ **FIGURE 57–9 A,** Anterolateral paddle placement for external countershock. External paddles are placed at the second right intercostal space and at the anterior axillary line in the fifth left intercostal space. **B,** Ventricular fibrillation converted to normal sinus rhythm.

most common bypass tract is an accessory atrioventricular (AV) pathway otherwise known as a Kent bundle. This is the anomaly seen in *Wolff-Parkinson-White syndrome* (WPW).

Three basic ECG abnormalities are seen as a result of pre-excitation syndromes: (1) a P-R interval less than 120 milliseconds during sinus rhythm; (2) a QRS complex duration exceeding 120 milliseconds with a slurred, slowly rising QRS complex (delta wave) with the remainder of the QRS complex being normal; (3) secondary ST segment and T-wave changes that are usually directed in the opposite direction of the delta wave and QRS complex vectors.[3] Of the several types of disorders in this category, *Wolff-Parkinson-White syndrome* (WPW) appears most frequently. In clients with WPW, attacks of very rapid supraventricular dysrhythmias suddenly develop. Most adults with WPW have normal hearts, but if the tachydysrhythmias occur persistently, myocardial fatigue and ventricular failure may result.

Management

Clients with WPW do not require intervention unless they experience recurring tachydysrhythmias. In this instance, the physician may elect to use vagotonic maneuvers; cardioversion, adenosine, propranolol, amiodarone, and sotalol can affect both the AV node and the accessory pathway. The use of lidocaine or verapamil can increase the ventricular rate and can precipitate ventricular fibrillation. Electrophysiologic evaluation is recommended for appropriate drug therapy and possible accessory pathway radiofrequency ablation (an interventional procedure that destroys the accessory pathway).[3,6]

DISTURBANCES IN CONDUCTION

VENTRICULAR ASYSTOLE

Ventricular asystole (cardiac standstill) represents the total absence of ventricular electrical activity (Figure 57-8, *C*). The client has no palpable pulse (no cardiac output), and a rhythm is absent if the client is monitored. The occurrence of sudden ventricular asystole in a conscious person results in dizziness followed within seconds by loss of consciousness, seizures, and apnea. If the dysrhythmia remains untreated, death ensues. Ventricular asystole must be treated immediately.[3,6]

Cardiac standstill can occur as a primary event, or it may follow VF or pulseless electrical activity. Asystole can occur also in clients with complete heart block (CHB) in whom there is no escape pacemaker. Possible causes include the following:

- Hypoxia
- Hyperkalemia and hypokalemia
- Pre-existing acidosis
- Drug overdose
- Hypothermia

Management

The treatment of choice consists of CPR, epinephrine, atropine, transcutaneous pacing, and correction of the cause.[3,5,6]

PULSELESS ELECTRICAL ACTIVITY

Pulseless electrical activity (PEA), formerly called electromechanical dissociation (EMD), represents the presence of electrical activity in the heart, as seen on the monitor; however, a pulse cannot be detected by palpation of any artery. Thus the ventricles fail to produce an effective contraction despite continued electrical activity. Common causes include end-stage cardiac disease, cardiac tamponade, massive pulmonary embolus, tension pneumothorax, severe hypovolemia, prolonged cardiac resuscitation, exsanguination, or acute malfunction of a prosthetic valve.[3]

Management

Rapid searching for the cause is imperative. Until the cause is located, CPR is initiated in conjunction with advanced cardiac life support measures.

SUDDEN CARDIAC DEATH

Sudden cardiac death is defined as death resulting from an abrupt loss of heart function (cardiac arrest). The victim may or may not have known heart disease. The time and mode of death are unexpected, and death occurs within minutes after the manifestations appear. More than 163,000 deaths occur annually because of sudden cardiac death, with an annual incidence of 0.55 per 1000.[1]

OUTCOME MANAGEMENT OF LIFE-THREATENING DYSRHYTHMIAS

Medical Management

The goal of management is to stop the dysrhythmia immediately and to restore normal sinus rhythm. Remember, because there is inadequate or no perfusion of blood during these dysrhythmias, CPR with advanced cardiac life support measures are performed. Finally, the cause of the dysrhythmia is identified and treated.

Life-threatening dysrhythmias can often be effectively controlled by defibrillation. The most crucial element for survival after cardiac arrest is the time interval from collapse to care, especially defibrillation. With each passing minute, the chances of survival decline as much as 10%.

Electrical intervention can (1) abruptly stop the heart's erratic electrical discharge or (2) restore the flow of electrical current where there is none. Methods of electrical therapy include defibrillation and cardioversion.[3,6]

Defibrillation

The use of defibrillation delivers an electrical biphasic current (shock) of preset voltage to the heart through paddles or special patches placed on the chest wall (closed chest procedure). This current causes the entire myocardium to depolarize completely at the moment of shock, thus producing transient asystole and allowing the heart's intrinsic pacemaker to regain control. The amount of energy required to produce this effect is determined largely by the client's *transthoracic impedance,* or resistance to current flow. Because of this factor, the amount of energy that reaches the heart is less than the amount that the defibrillator is charged to deliver.[10]

The procedure is associated with potential hazards, particularly myocardial damage. The higher the amount of energy or frequency of the shocks, the greater the risk of injury. Advances in the equipment now allow measurement of transthoracic impedance. Once impedance is determined, the defibrillator automatically selects the amount of biphasic current needed that can restore rhythm and cardiac output. It is expected this mode of defibrillation will reduce the risk of complications.[3,6]

The degree of transthoracic resistance depends on several variables:

1. *Energy level.* The higher the energy level that is selected, the more current will follow.
2. *Number and frequency of shocks.* The more shocks administered and the shorter the time between them, the lower the transthoracic resistance.
3. *Ventilation phase.* Resistance is lower when shocks are delivered during exhalation, when there is less air (and therefore smaller diameter) in the lungs.
4. *Paddle or patch size.* The larger the paddle, the lower the resistance.
5. *Chest size.* The smaller the distance between the defibrillator electrodes once they are in place, the lower the resistance.
6. *Paddle-skin or patch-skin interface material.* Conductive material between the skin and paddles/patches reduces transthoracic impedance.
7. *Paddle or patch pressure.* Applying firm pressure increases contact between the skin and the paddles/patches, helping to overcome transthoracic resistance. Exert about 25 pounds of pressure on each paddle.
8. *Paddle or patch placement.* Place one paddle on the upper chest, to the right of the sternum; place the other paddle on the lower left chest, to the left of the nipple, with the center of the paddle in the midaxillary line. If patches are used, they can be placed in a similar fashion or in an anterior-posterior fashion.

If the client has a permanent pacemaker or an internal cardiac defibrillator, place the paddles or patches at least 5 inches away from the generator to avoid damaging it. If a temporary pacing system is in use, disconnect the pacing lead from the pulse generator immediately before defibrillation and reconnect it after the shock.[4,10]

Most defibrillators can be used to perform either *synchronized* cardioversion or *unsynchronized* cardioversion (commonly called *defibrillation*). Defibrillation (unsynchronized) is always indicated in VF and is also used in VT when the client is unconscious and pulseless. Specially trained nurses, emergency medical technicians, and physicians perform this procedure in acute settings.[3]

Care Before Defibrillation

Immediately before defibrillation, assess the client's responsiveness and do the following: SAFETY ALERT

1. **If the client is not responsive, call for immediate assistance (or activate the EMS system).**
2. **Call for the defibrillator and crash cart.**
3. **Assess the client's airway, breathing, and circulation (ABCs). Open the airway. Look, listen, and feel.**
4. **If the client is not breathing, give two slow breaths.**
5. **Assess the client's circulation; if no pulse is present, start CPR.**
6. **Perform CPR until the defibrillator is in place.**
7. **Check the ECG to verify the presence of VF or pulseless VT; confirm in two leads.**
8. **Check leads for any loose connections.**
9. **Remove any nitroglycerin patch.**

On confirmation of the emergency, the code is announced overhead so that the physician and ancillary and support staff can be present to assist with advanced cardiac life support measures. Continue CPR measures and ensure that intravenous access is available. Once the physician arrives, he/she will take charge of the situation and guide further management.

Care During Defibrillation. When VF develops, clinicians must attempt defibrillation at the earliest opportunity. The paddles are lubricated with electrode gel or conducting pads to enhance conduction and prevent burning of the skin. The gel should not extend beyond the paddles, and the paddles must lie flat against the body to avoid current arching or burns. The clinician places the paddles firmly against the chest. A transverse (anterolateral) position for paddle placement is used. One paddle is placed at the second intercostal space, at the right of the sternum, and the other paddle is positioned at the fifth intercostal space on the anterior axillary line (see Figure 57-9, *A*).

To ensure safe defibrillation, people who perform defibrillation must always announce when they are about to shock. The phrase "One. I'm clear. Two. You're clear. Three. All clear" is recommended. Because electricity is SAFETY ALERT

carried along metal devices and the client, all personnel, including the clinician administering the shock, must stand back from the bed. Open chest defibrillation occurs when electrical current is applied directly to the heart.

Care After Defibrillation. The clinician immediately assesses the ECG and pulse after defibrillation. If the first countershock is unsuccessful, immediate defibrillation must be performed again at a higher energy level (300 and 360 J). Monophasic defibrillation may be applied up to three times (200, 300, 360 J) if needed for persistent VF or pulseless VT. Defibrillators are frequently equipped with paddles that can monitor the ECG, even immediately after defibrillation. Therefore if the paddles are left in place after the shock has been delivered, the cardiac response can be quickly evaluated.

If the three defibrillations have not been successful, CPR should be continued. A successful response is indicated by cessation of fibrillation, restoration of sinus rhythm, and palpation of a regular pulse (see Figure 57-9, *B*). After successful defibrillation, continuous ECG monitoring is required. The client's vital signs and neurologic status must also be continuously assessed.

For clients with a pacemaker or an automatic implantable cardioverter-defibrillator (AICD), a programmer-analyzer should be available to examine the system for damage and erroneous reprogramming after defibrillation. Continue to monitor for pacemaker or AICD malfunction for at least the next 24 hours.

In documenting the outcome of defibrillation, record the following points:

- Preprocedure rhythm
- Times and voltage of shocks delivered
- Post-defibrillation rhythm pattern
- Names, times of administration, and doses of administered medications
- Other hemodynamic data available before, during, and after defibrillation

Automated External Defibrillator. An automated external defibrillator (AED) delivers biphasic electrical shocks to a client after it "auto-analyzes" VT or VF through an internal microprocessor-based detection system that analyzes the rhythm for the characteristics of VF or VT. The device is attached to the client with adhesive sternal-apex pads on flexible cables, which allows "hands-free" defibrillation, a feature available with conventional defibrillation as well. When VF or VT is present, the AED "advises" the operator to deliver a shock. This device was a milestone development in the fight against sudden cardiac death, and was designed for use by non-medical personnel with little or no medical training.[3]

The most common cause of unconsciousness in an adult is VF. Defibrillation is the only effective treatment.

AEDs are present in emergency response units and have been placed in many public settings because of the ease in using them and their impact on sudden cardiac death.

🪔 Termination of Resuscitation

In general, if an organized rhythm and pulse have not returned, the advanced cardiac life support team leader can cease efforts to resuscitate clients from confirmed and persistent asystole when the client has received successful endotracheal intubation, successful IV access, suitable CPR and advanced cardiac life support measures, and all rhythm-appropriate medications. Always consider any pre-existing problems that may make the client less responsive to defibrillation (acidosis, hypokalemia, hyperkalemia, hypoxia, hypovolemia), and treat them appropriately. In many cases clients may have other, noncardiac, disorders that make resuscitation attempts futile.

The American Heart Association guidelines for emergency cardiac care do not state a specific time limit beyond which rescuers cannot have a successful resuscitation. Cardiac arrests in special situations such as hypothermia, electrocution, and drug overdose present exceptions to any rules. Special situations call for common sense and clinical judgment.[5]

Interventional Medical Management

Ablating Conduction Pathways

A variety of procedures can be used to treat dysrhythmias when medications are not successful in bringing about conversion of the abnormal rhythm to a normal rhythm. Interventions include (1) chemical and mechanical ablation and (2) radiofrequency ablation of the abnormal pathway. These procedures involve risk to normal conduction tissue, and a pacemaker may be needed either temporarily or permanently.[3]

Chemical Ablation. Alcohol or phenol is inserted into involved areas of the myocardium through an angioplasty catheter leading to myocardial necrosis. Recurrences of tachycardia after successful chemical ablation are common. Chemical ablation is used only when other ablative approaches have failed and no other options are available. Postprocedural care is the same as that for angioplasty, with the exception of expected cardiac enzyme elevation following chemical ablation.[3]

Mechanical Ablation. The abnormal pathway is surgically removed or treated with a cryoprobe to interrupt its effect on heart rhythms. SVT, atrial fibrillation, atrial flutter, and WPW syndrome may be treated with this method when the client does not respond to medication. Before the procedure the myocardium is mapped to determine whether other forms of surgery (e.g., coronary bypass grafting, valve replacement) might correct the dysrhythmia. Mapping also isolates the area to be treated. The procedure may be performed through open-heart or closed-heart methods.[3] Postprocedure care and recovery are similar to those following cardiac catheterization.

Radiofrequency Ablation. Radiofrequency catheter ablation (RFA) is used primarily for SVT associated with WPW or AV nodal reentry, although it has also been used successfully to treat refractory VT. A steerable pacing catheter directs low-power, high-frequency current to a localized accessory pathway and necroses a small portion of myocardium along that pathway. When radiofrequency current is applied, the temperature of the contact tissue rises, water is driven out, and coagulation necrosis results. The amount of tissue injury depends on the amount of energy delivered (5 to 50 W), the length of time it is delivered (10 to 90 seconds), and the resistance at the end of the catheter. RFA produces lesions that are smaller and more controllable than DC catheter ablation lesions.[3]

The major advantage of RFA is the high rate of success, especially with SVT, and low morbidity. RFA can be more successful with AV node reentry or AV reentry tachycardia than conventional drug therapies.

Although RFA is a relatively safe procedure, the following complications can occur:

- Cardiac tamponade (1%)
- Deep vein thrombosis (1%)
- Trauma to vessel (1%)
- Transient ischemic attack or stroke (0.5%)
- Perforation of AV leaflet (extremely rare)
- Hematoma at introducer site (common)
- Unintentional AV block requiring pacemaker implantation (up to 10%)

Postprocedure nursing care and recovery are similar to those following cardiac catheterization. Specific nursing responsibilities include (1) preprocedure education of client and family, (2) interventions to reduce anxiety before and during the RFA procedure, (3) monitoring of vital signs and lower-extremity perfusion during and after the procedure, and (4) discharge instructions. Clients are usually discharged within 24 hours after RFA and are instructed to resume normal activities gradually but to avoid strenuous activities for 7 to 10 days. ECGs are obtained routinely at 1, 3, 6, and 9 months after RFA.[3]

Surgical Management

Clients with persistent heart rhythm problems may benefit from implanted devices to control their rhythm to control abnormal impulses or generate an impulse.

Controlling Impulses

Automatic Implantable Cardioverter-Defibrillator

Abnormal impulses can be controlled with an implanted device to cardiovert or defibrillate the heart. Before the development of the automatic implantable cardioverter-defibrillator (AICD), antidysrhythmic drugs were the standard of treatment for recurrent VT and VF; however, these drugs had dangerous side effects including a propensity to cause dysrhythmias. Antidysrhythmic drug therapy is now primarily used for clients with a low risk of sudden cardiac death or for clients with supraventricular dysrhythmias, while AICDs are the standard of treatment for clients at high risk for sudden cardiac death. Therefore the primary purpose of the AICD is detection and termination of VT and VF. The MADIT II trial outlines inclusion criteria for clients needing AICD implantation, including (1) post-myocardial infarction, (2) ejection fraction of equal to or less than 30%, (3) greater than 10 PVCs per hour.[11]

The AICD consists of a pulse generator and leads (Figure 57-10). The generator consists of electronic circuits that monitor the cardiac rhythm, analyze

FIGURE 57-10 A, An automatic implanted cardioverter-defibrillator (ICD) from Medtronic. **B,** The device can be implanted in the upper chest or in the abdomen. It detects dysrhythmias and delivers an electrical shock to the heart muscle.

dysrhythmias, and begin appropriate treatment; a capacitor that charges and discharges; batteries; and information storage so that the device can be interrogated and its history obtained. The device also has a "back-up" pacemaker as postshock bradycardia is common. Compared with external defibrillation, this implanted system does not require as much energy because less energy is lost when the impulse is applied directly to the heart. Interrogation of the AICD provides information regarding manufacturer, model, settings, recorded events, battery life, and lead parameters.[3]

The AICD is usually implanted surgically into a pouch below the left clavicle (similar to implantation of a permanent pacemaker) for two types of conditions.[3,11]

1. Survival of one or more episodes of sudden cardiac death resulting from VT or VF
2. Recurrent, refractory, life-threatening ventricular dysrhythmias that can develop into VT or VF, or both, despite antidysrhythmic therapy

Clients who require AICDs have a great deal of anxiety. Anxiety can develop from past episodes of near death as well as from feelings of not ever being able to die. Other clients may fear that the AICD will not be able to reverse the dysrhythmia. Be sensitive to these thoughts, and facilitate their discussion.[4,10]

Restoring Impulse Generation

Pacemakers

Pacemakers provide an artificial SA node and/or Purkinje system. A pacemaker is indicated if the conduction system fails to transmit impulses from the sinus node to the ventricles, to generate an impulse spontaneously, or to maintain primary control of the pacing function of the heart. Many conditions can affect the ability of the heart's conduction system to function normally, creating circumstances that warrant pacing (Box 57-3). Pacemakers can be *permanent* or *temporary*. Pacemakers can be used temporarily or prophylactically until the condition underlying the disturbance resolves. Pacemakers also can be used on a permanent basis if the client's condition persists despite adequate therapy.

BOX 57-3 **Conditions That May Necessitate a Pacemaker**
▪ Ablation
▪ Acute myocardial infarction
▪ Autonomic nervous system failure
▪ Cardiac surgery
▪ Drug toxicity (antidysrhythmics)
▪ Electrolyte imbalance
▪ Myocardial ischemia

Pacemaker Design. A pacemaker provides an external energy source for impulse formation and delivery. Whereas numerous pacemaker models are available, each with unique capabilities, every pacemaker consists of a pulse generator with circuitry, the lead(s), and the electrode system. *Single-chamber* pacemakers pace either the atria or the ventricles; *dual-chamber* pacemakers pace both the atria and the ventricles.

The pulse generator is essentially the pacemaker's power source. It houses the electronic circuitry responsible for sending out appropriately timed signals and for sensing the client's cardiac activity. The pulse generator can be external or internal. The external unit is designed for temporary pacing, primarily for support of transient dysrhythmias that impair cardiac output. The unit is the size of a small transistor radio and operates by dry-cell batteries (Figure 57-11). It has dials for the adjustment of power, rate of discharge, and mode. A pulse generator can also be permanently implanted. The surgeon places the permanent pulse generator into a small tunnel burrowed within the subcutaneous tissue below the right or left clavicle. The pulse generator is small (about the size of a vanilla wafer) and contains a sealed lithium battery. Pacemaker generators can be reprogrammed after insertion as

A

B

▪ **FIGURE 57-11** A permanent pacemaker. The pulse generator is placed under the pectoralis muscle (but above the breast). This is a dual-chamber pacemaker with leads in both the right atria and the ventricle.

needed. The output circuit controls the current pulse delivery rate, pulse duration, and refractory period. The sensing circuit is responsible for identifying and analyzing any spontaneous intrinsic electrical activity and responding appropriately.

The lead delivers the electrical impulse from the pulse generator to the myocardium. The lead(s) consist(s) of flexible conductive wires enclosed by insulating material. The electrode is the end of the lead that delivers the impulse directly to the myocardial wall. It is usually made of platinum-iridium, a highly conductive material that also deters the adherence of platelets. This system not only delivers electrical impulses but also relays information about spontaneous impulses back to the sensing circuit within the pulse generator.

Electrodes can be *unipolar* or *bipolar.* Unipolar designs incorporate the cardiac electrode as the negative terminal of the electrical circuit; the metallic shell or second wire of the impulse generator is the positive electrode. Bipolar systems use two wires, each ending in an electrode a short distance apart.

Pacemaker Methods. Impulses can be delivered to myocardial tissue by three major modes of artificial pacing: external, epicardial, and endocardial.

External (Transcutaneous) Pacing. The heart is stimulated externally through large, gelled electrode pads placed anteriorly and posteriorly and connected to an external transcutaneous pacemaker. Transcutaneous pacing is the treatment of choice in emergency cardiac care because it can be started quickly while a temporary transvenous pacemaker is being inserted or as prophylaxis against dysrhythmias. It is also the least invasive pacing technique. Because no vascular puncture is needed for electrode placement, transcutaneous pacing is preferred in clients who are receiving anticoagulation therapy or who might require thrombolytic therapy. However, many clients feel extreme discomfort with each paced beat; this is a significant limitation to transcutaneous pacing.

Because the anterior electrode is placed to the left of the sternum and centered close to the point of maximal impulse (PMI), excessive chest hair must be shaved to ensure good contact, or alternative pacing electrode positions must be used. The pacing device is usually activated at a rate of 70 beats/min. Electrical capture is characterized by widening of the QRS complex and broadening of the T wave.

Opioid analgesia and sedation may be given to clients who are conscious or who regain consciousness to reduce discomfort and anxiety. Additional complications of external transcutaneous pacing can include skin burns, muscle twitching, psychological reactions, failure to "capture" (inability of the impulse to initiate a contraction), and failure to "sense" (inability of the pacemaker to sense intrinsic electrical activity) (Table 57-3).

Epicardial (Transthoracic) Pacing. With this method of artificial pacing, the electrical energy travels through lead wires from an external pulse generator through the thoracic muscles directly to the epicardium. Epicardial pacing is most commonly used during and immediately after open-heart surgery because there is direct access to the epicardium at this time.

Some occasional complications include lead dislodgment, microshock, cardiac tamponade, infection, psychological reactions, failure to capture, and failure to sense.   SAFETY ⚠ ALERT

Endocardial (Transvenous) Pacing. Endocardial pacing is the most common mode of pacing the heart in emergency situations. The cardiologist inserts the pacing electrode via the transvenous route (the antecubital, femoral, jugular, or subclavian vein) and then threads the electrode into the right atrium or right ventricle so that it comes into direct contact with the endocardium (Figure 57-12). This procedure can be done at the bedside under fluoroscopic control or in a cardiovascular laboratory.

Major drawbacks include thrombophlebitis, infection at the insertion site, sepsis from nonsterile technique, increased chance of lead displacement as the client changes position, and the discomfort of having the extremity nearest the insertion site immobilized.   SAFETY ⚠ ALERT

Other additional complications occasionally seen are pacer-induced dysrhythmias, hiccups, abdominal twitching, myocardial irritability, perforation of chamber or septum, failure to capture, and failure to sense.

Temporary Pacing. Temporary pacing can be used in emergent or elective situations that require limited, short-term pacing (less than 1 week). The pulse generator is external. Temporary pacemakers are most commonly inserted transvenously, but they can be applied transcutaneously and can be inserted transthoracically.

Nursing Management

Although the principles of cardiac pacing are the same for temporary and permanent pacemakers, each type presents distinct issues for nurses to assess and to teach to the client and family. Clients with a temporary pacemaker need the following:

- An explanation about the pacemaker
- Monitoring for response to the pacemaker
- Maintenance of electrical safety
- Monitoring for pacing parameters (sensing, capturing, threshold)
- Protection against injury and infection

TABLE 57–3   Pacemaker Malfunctions and Nursing Interventions

Problem	Possible Cause	Nursing Interventions*
Failure to Pace Properly		
Intermittent or complete absence of pacing artifact	Battery failure A break or loose connection anywhere along system	Replace pulse generator. Replace battery unit.
Rapid, inappropriate firing of pacemaker (pacemaker-mediated tachycardia)	Pulse generator failure Circuitry failure "Oversensing" or "undersensing" by pacemaker	Check and tighten all connections between pulse generator and leads. Reduce or increase sensitivity threshold of pacemaker unit. Assess client's tolerance of pacemaker failure; have emergency drugs on hand; perform CPR[†] as indicated.
Failure to Capture		
Pacing artifact present but not followed by QRS complex or P wave	Increased pacing threshold; can be related to electrolyte imbalance, ischemia, drug toxicity, perforation, or excessive fibrosis of tissue at electrode site	Increase voltage by 1-2 mA (temporary pacemaker). Increase amplitude of pacemaker output/pulse width. Reposition client to either side in attempt to improve contact of electrode with endocardium; in temporary pacemaker, try moving arm if lead wire is inserted in antecubital area.
	Lead displacement caused by migration, or idle manipulation of pulse generator ("twiddler's syndrome")	Obtain chest film to determine pacemaker position. Have emergency drugs on hand; initiate CPR if necessary.
Failure to Sense		
Pacing artifact present despite presence of QRS complexes and P waves A competitive rhythm may develop	Sensitivity threshold set too low Intrinsic beats are of too-low voltage and go undetected by pacemaker's sensing mechanism	Increase sensitivity threshold on pulse generator. Reposition client. If client's intrinsic rhythm or rate is adequate, turn off pacemaker. Increase pacing rate to overdrive client's intrinsic heart rate.
	Dislodged or fractured lead Circuitry failure Electromagnetic interference	Give antidysrhythmics to decrease ectopy. Notify physician. Obtain chest x-ray to determine electrode placement.
Oversensing		
Results from inappropriate sensing of extraneous electrical signals or myopotentials (which should be ignored)	Sensitivity threshold set too high T wave sensing myopotentials Electromagnetic interference Two leads touching	Decrease sensitivity threshold. Correct conditions that produce large T waves.

*For all problems document malfunction by an electrocardiogram. If the pacemaker is programmable, have the reprogramming machine available. Monitor the client's tolerance to pacemaker malfunction (vital signs, chest pain).
[†]CPR, Cardiopulmonary resuscitation.
From Urden, L.D., Stacy, K.M., Lough, M.E. (Eds.), (2007) *Thelan's critical care nursing: Diagnosis and management* (4th ed.). St. Louis: Mosby.

Before the procedure, explain the purpose of the temporary pacemaker to the client and family. Ensure that a permit for the procedure has been signed and that all questions have been answered. Necessary equipment is gathered, and the external generator is checked (battery and sense and pace modes). Assess the client's vital signs and oxygen saturation; obtain a rhythm strip. Assess the need for sedation or analgesics, the client's level of anxiety, and the risk for bleeding.

During the procedure, monitor the client's ECG and vital signs continuously. Large P waves are seen as the catheter passes through the atrium, and larger QRS complexes are seen in the ventricles. Set and maintain the stimulus and sensitivity settings according to the physician's orders. Tape or suture the electrode at the insertion site.

After the procedure assess vital signs and peripheral pulses routinely along with emotional reactions to the procedure and pacing. Clients with temporary pacemakers must be placed on a cardiac monitor. Document the location and type of pacing lead. Note the pacing mode, stimulus threshold, sensitivity setting, pacing rate and intervals, and intrinsic rhythm. Pacing intervals are shown in Figure 57-13. Secure and check all

■ **FIGURE 57–13** Pacing intervals. The atrioventricular (A-V, delay) interval can be thought of as an artificial P-R interval. The programmed pacing rate, or *interval*, is also called the ventriculoventricular (V-V) interval. Ventricular pacing occurs if intrinsic ventricular activity does not occur within the V-V interval. (*From* Symbiotics series: Selecting the DDD patient [1984]. Minneapolis: Medtronic.)

■ **FIGURE 57–12** Transvenous temporary endocardial pacing is routine for most cardiac surgical procedures. This can be established by insertion of electrode wires through a vein (subclavian or internal jugular) and into the right atrium or right ventricle. Temporary pacing wires can also be advanced through pulmonary artery catheters.

PERMANENT PACING

Permanent pacing is indicated for chronic or recurrent dysrhythmias that are severe, unresponsive to antidysrhythmic medication, and caused by AV block or sinus node malfunction. The need for permanent pacemakers is confirmed through ECGs, Holter monitoring, and electrophysiology studies. Indications for permanent pacemakers have been grouped into three classes. Class I criteria are identified in Box 57-4.[8] 🪔

Clinical manifestations that are directly attributable to the slow heart rate include transient dizziness, lightheadedness, near syncope or frank syncope as manifestations of transient cerebral ischemia, and more generalized manifestations such as marked exercise intolerance or frank heart failure.[3,5,6]

Pacemaker Modes

There are two basic types of pacemakers:

1. *Fixed-rate* (non-demand or asynchronous). Fixed-rate pacemakers are designed to fire constantly at a preset rate without regard to the electrical activity of the client's heart. This mode of pacing is appropriate in the absence of any electrical activity (*asystole*) but is dangerous in the presence of an intrinsic rhythm because of the potential of the pacemaker to fire during the vulnerable period of repolarization and initiate lethal ventricular dysrhythmias.

2. *Demand* pacemakers contain a device that senses the heart's electrical activity and fires at a preset rate only when the heart's electrical activity drops below a predetermined rate (Figure 57-14).

In addition to a variety of capabilities, permanent pacemakers now have special programmable and antitachydysrhythmic functions that are quite complex. To communicate all the functions of the individual

connections. Monitor battery and control settings. Clean and dress the incision site according to protocols.

SAFETY ⚠ ALERT **Keep the generator dry and protect the controls from mishandling. The client must be protected from electrical microshocks and electromagnetic interference. Wear rubber gloves when exposed wires are handled. Check electrical equipment for adequate grounding.**

Limit the motion of the extremity at the insertion site. Stabilize the arm, catheter, and pacemaker to an arm board and avoid movement of the arm above shoulder level. Do not lift the client from under the arm. If the leg is the insertion site, limit its motion, especially hip flexion by limiting elevation of the head of the bed.

pacemakers, international codes were developed. Pacemakers are identified with a five-digit letter code. Although the last two letters contain pertinent information, commonly a pacemaker is referred to only by its first three letters (Box 57-5).

Pacemaker Function

Because there are many types of pacemakers with more than 250 programs, the general functions are discussed first. A simple demand pacing system works in the following manner. The cardiac cycle normally begins with the client's own beat. The pacemaker's sensor senses whether the intrinsic beat has occurred; if not, the pacer sends out an impulse to begin myocardial depolarization through a pulse generator. The impulse generator is said to "capture" the myocardium and thereby maintain heart rhythm.

ELECTRONIC PACEMAKER SPIKES

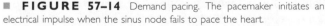

■ **FIGURE 57–14** Demand pacing. The pacemaker initiates an electrical impulse when the sinus node fails to pace the heart.

For a predetermined amount of time after the pacemaker impulse, the pacemaker cannot sense incoming signals. This feature prevents the pacer from sensing its own generated electrical current and from acting again. The *refractory period* is followed by the *noise-sampling period.* If any electromagnetic interference is sensed during this phase, the pacemaker goes into a fixed-rate mode of operation and remains in this mode until the source of interference is removed. At the end of the noise-sampling period, the *alert period* begins and the cycle starts again. If a PVC or PAC occurs during the alert period, the pacemaker can sense it and start its cycle again without emitting any impulse.

Electrocardiography of Paced Beats

In order to "turn on" a pacemaker and record its impulse generation and conduction, place a magnet over the pacemaker. The magnet disables the sensing mechanism, causing the pacemaker to fire at its programmed rate, regardless of the underlying cardiac rhythm.

Never place a magnet over an AICD as the magnet will suspend detection of VT and VF by the AICD, thus preventing the AICD from firing when VT or VF is present.   SAFETY   ALERT

The ECG appearance of a paced rhythm differs from that of a normal sinus rhythm. A pacing artifact is seen. With atrial pacing, a P wave follows the artifact but is hidden in some leads. Examination of leads II and V_1 is best for deciding whether a P wave follows a pacer spike. The QRS complex appears normal with atrial pacing; the impulse travels through the usual conduction system.[3]

The ECG with ventricular pacing shows an abnormal QRS complex because the impulse begins in the ventricle. With right ventricular endocardial pacing, a pseudo-LBBB wave is created on ECG. If the left ventricle is paced, a pseudo-RBBB is created.

Assess the ECG strip for pacer spikes followed by the expected appearance of a P wave or QRS complex. Spikes not followed by depolarization waves or paced beats that appear too early or too late may signal pacemaker failure.

Pacemaker Failure

Malfunctions can occur in the pacemaker's sensor or pulse generator. Complications associated with the components of the pacemaker system itself (see Table 57-3) may include the following:

1. *Failure to sense*—an inability of the sensor to detect the client's intrinsic beats; as a result, the pacemaker sends out impulses too early (Figure 57-15, *A*). The failure may be due to improper position of the catheter, tip or lead dislodgment, battery failure, the sensitivity being set too low, or a fractured wire in the catheter.

BOX 57-5   Classification System for Pacemakers

FIRST LETTER: CHAMBER PACED

Indicates which chamber(s) of the heart will be stimulated:

- V = Ventricle
- A = Atrium
- D = Dual-chamber (both atria and ventricles stimulated)

SECOND LETTER: CHAMBER SENSED

Indicates the chamber(s) of the heart in which the lead is capable of recognizing intrinsic electrical activity:

- V = Ventricle
- A = Atrium
- D = Dual-chamber (sensing capabilities in atria and ventricles)
- O = No sensing capability

THIRD LETTER: MODE OF RESPONSE

Indicates how the pacemaker will act based on the information it senses:

- T = Triggered (may have energy output triggered)
- I = Inhibited (pacing output inhibited by intrinsic activity)
- D = Dual-chamber (may be either inhibiting or triggering of both chambers)

FOURTH LETTER: PROGRAMMABLE FUNCTIONS

Indicates ability to change function once the pacemaker has been implanted:

- P = Programmable for one or two functions
- M = Multiprogrammable ability to change functions other than the rate or output

FIFTH LETTER: TACHYDYSRHYTHMIC FUNCTIONS

Indicates specific methods of interrupting tachydysrhythmias:

- B = Bursts of pacing
- N = Normal rate competition
- S = Scanning

EXAMPLES

Pacing Modes Within Single-Chamber Pacemakers

- *Atrial demand pacemaker (AAI).* A pacemaker that senses spontaneously occurring P waves and paces the atria when they do not appear.

- *Atrial fixed-rate pacemaker (AOO).* A pacemaker that paces the atria and does not sense.
- *Ventricular demand pacemaker (VVI).* A pacemaker that senses spontaneously occurring QRS complexes and paces the ventricles when they do not appear.
- *Ventricular fixed-rate pacemaker (VOO).* A pacemaker that paces the ventricles and does not sense.

Pacing Modes Within Dual-Chamber Pacemakers

- *Atrial synchronous ventricular pacemaker (VDD).* A pacemaker that senses spontaneously occurring P waves and QRS complexes and paces the ventricles when QRS complexes fail to appear after spontaneously occurring P waves, as in complete atrioventricular (AV) block. In this type of pacemaker, the pacing of ventricles is synchronized with the P waves so that the ventricular contractions follow the atrial contractions in a normal sequence. A major benefit is that it permits the heart rate to vary, and AV synchrony occurs, depending on the physiologic demands of the body. A built-in safety mechanism causes ventricular depolarizations to occur at a fixed rate should atrial rates become too fast.
- *AV synchronous pacemaker (VAT).* A pacemaker that has ventricular pacing, atrial sensing, and triggered response to sensing. The ventricular pacing stimulus will fire at a set time after sensing a spontaneous atrial depolarization.
- *AV sequential pacemaker (DVI).* A pacemaker that senses spontaneously occurring QRS complexes and paces both the atria and ventricles (the atria first, followed by the ventricles after a short delay) when QRS complexes do not appear.
- *AV sequential fixed-rate pacemaker (DOO).* A pacemaker that paces both the atria and ventricles but does not sense.
- *Optimal sequential pacemaker (DDD).* A pacemaker that senses spontaneously occurring P waves and QRS complexes and (1) paces the atria when P waves fail to appear, as in sick sinus syndrome; and (2) paces the ventricles when QRS complexes fail to appear after spontaneously occurring or paced P waves. In this type of pacemaker, like the VDD pacemaker, the pacing of ventricles is synchronized with the P waves so that the ventricular contractions follow the atrial contractions in a normal sequence.

---

2. *Failure to pace*—a malfunction of the pulse generator. The ECG shows an absence of any impulse (Figure 57-15, *B*). Component failure to discharge (pace) can be due to battery failure, lead dislodgment, fracture of the lead wire inside the catheter, disconnections between catheter and generator, or a sensing malfunction.

3. *Failure to capture*—a disorder in the pacemaker electrodes; the impulse does not generate depolarization (Figure 57-15, *C*). This complication can result from low voltage, battery failure, faulty connections between the pulse generator and catheter, improper position of the catheter, catheter wire fracture, fibrosis at the catheter tip, or a catheter fracture.

Clinical manifestations associated with pacemaker malfunctioning include syncope, bradycardia or tachycardia, and palpitations. When these manifestations occur, the malfunctioning leads or pacemaker must be replaced.

Teach the client and family how to care for the pacemaker and the precautions to follow (see the Client Education Guide feature on the Client with a Permanent Pacemaker, p. 1480).[12]

FAILURE TO SENSE

A   The pacemaker fails to recognize normal beats and generates an unnecessary pacemaker spike.

FAILURE TO PACE

B   The pacemaker fails to generate a pacemaker spike when needed.

FAILURE TO CAPTURE

C   The pacemaker generates a pacemaker spike but fails to produce a QRS.

FUSION BEAT

D

■ **FIGURE 57–15**   Pacemaker failures. **A,** Failure to sense. **B,** Failure to pace. **C,** Failure to capture. **D,** Fusion beat.

Nursing Management of Clients with Pacemakers

Assessment. Assess the client for *subjective* clinical manifestations of dysrhythmias and alterations in cardiac output: palpitations, syncope, fatigue, shortness of breath, chest pain, or skipped beats felt in the chest. The client may also feel anxiety about the heart disorder and may manifest nervousness, fear, sleeplessness, uncertainty, or hopelessness. *Objective* clinical manifestations may include diaphoresis, pallor or cyanosis, variations in radial and apical pulse rates such as bradycardia or tachycardia, rhythm changes, hypotension, crackles, and decreased mental acuity. The client may be fearful of being left alone. Monitoring is begun, and the heart rhythm is observed continuously by a nurse, a computer, and an ECG technician. Rhythm strips are examined at least every shift.

Explain the purpose of the pacemaker and the experience of having a pacemaker inserted to the client and family. Most permanent pacemakers are inserted transvenously. Try to keep the ECG leads off the possible insertion site. The insertion site is prepared according to hospital policy.

A preoperative ECG is obtained, and a patent IV line is maintained. Prophylactic antibiotics may be given.

After insertion, monitor vital signs and pacemaker function. Pain can usually be managed with oral analgesics if the transvenous approach has been used. Initially instruct the client to avoid excessive extension or abduction of the arm on the operative side. Perform passive range-of-motion exercises on the arm.

Obtain paced and nonpaced ECGs. A magnet can be placed over the pulse generator, converting it to a fixed-rate pacing mode, so that the client's intrinsic rhythm can be determined. The location of the pacemaker electrodes is determined by x-ray. The model and serial numbers of the pulse generator and leads, along with the date of implantation and programmed functions of the initial implant, are recorded.

Transtelephonic Pacemaker Monitoring. Special telephone monitoring of the client's pacemaker can be done on a routine outpatient basis. Telephone ECG systems are designed for follow-up monitoring of clients with pacemakers. Via finger tip, wrist, or ankle electrodes, the transmitter detects, amplifies, and converts a client's

CLIENT EDUCATION GUIDE

Client With a Permanent Pacemaker

WOUND CARE

1. Assess your wound daily, and keep the incision clean and dry until it heals.
2. Report any fever, redness, drainage, warmth, discoloration, or swelling to the physician.
3. Avoid constrictive clothing (e.g., tight brassiere straps), which puts excessive pressure on the wound and the pulse generator.
4. Avoid extensive "toying" with the pulse generator because this may cause pacemaker malfunction and local skin inflammation.

PACEMAKER MANAGEMENT

1. Measure your pulse rate as instructed by your physician in your wrist or on your neck. You will be taught how to do this before leaving the hospital.
2. Notify the physician if your pulse rate is slower than the set rate; also report sensations of feeling your heart "racing," beating irregularly, fatigue, or dizziness.
3. Avoid being near areas with high voltage, magnetic force fields, or radiation; this can cause pacemaker problems.
4. Avoid being near large running motors (gas or electric) and standing near high-tension wires, power plants, radio transmitters, large industrial magnets, and arc welding machines. Riding in a car is safe, but do not bring the pacemaker to within 6 to 12 inches of the distributor coil of a running engine.
5. You can continue to operate safely most appliances and tools that are properly grounded and in good repair, including microwave ovens, televisions, video recorders, AM and FM radios, electric blankets, lawn mowers, leaf blowers, and cars.
6. You can safely operate office and light industrial equipment that is properly grounded and in good repair, such as electric typewriters, copying machines, and personal computers.
7. An airport's metal detector can be triggered by the pacemaker's metal casing and the programming magnet. Mention your pacemaker to security guards. The metal detector itself does not harm the pacemaker.
8. At all times carry a pacemaker identity card (including programming information, pacemaker manufacturer, emergency phone numbers). Wear a medical alert bracelet.
9. Avoid activity that might damage the pulse generator, such as playing football or firing a rifle with the butt end against the affected shoulder.
10. Some stores sell antitheft devices that may affect pacemaker function. If you suddenly become dizzy, move away from the area and notify the store clerk about the pacemaker.
11. If radiation therapy has been prescribed to the area in which the pulse generator was implanted, the pulse generator must be relocated.
12. Do not lift more than 5 to 10 pounds (equivalent to a full grocery sack or a gallon of milk) for the first 6 weeks after surgery. Do not move your arms and shoulders vigorously for the first 6 weeks. Normal activities (including sexual activity) can be resumed in 6 weeks.
13. Discuss with the nurse the purpose, dose, schedule, and possible side effects of prescribed medications. Consult your written information sheets to reinforce learning.
14. Plan to see your physician to test your pacemaker. Your cardiologist periodically will reevaluate pacemaker function and can reprogram it if needed. You may also be able to check your pacemaker by telephone. If this is possible, you will receive instructions.

---

electrical activity and pacemaker artifacts to frequency-modulated audio tones for transmission, via the telephone, to an ECG receiver. From the transmitted signals, the ECG receiver provides an ECG strip recording and printout of the rate and pulse width of a client's implanted pacemaker.

Self-Care

It may be necessary to teach about the nature of the dysrhythmia several times because the client's attention span may be shorter than normal as a result of severe anxiety.

SAFETY ALERT

Before discharge, make certain that clients appreciate the importance of taking antidysrhythmic agents as prescribed. Include details about medication administration, dosage, and side effects in the discharge plan. If discharged too early and in an unstable condition, many clients risk further exacerbations or additional complications. Make sure that nursing discharge criteria are met and documented.

Clients who have experienced cardiac dysrhythmias while at a health care facility may be apprehensive about leaving the facility. Those who have experienced innocuous dysrhythmias may need only calm reassurance and an explanation of the cause of the disorder. Clients with recurring life-threatening dysrhythmias, such as VT, require comprehensive and specialized attention. These clients may have experienced frightening events in the course of their hospitalization.

When a client is at risk for development of a life-threatening dysrhythmia, ascertain whether the client's housemates and significant others know how to perform CPR. Refer them to community agencies that provide CPR training (e.g., the American Heart Association, the American Red Cross, local fire department, local hospital).

Sometimes clients with serious, chronic, or potential dysrhythmias use portable telemetry units for self-monitoring at home after discharge. This allows resumption of daily activities while providing continuous 24-hour surveillance of cardiac rhythm. Nurses are often responsible for instructing clients in the use of these units.

Ask the client to keep a diary of daily activities so that clinicians can correlate factors in the client's life that are contributing to the development of dysrhythmias.

Finally, instruct clients about the importance of regular medical follow-up. Advise them to keep regular appointments with their physician after discharge. Explain to the client and his or her significant others about how to obtain emergency medical attention if it becomes necessary.

Living under the constant threat of sudden death provokes anxiety, depression, and occasionally dependent behavior. In some cases psychological counseling can bolster coping resources. Recommend community and private counseling services for the client and the client's significant others.

CONCLUSIONS

Cardiac dysrhythmias can vary from benign to life-threatening, and the cardiac rhythm can change as quickly as a heartbeat and without warning. It is imperative to be aware of life-threatening dysrhythmias and immediate nursing interventions, including client assessment, CPR, and activation of colleagues or the EMS. Treatment methods may include temporary pacemaker insertion or application, permanent pacemaker implantation, a prescribed medical regimen, ablation therapy, or AICD implantation. Client education regarding taking medications as directed, reporting any manifestations or side effects, caring for the device wound, and following up with the cardiologist is necessary before discharge to complete client care regarding dysrhythmias.

THINKING CRITICALLY

1. You are walking with a client in the hospital. He is recovering from an MI. A dysrhythmia develops. What assessments should you perform? What care does the client need?

1 NOV 1400:20

9270-0980   MEDI-TRACE ®

Factors to Consider. What is the usual heart rhythm response to activity? How can you assess if your client is tolerating this rhythm? How should the client be returned to his room?

2. An 82-year-old woman is brought to the emergency department by her son after losing consciousness and hitting her head after falling. She is now awake and states that she has been having periods of dizziness and blackouts for the past few weeks. During your physical examination, you notice what appears to be a pacemaker device implanted under her left clavicle. What additional assessments should you make? What information should you obtain about the pacemaker?

Factors to Consider. What might have happened to the pacemaker during the fall? Could a faulty pacemaker be responsible for the loss of consciousness?

Discussions for these questions can be found on the website. **evolve**

BIBLIOGRAPHY

Citations appearing in red refer to primary research.

Citations appearing in blue refer to evidence-based practice guidelines and protocols.

1. American Heart Association. (2006). Heart disease and stroke statistics—2006 update: A report from the American Heart Association statistics committee and stroke statistics subcommittee. *Circulation, 113*(6), 85-151.
2. AHA scientific statement: Practice standards for electrocardiographic monitoring in hospital settings: An AHA scientific statement from disease in the young: Endorsed by the International Society of Computerized Electrocardiology and the American Association of Critical-Care Nurses. (2005). *Journal of Cardiovascular Nursing, 20*(2), 76-106.
3. Braunwald, E., Zipes, D.P., Libby, P., et al.. (2005). *Braunwald's heart disease: A textbook of cardiovascular medicine* (7th ed.). Philadelphia: Elsevier Saunders.
4. Conover, M.B. (2003). *Understanding electrocardiography* (8th ed.). St. Louis: Mosby.
5. Cummings, R. (2001). *ACLS provider manual.* Dallas, Tex: American Heart Association.
6. Fink, M.P., Abraham, E., Vincent, J., et al. (2005). *Textbook of critical care* (5th ed.). Philadelphia: Elsevier Saunders.
7. Greenberg, H., Case, R.B., Moss, A.J., et al. (2004). Analysis of mortality events in the Multicenter Automatic Defibrillator Implantation Trial (MADIT-II). *Journal of the American College of Cardiology, 43*, 1459-1465.
8. Gregoratos, G., Abrams, J., Epstein, A.E., et al. (2002). ACC/AHA/NASPE 2002 Guideline update for implantation of cardiac pacemakers and antiarrhythmia devices: Summary article: A report of the American College of Cardiology/American Heart Association task force on practice guidelines (ACC/AHA/NASPE Committee to update the 1998 pacemaker guidelines). *Circulation, 106*(16), 2145-2165.
9. Massie, B.M., & Amidon, T.A. (2004). Conduction disturbances. In L.M. Tierney, et al.. (Eds.), *Current medical diagnosis and treatment* (43rd ed.). Stamford, Conn: Appleton and Lange.
10. Massie, B.M., & Amidon, T.A. (2004). Disturbances in rate and rhythm. In L.M. Tierney, et al. (Eds.), *Current medical diagnosis and treatment* (43rd ed.). Stamford, Conn: Appleton and Lange.
11. McCabe, P.J. (2005). Spheres of clinical nurse specialist practice influence evidence-based care for patients with atrial fibrillation. *Clinical Nurse Specialist, 19*(6), 308-317.

12. Morton, P.G., Fontaine, D., Hudak, C., et al.. (2003). *Critical care nursing: A holistic approach* (8th ed.). Philadelphia: Lippincott Williams & Wilkins.

13. Shah, M., Akar, F.G., Tomaselli, G.F., et al. (2005). Molecular basis of arrhythmias. *Circulation, 12*(16), 2517-2529.

14. Surawicz, B. (2003). Brief history of cardiac arrhythmias since the end of the nineteenth century: Part 1. *Journal of Cardiovascular Electrophysiology, 14*, 1365-1371.

evolve *Did you remember to check out the bonus material on the Evolve website and the CD-ROM, including NCLEX®-Examination Style Review Questions, Open-Book Quizzes, and Chapter Review Audio Podcasts?*

http://evolve.elsevier.com/Black/medsurg

CHAPTER 58

Management of Clients with Myocardial Infarction

PATRICIA A. KERESZTES AND MARY WCISEL

The heart requires a balance between oxygen supply and oxygen demand in order to function properly. The integrity of the coronary arteries is an important determinant of oxygen supply to the heart muscle. Any disorder that reduces the lumen of one of the coronary arteries may cause a decrease in blood flow and oxygen delivery to the area of the myocardium supplied by that vessel and lead to acute coronary syndromes of angina, acute myocardial infarction (AMI), and sudden cardiac death.

Coronary heart disease (CHD) is the primary underlying cause of these syndromes and is the single largest killer of American men and women. The clinical syndromes associated with CHD are familiar to most Americans. Almost every day, the news media cover a story on a celebrity who has suffered from or was treated for chest pain, heart attack, or cardiac arrest. Turn on any television hospital drama and you will see someone seeking treatment for an episode of chest pain. Many of us also have had personal experience with CHD through the illness of a relative or close friend.

It is estimated that 1 million Americans will have a new or recurrent acute coronary syndrome this year. Acute coronary syndromes are responsible for more than 250,000 deaths annually and result from a progressive atherosclerotic process that culminates in rupture of atherosclerotic plaques and thrombus formation. This chapter reviews the risk factors, pathophysiology, clinical manifestations, and medical and nursing interventions for the acute coronary syndromes of angina pectoris (a type of chest pain) and AMI.

ANGINA PECTORIS

Angina pectoris is chest pain resulting from myocardial ischemia (inadequate blood supply to the myocardium). It is a common manifestation of CHD and affects about 6,400,000 Americans—2,400,000 men and 4,000,000 women. According to the Framingham Heart Study, approximately 400,000 new cases of angina occur each year. Angina can also occur in clients with normal coronary arteries, but it is less common. Clients with aortic stenosis, hypertension, and hypertrophic cardiomyopathy can also have angina pectoris.

Etiology and Risk Factors

Angina pectoris is associated with atherosclerotic lesions and is a manifestation of CHD (see Chapter 56). Angina can be caused either by chronic or acute blockage of a coronary artery or by coronary artery spasm. Chronic blockages are associated with fixed calcified (type Vb) or fibrotic (type Vc) atherosclerotic lesions that occlude more than 75% of the vessel lumen.

When fixed blockages are present in the coronary arteries, conditions that increase myocardial oxygen demand (e.g., physical exertion, emotion, exposure to cold) may precipitate episodes of angina. Because the severely stenosed arteries cannot dilate to deliver enough oxygen to meet the increased demand, ischemia results. In contrast, acute blockage of a coronary artery results from rupture or disruption of vulnerable atherosclerotic plaques that cause platelet aggregation and thrombus formation (see Etiology and Risk Factors under Acute Myocardial Infarction). Acute blockages are associated with unstable angina and AMI.

---

evolve **Web Enhancements**

Case Management Acute Myocardial Infarction

Case Study Cardiogenic Shock, Tachycardia, and Heart Failure

Concept Map Understanding Myocardial Infarction and Its Treatment

Tables Differential Diagnosis of Chest Pain

Be sure to check out the bonus material on the Evolve website and the CD-ROM, including free self-assessment exercises. **http://evolve.elsevier. com/Black/medsurg**

Primary prevention is through the lifelong commitment to reducing the risk factors of CHD (see Chapter 56). Secondary prevention is through recognition and early treatment of anginal attacks (see the Critical Monitoring feature below). Tertiary prevention consists of resolution of angina before myocardial damage occurs.

Pathophysiology

Three coronary arteries normally supply the myocardium with blood to meet its metabolic needs during varying workloads. The right coronary artery supplies arterial blood to the right side of the heart; the left coronary artery divides into the left circumflex artery, which feeds the posterior heart muscle, and the anterior descending artery, which supplies the anterior myocardium, especially the left ventricle. The coronary vessels are usually efficient and perfuse the myocardium during diastole. When the heart needs more blood, the vessels dilate. As the vessels become lined and eventually occluded with atherosclerotic plaques and thrombi, the vessels can no longer dilate properly.

If the coronary vessels slowly become occluded, collateral vessels develop to provide the myocardium with needed arterial blood. Collateral vessels are more common in clients with long-term coronary artery disease.

Myocardial ischemia develops if the blood supply through the coronary vessels or oxygen content of the blood is not adequate to meet metabolic demands. Disorders of the coronary vessels, the circulation, or the blood may lead to deficits in supply.

Disorders of the coronary vessels include atherosclerosis, arterial spasm, and coronary arteritis. Atherosclerosis increases resistance to flow. Arterial spasm also increases resistance. Coronary *arteritis* is inflammation of the coronary arteries caused by infection or autoimmune disease.

Disorders of circulation include hypotension and aortic stenosis and insufficiency. Hypotension may be a result of spinal anesthesia, potent antihypertensive drugs, blood loss, or other factors that result in decreased blood return to the heart. Aortic valve stenosis or insufficiency results in decreased filling pressure of the coronary arteries.

Blood disorders include anemia, hypoxemia, and polycythemia. Anemia and hypoxemia result in decreased oxygen flow to the myocardium. Polycythemia increases blood viscosity, which slows blood flow through the coronary arteries.

The opposite of supply is demand, and increased demands can be placed on the heart. Conditions that increase demands on the myocardium are those that increase cardiac output or increase myocardial need for oxygen (Box 58-1).

Myocardial ischemia occurs when either supply or demand is altered. In some people, the coronary arteries can supply adequate blood when the person is at rest;

CRITICAL MONITORING

Angina from Impending Myocardial Infarction

- Continuous, enduring, severe chest pain lasts more than 20 minutes.
- Pain is usually felt in the retrosternal area, possibly radiating to the arms (the pain is most common in the left shoulder and arm), back, neck, or lower jaw.
- Pain is described as squeezing, pressing, or a sensation of heaviness.
- Deep breathing or changing posture does not change the severity of the pain.
- Pain may occur in the upper abdomen, accompanied by nausea and vomiting.
- Pain is relieved by nitroglycerin; pain is not relieved by antacids or food.
- ECG often shows ischemic changes.
- Chest radiograph is normal for client.

BOX 58-1 Factors Influencing Myocardial Supply and Demand

FACTORS THAT DECREASE SUPPLY

Coronary Vessel Disorders

- Atherosclerosis
- Arterial spasm
- Coronary arteritis

Circulation Disorders

- Hypotension
- Aortic stenosis
- Aortic insufficiency

Blood Disorders

- Anemia
- Hypoxemia
- Polycythemia

FACTORS THAT INCREASE DEMAND

Increased Cardiac Output

- Exercise
- Emotion
- Digestion of a large meal
- Anemia
- Hyperthyroidism

Increased Myocardial Need for Oxygen

- Damaged myocardium
- Myocardial hypertrophy
- Aortic stenosis
- Aortic insufficiency
- Diastolic hypertension
- Thyrotoxicosis
- Strong emotions
- Heavy exertion

when the person attempts activity or is taxed in some other manner, however, angina develops. Myocardial cells become ischemic within 10 seconds of coronary artery occlusion. After several minutes of ischemia, the pumping function of the heart is reduced. The reduction in pumping deprives the ischemic cells of needed oxygen and glucose. The cells convert to anaerobic metabolism, which leaves lactic acid as a waste product. As lactic acid accumulates, pain develops. Angina pectoris is transient, lasting for only 3 to 5 minutes.[3,13] If blood flow is restored, no permanent myocardial damage occurs.

Clinical Manifestations
Characteristics of Angina
Angina is a clinical syndrome characterized by discomfort in the chest, jaw, shoulder, back, or arm. Angina pectoris produces transient paroxysmal attacks of substernal or precordial pain with the following characteristics:

- *Onset.* Angina can develop quickly or slowly. Some clients ignore the chest pain, thinking that it will go away or that it is indigestion. Ask what the client was doing when the pain began.
- *Location.* Nearly 90% of clients experience the pain as retrosternal or slightly to the left of the sternum.
- *Radiation.* The pain usually radiates to the left shoulder and upper arm and may then travel down the inner aspect of the left arm to the elbow, wrist, and fourth and fifth fingers. The pain may also radiate to the right shoulder, neck, jaw, or epigastric region. On occasion, the pain may be felt only in the area of radiation and not in the chest. Rarely is the pain localized to any one single small area over the precordium.
- *Duration.* Angina usually lasts less than 5 minutes. However, attacks precipitated by a heavy meal or extreme anger may last 15 to 20 minutes.
- *Sensation.* Clients describe the pain of angina as squeezing, burning, pressing, choking, aching, or bursting pressure. The client often says the pain feels like gas, heartburn, or indigestion. Clients do not describe anginal pain as sharp or knife-like.
- *Severity.* The pain of angina is usually mild or moderate in severity. It is often called "discomfort," not "pain." Rarely is the pain described as "severe."
- *Associated characteristics.* Other manifestations that may accompany the pain include dyspnea, pallor, sweating, faintness, palpitations, dizziness, and digestive disturbances.
- *Atypical presentation.* Women, older adults, and clients with diabetes may have atypical presentations of CHD that are equivalent to angina. In women, CHD may be manifested as epigastric pain, dyspnea, or back pain, whereas older adults frequently experience dyspnea, fatigue, or syncope.
- *Relieving and aggravating factors.* Angina is aggravated by continued activity, and most anginal attacks quickly subside with the administration of nitroglycerin and rest. The typical "exertion-pain, rest-relief" pattern is the major clue to the diagnosis of angina pectoris.
- *Treatment.* Treatments to reduce the demand on the heart, such as rest, or treatments that dilate the coronary arteries will commonly reduce the pain. The client may have used nitroglycerin and the client should be asked if the angina subsided.

An important aspect of assessing angina is to determine quickly and accurately if the pain is indeed angina. Other conditions also lead to chest pain, such as pulmonary embolism, pleurisy, and pneumonia (see the table on Differential Diagnosis of Chest Pain on the website).

SAFETY
ALERT
evolve

As vessels become lined with atherosclerotic plaques, plaques may be disrupted and thrombi may form, leading to clinical manifestations of inadequate blood supply in the tissues supplied by these vessels. Problems such as stroke, claudication, and angina develop. Stroke is described in Chapter 70 and claudication is discussed in Chapter 53.

Patterns of Angina
Classic angina pectoris can be subdivided into the following basic patterns:

- *Stable angina.* Stable angina is paroxysmal chest pain or discomfort triggered by a *predictable* degree of exertion (e.g., walking 20 feet) or emotion. Characteristically, a stable pattern of onset, duration, severity, and relieving factors is present. Normally, stable angina is relieved with rest or nitroglycerin, or both.
- *Unstable angina.* Unstable angina (preinfarction angina, crescendo angina, or intermittent coronary syndrome) is paroxysmal chest pain triggered by an *unpredictable* degree of exertion or emotion, which may occur at night. Unstable angina attacks characteristically increase in number, duration, and severity over time. If unstable angina occurs, it must be treated as a medical emergency with the client receiving immediate medical attention.
- *Variant angina.* Variant angina *(Prinzmetal's angina)* is chest discomfort similar to classic angina but of longer duration; it may occur while the client is at rest. These attacks tend to happen between midnight and 8 AM. Variant angina results from coronary artery spasm and may be associated with elevation of the ST segment on the electrocardiogram (ECG).
- *Nocturnal angina.* Nocturnal angina is possibly associated with rapid eye movement (REM) sleep during dreaming.
- *Angina decubitus.* Angina decubitus is paroxysmal chest pain that occurs when the client reclines and lessens when the client sits or stands up.

■ *Intractable angina.* Intractable angina is chronic incapacitating angina that is unresponsive to intervention.

■ *Postinfarction angina.* Pain occurs after MI, when residual ischemia may cause episodes of angina.

Diagnostic Tests

Initial laboratory testing and noninvasive testing of clients with suspected angina include resting ECG, chest radiography, hemoglobin, fasting glucose, and fasting lipid profile. Enzymes may be drawn for the more severe forms of angina in order to rule out myocardial infarction. Further testing is based on initial results of these and individual risk factors for CHD. The following modalities are described in Chapter 54.

Electrocardiography

The ECG tracings remain normal in more than 50% of clients with angina pectoris at rest. An ECG recorded in the presence of pain may document transient ischemic attacks with ST-segment elevation or depression. An ECG recorded during an episode of pain also suggests coronary artery involvement and the extent of cardiac muscle affected by the ischemic event.

Exercise Electrocardiography

During a *stress test,* the client exercises on a treadmill or stationary bicycle until reaching 85% of maximal heart rate. ECG or vital sign changes may indicate ischemia. Exercise electrocardiography is less sensitive in women and older adults.

Radioisotope Imaging

Various nuclear imaging techniques are used to evaluate myocardial muscle. Regions of poor perfusion or ischemia appear as areas of diminished or absent activity (cold spots).

Electron-Beam (Ultrafast) Computed Tomography (EBCT)

This noninvasive method enables detection of the amount of calcium in coronary arteries. Because calcification occurs with atherosclerotic plaque formation, measurement of coronary calcium may reflect the extent of coronary atherosclerosis. High coronary calcium values have been associated with obstructive coronary disease.

Coronary Angiography

Angiography remains the most accurate test to diagnose the percentage of blockage in coronary arteries because of atherosclerosis.

Chest X-Ray

Chest x-rays are an inexpensive technique that allows detection of cardiomegaly and noncardiac causes of chest pain (e.g., pleuritis or pneumonia).

OUTCOME MANAGEMENT

The aims of therapy in the treatment of chronic stable angina are to reduce manifestations and ultimately to reduce the risk of mortality and morbid events. These goals are accomplished through (1) antianginal pharmacologic intervention, (2) education and risk factor modification to control or eliminate known cardiovascular risk factors, and (3) in some instances, revascularization through interventional cardiology or coronary artery bypass graft (CABG) surgery. Smoking cessation after 1 year decreases the risk of CHD by 50%, a 10% reduction in cholesterol level lowers the risk of CHD by 20%, and a 6 mm Hg reduction in diastolic blood pressure lowers the risk of CHD by 10%. The American Heart Association (AHA) recommends that people with angina control their modifiable risk factors and seek prompt treatment for episodes of chest pain. The mnemonic "A, B, C, D, E" is promoted for health care professionals and clients alike in aiding to reduce manifestations and control risk factors:

■ *A* for aspirin and antianginal therapy
■ *B* for beta-blocker therapy and blood pressure control
■ *C* for cigarettes and cholesterol
■ *D* for diet and diabetes
■ *E* for education and exercise

Clients with chronic stable angina (CSA) are usually managed effectively with risk factor reduction and pharmacologic therapy. Revascularization through interventional cardiology procedures or CABG surgery is reserved for those clients with triple-vessel (all three coronary arteries) or left main coronary artery disease, with left ventricular dysfunction, or whose manifestations are not adequately controlled by pharmacologic therapy. Revascularization is used most often for clients with unstable angina or AMI. Interventional cardiology procedures and CABG are discussed in Chapter 56.

Medical Management

Medical management of clients with angina pectoris focuses on three goals: (1) relieve the acute pain, (2) restore coronary blood flow, and (3) prevent further attacks to reduce the risk of AMI.[13]

The diagnosis of angina pectoris is confirmed by history and various tests. A complete history of the pain and its pattern is collected to discriminate angina from other causes of chest pain. Clients are encouraged to describe the pain in their own words. Record a complete analysis of manifestations. This description provides a baseline that can be used in ongoing care.

Most physical findings are transient. The client exhibits pallor or has cold, clammy skin. Tachycardia and hypertension may be recorded. Pulsus alternans (the force of each beat varies) may be present at the onset of ischemic attacks. On auscultation, an S_3 or S_4 gallop or a paradoxical split of S_2 may be noted. If mitral regurgitation is present because of ischemia of the papillary muscle, a murmur can be heard.

Relieve Acute Pain and Restore Coronary Blood Flow

The primary goal of pharmacologic treatment of angina is to balance myocardial oxygen supply and demand by altering the various components of the process, thereby increasing oxygen supply to the myocardium or reducing myocardial oxygen demand. The components of myocardial oxygen consumption that can be pharmacologically treated are (1) blood pressure, (2) heart rate, (3) contractility, and (4) left ventricular volume. Drugs used in the treatment of angina and associated nursing implications are listed in the Integrating Pharmacology feature below.

The major types of medications used to treat the acute attack in angina pectoris are as follows:

- *Opiate analgesics* are used to relieve or reduce acute pain. By reducing pain, the heart rate often lowers and the need for oxygen by the myocardium also is reduced.
- *Vasodilators* help reduce acute pain and prevent further attacks by widening the diameter of coronary arteries and increasing the supply of oxygen to the myocardium. *Nitroglycerin,* a *short-acting* nitrate, has been the treatment of choice against anginal attacks since 1867. Administered sublingually, per tablet, or via translingual spray, nitroglycerin helps relieve or reduce anginal pain within 1 to 2 minutes. *Long-acting* nitrates, given orally or transdermally, help maintain coronary artery vasodilation, thereby promoting greater flow of blood and oxygen to the heart muscle.
- *Beta-adrenergic blockers* help reduce the workload of the heart, decrease myocardial oxygen demand, and may decrease the number of anginal attacks.
- *Calcium-channel blockers* are used to dilate coronary arteries, thereby increasing oxygen supply to the myocardium.
- *Antiplatelet* agents inhibit platelet aggregation and reduce coagulability, thus preventing clot formation.

Prevent Further Attacks

Education and counseling regarding modification of risk factors are necessary to reduce the progression of CHD and to prevent further attacks. Recommendations

---

INTEGRATING PHARMACOLOGY

Treatment of Angina

Angina is ischemic pain in the myocardium. The medications used to treat acute angina episodes are vasodilators designed to restore arterial flow (supply) or reduce oxygen consumption (demand).

Nitroglycerin is the most common medication used and should be given to clients with known ischemic heart disease who report manifestations of angina. Because of its potent vasodilatory effect, assess the blood pressure before beginning treatment and 5 minutes after each dose. The most common practice is to give three doses of sublingual nitroglycerin 5 minutes apart as long as the client does not become severely hypotensive. If the pain is not relieved, notify the physician immediately; morphine may be required. If the client does not have a history of ischemic heart disease, collect a thorough assessment of the pain and notify the physician immediately if there are any indications of serious forms of chest pain. Some physicians order simultaneous liquid antacids and nitroglycerin to reduce both cardiac and gastrointestinal pain. If the medications are given 5 minutes apart, it may help with clinical decision making about the cause of the pain. Concurrent use of sildenafil (Viagra) may cause severe hypotension and death.

Clients with long-standing angina may also use topical nitroglycerin of extended-release forms. These forms of nitroglycerin provide continuous vasodilation. Tolerance to the medication can develop, especially in doses with longer half-lives; hence topical nitroglycerin is removed during the night to restore efficacy. Assessment of nocturnal angina, especially during REM sleep, is needed.

A second method of controlling pain is to reduce the myocardial need for oxygen. Beta-blocking agents reduce myocardial oxygen consumption by controlling the high-oxygen demands from the effects of the sympathetic nervous system. Original forms of beta-blocking agents contained both $beta_1$ and $beta_2$ antagonists and therefore could prompt bronchoconstriction. Newer forms are selective $beta_1$ antagonists only.

Aspirin is commonly used in acute events and to promote blood flow through narrowed and tortuous coronary arteries, where slowed blood is likely to clot and prevent forward flow of blood. Aspirin prevents platelets from aggregating (collecting) by blocking prostaglandin synthesis. Aspirin is irritating to the gastrointestinal tract and should be given with food. It also leads to increased bleeding risk from all invasive procedures. Concurrent use of other medications that also slow clotting must be carefully monitored.

Other medications for the treatment of angina are the same as the medications used for the treatment of coronary artery disease (see Chapter 56).

should follow the guidelines established by the AHA for primary and secondary prevention of CHD. Specific recommendations for risk factor modification are described in Chapter 56.

Nursing Management of the Medical Client

🔔 Relieve Acute Pain and Restore Coronary Blood Flow

In addition to documenting the clinical manifestations of angina, ascertain how long the client has had angina, whether risk factors for CHD are present, and the client's emotional reaction to chest pain. Start cardiac monitoring, obtain a 12-lead ECG, and control ongoing angina. Until the angina is controlled and coronary blood flow is reestablished, the client is at risk for myocardial damage from myocardial ischemia. If the client reports angina, assess the pain and ask the client whether the pain is the same as that experienced in the past. Note new characteristics or increased pain. The phrase "all clients with chest pain get MONA" is used to guide treatment of clients with chest pain:

- *M,* morphine sulfate
- *O,* oxygen therapy
- *N,* nitrates
- *A,* aspirin

Give sublingual nitroglycerin tablets or spray as prescribed. Nitroglycerin dilates coronary arteries, reducing pain and restoring coronary blood flow. Because nitroglycerin causes vasodilation and hypotension, monitor blood pressure. If the pain is not relieved after three nitroglycerin tablets, each taken 5 minutes apart, or after morphine, notify the physician. In addition, an environment that provides rest and security as well as allays fear and anxiety helps reduce pain. Oxygen therapy is used to ensure adequate oxygenation. Aspirin is given for its antiplatelet activities.

Self-Care

The client must be knowledgeable about the care of episodes of angina and how to reduce the risk factors that exacerbate the process. Use the following information to help clients control risk factors for angina pectoris:

- Educate the client to avoid activities or habits that precipitate angina (eating large meals, drinking coffee, smoking, exercising too strenuously, going out in cold weather, becoming anxious and stressed). If an attack begins, the client should stop the activity and sit down. An antianginal medication (e.g., nitroglycerin) should be taken. Three pills can be taken sublingually 5 minutes apart. If the pain does not subside, worsens, or radiates, the client should take an aspirin. The client should call "911" and explain that he or she is experiencing chest pain;

the client would then be taken promptly to the emergency department. Emphasize this point, because if the client is experiencing an AMI, the sooner treatment is initiated, the lower the death rate. Family members should not drive the client to the hospital because of the risk for sudden death precipitated by ventricular fibrillation. If the client is taken by ambulance, defibrillators are available in case of ventricular fibrillation.

- Explain the importance of daily management of hypertension. Advise the client to take daily medication even if no clinical manifestations are evident (see Chapter 52).
- Encourage and help plan a regular program of daily exercise to promote improved coronary circulation and weight management.
- Instruct clients who smoke to quit smoking at once. Smoking cigarettes raises carboxyhemoglobin levels in the blood, which reduces the amount of oxygen available to the myocardium. Clients with angina pectoris exposed for 2 hours to cigarette smoke have elevations in carboxyhemoglobin concentration, decreased exercise tolerance, increased heart rate, and elevated blood pressure. Advise clients to avoid "passive smoking" (i.e., being with a smoker or in a smoke-filled room).
- Urge overweight clients to lose excess weight. Explain that weight reduction may also reduce blood pressure, cholesterol level, and the incidence of adult-onset diabetes. Encourage them to eat small meals, avoid high-calorie and high-cholesterol diets, abstain from gas-forming foods, and rest for short periods after meals. In addition, recommend a high-fiber diet, which not only may prevent constipation and other intestinal tract ailments but also may decrease the number and severity of anginal attacks. Diets high in fiber may also help lower serum cholesterol and triglyceride levels. CHD is less common among clients with a high intake of dietary fiber than in those with a low intake. High-fiber diets can also decrease hypertension.
- Help the client who leads an active, hectic life to adjust activities to a level below that which precipitates anginal attacks. Encourage brief rest periods throughout the working day, an early bedtime, and longer or more frequent vacations. Advise clients who are anxious and nervous to consider counseling. Relaxation techniques may also be used.

ACUTE MYOCARDIAL INFARCTION

Acute coronary syndrome refers to the clinical manifestations that are compatible with AMI. An AMI is also known as a heart attack, coronary occlusion, or simply a "coronary," which is a life-threatening condition characterized by the formation of localized necrotic areas within the myocardium. AMI usually follows the sudden occlusion of a coronary artery and the abrupt cessation of blood and oxygen flow to the heart muscle. Because the heart muscle must function continuously, blockage of blood to the muscle and the development of necrotic areas can be lethal.

AMI is the leading cause of death in America and is responsible for an estimated 529,000 deaths each year. Every year about 1.1 million Americans have AMIs. Every 29 seconds an American suffers a coronary event and approximately every 1 minute someone dies of a coronary event. About 250,000 people a year die before they reach the hospital. Studies indicate that half of all AMI victims wait more than 2 hours before getting help. On the basis of data from the Framingham study, about 45% of all AMIs occur in people younger than age 65 years and 5% occur in those younger than age 40. Eighty-five percent of people who die of AMI are 65 years of age or older. Women have higher in-hospital mortality than men. The difference may result from differences in treatment for men and women. In studies of women with AMI, aspirin, beta-blocking drugs, coronary thrombolysis, acute cardiac catheterization, percutaneous transluminal coronary angioplasty (PTCA), and CABG surgery were used less often than in men with AMI. Death rates for CHD are higher for African Americans, Hispanics, and American Indians than for Caucasians.

Etiology and Risk Factors

The most common cause of AMI is complete or nearly complete occlusion of a coronary artery, usually precipitated by rupture of a vulnerable atherosclerotic plaque and subsequent thrombus formation. Plaque rupture can be precipitated by both internal and external factors.

Internal factors include plaque characteristics, such as the size and consistency of the lipid core and the thickness of the fibrous cap, as well as conditions to which it is exposed, such as coagulation status and degree of arterial vasoconstriction. Vulnerable plaques most frequently occur in areas with less than 70% stenosis and are characterized by an eccentric shape with an irregular border; a large, thin lipid core; and a thin, fibrous cap.

External factors result from actions of the client or from external conditions that affect the client. Strenuous physical activity and severe emotional stress, such as anger, increase sympathetic nervous system responses, that may lead to plaque rupture. At the same time, sympathetic nervous system responses increase myocardial oxygen demand. Scientists have reported that external factors, such as exposure to cold and time of day, also affect plaque rupture. Acute coronary events occur more frequently with exposure to cold and during the morning hours. Researchers hypothesize that the sudden increases in sympathetic nervous system responses associated with these factors may contribute to plaque

rupture. The role of inflammation in triggering plaque rupture is currently being studied.

Regardless of the cause, rupture of the atherosclerotic plaque results in (1) exposure of the plaque's lipid-rich core to flowing blood, (2) seepage of blood into the plaque, causing it to expand, (3) triggering of thrombus formation, and (4) partial or complete occlusion of the coronary artery.

Unstable angina is associated with short-term partial occlusion of a coronary artery, whereas AMI results from significant or complete occlusion of a coronary artery that lasts more than 1 hour. When blood flow ceases abruptly, the myocardial tissue supplied by that artery dies. Coronary artery spasm can also cause acute occlusion. The risk factors that predispose a client to a heart attack are the same as for all forms of CHD (see Chapter 56).

Pathophysiology

AMI can be considered the end-point of CHD. Unlike the temporary ischemia that occurs with angina, prolonged unrelieved ischemia causes irreversible damage to the myocardium. Cardiac cells can withstand ischemia for about 15 minutes before they die. Because the myocardium is metabolically active, manifestations of ischemia can be seen within 8 to 10 seconds of decreased blood flow. When the heart does not receive blood and oxygen, it converts to *anaerobic metabolism,* creating less adenosine triphosphate (ATP) and more lactic acid as a by-product. Myocardial cells are very sensitive to changes in pH and become less functional. Acidosis causes the myocardium to become more vulnerable to the effects of the lysosomal enzymes within the cell. Acidosis leads to conduction system disorders, and dysrhythmias develop. Contractility is also reduced, decreasing the heart's ability to pump. As the myocardial cells necrose, intracellular enzymes are introduced into the bloodstream, where they can be detected by laboratory tests.

Figure 58-1 illustrates the depth of various types of infarctions in the wall of the ventricle. Cellular necrosis

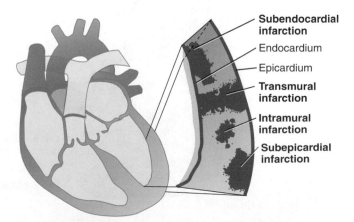

■ FIGURE 58–1 Depth of infarction in the wall of the ventricle. Subendocardial, intramural, and subepicardial injuries are only in one layer. Transmural infarction extends through all three layers.

occurs in one layer of myocardial tissue in subendocardial, intramural, and subepicardial infarctions. In a transmural infarction, cellular necrosis is present in all three layers of myocardial tissue. The infarct site is called the *zone of infarction and necrosis.* Around it is a zone of hypoxic injury, also called a penumbra. This zone can return to normal but may also become necrotic if blood flow is not restored. The outermost zone is called the *zone of ischemia;* damage to this area is reversible.

Within the first few hours of AMI, the necrotic area stretches in a process called *infarct expansion.* This expansion is furthered by the neurohormonal activation that occurs with AMI. Increased heart rate, ventricular dilation, and activation of the renin-angiotensin system increase preload during AMI in order to maintain cardiac output. Transmural infarctions heal by scar formation of the left ventricle, called *remodeling.* Expansion may continue for up to 6 weeks after an AMI and is accompanied by progressive thinning and lengthening of infarcted and noninfarcted areas. The gene expression of remodeled cardiac cells changes, causing permanent structural changes to the heart. Remodeled tissue does not function normally and can result in acute or chronic heart failure with left ventricular dysfunction and increases in ventricular volumes and pressures. Remodeling may continue for years after an AMI (see Chapter 56).

The most common site of an AMI is the *anterior wall* of the left ventricle near the apex, resulting from thrombosis of the descending branch of the left coronary artery (Figure 58-2). Other common sites are (1) the *posterior wall* of the left ventricle near the base and behind the posterior cusp of the mitral valve and (2) the *inferior (diaphragmatic) surface* of the heart. Infarction of the posterior left ventricle results from occlusion of the right coronary artery or circumflex branch of the left coronary artery. An inferior infarction occurs when the right coronary artery is occluded. In nearly 25% of inferior wall AMIs, the right ventricle is the site of infarction. Atrial infarctions develop less than 5% of the time. The Concept Map on p. 1491 further outlines the cellular effects that occur during an MI.

Clinical Manifestations

The clinical manifestations associated with AMI result from ischemia of the heart muscle and the decrease in function and acidosis associated with it. The major clinical manifestation of AMI is chest pain (Figure 58-3), which is similar to angina pectoris but more severe and unrelieved by nitroglycerin. The pain may radiate to the neck, jaw, shoulder, back, or left arm. The pain also may present near the epigastrium, simulating indigestion. AMI may also be associated with less common clinical manifestations, including the following:[3]

SAFETY
⚠
ALERT

- **Atypical chest, stomach, back, or abdominal pain**
- **Nausea or dizziness**
- **Shortness of breath and difficulty breathing**
- **Unexplained anxiety, weakness, or fatigue**
- **Palpitations, cold sweat, or paleness**

Women experiencing AMI frequently present with one or more of the less common clinical manifestations.

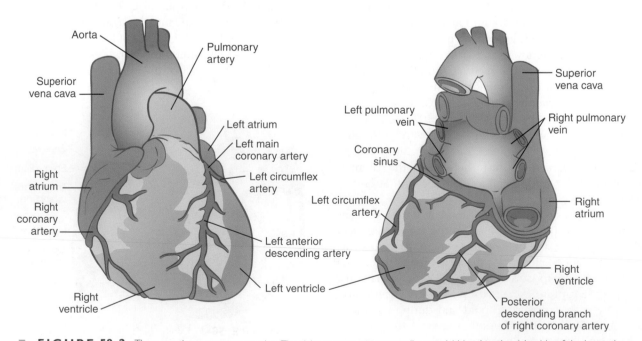

■ **FIGURE 58–2** There are three coronary arteries. The right coronary artery supplies arterial blood to the right side of the heart; the left coronary artery divides into the left circumflex artery, which feeds the posterior heart muscle, and left anterior descending artery, which supplies the anterior myocardium

Understanding Myocardial Infarction and Its Treatment

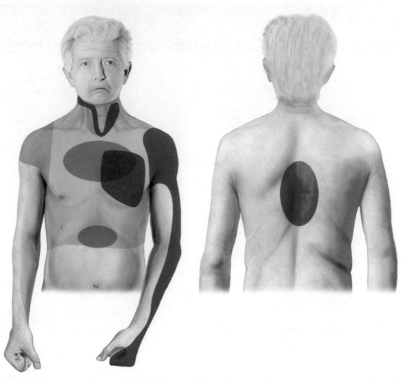

■ **FIGURE 58–3** Possible pain patterns with myocardial infarction. The red area is the most common location of pain. Orange areas are areas of referred pain and the location of pain in women. However, pain can develop in any area of the chest (yellow).

🪔 Diagnostic Evaluation

Guidelines recommend that within 10 minutes of arrival in the emergency department all clients with a suspected AMI (ischemic-type chest discomfort) ingest aspirin and have baseline cardiac serum markers drawn and a 12-lead ECG taken. Based upon appropriate triage, 30-day survival rates, and cost-effectiveness, recommended methods of identifying acute cardiac ischemia in emergency departments are troponin T serum levels and echocardiography. The Acute Cardiac Ischemia Time-Insensitive Predictive Instrument (ACI-TIPI), an algorithm based on questions and 12-lead ECG findings, is also accurate and of low cost.

Electrocardiography

The 12-lead ECG can be used to determine the location of the infarct. Leads V_1 and V_2 face the septum of the heart, leads V_3 and V_4 face the anterior wall of the left ventricle, and V_5 and V_6 face the lateral wall of the left ventricle. When blood flow to the heart is decreased, ischemia and necrosis of the heart muscle occur. These conditions are reflected in altered Q wave, ST segment, and T wave on the 12-lead ECG (Figure 58-4). Twelve-lead ECG examines the heart from 12 views, and in general the more leads with Q waves and ST segment changes the larger the infarct and the worse the prognosis (Figure 58-5). The Q-wave change is significant; normally the Q wave is small or absent. AMI from total occlusion of a coronary

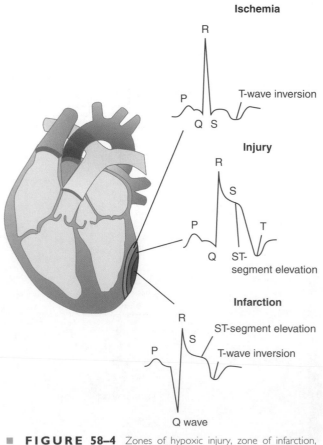

■ **FIGURE 58–4** Zones of hypoxic injury, zone of infarction, zone of necrosis, and the electrocardiographic patterns accompanying these changes during myocardial infarction.

■ **FIGURE 58–5** A 12-lead ECG showing sinus tachycardia and ST elevation consistent with acute myocardial infarction.

■ **FIGURE 58–6** Isoenzyme alterations in acute myocardial infarction. *(From Wong, S.S. [1996]. Strategic utilization of cardiac markers for the diagnosis of acute myocardial infarction. Annals of Clinical Laboratory Science, 26, 301-312. Copyright 1996 by the Institute for Clinical Science, Inc.)*

artery causes a visible Q wave on the ECG; AMI with less than total occlusion does not lead to Q wave changes. Ischemic tissue produces an elevation in the ST segment and a peaked T wave or inversion of the T wave. ST-segment elevation is considered significant if greater than 1 mm. Through the course of an MI, changes occur first in the ST segment, then the T wave, and finally the Q wave. As the myocardium heals, the ST segment and T wave return to normal, but the Q-wave changes persist. However, an ECG can be completely normal in a client with AMI, especially in the early hours following infarct.

💡 Laboratory Tests

Laboratory findings include elevated levels of serum creatine kinase (CK)-MB isoenzyme, myoglobin, cardiac troponin T, and cardiac troponin I. Historically, elevations in lactate dehydrogenase (LDH) M1 isoenzyme, serum aspartate transaminase (AST), leukocytes (leukocytosis), and erythrocyte sedimentation rate (ESR) have aided in the diagnosis of AMI. Although serum levels of these substances can be drawn, isoenzymes are used today to diagnose AMI. Isoenzyme changes in AMI follow a typical pattern (see Figure 58-6). Knowing the typical pattern allows an estimation of the time of the actual injury.

Troponin. The cardiac troponin complex is a basic component of the myocardium that is involved in the contraction of the myocardial muscle. Positive levels of troponin are considered virtually diagnostic of AMI.

Cardiac *troponin T* is similar to CK-MB with regard to sensitivity, and levels increase within 3 to 6 hours after pain has started. Levels remain elevated for 14 to 21 days. This is useful (and more accurate than LDH) in confirmation of distant AMI.[15,21]

Cardiac *troponin I* levels increase 7 to 14 hours after AMI. This is a very specific and sensitive indicator of AMI and is not affected by any other disease or injury to any other muscle except cardiac muscle. Elevation persists for 5 to 7 days.

Myoglobin. Myoglobin is a heme protein found in striated muscle fibers. Myoglobin is rapidly released when myocardial muscle tissue is damaged. Because of the rapid release, it can be detected within 2 hours after AMI. Although many other factors can raise the serum myoglobin level (e.g., strenuous exercise, heavy ethanol use), myoglobin is a highly sensitive indicator of AMI if serum levels double when a second sample is drawn within 2 hours of the first. Conversely, it is reliable to exclude the diagnosis of AMI if the levels do not increase every 2 hours. The diagnostic window ends 24 hours after an AMI.[21]

CK-MB. Serum levels of CK-MB (an isoenzyme of CK found primarily in cardiac muscle) increase 3 to 6 hours after the onset of chest pain, peak in 12 to 18 hours, and return to normal levels in 3 to 4 days.

LDH. The LDH$_1$ subunit is plentiful in heart muscle and is released into the serum when myocardial damage occurs. Serum levels of LDH elevate 14 to 24 hours after onset of myocardial damage, peak within 48 to 72 hours, and slowly return to normal over the next 7 to 14 days. Figure 58-6 illustrates the pattern of enzyme changes after AMI.

AST. Serum levels of AST increase within several hours after the onset of chest pain, peak within 12 to 18 hours, and return to normal within 3 to 4 days.

Leukocytosis. Leukocytosis ($10,000/mm^3$ to $20,000/mm^3$) appears on the second day after AMI and disappears in 1 week. Myeloperoxidase, a leukocyte enzyme, was recently shown to be predictive of AMI even in clients without elevations in troponin T level.

Imaging Studies

Radionuclide imaging studies provide information on the presence of coronary artery disease as well as the location of ischemic and infarcted tissue. Cardiac imaging studies have been used to provide information for management decisions of clients who present to the emergency department with acute chest pain.

When a client experiences acute chest pain, perfusion imaging with agents such as thallium, sestamibi, and teboroxime can be used to identify ischemic and infarcted tissue. Perfusion imaging is sometimes called "cold spot" imaging because the radioisotope in the bloodstream is not taken up by ischemic or infarcted tissue.

Infarct, or "hot spot" imaging, is useful in confirming AMI in clients who present to the hospital several days after an AMI. Technetium 99 m–tagged pyrophosphate binds with calcium in areas of myocardial necrosis. Areas of uptake (hot spots) seen on nuclear imaging indicate areas of infarction. Because this test does not give positive results for 24 hours, however, it cannot be used to identify an acute, early-stage MI. Radiolabeled antimyosin is also used for hot spot imaging, but its diagnostic value is limited because it cannot differentiate between a new infarct and a scar from an earlier infarct.

Positron Emission Tomography. Positron emission tomography (PET) is used to evaluate cardiac metabolism and to assess tissue perfusion. It can also be used to detect CHD, assess coronary artery flow reserve, measure absolute myocardial blood flow, detect AMI, and differentiate ischemic from nonischemic cardiomyopathy. It may also be used to assess myocardial viability to determine which clients can benefit from CABG.

Magnetic Resonance Imaging. Magnetic resonance imaging (MRI) helps identify the site and extent of an MI, assess the effects of reperfusion therapy, and differentiate reversible and irreversible tissue injury. Its use as a diagnostic tool for coronary artery disease is increasing, although MRI cannot be used in clients with implanted metallic devices, such as pacemakers or defibrillators.

Echocardiography. Echocardiography is useful in assessing the ability of the heart walls to contract and relax. The transducer is placed on the chest, and images are relayed to a monitor screen. Wall motion is abnormal in ischemic or infarcted areas. Complications such as mitral regurgitation, rupture of the left ventricle, and pericardial effusion can be detected.

Transesophageal Echocardiography. Transesophageal echocardiography (TEE) is an imaging technique in which the transducer is placed against the wall of the esophagus. The image of the myocardium is clearer when the esophageal site is used because no air and no ribs are between the transducer and the heart. This technique is particularly useful for viewing the posterior wall of the heart.

OUTCOME MANAGEMENT

Since the advent of coronary care units and devices that aid in promptly recognizing and treating life-threatening dysrhythmias, 70% to 80% of people experiencing an AMI survive the initial attack. Chances for survival greatly diminish with the presence of the following:

- Older age (clients 80 years or older have a 60% death rate)
- Manifestations of heart failure
- ST-segment elevation
- Elevation of cardiac markers
- Hypotension (systolic blood pressure less than 55 mm Hg on admission has a 60% death rate)
- More than three coronary risk factors
- More than two anginal events within 24 hours

Deaths generally result from severe dysrhythmias, cardiogenic shock, heart failure, rupture of the heart, and recurrent AMI. Clients who avoid complications after AMI still require 6 to 12 weeks for complete recovery. However, 25% of men and 38% of women die within 1 year after having AMI and 22% of men and 46% of women are disabled with heart failure within 6 years of an AMI.

Medical Management

Major goals of care for clients with AMI include the following:

- Initiating prompt care
- Determining the type of AMI (STEMI vs. NSTEMI)
- Reducing pain
- Delivering successful treatment for the acute pain and reperfusion of the myocardium
- Preventing complications
- Preventing remodeling and heart failure
- Rehabilitating and educating the client and significant others

Treat the Acute Attack Immediately

Clients with manifestations of AMI must receive immediate treatment. Delays may increase damage to the heart and reduce the chance of survival. The goal for treatment of AMI is "door to needle" in less than 30 minutes, or specifically from onset of pain till thrombolytic therapy within 30 minutes or percutaneous angioplasty within 1 hour.

SAFETY ⚠ ALERT

Most communities have an emergency medical system (EMS) that responds quickly (call "911"). Until EMS personnel arrive, keep the client quiet and calm. It is recommended that, if conscious, a client chew an aspirin at the onset of manifestations, because mortality is reduced 23% with this action alone.[1]

Many people who experience manifestations of AMI delay calling for help because they misinterpret what they are sensing. Their expectations of what AMI should feel like and their experience are not the same. In women, this delay may even be longer. Community education to "call first, call fast" is important.

While waiting for EMS to arrive, elevate the client's head and loosen any tight clothing around the neck. Once EMS workers arrive, the client is assessed and transported quickly to an emergency department. EMS workers are trained to respond to possible AMI clients with protocols to ensure quick and proper treatment. Sudden death from AMI caused by ventricular tachycardia degenerating first to ventricular fibrillation and later to asystole is the most common cause of sudden cardiac death. The client is given oxygen; an intravenous (IV) line is inserted, and the client is connected to a heart monitor. Portable automatic external defibrillators (AEDs) are becoming standard in public places. These devices can guide amateurs on how to resuscitate a person with chest pain who is having a dysrhythmia. Clients who become unconscious before reaching the emergency department may require defibrillation or cardiopulmonary resuscitation (CPR).

The client experiencing AMI needs immediate admission to a hospital with a coronary care unit if possible. The first 24 hours after AMI is the time of highest risk for sudden death. There is a significant benefit if treatment is administered within the first hour of onset of manifestations. The first hour after the onset of pain is the crucial time frame for salvage of the myocardium. Therefore efforts have been made to decrease the time for initial treatment. All emergency departments treat AMI clients within 30 minutes of presenting to the hospital. The mnemonic *4D's* (*d*oor, *d*ata, *d*ecision, and *d*rug), along with treatment algorithms, has been adopted by many emergency departments to treat those with AMI and remains current. Equally important is for everyone to have 911 access for EMS personnel who are trained in triage of chest pain and defibrillation.

Determining the Type of AMI

For purposes of determining appropriate treatment, AMI is viewed as part of a spectrum of coronary syndromes, which includes (1) ST-segment elevation myocardial infarction (STEMI), (2) non–ST-segment elevation myocardial infarction (NSTEMI), and (3) unstable angina. Clients with persistent ST elevation should be considered for reperfusion therapy (thrombolysis or primary percutaneous coronary interventions [PCIs]). Those without ST elevation will be diagnosed either with NSTEMI if cardiac markers are elevated or with unstable angina if serum cardiac markers provide no evidence of myocardial injury. Clients with no ST-segment elevation are not candidates for immediate thrombolytics but should receive anti-ischemic therapy and may be candidates for PCI urgently or during admission. Confirmation of

the diagnosis of NSTEMI requires waiting for the results of cardiac markers. In the case of unstable angina, diagnosis may await further diagnostic studies such as coronary angiography or imaging studies to confirm the diagnosis and to distinguish it from noncoronary causes of chest pain.

The initial focus should be on identifying clients with STEMI. An ECG should be performed and read within 10 minutes of ED arrival. If STEMI is present, the decision as to whether the client will be treated with thrombolysis or primary PCI should be made within the next 10 minutes. The goal for clients with STEMI should be to achieve a door-to-drug time of within 30 minutes and a door-to-balloon time of within 90 minutes. If STEMI is not present, then the workup proceeds looking for unstable angina or NSTEMI and for other causes of chest pain.

Reduce Pain

Upon admission, the client who complains of chest pain is admitted to the emergency department, given oxygen therapy, and placed on ECG monitoring. An IV line is placed, serum cardiac markers are drawn, and a 12-lead ECG is undertaken within 10 minutes. Pain control is a priority, and pain is usually treated with IV morphine. Continued pain is a manifestation of myocardial ischemia. Pain also stimulates the autonomic nervous system and increases preload, which in turn increases myocardial oxygen demand. Oxygen is used to treat tissue hypoxia.

Monitor Heart Rhythm

Because dysrhythmias are common, ECG monitoring is essential and antidysrhythmic medications should be on hand. A two-dimensional echocardiogram and test may be performed in the emergency department to aid in ruling in or ruling out AMI.

Improve Perfusion

The general principles of pharmacologic treatment of AMI consist of anti-ischemic and antithrombotic therapies, which are outlined in the Integrating Pharmacology feature on p. 1496.[1] Anti-ischemic therapy usually consists of beta-blockade and IV nitroglycerin. Antithrombotic therapy and the combination of different antithrombotic agents are being studied widely. Antithrombotic therapy is usually initiated with the administration of an aspirin if the client has not taken one before reaching the emergency department. Heparin therapy is the next step.

Antithrombotic therapy continues with medications that lyse (dissolve) the clot that forms part of the blockage of the coronary artery. Thrombolytic therapy includes streptokinase, urokinase, tissue-type plasminogen activator (t-PA), anisoylated plasminogen-streptokinase activator complex (anistreplase, APSAC), alteplase,

INTEGRATING PHARMACOLOGY

Medications for Myocardial Infarction

The portion of the coronary artery occluded by a thrombus can be opened by using various medications that dissolve the clot or prevent new clots from forming or extending. Non–clot-specific thrombolytic agents (streptokinase, urokinase) can be infused over 60 minutes after the client is premedicated with a steroid and diphenhydramine to prevent allergic responses. For large or anterior infarcts, clot-specific agents are more common forms of plasminogen activator. This medication is given in a bolus followed by an infusion. Several relative and absolute contraindications exist for thrombolytic therapy (see Box 58-2).

Heparin is also used in combination with the thrombolytic to prevent new clot formation. The dose of heparin is based on lean body weight and adjusted to the partial thromboplastin time. Heparin is contraindicated in clients with known bleeding conditions or recent stroke. Low-molecular-weight heparin is more commonly used because of ease of administration.

Preventing platelet aggregation is an important component of therapy. Aspirin continues to be used routinely in coronary angioplasty and to treat clients with myocardial infarction or unstable angina. The advantages of early aspirin administration are clear; it is strongly advised that aspirin be consumed early in care. Glycoprotein (GP) IIb/IIIa serves as the receptor on platelets that permits platelet aggregation. Agents that block this final common pathway by blocking the binding of adhesive proteins to GP IIb/IIIa, termed *GP IIb/IIIa antagonists,* are currently considered the most powerful specific inhibitors of platelet participation in acute thrombosis.

Pain is managed with morphine or intravenous nitroglycerin. Nitroglycerin is a coronary vasodilator used to reduce preload and afterload. Other medications, beta-blockers, ACE inhibitors, and statins are discussed in Chapter 56.

BOX 58-2 Absolute and Relative Contraindications for Thrombolytic Therapy

ABSOLUTE CONTRAINDICATIONS

- Any prior intracranial hemorrhage
- Ischemic stroke within 3 months *except* acute ischemic stroke within 3 hours
- Known structural cerebral vascular lesion (i.e., AVM)
- Known malignant intracranial neoplasm (primary or metastatic)
- Active bleeding or bleeding diathesis excluding menses
- Suspected aortic dissection
- Significant closed head trauma or facial trauma within past 3 months

RELATIVE CONTRAINDICATIONS

- History of chronic, severe, poorly controlled hypertension
- Severe uncontrolled hypertension on presentation (SBP >180 or DBP >100 mm Hg)
- History of prior ischemic stroke >3 months
- Dementia
- Known intracranial pathology not covered in contraindications
- Traumatic or prolonged CPR or major surgery in last 3 weeks
- Noncompressible vascular punctures
- Pregnancy
- Active peptic ulcer
- Current use of anticoagulants, the higher the INR the greater the risk
- Prior exposure (>5 days ago) to streptokinase/anistreplase
- Allergic reaction to streptokinase or anistreplase

---

urokinase plasminogen activator, and reteplase. For best efficacy, thrombolytic agents should be given within an hour after the onset of chest pain. However, new AHA guidelines advise that thrombolytic agents can still be given for up to 12 hours after the onset of chest pain. The choice of thrombolytic agent is not as important as the speed with which it is given. After the thrombolytic agent is administered, IV heparin or a glycoprotein IIb/IIIa is usually continued. All of these thrombolytic agents can be given intravenously.

Not all clients with AMI are suitable candidates for thrombolytic therapy (Box 58-2). History of recent cerebral vascular accident, surgery, pregnancy, and use of anticoagulants are contraindications for thrombolytic therapy. Complications of thrombolytics include bleeding, allergic reactions, and stroke. Successful reperfusion of the coronary arteries is evidenced by (1) return of ECG changes to normal, (2) relief of chest pain, (3) presence of reperfusion dysrhythmias, usually sudden onset of frequent premature ventricular contractions (PVCs) or short runs of PVCs, and (4) a rapid, early peak of the CK-MB isoenzyme ("washout"). If reperfusion is not attained or if the client is not a candidate for thrombolytic therapy, then primary angioplasty, stenting, or CABG may be performed. Interventional cardiology procedures and bypass surgery are discussed in Chapter 56. If ST elevation is present, reperfusion strategies are to be promptly initiated.[1] Guidelines suggest that thrombolytic therapy should be initiated within 30 minutes or PTCA should be initiated within 60 minutes. PTCA may be considered before thrombolytic therapy in institutions that have cardiac surgery capabilities, that have skilled physicians in PCTA, and that perform more than 200 PTCA procedures per year.

Antidysrhythmic agents are initiated. Clinicians begin beta-blockade and angiotensin-converting enzyme (ACE) inhibitors within 72 hours of onset to reduce ventricular remodeling and reduce mortality. Stool softeners are used to relieve constipation and to lower the risk of bradycardia from straining that stimulates the vagus nerve.

Determine the Location of the Myocardial Infarction

Determining the exact coronary vessel that has infarcted is done through analysis of the 12-lead ECG and is validated with coronary angiography to determine the degree of occlusion (expressed in percentage of blockage of each coronary artery). Determining the exact artery that is involved is important so potential complications can be assessed and minimized (Table 58-1). Knowledge of the area of the heart with infarct can prevent complications and allow diagnosis of AMI when ECG changes are not present.

Monitor for Complications

The possibility of death from complications always accompanies an AMI. Thus prime collaborative goals include the prevention of life-threatening complications or at least recognition of them.

Dysrhythmias. Dysrhythmias are the cause of 40% to 50% of deaths after AMI. Ectopic rhythms arise in or near the borders of intensely ischemic and damaged myocardial tissues. Damaged myocardium may also interfere with

the conduction system, causing dissociation of the atria and ventricles *(heart block)*. Supraventricular tachycardia (SVT) sometimes occurs as a result of heart failure. Spontaneous or pharmacologic reperfusion of a previously ischemic area may also precipitate ventricular dysrhythmias.

Provide continuous cardiac monitoring and frequent counts of PVCs (many monitoring systems count continuously). Notify the physician if more than six PVCs occur per minute and the client is symptomatic (e.g., hypotension, chest pain). For *dysrhythmias,* provide prompt intervention per protocol or orders. For new-onset, symptomatic *ventricular ectopy* (runs, couplets), administer amiodarone or lidocaine per order or protocol. For *ventricular tachycardia,* administer amiodarone or lidocaine; if pulseless ventricular tachycardia occurs, provide synchronized cardioversion. For *ventricular fibrillation,* provide immediate defibrillation coupled with CPR and administration of epinephrine or vasopressin. For *supraventricular tachycardia (SVT),* administer a vagal maneuver, adenosine, diltiazem, or amiodarone,

---

TABLE 58-1 **Clinical Manifestations Based on Location of Acute Myocardial Infarction**

Area	ST-Segment Elevation and Q Waves on 12-Lead ECG	Common Dysrhythmias	Other Manifestations	Complications
Left anterior descending (LAD)	V_1-V_6 depending on branch	Ventricular tachycardia Bundle branch blocks (BBBs) Premature ventricular contractions (PVCs) Atrial fibrillation or flutter	Severe heart failure Low CO, BP Elevated pulmonary artery diastolic pressure (PAD), pulmonary capillary wedge pressure	Cardiogenic shock Myocardial rupture High mortality with this location
Circumflex/V_5	I, aV_L, V_5, V_6 ST depression of V_1-V_4 (reciprocal)	AV nodal blocks (especially Mobitz 1)	Heart failure and left ventricular dysfunction Bradycardia	Papillary muscle dysfunction Aneurysms
Right circumflex artery (RCA)	II, III, and aV_F	Premature atrial contractions (PACs) and atrial fibrillation Atrioventricular (AV) block (all types)	Hypotension resulting from decreased right ventricle ejection, especially when client is given nitroglycerin or morphine sulfate Requires large volumes of fluids to maintain BP	Ventricular tachycardia/ventricular fibrillation
Inferior wall	II, III, aV_F	Atrial dysrhythmias	Hiccups, nausea, vomiting	Papillary muscle rupture Septal rupture
Anterior wall	V_3, V_4	Second-degree AV block Sinus tachycardia		Cardiogenic shock Extension of infarct to lateral wall
Septal wall	V_1, V_2	Infranodal BBB and second- and third-degree heart block		Septal rupture
Lateral wall	I, aV_L, V_5, V_6	AV nodal blocks		Cardiogenic shock and heart failure
Posterior wall	ST-segment depression V_1-V_4	Bradycardia	Nausea	Papillary muscle dysfunction Aneurysms

* The classic pattern of ECG changes with AMI begins with an abnormal T wave that is prolonged and peaked. This is followed within minutes by ST-segment elevation in the leads facing the area of injury with reciprocal changes of ST-segment depression in the opposite leads. Q-wave formation follows, and the Q-wave changes only disappear over months. The classic evolution of ST-segment elevation and Q-wave formation is often diagnostic of AMI. Knowledge of the area of the heart with infarct can prevent complications and allow diagnosis of AMI when ECG changes are not present.

BP, Blood pressure; *CO,* cardiac output.

and prepare for possible elective cardioversion. For *heart block or symptomatic bradycardia,* administer atropine and prepare for use a temporary pacemaker. Dysrhythmias are discussed in Chapter 57.

Cardiogenic Shock. Cardiogenic shock accounts for only 9% of deaths from AMI, but more than 70% of clients in shock die of it.[2] Causes include (1) decreased myocardial contraction with diminished cardiac output, (2) undetected dysrhythmias, and (3) sepsis. Clinical manifestations include systolic blood pressure significantly below the client's normal range, diaphoresis, rapid pulse, restlessness, cold and clammy skin, and grayish skin color. Shock can be prevented with sufficient IV fluids to prevent circulatory collapse and the identification of dysrhythmias.

Vasopressors are administered (dopamine, dobutamine) to raise blood pressure by increasing peripheral resistance. In other cases, vasodilators (nitroprusside, nitroglycerin) promote better blood flow in the microcirculation and reduce afterload. Positive inotropic agents (dobutamine, epinephrine, milrinone) increase cardiac contractility and cardiac output and improve tissue perfusion. Administer oxygen therapy and antidysrhythmic agents as prescribed, and continuously monitor arterial and pulmonary artery pressures. Analgesics such as morphine sulfate should be given to ensure client comfort. Chapter 81 explains shock in detail.

Heart Failure and Pulmonary Edema. The most common cause of in-hospital death in clients with cardiac disorders is heart failure. Heart failure disables 22% of male clients and 46% of female clients who experience an AMI and is responsible for one third of deaths after an AMI.

Heart failure may develop at the onset of the infarction or may occur weeks later. Clinical manifestations include dyspnea, orthopnea, weight gain, edema, enlarged tender liver, distended neck veins, and crackles. It is managed by correcting the underlying cause, relieving clinical manifestations, and enhancing cardiac pump performance.[22,24,27] Heart failure is discussed in Chapter 56, in *evolve* the Case Study feature above, right, and on the website.

Pulmonary Embolism. Pulmonary embolism (PE) may develop secondary to phlebitis of the leg or pelvic veins (venous thrombosis) or from atrial flutter or fibrillation. PE occurs in 10% to 20% of clients at some point, during either the acute attack or convalescence. PE is discussed in Chapter 61.

Recurrent Myocardial Infarction. Within 6 years after an initial AMI, 18% of men and 35% of women may experience recurrent MI. Possible causes include overexertion, embolization, and further thrombotic occlusion of a

Cardiogenic Shock, Tachycardia, and Heart Failure

Mr. Borg is a 70-year-old retired African-American man who was admitted to the emergency department (ED) after arriving by rescue squad. According to his wife, he had been vomiting and experiencing progressive weakness earlier in the day. When the rescue squad arrived at his home, he was in supraventricular tachycardia with a heart rate more than 180 beats/min. The squad administered adenosine (Adenocard) 6 mg IV, followed by an additional 12 mg 3 minutes later. En route he denied chest pain or shortness of breath, but he was becoming cyanotic and his heart rhythm was again becoming tachycardic. . . . *Case Study continued on the website and the CD-ROM with discussions, multiple-choice questions, and a nursing care plan.* *evolve*

coronary artery by an atheroma. The clinical manifestation is the return of angina. Management is the same as that for AMI.

Complications Caused by Myocardial Necrosis. Complications that are due to necrosis of the myocardium include ventricular aneurysm, rupture of the heart (*myocardial rupture*), ventricular septal defect (VSD), and ruptured papillary muscle. These complications are infrequent but serious, usually occurring about 5 to 7 days after MI. Weak, friable necrotic myocardial tissue increases vulnerability to these complications (Figure 58-7).

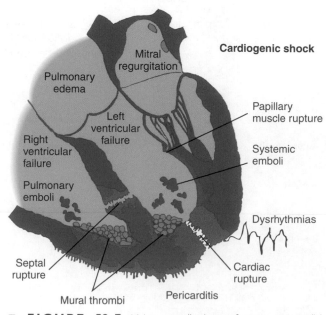

■ **FIGURE 58-7** Major complications of acute myocardial infarction.

Manifestations of heart failure develop with ventricular aneurysm, rupture of the ventricular septum, and rupture of the papillary muscle. Manifestations of severe mitral insufficiency often develop when the papillary muscle of the left ventricle ruptures. Ventricular dysrhythmias (e.g., frequent PVCs and ventricular tachycardia) occur often in the presence of a ventricular aneurysm (the necrotic tissue is very irritable). Manifestations of cardiac tamponade develop with rupture of the heart.

The goal of treatment is to decrease the workload of the heart and increase the oxygen supply to keep the area of infarction and necrotic tissue as small as possible. Surgery is performed to (1) excise the ventricular aneurysm, (2) replace the mitral valve if the papillary muscle is ruptured, or (3) repair the VSD. Pericardiocentesis and immediate surgery help relieve cardiac tamponade that occurs after rupture of the heart.

Pericarditis. In up to 28% of clients with an acute transmural MI, early pericarditis develops (within 2 to 4 days). The inflamed area of the infarction rubs against the pericardial surface and causes it to lose its lubricating fluid. A pericardial friction rub can be auscultated across the precordium. The client complains that chest pain is worse with movement, deep inspiration, and cough. The pain of pericarditis is relieved by sitting up and leaning forward.

Frequent assessment may lead to early identification and intervention. Relieve pain with analgesics, such as acetaminophen, nonsteroidal anti-inflammatory drugs (NSAIDs), or other anti-inflammatory agents. Reduce the client's anxiety by differentiating the pain of pericarditis from the pain of AMI.

Dressler's Syndrome (Late Pericarditis). Dressler's syndrome, a form of pericarditis, can occur as late as 6 weeks to months after AMI. Although the etiologic agent is unknown, an autoimmune cause is suggested. The client usually presents with a fever lasting 1 week or longer, pericardial chest pain, pericardial friction rub, and occasionally pleuritis with pleural effusions. This is a self-limiting phenomenon, and no prevention is known. Treatment includes aspirin, prednisone, and opioid analgesics for pain. Anticoagulation therapy may precipitate cardiac tamponade and should be avoided in these clients.

Nursing Management of the Medical Client

The goals of nursing management after AMI are as follows:

- Recognize and treat cardiac ischemia.
- Administer thrombolytic therapy as ordered, or ready client for PTCA and observe for complications.
- Recognize and treat potentially life-threatening dysrhythmias.
- Monitor for complications of reduced cardiac output.
- Maintain a therapeutic critical care environment.
- Identify the psychosocial impact of AMI on the client and family.
- Educate the client in lifestyle changes and rehabilitation.
- A care plan on care of the client with AMI lists specific nursing diagnoses, interventions with rationale and evaluation outcomes.

Rehabilitation and Education

Cardiac rehabilitation following AMI is an essential component of professional and personal management. The following are recommendations for managing rehabilitation of clients who have suffered an AMI:

- All clients with cardiovascular disease should adopt a cardioprotective dietary pattern.
- Intensive dietary advice, compliance checks, and long-term follow-up should be given, preferably by a dietitian.
- There is insufficient evidence to recommend nutritional supplements of antioxidant vitamins, minerals, or trace elements for the prevention of cardiovascular disease.
- Fish and fish oil supplements may reduce the risk of sudden cardiac death.
- For overweight and obese clients with CHD, the combination of reduced-carbohydrate diet and increased physical activity is recommended.
- Initial goal of weight loss therapy should be to reduce the client's weight by 10%.
- All clients with cardiovascular disease should be advised to quit smoking and should be supported to stop smoking as a priority measure.
- All clients with CHD should consider having standard pharmacotherapy with aspirin, beta-blocker, ACE inhibitor, and a statin unless contraindicated.
- Comprehensive cardiac rehabilitation should embrace a case management approach.

Strengthen the Myocardium. A successful rehabilitation program begins the moment the client enters the coronary care unit for emergency care and continues for months and even years after discharge from the health care facility. The overall goal of rehabilitation is to help the client live as full, vital, and productive a life as possible while remaining within the limits of the heart's ability to respond to increases in activity and stress. Six important subgoals of the rehabilitation process are as follows:

- Developing a program of progressive physical activity
- Educating the client and significant others about the cause, prevention, and treatment of CHD
- Helping the client accept the limitations imposed by illness

- Aiding the client in adjusting to changes in occupational goals
- Lessening the exposure to risk factors
- Changing the psychosocial factors adversely affecting recovery from CHD

Cardiac rehabilitation is a comprehensive, long-term program that involves periodic medical evaluation, prescribed exercises, and education and counseling about cardiac risk factor modification. Cardiac rehabilitation is a multifactorial program that begins when the client is still hospitalized and continues throughout recovery. Cardiac rehabilitation consists of four phases: phase I (inpatient), phase II (immediate outpatient), phase III (intermediate outpatient), and phase IV (maintenance outpatient).

Phase I (Inpatient). Phase I begins with admission to the coronary care unit. After AMI, clients usually remain on bed rest for less than 24 hours unless complications such as heart failure or dysrhythmias develop. Although the myocardium must rest, bed rest puts the client at risk for hypovolemia, hypoxemia, muscle atrophy, and pulmonary embolus. Thus the client must avoid both invalidism and reckless overexertion. These considerations are outlined in the Care Plan on pp. 1502-1509. Case managers may be assigned to coordinate care. See the Case Management feature on Acute Myocardial Infarction on the website.

Provide complete bed rest for the first day or two with use of a bedside commode for bowel movements. Most clients receive a 2-g sodium diet. If the client is nauseated, provide a clear liquid diet until nausea subsides. A coronary care nurse or physiotherapist should start passive exercises. As the client regains strength, have the client sit for brief periods on the side of the bed and dangle the feet. Allow the client to ambulate to a bedside chair for 15 to 20 minutes after the first day if dangling has been tolerated without development of chest pain, dysrhythmias, or hypotension. When the client is transferred from the coronary care unit to an intermediate or regular unit, bathroom privileges and self-care activities are encouraged. Wireless heart monitoring (telemetry) may continue. Allow brief walks in the hall with supervision. The length and duration of these walks are increased progressively, working up to 5 to 10 minutes according to the client's endurance. The client loses 10% to 15% of skeletal muscle and contractile strength within the first week of bed rest and 20% to 25% after 3 weeks of bed rest. The client must increase activities gradually to avoid overtaxing the heart as it pumps oxygenated blood to the muscles. The metabolic equivalent test (MET) provides one way of measuring the amount of oxygen needed to perform an activity:

$$1 \text{ MET} = 3.5 \text{ ml of } O_2/\text{kg/min}$$

One MET is about equivalent to the oxygen uptake a client requires when resting. Early mobilization activities after AMI should not exceed 1 to 2 METs, as from shaving, washing, and self-feeding. (Later activities can increase to 10 or 11 METs, such as cycling or running.)

With each activity level increase, monitor the heart rate, blood pressure, and fatigue level, adjusting the client's activity level accordingly. During early activities, the heart rate should not increase more than 25% above resting level. Blood pressure must not increase more than 25 mm Hg above normal.

SAFETY
⚠
ALERT

Help the client avoid fatigue. Dyspnea, chest pain, tachycardia, and a sense of exhaustion warn that the client is attempting to do too much. Instruct the client regarding these warning signs of overexertion. Include family members in these discussions; family members may fear that allowing the client to become active again will precipitate another AMI and while attempting to help, they may discourage autonomy.

During phase I, client education should include cardiac anatomy and physiology risk factors and management of CHD, behavioral counseling, and home activities.

Phase II (Immediate Outpatient). If no complications arise, the physician discharges the client to the home after a week. Nearly 50% of clients after AMI have an uncomplicated hospital course without evidence of angina, heart failure, or major dysrhythmias. There is a growing trend toward early discharge of clients with uncomplicated AMI. A team at one health care facility discharges post-AMI clients at the end of the fourth day but allows clients to go home early only if the household has adequate help and is conducive to rest. Such clients are followed up carefully by trained nurse-clinicians who visit the home and supervise physiologic status, exercise, and diet every other day. The Bridge to Home Health Care feature on p. 1501 discusses how to promote heart-healthy living after an AMI. Researchers believe that earlier discharge after AMI reduces depression as well as hospital expenses.

Resuming sexual activity may be one of the most difficult aspects of returning to normal life after AMI. Sexual intercourse usually may resume 4 to 8 weeks after an AMI. The client should be able to climb two flights of stairs before resuming sexual activity. Caution clients not to eat or drink alcoholic beverages immediately before intercourse. Taking nitroglycerin before intercourse may help prevent exertional angina. However, clients cannot take sildenafil (Viagra) while taking nitroglycerin; both medications are vasodilators.

Advise the client to stop smoking. Encourage frequent walks, but warn against strenuous activities, such as shoveling snow. The walking program aims for a goal of 2 miles in less than 60 minutes.

BRIDGE TO HOME HEALTH CARE

Heart-Healthy Living After an Acute Myocardial Infarction

The role of the home health nurse is to teach heart-healthy living to clients who had an AMI so that they can adjust their lifestyle. Focus your teaching on areas that will help clients become responsible for self-care. Assume that you need to repeat health education that was provided in the hospital during the AMI episode. When stress is high, clients usually recall little of what was taught.

Instruct the client and significant other or family member to monitor for clinical manifestations that may indicate extensions and recurrences of the AMI. Clients need to report indigestion, shortness of breath, increased edema, and palpitations. Learning when to call the physician or nurse for these physical problems is important.

Determine what your clients know about their medications. Knowing what the medication is called, its function, the schedule for taking it, and its side effects is required for client safety. Generally, multiple medications are prescribed, and you need to give the client written instructions and information about each medication. Many pharmacists provide a computer printout of medications and interactions for the client to keep. Medication planners that have compartments for various times of day allow the client to prefill medications for a week at a time and may prevent errors.

The convalescence period for the client and family creates anxiety about daily activities. Instruct the client to avoid prolonged baths or showers to prevent vasodilation. Use tepid water and a stool or bath chair in the shower. Encourage the use of energy-conservation techniques, such as keeping the arms at waist level and getting enough rest to prevent fatigue. Routine household activities and mild recreational activities, such as playing golf, are usually permitted.

Climbing more than two flights of stairs and lifting more than 20 pounds are restricted. If clients do not ask about resuming sexual relations, consider introducing the topic. They may be too timid to consult their physicians about this subject.

An appropriate unsupervised exercise is a prescribed indoor walking program. Exercising after a heavy meal or during mild illness is contraindicated. Instruct the client to begin each exercise session with a warm-up period that may last as long as 15 minutes and to end the session with a cool-down period. Walking should be constant and should last long enough to increase blood flow to the muscles.

The client or caregiver should have an emergency plan that includes having someone available to drive if a ride is needed and someone in the home who knows basic cardiopulmonary resuscitation (CPR). A personal emergency response system may be appropriate for clients who live alone. Some emergency response systems are worn around the neck, and the push of a button summons medical assistance. Caregiver stress, communication problems, and fear of the unknown are valid concerns. Community resources and additional information can be obtained by calling the American Heart Association's toll-free number: 1-800-242-8721.

A monitored group program may help the client achieve the best possible physical conditioning. These programs typically last from 10 to 12 weeks and are implemented in a supervised setting. They offer various training devices, such as treadmills, stationary bicycles, and rowing machines. During phase II, the client performs large-muscle exercises for at least 20 to 30 minutes three or four times a week. In addition, clients are trained in warm-up and stretching exercises. During the sessions, cardiac rehabilitation staff monitors cardiac rhythm, heart rate, and blood pressure before exercise, at peak exercise, and during recovery. Clients also report their level of perceived exertion several times during the exercise session.

Some clients may be able to return to work at the end of 8 or 9 weeks if they remain asymptomatic. Clients with less physically strenuous jobs can sometimes resume a full-time schedule, but manual laborers may have to work part time or find less taxing work. Occupational evaluations can be done to assess cardiac impairment in relation to job requirements and client skills.

Between the eighth and tenth weeks, the client requires a complete physical examination, including ECG, exercise stress tests, lipid analysis, and chest x-ray study. Clinicians must correct pre-existing health problems that might have contributed to the development of CHD (e.g., hypertension, anemia, hyperthyroidism).

Recovery after AMI may be lengthy and difficult. The client may have undergone surgery or may have been managed medically. In either case, a serious threat to integrity has occurred. Initially after AMI, clients may attempt to prove that they are not seriously ill. Coping strategies include denial and minimization. Some clients conceal the recurrence of chest pain. As recovery continues, clients begin to comprehend that a heart attack has really occurred, to understand why it happened, and to consider its impact on the future. Clients begin the process of life adjustment to find a lifestyle that can be tolerated and maintained while preserving a sense of self-worth. Several strategies are used to regain self-control, such as gauging progress, seeking reassurance, learning about health, and being cautious. Eventually, most clients come to terms with the fact that they will not be living life to the fullest. Clients learn to accept limitations and to refocus on other aspects of life. Some clients are unable to adjust. Sometimes clients find that they have had too many setbacks and are powerless to make changes or gain control. The education and counseling that accompany a structured cardiac rehabilitation program can help improve psychological well-being, social adjustment, and functioning.

Phase III (Intermediate Outpatient). The extended outpatient phase of cardiac rehabilitation lasts from 4 to 6 months. Exercise sessions continue to be supervised, and clients are taught how to monitor their exercise intensity by measuring their pulse rate or, if in a walking

The Client with Acute Myocardial Infarction

Nursing Diagnosis: Acute Pain related to myocardial ischemia resulting from coronary artery occlusion with loss or restriction of blood flow to an area of the myocardium and necrosis of the myocardium.

Outcomes: The client will experience improved comfort in the chest, as evidenced by a decrease in the pain rating, the ability to rest and sleep comfortably, have less need for analgesia or nitroglycerin, and have reduced anxiety.

NOC OUTCOMES Comfort Level, Pain Control, Pain: Disruptive Effects, Pain Level

Interventions	NIC INTERVENTIONS	Rationales
1. Assess the characteristics of chest pain, including location, duration, quality, intensity, presence of radiation, precipitating and alleviating factors, and associated manifestations. Have the client rate pain on a scale of 0 to 10, and document findings in nurses' notes.	Pain Management Cardiac Care: Acute	1. Pain is an indication of myocardial ischemia. Assisting the client in quantifying pain may differentiate pre-existing and current pain patterns as well as identify complications. Usually a scale of 0 to 10 is used, with 10 being the worst pain and 0 being none.
2. Assess respirations, blood pressure, and heart rate with each episode of chest pain.	Cardiac Care: Acute	2. Respirations may be increased as a result of pain and associated anxiety. Release of stress-induced catecholamines increases heart rate and blood pressure.
3. Obtain a 12-lead electrocardiogram (ECG) on admission and then each time chest pain recurs for evidence of further infarction.	Cardiac Care: Acute	3. Serial ECGs and stat ECGs record changes that can give evidence of further cardiac damage and location of myocardial ischemia.
4. Monitor the response to drug therapy. Notify the physician if pain does not abate within 15-20 minutes.	Pain Management Analgesic Administration	4. Pain control is a priority because it indicates ischemia.
5. Provide care in a calm, efficient manner that reassures the client and minimizes anxiety. Stay with the client until discomfort is relieved.	Cardiac Care: Acute Anxiety Reduction	5. External stimuli may worsen anxiety and increase cardiac workload as well as limit coping abilities.
6. Limit visitors as the client requests.	Cardiac Care: Acute Anxiety Reduction	6. Limiting visitors prevents overstimulation and promotes rest.
7. Administer morphine as ordered.	Pain Management Analgesic Administration	7. Morphine is an opiate analgesic and alters the client's perception of pain and reduces preload time vasoconstriction.
8. Administer nitrates as ordered.	Cardiac Care: Acute Medication Administration	8. Nitrates relax the smooth muscles of coronary blood vessels, decreasing ischemia and hence decreasing pain.

Evaluation: The client should be pain-free within 15 to 20 minutes after administration of drug therapy. The client will verbalize relief of pain and will not exhibit associated manifestations of pain.

Nursing Diagnosis: Ineffective Tissue Perfusion (Cardiopulmonary) related to thrombus in coronary artery, resulting in altered blood flow to myocardial tissue.

Outcomes: The client will demonstrate improved cardiac tissue perfusion, as evidenced by a decrease in the rating of pain and resolving ST segments.

NOC OUTCOMES Cardiac Pump Effectiveness, Circulation Status

Interventions	NIC INTERVENTIONS	Rationales
1. Keep the client on bed rest with a quiet environment.	Cardiac Care: Acute Hemodynamic Regulation, Circulatory Care: Arterial Insufficiency	1. Stress activates the sympathetic nervous system and increases myocardial oxygen needs.
2. Administer oxygen as ordered.	Cardiac Care: Acute Hemodynamic Regulation, Circulatory Care: Arterial Insufficiency	2. Oxygen increases myocardial supply of oxygen.
3. Administer thrombolytics or send the client for angioplasty as ordered.	Cardiac Care: Acute Circulatory Care: Arterial Insufficiency Medication Administration	3. Thrombolytic therapy or angioplasty can break apart the thrombus and increase myocardial tissue perfusion.
4. Monitor ST segments.	Cardiac Care: Acute Dysrhythmia Management	4. ST-segment elevation indicates myocardial tissue injury; ST-segment depression indicates decreased myocardial perfusion.

Evaluation: The return of ST segments to baseline is dependent on the degree of ischemia and rapidness of treatment.

Collaborative Problem: Dysrhythmias related to electrical instability or irritability secondary to ischemia or infarcted tissue, as evidenced by an increase or decrease in heart rate, change in rhythm, and atrial or ventricular dysrhythmias.

Outcomes: The client will have no dysrhythmias, as evidenced by normal sinus rhythm or return to the client's own baseline rhythm.

NOC OUTCOMES   Cardiac Pump Effectiveness, Circulation Status (NOC)

Interventions	NIC INTERVENTIONS	Rationales
1. Teach the client and family about the need for continuous monitoring. Keep alarms on and limits set at all times.	Dysrhythmia Management Cardiac Care: Acute Anxiety Management	1. Continued monitoring keeps staff aware of rhythm changes. Family anxiety is decreased when explanations are provided.
2. Assess the apical heart rate. Auscultate for change in heart sounds (murmurs, rub, S_3, and S_4).	Dysrhythmia Management Cardiac Care: Acute Circulatory Care: Arterial Insufficiency	2. The apical heart rate suggests early cardiac decompensation and potential loss of cardiac output.
3. Document the rhythm strip every shift and prn (as needed) if dysrhythmias occur. Measure the pulse rate, QRS, PR, and QT segments with each strip. Note and report any deviations from the client's baseline values.	Dysrhythmia Management Cardiac Care: Acute Circulatory Care: Arterial Insufficiency	3. Dysrhythmias are the most common complication after AMI.
4. Report six or more multifocal premature ventricular contractions (PVCs) per minute to the physician.	Dysrhythmia Management Cardiac Care: Acute Circulatory Care: Arterial Insufficiency	4. Multifocal PVCs indicate ventricular irritability, which decreases cardiac output and may lead to life-threatening dysrhythmias.
5. Give antidysrhythmic agents as ordered.	Dysrhythmia Management Cardiac Care: Acute Medication Administration	5. Antidysrhythmic drugs reduce myocardial irritability.
6. Monitor the effects of antidysrhythmic agents.	Dysrhythmia Management Cardiac Care: Acute Medication Administration	6. The desired results are increased diastolic threshold potential and decreased action potential duration.
7. Monitor serum potassium levels.	Dysrhythmia Management Cardiac Care: Acute	7. Altered potassium levels can affect cardiac rhythms.
8. Maintain a patent intravenous (IV) line or heparin lock at all times.	Dysrhythmia Management Cardiac Care: Acute Medication Administration	8. This measure is for emergency administration of IV cardiac medications.
9. Monitor ST segments, and document changes.	Dysrhythmia Management Cardiac Care: Acute	9. ST depression indicates myocardial ischemia, and ST elevation indicates injury; either may precipitate dysrhythmias.

Evaluation: Within 24 hours of admission, the client's cardiac rhythm will remain stable and the client will exhibit no manifestations of rhythm disturbance.

Nursing Diagnosis: Decreased Cardiac Output related to negative inotropic changes in the heart secondary to myocardial ischemia, injury, or infarction, as evidenced by change in the level of consciousness, weakness, dizziness, loss of peripheral pulses, abnormal heart sounds, hemodynamic compromise, and cardiopulmonary arrest.

Outcomes: The client will have improved cardiac output as evidenced by normal cardiac rate, rhythm, and hemodynamic parameters; dysrhythmias controlled or absent; and absence of angina.

NOC OUTCOMES   Cardiac Pump Effectiveness, Circulation Status

Interventions	NIC INTERVENTIONS	Rationales

Assess for and document the following as evidence of myocardial dysfunction with decreasing cardiac output:

Interventions	NIC INTERVENTIONS	Rationales
1. Mental status—be alert to restlessness and decreased responsiveness.	Cardiac Care: Acute, Hemodynamic Regulation Acid-Base Management Shock Management: Cardiac	1. Cerebral perfusion is directly related to cardiac output and aortic perfusion pressure and is influenced by hypoxia and electrolyte and acid-base variations.
2. Lung sounds—monitor for crackles and rhonchi.	Shock Management: Cardiac Cardiac Care: Acute, Hemodynamic Regulation Airway Management	2. Crackles may develop, reflecting pulmonary congestion related to alterations in myocardial function.
3. Blood pressure—monitor for hypertension or hypotension.	Shock Management: Cardiac Cardiac Care: Acute, Hemodynamic Regulation	3. Hypotension related to hypoperfusion, vagal stimulation, dysrhythmias, or ventricular dysfunction may occur; it may be related to pain, anxiety, catecholamine release, or pre-existing vascular problems.
4. Heart sounds—note the presence of gallop, murmur, and increased or decreased heart rate.	Shock Management: Cardiac Cardiac Care: Hemodynamic Regulation	4. Bradycardia may be present because of vagal stimulation or conduction disturbances related to the area of myocardial injury. Tachycardia may be a compensatory mechanism related to decreased cardiac output. A gallop may be related to fluid volume overload or heart failure, and a murmur may be present if ruptured chordae tendineae occurred.

(Continued)

CARE PLAN *evolve*

The Client with Acute Myocardial Infarction—Cont'd

5. Urine output—be alert to output less than 0.5 ml/kg/hr.	Shock Management: Cardiac, Hemodynamic Regulation Circulatory Care: Arterial Insufficiency	5. Urine output less than 0.5 ml/kg/hr may reflect reduced renal perfusion and glomerular filtration as a result of reduced cardiac output.
6. Peripheral perfusion—monitor for pallor, mottling, cyanosis, coolness, diaphoresis, and peripheral pulses.	Shock Management: Cardiac, Hemodynamic Regulation Circulatory Care: Arterial Insufficiency	6. Decreased peripheral pulses may indicate a decrease in cardiac output.
7. Monitor arterial blood gas (ABG) levels.	Shock Management: Cardiac, Hemodynamic Regulation, Acid-Base Management	7. Acidosis may cause dysrhythmias and depressed cardiac function and some cardiac medications increase oxygen demand and may cause hypoxia.
8. If a pulmonary artery catheter is used, record hemodynamic parameters every 2 to 4 hours and as required (prn). Be alert to pulmonary capillary wedge pressure (PCWP) greater than 18 mm Hg, cardiac output less than 4 L/min, and cardiac index less than 2.5 L/min.	Shock Management: Cardiac, Hemodynamic Regulation	8. A PCWP greater than 18 mm Hg may indicate fluid volume overload or heart failure. A cardiac output less than 4 L/min and a cardiac index less than 2.5 L/min indicate heart failure or decrease in cardiac output. Use hemodynamic monitoring to assess drug therapy and for prevention or early detection of complications of AMI (i.e., extension, heart failure, cardiogenic shock).
9. Maintain hemodynamic stability by monitoring the effects of beta-blockers and inotropic agents.	Shock Management: Cardiac, Hemodynamic Regulation, Medication Management	9. Assess the effect of drug therapy on myocardial contractility and function.
10. Monitor and assess angina for type, severity, and duration.	Shock Management: Cardiac, Hemodynamic Regulation	10. Angina indicates myocardial ischemia, which may decrease cardiac output.

Evaluation: Within 2 to 3 days of admission, the client should have normal hemodynamic pressures, normal vital signs, clear breath sounds, no shortness of breath, normal ABG values, and normal sinus rhythm with rate between 60 and 100 beats/min.

Nursing Diagnosis: Impaired Gas Exchange related to decreased cardiac output, as evidenced by cyanosis, impaired capillary refill, reduced arterial oxygen tension (Pao_2), and dyspnea.

Outcomes: Tissue Perfusion: The client will demonstrate improved gas exchange, as evidenced by absence of cyanosis, brisk capillary refill, absence of dyspnea, and ABG levels within normal limits.

NOC OUTCOMES   Pulmonary

Interventions	NIC INTERVENTIONS	Rationales
1. Administer oxygen as ordered; maintain continuous oximetry.	Oxygen Therapy Respiratory Monitoring	1. Increases amount of oxygen available for myocardial uptake; measures peripheral oxygen saturation.
2. Monitor ABGs as ordered.	Oxygen Therapy Respiratory Monitoring Acid-Base Management	2. The presence of hypoxia indicates a need for supplemental oxygen. Monitoring provides data on the adequacy of tissue perfusion and oxygenation.
3. Continue to assess the client's skin, capillary refill, and level of consciousness every 2-4 hours and prn.	Respiratory Monitoring Cardiac Care	3. Cyanosis (circumoral or in extremities) indicates hypoxia. Capillary refill greater than 3 seconds indicates poor perfusion and possibly hypoxia.
4. Assess respiratory status for dyspnea and crackles.	Oxygen Therapy Respiratory Monitoring	4. Dyspnea may indicate inadequate oxygenation, and the presence of crackles may impair gas exchange because of decreased exchange of oxygen and carbon dioxide through fluid in alveoli.
5. Prepare for intubation and mechanical ventilation if hypoxia increases.	Oxygen Therapy Respiratory Monitoring Airway Management	5. With increasing hypoxia, mechanical ventilation may be necessary to oxygenate the client adequately.

Evaluation: Within 2 to 3 days of admission, client's breath sounds will be clear, and ABG values will be within normal limits.

Collaborative Problem: Risk for Bleeding related to coagulopathies associated with thrombolytic therapy or arterial puncture after angioplasty.

Outcomes: The nurse will monitor for bleeding and reduce bleeding risk. If bleeding does occur, it will be recognized and treated at once.

NOC OUTCOMES   Blood Loss Severity

Interventions	NIC INTERVENTIONS	Rationales
1. Obtain coagulation studies as ordered. Follow protocols for adjustments of anticoagulants	Bleeding Precautions	1. Coagulation studies can help determine the tendency to bleed and if adjustments in anticoagulant medications are needed.
2. Monitor invasive line sites for active bleeding.	Bleeding Precautions	2. Thrombolytic therapy disrupts the normal coagulation process, and bleeding may occur at any invasive site.
3. Inspect all body fluids for presence of blood.	Bleeding Precautions	3. Internal bleeding may be manifested in urine, sputum, and gastrointestinal drainage.
4. Hold pressure on any discontinued lines for 15 minutes; if arterial, hold for 30 minutes.	Bleeding Precautions, Bleeding Reduction	4. Pressure is used to achieve hemostasis at catheter sites.
5. If the client has had an angioplasty, monitor puncture site frequently for hemorrhage.	Bleeding Precautions	5. Active bleeding may occur after angioplasty.
6. Observe neurologic status.	Bleeding Precautions	6. A change in neurologic status may indicate intracranial bleeding.
7. Avoid intramuscular (IM) injections.	Bleeding Precautions, Bleeding Reduction	7. IM injections may cause bleeding.
8. Assess for back or flank pain.	Bleeding Precautions	8. Flank or back pain may suggest retroperitoneal bleeding.
9. Keep IV line patent.	Bleeding Precautions, Bleeding Reduction Fluid Management Hypovolemia Management	9. In case of active bleeding, a patent line must be maintained to transfuse blood products.
10. Maintain an active type and crossmatch on the client.	Bleeding Precautions, Bleeding Reduction Fluid Management Hypovolemia Management	10. If the client requires blood or blood products, an active type and crossmatch helps eliminate any delay in treatment.

Evaluation: The nurse will monitor for and prevent bleeding.

Nursing Diagnosis: Powerlessness related to a near-death experience and anticipated lifestyle changes, as evidenced by verbalized "feelings of doom," crying, and anger.

Outcomes: The client will regain a sense of "control," as evidenced by feeling able to express feelings of powerlessness over the present situation and future outcomes.

NOC OUTCOMES   Fear Level

Interventions	NIC INTERVENTIONS	Rationales
1. Provide opportunities for the client to express feelings about oneself and the illness.	Coping Enhancement	1. These opportunities create a supportive climate and send the message that caregivers are willing to help.
2. Explore reality perceptions, and clarify if necessary.	Coping Enhancement	2. Listening to the client's feelings and words can help the client acquire a more hopeful outlook.
3. Eliminate the unpredictability of events by allowing adequate preparation for tests and procedures.	Coping Enhancement Anxiety Reduction	3. Information helps the client and family feel more hopeful and be more willing to participate in care.
4. Reinforce the client's right to ask questions.	Coping Enhancement	4. Maintain a supportive climate to let the client feel free to ask questions or have information repeated.
5. Allow choices when possible.	Coping Enhancement Decision-Making Support	5. Self-care allows the client to feel independent.
6. Provide positive reinforcement for increased involvement in self-care.	Coping Enhancement	6. When clients participate in planning for care, they are more likely to feel a sense of control and to follow through with actions.
7. Help the client identify strengths and areas of control.	Coping Enhancement	7. Self-confidence and security come with a sense of control; foster full client participation.

Evaluation: Within 24 hours of admission, client will verbalize a feeling of control over the situation and will actively participate in decisions regarding care.

(Continued)

CARE PLAN evolve

The Client with Acute Myocardial Infarction—Cont'd

Nursing Diagnosis: Anxiety and Fear related to hospital admission and fear of death, as evidenced by client and family appearing restless, hostile, or withdrawn; client and family verbalize fatalism or act extremely emotional as if in the grieving process.

Outcomes: The client will have reduced feelings of anxiety and fear, as evidenced by demonstrating appropriate range of feelings and initial manifestations of effective coping (participating in the treatment regimen), being able to rest, and asking fewer questions.

NOC OUTCOMES Anxiety Level		
Interventions	**NIC INTERVENTIONS**	**Rationales**
1. Limit nursing personnel; provide continuity of care.	Anxiety Reduction Coping Enhancement	1. Continuity of care promotes security and development of rapport with and trust of health care providers.
2. Allow and encourage the client and family to ask questions; do not avoid questions. Bring up common concerns.	Anxiety Reduction Coping Enhancement Decision-Making Support	2. Accurate information about the situation reduces fear, strengthens the client-nurse relationship, and assists the client and family to face the situation realistically.
3. Allow the client and family to verbalize fears.	Anxiety Reduction Coping Enhancement Decision-Making Support	3. Sharing information elicits support and comfort and can relieve tension and unexpressed worries.
4. Stress that frequent assessments are routine and do not necessarily imply a deteriorating condition.	Anxiety Reduction	4. The client may feel reassured after learning that frequent assessments may prevent development of more serious complications.
5. Repeat information as necessary because of the reduced attention span of the client and family.	Anxiety Reduction	5. The client's attention span is short, and time perception may be altered. Anxiety decreases learning and attention.
6. Provide a comfortable, quiet environment for the client and family.	Anxiety Reduction Coping Enhancement	6. A comfortable environment enhances coping mechanisms and reduces myocardial workload and oxygen consumption.

Evaluation: Coping is very individualized. Base the timing of outcomes on the client's demonstrated behaviors and statements.

Nursing Diagnosis: Risk for Constipation related to bed rest, pain medications, and NPO (nothing by mouth) or soft diet, as evidenced by subjective feeling of fullness, abdominal cramping, painful defecation, and palpable impaction.

Outcomes: The client will have improved bowel elimination, as evidenced by eliminating a stool without straining or having a vasovagal response (bradycardia).

NOC OUTCOMES Bowel Elimination		
Interventions	**NIC INTERVENTIONS**	**Rationales**
1. Ensure that the client has adequate bulk in diet and adequate fluid intake (without violating fluid restrictions).	Constipation/Impaction Management	1. Bulk and fluid within the colon prevent straining.
2. Monitor the effectiveness of softeners or laxatives. Instruct the client on prevention of straining and avoiding Valsalva (vasovagal) maneuver.	Constipation/Impaction Management Medication Management	2. Stool softeners decrease the myocardial workload of straining. The Valsalva maneuver causes bradycardia, decreasing the cardiac output.
3. Encourage the client to use a bedside commode rather than a bedpan.	Constipation/Impaction Management	3. Use of bedpans necessitates more straining and increases the vasovagal response.

Evaluation: Within 2 to 3 days of admission, client should have normal bowel function.

Nursing Diagnosis: Ineffective Health Maintenance related to AMI and implications for lifestyle changes.

Outcomes: The client and family will learn about the medical regimen and lifestyle changes, as evidenced by verbalizing an understanding of a heart attack and the necessary lifestyle changes regarding diet, medications, stress reduction, quitting smoking, and cholesterol, weight, and blood pressure reduction.

NOC OUTCOMES Knowledge: Treatment Regimen		
Interventions	**NIC INTERVENTIONS**	**Rationales**
1. Explain the following, providing both oral and written instructions: anatomy and functions of heart muscle and atherosclerotic process; definition of a "heart attack"; healing process of the heart; and role of collateral circulation.	Teaching: Disease Process, Coping Enhancement	1. Use of multiple learning methods enhances retention of material; information helps the client understand the underlying coronary arteries, problems of overall heart functions.

Interventions	NIC Interventions	Rationales
2. Assist the client with identifying personal risk factors.	Teaching: Disease Process, Coping Enhancement	2. Risk factor identification is the first step before changes can be implemented.
3. Assist the client in devising a plan for risk factor modification (e.g., diet; smoking cessation; cholesterol, stress, and blood pressure reduction).	Teaching: Disease Process, Coping Enhancement Decision-Making Support	3. This information is helpful in providing opportunity for the client to identify risk factors, assume control, and participate in treatment regimen.
4. Provide guidelines for a diet low in cholesterol and saturated fat. Arrange for dietary consultation before hospital discharge.	Teaching: Prescribed Diet, Coping Enhancement	4. Consultation with other health professionals enhances client learning from others. Guidelines developed with the client and family before discharge help once they are home.
5. Teach the client and family about medications that will be taken after hospital discharge (name, purpose, dosage, schedule, precautions, potential side effects).	Teaching: Prescribed Medications, Coping Enhancement	5. The more clients understand the medical regimen and potential side effects, the more adept they will be in monitoring for them.
6. Discuss post-AMI activity progression; arrange for a cardiac rehabilitation consultation.	Teaching: Prescribed Activity/Exercise, Coping Enhancement	6. Continued follow-up will let clients know how they are doing; outpatient cardiac rehabilitation supports and assists clients in the lifestyle changes necessary for a healthy recovery and life.
7. Use other professionals to collaborate in the care of the client.	Teaching: Disease Process Teaching: Prescribed Activity/Exercise Teaching: Prescribed Diet, Coping Enhancement	7. Dietitians can assist in diet education; social services can identify assistance in the area of finances and home help; cardiac rehabilitation personnel can assist in exercise regimens; clergy can assist in coping strategies; and support groups can assist in social support.

Evaluation: Adaptation to new self-care strategies is very individualized. Plan the projected time frame once the client's learning style is known.

Nursing Diagnosis: Risk for Activity Intolerance related to an imbalance between oxygen supply and demand, as evidenced by weakness, fatigue, change in vital signs, dysrhythmias, dyspnea, pallor, and diaphoresis.

Outcomes: The client will have improved activity tolerance, as evidenced by participating in desired activities, meeting activities of daily living (ADL), reduced fatigue and weakness, vital signs within normal limits during activity, and absence of cyanosis, diaphoresis, and pain.

NOC OUTCOMES   Activity Intolerance

Interventions	NIC INTERVENTIONS	Rationales
1. Monitor vital signs before and immediately after activity and 3 minutes later. If blood pressure decreases and heart rate increases, cardiac decompensation is suggested and activity should be decreased.	Cardiac Care: Rehabilitative	1. Vital signs should return to baseline levels in 3 minutes. The development of cardiac decompensation chest pain or dyspnea may indicate a need for an alteration in exercise regimen or medication.
2. Monitor for tachycardia, dysrhythmias, dyspnea, diaphoresis, weakness, fatigue, or pallor after activity.	Cardiac Care: Rehabilitative Oxygen Therapy Respiratory Monitoring	2. These indicators of myocardial oxygen deprivation may call for decreased activity, changes in medications, or use of supplemental oxygen.
3. Encourage verbalization of feelings or concerns regarding fatigue or limitations.	Cardiac Care: Rehabilitative Coping Enhancement	3. Knowing limitations prevents exertion and increasing myocardial workload.
4. Provide assistance with self-care activities, and provide frequent rest periods, especially after meals.	Cardiac Care: Rehabilitative	4. Large meals may increase myocardial workload and cause vagal stimulation, with resultant bradycardia or ectopic beats; caffeine, a cardiac stimulant, increases heart rate.
5. Increase activity per cardiac rehabilitation nurse and physician orders.	Cardiac Care: Rehabilitative	5. Gradual increase in activity increases strength and prevents overexertion, enhances collateral circulation, and restores a normal lifestyle as far as possible.

Evaluation: With stable acute myocardial infarction, the client should progress normally through steps of phase I cardiac rehabilitation without manifestations of exercise intolerance in 3 to 4 days.

(Continued)

The Client with Acute Myocardial Infarction—Cont'd

Collaborative Problem: Risk for Heart Failure related to disease process, as evidenced by tachycardia, hypotension or hypertension, S_3 or S_4 heart sounds, dysrhythmias, ECG changes, decreased urine output, decreased peripheral pulses, peripheral edema, cool ashen skin, diaphoresis, crackles, jugular vein distention, edema, and chest pain.

Outcomes: The nurse will monitor for clinical manifestations of heart failure by assessing cardiac rate, rhythm, hemodynamic parameters, skin perfusion, and CNS perfusion.

NOC OUTCOMES   Cardiac Pump Effectiveness

Interventions	NIC INTERVENTIONS	Rationales
1. Auscultate the apical pulse.	Cardiac Care: Acute Shock Management: Cardiac, Hemodynamic Regulation	1. Atrial (S_3) or ventricular (S_4) gallop rhythms are common and reflect tissue noncompliance or distention of chambers.
2. Assess heart rate and rhythm.	Cardiac Care: Acute Shock Management: Cardiac, Hemodynamic Regulation Dysrhythmia Management	2. Sinus tachycardia, paroxysmal atrial contractions, paroxysmal atrial tachycardia, multifocal atrial tachycardia, and PVCs are commonly seen with heart failure.
3. Document dysrhythmias, if present, as necessary.	Dysrhythmia Management Cardiac Care: Acute	3. Dysrhythmias reduce ventricular filling time, decrease myocardial contractility, and increase myocardial oxygen demands, which further compromises cardiac output.
4. Note lung sounds every 2 to 4 hours and as needed.	Cardiac Care: Acute, Respiratory Monitoring	4. Crackles may develop; ineffective cardiac output causes pulmonary venous congestion that leaks into the alveolar tissue, resulting in congestion.
5. Palpate peripheral pulses every 2 to 4 hours and as necessary.	Cardiac Care: Acute Circulatory Care: Arterial Insufficiency	5. Pulses may be weak, thready, or difficult to obtain when cardiac output is decreased.
6. Monitor blood pressure every 2 to 4 hours and as needed.	Cardiac Care: Acute	6. Hypotension related to hypoperfusion, vagal stimulation, or ventricular dysfunction may occur. Hypertension may be related to pain, anxiety, catecholamine release, or pre-existing vascular problems.
7. Inspect skin for pallor, cyanosis, and diaphoresis every 2 to 4 hours and as needed.	Cardiac Care: Acute Circulatory Care: Arterial Insufficiency	7. Pallor is associated with vasoconstriction, reduced cardiac output, and anemia. Cyanosis may develop during severe episodes of pulmonary edema. Dependent areas are often blue or mottled with increased venous congestion.
8. Monitor urine output, noting changes or decreasing output and dark or concentrated urine, every 2 to 4 hours and as needed.	Fluid Management Cardiac Care: Acute	8. Urine output less than 0.5 ml/kg/hr may reflect reduced renal perfusion and glomerular filtration as a result of reduced cardiac output.
9. Assess for chest pain.	Cardiac Care: Acute Pain Management	9. Chest pain may indicate inadequate cardiac perfusion related to the hypertrophied myocardium.
10. Assess for peripheral edema.	Cardiac Care: Acute	10. In heart failure, especially right-sided, the inability to pump blood forward results in venous pooling and increased pressure in the vascular space that leaks in the interstitium, presenting as peripheral edema.
11. Assess changes in sensorium.	Cardiac Care: Acute Circulatory Care: Arterial Insufficiency	11. Cerebral perfusion is directly related to cardiac output, and mentation may be a sensitive indicator of deterioration.
12. Provide frequent rest periods.	Cardiac Care: Acute	12. Physical rest decreases the production of catecholamines, which increases heart rate, myocardial oxygen demand, and blood pressure.
13. Instruct the client on avoidance of activities that increase cardiac workload.	Teaching: Disease Process Teaching: Prescribed Activity/Exercise	13. Avoidance of activities provides an opportunity for myocardial recovery and decreases workload and myocardial oxygen consumption.
14. Provide a bedside commode. Avoid the Valsalva maneuver.	Cardiac Care Teaching: Disease Process	14. The Valsalva maneuver stimulates the vagus nerve and causes bradycardia that temporarily decreases cardiac output.
15. Elevate the client's legs and avoid pressure under the knees. Permit increase in activity as tolerated and observe for breathing difficulty.	Teaching: Disease Process Teaching: Prescribed Activity/Exercise Cardiac Care	15. This position enhances venous return, reduces dependent swelling, decreases venous stasis, and may reduce the incidence of thrombus and embolus formation. If the left heart cannot pump blood forward, it may become trapped in the lungs/
16. Administer medications as ordered.	Medication Administration Cardiac Care	16. ACE inhibitors and beta-blockade were shown to help reduce the incidence of heart failure after AMI in clinical trials.[21]

Evaluation: The nurse will monitor for heart failure and report manifestations promptly.

Nursing Diagnosis: Excess Fluid Volume related to reduced glomerular filtration rate (GFR), decreased cardiac output, increased antidiuretic hormone (ADH) production, and sodium and water retention, as evidenced by orthopnea, S_3 heart sound, oliguria, edema, jugular neck vein distention, increased weight, increased blood pressure, respiratory distress, and abnormal breath sounds.

Outcomes: The client's fluid volume balance will be adequate, as evidenced by balanced intake and output (I&O), clear or clearing breath sounds, vital signs within normal limits, stable weight, and minimal edema.

NOC OUTCOMES	Fluid Overload Severity

Interventions	NIC INTERVENTIONS	Rationales
1. Monitor I&O (especially note color, specific gravity, and amount) every 2 to 4 hours, and as needed, and 24-hour totals.	Fluid Management	1. Intake greater than output may indicate fluid volume excess. If client receives diuretic therapy, an increase in output is expected.
2. Maintain chair or bed rest in the semi-Fowler position.	Cardiac Care Fluid Management	2. This position promotes diuresis by recumbency-induced increased GFR and reduced ADH production.
3. Involve the client and family in fluid schedules, especially if there are restrictions, and provide frequent oral care.	Coping Enhancement Teaching: Disease Process Fluid Management	3. Involving the client in the therapy regimen may enhance a sense of control and fosters cooperation with restrictions. Fluid restrictions dry the oral mucous membranes.
4. Weigh the client daily.	Fluid Management	4. Daily weights can show the increase or decrease in congestion and edema in response to therapy. A gain of 5 pounds represents about 2 L of fluid.
5. Assess for jugular neck vein distention, edema, peripheral pulses, and presence of anasarca.	Cardiac Care, Fluid Management	5. Excessive fluid retention may be demonstrated by venous engorgement and edema formation. Peripheral edema often begins in the feet and ascends upward as heart failure worsens.
6. Auscultate breath sounds. Note adventitious sounds, increased vascular volume, and pulmonary hypertension or worsening of heart failure.	Respiratory Monitoring Cardiac Care	6. These manifestations of pulmonary congestion reflect and monitor for dyspnea or tachypnea.
7. Monitor for sudden extreme shortness of breath, and feelings of panic.	Respiratory Monitoring Cardiac Care	7. These are manifestations of pulmonary edema.
8. Palpate for hepatomegaly. Note complaints of right upper quadrant pain or tenderness.	Cardiac Care	8. Advancing heart failure leads to venous congestion, which results in liver engorgement and altered liver function (i.e., impaired drug metabolism, prolonged drug half-life).
9. Evaluate the effectiveness of diuretics and potassium.	Fluid Management Medication Management Cardiac Care	9. Fluid shifts and use of diuretics can alter electrolytes, especially potassium and chloride supplements, which affects cardiac rhythm and contractility.
10. Note increased lethargy, hypotension, and muscle cramping.	Cardiac Care	10. These are manifestations of hypokalemia and hyponatremia that may occur because of fluid shifts and diuretic therapy.
11. Assess the need for dietary consultation as needed.	Cardiac Care Teaching: Prescribed Diet	11. Restrictions of foods high in sodium may be necessary. The client may need to eat foods enriched with potassium when taking loop diuretics.

Evaluation: Depending on the degree of heart failure, fluid volume excess may be slow to resolve. Initially, there may be a resolution of manifestations after diuresis. Fluid balance adjustments may then be made daily.

Nursing Diagnosis: Risk for Impaired Skin Integrity related to bed rest, edema, and decreased tissue perfusion, as evidenced by reddened areas and the presence of areas of breakdown.

Outcomes: The client will have intact skin integrity, as evidenced by an absence of reddened areas and no areas of breakdown.

NOC OUTCOMES	Tissue Integrity: Skin and Mucous Membranes

Interventions	NIC INTERVENTIONS	Rationales
1. Inspect the client's skin; note bony prominences, edema, altered circulation, pigmentation, obesity, and emaciation.	Pressure Ulcer Prevention	1. Altered skin color in isolated areas suggests damage caused by pressure or decreased circulation.
2. Assist with active or passive range-of-motion (ROM) exercises.	Pressure Ulcer Prevention	2. ROM exercises enhance venous return. Isometric exercises may adversely affect cardiac output by increasing myocardial work and oxygen consumption.
3. Reposition the client every 2 hours in a bed or chair.	Pressure Ulcer Prevention	3. Repositioning increases circulation and reduces the time that weight deprives any one area of blood flow.
4. Provide pressure-reducing devices, sheepskin, elbow protectors, and heel elevation if needed.	Pressure Ulcer Prevention	4. These devices reduce pressure to bone prominences and maintain skin integrity.
5. Assess and provide special air or flotation beds for clients at high risk for pressure ulcers.	Pressure Ulcer Prevention	5. These beds reduce pressure to skin and may improve circulation.
6. Pad the chair with a pressure reduction pad or 4 inches of foam.	Pressure Ulcer Prevention	6. Weak clients do not move spontaneously. Pressure reduction surfaces can prevent pressures in excess of capillary filling pressures.

Evaluation: Skin impairment may be evident within 48 hours of admission or a significant change in condition.

program, by counting the number of steps they take in a 15-second interval. Clients with dysrhythmias are monitored more closely, and intermittent rhythm strips may be taken. For clients who prefer to exercise at home, clinicians trained in cardiac rehabilitation can provide detailed, written instructions for a long-term exercise program. Various methods are used to determine the appropriate exercise routines. Periodic evaluation is necessary to assess the client's endurance and tolerance to the prescribed exercise program.

Phase IV (Maintenance Outpatient). Phase IV, the final phase of cardiac rehabilitation, usually takes place in the home or community and is unsupervised. The client maintains a program of regular exercise and other lifestyle modifications to modify cardiac risk. Clients should undergo an exercise testing and risk factor assessment annually.

CONCLUSIONS

CHD is a progressive occlusive disorder that commonly results in reduced coronary blood flow. This reduction in blood flow is manifested clinically by angina and AMI. AMI, permanent damage to the myocardium, may be the first indicator of the seriousness of the heart disease. Your responsibilities in the care of these clients are to educate them about the warning signs of AMI, to monitor their response to therapy, to prevent complications, and to promote rehabilitation.

THINKING CRITICALLY

1. Mrs. Polk, a 62-year-old housewife who cares for her two grandchildren, is admitted to the emergency department with complaints of chest pain. She is diaphoretic and pale and complains of pain "under my left breast that pushes to my back." She rates the pain as an 8 on a scale of 1 to 10. Her ECG shows an elevated ST segment. She is placed on oxygen therapy, and an IV line is inserted. Cardiac serum markers are drawn and sent to the laboratory. Her vital signs are temperature 36.9° C, apical pulse rate 110 beats/min, and blood pressure 108/68 mm Hg.

Factors to Consider. What additional testing is necessary to rule in or rule out an acute MI? What other information from Mrs. Polk's history might aid in the diagnosis?

2. The physician immediately orders reteplase, a thrombolytic agent, for Mrs. Polk.

Factors to Consider. What information must be obtained from Mrs. Polk to safely initiate thrombolytic therapy?

3. You administer the thrombolytic therapy as ordered. Mrs. Polk states her pain is now a 1 on a scale of 1 to 10. ST segments are resolving, and she is no longer diaphoretic.

Factors to Consider. What effects from the thrombolytic therapy appear to be occurring? Which side effects of the therapy should you anticipate?

4. A client with long-standing coronary artery disease experiences severe chest pain unrelieved by nitroglycerin. He is admitted with an acute MI to the coronary care unit. What are the priorities on admission? What medical treatment may be instituted in the first hours following the infarction?

Factors to Consider. What time frame is considered most crucial to the salvage of myocardial muscle? What care is given to the newly admitted client?

Discussions for these questions can be found on the website. **evolve**

BIBLIOGRAPHY

Citations appearing in red refer to primary research.

Citations appearing in blue refer to evidence-based practice guidelines and protocols.

1. American Heart Association. (2005). 2005 American Heart Association guidelines for cardiopulmonary resuscitation and emergency cardiovascular care. Part 8: Stabilization of the patient with acute coronary syndrome. *Circulation, 112*(Suppl IV), IV89-111.
2. American Heart Association (2006). *2006 Heart disease and stroke statistics: 2006 Update.* Dallas, Tex: American Heart Association. Available at www.americanheart.org/.
3. American Heart Association. (2002). *Heart attack, stroke & cardiac arrest warning signs.* Available at www.americanheart.org/.
4. Antman, E., et al. (2000). The TIMI risk score for unstable angina/non-ST elevation MI: A method for prognostication and therapeutic decision making. *Journal of the American Medical Association, 284*(7), 876-878.
5. Antman, E., et al. (2006). ACC/AHA guidelines for the management of patients with ST-segment elevation myocardial infarction: Executive summary. *Circulation, 110*(5), 588-636.
6. *Best practice evidence-based guideline—Cardiac rehabilitation.* (2002)The New Zealand Guideline Group. Available at www.nzgg.org.nz/library/gl-complete/Cardiac-Rehab/index.cfm.
7. Beattie, S. (1999). Management of chronic stable angina. *Nurse Practitioner, 24*(5), 44, 49, 53, 56, 59-61.
8. Braunwald, E., et al. (2002). ACC/AHA 2002 guideline update for the management of patients with unstable angina and non-ST-segment elevation myocardial infarction: A report of the American College of Cardiology/American Heart Association Task Force on Practice Guidelines. Available at www.acc.org/clinical/guidelines/unstable/unstable.pdf.
9. Brennen, M.L., et al. (2003). Prognostic value of myeloperoxidase in patients with chest pain. *New England Journal of Medicine, 349*(17), 1595-1604.
10. Cummings, R. (2001). *ACLS provider manual.* Dallas, Tex: American Heart Association.
11. Doering, L.V. (1999). Pathophysiology of acute coronary syndromes leading to acute myocardial infarction. *Journal of Cardiovascular Nursing, 13*(3), 1-20.
12. Dracup, K., & Cannon, C. (1999, April). Combination treatment strategies for management of acute myocardial infarction. *Critical Care Nurse Supplement,* 1-17.
13. Gibbons, R.J., et al. (2003). ACC/AHA 2002 guideline update for the management of patients with chronic stable angina: A summary article. *Circulation, 107,* 149-158.
14. Gibbons, R., et al. (2002). ACC/AHA 2002 guideline update for exercise testing: Summary article. *Circulation, 106,* 1883-1890.
15. Hudson, M., et al. (1999). Cardiac markers: Point of care testing. *Clinica Chimica Acta, 28*(4), 223-237.

16. Huikuri, H., et al. (2001). Sudden death due to cardiac arrhythmias. *New England Journal of Medicine, 345*(20), 1473-1482.

17. Lau, J., et al. (2001). Evaluation of technologies for identifying acute cardiac ischemia in emergency departments. *AHRQ Publication Evidence Report/Technology Assessment Number 26.* Available at www.ahrq.gov/.

18. Lee, T.H., & Goldman, L. (2000). Evaluation of the patient with acute chest pain. *New England Journal of Medicine, 342*(16), 1187-1193.

19. Libby, P., Ridker, P., & Maseri, A. (2002). Inflammation and athero-sclerosis. *Circulation, 105,* 1135-1143.

20. McAvoy, J. (2004). Case studies of ST-segment elevation before and after percutaneous coronary intervention in patients with acute myocardial infarction. *Critical Care Nurse, 21*(6), 32-39.

21. Murphy, M., & Berding, C. (1999). Use of myoglobins and cardiac troponins in the diagnosis of acute myocardial infarction. *Critical Care Nurse, 19*(1), 58-65.

22. O'Connor, C.M., Gattis, W.A., & Swedberg, K. (1999). Current and novel pharmacologic approaches in advanced heart failure. *Heart and Lung, 28,* 227-239.

23. Peeters, A., et al. (2002). A cardiovascular life history—A life course analysis of the original Framingham Heart Study cohort. *European Heart Journal, 23*(6), 795-799.

24. Rich, M.W. (1999). Heart failure disease management: A critical review. *Journal of Cardiac Failure, 5*(1), 64-75.

25. Rosenfeld, A. (2006). State of the heart: Building science to improve women's cardiovascular health. *American Journal of Critical Care, 15,* 556-567.

26. Smith, S., et al. (2006). ACC/AHA guidelines for secondary prevention for patients with coronary and other atherosclerotic vascular diseases: 2006 update. *Journal of American College of Cardiology, 47,* 2130-2139.

27. Soran, O., Schneider, V.M., & Feldman, A.M. (1999). Basic therapy for congestive heart failure: Current practice, new prospects. *Journal of Critical Illness, 14*(2), 78-89.

28. Thygesen, K., et al. (2000). Myocardial infarction redefined. A consensus document of the Joint European Society of Cardiology/American College of Cardiology Committee for the Redefinition of Myocardial Infarction. *Journal of American College of Cardiology, 36*(3), 959-969.

evolve   *Did you remember to check out the bonus material on the Evolve website and the CD-ROM, including NCLEX®-Examination Style Review Questions, Open-Book Quizzes, and Chapter Review Audio Podcasts?*

http://evolve.elsevier.com/Black/medsurg

UNIT 14

OXYGENATION DISORDERS

ANATOMY AND PHYSIOLOGY REVIEW:

The Respiratory System

Robert G. Carroll

Our body needs a constant supply of oxygen to support metabolism. The respiratory system brings oxygen through the airways of the lung into the alveoli, where it diffuses into the blood for transport to the tissues. This process is so vital that difficulty in breathing is experienced as a threat to life itself. Whether death is a real possibility or not, people with respiratory disorders are often anxious and fearful that they may die, perhaps agonizingly.

The respiratory system also has other essential functions:

- Expels carbon dioxide (CO_2), a metabolic waste product that is transported from the tissues to the lungs for elimination
- Filters and humidifies air that enters the lungs
- Traps particulate matter in the mucus of the airways and propels it toward the mouth for elimination by coughing or swallowing
- Prevents the entry of inhaled pathogens by activating the immune system

Respiratory control is tied most closely to arterial blood and brain CO_2 levels as well as to arterial blood oxygen levels. Respiration is also controlled by higher cortical centers. For example, an increase in ventilation accompanies exercise and keeps arterial blood gases within the normal range.

Respiratory problems are widespread. Acute disorders range from minor inconveniences (colds or flu) to more life-threatening problems (asthma, some types of pneumonia, and chest trauma). Chronic disabling conditions include *chronic airflow limitation* (also called chronic obstructive pulmonary disease) and certain restrictive lung diseases. Chronic respiratory problems affect many people, often causing them to make radical lifestyle changes, such as retiring from work earlier than they wish.

Respiratory problems are associated with many causes: allergies, occupational factors, genetic factors, smoking and tobacco use, infection, neuromuscular disorders, chest abnormalities, trauma, pleural conditions, and pulmonary vascular abnormalities. The most significant factor in chronic respiratory illness and lung cancer is cigarette smoking.

STRUCTURE OF THE RESPIRATORY SYSTEM

UPPER AIRWAYS

The airways are the regions through which air passes on its way to the exchange areas of the lungs. The upper airways consist of the nasal cavities, pharynx, and larynx.

Nasal Cavity

The nose is formed from both bone and cartilage. The nasal bone forms the bridge, and the remainder of the nose is composed of cartilage and connective tissue (Figure A&P14-1). Each opening of the nose on the face (*nostrils* or *nares*) leads to a cavity (*vestibule*). The vestibule is lined anteriorly with skin and hair that filter foreign objects and prevent them from being inhaled. The posterior vestibule is lined with a mucous membrane, composed of columnar epithelial cells, and goblet cells that secrete mucus. The mucous membrane extends throughout the airways, and cilia (hair-like projections) propel mucus to the pharynx for elimination by swallowing or coughing. The portion of the mucous membrane that is located at the top of the nasal cavity, just beneath the cribriform plate of the ethmoid bone, is specialized (*olfactory*) epithelium, which provides the sense of smell. Because the olfactory epithelium does not lie along the usual path of air movement, smell is enhanced by sniffing.

Along the sides of the vestibule are *turbinates,* mucous membrane–covered projections that contain a rich blood supply from the internal and external carotid arteries. They warm and humidify inspired air.

Paranasal sinuses, open areas within the skull, are named for the bones in which they lie: frontal, ethmoid, sphenoid, and maxillary. Passageways from the paranasal sinuses drain into the nasal cavities. The nasolacrimal ducts, which drain tears from the surface of the eyes, also drain into the nasal cavity.

The mouth is considered part of the upper airway but only because it can be used to deliver air to the lungs

FIGURE A&P14–1 Structures of the upper airway. Air enters the body through the nares or mouth and is filtered and humidified while passing toward the alveoli. The epiglottis directs air into the trachea during respiration and directs food into the esophagus during swallowing. Dashed arrows indicate passage of air into sinuses.

when the nose is obstructed or when high volumes of air are needed, such as during exercise. The mouth does not perform the nasal functions efficiently, especially those of warming, humidifying, and filtering air.

Pharynx

The pharynx is a funnel-shaped tube that extends from the nose to the larynx. It can be divided into three sections.

The *nasopharynx* is located above the margin of the soft palate and receives air from the nasal cavity. From the ear, the eustachian tubes open into the nasopharynx. The pharyngeal tonsils (called *adenoids* when enlarged) are located on the posterior wall of the nasopharynx.

The *oropharynx* serves both respiration and digestion. It receives air from the nasopharynx and food from the oral cavity. Palatine (faucial) tonsils are located along the sides of the posterior mouth, and the lingual tonsils are located at the base of the tongue.

The *laryngopharynx (hypopharynx)*, located below the base of the tongue, is the most inferior portion of the pharynx. It connects to the larynx and serves both respiration and digestion.

Larynx

The larynx is commonly called the *voice box*. It connects the upper (pharynx) and lower (trachea) airways. The larynx lies just anterior to the upper esophagus. Nine cartilages form the larynx: three large unpaired cartilages (epiglottis, thyroid, cricoid) and three smaller paired cartilages (arytenoid, corniculate, cuneiform). The cartilages are attached to the hyoid bone above and below the trachea by muscles and ligaments, all of which prevent the larynx from collapse during inspiration and swallowing.

The larynx consists of the endolarynx and a surrounding triangle-shaped bone and cartilage. The endolarynx is formed by two paired folds of tissue, forming the false and the true vocal cords. The slit between the vocal cords forms the *glottis*. The *epiglottis,* a leaf-shaped structure immediately posterior to the base of the tongue, lies above the larynx. When food or liquids are swallowed, the epiglottis closes over the larynx, protecting the lower airways from aspiration.

The thyroid cartilage protrudes in front of the larynx, forming the "Adam's apple." The cricoid cartilage lies just below the thyroid cartilage and is the anatomic site for an artificial opening into the trachea (tracheostomy, or cricothyroidotomy). The internal portion of the larynx is composed of muscles that assist with swallowing, speaking, and respiration and that contribute to the pitch of the voice. The blood supply to the larynx is through the branches of the thyroid arteries. The nerve supply is through the recurrent laryngeal and superior laryngeal nerves.

LOWER AIRWAYS

The lower airway, or tracheobronchial tree, is composed of the trachea, right and left mainstem bronchi, segmental bronchi, subsegmental bronchi, and terminal bronchioles (Figure A&P14-2). Smooth muscle, wound in overlapping clockwise and counterclockwise helical bands, is found in all of these structures. This arrangement allows contraction of the smooth muscle to decrease the diameter of the airways, increasing the resistance to air flow. This muscle is subject to spasm in many airway disorders. The lower airways continue to warm, humidify, and filter inspired air as it flows toward the lungs.

Trachea

The trachea (windpipe) extends from the larynx to the level of the seventh thoracic vertebra, where it divides into two main *(primary)* bronchi. The point at which the trachea divides is called the *carina*. The trachea is a flexible, muscular, 12-cm-long air passage with C-shaped cartilaginous rings. Along with all other regions

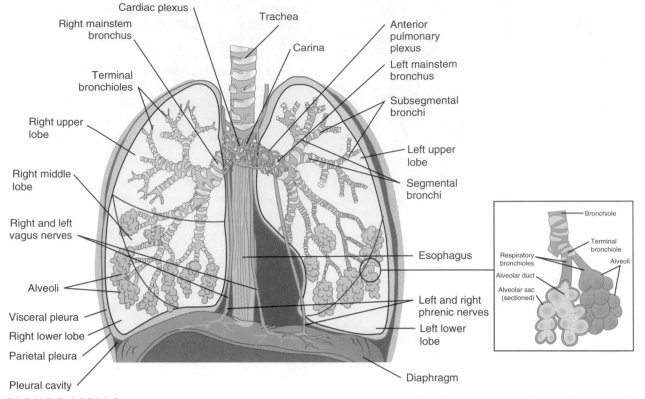

■ **FIGURE A&P14–2** Structures of the lower airways. Air passes from the trachea through bronchi and bronchioles before reaching the alveoli. Cartilage in the bronchi and trachea prevents airway collapse during forced expiration. *Inset:* Gas exchange occurs in the respiratory zone, which consists of the respiratory bronchioles, alveolar ducts, and alveolar sacs.

of the lower airways it is lined with pseudostratified columnar epithelium that contains goblet (mucus-secreting) cells and cilia (Figure A&P14-3). Because the cilia beat upward, they tend to propel foreign particles and excessive mucus away from the lungs to the pharynx. No cilia are present in the alveoli.

Bronchi and Bronchioles

The right mainstem bronchus is shorter and wider, extending more vertically downward, than the left mainstem bronchus. Thus foreign bodies are more likely to lodge there than in the left mainstem bronchus. The *segmental* and *subsegmental bronchi* are subdivisions of the main bronchi and spread in an inverted, tree-like formation through each lung. Cartilage surrounds the airway in the bronchi, but the bronchioles (the final pathway to the alveoli) contain no cartilage and thus can collapse and trap air during active exhalation.

The *terminal bronchioles* are the last airways of the conducting system. The area from the nose to the terminal bronchioles does not exchange gas and functions as *anatomic dead space*. The lack of gas exchange means that the first air out of the mouth during exhalation resembles room air, but the last air out (end-tidal air) resembles alveolar air.

LUNGS AND ALVEOLI

Lungs

The lungs lie within the thoracic cavity on either side of the heart (see Figure A&P14-2). They are cone-shaped, with the apex above the first rib and the base resting on the diaphragm. Each lung is divided into superior and inferior lobes by an oblique fissure. The right lung is further divided by a horizontal fissure, which creates a middle lobe. The right lung, therefore, has three lobes; the left lobe has only two. In addition to these 5 lobes, which are visible externally, each lung can be subdivided into about 10 smaller units *(bronchopulmonary segments)*. Each segment represents the portion of the lung that is supplied by a specific tertiary bronchus. These segments are important surgically, because a diseased segment can be resected without the need to remove the entire lobe or lung. The two lungs are separated by a space (the *mediastinum*) where the heart, aorta, vena cava, pulmonary vessels, esophagus, part of the trachea and bronchi, and the thymus gland are located.

The lungs contain gas, blood, thin alveolar walls, and support structures. The alveolar walls contain elastic and collagen fibers; these form a three-dimensional, basket-like structure that allows the lung to inflate in all directions. These fibers are capable of stretching when a

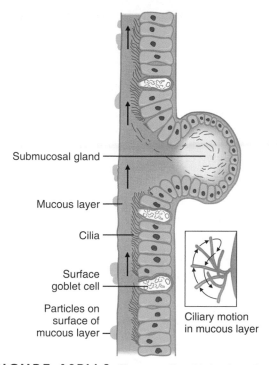

■ **FIGURE A&PI4-3** The mucociliary blanket is an important respiratory defense mechanism. Mucus is secreted by surface goblet cells. About 100 ml of mucus is normally secreted each day by the submucosal glands. Mucus covers the epithelial lining of the tracheobronchial tree in two layers: the watery solution layer close to the mucosal surface and the thicker gel layer. The cilia (hair-like projections) beat in an upward direction toward the upper airway. Particulate matter is trapped on the mucous layer and moved upward by the cilia. Debris-laden mucus is then either swallowed or expectorated as sputum.

pulling force is exerted on them from outside of the body or when they are inflated from within. The elastic recoil helps return the lungs to their resting volume.

Branches of the pulmonary artery provide most of the blood supply to the lungs. The blood is oxygen-poor, but oxygen is supplied by inspired air. The trachea and bronchioles, which are not part of the oxygen exchange surface, receive oxygen-rich blood from branches of the aorta.

Lung Volumes

The lungs of an average 19-year-old man have a total capacity of about 5900 ml. However, a person cannot exhale all the air from the lungs, and about 1200 ml of air always remains, no matter how forceful the expiration. This remaining volume *(residual volume)* prevents the collapse of the lung structures during expiration. The volume of air that moves in and out with each breath is called the *tidal volume.* During quiet breathing, tidal volume is about 500 ml. When a person takes a deep breath, the lung is more fully expanded. The amount of extra air inhaled, beyond the tidal volume, is called the *inspiratory reserve volume;* the extra air that can be exhaled after a forced breath is called the *expiratory reserve volume.*

Lung volumes are often combined into capacities:

- *Total lung capacity:* all four volumes
- *Vital capacity:* all volumes except residual volume, which is the amount a person can ventilate
- *Functional reserve capacity:* expiratory reserve plus residual volumes
- *Inspiratory capacity:* tidal volume plus inspiratory reserve volume

The rate at which air can be expelled from the lungs also provides diagnostic information. The "timed" forced expiratory volume (FEV) is obtained by having the client perform a maximum inspiration (to total lung capacity) followed by a maximal exhalation (to residual volume). The total amount of air exhaled is the vital capacity. FEV_1 indicates the volume of air exhaled during the first second, usually about 80% of vital capacity, and FEV_3 indicates the volume of air exhaled during 3 seconds, usually about 95% of vital capacity.

These volumes and capacities are frequently altered by disease. The pattern and severity of the change correlate with the severity of the disease processes. Lung volumes as measured by spirometry are shown in Figure A&PI4-4. Pulmonary function tests are described in Chapter 59.

Alveoli

The lung parenchyma, which consists of millions of alveolar units, is the working area of the lung tissue. At birth, a person has approximately 24 million alveoli; by age 8 years, a person has 300 million. The total working alveolar surface area is approximately 750 to 860 square feet. The blood supply flowing toward the alveoli comes from the right ventricle of the heart.

The entire alveolar unit (respiratory zone) is made up of respiratory bronchioles, alveolar ducts, and alveolar

■ **FIGURE A&PI4-4** Lung volumes and capacities as measured by spirometry. The four volumes of the lungs (identified on the left) are combined to form four capacities (identified on the right).

sacs (see Figure A&P14-2). The alveolar walls are extremely thin, with an almost solid network of interconnecting capillaries. Because of the extensiveness of the capillary system, the flow of blood in the alveolar wall has been described as a "sheet" of flowing blood.

Oxygen and CO_2 are exchanged through a respiratory membrane, about 0.2 mm thick (Figure A&P14-5). The average diameter of the pulmonary capillary is only about 5 μm, but red blood cells (7 μm in diameter) must squeeze through, actually touching the capillary wall. Thus the distance across which oxygen and CO_2 must diffuse is greatly reduced. Thickening of the respiratory membrane (e.g., with pulmonary edema or fibrosis) may interfere with normal exchange of gases.

The alveolus comprises two cell types: *type I pneumocytes,* which line the alveolus, are thin and incapable of reproduction but are effective in gas exchange. *Type II pneumocytes* are cuboidal and do not exchange oxygen and CO_2 well. They produce surfactant and are important in lung injury and repair because they differentiate into alveolar macrophages. They differentiate into type I cells; oxygenation is impaired during the transition from type II to type I cells.

THORAX

The bony thorax provides protection for the lungs, heart, and great vessels. The outer shell of the thorax is made up of 12 pairs of ribs. The ribs connect posteriorly to the transverse processes of the thoracic vertebrae of the spine. Anteriorly, the first seven pairs of ribs are attached to the sternum by cartilage. The 8th, 9th, and 10th ribs *(false ribs)* are attached to each other by costal cartilage. The 11th and 12th ribs *(floating ribs)* allow full chest expansion because they are not attached in any way to the sternum.

DIAPHRAGM

Breathing is accomplished by skeletal muscle alteration of the thoracic space. The diaphragm is the primary muscle of breathing and serves as the lower boundary of the thorax (Figure A&P14-6). The diaphragm is dome-shaped in the relaxed position, with central muscular attachments to the xiphoid process of the sternum and the lower ribs. Contraction of the diaphragm pulls the muscle downward, increasing the thoracic space and actively inflating the lungs. The nerve supply of the diaphragm

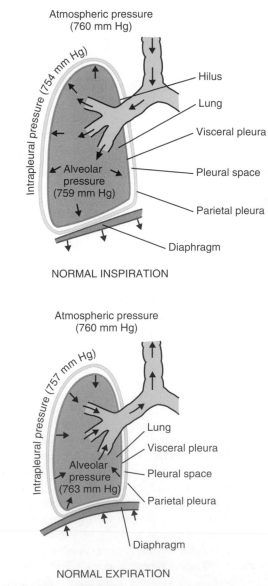

NORMAL INSPIRATION

NORMAL EXPIRATION

■ **FIGURE A&P14-6** Normal inspiration and expiration. Contraction of the diaphragm increases the size of the thoracic cavity, and reduces alveolar pressure to below atmospheric pressure. Relaxation of the diaphragm allows the elastic recoil of the lungs to diminish the size of the thoracic cavity, increasing alveolar pressure to greater than atmospheric pressure.

■ **FIGURE A&P14–5** The ultrastructure of the respiratory membrane where oxygen is exchanged. Accumulation of fluid in the interstitial space (pulmonary edema) diminishes the diffusion of oxygen into the pulmonary capillary.

(phrenic nerve) comes through the spinal cord at the level of the third cervical vertebra. Thus spinal injuries at C3 or above can impair ventilation.

PLEURAE

The pleurae are serous membranes that enclose the lung in a double-walled sac. The *visceral* pleura covers the lung and the fissures between the lobes of the lung. The *parietal* pleura covers the inside of each hemithorax, the mediastinum, and the top of the diaphragm; it joins the visceral pleura at the *hilus* (a notch in the medial surface of the lung, where the mainstem bronchi, pulmonary blood vessels, and nerves enter the lung).

Normally, no space exists between the pleurae; the *pleural space* is a potential space between the two layers of pleura. A thin film (only a few milliliters) of serous fluid acts as a lubricant in the potential space. The fluid also causes the moist pleural membranes to adhere, creating a pulling force that helps to hold the lungs in an expanded position because the parietal pleura is attached to the rib cage. The action of the pleurae is analogous to coupling two sheets of glass with a thin film of water. It is extremely difficult to separate the sheets of glass at right angles, yet they readily slide along each other. Because of the nature of this coupling, the movement of the lungs closely follows the movement of the thorax. If air or increased amounts of serous fluid, blood, or pus accumulate in the thoracic space, the lungs are compressed and respiratory difficulties follow. These conditions constitute *pneumothorax* (air in the pleural space) or *hemothorax* (blood in the pleural space) and pleural effusion (fluid in the pleural space).

FUNCTION OF THE RESPIRATORY SYSTEM

The respiratory system enhances gas exchange. Inspiration brings oxygen-rich air into the alveoli. The upper and lower airways filter and humidify inspired air. Gas exchange between the air and the blood occurs in the alveolus. Oxygen diffuses into the blood, and CO_2 diffuses from the blood into the alveolar air. The CO_2-enriched air is removed from the body during expiration. The large number and large surface area of alveoli are necessary to meet both resting and exercise gas exchange requirements.

The thorax and diaphragm alter pressures in the thorax to drive air movement. The movement of air depends on pressure gradients between the atmosphere and the air in the lungs, with air flowing from regions of higher pressure to regions of lower pressure. On inspiration, the dome of the diaphragm flattens and the rib cage lifts. As thoracic and lung volumes increase, alveolar pressure decreases and air is drawn into the lungs.

Airway resistance also affects air movement and is affected primarily by the diameter of the airways. Decreasing the diameter by half results in a 16-fold increase in airway resistance. Thus a decreased diameter of the airways caused by bronchial muscle contraction or by secretions in the airways increases resistance and decreases the rate of air flow. This is a common finding in obstructive airway diseases such as asthma.

During quiet breathing, expiration is usually passive, that is, does not require the use of muscles. The chest wall, in contrast to the lungs, tends to recoil outward. The opposing forces of lung and chest wall create a subatmospheric (negative) force of about −5 cm of water in the intrapleural space at the end of quiet exhalation. Exhalation is also a result of elastic recoil of the lungs.

VENTILATION

Ventilation, the movement of air in and out of the lungs (especially the removal of carbon dioxide from the lungs), involves three forces: (1) compliance properties of the lung and the thorax (chest wall), (2) surface tension, and (3) the muscular efforts of inspiratory muscles.

Compliance

Compliance refers to the ease with which the lung expands and indicates the relationship between the volume and the pressure of the lungs. The lungs are elastic structures that tend to recoil to a volume slightly less than *residual volume* (the volume of gas remaining in the lungs after a full exhalation). The force required to distend the lungs is the difference between the alveolar pressure and the intrapleural pressure. Diseases that cause fibrosis of the lungs result in "stiff" lungs with low compliance; stiff lungs require high inspiratory pressures to achieve a set volume of gas. In contrast, diseases such as emphysema that damage the elastic structure of the alveolar walls result in "floppy" lungs with greater compliance but poor recoil. Relatively low pressures can achieve the same volume of air during inspiration. Passive exhalation, normally a function of elastic recoil, is impaired.

Surface Tension

Changes in the surface tension of the liquid film lining the alveoli also affect compliance by changing resistance. *Surface tension,* the result of the air-liquid interface at each alveolus, restricts alveolar expansion on inspiration and aids alveolar collapse on expiration. Surfactant produced by type II cells in the alveolar lining lowers surface tension and thus increases compliance and aids ventilation and oxygenation. A deficiency of surfactant results in stiff lungs. Premature babies lacking surfactant may suffer infant respiratory distress syndrome, formerly called hyaline membrane disease.

Muscular Effort

Ventilation also requires muscular effort. For inspiration to occur, the pressure within the alveoli must be less than atmospheric pressure. Contraction of the diaphragm and the external intercostal muscles enlarges the size of the thorax. The external intercostal muscles pull the ribs upward and forward, thus increasing the transverse and anteroposterior diameter. Two accessory muscles of inspiration—the scalene and sternocleidomastoid muscles—elevate the first and second ribs during inspiration to enlarge the upper thorax and stabilize the chest wall. The sternocleidomastoid muscle elevates the sternum. The expanding thorax creates a more negative intrapleural pressure, which expands the lungs. When the alveolar pressure becomes lower than the atmospheric pressure, air flows into the lungs.

During exhalation, the inspiratory muscles relax. The elastic recoil of the lung tissue increases alveolar pressure above atmospheric pressure and causes air to move out of the lungs. Air flow stops when the recoil pressure of the lungs balances the muscular and elastic forces of the chest (see Figure A&P14-6).

Although expiration is usually passive, forced expiration and coughing employ accessory muscles to decrease the size of the thoracic space and cause expiration. Contraction of the abdominal muscles forces the diaphragm upward to its dome-shaped position. Contraction of the internal intercostal muscles pulls the ribs inward, thus decreasing the anteroposterior diameter of the chest wall.

Work of Breathing

Respiratory muscle contraction represents a significant metabolic load. Tidal volume and respiratory rate are adjusted to minimize the workload on the body. For example, clients with obstructive lung disease use slower but deeper breaths to maintain appropriate alveolar ventilation. Clients with restrictive lung disease use frequent, shallow breaths to maintain alveolar ventilation.

RESPIRATORY CONTROL

Human metabolism is not one of steady state. The oxygen needs of the tissues change with changing metabolic demands. Respiratory control mechanisms match the elimination of CO_2 and supply of oxygen to the metabolic needs. The lungs have no intrinsic control of themselves; instead, they are controlled by the central nervous system.

Central Nervous System Control

The medulla has several levels of respiratory centers. The dorsal respiratory group primarily provides for inspiration. The ventral respiratory group is normally quiet unless increased ventilation is needed or if active exhalation is performed. The pons has an apneustic center, which contains both expiratory and inspiratory neurons. The upper pons contains the pneumotaxic center, which fine-tunes breathing. For example, the pneumotaxic center allows for talking and breathing.

Output from the respiratory neurons, located in the medulla, descends via the ventral and lateral columns of the spinal cord to phrenic motor neurons of the diaphragm and intercostal motor neurons of the intercostal muscles. The result is rhythmic respiratory movements.

The cortex also allows voluntary control of breathing (holding our breath or altering the rate or depth of breathing).

Reflex Control

The cough reflex is a neural reflex stimulated by mechanical stimuli (Table A&P14-1). Inhaled irritants and mucus (mechanical stimuli) excite rapidly adapting pulmonary stretch receptors concentrated in the region of the carina and the large bronchi. The stimulation of the receptors results in high-velocity expiratory gas flow (cough).

Peripheral Control

Peripheral control of respiration is due to the sensing of the partial pressure of oxygen (Po_2) and the partial pressure of CO_2 (Pco_2) in the blood. In the blood, CO_2 is an acid. An increase in Pco_2 causes acidosis, and a decrease in pH. Receptors that are responsive to changes in oxygen, CO_2, and pH are located in the brain and in structures adjacent to blood vessels. Arterial blood oxygen and CO_2 pressures are sensed by receptors in the carotid body and the aortic body. The carotid body receptors are located close to the carotid sinus, and the aortic

TABLE A&P14–1	Physiologic Elements of a Cough
Deep inspiration	Inhaled volume of air must be sufficient to increase lung volume, to increase diameter of bronchi and bronchioles, and to move mucus up and out of airways
Inspiratory pause	Allows a buildup and distribution of air and pressure distal to mucus
Closed glottis	Intact muscles and nerves supplying larynx required; allows development of high intrapleural pressures, resulting in a high air flow velocity to propel mucus out of airway
Abdominal muscles	Increase intra-abdominal pressure, which forces diaphragm upward to increase intrapleural pressure against closed glottis
Open glottis	After intrapleural pressures increase, glottis opens suddenly to allow a high velocity of air to leave lungs; flow rates may be as high as 300 L/min
Mucus is expelled	Expulsion caused by high velocity of air leaving airway

bodies are located near the aortic arch. Chemoreceptors are also located on the brain side of the blood-brain barrier. These receptors respond only to P_{CO_2} (or pH). An elevated P_{CO_2} in arterial blood is the normal stimulus to increase ventilation. Low levels of partial pressure of oxygen in arterial blood (Pao_2) can stimulate ventilation, but only when Po_2 drops below 70 mm Hg. There is a powerful synergism between these respiratory stimuli, with the greatest ventilatory drive caused by a simultaneous increase in P_{CO_2} and decrease in Po_2.

GAS EXCHANGE AND TRANSPORT

The exchange of gases occurs between air and blood in the respiratory membrane. Respiration is the exchange of oxygen and CO_2 at the alveolar-capillary level (*external respiration*) and at the tissue-cellular level (*internal respiration*). During respiration, body tissues are supplied with oxygen for metabolism and CO_2 is released.

In the earth's atmosphere, air contains 20.84% oxygen, 78.62% nitrogen, 0.04% CO_2, and 0.50% water vapor. Each gas exerts a pressure (*partial pressure*) as if it were the only gas present. The sum of the partial pressures is the *barometric pressure*. When a liquid is exposed to a gas, gas enters the liquid in proportion to the individual pressures. Po_2 in the alveoli is about 104 mm Hg, and P_{CO_2} is about 40 mm Hg. Venous blood has a Po_2 of 40 mm Hg and a P_{CO_2} of about 45 mm Hg. These differences in concentration result in the movement of oxygen into the pulmonary capillary bloodstream and of CO_2 out of the pulmonary capillary bed into the alveoli (Figure A&P14-7).

The high Po_2 gradient between the alveolar air and blood is necessary because oxygen is less soluble than CO_2. Diseases that decrease gas diffusion generally alter oxygen exchange before altering carbon dioxide exchange.

Oxygen Transport

After diffusing into the pulmonary capillaries, oxygen is transported throughout the body by the circulatory system. The oxygen is dissolved in the plasma (3%) or bound in the ferrous iron–containing protein hemoglobin (97%). The combination of hemoglobin and oxygen forms *oxyhemoglobin*, which greatly increases the

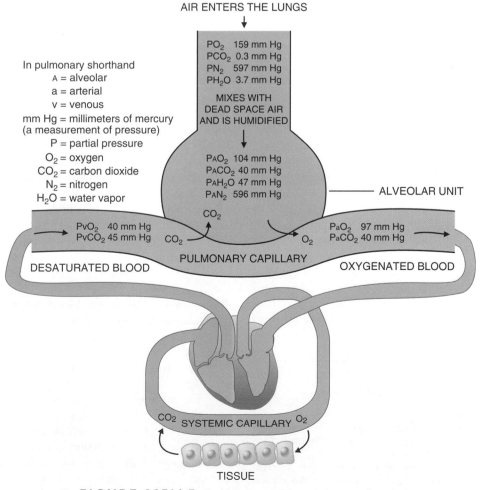

■ FIGURE A&P14–7 Partial pressures of gases during normal respiration.

oxygen content of the blood above that dissolved in plasma. Tissues take up oxygen at varying rates; the rate of oxygen consumption creates an oxygen pressure gradient between the blood and the mitochondria. Carbon monoxide (CO) and other chemicals impair the ability of hemoglobin to transport oxygen in the blood.

The *oxyhemoglobin dissociation curve* represents the relationship between Pao_2 and the saturation of hemoglobin. This saturation reflects the amount of oxygen available to the tissues. For a normal curve, it is assumed that the client's temperature is 37° C, pH is 7.40, and Pco_2 is 40 mm Hg. The oxyhemoglobin dissociation curve is affected by a number of factors, including (1) temperature, (2) pH, (3) Pco_2, (4) substances in the red blood cell (2,3-diphosphoglycerate [2,3-DPG]), (5) presence of CO, and (6) abnormal hemoglobin. Changes in the affinity of oxygen for hemoglobin cause the oxyhemoglobin curve to move from its normal contour, or to *shift* (Figure A&P14-8).

A *shift to the left* of the oxyhemoglobin dissociation curve increases the affinity of the hemoglobin molecule for oxygen. It is easier for oxygen to bind to hemoglobin, but oxygen is not easily released at the tissues. Thus at any Po_2 level, oxygen saturation is greater than normal but tissue hypoxia is present. Clinical situations that diminish the tissue delivery of oxygen include alkalosis, hypocapnia, hypothermia, decreased 2,3-DPG levels, and CO poisoning.

A *shift to the right* indicates an easier release of oxygen at the tissue level but more difficulty in binding in the lungs. This shift protects the body by allowing oxygen attached to hemoglobin to be released in the tissues to maintain adequate tissue oxygenation. Exercise improves the delivery of oxygen to the tissues, as do a number of clinical situations, including acidosis, hypercapnia, hyperthermia, hyperthyroidism (which increases 2,3-DPG levels), anemia, and chronic hypoxia.

Alternatively, shifts in the oxyhemoglobin dissociation curve can be expressed by a single numerical value—the P_{50}. The P_{50} represents that oxygen partial pressure at which 50% of the hemoglobin is bound to oxygen, that is, the 50% saturation point. If the affinity of hemoglobin for oxygen is decreased (shifted to the right), then a higher oxygen partial pressure is needed to bind 50% of the hemoglobin and the P_{50} is increased. Conversely, a decrease in the P_{50} represents a leftward shift in the curve, or an increase in the affinity of hemoglobin for oxygen (see Figure A&P14-8).

Carbon Dioxide Transport

CO_2, the waste product of tissue metabolism, is carried by the blood in the following ways: (1) combined with water as carbonic acid (70%), (2) coupled with hemoglobin (23%), or (3) dissolved in plasma (7%). Red blood cells contain the enzyme carbonic anhydrase, which rapidly breaks down CO_2 into hydrogen ions and bicarbonate ions. When venous blood enters the lungs for gas exchange, this reaction reverses, forming CO_2, which is then exhaled.

Relationship Between Ventilation and Perfusion

The relationship between *ventilation* (air flow) and *perfusion* (blood flow) determines the efficiency of gas exchange. Figure A&P14-9 illustrates ventilation with perfusion (unit of dead space), lack of ventilation of an alveolar unit with continued perfusion (a shunt), and total blockage with collapse of alveoli (atelectasis). Low ventilation-perfusion ($\dot{V}/\dot{Q}$) ratios and high $\dot{V}/\dot{Q}$ ratios both result in lower oxygen delivery to the body.

The ventilation-perfusion balance differs from the top to the base of the lung. Blood flow and (to a lesser extent) ventilation are greater in the more dependent lung segments at the base of the lung. Consequently,

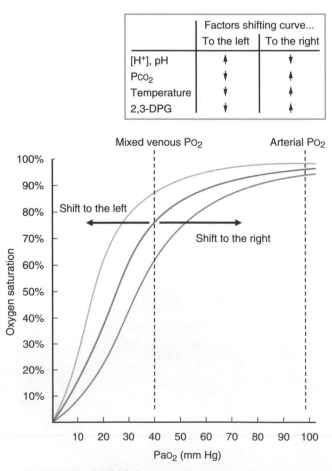

■ **FIGURE A&P14-8** The normal oxyhemoglobin dissociation curve, showing how changes in the affinity of oxygen for hemoglobin shift the curve to the right or the left. Changes in the Pao_2 at the flattened top portion of the curve result in small changes in oxygen saturation. The opposite is true as the slope of the curve becomes steeper. At the steepest portion of the curve, with the Pao_2 below 60 mm Hg, small changes in the Pao_2 result in large decreases in oxygen saturation.

NORMAL
A normally functioning alveolus and normal pulmonary capillary flow. Ventilation and perfusion match.

DEAD SPACE UNIT
When there is ventilation without perfusion, a dead space unit exists. Example: Pulmonary embolus preventing blood flow through the pulmonary capillary.

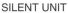

SHUNT UNIT
When there is no ventilation to an alveolar unit but perfusion continues, a shunt unit exists, and unoxygenated blood continues to circulate. Examples: atelectasis, pneumonia. The alveoli collapse.

SILENT UNIT
When there is neither ventilation nor perfusion, a silent unit develops. Example: Pulmonary embolus combined with ARDS (adult respiratory distress syndrome). The alveoli collapse.

■ **FIGURE A&PI4–9** Relationships between ventilation (air flow) and perfusion (blood flow).

the base of the lung has the lowest $\dot{V}/\dot{Q}$ ratio, and the apex of the lung has the highest $\dot{V}/\dot{Q}$ ratio.

The $\dot{V}/\dot{Q}$ balance is controlled at both the airway and vascular levels. Hypoxia, resulting from underventilation of an alveolar region, causes vasoconstriction, which redirects blood to well-ventilated alveoli. CO_2 in the airways dilates the airway smooth muscle. Poorly perfused alveoli have low CO_2 levels, and the resultant airway constriction directs ventilation to better perfused alveoli.

REGULATION OF ACID-BASE BALANCE

The lungs, through gas exchange, have a key role in regulating the acid-base balance of the body. Pulmonary disorders that change the CO_2 level in the blood cause either respiratory acidemia or respiratory alkalemia. Insufficient ventilation causes *hypercapnia,* a respiratory acidemia caused by retention of excessive amounts of CO_2. Hyperventilation, conversely, causes *hypocapnia,* a respiratory alkalemia caused by the low amounts of CO_2 in the blood.

The effectiveness of ventilation is best measured by the P_{CO_2} in the arterial blood (Pa_{CO_2}). Because the respiratory system normally maintains a Pa_{CO_2} between 35 and 45 mm Hg at sea level, a Pa_{CO_2} above this range represents *hypoventilation.* Anesthetic agents, sedatives, and opioids all tend to increase the resting Pa_{CO_2}. (Acid-base balance is detailed in Chapter 13.)

REACTION TO INJURY

The elaborate defense mechanisms of the lungs involve clearance mechanisms, defense by the respiratory epithelium, and immunologic responses in the lungs. Any injury to the lung affects the barrier between the atmosphere and the bloodstream. This barrier, which lies within the alveolar septum, is made up of epithelial (types I and II pneumocytes) and vascular endothelial cells. Injury resulting from airborne or blood-borne agents may increase vascular permeability and cause pulmonary edema. Inflammatory cells (e.g., neutrophils) arrive soon after acute injury. Then the proportion of lymphocytes, monocytes, and macrophages increases following a typical inflammatory process.

The basic lung repair processes include lymphatic drainage of excess fluid and phagocytic removal of protein and debris. This action generally restores lung function and structure. More severe injury requires endothelial and epithelial cell regeneration and proliferation of interstitial cells (fibroblasts). Type II cells that are generated for defense eventually differentiate into thin type I cells, which permit gas exchange. The lung's ability to recreate alveolar septa determines the degree to which normal lung function and structure are restored.

Defense by Clearance Mechanisms

The *upper airways* filter particles. Because the nose has a larger surface-volume ratio and a much more tortuous pathway for airflow than the mouth, particle deposition and conditioning of the air are more efficient when a person breathes through the nose. Larger particles (>10 mm) are generally trapped; smaller particles (<1 mm) may readily enter the lower airways.

There are four clearance mechanisms of the lower airways and alveoli:

- Cough (first five to eight bronchial generations)
- Mucociliary system (to terminal bronchioles)
- Macrophages (alveoli and respiratory bronchioles)
- Lymphatics (alveoli and interstitium)

The cough, an automatic protective reflex used to clear the trachea, occurs most rapidly in the clearing process (see Table A&PI4-1). If the swallowing reflex is delayed or absent, a cough may be stimulated to avoid aspiration of particles into the lower airways.

Defense by the Respiratory Epithelium

Unlike the upper and lower airways, the alveoli lack a mucous layer to trap foreign particles and cilia to propel them to the pharynx for elimination. The alveolar lining is made up of flat, membranous pneumocytes (type I cells) and rounded granular (type II) cells. The type II cells are resistant to injury and cover most of the alveolar surface after exposure to infectious agents. Alveolar macrophages, derived from type II pneumocytes, are also found over the surface of the alveoli. Alveolar macrophages are active phagocytes that remove dead cells and protein and that synthesize and secrete substances that regulate the immune system. They leave the lung by the mucociliary system or the lymphatic system.

Defense by Immunologic Mechanisms

The systemic immune system responds to the lung during inflammatory processes by mobilizing blood neutrophils and monocytes. Recruited thymus-dependent (T) and thymus-independent (B) lymphocytes contribute to local cell-mediated immune reactions and the production of specific antibodies within the alveoli. Cell-mediated immunity is a key determinant in resistance to organisms such as *Mycobacterium tuberculosis* and *Pneumocystis (carinii) jiroveci*. Immune mechanisms are generally a host defense function. However, hypersensitivity immune reactions lead to tissue injury and are responsible for clinical conditions such as asthma, granuloma formation, and lung transplant rejection. (Chapter 76 describes types I, II, III, and IV hypersensitivity reactions.)

EFFECTS OF AGING

Most of the changes that occur with aging affect the lower airway. Movement of cilia in the upper airway slows and becomes less effective. This change predisposes older clients to a greater number of respiratory tract infections.

Lung structure also changes with age. The lungs become rounder as a result of increased anteroposterior diameter, circumference, area, and height of the lung. The proportion of the lung formed by alveolar duct air increases, and alveolar air decreases. Loss of alveolar wall tissue and its elastic tissue fibers is seen. The result is a deterioration of lung function.

The air spaces enlarge, although this is not referred to as emphysema because it is not a result of disease. These changes may be due to environmental pollutants rather than to aging alone. An increased incidence of true emphysema and a greater prevalence of chronic cough and sputum production are seen in older adults. These findings suggest that environmental or occupational pollutants, in addition to the normal aging process, may be a component in the decline of lung function.

CONCLUSIONS

The primary function of the lungs is gas exchange. The physical structure of the airways allows air to be warmed, filtered, and humidified as it enters the body. In the alveolar sacs, oxygen is exchanged for CO_2. The mechanics of breathing are coordinated by the ribs, diaphragm, pleural space, elastic recoil of the lungs, and the nervous system. The respiratory system also helps regulate acid-base balance. Alterations in structure and function can result in various disorders.

BIBLIOGRAPHY

1. Berne, R., et al. (2004). *Physiology* (5th ed.). St. Louis: Mosby.
2. Carroll, R.G. (2007). *Elsevier's integrated physiology*. Philadelphia: Saunders.
3. Kierszenbaum, A.L. (2007). *Histology and cell biology: An introduction to pathology* (2nd ed.). St. Louis: Mosby.
4. Guyton, A., & Hall, J. (2006). *Textbook of medical physiology* (11th ed.). Philadelphia: Saunders.
5. Silverthorn, D. (2006). *Human physiology* (4th ed.). San Francisco: Pearson Benjamin Cummings.

CHAPTER 59

Assessment of the Respiratory System

DIANA MOXNESS AND SUSANNE A. QUALLICH

Nurses who care for clients experiencing respiratory disorders perform and interpret a variety of assessment procedures. This chapter discusses history and physical assessment as well as diagnostic procedures used to plan care for clients with respiratory disorders.

HISTORY

Biographical Data

Note the client's biological age and compare it with the client's appearance. Does the client look his/her stated age? Chronic respiratory disorders such as lung cancer or chronic obstructive pulmonary disease often make the client appear older.

Current Health
Chief Complaint

The client's clinical manifestations, sometimes described as the chief complaint, help to establish priorities for medical and nursing intervention. In emergency or acute situations, brief and simple questions regarding the chief complaint(s) are asked until the client's condition is stabilized.

Clinical Manifestations

Common clinical manifestations related to the respiratory system include noncardiac chest pain, dyspnea (difficulty breathing), cough, hemoptysis (bloody sputum), wheezing, stridor, and complaints related to the nose and sinuses. Figure 59-1 summarizes the assessment data that should be collected regarding common respiratory clinical manifestations. Note the onset, location, duration, characteristics, aggravating and relieving factors, associated manifestations, timing, setting, and severity of the problem. Some students use the mnemonic OLD CARTS to remember assessment data to collect from the client.

Noncardiac Chest Pain. Chest pain may be associated with pulmonary, cardiac, or gastrointestinal problems, and being able to distinguish between the three is important. Determine the location, duration, and intensity of the chest pain to provide early clues to the cause. Ask the client what instigates the pain (e.g., activity, coughing, movement) and what relieves the pain (e.g., nitroglycerin, splinting the chest wall, heat).

Pleuritic chest pain is commonly a sharp, stabbing pain that occurs at one site on the chest wall and increases with chest wall movement or deep breathing. Retrosternal (behind the sternum) pain is usually burning, constant, and aching. Pain can also originate in the bony and cartilaginous parts of the thorax.

Angina pectoris (pain of the chest) is cardiac in origin and may be associated with decreased blood flow to the heart and is a potentially life-threatening problem. Cardiac chest pain is usually described as an aching, heavy, squeezing sensation with pressure or tightness in the substernal area and can radiate into the neck or arms

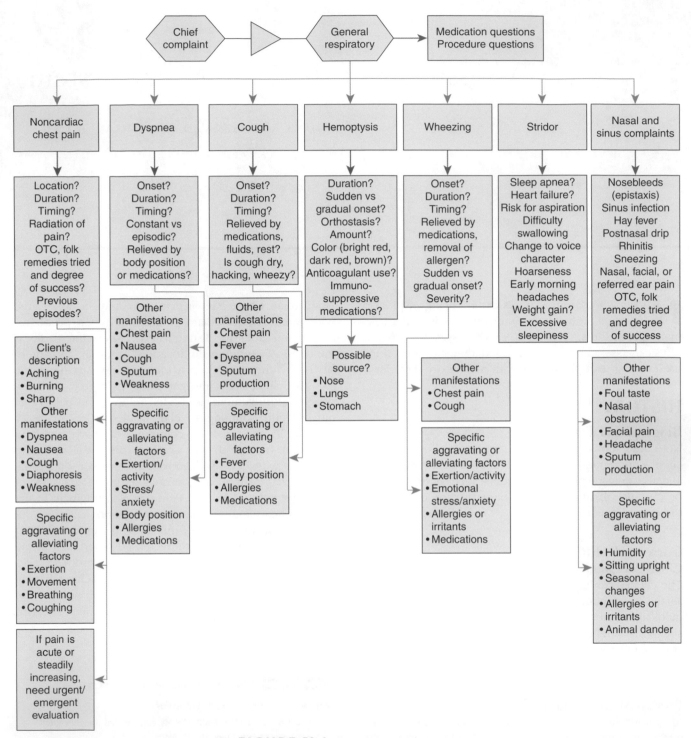

■ **FIGURE 59–I** Expanded respiratory assessment.

(see Chapters 54 and 56 for more information related to cardiac chest pain).

Clients with esophageal problems such as esophagitis, gastrointestinal reflux disease (GERD), and hiatal hernias may complain of chest pain. See Chapter 28 for more information related to assessment of these disorders.

Dyspnea. Dyspnea (difficulty breathing) is a common manifestation experienced by clients with pulmonary and cardiac disorders. It is a client's subjective assessment of the degree of work of breathing exerted for a given task or effort. Clients may define dyspnea as shortness of breath, suffocation, tightness, being winded, or being breathless. The subjective nature of dyspnea makes it difficult to quantify objectively.

Several methods are used to assess accurately the level of dyspnea experienced by a client. The Visual Analogue Scale (Figure 59-2) is used to quantify breathlessness by

How short of breath are you right now?

None

Extremely
severe

■ **FIGURE 59–2** The Visual Analogue Scale of dyspnea. Although the scale can be in the form of either a vertical or a horizontal line, the most commonly used scale consists of a 100-mm horizontal line, like the one shown here.

using the client's response to particular questions. It is easy to understand, and the amount of dyspnea during various activities can be assessed. The modified Borg Category Ratio Scale for assessment of dyspnea (found on the website) is used to rate the intensity of dyspnea. The scale is simple, and results have been reproduced in several populations.

In addition to a subjective assessment, document the characteristics of the dyspnea. Assess all the characteristics because many respiratory and nonrespiratory causes can result in dyspnea. The Integrating Diagnostic Testing feature below further details the evaluation of dyspnea.

Cough. Note when and how the cough began (suddenly or gradually) and how long it has been present. Determine the frequency of the cough and the time of day when the cough is better or worse (early morning, late afternoon, nighttime). The client may describe the cough as hacking, dry, hoarse, congested, barking, wheezy, or

bubbling. The Integrating Diagnostic Testing feature on p. 1528 further details the evaluation of a client with a cough.

Determine which medications or treatments the client has used for the cough (antitussives, codeine, inhalers, nebulizers, rest, sitting up).

Find out what precautions are used to prevent the spread of infection (if it is present).

SAFETY

⚠

ALERT

Sputum is the substance expelled by coughing or clearing the throat, but sputum production with coughing is not normal. The tracheobronchial tree normally produces about 3 ounces of mucus a day as part of the normal cleaning mechanism. Question the client about sputum color (clear, yellow, green, rusty, bloody), odor, quality (watery, stringy, frothy, thick), and quantity (teaspoon, tablespoon, cup) and document any changes. Ascertain whether sputum is produced only after the client is lying in a certain position. Sputum may also be a

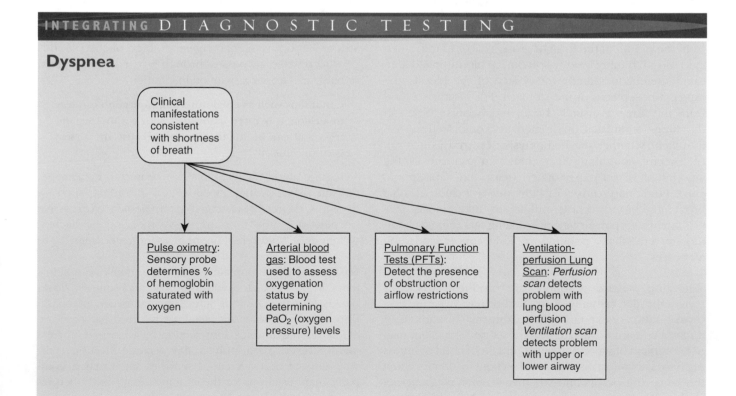

INTEGRATING DIAGNOSTIC TESTING

Dyspnea

Clinical manifestations consistent with shortness of breath

Pulse oximetry: Sensory probe determines % of hemoglobin saturated with oxygen

Arterial blood gas: Blood test used to assess oxygenation status by determining PaO$_2$ (oxygen pressure) levels

Pulmonary Function Tests (PFTs): Detect the presence of obstruction or airflow restrictions

Ventilation-perfusion Lung Scan: *Perfusion scan* detects problem with lung blood perfusion *Ventilation scan* detects problem with upper or lower airway

INTEGRATING D I A G N O S T I C   T E S T I N G

Cough

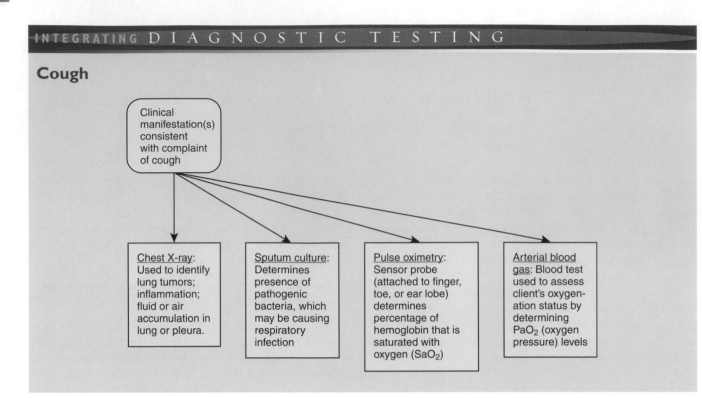

secretion from the oral or nasopharyngeal area or sinuses rather than from the tracheobronchial tree. For example, draining sinuses may provoke a productive cough.

Hemoptysis. Hemoptysis refers to blood expectorated from the mouth in the form of gross (visible to the naked eye) blood, frankly bloody sputum, or blood-tinged sputum. Attempt to identify the source of the blood—the lungs, a nosebleed, or the stomach. For instance, blood from the lungs is usually bright red because blood in the lungs stimulates an immediate cough reflex. Ask the client whether the hemoptysis occurred as a result of forceful coughing. Also obtain an estimate of the amount of blood expectorated (teaspoon, tablespoon, cup). Pulmonary causes of hemoptysis include chronic bronchitis, bronchiectasis, pulmonary tuberculosis, cystic fibrosis, upper airway necrotizing granulomas, pulmonary embolism, pneumonia, lung cancer, and lung abscesses.

Wheezing. Wheezing sounds are produced when air passes through partially obstructed or narrowed airways on inspiration or expiration. Wheezing may be audible, or it may be heard only with a stethoscope. The client may not complain of wheezing but complain of chest tightness or chest discomfort instead. Ask the client to identify when the wheezing occurs and whether it resolves spontaneously or medication is required for relief. Not all wheezing

is caused by asthma; wheezing can be caused by mucosal edema, airway secretions, collapsed airways resulting from loss of elastic tissue, and foreign objects or tumors partially obstructing air flow.

Stridor. Stridor is the name given to high-pitched sounds produced when air passes through a partially obstructed or narrowed upper airway on inspiration.

> **Conditions such as epiglottitis and aspiration can lead to stridor; it is often associated with respiratory distress and can be life-threatening because the airway is compromised.**   SAFETY ⚠ ALERT

Inquire about changes in voice character, hoarseness, difficulty swallowing, sleep-related disorders such as insomnia, degree of snoring, hypersomnolence (excessive sleepiness) in the morning, early morning headaches, weight gain, fluid retention, apnea, and restlessness.

Nasal and Sinus Complaints. There are many complaints that can be associated with the nose and sinuses. Nosebleeds (epistaxis), sinus infection, hay fever, postnasal drip, rhinitis, and nasal, facial, or referred ear pain are all common examples. Obstruction by engorged mucous membranes or nasal polyps may occlude the upper airway. Loss of or a decreased sense of smell may accompany manifestations of the common cold and allergies or may signal a more serious neurologic problem.

Inquire whether the client has experienced these manifestations previously and, if so, under what conditions. Ask the client about attempts at self-treatment, such as nasal sprays, decongestants, antihistamines, and other over-the-counter and herbal cold and allergy medications.

Ask the client about factors that alleviate or worsen the manifestations and any other conditions that seem to be related. This includes increased humidity, sitting upright, lying supine, weather and seasonal changes, or allergies. Nasal and sinus problems may be allergy related and provoked by pollen, fumes, smoke, animal dander, or dust particles. A foul taste in the mouth, unpleasant breath odor (halitosis), nasal obstruction, and facial pain (particularly over the frontal and maxillary sinuses) may accompany sinusitis. Chronic sinusitis may be accompanied by headache or facial pain present on awakening and diminishing during the day as the sinuses drain.

Review of Systems

In addition to the common clinical manifestations, the client may report other complaints that may be directly or indirectly related to a respiratory condition. These symptoms include fever, hoarseness, night sweats, anorexia, weight loss, dependent edema, recent or frequent colds, nasal discharge, sinus pain or pressure, and epistaxis (nosebleed). In addition, coughing may result in stress incontinence; you may want to ask female clients about this problem. Figure 59-3 provides a summary of specific history data that should be collected for a client with respiratory complaints.

Past Medical History

Review the past health history of the client and family members for data related to the upper and lower respiratory systems, which are common sources of both acute and chronic health problems. Assess clients with chronic conditions for changes in their ongoing respiratory manifestations as these changes provide clues to the cause of the new problem.

In addition to obtaining data regarding common childhood diseases and vaccinations, ask the client about the occurrence of tuberculosis, bronchitis, influenza, asthma, and pneumonia and the frequency of lower respiratory tract infections after upper respiratory tract infection. Determine the existence of congenital problems, such as cystic fibrosis and premature birth history, which can be associated with respiratory complications in the adult client. Inquire about vaccination against pneumonia and influenza. A one-time administration of the polyvalent pneumococcal vaccine Pneumovax provides lifelong immunity against pneumococcal pneumonia in most clients. However, revaccination has been a topic of discussion in recent years and may be necessary with some clients. Influenza or "flu" shots must be received annually in the fall of the year.

Ask about the date and results of the client's most recent chest x-ray or other pulmonary diagnostic tests. These test results can provide baseline data for the evaluation of the current problem. Inquire about previous injuries to the mouth, nose, throat, or chest (e.g., blunt trauma, fractured ribs, or pneumothorax).

Surgical History

Discuss the client's history of any procedure or surgery that pertains to the upper or lower respiratory system, such as biopsies or procedures to directly visualize the structures.

Allergies

Question the client about a history of allergies and timing of manifestations to help identify a possible allergic basis for the condition. Has the client been tested for allergies? When? Are medications (including allergy shots) taken prophylactically or on an as-needed basis to provide relief from manifestations?

Ask about precipitating and aggravating factors, such as foods, medications, pollens, smoke, fumes, dust, and animal dander. Ask the client to describe the allergic manifestations experienced (chest tightness, wheezing, cough, rhinitis, watery eyes, scratchy throat) and their severity. Determine the age at which allergies first occurred and whether they have become progressively more severe.

Medications

Obtain detailed information regarding both prescribed and over-the-counter medications, including herbal remedies, because many products affect the respiratory system. The client may routinely require antibiotics, bronchodilators, or steroids for respiratory tract infections. Specify the route of administration (pill, liquid, or inhalation). Many respiratory medications are inhaled through a metered-dose inhaler (MDI) or mini-nebulizer. Some medications can affect smell and taste; these include metronidazole, local anesthetics, clofibrate, some antibiotics, some antineoplastics, allopurinol, phenylbutazone, levodopa, codeine, morphine, carbamazepine, lithium, and trifluoperazine.

Herbal medicines for respiratory problems include remedies for nasal discharge and congestion, cough, sore throat, fever and headache, and possible immunostimulants. Expectorants include anise (*Pimpinella anisum*), coltsfoot (*Tussilago farfara*), and horehound (*Marrubium vulgare*). Coltsfoot and horehound are also believed to have antitussive action. Sore throat remedies include mint (*Mentha piperita* [peppermint], *Mentha spicata* [spearmint]) and slippery elm (*Ulmus rubra*). Remedies for the fever and headache that may accompany colds and influenza include boneset (*Eupatorium perfoliatum*), feverfew (*Tanacetum parthenium*), and white

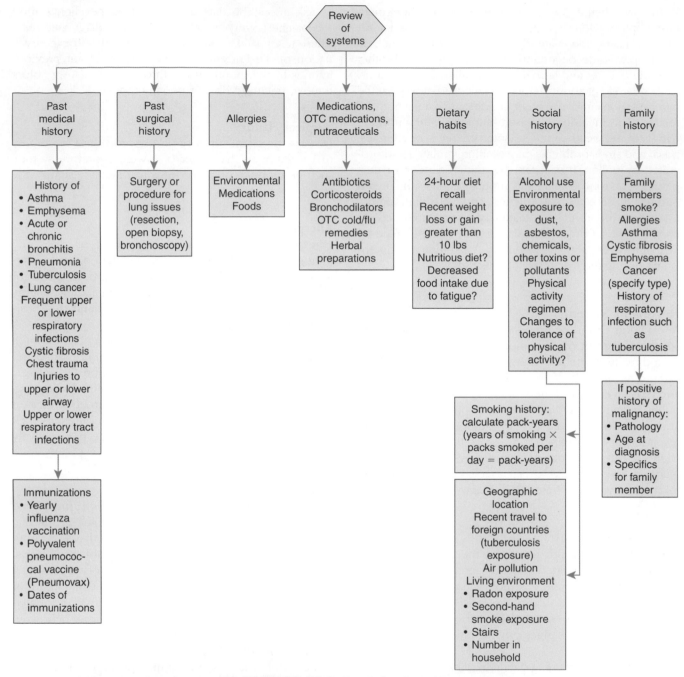

FIGURE 59–3 Expanded respiratory history.

willow *(Salix purpurea, Salix fragilis)*. Stimulants of the immune system, believed to help ward off colds and flu, include *Echinacea (E. angustifolia, E. pallida, E. purpurea)* and goldenseal *(Hydrastis canadensis)*. Refer to Chapter 4 for further discussion.

Dietary Habits

Maintaining a nutritious diet is important for clients with chronic respiratory disease, which can result in decreased lung capacity and greater workload for the lungs and cardiovascular system. The added workload increases caloric expenditure, and weight loss may occur. Clients may

become anorectic because of the effects of medications and fatigue. The client may not have enough energy to consume the needed calories to maintain body weight. Ask the client to recall intake for the last 24 hours. Assess the amount of protein, kilocalories, and sodium intake (see Chapter 28).

Social History

Respiratory status is affected by numerous factors that may lead to acute problems or that may affect the client's coping with chronic respiratory problems. Identify any environmental agents that might be contributing to the client's condition. Ask specifically about the work environment and hobbies. Focus on exposure to dust, asbestos, beryllium, silica, and other toxins or pollutants. Farmers are exposed to airborne particles such as grain dust, fertilizers, and animal dander. Hobbies may involve chemicals, heat, dust, and airborne particles from grinding, soldering, or welding.

Ask about recent travel to areas where respiratory diseases are prevalent, such as Asia (tuberculosis), the Ohio River valley (histoplasmosis), or the San Joaquin valley (valley fever). Polluted city air has also been related to increasing incidence and severity of asthma.

Ask about the client's living conditions. Assess for environmental hazards such as stairs or poor air circulation. A client with a chronic respiratory condition may have difficulty climbing stairs or breathing unfiltered air. How many people are in the household? Crowded living conditions increase risk of exposure to infectious respiratory diseases such as tuberculosis and cold viruses. Recent exposure to continuous air conditioning in a hotel or motel setting may be related to Legionnaires' disease.

Inquire about any history of smoking tobacco products and of drinking alcohol. Smoking has been associated with decreased ciliary function of the lungs, increased mucus production, and the development of lung cancer and chronic lung problems. Ask the client about the use of smokeless tobacco (snuff, chewing tobacco) and smoking non-tobacco substances (marijuana and clove cigarettes). The pack-year history, which helps quantify the smoking history, is determined by using the following equation:

$$\text{Years of Smoking} \times \text{Packs Smoked per Day} = \text{Pack-Years}$$

Ciliary action is slowed by alcohol, which reduces mucus clearance from the lungs. Heavy alcohol ingestion depresses the cough reflex and increases risk of aspiration.

Clients who are active may describe the onset of coughing and wheezing during exercise. These clients need to be further evaluated for exercise-induced asthma before continuing workouts. Clients with chronic respiratory conditions often do not have the lung capacity to sustain even mild forms of exercise and subsequently become dyspneic. Has tolerance for activity decreased or remained stable? Ask the client to describe typical activities, such as walking, light housekeeping chores, or grocery shopping, that are tolerated or, conversely, that result in shortness of breath.

Family Health History
Question the client about the family history of respiratory diseases. Identify blood relatives (in regard to genetically transmitted diseases) and family members (in regard to infectious conditions) who have had asthma, cystic fibrosis, emphysema, chronic obstructive pulmonary disease (COPD), lung cancer, respiratory tract infections, tuberculosis, or allergies. List the age and cause of death of each deceased family member. Do any household members smoke cigarettes, pipes, or cigars? Secondary inhalation of smoke often precipitates or worsens respiratory manifestations.

PHYSICAL EXAMINATION

Hypoxia as a result of respiratory conditions may precipitate subtle neurologic alterations, such as restlessness, fatigue, disorientation, and personality changes. Tachycardia usually accompanies respiratory problems as the body attempts to compensate for decreased oxygen delivery. Anorexia and weight loss are seen in many chronic respiratory conditions. Please refer to the normal findings as described in the Physical Assessment Findings in the Healthy Adult feature below. Refer to a physical assessment text for the details of a complete respiratory system assessment.

Physical Assessment Findings in the Healthy Adult

The Respiratory System

INSPECTION
Nose. Nose straight, without flaring or discharge; nares patent; mucosa pink and moist; septum midline, without masses or perforation.
Sinuses. Transilluminate.
Thorax. Even color; regular, even contour; respirations quiet, unlabored, of even depth, and without retractions, bulges, masses, or use of accessory muscles; anteroposterior-transverse diameter ratio 1:2.
Digits. Clubbing absent; nail beds pink; immediate capillary refill on blanching.

PALPATION
Nose. Nontender, without masses or lesions.
Sinuses. Nontender, without swelling or bogginess.
Trachea. Midline and mobile without crepitus.
Thorax. Chest wall symmetrical, smooth, without lumps, masses, tenderness, or crepitus; thoracic excursion symmetrical; tactile fremitus present.

PERCUSSION
Sinuses. Nontender.
Thorax and Lungs. Resonant throughout peripheral lung fields; cardiac dullness; diaphragmatic excursion ranges from 3 to 6 cm for each hemidiaphragm; with the right side slightly higher than the left.

AUSCULTATION
Thorax and Lungs. Vesicular sounds throughout peripheral lung fields; bronchovesicular sounds over the area of tracheal bifurcation, both anteriorly and posteriorly; bronchial sounds over the trachea anteriorly; adventitious sounds absent; vocal resonance absent.

General Assessment

Assess the client's level of consciousness and orientation. Note the skin and lip color. Assess the nail beds for color and the presence of clubbing, which occurs as a compensatory measure for chronic hypoxia. The Shamroth technique is a useful assessment for the presence of clubbing (Figure 59-4).

Nose and Paranasal Sinuses

External Nose

Inspect and palpate the external nose for deviations from normal alignment, symmetry, color, discharge, nasal flaring, lesions, and tenderness. The client should be able to breathe quietly through the nose rather than breathe through the mouth. Check the nasal canals for patency by asking the client to occlude one naris with a finger and to breathe through the open naris while closing the mouth. Ask the client to tip the head back, and inspect the outer nares for crusting, bleeding, or dryness, which should be absent.

Internal Nose

Next inspect the vestibules with a penlight while the client's head is tipped back. Normal findings include coarse hairs, dark red nasal mucosa, a clear passage without discharge, and a midline septum. Further examination of the internal nose requires the use of a nasal speculum and is not conducted unless indicated. Inspection may be hampered by nasal congestion.

Paranasal Sinuses

Palpate and percuss the frontal and maxillary sinuses to assess for swelling and tenderness, which are normally absent. Palpate the frontal sinuses simultaneously by placing the thumbs above the eyes, just under the bony ridge of the eye orbits, and apply gentle pressure. Palpate the maxillary sinuses by using either the index and third fingers or the thumbs to press gently on each side of the nose just under the zygomatic bones. Use direct percussion over the eyebrows for the frontal sinuses and on either side of the nose below the eyes in line with the pupils for the maxillary sinuses.

Smell

The senses of taste and smell are closely related. Smell is perceived mainly via the olfactory nerves, although some smell is perceived through the trigeminal nerves. Many conditions affect taste and smell, such as viral infections, normal aging, head injuries, and local obstruction. Smell impairment may be (1) hyposmia (a decrease in smell sensitivity) or (2) anosmia (bilateral and complete absence of smell sensitivity). Assess smell by having the client identify various odors by testing each nostril separately.

Thorax and Lungs

Accurate physical examination of the thorax and lungs requires being familiar with the anatomic landmarks of the posterior, anterior, and lateral thorax (see the figure of Thoracic Landmarks and Underlying Structures on the website). Use these landmarks to identify the underlying structures, particularly the lobes of the lung and the heart. When performing inspection, palpation, percussion, and auscultation of the respiratory system, the examiner should compare one side of the thorax to the other side to help determine the presence or absence of abnormalities (Figure 59-5).

■ **FIGURE 59–4** Clubbing. **A,** A normal digit, with an angle of 160 degrees. **B,** A flattened angle between the nail and the skin, exceeding 180 degrees. **C,** Advanced clubbing with a rounded nail. **D,** Assess clubbing with the use of the Shamroth technique. Instruct the client to place the nails of the fourth (ring) fingers together while extending the other fingers and to hold the hands up. A diamond-shaped space between the nails is a normal finding and indicates the absence of clubbing.

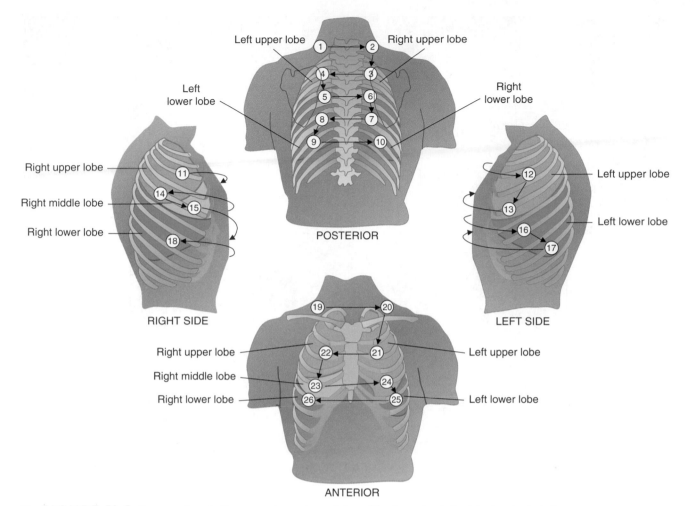

FIGURE 59-5 Sequence for palpation, percussion, and auscultation of the thorax (posterior, lateral, and anterior).

Inspection

Note the client's rate, rhythm, and depth of respirations. The normal respiratory rate for an adult is 14 to 20 breaths per minute. The Assessing Respiratory Patterns figure on the website describes examples of normal and abnormal respiratory patterns. Observe for signs of respiratory distress, such as nasal flaring or retractions, and bulging of intercostal or sternocleidomastoid muscles to facilitate breathing. Inspect the chest wall configuration by comparing the anteroposterior (AP) diameter to the transverse (lateral) diameter; the lateral diameter is normally twice the AP diameter. Figure 59-6 provides information about chest deformities.

Palpation

Palpate the trachea for midline position and slight movability. Palpate the chest wall for symmetrical thoracic excursion during inspiration and expiration (see Assessment of Thoracic Excursion figure on the website). Palpate costal angle (angle at the base of the rib cage); the costal angle should be less than 90 degrees. A costal angle greater than 90 degrees with an AP/lateral

diameter ratio of 1:1 indicates an abnormal barrel chest wall shape, as seen in clients with chronic obstructive pulmonary disease. Additionally, palpate for tactile fremitus, which involves palpating the posterior chest wall while the client says "ninety-nine"; compare the intensity of the vibrations on both sides for symmetry.

Percussion

Percussion over healthy lung tissue produces a resonant (low-pitched, hollow) sound. The pitch and qualities of other percussion sounds can be summarized as follows: (1) tympany (high-pitched, hollow, drum-like); (2) flat (high-pitched, soft); (3) dull (medium-pitched, thud-like). Figure 59-7 illustrates the location of various thoracic percussion sounds and the associated anatomic structures that produce the various sounds.

Auscultation

Lung auscultation provides critical assessment data in terms of a client's respiratory health. Auscultate in a pattern that compares the right side of the thorax to the left side. Auscultate all areas of the lungs over a bare chest in order to

■ **FIGURE 59–6** Chest deformities. **A,** Normal adult, for comparison. The ratio of anteroposterior diameter to transverse diameter can be seen here as 1:2. **B,** Barrel chest. The anteroposterior-transverse diameter ratio is 1:1. **C,** Pigeon chest (pectus carinatum). **D,** Funnel chest (pectus excavatum). **E,** Thoracic kyphoscoliosis.

achieve accurate findings. At each auscultation location, listen for a full respiration cycle of inspiration and expiration as the client breathes through the mouth. Auscultate for the type or character of the breath sounds and the presence of adventitious (extra) sounds. Table 59-1 describes

the characteristics of normal breath sounds, and Figure 59-8 illustrates the normal anatomic location of these sounds. Bronchovesicular or bronchial breath sounds heard in the peripheral lung fields can indicate consolidation of the lung resulting from inflammation and infection. Absent

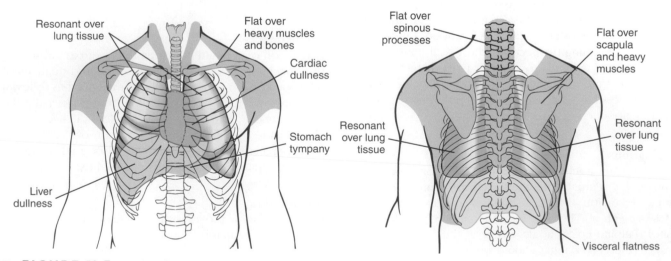

■ **FIGURE 59–7** Location of thoracic percussion sounds and their associated structures.

TABLE 59–1   Characteristics of Normal Breath Sounds

	Pitch	Amplitude	Duration	Quality	Normal Location
Bronchial (tracheal)	High	Loud	Inspiration < expiration	Harsh, hollow, tubular	Trachea and larynx
Bronchovesicular	Moderate	Moderate	Inspiration = expiration	Mixed	Over major bronchi where fewer alveoli are located: posterior, between scapulae, especially on right; anterior, around upper sternum in first and second intercostal spaces
Vesicular	Low	Soft	Inspiration > expiration	Rustling, like sound of wind in trees	Over peripheral lung fields where air flows through smaller bronchioles and alveoli

From Jarvis, C. (2006). *Physical examination and health assessment* (4th ed.). Philadelphia: Saunders.

or diminished breath sounds can also indicate lung disease. Table 59-2 provides a summary of adventitious lung sounds and the associated abnormal client conditions. Refer to a physical assessment textbook for additional details.

DIAGNOSTIC TESTING

Noninvasive Tests
Diagnostic procedures facilitate the assessment and diagnosis of client respiratory disorders. Commonly available diagnostic tests include pulmonary function tests, arterial blood gas analysis, pulse oximetry, ventilation-perfusion scan, chest x-ray, and sputum cultures.

Pulse Oximetry
The pulse oximeter passes a beam of light through the tissue, and a sensor attached to the finger tip, toe, or ear lobe measures the amount of light absorbed by the oxygen-saturated hemoglobin. The oximeter then gives a reading of the percentage of hemoglobin that is saturated with oxygen (SaO_2). SaO_2 is closely correlated with the saturations obtained from the pulse oximeter if it is greater than 70% (Table 59-3).

Pulmonary Function Testing
Pulmonary function tests (PFTs) provide information about respiratory function by measuring lung volumes, lung mechanics, and diffusion capabilities of the lungs. PFTs performed in a pulmonary function laboratory can measure respiratory volumes and capacities. PFTs done outside a laboratory are modified to include ventilation tests of forced expiratory volume, vital capacity, and maximal voluntary ventilation measures. Refer to the table Pulmonary Function Test (PFT) Components and the table Categorization of Obstructive and Restrictive Pulmonary Disorders and Pulmonary Function Test (PFT) Findings on the website for an explanation of the PFT recordings and results that indicate obstructive and restrictive lung disease.

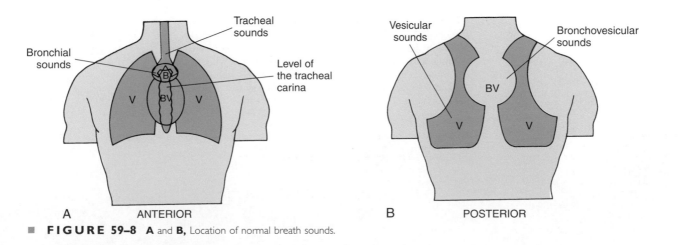

■ **FIGURE 59–8   A** and **B,** Location of normal breath sounds.

TABLE 59–2 Adventitious Breath Sounds

Sound*	Description	Mechanism	Clinical Example
Discontinuous Sounds			
Crackles—fine (rales, crepitations) Inspiration Expiration	Discontinuous, high-pitched, short crackling, popping sounds heard during inspiration that are not cleared by coughing; this sound can be simulated by rolling a strand of hair between fingers near the ear or by moistening thumb and index finger and separating them near the ear	Inhaled air collides with previously deflated airways; airways suddenly pop open, creating a crackling sound as gas pressures between two compartments equalize	*Late inspiratory crackles* occur with restrictive disease: pneumonia, heart failure, and interstitial fibrosis *Early inspiratory crackles* occur with obstructive disease: chronic bronchitis, asthma, and emphysema
Crackles—coarse (coarse rales)	Loud, low-pitched, bubbling, and gurgling sounds that start in early inspiration and may be present in expiration; may decrease somewhat by suctioning or coughing but will reappear shortly; sound like opening a self-fastening tape (Velcro) fastener	Inhaled air collides with secretions in trachea and large bronchi	Pulmonary edema, pneumonia, pulmonary fibrosis, and in terminally ill who have a depressed cough reflex
Atelectatic crackles (atelectatic rales)	Sound like fine crackles but do not last and are not pathologic; disappear after first few breaths; heard in axillae and bases (usually dependent) of lungs	When sections of alveoli are not fully aerated, they deflate and accumulate secretions; crackles are heard when these sections reexpand with a few deep breaths	In aging adults, bedridden people, or in people just aroused from sleep
Pleural friction rub	Very superficial sound that is coarse and low-pitched; it has a grating quality as if two pieces of leather are being rubbed together; sounds just like crackles, but *close* to the ear; sounds louder if stethoscope is pushed harder onto chest wall; sound is inspiratory and expiratory	Caused when pleurae become inflamed and lose their normal lubricating fluid; their opposing roughened pleural surfaces rub together during respiration; heard best in anterolateral wall where there is greatest lung mobility	Pleuritis, accompanied by pain with breathing (rub disappears after a few days if pleural fluid accumulates and separates pleurae)
Continuous Sounds			
Wheeze—high-pitched (sibilant rhonchi)	High-pitched, musical squeaking sounds that predominate in expiration but may occur in both expiration and inspiration	Air squeezed or compressed through passageways narrowed almost to closure by collapsing, swelling, secretions, or tumors; passageway walls oscillate in apposition between closed and barely open positions; resulting sound is similar to a vibrating reed	Obstructive lung disease such as asthma or emphysema
Wheeze—low-pitched (sonorous rhonchi)	Low-pitched, musical, snoring, moaning sounds; they are heard throughout cycle, although they are more prominent on expiration; may clear somewhat by coughing	Air flow obstruction as described by vibrating reed mechanism above; pitch of wheeze cannot be correlated with size of passageway that generates it	Bronchitis

*Although nothing in clinical practice seems to differ more than the nomenclature of adventitious sounds, most authorities concur on two categories: (1) discontinuous, discrete crackling sounds and (2) continuous, coarse, or musical sounds.

Modified from Jarvis, C. (2006). *Physical examination and health assessment* (4th ed.). Philadelphia: Saunders.

TABLE 59–3 Comparing Oxygen Saturation to Partial Pressure of Arterial Oxygen (Pao_2)

Oxygen Saturation (%)	Pao_2 (mm Hg)	Client Status
50	25	Life-threatening hypoxemia
75	40	Moderate hypoxemia
90	55	Mild hypoxemia

Chest X-Ray

Chest x-rays (Figure 59-9) provide information about the chest that may not be available through other assessment means and may be able to illustrate graphically the cause of respiratory dysfunction. Chest films may reveal abnormalities when there are no physical manifestations of pulmonary disease. Chest x-ray studies may be performed for a variety of reasons, including the following: as part of a routine screening procedure; when pulmonary disease is suspected; to monitor the status of respiratory disorders and abnormalities (pleural effusion, atelectasis, tubercular lesions); and to confirm endotracheal or tracheostomy tube placement.

Ventilation-Perfusion Scan

Ventilation-perfusion ($\dot{V}/\dot{Q}$) scans are used to assess lung ventilation and lung perfusion. $\dot{V}/\dot{Q}$ scans are used to confirm pulmonary embolism, pulmonary infarction, emphysema, fibrosis, and bronchiectasis. Although pulmonary angiography is the most specific diagnostic tool for pulmonary emboli, it is invasive; the $\dot{V}/\dot{Q}$ scan is less invasive and less dangerous. Quantitative perfusion scans may be helpful in preoperative assessment of clients undergoing surgical resection of thoracic malignancy.

Computed Tomography and Magnetic Resonance Imaging

Computed tomography (CT) provides more sophisticated tomography than is possible with conventional x-ray equipment. The CT scan is particularly helpful in identifying peripheral (pleural) or mediastinal disorders. Special techniques can be used to view pulmonary nodules. Thin cuts of CT scans are used in diagnosing interstitial lung disorders such as pulmonary fibrosis and bronchiectasis. Spiral or helical CT scan of the chest is an alternative to the lung scan for identifying pulmonary emboli.

Magnetic resonance imaging (MRI) employs magnetic fields rather than radiation to create images of body structures. MRI is used in much the same way as CT, although MRI is more definitive than CT because it creates more detailed images of anatomic structures.

Invasive Tests

The following paragraphs briefly describe other diagnostic tests used to detect pulmonary disorders. For a complete description of tests used to aid in the diagnosis of pulmonary disease, consult a diagnostic and laboratory tests textbook for more information related to pre- and postprocedure nursing care.

Laryngoscopy

Laryngoscopy is visual examination of the larynx and is used to diagnose laryngeal papillomas, nodules, polyps, or cancer. Laryngoscopy can be performed during bronchoscopy or as a separate procedure. Figure 59-10 shows a tumor on the vocal cord as seen via laryngoscopy.

Bronchoscopy

Bronchoscopy (Figure 59-11) is a test used for diagnostic and therapeutic uses. A flexible fiberoptic bronchoscope or a rigid bronchoscope permits visualization of the larynx, trachea, and bronchi. A bronchoscopy is useful for the diagnostic detection of tumors, inflammation, or strictures as well as to obtain tissue biopsies. Therapeutic uses of bronchoscopy include the removal of retained secretions or foreign bodies blocking air passages and to control bleeding within the bronchus.

■ **FIGURE 59–9** A normal chest x-ray film taken from the postero-anterior view. The backward L in the upper right corner is placed on the film to indicate the left side of the client's chest. **A,** Diaphragm; **B,** costophrenic angle; **C,** left ventricle; **D,** right atrium; **E,** aortic arch; **F,** superior vena cava; **G,** trachea; **H,** right bronchus; **I,** left bronchus; **J,** breast shadows.

■ **FIGURE 59–10** Large granular cell tumor of the true vocal cord, as seen during laryngoscopy. *(From Fu, Y.S., et al. [2001]. Head and neck pathology—With clinical correlations. New York: Churchill Livingstone.)*

Thoracentesis and Pleural Fluid Analysis

Thoracentesis is an invasive procedure that involves insertion of a needle into the pleural space for removal of pleural fluid or air (Figure 59-12). Pleural fluid is removed to therapeutically relieve pain or shortness of breath caused by excessive pleural pressure. A thoracentesis and pleural fluid analysis can also be a diagnostic tool to detect various disorders, such as inflammatory, infectious, or cancerous conditions.

A

■ **FIGURE 59–11** Bronchoscopy.

B

■ **FIGURE 59–12** Thoracentesis. **A,** Correct position of the client for the procedure. The arms are raised and crossed. The head rests on the folded arm. This position allows the chest wall to be pulled outward in an expanded position. If an institutional over-bed table is not available, you may leave the client's arms down, but position them toward the client's hips or cross them in front of the chest. **B,** Usual site for insertion of a thoracentesis needle for a right-sided effusion. The actual site varies, depending on the location and volume of the effusion. The needle is kept as far away from the diaphragm as possible but is inserted close to the base of the effusion so that gravity can help with drainage.

Median antebrachial vein

Radial artery ——   —— Ulnar artery

Veins from hand ——   —— Arterial volar arch

A

B

C

D

■ **FIGURE 59–13**   Obtaining a sample of arterial blood by arterial puncture. First, perform Allen's test, a quick assessment of collateral circulation in the hand. This test is essential before radial artery puncture. **A,** Occlude both the radial and the ulnar arteries with your fingers. Ask the client to close the hand into a fist. **B,** When the client opens the hand with the arteries still occluded, the hand is pale. **C,** When you release either the radial or the ulnar artery, the client's hand should become pink because of collateral circulation. Assess the patency of each of the two arteries in this way, one at a time. **D,** If collateral circulation is adequate, you can draw arterial blood from the radial artery with a heparinized needle and syringe as shown.

Biopsy

Biopsy of the lung or pleura requires a surgical excision of tissue. The tissue is examined for abnormal cellular structure (cancer cells) or infection.

Laboratory Tests
Sputum Culture

An infectious process can lead to excessive production of mucus (commonly called sputum). Assessment of sputum for bacteria, fungi, or cellular elements guides the treatment of an underlying infection. If possible, sputum should be collected before antimicrobial treatment is begun.

Nose and Throat Cultures

The throat and nose normally contain many organisms. Using a flexible sterile cotton swab, cultures of these areas are taken to identify certain pathogens, such as *Streptococcus* species, *Bordetella pertussis, Corynebacterium diphtheria, Haemophilus influenzae,* or respiratory syncytial virus (RSV). Bacteria in the nose and throat can be identified by culture during assessment of the upper airway. Some bacteria are normally present (streptococci, staphylococci, pneumococci, *Haemophilus influenzae,* and *Klebsiella pneumoniae*). Other organisms are abnormal (those causing diphtheria or tuberculosis). The culture should be collected before antimicrobial treatment is begun.

Arterial Blood Gases (ABGs)

The ABG analysis involves the use of arterial, rather than venous, blood to measure PaO_2, $PaCO_2$, and pH directly (Figure 59-13). Bicarbonate concentration (HCO_3^-) and SaO_2 are calculated as well. PaO_2 reflects the efficiency of gas exchange, whereas $PaCO_2$ reflects the effectiveness of alveolar ventilation. The acid-base status of the body (see Chapter 13) is indicated by the pH of arterial blood. ABG analysis is helpful in the assessment of clients who are acutely ill with either pulmonary or nonpulmonary disorders, who require an artificial airway, who are dependent on mechanical ventilation, or who are experiencing chronic respiratory disease.

CONCLUSIONS

The nurse's involvement in a general respiratory assessment includes a variety of interventions. The nurse must obtain specific history data, including information about smoking history and other environmental hazards. The physical examination includes the assessment techniques of inspection, palpation, percussion, and auscultation. In addition, the nurse also monitors and reports the results of various diagnostic tests used to evaluate the client's respiratory status.

BIBLIOGRAPHY

1. Bickley, L.S. (2003). *Bates' guide to physical examination and history taking* (8th ed.). Philadelphia: Lippincott Williams & Wilkins.
2. Hardin, K.A., Tharratt, R.S., & Louie, S. (2005). Asthma in adulthood: different and complex. *The Clinical Advisor, 8*(10), 34-40.
3. Infectious Disease Leadership Council. (2005). Management of respiratory tract infections: Practical approaches. *Clinical Advisor Supplement, 8*(4).
4. Jarvis, C. (2004). *Physical examination and health assessment* (4th ed.). Philadelphia: Saunders.
5. Pagana, K.D., & Pagana, T.J. (2005). *Mosby's diagnostic and laboratory test reference* (7th ed.). St. Louis: Mosby.
6. Regueiro, C.R. (2004). The latest approaches to managing pneumonia. *The Clinical Advisor, 7*(11), 25-31.

evolve *Did you remember to check out the bonus material on the Evolve website and the CD-ROM, including NCLEX®-Examination Style Review Questions, Open-Book Quizzes, and Chapter Review Audio Podcasts?*

http://evolve.elsevier.com/Black/medsurg

CHAPTER 60

Management of Clients with Upper Airway Disorders

MARGARET M. ECKLUND

The upper airway is considered to be the nasal passages, sinuses, and trachea. The initial complaint for clients with disorders of the upper airway is a problem with breathing. Obstructions to nasal breathing are observed in clients with nasal polyps, deviated nasal septum, or nasal fractures. Sinus infections create inflammation and congestion. Laryngeal disorders may also result in breathing problems. Tumors of the larynx create obstruction to air entering the trachea, as well as to air being exhaled. Vocal cord paralysis and laryngospasm may also affect the passage of air through the larynx and vocal cords. Because of the priority need to have a patent airway, the chapter will begin with maintaining the airway.

METHODS OF CONTROLLING THE AIRWAY

Airway obstruction can be prevented or treated with many modalities, depending on the underlying cause. Antihistamine treatment is discussed in Chapter 76. Intubation to support ventilation and oxygenation is discussed in Chapter 63. This chapter begins with a discussion of tracheostomy because it is a strategy of airway management in hospitalized clients, creating a portal to manage secretions, relieve obstruction, or provide ongoing mechanical ventilation.

Tracheostomy

A *tracheotomy* is a surgical incision into the trachea through overlying skin and muscles for airway management. A *tracheostomy* is the surgical creation of a stoma, or opening, into the trachea through the overlying skin (Figure 60-1). These terms are often used interchangeably. For simplicity, the term *tracheostomy* is used here.

Tracheostomy can be performed as an emergency procedure or as an elective procedure, depending on the indication. A competent provider can perform a percutaneous tracheostomy at the bedside in critical care

units. This method is cost-effective as it avoids the operating room cost, saves time, and avoids transporting critically ill clients to the operating room. The surgical approach, done as an open procedure in the operating room, includes removal of a portion of the tracheal ring to facilitate creation of a stoma for the tube placement. Surgically created tracheostomies may have sutures holding the tube in place for the first few postoperative days. A tracheostomy provides the best route for long-term airway maintenance. There are many indications for this procedure, including the following:

- Relief of acute or chronic upper airway obstruction, such as obstructive sleep apnea, trauma, bleeding, tumors, tissue swelling, infections, or burns (chemical or inhalation)
- Access for continuous mechanical ventilation, with the inability to wean (broadly defined as greater than 2 weeks of ventilation)
- Promotion of pulmonary hygiene by accessing airway for secretion removal
- Bilateral vocal cord paralysis
- Inability to protect own airway

---

evolve **Web Enhancements**

Bridge to Home Health Care   Living with a Tracheostomy

Client Education Guide   Swallowing Technique After a Partial Laryngectomy (Spanish Translation)

Care of a Tracheoesophageal Puncture Wound (English Version and Spanish Translation)

Exercises After Radical Neck Surgery (English Version and Spanish Translation)

Ethical Issues in Nursing   What Type of Client Education Is Needed for Informed Consent to Radical Procedures?

Be sure to check out the bonus material on the Evolve website and the CD-ROM, including free self-assessment exercises. **http://evolve.elsevier.com/Black/medsurg**

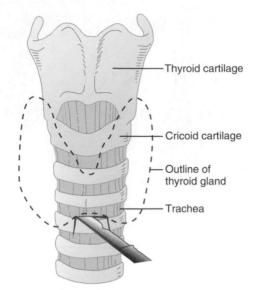

- **FIGURE 60–1**   Incision for a tracheostomy is made through the fibrous tissue above the third tracheal cartilage. Two small vertical incisions create a flap that can be closed later.

Labels on figure: Thyroid cartilage; Cricoid cartilage; Outline of thyroid gland; Trachea

A tracheostomy is by far the most satisfactory artificial airway. It bypasses the upper airway and glottis, making stabilization, suction, and the attachment of respiratory equipment much easier than with other types of artificial airways. The client has the potential to eat and, depending on the type of tube placed, talk, which can improve quality of life. Advantages to placement of tracheostomy tubes in critically ill clients include the need for less sedation, increased mobility, and reduced complications from immobility.

Tracheostomy Tubes

The tracheostomy opening is fitted with a tube to maintain airway patency. Tracheostomy tubes vary in their composition, number of separate parts, shape, and size. Tracheostomy tubes are chosen specifically for each client. Incorrectly fitted tubes can precipitate permanent or life-threatening damage.

The diameter of a tracheostomy tube must be smaller than the trachea so that it lies comfortably within the tracheal lumen. Air should be able to pass between the outer wall of the tracheostomy tube and the tracheal mucosa, and allow adequate perfusion to tracheal tissue. Although there is no standard tracheostomy tube sizing system, all packages indicate the inner and outer diameters in millimeters. Common size range for adult tracheostomy tubes is 6 to 8 mm. Tracheostomy tubes are made of various substances, such as nonreactive plastic, stainless steel, sterling silver, or silicone. Plastic tubes are disposable and used for only one person. Metal tubes may be reused after being sterilized. A tube must have a 15-mm hub for attachment to mechanical ventilation circuits, or manual resuscitation bags.

The length and curve of a tracheostomy tube are important to note. Tracheostomy tubes may be long or short. They may be angled, with the angle ranging from 50 to 90 degrees. Short to moderately short tubes with an angle of about 60 degrees are most often used. A tube must be long enough to avoid dislodgment into paratracheal tissue when the client coughs or turns his or her head. The lower end of a tracheostomy tube should be located above the carina. The curve of the tube must allow the tip to be in a straight line with the trachea, rather than pressing on the anterior or posterior tracheal wall. Tubes vary in material, and manufacturers produce standard as well as custom-made tubes to meet clients' needs. The ear, nose, and throat (ENT) surgeon selects the tube based on need, but as time progresses, it may be the bedside caregiver team of nurse, respiratory therapist (RT), and provider who determines the tube best suited for a client's needs. Tubes may have a single cannula, or may have an inner cannula. Inner cannulas will need to be removed periodically for cleaning; they may be reusable or disposable.

Tracheostomy tubes may be cuffed or uncuffed. An inflated cuff permits mechanical ventilation. Inflated cuffs deter secretions from the upper airway leaking into the lower airway, but do not create an absolute barrier. (Box 60-1). Tracheostomy cuffs do not hold the tube in place. Cuffs may be inflated with air, sterile water, or foam.

Standard Tracheostomy Tube. A standard tracheostomy tube (Figure 60-2) has (1) an outer cannula with cuff, flange, and pilot balloon and (2) an obturator. The parts fit together as one unit and may not be interchanged with other units. The tube fits in the tracheostomy stoma to keep it open. The tracheostomy tube has a flange or neckplate that fits flush with the neck and has holes on each side to attach the securing tapes or ties. A tracheostomy tube must be secured in place to prevent accidental extubation, excessive motion, or misalignment. Cloth tape or commercially available self-fastening (Velcro) ties may be used.

The obturator is placed into the outer tube before insertion. Its rounded tip smooths the end of the cannula and facilitates nontraumatic insertion of the tube into the stoma, with the aid of sterile lubricating jelly. The obturator is removed immediately after insertion to open the tube. Place the obturator in a plastic bag and tape it to the head of the client's bed in a conspicuous place. If the tracheostomy tube is accidentally displaced, the obturator can be immediately placed into the outer cannula for quick reinsertion.

A spare tube of the same type kept at the bedside is an important safety strategy. Accidental decannulation in the initial postoperative period may be considered an airway emergency. If the tube cannot be placed back in the stoma, the client may need urgent reintubation with an endotracheal tube. As the stoma matures postoperatively, the tube can be placed with greater ease.

SAFETY
ALERT

BOX 60-1 Inflation and Deflation of Tracheostomy Tube Cuff*

INFLATION (MINIMAL LEAK TECHNIQUE)

Objective

Inflate the cuff with the minimum volume of air required to adequately seal the trachea during positive-pressure ventilation and to prevent aspiration of foreign material while exerting the lowest possible cuff-to-tracheal wall pressure.

Intervention

1. Withdraw all residual air from the cuff.
2. Place 6 ml of air in a syringe.
3. Place the diaphragm of a stethoscope over the client's neck in the area of the tracheostomy tube cuff.
4. On inhalation, slowly inject air through the one-way valve into the pilot line in 1-ml increments.
5. Auscultate the neck area over the cuff.
6. Apply positive pressure to the tracheostomy tube with a manual self-inflating bag. An audible air leak can be heard via the stethoscope unless the cuff is inflated.
7. Continue slowly injecting air until the air leak is no longer present during inhalation.
8. When a leak is no longer auscultated, withdraw a small amount of air from the cuff until a very small leak is heard. This is called a *minimal leak*.
9. Note the amount of air necessary to achieve the minimal leak. This is the *minimal occluding volume* (MOV).
10. Once minimal leak is attained, measure the cuff pressure with a manometer.
11. Routinely measure and document cuff pressures.

DEFLATION

Objective

Allow air to flow around the tracheostomy tube to permit phonation and to provide an opportunity to blow secretions above the cuff into the oropharynx, where they can be removed by suctioning.

Intervention

Routinely deflating the cuff is not necessary provided that safe cuff inflation and cuff pressure measurements are performed.

1. Remove the ventilator assembly (if present) and attach a self-inflating bag to the 15-mm adapter on the inner cannula.
2. Hyperoxygenate, hyperinflate, and suction the trachea to remove secretions below the cuff. Remove secretions above the cuff by gently applying suction deep into the oropharynx.
3. Insert an empty syringe into the one-way valve, and pull back on the plunger to remove the air in the cuff. At the same time, apply positive pressure with the manual self-inflating bag. This maneuver blows secretions lying directly above the cuff into the mouth, which prevents secretions accumulated above the cuff from draining into the trachea and lower airway.
4. Suction the oropharynx again.
5. If the person is ventilator-dependent, remember that with the cuff "down" or deflated, a portion of ventilation volume will not reach the lungs. Air will escape through the upper airway, which may compromise the person's respiratory status. This volume loss creates an audible leak. Phonation is possible during the exhalation phase of ventilation.

*The same procedure is used for inflation and deflation of endotracheal tube cuffs.

Once the obturator is removed, the inner cannula is placed into the outer cannula. Lock it into place to prevent accidental removal (e.g., when the client coughs). Frequent removal and cleaning of the inner cannula are necessary to maintain airway patency. At the distal end, most inner cannulas have a standard 15-mm adapter that fits respiratory therapy and anesthesiology equipment.

Single-Cannula Tracheostomy Tube. A single-cannula tracheostomy tube is slightly longer than the standard tube and does not have an inner cannula. The longer single-cannula tube is used in the client with a thick neck or with an altered airway in whom a standard tracheostomy tube would be too short. Single-cannula tubes may have cuffs of variable types, or no cuff. Air-cuffed tubes may not be safely plugged because of the bulk of cuff within the airway. Silicone tubes with "tight to shaft" cuffs that inflate with sterile water offer safe options for plugging if the client has adequate air flow. Clients in whom a single-cannula tube is used must have continuous supplemental humidification to prevent obstruction by accumulated secretions.

Double-Cannula Tracheostomy Tube. Tubes with inner cannulas may be cuffed or uncuffed. Inner cannulas can be used when intermittent manual cleaning is desired. Inner cannulas are removed, inspected, cleaned, and put back in place or, if disposable, exchanged. Both inner and outer cannulas may have fenestrations.

Fenestrated Tracheostomy Tube. A fenestrated tracheostomy tube has one large opening (Latin, *fenestra*), or several small ones, on the curvature of the posterior wall of the outer cannula. Fenestrated tubes have an inner cannula and may be cuffed or cuffless. When the inner cannula is removed, the fenestration permits air to flow through both the upper airway and the tracheostomy opening. This may facilitate speech and more effective coughing. This tube may be used while a client is being weaned from a tracheostomy and for a client in whom use of the tracheostomy is expected to be prolonged. When the inner cannula is in place, the fenestration may be closed.

Foam Cuff Tracheostomy Tube. Tubes with a single cannula are for specialized needs. The cuff on the tube is

■ **FIGURE 60–2** Parts of a tracheostomy tube. *(Courtesy of Shiley, Inc., Irvine, Calif.)*

made of foam, so the cuff passively inflates to the desired size at atmospheric pressure. This design is intended to prevent injury to the trachea from over-inflated cuffs and used for clients who may have erosion of the airway or tracheomalacia.

Tracheostomy Speaking Valves. A speaking valve is a one-way plastic valve attached to the 15-mm end of a tracheostomy tube. This modification permits talking without the need to plug the tracheostomy tube. The one-way valve allows air (and the aerosol of supplemental humidification and oxygen) to flow into the tube during inspiration. On exhalation, the one-way valve closes, directing air from the lungs up through the vocal cords and upper airway. Phonation and effective coughing are facilitated by this normal passage of air.

SAFETY
⚠
ALERT

A talking tracheostomy is never used unless there is enough room around the tracheostomy tube to permit sufficient air flow for breathing. Always deflate a cuffed tracheostomy tube before the client uses the talking tracheostomy adapter. Cuff inflation prevents exhalation, potentially causing suffocation.

An important first step is assessment of the air flow initially with cuff deflation while monitoring the client with oximetry. Speech therapists are important team members to collaborate with respiratory care nurses and providers to ensure safety and quality for speaking valve use. Individuals may eat with valves on, and may have improved intake with better ability to smell. Because of the risk of airway occlusion, individuals should not sleep with speaking valves in place.

Talking Tracheostomy Tube. This tracheostomy tube allows speech by coordination of phonation efforts. Ventilation and phonation are separated because of different air sources. With this device, an air flow tube (that looks like a second pilot tube) runs outside the pilot (main) tube and opens just above the cuff. There is a port at the distal end of the air flow tube. When the port is occluded by a finger and compressed air or oxygen is directed through the air flow tube, a current of air is generated up through the vocal cords. With practice, the client learns to use this air flow for speech, although the "voice" produced in this way does not sound normal. Mucosal irritation may develop from the forced flow of air or oxygen into the upper airway. The portal can clog with mucus, creating less effective air flow and no vocalization.

Tracheostomy Button. Use of a tracheostomy button is sometimes indicated during weaning as an intermediate measure between using a standard tracheostomy tube and extubation. A button is a short, straight, plastic cylinder secured by a flange to the anterior tracheal wall but is not deep enough to enter the tracheal lumen. It has a removable cap with a one-way flap inside that permits inhalation but not exhalation. Exhalation occurs through the normal upper airway. When the cap is on, the client can talk. Without a 15-mm hub, the button cannot be used for ventilation.

It can replace a standard tracheostomy tube for clients with retained secretions who do not require ventilatory assistance. A button creates less airway resistance than that produced by a plugged standard tracheostomy tube; hence, breathing is easier. Artificial humidification of inspired air is necessary with a button (as with any tracheostomy tube), because the natural airway is bypassed.

Metal Tracheostomy Tube. Metal tracheostomy tubes are made of sterling silver or stainless steel. The most popular type is the Jackson tracheostomy tube. Metal tubes are cuffless and most often used in clients who have a permanent tracheostomy or laryngectomy. The inner cannula locks together with the outer cannula. Because metal tubes do not have a standard 15-mm adapter, rapid adaptation to respiratory or anesthesia equipment is impossible unless a specific adapter is available. The Hollinger tube is also made of metal and is similar to the Jackson tube. A plastic decannulation stopper, or plug, allows communication and upper airway breathing.

Permanent Tracheostomy. Most clients with a permanent tracheostomy use a cuffless tracheostomy tube. For appearance's sake, many clients prefer a low-profile inner cannula. This design does not incorporate a 15-mm adapter. Instead, the inner cannula fits into the outer cannula and lies flush with the neck. If the client has had a total laryngectomy, the cut end of the trachea is sutured to the skin, creating a permanent stoma. Once the stoma is healed, most laryngectomy clients do not need a tube.

🫖 Potential Problems Associated with Tracheostomy Tubes and Cuffs

The presence of an artificial airway bypasses the normal mechanism for protection against infection. Breathing that bypasses the upper airway does not permit the nose and mouth to warm or moisten inspired air. To prevent complications, caregivers must provide attention to aseptic technique and adequate humidification.

SAFETY ⚠ ALERT **The oral cavity becomes colonized with nosocomial bacteria within 48 hours of admission. Oral care, including plaque removal from teeth, even in clients who are nothing by mouth (NPO), helps prevent hospital-acquired pneumonia. Clients with artificial airways are at highest risk for this complication.**

Airway Obstruction. The flow of air through a tracheostomy tube may become occluded for several reasons. The tracheostomy tube may be misaligned so that its opening lies against the tracheal wall, preventing air flow. Cuff overinflation causes the cuff to herniate over the tip of the tube, obstructing air flow. Without adequate airway care, the inner cannula can become occluded with dried secretions or excessive bronchial secretions. Collaborate with respiratory care therapists to ensure adequate humidification is delivered to the airway. Heating and humidifying the inspired air will help keep mucus thin.

Infection. Tracheostomies increase the risk of bronchopulmonary infection because they (1) bypass upper airway protective mechanisms (i.e., filtering, warming, and humidifying) and (2) decrease mucociliary transport and coughing, thus increasing retained secretions. Stoma site infection may occur as well.

SAFETY ⚠ ALERT **Nosocomial infection is also a potential problem. The lower airway (below the larynx) is normally sterile. Therefore all solutions and equipment entering the trachea must be sterile. Organisms (e.g., *Pseudomonas aeruginosa* and other gram-negative bacteria) grow readily in respiratory equipment, which can then contaminate the lower airway. In addition, some bacteria may colonize a tracheostomy without causing infection.**

Ventilator-associated pneumonia (VAP) prevention strategies are implemented, including head-of-bed positioning greater than 45 degrees and frequent oral care for all clients with mechanical ventilation or artificial airways. Nurses need to be aggressive when performing oral care and clean the entire mouth, not just the lips and in front of the teeth.

Stoma care, including cleaning and skin care, should begin at its creation. Stoma maintenance promotes adequate skin integrity and provides a barrier to infection.

Changing Tracheostomy Tubes. Recommendations for changing tracheostomy tubes vary and therefore most physicians and health care facilities have established protocols. No standards exist in the literature. Each client has a unique set of circumstances that dictate the frequency of tracheostomy tube changes. Change of the tube based on need may be the best strategy to minimize risk and discomfort for the client. Tracheostomy care is discussed in a fundamentals of nursing textbook.

Accidental Decannulation. A tracheostomy tube that is not properly secured may be accidentally dislodged from the stoma. Because most new tracheostomy tubes are sutured in place, decannulation is rare, but it is serious nonetheless. Decannulation may occur while the ties are being changed. Manipulation of a tracheostomy tube or suctioning often produces vigorous coughing, which can expel the tube from the stoma unless the tube is held firmly. A stoma less than 4 days old may also close because a tract is not yet formed. If extubation occurs, call for help immediately and follow the steps in Box 60-2.

Maintain ventilation and oxygenation by bag and mask. If ventilation is impossible, you must reinsert the tube. To do so, deflate the cuff, remove the inner cannula of the tube, insert the obturator in the outer cannula, elevate the client's shoulders with a pillow, and gently hyperextend the neck. If accidental decannulation occurs once a tract has formed following a tracheostomy, the same procedure is used, but reinsertion of the tube is generally easier. If bleeding occurs or the airway is obstructed, use emergency measures as indicated earlier. If the tube cannot be reinserted, it should be considered an airway emergency and preparation for reintubation begun. **SAFETY ⚠ ALERT**

Tracheal Wall Necrosis. Necrosis of the tracheal wall can lead to the formation of an opening between the posterior trachea and the esophagus, called a *tracheoesophageal fistula*. The fistula allows air to escape into the stomach, causing distention. It also promotes aspiration of gastric contents. Fistulae most often develop when a

PREPARE FOR POTENTIAL DECANNULATION

Keep the following equipment at the client's bedside:
- Extra tracheostomy tubes of the same size and one size smaller
- Obturator belonging to the existing tube
- Tracheal dilator (spreader)
- Oxygen source
- Suction catheters and suction source
- Resuscitation bag

IF DECANNULATION OCCURS
- Call for help.
- Hyperextend the client's neck to facilitate tube reinsertion.
- Assess the presence of tracheal retention sutures and use them to maintain an airway:
  - Pull top suture upward and outward.
  - Pull lower suture downward and outward.
- If retention sutures are not present, insert the tracheal dilator into the tracheostoma to open the airway.
- Place the obturator into the outer cannula and reinsert the tracheostomy tube into the tracheostoma. If the replacement tube is cuffed, deflate the cuff before insertion.
- Secure the tube with ties or Velcro strap.
- Assess tube placement by auscultating for breath sounds. Insert the inner cannula and reconnect oxygen/ventilation equipment.
- If the tracheostomy tube cannot be reinserted in 1 minute, call a code.

cuffed tube is used in conjunction with a standard nasogastric (NG) tube. Use of small-lumen NG tubes can decrease the risk of fistula formation. Necrosis of the anterior trachea can lead to the rare but life-threatening complication of hemorrhage resulting from erosion into the innominate artery. This complication is manifested by bleeding in and around the tracheostomy or by pulsation of the tracheostomy tube. Immediate intervention is mandatory because exsanguination can occur.

Most tracheostomy tube cuffs are designed to exert a low pressure against the tracheal wall. These cuffs are easily distensible, so that they accept a high volume of air without generating excessive force (i.e., high-volume, low-pressure cuffs). Low cuff pressure is necessary to prevent damage to the tracheal mucosa. The volume of air in the cuff determines the pressure exerted on the tracheal mucosa. Cuff pressures should not exceed 20 cm H_2O. With pressures greater than 42 cm H_2O, circulation to the tracheal mucosa is impaired, resulting in ischemia and necrosis. This is because the normal pressure within tracheal arteries is 42 cm H_2O. In the veins and lymphatic vessels, the normal pressures are 24 and 7 cm H_2O, respectively. Tracheal damage from cuff pressure is a frequent complication of intubation. Cuffed tubes can cause tracheal damage in as few as 3 to 5 days.

Tracheal Dilation. Prolonged intubation can lead to dilation of the trachea from the cuff. This complication should be suspected when increasing amounts of air are needed to seal the cuff or when bulging of the tracheal wall is seen on x-ray films.

Tracheal Stenosis. Tracheal stenosis is narrowing of the trachea and may be noted 1 week to 2 years after intubation. It results from chronic inflammation, fibrosis, and necrosis, which cause scar formation in the inflamed trachea. It can also result from excessive movement of the tracheostomy tube from ventilator tubing. The severity of stenosis can be prevented by choosing the right size of tube, maintaining adequate cuff pressure, keeping intubation time short, preventing infection, and reducing movement of the tube. Tracheal stenosis is a potential complication of long-term tracheostomy and may require tracheal resection.

Tracheomalacia. Tracheomalacia is a softening of the trachea resulting from secretions pooling above the cuff and thinning the cartilage. This weakened area of the trachea collapses on deep inspiration, impeding air flow and making it difficult to achieve an adequate seal. This problem may be managed by using a foam cuff tracheostomy tube. This tube has a sponge-like consistency. The cuff is foam-filled and self-expands with air after insertion, conforming to the size and shape of the client's trachea, and reducing pressure on the tracheal wall.

Subcutaneous Emphysema. Subcutaneous emphysema develops when air escapes from the tracheostomy incision into the tissues, dissects fascial planes under the skin, and accumulates around the face, neck, and upper chest. These areas appear puffy, and slight finger pressure produces a crackling sound and sensation. Generally this is not a serious condition; the air is eventually absorbed. The underlying cause determines the serious nature of the treatment.

Weaning, Removal, and Rescue Breathing
Weaning from a Tracheostomy Tube

Clients can be weaned from mechanical ventilation if they can clear their secretions by mouth with an adequate cough, maintain oxygenation, and have a functional upper airway without obstruction. The multidisciplinary team collaborates for this assessment.

A tracheostomy tube is usually plugged by inserting a tracheostomy plug (decannulation stopper) into the opening of the outer cannula if the tube has a "tight to shaft" cuff, fenestration, or no cuff. This closes off the tracheostomy, allowing air flow and respiration to occur normally through the nose and mouth.

When a cuffed tracheostomy tube is plugged, the cuff must be deflated. If the cuff remains inflated, ventilation cannot occur, and respiratory arrest could result.

Air-cuffed tubes without fenestrations may not be safely capped.

Explain the process to the client and family. Most clients are anxious about weaning because they fear they may not be able to breathe. Constant, supportive observation during weaning is necessary. Encourage the client to begin to think about breathing through the nose again. This breathing is a strange sensation for people who have used a tracheostomy tube for a long time. Explain ways to facilitate optimal respiration and to maintain control of breathing (e.g., inhale slowly and completely through the nose; avoid holding the breath).

Arterial blood gas (ABG) analysis and measurement of spontaneous respiratory mechanics (respiratory rate, tidal volume, vital capacity, inspiratory effort, expiratory effort) are important assessments during the decannulation process. Oximetry and other noninvasive assessment modes may also be used once baseline ABG values are established. During weaning from tracheostomy, assess for indications of respiratory distress or ventilation impairment and suction frequency. Clinical manifestations of problems may include the following:

- Abnormal respiratory rate and pattern
- Use of accessory muscles to assist breathing
- Abnormal pulse and blood pressure measurements
- Abnormal skin and mucous membrane color
- Abnormal ABG levels or decreased oxygen saturation

Inability to Clear Mucus. Remove the tracheostomy plug immediately if any manifestation of respiratory distress or ventilation impairment appear. Also assess the client's quality of phonation and ability to deep-breathe and cough effectively. If oxygen has been administered via the tracheostomy, administer it at the prescribed rate of flow using nasal prongs. Prepare for possible return to mechanical ventilation, and have a manual resuscitation bag available at the bedside.

Removing a Tracheostomy Tube

A tracheostomy tube is removed after resumption of normal respirations as indicated by the client's ability to breathe comfortably with the tracheostomy plugged, to cough and expectorate secretions, and to maintain normal ABG values or oxygen saturation. Gradually increase the length of plugging sessions until the client is comfortable and confident with the tube plugged continuously for at least 24 hours.

After a tracheostomy tube is removed, place a petroleum gauze pad covered by a sterile dressing over the stoma. Providing an occlusive dressing minimizes air leak during the stoma healing process. Initially, every 8 hours, clean the skin around the stoma, remove mucus with hydrogen peroxide, rinse the area with normal saline, and apply a fresh, dry dressing over the healing stoma. Document the condition of the stoma and the surrounding skin. If either appears irritated or infected, notify the physician. Topical antibiotic ointment may be prescribed. A tracheostomy stoma closes gradually (over a period of several days). As long as the stoma is open, an air leak is present. Instruct the client to place clean fingers firmly over the dressing to facilitate normal speech and coughing.

After decannulation, ongoing assessment of respiratory function is necessary. Some complications of tracheostomy, such as tracheal stenosis, can appear months after tracheostomy tube removal.

Performing Rescue Breathing

Emergency rescue breathing in the bag-to-neck mode (i.e., mouth to tracheostomy or mouth to stoma) may be necessary if a client who has a tracheostomy or laryngectomy experiences respiratory depression or respiratory arrest. If a tracheostomy tube is in place, provide ventilation by attaching a manual self-inflating bag to the standard 15-mm adapter on the inner cannula. Some volume is lost from an uncuffed tube. Compensation of adequate ventilation can often be accomplished by altering the usual method of manual inflation (e.g., compress the bag more forcefully and quickly). If the tracheostomy tube is cuffed, inflate the cuff and maintain ventilation at the correct rate—that is, 12 to 16 breaths/min for an adult. If inflation of the cuff impedes ventilation, immediately deflate the cuff, and attempt to compensate for volume loss by compressing the bag more forcefully or quickly.

Nursing Management of the Client with a Tracheostomy

Preoperative Care

For clients who are to undergo elective tracheostomy, reinforce education provided by the physician. You may delegate some respiratory assistance tasks to other staff members, as discussed in the Management and Delegation feature on p. 1548. The client's understanding of the tracheostomy tube may be enhanced by looking at anatomic diagrams and by handling a tracheostomy tube. The postoperative changes in ability to speak and eat should be explained. If the tracheostomy is expected to be permanent, information about living a productive life with modifications in clothing can be provided. A visit by a client with a permanent tracheostomy may be desirable.

When an emergency tracheostomy is needed, precious seconds may be all the time available for teaching.

MANAGEMENT AND DELEGATION

Assisting with Respiratory Care

Assisting with respiratory care is one of the more controversial areas involving the use of assistive personnel. Opinions differ widely on the role of assistive personnel in caring for clients who need respiratory care. The performance of suctioning in particular is central to this debate. Your clinical facility should provide you with clear guidelines about the role of assistive personnel in this aspect of care.

The following aspects of respiratory care are commonly delegated to unlicensed assistive personnel:

- Setting up oxygen delivery equipment and suction equipment
- Stocking routine respiratory care supplies at the bedside
- Assisting clients with the use of an incentive spirometer (after client instruction from a nurse or respiratory care clinician)
- Assisting clients with coughing and deep-breathing (after client instruction from a nurse or a respiratory care clinician)
- Measuring and recording peripheral oxygen saturation (Spo_2)

Before the delegation of any aspect of respiratory care, consider the following:

- What is the client's respiratory status? Complete a thorough respiratory assessment.
- What is the indication for respiratory care? Is the client's condition stable? A client with acute respiratory compromise should receive your full attention and care; the care of such a client should not be delegated.
- Is your client receiving oxygen therapy? Oxygen is a type of medication for your client. All guidelines that pertain to medications also apply to oxygen. You may delegate the setup of oxygen delivery equipment to assistive personnel. However, you are responsible to verify that the ordered amount (dose) of oxygen is actually being delivered to the client.
- Does this client have a new or long-term tracheostomy? The tracheostomy tube that has been placed through a new surgical incision should be evaluated as for any other fresh postoperative site.
- Have the client and family members managed this tracheostomy at home? This is an opportunity to evaluate their sterile technique, to provide reinforcement, and to review instructions with the client and family. After doing so, you may choose to delegate suctioning for this client to assistive personnel.

Findings that are immediately reportable to you, the registered nurse, should be described for the assistive personnel. These include any change or difficulty that the caregiver or the client experiences during the provision of care, changes in the respiratory rate or pattern, and changes in the consistency, color, and quantity of respiratory secretions.

The client may be anxious or even unconscious. Education is often provided to the family to provide support to the individual.

Postoperative Care

Assessment. After tracheostomy, usual frequent assessment is required, including assessing amount, color, and consistency of secretions; and observing for indications of shock, hemorrhage, respiratory insufficiency, or complications related to the client's general condition or the surgical intervention.

Diagnosis, Outcomes, Interventions

Diagnosis: Ineffective Airway Clearance. Numerous factors can lead to ineffective airway clearance in clients with tracheostomy—for example, dehydration, fever, anesthesia, anticholinergic drugs, sedatives, and immobility.

Outcomes. The client will have effective airway clearance, as evidenced by no retained secretions, clear (or clearing) lung sounds, and no fever.

Interventions. Promote airway clearance and pulmonary aeration by changing the client's position frequently, providing humidification and hydration, using sedatives cautiously, and performing frequent hyperinflation and suctioning to promote lung expansion and reduce the risks of atelectasis, pulmonary infection, and ineffective gas exchange. Hyperinflation creates an "artificial sigh," improving lung aeration and facilitating removal of tracheobronchial secretions by enhancing the cough effort. When the client's condition is stabilized sufficiently, coughing may be enhanced by having the client place a finger over the tracheostomy tube opening while attempting to cough, if the tube is cuffless or the cuff is deflated. It is important that the client wash his or her hands before doing this. Have the client cough into clean gauze squares and dispose of them carefully. Paper tissues are not recommended for use with a tracheostomy.

Perform Suctioning. When a cuffed tracheostomy tube is used, secretions collect above the cuff. It is difficult to remove such secretions by oropharyngeal suctioning. Oral suction devices allow pharyngeal suctioning.

Suction clients' secretions based on assessment, not routinely, using sterile technique, preoxygenation, and hyperinflation, without routine instillation of normal saline. Routine suctioning increases airway trauma, and routine instillation of normal saline for suctioning increases the risk of pulmonary edema. Use proper technique to reduce mucosal trauma, which can lead to tracheal infection. SAFETY ALERT

Mucosal trauma is indicated by tracheal irritation, tracheitis, and bloody tracheal secretions.

If the client is unable to cough, suction the airway through the tracheostomy tube. See the Management and Delegation feature on p. 1548 before delegating activities to unlicensed assistive personnel.

Provide Tracheostomy Care. Tracheostomy care is detailed elsewhere in fundamentals of nursing textbooks. Reinsertion of the clean inner cannula is shown in Figure 60-3.

Provide Adequate Hydration. The normal hydrating mechanisms of the upper airway are bypassed by a tracheostomy. Hydration can be provided by an oral, parenteral, or inhalation route. Inhalation techniques include increasing the humidity of room air with a room humidifier and administering oxygen with heated humidification via a ventilator circuit or aerosol device and sterile water.

If humidification is insufficient, the body tries to compensate for the deficit by using its own water stores. The result is tenacious (very thick) mucus, which can compromise airway patency and increases the risk of secretion pooling and subsequent infection. Dried mucus also occludes air passages and leads to atelectasis, pneumonia, and potentially severe gas exchange abnormalities.

Prevent Tube Movement. Secure a tracheostomy tube in midline tracheal alignment. Support ventilator and aerosol tubing to prevent pulling on the tracheostomy tube. Be careful not to disconnect tubing when turning the client. If cloth tape is used to secure the tube, tie a square knot, allowing room for two fingers to slide comfortably under the tape. Avoid placing the knot over the client's carotid artery or spine. Inspect the skin under the securing tape for skin irritation. When a tracheostomy is required for prolonged periods, the use of fastening devices such as padded straps with self-adhesive fasteners promotes comfort.

Diagnosis: Risk for Impaired Gas Exchange. After tracheostomy, impaired gas exchange may occur because of various factors. Factors affecting oxygen delivery include (1) aspiration of blood, oral secretions, or gastric contents; (2) restricted lung expansion from immobility; (3) excessive tracheobronchial secretions; (4) inability to cough and deep-breathe; and (5) pre-existing medical conditions (e.g., obesity, fever, inadequate hydration, pneumonia, tracheal injury such as from burns).

Factors affecting the removal of carbon dioxide include (1) the use of sedatives or anesthetic agents, (2) deteriorating level of consciousness, and (3) any other condition potentially affecting ventilatory efficiency and leading to hypoventilation and retention of carbon dioxide.

Outcomes. The client will have adequate gas exchange, as evidenced by maintaining oxygen saturation at greater than 90% (or ABG values within normal limits) and having no manifestations of respiratory distress.

Interventions. Assessment of gas exchange by ABG analysis is important immediately after tracheostomy and whenever there is a change in the client's condition or a change in treatment. Continuous noninvasive monitoring with pulse oximetry is also used. If shock or hypotension exists, or if peripheral vasoconstrictive drugs are used, data obtained by transcutaneous monitoring may be incorrect because of vasoconstriction and probes should be placed on the ears if the fingers are cool.

> **Do not allow smoking in the room of a person who has a tracheostomy. Do not use aerosol spray cans (e.g., room deodorizers) near the person. Do not shake bedding or create dust clouds. Be careful when shaving or tending the person's hair that whiskers or hair does not fall into the trachea. Cover the tracheostomy with a thin cloth towel during shaving.**
>
> SAFETY ⚠ ALERT

Diagnosis: Risk for Infection. The tracheostomy bypasses normal upper airway protective mechanisms. The client also has an incision. Both areas can become infected.

Outcomes. The client will exhibit no indications of infection, as evidenced by the absence of fever and by having a clean and dry tracheostomy site, healing incisions, and clear sputum.

Interventions

> **Use aseptic technique when working with the tracheostomy. This includes performing careful hand-washing; appropriately using gloves, sterile supplies, and solutions; and changing and decontaminating respiratory equipment per CDC standards. Create a "loop" in the aerosol or ventilator tubing assembly; that is, let the tube loop down to catch condensate. Drain water and condensate in the tubing away from the tracheostomy into a receptacle.**
>
> **Clean and inspect the skin around the stoma and the stoma itself. Observe for indications of irritation, inflammation, skin breakdown, and purulent**
>
> SAFETY ⚠ ALERT

■ **FIGURE 60–3**   Reinserting a cleaned inner cannula.

drainage. Use a topical barrier to deter moisture, such as vitamin A and D ointment. If skin or stomal infection does occur, a topical antibacterial ointment may be prescribed.

Tracheostomy dressings (Figure 60-4) are often used, especially in the early postoperative stage. Damp blood and mucus-soaked dressings constitute a perfect medium for the growth of microorganisms. These conditions promote tissue irritation and breakdown. Change dressings whenever they are soiled or damp. Using normal saline and cotton-tipped applicators, carefully clean the skin each time the dressing is changed. Do not use plastic-backed or waterproof dressings. Moisture, secretions, and blood may seep behind the dressings, which retain warmth and moisture. Skin then becomes irritated and macerated.

Diagnosis: Risk for Aspiration. The presence of a tracheostomy increases the risk of aspiration because the tubes tether the larynx, preventing normal upward movement of the larynx and closure by the epiglottis on swallowing.

Outcomes. The client will exhibit no evidence of aspiration—that is, the client will have clear lung sounds, no fever, and no choking with swallowing.

Interventions. Intravenous fluids are usually given during the first 24 hours after tracheostomy. Then, if the client is alert and if swallowing and gag mechanisms are intact, oral intake of fluid and food may be attempted. Speech therapists can provide assessments and contributions to the plan of care. If a cuffed endotracheal tube was used before the tracheostomy, assess for the presence of tracheoesophageal fistula before permitting oral feedings. A client in whom normal swallowing is not

■ **FIGURE 60–4** Tracheostomy dressings. If there is significant bleeding or tracheal secretions, cleaning the skin and changing the dressing frequently may prevent infection and skin breakdown. Manufactured dressing with a precut slit has no fine threads that could unravel and enter the stoma. Place the dressing around the tracheostomy tube with the slit downward, as shown, or upward.

expected to return for some time, or in whom the swallowing mechanism is permanently impaired (e.g., after a stroke), requires gastrostomy feedings or a permanent feeding tube (see Chapter 30). Tube feedings may cause reflux, and the formula may be aspirated into the trachea. Before administering tube feedings, inflate the cuff of the tracheostomy tube. Leave it inflated for at least 1 hour after feeding. Suction above the cuff before deflating it to remove any tube-feeding material.

When feeding a client with a tracheostomy, have the client sit upright. Often, food and fluids with semi-solid consistency (e.g., pudding) are easier to swallow than water. Overinflation of the cuff causes swallowing difficulty. If oral fluid intake is limited, continue intravenous fluids or enteral feedings.

Diagnosis: Impaired Verbal Communication. Because the vocal cords are bypassed by the tracheostomy tube, the client cannot talk. The nursing diagnosis of *Impaired Verbal Communication* may need to be combined with the nursing diagnosis of *Fear* or *Anxiety* if the client feels afraid of not being able to summon help.

Outcomes. The client will have a satisfactory method of communicating with the nursing staff, as evidenced by being able to summon help and have needs met.

Interventions. Make sure the client can always reach an emergency call system to summon help. Be sure all staff members who may be answering the call system are aware that the client is unable to talk. Make a written list of common needs, words, and phrases that the client can point to (e.g., "I want to pass urine," "I am thirsty," or "I have pain") to communicate needs. Provide paper and pencil or a picture communication board to facilitate communication. Clients can seldom write clearly and it may be difficult to comprehend their written messages. When possible, assess the client's reading ability preoperatively and select appropriate communication tools to be used postoperatively. Other options include using a speaking valve, plugging of an appropriate tube, or using an electrolarynx.

Diagnosis: Risk for Constipation. When the glottis and vocal cords are bypassed (as with tracheostomy), the client cannot perform a Valsalva maneuver. This deficit impairs the person's ability to defecate.

Outcomes. The client will have regular bowel movements (according to a usual schedule).

Interventions. Assess for most recent bowel movement. Elimination is a frequently overlooked area of client care. Use prescribed stool softeners, laxatives, and even enemas or suppositories as necessary.

Diagnosis: Anxiety and Fear. Anxiety and fear are caused by various factors affecting the client with a tracheostomy—for example, inability to talk, fear of suffocating, anxiety about diagnosis, or fear that the tracheostomy tube will come out.

Outcomes. The client will have decreasing manifestations of anxiety and fear, as evidenced by a pulse rate within normal limits, a calm facial expression, the ability to communicate, and no expressed fears.

Interventions. Frequent observation is essential. Your presence and skilled nursing care are reassuring. Be certain to allow the client adequate time to communicate needs and concerns. Assist the family in reassuring the client that nurses are present and that the client is not alone.

Diagnosis: Risk for Ineffective Therapeutic Regimen Management (Individuals) and Risk for Ineffective Family Therapeutic Regimen Management. The client and family members need a lot of new information about permanent or long-term tracheostomy care.

Outcomes. Before discharge from the health care facility, the client and significant others will be confident in performing tracheostomy care, suctioning, and preoxygenation and will demonstrate proper use of safety measures, emergency airway management, aerosol therapy, and other aspects of the client's airway maintenance regimen.

Interventions. Learning self-care is important for the client with a permanent tracheostomy. It provides a sense of self-control and reduces dependency on others. The client and significant others should begin performing self-care procedures as soon as possible postoperatively in order to allow sufficient time for learning. Multimedia resources, videotape, and booklets should be used to supplement the demonstrations and teaching. Follow-up telephone calls, contact through the physician's office, and home health nursing care (see the Bridge to Home Health Care website feature on Living with a Tracheostomy) are necessary to identify the effectiveness of the teaching.

Significant others must also be able to provide tracheostomy care and other components of airway management. Teach family members how to provide rescue breathing using the information presented previously.

The client and significant others are often anxious about home management. Send home a duplicate tracheostomy tube for use in changing the tube or in the event of accidental decannulation. Close follow-up is essential. Arrange for home equipment and follow-up visits by a home health agency or community health nurse with expertise in caring for people with complex airway needs. Involve a tracheostomy nurse specialist in client teaching when available. Order home health care equipment from medical suppliers who employ respiratory therapists or nurses. Ideally, have the equipment initially delivered to the hospital, so that the client and significant others can learn its use under the supervision of professionals.

Evaluation. Nursing diagnoses related to airway management should be resolvable within a few days. Problems with communication, infection, constipation, and eating remain areas of concern and require long-term planning.

NEOPLASTIC DISORDERS

BENIGN TUMORS OF THE LARYNX

Papillomas are one type of benign tumor of the larynx. They are small, wart-like growths believed to be viral in origin. Papillomas may be removed by surgical excision or laser. Surgery must be exact, because the nondiseased portion of the vocal cords needs to be retained for function. Other benign tumors of the larynx are *nodules* and *polyps*. Nodules and polyps frequently occur in people who abuse or overuse their voice.

CANCER OF THE LARYNX

Cancer of the larynx accounts for 2% to 3% of all malignancies. Care of the client with cancer of the larynx presents a unique challenge to the nurse because of the cosmetic and functional deformities commonly resulting from the disorder and its treatment. Benign and early malignant tumors may be treated with limited surgery, and the client recovers with little functional loss. Advanced tumors require extensive treatment, including surgery, radiation treatments, and chemotherapy. When a total laryngectomy is required, postoperatively the client is unable to speak, breathe through the nose or mouth, or eat normally. In addition, the creation of a permanent tracheostoma resulting from surgery has a tremendous impact on the client's functional ability and quality of life.

Laryngeal cancer is classified and treated by its anatomic site. Cancer of the larynx (voice box) may occur on the glottis (true vocal cords), the supraglottic structures (above the vocal cords), or the subglottic structures (below the vocal cords) (Box 60-3).

The American Cancer Society estimates 8900 new cases of laryngeal cancer each year, most occurring in men. However, the incidence of cancer of the larynx in women is increasing. If untreated, cancer of the larynx is inevitably fatal; 90% of untreated people die within 3 years. It is potentially curable if diagnosed and treated early.

Etiology and Risk Factors

The primary etiologic agent in laryngeal cancer is cigarette smoking. Three of four clients in whom laryngeal cancer develops have smoked or currently smoke. Alcohol appears to act synergistically with tobacco to increase the risk of development of a malignant tumor in the upper airway. Additional risk factors include occupational exposure to asbestos, wood dust, mustard gas,

BOX 60-3 Clinical Manifestations of Laryngeal Cancer

GLOTTIC TUMOR

True glottic tumors interfere with normal closure and vibration of the vocal cords

Manifestations

- *Early:* Voice change, hoarseness, hemoptysis
- Dyspnea, respiratory obstruction, dysphagia, weight loss, pain
- *Metastasize:* Through regional lymph nodes (rare except in superior or inferior tumors)

SUPRAGLOTTIC TUMOR

Carcinoma of the false cord partially hiding the true cord

Manifestations

- *Early:* Aspiration on swallowing (especially liquids), persistent unilateral sore throat, foreign-body sensation, dysphagia, weight loss, neck mass, hemoptysis (expectoration of blood)
- *Late:* Dyspnea, pain in the throat or referred to the ear

SUBGLOTTIC TUMOR

Subglottic polyp; this type of polyp can be single and smooth or lobulated as shown

Manifestations

- *Early:* None
- *Late:* Dyspnea, airway obstruction, dysphagia, weight loss, hemoptysis

Top and bottom figures from DeWeese, D.F., & Saunders, W.H. (1982). *Textbook of otolaryngology* (6th ed). St. Louis: Mosby; middle figure from Del Regato, J.A., et al. (1985). *Ackerman and Del Regato's cancer* (6th ed.). St. Louis: Mosby.

and petroleum products and the inhalation of other noxious fumes. Chronic laryngitis and voice abuse may also contribute to the disorder. Research points to a link between tobacco exposure and mutation of the *p53* gene in squamous cell carcinoma of the head and neck.

Pathophysiology

Squamous cell carcinoma is the most common malignant tumor of the larynx, arising from the membrane lining the respiratory tract. Metastasis from cancer of the glottis is unusual because of the sparse lymphatic drainage from the vocal cords. Cancer elsewhere in the larynx spreads more quickly because there are abundant lymphatic vessels. Metastatic disease often may be palpated as neck masses. Distant metastasis may occur in the lungs. Patterns of spread of head and neck cancer are shown in Figure 60-5.

Clinical Manifestations

The earliest clinical warning signs of laryngeal cancer are dependent on the location of the tumor. In general, hoarseness that lasts longer than 2 weeks should be evaluated. Hoarseness occurs when the tumor invades muscle and cartilage surrounding the larynx, causing fixation of the vocal cords. Most clients wait before seeking a diagnosis for chronic hoarseness.

Tumors on the glottis prevent glottic closure during speech, which causes hoarseness or a voice change. Supraglottic tumors may cause pain in the throat (especially with swallowing), aspiration during swallowing, a sensation of a foreign body in the throat, neck masses, or pain radiating to the ear by way of the glossopharyngeal and vagus nerves. Subglottic tumors have no early

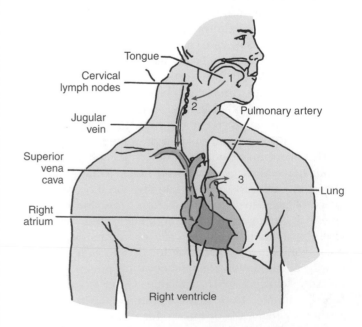

■ **FIGURE 60–5** Pattern of spread of head and neck cancer. *(From Black, J. [1991]. Reconstructive surgery in the elderly. Plastic Surgical Nursing, 11, 157.)*

manifestations; clinical evidence does not appear until the lesion grows to obstruct the airway.

Diagnostic Findings

The diagnosis of laryngeal cancer is made by visual examination of the larynx using direct or indirect laryngoscopy. The nasopharynx and posterior soft palate are inspected indirectly with a small mirror or an instrument resembling a telescope. While the mirror is inserted, slight pressure is applied to the tongue, and the client is instructed to say "a" and then "e," which elevates the soft palate. The instrument should not touch the tongue, or the client will gag. The nasopharynx is then inspected for drainage, bleeding, ulceration, or masses. Direct visualization of the larynx may be accomplished with use of several different instruments; most devices used are lighted endoscopes. The client is instructed to protrude the tongue, and the examiner *gently* holds the tongue with a gauze sponge and pulls it forward. A laryngeal mirror or telescopic endoscope is inserted into the oropharynx; again, contact with the tongue is avoided. The client is instructed to breathe in and out rapidly through the mouth, or to "pant like a puppy." Panting decreases the gagging sensation caused by the examination. During quiet respiration, the base of the tongue, epiglottis, and vocal cords are examined for manifestations of infection or tumor. The client is instructed to vocalize a high-pitched *eee* to approximate (close) the vocal cords. The examiner observes the movement of the cords, the color of the mucous membranes, and the presence of any lesions. If the client is unable to cooperate as described, the examination may be performed with a fiberoptic endoscope inserted through the nose.

Before any definitive treatment for tumor is initiated, a panendoscopy and biopsy are performed to determine the exact location, size, and extent of the primary tumor. Computed tomography (CT) or magnetic resonance imaging (MRI) is used to assist with this process. Laboratory analysis includes a complete blood count, determination of serum electrolytes including calcium, and kidney and liver function tests. These data help determine the physiologic readiness of the client for surgery. Because the airway will be altered after surgery, the client requires a thorough pulmonary assessment with ABG analysis for identification of any pre-existing pulmonary disorders that would interfere with breathing. Clients who are to undergo partial laryngectomy must have an adequate pulmonary reserve in order to produce an effective cough postoperatively. The operation is associated with an increased risk of aspiration, and the client must be able to cough to rid the airway of aspirated secretions. Finally, for ascertaining possible tumor spread or other primary tumors, a chest radiography and barium swallow study or esophagography are performed.

Once the tumor has been identified and a biopsy performed, the tumor can be staged. Staging has important implications for treatment choice and outcome. It is essential to determine the extent of the primary tumor in order to select the most appropriate intervention. Staging is accomplished by (1) measuring the size of the primary tumor, (2) determining the presence of enlarged lymphatic nodes, and (3) determining the presence of distant metastasis. This system of staging is called the TNM (tumor-node-metastasis) classification system (see Chapter 17).

OUTCOME MANAGEMENT

Medical Management

Tumor Ablation

The goal of client care is ablation of the tumor, with sparing of undiseased tissue when possible. The choice of treatment for glottic cancer depends on the degree of tumor involvement. If the tumor is limited to the true vocal cord, without causing limitation of the cord's movement, radiation therapy is usually the best treatment, with cure rates of 85% to 95%. The radiation dose depends on the size and location of the tumor; it is usually a minimum dose of 5500 to 6000 centigray (cGy; *gray* is a more accurate unit than *rad*) over 5 to 7 weeks. Hyperfractionation (delivery of radiation twice a day) may be done to improve tumor control. During radiation therapy, the client needs to be assessed for manifestations of destruction of normal tissue, ability to eat, airway distress, and other side effects. The complications of radiation therapy to the larynx include skin irritation, xerostomia, mucositis, laryngeal edema, and delayed healing. Radiation therapy is discussed in Chapter 17.

Supraglottic tumors may be treated with radiation therapy or a partial laryngectomy, with or without lymph node dissection. Subglottic tumors are usually more advanced carcinomas in which the tumor has spread to surrounding tissues. Metastasis is common. Treatment requires a total laryngectomy with or without radical neck dissection on the same or both sides of the tumor (see later discussion). The operative site may require reconstruction with pectoralis myocutaneous flaps (see Chapter 49).

Chemotherapy alone is not considered to be curative in treating head and neck cancers but it is now integrated into standard therapy for head and neck cancer. It may be administered preoperatively to reduce tumor size, concurrently with radiation therapy, postoperatively to reduce the risk of metastasis, or as palliative treatment. Larynx preservation may be possible with induction chemotherapy followed by radiation. Chemotherapy is generally not effective in advanced laryngeal cancer, but it may control the development of new primary tumors through a process called *chemoprevention.*

Clients with laryngeal tumors often present in a compromised nutritional state because of dysphagia and weight loss. In addition, surgery, radiation therapy, and chemotherapy can directly affect oropharyngeal structures and impair swallowing. Nutritional intervention should begin before treatment to prevent malnutrition, thereby improving the overall prognosis.

Nursing Management of the Medical Client

The client undergoing radiation therapy for laryngeal cancer should be taught about the procedure and how to assess for and manage any expected problems at home. Written material is usually best, so that the client and family can refer to it as needed. Skin care for the irradiated site should include using prescribed creams and sunscreens, which are "patted" onto the skin; avoiding extremes of temperature; avoiding rough or tight garments; and avoiding rubbing or scratching the area.

Surgical Management

The goals of surgical intervention for laryngeal cancer are to (1) remove the cancer, (2) maintain adequate physiologic function of the airway, and (3) achieve a personally acceptable physical appearance. Many clients require tracheostomy for airway management (see earlier discussion). Most clients with advanced laryngeal cancer also have malnutrition from obstruction to swallowing by the tumor, as well as from the effects of the cancer. Before surgery, supplemental nutrition may be provided by NG tube feedings or gastrostomy feedings. If long-term difficulty in swallowing is anticipated, a gastrostomy tube may be inserted at the time of surgery.

Laser Surgery
Small tumors can often be eradicated with the use of laser. Laser surgery for vocal cord tumors can preserve much of the normal glottis, leaving the client with a usable voice. Sometimes laser surgery is combined with radiation therapy.

Partial Laryngectomy
For cancer involving one true vocal cord, or one cord plus a portion of the other, a partial laryngectomy is feasible. This procedure is also called a vertical partial laryngectomy and involves the removal of half or more of the larynx (Figure 60-6). A horizontal neck incision is made, and the diseased portion of the vocal cord is removed. Sometimes up to one third of the contralateral cord is also removed. This operation is generally well tolerated, and the client has only mild difficulty swallowing and an altered but adequate voice.

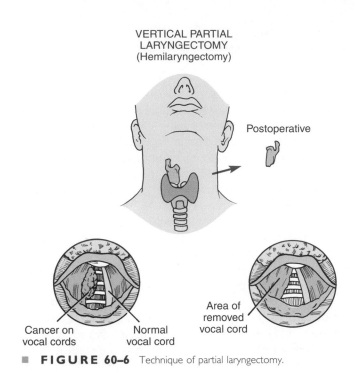

VERTICAL PARTIAL LARYNGECTOMY (Hemilaryngectomy)

Postoperative

Cancer on vocal cords

Normal vocal cord

Area of removed vocal cord

■ **FIGURE 60–6** Technique of partial laryngectomy.

Another form of partial laryngectomy is the supraglottic laryngectomy. This procedure is performed for cancer of the supraglottis. The surgeon removes the superior portion of the larynx from the false vocal cords to the epiglottis and may also remove a portion of the base of the tongue. Lymph node dissection also may be performed. Because the true vocal cords are preserved, voice quality is maintained. The major postoperative problem is risk of aspiration, because the epiglottis, which normally closes over and protects the larynx, has been removed. The airway is managed with a tracheostomy after surgery; when the edema subsides in surrounding tissues, the tracheostomy tube can usually be removed and the stoma allowed to heal. The client then needs to be taught how to swallow to avoid aspiration.

For selected confined transglottic carcinomas, a supracricoid partial laryngectomy may be indicated. This conservative procedure preserves functional speech and swallowing without a permanent tracheostomy.

Total Laryngectomy
For large glottic tumors with fixation of the vocal cords, a total laryngectomy is required. The larynx is the connection of the pharynx (upper airway) and the trachea (lower airway) (Figure 60-7, *A*). When the larynx is removed, a permanent opening is made by suturing the trachea to the neck. The esophagus remains attached to the pharynx (Figure 60-7, *B*). Because no air can enter the nose, the client loses the sense of smell. The biggest problem for the client after laryngectomy is loss of voice.

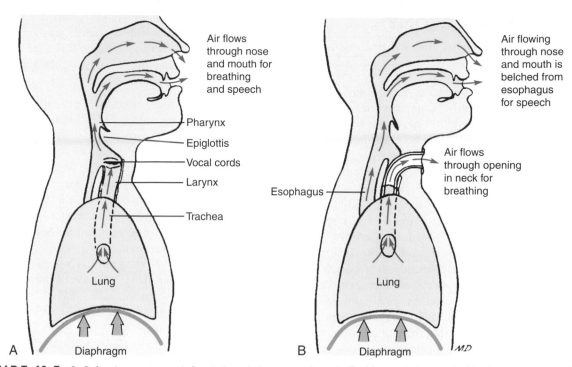

■ **FIGURE 60–7 A,** Before laryngectomy, air flow is through the nose and mouth. **B,** After surgical removal of the larynx, a new opening must be made for air passage. The trachea and esophagus are separated.

The client should be made aware that without surgery, the voice quality worsens as the tumor enlarges, but in any case the loss of voice constitutes a serious psychological issue. Because the trachea and esophagus are permanently separated by surgery, there is no risk of aspiration unless a fistula forms from the trachea to the esophagus. Besides this, the potential complications of the total laryngectomy are the same as those for the partial laryngectomy (see earlier discussion).

Cervical Lymph Node Dissection

Metastasis to the cervical lymph nodes is common with tumors of the upper aerodigestive tract. Surgical management of laryngeal tumors often includes neck dissection. Radical neck dissection (also called en bloc) involves the removal of lymphatic drainage channels and nodes, the sternocleidomastoid muscle, the spinal accessory nerve, the jugular vein, and tissue in the submandibular area. A modified radical neck dissection spares the spinal accessory nerve, and a selective neck dissection removes only the lymph nodes within the area of anticipated spread.

Complications

Possible complications after laryngeal surgery are airway obstruction, hemorrhage, carotid artery rupture, and fistula formation. Airway obstruction is due to edema in the surgical site, bleeding into the airway, or loss of airway from a plugged tracheostomy tube. Airway obstruction constitutes an emergency and requires immediate intervention for restoration of the airway.

Hemorrhage is usually the result of inadequate hemostasis during surgery. Some blood-tinged sputum is expected in the tracheal secretions for the first 48 hours, but frank bleeding from the tracheotomy site or tube is a manifestation of hemorrhage and must be reported to the physician immediately. Also assess the client for other manifestations of bleeding such as evident hematoma or unilateral swelling, tachycardia, hypotension, and changes in respiratory patterns.

Carotid artery rupture is usually a late complication and is related to poor condition of the neck tissue. It may be the result of previous radiation therapy to the area, pharyngocutaneous fistula, recurrent tumor, or infection. This condition is also a life-threatening emergency and carries an extremely high mortality. Mild bleeding from the oral cavity, neck, or trachea may precede impending rupture by 24 to 48 hours. A pulsating tracheostomy tube may indicate that the tip of the tube is resting on the innominate artery, which may cause injury to the artery and result in hemorrhage.

Fistulae between the hypopharynx and the skin may also develop. Many fistulae heal on their own, but treatment may require surgery, depending on the location and size.

PARTIAL LARYNGECTOMY
Nursing Management of the Surgical Client

Preoperative Care

In addition to the usual preoperative assessments, assess the client's nutritional status. Compare current body weight with ideal body weight, usual caloric intake, total lymphocyte count, albumin levels, and hemoglobin value and hematocrit. In addition, assess dentition and the oral cavity. Because many of these clients have abused tobacco and alcohol, the dentition and oral cavity are frequently in poor condition. In addition, if the client is an active alcoholic, plans should consider support through the period of alcohol withdrawal. The ideal plan of care would allow some nutritional support and oral care before surgery. Currently, few clients can be admitted before surgery; therefore such supportive care must be accomplished before hospital admission.

The client's work history and financial concerns should also be investigated during this initial assessment. Inability to purchase medical insurance or to pay for health care services may account for the client's lack of personal and medical care.

The client's usual coping strategies and family support should also be evaluated. Some degree of cosmetic (aesthetic) change will result after surgery, and the client will be unable to speak for some time. Preoperative plans should consider alternative methods of communication and family support networks. Preoperative education by rehabilitated laryngectomees is important for these clients.

Because of the multiple problems common in these clients, a team approach to their care is used. Members of the team usually include the primary physician or surgeon, nurses, a social worker, a dietitian, a speech or swallowing therapist, a physical therapist, a respiratory therapist, and home health care nurses. If extensive surgery is required, a plastic surgeon and a maxillofacial prosthodontist may also care for the client during reconstruction.

Postoperative Care

Assessment. In addition to the routine postoperative assessments, after a partial laryngectomy the client needs to undergo careful assessment of the airway, lung sounds, and position of the tracheostomy tube, as well as checking for potential complications related to the surgical procedure and the tracheostomy tube (see earlier discussion).

Diagnosis, Outcomes, Interventions

Diagnosis: Risk for Aspiration. Because of the removal of the epiglottis (which normally acts as a trap door to close the airway and prevent aspiration) and because secretions are excessive after surgery, the client is at very high risk for aspiration. This is a priority diagnosis.

Outcomes. The client will have reduced risk of aspiration, as evidenced by clear breath sounds throughout the chest, normal (for age) respiratory rate and rhythm, chest secretions that are clear or only slightly blood-tinged, and ability to cough.

Interventions. In the immediate postoperative period, priority is given to management of the upper airway. The client should be positioned in a greater than 45-degree angle to decrease edema of the airway, facilitate breathing, and improve comfort.

A cuffed tracheostomy tube is generally inserted during surgery and is maintained for the first several days after surgery to minimize aspiration of secretions and for assisted or controlled ventilation. Secretions collect above the cuff. For removal of secretions, the cuff should be deflated during exhalation. The client should be instructed to cough during deflation of the cuff. If the client cannot cough, suctioning should be used to prevent secretions from being aspirated. The cuff should be reinflated during inspiration.

When the edema has subsided, the tracheostomy tube may be removed. The decannulation process is slow and begins with observation of the client for aspiration, as follows. The cuff of the tube is deflated, and the client is observed for the ability to swallow saliva and other secretions without coughing or requiring additional suctioning. If increased secretions are present through and around the tracheostomy tube, aspiration is occurring and the cuff should be reinflated. If no aspiration is occurring, the tracheostomy tube can be replaced with a smaller, uncuffed tube. If the uncuffed tube is tolerated without aspiration, the tube is capped (plugged) to determine the client's ability to breathe through the upper airway. If the client can breathe through the upper airway for 24 hours, the tracheostomy tube is removed, and the stoma is taped closed and covered with an occlusive dressing.

Diagnosis: Ineffective Airway Clearance. The physical alteration in the airway and the presence of a tracheostomy tube interfere with normal movement of mucus up and out of the bronchial tree. In addition, as a result of prior smoking, the cilia have become ineffective. *Ineffective Airway Clearance* is also a priority nursing diagnosis for several days.

Outcomes. The client will have improved airway clearance, as evidenced by effortless, quiet respirations at baseline rate and clear breath sounds.

Interventions. The client may have copious secretions because of the presence of the tracheostomy tube, a history of chronic obstructive lung disease, and aspiration. There may also be oral secretions that cannot be swallowed. Oral secretions accumulate because of the disruption of normal air flow, and swallowing may be impaired as a result of surgery. In the alert and conscious client, coughing and deep-breathing mobilize and eliminate many of these secretions. However, in the client who has undergone head and neck surgery and is just emerging from anesthesia, these measures may not be possible. Suctioning of the trachea is needed for the first 24 to 48 hours after surgery. The frequency of suctioning depends on the client's needs, but suctioning every hour or more often is common for the first 24 hours. Suctioning techniques can be found in fundamentals of nursing textbooks.

SAFETY
⚠
ALERT
Sterile technique must be used to avoid introducing microorganisms into the tracheobronchial tree in a client with impaired immune defenses resulting from malignancy and surgery.

If present, the inner cannula of the tracheostomy tube should be cleaned as often as necessary to provide a clear airway. In the immediate postoperative phase, the inner cannula is cleaned after suctioning. Once the client is ambulatory and can handle secretions safely, the cannula can be cleaned three times a day and as necessary.

Aerosol administration of bronchodilators into deeper parts of the respiratory tract is recommended to prevent pulmonary complications. These treatments are performed every 4 hours for the first few days after surgery and then usually decreased to four times a day once the client can ambulate.

Diagnosis: Risk for Impaired Gas Exchange. Like other postoperative clients, clients with neck surgery have a high risk for atelectasis related to low tidal volume breathing secondary to pain, sedation, and increased mucus production.

Outcomes. The client will have adequate oxygenation, as evidenced by pulse oximetry values above 90%, ABG values within normal limits (that take into consideration any pre-existing lung disorders, such as emphysema), no air hunger, and clear lung sounds.

Interventions. Oxygenation is assessed through ABG analysis or pulse oximetry and the fraction of inspired oxygen (Fio_2) may be adjusted. If the client has pre-existent chronic air flow limitations, oxygen may have to be delivered at lower percentages or not at all. Compressed air with high humidity may be substituted in such cases.

Diagnosis: Impaired Nutrition: Less Than Body Requirements. A combination of the pre-existing malignancy and swallowing difficulties sets the stage for malnutrition. In addition, concomitant lung disorders and alcoholism, which are common in this population, increase the tendency for malnutrition.

Outcomes. The client will have an improved nutritional status, as evidenced by maintaining baseline body weight or losing less than 5 pounds; consuming adequate fluid, protein, fat, and carbohydrate each 24 hours; swallowing without aspirating or choking; and maintaining hemoglobin, hematocrit, albumin, and total lymphocyte values within normal limits.

Interventions. Immediately after surgery, typically an NG tube is inserted for removal of gastric secretions until postoperative ileus subsides. If long-term difficulty in swallowing is anticipated, a gastrostomy tube may be inserted at the time of surgery. Assess for hunger and passage of flatus as manifestations of returning gastrointestinal function; bowel sounds may or may not be present In some clients, tube-feeding with commercial supplements is indicated. Continually ascertain the correct position of the tube before each feeding. (Techniques for checking feeding tube placement can be found in fundamentals of nursing textbooks.) The tube-feeding can be administered by pump, slow drip, or bolus feeding, depending on the client's tolerance. Aspiration remains a high risk with partial laryngectomy, and precautions to guard the client from this event with its untoward results are critical.

When the epiglottis has been removed, the timing for resumption of oral feeding after a partial laryngectomy is controversial. One approach is to begin oral feedings with the tracheostomy tube in place when edema has subsided and the client is able to swallow secretions. The advantage of this technique is that aspirated liquid can be suctioned. A second technique is to delay oral feeding until the client has been decannulated and the stoma has healed. The advantage of this technique is that with a closed stoma, the client is able to increase intrathoracic pressure and remove any aspirated material through an effective cough.

Whenever the client eats, eating should be evaluated with a speech therapist. The Client Education Guide on p. 1558 lists precautions to teach clients undergoing a partial laryngectomy. Once swallowing can be accomplished without aspiration, carbonated beverages may be added. Thin liquids should be withheld until the risk of aspiration is minimal.

Diagnosis: Risk for Infection. The loss of primary defenses of the skin and delayed healing attributable to pre-existing malignancy and malnutrition make *Risk for Infection* a common nursing diagnosis.

Outcomes. The client will have no clinical manifestations of wound infection, as evidenced by continued approximation of incisional edges; decrease in the amount of wound drainage; absence of purulent drainage; absence of redness, swelling, tenderness, or warmth beyond the suture lines; absence of fever; and a white blood cell count within normal limits.

Swallowing Technique After a Partial Laryngectomy

- Begin with soft or semi-solid foods.
- Stay with a nurse or swallowing therapist during meals until you master the technique of swallowing without choking.
- Be patient; learning to swallow again is frustrating.
- Follow these steps in sequence:
  1. Take a deep breath.
  2. Bear down to close the vocal cords.
  3. Place food into your mouth.
  4. Swallow.
  5. Cough to rid the closed cord of accumulated food particles.
  6. Swallow.
  7. Cough.
  8. Breathe.

Interventions. During surgery, a wound drain is placed into the surrounding tissues of the neck and attached to constant suction. A closed wound drainage system is attached to the client's gown to prevent accidental dislodgment. Using standard precautions, assess the amount and color of the drainage every 4 hours for the first 24 hours. Assess the wound for manifestations of hematoma or seroma formation by noting whether the amount of drainage is increasing or whether there is a change in the color or consistency of the drainage. Also assess the color of the surgical incisions. If the amount of drainage is decreasing, the drain may be removed by the physician. Dressings are placed over the drain puncture sites on the skin. Small to moderate amounts of serosanguineous drainage should be expected for another 48 to 72 hours.

The suture lines should be cleaned at least twice daily with saline rinse. A thin film of a protective barrier ointment may be applied to the suture line to prevent crusting of secretions and to promote healing.

Evaluation. Expect the problems with airway management to resolve within a few days. Infection, apart from atelectasis, does not arise for about 72 hours. Nutritional problems and problems with healing may require several weeks to resolve.

Self-Care

The client who has undergone partial laryngectomy may be discharged from the hospital before completion of wound healing. If upper airway edema has not subsided, the client is discharged with a temporary tracheostomy. The client and significant others should understand and demonstrate proper care of the tube, including inner cannula care, technique for insertion of the entire tube in case of accidental decannulation, suctioning, humidification techniques, and emergency resuscitation measures.

Once decannulation has been performed, the stoma must be cleansed and an occlusive dressing applied at least once a day. Additional wound care includes cleaning the incision area with hydrogen peroxide and water and applying an antibiotic ointment. All instructions given to the client should be in writing, with additional teaching materials used as available. Ongoing assessment for healing, recurrent tumor, or a new tumor is required.

TOTAL LARYNGECTOMY

Nursing Management of the Surgical Client

The nursing management of the client after a total laryngectomy is the same as the care given to a client with a partial laryngectomy, except for feeding and teaching about permanent stoma care. Clients who have a total laryngectomy have a permanent tracheostomy and need to learn how to speak using alternative methods.

Nutrition

Immediately after surgery, the client's nutrition is supplemented with tube feedings. The client continues to receive tube feedings until edema has subsided and suture line healing has occurred. When the client can swallow saliva, oral feedings can begin. The diet usually begins with liquid or semi-soft foods and progresses as healing occurs.

Communication

For the first few days after surgery, the client should communicate by writing. If the client is very fatigued, requests such as "I need something for pain" may be expressed by using a communication board so that the client can just point to the statement. Even though the client cannot speak, conversation should still include the client's input through nodding and pointing and not be directed only to others, such as the family. Avoiding conversation with the client because of difficulty in communication is demeaning to the client and leads to frustration.

Artificial Larynx

An artificial larynx may be used as early as 3 to 4 days after surgery. These battery-operated speech devices are held alongside the neck or can be adapted with a plastic tube that is inserted in the mouth. The air inside the mouth is vibrated, and the client articulates as usual (Figure 60-8). The speech quality is monotone and mechanical-sounding but intelligible.

Esophageal Speech

Esophageal speech is a technique that requires the client to swallow and hold air in the upper esophagus. By

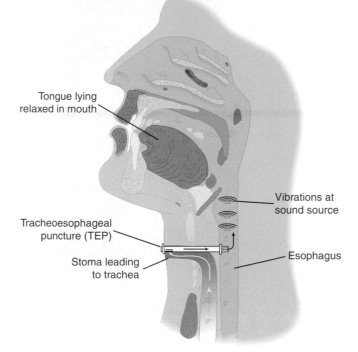

Tongue lying
relaxed in mouth

Vibrations at
sound source

Tracheoesophageal
puncture (TEP)

Esophagus

Stoma leading
to trachea

■ **FIGURE 60–9** Tracheoesophageal puncture for voice rehabilitation after laryngectomy. A prosthesis is inserted into a fistula created in the neck. The prosthesis has a one-way valve that permits air to pass into the esophagus but prevents accidental aspiration. To speak, the client occludes the prosthesis with a finger or attachment. Exhaled air is then shunted through the prosthesis, where it vibrates, and exits the mouth as a spoken word.

■ **FIGURE 60–8** Artificial larynx. This hand-held, battery-powered speech aid is placed against the neck. **A,** When the artificial larynx is activated, it creates a vibration that is transmitted to the neck and into the mouth. Words silently formed by the mouth become sounds from the vibrations emitted by the device. Any type of artificial larynx requires muscle and tongue control and hand strength; usually, such a device is not used until immediate postoperative neck tenderness has subsided. **B,** Electronic speech aid allows the client to adjust tone, pitch, and volume. An oral connector permits speech without the necessity of placing the device against the neck. This is an advantage immediately after surgery, when the neck is too sensitive for a neck-vibrating device.

controlling the flow of air, the client can pronounce as many as 6 to 10 words before stopping to swallow more air. The voice is deep but is loud and effective once the technique is mastered.

Tracheoesophageal Puncture

Tracheoesophageal puncture (TEP) is a surgical technique that also restores speech (Figure 60-9). A small puncture is made into the upper tracheostoma to the cervical esophagus for creation of a fistula. After the fistula tract has healed, a small one-way valve, or voice prosthesis, is inserted. By occlusion of the prosthesis, air can be shunted into the esophagus and used to produce speech. The TEP may be done concurrently with a total laryngectomy or as a secondary procedure after healing and radiation therapy. These devices require maintenance; therefore only clients who are highly motivated, who are able to perform self-care, and who have good manual dexterity are eligible for this procedure. Care of the TEP surgical wound is presented in the Client Education Guide feature on the website.

evolve

Self-Care

Clients should be discharged with an extra tracheostomy tube to allow tube changes at home (Figure 60-10). To provide supplemental humidification, normal saline may be instilled into the stoma several times each day to stimulate coughing, moisten the mucosa, and loosen dried secretions and crusts. Use of a bedside humidifier or vaporizer also aids in humidifying the inspired air. A stoma bib or covering should be worn to warm and filter inspired air and to prevent foreign bodies from entering the stoma.

■ **FIGURE 60-10** Insertion of a laryngectomy tube into a permanent tracheostoma. The obturator or guide is inserted into the outer cannula. After the tube is lubricated with water-soluble ointment, the client takes a deep breath and the lubricated tube is inserted. The obturator is removed, and the tube is tied in place.

These coverings can be purchased, or the client may improvise by using a scarf, necktie, or turtleneck shirt.

The client must be encouraged to continue speech therapy as begun in the hospital. The techniques to restore speech require much time for mastery; the client is seen by a speech therapist after dismissal from the hospital. Community support groups for clients after laryngectomy such as the Lost Cord Club and the International Association of Laryngectomees offer needed reassurance. Much patience is required by the client and family while the client is relearning to speak. The process is time-consuming and frustrating, and progress may sometimes be slow. Encourage the family to give the client enough time to formulate the words and not speak for the client.

Once the incision has completely healed, the tracheostomy tube is no longer required (Figure 60-11). This process varies but usually takes about 6 to 8 weeks. Occasionally, the tube may be required at night, if the

■ **FIGURE 60-11** Healed tracheostomy incision.

stoma is small or the client does not get adequate air exchange during sleep. Once the tracheostomy tube has been removed, the client can disguise the stoma with clothing and begin to regain a sense of normalcy.

Tub baths or showers are permitted, but the client must use caution to prevent introduction of water into the stoma, aiming the water spray at midchest. Commercial stoma shower covers are available. Water sports are prohibited. The client should wear a medical alert bracelet and carry an emergency wallet card to identify the fact that resuscitation cannot be performed through the mouth. Information about obtaining these forms of identification is available from the American Cancer Society. The use of mouth-to-stoma rescue breathing is imperative when resuscitation is needed in these clients. Family members should be directed to a community program that teaches mouth-to-stoma resuscitation. For additional security, a wireless "beeper" or automatic response monitoring device can be useful.

The client may require a nutritional plan for the first few weeks at home. The dietitian should work with the client and family to determine the consistency of food easiest to swallow as well as the kinds of foods required to obtain needed protein and calories.

It is essential that the client not smoke so that lung function is preserved and the risk of other cancers reduced. For some clients after laryngectomy, the process of smoking cessation seems pointless. Some clients continue to smoke by inhaling the cigarette smoke through the stoma. The attitude is one of "Why quit now? What else could happen to me?" Use extra support and encouragement with the client, remembering to be an advocate of the client's choice as well as providing assurance that the quality of life after smoking cessation improves.

Follow-up care is important to assess the healing process, to evaluate coping mechanisms, and to examine the client for possible metastasis or new tumors. The client should be taught to report any of the following manifestations to the physician:

■ A lump anywhere in the neck or body
■ Persistent cough, sore throat, or earache
■ Hemoptysis
■ Sores around the stoma or within the trachea that do not heal
■ Difficulty swallowing or breathing

NECK DISSECTION

Nursing Management of the Surgical Client

Preoperative Care

Before surgery, the client's understanding of the plans for surgery should be assessed. Determine what the surgeon has told the client and how much information has been retained or lost because of anxiety. In addition, address the fears the client has about the diagnosis of cancer and fears of deformity after surgery. Assist the client to understand the anatomic and physiologic alterations that will occur as a result of radical surgery. Explain to the client and family what to expect after surgery (e.g., placement in the intensive care unit, tracheostomy, drainage tubes) and review postoperative care (e.g., communication techniques to be used if a tracheostomy is to be placed).

The client's support systems and degree of coping should be assessed. If the client is an alcoholic, alcohol may be the usual coping tool. Because alcohol will not be available, assess the other coping mechanisms available to the client, and encourage the client to use them. Sources may include friends and family. Identify new support systems, if needed, such as interaction with people who have had the same surgery or diagnosis.

Postoperative Care

After surgery, the usual postoperative assessments are performed, with special attention given to the airway. Airway patency can be lost as a result of edema of the neck or bleeding within the area. Assess the client for manifestations of airway edema or bleeding. Auscultate lung sounds every 2 hours for the first 24 hours. Report manifestations of airway obstruction immediately.

Position the client with the head of bed elevated greater than 45 degrees to minimize postoperative edema. Monitor neck drainage for volume and color. Sanguineous or serosanguineous drainage is expected for the first 72 hours after surgery. Once drainage has stopped, the wound drains are removed.

Pressure dressings may be used in the immediate postoperative period, depending on physician preference. If a dressing is used, it should be reinforced as needed and observed for any drainage. If musculocutaneous flaps were needed for coverage, pressure dressings are not used, and special flap care is required. (See Chapter 49 for specific care of flaps.)

If the surgical defect was repaired with musculocutaneous flaps, the flap should be assessed for arterial inflow and venous outflow. Flap temperature, color, and blanching should be noted every hour for the first 24 hours and every 4 hours after that time. Other means of monitoring flap perfusion (Doppler signals) may be used.

Because of the disruption of the sensory nerve fibers from the incisions used, most clients report only minimal pain at the surgical site. If an en bloc radical neck dissection has been performed, postoperative shoulder dysfunction is the rule, with forward rotation and dropping of the shoulder. Sectioning of the spinal accessory nerve during neck dissection also interrupts innervation to the upper trapezius muscle.

Exercises to increase range of motion and muscle strength, shown in the Client Education Guide website feature on Exercises After Radical Neck Surgery, are encouraged to prevent a "frozen shoulder" and to restore full movement. If a selective or modified neck dissection has been performed, minimal alterations in range of motion and muscle strength are anticipated. Encourage use of exercise to prevent permanent disability.

Self-Care

After neck dissection, caution clients about the potential for injury to neck tissue because of lack of sensation. The use of a heating pad or exposure to temperature extremes may result in tissue injury (burns, frostbite) in a client who cannot feel these temperatures. Clients who have a tracheostomy need specific instructions for its management. Explain ongoing evaluations and follow-up.

INFECTIOUS, INFLAMMATORY, AND HEMORRHAGIC DISORDERS

SINUSITIS

Sinusitis is a common infection that may occur in any of the paranasal sinuses. *Pansinusitis* is infection of more than one sinus. The term *rhinosinusitis* is thought to more accurately describe respiratory manifestations referable to an inflammatory disease of the nose or sinuses. However, the terms *rhinitis* and *sinusitis* may still be used.

Sinusitis is a common medical condition that affects an estimated 35 million people a year. The sinuses are protected against infection by mucociliary action. The normal mucus produced by the sinuses is removed through small openings in the nose called *ostia*. When the ciliary action is impaired or the ostia are obstructed, mucus can accumulate in the sinus, which may then become infected. Blockage of the ostia may be due to a deviated nasal septum, bony abnormalities, congenital malformations, infections, or allergy.

A medical diagnosis of sinusitis is suggested by the client's clinical manifestations and confirmed by x-ray findings. Fever and chills along with headaches and facial pain exacerbated with bending, pain or numbness in the upper teeth, and a purulent or discolored nasal discharge may be present. Sinus radiographs or CT scans may show opacification of the sinus, thickened mucous membranes, and an air-fluid level (attributable to accumulation of secretions in the sinus), all indicative of sinusitis.

OUTCOME MANAGEMENT

Medical Management

Medical management of sinusitis includes (1) use of the appropriate antibiotic to manage the bacterial infection,

(2) decongestants to reduce nasal edema, (3) corticosteroid nasal sprays to reduce mucosal inflammation, and (4) humidification by use of normal saline solution irrigations or a vaporizer or humidifier to prevent nasal crusting and to moisten secretions.

Antibiotics are not prescribed routinely, because many cases of sinusitis are viral. Initial selection of antibiotics is based on the likely causative organisms indicated by the manifestations and the probability of resistant strains within a community. First-line therapy at most centers is amoxicillin for 14 days.

Medical means of providing drainage include topical and systemic vasoconstrictors. Oral alpha-adrenergic vasoconstrictors, including pseudoephedrine and phenylephrine, can be used for 10 to 14 days, allowing for restoration of normal mucociliary function and drainage. They may be contraindicated in clients with cardiovascular disease because they may cause hypertension and tachycardia. They also may be contraindicated in competitive athletes because of rules of competition.

Mucolytic agents, such as guaifenesin and saline lavage, have been shown to decrease the duration of sinus infections and can be performed by the client at home. Intranasal steroids are also commonly prescribed.

Antihistamines are beneficial for reducing osteomeatal obstruction in clients with allergies and acute sinusitis.

Antral irrigation or sinus lavage may be performed in clients who are not responding to treatment or who have increased purulent exudate in the maxillary sinus. Antral irrigation is performed with the use of a local anesthetic. A trocar (a sharp metal instrument) is inserted through the ostium in the lateral wall of the nose into the sinus. Prepare the client for the procedure with thorough explanations of the anesthetic procedure, the sensation of passage of the trocar through the ostium, and feelings of pressure. Normal saline solution is then injected through the cannula to rinse the sinus of purulent exudate. The client is placed in a sitting position, leaning slightly forward with the mouth open to allow drainage of the irrigating solution through the nose and mouth. A specimen of the exudate may be obtained for culture to determine the causative organism for prescription of an appropriate antibiotic. Sinus irrigations with normal saline can be performed by the client at home also.

Surgical Management

Functional Endoscopic Sinus Surgery

If nonoperative measures fail, functional endoscopic sinus surgery (FESS) may be necessary. The major objective of FESS is the reestablishment of sinus ventilation and mucociliary clearance. FESS is usually performed as an outpatient surgical procedure using local anesthesia (with or without conscious sedation) or with the client under general anesthesia. Small fiberoptic endoscopes are passed through the nasal cavity and into the

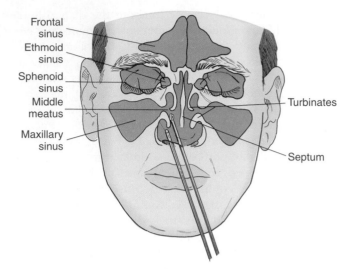

FIGURE 60–12 Functional endoscopic sinus surgery. The middle meatus is the site to which most of the sinuses drain; if it is plugged, drainage is obstructed. With an endoscope, the sinuses can be seen and obstructions removed.

sinuses to allow direct visualization of the sinuses in order to remove diseased tissue and to enlarge sinus ostia (Figure 60-12).

Possible complications of FESS include nasal bleeding, pain, scar formation, and, rarely, cerebrospinal fluid leak and blindness resulting from intraorbital hematoma formation or direct injury to the optic nerve. After FESS, nasal packing may be inserted to minimize nasal bleeding. Packing is removed within a few hours of the surgical procedure.

External Sphenoethmoidectomy

External sphenoethmoidectomy is a surgical procedure performed to remove diseased mucosa from the sphenoidal or ethmoidal sinus. A small incision is made over the ethmoidal sinus on the lateral nasal bridge, and the diseased mucosa is removed. Nasal and ethmoidal packing is then inserted. An eye pressure patch is usually applied to decrease periorbital edema.

Nursing Management of the Surgical Client

For the first 24 hours after sinus surgery, observe the client for profuse nasal bleeding, respiratory distress, ecchymosis, and orbital and facial edema. Apply ice compresses to the nose and cheek to minimize edema and control bleeding. Place the client in a position with the head of the bed greater than 45 degrees for 24 to 48 hours after surgery to minimize postoperative edema. The nasal packing is generally removed the morning after surgery; however, antral packing may remain in place for 36 to 72 hours. Give mild analgesics to the client to minimize discomfort postoperatively and before removal of the packing.

Instruct clients to increase fluid intake, which maximizes the water content of secretions. Although there may be some pain, a mild analgesic is usually all that is required. Minor nasal bleeding is expected for 24 to 48 hours after surgery. Use of a drip pad under the nose may eliminate the need for constant wiping (Figure 60-13). Instruct clients to avoid blowing the nose for 7 to 10 days after surgery; tell them to sniff backward or spit, not blow. Teach the client to sneeze only with the mouth open. Nasal saline sprays may be started 3 to 5 days after surgery to moisten the nasal mucosa. Explain that the client is to engage in minimal physical exercise and to avoid strenuous activity, lifting, and straining for approximately 2 weeks. After FESS, the client needs to return to the physician's office for removal of crusts and debris and for examination of the nose.

PHARYNGITIS

Pharyngitis is inflammation of the pharynx (tonsils, palate, uvula) and may be viral, bacterial, or fungal in origin. Beta-hemolytic streptococci are the most common infecting organisms. Clients may complain of a sore throat, difficulty in swallowing, fever, malaise, and cough and have an elevated white blood cell count. A culture of the pharyngeal mucosa is sometimes indicated before treatment is started. Treatment of pharyngitis depends on the causative agent. Both viral pharyngitis and bacterial pharyngitis are contagious by droplet spread. Good hand-washing technique is essential, and the use of a mask may prevent spread. Antibiotics are used to treat the bacterial

■ **FIGURE 60–13** A nasal drip pad is taped beneath the nares to absorb drainage after nasal or sinus surgery. The usual technique consists of folding 4 × 4 dressings into thirds and taping them in place. These dressings can be changed at the nurse's discretion.

pharyngitis, antifungal agents are used to treat fungal infections, and use of comfort measures is required for viral types. Bed rest, fluids, warm saline irrigations or gargles, analgesics, and antipyretics are recommended until the clinical manifestations are alleviated.

Chronic pharyngitis (chronic pharyngeal inflammation) is most common in people who habitually use tobacco and alcohol, have a chronic cough, are employed or live in dusty environments, or use their voices excessively. Clinical manifestations vary according to the degree of irritation and inflammation.

EPISTAXIS

Epistaxis (nosebleed) may result from irritation, trauma, infection, foreign bodies, or tumors. Epistaxis may also be the result of systemic disease (e.g., atherosclerosis, hypertension, blood dyscrasias) or systemic treatment (e.g., chemotherapy or anticoagulants), or it may be idiopathic.

OUTCOME MANAGEMENT

Medical Management

Anterior epistaxis is initially treated by assisting the client to a sitting position. Apply pressure by pinching the anterior portion of the nose for a minimum of 5 to 10 minutes. This maneuver is often successful because the most common source of epistaxis is the anterior part of the septum in an area known as Kiesselbach's plexus, a venous plexus vulnerable to trauma. In addition, the application of ice compresses to produce vasoconstriction may also reduce bleeding. If more definitive treatment is necessary, anterior epistaxis can usually be controlled by cauterization of the bleeding vessel with applications of silver nitrate. If these measures do not stop the bleeding, nasal packing may be inserted unilaterally or bilaterally. Antibacterial ointment is applied to 0.5-inch gauze, which is then gently but firmly inserted into the anterior nasal cavities to apply pressure to the bleeding vessels. The use of petrolatum gauze packing should be avoided, because it has no antimicrobial properties, and a malodorous discharge may develop within 1 to 2 days of insertion. Nasal packing should remain in place for a minimum of 48 to 72 hours.

Ten percent of nosebleeds are posterior, usually occurring in people older than 50 years. Posterior bleeding tends to cause increased swallowing of blood, which can be noted in the pharynx. For clients with posterior epistaxis, a *posterior plug* may be necessary in addition to the anterior nasal packing (Figure 60-14). Insertion of a posterior plug is very uncomfortable, and a mild analgesic may be required to reduce anxiety and discomfort. A small, red rubber catheter is passed through the nose into the oropharynx and mouth. A gauze pack

■ **FIGURE 60–14** Instillation of a posterior nasal pack (plug), typically used in an emergency. A catheter can also be used with the balloon placed to tamponade the bleeding.

is tied to the catheter, and the catheter is withdrawn; this moves the pack into proper placement in the nasopharynx and posterior nose to apply pressure. The nasal cavity is packed with 0.5-inch gauze, and the strings from the posterior pack are tied around a rolled gauze or bolus to maintain its position outside the nasal vestibule. The ties from the oral cavity are taped to the client's face to prevent loosening or dislodgment of the plug. A nasal balloon may be substituted for the traditional nasal pack. When the balloon is inflated with normal saline, pressure is applied to the lateral nasal wall.

Nursing Management of the Medical Client

Clients with a posterior plug and anterior nasal packing may be admitted to the hospital and monitored closely for hypoxia. The presence of posterior packing may alter consciousness and respiratory status, especially in older

adults. Because hypertension is frequently cited as a risk factor for epistaxis, monitor the client's blood pressure. General comfort measures, such as humidification, the use of a drip pad to collect bloody drainage and mucus, and application of water-soluble ointment around the nares to provide lubrication, help alleviate the discomfort. Monitor the client closely for any manifestations of airway obstruction and bleeding from the anterior or posterior nares. Inspect the oral cavity for the presence of blood, soft palate necrosis, and proper placement of the posterior plug. If the posterior plug is visible, notify the physician for readjustment of the packing. Posterior nasal packs remain in place for 5 days. Prophylactic antibiotics are used to prevent toxic shock syndrome and sinusitis.

Surgical Management

If anterior and posterior packs fail to control epistaxis, internal maxillary or ethmoidal surgical *artery ligation* may be required. An incision is made in the gum line above the incisor on the affected side, and the maxillary sinus is entered. The artery that supplies the area of bleeding is identified, and a metal clip or suture is used to ligate the artery.

Nursing Management of the Surgical Client

The nasal packing inserted to control epistaxis remains in place for a minimum of 24 hours, during which time the client must be observed for additional bleeding, evidence of hypertension or hypotension, and infection. Upon discharge, the client is instructed to minimize activity for approximately 10 days, such as avoiding strenuous exercise; not blowing the nose; sneezing with the mouth open; and not lifting, stooping, or straining. The use of water-soluble ointment around the nares may provide comfort, and mouth rinses of half-strength hydrogen peroxide mixed with water or saline should be provided for oral hygiene. The use of a humidifier or vaporizer adds supplemental moisture to prevent dryness and crusting of secretions.

RHINITIS

Rhinitis, or rhinosinusitis, is inflammation of the nasal mucosa. The classic manifestations of rhinitis are increased nasal drainage, nasal congestion, and paroxysmal sneezing. Normally, nasal drainage is composed of clear mucus. If the infection spreads to the sinuses, however, drainage may become yellow or green. Rhinitis may be classified as acute, allergic, vasomotor, or drug-related (rhinitis medicamentosa).

Acute rhinitis is also known as the common cold, or coryza. Acute rhinitis may be bacterial or viral in origin; it is treated symptomatically. Acute rhinitis usually lasts

5 to 7 days, with or without treatment. Common interventions for acute rhinitis are symptomatic and include supplemental humidification, decongestants to reduce the edema of the nasal mucosa, increased fluids to prevent dehydration, and analgesics to relieve the generalized myalgia. Sometimes antibiotics are given to prevent a secondary infection by bacteria.

Allergic rhinitis affects between 15% and 20% of the American population and occurs most often as a seasonal disorder. In addition to obstruction to nasal breathing, the client may also experience irritation of other mucous membranes (e.g., the conjunctiva, causing tearing and edema of the eyelids). There is a broad association between allergic rhinitis and disease affecting other body systems. Treatment is symptomatic. A complete allergy evaluation may be required to determine the offending allergen. Most clients are placed on a desensitization program and instructed to avoid the antigen (substance that causes the allergic reaction); treatment is with antihistamines, steroids, or mast cell–stabilizing sprays.

Vasomotor rhinitis causes the same manifestations as those of acute and allergic rhinitis but has no known cause. Clients with vasomotor rhinitis in whom results of bacterial culture and allergy evaluation are negative are given symptomatic treatment. If medications have been prescribed for the treatment of rhinitis (especially nasal sprays), the client must be taught the use of medications, including side effects and possible interactions with other medications.

Rhinitis medicamentosa is caused by abuse or overuse of topical nasal decongestant sprays or intranasal cocaine. These substances initially cause vasoconstriction. When used frequently, however, the initial decongestion is followed by severe mucosal edema. The edema is self-treated with more medication, and the rhinitis becomes cyclic. Management of rhinitis medicamentosa consists of avoidance of the causative agent and evaluation and treatment of the original problem.

LARYNGITIS

Laryngitis may be caused by an inflammatory process or vocal abuse. The laryngeal membrane is continuous with the lining of the upper respiratory tract, and infections in other areas of the nose and throat may include the larynx. Edema of the vocal cords caused by the chronic irritation of an upper respiratory tract infection inhibits the normal mobility of the vocal cords, which causes an abnormal sound.

Laryngitis may also be the result of gastroesophageal reflux disorder (GERD). In this syndrome, the cardiac sphincter between the stomach and the esophagus relaxes, and gastric acid is allowed to enter the esophagus. Reflux of gastric secretions, especially during sleep, may result in the aspiration of gastric secretions into the larynx, causing a chemical irritation or burning of the mucous membrane lining the larynx. Clients with gastroesophageal reflux may complain of hoarseness from the chemical irritation of the gastric acid on the vocal cords, increased mucus production from the body's natural tendency to protect the irritated membrane, foreign body sensation, or sore throat. Chronic cough and asthma may also be associated manifestations of GERD.

Hoarseness is a common manifestation of disorders of the larynx and may be caused by inflammation of the vocal cords, abnormal movements of the vocal cords, or a benign or malignant tumor of the vocal cords. All of these problems interfere with normal mobility of the vocal cords, which produces a change in sound. Abnormal voice may also be the result of vocal abuse. Screaming, shouting, and loud speaking over a period of time may produce edema of the vocal cords and the formation of nodules or polyps—outpouchings of inflamed mucous membranes.

The treatment of laryngitis is aimed at the causative factors. If inflammatory laryngitis is suspected, the inflammation should be treated. Antibiotics may be used if a bacterial infection is suspected. In severe cases, systemic steroids (e.g., methylprednisolone [Medrol]) may be prescribed to reduce inflammation and edema. Supplemental humidification may add increased moisture to liquefy secretions, and mucolytic agents may be prescribed to thin and mobilize mucus. The client with laryngitis may also be placed on voice rest to allow the edema of the vocal cords to subside without added strain. Caution the client to avoid whispering, which also causes excessive vocal cord strain.

Gastroesophageal reflux is initially treated symptomatically. The client is instructed to elevate the head of the bed 6 to 10 inches to minimize reflux; to avoid lying on the right side; to avoid eating or drinking for 2 to 3 hours before going to sleep; to avoid caffeine, alcohol, and tobacco, which are known to increase gastric secretions; and to use antacids and histamine-2-receptor blockers (famotidine [Pepcid], ranitidine [Zantac], omeprazole [Prilosec]) to neutralize and decrease acid production.

Chronic laryngitis may stem from repeated infections, allergy, chronic irritant exposure, long-term voice abuse, or reflux esophagitis of acidic gastric contents. Chronic laryngitis is manifested as a tickling sensation in the throat, voice huskiness, and painful or difficult phonation. Management involves correction or removal of the irritation, in addition to measures to increase comfort. Long-term voice retraining may be necessary if improper use or overuse of the voice is the main cause of chronic laryngitis. This retraining includes (1) learning to use the voice without straining and (2) forming and projecting words to use the diaphragm without shouting.

OBSTRUCTIONS OF THE UPPER AIRWAY

ACUTE LARYNGEAL EDEMA

Acute laryngeal edema may be associated with inflammation, injury, or anaphylaxis. This condition is manifested by hoarseness and dramatic shortness of breath of acute onset. Dyspnea progresses rapidly, and unless a patent airway is established, respiratory arrest occurs. Endotracheal intubation may be very difficult because the larynx is edematous and is likely to bleed. Emergency tracheostomy may be required. If anaphylaxis is the precipitating cause, subcutaneous epinephrine 1:1000 is given. Intravenous corticosteroids are also used.

CHRONIC LARYNGEAL EDEMA

Chronic laryngeal edema may occur when lymph drainage is obstructed, as with infection or tumor or after radiation therapy. If the edema is significant, an artificial airway may be required (either a tracheostomy or an endotracheal tube). The choice of route depends on the severity of the edema.

LARYNGOSPASM

Laryngospasm (spasm of the laryngeal muscles) may occur (1) after administration of some general anesthetic agents, (2) after repeated and traumatic attempts at endotracheal intubation, (3) as a response to some inhaled agents and foreign material, such as industrial fumes, dusts, and chemicals, and (4) from hypocalcemia.

Management is directed at reestablishing the airway as quickly and efficiently as possible. Administer 100% oxygen until the airway is fully reestablished and the larynx relaxes and spasms stop. Titrate Fio_2 according to ABG or pulse oximetry values. If the laryngospasm persists, paralysis with neuromuscular blocking agents, such as succinylcholine, may be required to allow intubation until the spasm subsides. Manual or mechanical ventilation is then necessary until the effects of the paralyzing agent have worn off. Occasionally, emergency cricothyroidotomy or tracheotomy may be necessary and should not be delayed.

LARYNGEAL PARALYSIS

Laryngeal paralysis may be the result of neck surgery, peripheral disorders, central nervous system (CNS) disorders, tumor, or viral infections; or it may be of unknown cause. One of the most common causes of laryngeal paralysis is trauma to the recurrent laryngeal nerve during thyroidectomy. Other causes of laryngeal paralysis are aortic aneurysm; mitral stenosis; thoracic surgery; thyroid gland carcinoma; neck injuries; tuberculosis; tumors of the bronchi, lungs, and mediastinum; metallic poisons (e.g., lead); and infection (e.g., diphtheria). CNS disorders that may lead to laryngeal paralysis include stroke and myasthenia gravis. Bilateral laryngeal paralysis is rare, and when it occurs, the client usually exhibits difficulty in breathing or stridor.

With unilateral vocal cord paralysis (in which only one vocal cord is affected), the airway is usually not impaired and the primary manifestation is hoarseness. The client may have a breathy quality of the voice. Aspiration of food or saliva may occur until the normal, moving cord compensates by approximating the paralyzed cord (bringing the cords together). The client must be observed for manifestations of aspiration such as coughing upon swallowing, ineffective cough, decreased breath sounds, and crackles, rhonchi, or wheezes. The client with bilateral vocal cord paralysis can have a near-normal voice if the vocal cords are paralyzed in the adducted position. However, the major concern is airway compromise, especially on exertion. Dyspnea, intercostal muscle retraction, and stridor may occur with activity or upper airway infections.

If the paralyzed cords are bilaterally adducted, an emergency tracheotomy may be required. Surgery, such as arytenoidectomy, in which one or both arytenoid cartilages are removed and the vocal cords are held in an open position, may be used to open the glottis.

Injection of absorbable sponge (Gelfoam), as a temporary measure, or of polytetrafluoroethylene (Teflon), for permanent correction, may be used if the client with unilateral vocal cord paralysis exhibits manifestations of aspiration or requires strength or projection of the voice. The injected material is placed into the paralyzed cord to add bulk and to allow better approximation with the functioning cord.

Type I thyroplasty is recommended for permanent unilateral vocal cord paralysis. For this procedure, a window is made in the thyroid cartilage through an external incision, and a stent is inserted to move the paralyzed vocal cord into a midline position. The client may show manifestations of airway edema from both the injection and the thyroplasty and should be observed for respiratory distress.

LARYNGEAL INJURY

Laryngeal injury most often results from trauma during a motor-vehicle accident, when the driver's neck strikes the steering wheel. Other causes include inhalation of hot gases and aspiration of caustic liquids. If complete airway obstruction does not occur, carefully assess for post-traumatic edema, which may lead to complete obstruction. Few outward manifestations may be present. It is often easy to overlook potential problems in the neck structures while focusing on other, possibly more dramatic injuries. Observe for increased dyspnea, intercostal muscle retraction, neck swelling, laryngeal tenderness, dysphagia, stridor, inability to speak, and change in respiration patterns.

The thyroid cartilage may be fractured. This problem leads to soft tissue and laryngeal edema as well as hematoma formation. If airway obstruction occurs, tracheostomy may be necessary. Indications of a fractured thyroid cartilage include (1) a tender, swollen ecchymotic neck, (2) stridor, (3) cyanosis in some cases, and (4) subcutaneous emphysema in some cases.

Damage to the larynx above the cricoid cartilage may lead to tracheal stenosis. The cricoid cartilage forms the only complete circle of cartilage in the upper airway, and it maintains the open lumen of the upper end of the airway.

CHRONIC AIRWAY OBSTRUCTION

NASAL POLYPS

Nasal polyps are outpouchings of mucous membrane lining the nose or paranasal sinuses and may occur as solitary or multiple lesions. Polyps may be exacerbated by allergic manifestations, although they are not caused by allergies. Most people who have symptomatic polyps seek medical attention for obstruction to nasal breathing.

The medical management of clients with nasal polyps is symptomatic. Attempts are made to reduce the size of the polyps by eliminating or treating the causative factor (i.e., allergy). In many clients, surgery is needed to remove nasal polyps in order to restore nasal breathing before allergy treatment. Nasal polypectomy (removal of nasal polyps) can be done in the physician's office or in the operating room. Nasal polypectomy is usually performed with use of a local anesthetic. The anesthetic (commonly lidocaine with epinephrine) eliminates discomfort while also producing vasoconstriction to minimize bleeding during the procedure. A snare-like instrument is used to remove the polyps. The bleeding sites are cauterized, and intranasal packing is inserted. Intranasal splints can be used to prevent formation of adhesions. The nasal packing is maintained for several hours to minimize the possibility of postoperative bleeding and is generally removed before discharge of the client from the health care facility.

Because of the presence of nasal packing and edema, clients need to breathe through their mouth for the first 24 to 48 hours. The use of humidification, frequent mouth care, and increasing oral fluids minimize the dryness and oropharyngeal discomfort. Inspect the oral cavity frequently to evaluate the effectiveness of these measures. Clients with polyps frequently also have asthma (when combined with aspirin allergy, this is called *triad disease*). Asthmatic manifestations may be exacerbated after surgery.

The client is positioned with the head of the bed greater than 45 degrees after surgery to minimize edema. In addition, continuous use of ice compresses is recommended for the first 48 hours to reduce edema and to control bleeding. With the proper application of nasal packing at the time of surgery and the use of ice compresses in the immediate postoperative period, nasal bleeding should be minimal. However, the client should be assessed for changes in vital signs and the oropharynx should be inspected for the presence of blood. Because the nasal packing absorbs anterior bleeding, it is essential to observe the client for posterior nasal bleeding. Manifestations of active posterior bleeding include frequent swallowing and the presence of blood in the throat.

Most clients experience only minimal discomfort after a nasal polypectomy. Mild analgesics may be given for any postoperative discomfort. The use of aspirin and aspirin-containing products should be avoided because of their anticoagulant effects. Instruct the client not to blow his or her nose and to refrain from sneezing if possible. When the stimulus to sneeze cannot be overcome, the client should sneeze through an open mouth.

DEVIATED NASAL SEPTUM AND NASAL FRACTURE

The nasal septum (the dividing structure of the nose) is usually straight and separates the nose into two equal chambers. After trauma, the septum may become deviated, creating asymmetrical breathing passages. For some clients, the deviation may cause an obstruction to nasal breathing, dryness of the nasal mucosa leading to bleeding, and occasionally a cosmetic deformity. A deviated nasal septum changes the velocity of air, altering normal nasal activity and resulting in dryness, crusting, nasal bleeding, and changes in the membranes lining the nose.

If a nasal fracture occurs, immediate medical management is advised. Within several hours of nasal injury, severe edema may occur, which causes difficulty in reducing the fracture. Immediately after the injury, ice should be applied. A simple nasal fracture may be reduced in an emergency facility with use of local anesthesia. If immediate reduction of the nasal fracture is not possible, it is advisable to wait several days until edema subsides but before healing begins.

For correction of a deviated nasal septum, reconstruction of a cosmetic deformity of the nose, and reduction of a nasal fracture, the principles of surgical management are similar. All three procedures are usually performed with use of local anesthesia combined with mild sedation. Because of the vasoconstrictor properties of local anesthetics, these agents reduce bleeding during and immediately after surgery. Surgery to correct a deviated nasal septum is known as a nasal septoplasty and consists of making an incision on either side of the septum, elevating the mucous membrane, and straightening or removing the offending portion of the cartilage. If a cosmetic deformity is also of concern or if the deformity interferes with septal reconstruction, a rhinoplasty (reconstruction of the external nose) may be done in conjunction with the nasal septoplasty or as a separate procedure. (See also Chapter 49.)

After these three procedures, intranasal packing and internal splints may be used to maintain the position of the septum, to control bleeding, and to prevent hematoma formation. If the client has undergone rhinoplasty or reduction of a nasal fracture, an external splint and a small dressing may also be applied. Postoperative care is directed at airway management, control of edema and hemorrhage, pain reduction, client education, and emotional support. Because of the presence of bilateral nasal packing, clients require the same care as discussed for the client who has undergone nasal polypectomy.

CONCLUSIONS

Disorders of the upper airway range from the common cold to cancer of the larynx. This chapter presents care of clients most commonly hospitalized with upper airway disorders. Nursing management ranges from assessment of life-threatening airway obstruction to teaching techniques that reduce the spread of infection.

THINKING CRITICALLY

1. The client has a temporary tracheostomy after undergoing a supraglottic laryngectomy. On the second postoperative day, the client indicates to you that he is having trouble breathing. How should you evaluate the client and eliminate the problem?

Factors to Consider. What principles are used as the basis of tracheostomy care? How does evaluation of pulse oximetry contribute to decision making for care?

2. You walk into the room of a client who underwent total laryngectomy 12 hours ago. The client is complaining of severe nausea but has not vomited. What are the client's risks following this type of surgery? How should you respond to the present problem?

Factors to Consider. What risks are inherent in the occurrence of tracheal interruption? How well can the client communicate with you at this time?

3. You enter the room of a client in whom a nosebleed has developed. Bright red blood is seeping continuously from the nares, and the client states that it feels like some blood is going down the back of his throat. What is the priority intervention? What are the implications if the bleeding continues?

Factors to Consider. What are the causes of epistaxis? What are the psychological effects of a nosebleed?

Discussions for these questions can be found on the website. **evolve**

BIBLIOGRAPHY

Citations appearing in red refer to primary research.

Citations appearing in blue refer to evidence-based practice guidelines and protocols.

1. AACN Practice Alert: Ventilator-associated pneumonia. (2005). *AACN Clinical Issues, 16,* 105-109. Accessed 08/04/06 at www.aacn.org />clinical practice>practice alerts.
2. American Cancer Society. (2002). *Cancer facts and figures 2002.* Atlanta, Ga: Author.
3. Branson, R.D., Campbell, R.S., Chatburn, R.L., et al. (1992). AARC Clinical Practice Guideline: Humidification during mechanical ventilation. *Respiratory Care, 37,* 887-890. Accessed 08/03/06 at www.rcjournal.com/online_resources/cpgs/hdmvcpg.html.
4. Britton, D., Jones-Redmond, J., & Kasper, C. (2001). The use of speaking valves with ventilator dependent and tracheostomy patients. *Current Opinions in Otolaryngology and Head and Neck Surgery, 9,* 147-152.
5. Cady, J. (2002). Laryngectomy: Beyond loss of voice: Caring for the patient as a whole. *Clinical Journal of Oncology Nursing, 6*(6), 347-351.
6. Ch'ien, A.P.Y., et al. (2002). Managing gastroesophageal reflux disease. *The Nurse Practitioner: The American Journal of Primary Health Care, 27*(5), 36-53.
7. Chulay, M. (2005). Suctioning: Endotracheal or tracheostomy tube. In D.L.M. Wiegand, & K. Carlson (Eds.), *AACN procedure manual for critical care* (4th ed., pp. 62-70). Aliso Viejo, Calif: American Association of Critical-Care Nurses.
8. Coltart, L., Elder, F., & Grant, F. (2003). Caring for the patient with a tracheostomy: Best practice statement. *2003 NHS Quality Improvement Scotland.* Accessed 05/19/06 at www.nahshealthquality.org.
9. Cutler, C.J., & Davis, N. (2005). Improving oral care in patients receiving mechanical ventilation. *American Journal of Critical Care, 14,* 389-394.
10. Devine, P., & Doyle, T. (2001). Brachytherapy for head and neck cancer: A case study. *Clinical Journal of Oncology Nursing, 5*(2), 55-57.
11. Dropkin, M.J. (1999). Body image and quality of life after head and neck cancer surgery. *Cancer Practice, 7*(6), 309-313.
12. Gaziano, J.E. (2002). Evaluation and management of oropharyngeal dysphagia in head and neck cancer. *Cancer Control, 9*(5), 400-409.
13. Gosselin, T.K., & Pavilonis, H. (2002). Head and neck cancer: Managing xerostomia and other treatment induced side effects. *ORL—Head and Neck Nursing, 20*(4), 15-22.
14. Hahn, M.J., & Jones, A. (2000). *Head and neck nursing.* London: Churchill Livingstone-Harcourt Publishers.
15. Heffner, J.E. (2001). The role of tracheotomy in weaning. *Chest, 120,* 477-481.
16. Higgins, T.S., et al. (1998). Nasal cavity, paranasal sinuses, nasopharynx conditions and care. In L.L. Harris & M.B. Huntoon (Eds.), *Core curriculum for otorhinolaryngology and head-neck nursing* (pp. 169-206). New Smyrna Beach, Fla: Society of Otorhinolaryngology and Head-Neck Nurses.
17. Jemal, A., et al. (2002). Cancer statistics, 2002. *CA: A Cancer Journal for Clinicians, 52*(1), 23-45.
18. Kearney, K. (2001). Epiglottitis. *American Journal of Nursing, 101*(8), 37-38.
19. Koch, W.M., et al. (1999). Head and neck cancer in nonsmokers: A distinct clinical and molecular entity. *Laryngoscope, 109,* 1544-1551.
20. Krouse, J.H. (1999). Introduction to sinus disease: I. Anatomy and physiology. *ORL—Head and Neck Nursing, 17*(2), 7-12.
21. Krouse, J.H., & Krouse, H.J. (1999). Introduction to sinus disease: II. Diagnosis and treatment. *ORL—Head and Neck Nursing, 17*(3), 6-16.

22. Krouse, J.H., & Krouse, H.J. (2002). Allergic disease and associated concurrent medical illnesses. *ORL—Head and Neck Nursing, 20*(4), 10-14.

23. McKenna, M. (1999). Postoperative tonsillectomy/adenoidectomy hemorrhage: A retrospective chart review. *ORL—Head and Neck Nursing, 17*(3), 18-21.

24. St. John, R.E., & Seckel, M.A. (2007). Airway management. In S.M. Burns (Ed.), *AACN protocols for practice: Care of mechanically ventilated patients* (2nd ed., pp. 1-57). Sudbury, Mass: Jones and Bartlett.

25. Scott, J.M., & Vollman, K.M. (2005). Endotracheal tube and oral care. In Lynn-McHale, D. Wiegand, & K. Carlson (Eds.), *AACN procedure manual for critical care* (4th ed., pp. 28-33). Aliso Viejo, Calif: American Association of Critical-Care Nurses.

26. Skillings, K.N., & Curtis, B.L. (2005). Tracheal tube care. In D.L.M. Wiegand, & K. Carlson (Eds.), *AACN procedure manual for critical care* (4th ed., pp. 79-86). Aliso Viejo, Calif: American Association of Critical-Care Nurses.

27. Skillings, K.N., & Curtis, B.L. (2005). Tracheal tube cuff care. In D.L.M. Wiegand, & K. Carlson (Eds.), *AACN procedure manual for critical care* (4th ed., pp. 71-78). Aliso Viejo, Calif: American Association of Critical-Care Nurses.

28. Skillings, K.N., & Curtis, B.L. (2005). Extubation/decannulation. In D.L.M. Wiegand, & K. Carlson (Eds.), *AACN procedure manual for critical care* (4th ed., pp. 34-37). Aliso Viejo, Calif: American Association of Critical-Care Nurses.

29. Sparacino, L.L. (2000). Epistaxis management: What's new and what's noteworthy. *Lippincott's Primary Care Practice, 4*(5), 498-507.

30. Spaulding, M.B. (2002). Recent advances in the treatment of head and neck cancer: A patient care perspective. *ORL—Head and Neck Nursing, 20*(1), 9-18.

31. Stapleton, E.R., et al. (Eds.) (2001). *BLS for healthcare providers.* Dallas: American Heart Association.

32. Steyer, T.E. (2002). Peritonsillar abscess: Diagnosis and treatment. *American Family Physician, 65*(1), 93-96.

33. Sue, R.D., & Susanto, I. (2003). Long-term complications of artificial airways. *Clinics in Chest Medicine, 24*, 457-471.

34. Wilkinson, J.M. (2000). *Nursing diagnosis handbook with NIC interventions and NOC outcomes.* Upper Saddle River, NJ: Prentice Hall.

evolve *Did you remember to check out the bonus material on the Evolve website and the CD-ROM, including NCLEX®-Examination Style Review Questions, Open-Book Quizzes, and Chapter Review Audio Podcasts?*

http://evolve.elsevier.com/Black/medsurg

CHAPTER 61

Management of Clients with Lower Airway and Pulmonary Vessel Disorders

SHERILL NONES CRONIN AND KIM MIRACLE

A distinguishing feature of lower airway and pulmonary vessel disorders is the presence of dyspnea. *Dyspnea* (shortness of breath) is a subjective experience that results when air flow, oxygen exchange, or both are impaired. The sensation of uncomfortable breathing can be as distressing as pain and can lead to severe functional disability. The intensity and frequency of dyspnea as well as its association with specific activities must be assessed to develop realistic expectations of treatment outcomes. Because the experience of dyspnea is associated with much anxiety, nursing interventions to relieve this manifestation are essential to the care of clients with conditions of the lower airways and pulmonary vessels.

DISORDERS OF THE LOWER AIRWAYS

ASTHMA

Asthma is a disorder of the bronchial airways characterized by periods of reversible bronchospasm (spasms of prolonged contraction of the bronchial airways). Asthma is often called *reactive airway disease.* This complex disorder involves biochemical, immunologic, endocrine, infectious, autonomic, and psychological factors. In 2005 approximately 22.2 million Americans were diagnosed with asthma, with 12.2 million having an asthma attack. The annual financial impact of this disease is approximately $16.1 billion in direct care and lost productivity.

Etiology and Risk Factors

Asthma occurs in families, which suggests that it is an inherited disorder. Apparently, environmental factors (e.g., viral infection, allergens, pollutants) interact with inherited factors to produce disease. Other inciting factors can include excitatory states (stress, laughing, crying), exercise, changes in temperature, and strong odors. Asthma also is a component of *triad* disease: asthma, nasal polyps, and allergy to aspirin.

Pathophysiology

Asthma involves a chronic inflammatory process that produces mucosal edema, mucus secretion, and airway inflammation (Figure 61-1). When people with asthma are exposed to extrinsic allergens and irritants (e.g., dust, pollen, smoke, mold, medications, foods, respiratory tract infections), their airways become inflamed, producing shortness of breath, chest tightness, and wheezing. Initial clinical manifestations, termed *early-phase reaction,* develop immediately and last about an hour.

When a client is exposed to an allergen, immunoglobulin E (IgE) is produced by B lymphocytes. IgE antibodies attach to mast cells and basophils in the bronchial walls. As shown in the Concept Map feature on p. 1572, the mast cell empties, releasing chemical mediators of inflammation, such as histamine, bradykinin, prostaglandins, and slow-reacting substance of anaphylaxis (SRS-A). These substances induce capillary dilation,

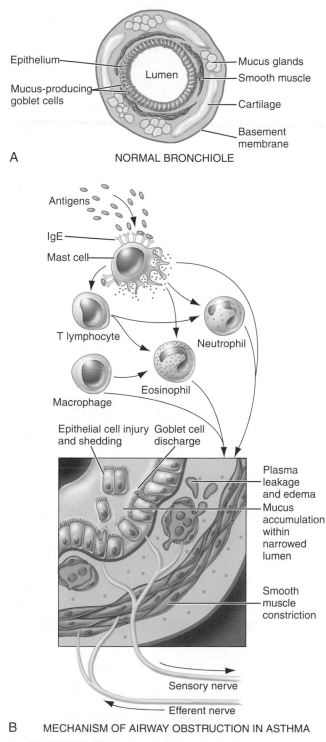

A NORMAL BRONCHIOLE

- Epithelium
- Lumen
- Mucus-producing goblet cells
- Mucus glands
- Smooth muscle
- Cartilage
- Basement membrane

- Antigens
- IgE
- Mast cell
- T lymphocyte
- Neutrophil
- Macrophage
- Eosinophil
- Epithelial cell injury and shedding
- Goblet cell discharge
- Plasma leakage and edema
- Mucus accumulation within narrowed lumen
- Smooth muscle constriction
- Sensory nerve
- Efferent nerve

B MECHANISM OF AIRWAY OBSTRUCTION IN ASTHMA

■ **FIGURE 61–1** Common bronchial wall changes in asthma are hypertrophied smooth muscle, edema, mucus gland hypertrophy, and mucus in the lumen. *(From Copstead, L.C., & Banasik, J.L. [2000]. Pathophysiology: Biological and behavioral perspectives. Philadelphia: Saunders.)*

leading to edema of the airway in an attempt to dilute the allergen and wash it away. They also induce airway constriction in an attempt to close the airway to prevent inhalation of more allergen.

About half of all asthma clients also experience a *delayed (late-phase) reaction*. Although clinical manifestations are the same as those in the early phase, they do not begin until 4 to 8 hours after exposure and may last for hours or days.

In both phases, the release of chemical mediators produces the airway response. In the late-phase response, however, the mediators attract other inflammatory cells and create a self-sustaining cycle of obstruction and inflammation. This chronic inflammation produces hyperresponsiveness of the airways. This hyperresponsiveness causes subsequent episodes in response not only to specific antigens but also to stimuli such as physical exertion and breathing cold air. Clinical manifestations may occur with increasing frequency and severity.

Both alpha-adrenergic and beta-adrenergic receptors of the sympathetic nervous system are found in the bronchi. Stimulation of alpha-adrenergic receptors causes bronchoconstriction; conversely, stimulation of beta-adrenergic receptors causes bronchodilation. Cyclic adenosine monophosphate (cAMP) balances the two receptors. Some theories suggest that asthma may be a result of lack of beta-adrenergic stimulation.

Clinical Manifestations

During asthma attacks, clients are dyspneic and have marked respiratory effort. Manifestations of marked respiratory effort include nasal flaring, pursed-lip breathing, and use of accessory muscles. Cyanosis is a late development.

Auscultation of breath sounds usually reveals wheezing, especially during expiration. The inability to auscultate wheezing in an asthmatic client with acute respiratory distress may be an ominous sign. It may indicate that the small airways are too constricted to allow any air flow. The client may require immediate, aggressive medical intervention. In addition, bronchospasm may lead to almost continuous coughing in an attempt to exhale and clear the airway.

The diagnosis of asthma is based on clinical manifestations, spirometry results, and response to treatment. Spirometry reveals decreased peak expiratory flow rate (PEFR), timed forced expiratory volume (FEV), and forced vital capacity (FVC). Functional residual capacity (FRC), total lung capacity (TLC), and residual volume (RV) are increased because air is trapped within the lungs. A 12% improvement in forced expiratory volume in 1 second (FEV_1) after inhaled administration of a beta-agonist bronchodilator implies a reversible air flow obstruction, that is, by definition, asthma. Figure 61-2 shows a peak flowmeter for monitoring air flow.

Baseline assessment of pulmonary status also may include pulse oximetry and arterial blood gas (ABG) analysis. Pulse oximetry usually reveals low oxygen

CONCEPT MAP

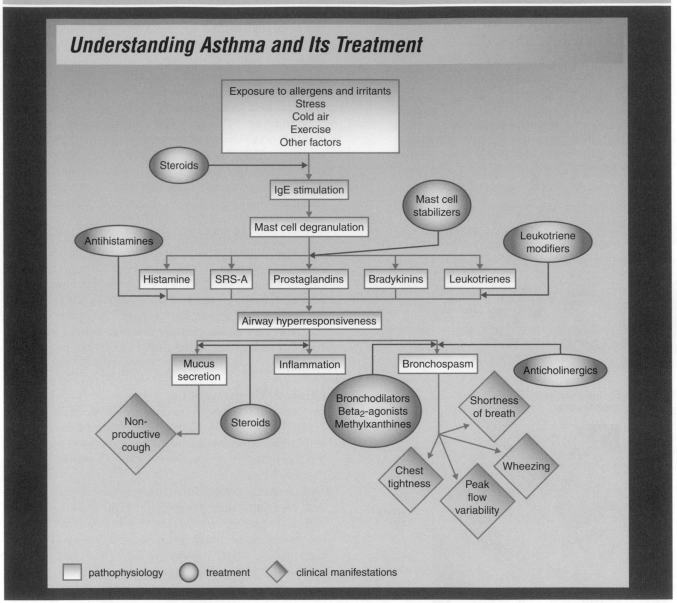

Understanding Asthma and Its Treatment

saturation. ABG results often show some degree of hypoxemia, with elevated partial pressures of arterial carbon dioxide ($Paco_2$) in severe cases.

Status asthmaticus is a severe, life-threatening complication of asthma. It is an acute episode of bronchospasm that tends to intensify. With severe bronchospasm, the workload of breathing increases 5 to 10 times, which can lead to acute cor pulmonale (right-sided heart failure resulting from lung disease). When air is trapped, a severe paradoxical pulse (i.e., drop in blood pressure >10 mm Hg during inspiration) develops as venous return is obstructed. Pneumothorax commonly develops. If status

asthmaticus continues, hypoxemia worsens and acidosis begins. If the condition is untreated or not reversed, respiratory or cardiac arrest ensues.

OUTCOME MANAGEMENT

Medical Management

Many disorders can cause wheezing, such as sinusitis, gastroesophageal reflux disease (GERD), heart failure, bronchitis, and lung tumors. These conditions are ruled out before an asthma diagnosis is given.

■ **FIGURE 61–2** Peak flowmeters. Several types of portable meters are available for self-monitoring of air flow.

Management of asthma is based on the severity of the disease (Table 61-1) and is directed at reversing airway spasm. The general goals of asthma therapy include the following:

- Prevention of chronic asthma and asthma exacerbations
- Maintenance of normal activity levels
- Maintenance of normal or near-normal lung function
- Minimal or no side effects while receiving optimal medications
- Client satisfaction with asthma care

Emphasis has moved away from episodic treatment of manifestations after they occur to long-term control through inhaled corticosteroids to prevent asthma whenever possible.

Reverse Airway Spasm

A severe asthma episode may constitute a medical emergency. Medical intervention for such episodes is aimed primarily at the following:

- Maintaining a patent airway by relieving bronchospasm and clearing excess or retained secretions
- Maintaining effective gas exchange
- Preventing complications, such as acute respiratory failure and status asthmaticus

Emergency management of the client begins with inhaled $beta_2$ agonists. $Beta_2$ agonists stimulate the beta-adrenergic receptors and dilate the airways. If the spasm does not abate (i.e., if FEV_1 remains <50% of predicted), nebulized atropine sulfate or intravenous (IV) steroids may be given. Atropine is an anticholinergic that blocks the effect of the parasympathetic system. When the vagus nerve is stimulated, bronchial smooth muscle tone increases. If these treatments do not reverse the clinical manifestations, the client usually is admitted to the hospital for further treatment.

If the client has an acute asthma attack and no medications are nearby, the attack sometimes can be lessened by *pursed-lip breathing*, which increases pressure in the airways so that they remain open and trapped air can be exhaled more easily.

SAFETY
ALERT

Supplemental oxygen is indicated if Pao_2 levels decrease to less than 60 mm Hg. Monitor the client closely for clinical manifestations of increasing anxiety, increased work of breathing, and indications of tiring. Endotracheal intubation and mechanical ventilation may be necessary. Sedation, and in rare cases administration of paralytic agents, may be necessary to blunt the client's respiratory effort and to prevent further air trapping and pressure increases. Status asthmaticus is treated

TABLE 61–1	Classifying Asthma Severity		
	Symptoms	**Nighttime Symptoms**	**Lung Function**
Step 4 Severe persistent	Continual symptoms Limited physical activity Frequent exacerbations	Frequent	FEV_1 or PEF ≤60% predicted* PEF variability >30%
Step 3 Moderate persistent	Daily symptoms Daily use of inhaled short-acting $beta_2$ agonist Exacerbations affect activity Exacerbations ≥2 times a week; may last days	>1 time a week	FEV_1 or PEF >60% to <80% predicted PEF variability >30%
Step 2 Mild persistent	Symptoms >2 times a week but <1 time a day Exacerbations may affect activity	>2 times a month	FEV_1 or PEF ≥80% predicted PEF variability 20%-30%
Step 1 Mild intermittent	Symptoms ≤2 times a week Asymptomatic and normal PEF between exacerbations Exacerbations brief (from a few hours to a few days); intensity may vary	≤2 times a month	FEV_1 or PEF ≥80% predicted PEF variability <20%

*FEV_1, Forced expiratory volume in 1 second; *PEF*, peak expiratory flow.
Data from National Institutes of Health. (1997). *Guidelines for the diagnosis and management of asthma* (NIH Pub No. 97-4051). Washington, DC: Author; and National Institutes of Health. (2002). *The NAEPP Expert Panel report: Guidelines for the diagnosis and management of asthma—Update on selected topics 2002* (NIH Pub No. 02-5075). Washington, DC: Author.

with aggressive use of IV corticosteroids and frequent administration of inhaled beta-adrenergic medications to avoid intubation and mechanical ventilation.

✺ Control Inflammation

Mucosal inflammation is controlled through the use of inhaled corticosteroids. Steroids prevent the mast cell from emptying, reducing the edema and spasm.

Mast cell stabilizers and leukotriene modifiers are included in special circumstances. Mast cell stabilizers, such as cromolyn (Nasalcrom, Intal) and nedocromil (Tilade), suppress the release of bronchoconstrictive substances during antigen-antibody reactions. Leukotriene modifiers are used in the treatment of both acute and chronic asthma. The release of leukotrienes into the asthmatic airways causes smooth muscle constriction, increased vascular permeability, edema of the airway mucosa, mucus release, and inhibited mucus clearance. Leukotrienes also attract eosinophils to the airway mucosa, which subsequently promote inflammation. Drugs that block leukotriene receptors mediate the actions of leukotrienes and serve as a useful addition to other therapies during an exacerbation. Leukotriene modifiers have also become an important component of therapy for chronic asthma, offering another class of medications for long-term asthma control. A growing body of evidence indicates that leukotriene modifiers are effective, are well tolerated, and have a low risk of adverse effects. Clinical trials have addressed the effectiveness of these drugs in clients with asthma. These medications have shown improvement in the FEV_1, a decreased need for rescue inhalers, and improvement in asthma symptoms. Leukotriene modifiers are not listed as preferred first-line treatment, yet they do have a potential role in the treatment of asthmatics of all severities. The concept of anti-IgE therapies is continuing to be explored as another therapy since there is a significant association between asthma and atopy, and since IgE plays a central role in the pathogenesis of atopy. However, no formal recommendations have been made thus far.

Nursing Management

Assessment

SAFETY ALERT

Initially, assess the client for clinical manifestations of airway distress. If present, they constitute an emergency that must be managed before a detailed history of the disease or other health problems is obtained. The Critical Monitoring feature above, right, lists manifestations of acute airway distress caused by asthma.

Asking clients to rate dyspnea on a scale of 0 to 10 is an easy and effective measure of present dyspnea and may help to monitor and evaluate dyspnea in clinic and home care settings: "On a scale of 0 to 10, indicate

how much shortness of breath you are having right now, with 0 meaning no shortness of breath and 10 meaning shortness of breath as bad as can be."[18]

Determine any known medication allergies so that they can be avoided during treatment. Ascertain whether the client has a history of cardiac disease because nonselective $beta_2$ agonists can produce tachycardia and stress a diseased heart.

Once the acute episode is controlled, explore the history of the client's asthma. Assist the client to determine whether there is a pattern to the manifestations in order to help identify a trigger that precipitates the asthma. If an extrinsic trigger can be identified, it may be possible to reduce or eliminate it. For example, if the client is allergic to mold, common sources of mold can be avoided. Ask about current medications. Some clients are inadvertently given medications that may induce bronchospasms. For example, a noncardioselective beta-blocker, such as propranolol (Inderal), prescribed for hypertension may cause bronchospasm.

Within the psychosocial domain, ask about the client's ability to manage the asthma as well as the client's general adaptation to the illness. Denial of the illness can interfere with early treatment. Determine whether the client feels control over the illness and feels capable of managing it. Clients who have this feeling of control show better compliance with treatments. Determine whether the client is experiencing an increased number of stressors. A stressful lifestyle may exacerbate asthma.

Assess the attitude of the family. The family can be a great source of support and can assist the client in recognizing early manifestations. In contrast, an unsupportive family may contribute to denial or may be an additional source of stress to the client. Involve the case manager (see the Case Management website feature on Chronic Obstructive Pulmonary Disease).

The client with a new diagnosis of asthma may be asked to assess the home and work environment for likely triggers of the clinical manifestations. In addition, skin testing for allergy may be performed.

Diagnosis, Outcomes, Interventions

Diagnosis: Ineffective Breathing Pattern. Because of airway spasm and edema, the client cannot move air in and out of the lungs as needed to maintain adequate tissue oxygenation. The correct nursing diagnosis would be *Ineffective Breathing Pattern related to impaired exhalation and anxiety*. Anxiety with dyspnea is another cause of breathing pattern problems.

Outcomes. The client will have improved breathing patterns, as evidenced by (1) a decreasing respiratory rate to within normal limits; (2) decreased dyspnea, less nasal flaring, and reduced use of accessory muscles; (3) decreased manifestations of anxiety; (4) a return of ABG levels to normal limits; (5) oxygen saturation greater than 95%; and (6) vital capacity measurements within normal limits or greater than 40% of those predicted.

Interventions. Assess the client frequently, observing respiratory rate and depth. Assess the breathing pattern for shortness of breath, pursed-lip breathing, nasal flaring, sternal and intercostal retractions, or a prolonged expiratory phase. During an acute asthma attack, these assessments can be conducted continuously.

Place the client in the Fowler position, and give oxygen as ordered. Monitor ABGs and oxygen saturation levels to determine the effectiveness of treatments. Compare pulmonary function test results with normal levels. The degree of dysfunction assists in planning client activity.

Diagnosis: Ineffective Airway Clearance. The excessive production of mucus and spasm in the airway makes it difficult to keep the airway patent. The nursing diagnosis *Ineffective Airway Clearance related to increased production of secretions and bronchospasm* is appropriate.

Outcomes. The client will have effective airway clearance, as evidenced by (1) decreased inspiratory and expiratory wheezing; (2) decreased rhonchi; and (3) decreasing dry, nonproductive cough.

Interventions. If the airway is compromised, the client's secretions may require suctioning. Some clients experience asthma episodes as a result of pulmonary infection. Monitor the color and consistency of the sputum, and assist the client to cough effectively. Encourage oral fluids to thin the secretions and to replace fluids lost through rapid respiration. The humidity in the room may be increased slightly. If chest secretions are thick and difficult to expectorate, the client may benefit from postural drainage, lung percussion and vibration, expectorants, and frequent position changes. Give frequent oral care, every 2 to 4 hours, to remove the taste of the secretions and remoisten the oral mucous membranes that have dried from mouth breathing.

The approach to pharmacologic therapy often is referred to as *step care,* meaning that the medications ordered and the frequency of administration are adjusted according to the severity of the client's asthma. Asthma medications are categorized into two major classes: (1) *long-term–control* medications, used to achieve and maintain control of persistent asthma; and (2) *quick-relief* medications, used to treat acute air flow obstruction and its accompanying manifestations. The most effective long-term–control medications are those that reduce inflammation, with inhaled steroids being the most potent. Quick-relief medications include short-acting inhaled $beta_2$ agonists and oral steroids.

For clients who respond poorly to inhaled agents, theophylline and aminophylline are still used at times. These medications are regarded as weak bronchodilators. Wide variations exist in their rates of metabolism, and these medications have a high potential for toxicity; for these reasons, their use is declining. Theophylline levels must be monitored to evaluate effectiveness and possible toxicity.

Figure 61-3 depicts a stepwise approach for managing asthma in adults. All clients with asthma require a short-acting inhaled $beta_2$ agonist as needed for acute manifestations. Clients with mild, moderate, or severe persistent asthma require daily long-term–control medications. The preferred treatment strategy is to start with more intensive therapy to achieve rapid control and then "step down" to the minimum therapy needed for maintenance.

Diagnosis: Impaired Gas Exchange. When air is trapped within alveoli, the alveoli are eventually drained of oxygen and the client can become hypoxic. The nursing diagnosis is *Impaired Gas Exchange related to air trapping*.

Outcomes. The client will have adequate gas exchange, as evidenced by (1) decreased inspiratory and expiratory wheezing; (2) decreased rhonchi; (3) oxygen saturation >90%; (4) Pao_2 greater than 60 mm Hg; (5) $Paco_2$ equal to or less than 45 mm Hg; (6) pH of 7.35 to 7.45; (7) usual skin color (no cyanosis); and (8) decreasing dry, nonproductive cough.

Interventions. Assess lung sounds every hour during acute episodes to determine the adequacy of gas exchange. Assess skin and mucous membrane color for cyanosis. Cyanosis is a late manifestation of hypoxia and an indication of serious gas-exchange problems. Monitor pulse oximetry for oxygen saturation levels. Administer oxygen as ordered to maintain optimal oxygen saturation.

Stepwise Approach for Managing Asthma in Adults and Children Older Than 5 Years of Age: Treatment

Classify Severity: Clinical Features Before Treatment or Adequate Control			Medications Required to Maintain Long-Term Control
	Symptoms/Day Symptoms/Night	PEF or FEV$_1$ PEF Variability	Daily Medications
Step 4 Severe Persistent	Continual Frequent	≤60% >30%	■ Preferred treatment: – High-dose inhaled corticosteroids AND – Long-acting inhaled beta$_2$-agonists AND, if needed, – Corticosteroid tablets or syrup long term (2 mg/kg/day, generally do not exceed 60 mg/day). (Make repeat attempts to reduce systemic corticosteroids and maintain control with high-dose inhaled corticosteroids.)
Step 3 Moderate Persistent	Daily >1 night/week	>60% – <80% >30%	■ Preferred treatment: – Low-to-medium dose inhaled corticosteroids and long-acting inhaled beta$_2$-agonists. ■ Alternative treatment (listed alphabetically): – Increase inhaled corticosteroids within medium-dose range OR – Low-to-medium dose inhaled corticosteroids and either leukotriene modifier or theophylline.
			If needed (particularly in patients with recurring severe exacerbations): ■ Preferred treatment: – Increase inhaled corticosteroids within medium-dose range and add long-acting inhaled beta$_2$-agonists. ■ Alternative treatment: – Increase inhaled corticosteroids within medium-dose range and add either leukotriene modifier or theophylline.
Step 2 Mild Persistent	>2/week but <1 time/day >2 nights/month	≥80% 20%-30%	■ Preferred treatment: – Low-dose inhaled corticosteroids. ■ Alternative treatment (listed alphabetically): cromolyn, leukotriene modifier, nedocromil, OR sustained-release theophylline to serum concentration of 5-15 mcg/ml.
Step 1 Mild Intermittent	≤2 days/week ≤2 nights/month	≥80% <20%	■ No daily medication needed. ■ Severe exacerbations may occur, separated by long periods of normal lung function and no symptoms. A course of systemic corticosteroids is recommended.

Quick Relief All Patients	■ Short-acting bronchodilator: 2-4 puffs short-acting inhaled beta$_2$-agonists as needed for symptoms. ■ Intensity of treatment will depend on severity of exacerbation; up to 3 treatments at 20-minute intervals or a single nebulizer treatment as needed. Course of systemic corticosteroids may be needed. ■ Use of short-acting beta$_2$-agonists >2 times a week in intermittent asthma (daily, or increasing use in persistent asthma) may indicate the need to initiate (increase) long-term control therapy.

⬇ **Step down**
Review treatment every 1 to 6 months; a gradual stepwise reduction in treatment may be possible.

⬆ **Step up**
If control is not maintained, consider step up. First, review patient medication technique, adherence, and environmental control.

Goals of Therapy: Asthma Control

■ Minimal or no chronic symptoms day or night
■ Minimal or no exacerbations
■ No limitations on activities; no school/work missed

■ Maintain (near) normal pulmonary function
■ Minimal use of short-acting inhaled beta$_2$-agonist (<1 time/day, <1 canister/month)
■ Minimal or no adverse effects from medications

Note
■ The stepwise approach is meant to assist, not replace, the clinical decision making required to meet individual patient needs.
■ Classify severity: assign patient to most severe step in which any feature occurs (PEF is % of personal best; FEV$_1$ is % predicted).
■ Gain control as quickly as possible (consider a short course of systemic corticosteroids); then step down to the least medication necessary to maintain control.
■ Provide education on self-management and controlling environmental factors that make asthma worse (e.g., allergens and irritants).
■ Refer to an asthma specialist if there are difficulties controlling asthma or if step 4 care is required. Referral may be considered if step 3 care is required.

■ **FIGURE 61–3** Stepwise approach for managing asthma in adults and children older than 5 years of age. *(From National Institutes of Health. [2002]. The National Asthma Education and Prevention Program Expert Panel report: Guidelines for the diagnosis and management of asthma—Update on selected topics [NIH Pub No. 02-5075]. Washington, DC: Author.)*

Nursing Diagnosis: Knowledge Deficit. If the client has just been diagnosed with asthma, the diagnosis of *Knowledge Deficit* may be used to identify specific topics needing education. State the diagnosis as *Knowledge Deficit related to use of inhaled and nebulized medications.*

Outcomes. The client will have increased knowledge about how and when to use nebulized medications as evidenced by explaining the manifestations to be treated with nebulized medications and the outcomes expected as well as how to hold the devices.

Interventions. Nebulized medications can be difficult to learn to use. The client must coordinate inhalation with compression of the metered-dose inhaler canister (Figure 61-4). The Client Education Guide on p. 1578 provides directions for using an inhaler. Observe the client's use of the nebulizer to ascertain whether the medication is entering the airway. Be certain the client knows what manifestations require the use of the nebulizer; also see the Self-Care section on this page.

Nursing Diagnosis: Risk for Decisional Conflict. This nursing diagnosis is related to allergens present in the environment and fits the client who must change a previous lifestyle or make an environmental change to reduce the risk of asthma.

Outcomes. The client will express an understanding of the conflict involved with maintaining the present lifestyle and its effect on asthma.

Interventions. The presence of pets that shed hair or dander, cigarette smoke, or occupational exposure to other allergens may require some lifestyle changes. In many cases, the pets can remain in the house but cannot sleep with the asthmatic client. Encourage clients to stop smoking, and teach clients and others about the dangers of second-hand smoke. Elimination of irritants is generally performed in a reasonable fashion, such as removing exposure to one allergen at a time. Potential improvements in a client's manifestations that might result from a major lifestyle change, such as job change or loss of a pet, may be offset quickly by the stress felt from such a change.

See the Care Plan feature on pp. 1582-1585 when working with COPD clients who have diagnoses of *Activity Intolerance, Anxiety, Imbalanced Nutrition,* or *Disturbed Sleep Pattern.*

Evaluation. Generally, asthma episodes can be reversed quickly if there is no underlying problem, such as infection. Expect the client to be hospitalized only briefly; plan a coordinated approach to assessment and follow-up.

Self-Care

Through appropriate use of the peak flowmeter and medications, clients with asthma should be able to anticipate most exacerbations and enhance their quality of life. Peak flow values fall about 24 hours before manifestations develop. Clients should be taught to increase their routine medications in anticipation of asthma exacerbations. Many clients can manage their asthma effectively with a thorough action plan to guide their decisions. An action plan for asthma is presented in Figure 61-5. It is recommended that a written plan be used as part of the overall effort to educate the client in self-management.

Changes in the treatment plan may be needed as asthma severity and control vary over time. Follow-up visits every 1 to 6 months are recommended to monitor the disease and to maintain control. The presence of one or more indicators of poor control (i.e., awakening at night with dyspnea or coughing, increased use of short-acting inhaled beta$_2$ agonists, increased urgent care visits) may suggest a need to "step up" therapy. Before increasing medications, however, consider other possible reasons for poor control (Table 61-2).

CHRONIC OBSTRUCTIVE PULMONARY DISEASE

Also known as *chronic obstructive lung disease,* chronic obstructive pulmonary disease (COPD) refers to several disorders that affect the movement of air in and out of the lungs. Although the most important of these—obstructive bronchitis, emphysema, and asthma—may occur in a pure form, they most commonly coexist with overlapping clinical manifestations. COPD can occur as a result of increased airway resistance secondary to bronchial mucosal edema or smooth muscle contraction. It may also be a result of decreased elastic recoil, as seen in emphysema. Elastic recoil, similar to the recoil of a stretched rubber band, is the force used to passively

■ **FIGURE 61–4** A client using a metered-dose inhaler with a spacer.

Asthma

CLIENT INSTRUCTIONS

Asthma may be triggered by pollen, dust, animal dander, molds, smoke, or other allergens. Learn what triggers your asthma and minimize your exposure to it.

Monitor the pollution index and pollen counts. Limit outdoor activities when these indicators are high.

Take all medications as prescribed by your physician. If you are taking both a bronchodilator and a steroid via inhaler, take the bronchodilator first to open the airways.

Use your peak flowmeter daily.

Follow these directions on how to use a peak flowmeter:

- Attach the mouthpiece and set the pointer to zero (0).
- Stand up and take a deep breath.
- Put the mouthpiece in your mouth, and close your lips tightly around it.
- Blow into the mouthpiece as hard and as fast as you can.
- Record the value and reset the meter.
- Repeat the procedure for a total of three readings.
- Record the highest value on your record sheet.
- Monitor peak flow daily; know your "green zone," when air flow is normal; the "yellow zone," when values have fallen and you need to increase your routine medications; and the "red zone," when you need to increase your rescue medications and notify your doctor.

Use these directions for using an inhaler:

- Remove the cap and shake the inhaler well.
- Hold the canister upright with your index finger on the top and your thumb on the bottom.

- Breathe out through your mouth.
- Place the mouthpiece 1 to 2 inches away from your opened mouth (unless using a spacer).
- Begin with a slow, deep breath. As you breathe in, press the canister down with your finger to give yourself one puff of medication.
- Hold your breath in for at least 5 to 10 seconds.
- Slowly breathe out, holding your lips tight (pursed).

If your physician has prescribed more than one puff, wait 1 minute between puffs to let the medication open up the upper airway. That way, the next puff can reach lower into your lungs.

Pursed-lip breathing, progressive muscle relaxation, and tripod positioning (i.e., leaning on your arms positioned in front of you) may improve your breathing during asthma episodes.

Unless your physician has told you to limit fluids, drink 8 to 10 glasses of water every day. Water helps to thin your sputum so that you can cough it up more easily.

Some forms of asthma may be triggered by exercise. Before starting an exercise program, discuss the exercise plan with your physician.

Call your physician if you experience any of the following manifestations:

- Wheezing and shortness of breath, even though you are taking your medications as prescribed
- Fever, muscle aches, chest pain, or thickening of sputum
- Sputum color changes to yellow, green, gray, or red (bloody)
- Problems that may be related to your medications (e.g., rash, itching, swelling, or trouble breathing)

---

deflate the lung and exhale. Decreased elastic recoil, analogous to an overstreched and weak rubber band, results in a decreased driving force to empty the lung.

COPD is a widespread disorder, 11.4 million U.S. adults (age 18 and over) are estimated to have the disease. However, close to 24 million have evidence of impaired lung function, suggesting an under-diagnosis of the condition. It is the fourth leading cause of death in America, claiming the lives of 122,283 Americans in 2003. Caring for clients with COPD has been estimated at $20.9 billion annually in direct care costs alone; however, the burden of COPD is even greater from a global perspective, where it is projected to rank fifth in 2020 in burden of disease caused worldwide.

Etiology and Risk Factors

Smoking is the primary risk factor for COPD. The numerous irritants found in cigarette smoke stimulate excess mucus production and coughing, destroy ciliary function, and lead to inflammation and damage of bronchiolar and alveolar walls. Other risk factors include air pollution, second-hand smoke, a history of childhood respiratory tract infections, and heredity. Occupational exposure to certain industrial pollutants may also increase risk.

Pathophysiology

COPD is a combination of chronic obstructive bronchitis, emphysema, and asthma. The pathophysiology of bronchitis and emphysema is presented here (see earlier discussion of pathophysiology of asthma).

Chronic Obstructive Bronchitis

Chronic obstructive bronchitis results from inflammation of the bronchi, leading to increased mucus production, chronic cough, and eventual scarring of the bronchial lining. In contrast to those of acute bronchitis, the clinical manifestations of chronic bronchitis continue for at least 3 months of the year for 2 consecutive years. Additionally, if the client has a post-bronchodilator FEV_1/FVC ratio of less than 70% and chronic bronchitis, the client is said to have chronic *obstructive* bronchitis, indicating that the client has obstructive lung disease combined

FIGURE 61–5 Asthma action plan. *(From National Institutes of Health. [1997]. Practical guide for the diagnosis and management of asthma [NIH Pub No. 97-4053]. Washington, DC: Author.)*

TABLE 61–2 Possible Reasons for Poor Asthma Control—"ICE"

Possible Reasons	Interventions
Inhaler technique	Check client's technique
Compliance	Ask when and how much medication the client is taking
Environment	Ask client whether something in the environment has changed
Also consider	Assess client for the presence of
Alternative diagnosis	concomitant upper respiratory disease or alternative diagnosis

From National Institutes of Health. (1997). *Practical guide for the diagnosis and management of asthma* (NIH Pub No. 97-4051). Washington, DC: Author.

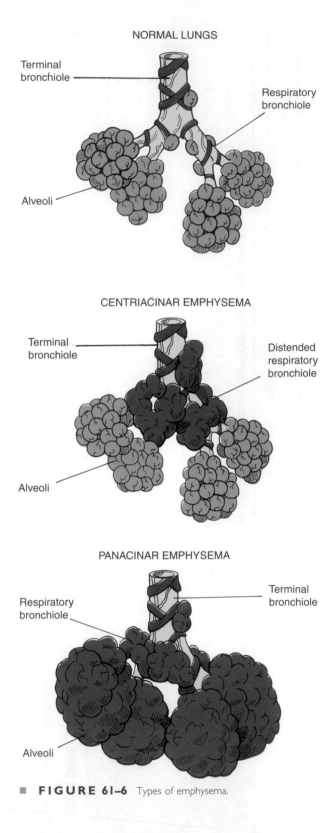

■ **FIGURE 61–6** Types of emphysema.

with chronic cough. Chronic bronchitis is characterized by the following:

■ An increase in the size and number of submucous glands in the large bronchi, which increases mucus production

■ An increased number of goblet cells, which also secrete mucus

■ Impaired ciliary function, which reduces mucus clearance

The lung's mucociliary defenses are impaired, and there is increased susceptibility to infection. When infection occurs, mucus production is greater, and the bronchial walls become inflamed and thickened. Chronic bronchitis initially affects only the larger bronchi, but eventually all the airways are involved. The thick mucus and inflamed bronchi obstruct the airways, especially during expiration. The airways collapse, and air is trapped in the distal portion of the lung. This obstruction leads to reduced alveolar ventilation. An abnormal ventilation-perfusion $\dot{V}/\dot{Q}$ ratio develops, with a corresponding fall in Pao_2. Impaired ventilation may also result in increased levels of $Paco_2$. As compensation for the hypoxemia, polycythemia (overproduction of erythrocytes) occurs.

Emphysema

Emphysema is a disorder in which the alveolar walls are destroyed. This destruction leads to permanent overdistention of the air spaces. Air passages are obstructed as a result of these changes, rather than from mucus production as in chronic bronchitis. Some forms of emphysema may result from a breakdown in the lung's normal defense mechanisms (alpha$_1$-antitrypsin [AAT]) against certain enzymes. Research has shown that the enzymes protease and elastase can attack and destroy the connective tissue of the lungs. Difficult expiration in emphysema is the result of destruction of the walls (septa) between the alveoli, partial airway collapse, and loss of elastic recoil. As the alveoli and septa collapse, pockets of air form between the alveolar spaces (blebs) and within the lung parenchyma (bullae). This process leads to increased ventilatory dead space from areas that do not participate in gas or blood exchange. The work of breathing is increased because there is less functional

■ **FIGURE 61–7** A client with chronic obstructive bronchitis. Note the stocky build and the presence of pursed-lip breathing. The slight gynecomastia is a side effect of corticosteroid therapy. The client's shoulders are raised because of shortness of breath and increased work of breathing.

■ **FIGURE 61–8** A client with emphysema. Note the thin appearance and the presence of continuous oxygen therapy. The use of accessory muscles of respiration (neck and shoulder muscles) reflects the client's shortness of breath and increased work of breathing necessary to increase minute ventilation and to maintain adequate arterial blood gas values.

■ **FIGURE 61–9 A,** Preoperative chest x-ray of a client with emphysema. Note the flattened diaphragm and the laterally hyperexpanded chest walls. **B,** Postoperative chest x-ray after lung volume reduction surgery. The right side of the diaphragm is rounded and no longer flattened by emphysematous lung tissue. *(From Allen, G. [1996]. Surgical treatment of emphysema using bovine pericardium strips. AORN Journal, 63[2], 373-388.)*

The Client with Chronic Obstructive Pulmonary Disease

Nursing Diagnosis: Impaired Gas Exchange related to decreased ventilation and mucus plugs.
Outcomes: The client will maintain adequate gas exchange as evidenced by arterial blood gas (ABG) values (i.e., Pao_2 of at least 60 mm Hg, pH within normal limits, and $Paco_2$ at baseline) or oxygen saturation greater than 90%, mental status at baseline, minimal anxiety.

NOC OUTCOMES Electrolyte and Acid-Base Balance, Respiratory Status: Gas Exchange, Respiratory Status: Ventilation, Tissue Perfusion: Pulmonary, Vital Signs Status

Interventions	NIC INTERVENTIONS	Rationales
1. Regularly monitor the client's respiratory rate and pattern, pulse oximetry, ABG results, and manifestations of hypoxia or hypercapnia. Report significant changes or a lack of response promptly.	Respiratory Monitoring	1. Prompt recognition of deteriorating respiratory function can reduce potentially lethal outcomes.
2. Administer low-flow oxygen therapy (1 to 3 L/min on 24% to 31% Fio_2) as needed via nasal prongs or a high-flow Venturi mask.	Oxygen Therapy	2. Oxygen corrects existing hypoxemia.
3. Assist the client into the high-Fowler position.	Positioning	3. The upright position allows full lung excursion and enhances air exchange.
4. Administer bronchodilators if ordered. Monitor for side effects.	Medication Administration: Inhalation	4. Bronchodilators relax bronchial smooth muscle, facilitating air flow. Common side effects include tremor, tachycardia, and other cardiac dysrhythmias.
5. Use caution when administering opioids, sedatives, and tranquilizers.	Medication Management	5. These medications are respiratory depressants and can further impair ventilation.

Evaluation: Bronchospasm is fairly quickly reversible with inhaled bronchodilators and steroids, but until the underlying trigger is controlled, it may quickly recur.

Nursing Diagnosis: Ineffective Airway Clearance related to excessive secretions and ineffective coughing.
Outcomes: The client will have improved airway clearance as evidenced by effective coughing techniques and a patent airway.

NOC OUTCOMES Respiratory Status: Airway Patency, Respiratory Status: Ventilation, Vital Signs Status

Interventions	NIC INTERVENTIONS	Rationales
1. Monitor lung sounds every 4 to 8 hours and before and after coughing episodes.	Respiratory Monitoring	1. Rhonchi present in the large airways may impair airway patency.
2. Teach the client to maintain adequate hydration by drinking at least 8 to 10 glasses of fluid per day (if not contraindicated) and increasing the humidity of the ambient air.	Fluid Management	2. Hydration helps to thin secretions.
3. Teach and supervise effective coughing techniques.	Airway Management	3. Proper coughing techniques conserve energy, reduce airway collapse, and lessen client frustration.
4. Teach and supervise incentive spirometer techniques 10 times per hour while awake.	Ventilation Assistance	4. Incentive spirometer is an objective measure of the depth of inhalation to promote lung expansion.
5. Perform chest physical therapy, if needed, and instruct the client and significant others in these techniques.	Airway Management	5. Chest physical therapy techniques use forces of gravity and motion to facilitate secretion removal.
6. Assess the condition of the oral mucous membranes and perform or offer oral care every 2 hours.	Oral Health Maintenance	6. Thick secretions line the mouth when the client coughs; oral care removes them.

Evaluation: The client will often require 48 or more hours to clear severely congested lungs.

Nursing Diagnosis: Anxiety related to acute breathing difficulties and fear of suffocation.
Outcomes: The client will express an increase in psychological comfort and demonstrate the use of effective coping mechanisms.

NOC OUTCOMES Aggression Control, Anxiety Reduction, Coping, Impulse Control

Interventions	NIC INTERVENTIONS	Rationales
1. Remain with the client during acute episodes of breathing difficulty, and provide care in a calm, reassuring manner.	Anxiety Reduction	1. Reassures the client that competent help is available if needed. Anxiety can be contagious; remain calm.
2. Provide a quiet, calm environment.	Environmental Management	2. Reduction of external stimuli helps promote relaxation.
3. During acute episodes, open doors and curtains and limit the number of people and unnecessary equipment in the room. Provide a fan if the client perceives a benefit from the moving air.	Environmental Management	3. Environmental changes may lessen the client's perceptions of suffocation.

Interventions	NIC INTERVENTIONS	Rationales
4. Encourage the use of breathing retraining and relaxation techniques.	Calming Technique	4. A feeling of self-control and success in facilitating breathing helps reduce anxiety.
5. Give sedatives and tranquilizers with extreme caution. Nonpharmaceutical methods of anxiety reduction are more useful.	Medication Management	5. Oversedation may cause respiratory depression.

Evaluation: Anxiety can usually be controlled quickly but may recur with each episode of dyspnea and requires both short-term and long-term interventions.

Nursing Diagnosis: Activity Intolerance related to inadequate oxygenation and dyspnea.

Outcomes: The client will have improved activity tolerance as evidenced by maintaining a realistic activity level (specify based on underlying condition and baseline activity) and demonstrating energy conservation techniques.

NOC OUTCOMES	Activity Tolerance, Endurance, Energy Conservation

Interventions	NIC INTERVENTIONS	Rationales
1. Monitor the severity of dyspnea and oxygen saturation with and following activity	Respiratory Monitoring	1. Activity increases the demand for oxygen, and the inability to meet the demand may result in dyspnea and desaturation.
2. Stop or slow any activity that leads to a significant change in respiratory rate, failure of pulse to return to near resting rate within 3 minutes of activity, and/or changes in mental status.	Energy Management	2. Significant changes in respiratory, cardiac, or circulatory status signal activity intolerance.
3. Maintain supplemental oxygen therapy as needed during activity.	Oxygen Therapy	3. Supplemental oxygen helps alleviate exercise-induced hypoxemia, thus improving activity tolerance.
4. Schedule active exercise after respiratory therapy or treatment (e.g., bronchodilator in metered-dose inhaler).	Exercise Promotion	4. Lung function is maximized during peak periods of medication and drug effect.
5. Assist the client in scheduling a gradual increase in daily activities and exercise.	Activity Therapy	5. Gradual increases in physical activity improve respiratory and cardiac conditioning, thus improving activity tolerance.
6. Advise the client to avoid conditions that increase oxygen demand, such as smoking, temperature extremes, excess weight, and stress.	Teaching: Disease Process	6. These factors increase peripheral vascular resistance, which increases cardiac workload and oxygen requirements.
7. Instruct the client in energy conservation techniques, such as pacing activities throughout the day, interspersed with adequate rest periods, and alternating high-energy and low-energy tasks.	Energy Management	7. Conservation techniques allow the client to accomplish more tasks with a limited energy supply.
8. Teach the client to use pursed-lip and diaphragmatic breathing techniques during activities.	Teaching: Prescribed Activity/Exercise	8. Breathing retraining ensures maximal use of available respiratory function. Pursed-lip breathing leaves positive end-expiratory pressure in the lungs and helps keep airways open.

Evaluation: Depending on the degree of underlying lung disease, activity intolerance may be slow to be correctable, and this goal should be long term for complete resolution.

Nursing Diagnosis: Imbalanced Nutrition: Less Than Body Requirements related to reduced appetite, decreased energy level, and dyspnea.

Outcomes: The client will eat 75% of served foods during the acute phase and maintain body weight within normal limits for gender and body build, and hemoglobin, prealbumin, and albumin levels will be within normal ranges.

NOC OUTCOMES	Nutritional Status, Nutritional Status: Food and Fluid Intake, Nutritional Status: Nutrient Intake, Weight Control

Interventions	NIC INTERVENTIONS	Rationales
1. Assist the client with mouth care before meals and as needed.	Oral Health Maintenance	1. Coughing and sputum production may impair appetite. Mouth-breathing dries mucous membranes.
2. Advise the client to eat small, frequent meals (e.g., six meals a day) that are high in protein and low in carbohydrates.	Nutrition Therapy	2. Large meals may create an excessive feeling of fullness that may make breathing uncomfortable and difficult. Protein is needed to maintain nutritional status because of the increased work of breathing. Carbohydrate intake should be reduced because they produce carbon dioxide.
3. Advise the client to avoid gas-producing foods, such as beans and cabbage.	Teaching: Prescribed Diet	3. Gas-forming foods may cause abdominal bloating and distention and thus impair ventilation.
4. Instruct the client in the use of high-calorie liquid supplements if indicated.	Teaching: Prescribed Diet	4. Liquid supplements provide high-calorie concentrations in a relatively small volume.
5. Advise hypoxemic clients to use oxygen via nasal cannula during meals.	Oxygen Therapy	5. Adequate oxygenation increases the energy available for eating.
6. Suggest methods to make meal preparation more convenient (e.g., Meals on Wheels program).	Nutritional Counseling	6. Reducing the energy expenditure of preparation maximizes the energy available for eating.

(Continued)

C A R E   P L A N   *evolve*

The Client with Chronic Obstructive Pulmonary Disease—Cont'd

7. Consult with the dietitian to assist with food choices that reduce the production of carbon dioxide.	Consultation Teaching: Disease Process	7. Clients with carbon dioxide retention benefit from foods that do not produce excess CO_2.
8. Monitor the client's food intake, weight, and serum hemoglobin, prealbumin, and albumin levels.	Nutritional Monitoring	8. Changes in body weight reflect the degree of nutrition or malnutrition. Hemoglobin, prealbumin, and albumin levels reflect protein intake.

Evaluation: Improving nutrition, lab values, and body weight are long-term goals. During an acute exacerbation of dyspnea, short-term goals such as the amount of dietary intake may be accomplishable.

Nursing Diagnosis: Disturbed Sleep Pattern related to dyspnea and external stimuli.
Outcomes: The client will report feeling adequately rested.

NOC OUTCOMES Rest, Sleep, Well-Being

Interventions	NIC INTERVENTIONS	Rationales
1. Promote relaxation by providing a darkened, quiet environment; ensuring adequate room ventilation; and following bedtime routines.	Sleep Enhancement	1. The hospital environment can interfere with relaxation and sleep. Using established bedtime rituals increases relaxation.
2. Schedule care activities to allow periods of uninterrupted sleep.	Sleep Enhancement	2. For most people, completing four to five complete sleep cycles (60 to 90 minutes) per night promotes a feeling of being rested.
3. Avoid the use of "sleeping pills."	Sleep Enhancement	3. Many forms of hypnotics, sedatives, and barbiturates impair sleep cycles.

4. Instruct the client in measures to promote sleep:
  a. Plan physical exercise during the day and passive, nonstimulating activities in the evening.
  b. Avoid stimulants, such as caffeine.
  c. Maintain a consistent bedtime and a regular bedtime routine.
  d. Eat a high-protein snack before bedtime.
  e. Use relaxation techniques (e.g., meditation, warm bath, massage, warm beverage).
  f. If the client awakens during the night, suggest a quiet, diverting activity, such as reading, in another room.
  g. If dyspnea is severe, a recliner chair or hospital bed may be more comfortable than a regular bed.
	Sleep Enhancement	4.
		  a. Activity increases the need for sleep and contributes to a feeling of tiredness.
		  b. Stimulants increase metabolism and inhibit relaxation.
		  c. Consistency promotes relaxation and prevents disruptions of the biologic clock.
		  d. Protein digestion produces tryptophan, an amino acid that may have a sedative effect.
		  e. Sleep is difficult unless the client is relaxed.
		  f. Frustration over being awake deters sleep efforts further. The bedroom should be associated mentally with sleep to enhance future sleep promotion.
		  g. The upright position facilitates ventilation.

Evaluation: During acute respiratory problems, sleep may be difficult because of interruptions and dyspnea. Short-term outcomes such as napping may be accomplishable. Long-term plans for sleep may have to be deferred until dyspnea is controlled.

Nursing Diagnosis: Interrupted Family Processes related to chronic illness of a family member.
Outcomes: The family will verbalize their feelings, participate in the care of the ill family member, and seek external resources as needed.

NOC OUTCOMES Caregiver Emotional Health, Caregiver Well-Being, Family Coping, Family Normalization

Interventions	NIC INTERVENTIONS	Rationales
1. Plan interventions considering the client and significant other as the unit of care. Encourage participation in the planning process.	Family Involvement Promotion	1. COPD affects the client and the client's significant others.
2. Assess family communication patterns, and intervene if they are ineffective. Family counseling may be needed.	Family Process Maintenance	2. Effective communication helps each member to understand his or her own and others' feelings. Counseling may facilitate healthy interaction.
3. Encourage as wide a social support network as feasible.	Family Support	3. The use of a wide support group prevents a few family members from being overloaded with responsibility.
4. Encourage the client and family to seek support from other sources (e.g., self-help groups and support groups, such as the Better Breathers clubs sponsored by the American Lung Association).	Support System Enhancement	4. Clients may benefit from opportunities to share common experiences and to learn from others in similar situations.
5. Provide the family with anticipatory guidance as the client's COPD progresses.	Teaching: Disease Process	5. Knowing what to expect facilitates family adjustment.

Evaluation: Coping with a family member's illness may require weeks or months to accomplish as the family learns to recognize and treat various exacerbations and live through various family events and activities with the disease (e.g., travel).

Nursing Diagnosis: Sexual Dysfunction related to dyspnea, reduced energy, and changes in relationships.
Outcomes: The client will report increased satisfaction with sexual function.

| NOC OUTCOMES | Sexual Functioning, Endurance |

Interventions	NIC INTERVENTIONS	Rationales
1. Provide an opportunity for the client to discuss concerns.	Sexual Counseling	1. Many people are embarrassed or reluctant to talk about sexual concerns.
2. Suggest measures that may facilitate sexual activity (e.g., alternative positions, use of bronchodilator therapy before beginning sexual activity, choosing a time of day when dyspnea is minimal).	Sexual Counseling	2. Such measures can reduce physical exertion and maximize available oxygen levels.
3. Encourage the client and partner to consider alternative forms of sexual expression (e.g., hugging, cuddling, stroking, kissing).	Sexual Counseling	3. Alternative methods require less energy expenditure compared with intercourse.
4. Recommend a professional sex therapist if appropriate.	Sexual Counseling	4. Talking with a skilled professional may assist the client with constructive problem-solving.

Evaluation: During an acute flare-up of dyspnea, the discussion of sexual activity should be introduced when appropriate. Resolution of the problems and issues is a long-term goal.

Nursing Diagnosis: Risk for Infection related to ineffective pulmonary clearance.
Outcomes: Client will have a decreased risk of infection as evidenced by health promotion behaviors and awareness of manifestations of pulmonary infection.

| NOC OUTCOMES | Knowledge: Infection Control, Tissue Integrity: Skin and Mucous Membranes |

Interventions	NIC INTERVENTIONS	Rationales
1. Teach the client to wash his or her hands after contact with potentially infectious material.	Infection Control	1. Hand-washing is the primary defense against the spread of infection.
2. Encourage the client to obtain a flu vaccination yearly and a pneumococcal vaccination every 5 years.	Infection Protection	2. Vaccination provides immunity for infections.
3. Teach the client and family how to care for and clean respiratory equipment used at home.	Infection Protection	3. Water in respiratory equipment is a common source of bacterial growth.
4. Teach the client and family the manifestations of pulmonary infections (change in color or volume of sputum, fever, chills, malaise, productive cough, confusion, increased dyspnea), and when to call the physician.	Infection Protection	4. Early recognition of manifestations can lead to a rapid diagnosis. Self-care with preplanned interventions (e.g., antibiotics) should be understood.

Evaluation: Risk reduction cannot be measured in a short period of time. Verbal statements of comprehension and plans to follow the instructions should be noted. Sometimes a reduction in the number of acute pulmonary infections or hospitalizations can be measured.

Nursing Diagnosis: Decisional Conflict related to smoking cessation.
Outcomes: The client and family will seriously consider the value of smoking cessation and develop a plan to stop smoking.

| NOC OUTCOMES | Decision Making, Participation: Health Care Decisions |

Interventions	NIC INTERVENTIONS	Rationales
1. Ask the client if he or she was smoking before hospitalization.	Smoking Cessation Assistance	1. Validates the frequency of smoking.
2. Advise the client and family on the benefit of smoking cessation.	Smoking Cessation Assistance	2. Many clients believe there is no benefit to stopping smoking now because lung damage is already present. Even though it is difficult to stop, most clients experience less dyspnea within a few weeks.
3. Assess if the client is ready to stop smoking now (or at dismissal).	Smoking Cessation Assistance	3. It is important for the client to determine if he or she is willing to try. Family may be helpful by discarding all remaining cigarettes.
4. Assist with plans for counseling and pharmacotherapy.	Smoking Cessation Assistance	4. Both cognitive and behavioral strategies are needed and can be provided by therapists.
5. Arrange follow-up care.	Smoking Cessation Assistance	5. Many clients benefit from nicotine patches or antidepressant medications to assist with smoking cessation.

Evaluation: Smoking cessation is a difficult problem. A short-term goal would be for the client to value the need to stop. The long-term goal would be the cessation of tobacco use.

lung tissue to exchange oxygen and carbon dioxide. Emphysema causes destruction of the pulmonary capillaries, further decreasing oxygen perfusion and ventilation.

The three types of emphysema are centriacinar, panacinar, and paraseptal (Figure 61-6). *Centriacinar* (or *centrilobular*) *emphysema,* the most common type, produces destruction in the bronchioles, usually in the upper lung regions. Inflammation begins in the bronchioles and spreads peripherally, but usually the alveolar sac remains intact. This form of emphysema occurs most often in smokers.

Panacinar emphysema destroys the entire alveolus and most commonly involves the lower portions of the lung. This form of the disease is generally observed in individuals with AAT deficiencies. Focal panacinar emphysema may also be seen at the lung bases in smokers with the centriacinar form.

Paraseptal (or *distal acinar*) *emphysema* primarily involves the distal airway structures, alveolar ducts, and alveolar sacs. The process is localized around the septa of the lungs or pleura, resulting in isolated blebs along the lung periphery. It is believed to be the likely cause of spontaneous pneumothorax. Giant bullae occasionally cause severe compression of adjacent lung tissue. The diagnosis of the disease, along with severity determination, is primarily accomplished through spirometry.

While all three disorders—asthma, chronic bronchitis, and emphysema—are present to some degree in clients with COPD, those individuals with chronic obstructive bronchitis as the major disease typically demonstrate a productive cough, decreased exercise tolerance, wheezing, shortness of breath, and prolonged expiration. As the chronic bronchitis progresses, copious amounts of sputum are produced and pulmonary infection is common. The client suffers from chronic hypoxemia and hypercapnia (Figure 61-7). The characteristic sitting position is leaning over a table with the shoulder girdle raised. Gait and walking pace correspond to the client's breathing with frequent rest periods to breathe.

Clients who have primary emphysema have progressive dyspnea on exertion that eventually becomes dyspnea at rest (Figure 61-8). The anteroposterior diameter of the chest is enlarged, and the chest has hyperresonant sounds to percussion. Chest films show overinflation and flattened diaphragms (Figure 61-9, *A*). ABG values are usually normal until later stages, when compensated respiratory acidosis is often evident. The client may have an enlarged heart and right ventricular lift. The electrocardiogram (ECG) shows right heart strain pattern and right axis deviation. Other manifestations may be cyanosis around the lips, neck vein distention, and pitting peripheral edema.

Complications

Respiratory tract infections commonly develop in clients with COPD. This situation is a result of alterations in the normal respiratory defense mechanisms and decreased immune resistance. Because respiratory status already is compromised, infection frequently leads to acute respiratory failure and is a common reason for hospitalization (see Chapter 63).

Spontaneous pneumothorax may develop from rupture of an emphysematous bleb. This rupture results in a closed pneumothorax and requires insertion of a chest tube for reexpansion of the lung (see Chapter 63).

Similar to asthma, chronic obstructive bronchitis and emphysema may worsen at night. Clients often report sleep-onset dyspnea and frequent or early-morning awakenings. During sleep, there is a decrease in the muscle tone and activity of the respiratory muscles. This decreased tone leads to hypoventilation, an increase in resistance of the airways, and $\dot{V}/\dot{Q}$ mismatch. Eventually, the client becomes hypoxemic.

OUTCOME MANAGEMENT

Medical Management

The treatment goals for the client with COPD are to improve ventilation, to facilitate the removal of bronchial secretions, to reduce complications, to slow the progression of clinical manifestations, and to promote health maintenance and client management of the disease. As in asthma, a step-care approach is used to guide medical intervention (Figure 61-10). The use of inspiratory muscle training may also be recommended in selected clients with COPD (see the Translating Evidence into Practice box on p. 1588).

Improve Ventilation

Bronchodilators remain the mainstay in the symptomatic management of COPD. These drugs reduce airway obstruction and are given on an as-needed basis or on a regular basis to prevent or reduce manifestations and exacerbations. They are usually administered via the inhalation route but in rare occasions may be given orally or administered intravenously. Regular treatment with long-acting bronchodilators is more effective and convenient than treatment with short-acting forms.

The principal bronchodilator treatments are beta$_2$ agonists, anticholinergics, and methylxanthines used singly or in combination. Beta$_2$ agonists are sympathomimetic drugs that act on the beta$_2$-adrenoceptors in the smooth muscles of the airways and cause bronchodilation. These drugs may also enhance mucus clearance and improve the endurance of respiratory muscles. Short-acting beta$_2$ agonists (e.g., albuterol) have minimal adverse effects, with rapid onset of action, a peak effect in 60 to 90 minutes, and duration of 4 to 6 hours. Side effects that may develop with the use of these drugs are tachycardia, tremor, nervousness, and nausea.

Summary of the GOLD guidelines				
Therapy at each stage of COPD				
Old	0: At risk	I: Mild	II: Moderate IIA IIB	III: Severe	
New	0: At risk	I: Mild	II: Moderate	III: Severe	IV: Very severe
Characteristics	Chronic symptoms Exposure to risk factors Normal spirometry	FEV_1/FVC <70% FEV_1 ≥80% With or without symptoms	FEV_1/FVC <70% 50% ≤FEV_1 <80% With or without symptoms	FEV_1/FVC <70% 30% ≤FEV_1 <50% With or without symptoms	FEV_1/FVC <70% FEV_1 <30% OR FEV_1 <50% predicted Plus chronic respiratory failure
	Avoidance of risk factor(s); influenza vaccination				
		Add short-acting bronchodilator when needed			
			Add regular treatment with one or more long-acting bronchodilators		
			Add rehabilitation		
				Add inhaled glucocorticosteroids if repeated exacerbations	
					Add long-term oxygen if chronic respiratory failure
					Consider surgical treatments

■ **FIGURE 61–10** Step-care approach to COPD care. *(From Global Initiative for Chronic Obstructive Lung Disease [GOLD]. [2006]. Global strategy for the diagnosis, management and prevention of COPD. Available at www.goldcopd.org.)*

Anticholinergic agents offer greater bronchodilator effect and fewer side effects than short-acting inhaled beta$_2$ agonists. These drugs work by blocking the cholinergic receptors located in the larger airways, resulting in bronchodilation. Ipratropium bromide (Atrovent) is the most commonly used drug in this category. When given by metered-dose inhaler, two puffs achieve maximal bronchodilation in 1.5 to 2 hours and last 6 to 8 hours. Adverse reactions from these drugs include dry mouth, nervousness, dizziness, fatigue, and headache.

Methylxanthines (e.g., theophylline, aminophylline), in both parenteral and oral forms, are also used to treat acute exacerbations. In addition to their bronchodilatory properties, methylxanthines enhance mucociliary clearance, stimulate the central respiratory drive, reduce pulmonary vascular resistance, and improve lung function during sleep. The level of benefit achieved with these agents is dose related, but there is no uniform relationship between the drug's effectiveness and serum blood levels. Age, smoking status, circulatory status, and hepatic function are factors that affect metabolism. Toxicity with methylxanthines may occur even at therapeutic levels, so blood levels of these agents need to be monitored closely. Several drugs also interfere with these agents even when administered in therapeutic levels. Side effects may include gastric upset, tachycardia, nausea and vomiting (possible toxicity), tremors, and nervousness.

Systemic glucocorticosteroids are used in the management of exacerbations of COPD. The exact mechanisms of action of these drugs in obstructive airway disease are poorly understood, but they shorten recovery time, improve lung function, and decrease hypoxemia. If used, corticosteroids should be administered either orally or parenterally, depending on the severity of the exacerbation. They should be used early in the course of treatment because their effect is not apparent for several hours. Clients who show a rapid response to parenteral steroids can be switched to oral forms on the third or fourth day of treatment, followed by a tapering course. The most common adverse effects are hypertension, peptic ulcer, dysphoria, hyperglycemia, cough, oral thrush, and fragile skin. A short course of corticosteroids may result in few adverse effects, but prolonged use does not result in greater efficacy and increases the risk of side effects.

🪔 Long-term oxygen therapy (>15 hours per day) has been shown to improve survival and quality of life in hypoxemic clients. Oxygen by nasal cannula should be provided at a flow rate sufficient to produce a resting Pao_2 of at least 60 mm Hg, or an Sao_2 greater than 89%. It

☞ TRANSLATING EVIDENCE INTO PRACTICE

Inspiratory Muscle Training in COPD

COPD is characterized by progressive deterioration of inspiratory muscle strength. A number of factors are suspected of contributing to this deterioration, including chronic hyperinflation of the lungs, loss of muscle mass, decline in nutritional status, effects of corticosteroid use, and aging.[2] Decreased inspiratory muscle strength worsens the sensation of dyspnea and places clients at risk for respiratory muscle fatigue and declines in functional status.[1]

General interventions, such as pulmonary rehabilitation, nutritional counseling, and client education to prevent acute exacerbations, help to improve overall muscle strength and reduce dyspnea. However, targeted training of the inspiratory muscles has been proposed as an approach for directly improving their strength and endurance. Inspiratory muscle training (IMT) is accomplished through resistance training techniques. These involve the use of commercially available hand-held devices that require the user to generate an increased inspiratory effort to allow inspiratory flow.

Although a significant amount of research has been done on IMT, its benefits have been debated.[4] This is largely due to methodological limitations of many of the studies.[3] In general, the evidence supports the effectiveness of the intervention when training is adequate in duration and frequency (for example, 20 to 30 minutes per day, 4 to 6 days per week) as well as intensity (40% to 70% maximal inspiratory pressure).[5] Current evidence-based guidelines for pulmonary rehabilitation issued by the American College of Chest Physicians and the American Association of Cardiovascular and Pulmonary Rehabilitation recommend the use of IMT in selected clients with COPD who have decreased inspiratory muscle strength and breathlessness despite receiving optimal medical therapy.[6] Supervision and monitoring during training are recommended to ensure that adequate training loads are generated and to evaluate client tolerance.

REFERENCES

1. Hill, K., Jenkins, S.C., Hillman, D.R., et al. (2004). Dyspnea in COPD: Can inspiratory muscle training help? *Australian Journal of Physiotherapy, 50*(3), 169-180.
2. Larson, J.L., Covey, M.K., & Corbridge, S. (2002). Inspiratory muscle strength in chronic obstructive pulmonary disease. *AACN Clinical Issues, 13*(2), 320-332.
3. Padula, C.A. (2006). Inspiratory muscle training: Integrative review. *Research and Theory for Nursing Practice, 20*(4), 291-304.
4. Ram, F.S.F., Wellington, S.R., & Barnes, N.C. (2006). Inspiratory muscle training for asthma. *Cochrane Library, 1,* CD003792.
5. Reid, W.D., Geddes, E.L., Brooks, D., et al. (2004). Inspiratory muscle training in chronic obstructive pulmonary disease. *Physiotherapy Canada, 56*(3), 128-142.
6. Reis, A.L., Bauldoff, G.S., Carlin, B.W., et al. (2007). Pulmonary rehabilitation: Joint ACCP/AACVPR evidence-based clinical practice guidelines. *Chest, 131,* 4-42.

is important to note that some clients with chronic hypercapnia (elevated $Paco_2$ level) may be oxygen sensitive; that is, their $Paco_2$ levels may rise when given supplemental oxygen, leading to suppression of the central nervous system and significant lethargy. This phenomenon is commonly known as *CO_2 narcosis*. There are several theories as to why supplemental oxygen increases hypercapnia in some CO_2 retainers and, in all likelihood, there are probably multiple factors involved. However, the key point is that clients with high $Paco_2$ levels who are receiving oxygen should be closely monitored to determine their response to therapy.

At times, the client may require mechanical ventilatory support for adequate oxygenation during exacerbations. Ventilatory support includes both noninvasive intermittent ventilation, using either negative- or positive-pressure devices, and invasive continuous ventilation via endotracheal tube or tracheostomy.

Remove Bronchial Secretions

Pulmonary hygiene is needed to rid the lungs of secretions and to reduce the risk of infection. In the hospital, the client may be treated with nebulized bronchodilators and positive-pressure air flow or positive end-expiratory pressure devices to increase the caliber of the airways. Postural drainage and chest physiotherapy may be prescribed to move the secretions from the small to the large airways, from which they can be expelled.

Reduce Complications

Deep venous thrombosis prophylaxis may be needed in clients who are immobilized, polycythemic, or dehydrated. Influenza vaccines can reduce serious illness. Pneumococcal polysaccharide vaccine is also recommended for clients 65 years and older and for those clients younger than age 65 with an FEV_1 <40% predicted.

Promote Exercise

All clients with COPD benefit from exercise programs, showing improvement in exercise tolerance and decreased dyspnea and fatigue. Aerobic exercise is used to enhance cardiovascular fitness and to train respiratory muscles to function more effectively. Exercise does not improve lung function, but respiratory muscles can be strengthened even when the lungs are diseased. Progressively increased walking is the most common form of exercise. Before a walking program is begun, ABGs should be assessed and compared with resting levels. Supplemental oxygen should be used during exercise if the client becomes severely hypoxemic.

Breathing exercises may also be prescribed. Encourage diaphragmatic breathing and pursed-lip breathing, and discourage rapid, shallow *panic* breathing.

Improve General Health

The most effective way to slow disease progression is for the client to stop smoking. Exposure to second-hand smoke, occupational dusts and chemicals, air pollution, and known allergens should also be minimized. All clients with COPD should avoid high altitudes, and supplemental oxygen may be required for air travel. No specific climate has been shown to alter the course of the disorder.

Adequate nutrition is essential to maintain respiratory muscle strength. Malnutrition is common and contributes to decreased respiratory muscle strength and reduced diaphragmatic mass. Consult a clinical dietitian to assist clients in modifying their diet to meet their caloric needs. Clients with COPD often have difficulty eating because of dyspnea. Offer the client frequent small meals rather than large meals. When the client must be tube-fed, substrate metabolism also may affect lung function. Normal carbohydrate metabolism produces carbon dioxide and water. Excess carbohydrate leads to increased production of carbon dioxide and can lead to respiratory distress. Enteral formulas are designed for pulmonary disease and provide more calories from fat, as discussed in the Case Study below. Adjust oxygen delivery devices so that the mouth is not obstructed but oxygen is delivered through the nose during eating.

Nursing Management of the Medical Client

Assessment. The nursing assessment should include a thorough exploration of the client's clinical manifestations. Determine the client's ability to recognize manifestations that require further care. For example, if a client says, "I knew I was developing an infection and went to the doctor," this statement indicates an understanding of the disorder. In contrast, if a client does not fully understand the reasons for hospitalization, educate the client about COPD. A review of past medical history helps to determine whether the client has other disorders, such as heart disease, that might affect treatment.

Complete a physical examination with an emphasis on the respiratory and cardiac systems. Note the degree of dyspnea, the presence of orthopnea, decreased breath sounds, and clinical manifestations of heart failure.

CASE STUDY   *evolve*

COPD with Nutritional Concerns

Bill Smith is a 55-year-old disabled car salesman who is cared for at home by his wife of 36 years. Bill is being seen in the office today for a routine visit. He reports that he has been coughing up more sputum than normal and that sometimes he feels as if he is choking. Bill's wife also reports that she is afraid he is not getting enough to eat, because she has noticed he has put three more holes in his leather belt to hold up his pants ....
Case Study continued on the website and the CD-ROM with discussions, multiple-choice questions, and a nursing care plan.

Evaluate mental status because confusion and restlessness may be early indicators of increasing hypoxia and hypercapnia. Record the client's baseline oximetry and the level of inspired oxygen. Ask if the client smokes and, if so, if he or she has interest in smoking cessation. Infection is a common cause of exacerbation of COPD. Note the presence of a productive cough, pain with coughing, fever, and the color and consistency of sputum.

Consider the impact of stressors that may have led to exacerbations of COPD. Possible factors include the progressive illness itself, marital or other family problems, and financial concerns. Review the client's usual coping strategies and determine effectiveness. Support systems, such as friends and family, also are important components of psychosocial stability. Determine the reliability of the client's support system.

The psychosocial impact of COPD is significant. Clients commonly have feelings of loss of control over their bodies and their social environment. These responses leave the client socially isolated and depressed and can severely affect quality of life. Psychosocial intervention is important.

A thorough history may need to be delayed until the client is able to breathe comfortably, or it may be taken over short periods of time or obtained through the family. Likewise, the physical examination should not tire the client. Protein-calorie malnutrition may be evident. Consult the dietitian for methods to improve the client's intake.

Evaluation. Dyspnea will be slow to improve. Expect several days for the client to return to baseline levels. Clients with COPD often continue to deteriorate despite medical care. It is difficult to cope with failing health that limits activity and employment. As much as possible, encourage the client to live an active life with daily exercise. The support of significant others is essential.

Diagnosis, Outcomes, Interventions. Common nursing diagnoses and interventions for the client with COPD are listed in the Care Plan for the client with COPD. Because COPD is common, many institutions use clinical paths or care maps to guide care. (See the Care Plan feature on pp. 1582-1585 and the Clinical Pathway on Chronic Obstructive Pulmonary Disease on the website.)   *evolve*

Surgical Management

In some clients, bullectomy (removal of large bullae, which compress the lung and add to dead space) may be of benefit. Lung transplantation may be used to provide relief of disabling manifestations and improve quality of life for clients with end-stage COPD, although its effect on survival remains unclear.

Lung volume–reduction surgery (LVRS) may improve work capacity and health-related quality of life for a select group of COPD clients. In this operation, portions of diffusely emphysematous lungs are removed to help restore more normal chest-wall configuration and to improve respiratory mechanics and functional capacity (see Figure 61-9, *B*). The ideal candidates for LVRS are individuals with severe upper-lobe emphysema and markedly reduced exercise capacity. In this group, the surgery may also improve survival.

Nursing Management of the Surgical Client

After surgery, monitor closely the client's ABG values. Chest assessment and radiographs help to determine whether the lungs are expanding. Assess the chest tubes for air leaks and drainage. Intensive pulmonary toilet is essential. Repeated coughing and deep breathing help to prevent pulmonary complications. Many clients have chest physiotherapy every 4 hours and nebulized aerosol treatments. Manage pain aggressively to promote activity and pulmonary hygiene.

After discharge, the client is assessed for adequate ventilation and tissue oxygenation (with pulse oximetry) and progressive wound healing. Pulmonary treatments may continue until lung sounds are clear. The client is weaned from oxygen and placed into a formal pulmonary rehabilitation program.

Modifications for Older Clients

The prevalence of COPD rises significantly in people in the middle to late adult years and is a leading cause of hospitalizations in older clients. The older client frequently has other problems that influence the treatment of COPD. For example, the client may have decreased exercise tolerance, impaired nutrition, or multiple co-morbid conditions. Also consider the possibility of drug interactions in older clients. Remember, too, that the older adult has special requirements when chronic conditions are exacerbated (see the Case Management feature on the Older Adult on the website).

Self-Care

Pulmonary rehabilitation is designed to reduce the toll of pulmonary disease for the client and the health care system. The goals of pulmonary rehabilitation are to reduce clinical manifestations, to improve quality of life, and to increase physical and emotional participation in everyday activities. Clients are taught how to administer medications, what side effects to look for and how to manage them, and the safe and correct use of oxygen. Lower-body exercise (walking, cycling) is commonly prescribed. Upper-body exercise is also used in some cases.

To facilitate self-care and adherence, the client and significant others need thorough information about the disease process. Review the manifestations of impending respiratory problems (e.g., increased confusion or drowsiness), respiratory tract infection, and right-sided heart failure (e.g., peripheral edema, distended neck veins) so that prompt intervention can be obtained if these complications develop. The need for routine respiratory follow-up should also be discussed. In your teaching, include a discussion of the hazards of infection and ways to decrease personal risk (i.e., avoid crowds during the flu and colds season, clean respiratory equipment well, obtain flu vaccines yearly). Review the need for lifestyle modifications, especially smoking cessation.

Clients with end-stage lung disease experience significant, intensely distressing manifestations, especially dyspnea. Whether care is provided in the home or in an extended-care facility, the focus is on minimizing dyspnea and making the client as comfortable as possible. The Bridge to Home Health Care feature on p. 1591 details client teaching and nursing interventions for the home setting.

BRONCHIECTASIS

Bronchiectasis, an extreme form of obstructive bronchitis, causes permanent, abnormal dilation and distortion of bronchi and bronchioles. It develops when bronchial walls are weakened by chronic inflammatory changes in the bronchial mucosa and occurs most often after recurrent inflammatory conditions. Any condition producing a narrowing of the lumen of the bronchioles, however, may result in bronchiectasis, including tuberculosis, adenoviral infections, and pneumonia.

Some forms of bronchiectasis are congenital and are associated with cystic fibrosis, sinusitis, dextrocardia (heart located on right side), and alterations in ciliary activity (Kartagener's syndrome). Bronchiectasis is usually localized to a lung lobe or segment rather than generalized throughout the lungs. At times, however, persistent, nonresolving infection may cause the disorder to spread to other parts of the same lung. Diagnosis may be confirmed by chest radiograph, bronchogram, or computed tomography (CT) scan.

Manifestations vary according to the etiologic agent. The main manifestations are cough and purulent sputum production in large quantities. Fever, hemoptysis, nasal stuffiness, and drainage from sinusitis also are common. The client may complain of fatigue and weakness. Clubbing of the fingers may be present.

OUTCOME MANAGEMENT

Management of bronchiectasis is the same as that for COPD. Most clients are managed medically to prevent progression of the disorder and to control clinical manifestations. Antibiotics, chest physical therapy, hydration, bronchodilators, and oxygen commonly are prescribed. Severe cases may be treated by surgical resection if the pathologic process is well localized in one lobe or two adjacent lobes and when no contraindications to surgery exist.

Conserving Oxygen with Chronic Obstructive Pulmonary Disease

Clients with chronic obstructive pulmonary disease (COPD) are challenged to make the most of their lives, given their available oxygen.

Usually, home health nurses are primarily responsible for monitoring manifestations; reviewing and reinforcing previously taught oxygen-conservation techniques; giving further instructions; and determining whether referrals to registered dietitians and occupational, physical, or respiratory therapists are needed. Evaluate what your clients already know, and proceed from there. Be certain that your clients understand the importance of using pursed-lip breathing, abdominal breathing, and metered-dose inhalers consistently and correctly. Have them demonstrate their technique.

Help your clients develop an oxygen-conservation plan that allows them to participate in activities that are most important to them. Ask them to keep a simple diary and to record their usual behavior during a 1- or 2-day period that includes all waking hours. When you analyze the diary, identify your clients' priorities. Help them relate specific activity to feelings of dyspnea during the day. In this way, you can teach specific oxygen-conservation techniques and pacing of activities to meet their priorities. To increase comfort, have your clients schedule the use of inhalers before activities and keep them within easy reach.

Encourage clients who are concerned about adequate oxygen for sexual activity to assume passive positions and to allow their partners to be more active. If winded, clients should use massage and other relaxation techniques as part of foreplay.

Adequate nutrition is essential to clients who have COPD; they may be malnourished because of respiratory muscle wasting. The diet should be high in protein and fat and low in carbohydrates. Answer your clients' questions, and determine whether they are willing or able to purchase, prepare, and eat the foods that were suggested. Encourage easy food preparation to prevent fatigue. Use foods that are prepackaged or can be heated in the microwave. Consider home-delivered meals. Use liquid food supplements to increase protein; many brands are available, including some that are specially formulated for people who have pulmonary problems.

Encourage clients to rest just before eating and to follow these suggestions. Eat in a relaxed and quiet area. Small, frequent meals are best. Schedule meals early in the day if fatigue increases as the day continues. Snack frequently. Schedule inhalers after meals because inhaler medications can taint the taste of food and make it more difficult to achieve adequate nutrition.

Clients who have COPD often feel isolated because of their decreased ability to leave their homes. Suggest that they and their families join local support groups where they can share their experiences and feelings about the disease and learn new techniques to improve their quality of life. Many hospitals sponsor groups. Another valuable resource is the American Lung Association, which has local offices throughout the United States; call for information about prevention and the latest developments in treatment.

DISORDERS OF THE PULMONARY VASCULATURE

PULMONARY EMBOLISM

Pulmonary embolism (PE) is an occlusion of a portion of the pulmonary blood vessels by an embolus. An embolus is a clot or other plug (thrombus) that is carried by the bloodstream from its point of origin to a smaller blood vessel, where it obstructs circulation. Depending on its size, an embolus can be lethal. It is estimated that in the United States more than 650,000 cases of pulmonary embolism are diagnosed annually.

Etiology and Risk Factors
Virtually all PEs develop from thrombi (clots), most of which originate in the deep calf, femoral, popliteal, or iliac veins. Other sources of emboli include tumors, air, fat, bone marrow, amniotic fluid, septic thrombi, and vegetations on heart valves that develop with endocarditis.

Major operations, especially hip, knee, abdominal, and extensive pelvic procedures, predispose the client to thrombus formation because of the reduced flow of blood through the pelvis. Traveling in cramped quarters for a long time or sitting for long periods is also associated with stasis and clotting of blood. Preventive measures, such as early ambulation, frequent leg exercises, sequential compression stockings, and anticoagulant prophylaxis, are essential.

Pathophysiology
When emboli travel to the lungs, they lodge in the pulmonary vasculature. The size and number of emboli determine the location. Blood flow is obstructed, leading to decreased perfusion of the section of lung supplied by the vessel. The client continues to ventilate the lung portion, but because the tissue is not perfused, a $\dot{V}/\dot{Q}$ mismatch occurs, resulting in hypoxemia (Figure 61-11).

If an embolus lodges in a large pulmonary vessel, it increases proximal pulmonary vascular resistance, causes atelectasis, and eventually reduces cardiac output. If the embolus is in a smaller vessel, less dramatic clinical manifestations follow but perfusion is still altered.

The arterioles constrict because of platelet degranulation, accompanied by a release of histamine, serotonin, catecholamines, and prostaglandins. These chemical agents result in bronchial and pulmonary artery

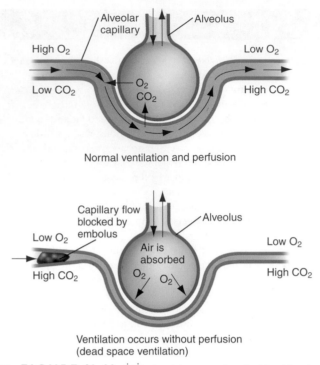

Normal ventilation and perfusion

Ventilation occurs without perfusion
(dead space ventilation)

■ **FIGURE 61–11** V̇/Q̇ mismatch occurs when the blood flow to a pulmonary arteriole is halted by a blood clot, but for a while air is still exchanged in the alveolus it serves. Because there is no blood to exchange oxygen for carbon dioxide, eventually the alveolus collapses.

constriction. This vasoconstriction probably plays a major role in the hemodynamic instability that follows PE.

Pulmonary embolism can lead to right-sided heart failure. Once the clot lodges, affected blood vessels in the lung collapse. This collapse increases the pressure in the pulmonary vasculature. The increased pressure increases the workload of the right side of the heart, leading to failure. Massive PE of the pulmonary artery can also result in cardiopulmonary collapse from lack of perfusion and resulting hypoxia and acidosis.

Clinical Manifestations

The clinical manifestations of PE are nonspecific and, in some clients, may not appear until late in the event. The most common manifestations of PE are tachypnea, dyspnea, anxiety or fretfulness, and chest pain. Hypoxemia may be present depending on the size of the embolism. Because these clinical manifestations are similar to those seen with myocardial infarction and other cardiovascular illnesses, overdiagnosis is as likely as underdiagnosis. Extensive differential diagnosis often is required. The pain usually experienced with PE is pleuritic in nature, caused by an inflammatory reaction of the lung parenchyma or by pulmonary infarction or ischemia, resulting from obstruction of small pulmonary arterial branches. Typical pleuritic chest pain is sudden in onset and exacerbated by breathing. The client is usually dyspneic, especially if the embolus has occluded major arteries or major portions of lung tissue. Apprehension, cough, diaphoresis, syncope, and hemoptysis may occur. The presence of hemoptysis indicates that the infarction or areas of atelectasis have produced alveolar damage.

Respirations typically increase. Crackles, an accentuated second heart sound, tachycardia, and fever may also develop. Less common findings include heart gallops, edema, heart murmur, and cyanosis.

Diagnostic Findings

When PE is suspected, the optimal strategy for diagnosis is an integrated approach that includes a thorough history and physical examination, supplemented by selective diagnostic tests. Pulse oximetry will be low and may be unresponsive to inhaled oxygen. ABG analysis indicates arterial hypoxemia (low Pao_2) and hypocapnia (low $Paco_2$) in massive PE. Severe respiratory alkalosis may occur. Lactate dehydrogenase (LDH) isoenzymes show an increase in LDH_3 if there is lung tissue injury. A chest radiograph may help to rule out other pulmonary diagnoses.

A noninvasive diagnostic test for PE is the V̇/Q̇ lung scan. A radioisotope lung scan is performed by IV injection of particles of human serum albumin that have been labeled with iodine 131 or technetium 99m. These particles are trapped in the pulmonary microvasculature and are distributed according to pulmonary flow. Both lungs are scanned with a scintillation counter, and the amount of radioactivity counted gives an indication of obstruction to flow. An alternative to lung scanning that is being used more frequently is spiral CT scan of the chest. This approach is particularly effective for identifying PE in the proximal pulmonary vascular tree and for clients who are unstable or have limited cardiopulmonary reserve.

Pulmonary angiography remains the definitive means of diagnosis of PE (Figure 61-12). A radiopaque contrast agent is injected into the right atrium and pulmonary artery via a catheter threaded through a peripheral vein. Visualization of any filling defects of the heart and right pulmonary artery is achieved by taking sequential radiographs. Because of the invasive nature of the test, pulmonary angiography typically is reserved for cases in which the index of clinical suspicion is high despite nondiagnostic findings on other tests.

The D-dimer plasma test helps exclude PE when the value is below 500 ng/L. It does not always help predict PE, however, because it is elevated from myocardial infarction, sepsis, and other systemic illnesses.

OUTCOME MANAGEMENT

Medical Management

Successful management of PE depends on having a high index of suspicion for manifestations such as dyspnea

■ **FIGURE 61–12** Angiogram showing a pulmonary embolus *(arrow).*

and anxiety in high-risk clients such as those who are immobile or have a malignancy. Prompt recognition of the condition and immediate treatment are essential. Goals are to stabilize the cardiopulmonary system and reduce the threat of a further PE with anticoagulation therapy or trapping with an umbrella in the vena cava. For some clients, the clot can be lysed.

Stabilizing the Cardiopulmonary System

Maintenance of cardiopulmonary stability is the first priority. Sometimes hypoxemia can be reversed with low-flow oxygen by nasal cannula. Other clients may require endotracheal intubation to maintain Pao_2 greater than 60 mm Hg. Hypotension is treated with fluids. If fluids do not raise the preload (right ventricular end-diastolic pressure) enough to raise blood pressure, inotropic agents may be required. Acidosis, which has a powerful vasoconstricting effect, is corrected with bicarbonate.

Anticoagulant Therapy

Typically, anticoagulation begins with IV standard (unfractionated) heparin sodium based initially on body weight and current level of anticoagulation to reduce the risk of further clots and to prevent extension of existing clots. *Anticoagulants do not break up existing clots,* but they do prevent extensions of existing clots. Clinical trials have shown that subcutaneously administered low-molecular-weight heparin is as safe and effective as standard heparin in the treatment of hemodynamically stable clients with PE. Anticoagulants are administered until a therapeutic partial thromboplastin time (PTT) is achieved. In general, the initial target International Normalized Ratio should be 2.5 to 3.0. Administration of sodium warfarin is begun about 3 to 5 days before heparin is stopped to provide a transition to oral anticoagulation. Because the half-life of warfarin is long, about 2 to 3 days is required to achieve adequate anticoagulation. Clients are maintained on warfarin for 3 to 6 months.

Fibrinolytic Therapy

The effectiveness of fibrinolytic therapy in the management of a massive PE is not clear, but it may be useful in clients who are hemodynamically unstable. Thrombolytic agents lyse the clots and restore right-sided heart function; however, some clinicians have found that although the clot dissolves, the death rate is not improved.

Nursing Management of the Medical Client

Monitor the client closely for hypoxemia and respiratory compromise, and assess vital signs and lung sounds frequently. Monitor ABG or oximetry values, and monitor the client for manifestations of right-sided heart failure. Auscultate heart sounds frequently, assessing for murmurs or extra heart sounds. Check for peripheral edema, distended neck veins, and liver engorgement.

To facilitate breathing, elevate the head of the bed and apply oxygen per physician's orders. Because the usual cause of a PE is thrombus from the lower legs, elevate the legs with caution to avoid severe flexure of the hips. Such flexure would slow blood flow and increase the risk of new thrombi.

The client typically experiences fear with the sudden onset of severe chest pain and inability to breathe. Anxiety, restlessness, and apprehension are common. Emotional support can reduce anxiety and lessen dyspnea. Stay with the client and give calm, yet efficient, nursing care.

Analgesics are given as needed to reduce pain and anxiety. Morphine is the most common agent. Anxiety and pain increase oxygen demand and dyspnea. Administer oral care with soft brushes or rinses while oxygen is in use, especially if the client breathes through the mouth.

Follow the anticoagulation protocols to achieve desired blood levels. Expect variations in PTT or INR during a 24 hour period with higher levels during the night and lower levels in the morning. Once

SAFETY

ALERT

anticoagulation is achieved, watch for manifestations of excess anticoagulation, such as blood in the urine, in the stool, or along the gums or teeth; subcutaneous bruising; or flank pain. When invasive studies, such as ABGs, are necessary, apply pressure to the puncture site for at least 10 minutes.

The client is discharged with oral anticoagulation therapy. Instruct the client about side effects, the importance of follow-up to monitor prothrombin times, the effect of diet on anticoagulation, and precautions to prevent bleeding. Review methods to reduce thrombophlebitis if that was the likely cause of the embolus (see Chapter 53).

Surgical Management

Surgical interventions that may be used in the treatment of PE include (1) vena caval interruption with the insertion of a filter (Figure 61-13) and (2) pulmonary embolectomy. The Greenfield filter, a basket-like cone of wires bent to look like an umbrella, is the most commonly used filter. The filter is inserted by threading it up the veins in the leg or neck until it reaches the vena cava at the level of the renal arteries. The filter allows blood flow while trapping emboli; however, vena cava filters are less effective than anticoagulation and may lead to deep vein thrombosis, and so these generally are used only when anticoagulants are contraindicated or ineffective.

Embolectomy is used in clients with significant hemodynamic instability caused by the embolus, especially those with unstable circulation and contraindications to thrombolytic therapy. An embolectomy involves surgical removal of emboli from the pulmonary arteries by either a thoracotomy or an embolectomy catheter.

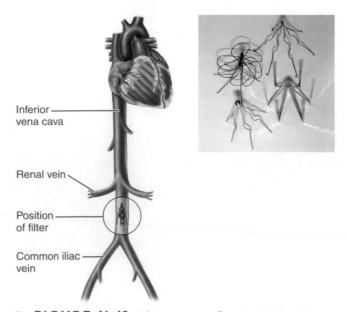

Inferior vena cava

Renal vein

Position of filter

Common iliac vein

■ **FIGURE 61–13**   Inferior vena cava filters inserted into the vena cava through the iliac vein, such as the Greenfield filter, prevent emboli from traveling to the lung.

Newly developed catheters use high-velocity jets of saline to draw the thrombus toward the catheter tip and pulverize it.

VENOUS AIR EMBOLISM

Venous air embolism (VAE) is the entry of air into the venous system. VAE may occur in any condition in which an open vein above the right atrium level is exposed to the atmosphere (e.g., trauma to a vein, insertion or removal of central venous catheters or pulmonary artery catheters, surgical procedures on the head and neck [e.g., craniotomy], pelvic operations in Trendelenburg position, and during gas insufflation in laparoscopy.

Entry of air into the venous system produces manifestations in the right ventricle, pulmonary circulation, or systemic circulation (if right-to-left shunts are present). Small amounts of air do not produce manifestations because air is removed from the circulation. Large boluses of air (3 to 8 ml/kg) can cause right ventricular outflow obstruction and result in cardiogenic shock and circulatory arrest.

Manifestations develop immediately following embolization and are similar to pulmonary thromboembolism. The severity of manifestations is related to the degree of air entry. Manifestations include dyspnea, chest pain, "mill wheel" murmur (a loud, churning, machinery-like murmur heard over the precordium), tachycardia, hypotension, decreased consciousness, circulatory shock, or sudden death (with severe VAE).

> **Reduce the risk of air embolus by carefully priming all intravenous tubing. Secure all connections in central lines and protect them from becoming dislodged when the client moves in bed or from the bed.**   SAFETY ⚠ ALERT

If VAE is suspected, any central line procedure in progress is immediately terminated and the line is clamped. Promptly place the client in Trendelenburg position and rotate toward the left lateral decubitus position. This maneuver helps trap air in the apex of the ventricle, prevents its ejection into the pulmonary arterial system, and maintains right ventricular output. The client is given 100% oxygen, and mechanical ventilation may be needed for significant respiratory distress or refractory hypoxemia. If a central venous catheter is present, aspirate from the distal port and attempt to remove air.

PULMONARY HYPERTENSION

Pulmonary hypertension is defined as a prolonged elevation of the mean pulmonary artery pressure (PAP) at or above 25 mm Hg (normal, 10 to 20 mm Hg) with a pulmonary capillary wedge pressure of 15 mm Hg or higher, both measured at rest. Forms of pulmonary hypertension are categorized according to the exact nature of the disease mechanism; i.e., those conditions that directly affect the pulmonary arterial tree (termed pulmonary arterial hypertension [PAH]), those that predominantly affect the venous circulation (pulmonary venous hypertension), and those conditions that affect the pulmonary circulation by altering respiratory structure or function (pulmonary hypertension associated with hypoxemia or chronic thromboembolic disease). PAH is further classified as either *idiopathic* or *familial* when supported by genetic investigation. The idiopathic form occurs in the absence of known causes. It occurs most often in young adults between the ages of 30 and 40 years, with women affected more often than men. A relationship with sleep-disordered breathing has also been found. The familial form is associated with an identified genetic mutation, increasing the risk among family members. The condition is relatively rare. However, increasing numbers of pulmonary hypertension–related hospitalizations and deaths seen among adults ages 65 and older suggest that as the U.S. population ages, pulmonary hypertension might become a more frequent diagnosis, particularly with accompanying chronic heart failure.

The pulmonary circulation is generally a low-pressure, low-resistance system. Increased cardiac output in a healthy person, as with exercise, causes minimal elevations in PAP because of the large pulmonary vascular reserve. When pulmonary vasoconstriction is present, however, pressure elevation occurs because the pulmonary vasculature cannot accommodate increased blood flow.

Milder forms of pulmonary hypertension are generally caused by pulmonary vasoconstriction resulting from chronic hypoxia, acidosis, or both. Administration of oxygen, correction of acid-base imbalance, and use of vasodilating medications in selected cases generally return PAP to normal, either completely or partially.

Clients with mild pulmonary hypertension may be relatively asymptomatic. In moderate to severe forms, the main (and occasionally only) manifestation is dyspnea. Fatigue, syncope, angina-like chest pain, palpitations, and muscular weakness also may occur.

A chest x-ray study shows right ventricular hypertrophy, enlarged pulmonary arteries, prominent hilar vessels, and normal or reduced intrapulmonary vascular markings. Right-heart cardiac catheterization is required to confirm the diagnosis and determine severity. Typical findings include elevated PAP and increased arteriovenous oxygen differences accompanied by normal systemic blood pressure and normal to low cardiac output.

OUTCOME MANAGEMENT

The overall prognosis in severe pulmonary arterial hypertension is poor, although treatment options are improving and survival rates are increasing. Supportive intervention with supplemental oxygen helps to reduce hypoxemia, whereas anticoagulants may be used to prevent thromboembolic events. Other conventional nonspecific therapy includes digoxin, diuretics, and high-dose calcium-channel blockade in those clients with acute vasoreactivity.

Vasodilator therapy is the cornerstone of pharmacologic management. Long-term prostacyclin (epoprostenol) therapy has been found to improve hemodynamic status and physical manifestations. Prostacyclin is a potent pulmonary vasodilator that also reduces right ventricular dilation, prevents tricuspid regurgitation from worsening, and has antithrombotic properties related to its effects on platelets. However, treatment with prostacyclin is expensive and difficult to manage because, among other drawbacks, it requires long-term, continuous central infusion. An oral endothelin-receptor antagonist, Bosentan, has been found to be just as effective in some clients. In addition, subcutaneous treprostinil and inhaled iloprost are prostacyclin analogs that have also shown some promising results.

Pulmonary thromboendarterectomy may provide a potential surgical cure in cases resulting from chronic thromboembolic disease. Some clients with severe pulmonary hypertension may undergo heart-lung or bilateral-lung transplantation. In addition, atrial septostomy may be performed in clients with severe PAH in whom other therapies either are unavailable or have failed, and who find themselves in need of palliative or bridging maneuvers. This procedure involves the creation of an intra-atrial right-to-left shunt to decompress the right atrium and right ventricle and augment left ventricle filling and cardiac output. This helps to increase tissue oxygenation delivery.

CONCLUSIONS

Lower-airway disorders include asthma, chronic air flow limitations, and inflammations of the airways. Nursing care centers on reversal of any airway spasms and education of the client about how to live with the disorder and how to reduce the risk of future problems. PE is a potentially life-threatening disorder that usually can be managed effectively with prompt recognition. Pulmonary hypertension is a disorder that is often difficult to diagnose and challenging to treat, although remarkable improvements in therapy have been made.

THINKING CRITICALLY

1. A 52-year-old woman is being treated at the neighborhood health clinic for chronic bronchitis. Her husband of 30 years smoked two to three packs of cigarettes a day. The client never smoked. During this exacerbation, she presents with shortness of breath; wheezing; a deep, throaty, productive cough when she tries to talk; and fatigue. Her blood pressure is 180/90 mm Hg, pulse is 90 beats/min, respirations are 28 breaths/min and labored, and

temperature is 99.4 ° F. She tells you that she tried to shovel the driveway on this cold winter day and did not wear a scarf over her mouth as she usually does. She further states that her inhalers did not seem to help her. She is taking a diuretic for hypertension, with blood pressure controlled at about 160/86 mm Hg. What is your priority nursing action? What teaching is appropriate at this time?

Factors to Consider. What are the clinical manifestations of chronic obstructive emphysema? What nursing assessments are in order?

2. An older client is recovering from pelvic surgery. Because of a previous stroke, she is hemiplegic. She has been on bed rest since the surgery. While the nursing assistant is giving her a bath, she notices the client grimacing as if in pain. The client responds to her question by pointing to her chest and nodding when asked if the pain is severe. The nursing assistant notifies you that the client is in distress. What is the priority assessment?

Factors to Consider. What complications of surgery and resulting bed rest might pose a risk for this client? How would you compare and contrast the clinical manifestations for pneumonia and pulmonary embolus?

3. You enter the room of the client from question 2 and discover that she is apprehensive. She is trying to hold her breath because it hurts to breathe. She is sweating, and there is frothy sputum on her lips. What nursing interventions are appropriate? What treatment might be ordered?

Factors to Consider. What are the clinical manifestations of pulmonary embolus? What diagnostic studies may be ordered?

evolve *Discussions for these questions can be found on the website.*

BIBLIOGRAPHY

Citations appearing in red refer to primary research.

Citations appearing in blue refer to evidence-based practice guidelines and protocols.

1. American Lung Association. (2006). *Asthma in adults fact sheet*. Available at www.lungusa.org.
2. American Lung Association. (2006). *Chronic obstructive pulmonary disease fact sheet*. Available at www.lungusa.org.
3. Benditt, J.O. (2006). Surgical options for patients with COPD: Sorting out the choices. *Respiratory Care, 51,* 173-178.
4. Brown, M.D., Rowe, B.H., & Reeves, M.J. (2004). The accuracy of the enzyme-linked immunosorbent assay D-dimer test in the diagnosis of pulmonary embolism: A meta-analysis. *Annals of Emergency Medicine, 40,* 133-144.
5. Burkstein, D., et al. (2005). Discussing the costs of asthma: Controlling outcomes, symptoms, and treatment strategies. *American Journal of Managed Care, 11*(11), s318-s328.
6. Capriotti, T. (2005). Changes in inhaler devices for asthma and COPD. *MEDSURG Nursing, 14*(3), 185-194.
7. Chu, E., & Drazen, J. (2005). Asthma: One hundred years of treatment and onward. *American Journal of Respiratory and Critical Care Medicine, 171*(11), 1202-1208.
8. Crompton, G.K. (2004). How to achieve good compliance with inhaled asthma therapy. *Respiratory Medicine, 98* (Suppl B), s35-s40.

9. Decramer, M., & Selroos, O. (2005). Asthma and COPD: Differences and similarities. *International Journal of Clinical Practice, 59*(4), 385-398.
10. Dolovich, M., et al. (2005). Device selection and outcomes of aerosol therapy: Evidence-based guidelines. *Chest, 127*(1), 335-371.
11. Doyle, R.L., McCrory, D., Channick, R.N., et al (2004). Surgical treatments/interventions for pulmonary arterial hypertension: ACCP evidence-based clinical practice guidelines. *Chest, 126* (Suppl 1), 63S-72S.
12. Geller, D. (2005). Comparing clinical features of the nebulizer, metered-dose inhaler, and dry powder inhaler. *Respiratory Care, 50*(10), 1313-1322.
13. Gift, A.G., & Narsavage, G. (1998). Validity of the numeric rating scale as a measure of dyspnea. *American Journal of Critical Care, 7*(3), 200-204.
14. Global Initiative for Chronic Obstructive Lung Disease (GOLD). (2006). *Global strategy for the diagnosis, management and prevention of COPD*. Available at www.goldcopd.org.
15. Hayashino, Y., Goto, M., et al (2005). Ventilation perfusion scanning and helical CT in a suspected pulmonary embolism: Meta analysis of diagnostic performance. *Radiology, 234,* 740-748.
16. Koschel, M. (2004). Pulmonary embolism. *American Journal of Nursing, 104*(6), 46-57.
17. National Heart, Lung, and Blood Institute. (2004). *Morbidity and mortality: 2004 chart book on cardiovascular, lung, and blood diseases*. Available at www.nhlbi.nih.gov/resources/docs/04_chtbk.pdf.
18. MacIntyre, N.R. (2006). Corticosteroid therapy and chronic obstructive pulmonary disease. *Respiratory Care, 51,* 289-296.
19. Mahler, D.A. (2005). Measurement of dyspnea: Clinical ratings. In D.A. Mahler & D.E. O'Donnell (Eds.), *Dyspnea: Mechanisms, measurement, and management* (pp. 147-165). Boca Raton, Fla: Taylor & Francis.
20. Mather, S., & Busse, W. (2006). Asthma: Diagnosis and management. *Medical Clinics of North America, 90*(1), 39-60.
21. Naunheim, K.S., Wood, D.E., Mohsenifar, Z., et al. (2006). Long-term follow-up of patients receiving lung-volume reduction surgery versus medical therapy for severe emphysema by the National Emphysema Treatment Trial Research Group. *Annals of Thoracic Surgery, 82,* 431-443.
22. O'Neill, B., Bradley, J.M., Macmahon, J., et al. (2004). Subjective benefit of inhaled therapies in patients with bronchiectasis: A questionnaire study. *International Journal of Clinical Practice, 58,* 441-443.
23. Rubin, L.J. (2004). Diagnosis and management of pulmonary arterial hypertension: ACCP evidence-based clinical practice guidelines. *Chest, 126*(Suppl 1), 4S-6S.
24. Simmons, P., & Simmons, M. (2004). Informed nursing practice: The administration of oxygen to patients with COPD. *MEDSURG Nursing, 13,* 82-85.
25. Tran, H., McRae, S., & Ginsberg, J. (2006). Anticoagulant treatment of deep vein thrombosis and pulmonary embolism. *Clinics in Geriatric Medicine, 22*(1), 113-134.
26. Wezel, S. (2005). Severe asthma in adults. *American Journal of Respiratory and Critical Care Medicine, 172*(2), 149-160.
27. Wick, J. (2006). Beyond the basics: Special issues in venous thromboembolism prevention. *Annals of Long-Term Care, 14* (1), 17-22.
28. Widlitz, A.C., McDevitt, S., Ward, G.R., et al. (2007). Practical aspects of continuous intravenous treprostinil therapy. *Critical Care Nurse, 27*(2), 41-50.
29. Young, B., & Flynn, T. (2005). Pulmonary emboli: The differential diagnosis dilemma. *Journal of Orthopedic & Sports Physical Therapy, 35*(10), 637-644.

evolve **Did you remember to check out the bonus material on the Evolve website and the CD-ROM, including NCLEX®-Examination Style Review Questions, Open-Book Quizzes, and Chapter Review Audio Podcasts?**

http://evolve.elsevier.com/Black/medsurg

CHAPTER 62

Management of Clients with Parenchymal and Pleural Disorders

NANCY L. YORK

The parenchyma of any organ, in this case the lung, is the tissue essential for the function of the organ. This chapter reviews disorders of the lung parenchyma, such as pneumonia, tuberculosis, cystic fibrosis, and cancer.

ATELECTASIS

Atelectasis is the collapse of alveoli or lung tissue. It develops when the alveoli become airless from absorption of their air without replacement of the air with breathing. Common causes of atelectasis include inhalation of irritating anesthetics, localized airway obstruction, insufficient pulmonary surfactant, or increased elastic recoil. Examples of each of these causes are given in Box 62-1. Atelectasis is particularly common after surgery, especially upper abdominal or thoracic procedures. Clients who are older, obese, or bedridden or who have a history of smoking are also more susceptible to atelectasis.

Atelectasis may be diagnosed through physical examination, although generally it is detected on chest radiograph. Some clients are asymptomatic. If significant hypoxemia is present, however, dyspnea, tachypnea, tachycardia, and cyanosis may occur. Chest auscultation may reveal bronchial or diminished breath sounds and crackles over the involved area. Temperature of less than 101° F (38.3° C) is common. However, older adults with atelectasis typically do not exhibit a fever.

If atelectasis is severe, physical assessment findings include the following:

- A dull percussion note over the affected lung area
- A decrease in tactile fremitus over the affected lung area
- Decreased chest movement on the involved side
- A tracheal shift toward the side of the atelectasis

None of these manifestations is specific for atelectasis, and the entire clinical picture must always be considered.

One of the primary goals of nursing intervention is to prevent atelectasis in the high-risk client. Frequent position changes and early ambulation help promote drainage of all lung segments. Deep-breathing and effective coughing enhances lung expansion and prevents airway obstruction. Incentive spirometry is an excellent means of encouraging a client to deep-breathe. Administration of pain medications may assist the client in taking deeper breaths; however, they should be used with caution to prevent respiratory depression from occurring.

If atelectasis develops, treatment is directed toward the underlying cause. If the client becomes hypoxic, oxygen should be administered as prescribed (e.g., per nasal cannula, 1 to 4 L/min). More aggressive measures to maintain airway patency, such as postural drainage, chest physiotherapy, and tracheal suctioning, may also be ordered. If an airway obstruction is causing atelectasis, bronchoscopy may be used to remove the material.

---

evolve Web Enhancements

Case Management Pneumonia

Client Education Guide Tuberculosis (English Version and Spanish Translation)

Clinical Pathway Pneumonia

Ethical Issues in Nursing How Should the Decision to End Continuous Mechanical Ventilation Be Made?

How Should the Federal Government Regulate Testing for Tuberculosis?

What is the Nurse's Obligation When Neuromuscular Blocking Agents Are Used?

Be sure to check out the bonus material on the Evolve website and the CD-ROM, including free self-assessment exercises. **http://evolve.elsevier.com/Black/medsurg**

BOX 62-1   **Causes of Atelectasis**

REDUCTION IN LUNG DISTENTION FORCES
- Pleural space encroachment (e.g., pneumothorax, pleural effusion, pleural tumor)
- Chest wall disorders (e.g., scoliosis, flail chest)
- Impaired diaphragmatic movement (e.g., ascites, obesity)
- Central nervous system dysfunction (e.g., coma, neuromuscular disorders, oversedation)

LOCALIZED AIRWAY OBSTRUCTION
- Mucus plugging
- Foreign body aspiration
- Bronchiectasis

INSUFFICIENT PULMONARY SURFACTANT
- Respiratory distress syndrome
- Inhalation anesthesia
- High concentrations of oxygen (oxygen toxicity)
- Lung contusion
- Aspiration of gastric contents
- Smoke inhalation

INCREASED ELASTIC RECOIL
- Interstitial fibrosis (e.g., silicosis, radiation pneumonitis)

INFECTIOUS DISORDERS

INFLUENZA

The term *flu* is often used inappropriately to describe many clinical manifestations and disorders. *Influenza* refers to an acute viral infection of the respiratory tract. Influenza usually occurs seasonally in epidemic form. People most at risk are very young children, older adults, people living in institutional settings, people with chronic diseases, and health care personnel. Influenza viruses have been identified as types A, B, and C. Type A is the most prevalent and is associated with the most serious epidemics. Type B outbreaks also can reach epidemic levels, but the disease produced is generally milder than that caused by type A. Type C viruses have never been connected with a large epidemic.

Clinical manifestations of influenza include fever, myalgias (muscular pain), and cough. Influenza predisposes to complications such as viral bronchitis or pneumonia, bacterial pneumonia, and superinfections (infections that occur during the course of antimicrobial therapy). Influenza differs from a common cold primarily in its sudden onset and widespread occurrence within the population. Conversely, colds have a slow onset of manifestations, usually do not cause fever, have malaise as a major manifestation, and commonly cause nasal manifestations.

In 2003 a large outbreak of influenza A (H5N1) or avian flu spread among poultry in Asia. By 2004 humans had become infected in nine countries; however, to date, no infection has been identified in the United States.

Spread of the avian influenza virus from an ill person to another person has been rarely reported. The majority of avian influenza infections in humans have resulted from direct or close contact with infected poultry or surfaces contaminated with secretions and excretions from infected birds. Symptoms can be mild but are more often severe and include cough, fever, acute respiratory failure, leukopenia, and thrombocytopenia. Death rates have been reported between 50% and 75%.

OUTCOME MANAGEMENT

Interventions for influenza are based on manifestations as they arise (i.e., supportive measures to relieve fever, myalgia, and cough). The Complementary and Alternative Therapy feature below summarizes research findings for certain supplements commonly used for respiratory tract infections. Antiviral medications can be prescribed for very early stages of influenza and may reduce the severity of the symptoms and shorten the duration of illness by 1 to 2 days. These drugs do not, however, replace the need for immunization.

COMPLEMENTARY AND ALTERNATIVE THERAPY

Vitamin E Supplements and Acute Respiratory Tract Infections in Older Adults

Older adults have a potentially increased risk of infectious diseases and related conditions because of reduced immune function. Therefore a randomized controlled trial was conducted to examine the effect of two capsules daily of one of the following: a multivitamin and mineral complex, vitamin E (200 mg/day), a multivitamin-mineral complex plus vitamin E, or a placebo for a maximum of 15 months. The primary outcomes measured were incidence and severity of acute respiratory tract infections. After a median study duration of 441 days, 1024 episodes of acute respiratory tract infections were reported by 68% of the participants. When the treatment groups were compared with the placebo group, results were similar for all aspects of incidence and severity of acute respiratory tract infection, except more clients in the multivitamin-mineral treatment arm experienced a significant reduction in activity restriction (34.8% versus 48.5%; $p = .04$, number needed to treat = 8). Individuals taking either multivitamin-mineral or vitamin E supplementation did not have a reduced incidence rate of acute respiratory tract infections. Interestingly, multivitamin-mineral supplementation had no effect on the severity of infection, whereas vitamin E supplementation was associated with illnesses of significantly greater severity.

REFERENCE

Gratt, J., Schouten, E., & Kok F. (2002). Effect of daily vitamin E and multivitamin-mineral supplementation on acute respiratory tract infections in elderly persons: A randomized controlled trial. *Journal of the American Medical Association, 288,* 715-721.

Influenza is a communicable disease spread by droplet infection.

SAFETY

⚠️

ALERT

Prevent the spread of this infection by encouraging clients with influenza to remain at home, practice frequent hand-washing, and cover the nose and mouth when sneezing or coughing.

Encourage clients at risk for influenza to obtain an annual immunization before the start of "flu season" each winter. Vaccination prevents influenza for many high-risk clients. Vaccination with the nasal-spray flu vaccine is now available for healthy people between the ages of 5 and 49 and who are not pregnant. However, clients who are severely allergic to eggs, have a history of Guillain-Barré syndrome, or are less than 6 months of age should not receive any type of influenza immunization.

PNEUMONIA

Pneumonia (pneumonitis) is an inflammatory process in lung parenchyma usually associated with a marked increase in interstitial and alveolar fluid. Advances in antibiotic therapy have led to the perception that pneumonia is no longer a major health problem in the United States. Among all nosocomial infections (hospital acquired), pneumonia is the second most common, but has the highest mortality.

Etiology and Risk Factors

There are many causes of pneumonia, including bacteria, viruses, mycoplasmas, fungal agents, and protozoa. Pneumonia may also result from aspiration of food, fluids, or vomitus or from inhalation of toxic or caustic chemicals, smoke, dusts, or gases. Pneumonia may complicate immobility and chronic illnesses. Pneumonia often follows influenza and together they rank as the seventh leading cause of death in the United States, and are the fifth leading cause in people older than 65.

Major risk factors for pneumonia include the following:

- Advanced age
- History of smoking
- Upper respiratory tract infection
- Tracheal intubation
- Prolonged immobility
- Immunosuppressive therapy
- A nonfunctional immune system
- Malnutrition
- Dehydration
- Homelessness
- Chronic disease states (such as diabetes, heart disease, chronic lung disease, renal disease, and cancer)

Additional risk factors are dysphagia; exposure to air pollution; altered consciousness (from alcoholism, drug overdose, general anesthesia, or a seizure disorder); inhalation of noxious substances; aspiration of food, liquid, or foreign or gastric material; and residence in institutional settings, where transmission of the disease is more likely. The Terrorism Alert feature on p. 1600 discusses the pneumonic plague.

Pathophysiology

Streptococcus pneumoniae, a major cause of bacterial pneumonia, generally resides in the nasopharynx and is carried asymptomatically in approximately 20%-50% of healthy individuals. It is the most common type of community-acquired pneumonia. Viral infections increase attachment of *S. pneumoniae* to the receptors on respiratory epithelium. Once inhaled into the alveolus, pneumococci infect type II alveolar cells. They multiply in the alveolus and invade alveolar epithelium. Pneumococci spread from alveolus to alveolus through the pores of Kohn, thereby producing inflammation and consolidation along lobar compartments. Inflamed and fluid-filled alveolar sacs cannot exchange oxygen and carbon dioxide effectively. Alveolar exudate tends to consolidate, so it is increasingly difficult to expectorate. Bacterial pneumonia may be associated with significant ventilation-perfusion mismatch as the infection grows.

Clinical Manifestations

The onset of all pneumonias is marked by any or all of the following manifestations: fever, chills, sweats, fatigue, cough, sputum production, and dyspnea. Less common symptoms include hemoptysis, pleuritic chest pain, and headache. Older clients may present not with fever or respiratory manifestations but with altered mental status and dehydration.

Chest auscultation reveals bronchial breath sounds over areas of *consolidation* (seen as dense white areas on the chest radiograph). Consolidated lung tissue transmits bronchial sound waves to outer lung fields. Crackling sounds (from fluid in interstitial and alveolar areas) and whispered *pectoriloquy* (transmission of the sound of whispered words through the chest wall) may be heard over affected areas. Tactile fremitus is usually increased over areas of pneumonia, whereas percussion sounds are dulled. Unequal chest wall expansion may occur during inspiration if a large area of lung tissue is involved; this is due to decreased distensibility in the affected area. Table 62-1 lists the most common types of pneumonia and their clinical manifestations.

A chest radiograph provides information about the location and extent of the pneumonia consolidation. Definitive diagnosis is usually determined through sputum culture analysis and sensitivity or serologic testing. Fiberoptic bronchoscopy or transcutaneous needle

TERRORISM ALERT

Pneumonic Plague

Plague is a life-threatening infectious disease caused by the *Yersinia pestis* bacteria. These bacteria are found in rodents, notably rats, and the fleas that feed on them. However, the bacteria can also be found in wild animals such as prairie dogs. Plague-causing bacteria exist in the environment today and intentional transmission through aerosol distribution is considered a potential bioterrorism tactic.

Yersinia pestis—also called the bubonic plague—leads to skin masses and necrosis and has been responsible for the deaths of thousands of people over time. A variant of plague is the pulmonary form, which is quickly fatal. Clinical manifestations occur anytime from 1 to 6 days after becoming infected. Bubonic plague should be suspected when a person develops flu-like symptoms including swollen glands, fever, chills, headache, and extreme exhaustion, and has a history of possible exposure to infected rodents, rabbits, or fleas. Once a person has the disease, he or she can spread the bacteria to others in close contact through droplets in the air during talking, coughing, or sneezing. The bacteria can be spread before the person even shows manifestations of the disease. Because of the delay between being exposed to the bacteria and becoming ill, people could travel over a large area—possibly infecting others—before showing manifestations of the disease.

When bubonic plague is left untreated, plague bacteria invade the bloodstream and can lead to pneumonic plague. Clinical manifestations of pneumonic plague include fever, weakness, and rapidly developing pneumonia with shortness of breath, chest pain, cough, and sometimes bloody or watery sputum. Nausea, vomiting, and abdominal pain may also occur. Without early treatment, pneumonic plague usually leads to respiratory failure, shock, and rapid death. The development of these severe respiration infection manifestations in a group of people should lead to the consideration of pneumonic plague. The bacterium used in an aerosol terrorism attack could cause the pneumonic form of plague.

Pneumonic plague is typically treated with the antibiotics gentamicin and streptomycin, which should be given within 24 hours of the first manifestations. People in direct and close contact with someone with pneumonic plague should wear tight-fitting disposable surgical masks. Clients with the disease should be immediately placed in isolation and medically supervised for at least the first 48 hours of antibiotic treatment. People who have been exposed to a contagious person can be protected from developing plague by receiving prompt antibiotic treatment.

REFERENCES

1. Snow, M. (2005). Preparing for a plague outbreak. *Nursing 2005, 35,* 14.
2. Weir, E. (2005). Plague: A continuing threat. *Canadian Medical Association Journal, 172,* 155.

(2) skin tests, if tuberculosis or coccidioidomycosis is suspected, and (3) blood and urine cultures to assess systemic spread.

Pneumonia may involve one or more lobe segments of the lungs *(segmental pneumonia),* one or more entire lobes *(lobar pneumonia)* (Figure 62-1, *A*), or lobes in both lungs *(bilateral pneumonia).* On the basis of location and radiologic appearance, pneumonias may be classified as bronchopneumonia, interstitial pneumonia, alveolar pneumonia, or necrotizing pneumonia. *Bronchopneumonia* (bronchial pneumonia) (see Figure 62-1, *B*) involves the terminal bronchioles and alveoli. *Interstitial (reticular) pneumonia* involves inflammatory responses within lung tissue surrounding the air spaces or vascular structures rather than the air passages themselves. In *alveolar* (or *acinar) pneumonia,* there is fluid accumulation in a lung's distal air spaces. *Necrotizing pneumonia* causes the death of a portion of lung tissue surrounded by viable tissue; x-ray examination may reveal cavity formation at the site of necrosis. Necrotic lung tissue, which does not heal, constitutes a permanent loss of functioning parenchyma.

OUTCOME MANAGEMENT

Medical Management

Treatment of pneumonia should include organism-specific antibiotic therapy, respiratory support as needed, nutritional support, and fluid and electrolyte management. Initial drug therapy should consist of empirical broad-spectrum antibiotics until the specific organism has been identified through sputum culture analysis. Oxygen should be administered as ordered, and bronchodilator medications, postural drainage, chest physiotherapy, and nasotracheal suctioning may be used to maintain airway patency. See the Clinical Pathway feature on Pneumonia on the website for a Care Map and *evolve* clinical guide to treating pneumonia.

Nursing Management of the Medical Client

Assessment. The nursing history should explore the following areas with the client in whom pneumonia is suspected or confirmed:

- Contact with other clients experiencing similar manifestations (suggests viral or mycoplasmal pneumonia)
- Factors suggesting the presence of noninfectious diseases that produce manifestations similar to those of pneumonia (e.g., pulmonary embolism, allergic reaction to drugs or other substances, cancer)
- Lowered levels of consciousness, which increase the risk of aspiration

aspiration/biopsy may be necessary for confirmation. Additional evaluation may consist of (1) transcutaneous oxygen level analysis or arterial blood gas (ABG) measurements to assess the need for supplemental oxygen,

TABLE 62–1   Assessment and Treatment of Pneumonia

Common Name	Clinical Manifestations
Pneumococcal pneumonia (caused by *Streptococcus pneumoniae*)	Sudden onset with a single shaking chill, high fever, stabbing pleuritic chest pain, malaise, weakness, occasional vomiting, tachypnea, dyspnea, and elevated WBC count
	Single or multiple lobar consolidation on chest x-ray film
	Cough productive of rusty brown or blood-streaked purulent sputum that turns yellow and mucoid
Staphylococcal pneumonia (caused by *Staphylococcus aureus*)	Sudden onset with fever, multiple chills, pleuritic pain, dyspnea, rales, decreased breath sounds, elevated WBC count, and exaggerated cough productive of purulent golden-yellow or blood-streaked sputum
	Chest x-ray film may show patchy infiltrates, empyema, abscesses, and pneumothorax
	Disease may start with headache, cough, and myalgia
Influenzal pneumonia (caused by *Haemophilus influenzae*)	Similar to those of pneumococcal pneumonia
	Cough productive of apple- or lime-green purulent sputum, which may be blood-tinged
Gram-negative bacterial pneumonia (most commonly caused by *Klebsiella pneumoniae*)	Sudden onset with high fever, multiple chills, pleuritic pain, dyspnea, cyanosis, and elevated WBC count
	Lobar consolidation and cavitation on chest x-ray film
	Cough productive of red sputum resembling currant jelly (mucoid, sticky, and difficult to expectorate)
Anaerobic bacterial pneumonia, hypostatic pneumonia (caused by normal oral flora)	Insidious onset with low-grade fever, dyspnea, crackles, cyanosis, hypertension, tachycardia, and elevated WBC count
	Patchy infiltrates in dependent lung segments on chest x-ray film
	Cough productive of purulent, greenish-yellow, foul-smelling sputum
Legionnaires' disease (caused by *Legionella pneumophila*)	Prodrome of 24-48 hours with fever, headache, and malaise followed by high fever with pulse-temperature dissociation, dyspnea, hypoxia, pleuritic pain, nausea, vomiting, diarrhea, confusion, and elevated WBC count
	Single or multilobar consolidation and small pleural effusions on chest x-ray film
	Dry cough productive of scant mucoid or blood-tinged sputum
Mycoplasma pneumonia (caused by *Mycoplasma* microorganisms)	Insidious onset with slowly rising fever, headache, myalgia, malaise, and normal WBC count
	Pulmonary infiltrate—sometimes extensive—on chest x-ray film
	Cough productive of scant mucoid sputum
	Client may show only minimal signs and symptoms
Viral pneumonia (caused by influenza A virus)	Prodrome with headache and myalgia followed by high fever, dyspnea, normal breath sounds with occasional wheezing and crackles, and normal or slightly elevated WBC count
	Diffuse, patchy infiltrates on chest x-ray film
	Dry cough with initial mucoid sputum that later turns purulent
	Cough may be unproductive
Fungal pneumonia (caused by histoplasmosis, blastomycosis, coccidioidomycosis, aspergillosis, candidiasis)	Usually asymptomatic
	When manifestations occur; they range from brief periods of malaise to severe, life-threatening illness
	Typical illness resembles influenza
Parasitic pneumonia (caused by protozoa, nematodes, platyhelminths); common organism is *Pneumocystis (carinii) jiroveci*	Clients who have *P. (carinii) jiroveci* pneumonia are invariably immunocompromised (HIV)
	Nonproductive cough, dyspnea, pleuritic chest pain, fever and night sweats, crackles
Aspiration pneumonia (caused by aspiration of gastric contents, food, or oropharyngeal secretions)	Often asymptomatic with minor aspiration
	Major aspiration may lead to tachypnea, apnea, cyanosis, hypotension, fever, adventitious lung sounds (crackles, rhonchi, wheezing), hypoxemia, respiratory failure, leukocytosis

HIV, Human immunodeficiency virus; *WBC*, white blood cell.

- Presence of tuberculosis or contact with others who have active tuberculosis
- Presence and character of any chest pain
- Presence and character of cough and sputum production

Perform respiratory assessments every 4 hours, including determination of the rate and character of respirations, auscultation of breath sounds, and assessment of skin and nail beds to determine the severity of hypoxia. In addition to the physical examination, transcutaneous oxygen level analysis or ABG measurements may be used to evaluate the need for oxygen support.

Diagnosis, Outcomes, Interventions. Nursing diagnoses common to pneumonia are described here. Other applicable nursing diagnoses are *Anxiety related to shortness of air; Deficient Fluid Volume related to fever, diaphoresis, and mouth breathing; Imbalanced Nutrition: Less Than Body Requirements related to dyspnea; Pain related to frequent coughing;* and *Impaired Oral Mucous Membranes related to mouth breathing and frequent*

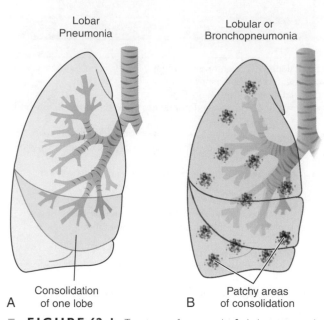

FIGURE 62–1 Two types of pneumonia. **A,** Lobar pneumonia with consolidation of one lobe of one lung. **B,** Lobular or bronchopneumonia with patchy consolidation throughout.

cough. Collaborative problems include risk of hypoxemia, respiratory failure, and sepsis.

Diagnosis: Impaired Gas Exchange. The nursing diagnosis is written as Impaired Gas Exchange related to retained secretions and inflammatory pulmonary infection.

Outcomes. The client will have improved gas exchange, as evidenced by maintaining oxygen saturations over 92% on decreasing amounts of inspired oxygen, having no manifestations of pallor or cyanosis, and retaining or improving baseline mental status.

Interventions. Titrate oxygen delivery rates to maintain oxygen saturations above 92% (or as ordered).

SAFETY
ALERT

If oxygen is administered, use needed safety precautions with oxygen and monitor oral mucous membranes.
  Assess the nares for signs of drying from oxygen use and assess the skin underneath the oxygen tubing for signs of pressure ulcers. Compare ongoing assessments of skin color and mental status; improvements in oxygen saturation should improve pallor and/or cyanosis and mental status to baseline.

Diagnosis: Ineffective Airway Clearance. Ineffective airway clearance is a common diagnosis and is related to excessive secretions and weak cough. The inflammation and increased secretions seen with pneumonia make it difficult to maintain a patent airway.

Outcomes. The client will maintain effective airway clearance, as evidenced by keeping a patent airway and effectively clearing secretions.

Interventions. Take measures to promote airway patency, such as increasing fluid intake, teaching and encouraging effective coughing and deep-breathing techniques, and frequent turning. Encourage clients to use their incentive spirometer every 2 hours while awake. Clients with an altered level of consciousness should be turned at least every 2 hours and should be placed in side-lying positions, unless contraindicated, to prevent aspiration. Only thickened liquids should be given to clients with dysphagia. Administer bronchodilating medications, if prescribed. If indicated, more aggressive measures to maintain airway patency may be required (e.g., chest physiotherapy, suctioning, artificial airway).

Diagnosis: Ineffective Breathing Pattern. This diagnosis is related to tachypnea. Many clients experience compensatory tachypnea because of an inability to meet metabolic demands. This occurs because affected alveoli cannot effectively exchange oxygen and carbon dioxide. Higher respiratory rates can also develop as a result of chest pain and increased body temperature.

Outcomes. The client will have improved breathing patterns, as evidenced by (1) a respiratory rate within normal limits, (2) adequate chest expansion, (3) clear breath sounds, and (4) decreased dyspnea.

Interventions. Position the client for comfort and to facilitate breathing (e.g., raise the head of the bed 45 degrees). Teach the client how to splint the chest wall with a pillow for comfort during coughing and about the use of incentive spirometry.

SAFETY
ALERT

Administer prescribed cough suppressants and analgesics cautiously because opioids may depress respirations more than desired. Routinely monitor respiratory rate/depth and transcutaneous oxygen levels, auscultate the chest, and document findings. Monitor ABG values, and observe for manifestations of hypoxemia, hypercapnia, and acid-base imbalance.

Diagnosis: Activity Intolerance. This diagnosis is related to decreased oxygen levels for metabolic demands. Depleted energy reserves, resulting from not eating during periods of dyspnea, and impairment of oxygen and carbon dioxide transport leave little oxygen to meet metabolic demands.

Outcomes. The client will have improved activity tolerance, as evidenced by an ability to perform activities of daily living and a progressive increase in physical activity without excessive dyspnea and fatigue.

Interventions. Assess the client's baseline activity level and response to activity. Note how well the client tolerates activity by assessing for changes in respiratory and pulse rates, marked dyspnea, fatigue, pallor or cyanosis, and dysrhythmias. Schedule activities after treatments or medications. Provide psychological support and a quiet environment to reduce anxiety and promote rest. Regulate nursing care and visitors as warranted by the client's condition. Gradually increase activity on the basis of tolerance. Balance activity with adequate rest periods.

SAFETY
⚠
ALERT

Teach the client to avoid conditions that increase oxygen demand, such as smoking, temperature extremes, weight gain, and stress. Pursed-lip and diaphragmatic breathing, which improve air flow, as well as techniques to lower energy use, should be reinforced. Activities that are tiring should be interspersed with rest

Diagnosis: Impaired Oral Mucous Membranes. The nursing diagnosis *Impaired Oral Mucous Membranes* may be indicated and is related to breathing through the mouth

Outcomes. The client will have improved oral mucous membranes as evidenced by improved oral assessment scores.

Interventions. Assess the oral mucous membranes every shift. If the client can swab the mouth, leave swabs and water on the over-bed table. If the client cannot moisten the mouth, swab the mouth for the client. Moisten the mouth and lips before meals.

Evaluation. Pneumonia should resolve quickly once the client is receiving organism-specific antibiotics, and as long as there are no immune disorders or malnutrition. Older clients may require additional time to fully recover.

ASPIRATION PNEUMONIA

Aspiration can lead to pneumonia. Healthy people aspirate during sleep, and an even higher proportion of severely ill clients aspirate routinely, which can lead to pneumonia. Tube-feeding and thin liquids can be aspirated, especially in clients with dysphagia. Reduce the risk of aspiration in clients with dysphagia by sitting them up to 90 degrees during eating. Tube-fed clients also need the head of bed elevated, at least 30 degrees. Furthermore, hold tube feedings when residual volume is high, and stop feeding 1 hour before treatments that require lowering the head of the bed (e.g., x-ray examination, chest physical therapy [CPT]). Recognize that when holding tube-feeding often, the client is not getting the needed calories, and the volumes administered at other times may need to be increased.

Self-Care

Clients with pneumonia who are ambulatory but have an ongoing health problem may require hospitalization. For clients with intact defense mechanisms and good general health, recuperation can often take place at home with rest and supportive treatment; the term *walking pneumonia* is sometimes used to describe this situation. Walking pneumonia is generally caused by the *Mycoplasma pneumoniae* organism.

LUNG ABSCESS

Lung abscess is a collection of pus within lung tissue. Single lung abscesses usually occur distal to a bronchial obstruction, commonly from aspirated foreign material (vomitus) or tumors. Multiple lung abscesses can follow pneumonia caused by necrotizing bacteria (such as *Staphylococcus aureus,* which creates necrotic lung tissue). Bacteria may also arise from septic emboli from infected foci, such as septic phlebitis. The body attempts to wall off the abscess with fibrous tissue. If the attempt is unsuccessful, the abscess ruptures into a bronchus, causing a cough that produces copious amounts of sputum.

Early clinical manifestations are similar to pneumonia (i.e., chills, fever, pleuritic pain, cough with abundant sputum). The sputum is purulent, foul-smelling, and foul-tasting. After bronchial rupture, hemoptysis often occurs. Chest auscultation reveals decreased breath sounds and dullness to percussion over the affected area. Crackles may be present when the abscess drains. The diagnosis is commonly confirmed by chest radiography or computed tomography (CT) scan. Sputum cultures assist with identification of the organism.

OUTCOME MANAGEMENT

Antibiotics are prescribed on the basis of culture results. The client's response to antibiotics is monitored. Caring for a client with a lung abscess is similar to caring for a client experiencing pneumonia (e.g., promoting hydration, teaching effective cough techniques, and administering postural drainage).

Lung abscesses produce copious volumes of sputum. Note the color, quantity, quality, and smell of the expectorated material, including the presence of blood. Use gloves when handling articles contaminated with sputum. The sputum may have a foul taste. Provide frequent opportunities for the client to use mouthwash, brush the teeth, and floss. Because long-term antibiotic administration is usually necessary, observe oral mucous membranes for indications of *Candida albicans* overgrowth (i.e., white patches). Encourage long-term dental care. Oral nystatin (which the client swishes around the mouth and swallows or spits) may be ordered.

Antibiotic therapy for a lung abscess may be needed for 8 weeks or longer. Clients with lung abscesses must understand the importance of compliance with the medication schedule. The entire course of antibiotics must be taken. Teaching about medications should cover (1) the reasons for taking them, (2) specific directions, such as time of day, frequency, and when to take in relation to food, (3) potential side effects, and (4) what to do if side effects occur. Reassessment after the antibiotic course is completed (e.g., with culture of sputum or chest films) is essential to evaluate the effectiveness of treatment.

PULMONARY TUBERCULOSIS

Tuberculosis (TB) is one of the two most prominent mycobacterial diseases known to humankind; the other is leprosy. The Centers for Disease Control and Prevention reports an estimated 2 billion people, or one third of the world's population, are infected with the bacterium that causes tuberculosis. Before the development of anti-TB drugs in the late 1940s, TB was the leading cause of all deaths in the United States. Drug therapy, along with improvements in public health and general living standards, resulted in a marked decline in incidence over the next 3 decades. However, between 1985 and 1992, the number of reported TB cases increased by 20%. This increase was attributed to the emergence of the human immunodeficiency virus (HIV) epidemic, drug misuse, influx of immigrants from developing countries, and deterioration of the nation's health care infrastructure.

In 2005 there were 14,093 reported cases of TB in the United States, a 3.8% decline from the previous year. However, two prevalent public health concerns remain about TB. First is the increase in the number of TB cases attributable to multi-drug-resistant organisms (MDR-TB) and extensive drug-resistant organisms (XDR-TB). These forms of TB have been found worldwide and are a threat to public health as a potential epidemic that is considered practically untreatable. Resistance to drugs has developed because of the long treatment course; and clients either stop taking their medication once they begin to feel well or are noncompliant with treatment as a result of other health problems, such as substance abuse.

The second public health concern is that clients with HIV infection are particularly susceptible to TB because *Mycobacterium tuberculosis,* the organism causing TB, is an extremely opportunistic pathogen. In some HIV-seropositive populations, the TB infection rate is 1000-fold higher than the annual rate in the United States. Clients infected with HIV are at greater risk for acquiring a new infection with rapid progression to active disease or for experiencing reinfection from dormant lesions.

Etiology and Risk Factors

TB is a communicable disease caused by *M. tuberculosis,* an aerobic, acid-fast bacillus (AFB). TB is an airborne infection and generally acquired by inhalation of a particle small enough (1 to 5 mm in diameter) to reach the alveolus. Droplets are emitted during talking, coughing, laughing, sneezing, or singing. Infected droplet nuclei may then be inhaled by a susceptible person (host). Before pulmonary infection can occur, the inhaled organisms must overcome the lung's defense mechanisms and penetrate lung tissue.

Brief exposure to TB does not usually cause infection. People most commonly infected are those who have repeated close contact with an infected person whose disease is not yet diagnosed. Such people may include anyone who has repeated contacts with medically underserved clients, low-income populations, foreign-born people, or residents of long-term care facilities or institutional settings. Other high-risk populations are intravenous drug users, homeless people, and people who are occupationally exposed to active TB (health care workers).

In countries that do not have public health programs and those in which TB commonly occurs in cattle, humans may experience bovine TB after drinking raw milk from infected cattle. This form of TB can be prevented by pasteurizing milk and maintaining tuberculin skin-testing programs for cattle.

Pathophysiology
Primary (First) Infection

The first time a client is infected with TB, the disease is said to be a *primary infection.* Primary TB infections are usually located in the apices of the lungs or near the pleurae of the lower lobes. Although a primary infection may be only microscopic (and hence may not appear on chest radiograph), the following sequence of events is typically observed.

A small area of bronchopneumonia develops in the lung tissue. Many of the infecting tubercle bacilli are phagocytosed (ingested) by wandering macrophages. However, before the development of hypersensitivity and immunity, many of the bacilli may survive within these blood cells and may be carried into regional bronchopulmonary (hilar) lymph nodes via the lymphatic system. The bacilli may even spread throughout the body. Thus the infection, although small, spreads rapidly.

The primary infection site may or may not undergo a process of necrotic degeneration, called caseation because it produces cavities filled with a cheese-like mass of tubercle bacilli, dead white blood cells (WBCs), and necrotic lung tissue. In time, this material liquefies, may drain into the tracheobronchial tree, and may be coughed up. Most primary tubercles heal over a period of months by forming scars and then calcified lesions, also known as Ghon's complex. These lesions may contain living bacilli that can be reactivated, especially if the client becomes immunocompromised, even after many years, and cause secondary infection.

Primary TB infections cause the body to develop an allergic reaction to tubercle bacilli or their proteins. This cell-mediated immune response appears in the form of sensitized T cells and is detectable as a positive reaction to a tuberculin skin test. The development of this tuberculin sensitivity occurs in all body cells 2 to 6 weeks after the primary infection. It is maintained as long as living bacilli remain in the body. This acquired immunity usually inhibits further growth of the bacilli and the development of active infection.

Approximately 10% of people infected with TB will eventually develop active disease within their lifetime. The reason active TB disease develops in some clients (instead of being controlled by the acquired immune response and thereby remaining dormant) is poorly understood. However, factors that seem to play a role in the progression from a dormant TB infection to active disease include the following:

- Repeated close contact with a person who has active TB
- Advanced age
- HIV infection
- Immunosuppression
- Prolonged corticosteroid therapy
- Living or working in a high-risk congregate areas (prison, long-term care facilities)
- Low body weight (10% or more below ideal weight)
- Substance abuse
- Presence of other diseases (e.g., diabetes mellitus, end-stage renal disease, or malignancy)

Secondary Infection

In addition to progressive primary disease, reinfection may also lead to a clinical form of active TB, or secondary infection. Primary sites of infection containing TB bacilli may remain latent for years and then may be reactivated if the client's resistance is lowered. Because reinfection is possible and because dormant lesions may be reactivated, it is extremely important for clients who have had a TB infection to be reassessed periodically for new evidence of active disease.

Clinical Manifestations

The detection and diagnosis of TB are achieved through subjective assessment findings and objective test results. The diagnosis can be difficult because TB mimics many other diseases and may occur concurrently with other pulmonary diseases. Nurses and other health care providers should maintain a high index of suspicion for TB in high-risk clients.

The history includes assessing the probability of recent or past exposure to TB as well as the client's occupation, other usual activities, and travel to or residence in countries with a high incidence of TB. A history of TB exposure is important, but most clients are unaware of exposure. It is advisable to determine whether the client has been previously tested for TB and to obtain the results of that testing. Typical findings in pulmonary TB are found in Box 62-2.

Primary TB infections may remain unrecognized because they are relatively asymptomatic. Calcified lesions

---

BOX 62-2   **Symptoms of Active Tuberculosis**

PULMONARY SYMPTOMS
- Dyspnea
- Nonproductive or productive cough
- Hemoptysis
- Chest pain that may be pleuritic or dull
- Chest tightness
- Crackles may be present on auscultation

GENERAL SYMPTOMS
- Fatigue
- Anorexia (loss of appetite)
- Weight loss
- Low-grade fever with chills and sweats (often at night)

---

on chest radiograph and a positive skin test reaction are frequently the only indications that a primary TB infection has occurred. Most clients harbor tubercle bacilli for life and never experience active disease because their body defenses are adequate to arrest primary infection. The tubercles heal through fibrosis and calcification. When an infected person develops the active disease, the following may occur: (1) the primary complex sites progress and worsen, (2) cavitation within the lung occurs, (3) active infection is spread, and (4) the client becomes clinically ill.

Diagnostic Findings

Tuberculin Skin Testing. Tuberculin skin testing, typically the Mantoux test, is performed on a routine basis in high-risk groups when active TB is suspected. Mantoux testing uses purified protein derivative (PPD) tuberculin to identify TB infection. A small amount (0.1 ml) of the derivative is administered intradermally to form a 6- to 10-mm wheal. The wheal must be examined ("read") in 48 to 72 hours by a trained professional. The presence of induration (a palpable, hard, raised formation), not erythema, indicates a positive test result. Table 62-2 shows how to interpret the TB skin test.

False-positive reactions to tuberculin skin testing can occur in clients who have other mycobacterial infections or who have received the bacille Calmette-Guérin (BCG) vaccination. False-negative reactions are also possible, especially in people who are immunosuppressed or anergic (impaired ability to react to antigens). For these clients, and for anyone who has a positive skin test reaction, the AFB sputum smear examination and chest radiograph are used to identify active disease. It is critical to initiate respiratory isolation of such clients until AFB sputum results are known.

The term tuberculin converter refers to a client who does not show radiologic or bacteriologic evidence of pulmonary TB but whose tuberculin skin test "converts" from a known negative reaction to a known positive

TABLE 62–2   Classifying Positive Tuberculosis Skin Test Reactions

Reaction ≥5-mm induration is considered positive in:	Reaction ≥10-mm induration is considered positive in:	Reaction ≥15-mm induration is considered positive in:
People suspected of having TB disease	Recent immigrants from high prevalence countries	People with no known risk factors for TB
HIV-infected people	IV drug users	
Recent contacts of infectious TB	Residents or employees of high-risk congregate areas	
People with fibrotic changes on chest x-ray consistent with prior TB	Mycobacteriology lab personnel	
Organ transplant recipients	Children <4 years, or children or adolescents exposed to adults at high risk	
People taking immunosuppressive therapy		

From Centers for Disease Control and Prevention. (2006) Prevention and control of tuberculosis in correctional and detention facilities: Recommendations from the CDC. *Morbidity and Mortality Weekly Report*, 55, 1-62.

reaction. The absence of a positive (reactive) tuberculin test result does not always mean that TB is absent.

QuantiFERON-TB Gold Test. The QuantiFERON-TB Gold Test is a newer diagnostic exam that was introduced in 2005. It is a blood test used to determine how a client's immune system reacts to *M. tuberculosis*. A positive QuantiFERON-TB Gold Test only tells that a person has been infected, and like the Mantoux skin test, does not confirm if a client has progressed to the active TB disease.

Acid-Fast Bacillus Smear and Culture. A more definitive diagnosis of TB is made from the AFB smear and culture. Three different sputum specimens are collected on three consecutive mornings. Sputum AFB smears are not extremely sensitive, but the positive result of a sputum AFB smear confirms active disease. A more reliable indicator is a positive culture for *M. tuberculosis*, which does confirm active TB; however, final culture results may not be available for 2 to 12 weeks. Although newer detection tests can generate faster results and show clinical promise, the increasing prevalence of MDR-TB and XDR-TB still mandates the use of traditional culture methods for diagnosis.

OUTCOME MANAGEMENT

Medical Management

Most people with newly diagnosed active TB are not hospitalized. If pulmonary TB is diagnosed in the hospitalized client, the client may be kept in the hospital until therapeutic drug levels are established. Some clients with active TB may be hospitalized for the following reasons:

- They are acutely ill.
- Concomitant diseases are present and acute.
- Their living situation is considered a high risk.
- They are thought to be noncompliant with therapy.

- They have a history of previous TB and noncompliance, and the disease has been reactivated.
- Improvement does not occur after treatment.
- The organisms are highly resistant, requiring second-line or third-line drugs, and brief hospitalization is required to monitor the effects and side effects of therapy.

Treatment of TB is a long-term process that should be initiated immediately upon suspicion of infection. Clients with a diagnosis of active TB are usually started on a minimum of four medications to ensure elimination of resistant organisms. The dose of some drugs may initially be large because the bacilli are difficult to kill. Treatment continues long enough to eliminate or substantially reduce the number of dormant or semidormant bacilli.

Medications used for TB may include *first-line* and *second-line* agents. *First-line* agents are almost always initially prescribed until results of culture and sensitivity tests are available. In clients with a previous history of incomplete TB treatment, resistant organisms may have developed and secondary agents are used.

The CDC currently recommends a two-phase approach for treatment, consisting of (1) an *induction* phase, using four drugs aimed at destroying large numbers of rapidly multiplying organisms, and (2) a *continuation* phase, usually using two drugs directed at eliminating remaining bacilli.

The recommended treatment regimen for previously untreated clients is 2 months of isoniazid (INH), rifampin (RIF), pyrazinamide, and ethambutol. This treatment, outlined in the Integrating Pharmacology feature on p. 1607, is followed by 4 or 7 months of a combination of INH with either rifampin or rifapentine. The length of time a client remains infectious varies. Sputum cultures and clinical responses (absence of fever and dyspnea, reduction in cough) are used to evaluate the effectiveness of the therapy.

If compliance with daily dosing is a problem, TB protocols call for administration of medications two or three

INTEGRATING PHARMACOLOGY

Tuberculosis Medications

Four medications are considered *first-line* for the treatment of tuberculosis: isoniazid, rifampin, pyrazinamide, and ethambutol. There are four different medication regimen choices using these drugs. Each regimen choice has an initial 2-month *induction* phase, followed by a *continuation* phase of either 4 or 7 months, depending upon laboratory findings.[1]

Isoniazid (INH) is the single most important drug used in treating TB. It is most frequently administered orally; however, other routes include intramuscular and intravenous administration. INH is low cost and can be given daily or two or three times weekly. It is metabolized by the liver and should be temporarily discontinued if liver enzymes are elevated to three times the normal range or if manifestations of hepatic toxicity (such as nausea, vomiting, anorexia, fatigue, or jaundice) occur. Typically INH is well tolerated by clients; however, the risk of developing hepatitis increases with age, alcohol consumption, and underlying liver disease.

Rifampin (RIF) is also a potent antituberculosis medication that can be given either orally or intravenously and is metabolized by the liver. Both INH and RIF are bactericidal and the combination of the two drugs allows action against active, slow, and intermittently growing organisms. A common side effect of RIF is that it colors the body fluids such as urine, sweat, saliva, sputum, and tears orange. Gastrointestinal upset is also a common side effect that can be decreased by dividing the dose in half and taking it twice a day with meals instead of once a day. Hepatotoxicity is rare but can occur.

Pyrazinamide and ethambutol provide adjunct effects that reduce the risk of acquired drug resistance while accelerating the client's response to treatment. Pyrazinamide is given to clients because of its effects of eliminating bacteria that are resistant to INH and RIF. Ethambutol is also given to clients until susceptibility to INH and RIF is demonstrated, at which time the drug can be discontinued.

Because of the duration of treatment, medication side effects, and lack of awareness of the severity of TB, noncompliance remains a serious problem. Local and national health initiatives, including providing medications at no cost, have been used to address these issues.

REFERENCES

1. Driver, C.R., Matus, S.P., Bayuga, S., et al. (2005). Factors associated with tuberculosis treatment interruption in New York City. *Journal of Public Health Management Practice, 11*, 361-368.
2. Sheff, B., & Hayes, D.D. (2005). Connecting the DOTS to treat pulmonary TB. *Nursing 2005, 35*, 24-25.

times a week rather than daily. If intermittent dosing is being used, clients should be assigned to receive *directly observed therapy* (DOT). Fixed-dose combinations of drugs are also available as a means to reduce clients' noncompliance to medical therapy. Rifamate (a combination of INH and RIF) and Rifater (a combination of INH, RIF, and pyrazinamide) combine drugs into one pill to decrease the risk of acquired drug resistance and medication errors because clients are required to take only a single daily dose. The Translating Evidence into Practice feature on p. 1608 describes how to assist with medication compliance among tuberculosis patients.

If the medication regimen does not seem effective (e.g., worsening manifestations, continued presence of AFB in sputum, increasing infiltrates or cavity formation on radiograph), then the treatment program needs reevaluation and the client's compliance should be assessed. At least two medications (never just one) are added to a failing TB treatment program.

Because medications used to treat TB have potentially serious side effects, baseline studies (depending on the specific drugs prescribed) are performed first. Drug toxicity can limit the treatment of TB. Drug tolerance, drug effect, and drug toxicity depend on factors such as the medication dosage, the time since last dosage, the medication's chemical formula, and the client's age, renal and intestinal function, and compliance with treatment.

Nursing Management of the Medical Client

Nursing management of the client with TB includes many interventions already discussed for the client with pneumonia, depending on the specific nursing diagnoses identified. Possible nursing diagnoses for the client with TB are as follows: *Anxiety; Ineffective Airway Clearance; Impaired Gas Exchange; Pain; Imbalanced Nutrition: Less Than Body Requirements; Ineffective Coping; Compromised Family Coping; Ineffective Health Maintenance; Deficient Knowledge related to treatment; Noncompliance;* and *Disturbed Sleep Pattern.*

Prevention of Transmission

During hospitalization, appropriate infection control and hospital employee health practices are essential. First, early identification of clients with TB is crucial. High-risk clients and clients with clinical manifestations of pneumonia should be placed immediately in airborne isolation until results of AFB smears and cultures are obtained. Private airborne isolation rooms should be maintained with negative pressure relative to the hallway; negative pressure keeps room air from flowing out into the hallway when the door is opened, thereby avoiding the spread of infectious particles outside the room. Negative-pressure ventilation sends room air directly to the outside, with at least six air exchanges per hour. Additional equipment, such as ultraviolet lamps (proven to kill mycobacteria) and high-efficiency particulate air (HEPA) filters, should also be used.

Personal protective equipment, called *particulate respirators,* is required for all health care workers entering a TB isolation room. When fitted properly,

SAFETY

⚠

ALERT

these respirators filter droplet nuclei; the fit of a particulate respirator should be reassessed if there is a change in the wearer's facial shape.

Monitoring health care workers' TB status is essential. Skin testing should be performed yearly in all health care workers who may be exposed to TB. Semi-annual testing should be completed in high-risk areas or where high rates of TB skin test conversion are occurring.

When a client is found to have TB, public health officials (often nurses) talk with the client and develop a contact list. Everyone with whom the client has had contact is then assessed with a tuberculin skin test and chest radiograph to evaluate for TB infection.

Preventive Therapy

Clients infected with *M. tuberculosis,* without the active TB disease, are considered to have a latent TB infection. These clients usually have a positive reaction to the tuberculin skin test; however, they are asymptomatic. Those with latent TB infection are not infectious and cannot spread TB infection to others, but approximately 10% will develop active TB disease in the future. Chemoprophylaxis may assist clients in avoiding active TB, as well as preventing initial infection in people recently exposed. Current recommendations for clients with latent TB infection include taking either isoniazid for 6 or 9 months or rifampin for 4 months.[15]

Self-Care

TB treatment is a long process. Nurses in clinics and public health facilities are often responsible for follow-up assessment and monitoring, including (1) determining medication compliance, (2) understanding the pharmacologic actions of medications, (3) monitoring unwanted side effects, (4) collecting follow-up sputum specimens, (5) obtaining serial chest radiographs, and (6) observing for reversal or worsening of initial assessment findings, all of which are part of the ongoing follow-up. It is essential that clients with TB, and their significant others, receive the information summarized in the Client Education Guide feature on Tuberculosis on the website. Providing complete information and ongoing support helps clients understand the long-term recovery process. The more information clients have and the more personal control they feel they have, the more likely they are to comply with treatment.

EXTRAPULMONARY TUBERCULOSIS

Extrapulmonary tuberculosis (XPTB) is TB that occurs anywhere outside the lungs. Pulmonary TB is the most common form of the disease, but after initial invasion, tubercle bacilli can spread throughout the body via the

---

☞ TRANSLATING EVIDENCE INTO PRACTICE

Directly Observed Therapy for Tuberculosis

Directly observed therapy (DOT) for tuberculosis (TB) is the practice of health care personnel observing or assisting clients as they take their prescribed medications. In addition, DOT allows health care personnel to provide immediate information and support to clients who require it. Directly observed therapy may be given in a variety of settings including a clinic, hospital, client's home, school, or workplace.

Directly observed therapy is the result of increasing nonadherence to the long-term treatment plan for TB. Nonadherence is a major problem facing health care providers and clients, and was a major contributing factor in the resurgence of TB in the 1990s. Clients who do not complete their drug regimen face an increased chance of spreading the disease to others, treatment failure, relapse of disease, emergence of drug-resistant forms of the disease, increased costs of therapy, disability, and even death.

Reasons for nonadherence are many. Factors relating to nonadherence include duration of treatment, medication side effects, homelessness, and cost. Additionally, lack of awareness of the severity of their TB disease has led to interruptions in clients completing their medication therapy.

Studies have documented the positive outcomes of DOT. Clients who participate in a DOT program demonstrate higher completion rates of therapy, lower relapse rates, less acquired drug resistance, and faster sputum conversion rates (from positive to negative). These outcomes ultimately lead to lower costs of treating TB for the client and society.

IMPLICATIONS

DOT is recommended by the CDC and is currently the basis for treating tuberculosis in the United States. If properly implemented, DOT can lead to successful cure rates, decrease spreading of the disease, decrease drug-resistant forms of the disease, and decrease costs to society. Nurses need to be aware of the positive outcomes of DOT and be able to educate clients on its purpose and results. Nurses need to conduct careful assessments to identify clients who are at risk or who do not adhere to their prescribed therapy. These clients need to be introduced immediately to DOT therapy until a cure is obtained.

REFERENCES

1. Driver, C.R., Matus, S.P., Bayuga, S., et al. (2005). Factors associated with tuberculosis treatment interruption in New York City. *Journal of Public Health Management Practice, 11,* 361-368.
2. Lobato, M.N., Wang, Y., Becerra, J.E., et al. (2006). Improved program activities are associated with decreasing tuberculosis incidence in the United States. *Public Health Reports, 121,* 108-115.
3. Sheff, B., & Hayes, D.D. (2005). Connecting the DOTS to treat pulmonary TB. *Nursing 2005, 35,* 24-25.

blood and lymph. *M. tuberculosis* thrives in oxygen-rich areas such as the cervical lymph nodes, pleura, renal cortex, bone growth plates, and meninges. It may also occur in the genitourinary tract, pericardium, abdomen, and endocrine glands.

Widespread dissemination throughout the body *(miliary tuberculosis)* involves the lungs and many other organs. It is more common in clients who are HIV-seropositive or are 50 years or older. Miliary TB may develop from delayed or late dissemination after immune system compromise in older people who were infected with TB many years earlier.

Despite the severity of the disease, XPTB is often difficult to detect. Weight loss, fatigue, malaise, fever, lymphadenopathy, and night sweats may or may not be present. The only physical finding that is specific for disseminated TB is a granuloma in the choroid of the retina. Clinical manifestations may precede changes in the chest radiograph.

The diagnosis and treatment of XPTB proceed similarly to those of pulmonary TB. However, the treatment period may be longer, and more medications may be used. Treatment depends on the extent, severity, course, and complications of the disease.

NONTUBERCULOUS MYCOBACTERIAL INFECTION

Nontuberculous mycobacteria (NTM), also known as MOTT (mycobacteria other than tubercle [bacilli]), are responsible for growing numbers of mycobacterial infections. Although NTM infection is still relatively uncommon, the following changes in disease patterns have appeared: (1) more cases, (2) wider geographical distribution, and (3) new groups of vulnerable hosts, most notably clients with HIV infection.

NTM are widely distributed in nature (i.e., in food, standing fresh water, saltwater, animal bedding, soil, animals, and birds), and most clients acquire their infections from environmental sources rather than from other diseased clients. Infection is common in the southeastern part of the United States and more prevalent in rural areas. The most commonly occurring NTM diseases are caused by *Mycobacterium avium* complex, *Mycobacterium kansasii,* and *Mycobacterium fortuitum.* The primary site of NTM disease is the lungs, although extrapulmonary sites (e.g., liver, spleen, lymph nodes, skin, joints) may occur. Disseminated disease with multiple organ involvement is also possible, most commonly in immunosuppressed clients.

Pulmonary NTM disease is similar to TB, although the clinical manifestations may be less severe. Clinical manifestations of the disease include (1) fever, (2) anorexia, (3) night sweats, (4) diarrhea, (5) abdominal pain, and (6) weight loss. Clients with pre-existing bronchopulmonary disease (e.g., bronchiectasis, chronic obstructive pulmonary disease [COPD], or healed pulmonary TB) are at highest risk of pulmonary involvement.

Diagnosis of NTM disease is often difficult because of the widespread distribution of the organisms in the environment. Definitive diagnosis of disease is possible only if NTM are isolated from specimens collected from normally sterile sites (e.g., blood, cerebrospinal fluid, bone marrow, lymph nodes) or through biopsy. However, NTM disease is strongly suspected when (1) a client presents with a clinical syndrome that is compatible with NTM, (2) no other pathogens can be identified, and (3) repeated sputum cultures reveal large numbers of NTM.

OUTCOME MANAGEMENT

The same medications used to treat TB are prescribed for NTM disease. However, NTM are considerably more resistant to drugs than *M. tuberculosis.* Consequently, combined drug regimens and treatment periods up to 24 months in duration are necessary. The more clients understand about the condition and its management, the more likely they will be to complete the full course of medication.

Other aspects of the nursing management of NTM disease are the same as for pulmonary TB (see earlier discussion). Because these diseases are not transmitted from person to person, isolation and measures to control infection, other than good hygiene, are not necessary.

SEVERE ACUTE RESPIRATORY SYNDROME

Severe acute respiratory syndrome (SARS), a coronavirus respiratory illness, was initially identified in 2003 in a unique risk group—previously healthy people. However, no new cases have been reported since late 2004. The incubation period for SARS is typically 2 to 7 days. The illness typically begins with a prodrome of fever (temperature >100.4° F [>38° C]) that is sometimes associated with chills, rigors, headache, diarrhea, malaise, and myalgia. Occasional mild respiratory manifestations are noted.

After 3 to 7 days, a lower respiratory phase begins with the onset of a dry, nonproductive cough or dyspnea, which can progress to hypoxemia requiring mechanical ventilation. As the condition progresses, chest radiograph shows focal interstitial infiltrates progressing to more generalized, patchy, interstitial infiltrates. In the late stages, chest radiograph shows areas of consolidation. Laboratory tests reveal leukopenia and thrombocytopenia or low-normal platelet counts. Early in the respiratory phase, elevated levels of both creatine phosphokinase (as high as 3000 international units/L) and hepatic transaminases (two to six times the upper limits of normal) have been noted. In most clients, renal function remains normal.

The virus is transmitted by close person-to-person contact, either when an infected person talks, coughs, or sneezes, exposing a non-infected person to respiratory droplets; or when a non-infected person touches a surface contaminated with infectious droplets and then touches their own mucous membranes. The majority of non-infected people who have close contact with a SARS-infected client remain well, while some people have reported a mild febrile illness without the severe respiratory manifestations. This suggests the illness does not always progress to the severe respiratory phase.

SAFETY ⚠ **ALERT**

However, because of the critical nature of the illness, SARS clients should be placed in airborne isolation rooms and health care workers should wear masks and gloves when in the client's room.

Treatment regimens currently are supportive and include antipyretics, oxygen, and ventilation. Antibiotics known to treat bacterial agents of atypical pneumonia have been found to be ineffectual. Initially, steroids were administered; however, no studies have supported their efficacy.

FUNGAL PULMONARY INFECTIONS

Most fungi that are pathogenic to humans limit their activities to the skin. However, the spores of some fungi become airborne and can be inhaled into the respiratory tract, causing pulmonary diseases that, in their chronic forms, produce granulomas similar to TB. The most common of these are coccidioidomycosis and histoplasmosis. Opportunistic fungal infections occur in clients with impaired immunity, including those who require long-term high-dose immunosuppressant therapy, have hematologic malignancies, or have undiagnosed HIV.

Coccidioidomycosis

Coccidioidomycosis is found in the Western hemisphere, primarily in the San Joaquin Valley of California, Utah, Nevada, New Mexico, Arizona, western Texas, and northern Mexico and South America. The disease is most likely to develop in people engaging in desert recreational activities or working in construction or other occupations that involve digging (e.g., archaeology, mining). The disease is mild and self-limiting in 60% of those affected. Such clients either are asymptomatic or have only mild upper respiratory tract assessment findings. The remaining 40% experience a syndrome similar to influenza, with cough, fever, pleuritic chest pain, myalgias, and arthralgias. *Erythema multiforme,* a flat, red rash that erupts with dark red papules, occurs in some people.

Histoplasma capsulatum

The causative organism of *histoplasmosis,* the fungus *Histoplasma capsulatum,* is endemic to the central and eastern portions of North America, most notably the Ohio River, Missouri River, and Mississippi River valleys.

It is also found in South and Central America, India, and Cyprus. This fungus lives in moist soil of appropriate chemical composition, in mushroom cellars, on the floors of chicken houses and bat caves, and in bird droppings, especially those from starlings, pigeons, and blackbirds.

H. capsulatum infections are usually asymptomatic or mild. Clinical manifestations include fever, fatigue, cough, dyspnea, and weight loss of 1 to 2 months' duration. A few clients may demonstrate disseminated or chronic forms of pulmonary fungal disease and have central nervous system, liver, spleen, gastrointestinal tract, or musculoskeletal involvement. Chronic disease may result in progressive changes similar to those seen with TB, including emphysema-like pulmonary structural changes.

OUTCOME MANAGEMENT

The diagnosis of fungal pulmonary diseases is usually based on history and clinical assessment findings. Skin testing is also used for coccidioidomycosis and can indicate exposure but not active infection. Chest radiographs may show hilar adenopathy (lymph gland enlargement), small areas of infiltrates, or manifestations of pneumonia. Sometimes, cavities and calcified nodules may form, usually remaining in the lungs as permanent indicators of previous infection. In addition to the pathogenic fungi, common fungal spores may cause serious, potentially fatal pulmonary disease in immunocompromised people. These fungi include *Aspergillus, Blastomyces dermatitidis, Candida,* and *Cryptococcus neoformans.*

Mild primary forms of fungal pulmonary disease usually do not require treatment. Progressive, disseminated, or chronic forms are usually treated with intravenous itraconazole or amphotericin B until the client is asymptomatic for 7 to 10 days. Initial treatment of clients diagnosed with HIV includes either itraconazole or amphotericin B. Amphotericin B is toxic and frequently causes acute reactions (e.g., chills, fever, vomiting, headache, decreased renal function) during infusion. Antiemetics, antihistamines, antipyretics, or hydrocortisone may be prescribed as premedications. To reduce the common problem of thrombophlebitis at the intravenous site, a small amount of heparin may be added to the infusion. If the disorder is not responsive to drug therapy, surgical removal of affected areas (e.g., lung cavities) may be necessary.

Nursing management in relation to fungal pulmonary infection consists of (1) providing preventive education to minimize exposure of clients to infectious fungi (i.e., learning to avoid high-risk situations and to recognize early indications of infection) and (2) offering appropriate support and education for infected clients and their significant others, along with symptomatic management of the disease. Education involves teaching not only about the disease and intervention measures but also about reportable indications of complications.

NEOPLASTIC LUNG DISORDERS

MALIGNANT LUNG TUMORS

Lung cancer is the malignant transformation and expansion of lung tissue, and is the most lethal of all cancers worldwide, responsible for 1.2 million deaths. Though declining, lung cancer remains the leading cause of cancer deaths in the United States, killing approximately 173,000 Americans annually.

There are three types of lung cancer based on the size and appearance of the cancer cells:

1. Non-small cell lung cancer (NSCLC) includes squamous cell carcinoma and adenocarcinoma. Squamous cell cancers start in the large bronchi and adenocarcinomas begin in the alveolus. Recently, specific oncogenes and inactivation of tumor suppressor genes have been found. The most important abnormalities detected are mutations involving the *ras* family of oncogenes.
2. Small cell carcinoma, also called "oat cell carcinoma," begins in the larger airways and becomes sizeable. It is linked to an oncogene called L-*myc*. The "oat" cell contains dense neurosecretory granules that often cause an endocrine/paraneoplastic syndrome. It is initially more sensitive to chemotherapy, but ultimately carries a worse prognosis and has often metastasized when initially found. This type of lung cancer is strongly associated with smoking.
3. Metastatic lung cancer is another common form of lung cancer. Tumors of the breast, colon, prostate, and bladder commonly metastasize to the lungs; however, any cancer has the capacity to spread to the lungs. Table 62-3 compares the types of lung cancer.

Etiology and Risk Factors

Cigarette smoking is by far the leading risk factor for lung cancer. People who smoke are 10 times more likely to develop lung cancer than nonsmokers. Approximately 90% of males and 80% of females who develop lung cancer are, or have been, smokers. The risk of lung cancer increases as the duration of smoking and the number of cigarettes smoked per day increases. The lung cancer death rate is directly related to the total amount (often expressed in "cigarette pack-years") of cigarettes smoked.

Second-hand smoke (SHS) is also a risk factor and has been classified by the Environmental Protection Agency as a group A carcinogen. Second-hand smoke is known

---

TABLE 62–3 Overview of Malignant Pulmonary Cancers

Cell Type	Approximate Incidence	Specific Characteristics	Growth Rate
Epidermoid (squamous cell)	30%	Arises from bronchial epithelium As growth occurs, cavitation may develop in lung distal to tumor; Pancoast's tumor arises in apex and upper lung zones Secondary infections distal to obstructive tumor in bronchioles commonly occur	Slow growth, with metastasis not common If metastasis occurs, usually to lymph, adrenals, and liver
Adenocarcinoma	45%	Majority arise from bronchial mucous gland Often subpleural; rarely cavitates; often arises in previously scarred lung tissue Incidence strongly linked to cigarette smoking Increasing incidence in women Bronchioloalveolar cell carcinoma is a subtype	Slow growth Can metastasize throughout lung or to other organs of body
Large cell	20%	More often peripheral mass, either single or multiple masses Cavitation common May be located centrally, midlung, or peripherally Rare hilar involvement Often grows to large tumor mass before diagnosis	Slow growth Metastasis may occur to kidney, liver, and adrenals
Small cell (oat cell)	15%	65%-75% manifest as hilar or central mass May compress bronchi Involvement of diaphragm through paralysis of phrenic nerve and hoarseness through paralysis of recurrent laryngeal nerve Pleural and pericardial effusions and tamponade often seen Does not form cavities	Rapid growth Metastasis to mediastinum and to thoracic and extrathoracic structures occurs early

to contain more than 60 cancer-causing compounds. There are no safe levels of SHS exposure for nonsmokers. Approximately 3000 lung cancer deaths are attributable to SHS annually in the United States.

People who develop lung cancer may also have a genetic predisposition. First-degree relatives of people with lung cancer have a two- to three-fold excess risk of lung cancer or other cancers, many of which are not smoking related. Age also has a role because lung cancer rarely occurs in people younger than 45 years. Tuberculosis and low levels of radiation, radon, and asbestos exposure also increase the risk of developing lung cancer. Recent studies have also suggested that smoking marijuana may increase the risk of developing lung cancer because of the high levels of tar and smokers' prolonged and deep inhalations.

Pathophysiology

Normal lung tissue is made up of cells that are programmed by genes to create lung cells of a certain size and shape that perform certain functions. Lung cancer develops when these cells mutate and reproduce excessively. The cancerous lung tissue cannot exchange oxygen and carbon dioxide and therefore performs no biological function. Furthermore, tumor cells grow and invade surrounding lung tissue. This will limit expansion of the affected lobes of the lung and interfere with gas exchange of oxygen and carbon dioxide. Airways are invaded, obstructing the flow of air. Cancerous cells invade local lymph nodes and the thoracic duct. Significant growth of the tumor and invasion may occur before diagnosis.

Clinical Manifestations

The warning signals of lung cancer are presented in Box 62-3. In many instances, lung cancer may mimic other pulmonary conditions. Extrapulmonary manifestations may occur before pulmonary manifestations. Specific clinical assessment findings vary according to tumor type, location, and extent as well as pre-existing pulmonary health.

BOX 62-3 Warning Signals of Lung Cancer

- Hoarseness
- Any change in respiratory patterns
- Persistent cough
- Sputum streaked with blood
- Frank hemoptysis
  - Rust-colored or purulent sputum
  - Fatigue
  - Chest, shoulder, back, or arm pain
  - Recurring episodes of pleural effusion, pneumonia, or bronchitis
  - Unexplained dyspnea, fever, or weight loss

Centrally located pulmonary tumors usually obstruct air flow, producing clinical manifestations such as coughing, wheezing, stridor, and dyspnea. As obstruction increases, bronchopulmonary infection often occurs distal to the obstruction. Chest, shoulder, arm, and back pain may develop as the tumor invades the perivascular nerves. Squamous and small cell tumors often cause hemoptysis. Small cell tumors may also extend into the pericardium, causing pericardial effusion and, possibly, tamponade. Cardiac dysrhythmias are also likely.

Peripheral pulmonary tumors often do not produce early assessment findings. In time, pleural pain develops that increases on inspiration, is sharp and severe, and is usually localized. Pleural effusion (see later) also occurs and, along with the pain, limits lung expansion.

Pancoast's tumor occurs in the apices of the lungs in both squamous cell and adenocarcinomatous cancers. The tumor is asymptomatic until it extends into surrounding structures. Clinical manifestations are caused by compression of the brachial plexus in the distribution from the eighth cervical nerve to the first two thoracic nerves. This results in arm and shoulder pain on the affected side along with atrophy of the arm and hand muscles. With continuing tumor growth, the ribs over the tumor (usually the first and second ribs) may be invaded, resulting in bone pain. Later, involvement of the cervical sympathetic nerve ganglia may lead to *Horner syndrome.* This syndrome consists of miosis (contraction of the pupil), partial ptosis (drooping upper eyelid), and anhidrosis (absence of sweating) on the affected side of the face.

Diagnostic Findings

Numerous diagnostic tests may be used to determine the presence and extent of lung cancer. Sputum cytologic study and chest radiograph may be initially used. Bronchoscopy may be used to biopsy a tumor located in the bronchial tree. Low-dose spiral CT scans detect involved lymph nodes and small (less than 1 cm) lung tumors in their early and treatable stages. A promising development in diagnosing lung cancer combines spiral CT screening with positron emission tomography (PET) scanning. Physiologic images show areas of accumulation in areas of the cancer. PET scans obtain images of the entire body and are used to determine whether lung cancer is isolated in one area or has metastasized.

Mediastinoscopy and thoracotomy are considered the "gold standard" for staging of lung cancer. Percutaneous transthoracic needle biopsy, esophageal endoscopic ultrasound, and endobronchial ultrasound for aspiration of involved nodes have also been used successfully to confirm the diagnosis of certain lung cancers. Radionuclide scans may be used to detect metastasis to the bone, liver, or brain. Central pulmonary tumors are easiest to locate and identify with fiberoptic bronchoscopy and sputum cytologic study. During bronchoscopy, bronchial washings or brushings are performed to obtain tumor cells for cytologic and pathologic study.

The appropriate staging of lung cancer is critical because treatment and prognostic information is based on both the type and stage of cancer. Table 62-4 explains the tumor-node-metastasis (TNM) classification scheme used for lung cancer staging, which is based on the anatomic extent of the disease (Figure 62-2). Staging information is valuable in helping clients and their families make treatment decisions and set appropriate short-term and long-term goals. Staging is primarily for non-small cell lung cancer only.

Metastasis

If tumors spread, by either direct extension or metastasis, further clinical manifestations may result. Direct extension to the recurrent laryngeal nerve produces hoarseness. Compression of the esophagus may cause dysphagia. Invasion or compression of the superior vena cava produces superior vena cava syndrome, a potentially life-threatening emergency. Obstruction of venous blood flow leads to clinical manifestations, including (1) shortness of breath, (2) facial, arm, and trunk swelling, (3) distended neck veins, (4) chest pain, and (5) venous stasis. Immediate palliative surgical treatment may be necessary.

Regional lymph node involvement may produce manifestations caused by impaired lymph drainage. Involvement of the mediastinal lymph nodes may result in vocal cord paralysis, dysphagia, diaphragmatic paralysis on the affected side (resulting from phrenic nerve compression), vena cava compression, and malignant pleural effusion (see later discussion). Usually, when mediastinal lymph nodes are involved, surgical excision of the pulmonary tumor is no longer possible.

OUTCOME MANAGEMENT

Early detection is the key to improving survival rates for clients with lung cancer. When premalignant changes begin, dysplastic cells are identifiable with fiberoptic bronchoscopy and sputum cytologic studies. At this stage, lesions are potentially curable. Unfortunately, a tumor must be at least 1 cm in diameter before it is detectable on a chest radiograph and typically invasion to surrounding tissues and metastasis have usually already occurred once the tumor reaches this size.

TABLE 62–4 Staging of Lung Cancer

Stage	Tumors	Node Involvement	Distant Metastasis Present
Occult carcinoma	TX	N0	M0
Stage 0	Tis	Carcinoma in situ	
Stage IA	T1	N0	M0
Stage IB	T2	N0	M0
Stage IIA	T1	N1	M0
Stage IIB	T2	N1	M0
Stage IIIA	T3	N0	M0
	T3	N1	M0
	T1-T3	N2	M0
Stage IIIB	Any T	N3	M0
	T4	Any N	M0
Stage IV	Any T	Any N	M1

T = extent of the size and location of the primary tumor; N = regional lymph node involvement; M = presence or absence of distant metastasis. Higher numbers indicate more advanced stages and/or spread of the disease. X indicates tumor cells are present; however, no tumor is visible on radiologic exam or bronchoscopy washings.

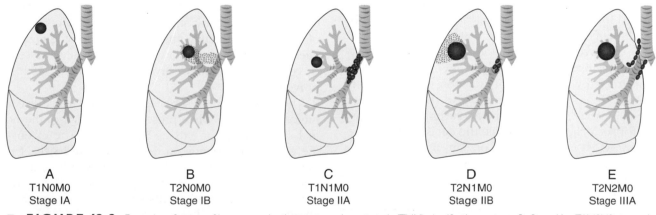

| A
T1N0M0
Stage IA | B
T2N0M0
Stage IB | C
T1N1M0
Stage IIA | D
T2N1M0
Stage IIB | E
T2N2M0
Stage IIIA |

■ **FIGURE 62–2** Examples of stages of lung cancer by the tumor-node-metastasis (TNM) classification system. **A,** Stage IA—T1N0M0: tumor is 3 cm or less in diameter with no metastases to regional lymph nodes and no distant metastasis. **B,** Stage IB—T2N0M0: tumor is greater than 3 cm in diameter or is any size that either invades the visceral pleura or has associated atelectasis or obstructive pneumonitis extending to the hilar region; however, there are no metastases to lymph nodes or distant metastasis. **C,** Stage IIA—T1N1M0: tumor is 3 cm or less in diameter with metastasis to lymph nodes in the peribronchial or ipsilateral hilar region, or both, without distant metastasis. **D,** Stage IIB—T2N1M0: tumor is greater than 3 cm in diameter or is any size that either invades the visceral pleura or has associated atelectasis or obstructive pneumonitis extending to the hilar region, with metastasis to lymph nodes in the peribronchial or ipsilateral hilar region, or both, without distant metastasis. **E,** Stage IIIA—T2N2M0: tumor is greater than 3 cm in diameter or is any size that either invades the visceral pleura or has associated atelectasis or obstructive pneumonitis extending to the hilar region, with metastasis to ipsilateral mediastinal or subcarinal nodes, without distant metastasis.

Medical Management

Management of the client with lung cancer depends on tumor type and stage as well as the client's underlying health status. Following diagnosis, primary treatment modalities are surgery, radiation therapy, and chemotherapy.

Radiation Therapy

Radiation therapy (radiotherapy) may potentially cure clients with locally advanced disease (1) for whom surgery poses an unacceptably high risk, (2) who have technically inoperable tumors, or (3) who refuse a thoracotomy. Radiotherapy may also be used in combination with surgery or chemotherapy to improve outcomes.

Radiation doses are limited by the presence of other structures in the treatment area and by normal tissue tolerance. Irreversible fibrotic changes and other pulmonary side effects may occur. To delineate precisely the area to be irradiated, CT scanning is often performed before treatment begins. This method also minimizes tissue damage to surrounding areas.

Radiotherapy may also be used in advanced cancers for palliation of manifestations such as chest pain, shortness of breath, cough, hemoptysis, and obstruction or compression of bronchi, blood vessels, or esophagus.

Chemotherapy

The response of lung cancer to chemotherapy depends on the tumor's cell type. SCLC responds to chemotherapeutic agents because of its rapid growth rate. Studies have demonstrated that survival in clients with SCLC can be improved with an intensive combination chemotherapy and radiotherapy to the mediastinum. However, because of the required escalating chemotherapy doses required for SCLC, toxicity often leads to discontinuation of the treatment course.

The effectiveness of chemotherapy in the treatment of NSCLC remains poor. This modality is commonly used in clients treated with surgery or radiation who experience recurrent disease or distant metastasis. However, large-scale studies have failed to demonstrate improved survival rates for such clients. As a result, the decision to use chemotherapy is usually made on an individual basis, depending on the client's previous history, current condition, and acceptance of the risks and side effects involved.

Nursing Management of the Medical Client

Diagnostic Phase

The client who is undergoing diagnostic tests for lung cancer faces an uncertain future. If the diagnosis is confirmed, the client can anticipate a variety of physical difficulties, potentially extensive medical treatment, and many emotional changes. The nursing assessment plays a critical role in developing a plan of care that will provide needed support.

The nursing history should include an exploration of the client's chief complaints, particularly cough (productive or nonproductive), fatigue, dyspnea, pain, weight loss, and recurrent infections. Ask the client about the presence of risk factors, such as a smoking history, exposure to occupational respiratory carcinogens, or a family history of the disease. Assess the client's socioeconomic situation and available social support because these factors affect subsequent management options.

Nursing management during the diagnostic phase focuses on emotional support and client education along with required physical care. Help clients maintain a sense of control by keeping them informed about all scheduled tests. Once a diagnosis of lung cancer is confirmed, nursing care must incorporate measures designed to help the client cope with anxiety and fear, family responses, financial considerations, absence from work and social activities, and possible changes in life goals.

Treatment Phase

Nursing care of the client receiving radiation and chemotherapy is detailed in Chapters 16 and 17.

Surgical Management

Surgical intervention is the treatment of choice in early-stage NSCLC. Cure is possible if the disease is still localized to the thoracic cavity and no distant metastases are present. However, few clients with NSCLC meet these criteria at the time of diagnosis. For clients who successfully undergo surgical resection, 15% will survive 5 years.

The role of surgical resection in the treatment of SCLC is limited because small cell cancer of the lung grows and metastasizes quickly. Surgery may be effective for clients with the early stages of SCLC, as a component of combined modality therapy with radiotherapy and chemotherapy. For clients with more advanced disease, surgery causes unnecessary risk and stress, with no proven benefits.

The primary aim of surgical resection is to remove the tumor completely while preserving as much of the normal surrounding lung tissue as possible. The extent of the operation depends on the location and size of the tumor and the severity of the underlying pathologic process. Clients with pre-existing pulmonary disease may not be able to tolerate extensive removal of lung tissue, anesthesia, or the risks of surgery.

Preoperative Management

Extensive pulmonary function testing may be performed before surgery to determine the client's ability to tolerate the proposed surgical intervention. Clients with impaired pulmonary function may be treated with antibiotics, bronchodilating medications, intermittent positive-pressure breathing procedures, and supervised breathing exercises to improve respiratory efficiency. Clients are encouraged to refrain from smoking during the preoperative period because smoking increases pulmonary secretions and diminishes blood oxygen saturation.

Surgical Procedures

Laser Surgery

Laser therapy is used as a palliative measure for relief of endobronchial obstructions that are not surgically resectable. However, the tumor must be accessible by bronchoscopy. Therefore tumors pressing on bronchial tissue from outside the bronchus are not amenable to laser therapy. Laser procedures do not produce systemic or cumulative toxic effects and are well tolerated. Laser therapy may be provided in an outpatient setting.

Pulmonary Resection

Complete resection of tumor remains the best chance of cure. Common pulmonary resection procedures are shown in Figure 62-3 and are discussed here.

Wedge Resection. In a wedge resection, a small, localized area of tumor near the surface of the lung is removed using special stapling devices. This operation can be performed either through a thoracotomy or by video-assisted thoracoscopic surgery (VATS). Because the resected area is small, pulmonary structure and function are relatively unchanged after healing. It is generally tolerated by most clients even if they have poor lung function.

Segmental Resection. Segmental resection is removal of one or more lung segments (a bronchiole and its alveoli). The remaining lung tissue overexpands to fill the previously occupied space.

Lobectomy. A lobectomy is the removal of an entire lobe of the lung. Postoperatively, the remaining lung overexpands to fill the open portion of the thoracic space. Clients with better lung function can tolerate removal of an entire lobe. A lobectomy is believed to be a better cancer operation since more surrounding normal lung tissue is removed. Therefore if there are microscopic cancer cells present, removal of more tissue is beneficial. A lobectomy is usually performed via a thoracotomy, but in some instances VATS can be used.

Pneumonectomy. Pneumonectomy is removal of an entire lung. Once the lung is removed, the involved side of the thoracic cavity is an empty space. To reduce the size of the cavity, the surgeon severs the phrenic nerve on the affected side to paralyze the diaphragm in an elevated position. A thoracoplasty, which is the removal of several ribs or portions of ribs to further reduce the thoracic space, may also be performed.

Closed-chest drainage is not used after pneumonectomy because there is no lung to reexpand. The empty chest can be filled with various products, such as balloons and implants to prevent shifting of the mediastinum, heart, and remaining lung.

Chest Tubes

Chest surgery causes a pneumothorax on the operated side. During a thoracotomy the parietal pleura is incised and the pleural space is entered. Atmospheric air enters the pleural space, changing the normally negative pressure in that pleural space to a positive pressure. As a result, the lung recoils to its unexpanded size and remains collapsed. Chest tubes are usually inserted in an operating room during chest surgery. However, in some emergencies, a chest tube may be inserted in a treatment room or at the bedside.

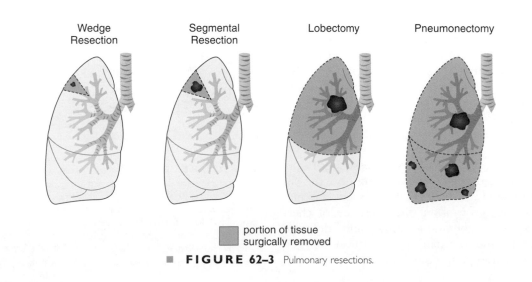

Wedge Resection   Segmental Resection   Lobectomy   Pneumonectomy

☐ portion of tissue surgically removed

■ **FIGURE 62–3** Pulmonary resections.

Two catheters are usually placed in the chest following resectional surgery (except pneumonectomy). One catheter (the upper [or anterior] tube) is placed anteriorly through the second intercostal space to permit the escape of air rising in the pleural space. The second catheter (the lower [or posterior] tube) is placed posteriorly between the sixth to ninth intercostal spaces in the midaxillary line to drain serosanguineous fluid accumulating in the lower portion of the pleural space. The lower tube may have a larger diameter than the upper tube, to enhance fluid drainage. Chest tubes are brought out of the chest wall through stab wounds made by the surgeon. The catheters are secured to the client's skin with sutures.

The two chest tubes may be joined to each other with a plastic Y-junction and then attached to one closed-chest drainage system. However, it is preferable to leave them separate and to attach them to separate drainage systems. This arrangement makes it possible to monitor air and fluid drainage from each tube separately and later to remove a non-draining tube without disrupting the rest of the system. Flexible drainage tubing connects the chest tube to the drainage collection apparatus. Usually, chest tubes are connected to a closed-chest drainage apparatus before the client leaves the operating room.

Nursing Management of the Surgical Client

Preoperative Assessment
Preoperative preparation of the client with lung cancer who is to undergo surgery is the same as for any surgical client but with greater emphasis on assessment and preparation of the respiratory system (see Chapter 14 for discussion of preoperative nursing care).

Preoperative Care
Nursing interventions during the preoperative period are aimed primarily at reducing the client's anxiety level. Anxiety results from fear of cancer and its prognosis as well as from fear of the surgical procedure and insufficient knowledge of surgical routines and postoperative self-care activities. The client and family are taught about the following issues:

The anticipated surgical procedure: Assess the client's (and family's) understanding, and provide further information as needed.

The early postoperative period: Discuss specifically what can be expected postoperatively and how the client can participate in recovery activities. Specific explanations should be given about the presence of chest tubes (except with pneumonectomy) and drainage tubes, intubation and mechanical ventilation, oxygen therapy, and available pain reduction measures.

Postoperative exercises: These include (1) respiratory exercises, such as the use of incentive spirometry (IS) to maintain effective pulmonary function, (2) splinting techniques to promote effective coughing and deep breathing (Figure 62-4), and (3) leg exercises to prevent thrombophlebitis. All of these exercises should be demonstrated preoperatively, and opportunity should be given for practice and return demonstration. Document the client's preoperative inspiratory capacity using the IS and use that volume as a target goal postoperatively.

Postoperative Assessment
During the immediate postoperative period a thorough assessment is essential. Make observations as often as the client's condition warrants. Frequency of observations is determined by the following factors:

- Amount of anesthesia received and the client's reaction to it
- Amount of intraoperative blood loss
- The client's preoperative condition (e.g., presence of pre-existing medical conditions, such as COPD, diabetes, and heart disorders)
- The client's response to pain
- Facility protocols

Postoperative Care
Nursing interventions are based on careful assessment and appropriate nursing diagnoses. General postoperative nursing measures are applicable (see Chapter 14). The Care Plan feature on pp. 1618-1621 discusses nursing management of the client undergoing thoracic surgery.

Maintain Closed-Chest Drainage. Clients have closed-chest drainage after all forms of chest surgery (except pneumonectomy) and some forms of chest trauma. The chest drainage system is airtight, or closed, to prevent

A   B   C

■ **FIGURE 62-4** Splinting techniques to promote effective coughing and deep breathing. Apply firm, even pressure after the client has taken a deep breath and during forced expiratory cough. Do not squeeze the chest or interfere with chest inspiratory expansion. **A,** Place one hand around the client's back and the other around the incisional area. **B,** Support the area below the incision with one hand while exerting downward pressure on the shoulder on the affected side with the other. **C,** Have the person hug a pillow during forced expiratory coughing.

the inflow of atmospheric pressure. Closed-chest drainage after a thoracotomy or chest trauma is used to do the following:

- Promote evacuation of air and serosanguineous fluid from the pleural space
- Prevent the reflux of atmospheric air into the pleural space
- Help reexpand the remaining lung tissue by reestablishing normal negative pressure in the pleural space
- Prevent mediastinal shift and pneumothorax by equalizing pressures on the two sides of the thoracic cavity

Two types of closed-chest drainage systems are available. The *wet suction control* systems have three main compartments (Figure 62-5, *A*):

- The *collection chamber* collects drainage and allows monitoring of the volume, rate, and nature of drainage from the pleural space.
- The *water-seal chamber* is used as a one-way valve so that air or fluids can drain from the client's chest but not return.
- The *suction-control chamber* uses suction to promote drainage from the pleural space (at a greater rate than achieved by gravity alone) and assist in reexpanding the lung.

The *dry suction control* systems have two main compartments (Figure 62-5, *B*). Regulating the level of suction is not performed through a column of water, but controlled with a self-compensating regulator using a spring or dial mechanism. Advantages of the dry system include ease in setup, no noise of bubbling water in the suction-control chamber, no evaporation of water over time, and provision of higher and more precise levels of suction. The collection chamber and water-seal chamber of a dry system are the same as for the wet systems.

Assess Chest Drainage. Measure and document the amount of drainage coming from the pleural space in the collection chamber. This record helps determine the amount of blood loss and the flow rate of drainage from the pleural space. Disposable systems are manufactured with a marked write-on surface on which to record the amount of drainage. Drainage rates and amounts are used in planning blood replacement therapy and assessing the client's status. As much as 500 to 1000 ml of drainage may occur in the first 24 hours after chest surgery. Between 100 and 300 ml of drainage may accumulate during the first 2 hours; after this time, the drainage should lessen. Excessive drainage or a sudden large increase may require further surgery to determine its cause.

Normally, chest drainage is grossly bloody immediately following surgery, but it should not continue to be so for more than several hours. Assess blood loss by monitoring the rising fluid level in the collection chamber. Suspect hemorrhage if the pulse rate becomes rapid and the blood pressure drops. Check fluid in the drainage collection chamber. If the fluid level has not risen, check the tubes for patency. Notify the surgeon if (1) the drainage remains frankly bloody for longer than the first few postoperative hours, (2) bleeding recurs after it has slowed, or (3) there are any other manifestations of hemorrhage.

■ **FIGURE 62–5**   Closed chest tube drainage systems. **A,** Three-chamber chest tube drainage system—wet suction control. **B,** Two-chamber chest tube drainage system—dry suction control.

C A R E   P L A N   *evolve*

The Client Undergoing Thoracic Surgery

Collaborative Problems: Potential complications of thoracic surgery: pulmonary edema; pneumothorax and mediastinal shift; subcutaneous emphysema; pulmonary embolism; cardiac dysrhythmias; hemorrhage, hemothorax, and hypovolemic shock; and thrombophlebitis.

Outcomes: The nurse will monitor for respiratory, cardiac, and vascular complications.

Interventions	NIC INTERVENTIONS	Rationales
1. Monitor for manifestations of acute pulmonary edema: a. Dyspnea b. Crackles c. Persistent cough d. Frothy sputum e. Cyanosis f. Decreased Sao₂ values	Monitoring	1. Circulatory overload may result from the reduced size of the pulmonary vascular bed because of surgical removal of pulmonary tissue and delayed reexpansion of the affected lung. Additionally, hypoxia increases capillary permeability, causing fluid to enter pulmonary tissue.
2. Monitor chest tube drainage system: a. Amount and color of drainage b. Water-seal chamber for tidaling and bubbling c. Suction-control chamber filled to appropriate level and bubbling d. Intact and occlusive dressing at insertion site	Monitoring	2. Chest tube drainage systems promote evacuation of air and drainage from the pleural space and assist in the reexpansion of lung tissue by reestablishing negative pressure in the pleural space after surgery.
3. Monitor for manifestations of tension pneumothorax: a. Severe dyspnea b. Tachypnea and tachycardia c. Extreme restlessness and agitation d. Progressive cyanosis e. Laryngeal and tracheal deviation to unaffected side f. Lateral or medial PMI shift	Monitoring	3. Postoperative tension pneumothorax can result from air leaking through pleural incision lines if closed-chest drainage fails to function properly.
4. Observe for subcutaneous emphysema around incision and in the chest and neck: a. Assess progression by periodically marking the chest with a skin-marking pencil at the outer periphery of emphysematous tissue; if neck involvement occurs, measure neck circumference at least every 1-2 hours b. Keep emergency tracheostomy tray at bedside	Monitoring	4. Subcutaneous emphysema may result from air leakage at the pulmonary incision site. a. Rapid progression (i.e., an increase of more than a hand's width in 1 hour) may indicate leakage through the bronchial stump b. Severe subcutaneous emphysema in the neck may compress the trachea and may require tracheostomy
5. Monitor for manifestations of pulmonary embolus: a. Chest pain b. Dyspnea and tachypnea c. Fever d. Hemoptysis e. Indications of right-sided heart failure	Monitoring	5. Pulmonary embolism is a serious potential complication after chest surgery and a significant cause of postoperative hypoxemia.
6. Assess cardiac monitor for the development of cardiac dysrhythmias, particularly atrial fibrillation, atrial flutter, and paroxysmal atrial tachycardia.	Monitoring	6. Cardiac dysrhythmias are fairly common after chest surgery. Rhythm disturbances result from a combination of factors, including increased vagal tone, hypoxia, mediastinal shift, and abnormal blood pH.
7. Monitor intravenous flow rates. Consult physician if fluid amounts (maintenance plus intermittent medications) exceed 125 ml/hr.	Monitoring	7. After chest surgery, intravenous fluids should not exceed 125 ml/hr because of possible circulatory overload (e.g., antibiotics).
8. Assess dressing and incisional area every 4 hours for evidence of bleeding (increase to every 1 to 2 hours if any bleeding develops). Assess drainage in closed-chest drainage system for manifestations of bleeding per hospital protocol.	Monitoring	8. Blood loss may be great with major thoracic surgery because blood vessels in the thorax are of large diameter and the incision is often large and produces considerable capillary oozing.
9. Monitor for manifestations of hypovolemic shock: a. Increased pulse rate b. Decreased blood pressure measurement c. Restlessness and decreased level of consciousness d. Decreased urine output (<0.5 ml/kg/hr) e. Cool, pale, clammy skin f. Increased respirations	Monitoring	9. The body compensates for lost blood volume by increasing blood flow (through increased heart rate) to vital organs and decreasing peripheral circulation.
10. Monitor for thrombophlebitis: a. Unilateral leg edema b. Calf tenderness, redness, unusual warmth	Monitoring	10. Anesthesia and immobility reduce vasomotor tone, leading to decreased venous return and peripheral pooling of blood.

	Monitoring	
11. Encourage client to perform leg exercises. Discourage placing pillows under knees, crossing the legs, or prolonged sitting. Apply elastic hose or pneumatic compression stockings, if ordered.		11. These measures prevent venous stasis, thus reducing the risk of thrombophlebitis.

Evaluation: Most complications occur early after surgery, except for pulmonary embolus.

Nursing Diagnosis: Ineffective Airway Clearance related to increased secretions and to decreased coughing effectiveness due to pain.

Outcomes: The client will demonstrate effective airway clearance, as evidenced by clear breath sounds, effective coughing, and adequate air exchange in the lungs.

NOC OUTCOMES	Airway Patency

Interventions	NIC INTERVENTIONS	Rationales
1. Once vital signs are stable, place the client in semi- or high-Fowler's position.	Airway Management	1. The upright position enhances lung expansion and facilitates ventilation with minimal effort.
2. Help the client cough and deep breathe every 1 or 2 hours (while awake) during the first 24 to 48 postoperative hours.	Cough Enhancement	2. Increasing the volume of air in the lungs promotes expulsion of secretions.
3. Instruct the client to take a deep breath slowly and to hold it for 3 to 5 seconds, then exhale; to take a second breath and then, while exhaling, to cough forcefully twice.	Cough Enhancement	3. Coughing helps move tracheobronchial secretions out of the lung. Deep breathing dilates the airways, stimulates surfactant production, and expands lung tissue.
4. When possible, schedule coughing and deep-breathing sessions at times when pain medication is maximally effective.	Cough Enhancement	4. The less postoperative pain a client experiences, the more effective are coughing and deep breathing.
5. Assess breath sounds before and after coughing. Provide support and reassurance: a. Explain that breathing exercises will not damage the lungs or the suture line b. Manually splint the incision area during coughing and deep breathing c. Offer sips of warm water d. Maintain adequate level of hydration and adequate humidity of inspired air e. Monitor results of chest radiographs f. Evaluate the need for suctioning	Cough Enhancement	5. This helps in evaluation of coughing effectiveness. a. Client's fear of "splitting open" the incision may hamper coughing efforts b. Physical support of the incision is both comforting and reassuring c. Warm water can aid relaxation and produce more effective coughing d. Fluids and moisture help thin secretions, making them easier to expectorate e. Frequent chest films help detect atelectasis and infection f. If coughing is ineffective, suctioning may be required to remove pulmonary secretions; suctioning should be performed cautiously so that disruption of pulmonary suture lines is avoided

Evaluation: The client will maintain clear and open airways, as evidenced by clear breath sounds, a normal rate and depth of respirations, and effective coughing. Outcomes on effective airway clearance may require days to achieve.

Nursing Diagnosis: Ineffective Breathing Pattern related to hypoventilation, pain, and decreased energy.

Outcomes: Effective breathing pattern as evidenced by a normal rate and depth of respirations, absence of dyspnea, and Sao_2 levels greater than 92%.

NOC OUTCOMES	Respiratory Status: Airway Patency, Respiratory Status: Ventilation

Interventions	NIC INTERVENTIONS	Rationales
1. Monitor for manifestations of ineffective breathing pattern: a. Tachypnea and tachycardia b. Dyspnea c. Use of accessory muscles or retractions d. Cyanosis e. Restlessness f. Decreased level of consciousness	Respiratory Monitoring	1. Postoperatively, ineffective breathing patterns may result from an altered level of consciousness because of anesthesia or decreased respiratory effort because of chest pain.
2. Monitor for and report a significant decrease in Sao_2 and Pao_2 levels and/or increased $Paco_2$ levels.	Respiratory Monitoring	2. Measuring Sao_2, Pao_2, and $Paco_2$ levels will assist in evaluating a client's respiratory status.
3. Provide interventions to reduce chest pain if present: a. Splint incisions b. Provide prescribed analgesics	Pain Control	3. A client with chest pain may take shallow breaths to prevent additional discomfort.
4. Maintain semi- to high-Fowler's positioning unless contraindicated.	Positioning	4. Fowler's positioning maximizes ventilation-perfusion

(Continued)

The Client Undergoing Thoracic Surgery—Cont'd

5. Implement measures to reduce client anxiety and fear: 　a. Provide reassurance 　b. Answer questions 　c. Maintain calm and supportive interactions with client and family 　d. Provide calm and restful environment 　e. Instruct client on relaxation techniques	Anxiety Reduction	5. Anxiety and fear may cause a client to breathe shallow or to hyperventilate

Evaluation: If interventions are successful, the client will demonstrate an effective breathing pattern with a normal rate and depth of respirations, absence of dyspnea, and Sao_2 levels greater than 92% within the first day postoperatively.

Nursing Diagnosis: Acute Pain related to surgical procedure.
Outcomes: The client will be more comfortable, as evidenced by verbalizing that discomfort is reduced, using less opioid medication, and increased participation in activities.

NOC OUTCOMES　Comfort Level

Interventions	NIC INTERVENTIONS	Rationales
1. Assess pain intensity using a self-report measurement tool.	Pain Management	1. Use of a consistent, valid tool promotes communication and evaluation of pain intervention effectiveness.
2. Administer pain medication as ordered.	Medication Management	2. Use of opioids is a common method of postoperative pain control. Opioids bind to opiate receptors, decreasing sensations of pain.
3. Observe for side effects of medication used.	Medication Management	3. Side effects are monitored.
4. Offer and instruct clients to ask for pain medication before pain becomes severe.	Medication Management	4. A preventive approach to pain control provides a more consistent level of relief and reduces client anxiety.
5. Assess medication effectiveness and avoid overmedication.	Pain Management	5. Adequate pain reduction must be obtained. However, overmedication can depress respirations and the cough reflex.
6. Use nonpharmacologic pain reduction measures concurrently.	Pain Management	6. Proper positioning and relaxation techniques and similar measures can augment effects of medications.

Evaluation: Pain will be most acute for the first 48 to 72 hours postoperatively, requiring opioids for pain control. Expect pain to subside after that time, and offer less potent opioids or analgesics.

Nursing Diagnosis: Impaired Physical Mobility related to pain, muscle dissection, restricted positioning, and chest tubes.
Outcomes: The client will maintain physical mobility in the arm and shoulder, as evidenced by regaining of preoperative arm and shoulder function.

NOC OUTCOMES　Joint Motion: Active

Interventions	NIC INTERVENTIONS	Rationales
1. Position client as indicated by phase of recovery and surgical procedure: 　a. Nonoperative side-lying position may be used until consciousness is regained 　b. Semi-Fowler's position (head of bed elevated 30 to 45 degrees) is recommended once vital signs are stable 　c. Avoid positioning client on operative side if a wedge resection or segmentectomy has been performed 　d. Avoid complete lateral positioning after pneumonectomy 　e. Avoid traction on chest tubes while changing client position; check for kinking or compression of tubing	Positioning	1. Repositioning maximizes lung expansion and drainage of secretions, promotes ventilation and oxygenation, and enhances comfort: 　a. This position prevents aspiration 　b. The upright position enhances lung expansion and facilitates chest tube drainage 　c. Lying on the operative side hinders expansion of remaining lung tissue and may accentuate perfusion of poorly ventilated tissue, thus further impeding normal gas exchange 　d. Because the mediastinum is no longer held in place on both sides by lung tissue, extreme turning may cause mediastinal shift and compression of the remaining lung 　e. Traction may dislodge the chest tubes; kinking or compression inhibits drainage and reestablishment of negative intrapleural pressure
2. Gently turn the client every 1 to 2 hours, unless contraindicated.	Positioning	2. Frequent turning promotes mobilization and drainage of air and fluid from the pleural space. Turning also improves circulation, promotes lung aeration, and enhances comfort.
3. Encourage regular ambulation, once the client's condition is stable. Maintain supplemental oxygen, if ordered.	Exercise Therapy: Ambulation	3. Early ambulation improves ventilation, circulation, and morale. Oxygen therapy is used to avoid hypoxia.

4. Begin passive ROM exercises of the arm and shoulder on the affected side 4 hours after recovery from anesthesia. Exercises should be performed two times every 4 to 6 hours through the first 24 postoperative hours, with progression to 10 to 20 times every 2 hours.

Exercise Promotion: Joint Mobility

4. ROM exercises help prevent adhesion formation in the operative area, which can lead to dysfunction syndrome (i.e., "frozen shoulder").

5. Active ROM exercises are begun once the client's condition permits.

Exercise Promotion

5. Active ROM exercises prevent adhesions of the incised muscle layers.

6. Encourage the client to use the arm on the affected side in daily activities (e.g., eating, reaching, grooming). Keep bedside stand on the operative side to encourage reaching. Teach the importance of continued use of the arm after discharge.

Exercise Promotion: Joint Mobility

6. Regular use of the affected arm and shoulder reduces the possibility of contractures.

Evaluation: Expect the client to be able to turn independently after 24 hours. Improvement in ROM requires a few days, until pain subsides and the chest tube is removed.

Nursing Diagnosis: Activity Intolerance related to difficulty in maintaining oxygenation secondary to pain and reduced lung volume.

NOC OUTCOMES	Activity Intolerance, Endurance

Interventions	NIC INTERVENTIONS	Rationales
1. Carefully assess client's response to activity and exercise. Observe for manifestations of dyspnea, fatigue, tachycardia, and tachypnea that do not subside in 3 minutes.	Monitoring	1. It may take time for the client's activity tolerance to increase, because the body must adjust to reduced respiratory capacity after resectional surgery.
2. Allow adequate rest periods between activities.	Energy Management	2. Adequate rest enables the client to cooperate more fully with activities.

Evaluation: The client's ability to tolerate activity is based on underlying lung disease, level of conditioning before surgery, and pain control. Expect the client to require several days to return to baseline.

Nursing Diagnosis: Risk for Ineffective Coping related to temporary dependence and loss of full respiratory function.

Outcomes: The client will use adaptive coping mechanisms, as evidenced by verbalizing feelings related to emotional state and taking appropriate actions to regain self-care capabilities.

NOC OUTCOMES	Coping, Information Processing, Role Performance, Social Support

Interventions	NIC INTERVENTIONS	Rationales
1. Provide opportunity for client to express feelings.	Emotional Support	1. Loss of normal body function and self-care capabilities can lead to feelings of powerlessness, anger, and grief. Open expression of these feelings can help client begin coping.
2. Encourage use of positive coping strategies that have been successful in the past.	Coping Enhancement	2. The use of effective coping actions can decrease feelings of hopelessness and helplessness.
3. Allow client to have as much control over daily activities and decision making as is possible.	Coping Enhancement	3. Active involvement in the plan of care gives the client a sense of control and promotes return to independence.
4. Support and praise all independent activities that promote recovery.	Emotional Support	4. Emotional support and encouragement help motivate the client to continue progress toward independence.

Evaluation: The use of effective coping mechanisms depends on prior coping strategies. This outcome may be met quickly if the client is able to cope with a diagnosis of cancer and has hope for recovery and a support system. On the contrary, coping in the face of a dreaded diagnosis, fear of pain, little hope for recovery, and limited support systems taxes the client's coping mechanisms.

Nursing Diagnosis: Knowledge Deficit related to self-care after discharge.

Outcomes: Client will be able to state or demonstrate discharge plans.

NOC OUTCOMES	Knowledge: Disease Process, Health Behaviors, Medication, Treatment Regimen

Interventions	NIC INTERVENTIONS	Rationales
1. Provide thorough instruction and preparation for hospital discharge:	Teaching: Procedure/ Treatment	1. Thorough understanding promotes compliance and enhances self-care capabilities.
a. Surgical wound and chest tube insertion site care		a. Wound care varies according to condition of incision and client
b. Continuation of exercise program		b. Continued exercise increases activity tolerance and prevents complications
c. Precautions regarding activity and environmental irritants		c. Heavy lifting should be avoided; return to work depends on the client's condition and type of job; however, it is usually possible to return to work within 4 to 6 weeks; environmental irritants can cause severe coughing episodes
d. Clinical manifestations to be reported to health care professionals		d. Evidence of infection, deteriorating respiratory status, or other complications should be reported promptly
e. Importance of regular follow-up care		e. The client should be monitored closely for manifestations of surgical complications, recurrence of malignancy, and metastasis
f. Community agencies that can provide resources, as needed		f. Community resources can facilitate home management

Evaluation: Client and family must demonstrate understanding of discharge teaching before leaving the hospital.

Assess Water-Seal Function. A water seal provides a one-way valve between atmospheric pressure and subatmospheric (negative) intrapleural pressure. It allows air and fluid to leave the intrapleural space but prevents the back-flow of atmospheric air into the chest.

On expiration, air and fluid in the pleural space travel through the drainage tubing. This air bubbles up through the water seal and enters atmospheric air. On inspiration, the water seal prevents atmospheric air from being sucked back into the pleural space (which would collapse the lung). The fluid in the water-seal compartment is not drawn into the chest cavity because the negative pressures generated during inspiration in the intrapleural space are not high enough to pull the fluid through the drainage tubing. However, fluctuation of the fluid occurs during respiration; this fluctuation is called *tidaling* (tidal movement) or *vacillation*.

A closed-chest drainage system must be airtight between the pleural space and the water-seal compartment. Any air leak allows the entry of atmospheric air into the pleural space during inspiration, creating a positive pressure that collapses the lung. All connections within the drainage system must be tight and secure. Securing of tubing connections should be done with waterproof tape. The water-seal chamber itself must have an air vent to provide an escape route for air passing through the water seal from the pleural space.

Observe the Water Seal. Fluid in the water-seal compartment should rise with inspiration and fall with expiration (tidaling). When tidaling occurs, the drainage tubes are patent and the apparatus is functioning properly. Tidaling stops when the lung has reexpanded or if the chest drainage tubes are kinked or obstructed. If tidaling does not occur:

1. Check to make sure the tubing is not kinked or compressed.
2. Change the client's position.
3. Have the client deep breathe and cough.
4. If these measures do not restore tidaling, notify the surgeon. (*Note:* Tidaling may not occur or may be minimal in systems not using suction.)

Observe for Bubbling in the Water-Seal Compartment. Bubbling in the water-seal compartment is caused by air passing out of the pleural space into the fluid in the chamber. *Intermittent* bubbling is normal on expiration and indicates that the system is accomplishing one of its purposes, that is, removing air from the pleural space.

Continuous bubbling during both inspiration and expiration, however, indicates that air is leaking into the drainage system or pleural cavity. Because air entering the system also enters the pleural space, this situation must be corrected in the following manner:

1. Locate the source of the air leak, and repair it if you can. Begin by inspecting the chest wall where the catheters are inserted.

2. If a chest catheter is loose or has been partially removed, gently squeeze the skin up around the catheter or apply sterile petrolatum gauze around the insertion site. Determine whether this measure stops the continuous bubbling in the chamber.
3. If the air leak continues, check the tubing, inch by inch, and all the connections. A break in the tubing or a loose connection may be found that can be sealed with tape.
4. If the leak still cannot be located, it may be necessary to replace the drainage system.

Rapid bubbling in the absence of an air leak indicates considerable loss of air, as from an incision or tear in the pulmonary pleura. When this occurs, notify the physician *immediately* so that appropriate measures can be taken to prevent collapse of the lung or mediastinal shift, such as (1) application of suction, (2) increase in the amount of suction, or (3) thoracotomy.

When caring for a client with water-seal drainage, find out whether this particular client's water-seal chamber should be bubbling. Having this knowledge facilitates accurate assessment of the drainage pattern (e.g., if intermittent bubbling changes to constant bubbling or if an apparatus that has not been bubbling begins to bubble).

Suction. Most clients who require a chest tube postoperatively need suction for 24 to 72 hours. Suction may be applied to a closed-chest drainage system for the following reasons:

- Gravity drainage is not adequate to pull air and fluid out of the pleural space through the chest catheters.
- The client's cough and respirations are too weak to force air and fluid out of the pleural space through the chest catheters.
- Air is leaking into the pleural space faster than it can be removed by a water-seal apparatus.
- The removal of air from the pleural space must be accelerated.

The amount of suction is typically 10 to 20 cm H_2O for a *wet suction control* system. This suction is regulated by the height of the water column in the suction chamber. The more water in the chamber, the more suction (subatmospheric pressure) is created. If there was no water in the chamber, atmospheric air would go straight from the air vent into the suction source as fast as the suction was applied. Passage of the air through water slows it, and the suction force is evenly controlled. Increasing the source of suction only causes more air to travel through the air vent. The suction applied to the client remains stable. An occluded atmospheric air vent is dangerous because it causes the suction to be applied directly to the pleural cavity.

For *dry suction control* systems, up to 40 cm H_2O of suction may be applied. Conditions requiring higher amounts of suction include a large air leak from the lung parenchyma, empyema, thick pleural effusions, or hemothorax. A suction force greater than 50 cm H_2O may cause parenchymal damage and should not be applied by any type of system.

Assess Suction Apparatus Function. Because most suction regulators can create potentially damaging amounts of suction, the amount of suction in the system must be controlled. Proper functioning of a wet suction control compartment is indicated by continuous bubbling in the suction-control chamber. Vigorous bubbling does not increase the amount of suction; rather, it causes the water in the bottle to evaporate more rapidly.

Absence of bubbling in a suction-control chamber means that the system is not functioning properly and that the correct level of suction is not being maintained. Possible reasons for malfunction of a mechanical suction apparatus include (1) large amounts of air leaking into the pleural space or into the drainage apparatus and (2) mechanical problems in the regulator (suction power source). The most serious problem is air leaking into the pleural space. Check for air leaks by briefly clamping the chest drainage tube close to the client's body and observing the chamber.

If bubbling begins in the suction-control chamber, there is nothing wrong with either the drainage apparatus or the regulator. The problem is therefore an air leak into the pleural space around the chest tubes. If the air leak cannot be sealed off (e.g., with petrolatum gauze), notify the surgeon immediately.

If bubbling does not begin in the suction-control chamber when the chest catheter is clamped, the problem is in the drainage connections or the regulator. Check the system carefully, looking for loose connections and for air leaks around compartment tops and in the tubing (e.g., split tubing). Make sure that the tubing is not kinked, is correctly positioned, and has no dependent loops. If the suction power source appears to be causing the problem, obtain another suction canister and regulator.

Because the chest catheter remains clamped during this inspection, observe the client closely for indications of tension pneumothorax (e.g., dyspnea, tachycardia, hypotension, tracheal shift). As soon as the problem is corrected, the fluid in the suction-control chamber begins to bubble. Immediately remove the clamps on the chest catheter.

Promote Chest Drainage. Closed-chest drainage systems must always be placed lower (preferably 1 to 2 feet) than the client's chest. Drainage by gravity is thus maintained, and fluid is not forced back into the pleural space. Chest drainage systems must be placed upright on the floor or hung from the foot of the bed.

If the drainage apparatus is on the floor, be careful not to lower a high-low bed or side rails onto it. If a client with closed-chest drainage is to be moved, always keep the chest drainage system below the level of the client's chest.

If the apparatus is placed above the level of the client's chest, even for a moment, fluid from the drainage chamber is siphoned back into the pleural cavity. If absolutely necessary, chest tubes may be clamped briefly during momentary movement of the apparatus above the level of the person's chest (e.g., when moving drainage apparatus from one side of the bed to the other if the tubing is not long enough to allow movement around an end of the bed).

Follow positioning orders carefully. If a client can be positioned on the side that has chest tubes, be sure the client is not lying on (compressing or kinking) the catheters or tubing. This may impair drainage, cause retrograde pressure (forcing drainage back into the pleural cavity), and increase the client's discomfort. Coil the drainage tubing (connecting the chest tube to the drainage apparatus) on the client's mattress so that it falls straight to the drainage apparatus, with no dependent loops. Dependent loops of tubing that contain fluid obstruct fluid flow and create back-pressure, thus impairing air or fluid drainage.

Drainage tubing should be neither too short nor too long. Excessive tubing length causes tangling and kinking. However, make sure the tubing is long enough to allow the person to turn and sit up without pulling on the chest tubes. Each time the client is turned or moved, check the chest tubes to make sure they are not being pulled or displaced. Check the drainage tubing to be certain it is properly positioned.

Tube patency is unlikely to be a problem when chest tubes are evacuating only air or when fluid or blood is draining well by gravity. However, if fragments of a blood clot or lung tissue are visible in the tube, *milking* a chest tube may be indicated. *Milking* entails compressing the tube intermittently using a twisting or squeezing motion. Theoretically, this technique will dislodge clot material from the tube lumen and propel it toward the drainage collection chamber.

Encourage Activity. Encourage a client with closed-chest drainage to cough and deep breathe frequently. In addition to clearing the bronchi of secretions, these activities promote lung expansion and the expulsion of air and fluid from the pleural space by increasing intrapulmonary and intrapleural pressures.

A client with a chest drainage system can sit up in bed, get in and out of bed, and ambulate without clamping of the chest tubes as long as the apparatus stays upright and below the level of the chest. Do not exert traction (pull) on the tubing. Various arrangements are used to hold a chest drainage system during ambulation. The device may be placed in a wheelchair in front of the client. Many disposable units have handles to allow for carrying. If the client's condition warrants, removal of suction during ambulation may be ordered, allowing gravity drainage.

Mobile Chest Tube Drainage Systems. Mobile chest drains (Heimlich valve, Tru-Close Thoracic Vent, Pneumostat Chest Drain Valve) are smaller chest tubes that use a mechanical one-way valve instead of a water-seal chamber; and do not have a suction-control chamber. Air is allowed to leave the chest on exhalation through the one-way collapsible flutter-type valve, which then prevents air from reentering on inhalation. Mobile chest drains are used for clients who require a chest tube but do not require suction to reinflate the lung and are not draining large amounts of fluid from the pleural cavity. They are used for clients who require long-term treatment for pleural effusions or persistent air leaks. Because of their small size and lack of large drainage collection system, clients are allowed to be more mobile earlier in their recovery.

Clamp Chest Drainage Tubing. In most situations, clamping of chest tubes is contraindicated. When the client has a residual air leak or pneumothorax, clamping the chest tube may precipitate a tension pneumothorax because the air has no escape route. If the tube becomes disconnected, it is best to immediately reattach it to the drainage system or to submerge the end in a bottle of sterile water or saline to reestablish a water seal; therefore one of these sterile solutions should be at the bedside at all times. If fluid is not readily available, it is preferable to leave the tube open because the risk of tension pneumothorax outweighs the consequences of an open tube.

There are occasions, however, when clamping is appropriate, such as the following:

- Assessing a persistent air leak
- Evaluating the client's readiness for removal of the drainage system
- Changing the drainage system

Except when clamping is clearly indicated, *never* clamp chest drainage tubes without an order to do so. If clamps must be used, the best time to apply them is after an exhalation. Then remove the clamps as soon as possible.

Remove Chest Tubes. The physician determines when to remove chest tubes and closed-chest drainage. One indication that the lung has reexpanded is the cessation of tidaling in the water-seal chamber (if suction is not applied). Chest auscultation, chest percussion, and chest radiographs confirm lung reexpansion.

Usually, a lung is fully reexpanded after 2 or 3 postoperative days of chest drainage. Chest tubes are generally left in place and connected to drainage systems for an additional 24 hours after all air and significant fluid drainage have stopped. The tubes may be temporarily clamped to determine how the client will tolerate their removal. Chest tubes may not be removed if the chest is draining more than 50 to 70 ml of fluid daily. The sooner the chest tubes can be removed, the better. Their presence often contributes to postoperative pain and inactivity. The longer the tubes are in place, the greater the risk of infection. Chest tubes used for treatment of empyema (see later discussion) may be in place longer than tubes placed after chest surgery.

Clients report removal of chest tubes is moderately to severely painful. The prescribed premedication for pain reduction should be administered approximately 30 minutes before the procedure. Assemble equipment as necessary, such as sterile scissors or a suture removal kit to cut sutures securing the tubes, sterile petrolatum gauze, 4-inch × 4-inch gauze to cover the wound, and occlusive waterproof tape.

If chest tubes are accidentally removed, cover the insertion site with sterile petrolatum gauze and notify the surgeon. Do not apply an occlusive dressing because it increases the client's risk of developing a tension pneumothorax. Observe the client closely and remove the petrolatum gauze to allow air to escape if respiratory distress develops.

SAFETY ALERT

BENIGN LUNG TUMORS

Benign pulmonary cancers account for approximately 2% to 5% of all primary pulmonary tumors. The term *benign* may be misleading because these tumors can mechanically interfere with lung function (e.g., obstruction of a major bronchus may occur), depending on the tumor's location. The most common benign lung tumor is the hamartoma, which usually arises in peripheral lung parenchyma. This tumor is more common in older men. Other benign tumor types are fibroma, hemangioma, lipoma, and papilloma.

Benign lung tumors are often difficult to diagnose because clients are generally asymptomatic. Unless there is pre-existing lung disease or major airway obstruction, pulmonary function study results and ABG values are usually within normal limits. The tumor may be first detected on chest radiograph or autopsy. Confirmatory diagnosis usually requires bronchoscopy or thoracotomy. Until the diagnosis is confirmed, most clients are anxious and fearful of the possibility of cancer. Emotional support is an important adjunct to the physical preparation required for diagnostic procedures.

Surgical intervention is the treatment of choice for all benign cancers. Tumor removal promptly alleviates any respiratory manifestations that may have resulted from pressure on lung structures. Postoperative management is the same as that after surgical treatment of malignant lung disease.

OCCUPATIONAL LUNG DISEASES

Occupational lung diseases are the leading cause of work-related illnesses in the United States. They are caused by the inhalation of various chemicals, dusts, and other particulate matter that are present in certain settings. Clients who are smokers or who have underlying lung disease are at a much greater risk of developing occupational lung diseases. The most commonly encountered occupational lung diseases are described in Table 62-5.

Acute respiratory irritation results from the inhalation of chemicals such as ammonia, chlorine, and nitrogen oxides in the form of gases, aerosols, or particulate matter. If such irritants reach the lower airways, alveolar damage and pulmonary edema can result. Although the effects of acute irritants are usually short-lived, some may cause chronic alveolar damage or airway obstruction.

Occupational asthma is often attributed to workplace exposure to allergens, such as plant and animal proteins (e.g., wheat flour, cotton, flax, and grain mites). In most cases, the asthma resolves after exposure is terminated. However, hyperactivity of the airways may persist for years.

Hypersensitivity pneumonitis, or allergic alveolitis, is most commonly due to the inhalation of organic antigens of fungal, bacterial, or animal origin. The nature of the exposure and the client's immunologic reactivity determine the pulmonary response. Nonatopic people (i.e., those with no history of allergies) demonstrate a pulmonary response to organic dusts more often than atopic people, although atopic people, too, may exhibit pulmonary reactions.

Pneumoconioses, or the "dust diseases," result from inhalation of minerals, notably silica, coal dust, or asbestos. These diseases are most commonly seen in miners, construction workers, sandblasters, potters, and foundry and quarry workers. Pneumoconioses usually develop gradually over a period of years, eventually leading to diffuse pulmonary fibrosis that diminishes lung capacity and produces restrictive lung disease. Early clinical manifestations are cough and dyspnea on exertion. Chest pain, productive cough, and dyspnea at rest develop as the condition progresses.

OUTCOME MANAGEMENT

Early detection is vital in preventing progression of occupational lung disease. The respiratory history should consist of (1) a complete occupational history and questions about the actual job performed rather than title or job description, (2) past as well as current occupations, (3) exposure to organic and inorganic substances in each job, and (4) smoking history. The physical examination should include assessment of respiratory pattern and effort, presence of cough, lung sounds, and other manifestations indicating potential lung disease. Some employers support ongoing assessment programs (e.g., routine pulmonary function studies or chest radiographs) for workers at risk for occupational lung disorders. Diagnosis

TABLE 62–5   Characteristics of Occupational Lung Disease

Disease	Onset of Symptoms	Diagnosis	Treatment	Clinical Course
Acute respiratory irritation	Immediate—within minutes of exposure Pulmonary edema may be delayed for hours	Consistent history Physical findings of respiratory tract irritation	Avoidance of exposure Respiratory support as needed	Resolves in hours to days Pulmonary edema may last days to weeks
Occupational asthma	Immediate—within minutes of exposure Can be delayed up to 6 hours	PFTs demonstrate reduced rates of FEV_1 to FVC Chest x-ray usually normal	Avoidance of exposure Asthma medication Steroids Bronchodilators	Resolves within hours Permanent loss of physiologic lung function may occur
Hypersensitivity pneumonitis	Within a few hours of exposure	Chest x-ray findings range from normal to fine or diffuse infiltrates PFTs demonstrate a reduction in vital capacity	Avoidance of exposure Steroids	Symptoms typically lessen in 48 hours Chest x-ray and PFT findings may last for weeks to months or may be permanent
Pneumoconiosis	Requires long-term exposure First manifestation is often cough progressing to dyspnea	Restrictive pattern on PFTs Chest x-ray with asbestosis shows interstitial markings in lower lobes and with silicosis shows opacities in upper lobes	Avoidance of exposure Cessation of smoking	Gradual worsening with fatigue, loss of appetite, chest pain, respiratory failure, and death

FEV₁, Forced expiratory volume in 1 second; *FVC,* forced vital capacity; *PFTs,* pulmonary function tests.

of occupational asthma allergens includes the nonspecific challenge test or skin-prick testing.

SAFETY

⚠

ALERT

Exposure precautions are essential for avoiding permanent pulmonary disability. Safety measures include adequate ventilation, the wearing of masks, and care in the handling of garments worn in dusty environments.

If occupational lung disease is significant, the client may qualify for a disability allowance. Refer clients to community resources, such as federal or state departments of labor, if they have questions about their eligibility for such allowances.

Nursing interventions for clients experiencing occupational lung diseases are similar to those for clients with other restrictive lung disorders (see the following discussion). Supportive measures can help clients adjust their lifestyles to their conditions.

RESTRICTIVE LUNG DISORDERS

Restrictive lung disorders constitute a major category of pulmonary problems. The category includes any disorder that limits lung expansion and produces a pattern of abnormal function on pulmonary function tests characterized by a decrease in total lung capacity (TLC). Restrictive lung diseases may result from conditions affecting lung tissues (intrapulmonary) or from extrapulmonary causes. Extrapulmonary causes include neurologic and neuromuscular disorders and disorders affecting the thoracic cage, pleura, and movement of the diaphragm. Obesity may also lead to restrictive lung disorders. Box 62-4 lists restrictive lung disorders.

Manifestations vary according to the cause of the restrictive disorder. For example, kyphosis, scoliosis, and kyphoscoliosis result in changes in the thoracic cage (Figure 62-6). Generally, clients with restrictive lung disease exhibit a rapid, shallow respiratory pattern. Chronic hyperventilation occurs in an effort to overcome the effects of reduced lung volume and compliance. Shortness of breath is experienced, at first only with exertion, but later at rest. As the disease progresses, respiratory muscle fatigue may occur, leading to inadequate alveolar ventilation and carbon dioxide retention. Hypoxemia is a common finding, especially in the later stages of restrictive lung disease.

Pulmonary function tests demonstrate impairment of the bellows' action of the lungs. Reduced total lung capacity (TLC) of less than 80% of expected value is the primary indicator of the restrictive lung disease. In addition, the ratio of forced expiratory volume in 1 second (FEV_1) to forced vital capacity (FVC), or FEV_1/FVC ratio, is normal or increased (i.e., 75% or more of expected values).

BOX 62-4   Restrictive Lung Diseases

Restrictive lung diseases are disorders affecting lung volumes and compliance of either chest wall or lung tissue. Their causes are classified as intrapulmonary or extrapulmonary.

INTRAPULMONARY

- Pulmonary fibrosis
- Sarcoidosis and other interstitial lung diseases
- Pneumonia
- Atelectasis
- Pneumoconiosis
- Surgical lung resection
- Neoplastic disease

EXTRAPULMONARY

- Head or spinal cord injury
- Amyotrophic lateral sclerosis
- Myasthenia gravis
- Muscular dystrophy
- Congenital chest wall deformity
- Acquired chest wall changes (e.g., kyphosis or scoliosis)
- Abdominal distention restricting diaphragmatic movement
- Sleep disorders
- Poliomyelitis
- Pleural effusion
- Pleurisy
- Excessive obesity

Often a specific diagnosis of restrictive lung disease is made only after extensive testing, including chest radiography, biopsy, immunologic testing, and testing to differentiate neurologic dysfunction, such as electromyography and cerebrospinal fluid analysis.

Spinal curvature

Cross section of thorax showing compression of lungs

■ **FIGURE 62–6** Thoracic scoliosis. Note the S shape of the spine. These thoracic deformities alter the chest cage space. Lung tissue may be compressed, producing altered lung function (restrictive lung disease).

OUTCOME MANAGEMENT

Management is based on the severity of impairment and the ability to reverse the condition. Clients with spinal deformities may be helped by corrective spinal surgery. Likewise, obese clients breathe better after weight loss. Selected clients may benefit from the use of transtracheal oxygen administration or nighttime mechanical ventilation with a mask or cuirass respirator (a device that covers the chest and moves the chest wall out and back through changes in pressure), especially clients who have postpoliomyelitis syndrome.

The primary goals of nursing management of the client with restrictive lung disease are (1) promotion of adequate oxygenation, (2) maintenance of a patent airway, and (3) achievement of the highest possible functional level. Interventions to attain these goals are similar to those used in the treatment of COPD (see Chapter 61). ABG analysis is important for monitoring oxygen needs, acid-base balance, and the effects of physical activity. $Paco_2$ values should be monitored because rising carbon dioxide level is an indicator of impending respiratory failure.

Most restrictive lung disorders are not reversible. End-stage disease is characterized by the development of pulmonary hypertension, cor pulmonale, severe hypoxemia, and eventual respiratory failure. Efforts should be made to maintain the client's functional status and quality of life at as high a level as possible.

CYSTIC FIBROSIS

Cystic fibrosis (CF) is a congenital restrictive lung disorder in which the secretions of the exocrine (mucus-producing) glands are abnormal. This disorder affects the sweat glands, respiratory system, digestive tract (particularly the pancreas), and reproductive tract. CF is the most common inherited genetic disease in the Caucasian population. There are approximately 30,000 people with CF in the United States, with almost 1000 new cases diagnosed each year. CF is an autosomal recessive trait, resulting from mutations at a single gene locus on the long arm of chromosome 7. CF used to be considered a "pediatric problem" because it was fatal in childhood. However, advances in early diagnosis and treatment, including antibiotics, chest physiotherapy, and nutrition programs, have extended the median life expectancy into the mid-30s.

Pathophysiology

A gene found on chromosome 7 is responsible for the function of the CF transmembrane conductance regulator (CFTR). When the CFTR is defective, both the rate of active ion transport and the resistance to ion flow across the superficial epithelium are altered. CF airway epithelia exhibit both raised transport rates (Na^+) and decreased Cl^- permeabilities. These abnormalities in the sodium and chloride transport alter water movement across the membrane, leading to thick secretions of mucoproteins that plug the airway. Furthermore, the mucociliary transport is slowed, which decreases the ability to clear the airways of mucus and leads to stasis of mucus and a medium for infection. Lung infections often develop from *Staphylococcus aureus* and *Pseudomonas aeruginosa* organisms, which seldom infect the lungs of healthy people.

The thick mucus also plugs the glands and ducts of the pancreatic acini, intestinal glands, intrahepatic bile ducts, and the gallbladder, causing dilation and fibrosis. These changes result in decreased production of pancreatic enzymes needed for digestion of carbohydrates, fats, and proteins. Sweat glands, salivary glands, and lacrimal glands are also affected, leading to high concentrations of sodium and chloride in these secretions.

Clinical Manifestations

The most common clinical manifestation is a persistent cough that is worse at night and upon arising. As CF progresses, the cough becomes productive and then paroxysmal, with gagging and emesis. Recurrent lung infections lead to tenacious purulent, often green sputum. Asthmatic wheezing is common. Because of the pancreatic involvement, clients may have steatorrhea.

Chest radiography shows hyperinflation, and pulmonary function tests reveal increased airway resistance. The airways are hyperreactive and clients often complain of dyspnea with cold air, smoke, and exercise. CF is diagnosed by elevated chloride levels in the sweat. Distal intestinal obstruction can occur, which presents as right lower quadrant pain, loss of appetite, occasional emesis, and often a palpable mass. The syndrome can be confused with appendicitis, which occurs frequently in clients with CF.

Delayed puberty is common in both males and females with CF. The delayed maturational pattern is likely secondary to the effects of chronic lung disease and inadequate nutrition on reproductive endocrine function. Most male clients with CF are azoospermic, reflecting obliteration of the vas deferens. Twenty percent of women with CF are infertile as a result of effects of chronic lung disease on the menstrual cycle. Thick, tenacious cervical mucus blocks sperm migration, and there are possible fallopian tube and uterine wall abnormalities in liquid transport. However, more than 90% of completed pregnancies produce viable infants, and women with CF are generally able to breast-feed infants normally.

OUTCOME MANAGEMENT

The goals of CF are to ensure a reasonable quality of life for as long as possible and to prevent or slow the decline in pulmonary functioning. Goals are achieved by removing secretions, improving aeration, promoting optimal nutrition, suppressing inflammation, and administering antibiotic agents.

Clearing tracheobronchial secretions is promoted by the following measures:

- Adequate hydration
- Bronchodilators and mucolytic aerosols
- Synthetic DNase—an enzyme that breaks down deoxyribonucleic acid (DNA) released from neutrophils and causes the "stickiness" of mucus
- Twice daily inhalation of hypertonic saline solution
- Effective coughing techniques

Additional interventions to assist clients with aeration and secretion removal include noninvasive ventilation such as positive expiratory pressure devices, postural drainage, and chest physiotherapy, percussion, and exercise. Oxygen is used if hypoxemia is present. Sitting erect also facilitates breathing.

Anti-inflammatory agents decrease inflammatory responses in the respiratory tract epithelium and improve pulmonary function. Short-term systemic corticosteroids are used during acute exacerbations and nonsteroidal anti-inflammatory drugs are often given long term.

Antibiotic therapy has played an important role in extending the life expectancy of clients with CF. Administration of intravenous antibiotics is essential during acute infections. Inhaled antibiotics provide a high concentration of drugs directly into the pulmonary system while minimizing systemic side effects. The choice of antibiotic should be determined by results of sputum culture and sensitivity testing. Sputum should be assessed for color, quality, and quantity.

SAFETY ⚠ ALERT **All respiratory equipment should be thoroughly cleaned on a routine basis to prevent reinfection from contaminated equipment.**

Persistent pulmonary infection with *Pseudomonas* organisms is common in the end stages of CF. Prolonged course of treatment with larger than normal doses of intravenous antibiotics is usually indicated. Moderate to severe hemoptysis can occur if the infection causes erosion of pulmonary blood vessels. Blood replacement and temporary cessation of postural drainage may be required.

Maintenance of adequate nutrition is critical. The majority of CF clients benefit from pancreatic enzyme replacement. The dose of enzymes is adjusted on the basis of weight gain, abdominal manifestations, and character of stools. Replacement of fat-soluble vitamins, particularly vitamins A, D, E, and K, is usually required.

Treatment of end-stage disease is primarily concerned with the management of severe complications. Obstruction of the airways leads to hyperinflation. In time, restrictive lung disease is superimposed on the obstructive disease. Pneumothorax (air in the chest cavity)

develops in 20% of all adult clients, requiring lung reexpansion with chest tubes.

Over time, pulmonary obstruction leads to chronic hypoxemia, hypercapnia, and acidosis. Pulmonary hypertension and, eventually, cor pulmonale may result. Treatment consists of digitalis, diuretics, and oxygen therapy. Clients with severely reduced lung function (FEV_1 <30% of predicted) whose disease no longer responds to maximal therapy and who are experiencing a decline in quality of life are often considered candidates for bilateral lung transplantation.

Attention to psychosocial concerns is a nursing priority throughout the course of the disease. In the adult client with CF, psychosocial concerns center on the following three major areas:

- Disease management (e.g., treatment compliance, sleep disturbance, hemoptysis, nutrition, and hospitalizations)
- Growth and development (e.g., daily activities, work, and sex and reproduction)
- Family relations (e.g., substance abuse, depression, anxiety, and marital problems)

Nursing intervention involves helping clients cope with these problem areas as well as providing emotional support to both clients and their families.

LUNG TRANSPLANTATION

Lung transplantation is the definitive therapy for many end-stage lung diseases that are unresponsive to medical therapy. Transplantation can involve replacement of one or both of the diseased lungs with lungs from a cadaver donor or lobar transplantation from a live donor. Lung transplantation is an accepted treatment modality for end-stage pulmonary diseases such as emphysema, cystic fibrosis, alpha$_1$-antitrypsin deficiency, drug-induced pulmonary fibrosis, sarcoidosis, and primary pulmonary hypertension. Although long-term survival after lung transplantation has improved, it still lags behind other solid organ transplants.

Preoperative Care

Preoperative assessment consists of both medical and psychosocial evaluation. After the severity of lung disease is established, a battery of tests is performed to rule out active infection and to evaluate cardiac, hepatic, hematopoietic, and renal functions. The client who smokes or has an active non-pulmonary infection, significant disease in other organ systems, or poor nutritional status will be ruled out as a transplant candidate. Psychosocial evaluation focuses on assessing the client's history of compliance with medical therapy, history of substance abuse, and ability to cope with stress.

Postoperative Care

Postoperatively, the client is observed for excessive bleeding. Vital signs, hemodynamic pressures, electrocardiograms (ECGs), ABG values, urine output, transcutaneous oxygen level analysis, and chest tube drainage are monitored hourly, or more frequently as the client's condition warrants. Pulmonary edema may develop in the denervated transplanted lung. Therefore the client will be placed on mechanical ventilation with positive end-expiratory pressure (PEEP) for 24 to 48 hours.

Serum electrolytes, complete blood counts, and chest radiographs are obtained at least daily. Fluids are restricted, lung sounds are auscultated, and the severity of peripheral edema is monitored. Pain control is important to allow deep breathing and coughing in addition to chest physiotherapy. Many clients benefit from epidural analgesia. Following extubation, maintain good pain control and help the client cough, deep breathe, and use incentive spirometry to expand the lung.

The client who has received a lung transplant is at risk for infection, organ rejection, pneumothorax, pleural effusions, pulmonary embolism, venous thromboembolism, lung hyperinflation, and phrenic nerve injury. Isolation is used to decrease inadvertent exposure to pathogens. Laboratory values are monitored frequently, especially the WBC and absolute neutrophil counts. Evaluate the client for clinical manifestations of infection, such as (1) changes in vital signs (especially fever), (2) local infections at intravenous access sites and incision lines, and (3) changes in respiratory status (excessive secretions, tachypnea, dyspnea, fatigue).

Rejection of the transplanted lung may manifest as dyspnea, development of infiltrates on chest radiograph, need for ventilatory support, and fatigue. Cyclosporin A is the most important immunosuppressive agent for lung transplant clients to prevent rejection. It is initially given IV and then converted to an oral route before the client's discharge.

Following the initial procedure, the client may experience alterations in self-concept related to changes in (1) appearance, from the side effects of medications such as steroids and immunosuppressants, (2) lifestyle, or (3) work ability and role performance. Be sensitive to these issues, and encourage the client and family to discuss their feelings and explore options.

Self-Care

Before discharge from the facility, teach the client about the medication regimen, and stress the need for daily medications despite a lack of any rejection manifestations. The client should report fever, dyspnea, cough, new or increased productive sputum, chest pain, reduced exercise tolerance, excessive weight gain, and fatigue to the physician. In addition, the client should begin a pulmonary rehabilitation program.

During follow-up visits, the client is monitored for manifestations of rejection, compliance with immunosuppressive therapy, and progress in functional status.

Lung transplantation offers some hope for extended life to clients with previously fatal conditions. However, it is a frightening and stressful surgery. Clients receiving lung transplants are always critically ill before surgery. In addition, they must undergo a radical, major surgical procedure and endure prolonged intensive care and isolation procedures. Clients with transplants also must adapt to an altered self-concept. The client and significant others need constant emotional support for achievement of a successful outcome.

Successful transplant outcomes can include markedly improved ABG levels 3 months after transplantation. Unilateral lung recipients may continue to have mild hypoxemia but rarely require supplemental oxygen. Pulmonary function studies have shown that some unilateral graft recipients can reach 60% to 65% of their predicted FVC and FEV_1 values. The values for bilateral lung recipients often approach normal predicted values, but these clients can have mild restrictive physiology.

Improved exercise capacity is also observed in recipients of both unilateral and bilateral lung transplants. Typically, transplant recipients can walk 100 to 120 m/min within 6 months of transplantation and are generally able to sustain this rate over time. Any limitations in exercise capacity appear to be related to muscle deconditioning and abnormalities in skeletal muscle oxidative capacity.

SARCOIDOSIS

Sarcoidosis is an inflammatory condition that affects many body systems. While the onset of sarcoidosis typically occurs between 20 and 40 years of age, it can be present in children and older adults. The disease is characterized by the formation of widespread granulomatous lesions. In addition to lung involvement, which occurs in more than 90% of cases, clients may present with clinical manifestations involving the peripheral lymphatic system, eyes, skin, liver, spleen, bones, salivary glands, joints, nervous system, and heart.

The cause of sarcoidosis remains unknown; it is suggested that a triggering agent (which may be genetic, infectious, immunologic, or toxic) stimulates enhanced cell-mediated immune processes at the site of involvement. A series of interactions between T lymphocytes and monocyte-macrophages leads to the formation of noncaseating (i.e., having no cheesy necrotic degeneration) granulomas, which are characteristic of the disease. Granuloma formation may regress with therapy or as a result of the disorder's natural course, but it may also progress to fibrosis and restrictive lung disease. In chronic cases, approximately 10% of clients die of the disease.

As many as half of clients are asymptomatic, and the diagnosis is confirmed by chest radiography. Clients with pulmonary manifestations usually present with a dry cough and shortness of breath. Chest pain, hemoptysis, or pneumothorax may also be present. Systemic manifestations include fatigue, weakness, malaise, weight loss, and fever. A definitive diagnosis of sarcoidosis is made from tissue biopsy. When lung involvement is suspected, bronchoscopy, bronchoalveolar lavage, mediastinoscopy, or open lung biopsy may be performed.

OUTCOME MANAGEMENT

Medical management is primarily determined by the extent to which the client's life is disturbed by the manifestations experienced. If the client with sarcoidosis is asymptomatic, management involves ongoing assessment for further disease progression, such as obtaining a chest radiograph every 6 months. When manifestations are present, medical treatment usually consists of systemic corticosteroids to suppress the immune process and often leads to dramatic improvement.

Nursing intervention in clients with sarcoidosis is the same as that in clients with other restrictive lung diseases and hypoxemia. Assess for drug side effects, especially adverse responses to corticosteroids (such as weight gain, change in mood, and development of diabetes mellitus). Also assess for manifestations of improvement, such as increased exercise tolerance, disappearance of initial assessment findings, improved pulmonary function studies, and better oxygenation. If assessment findings worsen, document them and notify the physician.

INTERSTITIAL LUNG DISEASE

Interstitial lung diseases (ILDs) comprise a group of chronic and diffuse inflammatory lower respiratory tract disorders. The term *interstitial* is used to indicate that the interstitium of the alveolar walls is thickened and has become fibrotic. The alveolar walls thicken as a result of the accumulation of inflammatory cells. The thickened alveolus becomes nonfunctional.

The cause of ILD is not clearly defined. It most commonly develops from idiopathic pulmonary fibrosis, sarcoidosis, and collagen-vascular disorders. ILD can also result from the inhalation of inorganic dust (such as crystalline silica, asbestos, and coal dust) or of organic dust from organisms encountered in farming, use of air conditioning, and animal husbandry. Other possible causes are radiation damage and infectious agents.

Manifestations of ILD are insidious and nonspecific, such as fatigue, progressive dyspnea, dyspnea at rest, and nonproductive cough. Because the clinical manifestations are nonspecific, ILD may remain undiagnosed for years.

The client's history plays a major part in diagnosis because it is important to determine the agents to which the client has been exposed. Physical examination may reveal reduced chest expansion, which is reflected as a decrease in TLC. Inspiratory and expiratory crackles are frequently heard. The crackles have a characteristic sound, like the sound of hook-and-loop tape (Velcro) being pulled apart. Clubbing of the finger tips may be present.

Diagnostic assessment includes gallium ventilation-perfusion scans. These scans usually reveal impaired perfusion in the lower lobes and multiple areas of impaired ventilation. The ventilation-perfusion mismatch results in hypoxemia and carbon dioxide retention. Bronchoscopy and biopsy may also be used to confirm ILD.

OUTCOME MANAGEMENT

Management of a client with ILD is based on the level of respiratory impairment. Inflammation is controlled with corticosteroids. Explain to the client that corticosteroids reduce further impairment but previously injured alveolar-capillary units are permanently damaged. Clients often show subjective improvement while taking steroids, the dosage of which can eventually be tapered and stopped. If the offending agent is known, the initial treatment is to remove the client from exposure to the agent. As the disorder progresses, inhaled corticosteroids and bronchodilators help mobilize secretions and provide oxygen during periods of exercise. Nursing management is the same as that for clients with restrictive lung disorders.

DISORDERS OF THE PLEURA AND PLEURAL SPACE

PLEURAL PAIN

Pleural pain is a common pulmonary manifestation arising from the parietal pleura, which is richly supplied with sensory nerve endings. Pleuritic pain indicates the presence of pleural inflammation (*pleurisy*) caused by pneumonia, pulmonary infarction, pleural effusion (see the following discussion), or pneumothorax, among others. It is often accompanied by a pleural friction rub that is discovered during chest auscultation.

Pleuritic chest pain often develops abruptly and is usually severe enough that the client seeks medical attention. It commonly occurs on only one side of the chest, usually in the lower lateral portions of the chest wall, and is aggravated by deep breathing or coughing. Often the client can point directly to the exact location of the pain. However, pleural pain may also be referred to the neck, shoulder, or abdomen. Because other types of chest pain (e.g., cardiac pain, chest wall pain) may be misinterpreted as pleuritic pain, careful assessment is necessary.

Pleuritic pain may restrict normal respiratory efforts, leading to problems with gas exchange and airway clearance. If pain-relieving measures, including administration of prescribed analgesics, do not relieve the pain, the physician may perform an intercostal nerve block (see Chapter 20).

PLEURAL EFFUSION

Pleural effusion is an accumulation of fluid in the pleural space. Pleural fluid normally seeps continually into the pleural space from the capillaries lining the parietal pleura and is reabsorbed by the visceral pleural capillaries and lymphatic system. Any condition that interferes with either secretion or drainage of this fluid leads to pleural effusion.

Causes of pleural effusion can be grouped into four major categories:

- Increased systemic hydrostatic pressure (e.g., heart failure)
- Reduced capillary oncotic pressure (e.g., liver or renal failure)
- Increased capillary permeability (e.g., infections or trauma)
- Impaired lymphatic function (e.g., lymphatic obstruction caused by tumor)

Clinical manifestations depend on the amount of fluid present and the severity of lung compression. If the effusion is small (i.e., 250 ml), its presence may be discovered only on a chest radiograph. With larger effusions, lung expansion may be restricted, and the client may experience dyspnea, primarily on exertion, and a dry, nonproductive cough caused by bronchial irritation or mediastinal shift. Tactile fremitus may be decreased or absent, and percussion notes dull or flat.

Thoracentesis (see Chapter 59) is used to remove excess pleural fluid. The removed fluid is analyzed to determine whether it is transudate or exudate. Transudates are substances that have passed through a membrane or tissue surface. They occur primarily in conditions in which there is protein loss and low protein content (e.g., hypoalbuminemia, cirrhosis, nephrosis) or increased hydrostatic pressure (e.g., heart failure). Exudates are substances that have escaped from blood vessels. They contain an accumulation of cells, have a high specific gravity and a high lactate dehydrogenase (LDH) level, and occur in response to malignancies, infections, or inflammatory processes. Exudates occur when there is an increase in capillary permeability. Differentiating between transudates and exudates helps establish a specific diagnosis. Diagnosis may also require analysis of the fluid for white and red blood cells, malignant cells, bacteria, glucose content, pH, and LDH.

Pleural fluid may be (1) hemorrhagic (or bloody), such as when a tumor is present or after trauma or pulmonary embolus with infarction; (2) chylous (or thick and white), such as after lymphatic obstruction or trauma to the thoracic duct; or (3) rich in cholesterol, such as in chronic, recurrent effusions caused by tuberculosis or rheumatoid arthritis. If there is a high WBC count and the pleural fluid is purulent, the effusion is called an empyema. An empyema of any volume requires drainage and treatment of the infection.

If the pus is not drained, it may become thick and almost solidified or loculated (containing cavities), a condition called fibrothorax. Fibrothorax may significantly restrict lung expansion and may require surgical intervention. The procedure, known as decortication, involves removal of the restrictive mass of fibrin and inflammatory cells. Decortication is usually not performed until the fibrothorax is relatively solid, so it can be easily removed.

After the thoracentesis, closed-chest drainage with suction is used to reexpand the lung rapidly and fill the pleural space. If the fibrous material has restricted the lung for some time, the lung may not reexpand effectively and further intervention (usually thoracoplasty) may be needed.

RECURRENT PLEURAL EFFUSIONS

In some cases, pleural effusions may recur despite repeated thoracenteses (e.g., malignancy-induced effusions), with resultant compromise of lung function or persistent pleural pain. Treatment of recurrent effusions is accomplished through obliteration of the pleural space. Methods of obliterating the pleural space are as follows:

- **Pleurectomy (pleural stripping):** Surgical stripping of the parietal pleura away from the visceral pleura, which produces an intense inflammatory reaction that promotes adhesion formation between the two layers during healing.
- **Pleurodesis:** Instillation of a sclerosing substance (e.g., unbuffered tetracycline, bleomycin) into the pleural space via a chest tube to create an inflammatory response that causes the pleura to adhere and sclerose to each other. During the instillation, the client is rolled side to side to spread the substance throughout the pleural space.

Because pleural space obliteration creates permanent changes, the client's existing and predicted postprocedure respiratory status must be carefully evaluated. If a large area is involved, significant alterations in ventilatory mechanics (e.g., deep breathing, coughing) may occur, leading to compromised respiratory function.

After the procedure, closely monitor lung function, including respiratory rate and ventilation pattern. Document alleviation or persistence of pleural pain and watch for indications of a return of the pleural effusion.

Pulmonary function studies (see Chapter 59) and ABG measurements should also be performed.

BRONCHOPLEURAL FISTULA

A bronchopleural fistula is a communication between the pleural space and a bronchus. It may occur when an undrained empyema erodes into a bronchus or when the pleural space does not heal spontaneously after removal of a chest tube. A bronchopleural fistula raises the risk of pleural infection and may compromise ventilation and oxygenation.

The management of clients with bronchopleural fistulas is complex because they are often slow to heal. The client may be discharged home with a chest tube still in place and connected to a collection drainage system. Teach the client and family how to care for the chest tube and collection system and to recognize both manifestations of irritation at the chest puncture site and changes in chest drainage (e.g., blood) that require the physician to be notified.

METASTATIC PLEURAL TUMORS

Primary tumors in the lungs and other organs often metastasize to the pleura. The primary tumor is usually in a lung but may occur in the breast, ovaries, liver, kidneys, uterus, testicles, or larynx or may result from leukemia or lymphoma. Metastatic pleural disease frequently causes pleural effusions. Assessment findings in malignant pleural effusion are the same as those in pleural effusion from other causes. Diagnosis of pleural effusion is by chest radiograph. The source of the effusion is determined from cytologic examination of pleural fluid obtained by thoracentesis. Intervention is the same as for any pleural effusion, along with treatment of the primary malignancy.

DISORDERS OF THE DIAPHRAGM

SUBDIAPHRAGMATIC ABSCESS

A subdiaphragmatic abscess can compromise a client's respiratory status or erode and perforate the client's diaphragm. Clinical manifestations include pleuritic pain or pain referred to the shoulder on the affected side. Dyspnea and poor or no diaphragmatic movement are common. Flank pain or tenderness and a palpable abdominal mass in the region of the abscess are noted. The client has fever, anorexia, weight loss, and vomiting. Chest radiograph shows the diaphragm is generally elevated on the affected side. Fluoroscopic studies of diaphragmatic movement reveal limitation or absence of diaphragmatic movement on the affected side. Pleural effusion also commonly occurs. Thoracentesis and analysis of the pleural fluid reveal an exudate.

Subdiaphragmatic abscesses are drained and treated with antibiotics. Supportive measures are used to maintain ventilation and respiratory status. An untreated subdiaphragmatic abscess is nearly always fatal. With treatment, the death rate is still high but drops to approximately 25%.

DIAPHRAGMATIC PARALYSIS

Diaphragmatic paralysis can involve either the entire diaphragm (bilateral) or one side (unilateral). The most common causes of bilateral paralysis include high spinal cord injury, thoracic trauma (including cardiac surgery), multiple sclerosis, tumor nerve compression, anterior horn disease, and muscular dystrophy. Unilateral paralysis of the diaphragm is much more common than is bilateral paralysis. The most common cause is nerve invasion from malignancy or trauma.

Although the diaphragm is the primary muscle of respiration, its role can be assumed in part by the accessory and abdominal muscles. As a result, unilateral diaphragmatic paralysis is often difficult to detect. The diagnosis is suggested by finding an elevated hemidiaphragm on the chest radiograph and is confirmed by fluoroscopy. During the fluoroscopic procedure, the client is asked to "sniff." If paralysis is present, the nonparalyzed side of the diaphragm descends during inspiration (the sniff), and the paralyzed side paradoxically rises. Clients with unilateral diaphragmatic paralysis usually experience dyspnea when lying on the affected side. Dyspnea on exertion is not usual unless there is underlying lung disease. Both TLC and vital capacity (VC) are reduced by about 20%. There is also less ventilation to the affected side, and mild hypoxemia occurs because of shifts of ventilation and blood flow. Pre-existing lung disease combined with unilateral diaphragmatic paralysis may be disabling, depending on the extent of the lung disease.

The effects of bilateral diaphragmatic paralysis are potentially much more severe. However, the problem is often subtle and overlooked, especially if the client has a neuromuscular disorder. Fatigue, disturbed sleep, and morning headache are frequently the only manifestations. Classic manifestations of bilateral paralysis of the diaphragm are increased dyspnea, paradoxical inward abdominal movement, and active use of accessory muscles when the client is lying supine. Functional residual capacity (FRC) is also decreased, as is lung compliance. In the side-lying position, ventilation is preferentially distributed to the uppermost lung tissue and away from blood flow, leading to a significant mismatch of ventilation and perfusion. Severe hypoxemia results. Reduced tidal volume leads to retention of carbon dioxide and respiratory acidosis.

Little can be done to treat diaphragmatic paralysis. Management is aimed at supporting ventilatory function as needed. If the phrenic nerve is intact, a phrenic nerve pacer may be surgically inserted. Use of a phrenic nerve pacer is useful primarily for clients with spinal cord injuries.

Nursing management focuses on maintenance of a patent airway and detection of deteriorating gas exchange. Because inspiration is impaired, the client may need assistance to cough and deep breathe effectively. Position the client on the unaffected side in the semi-sitting or sitting position. Suction secretions as necessary. Increase hydration to liquefy secretions. Administer oxygen as prescribed. If respiratory function declines significantly, the physician and client (or possibly significant others) must decide whether a permanent tracheostomy should be placed and whether mechanical ventilation or other assistance devices should be used.

CONCLUSIONS

Clients with lung disorders are a challenge to the nurse providing care. In addition to common nursing diagnoses centering on *Impaired Gas Exchange* and *Ineffective Airway Clearance,* the client is often anxious because of the feelings of dyspnea and air hunger. Management of lung disorders consists of methods to open the airway (bronchodilators), clear infection (antibiotics), and improve oxygenation (position, coughing and deep breathing, oxygen).

THINKING CRITICALLY

1. Your client, who has undergone a thoracotomy, has a pleural chest tube connected to water-seal drainage. While your client is being positioned for a bedside chest radiograph, the drainage tubing is inadvertently disconnected from the chest drainage apparatus. What actions should you take?

Factors to Consider. What happens to the normally negative pressure in the pleural space when it is exposed to room air? Is this a dangerous problem?

2. A client with exertional dyspnea is admitted to the unit with a diagnosis of pleural effusion. He has difficulty breathing during the transfer from the cart to bed. You are asked to prepare the client for a thoracentesis. How would you prioritize care? What preparations are necessary for a thoracentesis?

Factors to Consider. What is the purpose of a thoracentesis? How are complications avoided? What clients are at risk for pleural effusion?

Discussion for these questions can be found on the website.

BIBLIOGRAPHY

Citations appearing in red refer to primary research.

Citations appearing in blue refer to evidence-based practice guidelines and protocols.

1. Ahluwalia, G., Ahluwalia, A., Gupta, K., et al. (2005). Extrapulmonary tuberculosis, part 1: Pleura and lymph node disease. *Journal of Respiratory Diseases, 26,* 326-332.
2. Alberg, A.J., & Samet, J.M. (2003). Epidemiology of lung cancer. *Chest, 123,* 21S-49S.
3. American Cancer Society. (2006). *What are the key statistics about lung cancer?* Retrieved 12/01/06 from www.cancer.org/doc root/CRI/content/CRI_2_4_1x_What_Are_the_Key_Statistics_About_ Lung_Cancer_15.asp?sitearea=.
4. American Lung Association. (2006). *Lung disease data at a glance: Influenza and pneumonia.* Retrieved 12/10/06 from www.lungusa.org/site/pp.asp?c=dvLUK9O0E&b=316591.
4a. American Thoracic Society, Centers for Disease Control and Infectious Diseases Society of America. (2003). Treatment of tuberculosis. *Mortality and Morbidity Weekly Report, 52(RR11),* 1-77.
5. Anstead, G.M., & Graybill, J.R. (2006). Coccidioidomycosis. *Infectious Disease Clinics of North America, 20,* 621-623.
6. Arcasoy, S.M., & Wilt, J. (2006). Medical complications after lung transplantation. *Seminars in Respiratory and Critical Care Medicine, 27,* 508-520.
7. Barron, A., Brassell, S.A., & Shulman, L.P. (2005). Early cancer diagnosis: Present and future. *Patient Care, 39,* 27-30.
8. Bruce, E.A., Howard, R.F., & Franck, L.S. (2006). Chest drain removal pain and its management: A literature review. *Journal of Clinical Nursing, 15,* 145-154.
9. Centers for Disease Control and Prevention. (2006). Emergence of *Mycobacterium tuberculosis* with extensive resistance to second-line drugs—worldwide, 2000-2004. *Morbidity and Mortality Weekly Report, 55,* 301-328.
10. Centers for Disease Control and Prevention. (2006). Update: Influenza activity—United States, April 2-8, 2006. *Morbidity and Mortality Weekly Report, 55,* 421-448.
11. Centers for Disease Control and Prevention. (2006). *Testing for TB disease and infection—Tuberculin skin testing.* Core Curriculum on Tuberculosis. Retrieved 12/10/06 from www.cdc.gov/nchstp/ tb/pubs/corecurr/Chapter4/Chapter_4_Skin_Testing.htm.
12. Centers for Disease Control and Prevention. (2006). Trends in tuberculosis—United States, 2005. *Morbidity and Mortality Weekly Report, 55,* 301-328.
13. Couppie, P., Aznar, C., Carme, B., et al. (2006). American histoplasmosis in developing countries with a special focus on patients with HIV: Diagnosis, treatment, and prognosis. *Current Opinion in Infectious Diseases, 19,* 443-449.
14. Cystic Fibrosis Foundation. (2005). *Patient registry—Annual data report 2004.* Retrieved 12/05/06 from www.cff.org/ID=4573/ TYPE=2676/2004%20Patient%20Registry%20Report.pdf.
15. Davis, P.B. (2006). Cystic fibrosis since 1938. *American Journal of Respiratory and Critical Care Medicine, 173,* 475-482.
15a. Diagnosis and management of lung cancer: ACCP evidence-based guidelines. *Chest, 123* (15), 337S.
16. Driver, C.R., Matus, S.P., Bayuga, S., et al.. (2005). Factors associated with tuberculosis treatment interruption in New York City. *Journal of Public Health Management Practice, 11,* 361-368.
17. Dunn, L. (2005). Pneumonia: Classification, diagnosis, and nursing management. *Nursing Standard, 19,* 50-54.
18. Elkins, M.R., Robinson, M., Rose, B.R., et al.. (2006). A controlled trial of long-term inhaled hypertonic saline in patients with cystic fibrosis. *New England Journal of Medicine, 354,* 229-240.
19. Flanders, S.A., Collard, H.R., & Saint, S. (2006). Nosocomial pneumonia: State of the science. *American Journal of Infection Control, 34,* 84-93.
20. Gift, A.G., Jablonski, A., Stommel, M., et al. (2004). Symptom clusters in elderly patients with lung cancer. *Oncology Nursing Forum, 31,* 203-210.
21. Jett, J.R., & Miller, Y.E. (2006). Update in lung cancer 2005. *American Journal of Respiratory and Critical Care Medicine, 173,* 695-697.

22. Lawrence, V.A., Cornell, J.E., & Smetana, G.W. (2006). Strategies to reduce postoperative pulmonary complications after noncardiothoracic surgery: Systematic review for the American College of Physicians. *Annals of Internal Medicine, 144,* 596-608.

23. Leonard, M.K., Egan, K.B., Kourbatova, E., et al. (2006). Increased efficiency in evaluating patients with suspected tuberculosis by use of a dedicated airborne infection isolation unit. *American Journal of Infection Control, 34,* 69-72.

24. Lobato, M.N., Want, Y.C., Becerra, J.E., et al. (2006). Improved program activities are associated with decreasing tuberculosis incidence in the United States. *Public Health Reports, 121,* 108-115.

25. Mandell, L.A. (2005). Symposium on community-acquired pneumonia. Update on community-acquired pneumonia: New pathogens and new concepts in treatment. *Postgraduate Medicine, 118*(4), 35-46.

25a. Mandell, L.A., Bartlett, J.G., Dowell, S.F., et al. (2006). Update of guidelines for the management of community-acquired pneumonia in immunocompetent adults. *Clinics in Infectious Disease, 37,* 1405-1433.

26. Mapp, C.E., Miotto, D., & Boschetto, P. (2006). Occupational asthma. *La Medicina del Lavoro, 97,* 404-409.

27. Mehra, R., Moore, B.A., Crothers, K., et al. (2006). The association between marijuana smoking and lung cancer: A systematic review. *Archives of Internal Medicine, 166,* 1359-1367.

28. Moran, F., & Bradley, J. (2006). Non-invasive ventilation for cystic fibrosis. *Cochrane Library, 4,* 1-30.

29. O'Meara, E.S., White, M., Siscovick, D.S., et al. (2005). Hospitalization for pneumonia in the cardiovascular health study: Incidence, mortality, and influence on longer-term survival. *Journal of the American Geriatrics Society, 53,* 1108-1116.

30. Page, K.R., Sifakis, F., Montes de Oca, R., et al. (2006). Improved adherence and less toxicity with rifampin vs isoniazid for treatment of latent tuberculosis: A retrospective study. *Archives of Internal Medicine, 166,* 1863-1870.

31. Pirozynski, M. (2006). 100 years of lung cancer. *Respiratory Medicine, 100,* 2073-2084.

32. Trow, T.K. (2006). Clinical year in review: Occupational lung disease, pulmonary vascular disease, bronchiectasis, and chronic obstructive pulmonary disease. *Proceedings of the American Thoracic Society, 3,* 557-560.

33. United States National Institutes of Health. (2006). *Small cell lung cancer: Treatment.* National Cancer Institute. Retrieved 12/01/06 from www.cancer.gov/cancertopics/pdq/treatment/small-cell-lung/HealthProfessional/page1/print.

34. United States Department of Health and Human Services. (2006). *The health consequences of involuntary exposure to tobacco smoke: A report of the Surgeon General.* Atlanta, Ga: Department of Health and Human Services, Public Health Service, Centers for Disease Control and Prevention, National Center for Chronic Disease and Prevention and Promotion, Office of Smoking and Health.

35. Valdivia, L., Nix, D., Wright, M., et al. (2006). Coccidioidomycosis as a common cause of community-acquired pneumonia. *Emerging Infectious Diseases, 12,* 958-962.

36. van der Schans, C., Prasad, A., & Main, E. (2006). Chest physiotherapy compared to no chest physiotherapy for cystic fibrosis. *Cochrane Library, 4,* 1-21.

37. Vivek, N.A., & Kawut, S.M. (2005). Noninfectious pulmonary complications after lung transplantation. *Clinics in Chest Medicine, 26,* 613-622.

38. Westerdahl, E., Lindmark, B., Eriksson, T., et al. (2003). The immediate effects of deep breathing exercises on atelectasis and oxygenation after cardiac surgery. *Scandinavian Cardiovascular Journal, 37,* 363-367.

39. Williams, V.G. (2006). Tuberculosis: Clinical features, diagnosis and management. *Nursing Management, 20,* 49-53.

40. Yen, M.Y., Lin, Y.E., Su, I.J., et al. (2006). Using an integrated infection control strategy during outbreak control to minimize nosocomial infection of severe acute respiratory syndrome among healthcare workers. *Journal of Hospital Infection, 64,* 195-199.

CHAPTER 63

Management of Clients with Acute Pulmonary Disorders

LYNN WHITE

RESPIRATORY FAILURE

The most important function of the respiratory system is to provide the body tissues with oxygen and to remove carbon dioxide. The body relies primarily on the central nervous system (CNS), the pulmonary system, the heart, and the vascular system to accomplish effective respiration. Respiratory failure develops when one or more of these systems or organs fail to maintain optimal functioning. If the respiratory failure occurs so rapidly that the compensatory mechanisms cannot accommodate or if the compensatory mechanisms are overwhelmed, acute respiratory failure develops.

Respiratory failure is a broad, nonspecific clinical diagnosis indicating that the respiratory system is unable to supply the oxygen necessary to maintain metabolism or cannot eliminate sufficient carbon dioxide (CO_2). *Acute respiratory failure* is defined as a partial pressure of arterial oxygen (Pao_2) of 50 mm Hg or less on room air or a partial pressure of arterial CO_2 ($Paco_2$) of 50 mm Hg or more with a pH ≤ 7.25, along with clinical presentation. Some experts will also identify a pH of ≤ 7.35 as another indication of acute respiratory failure. In clients with chronic hypercapnia, $Paco_2$ elevations of 5 mm Hg or more from their previously stable levels indicate that acute respiratory failure has been superimposed on chronic respiratory failure.

Acute respiratory failure may be classified as hypoxemic or ventilatory failure with a rapid onset over minutes to hours or gradually over days. Clients with acute *hypoxemic* respiratory failure have severe arterial hypoxemia and are minimally responsive to supplemental oxygen despite adequate ventilation. Hypoxemic respiratory failure may be caused by diffuse problems such as pulmonary edema; near-drowning; adult (acute) respiratory distress syndrome (ARDS); or localized problems such as pneumonia, bleeding into the chest, or lung tumors.

Ventilatory or hypercapnic respiratory failure is when the client is unable to support adequate gas exchange leading to elevated $Paco_2$ levels that can result from CNS depression, inadequate neuromuscular ability to sustain breathing, or respiratory system overload. Conditions such as acute deterioration of chronic obstructive pulmonary disease (COPD), and status asthmaticus are other causes of ventilatory failure. Clients may have a combination of hypoxemic and hypercapnic respiratory failure.

HYPOXEMIC RESPIRATORY FAILURE

PULMONARY EDEMA

Pulmonary edema is the abnormal accumulation of fluid in the alveolar sacs and in the interstitial spaces surrounding the alveoli. Pulmonary edema is classified by its underlying causes: *Cardiogenic* causes include left ventricular failure, mitral valve stenosis, cardiogenic shock, hypertension, and cardiomyopathy. *Noncardiogenic* causes are shown in Box 63-1. Pulmonary edema can also develop after catastrophic injury to the CNS, such as head injury; this form of pulmonary edema is called *neurogenic* pulmonary edema.

Etiology

Normally, fluid moves into the interstitial space at the arterial end of the capillary as a result of hydrostatic pressure in the vessel and returns to the venous end of the capillary because of oncotic pressure and increases in interstitial hydrostatic pressure (see the Anatomy and

---

evolve **Web Enhancements**

Bridge to Home Health Care   Living with a Ventilator

Concept Map   Understanding ARDS and Its Treatment

Be sure to check out the bonus material on the Evolve website and the CD-ROM, including free self-assessment exercises. **http://evolve.elsevier.com/Black/medsurg**

- Aspiration of gastric contents, especially if a large amount of HCl is present
- Barotrauma (e.g., with PEEP with mechanical ventilation)
- Drugs (e.g., after administration of narcotics)
- Fluid overload from IV fluids or renal failure
- Hypoalbuminemia (e.g., nephrotic syndrome, hepatic disease, malnutrition)
- Sepsis
- Inhalation of toxic chemicals (e.g., sulfur dioxide, paraquat, phosgene, chlorine, nitrogen oxides)
- High altitudes (>8000 ft)
- Neurogenic stimulus (e.g., increased intracranial pressure, epileptic seizures, head trauma)
- Near-drowning syndrome
- Mechanical ventilation, oxygen toxicity, ARDS
- Malignancies blocking outflow of lymph within the lungs
- Pancreatitis
- Pneumonia
- Smoke inhalation (e.g., trapped in a burning building)
- Unilaterally, after reexpansion of collapsed lung (pneumothorax)

ARDS, Adult (acute) respiratory distress syndrome; *HCl,* hydrochloric acid; *IV,* intravenous; *PEEP,* positive end-expiratory pressure.

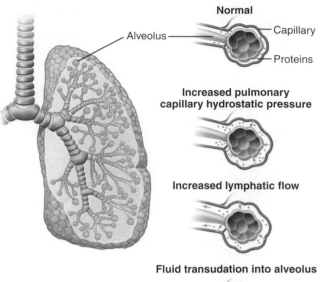

■ **FIGURE 63–1** Progression of pulmonary edema. Pulmonary edema occurs when capillary hydrostatic pressure is increased, promoting movement of fluid into the interstitial space of the alveolar-capillary membrane. Initially, increased lymphatic flow removes the excess fluids, but continued leakage eventually overwhelms this mechanism. Gas exchange becomes impaired by the thick membrane. Increasing interstitial fluid pressure ultimately causes leaks into the alveolar sacs, impairing ventilation and gas exchange.

Physiology Review for Unit 3). Fluid movement through the lung is no different; in fact, fluid in the interstitial spaces of the lungs is not uncommon. It normally escapes from the microcirculation and enters the interstitium, providing nutrients for the cells. The residual fluid is returned via the lymphatic system. Increased volume of fluid in the pulmonary arteries from obstruction of forward flow is the most common cause of pulmonary edema, and heart failure is the most common example of the obstruction of forward flow. Lung tumors can obstruct lymphatic flow and lead to pulmonary edema.

Pathophysiology

Increased hydrostatic pressure in the pulmonary vessels creates an imbalance in the Starling forces, resulting in an increase of fluid filtration into the interstitial spaces of the lung that exceeds the lymphatic capacity to drain the fluid away. Increasing volumes of fluid leak into the alveolar spaces (Figure 63-1). The lymphatic system attempts to compensate by draining excess interstitial fluid volume through the hilar lymph nodes and back into the vascular system. If this pathway becomes overwhelmed, fluid moves from the pleural interstitium into the alveolar walls. If the alveolar epithelium is damaged, the fluid begins to accumulate in the alveoli. Alveolar edema is a serious late manifestation in the progression of fluid imbalance.

Hypoxemia develops when the alveolar membrane is thickened by fluid hindering the exchange of oxygen

and CO_2. As fluid fills the interstitium and alveolar spaces, lung compliance decreases and oxygen diffusion is impaired. If pulmonary edema has developed because of left ventricular failure, right ventricular failure may occur because the pulmonary artery pressure is elevated. This elevation increases afterload for the right ventricle, resulting in increased workload of the heart and manifestations of right ventricular failure.

Clinical Manifestations

The manifestations of pulmonary edema are due to failure of the regulatory factors guiding fluid movement. Most manifestations are seen in the respiratory system and include marked dyspnea, tachypnea, weak and thready tachycardia, hypertension (if cardiogenic), orthopnea at less than 90 degrees, and the use of accessory muscles to aid breathing. The client's frequent coughing is an attempt to rid the chest of fluid. The sputum is thin and frothy because it is combined with water. If the hydrostatic pressure is very high, small capillaries break and sputum becomes pink tinged. The client may be anxious from dyspnea and restless from hypoxemia. Chest auscultation reveals crackles, wheezes, and the presence of an S_3 heart sound. A heart murmur may be noted if the cause is mitral valve disease. Pulse oximetry readings are commonly less than 85% and arterial blood gas (ABG) determinations may reveal an arterial Pao_2 of less than 50 mm Hg. Respiratory alkalosis is common because of the tachypnea. Pressure in the pulmonary artery and pulmonary artery wedge pressure (PAWP) are elevated. The chest x-ray shows areas of "whiteout" where fluid has replaced air-filled lung tissue, which normally appears black. Right ventricular failure may also be noted, with manifestations of hepatomegaly, jugular venous distention, and peripheral edema.

OUTCOME MANAGEMENT

Medical Management

Medical management concentrates on the following four areas: (1) correction of hypoxemia, (2) reduction in preload, (3) reduction of afterload, and (4) support of perfusion.

Correct Hypoxemia

It is imperative to maintain adequate oxygenation. Clients with severe pulmonary edema commonly require oxygen therapy at high Fio_2 levels and may require noninvasive positive- pressure ventilation (NPPV) such as continuous positive airway pressure (CPAP) or mechanical ventilation if they cannot meet the work of breathing. NPPV is any type of respiratory support that does not require endotracheal tube (ET) intubation.

Reduce Preload

The client is placed in an upright position. Usually, the client does not want to lie down because of orthopnea and a feeling of choking when supine. Diuretics are prescribed to promote fluid excretion. Nitrates, such as nitroglycerin, are used for their vasodilating properties, decreasing the workload of the heart muscle. Other management strategies consist of treating the underlying condition.

Reduce Afterload

Afterload is reduced to diminish workload on the left ventricle. Antihypertensive agents, including potent agents such as nitroprusside, are prescribed. Angiotensin-converting enzyme (ACE) inhibitors are considered essential in the treatment of pulmonary edema from congestive heart failure. ACE inhibitors reduce afterload and improve stroke volume and cardiac output. There is also a slight reduction in preload when renal perfusion is improved and diuresis begins. Morphine is prescribed to reduce the sympathetic nervous system response and to reduce anxiety from the dyspnea.

Support Perfusion

The left ventricle is supported by using inotropic medications such as dobutamine, dopamine, and norepinephrine. Nesiritide is also used to decrease PCWP, pulmonary artery pressure, right atrial pressure, and systemic vascular resistance while increasing cardiac output. Urine output is monitored closely to determine whether renal perfusion is adequate. An intra-aortic balloon pump (IABP) may be required with severe heart failure and pulmonary edema (see Chapter 55).

Nursing Management

Assessment. The client with pulmonary edema is assessed quickly on admission, concentrating on only the information and assessment findings essential to begin treatment. The client is typically anxious and having significant shortness of breath. Managing the client's anxiety and reducing the dyspnea are imperative. A complete assessment is carried out over the following hours, when the client can breathe more comfortably and answer questions. A baseline weight and lung assessment is essential, because these parameters will assist in determining the effectiveness of treatments.

Diagnosis, Outcomes, Interventions
Diagnosis: Impaired Gas Exchange. The fluid-filled alveoli block the exchange of gases. Use the nursing diagnosis *Impaired Gas Exchange related to capillary membrane obstruction from fluid* to plan care. This is the priority diagnosis.

Outcomes. The client will demonstrate improved gas exchange, as evidenced by rising Pao_2 to 55 or 60 mm Hg, oxygen saturation above 90%, normalizing pH, decreasing anxiety and dyspnea, and fewer crackles and wheezing within 12 hours.

Interventions. Monitor vital signs every 15 minutes initially, until the client is stable. Administer oxygen as ordered using a high-flow rebreather bag to maintain oxygenation. Titrate the actual liter flow of oxygen to maintain saturation above 90%.

> **Continuous assessment is needed because the client may not be able to tolerate the work of breathing and may quickly require NPPV or endotracheal (ET) intubation with mechanical ventilation. NPPV, mechanical ventilation, and intubation equipment should be readily available.**

SAFETY

ALERT

To reduce preload, position the client with the legs in a dependent position. Raising edematous legs increases venous return and will stress the overtaxed left ventricle. Preload is reduced with morphine and nitroglycerin. Because perfusion to the skin is often compromised, repositioning is important.

Air hunger can lead to panic and feelings of suffocation. Administering opioids (morphine) and anxiolytics to control both dyspnea and anxiety will relax the client and improve breathing. Stay with the client and use breathing techniques to support the client.

Diagnosis: Excess Fluid Volume. Accumulation of fluid from several causes leads to fluid overload. Use the nursing diagnosis *Excess Fluid Volume related to excess preload.*

Outcomes. The client will demonstrate improved fluid balance, as evidenced by diuresis (input less than output), decreased number of crackles and wheezes, eupnea, weight loss, resolving peripheral edema, decreased anxiety, and normalizing blood urea nitrogen levels.

Interventions. Administer a diuretic (furosemide is the most common) as prescribed to promote diuresis. Place an indwelling catheter to monitor response to diuretics. Monitor urine output hourly, weight, and potassium levels (potassium loss is a side effect of furosemide). Monitor blood pressure to determine whether the client can maintain perfusion without inotropic support. Because oral fluids are restricted, oral hygiene is completed every 2 hours.

Evaluation. If the previously described interventions are implemented immediately, a fairly rapid response to diuresis and oxygen therapy should be seen. It is not uncommon to diurese several liters of fluid, resulting in dramatic weight loss and reduction of dyspnea.

Self-Care

Consider the reasons for development of pulmonary edema when developing a plan for self-care. Clients may need further education on daily weights, dietary choices, and scheduling of medications. Instruct the client and family members on the early manifestations of fluid overload so that early intervention is possible.

ACUTE VENTILATORY FAILURE

Ventilatory failure is the inability of the body to sustain respiratory drive or the inability of the chest wall and muscles to mechanically move air in and out of the lungs. The hallmark of ventilatory failure is an elevated CO_2 level.

Etiology and Risk Factors

In acute ventilatory failure, the respiratory load placed on the lung to exchange oxygen and CO_2 is impaired by (1) problems of resistance to moving air in and out of the lung, (2) the ability of the lung to expand and contract (elastic recoil), and (3) conditions that increase the production of CO_2 or decrease the surface available for exchange of gases. The competence of the nerves and muscles coordinating the movement of the chest can also be impaired by loss of drive to breathe, impaired transmission of signals to the chest and diaphragm, and muscle fatigue.

Pathophysiology

Alveolar ventilation is maintained by the CNS acting through nerves and the muscles of respiration to drive breathing. Failure of alveolar ventilation leads to a ventilation-perfusion (expressed as $\dot{V}/\dot{Q}$) mismatch resulting in hypercapnia (rising CO_2 levels) and eventually acidosis develops. Left untreated, acute ventilatory failure leads to death.

Functional residual capacity (FRC) is the volume of air remaining in the lung after normal expiration. In obstructive forms of ventilatory failure, the residual pressure in the chest impairs inhalation and increases the workload of breathing. When end-expiratory alveolar volumes remain above their critical closing point, the alveoli remain open and functioning, allowing oxygen to diffuse into the bloodstream. If alveolar volumes fall below the closing point, the alveoli tend to collapse. When alveoli collapse, no oxygenation or blood flow to the alveoli occurs (Figure 63-2). In acute ventilatory failure, the residual volume and FRC are decreased, resulting in a true intrapulmonary shunt (perfusion without oxygenation) and decreased lung compliance.

Once alveolar collapse occurs, reinflation necessitates very high opening pressures, the generation of which significantly increases the work of breathing. The hypoxemia resulting from alveolar collapse and the increased oxygen consumption caused by the increased work of breathing may severely compromise the client.

Clinical Manifestations

To avoid frank apnea, recognizing impending ventilatory failure is critical. Continuous monitoring of high-risk clients concentrating on changes in respiratory rate and depth, mental status, and patterns of breathing is essential. The hallmark manifestations of hypercapnia are headache and dyspnea. The client may also verbalize that dyspnea is increasing despite treatment. Altered respiratory patterns can herald impending ventilatory failure. The client's respiratory rate can rise to 50 to 60 breaths/min, but the breaths are shallow and impaired by spasm of the airway. The rate can also fall to 4 to 6 breaths/min. Clients become confused and less conversant, and

■ FIGURE 63–2 Effects of positive airway pressure on the alveolus. **A,** The collapsed alveolus continues to be perfused with blood, but cannot exchange oxygen for carbon dioxide. **B,** The alveolus is opened by positive pressure.

are difficult to arouse. Electrolyte abnormalities, caused by a falling pH level, may cause cardiac dysrhythmias. If the cause of ventilatory failure is obstruction of the airway, the systolic blood pressure falls during inspiration as a result of intrathoracic resistance. This change, called *pulsus paradoxus,* is present when systolic blood pressure falls more than 10 mm Hg during inspiration. Pulse oximetry indicates steadily decreasing oxygen saturation values, and ABG analysis shows falling Pao_2 and rising $Paco_2$ values.

OUTCOME MANAGEMENT

Medical Management

Medical management is directed at reversing bronchospasm, maintaining oxygenation, treating the underlying problem, and providing ventilatory assistance. Mechanical ventilation is not used until other methods of maintaining ventilation have been tried.

Reverse Bronchospasm

Several forms of bronchodilators are used to treat obstructions to airflow in clients with COPD and asthma. These agents include inhaled beta$_2$-selective agonists (albuterol), ipratropium, corticosteroids, and rarely theophylline. If infection is the underlying cause, broad-spectrum antibiotics are given.

Maintain Oxygenation

Oxygen by mask may be adequate to support oxygenation. Using forms of NPPV such as CPAP reduces the workload of breathing by decreasing the force needed to overcome the pressure in the chest. Outcomes after mechanical ventilation with lower tidal volumes may be better than the traditional formula (10 to 15 ml of body weight per kilogram), which sometimes lead to stretch-induced lung injury.

Manage the Underlying Problem

There are many causes of ventilatory failure. Some of these causes can be quickly managed, such as reversing opiate overdose with naloxone, but others require more aggressive treatment. Supportive therapies are used to reverse or control the underlying problem.

Maintain Ventilation

Initially, NPPV should be used if the client is alert and can maintain the mask over the nose or mouth without becoming claustrophobic. NPPV keeps small airways open and improves gas exchange with the goal being to keep oxygen saturation above 90%. Frequent ABG readings may need to be taken to ensure that adequate oxygenation is being achieved. If NPPV is not successful,

mechanical ventilation is required and helps to minimize the work of breathing while effectively promoting gas exchange (oxygenation and ventilation). The client requires an artificial airway, usually by ET intubation and the use of positive-pressure ventilation (PPV). If prolonged intubation is required, the ET tube is replaced with a tracheostomy.

Endotracheal Intubation

Intubation

The ET tube is a long, slender, hollow tube usually made of polyvinyl chloride and is inserted into the trachea via the mouth or nose. In addition to providing a connection for ventilators, the ET tube provides a stable airway and facilitates removal of secretions. However, it allows the normal respiratory defenses to be bypassed and may reduce cough effectiveness. The ET tube also prevents verbal communication. It passes through the vocal cords, and the distal tip is positioned just above the bifurcation of the main stem of the bronchus (carina). Oral intubation is usually used for short-term airway management. Nasal intubation, a more secure method, is believed to be more comfortable because the tube does not move as much in the airway. However, nasal intubation is not being used much because of the risk of sinusitis. Before intubation, the client is supine, and all dental bridgework and plates and loose teeth are removed because these items can be jarred loose and aspirated during the procedure. The client's head is hyperextended, the lower aspect of the neck is flexed, and the mouth is opened (Figure 63-3). This position brings the mouth, pharynx, and larynx into a straight line. A laryngoscope is used to hold the airway open, expose the vocal cords, and serve as a guide for the tube into the trachea. ET tubes are inserted only by fully trained health care team members.

Intubation should not cause or exacerbate hypoxia. If the client's neck and mandible are mobile, the procedure usually takes about 30 seconds. Certain pre-existing conditions such as obesity with a stocky neck, a possible spinal cord injury, or rheumatoid arthritis of the neck can make intubation difficult. For clients with expected difficulty of intubation, an oxygen mask can be used to provide oxygen through the mouth. An oxygen saturation monitor may also be used to warn of hypoxemia.

A good practice to remember during difficult intubation is to hold your breath while intubation is attempted. If you must stop to breathe before the client is intubated, the intubation is taking too long. Stop the intubation, reoxygenate the client by mask, and reattempt intubation.

Immediately after ET tube insertion, tube placement is verified by auscultation and chest x-ray to ensure aeration of both sides of the chest. An end-tidal CO_2 monitor and assessment of oxygen saturation levels are also indications of correct ET tube placement. Record in the nurses' notes and on the respiratory flow sheet the point

■ **FIGURE 63-3 A,** A laryngoscope is used to visualize the vocal cords. **B,** The endotracheal tube is inserted with the client's head extended to align the airway.

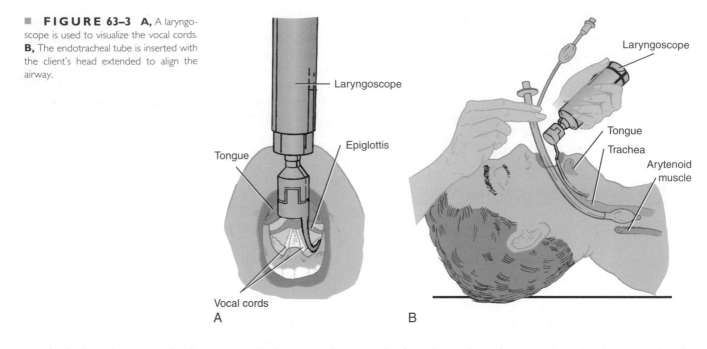

A

B

at which the tube meets the lips or nostrils by using the numbers listed on the side of the ET tube. If the tube slips, its correct position can be reestablished quickly. Secure the ET tube immediately after intubation with adhesive tape, twill tape, or specially designed ET tube holders (Figure 63-4). Current recommendations favor the use of commercial ET tube holders to minimize the

■ **FIGURE 63-4** Secured cuffed endotracheal tube with closed tracheal suction system. *(From Sill, J.R. [1991]. Respiratory care certification guide.* St. Louis: Mosby.)

risk of unplanned extubations. Retaping is required only if the tape becomes loose or soiled.

Cuff Inflation

The cuff of an ET tube seals the tube against the tracheal wall to facilitate PPV and protects the respiratory tract from aspiration of foreign material. The amount of air required to seal an ET tube cuff is reflected by the cuff pressure, which is usually maintained at less than 20 mm Hg. Most ET tubes are designed with soft plastic cuffs for use with high volumes of air at low pressures. Cuffs are inflated with a volume of air high enough to seal the trachea while exerting the lowest possible pressure on the tracheal wall. Low cuff pressure is necessary to prevent damage to the tracheal mucosa. Arterial pressures in the tracheal wall are approximately 20 to 25 mm Hg; venous pressures are 18 to 20 mm Hg. Therefore cuff pressures greater than 18 to 20 mm Hg impair circulation to the tracheal mucosa and necrosis may develop. Assess cuff pressures every 8 hours or as institutional policy dictates.

The most common method of cuff inflation *(minimal occlusion volume technique)* aims to provide an adequate seal in the trachea at the lowest possible cuff pressure. Slowly inject air into the cuff while auscultating with a stethoscope placed over the larynx (over the cuff) during a positive-pressure breath. At the point when sounds (from air movement) cease, inflation is stopped, indicating that the cuff is sealed against the tracheal wall.

Cuff Deflation

Generally, ET cuffs should remain inflated at all times. If cuff deflation is required for any reason, suction the trachea (with the client being hyperventilated and hyperoxygenated before and during this procedure) and clean the area above the cuff of secretions by gently suctioning deep into the oropharynx. Advance the suction catheter to the end of the ET tube and deflate the cuff while applying suction to the suction catheter so that any secretions lying above the cuff can be removed. If necessary, repeat pharyngeal suctioning.

Cuff Leaks

Cuff leaks can be a major problem. They may be caused by a rupture or tear in the cuff or pilot system or by a change in ET tube position in the trachea. There are several signs of a leak in or around the ET tube cuff, including the pilot balloon not filling when air is injected, the client can talk when the cuff is inflated, or air is heard leaking during positive-pressure breathing.

If the system is not functional, the ET tube may need to be replaced. Before replacement, increasing tidal volume may help maintain ventilation by compensating for the escaping gas. The client is at high risk for aspiration while the cuff is leaking.

Continuous Mechanical Ventilation

Normal respiration begins with the contraction of the diaphragm and respiratory muscles to create negative pressure in the chest: A vacuum is created and air flows in. When a ventilator is used, positive pressure (rather than negative pressure) forces air into the lungs. The positive pressure is necessary for gas exchange and to keep alveoli open. Unfortunately, positive-pressure forces can also damage the alveoli and may retard venous return and cardiac output. Trauma from high pressures in a ventilator is called barotrauma; the prefix "baro" means pressure. The high-risk groups for barotrauma include those clients with underlying lung disease.

The goals of continuous mechanical ventilation (CMV) are the following:

- To maintain adequate ventilation
- To deliver precise concentrations of Fio_2
- To deliver adequate tidal volumes to obtain an adequate minute ventilation and oxygenation
- To lessen the work of breathing in those clients who cannot sustain adequate ventilation on their own
- To prevent complications from the underlying problems

Modes of Ventilation

The ventilation mode refers to the way the client receives breaths from the ventilator. A control panel of one ventilator system is shown in Figure 63-5. Two common types of mechanical ventilation include volume-cycled and pressure-cycled. When selecting a mode of

■ **FIGURE 63–5**   Nellcor Puritan Bennett 760 Ventilator. *(Courtesy Mallinckrodt, Inc., Nellcor Puritan Bennett Ventilator Division.)*

ventilation, it is important to consider which mode will provide for adequate gas exchange while synchronizing with the clients own respiratory efforts, while decreasing the potential for barotrauma.

Pressure-cycled ventilation delivers a volume of gas to the airway using positive pressure during inspiration. This positive pressure is delivered until the preselected pressure has been reached. When the preset pressure is reached, the ventilator will cycle into passive exhalation. A disadvantage to this type of ventilation is that the volume delivered may not be sufficient depending on the compliance of the lung and the integrity of the ventilatory circuit (e.g., kinked tubing).

Volume-cycled (volume-controlled or *volume-limited) ventilation* delivers a preset tidal volume of inspired gas. The tidal volume has been preselected based on the ideal body weight, and is delivered to the client regardless of the pressure required to deliver this volume. The ventilator will automatically adjust the pressure needed to deliver the preset volume. If the client's breathing has become shallow, the ventilator will increase pressure to continue delivering the preset volume. A pressure limit can be set to prevent the occurrence of dangerously high airway pressures.

Table 63-1 describes several conventional modes of CMV. *Assist-control (A/C) ventilation* will deliver a preset volume of gas each time the client initiates a breath. If the client fails to initiate a breath within a preset amount of time, the ventilator will deliver a breath at a predetermined volume and rate. Each breath, whether client or ventilator generated, is delivered to a preset tidal volume or pressure limit. *Synchronous intermittent mandatory ventilation (SIMV)* delivers the preset volume or pressure breath for only those breaths that are ventilator initiated. Additional breaths are the result of the client's own efforts. The ventilator-delivered breaths are synchronized with the client's spontaneous breaths. This mode is often used for ventilator weaning.

When clients have special ventilation or oxygenation needs, a high-frequency ventilation mode may be indicated. High-frequency ventilation allows the delivery of smaller tidal volumes using a high-speed ventilation rate, up to as high as 360 breaths/min. The advantage of this mode is a decreased risk for alveolar trauma. Clients must be sedated to tolerate this type of ventilation. There are three types of high-frequency ventilation: high-frequency jet ventilation, high-frequency positive-pressure ventilation, and high-frequency oscillation. The most common indication for use is adult respiratory distress syndrome. It is also used in neonatal or pediatric clients.

Triggering Mechanisms

All breaths given to the client must be initiated or triggered. Triggering mechanisms can be based on (1) time, (2) negative pressure, (3) flow, or (4) volume.

Time-triggered inhalation is used to manage clients who cannot breathe on their own. The ventilator will trigger a breath after a preset time, serving as a backup in case a client's own breathing rate falls below a preset value.

Negative pressure inhalation is triggered by the initial negative pressure that begins inspiration. As soon as the client initiates a breath, the ventilator is triggered to produce inhalation. The sensitivity of the system is set to reduce the workload of breathing. Pressure fluctuations (e.g., hiccoughs, leaks) can cause premature triggering.

Flow-triggered inhalation occurs when the client can initiate a breath. The ventilator completes the breath by sensing the flow of air into the chest. This system works well in combination with positive end-expiratory pressure (PEEP).

Volume-triggered ventilation occurs when the ventilator completes the breath to maximize inhaled gas volumes.

TABLE 63–1 Modes of Mechanical Ventilation		
Mode of Ventilation	**Clinical Application**	**Nursing Implications**
Continuous mandatory ventilation (CMV), also known as assist control A/C, delivers gas at preset tidal volumes	Primary ventilatory mode in clients who are apneic or have weak respiratory efforts	May hyperventilate Sedation may be needed to control spontaneous breaths
Pressure controlled ventilation delivers gas at preset pressures over a set inspiratory time	Primary ventilatory mode for clients with changing pulmonary mechanics, such as airway resistance or lung compliance (e.g., ARDS)	Increased thoracic pressure may lead to decreased cardiac output for impaired venous return Requires sedation and/or paralysis
Pressure support ventilation	Primary ventilatory mode for clients with stable respiratory drive to overcome airway resistance from ET tube Primary weaning mode	Client should have less work to breathe Monitor for hypercapnia
Intermittent mandatory ventilation	Primary ventilatory mode for clients with decreased lung compliance or increased airway resistance Occasionally used for weaning	Monitor for hypercapnia

Safety and Alarms

Ventilators have several alarms to assist with their safe use.

SAFETY

⚠

ALERT

Alarms should be ON at all times to alert the caregiver to changes in the client's condition and hazardous situations such as unplanned extubation. Emergency equipment such as a hand-held resuscitation bag should be readily available. *High-pressure* alarms are triggered when there is increased airway resistance or decreased lung compliance. Increased airway resistance may be caused by secretions, bronchospasm, ET tube dislodgement or biting, coughing, or kinked ventilatory circuit tubing. Decreased lung compliance may be caused by pulmonary edema, pneumothorax, atelectasis, or acute respiratory distress syndrome. *Low-pressure* or *low-minute* volume alarms are caused by disconnected tubing, ET tube cuff leak, or apnea. An alarm should never be silenced until the cause has been investigated and corrected. If the source of the alarm cannot be determined, disconnect the client from the ventilator and use a hand-held resuscitation bag for manual ventilation with 100% oxygen until the problem can be resolved.

The Bridge to Critical Care feature on p. 1644 provides additional discussion of the alarm systems most commonly seen with ventilators.

Client-Ventilator Dyssynchrony

Ventilators breathe into the client through positive pressure (normal inhalation is through negative pressure), and this change in inhalation can lead to uncoordinated breathing. Ideally, the client should inhale and exhale when the ventilator inhales and exhales. When the client is not "in sync" with the ventilator, it appears that the client is "fighting" or "bucking" the ventilator. To avoid this problem, the ventilator is set to sense the client's own inhalation efforts and to support any spontaneous breathing. Also the patency of the ET tube should be confirmed by suctioning. If adjusting the ventilator settings does not help, the client may need to be sedated.

Positive End-Expiratory Pressure/Continuous Positive Airway Pressure

The techniques PEEP and CPAP are applied during expiration to prevent intrathoracic pressures from returning to ambient atmospheric pressure. CPAP is applied to a client with spontaneous respiration; PEEP is applied during mechanical ventilation. CPAP and PEEP are used to apply positive airway pressure that keeps the alveoli open and reduces the amount of shunting with the goal that the Fio_2 may be reduced to the lowest possible level to maintain gas exchange and to prevent oxygen toxicity. This increased pressure also increases functional residual capacity (FRC) and enhances oxygenation as a result of the enlarged surface area that is available for diffusion. In normal conditions, 10 cm H_2O is needed to keep the alveoli open. High tidal volumes and continuous cyclic expansion and collapse of the alveoli deplete surfactant in the alveoli and create the need for higher PEEP. Positive pressures of 10 to 25 cm H_2O are typically used in adults. Pressures may be adjusted until the level is found that produces the best Pao_2 without producing adverse effects. This level is called "best PEEP."

Risks of PEEP include overdistention of the alveoli, $\dot{V}/\dot{Q}$ mismatch, subcutaneous emphysema, and decreased cardiac output from increased intrathoracic pressure.

Physiologic Changes After Mechanical Ventilation

Many physiologic changes occur when a client is placed on mechanical ventilation. Decreased cardiac output is the most common of these. Normal unassisted respiration begins with subatmospheric pressure. Negative pressure increases during inhalation and decreases during exhalation. Positive pressure applied to the airway has the opposite effect. As positive pressure inflates the lungs, the pressure in the thorax builds, decreasing the flow of blood to the vena cava and to the right atrium of the heart. Exhalation is passive and pressures return to the normal resting subatmospheric level. Blood flow to and from the right ventricle is also decreased if PPV is continued for more than a few minutes. This, in turn, decreases the filling of the left ventricle, leading to a lowered cardiac output. The lowered cardiac output is reflected in the hypotension that clients commonly exhibit immediately after initiating mechanical ventilation. It is imperative that blood pressures be monitored closely.

Positive pressure may also briefly affect the left side of the heart by increased filling and output. This increase is due to the displacement of blood from the pulmonary system into the left ventricle. However, this effect is noted only immediately after institution of PPV.

PPV may lead to stretch injury in the alveoli and the release of inflammatory mediators. To minimize stretch injury, the lowest possible tidal volume and PEEP should be used.

Other body systems are also affected by PPV. During the inspiratory phase, the diaphragm descends into the abdomen, resulting in decreased blood flow to the splanchnic area, leading to ischemia of the gastric mucosa. Ischemia of the gastric mucosa may be one of the reasons that clients receiving PPV for an extended period have a high incidence of gastrointestinal bleeding and stress ulcerations. Decreasing blood flow to the splanchnic region also results in decreased blood flow to the kidneys. Decreased blood flow signals the posterior pituitary gland to increase secretion of vasopressin (antidiuretic hormone [ADH]). Elevated vasopressin levels lead to reabsorption of free water in the renal tubular cells, thereby increasing water retention. Lymphatic flow also decreases.

BRIDGE TO CRITICAL CARE

Troubleshooting Alarms

Display Message	Possible Cause	Remedy
High continuous pressure	Airway pressure higher than set PEEP plus 15 cm H_2O for more than 15 sec	Check client Check circuit Check ventilator settings and alarm limits
Check tubings	Disconnected pressure transducer (expiratory) Blocked pressure transducer (expiratory) Water in expiratory limb of ventilator Wet bacterial filter Clogged bacterial filter	Check ventilator internals on expiratory side Refer to service Replace filter Remove water from tubing and check humidifier settings (i.e., relative humidity) Check heater wires in humidifier (if present)
Airway pressure too high *Note:* If airway pressure rises 6 cm H_2O above set upper pressure limit, the safety valve opens Safety valve also opens if system pressure exceeds 120 cm H_2O	Kinked or blocked client tubing Mucus or secretion plug in endotracheal tube or in airways Client coughing or fighting ventilator Inspiratory flow rate too high Improper alarm setting	Check client Check ventilator settings and alarm limits
Limited pressure *Note:* Alarm is active only in PRVC and VS modes	Kinked or blocked client tubing Mucus or secretion plug in endotracheal tube or in airways Client coughing or fighting ventilator Improper alarm setting Client's lung/thorax compliance decreasing Client's airway resistance increasing	Check ventilator settings and alarm limits
Expired minute volume too high	Increased client activity Ventilator self-triggering (autocycling) Improper alarm limit setting Wet flow transducer	Check client Check trigger sensitivity setting Check alarm limit settings Dry the flow transducer
Expired minute volume too low	Low spontaneous client breathing activity Leakage in cuff Leakage in client circuit Improper alarm limit setting	Check client Check cuff pressure Check client circuit (perform leakage test if necessary) Check pause time and graphics to verify Consider more ventilatory support for client
Expired minute volume display reads 0	Flow transducer faulty Circuit disconnected from client	Replace flow transducer Connect Y-piece to client
Apnea alarm *Note:* If in VS, ventilator will revert to PRVC; back-up rate and time must be set	Time between two consecutive inspiratory efforts exceeds: Adult: 20 sec Pediatric: 15 sec Neonate: 10 sec	Check client Check ventilator settings
PEEP/CPAP and/or plateau pressure fails to be maintained	Leakage in cuff Leakage in client circuit Improper alarm limit setting	Check cuff pressure Check client circuit (perform leakage test if necessary) Check pause time and graphics to verify Consider more ventilatory support for client

Modified from *Servo Ventilator 300 operating manual 8.0* (1996). Solna, Sweden: Siemens-Elema AB. *CPAP,* Continuous positive airway pressure; *PEEP,* positive end-expiratory pressure; *PRVC,* pressure-regulated volume control; *VS,* volume support.

In addition, PPV can cause neurophysiologic changes. When the oxygenation levels improve in a client with respiratory failure, cerebral oxygenation also improves. A client with compensated *respiratory acidosis* (chronic CO_2 retention) may be adversely affected by positive-pressure breathing because too much CO_2 is exhaled, or "blown off." If acute respiratory alkalosis occurs, the client may exhibit dizziness, lightheadedness, and anxiety. If severe alkalosis persists, convulsions, cardiac dysrhythmias, and cerebral edema may occur. Cerebral edema may also contribute to intensive care unit (ICU) psychosis.

Oxygen toxicity can develop in clients who receive oxygen at concentrations greater than 70% for as little as 16 to 24 hours. Oxygen free radicals are produced in excess of their normal consumption by antioxidants; oxygen free radicals damage cell membranes, which increases the risk of pulmonary fibrosis. Manifestations of oxygen toxicity include fatigue, lethargy, weakness, restlessness, and nausea and vomiting. Later manifestations include severe dyspnea, coughing, tachycardia, tachypnea, crackles, and cyanosis. Because these manifestations are vague, oxygen concentration is limited to the minimal percentage and amount of time needed to maintain oxygenation.

Nursing Management

The nurse coordinates efforts of the health care team, teaches and supports the client and family, monitors the client's response to ventilation, intervenes to maintain oxygenation and ventilation, and ensures that the client's complex needs are met. The Care Plan feature on pp. 1646-1649 describes this coordinated care.

Neuromuscular Blocking Agents

Sedation with paralysis is often necessary to maintain ventilation by creating a synchronous respiratory pattern and reducing oxygen demand. In some clients, paralysis with neuromuscular blocking agents is also needed. The most common agents given are vecuronium (Norcuron) and pancuronium (Pavulon). Because neuromuscular blocking agents do not inhibit pain or awareness, they are combined with a sedative or an anxiolytic agent. Unfortunately, the use of paralytics has been linked to prolonged paralysis from either overdose of the medication or accumulation of active metabolites. Sedation assessment scales and/or bispectral index monitoring are techniques used to determine adequate sedation levels. Peripheral nerve stimulation, using a train-of-four (TOF) peripheral nerve stimulator, is commonly used to guide sustained paralysis. TOF delivers four low-energy impulses over a nerve; usually the ulnar nerve is used. When the ulnar nerve is stimulated, the response of the thumb is observed. The ideal response is two twitches of the thumb with four impulses. If no twitching is noted, the client is too paralyzed; if four twitches are noted, there is no

paralysis. There is some evidence that clients recall unusual dreams while under paralysis and sedation.

> **While necessary to provide comfort and facilitate treatment, careful monitoring to determine the minimum amount of sedation to meet treatment goals is important. Pain medication may also be required if the client has pain. If the client is awake, be aware of the anxiety or fear related to inability to breathe independently. Several nursing precautions are needed while these neuromuscular blocking agents are administered. Reorient the client often, and explain all procedures because the client can still hear but cannot move or see.**
>
> **Safety is a major concern because the client cannot verbalize or identify problems. Specific attention should be given to the eyes to prevent corneal abrasions and other eye injuries. Eye care with lubricating ointment is important.** SAFETY ⚠ ALERT

Suctioning

Because the client loses the ability to cough while on mechanical ventilation and secretions tend to pool and obstruct the airways, suctioning is often required.

> **The client should be suctioned through the ET tube only when needed to prevent hypoxemia and to prevent injury to bronchial and lung tissue. Priorities when suctioning a client include hyperoxygenation before suctioning and maintaining sterile technique including the use of the closed tracheal suction system (see Figure 63-4).** SAFETY ⚠ ALERT

See the nursing Care Plan on pp. 1646-1649 for additional guidelines for suctioning a client.

Complications of Mechanical Ventilation

There are several potential complications of mechanical ventilation. Ventilator-associated pneumonia (VAP) is a potentially avoidable nosocomial infection that occurs greater than 48 hours after mechanical ventilation. Clients that develop VAP are at increased risk of mortality as well as prolonged intubation times and increased ICU stays. The endotracheal tube provides a pathway for bacteria to enter the lower respiratory tract.

> **A major cause of VAP is colonization and aspiration of oropharyngeal secretions. Measures to prevent VAP include keeping the client's head of bed elevated at 30 degrees or higher and changing ventilator circuits only when visibly contaminated, providing frequent and thorough oral hygiene and meticulous suctioning techniques can prevent VAP.** SAFETY ⚠ ALERT

Other interventions found to be helpful in the prevention of VAP include stress ulcer and deep venous thrombosis prophylaxis. The Translating Evidence into Practice feature on p. 1650 describes additional nursing interventions to prevent or reduce this complication.

C A R E   P L A N   *evolve*

The Mechanically Ventilated Client

Nursing Diagnosis: Impaired Spontaneous Ventilation related to imbalance between ventilatory capacity and ventilatory demand.

Outcomes: The client will have a normal respiratory rate and pattern, return of arterial blood gases (ABGs) and pulse oximetry to normal, decreased dyspnea, absence of air trapping, and no complications after continuous mechanical ventilation (CMV).

| NOC OUTCOMES | Mechanical Ventilation Response |

Interventions	NIC INTERVENTIONS	Rationales
1. Check ventilator settings, Fio_2, alarms, connections, and endotracheal (ET) tube placement (use cm markings) at beginning of each shift, hourly thereafter, and after any changes. Ensure that alarms are functional.	Mechanical Ventilation	1. Determine baseline values, and validate that settings are accurate.
2. Assess lung sounds every 1-2 hours as indicated.	Mechanical Ventilation	2. Lung sounds should be present bilaterally (unless a previous change in lung sounds is known).
3. Check placement of the ET tube, and secure the tube. Check previous records for a mark that is visible (in cm).	Mechanical Ventilation	3. The visible portion of the ET tube should not change. Securing prevents dislodgment.
4. Use a bite block.	Mechanical Ventilation	4. A bite block prevents the client from chewing on the tube and ET tube compression.
5. Assess for pressure ulcers of skin or mucous membrane irritation every shift.	Skin Surveillance	5. Devices can cause pressure on the skin. ET tubes can place pressure on the lips and oral mucosa at the ET tube site.
6. Assess for agitation, distress, and "fighting" the ventilator.	Mechanical Ventilation	6. An incorrect ventilator setup may be providing less air than the client requires.
7. Assess for an obstructed airway. If it is obstructed, manually inflate lungs with a resuscitation bag and 100% oxygen and suction the airway.	Emergency Care	7. Airway obstruction with mucus may prevent oxygenation. Providing air to the client is imperative. A common cause of obstruction is retained secretions.
8. Sedate and paralyze the client if ventilator settings and oxygenation are adequate.	Mechanical Ventilation	8. Sedation and paralysis may be required to prevent mismatch.
9. Medicate the client if pain is present.	Comfort Care	9. Pain can lead to agitation.
10. Perform passive range-of-motion (ROM) or assisted ROM exercises and transfer the client to a chair when feasible.	Body Mechanics Promotion	10. Immobility leads to decreased respiratory muscle strength.

Evaluation: The timing of goal attainment will vary greatly because of underlying co-morbid conditions. Expect postoperative clients to require CMV for 24 hours or less. Clients with end-stage pulmonary disease may require prolonged ventilatory support.

Nursing Diagnosis: Impaired Gas Exchange and Ineffective Breathing Pattern related to underlying disease process and artificial airway and ventilator system.

Outcomes: The client will have improved gas exchange and breathing pattern, ventilation of both lungs, no manifestations of hypoxemia (O_2 saturation >90%, respiratory rate <24 breaths/min, no restlessness); arterial blood gases (ABGs) and acid-base balance will return to preintubation level or normal values.

| NOC OUTCOMES | Respiratory Status: Gas Exchange |

Interventions	NIC INTERVENTIONS	Rationales
1. Auscultate lung sounds and respiratory rate and pattern every 1 to 2 hours as needed.	Oxygen Therapy	1. Auscultation reveals the amount of fluid and secretion in the lungs, validates that the ET tube is placed correctly so that both lungs can be ventilated, and determines ventilatory effectiveness.
2. Provide adequate humidity via the ventilator or nebulizer.	Mechanical Ventilation	2. Replaces the function of the upper airway to warm and humidify the inspired air; thins secretions to facilitate their removal.
3. Turn and reposition the client every 2 hours.	Skin Integrity	3. Turning promotes the ventilation of both lungs and mobilization of secretions.
4. Monitor ABG values and pulse oximetry.	Oxygen Therapy	4. Degree of oxygenation can be indicated; lack of improvement in ABGs or falling oximetry may require a change in interventions.

Evaluation: If the client's underlying problem has been corrected by mechanical ventilation, these outcomes will be met quickly. If the client has a pre-existing pulmonary disease or is acutely ill, it may take several days for attainment of outcomes.

Nursing Diagnosis: Ineffective Airway Clearance related to inability to cough and stimulation of increased secretion formation in the lower tracheobronchial tree from the ET tube.

Outcomes: The client will have improved airway clearance, as evidenced by fewer crackles, fewer wheezes, and an absence of fever.

NOC OUTCOMES   Respiratory Status: Airway Patency

Interventions	NIC INTERVENTIONS	Rationales
1. Assess the need for suctioning: noisy, wet respirations; restlessness; increased pulse and respirations; visible mucus bubbling into the ET tube; and an increase in peak airway pressure.	Airway Suctioning	1. Detecting the need for suctioning early can prevent desaturation.
2. Thoroughly explain the procedure before starting, and provide reassurance to the client throughout.	Airway Suctioning	2. Suctioning can be an uncomfortable and frightening experience.
3. Airway suctioning is performed on an "as-needed" basis, not at regularly scheduled intervals.	Airway Suctioning	3. Suctioning can traumatize the airway and mucosa.
4. Select a catheter of appropriate size. The most common sizes for adults are 12F and 14F.	Airway Suctioning	4. The suction catheter should never exceed half the diameter of an artificial airway or the natural airway it is to enter.
5. Avoid excessive vacuum pressures that may traumatize the airway.	Airway Suctioning	5. The safe range of pressure for adults is 80 to 120 mm Hg.
6. Maintain sterility throughout the procedure. Use closed system for suctioning. Clean gloves can be used for closed suctioning; sterile gloves are needed for open suctioning.	Airway Suctioning	6. Usual cilia clearance and cough are suppressed. Closed systems avoid opening the ET tube and exposing the airway to the environment.
7. Hyperoxygenate before and after each suctioning attempt and after the procedure. Increase the Fio_2 on ventilator (remember to return to previous setting upon completion) or manually ventilate the client.	Airway Suctioning	7. Providing extra oxygen prevents desaturation from suctioning.
8. Instill saline infrequently and only when secretions are tenacious.	Airway Suctioning	8. Excess saline instillation before suctioning has been associated with pulmonary edema.

Evaluation: The ability to maintain a clear airway will require several days until the underlying problem (e.g., pneumonia) is stabilized and the client's strength returns.

Nursing Diagnosis: Anxiety related to dependence on CMV for breathing.

Outcomes: The client will exhibit decreased anxiety as evidenced by reduction in the level of stress or anxiety and decreased feelings of powerlessness.

NOC OUTCOMES   Anxiety

Interventions	NIC INTERVENTIONS	Rationales
1. Develop a means of communication.	Anxiety Reduction	1. Communication allows the client to have needs met.
2. Place a nurse-call device within the client's reach.	Anxiety Reduction	2. Anxiety is increased when fear of being alone is present.
3. Be available and visible.	Presence	3. The client's anxiety is alleviated when not alone.
4. Provide distractions (e.g., television, radio).	Calming Techniques	4. Anxiety is reduced because the client does not focus on the ventilator and noises.
5. Explain all procedures.	Anxiety Reduction	5. The client feels respected and fears are alleviated.
6. Medicate as necessary for anxiety.	Medication Administration	6. Antianxiety medications and opioids may be needed, but use them with caution during weaning because these drugs suppress respiratory drive.
7. Provide privacy.	Anxiety Reduction	7. Providing privacy demonstrates respect for the client.
8. Respect the client's rights and opinions.	Anxiety Reduction	8. The client feels respected and maintains dignity when included in discussion.
9. Provide a calm environment.	Calming Techniques	9. A frenzied environment engenders anxiety; if the client becomes anxious, ventilation is more difficult and oxygen needs increase.
10. Explain to the client and family that the client's vocal cords have been bypassed, which prevents talking; encourage them to use other modes of communication.	Emotional Support	10. Clients can hear and respond even though they cannot talk.

Evaluation: Expect the client to remain moderately anxious while receiving CMV.

(Continued)

The Mechanically Ventilated Client—Cont'd

Collaborative Problem. High Risk for Complications of CMV and Positive-Pressure Ventilation (PPV).
Outcomes: The nurse will monitor the client for pulmonary barotrauma, cardiovascular depression, inadvertent extubation, and improper positioning of the ET tube.

Interventions	NIC INTERVENTIONS	Rationales
1. Assess for acute, increasing, or severe dyspnea; agitation; panic; decreased or absent breath sounds; localized hyperresonance; increased breathing effort; tracheal deviation away from the side with abnormal findings; subcutaneous emphysema; and decreasing Pao_2 levels.	Mechanical Ventilation	1. Barotrauma can lead to pneumothorax or tension pneumothorax.
2. Assess for an acute or gradual fall in blood pressure, tachycardia (early manifestation), bradycardia (late manifestation), dysrhythmias, weak peripheral pulses, acute or gradual increase in pulmonary capillary wedge pressure (PCWP), and respiratory "swing" (depression) in arterial or pulmonary artery wave forms during inspiration.	Mechanical Ventilation	2. Cardiovascular depression can occur after an increase in tidal volume, positive end-expiratory pressure (PEEP), continuous positive airway pressure (CPAP), or with hyperinflation; positive pressure decreases venous return and cardiac output because of an increase in intrathoracic pressure.
3. Monitor for manifestations of inadvertent extubation: vocalization, low-pressure alarm, bilateral decrease in upper lobe airway sounds, gastric distention, clinical manifestations of inadequate ventilation; change in length of portion of ET tube that extends beyond the lip. If inadvertent extubation occurs, notify the physician, because reintubation may be necessary; manage ventilation and oxygenation with a self-inflating resuscitation bag.	Mechanical Ventilation	3. Inadvertent extubation can be obvious, as when the tube is found in the client's hand; it can also be obscure, as when the tube slips into the hypopharynx or esophagus.
4. Keep an intubation tray readily available.	Mechanical Ventilation	4. Intubation supplies may be needed quickly

Evaluation: Most complications of PPV occur within 48 hours after intubation. Inadvertent extubation can occur at any time.

Nursing Diagnosis: Risk for Infection related to impaired primary defenses in respiratory tract.
Outcomes: The client will remain free of infection, as evidenced by clear sputum, no fever, clear lung sounds, no increased difficulty with ventilation (e.g., increased peak inspiratory pressure), white blood cell (WBC) count within normal limits, and respiratory rate less than 24 breaths/min.

NOC OUTCOMES   Infection Severity

Interventions	NIC INTERVENTIONS	Rationales
1. Wash your hands thoroughly.	Infection Control	1. Hand-washing reduces spread of infection.
2. Use sterile technique for open suctioning.	Infection Control	2. The respiratory tract is considered sterile.
3. Monitor the client for increased breathing effort, localized changes on auscultation, and changes in Pao_2.	Respiratory Monitoring	3. Infected lung segments transmit sound differently (more solid) and do not permit gas exchange.
4. Provide oral care every 2 hours.	Infection Protection	4. The client's mouth becomes dry, and stomatitis may develop from lack of oral secretions.
5. Drain water from ventilator tubing; do not drain water back into the humidifier.	Infection Control	5. Water may become a source of contamination, especially from *Pseudomonas*.
6. Monitor laboratory values, WBC count, and differential.	Respiratory Monitoring	6. WBC count increases may indicate pulmonary infection.
7. Monitor sputum for changes in color, consistency, amount, and odor.	Respiratory Monitoring	7. Infection may cause sputum to increase, darken, thicken, and become malodorous.

Evaluation: Infection usually develops after 72 hours of intubation unless the client is immunosuppressed; then infection develops more rapidly.

Nursing Diagnosis: Imbalanced Nutrition: Less Than Body Requirements related to lack of ability to eat while on a ventilator and to increased metabolic needs.

Outcomes: The client will exhibit adequate nutritional intake, as evidenced by (1) stable weight or weight appropriate to height, (2) intake of adequate calorie levels, (3) no manifestations of catabolism, (4) wound healing, (5) absence of infection, (6) laboratory values within normal limits (prealbumin, total protein, transferrin), and (7) adequate muscle strength to breathe spontaneously.

NOC OUTCOMES	Nutritional Status	
Interventions	**NIC INTERVENTIONS**	**Rationales**
1. Provide adequate nutrition (high calorie intake, protein, vitamins, and minerals); provide a nutrition consult as needed.	Nutritional Therapy	1. Inadequate nutrition decreases diaphragmatic muscle mass, decreases pulmonary function, and increases mechanical ventilation requirements. Calorie and protein needs are calculated by a dietitian.
2. Begin tube-feeding as soon as it is evident that the client will remain on CMV for a length of time (usually 2-3 days).	Nutritional Therapy	2. The client should not be allowed to go into a catabolic state.
3. Avoid excessive carbohydrate loads.	Nutritional Therapy	3. Carbohydrate loads may increase carbon dioxide production to the point of producing hypercapnia.
4. Weigh the client daily.	Nutritional Monitoring	4. Changes in body weight are a reliable indicator of nutritional balance.
5. Monitor intake and output.	Nutritional Monitoring	5. Fluids are still required, and output should match intake.
6. Assess for complications of tube-feeding: aspiration, diarrhea, constipation. Position the client sitting upright for feeding, with the cuff inflated. Check for residual tube-feeding every 4 hours (continuous feeding) or before beginning another feeding (intermittent feeding).	Nutritional Therapy	6. Diarrhea is often caused by osmotic changes from an excessive concentration of tube-feeding or the use of sorbitol-based elixirs; consider reducing the concentration or changing to crushed pills. Constipation is caused by a lack of free water within the feeding; add 100 ml of water every 4 to 6 hours if allowable.
7. If the client cannot tolerate enteral feeding, consider parenteral nutrition to meet metabolic needs.	Nutritional Monitoring	7. Clients with decreased gastrointestinal function may require total parenteral feeding (TPN).
8. Monitor bowel sounds.	Nutritional Monitoring	8. Bowel obstruction and ileus present as changes in bowel sounds.
9. Before tube-feeding or between bolus feedings, obtain gastric pH and Hemoccult test every 8 hours.	Nutritional Therapy	9. A change in pH may indicate an increased risk of stress ulcer. A positive Hemoccult test indicates bleeding.

Evaluation: Malnutrition is preventable. Expect the client's weight to stabilize (unless there is fluid imbalance).

Nursing Diagnosis: Impaired Verbal Communication related to mute state when the ET tube is in place.

Outcomes: The client will be able to communicate with health care providers in order to have basic needs met.

NOC OUTCOMES	Communication	
Interventions	**NIC INTERVENTIONS**	**Rationales**
1. Help the client develop a means of communication. Keep a pencil and paper pad or a picture board readily available.	Communication Enhancement: Speech Deficit	1. With an ET tube passing through the vocal cords, the client cannot cough effectively or speak.
2. Be patient and willing to spend time communicating.	Communication Enhancement: Speech Deficit	2. Prevents feelings of frustration, and reduces anxiety.

Evaluation: Depending on pre-existing problems (language), disease-related problems (confusion), or treatment-related problems (restraints) affecting communication, the timing to develop effective communication may be long or short.

Nursing Diagnosis: Impaired Oral Mucous Membrane related to nothing by mouth (NPO) status.

Outcomes: The client's gums and mouth will remain moist and ulcer-free.

NOC OUTCOMES	Oral Hygiene	
Interventions	**NIC INTERVENTIONS**	**Rationales**
1. Provide oral hygiene every 2 hours, moistening the entire mouth and tongue.	Oral Health Restoration	1. Oral mucous membranes dry in 2 hours.
2. Moisten the mouth with solutions that do not contain alcohol or lemon.	Oral Health Restoration	2. Alcohol and lemon solutions dry mucous membranes.
3. Moisten lips with lubricant.	Oral Health Restoration	3. Lubricants prevent drying, cracking, and excoriation.
4. Brush the client's teeth twice daily.	Oral Health Restoration	4. Dental caries are prevented by saliva.
5. Suction oral secretions from mouth.	Oral Health Restoration	5. Secretions pool in the oropharynx because of the inflated tracheal cuff.
6. Assess for pressure areas from the ET tube and reposition daily.	Oral Health Restoration	6. ET tubes can lead to pressure ulcers on lips.

Evaluation: Oral mucous membranes can be restored to pink and moist within 24 hours. Oral care, however, is an ongoing need.

☞ TRANSLATING EVIDENCE INTO PRACTICE

Ventilator-Associated Pneumonia

Ventilator-associated pneumonia (VAP) is a nosocomial pneumonia that is a common problem in clients with ARDS, compared to other respiratory problems requiring mechanical ventilation. Bacteria may enter the respiratory tract from aspiration of oral-pharyngeal secretions or inhalation of aerosols containing bacteria. Aspiration is especially common in those clients who have decreased levels of consciousness, had devices or instruments in the lungs or gastrointestinal (GI) tract, or had surgery on the lungs or abdomen.

PREVENT GASTRIC REFLUX

Gram-negative bacillus infections from organisms originating in the GI tract are the most common. Usually bacteria are destroyed by acidic gastric pH, but when the pH is greater than 4 the bacteria can thrive. Tube feedings, histamines, and proton pump blockers contribute to lowering the gastric pH and have been associated with increased risk of pneumonias. Many ventilated clients have nasogastric tubes that predispose them to gastric reflux, which increases the risk of aspiration.[1] The most important intervention to prevent gastric reflux is elevation of the head of the bed. Unless medically contraindicated, the bed of a client on mechanical ventilation should remain elevated 30 to 45 degrees at all times.[2] Two studies have shown that head of bed elevation significantly decreases the incidence of VAP.[3,4]

PREVENT ASPIRATION

ET tubes prevent the glottis from closing, which leaves the airway exposed and allows oropharyngeal secretions that accumulate above the tube cuff to leak into the lungs. Mucus can accumulate on the top of the cuff of the ET tube and along the tube, where neither antibiotics nor white blood cells can reach the organisms to destroy them. Suctioning secretions from the ET tube cannot reach mucus on the top of the cuff. The CDC suggests using a particular type of ET tube, sometimes referred to as a continuous aspiration of subglottic secretions (CASS) tube.[5] It features an additional lumen that ends with an evacuation port just above the cuff, making it possible to remove secretions from above the cuff by applying continuous or intermittent suction through the extra lumen. Studies have found that the use of a CASS tube can significantly reduce the incidence of VAP.[2,6] Use only sterile fluid to clear a catheter that you are using to suction secretions from the client's lower respiratory tract if you are planning to reinsert it into the ET tube.[6]

Suction catheters are used to remove secretions in the ET tube. Two types exist: a closed system and an open system. Open suction systems are single use, and the frequency of changing closed systems is not clear. Studies have not shown significant differences in VAP and one study showed a significant reduction in days in the ICU.[7,8]

PROVIDE ORAL CARE

Although oral care has been linked to reduced VAP cases,[9] the frequency of oral care has not been described. Toothettes are the most common device used.

HAND-WASHING

Prevention of VAP is best accomplished through adequate hand-washing and wearing gloves when suctioning or manipulating the ET tube. Compliance with hand-washing is far from ideal and the use of alcohol gels may help increase compliance.[10,11]

IMPLICATIONS

VAP is a common complication in clients on ventilators because of changes in their risk profile for aspiration and lowered immune status. Nursing care can prevent or reduce the number of VAP cases.

REFERENCES

1. Kollef, M.H. (1999). The prevention of ventilator-associated pneumonia. *New England Journal of Medicine, 340*(8), 627.
2. Smulders, K., van der Hoeven, H., et al. (2002). A randomized clinical trial of intermittent subglottic secretion drainage in patients receiving mechanical ventilation. *Chest, 121*(3), 858.
3. Drakulovic, M.B., Torres, A., et al. (1999). Supine body position as a risk factor for nosocomial pneumonia in mechanically ventilated patients: A randomized trial. *Lancet, 354*(9193), 1851.
4. Ibanez, J., Penafiel, A., et al. (1992). Gastroesophageal reflux in intubated patients receiving enteral nutrition: Effect of supine and semirecumbent positions. *Journal of Parenteral and Enteral Nutrition, 16*(5), 419.
5. Centers for Disease Control and Prevention. (2004). *Guidelines for preventing health-care-associated pneumonia, 2003: Recommendations of CDC and the Healthcare Infection Control Practices Advisory Committee (HICPAC).* Retrieved 05/22/07 from www.cdc.gov/ncidod/hip/pneumonia/default.htm.
6. Valles, J., Artigas, A., et al. (1995). Continuous aspiration of subglottic secretions in preventing ventilator-associated pneumonia. *Annals of Internal Medicine, 122*(3), 179.
7. Johnson, K.L., Kearney, P.A., Johnson, S.B., et al. (1994). Closed versus open suctioning: Costs and physiologic consequences. *Critical Care Medicine, 22*(4), 658-666.
8. Cook, D., De Jonghe, B., Brochard, E., et al. (1998). Influence of airway management on ventilator associated pneumonia: Evidence from an randomized trial. *Journal of the American Medical Association, 279*(10), 781-787.
9. Mori, H., Hirasawa, H., Oda, S., et al. (2006). Oral care reduces incidence of ventilator-associated pneumonia in ICU populations. *Critical Care Medicine, 32*(2), 230-236.
10. Kim, P.W., Roghmann, M.C., et al. (2003). Rates of hand disinfection associated with glove use, patient isolation, and changes between exposure to various body sites. *American Journal of Infection Control, 31*(2), 97.
11. Sharir, R., Teitler, N., et al. (2001). High-level handwashing compliance in a community teaching hospital: A challenge that can be met!. *Journal of Hospital Infection, 49*(1), 55.

Dental or vocal cord trauma and tracheal mucosa damage from prolonged ET tube placement are a risk. Therefore tracheostomy may be used in clients who need long-term ventilation. Barotrauma may occur from excessive intra-alveolar pressure and is prevented by

careful PEEP adjustment and avoiding high tidal volumes if possible. Gastric complications include distention from air entering the gastrointestinal tract and stress ulcers from hyperacidity and inadequate nutrition. Aspiration of oral secretions or gastric contents can be prevented by maintaining head of bead elevation at >45 degrees, careful monitoring of gastric residuals, meticulous suctioning, and maintaining adequate cuff inflation. Medications that block production of gastric acids are often prescribed.

SAFETY

⚠️

ALERT

Self-extubation often occurs during times of agitation or turning and repositioning the client. Because the cuff is inflated, the tracheal wall can be damaged and bleeding can ensue. In most cases, the client requires reintubation, which must be done swiftly to prevent hypoxemia and to avoid inserting the ET tube through swollen tissues. Sometimes, the client can be monitored and not reintubated, especially if the time for extubation was approaching. Unplanned extubation often leads to increased duration of mechanical ventilation and longer ICU stays. Nursing interventions to prevent unplanned extubation are shown in Box 63-2.

Other complications that arise from extended mechanical ventilation include problems from limited mobility such as deep venous thromboembolism, skin breakdown, malnutrition, and stress and anxiety.

🪔 Weaning from a Ventilator

Weaning is the gradual withdrawal of mechanical ventilation. The criteria for weaning are shown in Box 63-3. The client's ability to breathe independently is the most important criterion for successful weaning. Minute ventilation and tidal volume are indicators that the client is meeting adequate tidal volume requirements; creating negative inspiratory force, which indicates inspiratory muscle strength; and generating positive expiratory pressure, which indicates respiratory muscle strength and ability to cough. The length of time required for successful weaning generally relates to the underlying disease process and to the client's state of health before the ventilator was used. For example, a young client who is recovering from an overdose of drugs can usually be weaned rapidly, but a client with COPD and acute

---

BOX 63-2   Strategies to Prevent Unplanned or Accidental Extubation

- Provide adequate sedation and pain control.
- Use wrist restraints according to hospital protocol.
- Secure the ET tube with tape or other commercial devices.
- Record the centimeter reference number at the lips.
- Assess the position of the ET tube routinely and after each position change.
- Support the ventilator tubes and suction tubing and keep them out of the client's reach.
- Use two staff members to reposition the ET tube.
- Explain the purpose of the tube and the need for restraints to the client and family.

ET, Endotracheal.

BOX 63-3   Criteria for a Ventilator Weaning Trial

- Reversal of underlying cause of respiratory failure
- Adequate oxygenation, indicated by the following:
  - Pao_2 ≥60 mm Hg on Fio_2 ≤40-50%
  - PEEP requirement ≤5-8 cm H_2O
  - pH ≥7.25
  - Pao_2/Fio_2 >150-300
- Heart rate ≤140 beats/min
- Stable BP with no or minimal vasopressive medications, such as dopamine or norepinephrine ≤5 mcg/kg/min
- No myocardial ischemia
- Temperature ≤100.4° F (38° C)
- Hemoglobin ≥8-10 g/dl
- Acceptable electrolyte values
- Adequate cough
- Capability to initiate inspiration/maximum inspiratory pressure less than or equal to −20 cm H_2O
- Adequate mentation without continuous IV sedation

From MacIntyre, N.R., Cook, D.J., et al. (2001). Evidenced based guidelines for weaning and discontinuing ventilatory support. A collective task force facilitated by the American College of Chest Physicians, the American Association for Respiratory Care and the American College of Critical Care Medicine. *Chest, 120*(6 Suppl), 375S.

---

respiratory failure with little or no pulmonary reserve often takes longer and requires much professional patience and skill. Weaning should be instituted after paralytics are discontinued, and sedation is tapered off. During the weaning process, the client should be observed for increased respiratory rate, shallow breathing, and decreased tidal volume, which may indicate muscle fatigue.

Techniques for Weaning

Spontaneous Breathing Trial. With the client still connected to the ventilator, the head of the bed is elevated and the client's ability to breathe on his or her own is measured. Most clients will be excited about coming off of the ventilator but at the same time concerned about being able to breathe on their own. Explain the weaning plan and assure the client you will remain at the bedside to monitor progress and problems with the trial.

Pressure Support Ventilation (PSV). Using this form of weaning, the ventilator delivers a set amount of positive pressure into the lungs with each breath initiated by the client. With PSV, the client controls both the length and the depth of each breath. This form of weaning is used for clients who have been on mechanical ventilation for longer periods of time.

Synchronized Intermittent Mandatory Ventilation (SIMV). With this mode of ventilation, the ventilator provides a set amount of breaths and tidal volumes in coordination with the client's efforts. As the client breathes more independently, the number of breaths by the ventilator decreases eventually to zero. This form of weaning is also used when more time is needed for weaning.

Difficulties in Weaning

A first weaning attempt may not be successful for several reasons, including decreased muscular strength caused by protein-carbohydrate malnutrition, underlying disease processes, or inability of respiratory muscles to sustain respiratory efforts as a result of disuse after prolonged CMV. Increased work of breathing caused by increased airway resistance, abdominal distention, a small-diameter artificial airway, upper airway obstruction, or unresolved acute lung diseases may also affect the success of the first weaning attempt. Other reasons include increased ventilation requirements, difficulty managing secretions, and psychological factors, such as fear and anxiety.

If the first attempt at weaning is not successful, determine the reasons and try to eliminate them in subsequent attempts. Clients who require prolonged ventilatory support and extended periods of weaning often do best in a setting that promotes rehabilitation concepts. These clients can usually be transferred to subacute or long-term acute care facilities.

Extubation

Extubation is the removal of the ET tube. Once the client has been weaned successfully, has demonstrated adequate ventilatory effort, and has maintained an acceptable level of consciousness to sustain spontaneous respiration, the ET tube may be removed. ET tubes are removed on physician's orders and only by health care team members qualified to reintubate if necessary. The occurrence of laryngospasm and tracheal edema after extubation may occlude the airway, requiring immediate reintubation.

The ET tube is suctioned, the cuff deflated, and the tube removed. Immediately after extubation, the client is usually placed on an oxygen mask. Assess the client for manifestations of respiratory distress and hypoxemia, as evidenced by restlessness, irritability, tachycardia, use of accessory muscles, and tachypnea. ABGs are obtained and monitored for decreased Pao_2 or increased $Paco_2$ levels, which indicate an inability to sustain ventilation. If these manifestations are noted, notify the physician and prepare for reintubation.

Dysfunctional Ventilatory Weaning Response

Some clients cannot adjust to lowered levels of mechanical ventilation, and the process of weaning them from the ventilator is delayed. The nursing diagnosis *Dysfunctional Ventilatory Weaning Response related to respiratory muscle fatigue or anxiety* was developed for these

situations. Manifestations of respiratory muscle fatigue include a respiratory rate more than 30 breaths/min, increased $Paco_2$ level, abnormal patterns of breathing, hemodynamic changes such as dysrhythmias, diaphoresis, anxiety, and dyspnea.

An unsuccessful attempt to wean the client may have taken place, resulting in reintubation. When the client cannot sustain ventilation independently, the ventilator is set at full ventilation; the client has no spontaneous breaths and therefore can rest. Once the client has rested, attempts at weaning should begin again. Some clients can never be weaned from mechanical ventilation. Those clients can be managed in less acute care units or at home for many years.

Ventilator-Dependent Clients

Some clients become stable and can be discharged from acute care and return home (see the website Bridge to Home Health Care feature titled Living with a Ventilator for ways to assist the ventilator-dependent client).

ADULT (ACUTE) RESPIRATORY DISTRESS SYNDROME

Adult (acute) respiratory distress syndrome (ARDS) is a sudden, progressive form of respiratory failure characterized by severe dyspnea, refractory hypoxemia, and diffuse bilateral infiltrates. It follows acute and massive lung injury that results from a variety of clinical states, often occurring in previously healthy people. The syndrome was first described in 1967 and has been referred to by several terms, including shock lung, wet lung, post-traumatic lung, congestive atelectasis, capillary leak syndrome, and adult hyaline membrane disease. Tremendous advances in the treatment of this condition have occurred over the last 2 decades.

Etiology and Risk Factors

ARDS develops as a result of ischemia in the alveolar capillary membrane during shock, oxygen toxicity, inhalation of noxious fumes or fluids (e.g., gastric acid), or inflammation from pneumonia or sepsis. There may be a direct insult to lung tissue or indirect injuries occurring in other body areas, with inflammatory mediators sent to the lung through the vascular system. Conditions leading to ARDS are listed in Box 63-4. Early recognition and treatment of these conditions may reduce the risk of ARDS.

Pathophysiology

The hallmark of ARDS is a massive inflammatory response by the lungs that increases permeability of the alveolar membrane, with resultant fluid movement into the interstitial and alveolar spaces. This leads to the

BOX 63-4 Risk Factors for Adult (Acute) Respiratory Distress Syndrome

DIRECT PULMONARY TRAUMA

- Viral, bacterial, or fungal pneumonias
- Lung contusion
- Fat embolus
- Aspiration (e.g., foreign material, drowning, vomitus)
- Massive smoke inhalation
- Inhaled toxins
- Prolonged exposure to high concentrations of oxygen

INDIRECT PULMONARY TRAUMA

- Sepsis
- Shock
- Multisystem trauma
- Disseminated intravascular coagulation
- Pancreatitis
- Uremia
- Drug overdose
- Anaphylaxis
- Idiopathic
- Prolonged heart bypass surgery
- Massive blood transfusions
- Pregnancy-induced hypertension
- Increased intracranial pressure
- Radiation therapy

development of noncardiogenic pulmonary edema, which decreases lung compliance and impairs oxygen transport. Three phases of ARDS have been described:[27]

1. *Phase 1 (exudative)* is seen approximately 24 hours after the initial insult and consists of damage to the capillary endothelium and leakage of fluid into the pulmonary interstitium. Microemboli also develop and cause a further increase in pulmonary artery pressures. Inflammatory responses accompany the pulmonary parenchymal damage, leading to the release of toxic mediators, the activation of complement, the mobilization of macrophages, and the release of vasoactive substances from mast cells. There is further damage to the basement membrane, interstitial space, and alveolar epithelium. Fibrin, blood, fluid, and protein exude into the interstitial spaces around the alveoli and increase the distance across the capillary membrane.

2. *Phase 2 (proliferative)* begins about 7 to 10 days later. Type I and type II alveolar cells are ultimately damaged, resulting in decreased surfactant production, alveolar collapse, and atelectasis, leading to further impairment in gas exchange. Significant hypoxemia is present because of decreased surfactant production, intrapulmonary shunting, and $\dot{V}/\dot{Q}$ mismatch.

3. *Phase 3 (fibrotic)* occurs in about 2 to 3 weeks. There is irreversible deposition of fibrin into the lung, resulting in pulmonary fibrosis, further decreasing lung compliance and worsening hypoxemia. The end

result is a significant $\dot{V}/\dot{Q}$ imbalance and profound arterial hypoxemia. (The Concept Map feature on Understanding ARDS and Its Treatment, p. 1654, illustrates these concepts.)

Clinical Manifestations

The initial insult of ARDS is followed by a period of apparently normal lung function that may last from 1 to 24 hours. Then hypoxemia rapidly develops and progresses along with decreasing lung compliance and development of diffuse lung infiltrates.

The earliest clinical manifestation of ARDS is usually an increased respiratory rate and profound dyspnea 12 to 24 hours after the initial injury. Breathing becomes increasingly labored; the client may exhibit air hunger and retractions. Chest auscultation may or may not reveal the presence of adventitious sounds. If present, abnormal sounds may range from fine inspiratory crackles to widespread coarse crackles. ABG analysis discloses increasing hypoxemia (Pao_2 <60 mm Hg) that does not respond to increased fractions of inspired oxygen levels (Fio_2 <40%) and compensatory hypocapnia. In the early stages, respiratory alkalosis is present because of hyperventilation. Later, metabolic acidosis develops from increased work of breathing and hypoxemia. The chest x-ray usually demonstrates diffuse, bilateral, and rapidly progressing interstitial or alveolar infiltrates (Figure 63-6).

Recommended diagnostic criteria include bilateral infiltrates seen on chest x-rays in the absence of fluid overload, ratio of Pao_2 (partial pressure of oxygen) to Fio_2 (fraction of inspired oxygen) less than or equal to 200 mm Hg (regardless of PEEP levels), and PAWP less than or equal to 18 mm Hg.[27] Additional diagnostic tests may be needed based on the underlying cause and include bronchial washing and biopsy to determine whether infection is present.

OUTCOME MANAGEMENT

The keys to successful management of ARDS are early detection and initiation of treatment. The goals of medical management are (1) respiratory and ventilatory support, (2) maintenance of hemodynamic stability, (3) treatment of the underlying cause, when possible, and (4) prevention of complications.

Medical Management

Support Respiration and Ventilation

Mechanical ventilation, ET intubation, and PEEP are usually required to maintain adequate blood oxygen levels. The goal of ventilatory support is to use the least amount of Fio_2 and PEEP possible to maintain oxygen saturation at or above 90% while decreasing the potential of

CONCEPT MAP

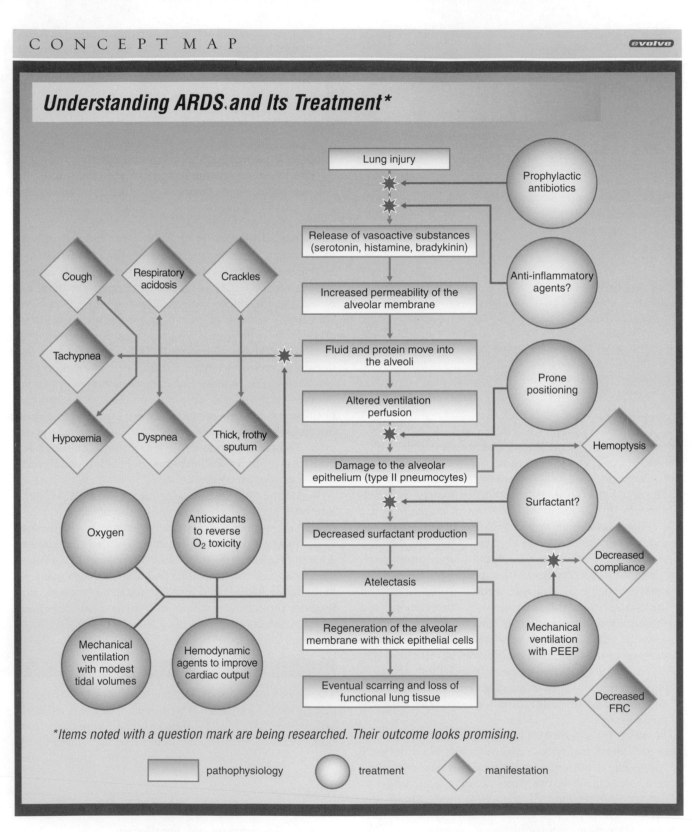

Understanding ARDS and Its Treatment*

*Items noted with a question mark are being researched. Their outcome looks promising.

pathophysiology   treatment   manifestation

oxygen toxicity. PEEP will also be used to decrease intra-pulmonary shunting and to recruit collapsed alveoli. Studies have shown that using smaller tidal volumes (permissive hypercapnia) and the least amount of PEEP possible can reduce the risk of lung injury (low levels of CO_2 [hypocapnia] have been shown to decrease lung compliance).[16,22] Additional studies have encouraged the use of inverse ratio ventilation (IRV) as one method of increasing mean airway pressure without creating further peak pressures in the alveolus from PEEP.[6] IRV

■ **FIGURE 63–6**   Adult (acute) respiratory distress syndrome (ARDS). This chest x-ray study shows massive consolidation from pulmonary edema following multisystem trauma. *(From Fraser, R.G., et al. [1990]. Diagnosis of diseases of the chest [3rd ed., p. 493]. Philadelphia: Saunders.)*

increases the inspiratory portion of each breath to more than half the respiratory cycle. Because IRV maintains a prolonged positive pressure through the ventilatory cycle, alveoli stay open and gas exchange is improved. Other alternative modes of ventilation (e.g., extracorporeal membrane oxygenation [ECMO] and partial liquid ventilation) may be used in some situations but are still considered investigational therapies. Surfactant therapy has been successful for neonates but to date has not had the same results in adults with ARDS.

Nitric oxide (NO) is now being used more often in the treatment of ARDS. NO causes selective vasodilation in the pulmonary vascular system and is a powerful bronchodilator. Inhaled NO dilates the capillary bed of the lungs, which in turn reduces the pressure in the pulmonary arteries without lowering systemic blood pressure.

Antioxidants, scavengers of oxygen free radicals, are also being used. *N*-Acetylcysteine and procysteine have been effective in reducing the degradative effect of the proteases. Pharmacologic efforts to inhibit the substances released by the endotoxins, neutrophils, and macrophages are also being explored. Prostaglandins are also being investigated as a possible treatment therapy for ARDS clients, especially those with sepsis and multiple organ failure. Steroids have been used with improvement in pulmonary function.

The prone position has been used to improve oxygenation by changing the distribution of perfusion. The belief is that ARDS does the greatest damage in the gravity-dependent parts of the lungs. By placing the client in a prone position, there is a change in the dependent portions of the lung, resulting in increased perfusion to the less damaged portions of the lungs and decreased pulmonary shunting. Prone positioning is also thought to

reduce compression of the lung by the heart, improve chest wall compliance, and result in better draining of bronchial secretions. Placing a client in a prone position requires coordination by many health care professionals to turn the client while maintaining equipment patency (e.g., ET tube) and decreasing client anxiety. Side effects include hypotension, desaturation, and dysrhythmias, although these appear to be short term. A plan for immediate repositioning in the event of deteriorating condition or cardiac or respiratory arrest should be in place before placing the client in the prone position. The prone position is shown in Figure 63-7 and is further discussed in the Translating Evidence into Practice feature on p. 1656.

Kinetic therapy via continuously rotating beds can also be used to improve ventilation. The constant postural drainage assists in removing airway plugs. To be effective, the movement must be at least 45 degrees from side to side, which is best accomplished by a rotation bed.

SAFETY ALERT

Shearing of the sacrum may develop, and therefore the client's skin should be completely assessed twice daily. Beds set to rotate at less than 40 degrees do not provide adequate pressure relief; if used at that degree, manual turning must also be completed. The nurse needs to stop the motion of the bed and inspect the skin to examine for shear and offload the sacrum for periods of time.

Maintain Hemodynamic Stability

Hemodynamic monitoring is used to observe the effect of fluids and degree of pulmonary edema. The use of pharmacologic agents in the treatment of ARDS varies according to the client's underlying disease process. Inotropic agents (e.g., dobutamine or dopamine) may be indicated to improve cardiac output and to increase systemic blood pressure. Fluids are carefully monitored to prevent systemic fluid overload.

■ **FIGURE 63–7**   Use of the prone position to improve ventilation-perfusion. *(Courtesy H.E.A.D. Prone, Inc., Cambridge, Mass.)*

🪔 TRANSLATING EVIDENCE INTO PRACTICE

Prone Positioning and Adult (Acute) Respiratory Distress Syndrome

Adequate perfusion and ventilation of lung tissue are important to provide adequate oxygenation to tissues and maintain life. Adult (acute) respiratory distress syndrome (ARDS) is typically characterized by decreased lung compliance and severe hypoxia. Using mechanical ventilation has long been accepted as a means to overcome the decreased compliance and to correct the life-threatening hypoxia. Additional studies are beginning to investigate the use of prone positioning with mechanical ventilation as another means to improve oxygenation while decreasing some of the complications associated with mechanical ventilation.

A meta-analysis completed by Curley identified 17 primary research studies that investigated the use of prone positioning.[3] Ryan and Pelosi presented findings from 11 studies investigating the use of prone positioning.[4] Although the studies all had different methodologies, each study met the criteria for scientific rigor and investigated the use of prone positioning to improve oxygenation. When combining the results of all 17 studies in the Curley meta-analysis, 69% of the clients (169 of 213 clients) responded positively to being placed in a prone position as demonstrated by an increase in the oxygenation saturation and Fio_2 ratio of 20% or more.[3] The studies reviewed by Ryan and Pelosi identified that 70% of the clients demonstrated improvement in oxygenation.[4] Various reasons were given for the improvements noted, including reexpansion of dependent portions of the lungs leading to atelectasis, changes in the $\dot{V}/\dot{Q}$ ratio, increase in functional residual capacity, and reduction in the amount of venous stasis.[4] As a result, the percentage of oxygen for mechanical ventilation could be decreased, thereby also decreasing the possibility of oxygen toxicity.

Several contraindications to the use of prone positioning included shock, hemorrhage, multiple trauma, spinal injury or instability, pregnancy, increased intracranial pressure, and recent abdominal surgery.[2,4] Both studies also identified complications associated with placing a client in a prone position, including the potential for impaired skin integrity, development of dependent edema in the face and anterior chest wall, damage to the eyes (corneal abrasions and ulcerations), nerve damage, and most importantly potential to dislodge extraneous tubes such as the endotracheal tube, venous and arterial lines, and Foley catheter. Care must be taken to prevent any of these complications. Strategies identified to prevent skin breakdown, eye injury, facial edema, and nerve damage included using padded cushions for bony prominences, repositioning the head every

2 hours, placing extremities in a functional position, inspecting the eyes and skin every 2 hours, and using pressure reduction devices.

To prevent loss of a line or the endotracheal tube when turning the client to and from a prone position, the nursing, respiratory therapy, and other health care professionals involved in the care of the client must work together in a coordinated effort for client safety and sense of security. Finally, a protocol must be in place for rapid response in the event the client goes into cardiopulmonary arrest while in the prone position.

SAFETY
⚠
ALERT

Another concern identified by the researchers was the use of tube feedings while the client is in the prone position. The increased potential for regurgitation and possible aspiration of feedings or stomach contents into the lungs was mentioned.[1] The need for caloric intake was recognized as important for the critically ill client. If the gastrointestinal function is confirmed, enteral feedings can be used with a client in the prone position with careful monitoring for potential aspiration.

None of the studies reported aspiration as a noted complication.

IMPLICATIONS

Additional studies need to be conducted on the effects of prone positioning for clients with adult (acute) respiratory distress syndrome. All the studies reviewed in the meta-analyses had small sample sizes (fewer than 30 clients in any one study). Consistent results of all the studies demonstrated the improved oxygenation of a majority of the clients. Prone positioning has been found to be an effective means to improve oxygenation in clients with adult (acute) respiratory distress syndrome, especially in the early stages of the adult (acute) respiratory distress syndrome when edema in the lungs and atelectasis are apparent.

REFERENCES

1. Balas, M. (2000). Prone positioning of patients with acute respiratory distress syndrome: Applying research to practice. *Critical Care Nurse, 20*(1), 24-36.
2. Breiburg, A., et al. (2000). Efficacy and safety of prone positioning for patients with acute respiratory distress syndrome. *Journal of Advanced Nursing, 32*(4), 922-929.
3. Curley, M. (1999). Prone positioning of patients with acute respiratory distress syndrome: A systematic review. *American Journal of Critical Care, 8*(6), 397-405.
4. Ryan, D., & Pelosi, P. (1996). Prone positioning in acute respiratory distress syndrome. *British Medical Journal, 312*, 860-861.

Treat the Underlying Condition

Antibiotics are administered if suspected or confirmed infection is present. Although controversial, the use of large doses of corticosteroids is also common. The rationale for steroid administration is to reduce inflammatory response and to promote pulmonary membrane stability; however, controlled clinical trials have not demonstrated

their effectiveness in ARDS. Indiscriminate use should be avoided.[6]

Monitor for Complications

In addition to lung fibrosis, other complications may arise during supportive management of the client with ARDS, such as cardiac dysrhythmias caused by hypoxemia, oxygen toxicity, renal failure, thrombocytopenia, gastrointestinal bleeding secondary to stress ulcers, sepsis from invasive lines, and disseminated intravascular coagulation (DIC) (see Chapter 75).

Prognosis

The outcome for any one client is difficult to predict. For most of the 1970s and 1980s, death rates seemed to be constant at 60% to 70%. In the 1990s, however, rates improved, and current rates are about 40%; however, a 90% death rate remains for clients with sepsis or multiple organ failure who develop ARDS.[8]

<h2 style="text-align:center">Nursing Management</h2>

The principles of nursing management of clients with pulmonary edema and care of the client requiring mechanical ventilation are appropriate in the care of the client with ARDS. Placing a client in prone position clearly is within the realm of nursing. Evaluation of the client's response to treatment as well as careful monitoring for potential complications is essential. Emotional support for the client's family and significant others is also important. The disease can progress very rapidly, leaving family members unprepared for the severity of the client's condition. Clear communications and frequent condition updates are essential to keeping the family adequately informed.

CHEST TRAUMA

The chest is a large, exposed portion of the body that is vulnerable to impact injuries. Because the chest houses the heart, lungs, and great vessels, chest trauma is frequently life-threatening. Injury to the thoracic cage and its contents can restrict the heart's ability to pump blood or the lungs' ability to exchange air and oxygenate blood. Major dangers associated with chest injuries are internal bleeding and punctured organs.

Chest injuries can range from relatively minor bumps and scrapes to severe crushing or penetrating trauma. Chest injuries may be *penetrating* or *blunt*.[30] Penetrating chest injuries may cause an open chest wound, permitting atmospheric air into the pleural space and disrupting the normal vacuum ventilation mechanism. Penetrating chest injuries may seriously damage the lungs, heart, and other thoracic structures. Blunt injuries are most commonly deceleration injuries associated with motor-vehicle crashes. Blunt chest trauma may also result from falls or blows to the chest.

Initial assessment is directed toward identifying and treating immediate life-threatening conditions. Any client with chest trauma should be considered to have a serious injury until proven otherwise. Airway patency, adequacy of breathing, and circulatory sufficiency (i.e., presence of shock), or ABCs, are always of primary concern.

Immobilization of a potential spinal cord injury should also be initiated.

Once initial emergencies have been addressed, assess the client more thoroughly (Box 63-5). A medical history helps to identify any pre-existing conditions that could further complicate the injury. A thorough physical examination should be performed, with care being taken not to focus only on obvious injuries. Information about the accident (obtained from the injured client or witnesses) assists in the diagnosis of regional as well as anatomic injuries. A chest x-ray and electrocardiogram (ECG) are obtained for detection of possible pulmonary or cardiac impairment.

OUTCOME MANAGEMENT

Initial management should focus on airway patency, ventilation, hemorrhage control, stabilization of any thoracic fractures, and immobilization of the spinal column. Clients are typically divided into two categories: stable

---

BOX 63-5   Chest Trauma: Assessment and Interventions

1. Assess "ABCs":
   a. Maintain *a*irway, *b*reathing, and *c*irculation.
   b. Ensure adequate air movement.
2. Obtain a quick history:
   a. What happened?
   b. What was the mechanism of injury?
   c. How long ago did it happen?
   d. Where is the pain? Does it radiate?
   e. Is there anything that makes the pain better or worse?
   f. What does the pain feel like?
   g. How severe is the pain on a scale of 1 to 10?
   h. Is there a significant medical history?
3. Perform a quick (1-minute) assessment for:
   a. Shortness of breath and cyanosis
   b. Vital signs
   c. Skin color and temperature
   d. Wound size and location
   e. Paradoxical chest movement
   f. Distended neck veins
   g. Tracheal deviation
   h. Respiratory stridor
   i. Bilateral breath sounds
   j. Use of accessory muscles
   k. Estimated tidal volume
   l. Subcutaneous emphysema
   m. Sucking chest wounds
   n. Heart sounds
   o. Dysrhythmias
4. Quickly intervene:
   a. Administer oxygen.
   b. Cover any open chest wound.
   c. Control flail segment.
   d. Prepare to insert a chest tube.
   e. Initiate a large-bore intravenous line.

and unstable. The stable client needs careful and continuous monitoring, and the unstable client requires immediate management of ventilation-perfusion imbalances, shock, and pain.

Ventilation-perfusion imbalances may result from atelectasis, hemopneumothorax, flail chest, aspiration, or pulmonary contusion. Oxygen or mechanical ventilation may be required. General respiratory status (e.g., rate and depth of respirations, chest movement, spontaneous vital volumes) and ABG values should be monitored closely. Deterioration of any of these parameters may indicate previously undetected injury or late-developing complications.

Therapeutic measures such as thoracentesis, chest tube insertion, bronchoscopic aspiration, video-assisted thoracic surgery (VATS), and thoracotomy (see Chapter 62) may be indicated. Management should focus on maintaining effective functioning of any equipment used (e.g., chest drainage system) and supporting the client and significant others to understand the procedures and the rationale for their use.

Monitor continually for clinical manifestations of shock. Shock often results from hypovolemia, but in the chest-injured client it may also be caused by cardiac tamponade, cardiac contusion, flail chest, or tension pneumothorax. Central vascular pressure readings (central venous pressure or pulmonary artery pressure) require careful interpretation. Once the cause of shock is determined, rapid treatment is crucial (see Chapter 81).

Excessive blood loss may further compromise oxygenation. Assess external bleeding carefully, and estimate blood loss. Internal bleeding may result from injuries to the thoracic or abdominal viscera, torn muscles, or fractures. Considerable bleeding (2 L or more) into the pleural space may occur. This is usually detected quickly as hypovolemic shock. Bleeding into areas such as the chest wall (e.g., from torn intercostal muscles) is more difficult to assess. A liter of blood can accumulate between the chest wall muscles without producing much swelling.

Fluid replacement is with blood and blood products, if indicated, or with crystalloid intravenous solutions (e.g., lactated Ringer's solution, normal saline). A chest-injured person may require large quantities of blood replacement. Until the results of typing and crossmatching are available, the client is given O-negative blood. The volume of blood replacement is determined through assessment of clinical findings, hemodynamic measurements, and laboratory results (e.g., hemoglobin and hematocrit). When possible, surgery is delayed until blood volume is restored.

Pain associated with chest injuries may cause the client to breathe rapidly and shallowly, which leads to atelectasis and pooling of tracheobronchial secretions. Analgesics minimize pain, permit periods of rest and relaxation, and allow the client to cough and to take deeper breaths.

Opioids are most effective if given via the intravenous route. Intercostal nerve blocks or epidural analgesia may be used in clients with underlying health problems. Splinting the chest may also be helpful.

SPECIFIC CHEST INJURIES

FRACTURED RIBS

Etiology and Risk Factors

Rib fractures are common chest injuries, particularly in older adults. Such fractures are usually associated with a blunt injury, such as a fall, a blow to the chest, coughing or sneezing, the impact of the chest against a steering wheel during rapid deceleration, or less obvious traumas, such as pushing furniture when osteoporosis is present. The fifth through the ninth ribs are most commonly affected.

Clinical Manifestations

Clinical manifestations include (1) localized pain and tenderness over the fracture area on inspiration and palpation, (2) shallow respirations, (3) the client's tendency to hold the chest protectively or to breathe shallowly to minimize chest movements, (4) sometimes bruising or surface markings from the trauma at the site of injury, (5) protruding bone splinters if the fracture is compound, and (6) a clicking sensation during inspiration when costochondral separation or dislocation is present.

Fractured ribs compromise ventilation by three mechanisms. Pain from the injury causes splinting, shallow breathing, and ineffective cough, which predisposes to atelectasis and pneumonia. Secretions accumulate and obstruct the bronchi, becoming a site of infection; shallow breathing reduces lung compliance.

> **Rib fractures can result in a flail chest, which interferes with the normal physiology of breathing, and bone splinters from fractured ribs may penetrate the lung or pleura, resulting in a pneumothorax or hemothorax.**
>
> SAFETY ⚠ ALERT

Chest x-rays are carefully reviewed for 24 to 48 hours after injury for indications of these complications. Bright-red sputum may be coughed up if the lung has been penetrated. Continuously assess the client for manifestations of pneumothorax or hemothorax, and report such findings promptly.[10]

OUTCOME MANAGEMENT 🪔

Fractured ribs are generally treated conservatively with good pulmonary physiotherapy, rapid mobilization, and proper pain management. Strapping the ribs with tape is no longer recommended because it restricts deep breathing and can increase the incidence of atelectasis and pneumonia.

Adequate pain control and splinting of the chest during coughing and deep breathing help the client with rib fractures to carry out painful but vital mobilization activities more comfortably. If pain is severe enough to impair ventilation significantly, a local anesthetic solution may be injected at the fracture site itself. Intercostal nerve blocks may also be used.[12] A client with an underlying chest or heart disease (e.g., COPD, heart failure) may benefit particularly from this type of pain management. A chest x-ray should be taken after this procedure to ensure that pneumothorax has not occurred. Hospitalization may be required, especially in older adults, whose vital capacity may be significantly compromised. The pain from fractured ribs usually lasts 5 to 7 days. Complete healing occurs in approximately 6 to 8 weeks.

FRACTURED STERNUM

Sternal fractures usually result from blunt deceleration injuries, such as impact from a steering wheel. About 40% to 60% of the clients with fractured sternums have other major injuries, such as flail chest; pulmonary and myocardial contusions; ruptured aorta, trachea, bronchus, or esophagus; and hemothorax or pneumothorax.[12]

Clinical manifestations include sharp, stabbing pain; swelling and discoloration over the fracture site; and crepitus. The main priority is to control associated injuries. A client with a nondisplaced fracture may need analgesics or intercostal nerve blocks for pain reduction. Surgical fixation may be required for severe sternal fractures.

FLAIL CHEST

Etiology and Risk Factors

Severe blunt injury to the chest often fractures multiple ribs and crushes the ribs onto lung tissue. By definition, a flail chest is one that has paradoxical movement of a segment of chest wall caused by fractures of 3 or more ribs anteriorly and posteriorly within each rib (Figure 63-8). The flail segment most commonly involves the lateral side of the chest. It is common for the end of a fractured rib to tear the pleura and lung surface (thereby producing *hemopneumothorax*) and for a crushed chest to have a flail segment. Pulmonary edema, pneumonitis, and atelectasis often develop rapidly with a crushed chest when fluids increase and collect at the injured site.

The "flail" segment no longer has bony or cartilaginous connections with the rest of the rib cage. Lacking attachment to the thoracic skeleton, the flail section "floats," moving independently of the chest wall during ventilation. This abnormality disrupts the normal bellows action of the thorax by causing *paradoxical motion,* during which the flail portion of the chest and its underlying lung tissue are (1) "sucked in" with inspiration (instead of expanding outward as normal) and (2) "blown out" with expiration (instead of collapsing normally inward).[12] This alteration in normal chest wall mechanics diminishes the client's ability to achieve an adequate tidal volume and to produce an adequate cough. Hypoventilation and hypoxia may result, leading to respiratory failure. Furthermore, mediastinal structures tend to swing back and forth (mediastinal flutter) with significant paradoxical

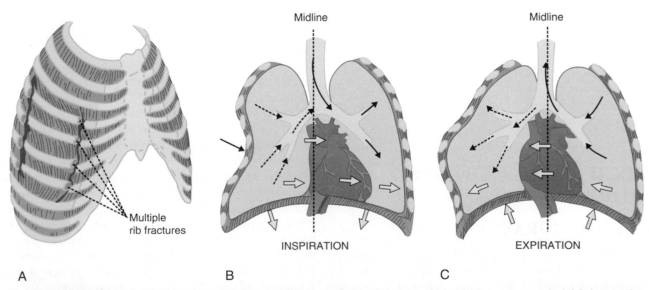

Midline

Midline

Multiple rib fractures

INSPIRATION

EXPIRATION

A   B   C

■ **FIGURE 63–8** Flail chest. *Solid and dashed arrows* indicate air movement; *open arrows* indicate structural movement. **A,** A flail chest consists of fractured rib segments that are unattached (free-floating) to the rest of the chest wall. **B,** On inspiration, the flail segment of ribs is sucked inward. The affected lung and mediastinal structures shift to the unaffected side. This compromises the amount of inspired air in the unaffected lung. **C,** On expiration, the flail segment of ribs bellows outward. The affected lung and mediastinal structures shift to the affected side. Some air within the lungs is shunted back and forth between the lungs instead of passing through the upper airway.

motion. These swings may seriously affect circulatory dynamics, producing elevated venous pressure, impaired filling of the right side of the heart, and decreased arterial pressure.

In addition, pulmonary contusion occurs, resulting in an accumulation of fluid in the affected alveoli, which leads to intrapulmonary shunting and further hypoxia. The full effects of pulmonary contusion may not be manifested until the height of the body's inflammatory response in 24 to 48 hours.

The client with a flail chest commonly experiences emotional and physical distress while trying to breathe despite excruciating pain. Respirations are usually rapid, shallow, and labored. Paradoxical movement of the chest wall is usually obvious if the client's bare chest is inspected. Breath sounds are absent or decreased on the affected side and crepitus may be heard or felt at the fracture site. Hypercapnia and hypoxia worsen as the effort necessary to breathe further depletes the already diminished oxygen supply. Frequent assessment of ABGs is needed to monitor respiratory effectiveness and to detect acidosis. Various factors produce metabolic and respiratory acidosis in chest-injured clients.

OUTCOME MANAGEMENT

Treatment is usually with intubation and mechanical ventilation, which can accomplish the following:

- Restore adequate ventilation, thus reducing hypoxia and hypercapnia
- Decrease paradoxical motion by using positive pressure to stabilize the chest wall internally
- Reduce pain by decreasing movement of the fractured ribs
- Provide an avenue for removal of secretions

Internal stabilization with continuous ventilation may require 21 days or more. Muscle relaxants or musculoskeletal paralyzing agents may be administered to reduce the risk of separation of the healing costochondral junctions. See earlier discussion in this chapter.

SPECIFIC PULMONARY INJURIES

PNEUMOTHORAX

Pneumothorax is the presence of air in the pleural space that prohibits complete lung expansion. Lung expansion occurs when the pleural lining of the chest wall and the visceral lining of the lung maintain negative pressure in the pleural space. When the continuity of this system is lost, the lung collapses, resulting in a pneumothorax.[24]

Pathophysiology

A pneumothorax may be closed or open. In a closed pneumothorax, air may escape into the pleural space from a puncture or tear in an internal respiratory structure such as the bronchus, bronchioles, or alveoli (Figure 63-9, *A*). Fractured ribs may also lead to closed pneumothorax. In an open pneumothorax, air may enter the pleural space directly through a hole in the chest wall or diaphragm (Figure 63-9, *B*).

A pneumothorax may be classified as spontaneous or traumatic, and either classification may result in a tension pneumothorax. A spontaneous pneumothorax may be idiopathic in that no cause can be found (primary) or as a result of another lung illness such as COPD, tuberculosis, or cancer (secondary). Whereas the chest wall remains intact, a bleb or bulla ruptures, leading to a collapsed lung. A traumatic pneumothorax results in a collapsed lung caused either by blunt force trauma to the chest wall or by the creation of an open sucking chest wound caused by a motor-vehicle accident, gun or knife wound, or a diagnostic procedure such as a thoracentesis. Additional risk factors for developing a pneumothorax are listed in Table 63-2.

A tension pneumothorax develops when air is trapped in the pleural space during inspiration and cannot escape during expiration. The intrapleural pressure becomes greater than the lung tissue pressure, resulting in compression of the lung and surrounding structures.

Clinical Manifestations

Clinical manifestations of *moderate* pneumothorax include tachypnea; dyspnea; sudden sharp pain on the affected side with chest movement, breathing, or coughing; asymmetrical chest expansion; diminished or absent breath sounds on the affected side; hyperresonance (tympany) to percussion on the affected side; restlessness; anxiety; and tachycardia.

Clinical manifestations of *severe* pneumothorax include all the preceding and distended neck veins; point of maximal impulse shift; subcutaneous emphysema; decreased tactile and vocal fremitus; tracheal deviation toward the unaffected side; and progressive cyanosis.

Chest x-ray may reveal a slight tracheal shift away from the affected side and retraction of the lung back from the parietal pleura. On chest x-ray, pneumothorax is expressed as a percentage. For example, a client may have a complete 100% to a partial 10% pneumothorax. The use of percentages allows for evaluation of progress on subsequent x-rays. If pneumothorax is suspected but respiratory distress is too severe to permit x-ray confirmation, the physician may insert an 18-gauge needle (emergency thoracentesis) into the second or third intercostal space in the midclavicular line. Aspiration demonstrates whether free air is present in the pleural space.

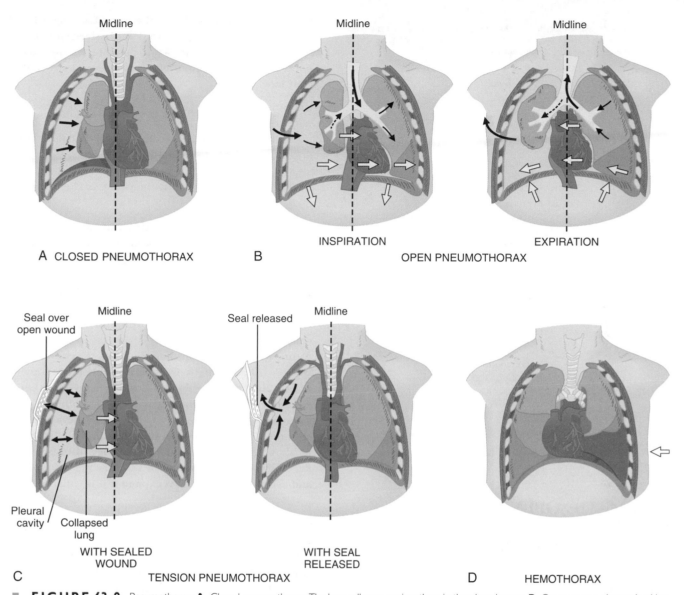

■ **FIGURE 63–9** Pneumothorax. **A,** Closed pneumothorax. The lung collapses as air gathers in the pleural space. **B,** Open pneumothorax (sucking chest wound). *Solid and dashed arrows* indicate air movement; *open arrows* indicate structural movement. A chest wall wound connects the pleural space with atmospheric air. During inspiration, atmospheric air is sucked into the pleural space through the chest wall wound. Positive pressure in the pleural space collapses the lung on the affected side and pushes the mediastinal contents toward the unaffected side. This reduces the volume of air in the unaffected side considerably. During expiration, air escapes through the chest wall wound, lessening positive pressure in the affected side and allowing the mediastinal contents to swing back toward the affected side. Movement of mediastinal structures from side to side is called mediastinal flutter. **C,** Tension pneumothorax. *Left,* If an open pneumothorax is covered (e.g., with a dressing), it forms a seal, resulting in tension pneumothorax with a mediastinal shift. A tear in lung structure continues to allow air into the pleural space. As positive pressure builds in the pleural space, the affected lung collapses, and the mediastinal contents shift to the unaffected side. *Right,* Tension pneumothorax is corrected by removing the seal (e.g., dressing), allowing air trapped in the pleural space to escape. **D,** Massive hemothorax *(arrow)* below the left lung, causing collapse of lung tissue.

OUTCOME MANAGEMENT

Most physicians prefer to insert a chest tube immediately into the pleural space via the fourth intercostal space at the midaxillary or anterior axillary line. The chest catheter is connected to closed-chest drainage (see Chapter 62). The catheter permits the continuous escape of air and blood from the pleural space, thus helping the lung expand by reestablishing negative subatmospheric pressure in the pleural space. Sometimes a thoracotomy is done to explore the chest surgically and to repair the site of origin of the pneumothorax or hemothorax. Surgical treatment may also be accomplished through VATS.[24] A thoracoscopy is completed with direct visualization of the defect in the chest that needs to be repaired. Because the VATS is less invasive than a thoracotomy, the client experiences less pain, has a smaller chest wound, and recovers faster and with fewer side effects, compared with a thoracotomy where the chest is opened.

TABLE 63–2   Risk Factors for Developing Pneumothorax

Type of Pneumothorax	Risk Factors
Spontaneous pneumothorax	Bleb or bulla
	Emphysema
	AIDS
	Asthma
	Cystic fibrosis
	Tuberculosis
	Sarcoidosis
	Malignancy
	Idiopathic pulmonary fibrosis
	Birt-Hogg-Dubé syndrome
	Necrotizing pneumonia
	Barotrauma or positive end-expiratory pressure
	High altitudes
	Decompression diving injuries
	Smoking
	Marfan syndrome
	Cocaine use
Traumatic pneumothorax	Chest surgery
	Insertion of central line
	Thoracentesis
	Gunshot wound
	Knife wound
	Penetrating foreign object
	Falls
	Motor-vehicle accidents
	Blunt chest trauma
	Fractured rib

Revised from Bucher, L., & Melander, S. (1999). *Critical care nursing.* Philadelphia: Saunders.

TRAUMATIC OPEN PNEUMOTHORAX AND MEDIASTINAL FLUTTER

A traumatic open pneumothorax occurs with sucking chest wounds. With this type of wound, a traumatic opening in the chest wall is large enough for air to move freely in and out of the chest cavity during ventilation (Figure 63-9, *B*). This abnormal movement of air through the chest wound produces a sucking noise that is audible in a quiet environment. Open sucking chest wounds may result from accidental injuries or surgical trauma. For example, if a chest drainage catheter is accidentally pulled out of a chest, the remaining puncture incision in the chest wall may become a sucking wound.

OUTCOME MANAGEMENT

SAFETY

⚠

ALERT

When an open sucking chest wound is detected, emergency intervention includes immediately covering the wound securely with anything available. An airtight covering usually prevents tension pneumothorax and preserves ventilation of the opposite lung. Do not waste time looking for a sterile gauze petrolatum dressing (the ideal covering for such a wound) if it is not immediately available. Cover the wound at once with whatever is at hand (e.g., a towel) until a sterile petrolatum dressing is available. When possible, fix the temporary dressing firmly in place with several strips of wide tape.

If the client is conscious and cooperative, ask the client to take a deep breath and to try to blow it out while keeping the mouth and nose closed. This pushing effort against a closed glottis helps push air out through the chest wound and reexpand the lung. When the client does this, apply the dressing before the client inhales again.

Stay with the chest-injured client after a dressing has been applied to a sucking wound. Carefully assess for indications of tension pneumothorax and *mediastinal shift* (contents of mediastinum [heart, great vessels, trachea, esophagus] are pushed to the unaffected side of the chest). These complications may develop if the air leak is in the lung or a bronchus; such a situation allows air to escape into the pleural space. In such instances, closing the chest wall wound with an airtight dressing prevents the outflow of escaping air, thereby accidentally converting an open pneumothorax into a tension pneumothorax. If a tension pneumothorax appears to be developing after the wound is sealed, immediately unplug the seal to allow the air to escape. Closed-chest drainage is necessary to (1) remove the air from the pleural space and (2) allow the lung to reexpand if it is collapsed.

SAFETY

⚠

ALERT

In addition to experiencing dyspnea and collapse of the lung on the affected side, the client with a traumatic open pneumothorax may experience *mediastinal flutter.* This complication results from air rushing in and out of the thoracic cavity on the affected side. With inspiration, the mediastinal structures (heart, trachea, esophagus) and collapsed lung are pushed toward the unaffected side. With expiration, these structures then move back toward the affected side. Fluttering back-and-forth movements of these vital mediastinal structures produce severe cardiopulmonary compromise, which is fatal if not treated promptly.

Chest tubes are inserted on the affected side away from the open wound. Surgical closure of the wound may follow. Supplemental high-flow oxygen should be administered.

TENSION PNEUMOTHORAX AND MEDIASTINAL SHIFT

Although it is dangerous to have air moving in and out of the pleural space with each respiration, the client is at even greater risk when air moves only into the pleural space and cannot move back out (tension pneumothorax). Tension pneumothorax (Figure 63-9, *C*) is a true emergency. Air enters the pleural space with each inspiration, becomes trapped there, and is not expelled during expiration (i.e., one-way valve effect). Pressure builds in the chest as the accumulation of air in the pleural space increases. Tension pneumothorax most commonly occurs with blunt traumatic injuries and is frequently associated with flail chest injuries.

If untreated, tension pneumothorax collapses the lung on the affected side as intrapleural pressure or tension increases, causing a mediastinal shift (mediastinal contents—heart, trachea, esophagus, great vessels—pushed or "shifted" toward the chest's unaffected side). Mediastinal shift may cause (1) compression of the lung in the direction of the shift (i.e., the lung opposite the pneumothorax) and (2) compression, traction, torsion, or kinking of the great vessels; thus blood return to the heart is dangerously impaired. The latter situation causes a subsequent decrease in cardiac output and blood pressure. Tension pneumothorax produces serious circulatory and pulmonary impairment that can be rapidly fatal. This is a high-priority emergency requiring prompt assessment and intervention.

Clinical Manifestations

Clinical manifestations of tension pneumothorax may include (1) marked, severe dyspnea; (2) tachypnea; (3) subcutaneous emphysema in the neck and upper chest; (4) progressive cyanosis; (5) acute chest pain on the affected side; (6) hyperresonance (tympany) upon percussion of the affected side; (7) tachycardia; (8) asymmetrical chest wall movement; (9) diminished or absent breath sounds on the affected side; and (10) extreme restlessness and agitation. Other manifestations include (1) neck vein distention; (2) laryngeal and tracheal deviation or shift to the unaffected side; (3) a feeling of tightness or pressure within the chest; (4) a point of maximal impulse (PMI) shift laterally or medially; (5) severe hypotension leading to shock; and (6) muffled heart sounds.

A suspected mediastinal shift may be confirmed by x-ray. Laryngeal and tracheal deviation toward the unaffected side can be detected by gentle palpation and with x-ray study. ABG analysis demonstrates hypoxia and respiratory alkalosis. When mediastinal shift is severe and not immediately corrected, respiratory acidosis may ensue.

OUTCOME MANAGEMENT

The immediate intervention is to convert a *tension* pneumothorax into an *open* pneumothorax, a less serious disorder. Large-bore chest tubes (36F to 40F) are inserted on the affected side at the fifth intercostal space anterior to the midaxillary line. Once tubes are inserted, suction drainage should be established. If a delay in the chest

tube insertion is anticipated, a 14- to 18-gauge needle may be inserted into the pleural space of the affected side at the level of the second intercostal space at the midclavicular line. Prompt thoracentesis to remove air may be life-saving. As trapped air rushes from a tension pneumothorax, the tension is relieved and the lung should reexpand; and if mediastinal shift is present, it corrects itself. Supplemental oxygen is administered.

HEMOTHORAX

Hemothorax may be present in clients with chest injuries. A small amount of blood (<300 ml) in the pleural space may cause no clinical manifestations and may require no intervention, with the blood being reabsorbed spontaneously. Severe hemothorax (1400 to 2500 ml) may be life-threatening because of resultant hypovolemia and tension (Figure 63-9, *D*). Massive hemothorax is associated with 50% to 75% mortality.

Clinical manifestations include respiratory distress, shock, and mediastinal shift. There is dullness upon percussion of the affected side. A chest film confirms a diagnosis of hemothorax. If the client is in severe distress, the physician may aspirate blood from the pleural space by inserting a 16-gauge needle into the fifth or sixth intercostal space at the midaxillary line. To drain intrathoracic accumulations of blood, the physician inserts a large-caliber (36F or larger) chest catheter, which is then connected to a drainage system. An initial drainage of 500 to 1000 ml is considered moderate, and additional treatment may not be required. An initial drainage of more than 1500 ml or continued large amounts of drainage (200 ml/hr) warrants immediate exploratory thoracotomy or the use of VATS to repair the site of active bleeding. Fluid replacement with O-negative blood or autotransfusion of blood should be used.

OTHER TRAUMATIC LUNG EVENTS

NEAR-DROWNING

Clients who initially survive suffocation after submersion in a water or fluid medium are said to have experienced a near-drowning or *immersion syndrome*. Immersion syndrome is the immersion into cold water that leads to cardiac dysrhythmias. Freshwater drowning (i.e., in a swimming pool) is more common than saltwater drowning. Risk factors that increase the potential for near-drowning are alcohol or drug ingestion, overestimation of swimming skills, hypothermia, hyperventilation, extreme fatigue, sudden acute illness (seizure or acute myocardial infarction), head or spinal cord injury from a diving mishap, and hypoglycemia.

Pathophysiology

Regardless of the fluid aspirated, the ultimate result is pulmonary edema. Both freshwater and saltwater wash out alveolar surfactant. Freshwater also changes the surface tension of surfactant. The loss of surfactant leads to alveolar collapse, intrapulmonary shunting, decreased lung compliance, and hypoxemia. Poor perfusion and hypoxemia result in acidosis and eventual pulmonary edema. Near-drowning also compromises the respiratory system and leads to hypoxia, hypercapnia, cardiac arrest, and severe alterations in fluid-electrolyte balance.

Clinical Manifestations

The client may be unconscious or awake but restless and complaining of chest pain or a headache. Vomiting often occurs. Hypothermia may also be present. Cardiac manifestations include tachycardia, hypotension, and dysrhythmias. Pink frothy sputum indicates that pulmonary edema is already present. Auscultation may reveal crackles, rhonchi, and wheezes. Hemoglobin, hematocrit, and electrolyte levels may be abnormal. White blood cell count may be elevated, especially if the water aspirated contained impurities.

OUTCOME MANAGEMENT

Begin assessment and interventions with the ABCs. If there is a possibility of spinal cord injury (such as with a diving injury), the spinal column should be immobilized. Basic cardiopulmonary resuscitation (CPR) should be initiated if necessary and continued, especially with hypothermic clients. Resuscitation efforts for clients with hypothermia have been successful long after typical CPR time guidelines would indicate to discontinue resuscitation efforts. Attempting to drain the fluid from the lungs is not advised.

Obtain a history of the submersion from the client or someone who has the information needed. Include the length of submersion, temperature of the water, any associated injuries, and type of water. Assess the level of consciousness. Note any respiratory efforts and adventitious sounds. Open the airway while maintaining spinal immobility. Look for manifestations of hypoxia, such as confusion, irritability, lethargy, or unconsciousness. Obtain a complete set of vital signs and assess for any additional injuries that may be present, including associated trauma, spinal cord injury from diving, air embolism from scuba diving, and seizures.

For respiratory insufficiency, intubate and ventilate with 100% oxygen and 5 to 10 cm of PEEP to prevent the alveoli from collapsing. If PEEP is used, slow and cautious removal of PEEP is required. Surfactant levels may remain low for up to 48 to 72 hours, especially after freshwater aspiration. If the client is breathing, provide respiratory support with a non-rebreather mask. Oxygen saturation should be maintained above 90%.[9]

Remove the client's wet clothing, and wrap the client in a warm blanket. Core rewarming may be indicated if the client is hypothermic. Rewarm the client slowly to avoid a rapid influx of anaerobic metabolites (lactic acid) that may be trapped in the cold extremities.

Once the vital functions are stabilized, correct any acid-base or electrolyte abnormalities. Diagnostic studies include ABG analysis, complete blood count, electrolytes, appropriate toxicology studies if alcohol or drug ingestion is suspected, and a chest film. Clients are at high risk for pulmonary edema even several hours after a near-drowning incident. Monitor neurologic status carefully. A deteriorating level of consciousness may indicate cerebral edema, severe acidosis, or increased hypoxia. Table 63-3 identifies factors associated with near-drowning outcomes.

CARBON MONOXIDE POISONING

Carbon monoxide (CO) is a colorless, odorless, tasteless gas that is formed by the incomplete combustion of any carbon fuel. Intoxication by CO is the leading cause of death by poisoning. CO preferentially binds to hemoglobin, with an affinity for hemoglobin 200 to 230 times greater than that of oxygen. CO displaces oxygen, leading to reduced supplies of oxygen in the arterial blood and development of tissue hypoxia. CO also shifts the oxygen-hemoglobin dissociation curve to the left, which further reduces the oxygen levels by decreasing the release of oxygen into the tissues.

Generally, there is a history of exposure to CO after being found in an enclosed space in the presence of gases or fire. Faulty furnaces are also associated with CO poisoning. If CO poisoning is due to smoke inhalation, manifestations such as hoarseness, stridor, burns, or soot on the mouth or nose may be present. Sputum may be black because of inhalation of soot.

TABLE 63–3 Factors Associated with Prediction of Outcome in Near-Drowning

Factors Suggestive of Favorable Outcome	Factors Suggestive of Poor Outcome
Submersion time <5 minutes	Submersion time >10 minutes
Immediate resuscitation	No resuscitation within first 10 minutes
CPR given <10 minutes	CPR given >25 minutes
Spontaneous cardiac rhythm in ED	Use of cardiotonic medications in field or ED
GCS score >6 on arrival at ED	GCS score <5
Spontaneous purposeful movement and intact brain stem function at 24 hours	No spontaneous purposeful movements 24 hours after submersion

CPR, Cardiopulmonary resuscitation; *ED,* emergency department; *GCS,* Glasgow Coma Scale.
From Shoemaker, W.C., et al. (2007). *Textbook of critical care* (5th ed.). Philadelphia: Saunders.

Clinical Manifestations

Clinical manifestations are vague until levels of CO bound to hemoglobin (carboxyhemoglobin, or COHb) are around 40%. With levels below 20%, manifestations include headache, vertigo, dizziness, nausea, and dyspnea on exertion. Above 20%, the client may have impaired concentration, clumsiness, and throbbing headache. Only when levels exceed 30% are manifestations more evident, including irritability, visual changes, impaired thought, and vomiting. At 40% vital signs change, and eventually seizures and coma ensue when levels are greater than 50%. The diagnosis is confirmed by measurement of carboxyhemoglobin levels in the blood. Pulse oximetry should not be used because the readings are unreliable because of the detection of carboxyhemoglobin as oxyhemoglobin.

OUTCOME MANAGEMENT

Removal of the CO from the body is imperative. When the client is breathing room air, the CO will be removed from the body in about 320 minutes. Administering 100% oxygen will shorten the half-life of CO to 80 minutes. Hyperbaric oxygen may be required to reduce the half-life of CO to minutes by forcing it off of the hemoglobin molecule for clients with severe CO poisoning. Hyperbaric oxygen will decrease the half-life of CO to 23 minutes.

Reasons for CO poisoning must be explored and interventions directed at correcting those problems should begin before hospital discharge. If the client's home furnace is faulty, it must be repaired. If the CO poisoning was a suicide attempt, crisis counselors should be used. Long-term neurologic and psychiatric consequences may develop, and the client should be observed and followed up by their usual health care provider.

CONCLUSIONS

Two forms of respiratory failure exist: hypoxemic and ventilatory. Hypoxemic failure includes problems that lead to failure to transport oxygen and CO_2 across the capillary. Ventilatory failure includes disorders that impair neurologic triggers to breathe and neuromuscular movement with respiration. Mechanical ventilation is a common method of treatment for both problems. Chest trauma involves life-threatening problems that demand prompt recognition and treatment.

THINKING CRITICALLY

1. You are caring for a client who is receiving mechanical ventilation. You have just suctioned the client's airway and begin to leave the room when the high-pressure alarm sounds. What should you do?

Factors to Consider. What changes in the client can trigger the high-pressure alarm? What changes in the ventilator can cause high pressure?

2. You are going to position the client prone to improve ventilation and perfusion. What considerations should be made before, during, and after the prone position is used?

Factors to Consider. How can the tubes be moved safely with the client? What complications might occur in a prone position? What procedures cannot be done while the client is prone?

Discussions for these questions can be found on the website. 〔evolve〕

BIBLIOGRAPHY

🔦 Citations appearing in red refer to primary research.

🔦 Citations appearing in blue refer to evidence-based practice guidelines and protocols.

1. Anas, N., & Lewis, K. (2000). Drowning and near-drowning. In A. Grenvik, et al. (Eds.), *The textbook of critical care* (4th ed., pp. 200-211). Philadelphia: Saunders.
2. Austan, F., & Polise, M. (2002). Management of respiratory failure with noninvasive positive pressure ventilation and heliox adjunct. *Heart and Lung, 31*(3), 214-218.
3. Balas, M. (2000). Prone positioning of patients with acute respiratory distress syndrome: Applying research to practice. *Critical Care Nurse, 20*(1), 24-36.
4. Ballard, N. (2006). Patients' recollections of therapeutic paralysis in the intensive care unit. *American Journal of Critical Care, 15*(1), 86-94.
5. Berenholtz, S., et al. (2004). Improving Care for the Ventilated Patient. *Joint Commission Journal on Quality and Safety, 30*(4), 195-204.
6. Brochard, L. (2000). Noninvasive ventilation. In A. Grenvik, et al. (Eds.), *The textbook of critical care* (4th ed., pp. 1302-1306). Philadelphia: Saunders.
7. Brower, R., et al. (2001). Treatment for ARDS [Electronic version]. *Chest, 120*(4), 1347-1367.
8. Burns, S. (1999). Making weaning easier: Pathways and protocols that work. *Nursing Clinics of North America, 11*(4), 465-479.
9. Burton, S., & Alexander, E. (2006). Avoiding the pitfalls and ensuring the safety of sustained neuromuscular blockade. *AACN Advanced Critical Care, 17*(3), 239-243.
9a. Centers for Disease Control and Prevention. (2004). *Guidelines for preventing health-care associated pneumonia.* Atlanta: CDC.
10. Chesnutt, M., & Prendergast, T. (2003). Lung. In L. Tierney, S. McPhee, & M. Papadakis (Eds.), *Current medical diagnosis and treatment* (pp. 306-311). New York: Lange Medical Books.
11. Cohen, R., & Moelleken, B. (2003). Disorders due to physical agents. In L. Tierney, S. McPhee, & M. Papadakis (Eds.), *Current medical diagnosis and treatment* (pp. 1549-1551). New York: Lange Medical Books.
12. Combes, A. (2007). Early predictors for infection recurrence and death in patients with ventilator-associated pneumonia. *Critical Care Medicine, 35*(1), 146-154.
13. Easter, A. (2001). Management of patients with multiple rib fractures [Electronic version]. *American Journal of Critical Care, 10*(5), 320-329.
14. Eutereuer, D. (2006). Health related quality of life in patients with chronic respiratory failure after long-term mechanical ventilation. *Respiratory Medicine, 100*(3), 477-486.
15. Fenstermacher, D., & Hong, D. (2004). Mechanical ventilation: What have we learned? *Critical Care Nursing Quarterly, 27*(3), 258-294.
16. Golden, P. (2000). Thoracic trauma [Electronic version]. *Orthopedic Nursing, 19*(5), 37-47.
17. Goll, C. (2001). Near drowning. In P. Swearingen & J. Hicks Keen (Eds.), *Manual of critical care nursing* (4th ed., pp. 136-140). St. Louis: Mosby.
18. Goll, C. (2001). Acute respiratory failure. In P. Swearingen & J. Hicks Keen (Eds.), *Manual of critical care nursing* (4th ed., pp. 243-246). St. Louis: Mosby.

19. Guerin, C. (2004). Effects of systematic prone positioning in hypoxemic acute respiratory failure. *Journal of the American Medical Association, 292*(17), 2379-2387.

20. Hardin, K.A. (2006). Sleep in critically ill chemically paralyzed patients requiring mechanical ventilation. *Chest, 129*(6), 1468-1477.

21. Hogarth, D.K., & Hall, J. (2004). Management of sedation in mechanically ventilated patients. *Current Opinion in Critical Care, 10*(1), 40-46.

22. Klein, D. (1999). Prone positioning in patients with acute respiratory distress syndrome: The Vollman Prone Positioner. *Critical Care Nurse, 19*(4), 66-71.

23. Lafferty, J., & Kavanagh, B. (2002). Hypocapnia. *New England Journal of Medicine, 347*(1), 43-53.

24. Lenart, S., & Garrity, J. (2000). Eye care for patients receiving neuromuscular blocking agents or propofol during mechanical ventilation. *American Journal of Critical Care, 9*(3), 188-191.

25. MacIntyre, N., et al. (2001). Evidence-based guidelines for weaning and discontinuing ventilatory support. *Chest, 120*(6), 375S-389S.

26. Markou, N., Myrianthefs, P., & Baltopoulos, G. (2004). Respiratory failure: An overview. *Critical Care Nursing Quarterly, 27*(4), 353-379.

27. Meade, M., & Herridge, M. (2001). An evidence-based approach to acute respiratory distress syndrome [Electronic version]. *Respiratory Care, 46*(12), 1368-1376.

28. Meduri, G.U. (2007). Methylprednisolone infusion in early severe ARDS: Results of a randomized controlled trial. *Chest, 131*(4), 954-963.

29. Moon, R., Dear, G., & Stolp, B. (2000). Hyperbaric oxygen in critical care. In A. Grenvik, et al. (Eds.), *The textbook of critical care* (4th ed., pp. 1534-1535). Philadelphia: Saunders.

30. Mortelli, M., & Manning, H. (2002). Acute respiratory distress syndrome [Electronic version]. *American Family Physician, 65*(9), 1823-1830.

31. Pierson, D. (2001). The future of respiratory care. *Respiratory Care, 46*(7), 705-718.

32. Rodger, M. (1999). Common respiratory problems: Pulmonary embolism, pneumothorax, and thoracic pulmonary surgery. In L. Bucher & S. Melander (Eds.), *Critical care nursing* (pp. 486-496). Philadelphia: Saunders.

33. Sakallaris, B. (1999). Acute respiratory failure. In L. Bucher & S. Melander (Eds.), *Critical care nursing* (pp. 411-445). Philadelphia: Saunders.

34. Sassoon, C., & McGovern, J. (2000). Oxygenation strategy. In A. Grenvik, et al. (Eds.), *The textbook of critical care* (4th ed., pp. 1308-1323). Philadelphia: Saunders.

35. Sole, M.L., Byers, J.F., Ludy, J.E., et al. (2003). A multi-site survey of suctioning techniques and airway management practices. *American Journal of Critical Care, 12*, 220-230.

36. Stacy, K. (2006). Pulmonary disorders. In L. Urden, K. Stacy, & M. Lough (Eds.), *Thelan's critical care nursing: Diagnosis and management* (5th ed., pp. 551-560, 570-573). St. Louis: Mosby.

37. Stacy, K. (2006). Pulmonary therapeutic management. In L. Urden, K. Stacy, & M. Lough (Eds.), *Thelan's critical care nursing: Diagnosis and management* (5th ed., pp. 587-613). St. Louis: Mosby.

38. Staudinger, T., et al. (2001). Comparison of prone positioning and continuous rotation of patients with adult respiratory distress syndrome: Results of a pilot study. *Critical Care Medicine, 29*(1), 51-56.

39. Tarizan, A.J. (2000). Caring for dying patients who have air hunger. *Journal of Nursing Scholarship, 32*(2), 137-143.

40. Taylor, R., & Trottier, S. (2000). Pathophysiology of acute lung injury. In A. Grenvik, et al. (Eds.), *The textbook of critical care* (4th ed., pp. 1382-1390). Philadelphia: Saunders.

41. The Acute Respiratory Distress Syndrome Network. (2000). Ventilation with lower tidal volumes as compared to traditional tidal volumes for acute lung injury and the acute respiratory distress syndrome. *New England Journal of Medicine, 342*(18), 1301-1308.

42. Voggenreiter, G., et al. (1999). Intermittent prone positioning in the treatment of severe and moderate posttraumatic lung injury. *Critical Care Medicine, 27*(11), 2375-2382.

evolve   *Did you remember to check out the bonus material on the Evolve website and the CD-ROM, including NCLEX®-Examination Style Review Questions, Open-Book Quizzes, and Chapter Review Audio Podcasts?*

http://evolve.elsevier.com/Black/medsurg

UNIT 15

SENSORY DISORDERS

ANATOMY AND PHYSIOLOGY REVIEW:

The Eyes and Ears

Robert G. Carroll

OVERVIEW

The visual, auditory, and olfactory systems are "distance" senses, bringing information about our environment to our perception. Each system detects the intensity and quality of stimuli, encodes and processes this information, and transmits it to various areas of the cerebral cortex. Together these senses provide much of the available information about our environment. This review covers vision and hearing; smell is described in Unit 7.

The *visual apparatus* is specialized to detect light. Light passes through the cornea, aqueous humor, lens, and vitreous humor before striking the retina. The visual receptors—rods and cones—encode data about the intensity and wavelength of light. This information is processed and transmitted through nerve cells of the retina, the optic nerve, and the thalamus before arriving at the visual cortex. The information is constructed in the primary and associated visual cortex into a conscious perception.

The *auditory apparatus* is specialized to detect sound. Sound waves pass through the pinna, through the auditory canal to the eardrum (tympanic membrane), through the bones of the middle ear, and then to the receptors in the cochlea. The auditory hair cells are arranged on the organ of Corti (the end organ for hearing) and are coded to detect the intensity and frequency of sound. This information passes through the auditory nerve through the lateral lemniscus and, finally, to the auditory cortex. Within the primary and secondary auditory cortex, auditory discrimination occurs.

VISUAL SYSTEM

STRUCTURE OF THE VISUAL SYSTEM

External Structures

The visual system is a complex group of structures that includes the eyeballs, muscles, nerves, fat, and bones. The *ocular adnexa* (Figure A&P15-1, *A*) are the accessory structures of the eye (muscles, fat, and bone) that support and protect it. The bony orbit (eye socket) surrounds and protects most of the eye so that only a small portion is visible. The orbit is formed from portions of the frontal, lacrimal, ethmoid, maxillary, zygomaticus,

sphenoid, and palatine bones. These bones are thin and fragile and break easily when pressure is applied to the eye (as in a fist fight). In addition to bone, the orbit also contains fat, various connective tissues, blood vessels, and nerves.

The *eyeball* is moved by six ocular muscles that are attached to the surface of the globe (Figure A&P15-2) and move the eye through six cardinal gazes. The four rectus muscles (the medial, lateral, superior, and inferior) move the eyes horizontally and vertically. The two oblique muscles (superior and inferior) rotate the eye in circular movements to allow vision at all angles.

The upper and lower *eyelids* are folds of skin that close to protect the anterior eyeball. When the eyelids close, they distribute tear film, which prevents evaporation and drying of the surface epithelium. The elliptic space between the two open lids is the *palpebral fissure*. The corners of the fissure are called the *canthi*. The medial, or inner, canthus is next to the nose; the lateral, or outer, canthus is the outside corner. Oil-secreting *meibomian glands* are embedded in both upper and lower lids (see Figure A&P15-1, *B*).

The *lacrimal gland*, in the upper lid over the outer canthus, produces tears that reach the eyeball through secretory ducts. Tiny openings *(puncti)* in both the upper and lower lids at the inner canthus direct tears to the lacrimal sac. The *nasolacrimal duct* directs the flow of tears into the nose. The tear film is composed of lipids secreted by the meibomian glands and dissolved salts, glucose, urea, protein, and lysozyme secreted by the lacrimal glands. The tear film lubricates, cleans, and protects the ocular surface. Mucus, secreted by goblet cells located in the lids, assists these processes.

Internal Structures

The *conjunctiva* is a thin transparent layer of mucous membrane that lines the eyelids and covers the eyeball (see Figure A&P15-1, *C*). The *cornea* is a transparent avascular structure with a brilliant, shiny surface. It is convex in shape, is about 0.5 mm thick, and acts as a powerful lens to bend and direct (refract) rays of light to the retina. The cornea is composed of five layers. It derives oxygen from the atmosphere. A rich network of nerve fibers in the outer layer (epithelium) produces a sensation of pain whenever the fibers are exposed or stimulated.

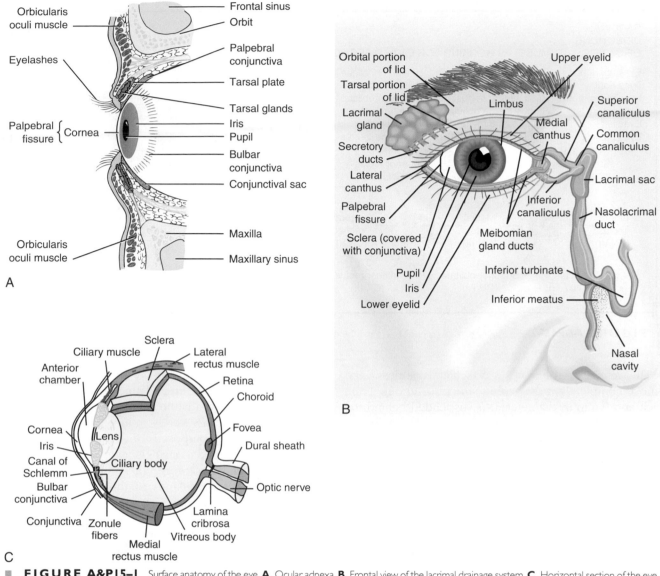

■ **FIGURE A&P15–1** Surface anatomy of the eye. **A,** Ocular adnexa. **B,** Frontal view of the lacrimal drainage system. **C,** Horizontal section of the eye.

The *sclera* is the fibrous protective coating of the eye. It is white, dense, and continuous with the cornea. In children, the sclera is thin and appears bluish because of the underlying pigmented structures. In old age, it may become yellowish from degeneration.

The *uveal tract,* the middle vascular layer of the eye that furnishes the blood supply to the retina, consists of three structures:

1. The *iris* is a thin, pigmented diaphragm with a central aperture, the pupil. Iris color is determined by the degree of pigmentation in the stromal melanocytes. The interaction of the two iris muscles (sphincter and dilator) determines pupil diameter. Expansion and contraction of the iris regulate the amount of light entering the eye.

2. The *ciliary body* produces and secretes *aqueous humor,* a clear alkaline fluid composed mainly of water that occupies the space between the iris and the cornea (the anterior chamber of the eye). The ciliary body is in direct continuity with the iris and is circular, surrounding the lens. Aqueous humor circulates from the posterior chamber through the pupil into the anterior chamber. The flow continues into the anterior chamber angle and is filtered out through the trabecular meshwork into Schlemm's canal. From there, the aqueous humor is channeled into a capillary network and into episcleral veins. Normal intraocular pressure is maintained as long as there is a balance between aqueous production and aqueous humor outflow.

3. The *choroid* is the posterior segment of the uveal tract between the retina and the sclera. It is composed of three layers of vessels and is attached to both the ciliary body and the optic nerve.

■ **FIGURE A&PI5–2**   The six cardinal directions of gaze and the muscles responsible for each.

The *lens* is a biconvex, avascular, colorless, and almost completely transparent structure, about 4 mm thick and 9 mm in diameter. It is suspended behind the iris by ligamentous fibers *(zonules),* which connect to the ciliary body. The sole purpose of the lens is to focus light on the retina. The change of focus from distant to near is called *accommodation.* There are no pain fibers or blood vessels in the lens. The lens is surrounded by a transparent envelope (the capsule). The lens of the eye consists of about 65% water and 35% protein.

The *vitreous body* is a clear, avascular, jelly-like structure. Vitreous fluid is thick and viscous, and occupies a space called the *vitreous chamber.* It fills the largest cavity of the eye, accounting for two thirds of its volume. It helps maintain the shape and transparency of the eye.

Retina

The retina is a thin, semitransparent layer of nerve tissue that forms the innermost lining of the eye. It consists of 10 distinct layers of highly organized, delicate tissue. The retina contains all the sensory receptors for the transmission of light and is actually part of the brain.

There are two types of retinal receptors: rods and cones. About 125 million *rods* are distributed in the periphery of the retina; they function best in dim light. Damage to these structures results in night blindness. The *cones,* numbering about 6 million and concentrated in the center of the retina, provide resolution of small visual angles, resulting in perception of fine details. They are also responsible for color vision.

The center of the retina *(macula)* is an area about 5 mm in diameter. In an ophthalmoscopic examination, it appears as a yellowish spot with a depressed center, the *fovea.* An area 1.5 mm in diameter where only cones are present, the fovea is the point of finest vision. Damage to the fovea can severely reduce central vision.

The retina is composed of many fine layers of neural tissue attached to a single layer of pigmented epithelial cells. The photoreceptor cells in the retina are nourished by the capillaries of the choroid layer just beneath the pigment epithelial cell layer. Oxygen supply to these delicate structures is crucial, because the conversion of visual stimuli into impulses that the brain records as images requires very active metabolic processes.

Optic Nerve and Neural Pathways

The optic nerve is located at the posterior portion of the eye and transmits visual impulses from the retina to the brain. The head of the optic nerve *(optic disc)* can be seen by ophthalmoscopic examination. The optic nerve contains no sensory receptors (rods or cones) and represents a blind spot in the eye. The nerve emerges from the back of the eye and extends for 25 to 30 mm, traveling through the muscle cone to enter the bony optic foramen, eventually joining the other optic nerve to form the optic chiasm. The optic nerve neurons synapse in the thalamus, and thalamic nerves then transmit the visual information to the occipital lobe of the cortex.

FUNCTION OF THE VISUAL SYSTEM

Vision requires accurate transmission of light to the photoreceptors of the retina, encoding of the wavelength and intensity by the retinal receptors, and interpretation of the coded signals by the visual cortex.

Transmission of Light

Light passes through the cornea, aqueous humor, lens, and vitreous humor before striking the retina. Blood vessels are opaque, and the cornea, lens, and fovea are sparsely vascularized, which enhances light transmission. The cornea and lens refract light, allowing it to converge to a focal point on the fovea of the retina. Refraction at the lens is regulated by contraction of the ciliary muscles.

Near vision is accomplished by contraction of the ciliary muscles, which increases curvature of the lens and brings near objects into focus on the retina. *Far vision* is accomplished by relaxing the ciliary muscles and flattening the lens. With age, lens elasticity decreases because of protein degeneration, reducing the ability to accommodate for near vision. Visual abnormalities are corrected by placing an appropriate refractor (eyeglasses or contact lens) in the light pathway.

Visual Receptors of the Retina: Cones and Rods

Three types of cones are sensitive to specific wavelengths of light, with peak sensitivities in the red, green, and blue wavelengths. Density of the cone receptors is highest in the fovea (the area of highest visual acuity). Bright light causes contraction of the iris, limiting the light entering the eye and focusing the light on the fovea. Exposure to light bleaches retinal photopigments, reducing the receptor responsiveness to subsequent exposure (light adaptation). However, prolonged exposure to dark allows the receptors to recover; cones recover completely in about 10 minutes.

Rods are sensitive to light in the green and yellow wavelengths and impart night *(scotopic)* vision. Rods are distributed throughout the retina, but few rods are in the fovea. In the dark, the iris dilates, admitting light to large portions of the retina. Consequently, night vision is enhanced by looking just to the side of the object of interest. After light exposure, rods recover slowly, taking about 20 minutes to return to peak sensitivity (dark adaptation). Because the rod photopigments are not sensitive to red light, exposure to red light does not interfere with dark adaptation.

Image Processing and the Visual Cortex

Interneurons in the retina process the receptor output and transmit information via the optic nerve to the thalamus. The thalamus processes information about the wavelength and intensity of the light and relays the information to the visual cortex. Visual space in the cortex is completely crossed; objects appearing on the left side of the body are represented on the right visual

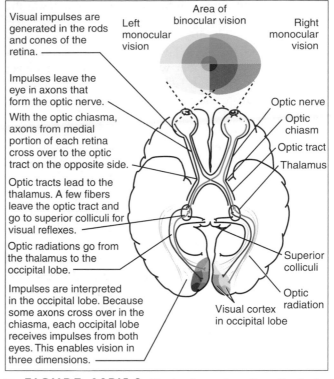

FIGURE A&P15–3 Visual pathways from the retina to the occipital lobe. The pathway is partially crossed, so that objects in the visual space of one side are interpreted in the contralateral visual cortex.

cortex and vice versa (Figure A&P15-3). The two eyes work together as one, focusing on the same point in space and fusing their images so that a single mental impression is obtained. The ability of the eyes to fuse two images into a single image is called *binocular vision,* accounting for one aspect of depth perception.

EFFECTS OF AGING ON VISION

Structural Changes

Several age-related changes occur in the structures of the eye and surrounding tissue. Eyebrows and eyelashes turn gray, and skin around the eyelids becomes wrinkled and loose because of loss of muscle tone and elasticity. Loss of orbital fat causes the eyes to sink deeper into the orbit and sometimes limits the upward gaze. Tear secretions may also diminish, resulting in the condition of dry eyes.

The most frequent and significant age-related change in the eye is the formation of a *cataract*. With age, the thickness and density of the lens increase and the lens becomes progressively yellowed and opaque. Throughout the life span, the lens continues to grow by forming new fiber cells. Although the rate of growth gradually diminishes, the accumulation of cells over time contributes to lens density. Loss of transparency also results from protein deterioration from absorption of ultraviolet radiation. The yellow material is associated with the development of abnormal fluorescent substances in the aging lens. The lens accommodation diminishes because of ciliary muscle atrophy.

The cells of the inner layer of the cornea (endothelium) decrease in number with age. Because this layer does not reproduce lost cells, the ability of this layer to heal after injury or surgery may be compromised. The corneal reflex also may be diminished or absent. Another phenomenon characteristic of aging is the *arcus senilis,* a grayish yellow ring found on the periphery of the cornea surrounding the iris. This ring is thought to be the result of the accumulation of lipids.

The ciliary body produces less aqueous humor during the aging process, but there is less outflow and intraocular pressure remains relatively stable or increases only slightly. The ciliary muscle tends to atrophy with age, and sometimes connective tissue replaces lost muscle tissue. The loss in muscle action along with lens thickening decreases the focusing ability of the lens. Decreasing ability to focus at near accommodation *(presbyopia)* is common.

Visual Changes

The major visual changes with aging include decreases in (1) visual acuity, (2) tolerance of glare, (3) ability to adapt to dark and light, and (4) peripheral vision. Each of these decreases is related to changes in the eye structure and each affects the quality and intensity of the light able to reach the retina.

Glare is a particular problem for older people. In combination with difficulty adjusting to dark and light, it is often the reason older adults stop driving at night. The lights from oncoming vehicles produce a glare when passing through both cornea and lens, which may make it very difficult to discern objects. Bright sunlight, either indoors or outdoors, causes an equally blinding glare. Indoor rooms should be lighted with soft incandescent lights, and sheer curtains can be used to diffuse bright sunlight.

Because the eye takes longer to adapt to changes from dark to light and vice versa, older people are at a greater risk for falls and injuries. Any place subject to sudden changes in lighting (e.g., inside a theater) can be dangerous. Getting up at night can be particularly hazardous for older adults. However, because red wavelengths are longer and are perceived by the cones, a red light in the bathroom at night allows enough vision to function without interfering with dark vision.

Peripheral vision decreases with age and may interfere with social interactions and physical activities. Older adults suffering from loss of peripheral vision may not notice someone sitting next to them. They may also have difficulty finding objects out of their range of vision.

The iris loses pigment with age, and older people may thus appear to have grayish or light blue eyes. The pupil becomes gradually smaller with age. A decrease in pupil size results in a smaller amount of light reaching the retina, meaning that the light must pass through the densest, most opaque area of the lens.

AUDITORY SYSTEM

STRUCTURE OF THE AUDITORY SYSTEM

The ear is housed in the *temporal bone* of the skull. The temporal bones are two of the eight cranial bones that form part of the base and lateral wall of the skull. The petrous portion of the temporal bone houses the otic capsule, the densest bone in the body. The temporal bone articulates with the sphenoid, parietal, and occipital bones.

External Ear

The ears are located on each side of the head at approximately eye level. The external ear is divided into the auricle *(pinna)* and the external auditory canal *(ear canal)*. The tympanic membrane *(eardrum)* separates the external ear from the middle ear.

Auricle (Pinna)

The *auricle* (pinna), the conspicuous part of the ear, is attached to the side of the head by skin at approximately a 20- to 30-degree angle. Except for the fat and subcutaneous tissue in the lobule, it is composed mostly of cartilage. The cartilage is held to the skull by small muscles (the posterior, anterior, and superior auricular muscles), which are innervated by the posterior auricular branch of the facial nerve.

The parts of the pinna are illustrated in Figure A&P15-4. The *helix,* the outer rim of the pinna, leads inferiorly to the

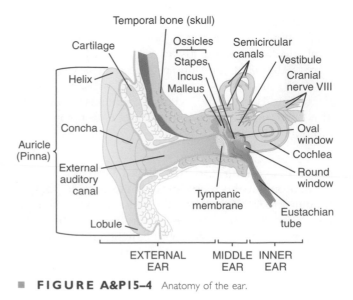

■ **FIGURE A&P15-4** Anatomy of the ear.

lobule. The *concha* is the deepest part, leading to the ear canal. The tragus and antitragus are triangular folds of cartilage that project over the entrance to the ear canal. Hair covers most of the ear, but it is usually rudimentary, except in the region of the tragus and antitragus.

In front of the external opening of the ear is the temporomandibular joint (TMJ). Often, TMJ problems produce referred pain to the ear (otalgia) because of their shared sensory nerve supply.

External Auditory Canal (Ear Canal)

The ear canal extends from the concha of the pinna to the tympanic membrane (see Figure A&P15-4). In adults, this slightly S-shaped canal is approximately 2.5 cm (1 inch) in length and follows an inward, forward, and downward path. The skeleton of cartilage in the outer third is continuous with the cartilage of the pinna. The inner two thirds is a bony canal entering the skull. The lumen of the ear canal is irregularly shaped and is narrowest where the transition from cartilage to bone occurs. The skin covering the cartilage portion is thick, containing sebaceous and ceruminous glands and hair follicles. The sebaceous and ceruminous glands secrete a golden to black substance called *cerumen* (wax). The skin covering the bony portion is very thin.

Tympanic Membrane

The tympanic membrane (eardrum) is an oval disk (approximately 1 cm in diameter); it covers the end of the auditory canal and separates the canal from the middle ear (see Figure A&P15-4). The eardrum is a thin, translucent, pearly gray membrane obliquely directed downward and inward, so that the posterior part is more accessible than the anterior part.

Middle Ear

The middle ear consists of the middle ear cleft and contents: ossicles, oval and round windows, eustachian tube, and facial nerve (see Figure A&P15-4). The middle ear lies between the ear canal and the *labyrinth* (inner ear). The middle ear cavity has a mucosal lining.

Ossicles

The middle ear contains the three smallest bones *(ossicles)* of the body, named according to their appearance. The outermost and largest ossicle is the *malleus* (hammer), which is firmly attached to the tympanic membrane. The innermost and smallest ossicle is the *stapes* (stirrup); its footplate occupies the oval window, in direct contact with the perilymph of the inner ear. The *incus* (anvil) lies between the other two and is shaped like a tooth with two roots (see Figure A&P15-4).

Windows

The middle ear contains two windows, whose names reflect their shape. The *round window* is an opening in the inner ear from which sound vibrations exit. The *oval window* is an opening in the inner ear into which sound vibrations enter. The oval window is not a true window because the footplate of the stapes bone covers it.

Eustachian Tube

The eustachian tube is a narrow channel approximately 35 mm (1½ inches) long and only 1 mm wide at its narrowest end. This tube connects the middle ear to the nasopharynx (see Figure A&P15-4). The structure consists mostly of fibrous tissue, cartilage, and bone; it extends downward, forward, and inward from each middle ear. The eustachian tube is lined with a mucous membrane that is continuous with the lining of the middle ear at one end and with the nasopharynx at the other end. A small section of this tube, originating in the middle ear, remains permanently open. Otherwise, the walls of the tube lightly oppose or touch each other, closing the tube to both the throat and ear and preventing the sound of normal nasal respiration and of one's own voice from passing up the eustachian tube.

Mastoid Bone

The mastoid section of the temporal bone includes the cone-shaped *mastoid process;* the *mastoid antrum,* a large cavity posteriorly continuous with the middle ear; and the *mastoid air cells,* which extend from the antrum and fill the temporal bone with air pockets.

The mastoid bone is a bony protuberance behind the lower portion of the pinna. The mastoid cavity is close to several important cranial structures: the dura of the temporal lobe, the cerebellar dura, the sigmoid sinus, and the jugular bulb. The middle ear is also bounded by the internal carotid artery. Therefore infection of the middle ear and mastoid cavities can also involve these structures.

Inner Ear (Labyrinth)

The inner ear or labyrinth is located deep within the petrous section of the temporal bone; it contains the sense organs for hearing and balance, which form the eighth cranial nerve (Figure A&P15-5). The inner ear is a complicated system of intercommunicating chambers and connecting tubes composed of two structures:

1. The *bony labyrinth* is the rigid capsule (otic capsule) that surrounds and protects the delicate membranous labyrinth. The *vestibule* connects the cochlea (for hearing) to the three semicircular canals (for balance). The *cochlea,* which looks like a snail shell with 2½ turns, is approximately 7 mm in diameter at the widest part and is structurally

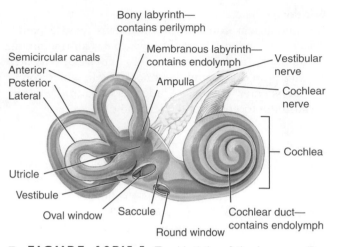

Bony labyrinth—
contains perilymph

Semicircular canals
Anterior
Posterior
Lateral

Membranous labyrinth—
contains endolymph

Ampulla

Vestibular
nerve

Cochlear
nerve

Cochlea

Utricle

Vestibule

Oval window

Saccule

Round window

Cochlear duct—
contains endolymph

■ **FIGURE A&P15–5** The labyrinths of the inner ear. *(From Applegate, E.J. [2000]. The anatomy and physiology learning system [2nd ed.]. Philadelphia: Saunders.)*

divided into 3 compartments (Figure A&P15-6). The upper compartment *(scala vestibuli)* leads from the oval window to the apex of the cochlear spiral. The lower compartment *(scala tympani)* leads from the apex of the cochlear spiral to the round window. The *scala media,* which contains the organ of Corti, lies between the scala vestibuli and scala tympani.

2. The *membranous labyrinth,* lying within but not completely filling the bony labyrinth, is bathed in a fluid called *perilymph,* which communicates with the cerebrospinal fluid (CSF) via the cochlear duct. The membranous labyrinth consists of the utricle, the saccule, the semicircular canals, the cochlear duct, and the *organ of Corti* (the end organ for

hearing). The membranous labyrinth contains a different fluid *(endolymph).* This fluid also protects the end organ because it acts as a cushion against abrupt movements of the head.

The three *semicircular canals* are at right angles to each other and are named the anterior (superior), posterior (inferior), and lateral (horizontal) canals. The horizontal canal lies closest to the middle ear. This arrangement allows detection of movement in all three dimensions.

FUNCTION OF THE AUDITORY SYSTEM

External Ear

The ears are a pair of complex sensory organs for both hearing and balance. Their location on either side of the head produces binaural hearing, allows the detection of sound direction, and aids in maintaining equilibrium. The temporal bone provides protection for the organs of hearing and balance. It houses (1) the external and internal auditory canals; (2) the mastoid air cells, which provide an air reservoir for the middle ear; (3) the blood vessels; (4) the facial, vestibular, and cochlear nerves; (5) the labyrinth; and (6) the cochlea.

Sound Wave Conduction

The head, pinna, and ear canal act as an integrated system to transmit sound vibrations to the eardrum. Sound is transmitted from the external ear through the middle ear (which amplifies the sound) to the inner ear (see

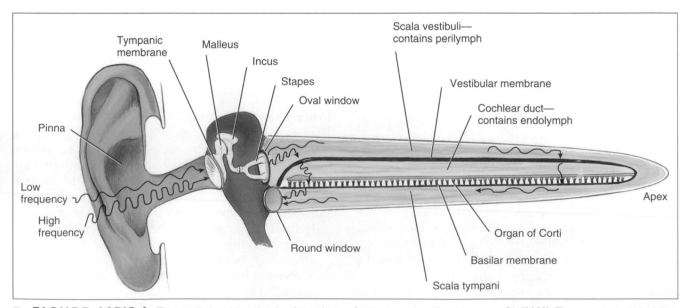

Tympanic
membrane

Malleus

Incus

Stapes

Oval window

Scala vestibuli—
contains perilymph

Vestibular membrane

Cochlear duct—
contains endolymph

Pinna

Low
frequency

High
frequency

Round window

Scala tympani

Organ of Corti

Basilar membrane

Apex

■ **FIGURE A&P15–6** The uncoiled cochlea, showing the pathway of pressure waves. *(From Applegate, E.J. [2000]. The anatomy and physiology learning system [2nd ed.]. Philadelphia: Saunders.)*

Figure A&P15-6). The funnel shape of the pinna collects and directs sound to the eardrum.

The tympanic membrane, a common membrane between the external ear canal and the middle ear space, protects the middle ear and conducts sound vibrations from the external ear to the ossicles. The tympanic membrane changes its tension to muffle sound. The sound pressure applied to the stapes (the smallest ossicle) in the oval window is 22 times greater than the sound pressure exerted on the eardrum. The pressure of the sound vibrations is increased as a result of transmission from a larger area to a smaller area, and the lever effect of the ossicular chain. The sound energy, after transformation, is carried by neural elements to the brain for decoding and, thus, hearing.

Wax Production

Cerumen (wax) protects the ear. Wax is to the ear what tears are to the eyes. The sticky consistency of the wax and the fine hairs of the ear canal help clean the ear canal of foreign matter and protect it from water damage. Impacted cerumen can cause hearing losses in clients of all ages. At times, wax must be mechanically removed.

Middle Ear
Sound Wave Conduction

The ossicles transmit sound vibrations mechanically (see Figure A&P15-6). The ossicles are held in place by joints, muscles, and ligaments, which also offer some protection from loud sounds. The light weight and the configuration of the ossicles provide an efficient means of transmitting sound vibrations from the air molecules of the external ear to the fluid molecules of the inner ear. Fluids offer more resistance than air and need more force to transmit movement. The ossicular chain produces and magnifies this force in order to move the inner ear fluids.

Ventilation and Pressure Regulation

The eustachian tube provides an air passage from the nasopharynx to the middle ear to equalize pressure on both sides of the eardrum. This tube regulates ventilation and pressure, both of which are necessary for normal hearing. During yawning, swallowing, and sneezing, the eustachian tube is opened by the *tensor veli palatini* muscle. The natural opening and closing of the eustachian tube also allows drainage of exudate from the middle ear mucosa. The tube can be forcibly opened by increasing nasopharyngeal pressure. This act is accomplished by attempting to blow air through the nose while holding the nose closed.

Inner Ear
Hearing

Sound waves are transmitted by the ossicles to the delicate membrane of the oval window (see Figure A&P15-6).

These vibrations move the perilymph in the scala vestibuli. The perilymph of the scala vestibuli is continuous with that of the scala tympani at the extreme tip of the "snail shell," called the *helicotrema*. The sound energy vibrations enter through the oval window and exit through the round window.

Vibrations in the perilymph of the scala vestibuli are transmitted through the vestibular membrane *(Reissner's membrane)* to the endolymph that fills the cochlear duct. The cochlear duct is located between the scala vestibuli and the scala tympani. The *organ of Corti,* which is bathed in the endolymph, lies on the basilar membrane in a spiral strip from the basal turn near the round window to the apex at the helicotrema. This organ transforms mechanical sound vibrations into neural activity and separates sound into different frequencies. The electrochemical impulse travels via the acoustic nerve to the brain stem. Auditory nerve input from both ears joins at the lateral lemniscus, reducing the possibility of unilateral deafness from central nervous system damage. The auditory nerves ascend through the thalamus to the cortex by a variety of pathways, reaching both the primary and secondary auditory regions of the temporal cortex of the brain. Efferent innervation via the acoustic nerve (eighth cranial nerve) reaches the cochlea and vestibule via the internal auditory canal, which also carries the facial nerve (seventh cranial nerve).

Sound is filtered by the ear components. Human auditory sensitivity ranges from 15 to 20,000 Hz. The auditory canal diminishes the passage of sounds with frequencies greater than 3500 Hz, the higher end of the human voice frequency. The middle ear diminishes passage of sounds with frequencies less than 1000 Hz, the lower end of human voice frequency. The muscles of the middle ear decrease sound transmission by uncoupling the ossicles. For example, contraction of the tensor tympani allows reflex adaptation to a noisy environment. Contraction of the stapedius decreases sound transmission while speaking.

Balance

The *utricle* and *saccule* are vestibular receptors that position the head as it relates to the pull of gravity. The utricle and saccule contain hair cells arranged in sheets (maculae). These hair cells detect changes in linear acceleration, including the force of gravity. The *semicircular canals* are arranged to sense rotational movements, such as movements or changes in position. Each of the semicircular canals connects with the utricle. Where the canals connect with the utricle is an enlarged portion *(ampulla)*. The ampulla contains a cluster of hair cells *(crista)* concerned with dynamic balance. For example, when head position is changed, movement of the endolymph stimulates the hair cells, initiating increased impulses that travel over the vestibular division of the acoustic nerve to the brain. Balance functions in the vestibular system, along with visual cues and musculoskeletal cues, combine to maintain balance. Hearing and balance are partially maintained with the loss of function of one ear.

EFFECTS OF AGING ON HEARING

Many physiologic changes lead to changes in hearing in older people. The hairs become coarser during the aging process; thus retention of wax is more of a problem. *Presbycusis,* a gradual sensorineural loss caused by nerve degeneration in the inner ear or auditory nerve, is a type of hearing loss that occurs with aging, even in people living in a quiet environment. Loss of auditory neurons in the organ of Corti and cochlear hair cell degeneration create an inability to hear high-frequency sounds. There may also be degeneration of the cochlear conductive membrane and decreased blood supply to the cochlea, leading to inability to hear at all (but especially higher) frequencies. Finally, a loss of cortical auditory neurons leads to diminished hearing and speech comprehension.

CONCLUSIONS

Vision and hearing are two senses that allow distance perception of the environment. Because we rely on these senses for communication with those around us, alterations in either sense can have a profound social and emotional impact. Some reductions in the ability to see or to hear are a normal part of age-related changes.

BIBLIOGRAPHY

1. Applegate, E.J. (2000). *The anatomy and physiology learning system* (2nd ed.). Philadelphia: Saunders.
2. Guyton, A.C., & Hall, J. (2007). *Textbook of medical physiology* (11th ed.). Philadelphia: Saunders.
3. Kandel, E.R., Schwartz, J.H., & Jessel, T.M. (2000). *Principles of neural science* (4th ed.). New York: McGraw-Hill.
4. McPhee, S.J., et al. (1999). *Pathophysiology of disease.* New York, McGraw-Hill.
5. Nolte, J. (2002). *The human brain* (5th ed.). St. Louis: Mosby.
6. Silverthorn, D. (2001). *Human physiology* (2nd ed.). Upper Saddle River, NJ: Prentice Hall.

CHAPTER 64

Assessment of the Eyes and Ears

SHARON LANZETTA AND LIANNE F. HERBRUCK

ASSESSMENT OF THE EYE

The eye is a unique organ because its external anatomy can be assessed easily. Internal eye structures, including blood vessels and central nervous system (CNS) tissue (the retina and optic nerve), are also easily visualized through the cornea without invasive procedures. The effects of many systemic problems, such as infections, cancer, and vascular and autoimmune disorders, can be detected during an internal eye examination. Clients may voice misconceptions about vision and the eyes (Box 64-1). If you encounter such misconceptions while conducting a physical examination, be prepared to address them.

HISTORY

A complete ophthalmic history includes demographic data, exploration of chief complaint and related manifestations, review of systems, past medical history, past surgical history, allergies and medications, dietary habits, psychosocial history and lifestyle, and family health history.

Biographical and Demographic Data

Demographic data relevant to ocular assessment include age and gender. The incidence of cataracts, dry eye, retinal detachment, glaucoma, esotropia (eyes turning inward), and exotropia (eyes turning outward) increases with age. Hereditary color vision deficits are more common in men than in women.

Current Health

As with many body systems, care must be taken when assessing ocular manifestations. Of the five senses, vision is the system that provides the most information. There may be a fear of vision loss or uncorrectable visual manifestations. Many disease processes, or their treatments, have potential to negatively impact visual health. Some eye issues, like wide-angle glaucoma, are usually found during routine eye examinations.

The four most common preventable causes of permanent vision loss in developed nations are (1) *amblyopia* (reduced visual acuity that is not correctable with glasses in the absence of anatomic defects in the eye or visual pathways), (2) diabetic retinopathy, (3) age-related maculopathy, and (4) glaucoma. Many of these ophthalmic disorders are asymptomatic, so routine eye examinations are therefore imperative.

Chief Complaint

The most common chief complaint is a change or loss of vision. The complaint may also be less specific, such as headache or eyestrain. Sometimes the client may be unable to verbalize a specific complaint, and the chief complaint could be as vague as "something is wrong with my eyes."

---

evolve Web Enhancements

Assessment Terms English and Spanish

Appendix B A Health History Format That Integrates the Assessment of Functional Health Patterns

Web Figures Snellen's Chart

An Otoscope

Weber and Rinne Tests for Hearing Impairment

Web Tables Constriction and Accommodation Tests for the Pupil

Tonometry and Slit-Lamp Examinations

Web Box Guidelines for Using an Ophthalmoscope

Be sure to check out the bonus material on the Evolve website and the CD-ROM, including free self-assessment exercises. **http://evolve.elsevier.com/Black/medsurg**

Clinical Manifestations

Ocular manifestations can be divided into three basic categories: (1) vision, (2) appearance, and (3) sensations of pain and discomfort. Whenever possible, characterize clinical manifestations according to onset, location, duration, and characteristics, such as frequency and severity. The circumstances surrounding onset as well as the client's response to treatment are important. Refer to Figure 64-1 for details on the initial assessment of the client with eye complaints.

Pain (Ophthalmalgia). Eye pain is often poorly localized. Nonspecific complaints include eyestrain, pulling, pressure, fullness, or generalized headache. The pain may be periocular, ocular, or retrobulbar (behind the globe). Foreign-body sensation produces a sharp superficial pain that can be relieved by topical anesthesia. Deeper internal aching may indicate glaucoma, inflammation, muscle spasm, or infection. The Integrating Diagnostic Testing feature on p. 1680 provides further cues for evaluation of the client with eye pain.

Abnormal Vision. Visual changes or loss of vision can be caused by abnormalities in the eye or anywhere along the visual pathway. Considerations may include refractive (focusing) error; lid ptosis (drooping eyelid); clouding or interference in the cornea, lens, or aqueous or vitreous space; and malfunction of the retina, optic nerve, or intracranial visual pathway. Refer to the Integrating Diagnostic Testing feature on p. 1681 for further details on the evaluation of the client with a visual changes complaint.

Abnormal Appearance. External changes in appearance include growths or lesions, edema, ptosis, and abnormal position. The most common abnormal appearance is a *red eye* (Box 64-2). Refer to the Integrating Diagnostic Testing feature on p. 1682 for further details on the evaluation of the client with a possible eye infection.

Abnormal Sensation. Adequate description of ocular sensation can help guide an appropriate diagnosis (Table 64-1 on p. 1683). Reflex spasm of the ciliary muscle and iris sphincter that occurs with inflammation may produce brow ache and *photophobia* (sensitivity to light) or a constricted pupil *(miosis)*. Itching is usually a sign of an allergic response. Dryness, burning, grittiness, and mild foreign-body sensation can occur with dry eyes or mild corneal irritation.

Review of Systems

The review of systems (ROS) information in Figure 64-2 on p. 1684 can be used as a guide to help determine underlying etiology of potential and realized visual issues. Many disease processes can affect vision. Vascular problems, such as hypertension, can impact blood flow to the eyes, causing changes in vision. Headaches with visual changes may indicate a tumor in the brain or be a cue to migraines. Obtaining the family visual history can alert the client to potential visual risks, and can assist the practitioner in helping the client to reduce these risks.

ROS relevant to ocular assessment includes asking about manifestations such as headaches and problems with sinusitis. Determine whether manifestations occur in association with pain or discomfort, visual changes, swelling, redness, or drainage from the eye. Record time of day and the season of year during which manifestations occur as well as any sensitivity to light.

Past Medical History

The past medical history focuses on systemic disorders commonly associated with ocular manifestations. Some of these illnesses, such as diabetes mellitus, rheumatoid arthritis, and thyroid disorders, may be recently acquired by adults, or may have occurred in the client's childhood. Inquire about childhood vaccinations, particularly for measles (rubella).

In addition to childhood and systemic diseases, ask about hypertension, multiple sclerosis, and myasthenia gravis. If the client wears eyeglasses or contact lenses, ask when the last eye examination took place and when the prescription was last changed. Hospitalizations related to the eyes or brain, including a history of head or eye trauma, must be assessed.

Surgical History

Record the client's surgical history. This may include corrective vision surgery such as laser-assisted in-situ keratomileusis (LASIK), radial keratotomy (RK), cataract removal, glaucoma treatment, or eye muscle correction. Some eye surgeries, such as those for glaucoma, can

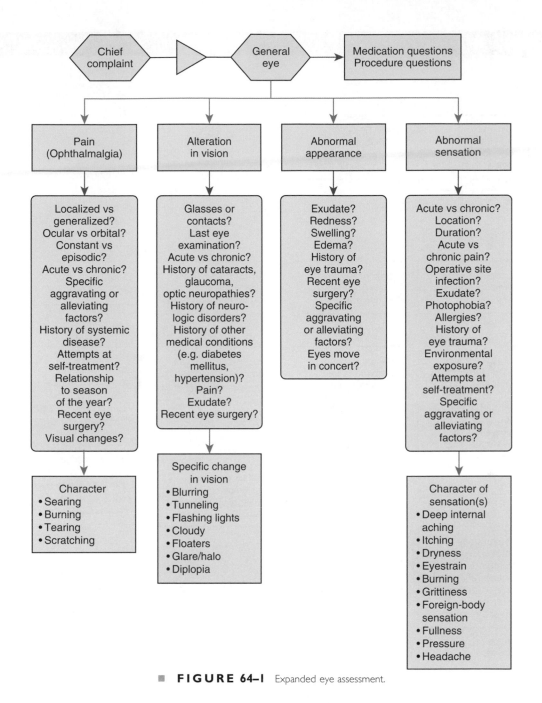

■ **FIGURE 64–1** Expanded eye assessment.

precipitate other eye issues (cataracts). History of brain or facial surgeries should also be assessed as these have the potential to affect vision.

Allergies

Note any allergies to medications (eye drops) and other substances, such as inhalants (dust, chemicals, or pollens) and environmental contacts (cosmetics or pollens). Allergic manifestations include eye redness, tearing, and itching.

Medications

Many medications, including prescription drugs, affect the eyes. Note the name, dose, and frequency the

medication is taken. Specifically ask about use of over-the-counter (OTC) eye drops, as those with antihistamines and decongestants can dry the ocular surface. Record current eye and systemic medications being used, and all other current and past ocular disorders.

Dietary Habits

Inquire about the use of herbal remedies and dietary supplements (vitamins). Some clients may consume large doses of vitamins, believing these substances will prevent the development of vision problems such as cataracts and macular degeneration. ▶ Studies have shown that diets rich in fruits, vegetables, and fish, or

INTEGRATING DIAGNOSTIC TESTING

Eye Pain

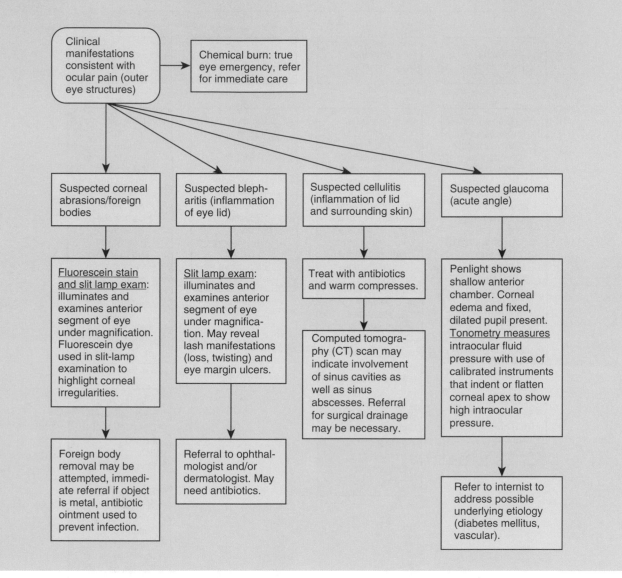

supplements of antioxidants C, E, and beta-carotene, have potential to reduce the incidence of visual problems like macular degeneration. However, many OTC preparations taken in too large a quantity can be harmful. Clients need to be aware of the risks and should be encouraged to be truthful about supplement ingestion.

Social History

Psychosocial history and lifestyle data significant to the ocular health history include occupational hazards, leisure activities and hobbies, and health management behaviors. Assess the client's work and/or hobbies that may include exposure to irritating fumes, smoke, or airborne particles. Also assess participation in activities that

increase the risk for eye or head trauma (such as football, racquetball, or baseball), as well as those that increase the risk of foreign-body injury or abrasion (e.g., hiking or gardening). Address client use of protective eye gear (such as safety goggles or sunglasses) when engaging in these activities.

Health management behaviors related to the eyes include self-care measures as mismanagement can negatively impact eye health. For example, is the diabetic client aggressively managing his/her disease? Is the client with contact lenses cleaning and storing them as recommended? Sunglasses are important as the ultraviolet rays of the sun can damage the eyes. Smoking is associated with increased risk of macular

INTEGRATING DIAGNOSTIC TESTING

Visual Changes

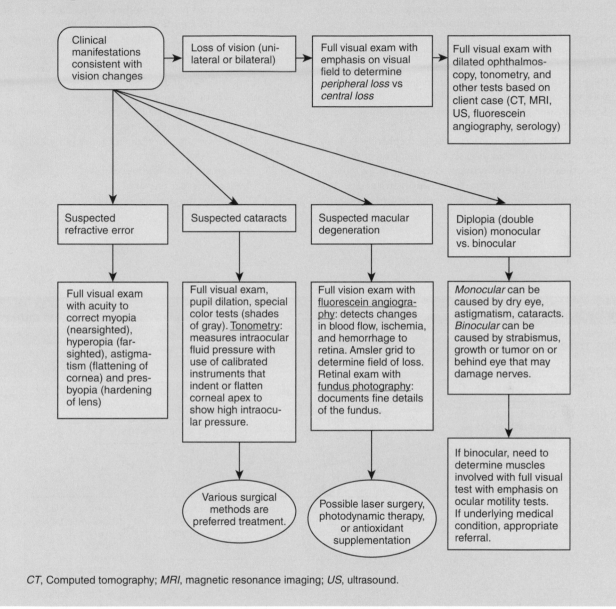

CT, Computed tomography; MRI, magnetic resonance imaging; US, ultrasound.

degeneration. Also, eating a healthy diet and getting adequate exercise can positively impact other disease processes, such as hypertension, which increases the odds of good visual health.

Visual ability is one of several capabilities necessary for a person to operate a motor vehicle. Use tact when reviewing a driving history for a client who may have impaired vision. Clients may not answer truthfully if they feel driving privileges may be lost.

The social stigma of blindness underlies the anxiety that clients experience with actual or potential vision loss. Loss of control in personal, family, and work situations can be devastating. Total loss of vision isolates a person within a different reality. Clients with actual or potential vision loss may be faced with barriers in their vocations that force an unwanted change, as not all work environments can be adapted for someone who is visually impaired. Issues of dependence versus independence are often a factor in the client's ability to cope with the stressors of vision loss.

Family Health History

Many ocular disorders tend to be familial (strabismus, glaucoma, myopia, hyperopia). Other conditions such as

---

BOX 64-2 Red Eye

Nurses often encounter a client whose chief complaint is a "red eye." The condition causing the eye to be red (engorgement of the conjunctival vessels) may be a subconjunctival hemorrhage that requires no treatment, or it may be a manifestation of a serious eye disorder, which requires immediate attention. Disorders involving red eye include the following:

Conjunctivitis—bacterial, viral, allergic, and irritative
Herpes simplex keratitis—inflammation of the cornea
Scleritis—inflammation of the sclera
Angle-closure glaucoma—sudden occlusion of the anterior chamber angle by iris tissue
Adnexal disease—stye, dacryocystitis, blepharitis, lid lesions (carcinoma), thyroid disease, and vascular lesions
Subconjunctival hemorrhage—accumulation of blood in the potential space between the conjunctiva and the sclera
Pterygium—abnormal growth of tissue that progresses over the cornea

Keratoconjunctivitis sicca—inflammation associated with lacrimal deficiency
Abrasions and foreign bodies—hyperemic response
Abnormal lid function—Bell's palsy, thyroid ophthalmopathy, or lesions that cause ocular exposure

To evaluate a red eye:
1. Check the client's visual acuity with a Snellen chart.
2. Inspect for a pattern of redness.
3. Observe for the presence of discharge.
4. Using a penlight or slit lamp, observe for corneal opacities.
5. Using fluorescein stain, observe for corneal defects.
6. Examine the anterior chamber for depth, blood cells, or pus.
7. Examine the pupils for irregularity.
8. Check intraocular pressure.
9. Observe for the pressure of proptosis or a lid disorder.

INTEGRATING DIAGNOSTIC TESTING

Eye Infection

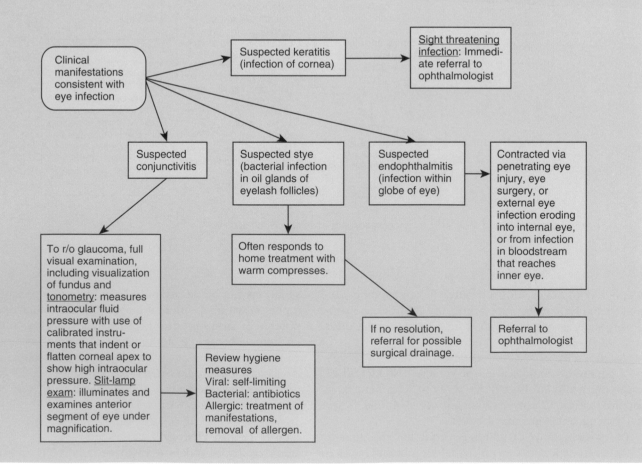

TABLE 64–1 Ocular Manifestations and Common Causes

Clinical Manifestation	Potential Cause
Blurring	Cataracts, iritis, macular degeneration, refractive error, eye fatigue, myopia, diabetes mellitus, corneal edema, optic neuritis or neuropathy
Eye numbness	Diabetes mellitus, peripheral neuropathy, conjunctivitis, stroke
Eye pain	Injury, infection, inflammation, glaucoma, foreign body, eye strain, sinusitis, corneal abrasions, hypertension, migraine, multiple sclerosis, tumor
Flashes	Retinal detachment, blow to the head, ocular migraine
Floaters	Red and white blood cells or gel-like clumps in the vitreous, retinal tear or detachment, normal part of aging
Foreign body	Object in eye, corneal scratches, abrasions or erosion, dry eye, conjunctivitis, contact lens issue, keratitis
Headache	Eyestrain, migraine headache, cluster headache, sinusitis, shingles, conjunctivitis, corneal abrasion or ulcer
Itching	Blepharitis (eyelid infection), conjunctivitis, contact lens issues, ocular allergy
Light sensitivity	Acute glaucoma, iritis, scleritis, corneal ulcer, thyroid disease, ectropion/entropion
Tearing	Blocked tear duct, dry eye, infection of lacrimal sac, ectropion (everted lid) or entropion (inverted lid)

diabetes mellitus, retinoblastoma, retinitis pigmentosa, and macular degeneration also tend to appear in families. Lack of a family health history does not rule out the possibility of a genetic disorder. Some clients do not know the ocular history of family members, and some may be embarrassed or hesitant to share the information. Accurate reporting of the family history can alert both client and caregiver to potential issues in the future.

PHYSICAL EXAMINATION

Basic physical examination of the eyes includes assessment of external structures via inspection and palpation. Other important assessments include testing of corneal reflexes, ocular motility (see the Snellen chart for assessment of visual acuity on the web and see Table 64-2 on p. 1685), visual acuity, and visual fields (Table 64-3 on p. 1686). It also includes examination of the internal eye structures with an ophthalmoscope. For an example of an assessment recording, see the Physical Assessment Findings in the Healthy Adult feature on p. 1687. For more in-depth physical examination explanations and techniques, please refer to a physical examination textbook.

External Eye

External eye structures include the eyebrows, eyelashes, eyelids, the lacrimal apparatus, anterior portion of the eyeballs, conjunctivae, sclerae, corneas, anterior chambers, pupils, and irides. Inspect and palpate these structures while the client sits at eye level. Table 64-4 on p. 1687 presents abnormal physical examination findings of the external eye.

Eye Position
Assess eye position for symmetry and alignment.

Eyebrows
Inspect the eyebrows for symmetry, hair distribution, skin conditions, and movement. The eyebrows normally move up and down smoothly under control of the facial nerves.

Eyelids and Eyelashes
Examine the eyelids and eyelashes for placement and symmetry. Normally, the sclerae are not visible above or below the irides when the eyelids are open. Elevate the eyebrows to inspect the upper lids for lesions. Inspect the lower lids by asking the client to open the eyes. Examine the skin of the eyelids and orbit by palpating for texture, firmness, mobility, and integrity of the underlying tissues. Assess the blink response. Blinking is an involuntary reflex that occurs bilaterally up to 20 times a minute.

Eyeballs and Lacrimal Apparatus
To palpate the eyeballs, instruct the client to close the eyes and look down. Place the tip of the index fingers on the upper eyelids, over the sclerae, and palpate gently. Normally, the eyeballs feel firm and symmetrical. Visualize the lacrimal apparatus by retracting the upper lid and having the client look down. The area should be free of swelling, edema, and excessive moisture, and there should be no regurgitation of fluid from the sac or puncta.

Conjunctivae and Sclerae
Inspect the conjunctivae and sclerae for color changes, texture, vascularity, lesions, thickness, secretions, and foreign bodies. The bulbar conjunctivae are colorless and transparent, allowing the sclerae to be seen. Small blood vessels may be visible. In Caucasians, the sclerae are white; in people with darker skin, they may appear light yellow. Retract the lower eyelids to expose the conjunctivae without applying pressure to the eyeballs. You (or the client) should gently push the lower lids down against the bony orbit while the client looks up. Healthy conjunctivae are pink to light red. If the lower palpebral conjunctivae are normal, the upper palpebral conjunctivae usually are not inspected. Wear gloves to inspect the palpebral conjunctivae, and wash your hands both before and after this portion of the examination.

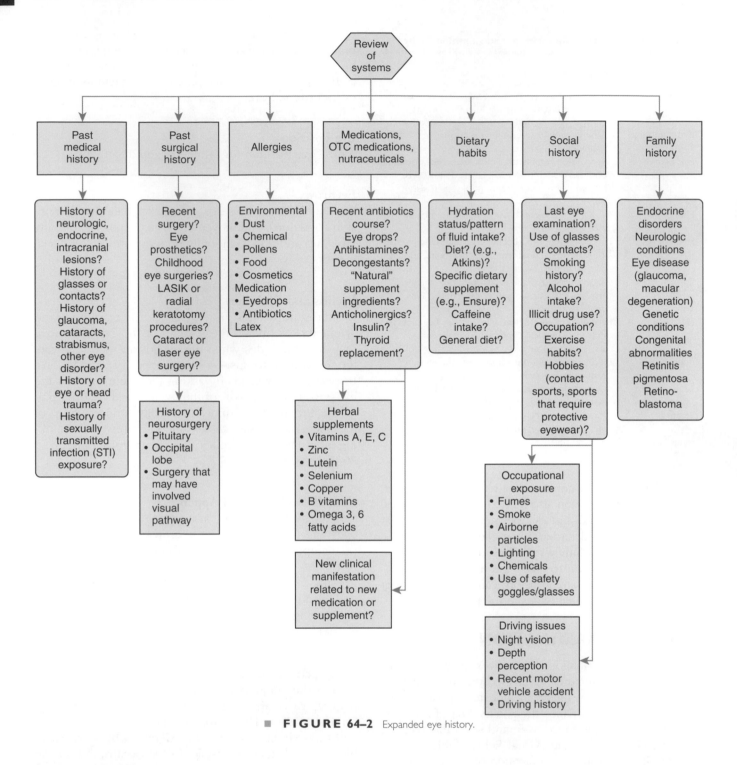

FIGURE 64–2 Expanded eye history.

Cornea and Anterior Chamber

Inspect the cornea and anterior chamber from an oblique angle while shining a penlight on the corneal surface. The irides are easily visible. In older adults, a thin, grayish white ring around the edge of the cornea (*arcus senilis*) may be seen. The anterior chambers should appear clear and transparent with no cloudiness or shadows cast on the irides. The depth of the chamber between the cornea and iris is normally about 3 mm.

Iris and Pupil

Inspect the iris and the pupil with the same oblique lighting from the penlight. The iris should light up and have a consistent color. The light should also cause the iris to constrict as the optic nerves are stimulated, causing the pupil to become smaller. Dim lighting causes the pupil to dilate. Pupils are normally black and round, have smooth borders, and are equal in size. Inspect the pupils for size, equality, shape, and ability to react to

TABLE 64-2   Physical Examination Tests of the Eye: *Reflexes and Motility*

Test	Purpose	Procedure	Results
Corneal reflex	Assesses function of fifth cranial nerve (trigeminal)	Client looks straight ahead; bring sterile cotton wisp from behind and lightly touch cornea; may also use syringe to puff air gently across cornea	Blinking and tearing indicate intact nerves
Corneal light reflex test (Hirschberg's test)	Determines eye alignment	Shine penlight 12-15 inches from bridge of nose with client staring straight ahead; observe light reflection from both corneas	Symmetrical reflection is normal Asymmetrical reflection can indicate strabismus, esotropia (deviates to nose), exotropia (deviates away from nose), hyperopia (vertical up), or hypotropia (vertical down)
Ocular motility	Gathers information about extraocular muscles; orbit; oculomotor, trochlear, and abducens nerves; brain stem connections; and cerebral cortex	Client tracks target with both eyes as it is moved through the 6 cardinal directions of gaze (see Fig. A&P15-2 in the Anatomy & Physiology Review). Nerve function testing: stand directly in front of client with penlight 12 inches from eyes; keeping head still, client follows light with eyes only; move in orderly fashion from center to outer edge of each of 6 cardinal directions	Eyes normally move parallel to each other in smooth unison Involuntary, rapid oscillating movement of eyeball (nystagmus) abnormal Eyes not parallel or eyelid covering more than a tiny portion of iris also abnormal
Cover-uncover test	Assesses eye muscle function and alignment for tropia (deviation of ocular alignment) and phoria (latent deviations with one eye covered)	Client stares at fixed point 20 inches away; cover one eye with opaque card and observe uncovered eye for lateral or medial movement as it focuses on fixed point; remove cover and observe that eye for movement as it focuses on fixed point Repeat for other eye	No movement is a normal finding Test may need to be repeated several times to confirm abnormal findings

light and accommodation. (See the table on the website titled Constriction and Accommodation Tests for the Pupil.) Pupil abnormalities may be caused by neurologic disease, intraocular inflammation, iris adhesions, systemic or ocular medication side effects, or surgical alteration.

Internal Eye

Internal eye structures are visible only with illumination such as that provided by a direct, or indirect, ophthalmoscope. These instruments are used to inspect the structures posterior to the iris, including the lens and fundus (which includes the retina, retinal vessels, choroid, optic disc, macula, and fovea). Using the ophthalmoscope requires considerable skill and practice. This section presents a brief overview of basic internal eye assessment. Please refer to a physical examination textbook for more in-depth discussion.

Direct Ophthalmoscopy

The direct ophthalmoscope uses a light source and reflective mirrors to provide a magnified (×15) image of the fundus (posterior portion of the eye) and a detailed view of the disc and retinal vascular bed. In a

darkened room, the instrument is held 1 to 2 inches away from the client's eye for examination (see the box on the website titled Guidelines for Using an Ophthalmoscope) (Figures 64-3 and 64-4). Retinal veins radiate from the disc and are darker, and slightly thicker, than arteries. They should not be pulsating, although as a normal variation you may see an occasional spontaneous pulsation. The retinal background is pink in Caucasian people and heavily pigmented in people with a dark complexion. Choroidal vessels may appear as linear orange streaks. The presence of a cataract, or cloudy cornea, may impair examination.

The fundus is the only site in the body where the vascular bed may be observed directly. Thus funduscopic examination yields information about many systemic diseases. Abnormal findings include an altered arteriovenous ratio, narrowed arteries, widened veins, pinched-off vessels, abnormal arterial light reflex, excessive tortuosity, numerous arteriovenous nicks, exudates, white patches, and focal hemorrhage.

Indirect Ophthalmoscopy

Indirect ophthalmoscopy provides a stereoscopic picture over a large area of the retina. The light source comes from a head-mounted light. The examiner holds a convex

TABLE 64–3 Vision Testing

Test	Purpose	Procedure	Results
Visual acuity	Determines clarity of cornea, lens, and vitreous; determines function of visual pathway from retina to brain. *For best corrected vision, allow client to wear glasses or contact lenses during exam.	1. Position client 20 ft in front of Snellen chart* (see website). 2. Client sits with one eye covered. 3. Ask client to read smallest line of print seen. 4. Credit client with line read with >50% accuracy; record results according to standardized numbers. 5. Assess with and without corrective lenses for both eyes.	Abnormal acuity implies uncorrected refractive error or pathology. *Normal is 20/20. *Myopia (nearsighted) is 20/30 or more. *Farsighted is 20/15 or less, but may be greater than average acuity. *20/200 with corrected vision is legal blindness.
Visual fields	To evaluate peripheral vision, you can use *confrontational method* (at right) or a computerized instrument. Computerized equipment permits more accurate detection and quantification of scotoma (area of decreased visual function).	1. Client sits 2 ft away from you, looking into your eyes. 2. Cover your right eye and client's left eye. 3. Hold a penlight equidistant between you and client, just out of view of peripheral visual field. Starting with superior field, bring object down until client states it is visible (you should also be able to see it). Repeat at 45-degree angles, through superior, temporal, inferior, and nasal fields. 4. Repeat for other eye.	Gross visual field abnormalities can be detected. If found, refer for further exam. Visual field alteration may be caused by CNS disorders (lesions, syphilis) or ocular disorders (glaucoma, retinal detachment).
Special Tests			
Color Vision			
Problems are genetic and more often seen in men (7%) than women (0.5%); also affected by nutrition, optic nerve disorder, fovea centralis problems	Not always common screening test. Detects those with altered color perception.	Common test involves use of color plates with numbers outlined in primary colors and surrounded by "confusion" colors.	Clients with color vision problems are unable to recognize figure presented.
Central Area of Blindness			
	Used to detect and follow development of central area blindness (scotoma), such as seen with macular degeneration.	Amsler grid: 20-cm square divided into 5-mm squares with dot in center. Holding the grid 12 inches from face, client fixes gaze on central dot and describes any areas of distortion or absence in grid.	If distortion or grid absence noted, refer for further exam.

Examples: 20/20 is normal; client reads at 20 ft what person with normal vision reads at 20 ft.
 20/60 means client reads at 20 ft what person with normal vision reads at 60 ft.
 20/15 means client reads at 20 ft what person with normal vision reads at 15 ft.
* Snellen chart: Generally placed at a distance of 20 feet, the distance at which rays of light from an object are practically parallel and little accommodation effort is needed. Sizes of symbols are identified according to the distances at which they are normally visible. For example, the largest symbols can be read 200 feet away by people with unimpaired vision.

lens in front of the client's eye and, through a viewing device attached to the headband, sees an inverted reversed image. The indirect ophthalmoscope provides for binocular visual inspection with depth perception and permits a wider field of view compared with the direct method.

Advanced Eye Assessment

Some common, but advanced, skills in internal assessment of the eye include tonometry, which is a method of measuring intraocular fluid pressure, and slit-lamp

examination, which examines the anterior segment of the eye under magnification (see the Tonometry and Slit-Lamp Examinations table on the website).

DIAGNOSTIC TESTING

There are many diagnostic tests to help determine the etiology of vision difficulties. A brief overview of some of these tests is presented in Table 64-5 on p. 1688. Please refer to diagnostic testing and physical examination textbooks for a more in-depth discussion of these tests.

Physical Assessment Findings in the Healthy Adult

The Eye

INSPECTION

Visual acuity 20/20. Eyebrows full, mobile. Eyelashes curve out and away from eyelids. Ptosis absent. Eyelids without lesions or inflammation. Eyes moist. Palpebral conjunctivae pink; bulbar conjunctivae clear. Scleral color even, without redness. Corneal light reflection symmetrical. PERRLA, directly and consensually. Cornea smooth; lens and anterior chamber clear. Irides evenly colored. EOMs full, without nystagmus. Conjugate movement. No strabismus. Visual fields full to confrontation.

PALPATION

Eyeballs firm. Orbits without edema. No regurgitation from puncta. Tenderness absent over lacrimal apparatus.

FUNDUSCOPIC EXAMINATION

Red reflexes visualized. AV ratio approximately 2:3. Vessels without tortuosity, narrowing, pulsation, or nicking. Disc margins clear, no cupping, cup-to-disc ratio 1:3. No evidence of retinal hemorrhage, patches, spots.

AV, Artery-to-vein; *EOM,* extraocular movement;
PERRLA, pupils equal, round, reactive to light and accommodation.

A

B

C

■ **FIGURE 64–3   A,** The examiner uses the right hand to hold the ophthalmoscope to the right eye to examine the client's right eye. The examiner uses the left hand when examining the client's left eye. Note the positioning of the examiner's free hand, which is placed to steady the client's head and to slightly retract the eyebrow. **B,** The examiner sees what appears in the angle of light through the viewing aperture. **C,** The actual area of retina visualized depends on the dilation of the pupil. Note the structures that may be examined.

TABLE 64–4   Abnormal Physical Examination Findings of the External Eye

Eye Structure	Abnormal Findings
Eye position	Sunken or protruding eyes, such as protrusion of one eye or both eyes (exophthalmos)
Lids	Sagging of upper lids that covers part of pupil (ptosis)
	Eyelids that turn inward (entropion) or outward (ectropion)
	Lid eversion and inversion
Blink	Rapid, infrequent, or asymmetrical blinking
Eyeball	Asymmetrical, hard, or soft
Lacrimal apparatus	Swelling, edema, excessive moisture, and regurgitation of fluid
Conjunctiva	Paleness or a bright red color
Cornea	Surface irregularity and cloudiness (opacity)
Anterior chamber	Shallow or deep chambers (3 mm is normal) are abnormal
	Cloudy or nontransparent
Iris	Bulging or uneven coloring
Pupil	Light intolerance (*photophobia*)
	Irregular or unequal pupils
	Pupils that do not react to light or accommodation

ASSESSMENT OF THE EAR

The otologic history can be an important assessment tool and should be obtained before audiometric testing. Certain behavioral cues can indicate hearing impairment (Box 64-3). Collect significant data by conducting a thorough interview. Include the specific items in the otologic history (Box 64-4).

HISTORY

An otologic history includes demographic data, current clinical manifestations, past health history, family health history, psychosocial history, and review of systems. Ear problems often result from childhood illnesses or abnormalities associated with adjacent structures. The history interview is essential for determining current problems related to the ear.

■ **FIGURE 64–4** A normal fundus. *(Courtesy Ophthalmic Photography at the University of Michigan W.K. Kellogg Eye Center, Ann Arbor, Mich.)*

BOX 64-3   Clues Suggesting Hearing Impairment

Any adult who exhibits one or more of the following traits may be experiencing hearing impairment:

- Is irritable, hostile, hypersensitive in interpersonal relations
- Has difficulty hearing upper frequency consonants (such as "sl" or "sh")
- Complains about people mumbling
- Turns up volume on television
- Asks for frequent repetition and answers questions inappropriately
- Loses sense of humor, becomes grim
- Leans forward to hear better or turns head to preferred side
- Shuns large-group and small-group audience situations
- Shuns areas with increased background noise
- Might appear aloof and "stuck up"
- Complains of ringing in the ears
- Has an unusually soft or loud voice

TABLE 64–5   Diagnostic Tests for the Eye

Test	Description
Fundus photography	Special retinal cameras are used to document fine details of the fundus for study and future comparison. Photographs are compared over time to identify subtle changes in disc shape and color (see Figure 64-4).
Exophthalmometry	Exophthalmometer is designed to measure forward protrusion of the eye. It provides a method of evaluation and record of progression/regression of the prominence.
Ophthalmic radiography	X-ray study, tomography, and computed tomography (CT) are useful in evaluation of orbital and intracranial conditions, as well as detection of foreign bodies.
Magnetic resonance imaging (MRI)	MRI allows multidimensional views to be obtained without repositioning client. MRI is used to image edema, areas of demyelination, and vascular lesions.
Ultrasonography (US)	US uses high-frequency sound waves transmitted through a probe placed directly on the eyeball. A-scan US measures axial length (distance from cornea to retina) to determine the refractive power of an intraocular lens in cataract surgery. B-scan US is used to evaluate lesions and their growth over time, or the presence of a foreign body.
Ophthalmodynamometry	Ophthalmodynamometry is a test that exerts pressure on the sclera with a spring plunger while the central retinal vessels emerging from the disc are observed. This instrument gives an approximate measurement of the relative pressures in the central retinal arteries and indirectly assesses carotid arterial flow on either side.
Electroretinography (ERG)	ERG measures the change in electrical potential of the eye caused by a diffuse flash of light through electrodes incorporated onto a contact lens that is placed directly on the eye.
Visual evoked response (VER)	VER is similar to ERG in that it also measures the electrical potential resulting from a visual stimulus. The entire visual pathway from the retina to the cortex can be evaluated through placement of electrodes on the scalp.
Fluorescein angiography (FA)	FA enhances fundus photography. The client receives an intravenous fluorescein dye injection, and the dye passes through the retinal and choroidal circulation, allowing those spaces to be visualized and photographed. A rapid sequence of photos captures perfusion of vessels and helps locate abnormalities, changes in flow, and hemorrhage.

BOX 64-4 Otologic History Assessment Guide

CURRENT PROBLEM

■ What changes are you having in your hearing?
■ Do you have any of the following manifestations?

■ Distortion of hearing	Yes	No
■ Differences in the pitch of sound	Yes	No
■ Noise in your ear	Yes	No
■ Fullness or pressure in your ear	Yes	No
■ Pain in your ear	Yes	No
■ Drainage from your ear	Yes	No

■ Have you ever had a hearing examination?
　■ If yes, why?
　■ What were the results?

USE OF HEARING AIDS

■ Are you wearing hearing aids now?	Yes	No
■ Are your hearing aids effective?	Yes	No
■ How old are your hearing aids?	L _____ yr	R _____ yr

ASSOCIATED PROBLEMS

■ Do you have any of the following manifestations?

■ Head noise or ringing	Yes	No
■ Feeling dizzy or unsteady	Yes	No
■ Blurred vision	Yes	No
■ Double vision	Yes	No
■ Numbness in the hands or feet	Yes	No
■ Weakness in the arms or legs	Yes	No
■ Tingling around the mouth or face	Yes	No
■ Loss of consciousness or blackouts	Yes	No
■ Fainting	Yes	No
■ Convulsions or seizures	Yes	No

RISK FACTORS

■ Have you ever worked around loud noises?	Yes	No
■ How long?	_____ yr	
■ Do you still work around loud noise?	Yes	No
■ Do you wear ear protection?	Yes	No

PAST HEALTH HISTORY

■ Did you have hearing problems as a child?	Yes	No
■ Did you have frequent ear infections as a child?	Yes	No
■ Did you ever have a perforation in your eardrum?	Yes	No
■ Did you ever get hit in the ear?	Yes	No
■ Have you had ear surgery?	Yes	No

■ If yes,

	Date	Operation	Surgeon
Right ear	_____	_____	_____
Left ear	_____	_____	_____

■ Do you have any food or medication allergies?
■ Please list and describe your reaction.

FAMILY HISTORY

■ Do you have family members who had difficulty hearing before 50 years of age?
　■ If yes, explain.

■ Have any members of your family ever had ear surgery?
　■ If yes, explain.

Biographical and Demographic Data

Demographic data relevant to otologic assessment include the client's age. Hearing impairment may occur as a consequence of the aging process (Table 64-6).

Current Health

Hearing problems can affect a client's ability to communicate as well as limit their social activities and job opportunities. A reduction in their physical, functional, and social activities, attributable to ear problems or hearing loss, can interfere with the client's independence, which can lead to isolation and depression. Hearing loss can result in feelings of frustration, embarrassment, and loneliness. It is important to assess both verbal and nonverbal feedback and to listen attentively. The nurse's communication style is adapted to the client. The nurse should face the client as directly as possible when speaking, speak slowly, and enunciate distinctly. This individualized approach will assist with the development of trust between the nurse and client that will provide a valid database.

Chief Complaint

When discussing ear complaints, ask about common clinical manifestations of the ear (Figure 64-5). The client may also complain of associated nausea or vomiting. Complete an analysis of clinical manifestations to determine the onset, duration, frequency, and precipitating and relieving factors. Explore the client's past health history to determine the chronicity of the problem and the probable cause (see Box 64-4).

Clinical Manifestations

The most common clinical manifestations of ear disorders are pain, hearing loss, vertigo, tinnitus, drainage, and infection. Systemic manifestations will also be described.

Pain (Otalgia). Pain may be perceived as a feeling of fullness in the ear. It may be intensified by movement and relieved by holding the head still or by applying heat. Ear pain may occur as a result of related problems of the nose, sinuses, oral cavity, pharynx, or temporomandibular joint (TMJ). Pain may occur in and around the ear and it may be intense. Fever, headache, nausea,

and vomiting may also be present. The Integrating Diagnostic Testing feature on p. 1692 describes the evaluation of a client with ear pain.

Hearing Loss. Hearing loss may occur suddenly or gradually and can accompany the normal aging process. The loss may be conductive, a result of damage to the middle ear or otosclerosis; sensory neural, a result of disease of the inner ear, nerve pathways or a result of loss of hair cells; or related to a CNS disorder. Central hearing loss may be due to brain tumors and lesions of the auditory pathway in the central nervous system. The client may report an inability to hear certain words or sounds or that sounds are muffled.

Vertigo. Vertigo is a sensation of motion while the person is not moving. A client may feel that either he or she or the room is moving. Sudden movement of the head may precipitate vomiting. Vertigo may last for hours or all day. *Dizziness* is a sensation of unsteadiness and a feeling of movement within the head or lightheadedness.

Tinnitus. Tinnitus (ringing in the ears) may be reported as high-pitched or low-pitched, roaring, humming, hissing, or loud and persistent. Tinnitus may occur more commonly at certain times of the day and may involve one or both ears. This sensory neural form of auditory disorder occurs even in the absence of sound waves.

Ear Drainage (Otorrhea). Ear drainage can be bloody (sanguineous), clear (serous), mixed (serosanguineous), or it may contain pus (purulent). Drainage may also be accompanied by odor and pain.

Infection. Ear infections in infants can impair their ability to hear spoken words and impede the development of the auditory nerve used for hearing and speech. The assessment of an adult client should also include a careful review of frequent ear infections as a child.

Systemic Manifestations

Hearing is essential in interacting with the environment. The ear is a special sensory receptor that is connected to specific areas of the cerebral cortex through the afferent pathways of the central nervous system (CNS). Clinical manifestations of the disease and treatment of the

TABLE 64–6 Changes in Auditory Acuity Caused by Aging

Anatomic Changes	Physiologic Changes
Degeneration of basilar conductive membrane of cochlea	Decreased ability to hear at all frequencies, with higher frequencies being most affected
Degeneration of cochlear hair cells	Decreased ability to hear high-frequency sounds
Decreased vascularity of cochlea	Loss of hearing equal at all frequencies
Loss of auditory neurons in spiral ganglia of organ of Corti	Loss of ability to hear high-frequency sounds
Loss of cortical auditory neurons	Diminished hearing and speech comprehension

■ **FIGURE 64–5** Expanded ear assessment.

underlying problem are important. Hearing loss, pain, infection, vertigo, tinnitus, and ear drainage are all principal manifestations attributed to the ears. Not all clients will present with the textbook common manifestations that are only related to the ears. Special consideration with emphasis on the nose, nasopharynx, and paranasal sinuses should also be included with the history and physical examination. Referred pain may also be from the teeth, tongue, tonsils, hypopharynx, larynx, salivary glands, and temporomandibular joint and should also be considered in the assessment.

Review of Systems

The past health history, family health history, and psychosocial history are integrated with the otologic history assessment (Figure 64-6). The nurse conducts a review of systems to provide focus for the physical examination. The review of systems related to the ear includes gaining information about problems or concerns that the client reports. Focus areas include asking about the location, quality, quantity, timing, precipitating factors, and aggravating or relieving factors.

Past Medical History

Common childhood diseases involving the ears include the following: acute middle ear infections (otitis media); eardrum perforations resulting from otitis media; complications of ear infections such as chronic otitis media, frequent upper respiratory tract infections, and acute and chronic sinus infections.

INTEGRATING DIAGNOSTIC TESTING

Ear Pain

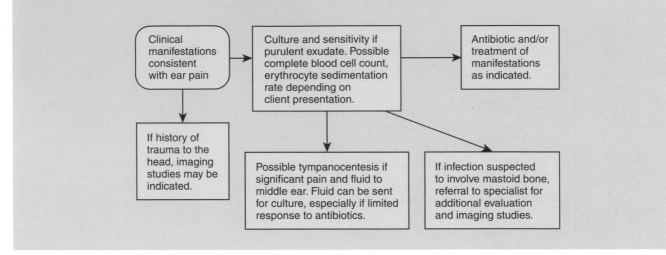

Clinical manifestations consistent with ear pain

Culture and sensitivity if purulent exudate. Possible complete blood cell count, erythrocyte sedimentation rate depending on client presentation.

Antibiotic and/or treatment of manifestations as indicated.

If history of trauma to the head, imaging studies may be indicated.

Possible tympanocentesis if significant pain and fluid to middle ear. Fluid can be sent for culture, especially if limited response to antibiotics.

If infection suspected to involve mastoid bone, referral to specialist for additional evaluation and imaging studies.

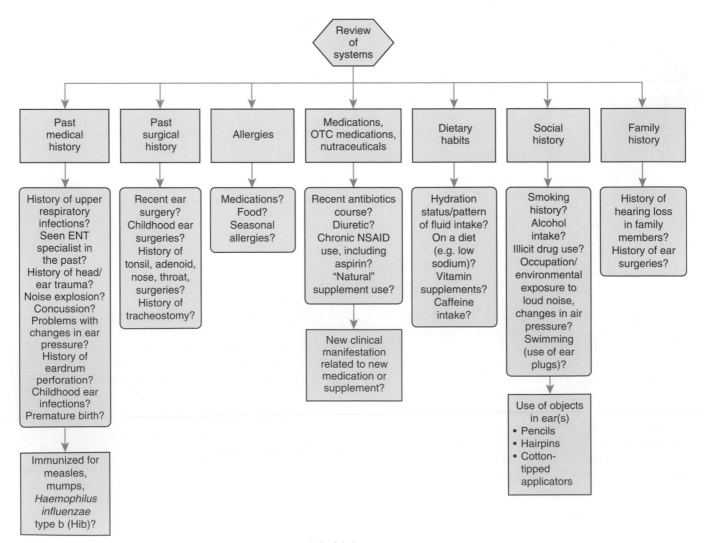

Review of systems

Past medical history

Past surgical history

Allergies

Medications, OTC medications, nutraceuticals

Dietary habits

Social history

Family history

History of upper respiratory infections? Seen ENT specialist in the past? History of head/ear trauma? Noise explosion? Concussion? Problems with changes in ear pressure? History of eardrum perforation? Childhood ear infections? Premature birth?

Recent ear surgery? Childhood ear surgeries? History of tonsil, adenoid, nose, throat, surgeries? History of tracheostomy?

Medications? Food? Seasonal allergies?

Recent antibiotics course? Diuretic? Chronic NSAID use, including aspirin? "Natural" supplement use?

Hydration status/pattern of fluid intake? On a diet (e.g. low sodium)? Vitamin supplements? Caffeine intake?

Smoking history? Alcohol intake? Illicit drug use? Occupation/environmental exposure to loud noise, changes in air pressure? Swimming (use of ear plugs)?

History of hearing loss in family members? History of ear surgeries?

Immunized for measles, mumps, *Haemophilus influenzae* type b (Hib)?

New clinical manifestation related to new medication or supplement?

Use of objects in ear(s)
• Pencils
• Hairpins
• Cotton-tipped applicators

■ **FIGURE 64–6** Expanded ear history.

Infectious diseases with ear sequelae include mumps, measles, and meningitis. Specifically inquire whether the client has been immunized for mumps, measles, and *Haemophilus influenzae* type b (Hib). In utero exposure to maternal influenza or rubella may result in congenital hearing loss in the child. Premature birth is also associated with hearing problems.

Inquire about a history of upper respiratory tract infections. Has the client had tonsil, adenoid, or other nose or throat surgery? Has the client ever consulted an ear specialist? Has the client suffered trauma to the head or ear, such as a severe blow or sustained loud noise exposure or concussion from sudden changes in air pressure (such as may occur in an explosion)? Does the history include chronic eardrum perforation?

Surgical History

A thorough surgical history is vital to the assessment of ear complaints. If the client has a history of ear diagnoses, inquire about any surgical procedures that may have been performed. This may include a mastoidectomy, tympanoplasty, stapedectomy, or a labyrinthectomy. Whenever possible, the date and the precise procedure should be documented, as there are various methods for performing a specific procedure, such as a myringoplasty for repair of perforation of the eardrum.

Allergies

In addition to asking about allergies to medications and other substances, inquire about allergies resulting in nasal stuffiness and congestion. Close proximity of the eustachian tubes to the nasal mucosa may result in edema, which obstructs the flow of air between the middle ear and nose so that air pressure cannot be equalized.

Medications

Obtain a complete medication history for prescription and over-the-counter drugs and herbal remedies. Determine the medication or supplement, and establish the dose, route, recent dosage changes, and length of time taken to ascertain if there is any relationship to the onset of the chief complaint.

Certain medications can damage the vestibulocochlear nerve (eighth cranial nerve), with resultant hearing loss, tinnitus, or disturbances in equilibrium. Aspirin is a common cause of tinnitus. Other drugs include aminoglycosides, analgesics, salicylates, quinine, chemotherapeutic agents, and antiprotozoal agents (Box 64-5).

Review the use of herbal remedies. Ginger *(Zingiber officinale)* is known for its antinausea effect and can be used for the relief of motion sickness. *Ginkgo biloba* has been used for tinnitus and vertigo.

Dietary Habits

Nutritional factors that describe the client's food and fluid consumption in relationship to the body's metabolic needs are important to assess. Adequacy of nutrient supply to local tissues should be considered. Inquire about dietary restrictions, use of food supplements (e.g., vitamins), ability to swallow and chew, and a history of any feeding problems. Ménière's disease may present with attacks of vertigo and tinnitus. Recent findings have indicated the use of a low-salt diet may be involved with the initial treatment of the disease.

Psychosocial History

Psychosocial and lifestyle factors that influence the incidence of hearing impairment include occupational hazards, environmental exposure, and leisure activities and hobbies. Leisure activities should include questions

---

BOX 64-5   Selected Ototoxic* Drugs

AMINOGLYCOSIDE ANTIBIOTICS
- Streptomycin
- Neomycin
- Gentamicin
- Tobramycin
- Amikacin
- Kanamycin
- Netilmicin

OTHER ANTIBIOTICS
- Vancomycin
- Viomycin
- Polymyxin B
- Polymyxin E
- Erythromycin
- Capreomycin
- Chloramphenicol
- Minocycline

OTHER DRUGS
- Chemotherapeutic agents (bleomycin, cisplatin, nitrogen mustard)
- Salicylates
- Quinine drugs
- Quinidine
- Chloroquine

DIURETICS
- Furosemide
- Ethacrynic acid
- Acetazolamide
- Bumetanide
- Mannitol

CHEMICALS
- Metals (lead, mercury, gold, arsenic)
- Alcohol
- Aniline dyes
- Caffeine
- Carbon monoxide
- Nicotine
- Potassium bromate
- Povidone-iodine

*Substances toxic to the ear.

about swimming. Contaminated water can provoke an external ear infection and, if the tympanic membrane is perforated, may lead to infection in the middle ear. Also, explore the client's ear hygiene habits to see if objects are used or inserted into the ear canal. Inserting objects into the ear canal to clean the ear may traumatize the ear canal and damage or perforate the tympanic membrane.

Ask about exposure to loud noises (Table 64-7), including the type, frequency, and duration. Sound intensity is measured in units known as *decibels (dB)*. Ordinary speech level measures about 50 dB; heavy traffic is about 70 dB; at above 80 dB noise becomes uncomfortable to the human ear. Exposure to levels greater than 85 to 90 dB for months or years causes cochlear damage.

Family Health History

Ask about a history of hearing loss or ear surgery among family members. Determine the age at onset for hearing loss or changes in hearing acuity.

PHYSICAL EXAMINATION

Physical examination of the ear includes assessment of hearing acuity, balance, and equilibrium. Because the external ear is completely visible, it is easy to identify anatomic landmarks and to assess abnormalities. Most of the middle ear and the entire inner ear, however, are inaccessible to direct examination; testing of auditory and vestibular function should be completed to help assess these structures. Refer to the Physical Assessment Findings in the Healthy Adult feature at right.

Inspection and Palpation
External Ear

Inflammation and infection are the most frequent conditions of the external ear seen by the nurse. In assessing the external ear, manipulation of the ear is important. Care must be exercised not to cause unnecessary pain.

Gross examination of both ears should precede individual examination of either ear. Use inspection and palpation to assess the external ear. Note the size, configuration, and angle of attachment to the head. Observe the configuration of the pinna for gross deformity. Note whether the ears protrude and, if so, the degree of protrusion; note the color of the skin of the ears; and determine whether additional skin tags are present. The skin of the ear should be smooth and without breaks or inflammation, especially in the crevice behind the ear. Note any lumps, skin lesions, or cysts, and record approximate size and location.

Perform palpation and manipulation of the pinna to detect tenderness, nodules, or *tophi* (small, hard nodules in the helix that are deposits of uric acid crystals characteristic of gout). During palpation, move the pinna, feel

---

Physical Assessment Findings in the Healthy Adult

The Ear

INSPECTION

Auricles symmetrical, superior portion level with outer canthus of eye. Outer canals clear. Preauricular and postauricular areas without swelling, masses, or lesions. AC > BC, bilaterally. No lateralization. Whisper heard at 3 feet.

PALPATION

Tenderness over tragus and mastoid absent. No masses.

OTOSCOPIC EXAMINATION

Soft cerumen present in canals. No discharge. TMs intact, gray. Cone of light at 4:00 in right ear and at 7:00 in left ear. Landmarks visualized. No retraction or bulging. TM freely movable with pneumatic pressure.

AC, Air conduction; *BC,* bone conduction; *TM,* tympanic membrane.

TABLE 64–7 Decibel (dB) Ratings and Hazardous Time Exposure of Common Noises

Typical Level* (dB)	Example	Dangerous Time Exposure
0	Lowest sound audible to human ear	
30	Quiet library, soft whisper	
40	Quiet office, living room, bedroom away from traffic	
50	Light traffic at a distance, refrigerator, gentle breeze	
60	Air conditioner at 20 ft, conversation, sewing machine	
70	Busy traffic, noisy restaurant (constant exposure)	Critical level begins
80	Subway, heavy city traffic, alarm clock at 2 ft, factory noise	More than 8 hr
90	Truck traffic, noisy home appliances, shop tools, lawnmower	Less than 8 hr
100	Chain saw, boiler shop, pneumatic drill	2 hr
120	Rock concert in front of speakers, sandblasting, thunderclap	Immediate danger
140	Gunshot blast, jet plane	Any length of exposure time is dangerous
180	Rocket launching pad	Hearing loss is inevitable

* Sound levels refer to intensity experienced at typical working distances. Intensity drops 6 dB with every doubling of distance from noise source.
Courtesy American Academy of Otolaryngology—Head and Neck Surgery, Washington, DC.

the mastoid area, and press on the tragus, noting any pain or discomfort, which may indicate inflammation or infection (see the Physical Assessment Findings in the Healthy Adult feature, p. 1694).

Ear Canal

Direct Observation. Inspection of the ear canal is carried out by direct observation, otoscopy, or microscopic examination. The extent and depth of the otology examination are determined by the nurse's skill level, training, and the health care setting. A basic understanding of the anatomy and physiology of the ear, and additional training by a health care professional, are required for the nurse to appreciate the wide range of normal findings. A physical examination text provides detailed instructions to perform direct observation of the ear canal.

Otoscopy. The eardrum is located at the end of the only skin-lined canal in the body. Proper visualization requires illumination and magnification for accurate assessment. An otoscope is portable, and otoscopic examination is the most commonly used method. An otoscope is a device (see the otoscope figure on the website and see Figure 64-7) that consists of a handle, a light source, a magnifying lens, and an attachment for visualizing the ear canal and eardrum. A pneumatic device attached to the otoscope is used for injecting air into the ear canal to test the mobility and integrity of the eardrum. Figure 64-8 shows a normal right eardrum.

Tests for Auditory Acuity

Assessment of the middle and inner ear for hearing is accomplished by sophisticated methods of indirect testing (audiometry and vestibular testing). A gross assessment of hearing can be made simply through conversation, by evaluating the logical sequence of replies, and the appropriateness of the responses. Gross assessments can be made at the bedside or in the office.

Test each ear separately to estimate hearing ability. Begin by occluding one of the client's ears with a finger. Then, standing 1 foot away, whisper two-syllable numbers softly toward the unoccluded ear and ask the client to repeat the numbers. Increase the intensity of your voice from a soft, medium, or loud whisper to a soft, medium, or loud voice. If you suspect that the client is lip-reading, turn the client's face to one side. Ask the client whether hearing is better in one ear than in the other ear. If auditory acuity between the two ears is different, test the ear that hears better first. Next produce noise in the better-hearing ear by rapidly but gently moving the finger in the client's ear canal while the other ear is tested.

Although the ticking of a watch can also be used to test hearing, it produces a higher-pitched sound, which is less relevant to functional hearing compared with the voice test.

■ **FIGURE 64–7** Use of the otoscope. **A,** Hold the otoscope handle between the thumb and fingers. Pull the pinna backward and upward in the adult to straighten the auditory canal. **B,** Carefully insert the speculum into the ear canal while allowing the back of the fingers that hold the otoscope handle to rest against the client's head. If a pneumatic bulb attachment will be used, position the bulb between thumb and otoscope handle to facilitate compression of the pneumatic bulb.

The tuning fork also provides a general estimate of hearing loss. A frequency of 512 Hz is recommended. The two major tuning fork tests date from the 19th century and are named after their originators: Weber and Rinne (see Table 64-8 and the figure of Weber and Rinne tests on the website).

Tests for Vestibular Acuity

Romberg Test. Assess the inner ear for balance by performing a Romberg test. The client stands with the

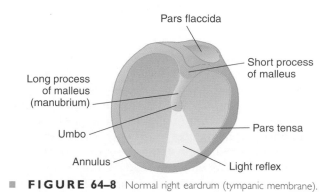

Pars flaccida

Short process of malleus

Long process of malleus (manubrium)

Pars tensa

Umbo

Annulus

Light reflex

■ **FIGURE 64–8** Normal right eardrum (tympanic membrane).

TABLE 64-8   Auditory Acuity Tests

Auditory Acuity Test	Purpose	Procedure	Interpretation
Weber	To assess conduction of sound through bone	Strike tuning fork on hand	Normal: sound is heard equally in both ears by bone conduction
		Place rounded tip of handle on center of client's forehead or nasal bone	Sensorineural (nerve) hearing loss: sound is heard in unaffected ear
		Placement on teeth, even false teeth, is reliable	Conductive (air conduction) hearing loss: sound is heard better in affected ear
		Ask if client can hear the tone in the center of the head, right ear, or left ear	
Rinne	Compares air conduction to bone conduction to help differentiate conductive from sensorineural hearing loss	Shift tuning fork between 2 positions: first against the mastoid bone (bone conduction) and second 2 inches from opening of ear canal (air conduction)	Normal: sound is heard twice as long or as loud by air conduction than by bone conduction
		Move tuning fork when client can no longer hear sound by bone conduction	Normal hearing: air conduction is greater than bone conduction = positive test
		Ask client to indicate if tone is louder in front or behind the ear	Conductive hearing loss: bone conduction sounds louder or longer than air conduction sound = negative test
		Ask client to state when tone is no longer heard by air conduction	Sensorineural hearing loss: client hears better by air conduction = positive test

feet together, arms by the sides, and eyes closed. Note the ability to maintain an upright posture with only a minimal amount of sway. Stand close to the client to offer balance support if it is needed. If the client loses his or her balance, this is a positive Romberg sign, suggesting a vestibular ear problem or cerebellar ataxia.

A *tandem* Romberg test should also be performed. Instruct the client to walk forward and backward, heel to toe. A peripheral vestibular lesion can cause marked swaying or falling. A client without pathologic vestibular change can usually maintain balance, depending on his or her age.

A *past-pointing test* can also indicate a labyrinthine disorder. While the client is seated, facing you with eyes open, hold out your index finger at the client's shoulder level. Instruct the client to touch your finger with the right index finger. Ask the client to lower the arm, close the eyes, and touch your finger again. Repeat the procedure, testing the client's left index finger. Observe and record the presence or absence as well as the degree and direction, of past-pointing. A labyrinthine disorder can lead to past-pointing when the eyes are closed. Cerebral lesions are indicated when past-pointing occurs whether the eyes are open or closed.

Test for Nystagmus. Nystagmus is involuntary, rhythmic oscillation of the eyes associated with vestibular dysfunction. Nystagmus occurs normally when a client watches a rapidly moving object or looks beyond 30 degrees laterally *(end-point nystagmus)*. To assess for *gaze nystagmus,* place your finger directly in front of the client at eye level. Ask the client to follow (track) the finger without moving the head. Starting at the midline, slowly move your finger toward the client's right ear and then the left ear, but not more than 30 degrees laterally, superiorly, or inferiorly. Observe the client's eyes for any jerking movements. For example, if the eyes jerk quickly to the left, and drift slowly back to the right, the client has left spontaneous *(horizontal)* nystagmus. Nystagmus is named for the direction of the fast phase. Nystagmus can be horizontal, vertical, or rotary.

DIAGNOSTIC TESTING

Noninvasive Tests
Tests for Aural Structure
The temporal bone and its structures can be examined easily by radiography (x-ray study). The oldest, but not necessarily most useful, study is x-ray examination of the mastoid bone. Radiographic techniques have largely been replaced by imaging studies, such as CT and MRI.

Computed Tomography
Computed tomography without contrast medium is the most commonly ordered CT scan for imaging of the temporal bone. Contrast is not generally needed because most bony structures are seen well. Contrast may be used to delineate vascular or soft tissue structures.

Magnetic Resonance Imaging
Magnetic resonance imaging reveals membranous organs as well as nerves and blood vessels of the temporal bone. MRI is the test of choice for tumors of the temporal bone. Contrast can be used for enhancement. For certain diagnostic assessments, both MRI and CT scans are obtained.

Invasive Tests
Arteriography
Arteriography is used to assess vascular abnormalities in the temporal bone.

Tests for Auditory Function
Audiometric Tests
Audiology may be broadly called the science of hearing. Audiometric tests are performed to measure hearing and comprehension. A hearing test is performed in a sound-proof booth by an *audiologist*. An *audiometer* is an electronic instrument used to test hearing by producing sounds of varying pure-tone frequencies. The client is asked to signal the audiologist by raising a hand or pressing a button when a tone is heard; the responses are plotted on a graph called an *audiogram*. Earphones are used for the audiogram.

Normal hearing is a range established nationally by testing the hearing levels of people of all ages. A client with normal hearing ability has 80% or more hearing, depending on the client's age.

Some audiometric tests are performed by computer-assisted instruments. The objective of these special tests is to reveal whether a disorder is in the cochlea, acoustic nerve, or brain stem (see Table 64-9).

Tests for Vestibular Function
Electronystagmography
The vestibular system can be tested by electrophysiologic means. Although the physical assessment of balance is important, the most common objective measurement of balance is accomplished by electronystagmography (ENG). The ENG instrument was developed to measure nystagmus (involuntary, rapid eye movement) in response to stimulation of the vestibular system. This stimulation includes testing the client at rest in different positions for both the eyes and the head and with different temperatures of air or water in the ear canals, thus stimulating the semicircular canals. The different test results give a recording (electronystagmogram) that reflects the status of each labyrinth and can indicate CNS disorders.

Platform Posturography
Platform posturography is another balance test that helps to identify, quantify, and localize the source of balance disorders. The client stands in a tall box-like device

---

TABLE 64–9 Auditory Function Tests

Tests for Auditory Function	Purpose	Procedure	Interpretation
Audiography	Components of hearing are tested through air conduction, bone conduction, and speech	Air conduction: tones presented through earphones Bone conduction: tones presented through bone conduction oscillator placed behind ear on mastoid bone	Difference between air and bone conduction signifies conductive hearing loss; if air and bone conduction are the same, either normal hearing or sensorineural (nerve) hearing loss exists
Tympanometry	Differentiates problems in middle ear Measures compliance (mobility) and impedance (opposition to movement) of tympanic membrane and ossicles of middle ear Also used to measure stapedius muscle reflex and its decay Also indicates function of acoustic nerve	Positive, normal, and negative air pressure is applied into external meatus and measures resultant sound energy flow; then traced on graph (tympanogram)	Abnormalities reveal dysfunction of middle ear, eustachian tube, and ossicles
Brain stem response	Assessment of auditory nervous system	Determined by presenting sound to ear and measuring response (computer averaging) in brain stem	Examiner obtains specific diagnostic information; imaging tests of the head are usually ordered to confirm abnormality
Electrocochleography	Measures response of cochlea and eighth cranial nerve to acoustic stimulation	Electrodes are placed through tympanic membrane onto promontory near round window or in ear canal, and acoustic stimulation is applied	Evaluates presence of Ménière's disease or perilymphatic fistula
Otoacoustic emissions (OAEs)	Low-level sounds produced by cochlea are involved in modulation of hearing mechanism	Can be measured quickly and are generally easier to obtain than test, especially in uncooperative and crying infants	Evoked OAEs can be observed in nearly all normal-hearing people; therefore serve as a useful screen for hearing acuity

while the floor moves. No visual cues are provided, and the response to correcting balance is recorded. Most people correct posture changes with adjustments in muscles (of the feet and ankles).

SAFETY ALERT

The client is strapped in for safety in case he or she loses balance.

This test can help to isolate the etiologic basis of balance disorders as vestibular, visual, or proprioceptive.

Rotary Chair Assessment

Rotary chair or harmonic acceleration can also be used. Rotation of the client in a chair in darkness provides information about vestibular dysfunction and the level of central compensation.

Laboratory Tests
Blood Tests

Blood tests that are diagnostic for systemic abnormalities are only secondarily significant for ear disease. For example, an elevated white blood cell (WBC) count suggests an infection but is not diagnostic of ear disease. In the presence of clinical manifestations of ear infection, and in the absence of other manifestations of infection, however, an elevated WBC count does suggest acute ear infection. Other blood tests are useful for diagnosis of autoimmune diseases and other systemic illnesses that can affect hearing and balance.

Cultures

Drainage samples from the ear canal are sometimes obtained for culture to identify an infecting organism. When long-term drainage is present, such as in chronic otitis media, cultures are more helpful because multiple pathogenic organisms can be present.

Tests for the Presence of Cerebrospinal Fluid

Clear drainage found in the ear presents a dilemma. Is this cerebrospinal fluid (CSF) or serous drainage? A fistula from the inner ear to the middle ear can drain CSF. This pathway can also lead to meningitis by retrograde contamination. Therefore an analysis of clear fluid drainage from the ear or nose is often helpful in the diagnosis.

Tissue Specimens

Biopsy specimens of abnormal tissue from the ear canal or from other tissue harvested during surgery are necessary to rule out a malignancy and to identify unusual problems. In an infected ear, abnormal tissue is readily identified by visual assessment.

CONCLUSIONS

Understanding the complexity of ocular structures and the physiology of vision is essential to providing comprehensive nursing care for clients with ocular disorders.

SAFETY ALERT

Hearing and balance are vital to a person's safety and independence. Understanding the physiology of hearing and balance is essential to providing comprehensive nursing care for clients with ear disorders.

Ophthalmic and otolaryngology registered nurses perform the roles of educator, technician, counselor, and coordinator in the diagnostic setting.

BIBLIOGRAPHY

Citations appearing in red refer to primary research.

Citations appearing in blue refer to evidence-based practice guidelines and protocols.

1. Eagle, R. (1999). *Eye pathology: An atlas and basic text*. Philadelphia: Saunders.
1a. Eskola, J., et al. (2001). Efficacy of a pneumococcal conjugate vaccine against acute otitis media. *New England Journal of Medicine, 344*(6), 403-409.
2. Folmer, R., Martin, W., & Shi, Y. (2004). Tinnitus: Questions to reveal the cause, answers to provide relief. *Journal of Family Practice, 53*(7), 532-540.
3. Goldblum, K. (Ed.) (2002). *Ophthalmic nursing core curriculum*. Dubuque, Iowa: Kendall.
4. Harris, L.L., & Huntoon, M.B. (Eds.) (1998). *Core curriculum for otorhinolaryngology and head-neck nursing*. New Smyrna Beach, Fla: Society of Otorhinolaryngology and Head-Neck Nurses.
5. Henry, J., Dennis, K., & Schechter, M. (2005). General review of tinnitus: Prevalence, mechanisms, effects, and management. *Journal of Speech, Language, and Hearing Research, 48*(5), 1204-1235.
6. Jarvis, C. (2004). *Physical examination and health assessment* (4th ed.). Philadelphia: Saunders.
7. Kanski, J. (2003). *Clinical ophthalmology* (5th ed.). Oxford: Butterworth Heinemann.
8. Rados, C. (2005). Sound advice about age-related hearing loss. *FDA Consumer, 39*(3), 20-27.
9. Scudder, S., et al. (2003). Predictive validity and reliability of adult hearing screening techniques. *Journal of the American Academy of Audiology, 14*(1), 9-19.
10. Vaughan, D., Asbury, T., & Riordan-Eva, P. (1999). *General ophthalmology* (15th ed.). Norwalk, Conn: Appleton & Lange.
11. Wilson, S., Giddens, J., & Thompson, J. (2004). *Health assessment for nursing practice* (3rd ed.). St. Louis: Mosby.
12. Woodson, G. (2001). *Ear, nose and throat disorders in primary care*. Philadelphia: Saunders.

evolve *Did you remember to check out the bonus material on the Evolve website and the CD-ROM, including NCLEX®-Examination Style Review Questions, Open-Book Quizzes, and Chapter Review Audio Podcasts?*

http://evolve.elsevier.com/Black/medsurg

CHAPTER 65

Management of Clients with Visual Disorders

SARAH C. SMITH

The role that vision plays in our lives is difficult to define because it is so deeply personal and intimate. It is the connection between the mind and the body and the rest of the world. The visual pathway is a multidimensional system with many structures and processes subject to trauma or disorders. When there is a failure of any part along the visual pathway, the result is loss of vision.

Loss of vision is closely associated with loss of independence. Even simple tasks become difficult to perform without assistance. Seeing what food is being served at the table; selecting clothes for color and design; avoiding objects while walking; and reading books, magazines, or personal mail are no longer possible. The visually impaired person must adapt to this loss to maintain control in the daily affairs of life.

The nursing diagnosis *Disturbed Sensory Perception (Visual)* is commonly identified for clients with visual problems or impairment. Nursing interventions focus on providing a safe environment and education for self-care. The most important assessment you can make, however, is to address your client's grieving process. Visual impairment is more than a physiologic deficit. It is a loss that has physical, emotional, and spiritual effects on the person afflicted. Even minor changes in vision can provoke feelings of anger and frustration in people who must rely on clear and sharp vision in their work (e.g., airline pilots, artists, photographers, architects). Permanent and profound loss of vision can result in morbid grieving in which an individual is unable to cope with or adapt to life changes.

Surveys have shown that most people are more afraid of going blind than dying of cancer. Although we have made some improvements in the way our society views and provides for people who are physically challenged, blind people are frequently regarded with pity. Loss of vision is a threat to a person's independence, self-esteem, and self-control.

GLAUCOMA

Glaucoma comprises a group of ocular disorders characterized by increased intraocular pressure, optic nerve atrophy, and visual field loss. It is estimated that more than 80,000 people in the United States are blind as a result of glaucoma. The incidence of glaucoma is about 1.5%, and in blacks between ages 45 and 65 years, the prevalence is at least five times that of whites in the same age group. In most cases blindness can be prevented if treatment is begun early.

Classification

Many terms are used to describe the various types of glaucoma:

- *Primary* and *secondary glaucoma* refer to whether the cause is the disease alone or another condition.
- *Acute* and *chronic* refer to the onset and duration of the disorder.
- *Open* (wide) and *closed* (narrow) describe the width of the angle between the cornea and the iris (Figure 65-1, *A*). Anatomically narrow anterior-chamber angles predispose people to an acute onset of *angle-closure glaucoma*.

Primary Open-Angle Glaucoma

Primary open-angle glaucoma, the most common form, is a multifactorial disorder that is often genetically

---

evolve *Web Enhancements*

Client Education Guide Care After Cataract Removal (Spanish Translation)

Be sure to check out the bonus material on the Evolve website and the CD-ROM, including free self-assessment exercises. **http://evolve.elsevier. com/Black/medsurg**

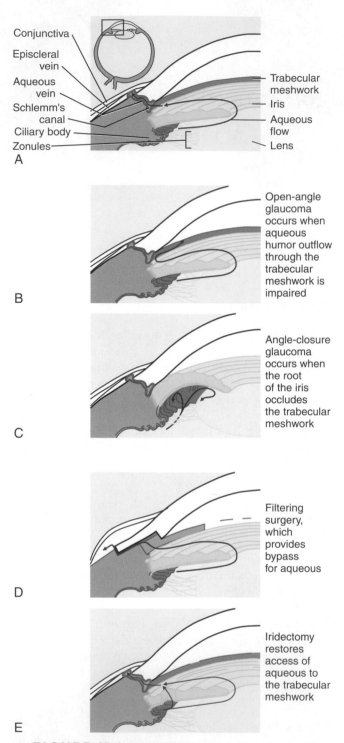

■ **FIGURE 65–1** **A,** Normal flow of aqueous humor. **B,** Open-angle glaucoma occurs when aqueous humor outflow is impaired by the trabecular meshwork. **C,** Angle-closure glaucoma occurs when the root of the iris occludes the trabecular meshwork. Filtering surgery **(D)** and iridectomy **(E)** restore the flow of aqueous humor through the trabecular meshwork.

determined, bilateral, insidious in onset, and slow to progress. This type of glaucoma is often referred to as the "thief in the night" because no early clinical manifestations are present to alert the client that vision is being lost. Aqueous humor flow is slowed or stopped because of obstruction by the trabecular meshwork (see Figure 65-1, *B*).

Angle-Closure Glaucoma

An acute attack of angle-closure glaucoma can develop only in an eye in which the anterior chamber angle is anatomically narrow. The attack occurs because of a sudden blockage of the anterior angle by the base of the iris (see Figure 65-1, *C*).

Other Forms of Glaucoma

Normal-tension glaucoma resembles primary open-angle glaucoma. In this type of glaucoma, the optic nerve is damaged even though intraocular pressure (IOP) is not high. *Secondary glaucoma* may occur as a result of trauma that can disrupt the flow pattern of aqueous humor.

Etiology and Risk Factors

About 90% of primary glaucoma occurs in people with open angles. Because there are no early warning clinical manifestations, it is imperative that regular ophthalmic examinations include tonometry and assessment of the optic nerve head (disc). The most common cause of chronic open-angle glaucoma is degenerative change in the trabecular meshwork, resulting in decreased outflow of aqueous humor. Hypertension, cardiovascular disease, diabetes, and obesity are associated with the development of glaucoma. Increased IOP also results from *uveitis* (inflammation of filtering structures). Encroachment by a rapidly growing tumor and chronic use of topical corticosteroids may also produce manifestations of open-angle glaucoma. Neither the causes of *low-tension glaucoma* nor the reasons optic nerves are damaged even though the IOP is "normal" (i.e., between 12 and 22 mm Hg) are known. People at higher risk for this form of low-tension glaucoma are those with a family history of normal-tension glaucoma, people of Japanese ancestry, and people with a history of systemic heart disease, such as irregular heart rhythm.

Secondary glaucoma develops from edema, eye injury *(hyphema)*, inflammation, tumor, or advanced cases of cataract or diabetes. Edematous tissue may inhibit the outflow of aqueous humor through the trabecular meshwork. Delayed healing of corneal wound edges may result in epithelial cell growth into the anterior chamber.

Pathophysiology

Intraocular pressure is determined by the rate of aqueous humor production in the ciliary body and the resistance to outflow of aqueous humor from the eye. IOP varies with diurnal cycles (the highest pressure is usually on awakening) and body position (increased when lying down). Normal variations do not usually exceed 2 to 3 mm Hg. IOP and blood pressures are independent of each other, but variations in systemic blood pressure may be associated with corresponding variations in IOP. Increased IOP may result from hyperproduction of aqueous humor or obstruction of outflow. As aqueous fluid accumulates in the eye, the increased pressure inhibits blood supply to the optic nerve and the retina. These delicate tissues become ischemic and gradually lose function.

Clinical Manifestations

Acute angle-closure glaucoma causes severe pain and blurred vision or vision loss. Some clients see rainbow halos around lights, and some experience nausea and vomiting. Secondary glaucoma has the same clinical manifestations as acute angle-closure glaucoma. Visual field defects are the result of the loss of blood supply to areas in the retina. The individual response to IOP varies; some clients sustain damage from relatively low pressures, whereas others sustain no damage from high pressure.

An ophthalmoscopic examination shows *atrophy* (pale color) and *cupping* (indentation) of the optic nerve head. The visual field examination is used to determine the extent of peripheral vision loss (see visual fields in Chapter 64). In chronic open-angle glaucoma, a small crescent-shaped *scotoma* (blind spot) appears early in the disease. In acute angle-closure glaucoma, the fields demonstrate larger areas of significant loss of vision.

In clients with angle-closure glaucoma, a slit-lamp examination may demonstrate an erythematous conjunctiva and corneal cloudiness. The aqueous humor in the anterior chamber may also appear *turbid* (hazy), and the pupil may be nonreactive. Increased IOP (>23 mm Hg) indicates the need for further evaluation. Gonioscopy is performed to determine the depth of the anterior chamber angle and to examine the entire circumference of the angle for any abnormal changes in the filtering meshwork.

OUTCOME MANAGEMENT

The goal of management is to facilitate the outflow of aqueous humor through remaining channels and to maintain IOP within a range that prevents further damage to the optic nerve. If the IOP is very high, it must be reduced to retain vision. If vision is lost, the goals are to restore independence for the client.

Medical Management

Reduce Intraocular Pressure (Promote Aqueous Flow)
Intraocular pressure can be reduced by increasing the outflow of aqueous fluids. In narrow-angle glaucoma

the pupil is constricted using topical miotics or epinephrine, which opens the canal of Schlemm and promotes drainage of aqueous humor. Further, the production of aqueous humor can be reduced by using topical beta-blocker or alpha-adrenergic agents or oral carbonic anhydrase inhibitors. Figure 65-2 shows the sites of action for various drugs.

Nursing Management of the Medical Client

Assessment. Nursing assessment includes establishing demographic data of age and race because open-angle glaucoma occurs most often in clients more than 40 years of age and in blacks. Determine whether there is a family history of glaucoma or other eye problems and whether the client has had ocular surgery, infections, or trauma. An accurate list of current medications is imperative because over-the-counter medications (such as antihistamines) may dilate the pupil, increasing the risk for angle-closure glaucoma. Always note a history of allergic reactions, particularly to medications or dyes.

Ask the client to describe any changes in vision. Although the manifestations of primary open-angle glaucoma are insidious, the client may describe blind spots in the periphery or an overall decreased visual acuity with loss of contrast sensitivity. Decreased, uncorrectable visual acuity usually occurs when there has been irreversible damage to the optic nerve.

If it has been previously established that the client has visual loss from glaucoma, assess how the client is coping with this loss. Although people adapt to the loss of vision

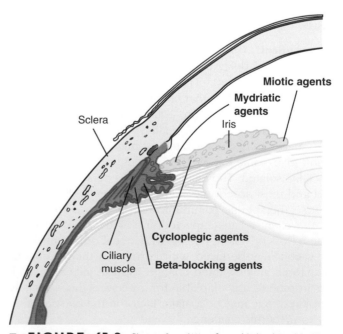

■ **FIGURE 65–2** Sites of action of mydriatic, beta-blocking, cycloplegic, and miotic agents.

in different ways, they usually manifest grief and loss at any stage of the disease process. Clients may be understandably anxious during examinations because they may fear discovery that further vision loss has occurred. Assess the client's perception of glaucoma and the effect it has on quality of life. Help the client identify effective coping skills that may have been used in the past.

Diagnosis, Outcomes, Interventions

Diagnosis: Disturbed Sensory Perception (Visual). The increased IOP alters the function of the optic nerve, decreasing vision. The nursing diagnosis *Disturbed Sensory Perception (Visual) related to recent loss of vision* may be appropriate if the loss of vision is a new problem for the client.

Outcomes. The client will maintain as much functional vision as possible, report no further loss of vision, adapt to any visual loss, be able to perform activities of daily living (ADL), and recognize clinical manifestations of complications.

Interventions. Reassure the client that although some vision has been lost and cannot be restored, further loss may be prevented by adhering to the treatment plan.

Diagnosis: Grieving. Vision lost to glaucoma is irreparable. Even with the most aggressive medical and surgical management, vision loss may progress. A typical nursing diagnosis would therefore be *Grieving related to loss of vision*. Significant loss of vision represents the need for compromise and adaptation for both the client and the client's family.

Outcomes. The client will express grief, describe the meaning of the loss, and share the grief with significant others.

Interventions. Assess the causative and contributing factors that may delay the work of grieving and promote family cohesiveness. The social stigma of blindness underlies the anxiety that clients experience with actual or potential loss of vision. Total loss of vision isolates a person within a different reality. Although most clients are successfully rehabilitated, some losses are permanent. Also, some people, for a variety of reasons, remain socially isolated. The image of a blind person who is pitied and must accept the charity of others is disturbing.

Use therapeutic communication to express empathy as the client relates expected and actual losses that are due to loss of vision. People with actual or potential loss of vision may be faced with barriers in their vocations that force an unwanted change. Not all jobs and work environments are adaptable for a person who is visually impaired. Age may be a major factor in the person's ability to meet this challenge.

Self-esteem is closely related to the roles of people in their particular lifestyle. Loss of control in personal,

family, and work situations can be devastating. The issue of dependence versus independence may also be a factor in the person's ability to cope with the stressors of vision loss.

Diagnosis: Risk for Ineffective Therapeutic Regimen Management (Individuals). The regimen for eyedrops and oral medications to control glaucoma ranges from simple to complex. This nursing diagnosis should be stated as *Risk for Ineffective Therapeutic Regimen Management (Individuals) related to complex medication schedule*.

Outcomes. The client will describe the disease process and the regimen for disease control and will relate how the medication routine will be incorporated into ADL.

Interventions. The client may need to instill as many as three or four different eyedrops from one to six times a day. Constricting eyedrops are usually prescribed four times a day, and beta-blockers are usually prescribed every 12 hours; however, the eyedrops may be needed every 4 to 6 hours. The schedule is designed to provide the best possible control of IOP around the clock.

Medications are an integral part of the treatment and care of a client with glaucoma, and nursing interventions must thus be directed at the client's ability to understand and comply with prescribed therapy. First, determine the client's current level of knowledge. Provide necessary information about glaucoma and its treatment in understandable terms. Diagrams may be helpful to the client and the client's significant others. Because treatment for glaucoma is often complex, involving both oral and topical ophthalmic medications, review a written plan of care in large print with the client and family. To maximize compliance, ensure that the plan of care fits into the client's lifestyle.

The administration of eyedrops is a critical component of self-care for the client with glaucoma. After instructing the client and family on the technique of instillation, validate the client's or the family's ability to instill eyedrops properly by asking for a return demonstration. Be sure to include discussion of medications and their side effects.

Evaluation. Independent self-care is the area for evaluation in the medically managed client. Evaluate the client's ability for self-care (a short-term outcome) and compliance with the medical regimen (a long-term outcome).

Modifications for Older Clients

Older clients with arthritic or shaking hands have difficulty instilling their own eyedrops. Instruct the client to lie down on a bed or sofa. Tilting the head back can lead to loss of balance. The eyedrop regimen for glaucoma requires accurate timing. Older clients may need visual reminders, such as a check-off list and may also need to use a timer or an alarm clock to help them remember.

Surgical Management

When maximal medical therapy fails to halt the progression of visual field loss and optic nerve damage, surgical intervention is recommended. Many procedures are used to improve aqueous humor outflow; however, no operation has been uniformly successful.

Laser Trabeculoplasty

The use of the laser to create an opening in the trabecular meshwork is often indicated before filtering surgery is considered. The laser produces scars in the trabecular meshwork, causing tightening of meshwork fibers. The tightened fibers allow increased outflow of aqueous humor. IOP is reduced through improved outflow in about 80% of cases. The effect of the laser treatment decreases with time, and the procedure may need to be repeated. Medical treatment with topical eyedrops is usually continued.

Trabeculectomy

Trabeculectomy is the creation of an opening through which the aqueous fluid escapes. A half-thickness scleral flap is loosely sutured over the created opening through which the fluid escapes, again resulting in subconjunctival absorption of aqueous humor (see Figure 65-1, C).

Filtering Procedures

Operations such as trephination, thermal sclerostomy, and sclerectomy create an outflow channel from the anterior chamber into the subconjunctival space (see Figure 65-1, D). Aqueous humor is absorbed through the conjunctival vessels. In about 25% of cases, the opening closes because of scar tissue formation and reoperation is necessary. Such filtering procedures are less successful in young and black clients, who tend to have an increased ability to produce thicker scar tissue. Topical corticosteroids are used postoperatively because their anti-inflammatory action inhibits proliferation of fibroblasts at the surgical site.

Iridotomy

Iridotomy is the creation of a new route for the flow of aqueous humor to the trabecular meshwork. The laser is used to create the new opening in the iris (see Figure 65-1, E).

Other Techniques

5-Fluorouracil (5-FU), mitomycin, and other antimetabolites are sometimes injected subconjunctivally because they also inhibit fibroblast proliferation and thereby reduce postoperative scarring. Ocular implantation devices (e.g., Molteno implant, Baerveldt seton) are sometimes used to control the flow of aqueous humor in clients with complicated types of glaucoma. A device is sutured to the outer surface of the eyeball on the sclera between the ocular muscles. A tiny probe is inserted under the scleral flap directly into the anterior chamber that directs the flow of aqueous humor more posteriorly than in the more common filtering procedures.

Cyclodestructive Procedures

When other surgical procedures have failed, *cyclocryotherapy* (application of a freezing tip) or cyclophotocoagulation (applied with a laser) may be used to damage the ciliary body and decrease production of aqueous humor.

Nursing Management of the Surgical Client

Preoperative Care

Preoperative nursing care includes preparing the client for a surgical procedure that may be performed in either an outpatient or an inpatient setting (see Chapter 14).

Laser therapy is most commonly performed in a clinic or office, including the use of a topical anesthetic. Explain both the expected outcome of the procedure and the "popping" sounds and flashing lights that the client will experience. Explain that there will be a waiting period (usually 1 to 2 hours) after the procedure to evaluate a possible rise in IOP. Because of the instability of the IOP, the client should arrange for a friend or family member to accompany him or her and to provide transportation.

Postoperative Care

Following surgery, the eye is covered with a patch and a metal or plastic shield for protection to protect from light and trauma. Instruct the client not to lie on the operative side to avoid pressure on the surgical site. When the effects of perioperative sedation have diminished, the client may ambulate and eat as desired.

Frequent monitoring of IOP is necessary because the surgical site is microscopic. Assess the client for continued or increasing pain, nausea, and decreased vision. Follow-up care is needed to monitor for delayed healing. The anterior chamber may fail to heal, or the wound may seal too tightly. Both situations warrant further surgery.

Self-Care

The postoperative plan must include client education and evaluation of the home environment and available care. Because the level of independence varies with each client, use information supplied by the client and family or friends to assess how much support may be needed. Although many clients with glaucoma undergo repeated surgical procedures, it is necessary to carefully review the information each time. The Client Education Guide on p. 1704 summarizes this essential information.

CATARACTS

A *cataract* is opacity of the lens. Some degree of cataract formation is to be expected in most people more than 70 years of age. Worldwide, cataract is the primary cause of reduced vision and blindness. More than 1 million cataract operations are now being performed annually in the United States. A person with a normal life span is more likely to undergo a cataract operation than any other major surgical procedure.

The most common cataract is the age-related or senile type. Senile cataracts usually begin around the age of 50 years and consist of cortical, nuclear, or posterior subcapsular opacities, which may coexist in various combinations. In cortical cataracts, spoke-like opacifications are found in the periphery of the lens. They progress slowly, infrequently involve the visual axis, and often do not cause severe loss of vision. Nuclear sclerotic cataracts are a result of a progressive yellowing and hardening of the central lens (nucleus). Most people older than 70 have some degree of nuclear sclerosis. Posterior subcapsular opacities occur centrally on the posterior lens capsule and cause visual loss early in their development because they lie directly on the visual axis.

Etiology and Risk Factors

The cumulative exposure to ultraviolet light over a person's life span is the single most important risk factor in cataract development. People who live at high altitudes or who work in bright sunlight, such as commercial fishermen, appear to experience cataract formation earlier in life. Glassblowers and welders who do not wear eye protection are also at higher risk.

Cataracts may develop as a result of many other systemic, ocular, and congenital disorders. *Systemic* disorders include diabetes, tetany, myotonic dystrophy, neurodermatitis, galactosemia, Lowe syndrome, Werner's syndrome, and Down syndrome. *Intraocular* disorders include iridocyclitis, retinitis, retinal detachment, and onchocerciasis. Infections (German measles, mumps, hepatitis, poliomyelitis, chickenpox, infectious mononucleosis) during the first trimester of pregnancy may cause *congenital* cataracts. Blunt trauma, lacerations, foreign bodies, radiation, exposure to infrared light, and chronic use of corticosteroids may also result in cataracts.

Pathophysiology

Cataract formation is characterized chemically by a reduction in oxygen uptake and an initial increase in water content followed by dehydration of the lens. Sodium and calcium contents are increased; potassium, ascorbic acid, and protein contents are decreased. The protein in the lens undergoes numerous age-related changes, including yellowing from formation of fluorescent compounds and molecular changes. These changes, along with the photoabsorption of ultraviolet radiation throughout life, suggest that cataracts may be caused by a photochemical process.

Cataracts progress in a predictable pattern. They begin as immature cataracts that are not completely opaque, and some light is transmitted through them, allowing useful vision. Mature cataracts are completely opaque (the former term for this stage was *ripe*). Vision is significantly reduced. Hypermature cataracts are those in which the lens proteins break down into short-chain polypeptides that leak out through the lens capsule. The pieces of protein are engulfed by macrophages, which may obstruct the trabecular meshwork, causing phacolytic glaucoma.

Clinical Manifestations

Blurred vision, sometimes monocular diplopia (double vision), photophobia (light sensitivity), and glare occur because the opacity of the lens obstructs the reception of light and images by the retina. Clients usually see better in low light, when the pupil is dilated, which allows for vision around a central opacity. There is no complaint of pain. A cloudy lens can be observed (Figure 65-3).

A cataract should be suspected when the red reflex seen with the direct ophthalmoscope is distorted or absent. Although cataracts can usually be easily identified with the direct ophthalmoscope, an accurate determination of the type and extent of the lens change requires a slit-lamp examination.

OUTCOME MANAGEMENT

Surgical Management

There is no known treatment other than surgery that prevents or reduces cataract formation. The role of diet

■ **FIGURE 65-3** The cloudy appearance of a lens affected by cataract. *(Courtesy Ophthalmic Photography at the University of Michigan W. K. Kellogg Eye Center, Ann Arbor, Mich.)*

The cataract is removed by making a small incision in the cornea. The cataract is broken into microscopic particles using an ultrasonic probe. The use of high-energy sound waves is called *phacoemulsification*. Then a folded intraocular lens (IOL) is inserted through the microincision, then unfolded, and locked into permanent position (Figure 65-4). The small incision is "self-sealing" and usually requires no stitches. It remains tightly closed by the natural outward pressure within the eye. This type of incision heals fast and provides a much more comfortable recuperation.

Complications

Postoperative infection, bleeding, macular edema, and wound leaks are possible; however, side effects after cataract surgery are rare. The incidence of retinal

is not clear. Some research, presented in the Complementary and Alternative Therapy feature below, suggests that egg yolks may improve vision. Unless other ocular complications or health factors exist, cataract surgery is performed on an outpatient basis. Preoperative eyedrops may include a dilating agent such as tropicamide (Mydriacyl) to facilitate the surgery. A cycloplegic cyclopentolate (Cyclogyl) may also be administered to paralyze the ciliary muscles. Cataract surgery is performed under topical anesthesia using eyedrops or regional anesthesia (retrobulbar injection of local anesthetic solution). The client is often given an intravenous sedative in addition.

COMPLEMENTARY AND ALTERNATIVE THERAPY

Egg Yolks and Better Vision

Two carotenoids may be deposited in the eye and prevent macular degeneration or cataracts (leading causes of blindness in older adults in the United States). These carotenoids are lutein and zeaxanthin, and they are found in large amounts in egg yolks. Researchers gave slightly more than 1 egg yolk per day to 11 individuals. About 1 month later, the researchers found significantly increased levels of the two carotenoids in the subjects' blood; however, the subjects' low-density lipoprotein (LDL, or bad cholesterol) levels also increased significantly. These carotenoids can also come from dark-green, leafy vegetables and corn; however, they are better absorbed when they come from egg yolks. In moderation (several times a week), egg yolks may prevent some eye problems, but clients must pay attention to cholesterol intake.

REFERENCE

Handelman, G., et al. (1999). Lutein and zeaxanthin concentrations in plasma after dietary supplementation with egg yolk. *American Journal of Clinical Nutrition, 70,* 247-251.

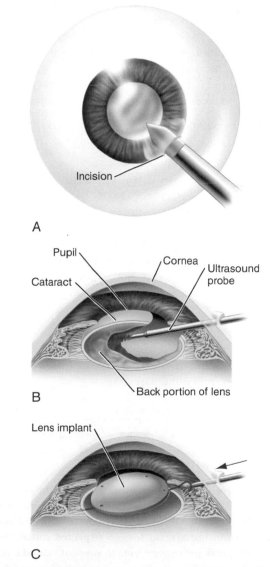

Incision

A

Pupil

Cornea

Cataract

Ultrasound probe

B

Back portion of lens

Lens implant

C

■ **FIGURE 65-4   A,** A small incision is made into the cornea for the insertion of the phacoemulsification tip. **B,** Using ultrasound, the cataract is dissolved. **C,** An artificial lens is inserted into the eye, which unfolds into place.

detachment is higher in the first 12 months after cataract surgery.

Nursing Management of the Surgical Client

Assessment. During the history and physical examination, ask the client about any predisposing factors (trauma, systemic diseases, medications such as corticosteroids, and other ocular problems). Visual acuity (both distant and near) in each eye is documented. Ask the client to describe visual disturbances. The client's visual acuity may be relatively close to normal ranges, and yet the client may experience difficulty in performing ADL. The client's individual perception of the quality of vision is an important factor in determining the need for surgery.

Diagnosis, Outcomes, Interventions
Diagnosis: Disturbed Sensory Perception (Visual). An IOL does not provide the same visual acuity as the natural lens of the eye. Although vision may be greatly improved, varying degrees of change in depth perception may remain. In addition, the eye is patched for protection, making vision monocular. Write the nursing diagnosis as *Disturbed Sensory Perception (Visual) related to lens extraction and replacement and use of eye patch.*

Outcomes. The client will have improved visual perception as evidenced by improved vision or adaptation to changes in visual acuity.

Interventions. Adaptation is the key issue in caring for the client having cataract surgery. Nursing interventions are based on assisting the client to gain or maintain as much independence as possible. Evaluate the client's lifestyle, abilities, and home environment. A 55-year-old client who is an architect and otherwise healthy may have an early cataract removed because it interferes with his work in areas where bright light is used. A 75-year-old diabetic client who is retired and mainly watches television has entirely different needs.

Evaluation. Adaptation to restored normal vision is usually rapid. Adaptation to limited vision requires more time based on individual variations.

Self-Care

After cataract surgery, clients are expected to return for a follow-up visit the next morning and again at 1 week and at 1 month.

SAFETY
⚠
ALERT

Postoperative care includes observation of the ocular dressing, if present, and assessment of the client's ability to perform ADL at the preoperative level. Nausea and vomiting are no longer expected outcomes of the surgical procedure but, if present, should be reported immediately. The eye patch is usually removed the next morning but may be removed after a few hours if the client has limited vision in the other

eye. Instruct the client to wear a metal or plastic shield to protect the eye from accidental injury and not to rub the eye.

Glasses may be worn during the day. The Client Education Guide below provides instructions for clients to follow.

Restrictions on postoperative activity vary according to the practice of the ophthalmologist. Generally, the client should avoid heavy lifting (>15 pounds) or straining in the early postoperative period.

Eye care for the client after cataract surgery is the same as that for glaucoma clients (see Glaucoma). Postoperative eye medications may include antibiotics, corticosteroids, or both. Assess the client's or the family's ability to instill eyedrops appropriately. Review the rationale and schedule for the medications with the client and family. Postoperative discomfort should be minimal to moderate and is usually relieved by acetaminophen. Clients commonly experience an itching sensation after cataract surgery. Instruct the client to report any pain that is unrelieved. Review the clinical manifestations of infection and increased IOP with the client and family.

Depending on the client's age, ability, and availability of assistance, make a referral for home health care if indicated. Adjustment to changes in vision also varies with the individual client.

RETINAL DISORDERS

RETINAL DETACHMENT

Retinal detachment is the separation of the retina from the choroid, a membrane dense with blood vessels that

---

CLIENT EDUCATION GUIDE ☰

Care After Cataract Removal

- Leave the eye patch in place.
- For 24 hours, limit your activity to sitting in a chair, resting in bed, and walking to the bathroom.
- Do not rub your eye.
- You can wear your glasses.
- Do not lift more than 5 pounds (the weight of a gallon of milk).
- Do not strain (or bear down).
- Do not sleep on the operative side of your body.
- Take your eyedrops.
- Take acetaminophen (e.g., Tylenol) as needed for pain or itching.
- DO NOT take aspirin or drugs containing aspirin.
- Report any pain that is unrelieved, redness around the eye, nausea, or vomiting.
- Wear an eye shield to protect your eye.

is located between the retina and the sclera ("white" of the eye). The retina is a thin layer of light-sensitive tissue that lines the back portion of the eye. When the retina detaches, it is deprived of its blood supply and source of nourishment and loses its ability to function. This can impair vision to the point of blindness.

Rhegmatogenous retinal detachment is the most common type and is due to a retinal hole. Liquid in the vitreous body seeps through the hole and separates the retina from its blood supply. Without intervention, the detachment continues to spread and the detached retina loses the ability to function. It may become increasingly detached over a period of hours to years.

Predisposing factors to retinal detachment include aging, cataract extraction, degeneration of the retina, trauma, severe myopia, previous retinal detachment in the other eye, and a family history of retinal detachment. Retinal holes and tears usually occur from spontaneous vitreous traction, but abnormal adhesions may be present between the retina and vitreous body secondary to diabetic retinopathy, injury, or other ocular disorders. Atrophy of the vitreous body may also result in a retinal tear.

Characteristic clinical manifestations of retinal detachment are described by clients as a shadow or curtain falling across the field of vision. Shadows or black areas in the field of vision are the result of separation of visual receptors from the neural pathway. No pain is associated with a detached retina. The onset is usually sudden and may be accompanied by a burst of black spots or floaters indicating that bleeding has occurred as a result of the detachment. The person may also see flashes of light caused by separation of the retina.

Visual field loss occurs in the opposite quadrant of the actual detachment. For example, a tear in the temporal region, which is affected more frequently, creates a visual defect in the nasal area. The extent of loss of vision is related to the portion of the retina involved. Giant retinal tears involving the entire retina may result in temporary blindness, whereas peripheral tears may not interfere with central vision at all.

The pupil must be widely dilated for a retinal examination. Tell clients that they will experience an extremely bright light and will be asked to change their gaze frequently to facilitate the ophthalmoscopic examination. A scleral depressor also may be used externally on the lid or conjunctiva to assist in rotating the eyeball and to indent the retina for increased viewing ability. Areas of detachment appear bluish gray as opposed to the normal red-pink color (Figure 65-5).

■ **FIGURE 65–5** Bluish gray appearance of areas of retinal detachment. *(Courtesy Ophthalmic Photography at the University of Michigan W. K. Kellogg Eye Center, Ann Arbor, Mich.)*

is to place the retina back in contact with the choroid and to seal the accompanying holes and breaks. Because retinal detachment repair may take several hours, general anesthesia is commonly used. The pupil must be widely dilated before the operation, and the client may be given a sedative.

Laser Photocoagulation

If the retina is torn or the detachment is slight, a laser can be used to burn the edges of the tear and halt progression. If the detachment is small, the laser can seal the retina against the choroid. Laser surgery is usually performed as an outpatient procedure under local anesthesia.

Cryopexy

Cryopexy uses nitrous oxide to freeze the tissue behind the retinal tear, stimulating scar tissue formation that will seal the edges of the tear. It is usually done as an outpatient procedure with the client under local anesthesia.

Pneumatic Retinopexy

Pneumatic retinopexy is most effective for detachments that occur in the upper portion of the eye. The eye is numbed with local anesthesia, and a small gas bubble is injected into the vitreous body. The bubble rises and presses against the retina, pushing it against the choroid. The gas bubble is slowly absorbed over the next 1 or 2 weeks. Cryopexy or laser is used to seal the retina into place.

Scleral Buckling

The surgical procedure to place the retina back in contact with the choroid is called *scleral buckling* (Figure 65-6). The sclera is actually depressed from the outside by

OUTCOME MANAGEMENT

Surgical Management

There is no known medical treatment for a detached retina. The goal of surgical repair of retinal detachment

■ **FIGURE 65–6** **A,** Detached retina. **B,** Scleral buckling to repair a detached retina. A silicone sponge implant is placed over the tear and held in place with an encircling band. An air or gas bubble may be used to apply pressure on the retina from the inside of the eye. When the buckle is tightened, the implant indents the sclera, holding the choroid and retina together.

rubber-like silicone (Silastic) sponges or bands that are sutured in place permanently. In addition to the buckling procedure, an intraocular injection of air or sulfur hexafluoride (SF6) gas bubble, or both, may be used to apply pressure on the retina from the inside of the eye. This holds the retina in place by gravitational force during the healing phase. Postoperative positioning of the client maximizes the tamponade effect of the air or gas bubble. The bubble is slowly absorbed.

Postoperative swelling of tissues and cells in the anterior chamber caused by the inflammatory process or compromise of the venous drainage system may result in increased IOP. Because of the fragility of the tissues involved in the repair, re-detachment of the retina may occur at any time. At times, the retina has been separated from its blood supply long enough that, even when reattached, it no longer has useful function and the client's vision does not improve significantly. Postoperative infection is also a risk.

The client should not expect immediate return of vision. Postoperative inflammation and the dilating drops interfere with vision. As healing takes place over weeks and months, vision may improve gradually.

Nursing Management

Nursing care focuses on helping the client cope with the fears and reality of loss of vision and to adapt to changes in vision. The client must be aware of the clinical manifestations of further loss of vision.

Following surgery, observe the eye patch for any drainage. Blood loss in retinal detachment surgery is minimal, and only serous drainage is expected on the postoperative dressing. Assess the level of pain and the presence of nausea.

Activity restrictions may be necessary if an air or gas bubble has been injected. The client needs to be positioned so that the bubble can apply maximal pressure on the retina by the force of gravity. This position, usually head down and to one side, is maintained for several days. Provide suggestions for comfort and support with the positioning (pillows under stomach, elbows, or ankles).

Encourage the client to resume a regular diet and fluids as tolerated. The eye patch and shield are removed the next morning. Redness and swelling of the lids and conjunctiva should be expected from the surgical manipulation. After several days, the swelling and ecchymosis of the lids subside, but the conjunctiva may remain red or pink for a few weeks.

Postoperative eye medications generally include an antibiotic-steroid combination eyedrop to prevent infection and reduce inflammation. Cycloplegic agents are prescribed to dilate the pupil and relax the ciliary muscles, which decreases discomfort and helps prevent the formation of iris adhesions to the corneal endothelium *(synechiae)*. Either warm or cold compresses may be applied for comfort several times a day.

Self-Care

Because retinal detachment surgery is often performed on an urgent basis, the client rarely has an opportunity to plan for the surgery. Evaluate the home environment, and assist the client and family in preparing for any necessary support. You may need to find help at home for independent living until sight returns or the client adapts to changes in vision. Although the eye patch is usually removed early in the postoperative period, clients commonly have decreased functional vision in the eye. The Bridge to Home Health Care feature on p. 1709 suggests ways to help clients cope with failing vision.

Instruct the client to clean the eye with warm tap water using a clean washcloth. Warm compresses may be continued at home. Either an eye shield or glasses should be worn during the day, and the shield should be worn during naps and at night. Advise the client to avoid vigorous activities and heavy lifting during the

BRIDGE TO HOME HEALTH CARE

Coping with Failing Vision

Providing a safe home environment for the client with failing vision is essential. Promoting an autonomous lifestyle is desirable. Assessing the client's ability to remain safely at home is an important responsibility of home health care nurses.

Basic emergency procedures can be implemented by the use of nationwide services such as Lifeline. This service provides a portable electronic device usually worn around the client's neck or wrist. By simply pushing the button, immediate contact is made with emergency personnel. The toll-free phone number is 1-800-852-5433.

Local telephone companies can provide special adaptive equipment for 9-1-1 access. Telephones that can be programmed and have lighted or large numbers are available in most retail stores.

Home safety precautions can be simple. Burns can be prevented by color-coding water faucets. Use red for hot water and blue for cold water. Marking the "Off" dials on stoves and microwave ovens with colored tape or paint reduces the chance of injury.

Adequate lighting is essential. During the day, natural light is preferable. Open drapes or shades to provide ample light. Replace light bulbs with the highest wattage recommended.

Removal of hazards, such as throw rugs, clutter, and unnecessary furniture, can promote unrestricted ambulation. Handrails can be installed in hallways, in bathrooms, and on steps to prevent falls. Equipment such as canes, walkers, raised toilet seats, and bathtub rails promote safety. These items are available at medical supply stores.

Many commercial products are now marketed that can be of great assistance in the home. Pill organizers are clearly marked boxes with the day of the week and the times pills are to be taken. These can be filled by family members for a week at a time. Electronic lamp timers and voice-activated switches will allow the client to function more independently.

Access to a television and a radio is important. Large-print newspapers and reading materials help keep the client in touch with current events. The local library and the American Association for the Blind can provide assistance in obtaining needed items.

Creativity and planning can allow the client to remain at home in a safe environment for as long as possible.

immediate postoperative period. If an air or gas bubble has been injected, it may take several weeks to be totally absorbed. Clients are advised to avoid air travel during this time because the gas and air expand at high altitudes.

DIABETIC RETINOPATHY

Diabetic retinopathy is a progressive disorder of the retina characterized by microscopic damage to the retinal vessels, resulting in occlusion of the vessels. As a result of inadequate blood supply, sections of the retina deteriorate and vision is permanently lost. Diabetic retinopathy is one of the leading causes of blindness worldwide. All diabetic people are at risk for retinopathy, although there appears to be a strong correlation between incidence and severity of retinopathy and duration of the disease and blood glucose control. About 30% to 40% of the diabetic population has some degree of retinopathy. Clients who have had diabetes for 15 to 20 years have an 80% to 90% risk for development of retinopathy. Recently a genetic predisposition to retinopathy was found in the Asian Indian population with diabetes. People with allele 210 bp have increased risk.

The two types of diabetic retinopathy are (1) background (*nonproliferative*) and (2) *proliferative*. In background retinopathy, the retinal vessels are hyperpermeable and weak. The capillaries develop microaneurysms, and the retinal veins become dilated and tortuous. Multiple hemorrhages occur from these defective vessels. Retinal edema is caused by leaking capillaries, and after the serous fluid is absorbed, a yellowish precipitate ("hard exudate") remains. Hemorrhages, exudates, and ischemia contribute to impaired vision, particularly if these occur on or around the macula. Progressive retinal ischemia stimulates the growth of new but ineffective blood vessels. These new and fragile blood vessels proliferate and grow into the vitreous body. These vessels leak, hemorrhage, and undergo fibrous changes that may form bands that pull on the retina, causing detachment. This process is called *proliferative retinopathy* (Figure 65-7). With increasing ischemia, microinfarcts of the nerve fiber layer, called "cotton-wool spots," appear.

Clinical manifestations are quite varied. Clients may report "spiders," "cobwebs," or tiny specks floating in their vision; dark streaks or a red film that blocks vision; vision loss, usually in both eyes, but more so in one eye; blurred vision that may fluctuate; a dark or empty spot in the center of the vision; poor night vision; or difficulty adjusting from bright light to dim light (Figure 65-8).

■ **FIGURE 65–7** Proliferative diabetic retinopathy. Neovascularization covers one fourth to one third of the optic disc (*arrow*).

OUTCOME MANAGEMENT

The two main treatments for diabetic retinopathy are photocoagulation and vitrectomy. In most cases, these treatments are effective and slow or stop the progression of the disease for some time.

Photocoagulation

The goal of photocoagulation is to stop the leakage of blood and fluid in the retina and thus slow the progression of diabetic retinopathy. In photocoagulation a high-energy laser beam creates small burns in areas of the retina with abnormal blood vessels to seal any leaks. The procedure can be done as an outpatient using local anesthesia. A medical contact lens is placed on the cornea to help focus laser light on the sections of the retina to be treated. Fluorescein angiographic photographs may serve as maps to show where the laser burns should be placed. For proliferative diabetic retinopathy, panretinal or scatter photocoagulation can be used to treat the entire retina except the macula. The treatment causes the abnormal new blood vessels to shrink and disappear. Thus it reduces the chances of vitreous hemorrhage. Panretinal photocoagulation is usually done in two or more sessions. The treatment significantly reduces the risk of severe vision loss.

Vitrectomy

Vitrectomy is removal of the blood-filled vitreous. A vitreous cutter cuts the tissue and removes it, piece by piece, from the eye. The volume of removed tissue is replaced with saline to maintain the normal shape and pressure of the eye. During a vitrectomy the surgeon

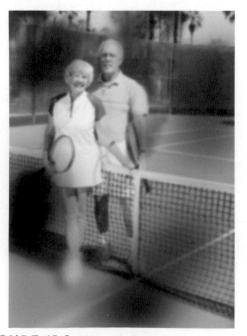

■ **FIGURE 65–8** Vision with diabetic retinopathy.

may also use a laser probe to perform a procedure called *panretinal photocoagulation* to prevent renewed growth of abnormal blood vessels and bleeding.

Nursing Management of the Surgical Client

Shortly after laser treatment, the client can usually return home driven by someone else. Vision will be blurry for about a day. Mild pain, headache, and sensitivity to light are expected and can be controlled with an eye patch and over-the-counter pain relievers. Immediately following laser surgery to treat macular edema, small spots caused by the laser burns may appear in the visual field. The spots generally fade and disappear with time. Follow-up care should be arranged before the client leaves; new areas of leakage may appear later and may require additional laser treatments.

RETINITIS PIGMENTOSA

Retinitis pigmentosa, described in the Genetic Links feature on p. 1711, is a genetic disorder that initially destroys the rods of the eye. Because the rods perceive black and white vision, the earliest manifestation is noticed during childhood as night blindness. Over the next several years, manifestations progress until a total loss of peripheral vision occurs. In time, central vision is also lost. No treatment is available to slow or stop this disorder. Genetic counseling is advised.

AGE-RELATED MACULAR DEGENERATION

Age-related macular degeneration (AMD) is a degenerative process that affects the macula and surrounding tissues, resulting in central visual deficits. AMD is found to some degree in most adults over 65 years of age. It is one of the most common causes of visual loss in older people. The exact cause is unknown, but the incidence increases with each decade in people over 50 years of age. It may be hereditary. It has been demonstrated that the blue rays of the spectrum (sunlight or its reflection in the ocean or desert) seem to accelerate macular degeneration more than other rays of the spectrum. There are two types of age-related macular degeneration: (1) nonexudative *(dry)* and (2) exudative *(wet)*. Both types are usually bilateral and progressive.

Nonexudative AMD is characterized by atrophy and degeneration of the outer retina and underlying structures. Seventy percent of clients have the dry form, which involves thinning of the macular tissues and disturbances in its pigmentation. Yellowish round spots *(drusen)* may be seen on the retina and macula with an ophthalmoscope. Drusen are deposits of amorphous material from the pigment epithelial cells of the retina. Over time, these spots increase, enlarge, and may calcify.

GENETIC LINKS

Retinitis Pigmentosa

DESCRIPTION

Retinitis pigmentosa (RP) describes a group of inherited disorders in which abnormalities of the photoreceptors (rods and cones) or the retinal pigment epithelium (RPE) of the retina lead to progressive visual loss. Clients initially experience "night blindness" (decreased night vision), followed by constriction of the peripheral visual field and eventually loss of central vision in the advanced stage of the disease. Most clients are legally blind by age 60. The prevalence of RP is approximately 1 in 3500 to 1 in 4000 individuals in the United States and Europe; it is considered the most common inherited cause of blindness.

GENETICS

RP can be inherited in an autosomal-dominant, autosomal-recessive, or X-linked recessive fashion. The molecular genetic causes of RP are unusually complicated. Many different genes may cause the same disease, and different mutations in the RP genes may cause different diseases. The mode of inheritance is determined by family history. To date, at least 34 different genes are known to cause RP; mutations in at least 12 genes cause autosomal-dominant RP, 16 genes cause autosomal-recessive RP, and 6 genes cause X-linked RP.

DIAGNOSIS/TESTING

The diagnosis of RP is based on documentation of progressive loss in photoreceptor function by electroretinography (ERG) and visual field testing. DNA testing is available for all the cloned genes causing RP on a research basis only. Routine genetic testing for RP is not available in clinical laboratories.

MANAGEMENT

RP is neither preventable nor curable, but therapy with high-dose vitamin A has been suggested to have a possible effect on slowing changes in retinal function. Various optical aids have been promoted for RP clients, and referral to agencies for the visually impaired can assist in providing vocational training, mobility training, and skills for independent living.

At the exudative stage of AMD, Bruch's membrane, which lies just beneath the pigment epithelial cell layer of the retina, becomes compromised. Thirty percent of clients have the wet form, which can involve bleeding within and beneath the retina, opaque deposits, and eventually scar tissue. The wet form accounts for 90% of all cases of legal blindness in clients with macular degeneration. It results in serous fluid leaks from the choroid, with accompanying proliferation of choroidal blood vessels. A dome-shaped retinal pigment epithelium may be seen when examining the fundus. These leaks produce a visual effect called metamorphopsia, which appears as distorted lines; the center of vision appears more distorted than the rest of the scene. A dark, blurry area or "whiteout" appears in the center of vision. Color perception changes or diminishes. Fundus photography and angiography may be performed on a regular basis to document and evaluate changes.

OUTCOME MANAGEMENT

Recent research findings, reviewed in the Complementary and Alternative Therapy feature below, have shown that the use of high-dose antioxidant vitamins C and E, beta-carotene, and zinc supplements may delay progression of AMD and vision loss. Currently there are several drugs that are injected inside the eye to halt the angiogenesis that causes the distortion and loss of central vision. VEGF (vascular endothelial growth factor) drives the production of blood vessels, and there are new drugs that block the release of VEGF.

The client with AMD is threatened with the loss of central vision (see the Bridge to Home Health Care feature on Coping with Failing Vision on p. 1709). To evaluate changes in vision, teach the client to use the Amsler chart at home. You may assist the client to maximize remaining vision with low-vision aids and community referral to a low-vision specialist and low-vision support groups.

CORNEAL DISORDERS

CORNEAL INJURY

The cornea can be injured in many ways, such as with direct trauma, over-worn contact lens, chips of flying metal or glass fragments, or even dirt. A client with a

COMPLEMENTARY AND ALTERNATIVE THERAPY

Macular Degeneration and Dietary Supplements

The largest randomized trial ($n = 3640$) of a combination daily dietary supplement (500 mg of vitamin C, 400 international units of vitamin E, 15 mg of beta-carotene, 80 mg of zinc, plus 2 mg of copper) compared with placebo for macular degeneration found a significant reduction in the risk of disease progression over the 6-year study. The only individuals who benefited, however, were those with intermediate to advanced stages of already diagnosed macular degeneration. Individuals at risk or with early stage macular degeneration did not benefit from taking this supplement combination over the study period. In addition, the supplement combination did not have any effect on cataract development or risk.

REFERENCE

Age-Related Eye Disease Study Research Group. (2001). A randomized, placebo-controlled, clinical trial of high-dose supplementation with vitamins C and E, beta carotene, and zinc for age-related macular degeneration and vision loss: AREDS report no. 8. *Archives of Ophthalmology, 119,* 1417-1435.

corneal injury will typically have a dramatic, painful, profusely lacrimating eye. The bulbar conjunctiva blood vessels will be prominent (injected).

 SAFETY ALERT

Treatment includes removing any imbedded items and then resting the eye (keeping it closed, using antibiotic ointments). Clients who are unconscious can also develop corneal dryness attributable to lack of blinking (Box 65-1).

CORNEAL DYSTROPHIES

Corneal dystrophies comprise a group of hereditary and acquired disorders of unknown cause, characterized by deposits in the layers of the cornea and alteration of the corneal structure. Corneal dystrophies are associated with all five layers of the cornea. Although the disease usually originates in the inner layers (Descemet's membrane, the stroma, and Bowman's membrane), the degeneration, erosion, and deposits affect all layers. Corneal endothelium constantly removes fluids from the cornea to maintain its clarity. As the endothelial cells are gradually lost, the dystrophy progresses. Once lost, the endothelial cells do not grow back but instead spread out to fill the empty spaces. The pump system becomes less efficient, causing corneal clouding, swelling, and eventually reduced vision.

OUTCOME MANAGEMENT

The goal of treatment is to restore visual clarity for both safety and improved quality of life.

Medical Management

Dystrophies cannot be cured; however, with certain medications, blurred vision resulting from corneal swelling can be controlled. Saline eyedrops or ointments are

---

BOX 65-1 Eye Care for Unconscious Clients

Unconscious, sedated, or paralyzed clients are at high risk of corneal injury because they cannot maintain normal lid closure. Normal lid closure during sleep is provided by tonic contraction of the orbicularis oculi muscle. The use of muscle relaxants reduces the tonic contraction of the muscle and leads only to passive closure of the eyelids. Further, the client may have lost the blink reflex when sedatives are used. Tears quickly evaporate from the eye and increase the risk of injury. Corneal abrasion has been reported in as little as 48 hours.

Eye protection and lubrication are important to preserve sight. The use of eyedrops or ointments is effective in maintaining eye moisture. Films that preserve humidity in the eye can also be used; however, the family may be alarmed by the client's appearance with these products.

Data from Joyce, N. (2002). *Eye care for intensive care patients. A systematic review.* Adelaide, South Africa: The Joanna Briggs Institute for Evidence Based Nursing and Midwifery.

---

often prescribed to draw fluid from the cornea and reduce swelling. Another simple technique that reduces moisture in the cornea is to hold a hair dryer at arm's length, blowing air into the face with the eyes closed. This technique draws moisture from the cornea, temporarily decreases swelling, and improves vision.

Surgical Management

Corneal Transplantation

Corneal transplantation *(keratoplasty)* is the use of donor corneas to improve the clarity of vision. Two depths of keratoplasty are performed. Penetrating keratoplasty indicates full-thickness corneal replacement; lamellar keratoplasty denotes a partial-thickness procedure. Because there is a direct relationship between age and health of the endothelial layer of the cornea, young donor tissue is preferred. Donor eyes are obtained from cadavers; donor eyes must be enucleated soon after death because of rapid endothelial cell death and must be stored in a preserving solution. Storage, handling, and coordination of donor tissue with surgeons are provided by a network of state eye-bank associations around the country.

Corneal transplantation surgery is usually performed with the client under local anesthesia. Figure 65-9, *A*, shows the eye after keratoplasty. Unlike cataract surgery, however, visual return after a corneal transplant is relatively slow and typically takes 6 to 12 months. The reason for the slow return of vision is that the sutures holding the new cornea in place tend to distort the vision, and they must be left in place for a considerable time before it is safe to remove them.

Rejection of donor tissue can occur following corneal transplantation from unsuitable storage of donor tissue, dystrophy of the donor's endothelium, surgical trauma, or immunologic rejection. Wound leakage, bleeding into the anterior chamber, glaucoma, cataract, and infection are other complications that may occur. At the first sign of graft rejection, when the cornea becomes cloudy and edematous and when there is an anterior chamber reaction (the presence of white blood cells or protein) (see Figure 65-9, *B*), topical steroids are prescribed in frequent doses to control the inflammatory response and to reverse the rejection reaction. In severe cases, a second transplantation may be necessary.

Nursing Management of the Postoperative Client

Corneal transplantation is usually performed as outpatient surgery. Postoperatively the client returns from the operating room with an eye patch and protective shield in place. Observe the patch for signs of drainage. No bleeding is expected with this procedure. The client should experience only mild to moderate discomfort, which should be relieved by acetaminophen. Unreduced

■ **FIGURE 65–9 A,** Clinical appearance of the eye after keratoplasty. **B,** Acute graft rejection. *(Courtesy Ophthalmic Photography at the University of Michigan W.K. Kellogg Eye Center, Ann Arbor, Mich.)*

pain may indicate a rise in IOP and should be reported to the surgeon. Because the eye patch is to be in place until the following morning, assess the client's ability for self-care and reinforce information on the hazards of monocular vision.

The eye is examined the next morning with the slit lamp. Depending on the extent of preoperative visual limitations, most clients experience improved vision immediately. Instruct clients, however, not to overestimate their expectations for full vision. Vision continues to improve gradually because the healing process may take up to a year or more. Glasses or contact lenses are usually needed to obtain the best result. Many months may be required for restoration of vision, and revisions in the care plan may be needed.

Self-Care

Postoperative eyedrops usually include an antibiotic and a corticosteroid. Topical corticosteroid therapy may

be needed indefinitely. Discharge instructions include the rationale for the medications and proper instillation technique.

> **It is important for the client to wear eye protection in the form of regular glasses, sunglasses, or a protective shield to prevent injury to the eye. Advise the client never to rub the eye. The area around the eye may be cleaned with warm tap water using a clean washcloth.**   SAFETY ALERT

Teach the client and family to recognize the clinical manifestations of increased IOP, infection, and graft rejection. A mnemonic tool may be useful in teaching the client to remember the signs of graft rejection (RSVP):

- R Redness
- S Swelling
- V Decreased vision
- P Pain

Advise the client to evaluate vision in the eye each day. A picture on the wall or some object in a well-lighted room should be selected as a point of reference. If a change in vision from the day before is noted, the client should reevaluate his or her vision in a few hours. If no improvement is noted or if vision is worse, the client should notify the physician. Because graft rejection may occur at any time (even years) after the surgery, advise the client to make the vision check a routine part of ADL for the rest of his or her life.

OCULAR MELANOMA

Although less than 1% of the people in the United States are affected by malignant ocular tumors, treatment of these tumors can be a challenge for both client and nurse. Choroidal melanomas are often detected during a routine ocular examination because there is no pain associated with the development of the tumor. By the time the tumor has grown large enough to obstruct vision, there may be involvement of the macula and metastasis.

OUTCOME MANAGEMENT

The goal of treatment is to care for the malignancy while preserving the eye.

Medical Management

When ocular melanoma is discovered early, radiation therapy alone may be the treatment of choice. Radiation therapy to the eye is accomplished through insertion of a tiny plate or plaque about the size of a dime that holds tiny seeds of radioactive iodine 125. The plaque is sutured to the sclera directly over the site of the tumor. It is left in place for several days, depending on the required dose, and then removed. Both insertion and removal are performed in the operating room. During treatment a lead shield is placed over the eye. Radiation exposure to the nurse who cares for the client is minimal—a small fraction of a chest x-ray study. Despite this extremely low exposure, the routine restrictions for hospital personnel and visitors are implemented for consistency. Hospitalization for treatment with radioactive iodine is required, depending on regulations.

SAFETY ALERT Follow the principles of radiation safety: reduce distance from the client, wear a lead shield and use a lead shield at the bedside, and limit time at the bedside by condensing assessments and interventions.

During the client's hospitalization for this treatment, provide support and encouragement for the client. The plaque is only mildly to moderately uncomfortable, and discomfort should be relieved with acetaminophen. The difficult challenge for clients is confinement to their room with limitations on visitors at a time when support is essential. Eye medications include a cycloplegic agent and an antibiotic-steroid eyedrop.

Surgical Management

Enucleation
The goal of surgical removal is to preserve life by removing the tumor. Removal of the entire eyeball *(enucleation)* has been the traditional method of treatment and may be combined with radiation treatments. *Exenteration* (removal of the eyeball and surrounding tissues and bone) may also be necessary. The goal for clients following enucleation is adaptation to monocular vision and return to their former level of independence.

Enucleation is usually performed with the client under general anesthesia, but IV conscious sedation may also be used. The ocular muscles are dissected from the eyeball, which is removed by severing the optic nerve and vessels at the back. An acrylic sphere covered by donor scleral tissue is usually placed within the capsule of tissue that formerly held the eyeball. Scleral tissue encourages fibrovascular ingrowth, which prevents migration and extrusion of the implant. A soft plastic scleral shell is placed in the visible outer portion of the socket as a support until a permanent prosthesis can be made. A newer type of implant, hydroxyapatite, which is made of the same inorganic material present in human bone, is now being used.

Several weeks later a central hole is drilled into the sphere and covering tissues. A peg (which later fits into a depression on the posterior surface of the artificial eye) is then inserted into the hole. The movement of the implant by the muscle cone is transferred directly to the prosthesis. With the artificial eye being primarily supported by the peg instead of the lids and socket tissues, fewer cosmetic and structural complications occur.

Nursing Management
The client undergoing enucleation for a malignant tumor is stressed not only by the threat of cancer but also by disfigurement of the face. Assess the client's response, home, and family for support mechanisms. Nursing interventions are focused on assisting the client to grieve for the lost body part and lost vision and to identify coping mechanisms that will facilitate rehabilitation.

Preoperative Care
Assist the client in preparing for the surgical procedure. Most often the client is made aware of the tumor at a routine office visit. Surgery is usually scheduled within a few days. Recognizing that the client is most appropriately in a state of shock and denial, carefully explain the perioperative events. Although it is possible to have an enucleation as an outpatient procedure, the client may stay overnight in the hospital.

Postoperative Care
Provide routine postoperative care. The client returns from the operating room with a pressure dressing over the eye. Assess the dressing for bleeding using standard postoperative routines. Clients are understandably anxious about the removal of the dressing the next morning. Prepare the client by explaining how the eye and conformer will appear. The socket and lids will be swollen, and the white plastic conformer is visible.

SAFETY ALERT Determine the client's or the family's ability to care for the wound postoperatively.

Some clients fear that their appearance will frighten others, especially children. In this case, an eye patch may be worn during the 4 to 6 weeks before the prosthesis is fitted but should not be worn continuously. Eventually the eye prosthesis can be worn and looks pleasingly normal (Figure 65-10). Refer to a fundamentals of nursing textbook for insertion and removal of the prosthesis.

The area around the lids may be cleaned with warm tap water with a clean washcloth. Soap and water should be kept away from the socket. If the plastic conformer accidentally comes out, it should be washed and replaced. Antibiotic ophthalmic ointment is usually ordered to be instilled in the socket once or twice a day.

Self-Care
Adjustment to monocular vision is a challenge the client begins to face immediately. Depth perception is altered, and the client needs to exercise caution in walking, crossing streets, and driving. Advise the client to practice ADLs until visual and body adjustments are made.

■ FIGURE 65–10 An ocular prosthesis. *(Courtesy Ophthalmic Photography at the University of Michigan W.K. Kellogg Eye Center, Ann Arbor, Mich.)*

SAFETY

⚠

ALERT

Emphasize the need for extra precaution with the remaining eye. Eye protection should be worn when engaging in any activity that might even remotely result in an injury. Many clients are advised to wear glasses even if no correction is needed.

EYELID, LACRIMAL, AND CONJUNCTIVAL DISORDERS

DRY EYE SYNDROME

Dry eye syndrome is a condition in which tear production is inadequate. It most commonly occurs in women between 50 and 60 years of age. Three primary causes are lacrimal gland malfunction, mucin deficiency, and mechanical abnormalities that prevent the spread of tears across the surface of the eye. The lacrimal gland can be genetically malformed or malformed because of injury or infection. Tear production is also decreased in Sjögren's syndrome, an autoimmune disorder that commonly accompanies rheumatoid arthritis. Facial nerve (seventh cranial nerve) palsy disrupts tear production. Mechanical abnormalities include problems with eyelid structure, eyeball extrusion, and misuse of contact lenses. Conjunctivitis and mumps can obstruct the gland. Some medications, such as antihistamines, atropine, and beta-adrenergic blocking agents, decrease tear production.

Manifestations include burning, itching eyes and a sensation of "something" in the eye. The term *keratoconjunctivitis sicca* is used to describe the problem.

Management includes determining the degree of injury to the cornea. Artificial tears (eyedrops and lubricants) can be used. In addition, some clients benefit from using airtight goggles at night to prevent tear evaporation. Postmenopausal women have found some relief from

estrogen replacement therapy. Surgery can be used to open the lacrimal duct or to repair lid problems.

Other eyelid, lacrimal, and conjunctival disorders are discussed in Table 65-1.

REFRACTIVE DISORDERS

Light is bent (refracted) as it passes through the cornea and lens of the eye. Refractive errors exist when light rays are not focused appropriately on the retina of the eye. Three basic abnormalities of refraction occur in the eye: (1) myopia, (2) hyperopia, and (3) astigmatism. Optical correction is important to distinguish between visual loss caused by disease and visual loss caused by refractive error. *Refractometry* is the measurement of refractive error and should not be confused with *refraction,* the method used to determine which lens or lenses (if any) will most benefit the client.

MYOPIA

Myopia, or *nearsightedness,* is a condition in which the light rays come into focus in front of the retina (Figure 65-11, *A*). In this case the refractive power of the eye is too strong and a concave, or minus, lens is used to focus light rays on the eye. In most cases myopia is caused by an eyeball that is longer than normal, which may be a familial trait. Transient myopia may occur with the administration of a variety of medications (sulfonamides, acetazolamide, salicylates, and steroids) and has been associated with other disorders, such as influenza, typhoid fever, severe dehydration, and large intakes of antacids (for stomach ulcers). Correction is accomplished with eyeglasses or contact lenses.

HYPEROPIA

The hyperopic, or *farsighted,* eye focuses light rays behind the eye, and consequently the image that falls on the retina is blurred (see Figure 65-11, *B*). Vision may be brought into focus by placing a convex, or plus, lens in front of the eye. The lens supplies the magnifying power that the eye is lacking. Hyperopia may be caused by an eyeball that is shorter than normal or a cornea that has less curvature than normal. Because children have a greater ability to accommodate, they are less often affected than adults. Demands for close work and reading usually instigate manifestations of headache or eyestrain. Correction is based on a person's age and individual needs and complaints.

ASTIGMATISM

Astigmatism is a refractive condition in which rays of light are not bent equally by the cornea in all directions

TABLE 65–1   Eyelid, Lacrimal, and Conjunctival Disorders

Disorder	Definition	Appearance	Management
Dacryocystitis	Inflammation of tear drainage system	Pus-like drainage or raised, red lump near puncta	Antibiotics, daily massage of lacrimal system
Hordeolum (stye)	Infection of glands of eyelids	Redness and swelling of localized area of eyelid	Warm compresses and antibiotics; may need to be incised and drained
Chalazion	Chronic granuloma of meibomian gland	Painless, localized swelling of lid margin	If cosmetically distracting, may be surgically removed
Blepharitis	Chronic, bilateral inflammation of eyelids	Itching and burning of eyes; eyes appear red; scales noted on lashes	Wash eyelids with baby shampoo, water, and cotton-tipped applicators; antibiotic ointments may be prescribed
Conjunctivitis	Inflammation of conjunctiva from various microorganisms	Redness, tearing, and exudation of eyelid; may progress to eyelid drooping, abnormal tissue growth	Antibiotic eyedrops
Entropion	Turning in eyelid margin	Inversion of lower eyelid; dry and irritated eyes	Surgical resection
Ptosis	Drooping of eyelid from several causes	Irritation of eye caused by drying, loss of tears	Artificial tears; surgical correction needed; sometimes glasses used to lift redundant skin
Lagophthalmos	Inadequate closure of eyelids	Irritation of eye caused by drying	Artificial tears, eye shields at night; surgical correction
Absence of blinking	Lack of blinking seen with Parkinson's disease and hyperthyroidism	Blinking fewer than 20 times/min	Artificial tears; eye shields at night

so that a point of focus is not attained (see Figure 65-11, *C*). In most instances, astigmatism is caused because the curvature of the cornea is not perfectly spherical. This is the cause of poor vision for both distant and near objects. Astigmatism is corrected with cylindrical lenses.

Surgical Management

Refractive Surgery
Laser in situ keratomileusis (LASIK) is the most commonly used corrective surgery for nearsightedness in the United States. An extremely thin layer of the cornea is peeled back for laser reshaping on the middle layer of the cornea, and then the thin layer is put back in place. There is little postoperative discomfort, rapid recovery of clear vision, and quick stabilization of refractive change. LASIK is performed in a surgeon's office or same-day surgery center and does not require a hospital stay. It takes about 10 to 15 minutes per eye. It has a high success rate and low complication rate for low to moderate nearsightedness and may also be used to correct more severe nearsightedness.

LASEK (laser epithelial keratomileusis) is a relatively new procedure that is technically a variation of others. Also called epithelial LASIK or E-LASIK, LASEK is used mostly for people with corneas that are too thin or too flat for LASIK. It was developed to reduce the chance of complications that occur when the flap created during LASIK is not the ideal thickness or diameter.

Corneal ring implants (In-tacs) are clear pieces of acrylic that can be surgically implanted into the cornea. The implants flatten the cornea and thereby reduce

nearsightedness. The implants are shaped like crescents or half-circles. Two implants are used for each eye, and the implants are inserted along the sides of the cornea *(corneal periphery)*. They do not cover the central

Myopia (nearsightedness)
A

Corrected with biconcave lens

Hyperopia (farsightedness)
B

Corrected with biconvex lens

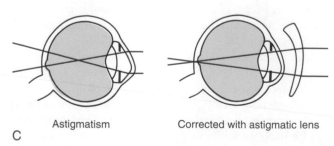

Astigmatism
C

Corrected with astigmatic lens

■ **FIGURE 65–11   A-C,** Common refractive disorders and their correction. *Dashed lines* in **A** and **B** indicate normal eye contour.

portion of the cornea. Corneal ring implants appear to be very effective for correcting mild nearsightedness.

Nursing Management of the Surgical Client

Clients are assessed preoperatively for degree of myopia or astigmatism. Clients with severe refraction problems may not achieve full correction. Surgery is performed on an outpatient basis with local anesthesia. Eye protection is used, such as goggles to prevent dry eyes. Vigorous activities, activities that could get water in the eye, and eye makeup are to be avoided.

The eye is treated with steroid eyedrops, and most clients report watering of the eyes and minimal pain. Refraction slowly stabilizes after surgery. There is a period of adjustment during which visual acuity waxes and wanes. Reduced contrast sensitivity in night vision and daytime glare is common. Some clients require re-treatment for scarring that is unresponsive to topical steroids.

OCULAR MANIFESTATIONS OF SYSTEMIC DISORDERS

ENDOCRINE DISORDERS: GRAVES' DISEASE

Graves' disease may exist with or without any clinical evidence of thyroid dysfunction. Ocular manifestations include retraction of both upper and lower lids, resulting in a staring or frightened expression (Stellwag's sign); and lid lag (Graefe's sign), the retarded lowering of the upper lid when looking down (Figure 65-12). When the gaze is changed from down to up, the globe then lags behind the upper lid. Other signs are infrequent blinking, marked fine tremor with lid closure, and jerky movements on lid opening.

■ **FIGURE 65–12** Graves' exophthalmos. *(Courtesy Ophthalmic Photography at the University of Michigan W.K. Kellogg Eye Center, Ann Arbor, Mich.)*

The globes enlarge because of the increased size of extraocular muscles, edema of tissues, and excess orbital fat. The eye develops *proptosis* (forward protrusion of the eyeballs), which is called *exophthalmos*. Subsequent degeneration of muscle tissue leads to fibrosis, which restricts muscle movement, resulting in double vision.

As a primary measure, adequate control of thyroid abnormalities is essential. Diuretics as well as steroid therapy and radiotherapy may be indicated. Surgical interventions include corrective lid surgery and tarsorrhaphy for lid retraction to protect the cornea. Decompression of the orbit, which usually involves removal of the inferior and medial walls of the orbit, may be necessary to accommodate proliferative orbital fat and enlarged ocular muscles. Ocular muscle surgery may also be indicated. If the surgery is extensive, suction drains may be placed at the operative sites. Drainage is usually serosanguineous.

It is important that the client sleep with the head elevated to reduce postoperative swelling.

Advise the client to expect redness, swelling, and ecchymoses around the eyes and lids. In the immediate postoperative period, check the client's visual acuity with a near-vision card every hour to monitor the possibility of pressure on the optic nerve (see Thinking Critically). Caution the client to modify normal activities for the first 2 weeks after surgery.

SAFETY

ALERT

RHEUMATOID AND CONNECTIVE TISSUE DISORDERS

Sjögren's syndrome includes keratoconjunctivitis sicca, a common condition in which tear secretion is reduced in association with a systemic disorder such as rheumatoid arthritis, psoriatic arthritis, connective tissue disorders, sarcoidosis, or Crohn's disease. Manifestations include ocular irritation and foreign-body sensation. Frequent instillation of lubricating eyedrops or ointment is effective in most cases.

Several ocular problems may be associated with systemic lupus erythematosus (SLE), a connective tissue disorder. The eyelids may be involved, with the discoid lesions characteristic of the disease. Punctate epithelial keratopathy and secondary Sjögren's syndrome may also occur. Retinopathy of SLE produces cotton-wool spots and increased retinal vessel fragility, as in diabetes. Optic neuropathy can also occur.

NEUROLOGIC DISORDERS

About 90% of clients with myasthenia gravis have ocular involvement. In most cases it is the presenting manifestation. *Ptosis* (drooping of the eyelid) is bilateral but may be asymmetrical. Diplopia is frequently in the vertical plane. Nystagmus is also present. Ocular myopathy and cranial nerve palsy may develop later, as may ophthalmoplegia (paralysis of all extraocular muscles). Medical treatment is supportive and includes systemic steroids.

There is also a close association between optic neuritis and multiple sclerosis. About three fourths of women and one third of men with optic neuritis have multiple sclerosis at 15-year follow-up. Typically an attack of optic neuritis starts with acute onset of loss of vision in one eye, with periocular discomfort made worse by movement of the eye. Visual impairment is progressive over 2 weeks and usually resolves after 4 to 6 weeks. Recovery may take longer and may be incomplete. Medical treatment consists of oral, IV, and retrobulbar steroids.

CIRCULATORY DISORDERS

The primary response of retinal arterioles to hypertension is a narrowing. In clients with chronic hypertension, the blood-retina barrier is disrupted in small areas, resulting in increased vascular permeability. Funduscopic examination reveals vasoconstriction, leakage, and arteriosclerosis. Hypertensive retinopathy is graded for severity on a scale of 1 to 4, with 4 the most severe. Systemic hypertension is also associated with an increased risk of retinal vein occlusion. There is no known treatment for retinal vein occlusion.

LYME DISEASE

Lyme disease *(Borrelia burgdorferi),* transmitted by the bite of a tick, consists of three stages. The initial stage involves a lesion and erythema around the bite, accompanied by regional lymphadenopathy, malaise, fever, headache, myalgia, arthralgia, and frequently conjunctivitis. Several weeks to months later, the second phase is associated with neurologic and cardiac problems. Along with these problems, there may be cranial nerve palsies, uveitis, optic neuropathy, keratitis, choroiditis, and exudative retinal detachments. Rheumatologic complications may develop in the third stage, which may occur over several years. Tetracycline and penicillin are effective in treating the initial infection and in preventing late complications.

CONCLUSIONS

To provide comprehensive nursing care for clients, it is essential to understand the complexity of ocular structures and the physiology of vision. The specialty practice of ophthalmic nursing is devoted to caring for clients with eye disorders. Ophthalmic registered nurses perform the roles of caregiver, advocate, educator, counselor, technician, coordinator, and researcher. Ophthalmic nursing care not only is directed at those biologic systems that are affected by an actual or potential deficit but also is an integration of how actual or potential visual deficits affect the individual as an entire being.

THINKING CRITICALLY

1. Your client is a 72-year-old retired carpenter who has undergone outpatient cataract surgery. He and his wife live an hour away from the surgery center, where they received instructions to call the emergency number if any unusual pain or nausea occurs. They have an appointment to return for a follow-up evaluation the next morning. After supper the client's wife calls to report that her husband has a headache. She says that her husband also has an upset stomach, but she thinks he feels queasy because he ate some spicy food. The client does not want his wife to drive him back at night and thinks she should not have bothered to call because they have an appointment in the morning. How would you proceed? What further assessment data are needed? What are the likely complications following cataract surgery, and what are their clinical manifestations?

Factors to Consider. Might the headache and upset stomach be related to the cataract surgery, or are they likely to be unrelated?

2. Your client, a 55-year-old woman with Graves' ophthalmopathy, has undergone surgery in the late afternoon today for a right orbital decompression. An incisional drain is in place at the right temple with a bulb attached for suction. The surgeon has ordered postoperative vision checks with a near-vision card every hour throughout the night. The surgery lasted more than 3 hours; general anesthesia was used, and the client is still sedated. Her right eye is extremely swollen; she is unable to open it to read the vision card. She winces and cries when her operative eye is touched, and she is so sleepy that she cannot respond by reading the vision card. What should you do to carry out the surgeon's postoperative orders?

Factors to Consider. Are such severe eye pain and swelling normal postoperative findings? How would you assess the eye? How would you rouse the client to perform these crucial eye assessments?

Discussions for these questions can be found on the website.

BIBLIOGRAPHY

Citations appearing in red refer to primary research.

Citations appearing in blue refer to evidence-based practice guidelines and protocols.

1. Age Related Eye Disease Study. (2001). Age-related eye disease study: A randomized, placebo-controlled clinical trial for high dose supplementation with vitamins C, E, and beta carotene for AMD and vision loss. *Archives of Ophthalmology, 119*(10), 1417-1436.
2. Banerjee, S. (2006). A review of developments in the management of retinal diseases. *Journal of the Royal Society of Medicine, 99*(3), 125-127.
3. Evans, J.R. (2006) Antioxidant vitamin and mineral supplements for slowing the progression of age-related macular degeneration. *Cochrane Database of Systematic Reviews* 2006, 19(2), CD000254. DOI: 10.1002/14651858.CD000254.pub2.

4. Garvican, L., Cloves, J., & Gillow, T. (2000). Preservation of sight in diabetes: Developing a national risk reduction program. *Diabetic Medicine, 17*(9), 627-634.

5. Goldblum, K. (Ed.) (2007). *Ophthalmic nursing core curriculum.* Dubuque, Iowa: Kendall Publishing.

6. Greenlee, E.C. (2005). Laser and surgical treatment for glaucoma: An overview. *Insight, 30*(4), 32-37.

7. Halle, C. (2002). Achieve new vision screening objectives. *Nurse Practitioner, 27*(3), 21-22, 25–26.

8. Kanski, J. (1999). *Clinical ophthalmology* (4th ed.). Oxford: Butterworth Heinemann.

9. Smith, S.C., Lamp, P., & Liu, J. (2005). Age-related macular degeneration: Answers to some common questions. *Insight, 30*(3), 17-21.

10. Smith, S. (2001). The dry eye: An introduction. *Plastic Surgical Nursing, 21*(3), 135-140.

11. Subramanian, M.L., & Topping, T.M. (2004). Controversies in the management of primary retinal detachments. *Ophthalmology Clinic 2004, 44*(4), 103-114.

12. Ticho, B.H., & Dreger, V. (2000). Enucleation: Indications, methods and prosthetic devices. *Insight, 25*(1), 23-27.

13. Vaughan, D., Asbury, T., & Riordan-Eva, P. (2004). *General ophthalmology* (16th ed.). Norwalk, Conn: Appleton & Lange.

14. Watkinson, S., & Chetram, N. (2005). A nurse-led approach to diabetic retinal screening. *Nursing Times, 101*(36), 32-34.

15. Whitaker, R., & Whitaker, V. (1999). Glaucoma: What the ophthalmic nurse should know. *Insight, 24*(3), 86.

evolve   *Did you remember to check out the bonus material on the Evolve website and the CD-ROM, including NCLEX®-Examination Style Review Questions, Open-Book Quizzes, and Chapter Review Audio Podcasts?*

http://evolve.elsevier.com/Black/medsurg

CHAPTER 66

Management of Clients with Hearing and Balance Disorders

HELENE J. KROUSE

HEARING IMPAIRMENT

Hearing impairment ranges from minor difficulty in understanding words or hearing certain sounds to total deafness. Hearing impairment is the nation's primary disability: 1 in 15 Americans is affected. By the year 2050, about 1 in 5 people in the United States will be 55 years or older; of these estimated 58 million people, 26 million are expected to have hearing impairment. Of the 10 million people in the United States with a hearing loss who are now 65 years or older, more than 90% have a sensorineural hearing loss. Because of fear, misinformation, lack of information, and vanity, many people do not admit that they have a hearing problem. Up to 80% of all hearing impairments are caused by hearing nerve disorders, for which no cure is currently available. Hearing impairments diminish the quality of life for one third of adults between 65 and 75 years of age.

Etiology and Risk Factors

Many factors influence the type and amount of hearing loss. Hearing loss is not an actual disorder but is a clinical manifestation of many possible problems. Both common and uncommon causes of hearing impairment are examined in this chapter. Hearing loss can be classified into three main areas:

- Conductive hearing loss (i.e., otosclerosis, trauma)
- Sensorineural hearing loss (i.e., presbycusis, noise-induced, and sudden hearing loss)
- Mixed hearing loss

Conductive hearing loss results from interference of sound transmission through the external ear and middle ear. It may be caused by (1) anything that blocks the external ear, such as wax, infection, or a foreign body; (2) thickening, retraction, scarring, or perforation of the tympanic membrane; or (3) any pathophysiologic changes in the middle ear that affect or freeze one or more of the ossicles (Figure 66-1).

Sensorineural hearing loss is caused by impairment of the function of the inner ear, the eighth cranial nerve, or the brain. Causes are congenital and hereditary factors, noise injury, aging and degenerative processes, Ménière's disease, and ototoxicity. Systemic disorders, such as autoimmune disease, syphilis, certain collagen disorders, and diabetes, may cause sensorineural hearing losses. Cigarette smoking and exposure to environmental tobacco smoke have been associated with age-related hearing loss. Many medications can be ototoxic; see the Integrating Pharmacology feature, p. 1721.

In a *mixed hearing loss,* conductive and sensorineural hearing components are present simultaneously. A client with a perforated eardrum and presbycusis has both conductive and sensorineural hearing losses.

Conductive Hearing Loss

Ear Obstructions

Obstruction of the ear is most commonly caused by impacted cerumen (wax). Although the ear canal is self-cleaning, cerumen may become impacted from a disorder or from improper cleaning. Older people are more susceptible to cerumen impaction because hair in the ear becomes coarser with age and traps the wax. Some people produce more cerumen in the ear canal

---

evolve Web Enhancements

Care Plan The Client with Vertigo

Client Education Guide Infection of the Tympanic Membrane, Middle Ear, or Mastoid Cavity (English Version and Spanish Translation)

Precautions After Ear Surgery (Spanish Translation)

Be sure to check out the bonus material on the Evolve website and the CD-ROM, including free self-assessment exercises. **http://evolve.elsevier.com/Black/medsurg**

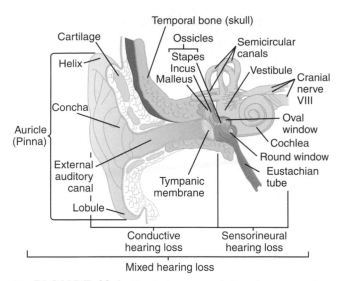

■ **FIGURE 66–I** Hearing loss can result from three causes. Conductive hearing loss occurs in areas of the outer ear when sound is conducted. Sensorineural hearing loss occurs in the inner ear where sound is transmitted by the nerves. In addition, both types can be present, called mixed hearing loss.

and require a regular routine for eliminating excessive buildup of wax in the ear canal. Insertion of cotton-tipped swabs into the ear canal can create further impaction of ear wax or can even traumatize the ear canal or perforate the eardrum.

Ear obstruction can also be caused by a wide array of foreign bodies that fit into the ear canal and impede conduction of sound waves. The most common foreign bodies found in the adult ear are pieces of cotton (such as cotton swabs) and insects. Foreign bodies commonly seen in children consist of small toys, beads, insects, and food, such as kernels of corn.

Infection

Many infections can lead to hearing loss. An infection of the inner ear, called *labyrinthitis,* can be either viral or bacterial in origin. Viral labyrinthitis can be associated with recent respiratory tract infections, measles, mumps, or rubella. Bacterial labyrinthitis, which is rare, is associated with otitis media or meningitis. Otitis media is a common disorder of the middle ear. Repeated infections or allergic inflammation can lead to fluid accumulation

INTEGRATING PHARMACOLOGY

Ototoxic Medications

Ototoxic medications are those drugs that have the potential to cause damage to the inner ear structures that may result in temporary or permanent loss of hearing or an aggravation of an existing sensorineural hearing loss. As a result of using ototoxic medications, the degree of hearing loss that occurs and the amount of recovery that follows depend upon the amount and duration of the use of that particular medication. A client receiving more than one ototoxic medication is even more vulnerable to developing a sensorineural hearing loss or aggravating an existing sensorineural hearing loss.

With high peak plasma concentrations, the aminoglycosides diffuse into the perilymph where their half-lives are five to six times longer than those in plasma. Diffusion out of the perilymph is enhanced when a low trough level occurs. Ototoxicity occurs because of hair cell destruction. They usually affect the sensory cells in the basal turn of the cochlea, first producing a high-frequency sensorineural hearing loss that can progress to involve the middle and lower frequencies. It is thought that aminoglycosides cause an imbalance in the ionic equilibrium of the inner ear by interfering with active transport systems. Damage can occur following a single administration of these drugs or after repeated doses. Clients who receive these medications must be monitored with peak and trough serum concentrations assessed for therapeutic and safe levels. The risk of ototoxicity is increased when more than one ototoxic medication is given.

Diuretics alter the electrolyte composition of the endolymph of the inner ear. Chemotherapeutic medications produce

permanent hearing loss. Cisplatin is a common cancer treatment and, unfortunately, it is cochleotoxic. The toxicity of cisplatin is synergistic with gentamicin, and high doses of cisplatin have been reported to cause total deafness. The other medications listed here produce transient hearing loss or tinnitus and some produce permanent hearing loss.

Ototoxic medications include these groups of medications.

Aminoglycoside antibiotics	Gentamicin, kanamycin, neomycin, streptomycin, tobramycin, amikacin
Antibiotics	Vancomycin, erythromycin, polymyxin B, polymyxin E, minocycline, chloramphenicol, Biaxin, Zithromax
Diuretics (loop)	Furosemide (Lasix), bumetanide (Bumex), ethacrynic acid (Edecrin)
Diuretics (osmotic)	Mannitol, acetazolamide
Analgesics/antipyretics/ NSAIDs and antimalarial drugs	Salicylates (aspirin compounds) Advil, Aleve, Anaprox, Clinoril, Feldene, Indocin, Lodine, Motrin, Nalfon, Naprosyn, Nuprin, Toradol, Voltaren, quinine, chloroquine
Antineoplastic drugs	Cisplatin, nitrogen mustard, vincristine, bleomycin
Miscellaneous	Alcohol, atropine, barbiturates, caffeine, ergot, gold, lidocaine, nicotine

behind the eardrum, causing dampening of the sound being conducted to the inner ear. In addition, drainage, perforation, or scarring of the tympanic membrane can result in a conductive hearing loss. Otitis media and other infectious ear processes are discussed later in the chapter under Otalgia.

Otosclerosis

Otosclerosis is a genetic disorder in which repeated resorption and redeposition of abnormal bone gradually leads to fixation of the footplate of the stapes in the oval window (Figure 66-2, *A*). The immobility of the footplate prevents transmission of sound vibration into the inner ear, leading to conductive hearing loss. This disorder occurs twice as often in women and is 10 times more prevalent in whites. The disorder is autosomally dominant with variable penetrance and therefore can be transmitted to offspring if only one parent has the disorder.

Tympanosclerosis

Tympanosclerosis is the result of repeated infection and trauma to the tympanic membrane. It consists of a deposit of collagen and calcium within the middle ear that can harden around the ossicles, causing a conductive hearing loss. Tympanosclerotic deposits can also be found mounded in the middle ear or as plaque on the tympanic membrane.

Trauma to the Tympanic Membrane

The tympanic membrane can be damaged by trauma. Increased pressure from a hand slap, falling in water, sports injuries, cleaning the ear with a sharp instrument, and industrial accidents involving welding sparks can rupture the thin membrane. Trauma to the tympanic membrane from a blast or blunt injury can involve the middle ear, causing a fracture or dislocation of the ossicles and tearing of the tympanic membrane. When the tympanic membrane is perforated, infection is a concern.

Sensorineural Hearing Loss

Presbycusis

Presbycusis is a progressive hearing loss found predominantly in older people. This degenerative process involves changes in the labyrinthine structures over time. The client initially experiences a decrease in high-frequency sound. At times, *tinnitus,* or the perception of noise in the ear, accompanies this decline in hearing.

Sudden Hearing Loss

Sudden (idiopathic) hearing loss (SHL) is a fairly common condition in which the client loses hearing in an ear within minutes or hours. This condition is almost exclusively unilateral. Prompt early intervention with oral corticosteroids has been shown to at least partially restore the lost hearing in many clients with sudden hearing loss.

Sensorineural hearing loss of abrupt onset can sometimes occur from discrete causes. Some of these specific causes are (1) rapid infectious processes, such as meningitis or mumps; (2) ototoxic agents; (3) trauma; (4) metabolic disturbances; and (5) immunologic disorders. In most cases of SHL, however, no specific cause is found.

Hearing Loss

Congenital episodes of sensorineural hearing loss are not uncommon. These losses can be severe and present at birth or can develop during childhood or early adulthood and gradually worsen with time. Congenital hearing loss often results in total deafness. It can occur either in a genetic pattern within families or spontaneously. Both autosomal-recessive and autosomal-dominant methods of transmission have been documented. In milder cases of congenital hearing loss, the individual may not be aware of a loss until hearing is screened for work or school. In families with a history of congenital hearing loss, infant screening is essential to allow early detection of the problem and rehabilitation of congenitally deaf infants.

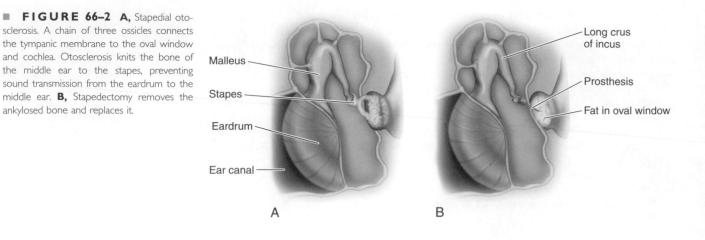

■ **FIGURE 66–2 A,** Stapedial otosclerosis. A chain of three ossicles connects the tympanic membrane to the oval window and cochlea. Otosclerosis knits the bone of the middle ear to the stapes, preventing sound transmission from the eardrum to the middle ear. **B,** Stapedectomy removes the ankylosed bone and replaces it.

Malleus

Stapes

Eardrum

Ear canal

Long crus of incus

Prosthesis

Fat in oval window

A

B

Noise-Induced Hearing Loss

Noise-induced hearing loss is a specific type of sensorineural hearing loss that most often occurs over time from repeated acoustic trauma from loud noise. The major causes are industrial noise, the use of firearms, and listening to loud music. Traumatic injury associated with a sudden loud noise, such as a blast, can also result in noise-induced hearing loss.

Benign and Malignant Tumors

Both benign and malignant tumors of the temporal bone can involve the inner ear and lead to sensorineural hearing loss. The most common benign tumor is an acoustic neuroma or schwannoma of the eighth cranial nerve. The tumor usually develops in the internal auditory canal, the bony channel through which the vestibular nerve passes as it leaves the inner ear. The tumor presses on the nerve, which then sends false signals to the brain. If the vestibular portion of the nerve is compressed, the client is unable to interpret stimuli about position and movement. If the cochlear branch is compressed, the client experiences tinnitus. The first clinical manifestation is often partial or complete sensorineural hearing loss followed by tinnitus. The client may also report dizziness.

Other tumors in the cerebellopontine angle likewise involve the seventh and eighth cranial nerves as they enter the internal acoustic meatus. Malignant tumors invade the entire inner ear, usually spreading from the middle ear and mastoid system.

Ménière's Disease

Ménière's disease is a disorder that affects both vestibular and auditory function. It is caused by excess endolymph (intracellular fluid in the membranous labyrinth of the inner ear) in the vestibular and semicircular canals. Hearing loss is fluctuant and usually subtle and reversible in the early stages. Later the hearing loss becomes permanent. Although Ménière's disease is associated with sensorineural hearing loss, the most prominent clinical manifestation is *vertigo* (feeling that the surroundings or one's own body is revolving). Therefore it is fully discussed in the section Balance Disorders.

Central Auditory Dysfunction

Central auditory dysfunction is a phenomenon whereby the central nervous system (CNS) cannot interpret normal auditory signals. Central auditory dysfunction, also known as *central deafness,* is a rare form of sensorineural hearing loss. Diseases that alter the CNS, such as strokes and tumors, can cause central deafness.

Mixed Hearing Loss

Some causes of hearing impairment can result in both sensorineural and conductive hearing losses. These types of losses are referred to as *mixed hearing loss.* Clients with mixed hearing loss present with clinical manifestations associated with both sensorineural and conductive hearing losses.

Pathophysiology

Conductive hearing loss is the result of interference of sound transmission into and through the external ear and middle ear. The inner ear is not affected in a pure conductive loss; therefore sound transmission from the inner ear to the brain is normal. Normal movement of sound vibrations through the ear canal, tympanic membrane, or ossicles is impeded because of the nature of the disease process involved in the conductive loss. Sound is perceived as faint or distant, but it remains relatively clear. Most conductive hearing losses are correctable by medical or surgical treatment.

Sensorineural hearing loss, however, results from disease or trauma to the organ of Corti or auditory nerve pathways of the inner ear leading to the brain stem. Normal reception and transmission of sound waves are disrupted. Sound is distorted and faint. Sensorineural hearing losses are usually permanent and are generally not correctable by medical or surgical treatment.

Clinical Manifestations

Most hearing loss is gradual and goes unnoticed by the client until several incidents of communication problems have occurred. Significant others and co-workers are usually aware of the client's hearing problem long before the client realizes or admits to the problem. Box 66-1 lists the manifestations of hearing loss.

The hearing impaired or "hard-of-hearing" client may repeat the information, even incorrectly, or may ask for clarification. Clients with a hearing loss can also experience distorted or abnormal sounds. Sometimes a sound is heard at different pitches for each ear; this is called *diplacusis.* A sound may cause a rapid increase in loudness; this is called *recruitment.* These abnormal sounds can cause discomfort.

BOX 66-1   Manifestations of Hearing Loss

- Failure to respond to oral communication
- Frequently asking others to repeat statements
- Inappropriate response to oral communication
- Failing to respond when not looking in the direction of the sound
- Excessively loud speech
- Abnormal awareness of sounds
- Strained facial expressions
- Tilting of head when listening
- Faulty speech articulation
- Listening to radio and television at increased volume
- Avoiding crowds and better understanding of speech when in small groups

The onset of a conductive hearing loss can be sudden or progressive. In cases of fluid in the middle ear, hearing loss is often bilateral but is usually restored with medical or surgical treatment. In other conductive processes, such as otosclerosis, clinical manifestations consist of slow progressive hearing loss with changes noted even in adolescence. Hearing loss is usually bilateral but may be asymmetrical. Other manifestations are mild tinnitus, recurrent vertigo, and postural imbalance. It is common for the client to speak in a soft voice.

If damage to the tympanic membrane is suspected, such as perforation, examination of the client may reveal a conductive hearing loss and serous drainage in the ear canal. The hearing loss found with a total perforation of the eardrum is approximately 35 dB (one third of the hearing range). With small perforations, no loss may be present. If a perforation is present, damage to the ossicles should be suspected. Diagnostic findings of conductive hearing loss include greater bone conduction than air conduction on the Rinne test. If hearing loss is greater in one ear, Weber's test shows lateralization to the more affected ear. Pure-tone audiometry confirms hearing loss. *Speech discrimination* (understanding of words) is usually maintained.

Noise-induced hearing loss is characterized by a greater loss in the higher frequencies. Sudden or fluctuating hearing losses are recognized as separate disorders from routine sensorineural hearing loss. Although fluctuating losses usually suggest syphilis or Ménière's disease, sudden sensorineural hearing losses are believed to be viral in origin. Recognition of these patterns is important because medical treatment of such disorders can result in significant improvements in hearing. A characteristic of a severe hearing loss is loss of discrimination. To some clients, a hearing loss feels like a blockage or fullness in the ear or an inability to distinguish the direction of sounds.

Tinnitus accompanies most sensorineural hearing losses and is annoying. *Tinnitus* literally means "ringing" but can actually sound like roaring, the chirping of crickets, or occasionally music. Tinnitus is not a disease but a distressing manifestation, and it is sometimes a warning sign of hearing loss or other, more serious problems. Ear noise that cannot be heard by an observer is classified as *subjective tinnitus,* which is the most common kind. Any ear noise that can be heard by someone other than the client is called *objective tinnitus.* In some clients the tinnitus becomes the problem, and the underlying cause may be forgotten.

The major nursing responsibility in a client with tinnitus is to perform a thorough history and assessment of the onset, frequency, constancy, and level of intensity of the tinnitus. Unilateral tinnitus merits a complete neuro-otologic evaluation with the goal of ruling out the possibility of a tumor, most likely an acoustic neuroma. The nurse must keep in mind that tinnitus is a manifestation of an underlying pathologic process that warrants further referral.

Table 66-1 presents the clinical manifestations of conductive and sensorineural hearing losses. Diagnostic measures include (1) testing for hearing of pure tones on audiometry, (2) speech reception and discrimination, (3) tympanometry, and sometimes (4) brain stem auditory evoked responses. Tones are presented using earphones (air conduction) and vibrators (bone conduction). The minimal level at which the client can hear is determined. The *speech reception threshold* is the lowest intensity at which the client can correctly repeat 50% of the words presented. The speech discrimination test is a measure of the client's ability to understand speech when it is presented at a volume that is easily heard.

OUTCOME MANAGEMENT

Medical Management

All health providers should teach clients how to prevent hearing loss and should screen for hearing loss in high-risk groups (Box 66-2). The goals for medical management of the client with hearing impairment are to (1) restore hearing, (2) assist hearing, (3) manage tinnitus, and (4) implement aural rehabilitation.

Restore Hearing

Hearing loss that results from blockage or fullness in the ear associated with an infectious process may be restored to normal with administration of antibiotics for bacterial infections. In the case of sudden hearing loss, prompt administration of oral corticosteroids is used in an attempt to lessen the progressive hearing loss or to reverse a sudden loss. Antiviral medications have been advocated for sudden sensorineural hearing loss, although they have not been shown in clinical trials to be of additional benefit. If ototoxicity is suspected, all ototoxic medications are discontinued.

TABLE 66-1 **Clinical Manifestations of Conductive and Sensorineural Hearing Losses**

	Conductive Hearing Loss	Sensorineural Hearing Loss
Voice quality	Soft voice	Loud voice
Effect of environmental noise on hearing	Hearing improved	Hearing made worse
Speech discrimination	Good	Poor
Ability to hear on telephone	Good	Poor
Lateralization on Weber's test	To diseased ear	To normal ear
Result of Rinne test	Negative, AC < BC	Positive, AC > BC

AC, Air conduction; BC, bone conduction.

BOX 66-2 Hearing Impairment: Prevention and Screening

Identification of clients at risk for hearing loss and adequate protection of the ears are important to maintain normal function.

PRIMARY PREVENTION

- Avoid ototoxic drugs.
- Recognize and treat infectious diseases such as meningitis, mumps, and measles.
- Wear protective headgear or helmets when participating in sports.
- Avoid insertion of hard instruments or objects into the ear canal.
- Wear earplugs and avoid prolonged exposure to noise levels in excess of 80 decibels (dB).

SECONDARY PREVENTION

- Perform hearing screenings in children and adults 65 years and older.
- Monitor blood levels of medications with ototoxic side effects, observing for vertigo, lessened hearing acuity, and tinnitus.

TERTIARY PREVENTION

- Encourage hearing-impaired clients to attend rehabilitation programs.
- Teach the proper use and care of hearing aids.
- Encourage family to continue to communicate with the hearing impaired.

Assist Hearing

Unfortunately, most hearing losses are permanent, and hearing cannot be restored. The use of hearing aids and assistive listening devices can greatly improve the client's ability to communicate and interact with others. Hearing aids amplify sound in a controlled manner. They are used by both *hearing-impaired* clients (those with slight or moderate hearing loss) and *deaf* clients (those with severe or profound hearing loss). Hearing aids make sound louder but do not improve the quality of sound. Therefore clients with decreased discrimination benefit less from a hearing aid. The hearing aid amplifies all background noises, such as hospital machinery, background conversation in restaurants, footsteps, and department store noises, as well as speech. These noises may mask conversation or confuse the hearing-impaired client, especially older adults.

A client should undergo a trial period before purchasing a hearing aid to see whether he or she can adapt to its use. In fact, in most states, such a trial period is mandatory. Bilateral (binaural) aids may be desirable. Hearing aids can be worn in the following locations: in the ear, in the ear canal, behind the ear (postauricular), in eyeglasses, and in the middle of the chest (body-worn aid).

Regardless of type, the hearing aid consists of four parts. The microphone receives sound waves from the air and changes sounds into electrical signals. The amplifier increases the strength of electrical signals. The receiver (loudspeaker) changes the electrical signals into sound waves, and the battery provides the electrical energy needed to operate the hearing aid. On all types of hearing aids except the body-worn type, all four components are housed in one small case. The louder sounds are then directed into the ear through a custom-molded earpiece.

The evolution in hearing aid design has led to smaller and more effective aids. Small hearing aids are available that fit into the ear canal. The latest advancements in hearing aids are digital processing and directional microphones, which enhance the voice of a speaker in front of the client and suppress background noise. Programmable hearing aids allow the selection of various amplification patterns by the user and may have some added benefit for clients. Hearing aid technology continues to advance in improving the person's quality of life.

Assistive listening devices help the hearing-impaired client hear the television or radio as well as use the telephone. Stationary devices called *teletypewriters* and a portable instrument called a *telecommunication device for the deaf* (TDD) are used for telephone communication by the profoundly deaf. A flashing light signals the presence of a dial tone, a busy signal, or a ring. When another teletypewriter or TDD is reached, messages are typed and displayed on a screen or printed. Other devices, such as flashing lights that alert a deaf person to a ringing doorbell, alarm clock, or smoke alarm, are available. Hearing dogs are trained to be sensitive to certain noises, such as the telephone, doorbells, and crying children. On hearing the sound, a hearing dog moves back and forth between the client and the sound to alert the client.

Manage Tinnitus

Tinnitus can be a distressing disorder associated with sensorineural hearing loss. Many approaches have been tried to alleviate this problem, including biofeedback, electrostimulation, hypnosis, medication, hearing aids, and tinnitus maskers. They have all met with minimal success. Tinnitus maskers appear similar to hearing aids except that they generate noise. The tinnitus masker is of benefit only while it is being used. Every approach for relief from tinnitus is only moderately successful, at best. Clients should be counseled to avoid unproved treatments for tinnitus. The nurse and the client's family must be alert to manifestations of depression if the tinnitus is chronic. The quality of the spouse's support of the client with tinnitus has been shown to be strongly correlated with role function. In addition, the nurse should be alert to spousal interaction and should facilitate problem-solving as needed.

Implement Aural Rehabilitation

Aural rehabilitation may improve communication if (1) hearing loss is irreversible or is not amenable to surgical intervention or (2) the client elects not to have surgery. The purpose of aural rehabilitation is to maximize the hearing-impaired client's communication skills.

Hearing is one of our primary modes of communication. Rehabilitation is directed toward teaching the client to use the other senses more effectively, those of vision, touch, and vibration, and to maximize the use of any remaining hearing ability. The outcome of rehabilitation is affected by all demographic variables and the severity of impairment. As with other forms of rehabilitation, success depends partly on the client's level of motivation.

Speech reading, the current term used for lip reading, is an important means of communication. Speech reading is the process of understanding vocal communication by the integration of lip movements with facial expressions, gestures, environmental clues, and conversation contexts. Speech reading is difficult without auditory cues for several reasons. Many movements for speech are rapid, many sounds are similar (*b, m, p*), and the production of certain sounds in any language is not visible. The hearing-impaired client must guess at a high percentage of words. Knowledge of this fact alone helps the nurse be more understanding of the client who is using this communication approach.

Because of reduced auditory feedback (the inability of hearing-impaired clients to monitor their own speech), the clearness, pitch quality, or rate of the client's speech may deteriorate. These changes may alter the efficiency of communication and reduce the intelligibility of speech. The goal of speech training is to conserve, develop, or prevent deterioration of speech skills.

Last, but still important, is sign language. Sign language allows communication by hand signals that represent different letters of the alphabet, words, and phrases.

Nursing Management of the Medical Client

Assessment. The client's ability to communicate may be informally assessed during the history. The nurse should assess the client's ability to follow conversation. During the interview, the nurse should look for answers to the following questions:

1. Does the client admit to having a hearing loss and difficulty communicating, or does the client blame other people for not speaking clearly?
2. In what settings does the client have more problems with hearing or communicating?
3. Are family members, co-workers, and friends aware of the hearing problem? Are they supportive of the client, making communication easier and including the client in conversation? Do others feel frustrated or angry when the client cannot hear correctly or

does not respond? Does the client feel left out or embarrassed?
4. Does the client try to understand spoken words? Or does the client withdraw or refuse to participate, letting others do the talking?
5. Does the client wear a hearing aid? Does it appear to work?

Occasionally, laboratory, radiologic, and vestibular examinations are used for assessment. In an otology office, the nurse may have the responsibility of performing the history, otologic examination, and screening audiometry. The history is often the most important part of the clinical assessment, as previously described (see Chapter 64, Box 64-4). The extent of assessment of the sensorineural hearing loss depends on the setting and the nurse's educational preparation and experience. Nurses should be able to inspect the outer ear and grossly assess auditory acuity.

Visualization of the ear canal and tympanic membrane is accomplished with the otoscope. Cerumen in the canal or on the eardrum can interfere with the examination and may need to be removed. The blind removal of ear wax with an ear syringe should be performed only if the ear is free of other abnormalities, such as an infection or perforation of the eardrum.

Impacted accumulations of ear wax may be softened and loosened for removal by alternating instillations of glycerin and hydrogen peroxide eardrops. The eardrops are warmed to body temperature and used daily as directed for 1 to 2 weeks. The ear is then irrigated gently with warm water for removal of the softened wax or cleaned under magnification with a cerumen spoon. Wax on the tympanic membrane should be removed by an otolaryngologist or an advanced-practice nurse in otorhinolaryngology.

Diagnosis, Outcomes, Interventions

Diagnosis: Impaired Verbal Communication. Clients who have lost their ability to hear are best described with the nursing diagnosis *Impaired Verbal Communication related to effects of hearing loss.*

Outcomes. The client will develop effective methods to communicate needs and will be included in conversation.

Interventions. When normal conversation is impossible, writing may be used successfully by clients who have good comprehension of English (or their primary language). Writing may cause frustration when the client's primary language is American Sign Language because it is grammatically different from standard English. Visual aids, such as pictures, diagrams, and models, may also improve the nurse's ability to explain medical terminology or procedures. An expert interpreter should be used when other attempts to communicate have failed or when speed and accuracy are critical. The National Registry of Interpreters for the Deaf (NRID) has local chapters and offers certification for qualified individuals. Box 66-3 lists common nursing interventions to improve communication with hearing-impaired clients. They can apply to all clients, regardless of the type or severity of hearing loss.

Many hearing-impaired clients live in the community. Nurses may see these clients for their hearing problems or for many other problems. The Bridge to Home Health Care feature at right addresses approaches to home care of hearing-impaired clients.

Diagnosis: Ineffective Coping. The individual with a loss of hearing goes through the same stages of grieving as others experiencing a loss. Rehabilitation cannot begin until some acceptance of the hearing loss has taken place, leading to the nursing diagnosis *Ineffective Coping related to recent loss of hearing*.

BOX 66-3   Common Nursing Interventions for Hearing-Impaired Clients

- Get the client's attention by raising your arm or hand.
- Stand with a light on your face; this helps the client to speech-read.
- Talk directly to the client while facing him or her.
- Speak clearly, but do not overaccentuate words.
- Speak in a normal tone; do not shout. Shouting overuses normal speaking movements and so may cause distortion and may be too loud for the client with sensorineural damage. If the client has conductive loss only, it is sometimes helpful to make the voice louder without shouting.
- If the client does not seem to understand what is said, express it differently. Some words are difficult to "see" in speech reading, such as "white" and "red."
- Move closer to the client and toward the better-hearing ear.
- Write out proper names or any statement that you are not sure was understood.
- Do not smile, chew gum, or cover the mouth when talking.
- Remember that a client's inattention may indicate tiredness or lack of understanding.
- Use phrases rather than one-word answers to convey meaning. State the major topic of the discussion first, and then give details.
- Do not show annoyance by careless facial expressions. Clients who are hard of hearing depend more on visual clues for understanding.
- Encourage the use of a hearing aid if it is available; allow the client to adjust it before speaking.
- In a group, repeat important statements, and avoid making asides to others in the group.
- Avoid the use of the intercommunication system because this may distort sound and cause poor communication.
- Do not avoid conversation with a client who has hearing loss. It has been said that to live in a silent world is much more devastating than to live in darkness, and clients with hearing loss appear to have more emotional difficulties than do those who are blind.

🏠 BRIDGE TO HOME HEALTH CARE

Living with a Severe Hearing Loss

People are often reluctant to admit that they have a hearing impairment. This reluctance results in difficulty with verbal communication, inability to follow instructions, and social isolation. To maximize communication, reduce background noise (turn off the television or radio), face the person, and speak clearly without shouting. Sometimes the only way to communicate is by writing. Develop written materials for repeated use. Include introduction materials (e.g., your name, your agency's name, the purpose of your visit), reportable problems, and treatment regimens.

In many cases, hearing loss is due to accumulation of cerumen. Use an otoscope to visualize the ear canal. If cerumen is present, a physician may need to remove it. If you are responsible for removing the cerumen, contact the physician to discuss a prescription for an ear irrigation solution, instill the solution, and evaluate the amount and color of drainage.

When people experience a hearing loss, they need a medical evaluation and a hearing aid evaluation. Many older adults are reluctant to wear a hearing aid for various reasons. It is a visual manifestation of an impairment, it is expensive, and it necessitates leaving home for evaluation, fitting, and follow-up appointments. If a client's reluctance is due to cosmetic reasons, show pictures of hearing aids and discuss individuals who wear hearing aids, such as former President George Bush. Newer hearing aids are available that are smaller, less noticeable, and more discreet.

If cost is a problem, consider a referral to a social worker to identify local resources. Currently Medicare pays for the cost of a hearing evaluation and little for the hearing aid; Medicaid usually pays for the hearing aid. Consider other financial resources, such as the American Association of Retired People and local hearing aid vendors. When leaving home is a problem, check whether a vendor will make a home visit. If this is not possible, suggest that the client use a head-set amplifier that can be purchased from a local electronics store.

Teaching is an important nursing intervention related to hearing impairment. It involves cleaning the devices and changing the batteries. Also, evaluate the client's ability to use the telephone and answer the door. Local telephone companies can equip the telephone with an adjustable volume control, hearing aid adapters, loud ringing signals, and a telecommunication device for the deaf (TDD). A TDD allows the hearing-impaired individual to communicate by typing information into a specially designed device. To receive information, the receiver must have a specific TDD telephone number. Teach the client with a TDD about TDD telephone numbers for an emergency response, and provide information about the home health agency and community resources.

It is important to involve informal caregivers, significant others, and family members in the management of a hearing impairment. Teach these people to maximize communication with a variety of techniques and adaptive equipment.

Outcomes. The client will discuss or will demonstrate problem-solving–based coping strategies, as evidenced by the following:

1. Taking the initiative to inform others of the hearing impairment and requesting that they assist with communication by using techniques that promote comprehension
2. Not experiencing feelings of embarrassment, frustration, or withdrawal
3. Not blaming others for failure to communicate effectively
4. Avoiding situations and environments, such as noisy areas, that impair hearing

Interventions. Work with the client and family on methods to enhance communication and thereby enhance coping. Encourage the client to role-play how he or she might tell people about the hearing impairment and indicate what techniques should be used to help hearing. Self-help groups, such as Self-help for Hard of Hearing People (SHHH), located in Bethesda, Maryland, can assist with resources, information, and support for clients and their families.

Diagnosis: Impaired Social Interaction. Clients with hearing losses can experience fears of inadequacy, feelings of inferiority, depression, and varying degrees of stress and isolation. The nursing diagnosis *Impaired Social Interaction related to perceived inability to interact with others secondary to hearing loss* can be used to guide interventions.

Outcomes. The client will exhibit a willingness to be involved in social situations as evidenced by (1) attempting to become a part of social events, (2) conversing with others, (3) indicating lessened feelings of inadequacy, and (4) responding appropriately to questions asked (not fabricating answers to cover hearing loss).

Interventions. The American Speech-Language Hearing Association (ASHA) urges that all clients with hearing impairments *not* be grouped into one category. Each client is unique and has an individual hearing problem. The nurse functions as a role model in accepting the client as an individual and demonstrating effective communication techniques.

Work with the client to enhance coping, encourage continued social involvement, and advocate the use of various organizations to their fullest extent. Many agencies and associations exist for the hearing-impaired client. Services are offered by audiology clinics and sponsored by universities, hospitals, community programs, state or local departments of health, the Department of Veterans Affairs (VA), and national organizations.

Diagnosis: Deficient Knowledge of Managing Hearing Loss. Clients with new hearing aids need information about their care and proper use. Therefore *Deficient Knowledge of managing hearing loss related to lack of previous exposure to a hearing aid* is an important nursing diagnosis.

Outcomes. The client will have greater knowledge about the hearing aid as evidenced by proper use and care of the aid.

Interventions. The hearing aid user should know how to care for the aid and what to do if the device does not work. Gain a basic knowledge of the hearing aid to help with insertion for clients who are ill. Encourage the client to use the hearing aid and to store it safely when not using it. Turn the device off before removal to prevent squealing feedback. The maintenance of a hearing aid is becoming less of a problem today. Usually the aid is returned to the dealer for factory repair while the client uses a "loaner" hearing aid. Unlicensed assistive personnel often care for clients with hearing aids. Delegation of care of the hearing aid and the hearing-impaired client is shown in the Management and Delegation feature on p. 1729.

Cost has been cited as a major factor in the non-use of hearing aids. Clients needing financial assistance should be referred to the state department of vocational rehabilitation, the local Lions Club, and, in some states, Medicaid.

Evaluation. A client with a new hearing loss or disorder needs frequent evaluation to determine the severity of hearing loss, coping strategies, and ability to communicate adequately. Because many forms of hearing loss are permanent or progressive, long-term evaluation should also be performed to be certain the client is adapting positively. Also determine whether the client has questions about the equipment used for hearing rehabilitation and the need for further education.

Surgical Management

Surgery is usually not warranted for sensorineural hearing loss; however, because mixed, conductive, and sensorineural hearing loss exists, surgery may be performed to (1) restore the conductive hearing loss, (2) remove a tumor, and (3) assist hearing in profoundly deaf people.

Restore Conductive Hearing Loss

The most common cause of conductive hearing loss is serous otitis media (see later discussion). Although most commonly seen in children, this disorder can occur at any age. In cases of serous otitis media and persistent conductive hearing loss that do not resolve after 2 to 3 months of medical management, an incision into the tympanic membrane and evacuation of fluid can be performed with the client sedated using local or general anesthesia. This procedure, known as *myringotomy*, will restore hearing. It is discussed later in this chapter.

Hearing Aids

Caring for hearing aids and helping clients with maintenance of these devices may be delegated to unlicensed assistive personnel. Clients with new hearing aids need individualized teaching provided by you, the registered nurse. You are to evaluate the client's understanding of the instruction. Before delegating hearing aid care, consider the following issues:

The client's learning needs. Is this a new hearing aid? Does the client have a new hearing loss disorder? If so, you should instruct the client to care for these devices and provide consistent teaching.

The competency level of the unlicensed assistive personnel who will potentially perform hearing aid care. Unlicensed assistive personnel may not provide the initial instruction but may reinforce the instructions you have provided.

Instruct unlicensed assistive personnel caring for the client with a hearing aid to achieve the following:

- Encourage the use of hearing aids and independent care by clients without cognitive impairment.
- Provide safe storage of the hearing aids when not in use (in the client's personal case or another small storage device). If the client is hospitalized, ensure that the case is labeled with the client's name and location.
- Turn the device off when it is not in use. If the aid is to be off for a prolonged duration (such as during the night or sleeping hours), open the battery compartment to avoid additional drainage of battery power.
- Cleanse the ear mold with mild soap and water each day or as needed.
- Completely dry the ear mold before reconnecting it to the hearing aid.
- Help the client insert the ear mold into the ear. If the hearing aid makes a whistling noise, the device is not inserted properly into the ear. At this point, it may be necessary for you to assess more completely placement in the ear canal.
- Allow the client to adjust the volume before speaking.
- Speak clearly in a normal tone to the client. Do not shout.
- Turn off the device before removing it to prevent squealing "feedback."

If the hearing aid fails to work:

- Check the on-off switch.
- Inspect the ear mold for cleanliness.
- Examine the battery for correct insertion.
- Examine the cord plug for correct insertion.
- Examine the cord for breaks.
- Replace the battery, cord, or both, if necessary. The life of batteries varies according to the amount of use and power requirements of the aid. Batteries last 2 to 14 days.

Findings that are immediately reportable to you are (1) difficulty with placement in the ear, (2) redness or drainage in the ear, (3) mechanical failure of the device, and (4) other issues of concern to the client.

Another type of conductive hearing loss that can be treated medically or corrected surgically results from otosclerosis. Because speech discrimination is usually unimpaired, simple amplification of sound is quite effective. People who are at high risk of otosclerosis or who are not candidates for surgery can be given medications in an attempt to reduce the severity of the bony fusion. The clinical efficacy of medical therapy remains unsubstantiated.

Stapedectomy

Surgical intervention for otosclerosis has been very successful. *Stapedectomy* is a surgical procedure whereby the damaged stapes is removed and replaced with a stainless-steel, polytetrafluoroethylene (Teflon), or plastic prosthesis (see Figure 66-2, *B*). The oval window is grafted with absorbable gelatin sponge (Gelfoam) or tissue grafts. Stapedectomy was once a common middle ear procedure; however, the pool of clients with otosclerosis is dwindling, and today stapedectomy is performed less often.

The client must be free of otitis externa and otitis media before surgery. To reduce the risk of bleeding, the client should use no aspirin or products with aspirin for 1 week before surgery. Preoperative and postoperative audiograms and tympanograms are performed to test hearing acuity levels.

After surgery the client is often instructed to lie on the nonoperative ear with the head of the bed elevated. This position helps reduce edema and prevent dislodgment of the prosthesis. Antibiotics are prescribed. The packing in the ear canal should not be disturbed. On discharge from the hospital, the client is told to report the acute onset of vertigo. To reduce the risk of development of a perilymph fistula (rupture of the oval window, which permits leakage of perilymph fluid), the client should avoid excessive exercise, straining, and activities that might lead to head trauma. If the client needs to blow the nose, it should be done gently, one nostril at a time. The client should sneeze with the mouth open. No airplane travel is allowed for 1 month.

Hearing aids may still be required after stapedectomy, and the client's hearing will need to be reevaluated. Complications of the operation include granuloma formation and perilymph fistula. Either complication may result in profound deafness and persistent vertigo. Hearing loss may also develop after surgery from middle ear adhesions or shifting of the prosthesis.

Tumor Excision

Surgery and gamma knife radiotherapy are current treatments of acoustic neuroma. Current microsurgical techniques often allow preservation of hearing and usually enable resection of the tumor without injury to the facial nerve. In older clients, especially those with total deafness in the affected ear, a more conservative, non-surgical approach is sometimes taken because acoustic neuroma is benign and very slow growing.

Assist Hearing in Profound Deafness

Use of implantable hearing devices (IHDs) may be appropriate in certain clients. There are three types of IHDs: cochlear implants, temporal bone stimulators, and middle ear implants.

Cochlear Implants. Cochlear implants provide auditory sensation to clients with severe to profound sensorineural hearing loss who cannot benefit from a hearing aid (Figure 66-3). The cochlear implant contains a small computer that changes the spoken word to electrical impulses. The impulses are transmitted across the skin to an implanted coil that carries the impulse to the hearing nerve endings in the cochlea by means of an electrode introduced through the round window. The most effective cochlear implants use multiple-frequency channels. In multichannel cochlear implants, up to 22 electrodes are inserted along the cochlear partition. The surgery for insertion of a cochlear implant is similar to mastoid surgery. The success of a cochlear implant varies widely, ranging from minimal improvement in auditory awareness to the ability to understand speech on the telephone. Preoperative vestibular testing is highly recommended for all clients in whom a cochlear implant is being considered.

Temporal Bone Stimulators (BAHA, Bone-Anchored Hearing Aid). In some cases of hearing loss, sound can be transmitted by applying stimulation directly to the temporal bone, thereby transmitting sound through the skull to the inner ear. For clients with a conductive hearing loss, a device is available in which the receiver is implanted under the skin into the skull. The external device transmits the sound through the skin. This device is worn above the ear rather than in the ear canal.

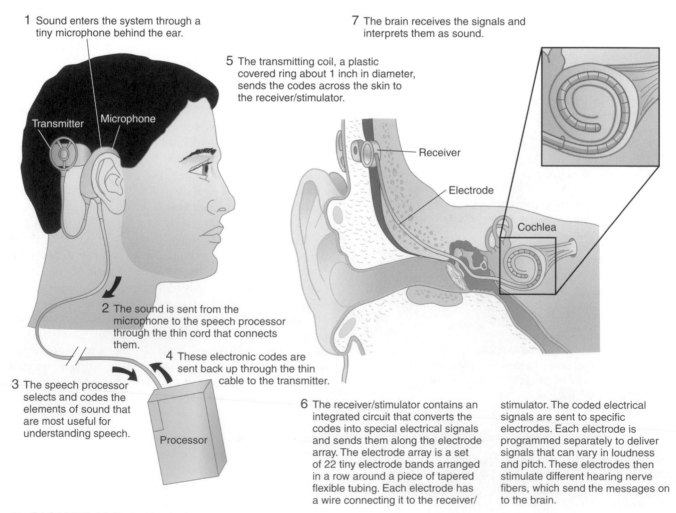

1 Sound enters the system through a tiny microphone behind the ear.

Transmitter   Microphone

2 The sound is sent from the microphone to the speech processor through the thin cord that connects them.

3 The speech processor selects and codes the elements of sound that are most useful for understanding speech.

Processor

4 These electronic codes are sent back up through the thin cable to the transmitter.

5 The transmitting coil, a plastic covered ring about 1 inch in diameter, sends the codes across the skin to the receiver/stimulator.

7 The brain receives the signals and interprets them as sound.

Receiver

Electrode

Cochlea

6 The receiver/stimulator contains an integrated circuit that converts the codes into special electrical signals and sends them along the electrode array. The electrode array is a set of 22 tiny electrode bands arranged in a row around a piece of tapered flexible tubing. Each electrode has a wire connecting it to the receiver/ stimulator. The coded electrical signals are sent to specific electrodes. Each electrode is programmed separately to deliver signals that can vary in loudness and pitch. These electrodes then stimulate different hearing nerve fibers, which send the messages on to the brain.

FIGURE 66–3 Cochlear implant to restore hearing.

Because some conductive hearing losses cannot be surgically repaired, the temporal bone stimulator may provide an alternative rehabilitative method to conventional hearing aids. It is not widely used at present.

Middle Ear Implants (Semi-Implantable Hearing Device).
A variety of IHD devices are being evaluated for sound amplification and quality for individuals with moderate to moderately severe sensorineural hearing loss. However, many challenges have to be met before a workable device is available. This method of hearing aid technology is still in the research stage.

OTALGIA

Otalgia is defined as pain in the ear, or earache. Otalgia can be primary in origin (i.e., coming from a disorder in the ear), infectious, or referred (i.e., coming from a disorder outside the ear). Otalgia from ear pain can be the result of infection in the external or middle ear or of trauma to the ear and head. Referred otalgia can be caused by disorders in the temporomandibular joint (TMJ), cranial nerves, face, scalp, pharynx, tonsils, thyroid, trachea, teeth, or cervical muscles.

Etiology and Risk Factors

Otalgia can be related to infectious processes in the external ear and middle ear. Bacterial contaminants can enter the ear through insertion of unclean articles, such as fingers or toys. Insertion of any sharp object into the ear canal can traumatize the skin and provide an open medium for infection. Instillation of contaminated solutions into the ear or swimming in polluted water raises the risk for development of ear infection and inflammation. Clients with recent upper respiratory tract infections, eustachian tube dysfunction, and allergies are also at increased risk for ear infections.

Infectious and neoplastic processes of the pharynx can also cause referred otalgia. It is not uncommon for clients with acute tonsillitis to complain of significant ear pain, even though the ears may be normal on examination. Otalgia following tonsillectomy is universal and is not a manifestation of infection. In clients with unilateral otalgia and a history of smoking, consideration must be given to a neoplastic process of the lateral pharynx, especially if concurrent manifestations, such as hoarseness or dysphagia, are present. Examination of the lower pharynx by means of a fiberoptic endoscope is necessary in the smoker with persistent hoarseness, and referral to an otolaryngologist is indicated.

Trauma to the head, temporal bone, and ear can also result in ear pain. Engaging in contact sports without protective headgear can result in severe trauma to the head, injuring the hearing apparatus. A blow to the ear by an object such as a ball or hand can cause local or diffuse pain in the area. Noise trauma from a blast or loud noise may create a ringing sensation that is perceived as painful and uncomfortable. Nerve damage may be accompanied by intolerance to even soft sounds, resulting in severe pain. Exposure to extremely hot or cold temperatures can lead to burns or severe frostbite, respectively, of the external ear.

Blockage of the eustachian tube and otalgia can be the result of enlarged adenoid tissue and tonsils in children, middle ear infections often associated with upper respiratory tract infections, and *barotrauma* (pressure injury to the middle ear). Acute blockage from altitude changes caused by flying or underwater diving will cause middle ear problems. Hyperbaric oxygen treatments can also cause barotrauma. Hyperbaric oxygen treatment is common for carbon monoxide poisoning as well as other disorders. The incidence of barotrauma is increased when an upper respiratory tract infection is present. *Aerotitis media* is a form of serous otitis media in which fluid or air is trapped in the middle ear during descent in an airplane. Any long-term blockage of the eustachian tube leads to serous otitis media and a hearing loss.

Mouth and gum pain, TMJ pain, cervical muscle tenderness, and pain from dental work can cause referred pain to the ear. TMJ arthralgia may result from teeth grinding, gum chewing, excessive talking, or biting down on hard objects. The resultant inflammation to this joint can be perceived by the client as an earache. Similarly, stress on the neck muscles can be referred to the ear.

External Ear Trauma

Auricular trauma is common because ears are prominent and unprotected. The pinna is subject to lacerations, blunt injury, abrasions, burns, and frostbite. A special concern with ear trauma is that a hematoma can quickly develop between the skin and cartilage (called *perichondrial hematoma*). The hematoma exerts pressure on the cartilage, impairing its healing. Such hematomas are common after blunt injuries such as occur in wrestling, fighting, or boxing and are responsible for so-called "cauliflower ear."

People can often avoid ear trauma by wearing headgear for contact sports, wide-brimmed hats in the summer, and earmuffs or hats in the winter; heavy pierced earrings should not be worn because they can lacerate the lobule.

Foreign Bodies

Surprisingly a wide array of foreign bodies fit into the ear canal. The most common foreign body found in the adult ear is either a piece of cotton or, most annoying, an insect.

Ear pain from obstruction usually results from the buildup of matter in the ear canal, which leads to pressure and pain. Clients may also report decreased hearing, a sense of fullness, a throbbing sensation, and itching. The onset, duration, frequency, and intensity of manifestations should be noted.

Eustachian Tube Disorders

Because the eustachian tube connects the middle ear to the nasopharynx, pharyngeal disorders also cause eustachian tube dysfunction and thus secondary middle ear problems. For example, in children a common disorder is blockage of the eustachian tube by enlarged adenoid tissue. In adults swelling of the mucosa in the eustachian tube during an upper respiratory tract infection can lead to serous otitis media (see later discussion). For persistent unilateral blocked eustachian tube, a malignant tumor must be ruled out as the cause.

Ear Infections

Otitis Externa. The most common problems found in the external ear are infections, primarily bacterial or fungal. The most frequent infection, called *external otitis,* involves the external ear canal. Infection begins when the protective waxy coating has been damaged by dryness, moisture, or treatment. Infection can lead to edema, which can occlude the canal. External otitis occurs more frequently in the summer than in the winter. The most common form of external otitis is also called *swimmer's ear,* because it is prevalent in clients in whom water remains in the ear canal after swimming. In addition, opportunistic fungal infections are common. When a debilitating systemic disease such as diabetes is present, the external otitis can spread aggressively through cartilage and bone and is then named *malignant external otitis; Pseudomonas aeruginosa* is the usual offending pathogen.

Occasionally infection involves only the cartilage of the pinna (chondritis), with resultant necrosis of the cartilage and loss of the distinctive shape of the pinna if the infection is not treated quickly. Frostbite of the pinna has findings similar to those of infection. Another form of infection is seen as an ear canal furuncle or abscess.

Tympanic Membrane Infection. Infections of the external ear canal can involve the surface of the tympanic membrane. A specific infection of the tympanic membrane is *bullous myringitis.* This inflammatory disease forms blisters or bullae between the layers of the eardrum, which are extremely painful. It is usually caused by the bacterium *Mycoplasma pneumoniae.* Holes or perforations of the tympanic membrane can be caused by infection and also can be accompanied by drainage.

Tympanic membrane disorders can lead to perforation of the membrane. A perforation may be acute, as seen in trauma and acute infection, or chronic, as seen in repeated infection. An acute perforation has a better chance of healing spontaneously than does a chronic perforation.

Otitis Media. Otitis media is the most prevalent disorder of the middle ear. It is most common in children but does occur in adults. When an infection is sudden in onset and short in duration, the diagnosis is acute suppurative otitis media. When the infection is repeated, usually causing drainage and perforation, the problem is chronic otitis media. Chronic otitis media is often caused by organisms such as *Pseudomonas, Staphylococcus,* and *Klebsiella.* Anaerobes such as *Bacteroides* have also been identified in culture analysis of specimens from the ear. Infection can cause swelling of the mucosa throughout the middle ear and eustachian tube. At times *serous otitis media* is found in conjunction with upper respiratory tract infections or allergies.

Chronic otitis media can lead to tympanic membrane retraction, adhesive otitis media, or necrosis of the tympanic membrane (perforations) or of the ossicles. Both problems create a conductive hearing loss. Necrosis of the bone covering of the facial nerve may cause facial paralysis. Because of the anatomy of the temporal bone, middle ear infection can also lead to brain abscesses that are life-threatening if not treated properly. Cholesteatoma, another complication, is discussed on p. 1733.

Subsequent to infectious otitis media or allergic disease, fluid may form in the middle ear, known as *serous otitis media.* This fluid is formed when a vacuum develops in the middle ear, caused by a blocked eustachian tube. When the swelling subsides, the fluid may be too thick to drain. Tympanometry is a useful diagnostic assessment to distinguish a normal ear from one with a middle ear effusion.

Mastoiditis. The mastoid system is a series of air cells contained within the temporal bone that communicate with the middle ear. Before the discovery of antibiotics, a mastoid infection was a life-threatening event. Now acute mastoiditis is rare, although chronic mastoiditis does sometimes occur. With repeated middle ear infections, the mastoid cavity becomes a significant part of the problem, increasing the amount of drainage. A chronic infection also leads to the development of cholesteatoma (see following section).

Drainage from the mastoid cavity via the ear canal is the most likely manifestation to appear. The drainage courses through the middle ear and out the tympanic membrane through a perforation. Tenderness over the mastoid cavity behind the ear points to an infection but usually is caused by an acute exacerbation of chronic mastoiditis rather than an acute mastoiditis. The protrusion of the pinna as a result of swelling over the mastoid may be part of this process.

Cholesteatoma. *Cholesteatoma* is a cyst in the middle ear or mastoid system that is lined with squamous epithelium and filled with keratin debris. Often infection is present in the mass of the cholesteatoma. Although cholesterol granules can be present in the specimen, yielding the term *cholesteatoma,* they are not the primary pathologic process.

Cholesteatoma most often results from chronic otitis media or marginal perforation of the tympanic membrane. Clients have conductive hearing loss and foul-smelling discharge from the ears. Although it is a benign growth, the cholesteatoma causes erosion of the surrounding structures, leading to other problems, such as brain abscesses, vertigo, and facial paralysis. Fortunately, these complications are uncommon.

Other Masses. Benign masses of the external ear canal are usually cysts that arise from a sebaceous gland or, more rarely, from the cerumen glands. Cysts can also be congenital in nature. Bony protrusions seen in the bony portion of the ear canal are called *exostoses.* The skin covering an exostosis is normal. If the skin is red, the mass is usually an abscess. Infectious polyps found in the ear canal arise from either the tympanic membrane or, more commonly, the middle ear, through a hole in the tympanic membrane.

Malignant tumors are also found in the external ear. The cutaneous carcinomas are most often basal cell carcinoma on the pinna and squamous cell carcinoma in the ear canal. If not treated, the carcinomas can invade underlying structures; squamous cell carcinoma may spread throughout the temporal bone. Rare tumors of the cerumen glands are of the adenoma cell type. Masses of the external ear are diagnosed through physical examination and biopsy to rule out malignancy. Surgical excision may be required.

Both benign and malignant tumors can involve the tympanic membrane, but they seldom arise from it; however, an infectious glandular polyp can be isolated to the tympanic membrane. Tumors in the middle ear can be seen through or protrude through the tympanic membrane.

The same tumors that arise in the middle ear can be found in the mastoid cavity. Because the mastoid cavity is connected to other air cells throughout the temporal bone and is close to the brain, malignant tumors at this location carry a poor prognosis.

Pathophysiology

Otalgia related to a problem in the ear is usually the result of an inflammatory process that can be caused by trauma or infection. Inflammation causes chemical mediators to be released into the tissue and the chemotaxis of leukocytes to the damaged area, resulting in tissue edema, pain, heat, and redness. This inflammatory process results in swelling of tissue that impinges on nerve endings and surrounding areas, causing the otalgia. Masses such as tumors grow and press on nearby tissue and nerves, causing pain. Sometimes the infection or mass erodes into tissue and bone as in cholesteatoma and causes further inflammation and pain.

Otalgia can also be caused by referred pain to the ear. In conditions such as TMJ or cervical adenopathy, the pain does not originate in the ear; however, the neuronal pain pathways for these processes cross over and are perceived in the ear. Although the perception of pain in the ear is real, the cause of the pain is not related to a pathologic process in that area.

Clinical Manifestations

In the case of head trauma and damage to the tympanic membrane, clients often report an episode of brief but intense otalgia. If the tympanic membrane is ruptured from barotrauma or otitis media, the client often notes a sudden reduction of pressure and pain. Pain is not usually elicited on palpation of the external ear; this phenomenon usually provides a differential diagnosis between problems of the external ear and middle ear. Disorders involving the tympanic membrane are painful, perhaps the most painful of all middle ear disorders. Hearing loss may be noted but is often reversible. Vertigo may also be present.

Ear pain from obstruction usually results from the buildup of matter in the ear canal, which leads to pressure and pain. Clients may also report decreased hearing, a sense of fullness, a throbbing sensation, and itching. The onset, duration, frequency, and intensity of manifestations should be noted.

Pain in the external ear is the most common clinical manifestation of infection. Pain ranges from mild to severe and is generally unilateral. Pain is more intense when the ear canal is swollen. Painful sites are tender because of the close proximity of bone (a hard surface) when the ear is palpated. A clue to early external otitis is tenderness when the pinna is gently pulled, in contrast to otitis media, in which touching the ear does not cause pain. A forerunner of pain in external otitis is itching in the ear canal. Inflammation (redness) is easily identified with an otoscope. At different stages of infection, drainage will be found from the ear canal. In early infectious disorders, the drainage may be clear rather than discolored by pus.

Manifestations of otitis media include ear pain and an immobile tympanic membrane. Because the tympanic membrane is a semitransparent membrane, what lies beneath it is visible. It can also become discolored or displaced. Therefore both fluid and infection can be seen in the middle ear. The tympanic membrane may be dull or red instead of the normal pearly gray. The eardrum may be normal, perforated, infected, retracted, or bulging depending on the disease process involved. In addition, the client may report bubbling, crackling, or popping sensations in the ear, especially during swallowing. There is a sense of fullness in the ear and conductive hearing loss that fluctuates.

Suppurative otitis media is invasion of the middle ear by virulent organisms and formation of pus, often accompanied by purulent *otorrhea* (drainage). Clinical manifestations include intense ear pain, fever, mild to moderate conductive hearing loss, thickened and bulging tympanic membrane, and occasional dizziness.

OUTCOME MANAGEMENT

Medical Management

The goals of medical management are to (1) promote healing, (2) alleviate pain, and (3) restore normal function of the ears.

Promote Healing

Ear Irrigation. The ear is commonly irrigated to cleanse the external auditory canal or to remove impacted wax, debris, or foreign bodies to promote healing. Irrigation is not used in clients with a history or clinical suspicion of perforated eardrum. Ear irrigation is performed as follows.

Warm the irrigating solution (usually water) to body temperature, and place it in the irrigating syringe. Dizziness is a common side effect of irrigating with fluids that are colder or warmer than body temperature. Protect the client's clothes with a plastic drape, and place a kidney-shaped basin below the ear to catch the irrigating solution. Have the client sit with the ear to be irrigated toward you and downward to drain the material. In the adult, pull the external ear upward and backward (or in children pull the external ear directly back), and direct the tip of the syringe along the upper wall of the ear canal (Figure 66-4). The canal should not be completely obstructed by the syringe to allow the back-flow of solution. When charting the ear irrigation, include the type of irrigation solution used and the nature of returned solution regarding amount, texture, color of cerumen, and type of debris. In addition, instruct the client to report pain, vertigo, or nausea during the procedure.

Sometimes the client is instructed to use a medicinal ear irrigation solution. The most common solution for ear irrigation is boric acid and alcohol, which is obtained by prescription. This solution cleanses the ear of debris and infection and provides a drying agent. A 2- or 3-ounce ear syringe is needed for irrigation. A family member performs the irrigation for the client. Usually the ear irrigation is followed by the use of eardrops.

Candling is a folk remedy that has gained popularity in recent years. In this technique, a candle is placed in

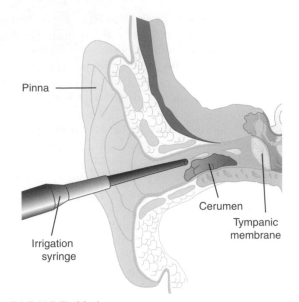

■ **FIGURE 66–4** Ear irrigation. The tip of the syringe is directed along the upper wall of the ear canal.

the ear canal. The wick is lighted and the candle is allowed to burn for a short period of time. Supposedly, the burning flame creates a vacuum at the other end of the candle, which can suck wax and other evil humors from the canal. When the candle is removed, the base of the candle typically will appear dark brown, leading the person to believe that their ear wax has been removed by candling. Candling has shown no benefit and, in fact, has been associated with harm. Hot wax can burn the external ear or tympanic membrane. It can also lead to perforation of the tympanic membrane.

Antibiotics. Local and systemic antibiotics are the cornerstone of preventing and managing infections of the ear canal; however, the first rule of treating infection is meticulous cleaning of the site so that the local antibiotic can reach the infected area. Suction, irrigation, or manual removal of matter with a cotton-tipped swab can be used. Regular application of antibiotic-steroid eardrops for a week is required.

If the ear canal is swollen shut, a wick may be inserted to allow the drops to penetrate the canal. Eardrops are placed directly on the wick. Commercially prepared wicks or single pieces of one-fourth-inch gauze can be used. The wick serves not only as a bandage but also as an excellent vehicle to medicate the ear canal. The wick is gently inserted into the ear canal by means of forceps while the external ear is gently pulled upward and backward. The wick is usually slightly less than 1 inch long (Figure 66-5). The client should lie on the unaffected side for 3 to 5 minutes to allow gravity to promote movement of the medication

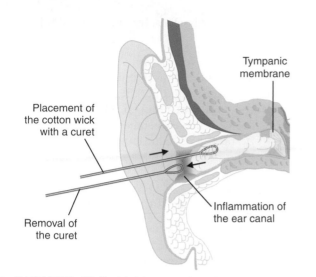

■ FIGURE 66–5 Administration of antibiotics for otitis externa. A curette with a cotton wick around it is placed in the ear canal. The wick is gently placed in the canal, and an antibiotic or treatment solution is added to the wick.

into the ear canal. If the infection is generalized or severe, systemic antibiotics are used. An infection that involves cartilage has to be treated aggressively and quickly with systemic antibiotics to avoid complications.

With any form of otitis media, appropriate antibiotic therapy may be necessary. If drainage is present, a specimen may be collected for culture analysis and sensitivity testing. Most episodes of acute otitis media, however, do not produce drainage, and the specific bacterial cause need not be identified. Otitis media is generally easily managed, but if it is not treated properly, it can lead to meningitis and brain abscess because of the proximity of the ear to these tissues.

Suppurative otitis media is managed with systemic antibiotics, topical antibiotic drops, and analgesics. If otitis media becomes chronic, myringotomy may be required to ventilate the middle ear and equalize pressure between the middle ear and external ear. Because infection starts in the middle ear, the problems in the mastoid cavity are avoided by early use of antibiotics with otitis media.

Alleviate Pain

Because external otitis is one of the most painful disorders of the ear, appropriate analgesics are required. Pain persists for 24 to 48 hours after treatment is initiated. Once the swelling and drainage are reduced by treatment, in about 48 hours the pain subsides.

Restore Normal Function and Remove Foreign Bodies

Removal of foreign bodies from the ear canal can be quite difficult. The nurse should not spend a long time attempting to remove an object from the ear without asking for help. The external auditory canal is an exquisitely sensitive, elliptical, cylinder-like structure. In adults, it is about 24 mm long and has two anatomic points of narrowing. Objects caught behind these narrow points create the greatest problems for removal. If perforation of the tympanic membrane is deemed unlikely and the object is not tightly wedged, you can irrigate the external canal with warm water. Direct the stream of water superiorly and anteriorly into the ear canal and around the object (see Figure 66–4). Water pressure builds up and forces the object outward. It often takes about 200 to 300 ml of water to remove an object. Do not irrigate vegetable foreign proteins, such as beans, because they swell and become even more difficult to remove.

For removal of a live insect, the ear canal is filled with mineral oil, lidocaine, or an ether-soaked cotton ball, *not water,* to kill or stupefy the insect. Water would cause the insect to swell and become more difficult to remove.

The least traumatic method of removing a foreign body is with the aid of an operating microscope. After removing the object, inspect the tympanic membrane and ear canal for manifestations of trauma. If trauma is noted, the client should be treated for external otitis and seen again in 4 to 5 days.

Nursing Management of the Medical Client

Assessment. When obtaining the history of the pain, ask the client about what events have triggered the ear pain, paying special attention to a recent history of upper respiratory tract infection, travel by airplane, exposure to loud noises, trauma to the head, and stressors that lead to teeth grinding or dental work.

The nurse first observes the external ear for redness, swelling, lumps, scaling, crusting, or drainage, either serous or purulent. During assessment of the external ear, manipulation of the ear is important. If the client complains of pain when any part of the ear is palpated, an abscess, a lesion, or some kind of inflammatory process of the ear canal is suspected. If an otoscopic examination is performed, care must be taken not to cause the client unnecessary pain. An abscess may be close to the opening of the canal, where the pressure of the speculum may cause greater pain.

During the physical examination, determine the presence of pain with swallowing, neck rotation, palpation of the face and head (over the sinuses), palpation of the mastoid process, and manipulation of the pinna. Assess the TMJ by inserting your index fingers into the external auditory canals and applying pressure anteriorly while the client opens and closes the mouth. TMJ syndrome may cause pain, clicking, or crepitation of the joint during movement.

Diagnosis, Outcomes, Interventions

Diagnosis: Risk for Infection. Because of tissue damage from trauma, foreign body, or pathogen, the nursing diagnosis *Risk for Infection related to tissue destruction* may be appropriate in the client with otalgia.

Outcomes. The client will have reduced risk of infection or will experience resolution of infection without complications.

Interventions. Monitor for clinical manifestations of infection, and administer antibiotics as prescribed. Other medications, such as antihistamines, decongestants, and steroid nasal sprays, may be ordered to reduce inflammation that can damage tissue. Teach the client to complete the entire prescription of the antibiotic even though manifestations may have cleared (see the Client Education Guide on Infection of the Tympanic Membrane, Middle Ear, or Mastoid Cavity on the website).

During an infectious process, instruct the client to avoid getting water in the ear while bathing or showering by using earplugs or placing cotton balls coated with petroleum jelly in the ear canal.

Eardrops may also be prescribed for bacterial or fungal infections, which are often seen in otitis externa. Various irrigations of the mastoid system and middle ear are used for chronic infections along with antibiotic eardrops or powders. In chronic otitis media with discharge, both broad-spectrum oral antibiotics and topical antibiotic drops are used.

Diagnosis: Acute Pain. Otalgia may be caused by a process in the ear or may be referred from a source outside the ear, resulting in the nursing diagnosis *Acute Pain related to inflammation in the external or middle ear or from referred pain in the head and neck area.*

Outcomes. The client will be able to reduce pain and achieve an acceptable comfort level.

Interventions. Otalgia is managed by treating the primary problem. Comfort can be promoted by using anesthetic ear solutions or systemic analgesics. After the physician has prescribed the analgesic therapy, instruct the client as to the amount, frequency, and duration. Other measures are the application of heat by warm compress, a soft diet, a quiet environment, and positioning of the client with the affected ear down.

The client with TMJ syndrome should avoid chewing and hyperextension of the jaw (e.g., during dental examination and care). The client should also try to stop grinding the teeth. A specially fitted mouth guard to be worn while sleeping can be helpful in preventing teeth grinding at night.

In the case of eustachian tube dysfunction or barotrauma, teach the client how to facilitate opening of the eustachian tube. Chewing gum, sucking hard candy and swallowing often, yawning, and blowing air out against closed nostrils (Valsalva maneuver) help open the tube.

Evaluation. The positive outcome for the client with otalgia depends on (1) the thoroughness of the instructions provided by the nurse and (2) the client's adherence to the prescribed treatment regimen. Ongoing assessment of the client to achieve resolution of infectious and inflammatory processes contributing to the otalgia is key to effective management.

Surgical Management

The surgical treatment of infections involves incision and drainage in the acute phase for abscesses and, at times, for perichondritis. Perichondrial hematomas are incised and drained and then dressed in large, bulky dressings. The most common surgical treatment is excision of cysts and cutaneous carcinomas. For conditions that occlude the ear canal, more extensive surgery that involves removal of bone and skin grafting, known as a *canaloplasty,* is performed.

Myringoplasty

Surgery can be performed on the tympanic membrane with use of an operating microscope for magnification. Closure of a simple perforation is called a *myringoplasty.*

Tympanoplasty

Tympanoplasty is the surgical correction of a perforated tympanic membrane. In tympanoplasty, a graft of temporalis fascia or other connective tissue is placed to restore the damaged tympanic membrane. The location of the graft depends on the original defect. Sometimes tympanostomy (ventilation) tubes are inserted.

Ossiculoplasty

The surgical procedure of ossicular reconstruction is called *ossiculoplasty.* Various methods of repositioning these tiny ear bones are now in use. In addition, various synthetic prostheses have been used to reconnect the ossicles to carry sound. In an attempt to prevent extrusion of the prostheses, tissue is combined with the prostheses to rebuild the ossicles (Figure 66-6).

Myringotomy

An incision into the tympanic membrane through which fluid is removed by suction is called *myringotomy.* To keep the incision open and to prevent a recurrence of fluid, various types of transtympanic tubes can be inserted into the incision. These tubes extrude by themselves in 3 to 12 months and rarely have to be removed. More permanent tubes (T tubes) with larger flanges may be used for clients who require repeated myringotomies.

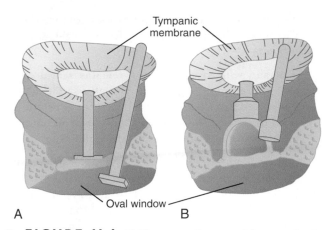

■ **FIGURE 66–6** Middle ear prostheses used for reconstruction. **A,** Ossicle columella prosthesis (total ossicular replacement). **B,** Ossicle cup prosthesis (partial ossicular replacement). *(Courtesy Arnold G. Shuring, MD.)*

Mastoidectomy

Radical mastoidectomy removes the contents of the mastoid bone for control of infection and cholesteatoma. Because the radical mastoidectomy sacrifices hearing, a modified radical mastoidectomy was developed to save the remaining middle ear structures. With the advent of antibiotics, simple mastoidectomy became possible, which maintained a normal-appearing ear canal. Because radical and modified mastoidectomies exteriorize the mastoid cavity to the external ear canal, they are known as *open* or *canal wall–down mastoidectomies. Closed* or *canal wall–up mastoidectomies* are simple mastoidectomies with modifications that are performed in conjunction with tympanoplasty and ossiculoplasty to retain or regain hearing. Today even the open mastoidectomy is performed with various tympanoplasties.

Nursing Management of the Surgical Client

Preoperative Care

The scope of nursing activities for the client undergoing ear surgery can be as broad as a preoperative assessment performed in an office or clinic or as limited as an assessment performed in the holding area of the surgical suite. Before surgery, an audiogram and tympanogram are obtained to assess preoperative hearing acuity. The client's level of knowledge about the procedure, expectations, and psychosocial readiness for surgery are evaluated along with the physiologic status.

The client undergoing ear surgery should be told what to expect during the procedure because local anesthesia with sedation is often used. Instructions should be given about the duration of the procedure, the estimated length of hospital stay, and immediate postoperative instructions.

Postoperative Care

Pain is not usually a major problem, but mild analgesia may be required. Vertigo or lightheadedness may occur when the client ambulates for the first time. Clients should be supervised when ambulating on the day of surgery to protect themselves from falling. Some clients who are quite vertiginous exhibit nystagmus (see Chapter 64) from stimulation of the inner ear. The vertigo usually passes very quickly and seldom requires medication.

Position the client as ordered; usually the client lies with operated ear up for several hours after surgery. The ear rarely bleeds after surgery. A small amount of serosanguineous drainage on a cotton ball is expected. The Client Education Guide below lists precautions for clients to take after ear surgery.

BALANCE DISORDERS

Vertigo is the perception that either oneself or one's surroundings are moving. Vertigo is often described as "dizziness." Dizziness, which can involve feelings of

---

CLIENT EDUCATION GUIDE

Precautions After Ear Surgery

To prevent injury and promote healing:
- Continue to blow your nose gently one side at a time and to sneeze or cough with your mouth open for 1 week after surgery.
- Avoid physical activity for 1 week and exercises or sports for 3 weeks after surgery.
- Return to work as recommended, usually 3 to 7 days after surgery (3 weeks if work is strenuous).
- Avoid heavy lifting, especially after stapedectomy.
- Change the cotton ball in your ear daily as prescribed.
- Keep your ear dry for 4 to 6 weeks after surgery.
- Do not shampoo for 1 week after surgery.
- Protect your ear when necessary with two pieces of cotton (outer piece saturated with petroleum jelly).
- Avoid airplane flights for the first week after surgery. For sensation of ear pressure, hold your nose, close your mouth, and swallow to equalize pressure.
- Wear noise defenders in loud environments.
- Report any drainage other than a slight amount of bleeding to the physician.
- Normal occurrences in the initial period after ear surgery may include the following:
  - Decreased hearing in operated ear from surgical packing (people may sound like they are talking in a barrel)
  - Noises in the ear, such as cracking or popping
  - Minor earache and discomfort in cheek and jaw
  - Ear swelling

disorientation in space or lightheadedness, is different, however. Vertigo results from imbalance of neural signals from the vestibular system in the ears. The imbalance of signals is interpreted by the brain as constant motion in space.

Disorders of balance and coordination result from problems of the vestibular system and "righting" reflexes. Balance can also be affected by problems outside the vestibular system. Few problems are more private than those involving one's sense of balance. Balance problems may be debilitating and may also cause embarrassing gait problems, which can jeopardize safety. More than 90 million Americans age 17 years or older have experienced vertigo or a balance problem. Vertigo is second only to chronic pain as the most common manifestation reported in America today.

Although vertigo and dizziness are not synonymous, they both relate to a sense of balance and equilibrium. Dizziness, vertigo, and syncope (fainting) are all manifestations of one of the following types of problems:

- Peripheral vestibular disorders (i.e., labyrinthine or inner ear)
- Central disorders (i.e., medullary, cerebellar, or cortical)
- Systemic disorders (i.e., cardiovascular or metabolic)

Peripheral vestibular disorders involve problems in the labyrinth or internal ear. Central disorders result from a problem in the brain or nerves, such as a tumor of the eighth cranial nerve (acoustic neuroma) or stroke. Systemic disorders begin in a nerve or organ outside the cranium (e.g., orthostatic hypotension, hypoglycemia). Examples of common causes of vertigo and dizziness, grouped by etiology, are presented in Box 66-4.

BOX 66-4 Disorders Associated with Vertigo and Dizziness

PERIPHERAL LABYRINTHINE (INNER EAR) DISORDERS
- Benign paroxysmal positional vertigo (BPPV)
- Labyrinthitis
- Ménière's disease
- Cholesteatoma

CENTRAL NERVOUS SYSTEM DISORDERS
- Cerebellar lesions
- Temporal lobe lesions
- Tumors of cranial nerve VIII (e.g., acoustic neuroma)
- Stroke
- Multiple sclerosis

SYSTEMIC DISORDERS
- Diabetes
- Postural hypotension
- Arthritis
- Hypoglycemia
- Allergies

Little can be done to reduce the risk of balance disorders. Clients should be treated early for manifestations of ear problems.

SAFETY ALERT

The person with vertigo usually remains seated or supine to prevent falling. Clients at high risk for falling as a result of vertigo should stand up slowly to prevent injury and should keep a light on at all times to enable visual cues to lessen the disequilibrium.

Finally, situations that lead to vertigo should be avoided. Motion sickness occurs normally if the provocative stimulus is present. Humans are not evolutionarily adapted to special environmental situations, such as deep-sea diving, high-speed flying, and space travel. Vertigo or dizziness may occur in these environments.

PERIPHERAL VESTIBULAR DISORDERS

Benign Paroxysmal Positional Vertigo

Benign paroxysmal positional vertigo (BPPV) is a common cause of vertigo. It tends to follow head injury and viral infections of the inner ear. BPPV is due to *cupulolithiasis,* the presence of calcium crystals in the semicircular canals. These crystals are normally deposited on small hair-like structures in the ear called *otoliths,* and they slow responses to head movement. When they are dislodged, head movement creates a hypersensitive response. BPPV is provoked when the head is placed in certain positions, usually hyperextended and to one side. Clinical manifestations usually consist of brief attacks of rotational vertigo, a rapid head tilt to the affected ear, and a lag time of 3 to 6 seconds between change of position and vertigo with nystagmus. It is usually self-limited and resolves spontaneously over weeks to months.

Labyrinthitis (Vestibular Neuronitis)

Labyrinthitis is infection or inflammation of the cochlear or vestibular portion of the inner ear or both. Causes are not fully understood, but the syndrome tends to occur in spring and early summer and to be preceded by an upper respiratory tract infection. A virus has therefore been implicated but has never been isolated. Three classic manifestations are reported: vertigo, nausea, and vomiting. There are no hearing changes. Vertigo is usually sudden in onset; it peaks in 24 to 48 hours and then gradually subsides over 1 to 2 weeks. Supportive treatment is usually given during the wait for the underlying problems to clear.

Ménière's Disease

Ménière's disease is caused by excess endolymph in the vestibular and semicircular canals. Normal vestibular activity depends on the stability of fluid pressure.

Ménière's disease causes hearing changes and vertigo. Ménière's disease is an episodic illness that waxes and wanes, often remaining quiescent for many years and then reappearing. A cluster of manifestations develops consisting of (1) paroxysmal whirling vertigo, (2) fluctuating hearing loss, (3) tinnitus, and (4) aural fullness. Only one or two manifestations may be present initially. Vertigo is characterized by remission and relapses without apparent cause, although the manifestations become less severe in time. The initial attacks consist of approximately 30 minutes of intense vertigo, which commonly provokes nausea and vomiting. Remaining stationary reduces vertigo. A sensorineural hearing loss (see Hearing Impairment) that may be reversible in the early stages is a serious consequence of Ménière's disease.

CENTRAL DISORDERS OF BALANCE

Dizziness may be a manifestation of a transient ischemic attack (TIA) ("small stroke"). A temporary loss of blood flow to the brain leads to several manifestations, depending on the brain area that is not being perfused. Clients can experience momentary losses of consciousness; transient numbness, tingling, and weakness; and changes in speech. TIAs should be reported and treated aggressively to prevent true ischemic changes.

SYSTEMIC DISORDERS LEADING TO VERTIGO

Physiologic Vertigo

Physiologic vertigo is involved in common disorders such as motion sickness. In these conditions, vertigo is minimal or absent, but autonomic manifestations are present. Motion sickness leads to perspiration, nausea, vomiting, increased salivation, yawning, and malaise. Physiologic vertigo can usually be suppressed by supplying sensory cues that come from other stimuli. For example, motion sickness from reading in a car can be reduced by looking out the window at the moving environment.

Presbyastasis

A disorder that is recognized more and more is *presbyastasis,* or disequilibrium of aging. Because of the generalized degenerative changes that occur in aging, balance and stability are affected. In addition to the labyrinth, balance also depends on the visual system and the proprioceptive changes in the muscles. Because all three systems are involved in aging, older adults have difficulty with stability, which results in falls and subsequent trauma.

Orthostatic Hypotension

Orthostatic hypotension is a sudden drop in blood pressure and dizziness on sitting or standing. The manifestations noted are lightheadedness and faintness, not vertigo, which is due to inadequate cerebral blood flow. Older adults are at high risk of orthostatic hypotension because of atherosclerosis and the use of medications that lead to diuresis or hypotension (e.g., furosemide, calcium-channel blockers). Orthostasis is diagnosed through assessment of positional blood pressure changes. Clients should be taught to change position slowly, and medications may require adjustment if blood pressure is too low.

Pathophysiology

The body maintains balance and equilibrium by responding to an intricate network of information. The ability to maintain balance depends on the intactness of four systems:

- Vestibular system (the labyrinth or inner ear)
- Visual system (the eyes)
- Proprioceptive system (the somatosensory nerves of joints and muscles)
- Cerebellar system (the coordinator)

The sensations transmitted from the ears, the eyes, and the somatosensory nerves are integrated in the brain stem and cerebellum and perceived in the cerebral cortex. Gradual interference of vestibular input causes compensatory changes that allow the brain to adjust slowly. Quick changes demand more adjustments than can be made. Infections can destroy the nerve and alter transmission of messages. Ménière's disease is an increase in the volume of endolymph with distention of the entire endolymphatic system. This distention and increased fluid results in permanent damage to both the vestibular and the cochlear apparatuses. Overproduction of endolymph can slow transmission of messages and lead to the perception that the body is in constant motion. Head trauma can shake free calcium carbonate crystals on the utricular macule and alter endolymph movement.

Clinical Manifestations

Vertigo is the most common clinical manifestation in a client with a balance problem. The clinical manifestations of balance disorders vary widely depending on (1) the cause, (2) the location (one or both ears), (3) the client's age at onset, (4) the extent of the loss of vestibular function, and (5) the rapidity with which damage occurs. Disease in the external ear, middle ear, and inner ear usually leads to vertigo that is sudden, transient, and accompanied by vagal manifestations (e.g., nausea, vomiting, sweating, pallor). The vertigo associated with cerebrovascular lesions does not follow a pattern; however, tinnitus and hearing loss are usually not present.

An important differentiation is whether the vertigo is associated with hearing loss. The close anatomic relationship between the balance and hearing systems

TABLE 66–2 Vestibular and Nonvestibular Vertigo

	Vestibular	Nonvestibular
Common descriptions	Spinning (environment moves), on a merry-go-round	Lightheadedness, feeling of being dissociated from body, swimming, giddiness, spinning inside (environment stationary)
Clinical manifestations	Drunkenness, tilting, motion sickness, off balance	
Course of illness	Episodic	Constant
Precipitating factors	Head movement, position change	Stress, hyperventilation, cardiac dysrhythmia, orthostatic hypotension
Associated manifestations	Nausea, vomiting, tinnitus, hearing loss, impaired	Perspiration, pallor, paresthesias, palpitations, vision, unsteadiness, syncope, difficulty concentrating, tension headache; anxiety

sometimes causes the sensation of vertigo in conjunction with a hearing loss. In most instances, vertigo is present without a hearing loss. It is also important to distinguish between vertigo from vestibular problems and other forms of vertigo. Table 66-2 differentiates the two forms of vertigo.

Dizziness is described by clients in such varied terms that it is almost impossible to define. Not all the terms listed here suggest true vertigo. The nurse should record the terms or description the client uses to help find the actual cause. Clinical manifestations are listed in Box 66-5.

For the client with vertigo, the differential diagnosis may be accomplished by means of a thorough medical assessment, including audiometry, vestibular tests, imaging evaluation, and, sometimes, laboratory studies. Clients who have had vertigo may become quite anxious when they think about experiencing it again. Even after the vertigo has abated, anxiety tends to persist. Because vertigo is only a clinical manifestation, the diagnosis and treatment of the underlying disease are important. Unlike with vision or hearing problems, no single organ is responsible for balance problems. Therefore the diagnosis, treatment, and rehabilitation of the client with a balance problem can be difficult as well as frustrating.

OUTCOME MANAGEMENT

Medical Management

Control of episodes of the disease is usually possible, although a cure is not yet available. Two main treatment goals guide the medical management of the client with vertigo. They are (1) suppression of the CNS and the vestibular system and (2) vestibular rehabilitation.

Suppress the Central Nervous System and Vestibular System

Treatment of acute vertigo involves several medicines, called *antivertigo agents*. These medicines tend to suppress the balance system or the CNS, allowing recovery over time. They should be used judiciously in clients with BPPV because they slow recovery of function.

A low-salt diet and a diuretic may reduce the frequency of attacks of Ménière's disease by decreasing the volume of endolymph. Other changes in lifestyle include avoiding caffeine, smoking, and alcohol. The client should try to reduce stress, get regular sleep, and remain physically active, but avoid excessive fatigue. If clients have had vertigo without warning, they should not drive. Safety may require they forego ladders, scaffolds, and swimming.

A recent treatment for manifestations associated with Ménière's disease is the application of low-pressure pulses through the ear canal to the middle ear. This airwave transmission passes through the external and middle ear structures to the fluids in the inner ear. The initial use of this device shows promise in relieving vertigo and improving hearing function during the early stages of Ménière's disease.

Promote Vestibular Rehabilitation

Vestibular rehabilitation is a recognized form of control for vertigo. Because the balance system can compensate,

BOX 66-5 Clinical Manifestations of Vertigo

- Staggering
- Giddiness
- Lightheadedness
- Disorientation
- Visual blurring
- Veering in one direction while walking
- Unsteadiness
- Reeling
- Faintness
- Wooziness
- Shakiness
- Instability
- Wobbliness
- Bewilderment
- Confusion
- Being dazed
- Clumsiness
- Sense of floating
- Sense of falling
- Weakness
- Vague feeling of uncertainty

head and total body exercises are performed by the client to hasten compensation. Vestibular rehabilitation consists of exercises that promote vestibular adaptation, habituation, and activities of daily living. Usually physical therapists are involved in structuring this treatment. Vestibular rehabilitation uses all three organ systems that provide balance.

The exercises included in vestibular rehabilitation are performed as follows:

1. While lying in bed, slowly and then quickly turn the eyes up, down, and from side to side, and the head forward, backward, and from side to side.
2. Perform the same exercises while sitting; in addition, bend forward and pick up objects from the ground.
3. While standing, perform the previously mentioned exercises; in addition, change from sitting to standing position with the eyes open and then closed, and turn around in between (i.e., change direction as well as position with eyes open and closed).
4. While moving about, walk up and down steps with the eyes open and then closed, or play games involving stooping and stretching, such as basketball.

It is believed that when vertigo is induced by these exercises, a tolerance for it is acquired. Clients should perform these exercises from the time of the acute attack and continue until they are free of manifestations for 2 consecutive days. Driving a car safely needs to be addressed with clients who have vertigo. Vestibular rehabilitation therapy has been found efficacious in treating vertigo associated with certain types of vestibular deficits. Several studies have found marked improvements in postural stability, walking, and symptom control in clients who have undergone vestibular rehabilitation therapy compared with those who have not participated in this treatment. Appropriateness of this therapy in treating vertigo in older clients has been evaluated in a few studies. As discussed in the Translating Evidence into Practice feature at right, initial findings indicate that vestibular rehabilitation is well tolerated and can be effective treatment for vertigo in the older person.

A specific intervention strategy that is currently being used involves a series of manipulative interventions known as the *Epley maneuvers*. These maneuvers, which are used specifically for BPPV, are designed to facilitate return of dislodged otoliths to their more normal position within the labyrinth. The Epley maneuvers are essentially a more direct, rapid method to restore normal function and are of variable efficacy.

Nursing Management of the Medical Client

Assessment. Nursing assessment of the client with a balance problem should consist of the following areas:

1. A client interview to obtain a health history and specific information about the onset and characteristics

---

TRANSLATING EVIDENCE INTO PRACTICE

Vestibular Rehabilitation in Older Adults

Vestibular rehabilitation therapy (VRT) provides a comprehensive approach to management of the vertiginous client, which includes exercises that promote stability and alleviate manifestations while improving daily functioning. VRT is implemented in phases. Initially the person performs vestibular adaptation exercises to promote compensatory processes in the central nervous system. These adaptation exercises focus on improving stability in different postural positions (supine, sitting, and standing) and facilitating performance of activities of daily living. Habituation exercises are instituted later in the process during the maintenance phase of treatment.

Vestibular rehabilitation (VR) intervention is effective in reducing manifestations and improving balance and postural control in clients with dizziness and vertigo. Clients with chronic vestibular disorders accompanied by unsteadiness, imbalance, or motion intolerance often experience significant symptom improvement and reduction in falls after receiving weekly sessions of VR designed for daily home use.

The effectiveness of VR treatment is strongly related to the client's strict adherence to the regimen of activities during the rehabilitation period. This involves ongoing support, instruction, and evaluation to obtain benefits from VR in managing vertigo. While performing these exercises, individuals often experience manifestations of vertigo and dizziness and may become unsteady. Older people commonly experience dizziness and unsteadiness as a result of age-related deterioration of the vestibular system. Along with the physical consequences of gait alteration and disequilibrium, the older person may feel anxious and less confident in functioning independently. Inclusion of general precautions and protective adaptations to prevent falls, such as the use of walkers and handrails, is included in the rehabilitation program, especially with older clients.

Vestibular rehabilitation can be an effective treatment in managing vertigo in certain vestibular disorders. It is beneficial in alleviating manifestations and improving function and activities in older adults. VR is well tolerated by the older client, especially with the inclusion of specific protective measures to reduce the risk of falls and injury. Maintaining positive, ongoing support of the client throughout the rehabilitation period can increase adherence and improve treatment outcomes.

---

of the balance problem and associated hearing problems. Attempt to distinguish the type of vertigo reported, and note aggravating conditions (e.g., head movement)

2. Assessment of the effect of the vertigo on the client's performance of activities of daily living
3. An interview with a family member to determine the effects of the client's balance problem on others

The importance of the history and interview cannot be overemphasized. An adequate description of vertigo should include information about the onset, exacerbating and alleviating factors, associated clinical manifestations, and predisposing factors in the medical history, as previously described. All clients bring some degree of anxiety regarding this illness to the examination. Balance problems can have devastating effects on a client's behavior. The disruption of the client's routine, the severity of the "attacks," and the fear of the unknown can make the client agitated, anxious, or depressed. The nurse must be aware of these feelings and must demonstrate self-confidence, patience, courtesy, and gentleness.

A structured questionnaire such as the one shown in Box 66-6 should be completed by the client. These questions can also be used to facilitate the interview; however, the interview should be guided by client cues. A gross assessment of the client's balance can be made by watching the client's gait. Evidence of instability may be noted if the client touches the wall or walks with a wide-based, waddling gait.

The same inspection, palpation, and otoscopic examination should be performed for the client with a balance problem as was performed for the client with hearing loss (see earlier discussion). The client must be questioned about the loss of hearing and tinnitus, which can accompany a balance problem.

Diagnosis, Outcomes, Interventions. Nursing care is detailed in the Care Plan feature on The Client with Vertigo on the website.

Surgical Management

About 5% or less of all clients with vertigo undergo surgical intervention.

Endolymphatic Sac Surgery

The endolymphatic sac procedures include decompression and various forms of shunts to the CNS or mastoid cavity. The intent of these procedures is to lessen the fluid pressure within the labyrinth and control the vertigo of Ménière's disease. A collective review of the results of 1800 cases of various surgical approaches to the endolymphatic sac found that 22% of clients had improved hearing, 53% had no change in hearing acuity, and 25% had worsened hearing as determined by the established guidelines. Refinement of surgical approaches and outcomes research on these techniques continues to be important.[16a]

Labyrinthectomy

Labyrinthectomy is a form of surgery designed to destroy the labyrinth and eliminate its abnormal input. It is performed through the oval or round window (membranous limits of cochlear and inner ear). This is a destructive procedure that removes the membranous labyrinth, either subtotally through the oval window or totally through the mastoid bone. Any remaining hearing is sacrificed.

In a nonsurgical approach to labyrinthectomy, an ototoxic drug can be injected through the tympanic membrane into the middle ear to destroy the hair cells of the vestibular system. This procedure is carried out over a series of visits and is designed to decrease the abnormal vestibular signal in the affected ear. A secondary and sometimes unavoidable effect is concurrent cochlear toxicity. Clients are treated until their vestibular manifestations improve significantly, with the goal of preserving as much hearing as possible.

Vestibular Nerve Resection

Vestibular nerve resection is a highly effective procedure performed to alleviate vertigo. Vestibular nerve resection

---

BOX 66-6   Assessment Guide for Clients with Balance Disorders

A. When you are dizzy, do you experience any of the following sensations? Please read the entire list first. Then circle the numbers of those sensations that describe what you experience most accurately.
  1. Lightheadedness
  2. Tendency to lose balance or to fall
  3. Objects spinning or turning around you
  4. Sensation that you are turning
  5. Headache
  6. Nausea or vomiting
  7. Pressure in the head
B. Please fill in the blank spaces.
  1. When did the dizziness first occur? _____
  2. Is your vertigo constant? _____
  3. Does it come in attacks? _____
  4. How often do attacks occur? _____
  5. How long are the attacks? _____
  6. Does vertigo occur only in certain positions?
    ▪ When upright?
    ▪ When lying flat?
    ▪ Turning to the right?
    ▪ Turning to the left?
  7. Have you ever stumbled or fallen because of vertigo?
  8. Do you know of anything that will stop the vertigo or make it better?
    Make your vertigo worse?
    Bring on an attack?
  9. Did you ever injure your head?
  10. Do you take any medications regularly (e.g., tranquilizers; oral contraceptives; barbiturates; a course of antibiotics, such as streptomycin, neomycin)?
  11. Do you use tobacco in any form?
    Alcohol?
  12. Have you worked for long in a noisy environment?
  13. Do you suffer easily from motion sickness?

can be performed through the labyrinth (sacrificing hearing) or around the labyrinth (saving hearing). The retrolabyrinthine surgical approach is the most common form of surgical control for vertigo today. This method preserves the inner ear structures and approaches the vestibular nerve from behind the semicircular canal. Alleviation of the client's vertigo is usually immediate. Because of the compensation by all the other structures related to maintaining balance, a client can function with only one labyrinth.

CONCLUSIONS

Nurses caring for clients with hearing and balance problems need to focus on safety and on promoting independence. Many hearing-impaired clients live a normal life with hearing augmentation and aural rehabilitation.

SAFETY

⚠️

ALERT

Clients who have diminished hearing or balance disorders are at increased risk for injury because of lack of awareness of the risks or from losing balance.

Infections of the ears remain common, but excellent antibiotics have reduced the incidence of chronic problems caused by infections. Tumors of the ear are rare, but when they occur, they are quite destructive.

THINKING CRITICALLY

1. A middle-age man comes to the health clinic with ear pain and difficulty hearing. He had some serous drainage 1 day ago but does not recall any recent infection (throat or ear). The problem has persisted intermittently over the past 6 months and is getting progressively more painful and occurring more frequently. If surgery were deemed necessary for this client, how would you prepare him? What discharge teaching might need to be completed for this client after ear surgery?

Factors to Consider. What preoperative assessments are needed? How should equal pressures be maintained on the tympanic membrane? What normal occurrences might the client expect in the initial period following surgery?

2. An older woman reveals a 10-year history of ear infection. She is experiencing sensorineural hearing loss associated with presbycusis, which affects older people. During her clinic appointment, she tells the nurse that her right ear is painful and is keeping her awake at night. She explains that she can hear most sounds, although sounds on the right side seem to be coming through a filter. She has been using her eardrops as directed but has stopped taking her oral antibiotic because she felt better 2 days ago. She requests information about daily medication or a surgical procedure that might alleviate the problem. How should you respond to the client's request? How do age-related changes contribute to her problem?

Factors to Consider. What is the assessment focus for this client? What is the prognosis for the client with presbycusis? What type of teaching does the client require?

Discussions for these questions can be found on the website. **evolve**

BIBLIOGRAPHY

Citations appearing in red refer to primary research.

1. Barreire, S.O. (2005). Spin cycle: Evaluation and management of dizziness and vertigo. *Advance Nurse Practitioner, 13*(3), 22-27.
2. Brackmann, D.E., Shelton, C., & Arriaga, M.A. (Eds.) (2001). *Otologic surgery.* Philadelphia: Saunders.
3. Chawla, N., & Olshaker, J.S. (2006). Diagnosis and management of dizziness and vertigo. *Medical Clinics of North America, 90*(2), 291-304.
4. Copeland, B.J., & Pillsbury, H.C. (2004). Cochlear implantation for treatment of deafness. *Annual Review of Medicine, 55,* 157-167.
5. Cummings, C.W., Haughey, B.H., Thomas, J.R., et al. (2004). *Cummings otolaryngology: Head and neck surgery* (4th ed.). St. Louis: Mosby.
6. Das, S., & Buchman, C.A. (2005). Bilateral cochlear implantation: Current concepts. *Current Opinions in Otolaryngology—Head and Neck Surgery, 13*(5), 290-293.
7. Ferrite, S., & Santana, V. (2005). Joint effects of smoking, noise exposure and age on hearing loss. *Occupational Medicine, 55*(1), 48-53.
8. Gates, G.A. (2006). Ménière's disease review 2005. *Journal of the American Academia of Audiology, 17*(1), 16-26.
9. Gottshall, K.R., Hoffer, M.E., Moore, R.J., et al. (2005). The role of vestibular rehabilitation in the treatment of Meniere's disease. *Otolaryngology—Head and Neck Surgery, 133*(3), 326-328.
10. Halmagyi, G.M. (2005). Diagnosis and management of vertigo. *Clinical Medicine, 5*(2), 159-165.
11. Hannon, S.A., Sami, F., & Wareing, M.J. (2005). Tinnitus. *British Medical Journal, 330*(7485), 237.
12. Harris, L.L., & Huntoon, M.B. (Eds.) (2008). *Core curriculum for otorhinolaryngology and head-neck nursing* (2nd ed.). New Smyrna Beach, Fla: Society of Otorhinolaryngology—Head and Neck Nurses, Inc.
13. Hol, M.K., Bosman, A.J., Snik, A.F., et al. (2005). Bone-anchored hearing aids in unilateral inner ear deafness: An evaluation of audiometric and patient outcome measurements. *Otology and Neurotology, 26*(5), 999-1006.
14. Macias, J.D., Massingale, S., & Gerkin, R.D. (2005). Efficacy of vestibular rehabilitation therapy in reducing falls. *Otolaryngology—Head and Neck Surgery, 133*(3), 323-325.
15. Meli, A., Zimatore, G., Badaracco, C., et al. (2006). Vestibular rehabilitation and 6-month follow-up using objective and subjective measures. *Acta Otolaryngology, 126*(3), 259-266.
16. Rosenfeld, R.M., & Bluestone, C.D. (Ed.) (2003). *Evidence-based otitis media* (2nd ed.). New York: Marcel Dekker.
16a. Moffat, D.A. (1994). Endolymphatic sac surgery: Analysis of 100 operations. *Clinical Otolaryngology 19*(3), 261-266.
17. Rosenfeld, R.M., Singer, M., Wasserman, J.M., et al. (2006). Systematic review of topical antimicrobial therapy for acute otitis externa. *Otolaryngology—Head and Neck Surgery, 134*(4 Suppl), S24-48.
18. Roy, D., & Chopra, R. (2002). Tinnitus: An update. *Journal of the Royal Society of Health, 122*(1), 21-23.
19. Semaan, M.T., Alagramam, K.N., & Megerian, C.A. (2005). The basic science of Ménière's disease and endolymphatic hydrops. *Current Opinions in Otolaryngology—Head and Neck Surgery, 13*(5), 301-307.
20. Sen, P., Georgalas, C., & Papesch, M. (2005). Co-morbidity of migraine and Ménière's disease—Is allergy the link? *Journal of Laryngology and Otology, 119*(6), 455-460.

21. Snik, A.F., Mylanus, E.A., Proops, D.W., et al. (2005). Consensus statements on the BAHA system: Where do we stand at present? *Annals of Otology, Rhinology, and Laryngology, 195*(Dec Suppl), 2-12.

22. Waddell, A. (2004). Tinnitus. *Clinical Evidence, 12,* 798-807.

23. White, J., Savvides, P., Cherian, N., et al. (2005). Canalith repositioning for benign paroxysmal positional vertigo. *Otology and Neurotology, 26*(4), 704-710.

evolve *Did you remember to check out the bonus material on the Evolve website and the CD-ROM, including NCLEX®-Examination Style Review Questions, Open-Book Quizzes, and Chapter Review Audio Podcasts?*

http://evolve.elsevier.com/Black/medsurg

UNIT 16

COGNITIVE AND PERCEPTUAL DISORDERS

ANATOMY AND PHYSIOLOGY REVIEW:

The Neurologic System

Robert G. Carroll

The nervous system is the body's most organized and complex structural and functional system. It profoundly affects both psychological and physiologic functions. This unit discusses the importance of the nervous system to human functioning and the major consequences of neurologic disorders.

CENTRAL NERVOUS SYSTEM

The brain and spinal cord are known collectively as the *central nervous system* (CNS). The CNS is divided into three major functional divisions:

1. Higher-level brain, or cerebral cortex
2. Lower brain level (basal ganglia, thalamus, hypothalamus, midbrain, pons, medulla, cerebellum)
3. Spinal cord

These structures are protected by a rigid bony encasement, three layers of membranes, a fluid cushion, and a blood-brain or blood–spinal cord barrier.

BRAIN

The brain is the largest and most complex part of the nervous system. It is composed of more than 100 billion neurons and associated fibers. The brain tissues have a gelatin-like consistency. This semi-solid organ weighs about 1400 g (approximately 3 pounds) in the adult human.

Cerebrum

The cerebrum is divided by a deep groove *(longitudinal fissure)* into two sections called *cerebral hemispheres.* A transverse fissure separates the cerebrum from the cerebellum. The outermost layer of the cerebrum, the *cerebral cortex,* is only 2 to 5 mm thick. Directly beneath the cerebral cortex are varying thicknesses of association tracts above the commissural tracts, known as the *corpus callosum* (Figure A&P16-1).

The cerebral cortex is composed of gray matter (predominantly nerve cell bodies and dendrites) formed into raised convolutions, or *gyri.* About 75% of the neuronal cell bodies in the brain are found in the cortex. The shallow grooves between the gyri *(sulci)* divide the cerebral cortex into five lobes: frontal, parietal, occipital, temporal, and central (insula) (Figure A&P16-2).

The term *neocortex* is often used to refer to the cerebral cortex. The neocortex includes all the cerebral cortex except the olfactory portions and the hippocampal regions.

Both the left cortex and the right cortex interpret sensory data, store memories, learn, and form concepts; however, each hemisphere dominates the other in many functions. In most people, for example, the *left* cortex has dominance for systematic analysis, language and speech, mathematics, abstraction, and reasoning. The *right* cortex has dominance for assimilation of sensory experiences, such as visual-spatial information, and activities such as dancing, gymnastics, music, and art appreciation.

In the frontal lobes, the precentral gyrus *(motor cortex)* controls voluntary motor activity. Most of these fibers cross to the opposite side of the brain at the medulla and descend via the spinal cord as the *lateral corticospinal tracts.* The area anterior to the precentral gyrus *(premotor area)* is also associated with voluntary motor activities. *Broca's area,* which lies anterior to the primary motor cortex and superior to the lateral sulcus, coordinates the complex muscular activity of the mouth, tongue, and larynx and makes expressive *(motor)* speech possible. Damage to this area leaves the client unable to speak clearly, a disorder called *Broca's aphasia.*

The *prefrontal areas* control (1) attention over time (concentration); (2) motivation; (3) the ability to formulate or select goals; (4) the ability to plan; (5) the ability to initiate, maintain, or terminate actions; (6) the ability to self-monitor; and (7) the ability to use feedback (called *executive functions*). These same areas are thought to contribute to reasoning, problem-solving activities, and emotional stability by inhibiting the limbic areas of the cerebrum (see later discussion).

Each *parietal lobe* is located posterior to the central sulcus of Rolando and contains a primary somatic (tactile) receptive area and the somatic (tactile) association areas. The post-central gyrus and the anterior portion of the parietal lobe are the primary receptive (interpretation) areas for tactile sensations (e.g., temperature, touch, pressure). The association areas occupy the remainder of the parietal lobe. Concept formation and abstraction are carried out by the parietal association areas. The right parietal areas are also dominant for spatial orientation and awareness of size and shapes *(stereognosis)* and body position *(proprioception).* The left parietal areas assist with right-left orientation and mathematics.

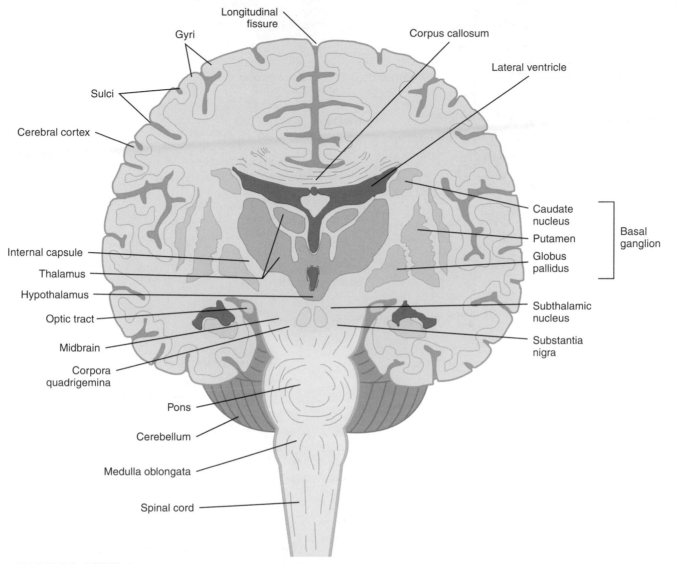

■ **FIGURE A&P16–1**   Structures of the brain (coronal section).

Each *occipital lobe* contains a primary visual receptive (interpretation) area and visual association areas. The primary visual cortex is on either side of the calcarine sulcus. The other areas of the occipital cortices are visual association areas. Visual memories are stored in these areas, which contribute to our ability to recognize visually and understand our environment.

Each *temporal lobe* is located under (inferior to) the lateral sulcus. The temporal lobe contains a primary auditory receptive area and secondary auditory association areas. Spoken language memories are stored in the left temporal auditory association areas. All other sound memories that are not language (e.g., music, various animal sounds, other noises) are stored in the right temporal lobe auditory areas. Damage to these areas would leave one unable to understand spoken or written language or to recognize music or other environmental sounds. Cells that facilitate understanding language reside in *Wernicke's area*.

The *central (insula) lobe* is located deep within the lateral sulcus and is surrounded by the frontal, parietal, and temporal lobes. Nerve fibers for taste pass through the parietal lobe to the insular lobe. Many association fibers leading to other parts of the cerebral cortex pass through this lobe.

Hippocampus

The hippocampus, a part of the medial section of the temporal lobe, plays an essential role in the process of *memory*, a complex phenomenon. Three levels of memory have been identified:

1. *Short-term (recent) memory* is lost after seconds or minutes.
2. *Intermediate memory* lasts days to weeks and eventually is lost.
3. *Long-term (remote) memory* is stored and lasts a lifetime.

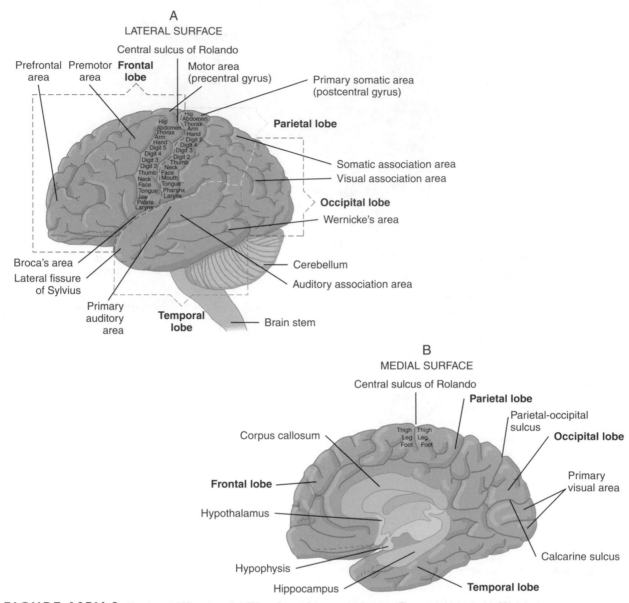

FIGURE A&P16–2   The lateral **(A)** and medial **(B)** surfaces of the cerebral cortex. The central lobe is the fifth lobe.

Theories about the physiologic basis of memory suggest that reverberating neuronal messages cause short-term memory and that actual neuronal structural changes lead to long-term memory. The hippocampus assists in the conversion of short-term memory into intermediate and long-term memory in the thalamus. The association fibers of the frontal, parietal, temporal, and occipital lobes as well as the diencephalon are important in long-term memory.

Basal Ganglia

The basal ganglia consist of several structures of subcortical gray matter buried deep in the cerebral hemispheres. These structures include the caudate nucleus, putamen, globus pallidus, substantia nigra, and subthalamic nucleus. The basal ganglia serve as processing stations that link the cerebral cortex to thalamic nuclei. Almost all the motor and sensory fibers connecting the cerebral cortex and the spinal cord travel through the white matter pathways near the caudate nucleus and putamen ganglia. These pathways are known as the *internal capsule*. The basal ganglia, along with the corticospinal tract, are important in controlling complex motor activity.

Diencephalon

The *diencephalon* is composed of the thalamus and the hypothalamus. The paired *thalami* lie between the cerebral hemispheres and superior to the brain stem. Its gray matter surrounds the lateral edges of the third ventricle. The *hypothalamus* forms the floor and portions of the wall of the third ventricle. Other important structures found in and near the diencephalon include (1) the optic tracts and optic chiasm, (2) the pituitary gland on the floor of the diencephalon, and (3) the pineal gland on the roof of the diencephalon.

The thalamus channels all ascending (sensory) information, except smell, to the appropriate cortical cells. The hypothalamus regulates autonomic nervous system (ANS) functions, such as heart rate, blood pressure, water and electrolyte balance, stomach and intestinal motility, glandular activity, body temperature, hunger, body weight, and sleep-wakefulness. It also serves as the regulator of the pituitary gland by releasing factors that stimulate or inhibit pituitary gland output.

Limbic System

The limbic system comprises many nuclei, including parts of the medial portion of the frontal and temporal lobes (hippocampus), thalamus, hypothalamus, and the basal ganglia. It is considered the center for feelings and control of emotional expression (fear, anger, pleasure, sorrow). The limbic system (the temporal lobe component) also receives nerve fibers from the olfactory bulbs and thus plays an essential role in the interpretation of smells.

Brain Stem

The brain stem is composed of the midbrain, pons, and medulla oblongata (Table A&P16-1). They are composed of ascending pathways, the reticular formation, cranial nerves and their nuclei, and descending autonomic and motor pathways.

Reticular Formation

The reticular formation is composed of a complex network of gray matter (nuclei), ascending reticular pathways, and descending reticular pathways. Its nuclei extend from the superior part of the spinal cord to the diencephalon and communicate with the basal ganglia, cerebrum, and cerebellum.

The reticular formation assists in regulation of skeletal motor movement and spinal reflexes. It also filters incoming sensory information to the cerebral cortex. About 99% of sensory information is disregarded as unessential. One component of the reticular formation, the *reticular activating system,* controls the sleep-wake cycle (see Chapter 22) and consciousness.

Cerebellum

The cerebellum is composed of gray and white matter. The *cortex* of the cerebellum is a thin layer of gray matter arranged in parallel long and deep gyri, called *folia,* and separated by cerebellar sulci (Figure A&P16-3). Deep fissures divide the cerebellum into three lobes, but the functional division of the cerebellum consists of a right and left hemisphere separated by a narrow band of white matter called the *vermis.* An extension of dura mater, the *falx cerebelli,* partially separates the hemispheres.

TABLE A&P16–1 Brain Stem Structures and Their Functions

Structures	Functions
Midbrain	
Corpora quadrigemina	
Superior colliculi	Visual reflexes
Inferior colliculi	Auditory reflexes
Cerebral aqueduct	
Origin of CN III and IV	
Ascending sensory pathways	
Reticular formation	
Red nuclei	Motor pathways to spinal cord, cerebellum
Substantia nigra	Part of basal ganglia
Descending motor pathways	
Pons	
Fourth ventricle	
Nuclei of inferior colliculus	Auditory processing
Nuclei of CN V, VI, VII	
Locus ceruleus	Secretes norepinephrine
Raphe nuclei	Secrete serotonin
Ascending sensory pathways	
Medical lemniscus, auditory pathway	Discriminative touch
Descending motor pathways	
Medial longitudinal fasciculi	Efferent pathway to spinal cord
Reticular formation	
Respiratory centers	
Pontine nuclei; pontocerebellar fibers	
Medulla Oblongata	
Fourth ventricle	
Central canal	
Raphe nuclei	Secrete serotonin
Ascending sensory pathways	
Medial lemniscal pathways	Discriminative tactile pathways
Spinothalamic and trigeminothalamic tracts	Pain pathways Tactile, temperature
Lateral lemnisci	Auditory pathways
Nuclei of CN VIII, IX, X, XI, XII	
Olive and vestibular-cerebellar systems	
Pyramids (corticospinal, corticobulbar, corticopontine)	Voluntary motor
Reflex centers: respiratory, vasomotor, cardiac, coughing, swallowing, sneezing, vomiting	
Reticular formation	
Descending motor pathways (pyramids)	Voluntary motor

CN, Cranial nerve.

The cerebellum integrates sensory information related to the position of body parts, coordinates skeletal muscle movement, and regulates muscle tension, which is necessary for balance and posture. Three pairs of nerve tracts (*cerebellar peduncles*) provide the communication pathways. The inferior peduncles are sensory (*afferent*)

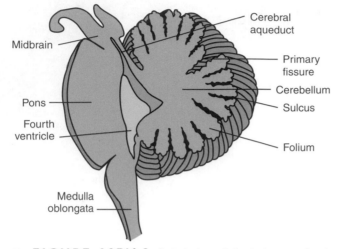

■ **FIGURE A&PI6–3** Sagittal view of the brain stem, fourth ventricle, and cerebellum.

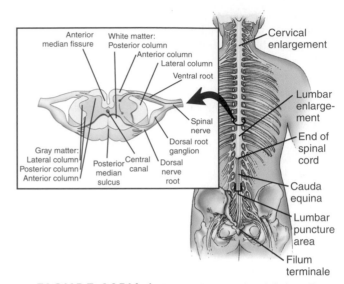

■ **FIGURE A&PI6–4** The spinal cord ends at L-2. *Inset,* Transverse section *(left)* of the spinal cord. *(Modified from Thibodeau, G., & Patton, K. [2007]. Anatomy and physiology [6th ed.]. St. Louis: Mosby.)*

pathways from the spinal cord and medulla, which carry information related to the position of body parts to the cerebellum. The middle peduncles carry information about voluntary *(purposeful)* motor activities from the cerebral cortex to the cerebellum. The cerebellum also receives sensory input from the receptors in the muscles, tendons, joints, eyes, and inner ear. After this information is integrated and analyzed, the cerebellum sends impulses via the superior peduncles *(efferent pathways)* to the brain stem, thalamus, and cortex.

Most of the tracts in the cerebellum travel through various nuclei without crossing. Therefore the right cerebellar hemisphere predominantly affects the right (ipsilateral) side of the body and vice versa.

SPINAL CORD

The *spinal cord,* that portion of the CNS surrounded and protected by the vertebral column, is continuous with the medulla and lies within the upper two thirds of the *vertebral canal* (the cavity within the vertebral column). The lower spinal cord terminates caudally in a cone-shaped structure known as the *conus medullaris* at the level of the first (L1) and second (L2) lumbar vertebrae. The spinal cord is subdivided into four areas: (1) cervical cord, (2) thoracic cord, (3) lumbar cord, and (4) sacral cord (conus medullaris) (Figure A&P16-4).

Within the spinal cord, butterfly-shaped gray matter (mostly unmyelinated) is surrounded by mostly myelinated white matter. The white matter consists of *ascending tracts* and *descending tracts* that conduct nerve impulses between the brain and the cells outside the CNS. The cell bodies in the gray matter are grouped into clusters of nuclei and *laminae* (a defined group or column of cells). The tracts in the white matter are arranged into three paired columns: posterior, lateral, and anterior (Figure A&P16-4, *inset*).

Ascending and Descending Pathways

The *ascending (sensory) pathways* carry sensory information through the spinal cord to the brain. For example, the spinothalamic tract carries sensory information from the spinal cord to the thalamus. After synapsing in the thalamus, information is relayed to regions of the brain such as the parietal lobe. *Descending (motor) pathways* carry mostly efferent signals to the spinal cord. The corticospinal tract *(upper motor neuron)* is a descending tract passing from the frontal lobe of the cerebral cortex to the motor neurons of the spinal cord. *Lower motor neurons* are cells that begin in the anterior horn of the spinal cord and pass through the spinal nerves to the muscle cells. *Propriospinal tracts* remain within the cord.

Table A&P16-2 summarizes the specific functions of the major brain and spinal cord tracts.

Many of the tracts communicating with the cerebral cortex cross (decussate), but not all cross at the same place. The term *contralateral* refers to the opposite side of the body and is used to describe tracts that cross (often at the medulla) and ascend or descend; *ipsilateral* (same-sided) tracts do not cross. For example, sensory tracts (including the anterior spinothalamic, posterior, and anterior spinocerebellar tracts) cross in the medulla as they ascend to the cerebral cortex. Therefore the sensory neurons in the cerebral cortex interpret sensory stimuli from the contralateral side of the body.

The lateral corticospinal spinal tract *(pyramidal tract)* crosses at the medulla as it descends from the frontal lobe of the cerebral cortex to the spinal cord. The posterior spinocerebellar tracts are ipsilateral tracts and thus coordinate muscular function on the same side of the body. The crossing of the lateral spinothalamic tract is unique.

TABLE A&P16–2 Major Nerve Tracts of the Spinal Cord

Tract	Location	Function
Ascending Tracts		
Fasciculus gracilis	Posterior column	Touch, pressure, body movement, position
Fasciculus cuneatus	Posterior column	Pain, temperature
Spinothalamic	Lateral and anterior columns	Light (crude) touch
Spinocerebellar		
Posterior	Lateral column	Coordination of muscle movements
Anterior	Lateral column	
Descending Tracts		
Corticospinal		
Lateral	Lateral column	Voluntary motor
Ventral	Anterior column	Voluntary motor
Reticulospinal		
Anterior	Anterior column	Muscle tone, sweat glands
Medial	Anterior column	
Rubrospinal	Lateral column	Coordination of muscle movements
Lateral	Lateral column	Autonomic nervous system fibers

PROTECTIVE AND NUTRITIONAL STRUCTURES

Cranium and Vertebral Column

Eight bones that fuse early in childhood compose the cranium. The fused junctions are called *sutures*. The cranium encloses the brain structures and serves as a source of protection.

The floor, or *basilar plate*, of the cranial vault has three depressions, called *fossae*. The frontal lobes lie in the anterior fossa. The temporal lobes and the base of the diencephalon lie in the middle fossa. The cerebellum rests in the posterior fossa.

The vertebral column, a flexible series of vertebrae, surrounds and protects the spinal cord. It consists of 7 cervical vertebrae, 12 thoracic vertebrae, 5 lumbar vertebrae, 5 sacral vertebrae fused into a sacrum, and 4 coccygeal vertebrae fused into a coccyx. Ligaments hold the vertebrae together, and disks between the vertebrae prevent the bones from rubbing together.

Meninges

The *meninges*, three membranes that envelop the brain and spinal cord, are predominantly for protection (Figure A&P16-5). Each layer—the pia mater, arachnoid, and dura mater—is a separate membrane.

The *pia mater* is a vascular layer of connective tissue that is so closely connected to the brain and spinal cord that it follows every sulcus and fissure. This layer serves as a supporting structure for blood vessels passing through to the tissues of the brain and spinal cord. The

■ **FIGURE A&P16–5** The meninges (coronal section through the superior sagittal sinus).

pia mater and astrocytes together form the membrane part of the blood-brain barrier (see Blood-Brain Barrier).

The *arachnoid,* a thin layer of connective tissue, extends from the top of each gyrus to the top of the adjacent gyrus; it does not extend into the sulci and fissures. The space between this layer and the pia mater is known as the *subarachnoid space.* Cerebrospinal fluid (CSF) flows through this space.

The cranial *dura mater* is a tough, nonstretchable vascular membrane with two layers. The *outer* dura mater is actually the membrane *(periosteum)* of the cranial bones. The *inner* dura mater forms the plates that separate the two cerebral hemispheres *(falx cerebri)*, the cerebrum and the brain stem and cerebellum *(tentorium cerebelli)*, and the cerebellar hemispheres *(falx cerebelli)*. The tentorium cerebelli is a landmark term that is often used by clinicians to separate parts of the brain; it is often referred to as *tentorium. Supratentorial* refers to the cerebrum and all the structures superior to the tentorium cerebelli; *infratentorial* refers to structures inferior to the tentorium cerebelli: the brain stem and the cerebellum.

Brain spaces that often fill with blood after head trauma include the potential space *(subdural space)* between the inner dura mater and the arachnoid and the *epidural space* between the dura mater and the periosteum.

The meninges anchor the spinal cord. The pia mater, which closely surrounds the spinal cord, continues from the tip of the conus as a thread-like structure *(filum terminale)* to the end of the vertebral column, where it is anchored into the ligament on the posterior side of the coccyx. The *denticulate ligaments* extend laterally from the pia mater to the dura mater to suspend the spinal cord from the dura mater.

Two common spaces that are commonly accessed by physicians are the subarachnoid space (for diagnostic studies) and the epidural space (for delivery of medications).

The *subarachnoid space* extends below the level of the spinal cord to the second sacral (S2) vertebral level, and the *epidural space* lies between the dural sheath and the vertebral bones.

Reflex Mechanisms

Our unconscious automatic responses to internal and external stimuli, known as *reflex responses,* provide many homeostatic functions. Although the spinal cord is often thought of as the reflex center, it is not the only site for reflex regulation. Many of the complex reflexes controlling heart rate, breathing, blood pressure, swallowing, sneezing, coughing, and vomiting are found in the brain stem.

Some intrinsic reflex circuits in the spinal cord create patterns of movement (flexion and extension) that are the basis for posture and forward progression. Other reflex circuits are the basis for spinal cord reflexes, which include the myotatic (deep tendon, stretch) reflex, the flexor withdrawal reflex, the crossed extension reflex, and the extensor thrust reflex. Visceral-somatic reflexes can also excite or inhibit the motor neurons, producing changes in muscle tone and even in movement.

Neuromuscular spindles monitor muscle stretch. As a muscle stretches, increased firing of spindles leads to contraction of the same muscle, commonly seen as the *knee-jerk reflex*. The Golgi tendon organs are sensory nerve endings that protect against excessive force developed during contraction.

Simple reflexes require only two or three neurons; for example, the *knee-jerk reflex* requires only a sensory neuron and a motor neuron. The *withdrawal reflex* helps prevent or decrease tissue injury when a body part touches a potentially harmful object. The harmful stimuli are sent via the sensory neuron to the interneuron in the spinal cord for interpretation, and the response message is sent via the motor neuron, resulting in the withdrawal response (Figure A&P16-6).

Cerebrospinal Fluid and the Ventricular System

The CSF is a clear, colorless fluid. About 100 to 160 ml of CSF circulates through the ventricles and within the subarachnoid space. When a person is lying in a horizontal position, the average CSF pressure is 100 to 180 mm Hg.

About two thirds of the CSF is made in the choroid plexus of the four ventricles, primarily in the lateral ventricles. Small amounts are produced by ependymal, arachnoid, and other brain cells. The *choroid plexus* is a network of blood vessels within the pia mater that is in direct contact with the lining of the ventricles. The choroid plexuses together produce about 500 ml of CSF per day. If CSF were allowed to accumulate, it would exert enough pressure to damage the brain. Normally, however, it is absorbed into the blood at the same rate at which it is formed.

The *ventricular system* is a series of cavities within the brain. CSF flows from each of the lateral ventricles via the foramen of Monro into the third ventricle (Figure A&P16-7). The third ventricle is midline just beneath the fornix. CSF drains from the third ventricle through the aqueduct of Sylvius into the fourth ventricle. The fourth ventricle is located in the brain stem just anterior to the cerebellum. From the fourth ventricle, CSF passes via one of three foramina (two foramina of Luschka and one foramen of Magendie) into a large

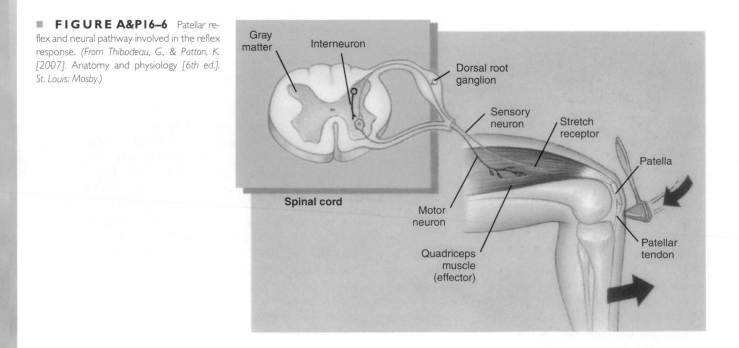

■ **FIGURE A&P16-6** Patellar reflex and neural pathway involved in the reflex response. *(From Thibodeau, G., & Patton, K. [2007]. Anatomy and physiology [6th ed.]. St. Louis: Mosby.)*

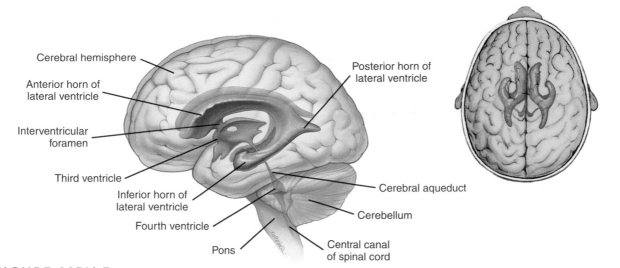

■ FIGURE A&P16–7 The ventricles of the brain produce and circulate cerebrospinal fluid. *(From Thibodeau, G., & Patton, K. [2007]. Anatomy and physiology [6th ed.]. St. Louis: Mosby.)*

subarachnoid space that lies behind the medulla and below the cerebellum, called the *cisterna magna*. The cisterna magna is continuous with the subarachnoid space, which surrounds the brain and spinal cord.

Eventually, the CSF circulates upward into the region of the superior sagittal sinus, where it is absorbed across the arachnoid villi. The arachnoid granulations are extensive tufts of pia-arachnoid that, along with the inner dura, extend into the superior sagittal sinus and permit one-way flow of CSF into the sinus.

Blood-Brain Barrier

Three brain barriers (blood-brain, blood-CSF, and brain-CSF) primarily regulate and maintain an optimal and stable chemical environment for neurons. Brain barriers are either physical barriers or physiologic processes (transport systems) that slow movement of certain substances from one CNS compartment to another by regulating ion movement between the compartments. Physical barriers include tight junctions of the endothelial cells lining the capillaries, pores of the capillaries of the choroid plexuses, the basement membrane (ependymal cells) next to the choroid plexuses, and the pial-glial membrane.

An intact blood-brain barrier may prevent some drugs from crossing into the brain, a fact that must be considered when medications are prescribed for nervous system disorders. Certain events, including dilutional hyponatremia, acute hypertension, high doses of some anesthetics, vasodilation, and hypercarbia, can increase the permeability of the blood-brain barrier.

BLOOD SUPPLY

The brain receives 20% of the cardiac output and uses 20% of the body's oxygen. Glucose is catabolized or burned for its energy. Gray matter has higher metabolic needs than white matter. Blood flow is regulated by levels of the metabolite carbon dioxide. An increase in neuronal metabolism produces an increase in carbon dioxide, leading to a local vasodilation. Local regulation of blood flow ensures that blood flow is proportional to neuronal metabolic needs.

The vertebral arteries and the internal carotid arteries (Figure A&P16-8) provide the arterial supply to the brain.

Arterial Supply

The *vertebral arteries* branch from the subclavian arteries, travel through the transverse foramina in the cervical vertebrae, and enter the cranial vault through the foramen magnum. The vertebral arteries are located on the anterolateral surface of the medulla. At the junction of the medulla and pons, the vertebral arteries join to form the basilar artery. The basilar artery bifurcates at the midbrain level to form two posterior cerebral arteries. The vertebral artery system supplies the brain stem, the cerebellum, the lower portion of the diencephalon, and the medial and inferior regions of the temporal and occipital lobes.

The *internal carotid arteries* branch from the common carotid arteries and enter through the carotid canals at the base of the skull. The internal carotid arteries bifurcate into the anterior and middle cerebral arteries.

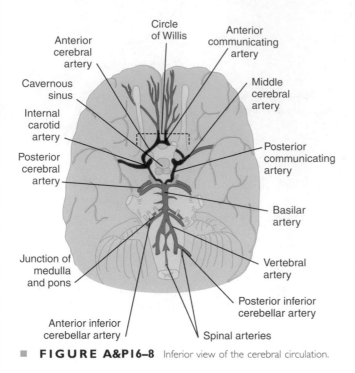

■ **FIGURE A&P16–8** Inferior view of the cerebral circulation.

Near this bifurcation, the *circle of Willis* (a ring of blood vessels at the base of the brain) is formed by the posterior cerebral arteries, posterior communicating arteries, internal carotid arteries, anterior cerebral arteries, and anterior communicating branches. The internal carotid arteries supply the upper diencephalon, basal ganglia, lateral temporal and occipital lobes, and parietal and frontal lobes. The middle cerebral arteries supply large portions of the frontal, parietal, temporal, occipital, and insular lobes and the basal ganglia, internal capsule, and thalamus. The anterior cerebral arteries supply the medial portions of the frontal and parietal lobes and the upper basal ganglia and internal capsule (see Figure A&P16-8).

The spinal cord derives its arterial blood supply from small spinal arteries that branch off larger arteries, including the vertebral, ascending cervical, deep cervical, intercostal, lumbar, and sacral arteries. These arteries and their branches form the three main arteries of the spinal cord—the anterior spinal artery and a pair of posterior spinal arteries, which extend the length of the cord.

Venous Supply

Most of the venous blood from the head returns to the heart through the internal jugular veins, the external jugular veins, and the vertebral veins.

Venous distribution is similar to arterial distribution of the spinal cord. The venous system drains into the venous sinuses located between the dura mater and the periosteum of the vertebral column.

CELLS OF THE NERVOUS SYSTEM

Structure

Nervous tissue consists mainly of *neuroglia* and *neurons* (as well as vascular and some connective tissues). Neurons are responsible for communication, and neuroglial cells provide support for the activity of neurons. The brain and spinal cord constitute the CNS.

Neuroglia

Glial cells, collectively called *neuroglia,* provide structure and support for neurons. They are plentiful, with a ratio of glial cells to neurons as high as 50 to 1. They also control ion concentrations within the extracellular space and contribute to the transport of nutrients, gases, and waste products between neurons and the vascular system and the CSF. Clinically, these cells are responsible for the development of many intracranial tumors. Four types of neuroglial cells exist (Figure A&P16-9).

In addition to these functions, each type of glial cell has specific functions.

1. *Astrocytes* supply nutrients to the neurons. They have specialized contacts with blood vessels in the pial-glial membrane and form part of the blood-brain barrier. Astrocytes appear to be the CNS cells that respond to brain trauma by forming scar tissue.
2. *Oligodendrocytes* are comparable to the Schwann cells in the peripheral nervous system (PNS). These cells wrap themselves around axons, and the spiraled part of their membrane is referred to as *myelin.* The outermost part of the Schwann cells also makes up the *neurilemma,* a sheath that surrounds the myelin sheath. The neurilemma is essential to nerve regeneration (see later discussion).
3. *Microglia* are phagocytic scavenger cells and are related to macrophages. They phagocytose products from injured neurons.
4. *Ependymal cells* line the ventricles, choroid plexuses, and the central canal that extends through the spinal cord. They create a one-cell-layered membrane that allows regulated diffusion of substances between the interstitial fluid and the CSF.

Neurons

A neuronal cell body *(soma)* is like other cells in that it contains most of the organelles seen in other cells. Unique structures in the neuron include *neurofibrils,* which are networks of thread-like structures supporting other structures. *Nissl bodies* are dark-staining sections of rough endoplasmic reticulum and are unique to the neuron.

Tree-like *dendrites* carry messages to the neuronal cell body; *axons* carry messages away from the cell body (Figure A&P16-10).

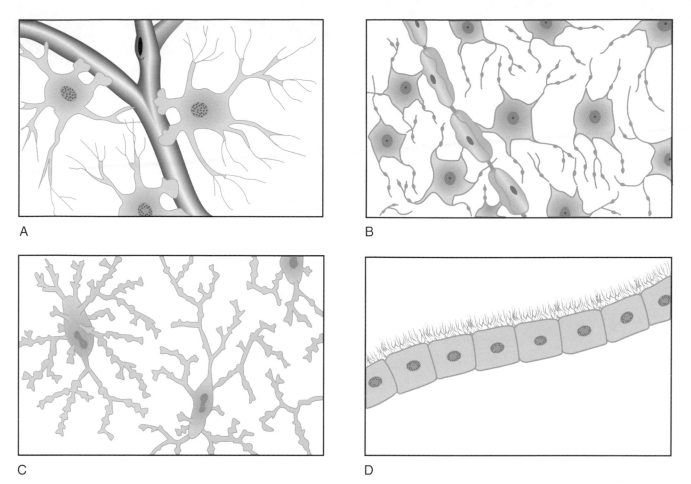

A

B

C

D

■ **FIGURE A&P16–9** Neuroglial cells. **A,** Astrocytes along the capillary. **B,** Oligodendrocytes along the nerves. **C,** Microglia (phagocytes). **D,** Ependymal cells form a sheet that lines fluid cavities in the brain.

Three types of neurons exist:

1. *Unipolar* neurons have only one nerve fiber leaving the cell body, but they branch to form a dendrite and axon. Unipolar neurons often send general sensory signals.
2. *Multipolar* neurons have numerous afferent synapses and axons that make multiple synapses.
3. *Bipolar* neurons are often utilized in the pathways of special sensory systems (eyes, nose, and ears).

Synapses, which are crucial to nerve function, are small spaces between neurons and their targets (other neurons, muscles, or glands). As a message travels down the neuron, it reaches a synapse that it must cross to "jump" to the next neuron. There are two types of synapses; *chemical* synapses dominate. In an *electrical synapse,* the electrical nerve impulses of two cells cross directly through a very small separation (called *gap junctions* or a *nexus*) from the presynaptic to the postsynaptic cell; this type of synapse is also found in smooth and cardiac muscle cells.

Chemical substances called *neurotransmitters* are discharged into the space *(cleft)* between two neurons and propel the message onto the next neuron. Transmitters

are manufactured in the cell body and transported anterograde to the terminals *(boutons),* stored, and secreted from the vesicles in the first neuron *(presynaptic neuron)* into the synaptic cleft (see Figure A&P16-10). The neurotransmitter excites, inhibits, or modifies signals to the second neuron *(postsynaptic neuron)* by interacting with the receptors on its membrane. More than 100 neurotransmitters have been identified. Box A&P16-1 lists the more common transmitters.

IMPULSE CONDUCTION

Resting Potential

A neuron not conducting a nerve impulse is said to be "resting." Although it is resting, it remains charged and potentially ready to fire. The potential to fire is produced by a difference in electrical charge between the interstitial fluid outside the neuron and the intracellular fluid within (Figure A&P16-11). The inside of the nerve cell is electrically negative, and the interstitial fluid is electrically positive. A resulting membrane potential, measured in millivolts (mV), results from this difference in electrical potential between the two compartments. The *resting*

Modified from Guyton, A.C., & Hall, J.E. (2007). *Textbook of medical physiology* (11th ed.). Philadelphia: Saunders.

■ **FIGURE A&P16–10** A neuron (the basic element of the nervous system) and a chemical synapse.

■ **FIGURE A&P16–11** Generation of nerve impulses. The resting membrane potential is shown at −70 mV.

membrane potential (RMP) of neurons is between −45 and −75 mV, somewhat less polarized than the −90 mV RMP of cardiac and skeletal muscle cells.

The cell is *depolarized* when an influx of sodium makes the membrane potential more positive (i.e., rising to zero). In most cells, this is due to an electrical stimulus transmitted by an adjacent cell.

As the membrane potential rises during depolarization, it reaches a specified level *(threshold)*. When threshold is reached, the excited cell is committed to full action potential because the cell follows an all-or-none phenomenon.

Repolarization is the restoration of the membrane polarity, and sodium and potassium are returned to their usual places via the sodium-potassium pump.

After an action potential is generated, no segment of the nerve fiber can conduct another action potential for a brief period of time (<1 ms). This interval is called the *absolute refractory period.* Sodium and potassium are returning to their original locations during this period, and sodium cannot enter the nerve cell. During the next period, called the *relative refractory period,* only a stimulus stronger than the ordinary one can produce an action potential. On average, a return to a resting potential takes approximately 10 to 30 ms.

Nerve Impulses

Because neurons are arranged in chain-like pathways, impulses must travel quickly from one cell to another. In nerve cells the impulse begins at the axon. When the action potential reaches the presynaptic knob at the dendrite, the membrane's permeability to calcium increases, allowing increased calcium influx. Calcium promotes fusing of the vesicles with the membrane and release of the neurotransmitters inside. Some neurotransmitters are transported back into the vesicles *(reuptake).* Others are decomposed by an enzyme process. For example, acetylcholinesterase decomposes acetylcholine at the postsynaptic membrane.

Myelin

Myelin surrounds most large nerve fibers and is separated by nodes of Ranvier. Action potentials are generated only at the nodes, and thus they skip between them rather than depolarize the entire membrane. This jumping characteristic is known as *saltatory conduction.* Conduction using this process is rapid. Neurons with their axons covered by myelin are called *myelinated nerve fibers;* neurons with little or no myelin are called *unmyelinated nerve fibers.* Myelinated fibers in the CNS constitute the *white matter* in the brain and spinal cord. *Gray matter* consists of cell bodies. The speed of the nerve impulse conduction is also related to the diameter of the fiber; the greater the diameter, the faster the impulse.

Receptors

Receptors are biologic transducers that use the stimulus of one form of energy—mechanical, electrical, chemical, thermal, or light—to initiate the "electrical" energy of the nerve impulse. Although sensory receptors may be stimulated by more than one form of energy, each receptor is especially sensitive to a particular form of energy.

Receptors exhibit a phenomenon known as *adaptation,* a decreased receptor sensitivity in response to steady continuous stimuli. Slow-adapting receptors can maintain the lower rate of discharge for minutes to even hours. Fast-adapting receptor bursts of impulses terminate less than 1 second after initiation of the stimulus. The mechanism of adaptation is not known.

Receptors respond more effectively to change than to continuous stimulation. This characteristic of nerve "fatigue" is protective.

PERIPHERAL NERVOUS SYSTEM

The PNS includes all neurons other than those in the brain and spinal cord. It consists of pathways of nerve fibers between the CNS and all outlying structures in the body. Included in the PNS are 12 pairs of cranial nerves and 31 pairs of spinal nerves.

Nerves that conduct impulses to the brain and spinal cord are called *sensory (afferent) neurons.* Nerves that conduct impulses away from the brain and spinal cord are called *motor (efferent) neurons.* Most nerves are mixed, having both sensory and motor components.

SPINAL NERVES

The spinal nerves develop from a series of nerve rootlets that collect laterally as spinal roots. Each spinal nerve consists of a *dorsal (sensory) root* and a *ventral (motor) root,* which unite to form a spinal nerve. The dorsal root emerges from the posterolateral cord. The ventral root emerges from the anterolateral spinal cord. There are 31 pairs of spinal nerves: 8 pairs of cervical nerves, 12 pairs of thoracic nerves, 5 pairs of lumbar nerves, 5 pairs of sacral nerves, and usually 1 pair of coccygeal nerves (see Figure A&P16-4). The specific area of sensory reception for each dorsal root is called a *sensory dermatome* (Figure A&P16-12).

The peripheral nerves that are formed into plexuses have specific names. There are three major plexuses:

1. The *cervical plexus* supplies the muscles and skin of the neck and branches to form the phrenic nerve, which innervates the diaphragm.
2. The *brachial plexus* supplies the muscles and skin of the shoulder, axilla, arm, forearm, and hand. It branches to form the ulnar, median, and radial nerves.
3. The *lumbosacral plexus* supplies sensory and motor impulses to the muscles and skin of the perineum, gluteal region, thighs, legs, and feet. Its many branches include the pudendal, gluteal, femoral, sciatic, tibial, and common fibular nerves.

CRANIAL NERVES

Twelve pairs of cranial nerves arise from the brain. Most of the cranial nerves are composed of both motor and sensory neurons, although a few cranial nerves carry only sensory impulses (Figure A&P16-13). Except for the olfactory and optic nerves, whose nuclei lie just below the cerebrum, all other cranial nerve nuclei lie within the brain stem. Table A&P16-3 presents the 12 pairs of cranial nerves.

■ **FIGURE A&P16–12** Dermatomes (segments of the spinal cord) indicate distribution of spinal nerves. *Solid lines* divide the regions of the spinal cord (i.e., cervical, thoracic, lumbar, sacral). *Dotted lines* indicate dermatomes. **A,** Torso and limbs. **B,** Anterior chest. **C,** Perineum. **D,** Feet. Dermatomes are used during assessment to identify specific areas of sensory impairment (e.g., touch, pain, temperature).

AUTONOMIC NERVOUS SYSTEM

The autonomic nervous system (ANS) is the part of the PNS that coordinates involuntary activities, such as visceral functions, smooth and cardiac muscle changes, and glandular responses. Although it can function independently, its primary control is from the brain and spinal cord. The ANS has two divisions: the *sympathetic* and *parasympathetic nervous systems*. The efferent ANS fibers travel within some cranial and spinal nerves. These two systems are highly integrated and interact with each other to maintain a stable internal environment.

Unlike the *somatic* neurons, which usually are single neurons linking the CNS to a muscle or gland, the ANS has a *two-neuron chain* leading to the effector organ. The terminal of the first neuron is located in the CNS and synapses with nerve fibers whose cell bodies are within an autonomic ganglion. The axon of the second neuron *(postganglionic fiber)* carries impulses to the target viscera. An exception is the adrenal medulla, which is innervated directly by preganglionic fibers.

The medulla is actually composed of postganglionic neurons that secrete epinephrine into the bloodstream during an "adrenaline rush."

The *sympathetic nervous system* coordinates activities used to handle stress and is geared for action as a whole for short periods. The preganglionic neurons of the sympathetic nervous system emerge from the spinal cord via the motor (ventral) roots of the thoracic and upper two lumbar spinal nerves (T1-L2) (Figure A&P16-14). Preganglionic axons are short; postganglionic axons are long.

The *parasympathetic nervous system* is associated with conservation and restoration of energy stores and is geared to act locally and discretely for a longer duration. The preganglionic fibers emerge from the brain stem via the cranial nerves and from the spinal cord via the sacral spinal nerves at S-4. These preganglionic fibers have long axons that synapse with the postganglionic neurons in ganglia close to or located within the organs to be innervated. Each postganglionic neuron has a relatively short axon. Most, but not all, organ systems have both parasympathetic and sympathetic innervation. About 75% of the parasympathetic fibers are in the vagus nerve.

■ **FIGURE A&P16–13** Ventral surface of the brain showing the attachment of the cranial nerves. *(From Thibodeau, G., & Patton, K. [2007]. Anatomy and physiology [6th ed.]. St. Louis: Mosby.)*

TABLE A&P16–3   Functions and Types of Cranial Nerves

	Name	Function	Type
I	Olfactory	Olfaction (smell)	Sensory
II	Optic	Vision	Sensory
III	Oculomotor	Extraocular eye movement	Motor
		Elevation of eyelid	
		Pupil constriction	Parasympathetic
IV	Trochlear	Extraocular eye movement	Motor
V	Trigeminal		
	Ophthalmic division	Somatic sensations of cornea, nasal mucous membranes, face	Sensory
	Maxillary division	Somatic sensations of face, oral cavity, anterior two thirds of tongue, teeth	Sensory
	Mandibular division	Somatic sensation of lower face	Sensory
		Mastication (chewing)	Motor
VI	Abducens	Lateral eye movement	Motor
VII	Facial	Facial expression	Motor
		Taste, anterior two thirds of tongue	Sensory
		Salivation	Parasympathetic
VIII	Vestibulocochlear		
	Vestibular	Equilibrium	Sensory
	Cochlear	Hearing	Sensory
IX	Glossopharyngeal	Taste, posterior third of tongue; pharyngeal sensation	Sensory
		Swallowing	Motor
X	Vagus	Sensation in pharynx, larynx, external ear	Sensory
		Swallowing	Motor
		Thoracic and abdominal visceral parasympathetic nervous system activities	Parasympathetic
XI	Spinal accessory	Neck and shoulder movement	Motor
XII	Hypoglossal	Tongue movement	Motor

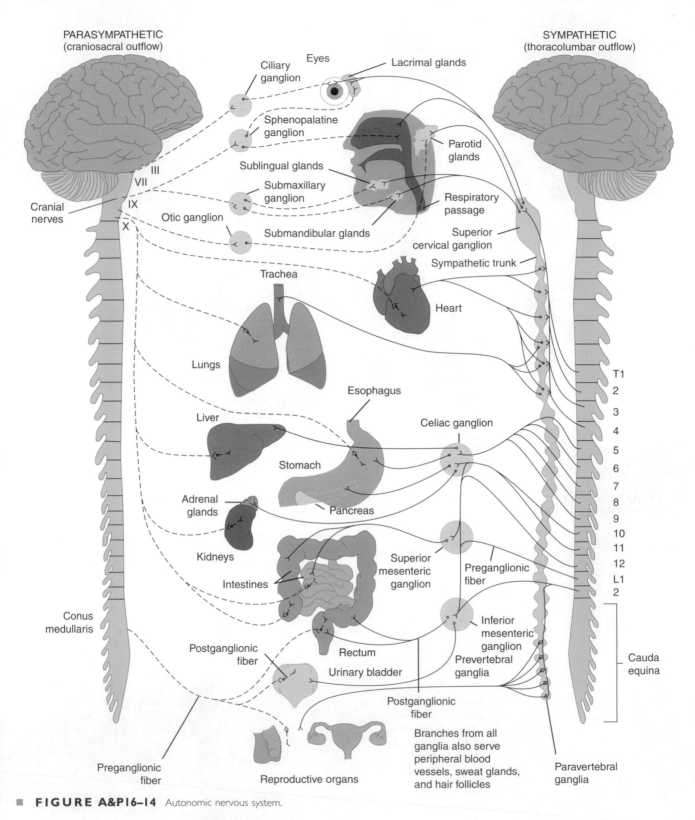

PARASYMPATHETIC
(craniosacral outflow)

SYMPATHETIC
(thoracolumbar outflow)

■ **FIGURE A&P16–14** Autonomic nervous system.

Table A&P16-4 lists the effects of both the sympathetic and parasympathetic nervous systems on different organs. These functions and responses are related to the type of neurotransmitter released. The preganglionic fibers of the sympathetic and parasympathetic nerves and the postganglionic fibers of the parasympathetic nerves release acetylcholine. The postganglionic fibers of the sympathetic nerves release norepinephrine. Fibers that secrete

TABLE A&P16–4   Effects of the Sympathetic and Parasympathetic Nervous Systems on Organs

Organ	Effect of Sympathetic Stimulation	Effect of Parasympathetic Stimulation
Eye		
Pupil	Dilation (alpha)	Constriction
Ciliary muscle	Slight relaxation (far vision)	Constriction (near vision)
Glands	Vasoconstriction and slight secretion	Stimulation of copious secretion (containing many enzymes for enzyme-secreting glands)
Nasal		
Lacrimal		
Parotid		
Submandibular		
Gastric		
Pancreatic		
Sweat glands	Copious sweating (cholinergic)	Sweating on palms of hands
Apocrine glands	Thick, odoriferous secretion	None
Heart		
Muscle	Increased rate ($beta_1$)	Slowed rate
	Increased force of contraction ($beta_1$)	Decreased force of contraction (especially of atria)
Coronaries	Dilated ($beta_2$); constricted (alpha)	Dilation
Lungs		
Bronchi	Dilation ($beta_2$)	Constriction
Blood vessels	Mild constriction	? Dilation
Gut		
Lumen	Decreased peristalsis and tone ($beta_2$)	Increased peristalsis and tone
Sphincter	Increased tone (alpha)	Relaxation (most times)
Liver	Gluconeogenesis, glycogenolysis ($beta_2$)	Slight glycogen synthesis
Gallbladder and bile ducts	Relaxation	Contraction
Kidney	Decreased output and renin secretion	None
Bladder		
Detrusor	Relaxation (slight) ($beta_2$)	Contraction
Trigone	Contraction (alpha)	Relaxation
Penis	Ejaculation	Erection
Systemic arterioles		
Abdominal viscera	Constriction (alpha)	None
Muscle	Constriction (alpha)	None
	Dilation ($beta_2$)	
	Dilation (cholinergic)	
Skin	Constriction	None
Blood		
Coagulation	Increase	None
Glucose	Increase	None
Lipids	Increase	None
Basal metabolism	Increase up to 100%	None
Adrenal medullary secretion	Increase	None
Mental activity	Increase	None
Piloerector muscles	Contraction (alpha)	None
Skeletal muscle	Increased glycogenolysis ($beta_2$)	None
	Increased strength	
Fat cells	Lipolysis ($beta_3$)	None

Modified from Guyton, A.C., & Hall, J.E. (2007). *Textbook of medical physiology* (11th ed.). Philadelphia: Saunders.

acetylcholine are called *cholinergic fibers;* fibers that secrete norepinephrine are called *adrenergic fibers*.

The complexity of the sympathetic and parasympathetic response also depends on the type of receptor that combines with the neurotransmitter. The sympathetic nervous system has five types of receptors: alpha$_1$, alpha$_2$, beta$_1$, beta$_2$, and beta$_3$. The parasympathetic nervous system has two general classes of receptors, muscarinic and nicotinic.

EFFECTS OF INJURY ON THE NERVOUS SYSTEM

REGENERATION

For many years it was thought that nerve cell bodies were not able to regenerate; however, it appears that CNS cortical neurons do attempt to regenerate. PNS regeneration can occur if only the axon in the PNS is injured. Initially there is breakdown of the myelin sheath and axon. The axon swells and fragments while the myelin sheath disintegrates distal to the injury. The cell body takes up water. Macrophages phagocytose the breakdown products. Neurilemma cells migrate into the emerging space (Figure A&P16-15).

The injured axon tip forms a new plasma membrane. A few days after injury, sprouts emerge from the tip. Peripheral nerve sprouts enter the distal stump and often come in contact with a neurilemma cord, which serves as a guide. The regenerating axon grows along the cord at a rate of 4 mm daily. Later the neurilemma cells encapsulate the regenerating nerve fibers. With time the axon and myelin sheath both thicken. Axons within the CNS sprout and form growing tips but appear unable to sustain the metabolic responses necessary for extensive regeneration. It is believed that the axon tip is not able to penetrate the glial scar formed at the injury site, such as after spinal cord injury.

An uninjured axon may sprout a collateral branch at a node of Ranvier that may enter into an adjacent denervated neurilemma cord. Collateral nerve regeneration occurs in both the PNS and the CNS, for example, after peripheral nerve trauma or inflammation of a peripheral nerve, as in Bell's palsy.

EFFECTS OF AGING ON THE NERVOUS SYSTEM

Neurons undergo senescence. Intracellular, cellular, and biochemical changes occur. Lipofuscin accumulates in the cell. Neurofibrillary tangles and senile plaques develop. After we reach 30 years of age, neurons decrease in number and neuroglial cells increase in size and number. The number of dendrites decreases, but the intrinsic dendritic changes are quite variable in hippocampal areas of the brain on postmortem examination in the normal aging population. Variations in dendrite length, stability, and growth have been attributed to compensatory response to death of dendrites.

Aging has little effect on sensory and primary memory but causes a decrease in working memory, including longer retrieval times for short-term memory, categorization, and episodic memory. Dendritic changes are quite pronounced in pathologic conditions such as Alzheimer's disease (see Chapter 72). The axons also change in normal aging; their diameters thin, and the number of receptors decreases.

CONCLUSIONS

The nervous system has three major divisions:

1. The CNS regulates higher-level processes, such as thought and vital functions.
2. The PNS provides pathways to the CNS.
3. The ANS coordinates involuntary activities such as digestion.

The *neuron* is the structural and functional unit of the nervous system. The typical neuron is composed of a cell body, one axon, and several dendrites. The impulses along the nerve are carried through the action of several electrolytes. Neurotransmitters carry the impulse from neuron to neuron.

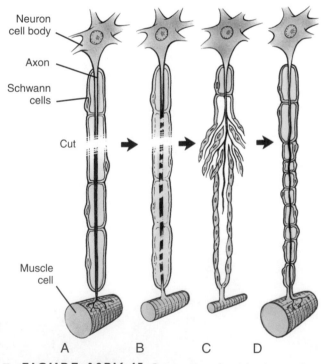

Neuron cell body
Axon
Schwann cells
Cut
Muscle cell

A B C D

■ **FIGURE A&P16–15** Regeneration of peripheral nerve tissue. **A,** An injury results in a cut nerve. **B,** Immediately after the injury, the distal portion of the axon degenerates, as does its myelin sheath. **C,** The remaining neurilemma cells tunnel from the point of injury to the effector. New Schwann cells grow within this tunnel, maintaining a path for regrowth of the axon. Meanwhile, several growing fibers reach the tunnel. **D,** The neuron's attachment is reestablished. *(From Thibodeau, G., & Patton, K. [2007]. Anatomy and physiology [6th ed.]. St. Louis: Mosby.)*

BIBLIOGRAPHY

1. Berne, R., et al. (2007). *Physiology* (5th ed.). St. Louis: Mosby.
2. Guyton, A.C., & Hall, J.E. (2007). *Textbook of medical physiology* (11th ed.). Philadelphia: Saunders.
3. Kandel, E.R., Schwartz, J.H., & Jessel, T.M. (2000). *Principles of neural science* (4th ed.). New York: McGraw-Hill.
4. Thibodeau, G., & Patton, K. (2007). *Anatomy and physiology* (6th ed.). St. Louis: Mosby.

CHAPTER 67

Assessment of the Neurologic System

CLARE M. SEKERAK

Assessment of a client experiencing a neurologic disorder is a challenge. Neurologic disorders range from simple to complex and can have profound consequences for activities of daily living (ADL) and survival. Neurologic assessment establishes baseline data that are used to compare ongoing assessments, diagnose actual and potential health problems, manage client care, and evaluate the outcome. Because of the complexity of the nervous system, neurologic assessment is both multifaceted and lengthy. A comprehensive history, a neurologic examination, and general or specific neurodiagnostic studies are the primary components of a neurologic assessment.

Neurologic assessment is both anatomic and functional. Continuous observations of the client are made and compared with baseline data. Astute observations are essential because many neurologic changes occur subtly. Nurses collect data on the client's ability to function physically (self-care deficit) and mentally (confusion and altered problem solving). Finally, because many neurologic disorders are serious, the nurse provides skillful, crisis-oriented support for the client and significant others.

This chapter presents basic neurologic assessment procedures. Additional assessment techniques for specific neurologic disorders are discussed throughout Unit 16. To avoid missing parts of a complex examination, novice practitioners should follow the assessment sequence described in this chapter. The sequence suggested in Table 67-1 integrates cranial nerve and reflex testing into motor and sensory examinations.

HISTORY

The history consists of biographical data, the chief complaint and clinical manifestation analysis, a review of systems, past medical history, surgical history, allergies, medications history, dietary habits, psychosocial history, and family health history.

The health history guides the physical examination. Some complaints require a complete neurologic examination while other complaints may require a more focused examination on a particular system or anatomic area. For example, a complaint of dizziness cues a focus on examination of the eyes, ears (vestibular nerve), and cerebellar function instead of motor and sensory functions. Detailed neurologic examination is indicated when the client reports behavioral changes, altered level of consciousness (LOC), growth and development problems, pain, changes in motor or sensory function, infection, or trauma.

Assess for neurologic problems that may be related to other problems, such as alcohol and recreational drug use, metabolic imbalances, and metastatic lesions.

Biographical and Demographic Data

Biographical data comprise demographic, administrative, and insurance information. Often included are (1) a personal profile or brief description of the client, (2) the source of the history (client or a significant other),

---

evolve Web Enhancements

Assessment Terms   English and Spanish

Appendix A   Religious Beliefs and Practices Affecting Health Care

Appendix B   A Health History Format That Integrates the Assessment of Functional Health Patterns

Web Figures   Cerebral Angiography

Electromyography

Web Tables   Normal Cerebrospinal Fluid (CSF) Values and Significance of Abnormal Values

Web Boxes   Terms Associated with Gait Disorders

Types of Electrical Brain Waves

Be sure to check out the bonus material on the Evolve website and the CD-ROM, including free self-assessment exercises. **http://evolve.elsevier.com/Black/medsurg**

TABLE 67-1 Neurologic Assessment Guidelines

Functional Category	Specific Category	Area of Nervous System Involved	Assessment Technique	Examples of Disorders
1. Consciousness (awareness of self and environment)	Arousal response to verbal, tactile, and visual stimuli	Reticular activating system (mesencephalon, diencephalon) Both hemispheres	Is client alert? What is attention span? Is there normal response to visual and auditory stimuli? Reaction to loud noises, shaking, deep pressure over eye orbits or sternum? Are vital signs, pupils, and reflexes normal?	Elevation: insomnia, agitation, mania, delirium Depression: somnolence, lethargy, semicoma, coma
2. Mentation	Thinking	Cerebral hemispheres plus specific regional functions	Is client oriented (time, place, person)?	Disorientation
	Insight, judgment, planning	Frontal lobe, with association fibers to other area of cerebrum	Does client recognize implication of illness? Are goals congruent with abilities? How would client respond to given situation (house on fire)?	Lack of judgment, inattention to grooming, appearance, and personal habits
	Fund of information	Basic biologic intellect (frontal lobe) integrated into other areas	Calculation ability, knowledge of current events consistent with educational level. Who is U.S. president?	Impairment—functioning not congruent with level of education
	Memory	Temporal lobe and association to most other areas of cortex		
	Recent	Hippocampus	What did client eat for breakfast? What happened yesterday?	Dementia
	Past	Frontal lobe	Recall past events during taking of history.	Lapses of memory for past events may coincide with past CNS problems (trauma, infection, psychic trauma)
	Feeling (affect) (congruence of response to stimulus)	Limbic system (usually involves both hemispheres)	Compare observed with expected reactions. Are emotions labile? Appropriate?	Blunted affect: hysteria, schizophrenia, bilateral frontal lobe lesions
	Perceptual distortions (illusions, hallucinations)	General and specific cortical areas in hallucinations	Observe for behavior indicating perceptual problems.	Irritative lesions of cortex may lead to hallucinations (occipital cortex → visual, postcentral gyrus → somatic sensation, uncus → smell)
3. Language and speech	Dysarthria (defects in articulation, enunciation, and rhythm in speech)	Impairment of muscles of tongue, palate, pharynx, or lips (may be due to impulses or incoordination) Brain stem, cerebellum, or extraneural causes; CN V, VII, IX, X, XII	Have client repeat a difficult phrase ("Susie sells seashells by the seashore").	Slurring, slowness, indistinctness, nasality, break in normal speech rhythm (speech of intoxication); amyotrophic lateral sclerosis; pseudobulbar palsy; myasthenia gravis; stroke
	Dysphonia (abnormal production of sounds from larynx)	Recurrent laryngeal nerve problems (part of vagus, CN X)	Is client's voice hoarse, strained, soft?	Parkinsonism, dystonia
		Many extraneural causes	Whispered voice is intact. Use indirect laryngoscopy findings.	Compression of recurrent laryngeal nerve by bronchogenic carcinoma of left mainstem bronchus
				Left atrial hypertrophy
		Medulla (area of nucleus of CN X)		Brain stem tumors, occlusion of posterior inferior cerebellar or vertebral artery

Aphasia (inability to use and understand written and spoken words)	Fluent (receptive): left temporal and parietal lobes (Wernicke's area)	Observe vocal expression, written expression, comprehension of spoken and written language, and gesture communication.	Stroke of middle cerebral artery Trauma, tumor, abscess in left temporal and parietal lobe areas
	Nonfluent (expressive): Broca's area (lateral) inferior portion of frontal lobe of dominant side		Damage to Broca's area or association fibers (stroke, tumor)
	Global (combined)		
Agnosia (inability to recognize objects or symbols by means of senses)	Primarily in parietal, temporal, and occipital areas	Sense organs intact? Can the client recognize objects by sight, touch, hearing?	Stroke
4. Motor function Expression (facial)	CN VII	Symmetry of smile, frown, raising of eyebrows	Central facial weakness (upper motor neuron dysfunction); weakness of lower half of face *Causes:* stroke, corticobulbar tract Peripheral facial weakness (lower motor dysfunction); weakness of entire half of face *Causes:* Bell's palsy, brain stem tumor, fracture of temporal bone
Eating (chewing, swallowing)	CN V, VII, IX, X, XII	Strength of masticator muscles, gag reflexes, ability to swallow	Tetanus, peripheral spasm of muscle; amyotrophic lateral sclerosis, medullary tumor; pseudobulbar palsy may be associated with dysarthria
Eye movements	CN III, IV, VI	Extraocular movement, pupil size, reactivity, pupils react equally to accommodation, diplopia, nystagmus	Cerebral peduncle pressure → CN III dysfunction, cavernous sinus thrombus → CN III, IV, VI problem Muscular problems (myasthenia gravis, hyperthyroid) Horner's syndrome (ptosis, constricted pupil), anisocoria
Moving	Motor precentral gyrus (pyramidal) and cerebellar systems, basal ganglia, CN XI, spinal cord, upper motor neuron (brain → spinal cord via corticospinal tract)	Gait, heel-to-toe walking, presence or absence of involuntary movements, coordination, muscle tone, mass, strength, Romberg's test, ability to shrug shoulders and to rise from chair	*Upper motor neuron:* Brain and cord-sparing anterior horn cell Tone ↑↑ (spastic) Bulk ↓ because of atrophy of disuse Reflexes ↑↑ because of loss of central inhibition No fasciculations Frequent clonus
	Lower motor neuron (motor cells of cranial and spinal nerves and anterior horn cells → peripheral muscles)		*Lower motor neuron:* Segment anterior horn cell peripheral nerve Tone ↓↓ (flaccid) Bulk ↓ because of tone loss Reflexes ↓ or absent from loss of anterior horn cell Fasciculations No clonus
	Involves cerebellum		*Cerebellar problem* → loss of coordination and balance

(Continued)

TABLE 67-1 Neurologic Assessment Guidelines —Cont'd

Functional Category	Specific Category	Area of Nervous System Involved	Assessment Technique	Examples of Disorders
5. Sensory function	Seeing	CN II: optic, occipital lobe	Acuity, visual fields, funduscopy	Field test: loss in retina or optic nerve → loss in eye involved, optic chiasm → bitemporal hemianopsia
				Optic tract → homonymous hemianopsia, parietal lobe → quadrant problems (inferior), temporal lobe → superior quadrant problems
				↑ Intracranial pressure → papilledema (raised disc → hemorrhage)
	Smelling	CN I: temporal lobe (uncus)	Ability to detect familiar odors	Usually ↓ smell from extraneural causes (upper respiratory tract infection, allergy, smoking); olfactory groove; meningioma, olfactory hallucinations
	Hearing	CN VIII: cochlear division, temporal lobe	Acuity of hearing, presence or absence of unusual sounds, Weber and Rinne tests	May have conductive (nerve OK) or neural hearing loss; Ménière's syndrome (tinnitus, hearing loss, vertigo, and nystagmus), basilar skull fracture → otorrhea
				Brain stem vascular dysfunction or tumors → ↓ hearing
	Taste	CN VII, IX: insular lobe	Ability to differentiate sweet, salt, sour, and bitter	Brain stem or insula lesions → ↓ taste; extraneural causes, smoking, poor oral hygiene
	Feeling (sensory)	Peripheral nerves → Dermatomes → Spinal cord → Tracts (leading to)	Pain: pinprick	Polyneuropathy (diabetes mellitus, anemia)
			Touch: cotton touched to skin	Spinal cord lesions → dermatome alterations
			Proprioception: check where digit is in space	Upper pons → thalamus, contralateral loss
		Pain-temperature-tactile, anterolateral system, proprioception, stereognosis, dorsal roots → thalamus leading to somasthetic area (postcentral gyrus, parietal lobe)	Vibration: place vibrating tuning fork on bony prominence	Thalamus → contralateral loss + paresthesias
			Temperature: test tubes of cold and warm water laid against skin; person identifies whether hot or cold	Thalamus → cortex → cortical sensory loss
6. Bowel and bladder function	Bowel function	Afferent Spinal nerve S3-5 External sphincter (voluntary control) Internal sphincter	Check for fecal impaction or incontinence	Fecal incontinence with lesions S3-5
			Check muscle tone	Anal anesthesia—conus medullaris and tabes dorsalis
		Autonomic nervous system		May be extraneural causes
		Cerebral cortex		Loss of inhibitory control (stroke)
	Bladder function	Autonomic nervous system	Feels when bladder is full, complete emptying	Urinary incontinence
			Does client have urgency, frequency?	
		Afferent Spinal nerve T9-L2, S2-4 Pudendal nerve		Flaccid bladder
		Efferent Spinal nerve T11-L2 External sphincter (voluntary) Spinal nerve S2-4 Cerebral cortex		Spastic bladder
				Loss of inhibitory control (stroke) May be extraneural causes

C, Cervical; CN, cranial nerve; CNS, central nervous system; L, lumbar; S, sacral; T, thoracic; ↑, increased; ↑↑, significantly increased; ↓, decreased; ↓↓, significantly decreased; →, may affect or lead to.

and (3) the client's mental status (indicating the reliability of the data). Neurologic problems often affect mental status, sometimes making it difficult to obtain an accurate history directly from the client.

Current Health

Ask about the client's current state of health. Neurologic disorders often affect the client's lifestyle. The history should begin with an open-ended and non-direct inquiry to allow the client to describe the problem. Allow the client to describe how current conditions impact daily life. Explore areas of concern for the client.

Chief Complaint

Obtain a detailed description of the events that have led the client to seek care. Avoid suggesting manifestations to the client, and use open-ended questions. Allow clients to describe the problem in their own words and try not to interrupt. When given the opportunity, often clients will disclose their real concerns as the history-taking proceeds. A client with a complaint of headaches may only be concerned about headaches or may be fearful of a more serious problem such as brain tumor or aneurysm. If the client feels rushed or interrupted, these concerns may not be revealed. Elicit a detailed report from the client regarding the issues that relate to the chief complaint (Figure 67-1).

Clinical Manifestations

Determine the onset and sequence of manifestations and their progress. Ask the client to describe neurologic disease processes accurately to facilitate the diagnostic process. Allow the client to describe manifestations using his or her own words. Use a systematic analysis to elicit the characteristics and progression of manifestations (see Chapter 2). Inquire about the frequency, duration, and location of manifestations. Ask about related complaints. For example, urinary retention and bowel incontinence can occur in spinal injuries. Ask the client what improves or aggravates the condition. Common clinical manifestations of neurologic problems include pain, dizziness, sensory and/or motor function complaints, and LOC issues. The chief complaint guides the discussion of the clinical manifestations.

Pain. Pain is a common complaint of clients presenting with neurologic problems. Discussion should focus on the site (headache, back pain, pain in extremities), onset (sudden, gradual), frequency, duration, and character (throbbing, achy, dull, or sharp). Does the pain go anywhere else? What are the precipitating factors (headaches: aura, walking, neck movement) and relieving factors (medications, stretching, rest, applying cold/heat)? Ask about injury or trauma, including previous neurologic

injuries. Inquiry should also include related manifestations (headache: nausea, back pain: muscle spasms). Refer to the Integrating Diagnostic Testing feature on p. 1769 for details of further diagnostic evaluation of the client with complaints related to suspected nerve root compression, a possible cause for pain of neurologic origin.

Dizziness. Many clients present with a complaint of dizziness. Ask the client to describe what is meant by "dizziness" (lightheaded vs. room spinning). Ask if it is related to postural changes (orthostatic blood pressure drop, positional vertigo). What head movements cause problems? What happens when the client turns rapidly or rolls over in bed? Does the client have vision problems? Does the client have ear problems such as hearing loss, ringing, or buzzing (tinnitus)? Does the dizziness improve or worsen when eyes are closed? Does visual fixation help? Inquire about other causes of dizziness (cardiac dysrhythmias, anxiety [panic attacks], history of diabetes mellitus [decreased blood glucose level], ear infection).

Sensory Complaints. Common sensory complaints of the neurologic client include alterations in the ability to see, taste, hear, smell, and feel (pain, numbness, tingling). Ask the client to describe the sensation and its quality (shooting, stabbing, dull, sharp) and its severity. Ask about the site of the sensory abnormality as well as the distribution (stocking glove, extremity). Inquire about onset, frequency, and duration of manifestations. What are the precipitating factors (walking, neck movement, chewing, exposure to cold)? What relieves the manifestations (rest, change of position, medications)? Refer to the Integrating Diagnostic Testing feature on p. 1770 for details of the evaluation of a sensory complaint.

Motor Complaints. Motor complains include weakness, problems with coordination (balance, clumsiness, and gait disturbances), and involuntary movements (tremor, tics). Inquire about the site, onset, frequency, and duration of any manifestations. What precipitates and what improves these conditions?

Loss of Consciousness/Alterations in Mental Status. Impaired consciousness level is a common neurologic problem. Inquire about onset (gradual or sudden) and duration (transient or persistent). If the client's LOC remains diminished at the time of the interview, other sources of information such as family, friends, and the ambulance team may need to be questioned. Refer to the Integrating Diagnostic Testing feature on p. 1771 for details of the evaluation of the client who presents with alterations in level of consciousness.

Is there a history of head trauma (immediately leading to admission or recent: within 6 weeks)? If there is a history of trauma, what type of trauma occurred (fall, blunt force, motor vehicle accident, sports injury with head

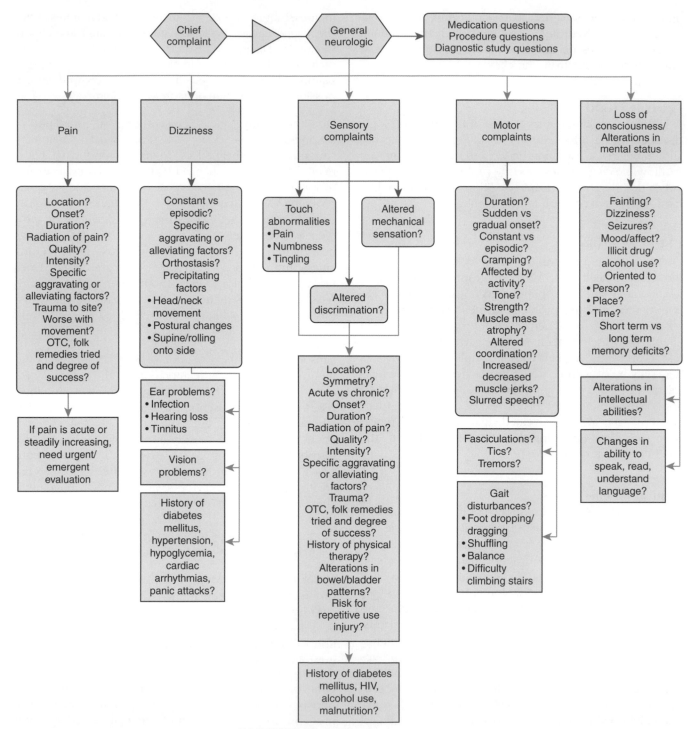

FIGURE 67–1   Expanded neurologic assessment.

impact)? Is there limb twitching and incontinence (seizure) associated with the episode of decreased level of consciousness? What precipitated the episode (injury, infection, fever, aura)? Does the client have a history of diabetes mellitus, alcoholism, drug abuse, psychiatric illness (drug overdose), or epilepsy?

Review of Systems

In contrast to the assessment of current health where the client is encouraged to give information through openended and general questions, the review of systems (ROS) uses direct questions. The purpose of the ROS is to gain more information about the client's presentation.

INTEGRATING DIAGNOSTIC TESTING

Nerve Root Compression

Clinical manifestations consistent with spinal cord and nerve root compression

Laboratory tests based on medical history (infection, fever, chills, IV drug use)

Diagnostic studies

Laboratory testing:
Infection:
CBC: WBC
ESR
C-reactive protein
Blood cultures
CSF: WBC and RBC

Subsequent management based on findings.
Options include:
• Acute/urgent/routine neurosurgical management
• Medical management
• Possible physical therapy

Spinal X-Ray: shows fractures, dislocation, compressions, curvature, erosion, narrowed spinal cord canal, congenital malformations, neoplasms, and degenerative processes.

Magnetic Resonance Imaging (MRI): Superior imaging of spinal cord, syrinx, tumors, and cysts. MRI without contrast is used when there is low suspicion for tumor, abscess, or history of prior spine surgery. Gadolinium contrast indicated if history of spine surgery or suspicion is high for tumor or abscess. Contraindicated with certain metal implants.

Myelography (CT myelogram): X-ray study in which contrast material is injected into subarachnoid space to examine spinal canal under CT guidance. A LP is performed and some CSF is removed. Used to visualize intradural nerve roots when MRI is contraindicated.

CBC, Complete blood cell count; *CSF*, cerebrospinal fluid; *ESR*, erythrocyte sedimentation rate; *IV*, intravenous; *LP*, lumbar puncture; *RBC*, red blood cells; *WBC*, white blood cells.

Do not repeat questions already asked earlier in the health history, but ask questions regarding topics not previously assessed (Figure 67-2 on p. 1772).

Neurologic disorders often subtly affect the ability to function in an integrated fashion. Ask the client to describe any neurologic manifestations, such as behavior changes, mood swings, loss of consciousness, seizures, headaches, dizziness, vertigo, memory deficits, speech or motor function problems (unstable balance or posture, gait changes, tics, tremors), and sensory function problems (vision changes, pain, paresthesia or tingling, paralysis). Has the client had any difficulty swallowing or a change in voice? Has the client experienced sexual difficulties such as erectile difficulties or loss of libido? Significant neurologic assessment data are listed in Box 67-1 on p. 1773. Detailed questions for the review of systems can be found on the website.

The client who has a neurologic problem may be unaware of its presence. Attempt to supplement and corroborate the history and review of systems by speaking with a family member or significant other who knows the client well. Ask specifically about mental or physical changes that have been noticed.

Past Medical History

Collect data regarding common childhood diseases and immunizations. Diseases associated with neurologic sequelae include rubella, rubeola, cytomegalovirus infection, herpes simplex, influenza, and meningitis. Ask whether the client has completed the recommended immunization schedule. Public health resources provide schedules for childhood immunizations as well as recommendations for travelers to foreign countries.

The growth and development history may help determine whether neurologic dysfunction was present at an early age. The perinatal history may contain data about maternal toxemia; neural tube defects; or in utero exposure to viruses (rubella), alcohol, tobacco, or other drugs, and radiation. Ask whether the client was born at full term. Premature birth increases the risk of neurologic damage from inadequate oxygenation and intracranial bleeding

INTEGRATING DIAGNOSTIC TESTING

Sensory Complaints

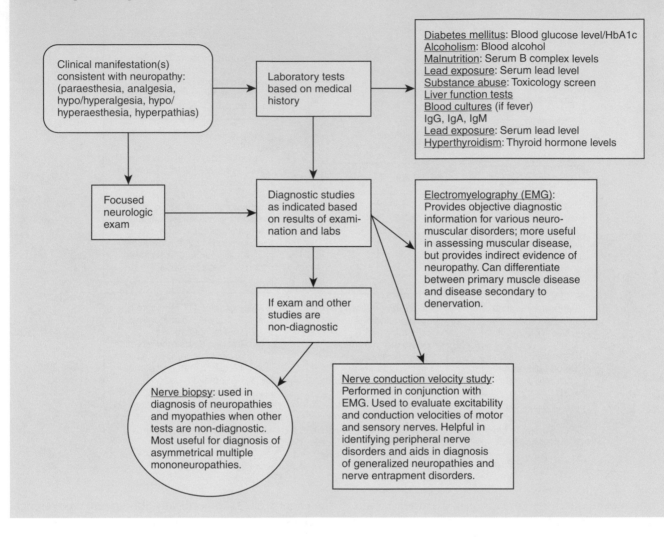

if ventilator support was used. A difficult or prolonged labor and delivery can result in hypoxia or use of forceps or vacuum extraction for delivery, with consequent central and peripheral neurologic damage.

At what age did the client accomplish major developmental tasks, such as walking and talking? Was the client able to participate in games, sports, and other childhood activities with peers? Did the client have any problems with coordination, balance, or agility?

A number of major illnesses are associated with neurologic changes, such as HIV, tuberculosis, diabetes mellitus, pernicious anemia, cancer, infections, shingles, and hypertension. Vascular disorders such as cardiac valve disease and atrial fibrillation are associated with transient ischemic attacks (TIAs) and stroke. Hypertension increases the risk of intracerebral bleeding. Systemic metabolic effects of advanced liver and renal diseases

can affect mental function. Inquire about injuries and hospitalizations for neurologic system problems such as head trauma, seizures, stroke, and crushing tissue injury.

Has the client undergone a neurologic diagnostic study, such as electroencephalography (EEG), electromyography (EMG), magnetic resolution imaging (MRI), or computed tomography (CT)? Results of such diagnostic studies provide valuable data for future comparison.

Past Surgical History

Inquire about the client's past surgeries, especially those related to neurologic problems such as spinal disorders, peripheral neuropathies, and cranial surgeries. Ask about surgical complications as some surgeries have a potential for nerve damage to surrounding tissue. Ask about past exposure to spinal and epidural anesthetics as well as any complications.

INTEGRATING DIAGNOSTIC TESTING

Altered Level of Consciousness

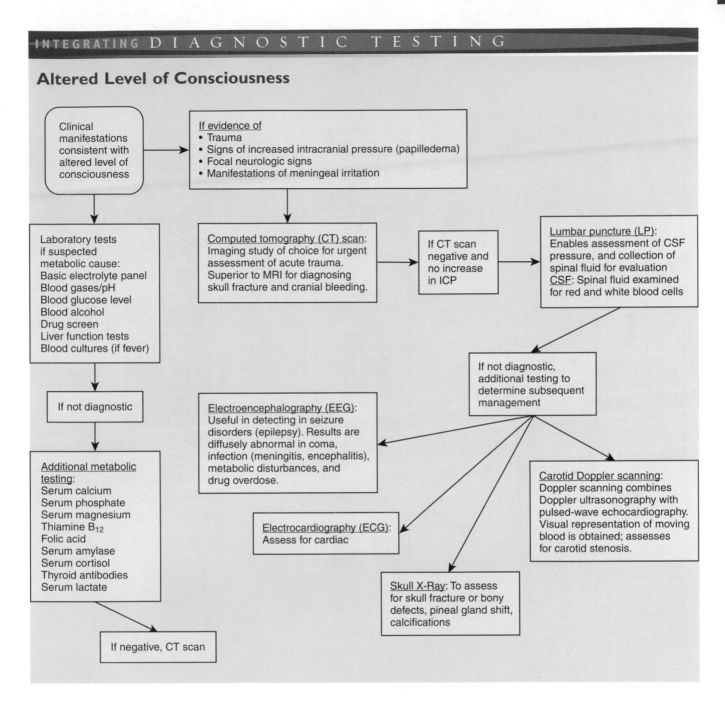

Clinical manifestations consistent with altered level of consciousness

If evidence of
• Trauma
• Signs of increased intracranial pressure (papilledema)
• Focal neurologic signs
• Manifestations of meningeal irritation

Laboratory tests if suspected metabolic cause:
Basic electrolyte panel
Blood gases/pH
Blood glucose level
Blood alcohol
Drug screen
Liver function tests
Blood cultures (if fever)

Computed tomography (CT) scan: Imaging study of choice for urgent assessment of acute trauma. Superior to MRI for diagnosing skull fracture and cranial bleeding.

If CT scan negative and no increase in ICP

Lumbar puncture (LP): Enables assessment of CSF pressure, and collection of spinal fluid for evaluation CSF: Spinal fluid examined for red and white blood cells

If not diagnostic, additional testing to determine subsequent management

If not diagnostic

Electroencephalography (EEG): Useful in detecting in seizure disorders (epilepsy). Results are diffusely abnormal in coma, infection (meningitis, encephalitis), metabolic disturbances, and drug overdose.

Additional metabolic testing:
Serum calcium
Serum phosphate
Serum magnesium
Thiamine B_{12}
Folic acid
Serum amylase
Serum cortisol
Thyroid antibodies
Serum lactate

Electrocardiography (ECG): Assess for cardiac

Carotid Doppler scanning: Doppler scanning combines Doppler ultrasonography with pulsed-wave echocardiography. Visual representation of moving blood is obtained; assesses for carotid stenosis.

Skull X-Ray: To assess for skull fracture or bony defects, pineal gland shift, calcifications

If negative, CT scan

Allergies

Ask the client about food and drug allergies, especially to antibiotics, shellfish, and IV contrast dye.

Medications

The medication history includes all medicines that the client is taking or has taken, both prescription and over-the-counter, including herbal preparations. Specifically ask about aspirin and other anticoagulants, anticonvulsants, antidepressants, antihypertensives, oral contraceptive pills, central nervous system (CNS) stimulants such as diet pills, and CNS depressants such as opioids, antibiotics, antimicrobials, antirheumatics, tranquilizers, and sedatives.

Many medications have side effects involving the parasympathetic or sympathetic nervous system. Medications can have side effects involving the central nervous system, such as confusion, sedation, or agitation. Diet pills have been linked to stroke.[13] Many preparations for allergies and colds contain ingredients that can cause drowsiness. There are many types of medications that can cause peripheral nerve damage. Steroids can cause myopathies. Chemotherapy is associated with neuropathies.

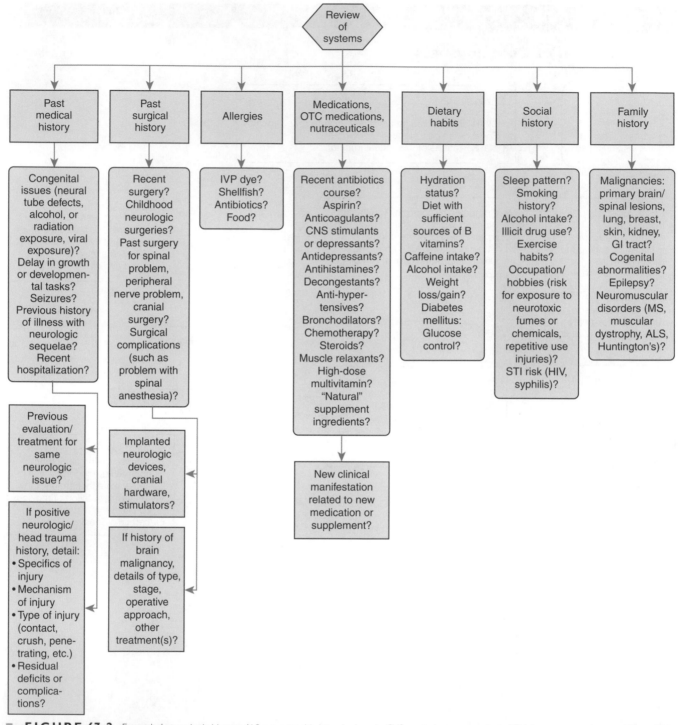

■ **FIGURE 67–2** Expanded neurologic history. *ALS,* amyotrophic lateral sclerosis; *CNS,* central nervous system; *IVP,* intravenous pyelogram; *MS,* multiple sclerosis; *STI,* sexually transmitted infection.

A number of medications may alter the sense of smell, such as antibiotics, antihistamines, decongestants, antihypertensives, bronchodilators, muscle relaxants, and psychiatric agents.

Clients are increasingly turning to herbal medications to treat neurologic problems, may not consider them to be medications, and fail to mention them unless specifically asked. Common herbal preparations used for neurologic problems are listed in Box 67-2.

Dietary Habits

Inquire about the client's dietary habits. Ask the client what was eaten in the previous 24 hours as an example of a typical day's diet. Specifically ask about intake of

---

BOX 67-1 Manifestations Related to Neurologic Assessment

EYE
- Vision and visual field loss
- Diplopia
- Ptosis
- Proptosis

EAR, NOSE, AND THROAT
- Infections
- Hearing loss
- Tinnitus
- Dizziness
- Vertigo
- Voice change
- Dysphagia
- Changes in taste or smell
- Experiences of unusual smells

CARDIOVASCULAR
- Syncope
- Palpitations
- Hypotension
- Hypertension
- Vertigo
- Transient ischemic attacks
- Stroke

NEUROLOGIC
- Weakness
- Numbness
- Paresthesias
- Headache
- Pain
- Altered thinking
- Speech difficulty
- Vomiting
- Vertigo
- Ataxia
- Fainting
- Seizures
- Any loss of consciousness
- Distortions of reality
- Use of consciousness-altering drugs
- Disorientation to time, place, or person
- Altered sleep patterns
- Changes in ability to speak, read, or understand language
- Changes in memory of recent or remote events
- Changes in ability to concentrate

SKIN
- Hair and nail changes

MUSCULOSKELETAL
- Tremor
- Weakness
- Altered coordination
- Staggering
- Difficulty climbing stairs

BOX 67-2 Common Herbal Preparations Used for Neurologic Problems

CNS stimulants: Betel nut *(Areca catechu);* ephedra *(Ephedra sinica, E. vulgaris, E. nevadensis),* also known as Ma Huang, and illegal in some areas; nutmeg *(Myristica fragrans)*

Sedatives/hypnotics: Chamomile *(Matricaria recutita, Chamaemelum nobile);* gotu kola *(Centella asiatica);* hops *(Humulus lupulus);* kava kava *(Piper methysticum);* St. John's wort *(Hypericum perforatum);* valerian *(Valeriana officinalis)*

Antidepressives: *Ginkgo biloba;* sage *(Salvia officinalis);* St. John's wort; sage can be used as an aid for dizziness, as can *G. biloba; G. biloba* has also been indicated for treating tinnitus, short-term memory loss, and headache

Analgesics: Cayenne *(Capsicum),* taken internally for headache and toothache or applied externally for neuralgia; feverfew *(Tanacetum parthenium),* used for prevention of migraine and cluster headaches; white willow *(Salix purpurea, S. fragilis, S. daphnoides),* used as an analgesic and antipyretic

Antihypertensive or anti-stroke effects: Garlic *(Allium sativum); G. biloba;* onion *(Allium cepa);* reishi mushroom *(Ganoderma lucidum)*

---

diabetes mellitus because neuropathies may be related to diabetes mellitus. Discuss weight loss and gain patterns.

whole grains and cereals. Deficiency of vitamin B_{12} causes central nervous system damage leading to polyneuritis and weakness. Deficiencies of B complex vitamins [B_1 (thiamine), B_2 (riboflavin), B_3 (niacin), B_5 (pantothenic acid), or B_6 (pyridoxine)] lead to peripheral nerve damage. Inquire about folic acid supplementation in female clients of childbearing age. Ask about the client's pattern of fluid intake and caffeine consumption. Review diet and blood glucose control of clients with

Social History

An understanding of personal psychosocial factors (educational background, level of performance, and personality changes) enhances assessment. Inquire about changes that have occurred in daily routines. Ask about changes in sleep patterns, exercise routines, perceived stressors, and sexual interest and performance. Ask about sexual history. Has the client engaged in sexual behaviors that increase risk of infections? Inquire about alcohol and tobacco intake. Ask about the client's hobbies, recreational activities, and occupation. Is there risk of exposure to neurotoxic fumes or chemicals such as pesticides, paints, or bonding agents (glue)? Does the client spend time in an inadequately ventilated living area or workspace? Inquire about the current or past use of recreational drugs, the type of drug, and the duration of use.

Family Health History

Ask about a family history of neurologic disorders to determine the presence of genetic risk factors. Inquire about epilepsy, Huntington's disease, amyotrophic lateral sclerosis, muscular dystrophy, hypertension, stroke, mental retardation, and psychiatric disorders. Inquire about family history of cancer such as primary brain or spinal lesions as well as other cancers. Common sources of metastatic brain tumors are cancers of the lung, breast, skin, kidney, and gastrointestinal tract.

PHYSICAL EXAMINATION

The physical examination is intended to detect abnormalities in neurologic functioning. Variations in client age, physical condition, and LOC determine how detailed an examination can be. The neurologic examination is described here. Adapt the examination to the client's severity of illness and ability to cooperate. Box 67-3 presents a guide for adapting the assessment in various situations. A suggested sequence for the physical examination is as follows:

1. Vital signs
2. Mental status (including language and communication)
3. Head, neck, and back
4. Cranial nerves (including pupils)
5. Motor system (including coordination and gait)
6. Sensory function
7. Reflexes
8. Autonomic nervous system

Neurologic findings are summarized in the Physical Assessment Findings in the Healthy Adult feature on p. 1775. For a detailed guide to neurologic assessment, consult a physical examination textbook.

Vital Signs

Assess vital signs first because neurologic disorders can cause life-threatening changes. Clients who have cervical spinal cord injuries exhibit a classic triad of hypotension, bradycardia, and hypothermia related to the loss of sympathetic nervous system function. Changes in vital signs can accompany the late stages of increased intracranial pressure (ICP) in an attempt to preserve brain tissue. *Cushing's response* consists of elevated systolic blood pressure, widened pulse pressure, and bradycardia. Respiratory rate and rhythm can be altered by increased ICP on the brain stem.

Mental Status

Assess and document general data about the client's mental status. The mental status examination includes assessment of level of consciousness (LOC), orientation, memory, mood and affect, intellectual performance,

---

BOX 67-3 The Initial Neurologic Examination in the Clinical Setting

The sequence in which the neurologic examination is performed and the amount of time devoted to each step are dictated by the client's situation. For example, assessment of the head-injured client in the emergency department requires evaluation of vital signs, pupil reactivity, level of consciousness, and motor response. These clients may not be stable or cooperative enough to allow completion of the cranial nerve and sensory response assessment. Spinal cord–injured clients, however, are usually coherent and able to participate in the sensory examination. The sensory assessment information is essential for documenting changes in the status of spinal cord–injured clients.

As clients become more stable and cooperative, the examination can be performed in more depth and with less frequency. Remember that neurologically impaired clients frequently experience fluctuations in status. Alter the assessment schedule and technique to detect and report these fluctuations.

Following are suggested modifications in the screening neurologic examination that may be made on the basis of the client's initial presentation:

Initial examination for diagnosis and triage:
- Client history based on chief complaint
- Physical examination, including vital signs
- Level of consciousness
- Pupillary response
- Brain stem function (corneal reflex)
- Motor and sensory functions in all four extremities

If the client is conscious and stable:
- Complete baseline neurologic examination
- Focused examinations at prescribed intervals

If the client is conscious and unstable:
- Quick baseline physical assessment
- Frequent focused examinations until client is stable
- Vital signs
- Level of consciousness
- Pupillary response
- Brain stem function
- Motor and sensory functions in extremities
- Spinal cord function

If the client is unconscious but stable:
- Vital signs
- Level of consciousness and ability to arouse
- Cranial nerve function
- Motor and sensory functions
- Pathologic reflexes

If the client is unconscious and unstable:
- Vital signs
- Level of consciousness
- Cranial nerve function
- Motor and sensory functions relative to the ability to test for them
- Pathologic reflexes
- Frequent focused examinations on ongoing basis (hourly or more often)

If spinal cord involvement is suspected:
- Motor functions in detail with testing of specific muscle groups
- Sensory function
- Reflexes
- Bowel and bladder functions
- Vital signs

The Neurologic System

INSPECTION

Mental Status. Oriented to person, place, time, and situation. No difficulty recalling recent and past events. Serial 7's deferred. Mood and affect congruent, cooperative, and pleasant. Thought process clear and logical. Demonstrates effective problem solving. Speech articulate, clear, and fluent.

Head, Neck, and Back. Normocephalic without obvious lesions. Maintains head position. Spine in straight alignment with normal cervical, thoracic, and lumbar curves. Neck and back have full range of motion.

CRANIAL NERVES

CN I. Discerns smell of coffee, cinnamon, alcohol.

CN II. Visual acuity per Snellen chart is OU = 20/20. Visual fields full to confrontation. Optic disc margins sharp, no cupping; cup-to-disc ratio is 1:3. Retina-arteriovenous ratio is 2:3, without nicking. Fovea visualized.

CN III, CN IV, CN VI. PERRLA, direct and consensual. Accommodation present. EOMs intact without nystagmus or strabismus. Cover-uncover test negative. Corneal light reflections symmetrical.

CN V. Opens and closes mouth; chews, clenches teeth, and moves jaw side to side voluntarily. Sensation intact to forehead, cheeks, and chin. Corneal reflexes present.

CN VII. Face movements symmetrical with smiling, frowning, eyebrow raising, lip pursing, and cheek puffing. Discerns sweet, salty, sour, and bitter tastes (also CN IX).

CN VIII. Gross hearing intact. Whisper heard at 3 feet. Air conduction greater than bone conduction bilaterally.

CN IX and CN X. Tongue and uvula midline. Uvula and soft palate rise in midline with phonation. Gag reflex present bilaterally. Swallows, coughs, and speaks without difficulty.

CN XI. Performs shoulder shrugs. Turns head against resistance. Maintains head position against resistance.

CN XII. Tongue protrudes midline without deviation; pushes side to side with equal strength.

Motor Function. Muscle groups symmetrical. Gross and fine motor coordination intact. Moves all extremities through range of motion. Romberg's test negative. Pronator drift absent. Gait smooth, steady. Maintains balance walking on toes and heels. Rapid alternating movements and point-to-point maneuvers performed without difficulty.

Sensory Function. Sensation to light touch, pain, and vibration intact distally and over trunk, neck, and face. Position sense of fingers and toes intact. Stereognosis and graphesthesia present bilaterally. Two-point discrimination: 2 mm on index fingers. Discerns 2-point simultaneous stimulation.

PALPATION

Head, Neck, and Back. Skull without lesions or tenderness; smooth and firm. Neck and paravertebral muscles firm, relaxed, and nontender. No pain or tenderness over spinous processes.

Motor Function. Muscle bulk full and tone firm; strength rated as 5/5 bilaterally.

PERCUSSION

Reflexes. Deep tendon reflexes rated 2+ (on a scale of 0 to 4+) in triceps, biceps, wrists, knees, and ankles. Plantar reflexes present bilaterally. Abdominal reflexes present in all four quadrants.

AUSCULTATION

Vascular Flow. Absence of bruit over carotid arteries bilaterally.

---

judgment and insight, and language and communication. Cultural and educational background of the client must be considered when evaluating mental status. 🪔 The mental status examination is summarized in Box 67-4.

Level of Consciousness

🪔 The level of consciousness (LOC) is the most sensitive indicator of changes in neurologic status. LOC refers to level of arousal and wakefulness and the ability to respond to the environment. Begin by observing spontaneous behavior before using stimuli. To be certain that you are assessing cerebral function, rather than spinal cord reflex, use central stimuli whenever possible. Noxious stimuli are discussed in Chapter 68. Document the location and type of stimuli applied along with the client's response.

The time between assessments should also be noted to assess how quickly changes occur. 🪔 The *Glasgow*

Coma Scale is an assessment tool designed to note trends in a client's response to stimuli in terms of eye opening, verbal response, and motor response (see Chapter 68). Many variations of this scale now exist for use with other client populations.

Orientation

Establish *orientation* to time, place, person (×3), and event or situation (×4). Orientation to time is usually lost first. Orientation to self (person) is usually maintained except in advanced dementia.

Memory

Identify gross deficits in long-term and short-term memory with simple tests. Test *long-term memory* when the client relates the past health history (of course, another source must be able to validate the data). Test *short-term memory* by asking the client to recall recent information.

BOX 67-4 Mental Status Examination

Level of consciousness (LOC): Most important part of assessment. (LOC is the most sensitive indicator of changes in neurologic status) Assess client's ability to respond to environment. Begin with least invasive stimuli; increase stimuli if no response. Document BEST response.

Types of stimuli: None, verbal, light touch, pain (use central stimuli: pressure on trapezius or pectoralis major muscle, sternal rub, supraorbital pressure).

Types of responses:
- Obeys simple commands.
- Localizes pain: Moves arm across the midline away from stimuli.
- Withdrawal: Movement to move away from stimuli but does not cross midline.
- Abnormal posturing: Only seen in coma, may be unilateral or bilateral.
  - (a) Flexion—arm abduction and elbow flexion, possibly with flexion of wrists, plantar flexion and extension of lower extremities
  - (b) Extension—arm adduction and elbow extension with flexion of wrists, rigid extension of lower extremities

Orientation:
- Person (usually not lost): What is your name?
- Time (usually lost first): What year is this?
- Place and event (or situation = orientation × 4): What kind of place is this? Where are you? What brought you to the hospital today?

Memory (must be able to verify information to evaluate for confabulation):
- Long-term memory (preserved except in advanced dementia): Past health history, historical dates such as date of high school graduation, birth date, names of family members.

- Short-term memory: Recent events: "What brings you here today?" "Tell me what you ate for breakfast."
- Ability to learn: Three words to remember (red, Broadway, three). Ask the client to say the words immediately, and then to repeat them after a few minutes.

Mood and affect: Ask the client to describe how he or she feels; observe facial expression. Is the client's affect appropriate to the situation?

Intellectual performance: Ability to identify commonly known people, places, current events, reversed *serial 7's* or *3's,* simple addition or subtraction problem.

Judgment and insight reasoning: Are the answers logical? Do they relate to the question? "What would you do if you lost your house keys?" Ask the client to explain a proverb such as "A rolling stone gathers no moss."

Language and communication:
- Expression: Evaluate speech for flow, choice of words, and completion of phrases or sentences. Assess speech quality. Assess speech for articulation problems (usually motor disorders) or comprehension or expression problems (aphasic disorders). Test comprehension in aphasic clients by asking *yes* or *no* questions or to follow simple verbal commands. Assess written expression by having the client write answers to simple questions on paper.
- Comprehension of spoken language: Ability to follow commands ("Stick out your tongue").
- Comprehension of written language: Ability to read several words or sentences and explain them. Have the client read a simple command and then perform the command.

Integrated sensory functions: Integration of cortical functioning (calculation) and visual recognition with expressive speech. Ask the client to identify common objects, such as a pen, a key, and a watch. Ask the client to write a sentence.

Mood and Affect

Facial expression may reveal emotions such as anxiety, distrust, and depression. Is the client's affect appropriate to the situation?

Intellectual Performance

Intellectual performance consists of the fund of knowledge and calculation ability. Ask the client to identify commonly known people, places, or current events.

Judgment and Insight

Judgment and insight include reasoning, abstract thinking, problem solving, and the client's perception of the situation. Assess reasoning, abstract thinking, and problem solving for indications of major problems with thought content. Listen to how the client answers questions. Can the client concentrate and remain focused, or is the client easily distracted?

Language and Communication

Language and communication assessment tests the ability to express and comprehend one's environment. Gross evaluation of *comprehension* and *expression* begins with the initial interview. Does the client initiate speech? Is speech fluent and appropriate? Assess speech quality. Assess speech for articulation problems (dysarthrias, usually motor disorders) or comprehension or expression problems (aphasic disorders).

Assess comprehension to both spoken and written language. If the client is expressively aphasic, test comprehension by asking *yes* or *no* questions or by having the client follow simple verbal commands.

Evaluate verbal expression as the client responds to questions that require more than a nod or a "yes" or "no" answer. Evaluate speech for flow, choice of words, and completion of phrases or sentences. Assess written expression by having the client write answers to simple questions on paper.

Integrated sensory functions involving language are often tested with this portion of the neurologic examination. Have the client perform simple addition or subtraction without writing or ask the client to orally identify common objects. These skills require integration of cortical functioning (calculation) and visual recognition with expressive speech.

Head, Neck, and Back

Examine the head, neck, and spine using inspection, palpation, percussion, and auscultation. Tumors, vascular disorders, traumatic disorders, and problems involving the vertebrae and surrounding muscles may be detected.

Inspection

Inspect the head for size, shape, contour, and symmetry. Note any ecchymosis (bruising) around the eyes or behind the ears. Anterior basilar skull fractures often result in "raccoon eyes," with periorbital ecchymosis and, occasionally, drainage of cerebrospinal fluid (CSF) from the nares. Middle fossa basilar skull fractures often result in ecchymosis over the mastoid process behind the ears (Battle's sign) and drainage of blood, CSF, or both from the ears. Assess the spine and back for symmetry. Look for skin tags, lipomas, hairy patch (hypertrichosis), or dermal sinus tract along the spine.

Palpation

Palpate the skull lightly for nodules or masses and to supplement inspection findings. The skull normally feels smooth and firm. Areas of bogginess or depressions are abnormal. Palpation of neck muscles may identify masses or tender areas. Ask the client to flex the neck with the chin touching the chest and look for nuchal (back of the neck) rigidity, which is a manifestation of meningeal irritation.

Inspect and palpate spine alignment. Note any deviation from the normal curvatures. Palpate the paravertebral muscles for masses, tenderness, and spasm (also see Chapter 25).

Percussion

Gentle percussion over the spinous processes may produce pain or tenderness, which are abnormal findings.

Auscultation

Auscultation of major neck and other vessels may reveal bruits or other sounds suggesting an abnormality. Use the bell of the stethoscope to auscultate the carotid arteries. Bruits result from turbulent flow, usually a manifestation of atherosclerotic disease.

Cranial Nerves

The cranial nerves are referred to by specific name or Roman numeral. Cranial nerve (CN) examination is important for two reasons. First, CN III through CN XII arise in the brain stem. Testing their function provides information about the brain stem and related pathways. Second, three reflexes involving cranial nerves are called *protective reflexes* (corneal, gag, and cough reflexes). The presence or absence of protective reflexes indicates the ability to protect the eye surfaces and airway. This is especially important in unconscious clients.

Normal cranial nerve reflexes require an appropriately received stimulus *(input)* that produces an appropriate response *(output)*. During testing of cranial nerves, the absence of a normal response may indicate (1) failure to receive stimuli (input failure), (2) failure to respond appropriately (output failure), or (3) a combination of input and output failure. Cranial nerves occur in pairs (right and left). Dysfunction may be unilateral or bilateral. The cranial nerves are part of the peripheral nervous system (PNS) and abnormalities may be a manifestation of a systemic neurologic disease (e.g., Guillain-Barré syndrome). Refer to Table 67-2 for details of cranial nerve testing.

Be aware that some abnormal findings are not clinically significant. Anosmia may develop in older people as a normal aging process. CN I cannot be accurately assessed in clients with upper respiratory infections (URI). In about 20% of the population, *anisocoria* (unequal pupils) is a normal finding. Older clients who have undergone cataract surgery with lens implants may have irregular, nonreactive pupils. This finding does not indicate neurologic damage.

Motor System

Assessing the motor system thoroughly involves numerous procedures. The following discussion focuses on the screening examinations and common abnormalities.

Muscle Size

Inspect all major muscle groups bilaterally for symmetry, hypertrophy, and atrophy.

Muscle Strength

Assess the power in major muscle groups against resistance (see Chapter 25). Assess and rate muscle strength on a 5-point scale in all four extremities, comparing one side with the other (Table 67-3 on p. 1781).

Next, test for subtle weakness in upper and lower extremities. For upper extremities, have the client hold the arms straight out in front with the palms up ("like holding a tray"). Ask the client to close the eyes and to maintain the position. A *pronator drift* is said to be present if one arm pronates and falls lower than the other. For the lower extremities, have the client walk on the heels and then on the toes to test dorsiflexion, plantiflexion, and balance.

Assessment of specific muscle groups evaluates deficits in certain areas, such as spinal cord disorders. Disorders of muscle strength may be exhibited as weakness

TABLE 67–2 Cranial Nerve Testing

Nerve	Function	Method for Assessment	Indication of Dysfunction	Causes of Dysfunction
Olfactory nerve (CN I)	Purely sensory Smell	Identify an aromatic, nonirritating odor (coffee, toothpaste) with each nostril separately and with eyes closed	Anosmia	Neurogenic: fracture of cribriform plate or ethmoid bone; tumor of frontal lobe or olfactory bulb/tract Nonneurogenic: sinus disorders or surgery, tobacco smoker, cocaine use, URI, advanced age
Optic nerve (CN II)	Purely sensory Vision: central and peripheral	Visual Acuity: Read Snellen chart or newspaper; or identify number and movement of fingers Visual fields: Confrontation: compare peripheral vision to examiner	Amaurosis (blindness): decreased or absent central vision Vision loss in one or more directions or in a portion of visual field (half of visual field, middle portion, or both sides)	Nonneurogenic: corneal defect or cataracts Neurogenic: trauma, stroke, occipital lobe lesion, diabetes mellitus, multiple sclerosis One eye: globe or anterior optic chiasm lesions Bilateral: optic chiasm or tract or occipital cortex Bitemporal: optic chiasm defect (pituitary tumor)
		Funduscopic and gross exam: inspect for trauma and cataracts Examine fundus with ophthalmoscope	Diabetic retinopathy; loss of venous pulsation; papilledema: optic disc swelling	Fracture of optic foramen; diabetes mellitus; laceration or blood clot in temporal, parietal, or occipital lobes; increased ICP
CN III, IV, VI assessed together: Oculomotor nerve (CN III)	Purely motor Eyelid elevation (III)		CN III: ptosis: upper eyelid droop	Horner's syndrome (unilateral ptosis and pupil constriction); myasthenia gravis (bilateral ptosis)
Trochlear nerve (CN IV) Abducens nerve (CN VI)	EOMs: nasally, up and temporal, up and nasally, down and temporal (III); downward and nasally (IV); far lateral gaze (VI)	EOMs: "six cardinal fields of gaze" (CN III, IV, VI) Nystagmus (involuntary eye movements), seen as fine, rhythmic eye movements that can be vertical, horizontal, or rotational	Inability of an eye to move nasally, up and nasally, up and temporally, or downward Double vision (diplopia)	Pressure on CN III, CN IV, or CN VI at brain stem because of fracture of orbit; increased ICP and tumor/trauma to base of brain, degenerative neurologic diseases such as multiple sclerosis, myasthenia gravis CN IV dysfunction
		Inability to look down or to walk down steps because of visual disturbance Inability of an eye to move laterally outward		CN VI dysfunction
	Pupil size at rest and pupil constriction (III)	Pupil constriction: shine light at eye from side Direct response: connection in midbrain of CN II and ipsilateral CN III consensual response (other eye): connection in midbrain of CN II and contralateral CN III	Irregular shaped pupils Anisocoria: unequal pupils; no or sluggish response to light or accommodation	Cataract surgery; glaucoma; COPD: large sluggish pupils because of hypoxemia CN III dysfunction: nerve damage Increased ICP or edema in uncus of temporal lobe Medications: opiates: small and sluggish; atropine: large and sluggish
		Accommodation: bring a pen or finger toward center of client's face		

		Assessment Techniques	Abnormal Findings	Associated Conditions
Trigeminal nerve (CN V)	Mixed Motor: masticator Innervates muscles for chewing	Clamp jaw shut, open mouth against resistance, open mouth widely, move jaw from side to side, and make chewing movements	Weakness (rare), aching, or spasm of masseter or temporal muscles	Jaw clenching; temporal arteritis, tetanus, parotitis, dystonic reaction to antipsychotic drugs
	Sensory: All sensations for entire face, scalp, cornea, and nasal and oral cavities	With client's eyes closed, test sensations on both sides of entire face: pain (sharp pin), touch (wisp of cotton), and temperature (hot and cold objects) Corneal reflexes: gently touch cornea with sterile wisp of cotton or gently stroke eyelash (CN V, sensory; CN VII, motor; eye blink)	Facial pain, paresthesias	Trigeminal neuralgia Medulla (loss of pain and temperature), pons (touch), and brain stem tumor or trauma, orbital fracture, and trigeminal neuralgia
Facial nerve (CN VII)	Mixed Motor: facial expression	Observe face for symmetry Assess facial muscles: smile, frown, raise forehead and eyebrows, tightly close eyes against resistance, whistle, show teeth, and puff out cheeks	Central deficits: affects lower half of face only; caused by CNS defect Peripheral deficit: deficit involving both upper face and lower face; caused by CN VII lesion Facial asymmetry loss of nasolabial fold, inability to close eye and blink reflexively, drooling, difficulty swallowing secretions, loss of tearing	Stroke (cerebral causes) Peripheral CN VII injury: facial weakness, Bell's palsy, temporal bone fracture, peripheral laceration or contusion of parotid region
	Sensory	Test taste on anterior part of tongue with eyes closed, eyes and tongue protruding Place taste substance on one side of anterior tongue Test taste on each side for sweet, salty, sour, and bitter	Loss of taste on anterior two thirds of tongue	
Vestibulocochlear or acoustic nerve (CN VIII)	Purely sensory Hearing (cochlear)	Auditory acuity: listen and respond to whispered words, fingers rubbing; test ears separately Air and bone conduction: Weber test: vibrating tuning fork placed midline on skull Rinne test: vibrating tuning fork placed on mastoid process; when client indicates it is no longer heard, move tuning fork by ear and have client indicate when no longer heard	Whispered words, fingers rubbing not heard correctly or equally Sound lateralized to one side (negative Weber); sound lateralizes toward side with hearing loss (conductive); sound lateralizes toward side without hearing loss (sensorineural) Bone conduction equal to or longer than air conduction (negative Rinne)	Conductive hearing loss: tympanic membrane damage, ear wax, otitis media Sensorineural hearing loss: possibly caused by medications (gentamicin), acoustic nerve tumor

(Continued)

TABLE 67-2 Cranial Nerve Testing —Cont'd

Nerve	Function	Method for Assessment	Indication of Dysfunction	Causes of Dysfunction
	Balance (vestibular)	Equilibrium tests Romberg: stands with feet together and eyes closed	Swaying, wide-based stance to maintain balance (positive Romberg)	Ménière's syndrome, acoustic neuroma
		Caloric tests: oculovestibular reflex (usually performed on comatose client only): inject cold or warm water into each ear and observe eye movement away from (cold) or toward (warm) stimulus	No response	Lesion in pons or lower brain stem: impending brain death
CN IX and X assessed together Glossopharyngeal nerve (CN IX)	Mixed *Motor:* swallow, gag, vocalization (IX, X); posterior pharynx muscles (IX); cough (X)	Say "Ahhh": soft palate and pharynx rise symmetrically, uvula is midline Assess voice: stimulate back of throat with tongue blade to check gag	Uvula deviates, palate fails to rise Hoarse voice Nasal voice No gag	Lower brain stem tumor or stroke, Guillain-Barré Vocal cord paralysis Palate paralysis
Vagus nerve (CN X)	*Sensory:* taste to posterior third of tongue, inner ear sensation (IX); decreases heart rate, increases GI motility (X)	Assess taste to back of tongue with sugar and salt, listen to heart rate and rhythm, bowel sounds	Weak cough Loss of taste, tachycardia, ileus	Brain stem trauma or tumor, neck trauma, stroke
Spinal accessory nerve (CN XI)	Purely motor Shoulder elevation and lateral head rotation	Shoulders symmetrical, shrugs shoulders against resistance, turns head laterally against resistance toward midline, able to lift head off pillow	Drooping of a shoulder, muscle atrophy, weak shoulder shrug, or weak turn of head	Possible causes of abnormal findings include neck trauma, radical neck surgery, and torticollis
Hypoglossal nerve (CN XII)	Purely motor Tongue movement	Stick out tongue, move it side to side and against inside of each cheek; says "**light, tight, dynamite**"	Deviation of tongue to weak side, atrophy, fasciculations, slurred speech (dysarthria)	Stroke, ALS, neck trauma with major blood vessel damage, multiple CN lesions: V, VII, XII

TABLE 67-3   Neuromuscular Strength Assessment

Movement	Test Against Resistance	Muscle	Spinal Cord Level
Shoulder elevation	Shrug shoulders	Supraspinatus	C4-5
Elbow flexors	Flex elbow: pull forearm to face	Biceps	C5-6
Elbow extensors	Straighten elbow	Triceps	C7-8
Wrist extensors	Flex wrist up	Extensor carpi radialis	C6-7
		Extensor carpi ulnaris	C7-8
Hand intrinsics	Spread fingers apart	Interossei	C8-T1
Hip flexors	Raise knee to chest	Iliopsoas	L1-3
Knee extensors	Bend knee 90 degrees and straighten knee	Quadriceps	L3-4
Ankle dorsiflexors	Pull ankle up/toes toward head	Tibialis anterior	L4-5
Ankle plantiflexors	Push ankle/toes down (press gas pedal)	Gastrocnemius	S1-2

on one side of the body, in both lower extremities, or in both upper and lower extremities. If asymmetry is detected, ask the client or family whether it is long-standing or recent. Consider the client's age, handedness, and physical condition when interpreting the results of muscle-strength testing.

Muscle Tone

Assess muscle tone while moving each extremity through its range of passive motion. When tone is decreased *(hypotonicity),* the muscles are soft, flabby, or flaccid; when tone is increased *(hypertonicity),* the muscles are resistant to movement, rigid, or spastic. Note the presence of abnormal flexion or extension posture.

Muscle Coordination

Assessment of muscle coordination consists of testing rapid alternating movements, point-to-point maneuvers, and maintenance of truncal balance and head position. Test *rapid alternating movements* by asking the client to touch (approximate) each finger to the thumb quickly in succession. Alternatively, ask the client to pat the thighs first with the palms, then with the back of the hands, and to repeat the patting quickly.

For *point-to-point testing,* hold up an index finger approximately 18 inches from the client. Ask the client first to touch his or her nose with a finger, then touch your index finger, and then touch the nose again. Repeat this several times while you move your index finger to different locations. Perform the test for the client's right and left hands. Test lower-extremity coordination by asking the client to place the heel of the foot below the other knee and then slide the heel down the shin toward the great toe. Repeat for the other leg.

Assess *truncal balance* with the client sitting. Can the client remain upright without support? Gently push the client to a leaning position. Can the client return to an upright position? Note *head position* by observing the ability to move the head while following your movements.

Disorders related to coordination indicate cerebellar or posterior column lesions. The defining characteristics of cerebellar dysfunction are (1) ataxia, (2) intention tremor (tremor upon nearing the object), (3) nystagmus, (4) ocular dysmetria (inability to gaze on an object), and (5) dysdiadochokinesia (arresting one motor impulse and substituting an opposite one).

Gait and Station

Assess gait and station by having the client stand still, walk, and walk in tandem (one foot in front of the other in a straight line). Walking involves the functions of motor power, sensation, and coordination. The ability to stand quietly with the feet together requires coordination and intact *proprioception* (sense of body position).

> **If the client has difficulty standing, assess further to determine whether the client is weak or unsteady. If the client is weak, protect the client from falling.**
>
> SAFETY ALERT

The box Terms Associated with Gait Disorders on the website lists and describes terms used to describe gait *evolve* disorders.

Movement

Examine the muscles for fine and gross abnormal movements. Examples of fine abnormal movements are *fasciculations* (involuntary ripples or twitches that occur while the client is relaxed), which may indicate lower motor neuron disease. Examples of more grossly abnormal movements, often representing extrapyramidal disease, are described in Box 67-5.

Move all joints through a full range of passive motion. Abnormal findings include pain, joint contractures, and muscle resistance.

Test for *apraxia* (the inability to carry out a learned movement on command in the absence of weakness or paralysis). Ask the client to perform a common activity, such as tying shoes or combing hair. Apraxia is present if a client can follow other commands (indicating intact comprehension), has the motor strength to move the extremity involved, but cannot carry out the command.

Motor Testing of the Unconscious Client

An unresponsive client can be tested only for response to painful stimuli (reflex withdrawal of limbs, wincing,

---

BOX 67-5 Abnormal Movements Associated with Extrapyramidal Disease

Akinesia: Reduced body movement in the absence of weakness or paralysis; habitual movements (swinging arms) limited or absent

Athetosis: Gross, writhing, worm-like movements of body, face, or extremities

Ballismus: A form of chorea; involuntary dramatic movements of arms and legs (**hemiballismus** involves only one side)

Bradykinesia: Slow movement

Chorea: Discrete, jerky, purposeless movements in distal extremities and face

Dystonia: Prolonged twisting movements or postures

Myoclonus: Sudden muscle contractions of varying intensity that may involve a small part of one extremity or the entire body; may violently fling a client to the floor

Spasms: Involuntary contraction of large muscle groups (arms, legs, neck)

Tic: Involuntary movement of groups of muscles in stereotypic patterns; may be physical or psychogenic in origin; pathologic causes of tics include Tourette's syndrome

Tremors: Involuntary trembling or quivering; may vary in direction, amplitude, rhythmicity, parts involved, speed, and timing in relation to rest or activity; types include parkinsonian, essential, and cerebellar

---

grimacing). Although a pain stimulus is used, the response is usually recorded as a motor system response. These responses are often incorporated into the motor scale of the Glasgow Coma Scale. (See Chapter 68 for further information.) Box 67-6 describes the most common responses to painful stimuli.

Sensory Function

Sensory assessment involves testing for touch, pain, vibration, position (proprioception), and discrimination. Assessment of hearing, vision, smell, and taste is also

---

BOX 67-6 Responses to Painful Stimuli

Localization: Reaches for the source of the stimulus and attempts to push the examiner away

Flexion withdrawal: Moves without purpose and may exhibit minimal movement, grimacing, or wincing

Abnormal flexion (decorticate posturing): Flexes, adducts, and internally rotates the wrists and arms to the chest and rigidly extends the legs (indicates damage in the corticospinal tracts near the cerebral hemispheres that has left the rubrospinal tract intact)

Abnormal extension (decerebrate posturing): Extends and pronates the arms while rigidly extending the legs (indicates damage in the upper brain stem)

No response: No visible reaction to painful stimuli

---

sensory assessment. Sensory assessment may identify dermatomes as having normal, absent, reduced, exaggerated, or delayed sensation. A complete sensory examination is possible only on a conscious and cooperative client. Always test sensation with the client's eyes closed. Help the client relax and keep warm.

Conduct sensory assessment systematically. Test a particular area of the body, and then test the corresponding area on the other side. Begin testing a selection of dermatomes that represent cervical, thoracic, lumbar, and sacral segments of the spinal cord. If you note a sensory loss, you can perform a more detailed testing of surrounding dermatomes. Sensation assessment may be documented on a body chart of dermatomes.

Superficial Sensation

Test superficial sensations by stimulating the skin in symmetrical areas on each side of the body according to dermatome distribution.

Test *superficial pain* by alternating the sharp and dull ends of a broken cotton applicator. The wooden broken end is pointed enough for testing sharp sensation, yet dull enough not to break the skin. The cotton swab end serves as the dull stimulus. Ask the client to close the eyes. Explain that the client will feel a sharp or a dull stimulus. Alternate the two stimuli inconsistently (so that the client cannot predict which is being used), and ask the client to distinguish sharp from dull.

Use a cotton wisp to assess *light touch*. Follow the same guidelines as for testing superficial pain sensation, stimulating symmetrical areas of the dermatomes.

Temperature is not assessed routinely. Where there is a loss of the sense of pain, test for awareness of temperature. Pain and temperature sensations travel on related pathways. Use two test tubes, one filled with warm water and one with cold water.

Mechanical Sensation

Mechanical sensations are assessed with vibration and proprioception. Use a tuning fork to test for *vibration*. Place the end of a vibrating tuning fork on a distal bony prominence, such as a finger or great toe joint. Ask the client to indicate when the vibration is felt and when it is no longer felt. Once the client indicates that the sensation has stopped, test your own joint to see whether you can feel vibration. You serve as the control. If the client reports that the sensation has stopped but you can still sense a clear vibration, the client has reduced vibratory sense.

Test *proprioception* by holding the side of the client's fingertips, then the great toes, between thumb and index finger. As each of the client's fingers and toes are gently flexed and extended, ask the client to state when movement is felt and in what direction. Test more proximal joints if impairment is detected.

Discrimination

Cortical discrimination depends on the ability to integrate and interpret sensory stimuli in the parietal lobe. Included are tests for stereognosis, graphesthesia, extinction phenomenon, and simultaneous two-point stimulation (Box 67-7).

Abnormalities of sensation are defined in Box 67-8, and Figure 67-3 summarizes patterns of sensory loss. Sensory changes are part of the normal aging process. Careful assessment of such changes is the basis of nursing intervention for older clients. Table 67-1 contains guidelines for assessment.

BOX 67-7   Tests for Cortical Discrimination

Stereognosis (discernment of the form and configuration of objects felt, or three-dimensional discrimination): Place three small, familiar objects (such as a coin, a key, and a paper clip) one at a time in the client's hands. Ask the client to identify each with the eyes closed.

Graphesthesia (recognition of the form and configuration of written symbols): Trace different separate letters and numbers on the client's palm with the blunt end of a pen. Ask the client to identify each with the eyes closed. Orient the figures so that they are right-side-up for the client.

Extinction phenomenon (simultaneous stimulation): Prick the client's skin at the same point on the two sides of the body at the same time. Ask the client to state whether one or two pricks are felt.

Two-point stimulation (two-point discrimination): Simultaneously prick the skin with two pins at varying distances apart to identify the smallest distance at which the client can perceive two pricks. Normal distances at which two-point discrimination is lost are as follows: upper arms, 75 mm; thighs, 75 mm; back, 40 to 70 mm; chest, 40 mm; forearms, 40 mm; palms, 8 to 12 mm; toes, 3 to 8 mm; fingertips, 2.8 mm; and tongue, 1 mm.

BOX 67-8   Abnormalities of Sensation

Dysesthesias: Well-localized, irritating sensations, such as warmth, cold, itching, tickling, crawling, prickling, and tingling

Paresthesias: Distortions of sensory stimuli (light touch may be experienced as burning or painful sensation)

Anesthesia: Absence of the sense of touch

Hypoesthesia: Reduced sense of touch

Hyperesthesia: Pathologic (abnormal) overperception of touch

Analgesia: Absence of the sense of pain

Hypalgesia: Reduced sense of pain

Hyperalgesia: Increased sense of pain

Agraphesthesia: Inability to identify symbols traced on the palm when the eyes are closed

Astereognosis: Loss of sense of three-dimensional discrimination

---

Reflex Activity

Reflex testing evaluates the integrity of specific sensory and motor pathways. Reflex activity assessment, always a part of neurologic assessment, provides information about the nature, location, and progression of neurologic disorders.

Normal Reflexes

Two types of reflexes are normally present: (1) superficial, or cutaneous, reflexes; and (2) deep tendon, or muscle-stretch, reflexes (Table 67-4).

Superficial (Cutaneous) Reflexes. Superficial (cutaneous) reflexes are elicited by stimulation of the skin or mucous membranes. The stimulus is produced by stroking a sensory zone with an object that will not cause damage. Superficial reflexes (abdominal, plantar, corneal, pharyngeal [gag], cremasteric, and anal) are absent in pyramidal tract disorders.

Deep Tendon (Muscle-Stretch) Reflexes. Deep tendon reflexes are also called muscle-stretch, or myotactic, reflexes because reflex muscle contraction normally results from rapid stretching of the muscle. This is produced by sharply striking a muscle tendon's point of insertion with a sudden, brief blow of a reflex hammer (Figure 67-4 and Box 67-9 on p. 1786). Reflexes commonly assessed include the biceps, triceps, brachioradialis, patella, and ankle jerk (Achilles tendon).

Other Normal Reflexes. Some normal reflexes involve structures other than skeletal muscles. For example, reflex mechanisms help maintain respiration and keep blood pressure within normal limits. Reflex salivation may follow the taste (or smell) of food. Flashing a light in an eye causes the pupils of both eyes to constrict *(light reflex* or *pupillary reflex)*.

Abnormal Reflexes

Pathologic reflexes indicate neurologic disorders, often related to the spinal cord or higher centers. These responses include Babinski's, jaw, palm-chin (palmomental), clonus, snout, rooting, sucking, glabella, grasp, and chewing reflexes. Babinski's reflex and clonus are discussed below. Box 67-10 on p. 1787 lists additional abnormal reflexes.

Babinski's Reflex. When exaggerated deep reflexes are present, superficial reflexes are usually diminished or absent and pathologic reflexes (Babinski's reflex) are observed. The presence of Babinski's reflex is indicative of an upper motor neuron lesion. Test for Babinski's reflex by gently scraping the sole of the foot with a blunt object. To elicit the reflex, start the stimulus at the

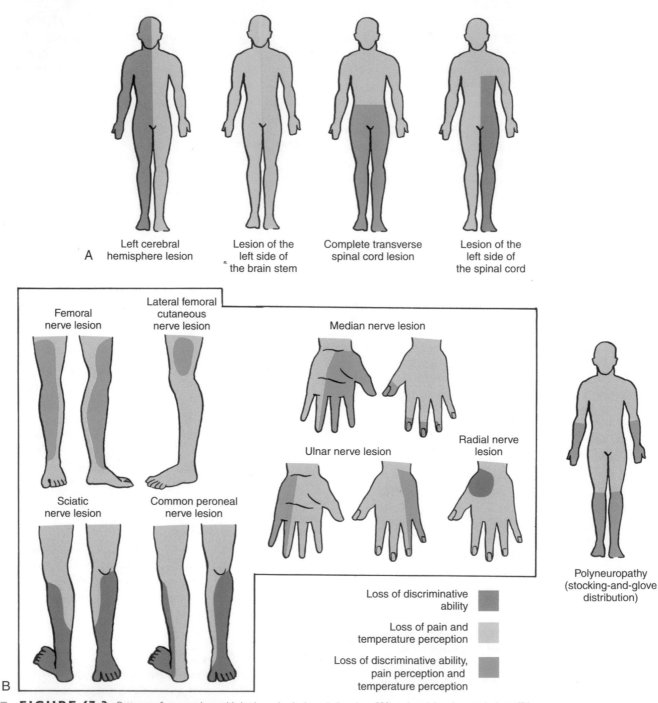

■ **FIGURE 67–3**   Patterns of sensory loss with brain and spinal cord disorders **(A)** and peripheral nerve lesions **(B).**

midpoint of the heel, and move upward and laterally along the outer border of the sole to the ball of the foot. Continue the stimulus across the ball of the foot (without touching the toes) toward the medial side and off the foot. Alternatively, start the stimulus at the midlateral sole and carry it down toward the heel. A normal response is plantar flexion of the toes. An abnormal response (presence of Babinski's reflex) is dorsiflexion of the great toe and, often, fanning of the other toes (Figure 67-5). In extreme circumstances, a Babinski reflex may be accompanied

by dorsiflexion of the foot at the ankle and flexion at the knee and hip (called *triple flexion*).

Clonus. Clonus consists of rapidly alternating joint flexions and extensions resulting from continuous rhythmic contractions of a stretched muscle. This is not like a normal stretch reflex, which typically produces one reflex action. With clonus, the action continues. Support the leg at the knee, and help the client relax the leg. Rapidly flex the foot, and hold it in a flexed position. The flexion

TABLE 67–4   Important Reflexes

Reflex	Assessment Technique	Expected Response	Pathway Involved*
Tendon Reflexes			
Biceps reflex	A blow on examiner's thumb placed over biceps tendon	Flexion of elbow	C5-6
Brachioradialis reflex (supinator)	Styloid process of radius is tapped while forearm is in semiflexion and semipronation	Flexion of elbow, fingers, and hand with supination of forearm	C5-6
Triceps reflex	Strike on triceps tendon just above olecranon	Extension of elbow	C6-8 (C7 primarily)
Patellar reflex (knee jerk)	Tap on patellar tendon	Leg extends	L2-4
Achilles reflex (ankle jerk)	Tap on Achilles tendon	Plantiflexion of foot	S1-2
Superficial Reflexes			
Corneal reflex	Light touch at corneoscleral junction	Closure of eyelids	CN V, VII
Palatal and pharyngeal reflexes	Light touch to soft palate and pharynx	Elevation of palate; gagging	CN IX, X
Abdominal reflexes	Stroke skin of upper, middle, and lower abdomen toward umbilicus	Contraction of abdominal wall toward stimulus	Upper: T7-9 Middle: T9-11 Lower: T11-12
Cremasteric reflex	Stroke medial surface of upper thigh	Elevation of ipsilateral scrotum and testicle	T12-L2
Anal reflex	Stroke perianal region	Contraction of external anal sphincter	S3-5
Plantar reflex (normal)	Stroke sole of foot	Plantar flexion of toes	L4-S2
Plantar reflex (pathologic; Babinski's sign)	Stroke sole of foot	Dorsiflexion of great toe and fanning of other toes	L4-S2

* C, Cervical; CN, cranial nerve; L, lumbar; S, sacral; T, thoracic.
Modified from Bader, M., & Littlejohns, L. (Eds.) (2004). *AANN core curriculum for neuroscience nursing* (4th ed.). Philadelphia: Saunders.

stretches the calf muscles and causes repeated "beats" of clonus if this reflex is present.

Grading Reflex Activity

Figure 67-6 shows the grading and documentation of superficial reflexes. Although 1+ or 3+ responses are not considered normal, they may not be significant findings. Asymmetrical responses are more significant. Abnormal reflexes may be present in both neurologic and metabolic disorders. See Table 67-4 for a summary of important reflexes.

Autonomic Nervous System

The autonomic nervous system cannot be examined directly. The autonomic nervous system innervates many body organs through sympathetic and parasympathetic pathways; thus its function is evaluated by a full body systems assessment. Clinical manifestations of autonomic nervous system disorders occur in many body systems. Unit 16 focuses on neurologic disorders (heat-stroke, autonomic dysreflexia). Disorders of other portions of the autonomic system are discussed in the cardiac, urinary, digestive, reproductive, and endocrine units of this book.

The following are examples of activity under autonomic nervous system influence:

- Increased or decreased heart rate
- Peripheral vasoconstriction or vasodilation
- Bronchoconstriction or bronchodilation
- Increased or decreased peristalsis
- Constriction or dilation of the pupil

Review medications the client is taking. Many medications have side effects involving the parasympathetic or sympathetic nervous system.

DIAGNOSTIC TESTING

Noninvasive Tests of Structure
Skull and Spinal X-Ray Studies

Skull x-ray studies reveal the size and shape of the skull bones, suture separation in infants, fractures or bony defects, erosion, calcification, sella turcica erosion, and pineal gland shift (>12 years of age). Spinal x-ray studies show fractures, dislocation, compressions, curvature, erosion, narrowed spinal cord canal, congenital malformations, cancers, and degenerative processes.

Computed Tomography

Computed tomography (CT) uses a computer to reconstruct a cross-sectional image from measurements of x-ray tissue penetration. The primary purpose of CT scanning is to detect intracranial bleeding, space-occupying lesions, cerebral edema, and shifts of brain structures (Figure 67-7). Infarctions, hydrocephalus, and cerebral atrophy can also be identified. It is especially useful in acute trauma not only because it can identify the extent

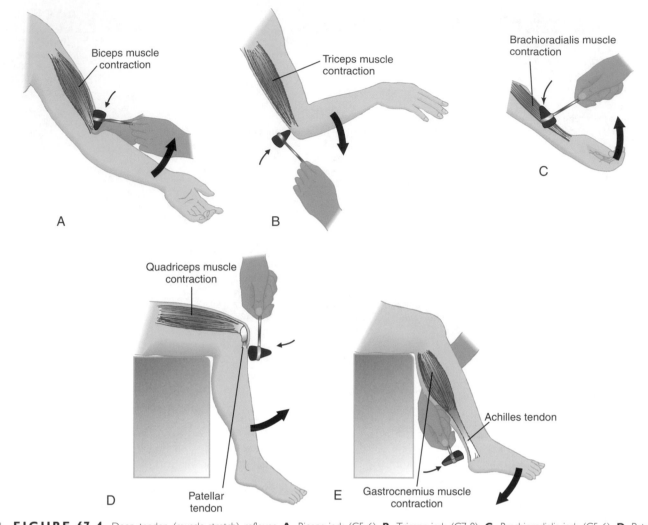

■ **FIGURE 67–4** Deep tendon (muscle-stretch) reflexes. **A,** Biceps jerk (C5-6). **B,** Triceps jerk (C7-8). **C,** Brachioradialis jerk (C5-6). **D,** Patellar reflexes (L2-4). **E,** Ankle jerk (S1-2).

BOX 67-9   Assessing Deep Tendon Reflexes

Use the following guidelines when assessing deep tendon reflexes:
1. Test deep tendon reflexes with the client either sitting or supine.
2. Support the joint where the tendon is being tested so that the attached muscle is relaxed.
3. Use the pointed end of a triangular reflex hammer to strike over small areas while you place your thumb over the biceps tendon. Use the flat end of the hammer to strike over larger areas, such as the Achilles tendon.
4. Hold the reflex hammer loosely between thumb and fingers so it can swing in an arc.
5. Swing the reflex hammer using only wrist motion, not the arm or elbow.
6. Tap the tendon briskly.
7. Note the speed, force, and amplitude of reflex responses.
8. Compare reflex responses on the two sides of the body.

9. Grade reflexes on a 0 to 4+ scale. Consider the strength of the reflex in relation to the bulk of the muscle mass.

Repeat testing of reflexes graded 0 or 1+ by using the technique of reinforcement (see next phase). Note in the record that *reinforcement* was used. Reinforcement is a maneuver used to enhance deep tendon reflex responses when they are graded 0 or 1+. Reinforcement maneuvers for various deep tendon reflexes are as follows:
1. Ask the client to perform isometric contraction of other muscles, which may increase the generalized reflex response.
2. For the upper extremities, have the client either clench the teeth together or contract the quadriceps muscles (push the thighs against the table).
3. For the lower extremities, have the client lock the fingers together and try to pull them apart at the same time you test the tendon.

BOX 67-10   Abnormal Reflexes

Jaw reflex. The jaw reflex is also called the *mandibular reflex* or *jaw jerk*. Have the client relax the mouth, leaving it open slightly. Then tap gently on the lower jaw below the mouth. The jaw normally contracts and closes the mouth as a result of downward tapping. This reflex is absent in most people but may be present in clients who have lesions in the corticobulbar tract above the mid-pons.

Palm-chin (palmomental) reflex. The palm-chin reflex is produced by vigorous, rapid irritation on the mound of the palm at the thumb's base with a blunt instrument, which causes the chin muscles to pull up on the same side.

Snout reflex. A brisk midline tap above or below the mouth results in pursing of the lips. This reflex is normal in infants but is abnormal in adults.

Rooting reflex. Stroking the side of the face causes the mouth to open and the head to turn to the stimulated side. This reflex is normal in infants but is abnormal in adults.

Sucking reflex. Touching the lips with a blunt object results in movement of the tongue, lips, and jaws. This reflex is normal in infants but is abnormal in adults.

Glabella reflex. Tapping the forehead between the eyebrows results in sustained closure of the eyelids.

Grasp reflex. Placing an object in the palm of the hand causes the fingers to curl around it.

Chewing reflex. A tongue blade placed between the teeth results in the tight closing of the jaws.

■ **FIGURE 67–5** Babinski's reflex. **A,** Test maneuver. Using a blunt point, scratch the sole of the foot as shown. **B,** Normal response (absence of Babinski's response) is plantiflexion of the toes. **C,** Abnormal response (presence of Babinski's response) is dorsiflexion of the big toe and often a fanning of the other toes.

■ **FIGURE 67–6** Documentation of muscle-stretch and superficial reflexes in left hemiparesis. Muscle-stretch reflex grades: 0, absent; 1, diminished; 2, normal; 3, brisker than normal; 4, hyperactive (clonus). Superficial reflex grades: 0, absent; ±, equivocal or barely present; +, normally active.

of injuries quickly but also because it is readily available at lower cost than other types of scans. It is superior to MRI for diagnosing skull fractures and subarachnoid hemorrhage.

Advances in technology have expanded the uses of CT. CT fluoroscopy combines CT with real time imaging, which is useful during interventional procedures such as surgery and spinal injections. Spiral CT uses injection of contrast material followed by rapid image sequencing to study movement of the contrast material through the cerebral blood vessels. Xenon CT uses inhaled xenon gas, which is absorbed into the bloodstream, to enhance views that depict regional cerebral blood flow. CT angiography is a noninvasive alternative to conventional angiography for viewing intracranial blood vessels in two-dimensional and three-dimensional format. The image can be rotated 360 degrees.

CT scans can be used for stereotactic procedures. Before the scan, a frame is applied to the client's head with pins inserted into the skull. The scan is performed with the frame in place. The computer marks reference measurements on the scan to guide the location of treatment.

Magnetic Resonance Imaging

Magnetic resonance imaging (MRI) combines radiofrequency (RF) waves and magnetic fields to provide more

■ **FIGURE 67–7** A computed tomography scan of the head. The brain tissue is gray, and the skull is white. The mass in the left frontal lobe *(arrow)* is blood from a head injury.

■ **FIGURE 67–8** Magnetic resonance imaging of the head. The eyes are evident at the top of the image. The client has a brain tumor (*arrow*).

anatomically detailed pictures than are available with CT (Figure 67-8). MRI has several advantages over CT. MRI can detect disorders in white matter pathways caused by loss of myelin, as in multiple sclerosis, better than CT. MRI can evaluate cerebral infarction within hours of the event; CT would not demonstrate the ischemic stroke for several days. MRI is the scan of choice for congenital brain malformations and spinal cord lesions. MRI with contrast material delineates blood flow through cerebral blood vessels in more detail than is possible with CT. MRI is contraindicated with certain metal implants, such as pacemakers.

Noninvasive Tests of Function
Electroencephalogram

An electroencephalogram (EEG) is a measurement of the electrical activity of the superficial layers of the cerebral cortex. The electrical potentials from neuron activity within the brain are recorded in the form of wave patterns. See the box Types of Electrical Brain Waves on the website for a description of the common types of brain wave patterns.

The EEG is used to assess seizure disorders. The results are diffusely abnormal in various metabolic disturbances, toxic conditions (drug overdose), coma, dementias, infections (meningitis and encephalitis), narcolepsy, and insomnia. The EEG may be used in the operating room to monitor cerebral activity during surgery on the blood vessels in the head or neck. Absence of waves on the recording ("flat lines") may be one of the criteria for defining brain death.

Evoked Potential Studies

Evoked potential (EP) studies measure evoked potentials or the brain's electrical response to various stimuli. EP studies assess the transit time of afferent pathways of the cerebral hemispheres and the brain stem. Typical stimuli are flashing lights, buzzing tones, and peripheral nerve stimulation. EP studies can be used to assess blindness, deafness, and brain stem injury. Evoked potential studies are carried out in the same fashion as EEG studies. EP studies can detect abnormalities in infants, children, and clients who are sedated or paralyzed with neuromuscular blocking agents.

Neuropsychological Testing

Neuropsychological testing involves a series of tests to evaluate cortical function by localizing the area and the extent of impairment and determining the rate of progression or recovery. The tests gauge many types of abilities, such as motor, perceptual, language, visuospatial, and cognitive. General measures of intelligence (Wechsler Adult Intelligence Scale) as well as tests of emotional and personal adjustment (the Minnesota Multiphasic Personality Inventory) are used. Test results can provide information regarding the extent of cognitive impairment and the effect it may have on functional ability and can aid in determining decision-making ability for legal and insurance matters. Test results may be used to make recommendations about treatment, including educational and vocational rehabilitation.

Magnetic Resonance Spectroscopy

Magnetic resonance spectroscopy (MRS) is a noninvasive MRI method of studying the distribution of chemicals or molecules in the body. MRS can detect abnormal amounts or those that are not normally present. The amount or presence of certain molecules or markers is associated with specific neurodegenerative diseases such as multiple sclerosis, Huntington's disease, dementia, and disorders of the mitochondria. Presently, MRS is mainly used in research.

Functional Magnetic Resonance Imaging

Similar to MRI, functional magnetic resonance imaging (fMRI) uses a strong magnet and radiofrequency waves to produce an image. Instead of lying still and quiet, the client performs cognitive, motor, or sensory tasks during the scan. The client may be asked to recite all the words they can remember that start with a certain letter or press a button at the sound of a noise. Certain areas of the brain are activated with each type of task. The fMRI detects changes in venous blood oxygenation and blood flow in activated areas. Blood flow increases in areas where neuronal activity increases. The fMRI is currently used more for experimental than diagnostic purposes. It increases understanding of the effects of stroke, hypoglycemia, and neurodegenerative diseases on specific areas of the brain. Clinically, it is useful for presurgical brain mapping to minimize damage to eloquent regions.

Positron Emission Tomography

Positron emission tomography (PET) enables visualization of physiologic function in body areas. Often the function of diseased tissue is different from that of normal tissues. PET has three primary uses: determining the amount of blood flow to specific body tissues; revealing how adequately tissues use blood or nutrients, such as oxygen; and mapping specific receptors, such as medications and neurotransmitters.

Cerebral blood flow, cerebral glucose metabolism, and oxygen extraction can be measured by PET. It is used in the diagnosis of stroke, brain tumors, and epilepsy and to chart the progress of Alzheimer's disease, Parkinson's disease, head injury, schizophrenia, and bipolar disorder.

A modification of the procedure, called single-photon emission computed tomography (SPECT), has been developed. SPECT uses less precise but more stable and more commercially available isotopes to measure cerebral blood flow rather than metabolic activity as measured with PET. SPECT is used to analyze blood flow in clients with ischemic stroke, subarachnoid hemorrhage, migraine, Alzheimer's disease, epilepsy, and other neurodegenerative diseases, such as Parkinson's disease.

Noninvasive Tests for Vascular Abnormalities

The noninvasive tests described here are useful in assessing cerebrovascular disorders.

Doppler Ultrasonography

Doppler ultrasonography may be used to measure blood flow (including direction and velocity) in the supraorbital region. In clients with occlusion or stenosis of the internal carotid artery, the direction of blood flow is altered (reversed) in the supraorbital artery, a change that may be detected by ultrasonography. Transcranial Doppler studies evaluate arterial flow in the circle of Willis and its major branches.

Doppler Scanning

Doppler scanning combines Doppler ultrasonography with pulsed-wave echocardiography. Visual representation of moving blood is obtained. Assessment of flow through carotid arteries is a common use of Doppler scanning.

Invasive Tests of Structure
Lumbar Puncture

In a lumbar puncture (LP), also known as a *spinal tap,* a needle is inserted into the subarachnoid space in the lumbar region of the spine below the level of the spinal cord. CSF can be withdrawn or substances can be injected into this space.

Lumbar puncture is performed for assessment and therapeutic purposes. LP enables assessment of CSF pressure and collection of CSF for evaluation. In adults, CSF can be assessed for WBCs, RBCs, chloride, glucose, protein, and lactate dehydrogenase (LDH) as well as pressure. Other tests that can be performed include serology for syphilis, glutamine, C-reactive protein, and a variety of cell stains. See the table Normal Cerebrospinal Fluid (CSF) Values and Significance of Abnormal Values on the website for common abnormalities seen on CSF analysis. *evolve*

Therapeutically, LP is used to administer spinal medications such as analgesics, antispasmodics, chemotherapy, and anesthetics. These medications can also be delivered via continuous infusion pump.

Myelography

A *myelogram* is an x-ray study in which contrast material is injected into the subarachnoid space to examine the spinal canal. A LP is performed and some CSF is removed. Myelography is used to visualize intradural nerve roots in selected clients in whom MRI cannot be performed.

Cerebral Angiography

Aneurysms and arteriovenous malformations (AVMs) are best detected by angiography. A *cerebral angiogram* consists of injection of contrast material into an artery to visualize intracranial circulation (see the Cerebral Angiography figure on the website). Angiography is the procedure used most often to visualize aneurysms, AVMs, major vessel displacement, vascular occlusion, and thrombi. *evolve*

Interventional Angiography

A polymer, glue, or small balloons are used to occlude feeding vessels in tumors or AVMs. Blocking the feeding vessels reduces the size and vascularity of the tumor or AVM, thus diminishing the need for, and the complications of, its surgical removal. Interventional angiography also enables balloon angioplasty to be performed to expand atherosclerotically narrowed cerebral vessels.

Digital Venous Angiography

Computerized digital video subtraction systems allow visualization of vascular structures. Much less contrast medium is required compared with that needed for cerebral angiography. A central venous line is necessary to inject the contrast medium. Indications for digital venous angiography include the following:

- Assessment for transient ischemic attacks
- Serial follow-up evaluations for known carotid stenosis
- Assessment of intracranial tumors
- Postoperative assessment of aneurysms
- Follow-up evaluations after extracranial or intracranial bypass procedures
- Assessment of dural venous sinuses

Invasive Tests of Function
Caloric Testing

The oculovestibular reflex, or *caloric test,* provides information about the function of the vestibular portion of CN VIII and pathways in the pons and midbrain. It aids in the differential diagnosis of brain stem lesions (see also Chapter 68).

The test is performed only in an unconscious client to determine the presence of brain stem function. Check that the ear canal is patent and that the tympanic membrane is intact. Ice-cold water is introduced into the auditory canal. If brain stem function is intact, the eyes move in a conjugate fashion away from the irrigated side and then quickly move back to midline. Irrigation with warm water results in the eyes moving toward the side where the ear is being irrigated. With brain stem death, this nystagmus pattern does not occur. Oculovestibular tests are contraindicated for clients with perforated eardrums or with acute labyrinthine disease.

Peripheral Nerve Studies

Electromyography. Electromyography (EMG) is used to measure and document electrical currents produced by skeletal muscles, called *muscle action potentials*. Small-needle electrodes are inserted into muscles. The electrical potentials of each muscle are amplified, transmitted to an oscilloscope, and displayed on a screen. The recording can be made audible and documented on *evolve* paper (see the figure Electromyography on the website).

EMG can differentiate between primary muscle disease and disease secondary to denervation. The results may indicate a transmission defect at the neuromuscular junction, such as myasthenia gravis. The procedure can be used to help to differentiate diseases of the anterior horn cells from those primarily of peripheral nerves.

Nerve Conduction Velocity Study. A nerve conduction velocity (NCV) study, often performed in conjunction with EMG, is used to evaluate the excitability and conduction velocities of motor and sensory nerves. It is helpful in identifying peripheral nerve disorders. A stimulating electrode and a recording electrode are placed to test specific nerves (usually on a limb). The time required for the passage of a nerve impulse from the point of stimulation to the point of recording is measured precisely.

Conduction velocity is calculated. Both motor and sensory modalities can be altered in peripheral nervous system disorders (carpal tunnel syndrome), whereas only motor fibers are affected in chronic disease of the anterior horn cell or motor nerve roots.

Muscle or Nerve Biopsy

When other tests are inconclusive, muscle and nerve biopsies are used in the diagnosis of myopathies and neuropathies. An EMG is helpful in locating those muscle areas that are most abnormal. It is important that areas that have been traumatized by needle electrodes be avoided when tissue is taken for biopsy. Different techniques are used to obtain the specimens, for example, open incision or needle biopsy.

Cellular Assessment

With analysis of the human genome, genetic testing has increased in importance in recent years. Chromosomes can be prepared for microscopic examination from tissue culture of cells obtained from peripheral blood, bone marrow, skin, chorionic villus, and autopsy specimens. Chromosome analysis assists diagnosis of some abnormal neurologic conditions and provides the basis for genetic counseling in families with evidence of congenital neurologic malformations and inherited neurologic diseases. Mental retardation and convulsive seizures may result from neurologic dysfunction associated with inborn errors of metabolism.

CONCLUSIONS

Neurologic assessment begins with the history of the disorder and proceeds to the physical examination. The physical examination can be lengthy because of the complexity of the CNS. The neurologic examination consists of assessments of cognition, sensation, motor function, and reflexes. The complexity and length of time required for the assessment may tempt you to omit portions to speed up the process. Before omitting portions, remember that the assessments provide baseline data for further evaluation and legal proof of a client's status. Diagnostic tests include LP, CT, MRI, and angiography. Understanding how a test is performed enables the nurse to provide adequate client preparation and to perform appropriate follow-up assessments.

BIBLIOGRAPHY

Citations appearing in red refer to primary research.

Citations appearing in blue refer to evidence-based practice guidelines and protocols.

1. Bader, M., & Littlejohns, L. (Eds.) (2004). *AANN core curriculum for neuroscience nursing* (4th ed.). Philadelphia: Saunders.
2. Blumenfeld, H. (2002). *Neuroanatomy through clinical cases.* Sunderland, Mass: Sinauer Associates.

3. Cipriano, J. (2003). *Photographic manual of regional orthopaedic and neurologic tests* (4th ed.). Atlanta: Lippincott Williams & Wilkins.

4. Estes, M. (2006). *Health assessment & physical examination* (3rd ed.). Australia: Delmar Thomson Learning.

5. Evans, R.W. (2003). *Saunders manual of neurologic practice*. Philadelphia: Saunders.

6. Goetz, C. (2003). *Textbook of clinical neurology* (2nd ed.). Philadelphia: Saunders.

7. Guyton, A., & Hall, J. (2006). *Textbook of medical physiology* (11th ed.). Philadelphia: Saunders.

8. Hickey, J.V. (2003). *Clinical practice of neurological and neuroscience nursing* (5th ed.). Philadelphia: Lippincott Williams & Wilkins.

9. Jarvis, C. (2004). *Physical examination and health assessment* (4th ed.). Philadelphia: Saunders.

10. Kernan, W., et al. (2000). Phenylpropanolamine and the risk of hemorrhagic stroke. *New England Journal of Medicine, 343*(25), 1826-1832.

11. Lindsay, K., & Bone, I. (2004). *Neurology and neurosurgery illustrated* (4th ed.). Edinburgh: Churchill Livingstone.

12. Lynn-McHale, D., & Carlson, K. (Eds.) (2005). *AACN procedure manual for critical care* (5th ed.). Philadelphia: Saunders.

13. Pagana, K., & Pagana, T. (2006). *Manual of diagnostic and laboratory tests* (3rd ed.). St. Louis: Mosby.

evolve *Did you remember to check out the bonus material on the Evolve website and the CD-ROM, including NCLEX®-Examination Style Review Questions, Open-Book Quizzes, and Chapter Review Audio Podcasts?*

http://evolve.elsevier.com/Black/medsurg

CHAPTER 68

Management of Comatose or Confused Clients

CHRISTINA STEWART-AMIDEI

Perhaps more than any other clients we encounter, clients who are comatose or confused need to be cared for in a holistic manner. All aspects of physiologic and psychological function need to be addressed. Even if clients cannot interact with their surroundings the nurse must care for them in a respectful and dignified manner. It is important for family members to see that their loved ones are spoken to and cared for in a professional and caring way. The term *patient* is used in this chapter to describe the client who is comatose. It is assumed that such a client cannot be an active participant in care and that the *family* serves as the *client* in these circumstances.

DISORDERS OF CONSCIOUSNESS

Consciousness is a state of being with two important aspects: (1) wakefulness and (2) awareness of self, environment (including place), and time. Wakefulness is the ability to maintain an awake state or to be easily aroused from sleep. *Awareness of self* means that the client can identify himself or herself. *Awareness of place* indicates that the client can identify his or her present location and reason for being there. *Awareness of time* indicates that a client knows the date, month, and year and can identify common current facts, such as the season.

Unconsciousness can be brief, lasting for a few seconds to minutes, or sustained, lasting for an hour or longer. To produce unconsciousness, a disorder must (1) disrupt the ascending reticular activating system, which extends the length of the brain stem and up into the thalamus; (2) significantly disrupt the function of both cerebral hemispheres; or (3) metabolically depress overall brain function, as in a drug overdose.

Coma is a state of sustained unconsciousness in which the patient (1) does not respond to verbal stimuli, (2) may have varying responses to painful stimuli, (3) does not move voluntarily, (4) may have altered respiratory patterns, (5) may have altered pupillary responses to light, and (6) does not blink. In general the longer the coma lasts, the more likely it is irreversible. Duration of coma is also associated with mortality and outcome; the longer the coma, the higher the mortality, and the poorer the neurologic outcome.

Etiology and Risk Factors

Two types of disorders produce coma (Table 68-1):
1. Structural lesions in the brain that place pressure on the brain stem or the structures within the posterior cranial fossa, including the cerebellum, midbrain, pons, and medulla. These types of lesions affect the reticular activating system (RAS).
2. Metabolic disorders and diffuse lesions, which impair wakefulness and awareness by reducing the supply of oxygen and glucose, by allowing waste products to accumulate in the brain, or by altering other cerebral metabolic processes.

Structural causes of coma include head trauma, ischemic or hemorrhagic stroke, and brain tumors. Automobile and motorcycle accidents, physical assaults, gunshot wounds, and falls are common causes of head injury.

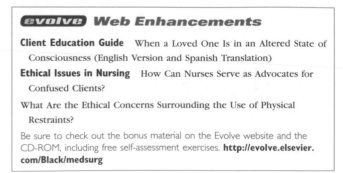

evolve **Web Enhancements**

Client Education Guide When a Loved One Is in an Altered State of Consciousness (English Version and Spanish Translation)

Ethical Issues in Nursing How Can Nurses Serve as Advocates for Confused Clients?

What Are the Ethical Concerns Surrounding the Use of Physical Restraints?

Be sure to check out the bonus material on the Evolve website and the CD-ROM, including free self-assessment exercises. **http://evolve.elsevier. com/Black/medsurg**

TABLE 68–1	Causes of Altered Consciousness
Type of Lesion	**Causes**
Structural Brain Lesions	
Supratentorial lesions (cause upper brain stem dysfunction)	Cerebral edema
	Brain tumor
	Brain abscess
	Cerebral hemorrhage
	Cerebral infarction (large)
	Epidural hematoma
	Subdural hematoma
Infratentorial lesions (compress or destroy reticular formation)	Cerebellar abscess
	Brain stem or cerebellar hemorrhage
	Brain stem or cerebellar infarction
	Brain stem or cerebellar tumor
Metabolic disorders and diffuse lesions	Diseases of other organs (e.g., heart, liver, lungs, endocrine glands, kidney)
	Poisons, alcohol, and drugs
	Fluid, electrolyte, acid-base imbalances
	Seizures
	Infections (e.g., encephalitis, meningitis)
	Severe nutritional deficiencies
	Hypoglycemia
	Ischemia or anoxia
	Syncope
	Temperature regulation disorders

The impact of the initial injury causes damage, but further damage can occur as a result of ischemic consequences of injury. Ischemic stroke occurs with interruption of blood supply to the brain. Ischemia can directly affect structures involved in consciousness or cause swelling of the brain, leading to coma. Hemorrhagic stroke can occur as a consequence of hypertension or from rupture of a vascular anomaly. Hemorrhage causes coma by placing pressure on brain tissue. Tumors may metastasize from other organs or arise from the brain itself. Increased intracranial pressure caused by the tumor may lead to coma.

There are many metabolic causes of coma. The term *metabolic* is used to describe any problem that alters brain metabolism. *Hypoxia* is a common cause of metabolic coma. Blood loss, high altitudes, or carbon monoxide poisoning may deprive the brain of oxygen. *Ischemia,* inadequate tissue levels of oxygen, may occur with cardiac disorders in which cardiac output is decreased, such as cardiac arrest or even fainting.

Of note is that coma may be purposely induced as a means to treat neurologic and other serious illnesses. In this situation, medication such as propofol is given to produce coma to rest the brain and hopefully prevent further injury to the brain. Induced or therapeutic coma may be considered for clients with extreme brain swelling secondary to brain injury, stroke, or metabolic disease. Therapeutic coma may be continued for days to a few weeks. Care for patients in induced coma is largely the same as for those who are comatose from some disease process. Full life support in an intensive care setting is required.

Pathophysiology

Consciousness is a complex function controlled by the RAS and its integrated components. The RAS begins in the medulla as the reticular formation (RF) (Figure 68-1). The reticular formation connects to the RAS, located in the midbrain, which then connects to the hypothalamus and thalamus. Integrated pathways connect to the cortex via the thalamus and to the limbic system via the hypothalamus. Feedback systems also connect at the brain stem level. The reticular formation produces wakefulness, whereas the RAS and higher connections are responsible for awareness of self and the environment. Diffuse cortical connections allow maximum integration of all conscious-related activities.

Disorders that affect any part of the RAS can produce coma. To produce coma, a disorder must affect both cerebral hemispheres or the brain stem itself. Disorders affect these areas in one of three ways:

1. Direct compression or destruction of structures responsible for consciousness. A tumor or hemorrhage in the brain stem or swelling in the cerebral hemispheres can cause coma in this manner.
2. Decrease in availability of oxygen or glucose, both of which are needed for cerebral metabolism. Hypoxia and ischemia are the most common causes; without oxygen and glucose, the brain cannot form the chemicals necessary to carry out its functions.
3. Toxic effects of substances on structures of the RAS. Toxic wastes from liver or kidney disease, bacterial invasion from meningitis, and metabolites from drug overdose are examples of such substances.

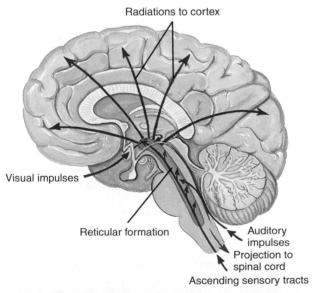

■ **FIGURE 68–1** The reticular activating system (RAS) consists of centers in the brain stem reticular formation along with fibers conducting to the centers from below and fibers conducting from the centers to widespread areas of the cerebral cortex. A functioning RAS is essential for consciousness. *(From Thibodeau, G., & Patton, K. [2003]. Anatomy and physiology [5th ed., p. 395]. St. Louis: Mosby.)*

The causes may overlap. The anatomic location and the severity of the problem determine the depth of coma.

Clinical Manifestations

Supratentorial lesions (located above the dura roofing the cerebellum) cause a fairly predictable set of clinical manifestations (Table 68-2). Such lesions can involve cortical or subcortical areas of the brain tissue, as with ischemia. The disorder may also be located in only one hemisphere, as with tumor or hemorrhage. These lesions produce manifestations such as headache, localized sensorimotor deficits, and seizures. The manifestations are related to the specific area of the brain affected.

For example, if the client has a mass in the frontal lobe, early clinical manifestations may consist of headaches, memory deficits and subtle motor deficits (unilateral arm drift), or partial seizures on the side of the body opposite the brain lesion. *Partial seizures* are seizures that occur in one area of the body, such as the hand. As the lesion expands, manifestations worsen because the lesion places pressure on nearby areas. This pressure may cause a more pronounced unilateral motor deficit (e.g., client cannot raise the right leg or arm), aphasia, or a deficit in the visual field (blind in one half of the visual field). The client usually has intact pupillary reflexes. The Critical Monitoring feature on p. 1795 describes these and other neurologic changes. If the lesion progresses, coma eventually develops. Coma indicates that the lesion has expanded and now compresses structures deep in the brain stem.

Disorders of the infratentorial area (located beneath the dura roofing the cerebellum) cause the client to lose consciousness suddenly either (1) by directly affecting the RAS or its pathways or (2) by invading the brain stem or reducing its blood supply. Infratentorial lesions may produce unusual respiratory patterns (Table 68-3). The brain stem houses the center for rhythmic breathing. This center's function is lost as consciousness decreases, and the lower brain stem begins to regulate breathing by responding to changes primarily in the carbon dioxide levels as well as in acid-base balance and oxygen levels. The result is a very irregular breathing depth and pattern. A lesion in the brain stem commonly compresses the cranial nerves, and various cranial nerve deficits can be seen. In particular, abnormal eye movements and loss of pupillary reactivity to light are noted. Specific patterns of pupil size and reactivity to light occur when pressure is exerted at various levels (see Table 68-3).

Coma caused by a metabolic disorder more often is manifested as the presence of bilateral or symmetrical findings because the disorder affects the entire brain. The client usually demonstrates confusion and stupor before any physical manifestations are noticed. Physical manifestations of coma caused by a metabolic disorder include tremor, asterixis (flapping tremors of the hands), *myoclonus* (a single, sudden jerking movement), and seizures. Pupillary response is usually normal unless the condition is related to drug overdose. Depending on the underlying cause, acid-base imbalances may be noted. For example, metabolic acidosis would be present in a patient with diabetic coma.

Level of consciousness is the single most important indicator of neurologic function. In the comatose patient, this indicator is lost and other indicators of neurologic function must be evaluated. Information about the time frame of onset, motor response, pupil size and reactivity to light, presence or absence of oculocephalic and oculovestibular responses and other cranial nerve functions, and breathing pattern can localize the level of involvement and determine the depth of coma. For further discussion about these indicators, see Chapter 73.

Diagnostic Findings

The neurologic examination is supplemented by diagnostic testing. Tests identify structural or physiologic abnormalities that affect brain function.

Computed Tomography and Magnetic Resonance Imaging

A computed tomography (CT) or magnetic resonance imaging (MRI) scan usually provides data that indicate a structural cause for the coma. In coma a CT scan is usually performed first because it is quicker. Tumors and areas of bleeding are evident on the scan. In metabolic

TABLE 68-2 Differential Manifestations of Structurally Induced and Metabolic Coma	
Mechanism	**Manifestations**
Supratentorial coma	History of progressive onset; initiating manifestation is usually focal cerebral dysfunction; neurologic manifestations at any given time point to one anatomic area (e.g., frontal lobes, thalamus)
	Signs of dysfunction progress cephalocaudad
	Motor manifestations are often symmetrical
Infratentorial coma	History of sudden onset of coma
	Localizing brain stem manifestations precede or accompany coma onset
	Cranial nerve palsies
	"Bizarre" respiratory patterns that appear at coma onset
Metabolic coma	Confusion and stupor commonly precede motor manifestations
	Motor manifestations are usually symmetrical
	Pupillary reactions are usually preserved
	Asterixis, myoclonus, tremor, and seizures are common
	Acid-base imbalances with hyperventilation or hypoventilation are common

CRITICAL MONITORING

Manifestations of Changes in Neurologic Status

"Change" is the key word. Notify the physician whenever there is a change in the patient's neurologic status. The following manifestations are listed in the order that indicates a *worsening* in the patient's condition. Remember, a patient may display a "transient" deterioration in neurologic responses that does not warrant calling a physician. For example, after you have just performed suctioning of the patient's airway or have turned the patient, you would anticipate a possible change in neurologic status. If you hyperoxygenate the patient and ensure proper positioning for venous return from the jugular veins and airway maintenance, however, any manifestations of increased deficit should last only a few seconds or no more than a few minutes. Worsening deficit that lasts longer than this increases the risk for irreversible brain injury and requires immediate attention.

NORMAL

- Alert, oriented to person, place, time
- Responds appropriately to verbal commands
- Eyes open spontaneously with any stimulus, unless in a deep sleep

ABNORMAL; CHANGES CAUSED BY ALTERED PERFUSION OF THE CEREBRAL CORTEX

- Altered level of consciousness
- Altered perception of time, then place, and lastly person
- Motor deficits (e.g., hemiparesis, hemiplegia)
- Speech deficits (e.g., expressive or receptive speech or both)
- Memory deficits (e.g., recent, intermediate, remote)
- Hyperreflexia
- Babinski's sign
- Seizures
- Decorticate rigidity
- Emotional lability
- Altered sensory interpretation
- Cheyne-Stokes respiration
- Headache, nausea, vomiting, papilledema

ABNORMAL; CHANGES CAUSED BY ALTERED PERFUSION JUST INFERIOR TO THE CORTEX

- Pupillary changes: asymmetry of size, shape, or time-responsiveness
- Loss of reaction to direct light
- Visual field changes (e.g., homonymous hemianopsia; see Chapter 70)

CN, Cranial nerve.

ABNORMAL; CHANGES CAUSED BY ALTERED PERFUSION OF THE DIENCEPHALON

- Altered temperature; first high fevers, then hypothermia
- Cheyne-Stokes respiration

ABNORMAL; CHANGES CAUSED BY ALTERED PERFUSION OF THE POSTERIOR PITUITARY GLAND

- Diabetes insipidus (decreased antidiuretic hormone)

ABNORMAL; CHANGES CAUSED BY ALTERED PERFUSION OF THE MIDBRAIN

- Dysfunction of CN III (loss of reaction to indirect or consensual light, disconjugate eye movement)
- Dysfunction of CN IV (disconjugate eye movement)
- Central neurogenic hyperventilation

ABNORMAL; CHANGES CAUSED BY ALTERED PERFUSION OF THE UPPER PONS

- Dysfunction of CN V (altered sensory function to cornea, nasal membranes, face, oral cavity, tongue, teeth, or altered mastication)
- Dysfunction of CN VI (altered lateral eye movement)
- Dysfunction of CN VII (altered facial expression, taste, and salivation)
- Central neurogenic hyperventilation
- Abnormal extension posture
- Pinpoint pupils

ABNORMAL; CHANGES CAUSED BY ALTERED PERFUSION OF THE LOWER PONS

- Apneustic breathing
- Flaccidity

ABNORMAL; CHANGES CAUSED BY ALTERED PERFUSION OF THE MEDULLA

- Dysfunction of CN VIII (altered equilibrium and hearing)
- Dysfunction of CN IX (altered taste, pharyngeal sensations, and cough and swallowing)
- Dysfunction of CN X (altered sensations in pharynx, larynx, external ear, and altered cough and swallowing; altered parasympathetic nervous system functions in thoracic and abdominal viscera)
- Dysfunction of CN XI (altered neck and shoulder movement)
- Dysfunction of CN XII (altered tongue movement)
- Projectile vomiting
- Cushing's triad (increased systolic blood pressure, wide pulse pressure, bradycardia)
- Ataxic (Biot's respiration)

---

coma the structures may appear unremarkable, or edema or diffuse nonspecific changes may be seen.

Lumbar Puncture

A lumbar puncture can be performed when it is known, from data provided by the CT or MRI scans, that the patient does not have an expanding intracranial mass.

Obtaining this information before lumbar puncture is done avoids the risk of herniation caused by sudden changes in cerebrospinal fluid (CSF) pressures (low in the spinal column and high in the ventricles). A lumbar puncture can assist in the diagnosis of infection or bleeding as a cause of coma. The CSF may be cloudy when the client has an infection or bloody when there is bleeding into the ventricles or the subarachnoid space.

TABLE 68–3 Eye Manifestations and Respiratory Patterns by Level of Involvement in Coma

Level of Involvement	Eye Manifestations	Respiratory Pattern
Supratentorial	Small reactive pupils	Cheyne-Stokes: regular respirations with regular periods of apnea
Upper midbrain	Fixed, dilated pupils (unilateral or bilateral) or midposition fixed pupils	Central neurogenic hyperventilation: regular, deep respirations
Upper pons	Midposition fixed or pinpoint pupils	Apneustic breathing: regular but deep inspiration and expiration with regular periods of apnea
Lower pons	Pinpoint pupils	Cluster breathing: clusters of irregular inspiration and expiration between periods of apnea
Medulla	Pinpoint or midposition fixed pupils	Ataxic breathing: completely irregular respirations with apneic periods

Electroencephalography

Electroencephalography (EEG) can be used to determine whether the patient is comatose because of continuous seizures. EEG results are abnormal in many patients with coma and do not serve as a clear diagnostic tool. A portion of the general population may have abnormal EEG results as well.

Laboratory Tests

Liver, endocrine, and kidney function may be evaluated through blood tests. A urine or blood toxicology screen may be useful in distinguishing drug-induced coma. Blood oxygenation tests may be used to evaluate for hypoxia. Other laboratory tests specific to the patient's situation may be ordered. Chapter 67 covers specific neurologic diagnostic tests.

Tests for Abnormal Ocular Reflexes

Oculocephalic Response

The oculocephalic response (OCR), also known as *doll's eye reflex*, is movement of the eyes in the direction opposite that in which the head is moved. For example, the doll's eye reflex is present if the eyes move to the right when the head is rotated to the left, and vice versa. This test can be performed only in unconscious patients because conscious patients have voluntary control over eye movements. The absence of the doll's eye reflex indicates that brain stem function is preserved. The reflex is present in patients with brain stem problems. The doll's eye test should never be performed in comatose patients with suspected or known cervical spine injury because the head movement required may produce permanent spinal cord damage.

The brain stem in a comatose patient may be functioning even in the absence of the doll's eye reflex. Patients in metabolic coma, except that caused by barbiturate or phenytoin (Dilantin) poisoning, retain ocular reflexes. Other agents and disorders can block the eye's response. Neuromuscular drugs, such as succinylcholine, and Ménière's disease, which destroys the labyrinth in the ear, obliterate the oculocephalic response. In the patient without Ménière's disease or evidence of neuromuscular drugs, however, absence of the oculocephalic response supports the diagnosis of brain death.[4]

Oculovestibular Response

If oculocephalic responses (OCRs) are absent, an oculovestibular response (OVR) (caloric) test can be performed to test cranial nerves III, IV, VI, and VIII (see Chapter 67). A normal response to instillation of iced water into one ear canal is seen as slow, smooth movement of both eyes toward the irrigated ear, followed by fast movement to the opposite side with nystagmus. Instillation of warm water results in slow eye movement away from the irrigated ear, followed by a fast movement to the same side with nystagmus. *Nystagmus* is the involuntary oscillation of the eyeballs; it may be horizontal, vertical, oblique, rotary, or mixed, with various rates of movement.

Failure to produce eye movement and nystagmus with the instillation of warm or cold water into the ear canal indicates an altered brain stem, with a few exceptions. The use of ototoxic drugs, barbiturates, sedatives, phenytoin, or tricyclic antidepressants or the presence of Ménière's disease may produce a false-negative caloric test result. In a patient without these conditions, the absence of an OVR supports the diagnosis of brain death.

Testing the OVR is contraindicated in a patient with a ruptured tympanic membrane (eardrum) or otorrhea (ear discharge). This test is usually performed only in comatose patients because awake patients may vomit in response to stimulation of cranial nerve VIII.

OUTCOME MANAGEMENT

Medical Management

The goals of medical management are to preserve brain function and to prevent additional brain injury. The primary focus is on maintaining the supply of oxygen and glucose to the brain.

The patient's airway, breathing, and circulation ("ABCs") must be maintained. A nasal or oral airway may be inserted for a short time. If the patient is breathing spontaneously, closely monitor the airway and respirations because the airway may become obstructed and aspiration may occur as consciousness decreases. If the patient is completely unresponsive or respiratory patterns become ineffective, an endotracheal tube is inserted, with care taken to avoid injury to the cervical spine (see also Chapter 63). Ventilation and supplemental oxygen are given.

Normal cerebral perfusion is promoted through monitoring blood pressure and maintenance of the systolic pressure between 100 and 160 mm Hg. Blood pressures lower or higher than these levels may alter cerebral perfusion pressure. Use of vasoactive agents may be required to keep the systolic pressure at 100 mm Hg or the *mean* systolic blood pressure above 80 mm Hg, or medications may be needed to lower the blood pressure. Blood pressure must be cautiously lowered, however, because high blood pressure may represent a compensatory mechanism to perfuse the brain.

Determine Level of Involvement

Once airway, breathing, and circulation are established, initial assessment of the comatose patient includes evaluation of the following factors:

1. Level of consciousness, through observation of response to stimuli.
2. Presence or absence of localizing neurologic manifestations, such as unilateral lack of movement or posturing, indicating focal intracranial disease.
3. Pupil size and reactivity to light.
4. Deep tendon and superficial reflexes (see Chapter 67). Superficial reflex assessment is particularly valuable in comatose patients because it provides objective information about brain stem function in the absence of consciousness. Assess the corneal reflex carefully to avoid corneal abrasion.
5. Response to noxious stimuli. First, loud verbal stimuli and then shaking are performed to produce a response. If none is noted, the examiner applies a painful stimulus, such as pressure to the sternum, nail beds, or supraorbital notch. Care must be taken not to damage skin underlying the areas where pressure is applied. Other aspects of sensory assessment are not possible or are unreliable in comatose patients.
6. Evidence of trauma. Trauma may be the result of coma rather than the cause of it (e.g., a tongue bite may result from a seizure). Examine the ears for ruptured eardrums and otorrhea.
7. Determination of serum oxygenation, blood alcohol, blood urea nitrogen, ammonia, and glucose levels if manifestations suggest a metabolic disorder.
8. History from significant others (or observers of what has happened), if possible.

Reverse Common Causes of Coma

Immediate interventions for the patient in a coma include treatment of common causes of coma while assessment of neurologic status and diagnostic testing continue. For example, after a blood specimen is drawn for testing, intravenous (IV) glucose is given to reverse potential insulin reactions. For comatose patients who appear malnourished and have a possible history of alcohol abuse, Wernicke's encephalopathy may occur. These patients are commonly given thiamine for prevention of Wernicke's encephalopathy, especially if they are given glucose.

If the patient is having repetitive seizures, coma and brain damage can follow. The patient is given IV diazepam or lorazepam to stop the seizures. If the patient is not intubated, closely monitor the airway because of the respiratory depressant effects of these medications.

Many metabolic causes of coma lead to acid-base, fluid, and electrolyte imbalances. The patient's acid-base balance should be restored quickly. Fluid imbalances should be restored slowly to prevent rebound fluid shifts into the brain (see Chapter 11). Isotonic saline is usually given if the patient is dehydrated, and fluids are withheld if the patient is fluid overloaded. If cerebral edema is present, osmotic diuretics may be used to promote shifting of extracellular brain fluid back into the plasma. Other medications, such as steroids, barbiturate therapy, and neuromuscular blocking agents, decrease intracranial pressure (ICP) through more indirect means. (Electrolyte imbalances are covered in Chapter 12.)

If infection is suspected, specimens for culture are obtained from the blood, urine, throat, and wounds (if present). Once such specimens have been collected, antibiotics are given. Body temperature should be normalized as much as possible by means of antipyretics, air circulation, and cooling blankets. Care must be taken to ensure that the patient does not shiver because shivering increases ICP.

Coma from drug overdose may be reversed by specific antidotes if the ingested drug can be identified. Often, however, the specific drug ingested is not known. A urine or blood specimen should be collected for a toxicity screen. Opioid overdose may be reversed with naloxone. Because the duration of action of naloxone is 2 to 3 hours shorter than that of most opioids, naloxone may need to be administered again. Seizures resulting from cocaine overdose can be treated with diazepam. Patients with cocaine overdose often have cardiac dysrhythmias and irregular respirations. Instillation of activated charcoal can be used to absorb medications. In rare circumstances, hemodialysis may be used to remove toxins from the blood.

Structural causes of coma may require surgery to decompress the cranial vault. Burr holes may be created to drain a subdural hematoma. A craniotomy may be performed to remove a tumor, abscess, or intracerebral hematoma. A ventricular catheter or shunt may be placed to relieve hydrocephalus.

To stimulate your thought process, see Thinking Critically at the end of this chapter for the description of a scenario involving a patient with coma from a hypertensive hemorrhage.

Prevent Complications

If the coma is prolonged, initiate enteral feeding to promote nutrition and prevent muscle wasting. Parenteral nutrition may be used if paralytic ileus is present. Take care to avoid hyperglycemia, which can exacerbate brain injury in the presence of ischemia. Brain cells have a high glucose need compared with other cells; however, supplying the necessary glucose without causing brain damage requires a delicate balance.

Prevent the complications of immobility, such as pneumonia and pressure ulcers, with frequent turning or the use of an oscillating bed. Continue to reposition the patient to relieve skin pressure unless the bed provides more than 40 degrees of rotation. The eyes may need to be taped closed to avoid corneal abrasion. Suctioning may be needed to keep the airway clear and prevent pneumonia. Passive range-of-motion exercises keep joints mobile and minimize muscle wasting. Position the extremities in correct alignment to prevent contractures. Use sequential compression stockings to prevent deep venous thrombosis (DVT); low-dose heparin may also be ordered. All these complications are continually assessed for and are treated promptly if they occur.

Outcomes. In the past, little information was available on which to base a prediction about the outcome for a patient in coma. Most of the time, a "wait-and-see" approach was taken. Today the family and the health care team should have some idea of the probable eventual outcome for the patient. It is discouraging and inappropriate to treat a patient vigorously who has no chance of recovery, but it is even more inappropriate to deny treatment to a patient with a reasonable chance of recovery.

Coma after head injury has a statistically better outcome than coma associated with medical illness. About 50% of patients in coma from head injury die, many instantly. Immediate treatment may improve the outcome somewhat for those who reach the hospital. Recovery in traumatic cases is closely linked to age; the younger the patient, the better the recovery. Severely abnormal neuro-ophthalmologic manifestations reflecting brain stem dysfunction imply a poor prognosis; about 90% of patients with such manifestations either die or remain in near-vegetative states.

The absence of pupillary, corneal, or oculovestibular responses during the early stages of coma is highly predictive of mortality or significant morbidity (e.g., persistent vegetative state). The recovery of these responses

and a return to purposeful movement correlate with a better prognosis. Patients who lapse into coma as a result of metabolic disorders have an extremely poor prognosis if the coma lasts longer than 1 week.

Some patients in coma awaken slowly and begin to respond normally. They often require physical, occupational, and speech therapy to return to maximal levels of function. Persistent unresponsiveness is caused by damage to any area of the brain that destroys the patient's ability to respond to the environment. The brain stem and cerebellum remain intact, however, so that vital functions, such as heart, lung, and GI functions, continue. Patients can remain unresponsive for years. Significant ethical and legal debates have arisen regarding the maintenance of nutritional intake for such a patient, particularly when a patient's family questions the rationale for artificial feeding.

Coma stimulation—application of planned meaningful, multimodality sensory stimulation—has been suggested as a measure to enhance outcome from coma. Clinical validity of coma stimulation has not been clearly established. The type of stimulation, timing of application, and outcomes measures used vary among studies, making it difficult to determine whether coma stimulation is of benefit.[2] Nonetheless the nurse is encouraged to interact with comatose patients through all their sensory systems.

Nursing Management of the Medical Client

Assessment. Frequent, systematic, and objective nursing assessment of the comatose patient, including neurologic status, is essential. Serial observations are important for comparison and to facilitate prompt reporting of even subtle changes in status. Even if assessment findings seem insignificant for long periods, documentation provides an objective pattern and an important baseline for future observations. Assessment of consciousness is most effective when the assessments are performed by a consistent nurse. The neurologic assessment is performed as often as every 15 minutes during the first few hours of coma. Depending on the patient's condition, assessments may need to be continued hourly for several days.

See the Critical Monitoring feature on Manifestations of Changes in Neurologic Status on p. 1795, which lists the neurologic manifestations of a person who is unconscious. Presenting manifestations are ordered according to the degree of seriousness. Remembering these subtle changes in assessment helps in early identification of a patient's improvement or worsening. A decrease in the patient's Glasgow Coma Scale (GCS) score also indicates worsening. The GCS is the most common neurologic assessment tool used in clinical practice (see Chapter 73).

Although neurologic assessment is the priority evaluation, the entire body of a comatose patient must be periodically observed because the patient is unable to offer any specific complaints. Complications of the initial condition causing coma, injuries sustained from other causes, and/or immobility can arise at any time during the course of care. If surgery has been performed, postoperative assessments must be performed as well.

Diagnosis, Outcomes, Interventions. This section describes interventions appropriate for all comatose patients regardless of the cause of the coma. Interventions specific to particular forms of coma are described elsewhere (e.g., hepatic coma in Chapter 47, and uremic coma in Chapter 36).

Comatose patients are completely dependent on others because their protective reflexes are impaired. Nursing intervention provides the safety normally afforded by protective reflexes. Coma is often life-threatening and requires aggressive medical intervention. Physicians are concerned with establishing a medical diagnosis and prescribing appropriate treatment; nurses are responsible for meeting basic human needs and preventing the complications associated with coma. Nurses are also responsible for assessing and intervening to reduce ICP.

Altered cerebral tissue perfusion is one of the highest risks for a patient with an altered level of consciousness. This outcome is often seen as a direct consequence of increasing ICP. Nursing management of this problem is described in Chapter 73.

Diagnosis: Risk for Suffocation. Patients who are unconscious cannot swallow because of loss or suppression of the gag or coughing reflex and thus are at risk for suffocation. Airway obstruction is the most common source of harm to patients with decreased consciousness. Write the nursing diagnosis as *Risk for Suffocation related to loss of gag reflex.*

Outcomes. The patient will exhibit no manifestations of accidental suffocation or airway obstruction as evidenced by (1) clear lung sounds; (2) equal lung expansion; and (3) the absence of stridor, cyanosis, and pallor.

Interventions. For initial airway management, an oral airway can be inserted in an unconscious patient. Endotracheal intubation, with the use of a ventilator, may be required to maintain airway patency or improve ventilation.

For extended airway management, a tracheostomy may be required to (1) allow long-term continuous mechanical ventilation, (2) facilitate removal of tracheobronchial secretions, and (3) separate the upper and lower airways (see Chapter 63).

Diagnosis: Risk for Aspiration. The lack of effective airway clearance and gag reflex puts the comatose patient at *very* high risk for aspiration. Write the nursing diagnosis as *Risk for Aspiration related to lack of effective airway clearance and loss of gag reflex.*

Outcomes. The patient will exhibit no manifestations of aspiration as evidenced by (1) clear lung sounds, (2) no stridor, (3) absence of fever, (4) minimal amounts of clear mucus on suctioning, and (5) clear lungs as demonstrated by chest x-ray.

Interventions. Monitor the results of arterial blood gas (ABG) analysis and pulse oximetry to determine the level of oxygenation provided by ventilators or oxygen. Assess breath sounds every 1 to 2 hours in acutely ill patients. Keep suctioning equipment available.

Perform tracheobronchial suctioning only as needed to prevent or decrease the accumulation of secretions from immobility, the lack of a cough and sigh reflex, or pneumonia. Failure to suction secretions of a person who cannot expectorate can cause hypoxia and result in neurologic damage. Suctioning should be gentle, and the catheter should not remain in the airway for longer than 10 seconds. While suctioning, observe the cardiac monitor for bradycardia and dysrhythmias (e.g., premature ventricular contractions) secondary to hypoxia. Hyperoxygenating the patient before, during, and after suctioning decreases the risk of dysrhythmias and cerebral desaturation. Limiting the suctioning time to 10 seconds also minimizes increased ICP associated with suctioning. Never suction the nasal passages in any patient with facial or skull base fractures because the suction catheter can enter the cranial cavity.

A comatose patient may lack pharyngeal reflexes and be unable to swallow. Pneumonia secondary to aspiration is a common cause of death in unconscious patients.

> **To reduce the risk of aspiration, never give a comatose patient fluids to swallow.**
>
> SAFETY
> ⚠
> ALERT

Secretions also accumulate in the posterior pharynx and may be aspirated. If the patient is intubated or has a tracheostomy, make sure the cuff is inflated. Suction the upper trachea and posterior pharynx as often as necessary to remove secretions. After tracheal suctioning, the same suction catheter can be used for oral or pharyngeal suctioning, but not vice versa. Also, turn the patient from side to side every 2 hours to facilitate drainage of secretions and prevent pneumonia; position the patient upright or prone periodically if the patient's condition permits.

As consciousness returns and the patient begins to respond to verbal stimuli and has a gag reflex, test the patient's ability to suck and to swallow liquids. Before the test, position the patient in high Fowler's position, and have suction equipment nearby in case it is needed. Use a thick juice, nectar, or ice chips rather than water; liquid of a thick consistency is easier to swallow. Place about 1 teaspoon of liquid into the back of the mouth. Observe for swallowing, and suction as needed to prevent aspiration. If a patient cannot suck through a straw or drink from a glass because of facial paralysis, place fluids in the unaffected side of the mouth with an irrigation syringe. Watch for difficulty in swallowing. Suction as needed.

If there is any question about a patient's ability to swallow, a formal swallow evaluation should be performed by a speech therapist. Patients who cannot swallow for long periods may require placement of a gastrostomy tube. Many rehabilitation and extended-care facilities require the use of gastrostomy tubes rather than nasogastric (NG) tubes because there is less risk of aspiration with gastrostomy tube feedings.

Patients with impaired swallowing require special instruction. Swallowing can be stimulated by having the patient lean the head forward and, after taking fluid, quickly tip the head backward. Stroking the anterior neck may also promote swallowing.

Once a patient can safely swallow, begin oral nutrition with small liquid feedings, progressing to a soft diet. Discontinue tube feedings only when the patient can take adequate nutrition orally. Many patients are fed orally during the daytime and tube-fed at night to maintain adequate nutrition.

When changing from tube-feeding to oral feeding, turn off the tube-feeding several hours before the meal. This will stimulate the appetite. When a patient begins to eat independently, allow adequate time and be reassuring and encouraging. Remind the patient to eat slowly and to swallow after each bite. Position the patient sitting up as tolerated.

Diagnosis: Impaired Oral Mucous Membrane. Several factors can impair oral mucous membranes. The comatose patient usually has an NPO (nothing by mouth) order, is unable to swallow, and breathes through the mouth. A possible nursing diagnosis might be *Impaired Oral Mucous Membrane related to mouth breathing*.

Outcomes. The patient will maintain intact oral mucous membranes as evidenced by oral and nasal mucous membranes that are pink, moist, and without lesions, crusts, or bloody drainage.

Interventions. Using a flashlight and tongue depressor, inspect the patient's mouth every 8 hours. Keep the patient's lips coated with a water-soluble lubricant to prevent encrustation, drying, and cracking. Carefully inspect a paralyzed cheek for crusts or other conditions that require intervention.

At least twice a day, brush the patient's teeth with a small or sponge toothbrush, and rinse the mouth. Place a comatose patient in a lateral position to prevent aspiration. If facial paralysis is present, keep the affected side uppermost. Keep the patient's mouth open by placing an oral airway or bite block between the teeth. Clean the oral mucous membranes (especially the roof of the mouth), tongue, and gums. Pay close attention to the roof of the mouth in patients who breathe through the mouth

for long periods. Crusts of dried mucus may form, break off, and be aspirated. Use of artificial moisturizers may help prevent crust formation; however, frequent oral care is the best prevention. Avoid using agents that contain lemon or alcohol because they dry the membranes. Suction excess secretions to prevent aspiration. Toothbrushes with suction attachments are now available in many health care agencies.

Nasal passages may become occluded because an unconscious patient is unable to sniff, blow, sneeze, or otherwise clear the nose. To clear the nasal passages of mucus and crust formations, gently swab the nose with an applicator moistened with water or normal saline. Then apply a thin coat of water-soluble lubricant with a cotton-tipped applicator. Do *not* clean the nasal passages or ears of a patient with a skull base fracture. If bleeding occurs from the ears or nose or if CSF (a watery discharge) appears to be draining from these areas, notify the physician.

Diagnosis: Risk for Impaired Skin Integrity. Normal reflexes reduce the risk of skin ischemia by signaling conscious (even sleeping) people to shift their body weight. Comatose patients have lost these protective reflexes and are completely immobile. Sometimes patients are agitated and can shear the skin with frequent nonpurposeful movements; this diagnosis also applies to these patients. Write the nursing diagnosis as *Risk for Impaired Skin Integrity related to immobility*.

Outcomes. The patient will have reduced risk of skin impairment, as evidenced by no reddened areas over bony prominences and no areas or manifestations of skin irritation or dryness.

Interventions. Provide nursing intervention for all self-care needs, including bathing and care of the hair, skin, and nails. Patients often scratch themselves as the depth of unconsciousness lessens; therefore keep the nails trimmed. Patients who are comatose for long periods may be lifted occasionally into a bathtub half-filled with warm water. It may be helpful to apply solutions high in fatty acids (e.g., castile soap, baby oil, or cold cream) daily and to bathe the patient weekly to prevent loss of cutaneous oils as well as skin irritation and dryness.

Perineal care should be performed at least every 8 hours and after every episode of incontinence. If perineal care is not effective for a woman with vaginal discharge or odor, consult the physician about the use of cleansing douches.

When the patient cannot respond to local tissue hypoxia from being in one position for an extended time, the risk of pressure ulcers increases. Patients should be turned at least every 2 hours. If turning is impossible because of the patient's medical condition, place the patient on a special mattress or bed (Figure 68-2). The use of a special bed, however, does not eliminate the

■ **FIGURE 68-2 A,** BioDyne, an oscillating-air support surface. **B,** Roto Rest, an oscillating bed. Both devices are used to prevent tissue hypoxemia and reduce the incidence of nosocomial pneumonia in patients that are unable to move or care for themselves. *(Courtesy Kinetic Concepts, Inc., San Antonio, Tex.)*

need to turn the patient and assess the skin. In addition, meet the nutritional needs of the patient to reduce the risk of pressure ulcers.

Diagnosis: Risk for Disuse Syndrome (Contractures). Normal movement and stretch are needed to prevent tightening of one group of muscles. When muscle groups are not used during periods of immobility, joint contractures can develop. Footdrop is of special concern. Write the nursing diagnosis as *Risk for Disuse Syndrome (Contractures) related to lack of voluntary movement.*

Outcomes. The patient will maintain full range of motion in any joint as evidenced by an absence of contractures.

Another outcome could be that the patient will have a reduced risk of contractures as evidenced by (1) a normal range of motion, (2) an absence of flexed arms and legs, and (3) no manifestations of footdrop.

Interventions. Prevent contractures by maintaining the patient's extremities in functional positions with proper support. Hand and forearm splints prevent flexion contracture of the fingers and wrists. Orthotic devices or high-top athletic shoes are used to support the feet. Remove the support devices every 4 hours to perform skin care and passive exercises. Assess the heel closely.

Diagnosis: Imbalanced Nutrition: Less Than Body Requirements. Comatose patients cannot eat and yet have normal or even increased metabolic needs; they can quickly become malnourished. Write the nursing diagnosis as *Imbalanced Nutrition: Less Than Body Requirements related to inability to eat and swallow.*

Outcomes. The patient will demonstrate the following manifestations of adequate nutrition: (1) stable weight; (2) adequate calories for age, height, and weight; (3) intake equaling output; (4) healing of incisions and wounds within 12 to 14 days; and (5) hemoglobin, blood urea nitrogen, total lymphocyte count, total protein, and serum albumin values within normal limits for age and gender.

Interventions. Intravenous fluids are begun on admission for comatose patients. Initially the IV site provides access to the circulatory system for the administration of medications. Because fluid intake is restricted and only limited amounts of glucose and few electrolytes are given by the IV route, an IV infusion cannot be considered nutritional support. Consider that 1 L of solution of 5% dextrose provides only 200 kilocalories!

Just because a patient is comatose, never assume that hunger is not present and that caloric needs are reduced. In fact, the opposite is true; such a patient's caloric needs are usually increased. Nutritional and fluid needs of comatose patients are usually met through enteral feedings because of the risk of aspiration with the oral route. If the patient does not have paralytic ileus or delayed gastric emptying and if bowel sounds are audible, start enteral feedings. The Management and Delegation feature on p. 1802 describes nursing considerations when administering or delegating enteral therapy.

The nutritional requirements of a patient in coma are complex; a complete nutritional assessment with comparison of height and weight charts, laboratory tests, and clinical examination is essential. Comatose patients may have a marked increase in metabolic needs. Malnutrition increases the morbidity and mortality of neurologically ill patients. Diarrhea and delayed gastric emptying may result from malabsorption. Healing cannot take place in the presence of a negative nitrogen state. Immunodeficiency, with increased risk of infection, sepsis, stress ulcers,

MANAGEMENT AND DELEGATION

Preparing Enteral Nutrition

Enteral nutrition may be delivered via oral, nasal, gastrostomy, or jejunostomy tubes. Gastrostomy or jejunostomy tubes are most commonly used because they pose a lower risk of aspiration. The delivery of enteral nutrition, including the verification of tube placement, is your responsibility. You may choose to delegate the reconstitution or preparation of enteral feedings to assistive personnel. Before delegating the preparation of tube-feeding or refilling the nutrition reservoir bag, consider the following:

- Your abdominal assessment does not reveal abdominal distention, pain, discomfort, or complaints of nausea. Your examination includes verification of tube placement and residual volume of less than 50% of the previous hour's intake. The presence of any of these findings would prompt you to delay the tube-feeding and notify the physician of your examination findings.
- You have checked the physician's order for the type and rate of tube-feeding to be delivered.
- Instruct assistive personnel in the proper dilution and handling of enteral feeding. (*Hint:* When mixing powdered enteral feedings, always place the powder in the mixing container before the water; this will ensure that the powder fully dissolves.)
- Instruct assistive personnel to place a 4-hour supply of feeding in the reservoir bag and to store the remaining mixture in a refrigerator for future use. Label the storage container with the patient's name, date on which mixture was prepared, and description of mixture.
- Although assistive personnel may prime the pump, you must set the pump and ensure that the flow rate matches the ordered flow rate.
- You are responsible for performing any irrigation of the tube.
- You may delegate care of gastrostomy and jejunostomy tube site to assistive personnel.
- You are responsible for monitoring fluid and nutritional balance via input and output and changes in weight.
- Describe findings that are immediately reportable to you for assistive personnel. They include any difficulty in preparing the enteral feeding and patient complaints of fullness, nausea, or vomiting.
- Verify the competence of assistive personnel in performing these tasks during orientation and annually thereafter.

weight loss, skeletal-muscle protein wasting, and lung tissue catabolism, leading to diaphragmatic weakness with respiratory reduction, results from prolonged calorie and protein deprivation. Starvation can lead to death.

Nursing responsibilities in tube-feeding of comatose patients are critical because these patients cannot communicate and may have lost protective cough and gag reflexes. The possible complications from enteral feeding, and their prevention, are described in the following list:

- Vomiting and aspiration if the stomach is overfilled or the head of the patient is below the level of the stomach, such as during chest physiotherapy. When tube-feeding a patient, elevate the head of the bed at least 30 degrees to minimize possible aspiration.
- Delayed gastric emptying. Check residual volumes every 4 hours. If the residual volume is more than 100 ml, delay the feeding for 1 hour and then reassess. Assess bowel sounds, and check for gastric distention; if this complication persists after several hours, notify the physician. If there is a high suspicion that the patient has a bowel obstruction, do not return the gastric residue to the stomach.
- Tube dislocation into the trachea or lungs, causing aspiration. Comatose patients are often restless. Tape the tube securely to prevent dislodgment. Aspiration may occur if a feeding tube is pulled out during a feeding session or whenever it is unclamped. During feeding sessions, cloth "wristlets" or wrist restraints may be needed.
- Verify NG tube placement by aspirating for gastric contents. Some agency policies and some manufacturers of small-bore tubes require checking tube placement by listening with a stethoscope for "whooshing" while instilling air through the tube. Never tube-feed a patient in the supine position unless all other positions are impossible to use. Leave the head of the bed elevated 30 degrees for at least 30 minutes after bolus feedings.
- Ulcerated or crusted nares caused by local pressure from the feeding tube.
- Tracheoesophageal fistula, that is, breakdown of the anterior esophageal wall from prolonged contact between the NG tube and a tracheostomy tube. This complication is manifested by gastric contents in tracheal secretions. Stop the feeding and notify the physician immediately.
- Trauma to the gastric mucosa if the tube's distal end hardens, as may happen over time.
- Fluid volume deficit if hypertonic tube feedings are given. To prevent this problem, ensure that the patient receives approximately 1 ml of fluid for every kilocalorie of feeding. Depending on the agency's policy, this intervention may require consultation with the dietitian or the physician.
- Constipation or diarrhea, which may develop from the osmolarity of the feeding, the use of liquid medications with a sorbitol base, or a too rapid infusion.
- Sacral pressure ulcers from continued positioning in the semi-Fowler position. Turn the patient 30 degrees lateral (to the side) with the head of the bed elevated to reduce pressure on the sacrum.

Diagnosis: Risk for Deficient Fluid Volume. The comatose patient cannot drink fluids or respond to normal thirst mechanisms. Such a patient is therefore at *Risk for Deficient Fluid Volume*. Recall that hypertonic tube feedings also increase this risk.

Outcomes. The patient will have reduced risk of deficient fluid volume as evidenced by (1) intake and output being equal for 24, 48, and 72 hours; (2) stable body weight; (3) absence of excessive perspiration, diarrhea, or vomiting; (4) serum glucose, hematocrit, BUN, creatinine, sodium, potassium, and chloride values within normal limits; and (5) moist oral mucous membranes with an absence of tongue furrows.

Interventions. Important aspects in maintaining fluid and electrolyte balance in unconscious patients are (1) accurate documentation of intake and output, (2) daily weights with comparison of trends, and (3) assessment and documentation of conditions that might increase fluid volume deficit (e.g., diaphoresis, polyuria, diarrhea, vomiting, hypertonic tube feedings).

Before fluid and electrolyte intervention is planned for a comatose patient, carefully assess the fluid-electrolyte status. The coma itself may have a fluid or electrolyte cause. Blood tests such as glucose, hematocrit, BUN, creatinine, sodium, potassium, chloride, and carbon dioxide measurements help determine fluid and electrolyte status (see Chapters 11 and 12). Dehydration and water intoxication (true hyponatremia) are common causes of electrolyte imbalance associated with coma.

Always avoid overhydration in a patient receiving IV fluids because of the risk of cerebral edema. Diuretics may be prescribed to correct fluid overload and reduce edema. Monitor the response to these medications. When evaluating the response to any diuretic, empty the indwelling catheter before administering the diuretic. Evaluation of the response should consider the diuretic given, the dose, and the patient's renal status.

Diagnosis: Risk for Injury. It may not be apparent that the comatose patient is at *Risk for Injury* because he or she does not move.

SAFETY ⚠ ALERT If the coma starts to lighten, however, the patient can move and without protection could fall or be injured. Seizures may also occur, leading to injury. Although loss of the corneal blink reflex, which increases the risk of corneal abrasions, is also a type of injury, it is addressed as a collaborative problem.

Nursing interventions for a loss of the corneal blink reflex are discussed in Chapter 65.

Outcomes. The patient will not sustain injury as evidenced by an absence of abrasions or bruises and experiencing no falls from bed.

Interventions

SAFETY ⚠ ALERT Keep the side rails up on the bed and the bed in the lowest position whenever the patient is not receiving direct care or is unattended. Observe seizure precautions for anyone who has a history of seizure or is at risk of seizure. Protect the patient from injury during seizures or periods of agitation (e.g., use padded side rails, keep the patient's nails short and filed). It is of utmost importance to protect the patient's head. Give the prescribed seizure medication on time to maintain a high seizure threshold. If a dose of the medication is missed for any reason (e.g., vomiting), notify the physician. Antiepileptic medication should not be withheld without a physician order.

Use caution when moving the patient, who cannot voice pain. Give adequate support to the limbs and head when moving or turning the unconscious patient. Limbs without tone may dislocate if they are allowed to fall unsupported. Always turn an unconscious patient toward you or someone else to prevent falls. Protect an unconscious patient from external sources of heat (e.g., heating pads).

Do not restrain the patient unless absolutely necessary because restraint is likely to worsen confused and combative behavior. If restraints are used, they must be released at least every 2 hours for range-of-motion exercises and skin checks. Do not leave unstable patients unattended. Attempt to manage the patient's behavior without restraints first. "Sitters," hospital volunteers, or family members or friends may be able to provide attendant services. Avoid oversedation because it may alter respirations, which increases ICP and masks changes in a patient's level of consciousness.

Diagnosis: Bowel Incontinence. Once a paralytic ileus is corrected, the patient will produce feces. Most patients are incontinent because voluntary control is required for the function of the external anal sphincter. Write the nursing diagnosis as *Bowel Incontinence related to inability to respond to normal cues about evacuation;* also consider *High Risk for Impaired Skin Integrity related to fecal incontinence.*

Outcomes. The patient will have reduced fecal incontinence, as evidenced by (1) a bowel movement every 2 to 3 days and (2) no manifestations of fecal impaction.

Interventions. Plan interventions to (1) control bowel movements, (2) maintain the patient's normal elimination schedule, and (3) prevent fecal impaction or constipation. As soon as the patient is able, begin a program of bowel retraining. Maintain a regular schedule, administering stool softeners and suppositories, and performing digital removal of stool at about the same times each day. Examine the abdomen frequently for distention.

Constipation and fecal impaction may occur. Small, frequent liquid stools may indicate impaction. If diarrhea or constipation persists, assess for possible causes, such as medications, enteral feedings, and intestinal bacterial infections.

SAFETY ALERT   **Consult with the physician before performing digital removal of stool in a patient with an altered level of consciousness. This intervention has been known to induce seizures and may increase ICP. Rectal application of an anesthetic jelly before the stimulus decreases this risk.**

Diagnosis: Interrupted Family Processes. Having a family member in a coma is a significant stressor. A possible nursing diagnosis is *Interrupted Family Processes related to uncertain future or impending death of a family member.* Individualize the etiology portion of the diagnosis to fit the specific patient and family.

Outcomes. Family members will exhibit positive coping behaviors as evidenced by (1) showing an ability to solve problems, (2) meeting the needs of other family members, and (3) asking questions about the patient that indicate understanding of previous teaching.

Interventions. The significant others of a comatose patient are often very distressed. It is difficult for family members when they cannot communicate with the patient. The uncertainty of not knowing whether the patient will recover is a major stressor. Include family members in the patient's care to the extent that they can and want to be involved. Family members need information and realistic hope.

It is important for the family to see the patient receiving high-quality, professional, and compassionate nursing care. For example, talk to the patient as though he or she can understand. Initially this behavior will seem awkward, but in time it will feel appropriate. Tell the patient that he or she will be turned to the side, bathed, and so on before performing the task. Depending on the depth of the coma, the patient's sense of hearing may still be intact. Therefore speak to the patient as if he or she can hear, and tell the family to do the same. Comatose patients have awakened and reported that they remember hearing specific voices.

The family is often in a state of shock, needing someone to recognize their needs and help them through this difficult situation. They may experience various conflicting feelings, such as guilt and anger. The Client Education Guide feature on When a Loved One Is in an Altered State of Consciousness on the website suggests ways for the patient's family members to cope with these feelings.

Allow significant others to stay with the patient when and where possible. At times family members may become zealous about attending and may stay at the patient's bedside continuously. Encourage family members to care for themselves also by eating regular meals and obtaining adequate sleep. Have them consider using external support systems (e.g., neighbors and church groups). Tell them they will be telephoned if any significant changes occur in their loved one's status, and ask them to leave a phone number where they can be reached. Encourage family members to phone if they have questions or concerns.

Social workers may be contacted to provide additional support. Some hospitals, especially tertiary care centers, have "family homes," where family members who must travel a long distance to the hospital may stay to be close to the hospital and the patient.

Evaluation. The patient may remain comatose for a few hours or even months. Some comatose patients (e.g., patients with diabetic coma) awaken and make a complete recovery while in the hospital. Therefore some expected outcomes have brief time frames (e.g., airway obstruction), whereas others are prolonged, requiring frequent reevaluation (e.g., family coping). Your evaluation may identify a need for revision of the care plan.

Modifications for Older Adults

The older patient in a coma requires the same quality of care as patients in other age groups; however, the older patient is at higher risk for all complications of immobility, especially pressure ulcers and pneumonia. Urinary retention is common in older men because of prostatic enlargement. Finally, fully assess the patient for the common disorders of aging (e.g., diabetes) that might be the cause of the coma.

Self-Care

The site to which a patient with coma is discharged from an acute care setting depends on (1) the condition of the patient, (2) the cause of the coma, and (3) the level of available family support. If the patient is recovering from coma, plan for placement in a rehabilitation center. Patients remaining in coma but showing slow recovery may be placed in an extended-care facility until they can participate in rehabilitation.[2,4] Coma stimulation programs, although not readily available, provide an alternative for the patient who is slow to recover.[2]

If the patient is in a coma and is not expected to awaken but may live for a time with nutritional support, placement in a skilled nursing center is common.[4] In these centers, supportive care is given. Family members usually specify how aggressively they wish the patient to be treated in the event of a deterioration in status. Your role in discharge of the comatose patient centers on communication with the receiving nurses and the family. If the patient is ventilator dependent or combative, special consideration is required for transport to the new facility. Provide a complete plan of care.

CONFUSIONAL STATES

Confusion is a mental state marked by alterations in thought and attention deficit, followed by problems in comprehension. It is accompanied by a loss of short-term memory and, often, irritability alternating with drowsiness. Confusion is a common clinical manifestation in many neurologic and metabolic disorders, and increases in incidence with age. Since confusion has been shown to increase both morbidity and length of hospital stay, this is of major concern.

Etiology and Risk Factors

Confusion has many causes. Common causes of acute confusion are alcohol withdrawal and drug ingestion. Confusion can also follow fever, head injury, and use of anesthetics. Other causes of confusion are decreased cerebral perfusion, hypoxia, hypoglycemia, severe fluid and electrolyte disorders, sepsis, liver or renal failure, poisons, and drug overdose.

Types of confusion include delirium and dementia. Delirium is an acute reversible form of confusion. Three features are common to all types of *delirium:*

- A disturbance of consciousness with a reduced ability to focus, sustain, or shift attention
- A change in cognition (memory, language, disorientation) or development of a perceptual disturbance that is not better accounted for by a pre-existing, established, or evolving dementia
- A change that develops over a short time (hours to days) and may fluctuate during the course of the day

Several classifications of delirium have each of the three common features but specific causes. They are (1) delirium related to a general medical condition, (2) delirium resulting from substance intoxication (prescribed drugs, over-the-counter medications, or street drugs), (3) delirium caused by substance withdrawal, (4) delirium with multiple causes, and (5) delirium "not otherwise specified."[6]

Sundowning is defined as agitation, confusion, and restlessness that occur after the sun sets; however, diurnal variations may be responsible for these changes as well.[3]

Dementia is the chronic form of confusion. Common features in dementia are the following:

- The development of multiple memory impairments
- One or more of the following cognitive disturbances: *aphasia* (problems with expressing speech or understanding sounds), *apraxia* (inability to convert a thought to action), *agnosia* (inability to recognize objects), and impaired executive functioning

- Significant impairment and decline in social or occupational functioning
- A gradual onset and continuing cognitive decline

The classifications of dementia include the four common features with variable causes and characteristics. There are many subtypes of dementia of the Alzheimer's type. Other types of dementia are (1) vascular dementia (multi-infarct), (2) dementia secondary to other general medical conditions, (3) substance-induced persisting dementia, (4) dementia with multiple causes, and (5) dementia "not otherwise specified."[7]

An in-depth discussion of the care related to specific types of delirium and dementia, as well as the memory changes that occur in patients with amnesic disorders and other cognitive disorders not meeting the criteria for any of the preceding classifications, is beyond the scope of this book. The reader should see a psychiatric textbook for this information. This discussion focuses on the general care of a patient with confusion; however, because dementia of the Alzheimer's type is a growing problem, Chapter 72 details the pathologic processes and care related to this type of degenerative disease.

Risk factors that lead to confusion vary with the specific etiologic factors. In general, the proper management of various diseases, such as diabetes mellitus, would reduce the incidence of confusion. Disorders such as Alzheimer's disease have no known prevention at this time, although new drugs may slow disease progression. Avoid the use of any medications that contribute to confusion in people who are at risk for confusion.

Pathophysiology

Three mechanisms account for the development of *acute confusional states:* (1) damage to the brain with swelling or loss of oxygen, blood, or both (functional disorder); (2) impairment of the action of the nervous system by chemicals or other substances (metabolic disorder); and (3) the rebound overactivity of a previously depressed center in the brain. Chemicals that cross the blood-brain barrier, such as alcohol, impair the metabolism of neuronal cells. When the drug action wears off or the drug is withdrawn from the patient, the lower centers in the brain are overactive. This overactivity accounts for the development of acute confusion, combativeness, and other abnormal behaviors.

Chronic confusional states are due to disorders that cause brain tissue destruction, biochemical imbalances, or compression of the brain. For example, people with Alzheimer's disease lack acetylcholine, a neurotransmitter that is necessary for short-term memory. Other disorders that cause chronic confusion may be inherited; may be secondary to a transmissible agent, as with Creutzfeldt-Jakob disease; or may follow diseases such as encephalitis.

Clinical Manifestations

The earliest manifestation of a confusional brain disorder is a *disorder of attention*. The patient may report the loss of concentration or may appear preoccupied. At the same time, restlessness, emotional lability, insomnia or drowsiness, and vivid nightmares may begin. Patients may appear anxious and may fear that they are "going crazy." As the disorder progresses, stupor and coma develop. Behaviors seen in the patient are reflective not of personality but of the cause of the disorder. For example, barbiturate or alcohol abuse and withdrawal and liver disorders cause agitated delirium. In contrast, anoxia and kidney and lung disorders are associated with a quieter response. Disorders that develop rapidly are more likely to cause an agitated response than those that develop slowly.

Fluctuations in cognition (the ability to think and reason) are common in patients with metabolic brain disorders. Patients may be totally irrational one moment and lucid the next. Some of the fluctuations are caused by the environment. Delirious patients become more disoriented at night, in unfamiliar surroundings, when they hear unfamiliar noises or see unfamiliar people, or when restraints are used. The lack of a window in the room has caused many patients to become disoriented.

Loss of memory for recent events is a hallmark of metabolic brain disorders. The patient commonly has difficulty with both immediate recall and abstract thought. Patients who are delirious quickly lose orientation to time. Normal people can readily recall six or seven digits forward and five or six backward and identify the commonalities between an orange and an apple or a tree and a bush; delirious patients cannot do these things. The patient's general intelligence level can affect the behaviors observed, however. If possible, the patient's level of education should be known before the assessment.

Perceptual errors (e.g., mistaking the nurse for a daughter) as well as hallucinations, illusions, and delusions are common accompaniments of delirium.

Hallucinations are sensations occurring in the absence of external stimuli. A patient may hear, see, feel, smell, or taste something that is not present. The patient may or may not realize that the experience is "not real." Unfortunately, the most common hallucinations involve rodents and unfriendly animals (e.g., snakes, spiders). These visions are terribly frightening.

Illusions differ from hallucinations in that illusions are the misinterpretation of something actually in the environment. For example, if a patient sees a shadow on the drape and mistakes it for a real person, the patient is experiencing an illusion.

Delusions are thoughts or beliefs that have no basis in fact. For example, a patient may think that he or she has been robbed or poisoned when there is no basis for this belief.

No specific diagnostic tests for confusion exist. The patient may undergo CT or MRI scanning to determine whether there is a structural cause for the confusion, such as a tumor or stroke. In addition, a series of laboratory studies may be performed to look for a metabolic cause. Common studies include a complete blood count, electrolyte measurements, determination of vitamin B_{12} and folate levels, thyroid and liver function studies, drug toxicity screening tests, and an EEG. A lumbar puncture may be performed for CSF analysis.

OUTCOME MANAGEMENT

Medical Management

In all care settings, the medical management of the confused patient begins by determining the cause of the confusion and correcting it, if possible.[3] When no specific cause is found, the medical management focuses on controlling manifestations. Sometimes medications can be given to calm agitation. Nutritional needs also must be monitored.

Nursing Management of the Medical Client

Assessment. A thorough history is required for assessment of the confused patient. The history should include the onset of the confusion, past medical illnesses, work and occupational history, and past injuries. Disorders such as diabetes or liver failure may be out of control and responsible for the confusion. The patient may have been exposed to heavy metals or toxic wastes at work. Record past injuries, especially head injury. Depending on the level of confusion, the patient may not be able to answer each question, and you may need to rely on the family or others who have been with the patient. Review medications, including over-the-counter drugs and nutritional supplements.

Specific questions about the patient's ability to handle routine financial transactions or home safety with tasks such as cooking, dressing, and driving will help determine whether the patient can be safely returned home or is in need of an alternative arrangement. At times the family will report a change in personality, such as apathy, social isolation, disinterest in current events, and irritability. Record these observations because they may be clinical manifestations of Alzheimer's disease or frontal lobe lesions.

The confused patient requires ongoing assessment with the Mini-Mental State Examination (see Chapter 67). This examination is much more sensitive than other tools for serial evaluations of confused patients.[7] Analyze the data collected to determine whether the confusion is improving, worsening, or unchanged.

The confused patient is often combative and argumentative. Observe for factors in the patient's environment that might affect confusion. Assess whether the patient is able to refrain from self-injury or injury to others. If not bedridden, the patient may wander about and become lost or injured if harmful items are not secured (e.g., knives).

Confusion can occur in patients of any age or culture and from variable causes. The nurse's role as a patient advocate supersedes personal bias related to any of these variables.

Diagnosis, Outcomes, Interventions. This section describes interventions appropriate to the confused patient, regardless of the cause, with an emphasis on the issue of safety.

Diagnosis: Disturbed Thought Processes. Use the nursing diagnosis *Disturbed Thought Processes related to failure in memory and lack of self-protective behavior to address needs for safety.*

Outcomes. The patient will have improved thought processes as evidenced by (1) higher scores on the Mini-Mental State Examination and (2) decreased frequency of hallucinations, illusions, and delusions.

Interventions. The confused patient will benefit from consistency in the environment and care routine. Keep objects, such as the tray table and bedside chair, in the same place. If possible, the same staff member should care for the patient. Give the patient short explanations as events occur, such as "You need an x-ray" and "Please sit in the wheelchair." Saying to a confused patient, "In 2 hours, an x-ray tech will be coming to take you for a CT scan," is useless because such a patient will neither understand nor remember it. Response time may be slowed in confusion; allow the patient time to respond.

Reorient the patient as often as necessary, but use caution about the specific communication used. Patients with chronic untreatable confusion do not benefit from reorientation and may become more agitated when you attempt to reorient them. For example, in one study in which a 92-year-old patient was told repeatedly that her mother or father could not possibly be alive, the patient reacted each time as if it was the first time she had been told and grieved deeply. For these selected patients, avoid reorienting, redirect their thoughts and agitation, or "go along" with the confusion. Of course, when the patient is at risk of injury, safety precautions are foremost. Clocks and calendars in the room also help with reorientation. The use of familiar objects is helpful when a patient's remote memory is intact. For example, the use of a quilt from home on the bed may help the confused patient recognize the bed as his or her own.

Promote reduction of unfamiliar noise because it adds to confusion. The patient's room should be quiet and softly lighted without producing shadows.

Consistency in the care of a patient with confusion requires communication among caregivers. This communication occurs not only through the oral reporting method but also in the care plan and documentation records.

Diagnosis: Risk for Injury. Confusion greatly increases risk of harm. The patient cannot interpret, or may not be able to respond to, environmental stimuli that precede danger. Write the nursing diagnosis as *Risk for Injury related to the unpredictable behavior and inability to interpret environmental stimuli.*

Outcomes. The patient will have reduced risk of injury and will not injure others.

Interventions

> **Assess patients at risk of falling often and toilet them every 2 hours. Falls are commonly due to attempting to reach the toilet.**
>
> SAFETY ⚠ ALERT

The patient must be protected from self-injury. The patient should be in a room near the nursing station so that assessments can be performed every 30 to 60 minutes. In addition, the bed should be in the low position. Structure the patient's environment to minimize injury; remove any extraneous equipment.

The routine use of physical restraints (e.g., side rails, cloth restraints) or chemical restraints (e.g., medication) is discouraged.[8] The use of side rails and restraints does not guarantee that patients will not fall and often either makes them more agitated or leads to more severe injury when they do fall. Alternatives to restraints include the use of sitters for ongoing observation and placement of the patient in an area permitting constant observation, such as the nursing station. Motion detection devices can be applied to the patient or the bed to signal the nursing staff when movement occurs. If all other alternatives have been unsuccessful and restraints are used, make frequent assessments and record the data. Cloth restraints must be removed every 2 hours to assess the skin beneath them and perform range-of-motion exercises. Chemical restraint (e.g., tranquilizers) can result in greater confusion and tremors (extrapyramidal symptoms). Net beds may be required for highly agitated clients. Follow manufacturer's recommendations and agency policy when using these beds.

The patient with brain alteration is not in control of his or her behavior. Behaviors may be unpredictable, irrational, or impulsive, or the patient may be frightened and suspicious. Never "punish" a confused patient for inappropriate behavior or remarks. Instead, remember that these personality changes are a result of brain lesions, and adjust the care plan accordingly. If a patient is agitated, provide reassurance and a calm environment. Redirect or distract the patient. Monitoring systems may be used for patients who wander.

SAFETY ALERT

Confused older patients are at increased risk for falls. A formal assessment of the risk of falls should be completed. Some institutions have programs for patients who are at risk for falling or who have fallen. These programs include frequent assessments, identification of risk on the door or door frame, routine toilet trips, bed and wandering monitors, and environmental changes (mattress on the floor, use of a lap buddy). Trying to ambulate to the bathroom is a common time for falls, and toilet trips should be offered routinely (every 2 hours).

Diagnosis: Disturbed Sleep Pattern. A common problem seen in confused patients consists of daytime napping and nighttime hallucinations. This problem is stated as *Disturbed Sleep Pattern related to alterations in usual sleep habits.*

Outcomes. The patient will have improved sleep patterns as evidenced by (1) sleeping 4 to 6 hours continuously at night and (2) not sleeping as often during the day.

Interventions. Plan nighttime interventions to allow 4 to 6 hours of uninterrupted sleep. Recall that a sleep cycle requires 1.5 to 2 hours, and the loss of rapid eye movement (REM) sleep can increase confusion. When you enter the room at night, assess the patient for REM. If REM is present, the patient should be allowed to complete the REM portion of the sleep cycle. You should return later to care for the patient.

Keep the patient active during the day so that there is some fatigue by nighttime. Daytime sleeping is a difficult pattern to break, and the patient may have to be kept awake for this pattern to be reversed. Bedtime routines should be developed. Avoid the use of caffeinated beverages and alcohol, which may prevent sleep. For the older patient, the normal changes in sleep with aging need to be considered, such as the greater use of short naps and less sleep during the night. Sleeping medications are seldom given to the confused patient because they often alter sleep cycles and rob the patient of REM sleep. See Chapter 22 for further information about sleep disorders.

Diagnosis: Risk for Caregiver Role Strain. The unfamiliar behavior of the confused patient or the stress of providing continual care for the patient at home may increase stress in the family and alter their ability to cope. This nursing diagnosis is stated as *Risk for Caregiver Role Strain related to long-term, stressful, and complex care required by family member.*

Outcomes. The patient's family members will maintain their own physical and psychological health as evidenced by (1) improved use of support systems, (2) obtaining of adequate equipment to provide care, (3) limited use of addictive substances for coping, (4) interaction with friends and extended family (as desired), and (5) appropriate analysis of the patient's condition.

Interventions. Teach the family to monitor for the effects of confusion. When confusion is a new problem for the patient, the family will be distressed by the behavior. Explain to the family that the patient is not able to control behavior or speech at this time. Assess whether the patient becomes calm or agitated when the family is present, and advise visitations accordingly. If possible, the need for and use of restraints should be explained to the family before they see a patient in restraints. The family may become very upset when they see their loved one "tied" to a bed. Advance explanations can avert some of this reaction. In some instances, patients have suffered injury because the family did not understand the purpose for the restraints and untied them. The Management and Delegation feature on p. 1809 describes goals and assessments related to physical restraints.

Planning discharge from the hospital for the confused patient varies with the cause of confusion. If the confusion is acute and full recovery is expected, the patient may be able to go home under the care of family members. If the confusion is chronic, the patient needs either care or supervision at home or placement in an extended-care facility. Some communities offer adult day care and respite services that give family members relief from the constant care of the confused person. See Chapter 72 for care of the patient with Alzheimer's disease at home.

Advise the family to have legal counsel determine the patient's competence and the need for guardianship or durable power of attorney. The family may also need to grieve the loss of the patient's previous functional role, personality, companionship, and so on. Assess for evidence of violence in the caregiver and the patient. Caregiver violence is possible, especially if the patient was violent toward the caregiver in the past.

Help the caregiver find respite care and personal time to meet his or her own needs and to learn stress management techniques. Female caregivers are especially vulnerable to social isolation.

Evaluation. Most of the time, confusion will require many months to abate. The diagnosis of a chronic, progressive condition such as Alzheimer's disease or dementia of the Alzheimer's type may require an entire change in care plan prioritization. These conditions are discussed in Chapter 72.

Modifications for Older Patients

It is common but incorrect to believe that older people naturally undergo a marked deterioration in mental function. In general, older people have difficulty recalling

MANAGEMENT AND DELEGATION

Physical Restraints

The use of physical restraints to protect a patient from self-harm or injury or to manage a patient at risk for disruption of medical therapies is a decision made collaboratively between you and the physician and may include consultation with other members of the interdisciplinary team. The serious decision to use physical restraints is made after your comprehensive assessment and evaluation of previous interventions and alternatives.

A clear goal is the use of the least restrictive device for the shortest interval possible. Regulatory agencies consider the use of restraints to be a high-risk intervention. Death and injury have been associated with restraint use in hospital environments. Your clinical site should provide you with clear guidelines regarding the use of restraints and the role of unlicensed assistive personnel in caring for restrained patients.

Before delegating care of the patient in physical restraints, consider the following:

- Have the patient and family been informed and educated regarding the need for restraints to protect the patient? Your education of the patient and family should include standards of care and discussion of what factors lead to discontinuation of restraints.
- Have you assessed the patient to determine the most appropriate type of restraint? The restraint must be the right size. Follow the manufacturer's recommendations for sizing. Never use anything other than a manufactured device that has been approved by the Food and Drug Administration.
- Have you obtained a physician's order for the use of restraints? In addition to the initiation order for restraints, there should be ongoing discussion of the need to continue restraint use with the interdisciplinary team and physician order updates every 24 hours.

Your assessment of the patient's safety and comfort needs must occur at regular intervals as defined by your institution. You are accountable for assessing and documenting the patient's condition, the patient's response to restraints, and the safety and comfort interventions provided.

Consider the following points when delegating components of care to assistive personnel:

- Be clear about the type of restraint being used. In addition to applying restraints according to the manufacturer's instructions, restraints are to be secured only to the bed frame or chair with slip knots.
- Explain that restraints are never used as a punishment.
- Patients with altered mental status experiencing unmet elimination needs may become agitated. Instruct assistive personnel to offer assistance with elimination at regular intervals.
- Provide specific expectations and a time schedule for observation of the patient.
- Provide instruction about how to remove restraints one at a time in agitated patients.
- Explain how to respond to patients who ask for the restraints to be "cut off" by re-explaining the need for them.

You may delegate these components of care to assistive personnel:

- Assistance with activities of daily living, such as bathing, grooming, and feeding.
- Active or passive range of motion.
- Turning and repositioning the patient. The assistive personnel should be instructed to resecure restraints after position changes.

Describe for the assistive personnel the findings that are immediately reportable to you. Such findings may include skin redness or irritation noted at points of contact with the restraint device, changes in color or movement of areas distal to the restraint, the patient's unplanned removal of a restraint, disruption of a medical therapy, and the patient's complaints of discomfort or distress. Verify the competency of assistive personnel in caring for restrained patients during orientation and in an ongoing manner thereafter.

---

new information, but their remote memory is intact. In addition, depression occurs in 20% to 30% of older people. Depression may follow the loss of friends, spouse, health, and independence and may lead to manifestations such as memory loss and confusion.

Older adults are particularly at risk for confusion during hospitalization.[3,6] They are dealing not only with the stress of being ill but also with the stress of an unfamiliar environment. Older patients may rely heavily on familiar landmarks and routines to help them maintain an independent lifestyle. These cues are often lost in the hospital or extended-care setting. A large percentage of the population in hospital and extended-care settings are older adults, who typically have other conditions that contribute to confusion. Confusion is best managed by using a team approach and teaching unlicensed assistive personnel to (1) introduce themselves at the beginning of a work shift; (2) use the same time for the patient's sleep, naps, and meals; (3) routinely place the patient on the toilet or commode; (4) talk to the patient about the past; (5) gently redirect lost or wandering patients; and (6) encourage self-care (eating, dressing, and so on).

CONCLUSIONS

Patients who are confused or comatose are vulnerable to many complications, including injury, aspiration, malnutrition, and skin breakdown. Nurses provide a lifeline for these patients, giving protection and promoting normal body functions. The families of these patients require therapeutic management because they face many difficult decisions.

THINKING CRITICALLY

1. A 48-year-old man is brought to the emergency department by ambulance. His wife states that he had been shaving in the bathroom when she heard a thud. She found him unresponsive on the floor. How do you intervene?

Factors to Consider. What was the patient's neurologic baseline when he was received in the emergency department? What other clinical manifestations did the patient display? Were there any physical manifestations of injury to his head or other parts of his body? Does he have any other significant medical history or allergies?

2. You are caring for a 72-year-old woman who recently underwent repair of a hip fracture. Her husband indicates that she had recently been confused, which led to her falling and fracturing her hip. How do you intervene?

Factors to Consider. What do you include in your assessment? What types of interventions do you need to consider? How do you involve her family?

evolve *Discussions for these questions can be found on the website.*

BIBLIOGRAPHY

Citations appearing in red refer to primary research.

Citations appearing in blue refer to evidence-based practice guidelines and protocols.

1. Bateman, D.E. (2001). Neurologic assessment of coma. *Journal of Neurology, Neurosurgery, Psychiatry, 71*(1), 13-17.
2. Hansen, L., Archbold, P.G., Stewart, B. et al. (2005). Family caregivers making life-sustaining treatment decisions: factors associated with role strain and ease. *Journal of Gerontological Nursing, 31* (11), 28-35.
3. Hickey, J.V. (2002). Management of the unconscious patient. In *The clinical practice of neurological and neurosurgical nursing* (5th ed., pp. 288-299). Philadelphia: J.B. Lippincott.
4. Hilgers, J. (2003). Comforting a confused patient: Learn how simple interventions and diversions can help. *Nursing, 33,* 48-50.
5. Laplante, J., & Cole, M.G. (2001). Assessment. Detection of delirium using the Confusion Assessment Method. *Journal of Gerontological Nursing, 27*(9), 16-23.
6. Miller, J., Campbell, J., Moore, K., Schofield, A. (2004). Elder care supportive interventions protocol: Reducing discomfort in confused, hospitalized older adults. *Journal of Gerontological Nursing, 30*(8), 10-18.
7. Neri, M., Bonati, P.A., Pinelli, M. et al. (2007). Biological, psychological and clinical markers of caregiver's stress in impaired elderly with dementia and age-related disease. *Archives of Gerontology and Geriatrics, 44,* Suppl (1), 289-294.
8. Oh, S., & Seo, W. (2003). Sensory stimulation programme to improve recovery in comatose patients. *Journal of Clinical Nursing, 12*(3), 394-404.
9. Park, M., & Tang, J.H. (2007). Evidence-based guidelines changing the practice of physical restraint use in acute care. *Journal of Gerontological Nursing, 33*(2), 9-16.
10. Rapp, C.G. (2001). Acute confusion/delirium protocol. *Journal of Gerontological Nursing, 28*(4), 21-33.
11. Wijdicks, E.F. (2000). Coma in the critically ill: Using neurologic findings and clinical context as clues to diagnosis. *Journal of Critical Illness, 15*(11), 609-610, 615-618.

evolve *Did you remember to check out the bonus material on the Evolve website and the CD-ROM, including NCLEX®-Examination Style Review Questions, Open-Book Quizzes, and Chapter Review Audio Podcasts?*

http://evolve.elsevier.com/Black/medsurg

CHAPTER 69

Management of Clients with Cerebral Disorders

CHRISTINA STEWART-AMIDEI[*]

SEIZURE DISORDERS

Seizures are sudden, abnormal electrical discharges from the brain that result in changes in sensation, behavior, movements, perception, or consciousness. A seizure may occur in isolation or with low blood glucose level, drug or alcohol withdrawal, or traumatic brain injury. *Epilepsy* is a chronic disorder of recurrent seizures. An isolated, single seizure does not constitute epilepsy.

EPILEPSY

Epilepsy is derived from the Greek *epilepsia,* meaning "seizure." In early times, epilepsy was viewed as being of divine origin and was called the "sacred disease" because someone with epilepsy was thought to be "seized" or struck down by the gods. An epileptic syndrome consists of recurrent episodes of one or more of the following manifestations: loss of consciousness, convulsive movements or other motor activity, sensory phenomena, and behavioral abnormalities. About 2.3 million Americans are known to have seizures or epilepsy. About 181,000 new cases of seizures are documented annually.

Etiology and Risk Factors

Epilepsy can be caused by any process that disrupts the stability of the neuronal cell membrane. A variety of conditions are associated with an extremely high likelihood of onset of a chronic seizure disorder. For example, severe, penetrating head trauma is associated with up to a 50% risk of the development of epilepsy. This association suggests that the injury results in a long-lasting pathologic change in the central nervous system (CNS) that transforms a presumably normal neural network into one that is abnormally hyperexcitable.

The identified mechanisms responsible for neuronal malfunction are unknown. Possible theories include neuronal cell membrane impairment, abnormalities involving the sodium-potassium pump, and changes in various neurochemicals. The neuronal cell membrane appears to be more permeable and more sensitive to various offending factors than other cell walls. An epileptogenic focus may develop at an area of altered cell membrane permeability, be limited to a specific area, or encompass the entire cortical surface.

Most seizures have no identifiable cause and are termed idiopathic. Idiopathic epilepsy most often begins before the age of 20 years and rarely begins after age 30. Seizures beginning in newborns and infants are often caused by congenital brain defects, birth injuries, or metabolic problems such as anoxia, hypoglycemia, or hypocalcemia. Although the underlying cause may be perinatal, seizures may not begin for many years, often with onset during puberty. Seizures may be induced by high temperatures in children who are otherwise normal and who never develop other neurologic problems, including epilepsy. After the age of 20 years, generalized seizures usually have an identifiable cause. Primary causes include traumatic brain injury, brain tumor, and infection. Other than in children younger than age 5 years, the highest

*The author thanks Melanie S. Minton for her contributions to this chapter in the seventh edition of *Medical-Surgical Nursing.*

---

evolve **Web Enhancements**

Client Education Guide Epilepsy (Spanish Translation)

Migraine Headache (Spanish Translation)

Be sure to check out the bonus material on the Evolve website and the CD-ROM, including free self-assessment exercises. **http://evolve.elsevier. com/Black/medsurg**

incidence of new-onset seizures is in people older than 65 years. In this age group, the increased risk is attributed to the increase in conditions that cause neurologic changes. These include cerebrovascular disease, tumor, delirium, Alzheimer's disease, infection, brain trauma, and chronic alcoholism, as well as the aging process itself.

Simulated convulsive episodes may occur in clients with psychiatric disorders. These are called "pseudoseizures." One key to differentiating between pseudoseizures and actual seizures is to look for stereotypical movements and a paroxysmal nature of the episodes. Clients with recurrent seizures exhibit the same stereotypic movements with each seizure. Clients exhibiting pseudoseizure make different movements with each seizure.

Pathophysiology

When the integrity of the neuronal cell membrane is altered, the cell begins firing with increased frequency and amplitude. When the intensity of the discharges reaches the threshold, the neuronal firing spreads to adjacent neurons, ultimately resulting in a seizure. Normally, excitatory messages from a single hypersensitive neuron in the cerebral cortex are modulated by deeper structures (e.g., thalamus and brain stem) (Figure 69-1). In epilepsy, these bursts of electrical activity from the cortex are not modulated. Eventually, inhibitory neurons in the cortex, anterior thalamus, and basal ganglia slow neuronal firing. Once inhibitory processes develop or the epileptogenic neurons are exhausted, the seizure stops. These later events depress CNS activity and impair consciousness. This period of impaired consciousness after a seizure, called a *postictal state,* may be manifested as sleep, confusion, or fatigue.

Seizure activity increases cerebral oxygen consumption and the need for adenosine triphosphate (ATP). Supplies of oxygen and glucose are rapidly consumed. To meet these demands, cerebral blood flow increases during a seizure. If the seizure is ongoing (as in status epilepticus), severe hypoxia and lactic acidosis occur and may result in brain tissue destruction.

Clinical Manifestations

Epilepsy may be classified according to the age at onset, cause, area of origin, abnormalities on the electroencephalogram (EEG), and clinical manifestations of seizure. The International Classification of Epileptic Seizures, used here, is based on the clinical seizure type and on EEG findings during seizures (the ictal period) and between seizures (the interictal period). According to this classification, there are two major categories of seizures. The neurologic abnormality may be limited to a specific part or focus of the brain, hence the term *partial* seizures. Additionally, the seizure may involve the entire cortical surface, to produce a *generalized* seizure.

■ **FIGURE 69-1 A,** Normally, excitatory messages from the cerebral cortex are modulated by deeper structures. **B,** In clients with epilepsy, bursts of activity from the cortex are not modulated and these bursts spread. *(From Devinsky, O. [1994]. Seizure disorders. Clinical Symposia, 46[1], 1-54. Modified from an original illustration in Clinical Symposia, illustrated by John Craig, MD, copyright by Ciba-Geigy Corp.)*

Partial Seizures with No Loss of Consciousness

Partial seizures are the most common type of epilepsy. The first clinical and electroencephalographic changes indicate initial activation of neurons in one part of the cerebral hemisphere. They are further classified according to whether or not consciousness is impaired. There are four types of simple partial seizures that do not impair consciousness. These include seizures with motor manifestations, those with somatosensory or "special senses" manifestations, those with autonomic manifestations, and those with psychic manifestations.

Motor Manifestations. Partial seizures with motor manifestations arise from a focus in the motor cortex. The resulting motor activity (seizure) occurs in the part of the body innervated by motor neurons originating in the affected region of the cortex. Because the hand and fingers have the largest cortical representation, many focal motor seizures begin with convulsive movement in the upper extremity. Involuntary movements may spread centrally and involve the entire limb, including one side of the face and lower extremity. This progression or spread is known as the "Jacksonian march." The client also may exhibit changes in posture or spoken utterances.

Somatosensory Manifestations. If the epileptogenic focus is in the parietal region, the client experiences sensory phenomena such as numbness and tingling in the affected area. If the focus is in the occipital region, the client may experience bright, flashing lights in the field of vision opposite the side of the focus. Likewise, the client can have changes in speech or taste with involvement of the posterior temporal area of the dominant hemisphere.

Autonomic Manifestations. Seizures of the autonomic system produce epigastric sensations, pallor, sweating, flushing, piloerection (goose flesh), pupillary dilation, tachycardia, and tachypnea.

Psychic Manifestations. Seizures arising in the anterior temporal lobe can begin with psychic manifestations. These seizures frequently begin with an aura, a subjective sensation that helps localize the focus. An aura may be a strange smell, noise, or sensation preceding a seizure, or a sense of "rising" or "welling up" in the epigastric region. Visual distortions and feelings such as déjà vu are common.

Complex Partial Seizures

There are two types of complex partial seizures: complex partial seizures with automatisms and partial seizures evolving into generalized seizures.

Complex Partial Seizures with Automatisms. The most characteristic features of a complex partial seizure are the accompanying *automatisms*. These automatic behaviors include purposeless repetitive activities such as lip-smacking, chewing, patting a part of the body, or picking at clothes while in a dreamy state. Inappropriate or antisocial behavior may also occur during the seizure. This unusual behavior may cause the client to be viewed as psychotic or otherwise mentally disturbed. However, abnormalities may be subtle and detected only by a trained observer.

Complex partial seizures with automatisms usually last 2 to 3 minutes but can last up to 15 minutes. The client is usually unaware of any activity during the seizure and may be confused or drowsy postictally. Attempts to restrain the client during a seizure may induce combative and uncooperative behavior.

Partial Seizures Evolving to Secondary Generalized Seizures. These seizures start from a particular focus, and then the electrical discharges spread throughout the brain. Clinically, the client first shows focal manifestations; for example, one side of the face moves, and then the whole body becomes involved. Consciousness is lost if the discharges spread throughout the brain.[46]

Generalized Seizures

Generalized seizures lead to a loss of consciousness. They can be convulsive or nonconvulsive. Generalized seizures involve both hemispheres. About one third of seizures are generalized. Types of generalized seizures are absence, myoclonic, clonic, tonic, tonic-clonic, and atonic.

Absence Seizures. Absence seizures are abrupt periods of staring and lapses of awareness lasting a few seconds to a few minutes. They occur in childhood and early adolescence. Tonic-clonic or partial seizures may develop at any time in clients who have had absence seizures.

Myoclonic Seizures. Myoclonic seizures involve sudden uncontrollable jerking movements of either a single muscle group or multiple groups, sometimes causing the client to fall. The client loses consciousness for a moment and then is confused postictally. These seizures often occur in the morning; clients often report that they spill their coffee with their seizure.

Clonic Seizures. The clinical manifestations of clonic seizures include rhythmic muscular contraction and relaxation lasting several minutes. Distinct phases of clonic seizures are not easily observed.

Tonic Seizures. Tonic seizures include an abrupt increase in muscular tone and muscular contraction. In addition, with tonic seizures there is a loss of consciousness and the presence of autonomic manifestations. Tonic seizures may last from 30 seconds to several minutes.

Tonic-Clonic Seizures. Formerly known as "grand mal" seizures, tonic-clonic seizures are the type of seizures most closely associated with epilepsy. However, this type of generalized seizure comprises only 10% of all seizures. A tonic-clonic seizure typically proceeds as follows:

1. An aura may or may not be present.
2. Sudden loss of consciousness may occur.
3. In the tonic phase, the entire body becomes rigid (Figure 69-2, *A*). If standing or sitting, the client falls stiffly to the floor. A cry may be uttered. Respirations are interrupted temporarily, and the

client may become cyanotic. The jaw is fixed and the hands are clenched. The eyes may be opened wide; the pupils are dilated and fixed. The tonic phase lasts 30 to 60 seconds. At the end of this phase the client breathes deeply.

4. The clonic phase begins next, with rhythmic, jerky contraction and relaxation of all body muscles, especially those of the extremities (see Figure 69-2, *B*). The client is usually incontinent and may bite the lips, tongue, or inside of the mouth. Excessive saliva is blown from the mouth, which creates frothing at the lips.

5. An entire tonic-clonic seizure may last from 2 to 5 minutes, after which the client enters the postictal phase, during which the client relaxes and remains totally unresponsive for a time (see Figure 69-2, *C*). The client may rouse briefly and then go into a postictal sleep lasting 30 minutes to several hours. This sleep may be followed by general fatigue, depression, confusion, or headache, all of which gradually resolve. The client has complete amnesia for the seizure episode and may feel nauseated, stiff, and sore. Bruising may occur as the result of falls. Petechial hemorrhages may develop on the face and chest due to the vasovagal responses.

SAFETY

⚠

ALERT

Tongue biting or falling during the seizure may cause other injury.

Tonic-clonic seizures vary in frequency from many times daily to once or twice a year. Tonic-only and clonic-only seizures may also occur.

Atonic Seizures. Atonic seizures are associated with a total loss of muscle tone. They may be mild, with the client briefly nodding the head, or the client may fall to the floor. Consciousness is impaired only briefly.

Diagnostic Tests

The major diagnostic tool for assessment of clients suspected of having epilepsy is the EEG (see Chapter 67). This test assists in (1) locating the focus of abnormal electrical discharges, if present, (2) establishing a diagnosis of epilepsy, and (3) identifying the specific type of seizures. The EEG records only the electrical activity of the cerebral cortex at the time it is taken. With this limitation, a normal EEG tracing does not always exclude a diagnosis of epilepsy, and EEG abnormalities do not always confirm the diagnosis. During a seizure, EEG abnormalities involve all parts of the cortex. Between seizures, clients with epilepsy may show EEG abnormalities not characteristic of seizure disorders. An ambulatory EEG study can be used to clarify suspected seizures that occur frequently. The monitor used is similar to a Holter monitor. Long-term video EEG monitoring may help classify seizures, and is also used to rule out pseudoseizures.

Occasionally, diagnostic tests such as computed tomography (CT) and magnetic resonance imaging (MRI) are used to rule out brain lesions that can trigger seizures. Positron emission tomography (PET) and single-photon emission computed tomography (SPECT) may be helpful to measure cerebral blood flow in clients undergoing surgery for epilepsy. A complete seizure profile and history is as important as the EEG and other diagnostic studies. The seizure profile includes a baseline neurologic examination

A

Tonic phase

B
Clonic phase

C
Postictal phase

■ **FIGURE 69–2 A,** Generalized convulsive seizures may begin with myoclonic jerks or, rarely, with absences. The tonic phase begins with flexion of the trunk and elevation and abduction of the elbows. Subsequent extension of the back and neck is followed by extension of arms and legs. This can be accompanied by apnea, which is secondary to laryngeal spasm. Autonomic signs are common during this phase and include increase in pulse rate and blood pressure, profuse sweating, and tracheobronchial hypersecretion. This stage lasts for 10 to 20 seconds. **B,** In the clonic phase, the tonic muscles relax intermittently, lasting for a variable period of time. During the clonic stage, a generalized tremor occurs at a rate of 8 tremors per second, which may slow down to about 4 tremors per second. The atonic periods gradually become longer until the last spasm. Voiding may occur at the end of the clonic phase as sphincter muscles relax. The atonic period lasts about 30 seconds. The client continues to be apneic during this phase. **C,** Postictal state includes a variable period of unconsciousness during which the client becomes quiet and breathing resumes. The client gradually awakens, often after a period of stupor or sleep, and often is confused, with some automatic behavior. Headache and muscular pain are common. The client does not recall the seizure itself.

and description of the seizure activity. Laboratory studies may rule out other causes for the seizure.

OUTCOME MANAGEMENT

Medical Management

The goals of management of clients with seizures and epilepsy are to prevent injury during seizures, eliminate factors that precipitate seizures, diagnose and treat the cause of the seizure, and control seizures to allow a desired lifestyle.

SAFETY

⚠

ALERT

During a seizure, the major goals are to maintain the airway, prevent injury to the client, observe the seizure activity, and administer appropriate anticonvulsant medications. In a hospital setting, suction equipment should be readily available.

The person experiencing a seizure usually requires protection from the environment. Objects should be moved out of the way so that the client does not strike his or her head or extremities. Any tight clothing around the person's neck is loosened. Put a pillow or folded blanket under the affected person's head, but do not flex the neck sharply or close the airway. Turning the person to his or her side displaces the tongue and usually opens the airway once the tonic phase has ceased. Do not attempt to open the airway with your fingers or an oral airway. A jaw thrust will open the airway without the potential to harm the client or the caregiver.

Factors that precipitate seizures should be eliminated, if possible. Eating a balanced diet, restricting excessive caffeine and alcohol intake, sleeping well, avoiding seizure triggers (e.g., flashing lights), and minimizing emotional stress may be helpful in preventing seizures.

Observers' descriptions of a seizure can be helpful in making a diagnosis, especially if the descriptions include details such as the sequence in which phenomena occurred. Instruct the family and unlicensed assistive personnel to make the following observations:

- How long did the seizure last?
- Where in the body did the seizure begin and how did it progress?
- Did the client's eyes or head deviate?
- Were the respirations labored or frothy?
- Was the client incontinent?
- Did the client lose consciousness?
- What were the types of movements and what body parts moved?

Medications are used to control seizures. Currently available antiepileptic drugs appear to act primarily by blocking the initiation or spread of seizures. Phenytoin, fosphenytoin sodium (Cerebyx), carbamazepine, valproic acid, and lamotrigine inhibit sodium-dependent action potentials, blocking the burst and firing of neurons. Phenytoin also appears to suppress seizure spread through inhibition of specific voltage-gated calcium channels.

Benzodiazepines and barbiturates augment inhibition by interacting with gamma-aminobutyric acid (GABA) receptors (see the Unit 16 Anatomy and Physiology Review). Valproic acid elevates the concentration of GABA in the brain, perhaps through interaction with enzymes involved in the synthesis (glutamic acid decarboxylase) and catabolism (GABA transaminase) of GABA. Gabapentin and pregabalin, which are structural analogs of GABA, appear to increase GABA levels by enhancing GABA synthesis and release, and may also cause a decrease in glutamate synthesis. The two most effective drugs for absence seizures, ethosuximide and valproic acid, probably act by reducing calcium conduction in thalamic neurons. Topiramate enhances GABA activity to facilitate seizure control.

Initial treatment begins with a single drug until either seizure control is attained or unacceptable side effects appear. Large doses of a single antiepileptic drug (AED) are often more helpful than smaller doses of several drugs. If side effects become intolerable before seizures are controlled, a second drug is added. Combining medications does carry the potential risk of drug-drug interactions, which can decrease effectiveness, as described in the Integrating Pharmacology feature on p. 1816. Nondrug therapies may also contribute to seizure control. The Complementary and Alternative Therapy feature on p. 1817 outlines a non-drug alternative for seizure control.

The use of AEDs is not without adverse effects. Although myriad adverse effects can occur, for the most part they can be grouped into three categories: idiosyncratic, dose-related, and allergic reactions. It is the responsibility of the nurse, as well as other health care team members, to instruct the client about the action, dosing, and possible side effects of the various AEDs. Developing a program of correctly prescribed AEDs requires weeks to months of medication adjustment by trial and error. (The desired outcome of pharmacologic management is monotherapy [use of one AED].)

Nursing Management of the Medical Client

The management of epilepsy does not usually involve hospitalization. However, a client may be hospitalized for a new-onset seizure for assessment, diagnosis, and education. Hospitalization may also be required if seizures become uncontrolled, for seizure monitoring, or if status epilepticus develops. Nurses have a role in assessing for ineffective health maintenance related to knowledge deficit or other barriers, anticipating risk of injury, and providing support for clients and their families who experience life changes related to seizure disorders.

INTEGRATING PHARMACOLOGY

Antiseizure Drugs

Many seizure disorders are controlled by various types of antiseizure drugs (sometimes called antiepileptic drugs). As well, different types of seizures require different medications. Epilepsy medication may be prescribed alone or in combination. If a client has more than one type of seizure, he or she may have to take more than one type of drug to gain control. More than 20 different antiepileptic drugs are available, all with different benefits and side effects. The choice of which drug to prescribe, and at what dosage, depends on many different factors, including the type of seizures, the person's lifestyle and age, how frequently the seizures occur, and, for a woman, the likelihood that she will become pregnant. People with epilepsy should follow their physician's advice and share any concerns they may have regarding their medication.

The first line of drug therapy is often phenytoin, carbamazepine, valproate, or levetiracetam, unless the epilepsy is a type that is known to require a different kind of treatment. For absence seizures, ethosuximide is often the primary treatment. For the client with stereotyped recurrent severe seizures that can be easily recognized by the person's family, the drug diazepam is available as a gel that can be administered rectally by a family member. This method of drug delivery may stop prolonged seizures before they develop into status epilepticus.

Most side effects of antiepileptic drugs are relatively minor, such as fatigue, dizziness, or weight gain. However, severe and life-threatening side effects such as allergic reactions can occur. Epilepsy medication also may predispose people to developing depression or psychoses. Clients with epilepsy should consult a physician immediately if they develop any kind of rash while on medication, or if they find themselves depressed or otherwise unable to think in a rational manner. Other danger signs that should be discussed with a physician immediately are extreme fatigue, staggering or other movement problems, blurring of vision, and slurring of words. Clients with epilepsy should be aware that their epilepsy medication can interact with many other drugs in potentially harmful ways. For this reason, people with epilepsy should always tell their treating physicians which medications they are taking. Women also should know that some antiepileptic drugs can interfere with the effectiveness of oral contraceptives, and they should discuss this possibility with their physicians.

Because older adults are more sensitive to medications, blood levels of medication are checked occasionally to determine whether the dose needs to be adjusted. The effects of a particular medication also sometimes wear off over time, leading to an increase in seizures if the dose is not adjusted.

DISCONTINUING MEDICATION

Some physicians advise clients with epilepsy to discontinue their antiepileptic drugs after 2 years have passed without a seizure. Others believe it is better to wait for 4 to 5 years. Discontinuing medication should only be done with a physician's advice and supervision. It is very important to continue taking epilepsy medication for as long as it is prescribed. Clients should ask their physician or pharmacist ahead of time what they should do if they miss a dose. Discontinuing medication without a physician's advice is one of the major reasons people who have been seizure-free begin having new seizures. Seizures that result from suddenly stopping medication can be serious and can lead to status epilepticus. Furthermore, there is some evidence that uncontrolled seizures trigger changes in neurons that can make it more difficult to treat the seizures in the future.

The chance that a client will eventually be able to discontinue medication depends on the person's age and his or her type of epilepsy. More than half of children who go into remission with medication can eventually stop their medication without having new seizures. One study showed that 68% of adults who had been seizure-free for 2 years before stopping medication were able to do so without having more seizures and that 75% could successfully discontinue medication if they had been seizure-free for 3 years. However, the odds of successfully stopping medication are not as good for clients with a family history of epilepsy, those who need multiple medications, those with partial seizures, or those who continue to have abnormal EEG results while taking medication.

Assessment. Assessment of clients not actively experiencing seizures includes the following:

- History, including prenatal, birth, and developmental history; family history; age at seizure onset; history of all illnesses and trauma; previous brain surgery or stroke; complete description of seizures, including precipitating factors; and presence of an aura
- Medication use and postictal (period of time following a seizure) manifestations
- Psychosocial assessment, including mental status examination

- Complete physical examination, focusing on neurologic manifestations (usually physical examination between seizures is normal)

Diagnosis, Outcomes, Interventions
Diagnosis: Risk for Injury. The diagnosis *Risk for Injury* is related to uncontrolled movement and/or loss of airway patency during a seizure.

Outcomes. The client will have reduced risk of injury and maintain a patent airway during a seizure as evidenced by showing no bruises or bumps following a seizure and by being able to regain adequate oxygenation following the seizure.

COMPLEMENTARY AND ALTERNATIVE THERAPY

Low-Carbohydrate or Ketogenic Diet for Seizures

The ketogenic diet (KD) is actually a non-drug therapy for children with epileptic seizures. It was developed in the 1920s and was based on the clinical observation that fasting suppresses seizures, probably through the induction of ketosis. Interestingly, the high-fat, low-carbohydrate KD tends to mimic the ketogenic effects of fasting and places the body into a constant state of ketosis. KD suppresses many different types of seizures, including those that do not respond to the conventional anticonvulsant drugs. The KD is given only after drug therapy has failed to provide adequate seizure control. KD is effective for tonic-clonic, absence, complex partial, and the multiple types of intractable seizures associated with Lennox-Gastaut syndrome.

REFERENCE

Likhodii, S., et al.. (2003). Anticonvulsant properties of acetone, a brain ketone elevated by the ketogenic diet. *Annals of Neurology, 54*, 219-226.

Interventions

SAFETY
⚠
ALERT

Seizure precautions should be implemented in all clients with a history of epilepsy and seizures. No oral temperatures should be taken; use axillary or rectal routes. The bedrails should be padded and up when the client is in bed. Seizure precautions also include inserting an intravenous needle for medication administration, and keeping oxygen with a nasal cannula and suction equipment, including suction catheters, at the bedside. Fall risk precautions are also needed.

See earlier discussion about assessments and how to maintain the airway during a seizure. After the seizure is completed, place the client in a lateral position and assess oxygen status.

Diagnosis: Risk for Impaired Adjustment. A diagnosis of epilepsy requires major modifications in lifestyle, and these changes are long term. Based on the assessment of the client's adaptation to the diagnosis, the nursing diagnosis is *Risk for Impaired Adjustment* related to complex and long-term health management needs, inability to be involved in high-risk activities, feelings of embarrassment about risk of seizing in public areas, or cost of treatments.

Outcomes. The client and family will state that they understand the need for ongoing treatments, safety awareness during high-risk activities, potential feelings of embarrassment or loss of control and/or costs of treatment.

Interventions. The major problem for clients with epilepsy is the unpredictability of the next seizure. For any activity, it is important to ask, "What would happen if I had a seizure while doing this?"

Five types of seizure precautions should be discussed with clients and their families. These lifestyle precautions are clearly more applicable to some clients than others.

1. Driving motorized vehicles: Generally no driving is allowed for 6 to 12 months following a seizure. However, state laws vary and also consider the pattern of seizures, for example, whether the client has seizures that occur exclusively during sleep. Consult current state and federal laws and regulations. For example, to resume commercial driving across state lines, a client must have a 5-year seizure-free period. The recommendation for driving cars and trucks extends to the operation of other motorized vehicles, such as boats, motorcycles, and others. Aircraft pilots are typically no longer permitted to fly.

2. Water precautions: Clients with seizures should ensure that they are in the presence of an adult lifeguard who can pull them out of the water if needed. Wearing a life jacket in a boat is important. Showers should be encouraged because taking a bath could lead to drowning with as little as 1 inch of water during the flaccid postictal phase.

3. Heights: Clients with seizures should not work at heights because they could fall and sustain injuries

4. Fire: Burns from injuries related to cooking are not uncommon. Teach clients to cook with other people present, and to avoid using the front burners.

5. Power tools: Caution with the use of power tools is required. In particular, supervision during their use is needed, and the use of safety devices, such as automatic shutoff switches, is recommended. Even the use of kitchen knives should be limited.

Diagnosis: Ineffective Health Maintenance. *Ineffective Health Maintenance* is the nursing diagnosis appropriate for clients who are having difficulty adjusting their life to their epileptic condition.

Outcomes. The client will have improved health maintenance as evidenced by maintaining routine dosing, consulting a physician whenever there is a problem, and wearing a medical alert identification tag or bracelet.

Interventions. Provide the client with verbal information and written reinforcement about (1) how AEDs prevent seizures, (2) the importance of taking prescribed medication regularly, and (3) care during seizures. Consult with the client to plan ways to make taking medication part of daily activities. Also, help the client to identify factors that precipitate seizures and ways of avoiding these factors. Such factors include increased stress, lack of sleep, emotional upset, and alcohol use. The Client Education Guide on p. 1818 lists other important client teaching information.

CLIENT EDUCATION GUIDE

Epilepsy

- Take prescribed dosages of medications to maintain your blood levels.
- Consult your physician if you are unable to take medication because of illness.
- Observe for side effects of antiepileptic drugs. Do not stop taking medications because of annoying side effects; this is very dangerous. Consult your physician first.
- Notify the physician if seizures are not controlled. Provide specific descriptions of the seizure activity.
- Do not take any over-the-counter medications without consulting your physician.
- Obtain a medical alert identification card (or bracelet or tag) with the name of the drug, dosage, and frequency; and your physician's name and phone number. Carry this identification with you at all times.

Evaluation. The short-term outcomes for the client who is experiencing a seizure are usually met within hours. An example is that the seizure stops and the client returns to the previous level of functioning. Nursing care of clients with confirmed epilepsy should focus on the long-term outcomes with self-care.

Modifications for Older Clients

With the increasing frequency of epilepsy in the older population, nurses need to be more aware of the changes in pharmacokinetics in this age group. Concurrent disease, foods, and drug-drug interactions affect absorption of anticonvulsant medication. A decrease in albumin, as is commonly seen in older adults, can increase the free plasma level of these drugs. Decreased metabolism can increase the half-life of these drugs, and decreased elimination can result in higher plasma levels.

Enteral feedings inhibit the absorption of phenytoin (Dilantin). Therefore the feeding should be turned off 2 hours before and after administration of phenytoin, or the dose should be adjusted based on plasma levels. Altered vitamin D metabolism with phenytoin increases the risk of osteoporosis. Carbamazepine (Tegretol) carries an increased risk of slowed cardiac conduction and heart failure; hyponatremia secondary to increased secretion of antidiuretic hormone, especially if the client is receiving a low-sodium diet; and altered cholesterol metabolism in the older population. Valproate (Depakene) carries an increased risk of causing hyperammonemia in older clients, leading to hepatic dysfunction, decrease in platelets, and toxicity related to its longer half-life in this population.

Surgical Management

For approximately 75% of clients with seizures, medical management with AEDs and follow-up evaluation suffices. The remaining 25% continue to have seizures. For about 5% of people with epilepsy, surgery is recommended to control the disease. A few years ago, the most common palliative surgery was anterior callosotomy. This surgery is still performed, but rarely. Several curative surgeries are possible, including lobectomy and lesionectomy.

Thorough assessment is necessary before surgery to determine the epileptogenic focus is located in the "dispensable" areas of the cerebral cortex. Dispensable areas are those for which there is a duplicative area in the cortex. A variety of neurologic tests are used, including video EEG, SPECT, or PET. Intelligence quotient (IQ) testing and psychological assessments are usually performed. Deep EEG electrodes may be surgically placed; this is done when surface electrodes are not sensitive enough to locate the seizure focus exactly. Electrodes are placed in the temporal and frontal lobes of the brain or in the subdural space. These techniques allow identification of deeper seizure foci. Intraoperative mapping may also be used to identify adjacent eloquent tissue that cannot be interrupted during seizure focus resection surgery. A *Wada test* simulates what may occur with surgery and may be used to determine hemispheric dominance, and the location of the speech and memory areas. An injection of amobarbital sodium (Amytal sodium) is given directly into the left internal carotid artery via a cerebral angiogram. If the left hemisphere is dominant, speech is arrested for 1 or 2 minutes, followed by misnaming and misreading for up to 8 to 9 minutes. After 30 minutes, the process is repeated in the right internal carotid artery. The physician looks for changes in sensation, abstract thought, and coordination. Postprocedural care is the same as that for cerebral angiography (see Chapter 67).

Operations for epilepsy include the following:

- Selective amygdalohippocampectomy: In this procedure the two structures within the temporal lobe that are commonly the genesis of seizure activity are removed.
- Temporal lobectomy: Focal resection of part of the temporal lobe, usually on the right side, is performed. If the dominant temporal lobe is removed, the client may experience language defects for a few weeks. Visual defects from loss of visual projection fibers are compensated for quickly. Other areas of the cortex (e.g., the frontal lobe) may also be resected, assuming there is either a defined structural abnormality or a highly localized seizure focus (Figure 69-3, *B*).
- Sub-pial resection: Fine cuts are made into the motor areas of the brain that do not control motor function, but do prevent the spread of the seizure.

- Resection: A cyst or lesion causing the seizures is removed.
- Hemispherectomy: An entire damaged side of the brain is removed; this procedure is performed to treat very severe epilepsy (see Figure 69-3, *C*).
- Corpus callosotomy: Fibers that connect the two halves of the brain are cut; this procedure is also done for treatment of severe epilepsy (see Figure 69-3, *A*).
- Vagal nerve stimulator implantation: The implantation of a vagal nerve stimulator (VNS) offers clients another treatment modality.

Although the underlying mechanism is not fully understood, the VNS is believed to provide a stimulus that desynchronizes the abnormal uncontrolled electrical discharge of the brain activity during a seizure. One study has reported that the benefits from VNS increase over time. For example, 40% to 45% of clients continue to experience a decrease in the frequency of seizures at 18 months after implantation of the VNS.

Nursing Management of the Surgical Client

Preoperative Care

The role of the nurse during the evaluation phase before surgery is to provide support and education. Clients who have epilepsy have been trying to control their seizures for most of their lives. Now, as part of the preoperative assessment, the health care team needs to observe the client during seizure activity. Therefore AEDs are stopped in the controlled hospital setting. This withdrawal period is often confusing and frightening. In addition, some clients are far from family and may be rethinking their decision to undergo surgery. Memory impairments are common because of both the side effects of medications and postictal states. Be certain to provide written material and reinforce education often.

Postoperative Care

Postoperative nursing care is the same as that for any client undergoing a craniotomy (see later discussion). The client is often placed in an intensive care unit (ICU) to facilitate frequent assessment. AEDs are continued after surgery and after leaving the hospital.

Self-Care

It is important for the client with epilepsy to live as normal a life as possible. The client and family members must learn to accept the condition and not exaggerate it or overprotect the client. The restriction on driving can be emotionally and economically devastating for clients of all ages and socioeconomic backgrounds.

A regular pattern of adequate diet, fluid intake, sleep, and moderate recreation and exercise is helpful. Many

clients find that skipping meals or not getting enough sleep lowers the threshold for seizures. Alcoholic beverages are contraindicated for two reasons. First, alcohol lowers the seizure threshold; second, alcohol is detoxified by the liver. Most AEDs are also metabolized by

Corpus callosotomy

Division of the corpus callosum disrupts the interhemispheric pathway for secondary generalization of partial seizures (unilateral seizure focus)

A

Temporal lobectomy

B   Area of resection   Hippocampus

Hemispherectomy

Basal ganglia

C   Area of resection

■ **FIGURE 69–3** Surgery for epilepsy can consist of corpus callosotomy **(A)**, temporal lobectomy **(B)**, or hemispherectomy **(C)**. *(From Devinsky, O. [1994]. Seizure disorders. Clinical Symposia, 46[1], 1-54. Modified from an original illustration in* Clinical Symposia, *illustrated by John Craig, MD, copyright by Ciba-Geigy Corp.)*

the liver. Consuming alcohol while taking an anticonvulsant places an increased strain on the metabolizing functions of the liver.

For some clients, the psychosocial impact of epilepsy is overwhelming. Because most seizures occur without warning, many clients spend their lives anticipating inappropriate behavior, embarrassment, and self-injury. Clients with epilepsy often have a poor self-image, feelings of inferiority, self-consciousness, guilt, anger, depression, and other emotional problems. Education and support groups can help clients deal with the emotional impact of epilepsy.

The client and family members should be taught that epilepsy is a chronic disorder that requires long-term management. Even though the client may have been seizure-free for some time, it is important to take medication as prescribed. Phenytoin, a common anticonvulsant, leads to excessive gingival (gum tissue) growth. Brushing two to three times daily helps retard gingival growth. Some clients have excess gingival tissue excised every 6 to 12 months. Medications may also cause diplopia, ataxia, sedation, and bone marrow depression. Most AEDs require periodic monitoring of serum drug levels, liver function, and complete blood counts. Clients with epilepsy should always wear or carry identification stating that they have epilepsy and providing the name and telephone number of their physician.

If the client is able to recognize that certain activities trigger the seizure, the activities can be avoided, or the client can be desensitized in some cases. For example, flickering lights can trigger seizures. Fluorescent lights and flickering shadows from trees on the road while driving during the late afternoon are common precipitants of seizures. If the client experiences an aura, precautions should be taken immediately to prevent self-injury from the impending seizure—for example, lying down on the ground or floor or, if driving a vehicle, pulling over to the side of the road and lying on the seat. Instruct clients to carry a large pillow in the vehicle or to use their arms to protect their heads.

Some clients with epilepsy cannot find employment if they admit to having seizures. However, falsifying job applications can result in dismissal from employment. These factors contribute to a higher incidence of depression among clients with epilepsy. Nurses can educate the public regarding epilepsy and help to dissipate prejudices. When discussing the long-term impact of epilepsy with the client, be empathetic but realistic. It is hoped the client can accept the lifestyle limitations of the disorder and not be overwhelmed by them.

SAFETY

⚠️

ALERT

The client's family needs to know what to do in the event of a seizure. The affected person should be protected from self-injury. Clothing should be loosened, the head protected from impact, and sharp objects in the environment removed. The person should not be forcibly restrained during a seizure but protected from self-injury. Hard objects or fingers should not be inserted into the mouth. People experiencing a seizure do not swallow the tongue—a common misconception. However, the tongue can occlude the airway, and positioning the head is important to protect the airway. After the head is protected from injury, the person should be placed in a side-lying position to displace the tongue and allow oral secretions to drain from the airway. Someone should stay with the person until full consciousness has returned. An ambulance should be called if the seizure lasts for longer than 10 minutes, if another seizure occurs before consciousness returns, if there is respiratory difficulty or evidence of injury, or if the person is pregnant. Sleepiness is common in the postictal period.

Various organizations exist that try to educate the public, introduce appropriate legislation, and assist people with epilepsy. In the United States, these include the Epilepsy Foundation of America and Epilepsy Services. Similar organizations exist in other countries.

STATUS EPILEPTICUS

Status epilepticus, a medical emergency, is a state in which a client has continuous seizures or seizures in rapid succession, without regaining consciousness, lasting at least 30 minutes. The most common cause of status epilepticus is the sudden withdrawal of AEDs. During a seizure, the brain's metabolic needs increase dramatically. If these heightened requirements continue without opportunity for the body to recover, the supply of glucose and oxygen to the brain becomes depleted, and permanent brain damage may occur.

OUTCOME MANAGEMENT

The major goals in managing a client with status epilepticus are to establish and protect the airway, to control the seizure, and to monitor for adverse outcomes.

The airway is maintained and aspiration prevented by placing the client in a side-lying position, suctioning the airway, and providing oxygen. Oxygen offers nothing to a client who is apneic; therefore intubation may be necessary to ventilate and oxygenate the client.

AEDs are given to terminate seizures and to prevent exhaustion. Intravenous (IV) infusion is begun immediately and maintained during treatment. Status epilepticus is treated with diazepam in doses of 5 to 10 mg (0.2 mg/kg) given every 10 to 20 minutes, for a total dose of up to 30 mg in an 8-hour period. Lorazepam (0.1 mg/kg) can also be administered in 4-mg doses given over 2 to 5 minutes, repeated every 10 to 15 minutes to a maximum of 8 mg (0.2 mg/kg). In addition, phenytoin can be given to a total dose of 15 to 18 mg/kg by slow IV push (no more than 50 mg/min). Assess the client for bradycardia and heart block while phenytoin is given. If this agent is not effective, diazepam or lorazepam can be used. Because each of these medications can depress respiration, emergency ventilation equipment should be readily available.

If diazepam or lorazepam is not effective, pentobarbital or propofol can be used to suppress brain activity. Inducing coma is used only after attempts with AEDs have failed. The client in drug-induced coma is ventilator-dependent and requires nursing care in an ICU for ventilatory assistance, continuous EEG monitoring, and hemodynamic monitoring.

Once status epilepticus has been controlled, the client may be unresponsive for a period of time. Clients may be in a postictal state or experiencing subclinical seizures. After the seizures have been controlled, maintenance AEDs are prescribed.

It is especially difficult for significant others to watch clients experiencing status epilepticus. The family needs support and information. Always explain to family members the treatment being given.[21,26,35,48-50]

BRAIN TUMORS

The Central Brain Tumor Registry for the United States (CBTRUS) estimated that 190,600 brain tumors would be diagnosed in the United States in 2005. Of that total, 43,800 were estimated to be primary brain tumors and the remainder to be secondary or metastatic. The overall incidence for primary brain and CNS tumors is 14 cases per 100,000 person years. The incidence of brain tumors appears to be increasing, but this may reflect improved and earlier diagnosis. CBTRUS notes that, as of 2000, approximately 359,000 people in the United States were living with a primary brain tumor, with 75% having benign tumors and 23% having malignant tumors.

Etiology

No clear etiologic factor has been established for any of the primary brain tumors. Although the type of cell that develops into the tumor can often be identified, the mechanism causing the cells to act abnormally remains unknown. Familial tendencies, immunosuppression, and environmental factors are being considered. The peak time for brain tumor development is the fifth to seventh decades of life; men are affected more commonly than women.

Pathophysiology
Intracranial Tumors

Brain tumors are described as "space-occupying lesions." This description means that the tumor displaces normal tissue. When normal brain tissue is compressed, blood flow is altered and ischemia develops. If unchecked, necrosis may occur. Tumors may also irritate surrounding tissue, producing considerable cerebral edema. Because little room is available for expansion of any of the intracranial contents, edema as well as the tumor cause progressively increased intracranial pressure (ICP), which leads to herniation of the brain (see Chapter 73). Both of these mechanisms can contribute to nonspecific neurologic deficits. Tumor location may produce deficits specific to the area of involvement.

Brain tumors are identified as primary or secondary lesions. Tumors arising from the brain or its supporting structures are called *primary* brain tumors; those metastasizing from other areas in the body to the brain are *secondary* tumors. Brain tumors may also be referred to as *intra-axial* or *extra-axial*. Intra-axial tumors are those that arise from within the cerebrum, cerebellum, or brain stem. Extra-axial tumors have their origin in the skull, meninges, or cranial nerves. Primary intracranial tumors may arise from the support cells (the neuroglial cells [gliomas]), from neurons (neuromas), or from supporting structures.

Glial Tumors. Gliomas are the most common type of glial cell tumor and can be found throughout the brain or spinal cord. These tumors occur in adults and children. Depending on the exact location, clinical manifestations may result in increased ICP or focal compression. Gliomas are often further classified based on their specific cell or origin. Astrocytomas arise from astrocyte cells, oligodendroglioma tumors arise from oligodendroglial cells, and ependymomas arise from ependymal cells (Table 69-1). Much confusion exists about pathologic and histologic nomenclature. Historically, staging or grading scales identified glial tumors as grade I (benign) through grade IV (malignant). The grade is assigned according to the degree of tumor cell differentiation. Tumors that are well-differentiated are classified as a lower grade while high-grade tumors are poorly differentiated.

Astrocytomas. These are tumors arising from the cells that repair and maintain the nervous system These are the most common of all primary brain tumors and can be found anywhere in the cerebral hemispheres. Peak age for occurrence is 50 to 60 years, but these tumors can afflict younger and older age groups. Their location determines the exact clinical manifestations.

Oligodendrogliomas. Oligodendrogliomas arise from cells that produce myelin and specifically affect myelinated (white matter) brain. They tend to develop in the cortex of the frontal and parietal lobes. This tumor is fairly slow-growing and calcifies, which makes it recognizable on x-ray studies. The calcification may contribute to the development of seizures as a presenting clinical manifestation. Oligodendrogliomas peak in clients

TABLE 69–1   *Schema for Classifying Brain Tumors**

Type of Tumor	Criteria
Astrocytoma	Increased number of astrocytes; mature astrocytes; normally developed astrocytes
Anaplastic astrocytoma	Increased number of less mature astrocytes; possibility of mitotic figures (mitotic figures represent increased cellular division and malignant changes)
Glioblastoma multiforme	Increased number of astrocyte cells; immature astrocytes; presence of mitotic figures; hemorrhage, necrosis, swelling, and obscure tumor margins

*This schema of astrocytoma, anaplastic tumor, and glioblastoma multiforme is also used for the astrocytoma, ependymoma, and oligodendroglioma.

between the ages of 30 and 50 years. Clinical manifestations in addition to seizures are headache, personality changes, and papilledema.

Ependymomas. These tumors arise from cells that line the ventricles and form the inner lining of the spinal cord. Although ependymomas may be found anywhere within the CNS, they are more commonly found adjacent to the fourth or lateral ventricles or within the spinal cord tissue. This tumor affects all age groups. Manifestations are caused by ventricular obstruction and include headache, vomiting, diplopia, dizziness, ataxia, vision changes, and motor and sensory abnormalities.

Neuromas. Neuromas can arise from any neuron but most commonly arise from the acoustic neurons. Neuromas account for only about 10% of all intracranial tumors.

Acoustic Neuromas. Acoustic neuromas are tumors of the Schwann cells of the eighth cranial nerve, the acoustic nerve. Manifestations are tinnitus, dizziness, and unilateral and permanent hearing loss. If the tumor is allowed to grow, it can displace the other cranial nerves—especially cranial nerves IV to X—and the brain stem. An excellent outcome can be expected with surgical resection or stereotactic radiosurgery, assuming the remaining cranial nerves are preserved. However, many clients experience at least temporary tinnitus, balance problems, and facial weakness after surgery or radiosurgery.

Pituitary Tumors. Pituitary tumors are usually slow-growing tumors that involve only the anterior lobe of the pituitary gland or extend into the floor of the third ventricle. Although histologically benign, they can reoccur after surgery. Manifestations can be related to hypofunctioning of the gland and include visual field defects, irregular or absent menstrual cycles, infertility, decreased libido, impotence, decreased body hair, and decreased production of pituitary-stimulating hormones; this decrease results in decreased thyroid and adrenal function. Hypersecretion can also occur and is related to the hormones that are in excess. Combinations of hyposecretion and hypersecretion can also be seen. Manifestations of pituitary tumors are often overlooked for months because they are so diverse. Clients are usually diagnosed by MRI scan and blood testing for the presence of pituitary-stimulating hormones. Visual abnormalities may also occur because of the proximity of the pituitary to the optic nerve. Tumor growth in this area may cause optic nerve compression, manifested as loss of visual field.

Meningiomas. Meningiomas are common benign tumors that may involve all meningeal layers; however, these tumors are believed to originate in the arachnoid cells (Figure 69-4). Most meningiomas are benign, but some tumors may become malignant.[14] Meningiomas may be found in the brain or spinal cord. They are slow-growing and occur at any age, most commonly at midlife and in women. Manifestations depend on location of the tumor and can be diverse. Outcomes are related to the site of the tumor. Recurrence is a concern.

Optic Nerve and Chiasm
Astrocytoma
Meningioma

Third Ventricle
Colloid cyst
Astrocytoma
Ependymoma
Metastatic tumors

Lateral Ventricle
Ependymoma
Meningioma
Choroid plexus papilloma
Subependymoma

Corpus Callosum
Astrocytoma
Glioblastoma
Lipoma

Cerebral Hemisphere
Astrocytoma
Glioblastoma
Oligodendroglioma
Meningioma
Sarcoma
Ependymoma
Metastatic tumors

Pineal Region
Germ cell tumors
Pineal cell tumors
Meningioma

Pituitary Region
Pituitary adenoma
Craniopharyngioma
Meningioma
Germ cell tumor
Sarcoma
Chordoma
Metastatic tumors

Brain Stem
Astrocytoma

Cerebellopontine Angle
Acoustic schwannoma
Meningiomas
Epidermoid cyst
Glomus jugulare tumor
Choroid plexus papilloma
Metastatic tumors

Cerebellum
Astrocytoma
Medulloblastoma
Hemangioblastoma
Metastatic tumors

Fourth Ventricle
Ependymoma
Choroid plexus papilloma
Medulloblastoma

■ **FIGURE 69–4** Common intracranial tumors and their usual locations. *(Modified from Osteen, R.T., Gansler, T & Lenhard, R.E. [2001]. American Cancer Society textbook of clinical oncology [3rd ed., p. 381]. Atlanta: American Cancer Society.)*

Metastatic Brain Tumors

Metastatic brain tumors are those with primary sites outside of the brain. Cancers of the lung, breast, and kidney and malignant melanoma are the major sources of metastatic brain cancers. Metastatic tumors to the brain are more commonly multiple, making them less amenable to therapy. The tumor location may be in the brain itself or in the meninges lining the brain. The common locations of brain tumors are shown in Figure 69-4.

Clinical Manifestations

Clinical manifestations may be nonspecific, caused by edema and increased ICP, or specific and related to a particular anatomic location.

Mental Status Changes

As in any neurologic or neurosurgical disorder, a change in the level of consciousness (LOC) or sensorium is often noted. Mental and emotional status changes such as lethargy and drowsiness, confusion, disorientation, and personality changes may be found.

Headaches

Headaches may be localized or generalized. They are usually intermittent, are of increasing duration, and may be intensified by a change in position or straining. Recurrent, severe headaches in a client who was previously free of headaches, or recurrent headaches in the morning, increasing in frequency and severity, may indicate an intracranial tumor and indicate the need for further assessment.

Nausea and Vomiting

The clinical manifestations of nausea and vomiting are believed to occur because of pressure on the medulla, where the vomiting center is found. The client often complains of a severe headache after lying flat in bed. As the headache increases in severity, the client may also experience nausea or spontaneous vomiting. During the episode of emesis, the client may hyperventilate, which decreases brain swelling, and after the vomiting episode may note that the headache is less severe.

Papilledema

Compression of the second cranial nerve, the optic nerve, may result in papilledema. The underlying pathophysiologic mechanism of papilledema is not clearly understood. Increased intracranial pressure obstructs venous return from the eye and backs up blood in the central retinal vein. Also known as "choked disc," papilledema is common in clients with intracranial tumors and may be the first manifestation of increased ICP. Early papilledema does not cause visual acuity changes and can be detected only through an ophthalmologic examination. Severe papilledema may be manifest by decreased visual acuity.

Seizures

Seizures, focal or generalized, are common in clients with intracranial tumors, especially cerebral hemisphere tumors (see earlier discussion). Seizures may be partial or generalized; partial seizures usually help localize tumor location.

Localized Manifestations

Localized clinical manifestations are caused by destruction, irritation, or compression of the part of the brain where the tumor is located. Table 69-2 lists specific clinical manifestations based on tumor location. Localized manifestations include the following:

- Focal weaknesses (e.g., hemiparesis)
- Sensory disturbances, including absence of feeling (anesthesia) or abnormal sensation (paresthesia)
- Language disturbances
- Coordination disturbances (e.g., staggering gait)
- Visual disturbance such as diplopia (double vision) or visual field deficit (monopia)

Despite the availability of extremely sensitive and sophisticated equipment, brain tumor diagnosis is often delayed because of difficulty recognizing early manifestations. No two adults with the diagnosis of brain tumor present with the same clinical manifestations. Older clients especially fail to report such problems during regular examinations because they forget or think that the manifestations are "just part of growing old."

Diagnostic Findings

If an intracranial tumor is suspected, noninvasive studies such as CT and MRI are performed (Figure 69-5). Other disorders may be ruled out with EEG, radionuclide scans, angiogram, or lumbar puncture. A stereotactic biopsy may confirm the diagnosis of a brain tumor and help in planning appropriate therapy. Three-dimensional imaging techniques help further localize the tumor in the brain and can assist with plans for resection. PET scans can also be used to study the biochemical and physiologic effects of the tumor.

OUTCOME MANAGEMENT

Medical Management

For the adult client with a brain tumor, there are many options for treatment. Regardless of which treatment modality is selected, the initial goal is to establish a

TABLE 69–2 Clinical Manifestations of Brain Tumors by Location

Location	Clinical Manifestations
Frontal lobe	Disturbed mental state, apathy, inappropriate behavior, dementia, depression, emotional lability, inattentiveness, inability to concentrate, indifference, loss of self-restraint and social behavior, impaired long-term memory, difficulty with abstraction, quiet but flat affect, dominant hemisphere expressive speech disturbance, impaired sphincter control with bowel and bladder incontinence, motor disorders, gait disturbances, paralysis, "frontal release signs," seizures
Temporal lobe	Receptive aphasia, generalized psychomotor seizures, visual field changes, personality changes, ataxia, headache, manifestations of increased ICP, tinnitus, recent memory impairment
Parietal lobe	Sensory deficits, motor and sensory focal seizures, agnosias, hypoesthesias, paresthesias, dyslexia, visual field cut, diminished appreciation of side opposite the tumor, headache, apraxia, tactile inattention, right/left disorientation
Occipital lobe	Headache, manifestations of increased ICP, visual impairment (homonymous hemianopsia), visual agnosia, cortical blindness, hallucinations, seizures
Cerebellar	Unsteady gait, falling, ataxia, incoordination, tremors, head tilt, nystagmus, CSF obstruction/hydrocephalus, truncal ataxia if vermis is tumor site
Brain stem	Vertigo, dizziness, vomiting, CN III-XII palsies/dysfunction, nystagmus, decreased corneal reflex, headache, vomiting, gait disturbance, motor and sensory deficits, deafness, intranuclear ophthalmoplegia, sudden death from cardiac and respiratory failure
Pituitary and hypothalamus	Visual deficits, headache, hormonal dysfunction, sleep disturbances, water imbalance, temperature fluctuations, imbalance in fat and carbohydrate metabolism, Cushing's syndrome
Ventricle	Obstruction of CSF circulation, hydrocephalus, rapid increase in ICP, postural headache

CN, Cranial nerve; *CSF,* cerebrospinal fluid; *ICP,* intracranial pressure.

■ **FIGURE 69–5** Magnetic resonance image revealing a midline frontal meningioma.

diagnosis. Most often this is accomplished through surgery; therefore surgical management is discussed first. Additional goals include managing increased ICP, controlling or preventing seizures, and monitoring for motor or sensory deficits and cranial nerve deficits.

Intervention depends on the type and location of the intracranial tumor and the client's medical condition. Management is always interdisciplinary, with several members forming a clinical team to support the client through care.

Surgical Management

Surgical intervention may range from biopsy to total removal of the brain tumor by way of a craniotomy. Surgical biopsy or resection confirms the histologic or pathologic diagnosis. Surgical resection also decreases the tumor burden, making other treatments and adjunctive therapeutic treatments more effective, and helps control increased ICP. With only a few exceptions, all clients with brain tumors require a craniotomy for surgical intervention.

Craniotomy

The term *craniotomy* means to surgically create an opening into the skull. A craniectomy (removal of a portion of the cranium) may be performed for decompression. There are many methods of removing the tumor, regardless of the type of tumor and the extent of tumor removed (Table 69-3).

Intraoperatively the client may be positioned in various ways to facilitate exposure and visualization. Such positions and head-supporting frames have the potential to cause skin pressure on the head, edema of the face, and muscle soreness, especially in the neck. Preoperatively or postoperatively, a ventriculostomy, in which a catheter is inserted through a burr hole into the ventricle, may be needed to drain cerebrospinal fluid (CSF) or blood. Drains may be used if a large area of dead space remains after tumor removal.

TABLE 69-3   Surgical Options for Brain Tumor Diagnosis and Excision

Procedure	Description
Preoperative Procedures to Locate and Map the Tumor and Nearby Structures	
Brain-mapping technique	Uses viewing wand to precisely identify location of specific anatomic functions (i.e., motor, sensory, and/or speech); methods developed include localizing tumors with ultrasound techniques and various wand-like devices
Cortical mapping	Intraoperative cortical EEG recording and monitoring, facilitating areas for greater accuracy of resection without loss of eloquent motor and/or sensory functions
Direct cortical stimulation	Electrical current is directed to specific area in brain, causing visible movement of corresponding body part
Frameless stereotactic localization systems	External devices are placed preoperatively and client's body is scanned using CT or MRI; localization systems scanning data are transferred to operating room, allowing determination of boundaries of lesion by means of a surgical "wand"
Intraoperative ultrasonography	Uses a hand-held device to differentiate tumors with a cystic component; ultrasound techniques allow identification of tumor margins
Somatosensory evoked potentials (SSEPs)	Measurement of electrical response of specific areas (e.g., visual, auditory, brain stem); after functions of such critical areas have been determined, these areas can be avoided during surgical manipulation
Surgical Techniques Used for Precise Location of the Tumor	
Intraoperative imaging techniques	Real-time CT or MRI for improved visualization
Stereotactic surgery	Localization of a specific target within three-dimensional space; with client stabilized in a head frame, tumor is imaged using either CT or MRI; data from scans are analyzed by a computer and a trajectory location is identified; stereotactic procedures may be used for biopsy or craniotomy
Treatment Options for Tumor Excision	
Embolization	Decreases blood supply to tumor; may be used in conjunction with surgical procedures
Laser surgery	Destroys tumor tissue using heat from laser without causing adjacent edema or damage
Neuro-endoscopic techniques	For treatment of third and/or lateral ventricle lesions; provides access to lesions in areas otherwise difficult to locate
Polymer wafer implants	Chemotherapeutic wafers are placed in tumor bed; carmustine is currently available, and other agents are being tested
Ultrasonic aspirator	Suction-like device used in removing solid tumors

CT, Computed tomography; *EEG*, electroencephalography; *MRI*, magnetic resonance imaging.

Nursing Management of the Surgical Client

Preoperative Care

More than at any other time, the role of the nurse caring for the client with the diagnosis of a brain tumor is diverse. The nurse in the neurosurgeon's office begins preoperative teaching. During the perioperative and postoperative periods, the nurse prepares the client for various transitions in the continuum of care.

Preoperative assessment includes the routine assessment data (see Chapter 2). In addition, a detailed history and physical examination provides a baseline for comparison of neurologic data. The nurse will obtain and record data on the following:

- Presenting clinical manifestations such as headache, nausea and vomiting, or focal deficits
- Vital signs, level of consciousness, and orientation to person, place, and time; ability to follow instructions; pupil equality, size, reactivity, accommodation, and reaction to light; extraocular eye movements; and cranial nerve function
- Limb strength, movement, and sensation; note limited or exaggerated movements, pronator drift, hand grip, dorsiflexion/plantiflexion, any paresis or paralysis, or sensory abnormalities
- Mental status—note any difficulties in problem-solving, limited memory, or behavior change

Preoperative interventions are similar to those for the care of other clients before surgery (see Chapter 14). The suddenness of the diagnosis and possibility of a cancer diagnosis may produce anxiety for both the client and family. Offer explanations and clarification as needed especially about placement in an intensive care unit and initial appearance altered by dressings, edema, and bruising. Be certain not to offer empty promises about recovery.

Postoperative Care

General postoperative complications after intracranial surgery do not differ from those after other forms of surgery. Ecchymosis and periorbital edema may be present after intracranial surgery but are transient. These changes affecting the appearance of the eyes and the face overall can be frightening to the client as well as to the family members.

Postoperative care of the client after craniotomy is shown in the accompanying Care Plan feature on pp. 1826-1828. See also the information on care of clients with increased ICP in Chapter 73.

C A R E   P L A N   *evolve*

The Client Who Has Undergone Craniotomy

Nursing Diagnosis: Risk for Ineffective Tissue Perfusion: Cerebral related to edema or bleeding after craniotomy.
Outcomes: The client will have intracranial pressure (ICP) less than 15 mm Hg, mean arterial pressure (MAP) greater than 70 mm Hg, cerebral perfusion pressure (CPP) greater than 50 mm Hg, neurologic assessments and vital signs at baseline values or improved, no clinical manifestations of increased ICP and/or herniation, and body temperature less than 38.5 ° C.

NOC OUTCOMES Cognitive Ability, Neurologic Status, Neurologic Status: Consciousness, Tissue Perfusion: Cerebral

Interventions	NIC INTERVENTIONS	Rationales
1. Assess neurologic status and vital signs frequently and compare with baseline values.	Neurologic Monitoring Vital Signs Monitoring	1. A change in level of consciousness is the first sign of increasing intracranial pressure (ICP).
2. Elevate head of bed to 30 degrees.	Cerebral Perfusion Promotion	2. Elevation facilitates venous drainage and reduces edema.
3. Maintain head and neck in neutral alignment.	Cerebral Perfusion Promotion	3. Neutral alignment facilitates venous drainage and reduces edema.
4. Change position slowly.	Cerebral Perfusion Promotion	4. Rapid changes in position increase cerebral blood flow and pressure.
5. Avoid Valsalva maneuver.	Cerebral Perfusion Promotion	5. Straining during coughing, movement in bed, or moving bowels increases ICP.
6. Monitor intake and output frequently.	Fluid Monitoring	6. Excess fluids can promote edema; dehydration can decrease cerebral arterial flow.
7. Monitor pulse oximetry and arterial blood gases.	Oxygen Therapy, Acid-Base Monitoring	7. The cerebrum is sensitive to lack of oxygen, and damage can occur within minutes after onset of hypoxia.
8. Reduce environmental stress by minimizing interruptions and stimuli.	Cerebral Perfusion Promotion Environmental Management	8. Noise and frequent interruptions may increase ICP.
9. Administer steroids as ordered.	Medication Administration	9. Steroids reduce cerebral edema.
10. Administer antiepileptic drugs as ordered.	Medication Administration Seizure Management	10. Seizures are common sequelae of brain surgery.

Evaluation: Depending on the etiology of edema or amount of bleeding, it may require hours to days to control ICP.

Nursing Diagnosis: Decreased Intracranial Adaptive Capacity related to neurologic changes from edema of surgical excision of sections of brain or tumor.
Outcomes: The client will have intracranial adaptive capacity as evidenced by controlled intracranial pressures.

NOC OUTCOMES Electrolyte and Acid-Base Balance, Fluid Balance, Neurologic Status: Autonomic, Neurologic Status: Cranial Sensory/Motor Function

Interventions	NIC INTERVENTIONS	Rationales
1. Perform Glasgow Coma Scale and other neurologic assessments q 1 hr. Compare findings to baseline, and report changes.	Neurologic Monitoring	1. Hourly observations allow early intervention when changes occur.
2. Maintain patent airway with Po_2 values greater than 85 mm Hg and Pco_2 between 25 and 30 mm Hg.	Cerebral Perfusion Promotion	2. Prevent cerebral hypoxia; hypercapnia increases cerebral blood flow.
3. Maintain sterile and patent CSF drain, keeping stopcock at level of tragus (or as specified). Monitor CSF color.	Cerebral Perfusion Promotion	3. CSF drainage is normally sterile. A plugged CSF drain would increase ICP. The tragus is level with the ventricles and allows normal intracranial pressures when maintained at that level.

Evaluation: Stabilizing the brain in order to reach normal levels of adaptation to changes in intracranial volume and pressures will require at least 72 hours depending upon the initial amount of edema and tissue injury.

Nursing Diagnosis: Ineffective Coping related to fear of changes in body image, role performance, or life expectancy.
Outcomes: The client will have improved individual coping, as evidenced by statements indicating feelings of self-worth, behaviors demonstrating self-worth, and less use of dependent behaviors.

NOC OUTCOMES   Aggression Control, Coping, Decision-Making, Impulse Control, Role Performance

Interventions	NIC INTERVENTIONS	Rationales
1. Encourage family members/significant others to assist in meeting need for close contact.	Support System Enhancement, Anxiety Reduction, Coping Enhancement	1. Family members may also fear that they will injure the client.
2. Anticipate needs.	Support System Enhancement, Anxiety Reduction, Coping Enhancement	2. Anxiety increases feelings of loneliness.
3. Offer praise and encouragement during ongoing assessment of client's readiness to move toward more competent coping.	Self-Esteem Enhancement, Anxiety Reduction, Coping Enhancement	3. Positive reinforcement helps to guide future steps toward independence.
4. Provide opportunities for expression and ventilation of feelings and issues.	Anxiety Reduction, Coping Enhancement, Emotional Support	4. Problem-solving coping styles are initiated by talking about feelings.
5. Utilize consistent personnel.	Support System Enhancement, Anxiety Reduction, Coping Enhancement	5. A therapeutic relationship is easier to maintain than to build.
6. Establish trust relationship; follow through on promises.	Support System Enhancement, Anxiety Reduction, Coping Enhancement	6. Feelings of fear and anxiety are reduced.

Evaluation: Coping skills will wax and wane over time. Expect periods of coping and periods of failure to cope with changes in prognosis.

Nursing Diagnosis: Anxiety related to uncertain future and prognosis.
Outcomes: The client will have decreased anxiety and express fears and concerns openly.

NOC OUTCOMES   Aggression Control, Anxiety Control, Coping

Interventions	NIC INTERVENTIONS	Rationales
1. Repeat information; provide information in different forms; encourage the client and/or significant other to write down questions and/or concerns.	Support System Enhancement, Anxiety Reduction, Coping Enhancement, Teaching: Individual	1. Depending on the type of tumor, the location of the tumor, and/or motor or sensory deficits, the client may be faced with the loss of specific functions and the possibility of having a malignancy. Appropriate interventions may help the client better understand the prescribed plan of care.
2. Encourage open communication between the client, significant others, and members of the health care team.	Support System Enhancement, Anxiety Reduction, Coping Enhancement	2. Having a diagnosis of brain cancer may immobilize all of the normal coping mechanisms of the client and significant others.
3. Involve the client's clergy or hospital chaplain if desired.	Spiritual Support	3. Spiritual support is crucial at times of serious illness for the client, family members, and significant others. The client need not be "religious" to gain support from clergy.

Evaluation: Anxiety should be controllable in a short time. However, changes in response to therapy or other outcomes will increase anxiety.

Nursing Diagnosis: Risk for Disturbed Thought Processes related to neurologic changes from edema or surgical excision of sections of brain or tumor.
Outcomes: The client will make decisions and process information at expected levels, express and identify anger, exercise control over own behavior, make appropriate choices, and/or cease hostile behavior.

NOC OUTCOMES   Cognitive Ability, Cognitive Orientation, Decision-Making

Interventions	NIC INTERVENTIONS	Rationales
1. Allow client to verbalize concerns, and channel these concerns to the appropriate person.	Emotional Support, Anxiety Reduction	1. Problem-solving coping begins with verbalization of concerns.

(Continued)

C A R E   P L A N   *evolve*

The Client Who Has Undergone Craniotomy—Cont'd

Interventions	NIC Interventions	Rationales
2. Offer reasonable choices to client.	Emotional Support, Anxiety Reduction	2. Feelings of control can be reestablished by offering choices to client. All options must be safe and implementable for the client.
3. Assist client to recognize alternatives and the implications of choices.	Emotional Support, Anxiety Reduction	3. This measure helps client with problem-solving abilities.
4. Report client's status to client, and allow for opportunity to make decisions about treatment or no treatment.	Client Rights' Protection	4. Do not keep facts from the client. The client has the right to know the diagnosis and to be a part of decisions about care.
5. Inform family about physiologic reasons for behavior, and teach them how to respond to client.	Family Support	5. The family needs to be informed about any abnormal behavior and how best to respond to it.
6. Use a consistent approach to inappropriate behavior; establish contracts if needed.	Anxiety Reduction, Behavior Management	6. Consistent approaches help the client relearn acceptable ways of personal expression.
7. Maintain nonjudgmental behavior.	Self-Esteem Enhancement, Emotional Support	7. The nurse realizes that the client's outbursts are not personal attacks but are due to the disease or feelings of loss of control.

Evaluation: Expect restoration of thought and behavior control to take weeks or months. Long-term coping by the family is important.

Nursing Diagnosis: Anticipatory Grieving related to potential loss of function, previous abilities, or life from brain cancer or surgery.

Outcomes: The client will have resolution of grief or progression through stages of grief, as evidenced by expressing feelings, maintaining hope, identifying problems with changes in body function, seeking help with anticipated problems, or developing realistic plans for the future.

NOC OUTCOMES   Aggression Control, Coping, Family Coping, Grief Resolution, Psychosocial Adjustment: Life Change

Interventions	NIC Interventions	Rationales
1. Acknowledge reality, but do not force its acceptance.	Truth Telling, Active Listening, Emotional Support	1. Denial is a powerful defense mechanism; clients will examine reality when they are ready.
2. Establish regular time to spend with client, family members, and/or significant others for the exclusive purpose of discussing feelings and concerns.	Family Support, Active Listening, Emotional Support	2. Discussions about feelings can be difficult; giving the client time to plan and prepare facilitates the discussion.
3. If denial is beneficial, respond by listening with and reflecting statements by client.	Active Listening, Emotional Support	3. It is important to understand that not all clients reach acceptance of their disease; some remain in complete denial.
4. Accept emotions and assist client, family members, and/or significant others to clarify them.	Active Listening, Emotional Support, Family Support, Counseling	4. This measure reinforces the ideas that emotional response is normal and that family members should be accepting of the client at all stages of grief.
5. Assess perceptions about realistic goals and the future.	Truth Telling, Active Listening, Emotional Support	5. Inaccurate perceptions about the future can prevent or stall planning.
6. Have the client list those activities he or she wants to perform/resume.	Hope Instillation, Normalization Promotion	6. Plans for the future can be uplifting.

Evaluation: Expect each client and family to cope differently with grief over losses or impending death. Clients may go through the "typical" stages in order or go back and forth between them.

Transsphenoidal Approaches to the Pituitary

Clients with tumors of the pituitary gland have surgical options for excision of the tumor. The most direct approach is the transsphenoidal approach, across the sphenoid bone at the base of the skull. This may be accomplished endoscopically, through the nose, or through an incision at the junction of the inner aspect of the upper lip and gingiva above the teeth. The floor of the sella turcica in the sphenoid bone is opened and the tumor is removed (Figure 69-6). Fat or muscle grafts, using tissue from the inside cheek, abdomen, or upper thigh, may be implanted at the surgical site to assist in healing of the wound. Nasal packing may or may not be used. Pituitary tumors that are not able to be accessed through the transsphenoidal approaches may require a craniotomy to resect the tumor.

Postoperative Care Following Pituitary Surgery

Postoperative care after pituitary surgery using a transsphenoidal approach includes protection of the oral/gingival or incision site. Frequent oral hygiene is provided, and a cool vaporizer mist may be used to keep oral mucous membranes moist. The nasal drip pad ("moustache" dressing) is assessed frequently for blood or clear fluid (CSF). The donor site and dressings are also assessed, and dressings are changed as needed. The client must be instructed to avoid nose blowing or sneezing if possible.

A serious complication of pituitary surgery is the development of diabetes insipidus (DI). In most clients, the DI is temporary; however, in clients in whom the stalk of the pituitary is removed or damaged, DI is permanent. DI results from a decreased secretion of antidiuretic hormone (ADH). The clinical manifestations of DI are polyuria (large urine volumes) and polydipsia (increased thirst). Clients with DI produce large volumes (2 to 15 L/day) of dilute urine with a specific gravity of 1.005 or less. These clients require laboratory assessment of serum and urine sodium levels and serum osmolalities. If left untreated, dehydration quickly occurs. Circulatory collapse (hypovolemic shock) and hypertonic encephalopathy occur as a result of fluid shifts in the brain. Usual treatment is with fluid replacement first, and then IV vasopressin (Pitressin) or inhalation or oral desmopressin (DDAVP) if DI persists. Long-acting forms of these agents can be used to treat chronic DI.

Medical Management

After surgery, when an exact histologic diagnosis has been obtained, the client may be offered adjuvant therapy, including radiation therapy and chemotherapy. These modes of cancer treatment are discussed in Chapters 16 and 17; this material is also applicable to the care of clients with brain cancer.

Radiation Therapy

Conventional radiotherapy delivers radiation using a linear accelerator. The standard dose for primary brain tumors is approximately 6000 Gy given five times a week for 6 weeks. For clients with metastatic tumors, a standard dose of radiation is approximately 3000 Gy. The exact dose depends on tumor characteristics, volume of tissue to be irradiated, and the goals of radiation therapy. Radiation treatments are usually given over shorter periods of time to allow for protection of normal surrounding tissues. The cancer cells in CNS tumors tend to be more slowly dividing; therefore the tumor response often takes longer. This concept is important for clients to understand, because they may be disappointed when they do not see effects during or immediately following irradiation.

As in many areas of medicine, new methods of treatment and improved delivery devices are helping clients daily. This is also the case with radiation therapy. Newer methods of delivery and more sophisticated machines are available. Table 69-4 lists examples of advances made in the area of radiotherapy for clients with brain tumors. A recent development is an inflatable balloon-filled catheter with radioactive iodine 125 placed directly in the tumor bed (GliaSite Radiation Therapy System). Additional forms of radiation therapy, although not considered conventional and, more important, not readily available, are heavy particle radiation therapy, fast neutron radiotherapy, photodynamic therapy, and boron neutron capture therapy. Despite its wide use, radiation therapy is not without consequences. Effects may be acute, early, delayed, or late delayed (see Chapter 17).

Chemotherapy

As part of a multimodal approach, chemotherapy may be given before, during, or after other therapies. There

■ **FIGURE 69–6** Transsphenoidal approach to the excision of pituitary tumors.

TABLE 69–4   Radiation Therapy Modalities for Treatment of Brain Tumors

Procedure	Description
Interstitial radiation (also called brachytherapy, tumor implants, tumor seeding, or radioactive pellets)	Temporary or permanent placement of radioactive substances in tumor bed Advantages: minimal effects to surrounding tissue Generally not advised in large tumors because of secondary swelling and edema Disadvantages: implantation requires a surgical procedure; because of radioactive substances, client must be protected and isolated to prevent exposure to family members and health care personnel
Stereotactic radiosurgery, stereotactic radiotherapy	Allows for a high dose of radiation beams to be directed precisely to a small brain tumor in a single session by localizing specific tumor site three dimensionally Gamma knife, Cyberknife, linear accelerator, or cyclotron is used to deliver radiation Best results when used on small, round, well-defined tumors Peacock technique incorporates stereotaxis, radiosurgery, and computers to deliver radiation exactly to tumor, skipping over vital areas that may be embedded in tumor such as nerves or blood vessels
Radiation sensitizing therapy	Use of various pharmacologic agents as "sensitizers" to make tumor more responsive to radiation therapy and other therapies
Intraoperative radiation	Direct irradiation of tumor while exposed in surgery; bypasses normal tissues
Conformal radiation	High or higher dose of external radiation "conformed" to match tumor's shape; goal is to deliver a uniform amount of radiation to entire tumor
Radioactive monoclonal antibodies	Antibodies that are cloned or mated to kill tumor cells

are several challenges in the use of chemotherapy in the treatment of brain tumors. The blood-brain barrier blocks chemotherapy from entering into the brain; however, some progress has been made. Recently, substances to open up the blood-brain barrier are being used. The osmotic diuretic mannitol may be used to disrupt the blood-brain barrier, allowing for greater drug concentration. There are also newer chemotherapeutic agents that cross the blood-brain barrier. Certain agents may enter and directly bind with the CSF or have a direct effect on the tumor. Brain tumor biology is still not well understood; hence it is difficult to find the optimal agent. Studies using newer agents have shown only minimal increase in survival, so research is ongoing.

Temozolomide is the most frequently used and effective chemotherapy agent for brain tumors. Nitrosoureas, for example, carmustine (BCNU) and lomustine (CCNU), are often used when temozolomide fails. Other agents are available. For the client with a brain tumor, the chemotherapy regimen may involve oral medication, IV solutions, intra-arterial routes, or intraventricular, intratumor, or epidural administration. Implanted devices, such as the Ommaya reservoir (see Chapter 17, Figure 17-3),[8] may also be used.

As with the treatment of any cancer invading the body and especially the brain, the hope lies in future research. Biologic response modifiers and modulation of the immune system are two of the keys that scientists hope may hold the answers.

The care of the client with a brain tumor is a challenging task for all involved. The client should not feel abandoned or uninformed during any portion of the care or treatment. To assist the client, family members, significant others, and the health care team, the American Cancer Society, the American Brain Tumor Association, and the National Brain Tumor Foundation are valuable resources.

SUBARACHNOID HEMORRHAGE

Subarachnoid hemorrhage (SAH) is bleeding into the subarachnoid space. Traumatic SAH develops from traumatic brain injury (TBI) (see Chapter 73). Spontaneous SAH is seen with intracranial aneurysms and arteriovenous malformations (AVMs). Other potential causes of spontaneous SAH include brain tumors (see earlier discussion), blood dyscrasias, and anticoagulant therapy.

Etiology
Spontaneous SAH occurs when an abnormal artery or vein ruptures and blood spills into the subarachnoid space or ventricles. In adults, aneurysms are the most common cause of SAH. Most intracranial aneurysms are either congenital or developmental.

Aneurysms
An intracranial aneurysm is a weakness in the tunica media, the middle layer of the blood vessel. The most common type of intracranial aneurysm is the saccular or berry aneurysm. The muscular walls of the artery weaken and lead to formation of a sac-like or berry-like structure.

Conditions that hasten the development of this type of aneurysm are smoking, hypertension, atherosclerosis, alcohol abuse, stimulant drug abuse, and the aging process. About 25% of all clients with intracranial aneurysms present with multiple intracranial aneurysms. Statistically, SAH is more common in females than in males.

Intracranial aneurysms are found more often in the anterior cerebral circulation (internal carotid artery and its branches—the anterior cerebral artery [ACA], the middle cerebral artery [MCA], and the posterior cerebral artery [PCA])—than in the posterior cerebral circulation, including the vertebral and basilar arteries. Intracranial aneurysms are found in locations where normal anatomic weaknesses occur—that is, in bifurcations and trifurcations.

Saccular aneurysms most commonly occur at the bifurcations of the large arteries at the base of the brain. Approximately 85% of aneurysms occur in the anterior circulation, mostly in the circle of Willis. The common sites include the junction of the anterior communicating artery with the ACA, the junction of the PCA with the internal carotid artery, and the bifurcation of the MCA. The top of the basilar artery, the junction of the basilar artery and the superior cerebellar artery or the anterior inferior cerebellar artery, and the junction of the vertebral artery and the posterior inferior cerebellar artery comprise most of the remaining sites of aneurysm formation.

Pathophysiology

As an aneurysm develops, it often forms a neck with a dome. The arterial internal elastic lamina disappears at the base of the neck. The media thins, and connective tissue replaces smooth muscle cells. At the site of rupture (most often the dome), the wall thins, and the tear that allows bleeding is often no more than 0.5 mm long. It is not possible to predict which aneurysms are likely to rupture, but limited data suggest that most ruptured aneurysms average 7 mm in diameter.

Blood byproducts from the SAH contribute to serious delayed effects. The most serious is vasospasm, defined as the constriction or narrowing of the cerebral vessels. In general, the more blood there is surrounding the arteries, the more likely there will be symptomatic vasospasm. Vasospasm causes ischemia and infarction and is the major cause of delayed morbidity or death following SAH.

Clinical Manifestations

Aneurysms found during incidental assessment, such as a work-up for headache, may be completely asymptomatic. More commonly, they are found after a SAH occurs. They may also produce symptoms without bleeding by placing pressure on adjacent structures as they enlarge. Once hemorrhage occurs, the symptoms are usually sudden and severe. The classic presentation is sudden onset of the "worst headache of my life." Hemorrhage is often accompanied by vomiting and generalized seizures may occur.

The client may lose consciousness immediately or may become confused and lethargic and gradually become comatose within hours, or the client may remain conscious and coherent. Manifestations of meningeal irritation (e.g., nuchal rigidity and pain, photophobia, back pain) are often present, caused by blood in the subarachnoid space. Depending on the location and size of the

aneurysm and the SAH, focal clinical manifestations may be noted (e.g., motor or sensory deficits, speech and cranial nerve deficits). Retinal hemorrhages may be present. Various grading scales have been developed. Table 69-5 presents criteria for the Hunt-Hess scale and the Fisher scale.

Manifestations of vasospasm appear 4 to 14 days after the hemorrhage, most frequently at about 7 days. The severity, duration, and distribution of vasospasm determine whether ischemia progresses to infarction. Manifestations of vasospasm vary according to the specific arterial territories involved. However, collateral blood flow may prevent the appearance of some expected manifestations. Spasm of the MCA typically causes contralateral hemiparesis and dysphasia (dominant hemisphere). Proximal ACA vasospasm causes bilateral leg weakness, abulia (faulty problem-solving), and incontinence, whereas severe vasospasm of the PCA causes hemianopia. Severe spasm of the basilar or vertebral arteries occasionally produces focal brain stem ischemia. All of these focal neurologic manifestations may develop over a few days, fluctuate, or present abruptly.

Diagnosis of SAH is usually based on history and physical examination. In about 80% to 90% of affected clients, enough blood is present to be visualized on a noncontrast CT scan. A small hemorrhage may not be seen on CT scan. If the scan fails to establish the diagnosis of SAH in the presence of symptoms, a lumbar puncture may be performed to look for the presence of subarachnoid blood. Lumbar puncture is contraindicated when ICP is elevated.

CT scan will also identify associated intracerebral clots, large clots surrounding an aneurysm, and the presence of hydrocephalus. Digital subtraction angiography or CT angiography is done to identify the presence,

---

TABLE 69–5 Grading Scales for Subarachnoid Hemorrhage

Grade	Clinical Criteria
Hunt-Hess Clinical Grading Scale for Clients with Aneurysmal Subarachnoid Hemorrhage	
I	Alert, minimal headache
II	Alert, moderate to severe headache (cranial nerve palsy allowed)
III	Lethargic or confused, or mild focal deficit
IV	Stuporous, moderate to severe hemiparesis, possibly early decerebrate rigidity
V	Deep coma, decerebrate rigidity, moribund appearance
Fisher Scale for CT Grading of Clients with Aneurysmal Subarachnoid Hemorrhage	
1	No SAH on CT scan
2	Thin SAH (<1 mm)
3	Thick SAH (>1 mm)
4	Intracerebral or intraventricular hemorrhage, with no or thin SAH (<1 mm)

CT, Computed tomography; *SAH,* subarachnoid hemorrhage.

location, and configuration of an aneurysm; these same tests may be ordered during the peak time of vasospasm to identify the extent of vasospasm. Transcranial Doppler is a useful bedside tool to identify increased blood velocity indicative of vasospasm.

OUTCOME MANAGEMENT

Medical Management

The client with an SAH resulting from an intracranial aneurysm presents a multidisciplinary challenge. SAH constitutes a medical emergency, and clients with SAH are critically ill, cared for in an ICU. Definitive treatment is often instituted within 24 hours of onset of manifestations. Recovery is variable; one third of SAH survivors may succumb to the disease and another one third may have permanent sequelae.

The goals for the management of a client with SAH include preventing rebleeding, maintaining cerebral perfusion pressure, controlling ICP, minimizing effects of vasospasm, managing hydrocephalus, and managing cardiac dysrhythmias.

Prevent Rebleeding

Rebleeding is prevented by the neurosurgeon or interventional radiologist securing the aneurysm. While waiting for a securing procedure, the nurse must keep the client quiet and comfortable. Reducing hypertension may minimize rebleeding risk as well. Ongoing neurologic assessment is essential regardless of the setting in which care is provided. For the first 24 to 72 hours, the nurse examines the serial data to note trends in the neurologic assessments that suggest changes or deterioration. The LOC is the most sensitive and early indicator of neurologic change, usually evident before pupillary changes, new hemiparesis, or changes in respiratory patterns are noted. The onset of lethargy or restlessness may be the first clinical manifestation of increased ICP, hydrocephalus, or vasospasm.

Cardiac and respiratory function is also closely monitored, particularly because of the direct role in providing adequate cerebral perfusion pressure (CPP) and oxygen supply to the brain. Because cardiovascular disease is common in people with aneurysms, and since SAH can have cardiac complications, continuous electrocardiographic monitoring is necessary to identify life-threatening dysrhythmias. Pulse oximetry is imperative to monitor peripheral oxygen saturation. In the ICU setting, most clients have a central IV line or a pulmonary artery catheter in place to monitor hemodynamic status for prescription of fluids and vasoactive medications. Central venous pressure or pulmonary capillary wedge pressure measurements are used for targeted therapy to manage fluid administration.

Reduce Vasospasm

To prevent vasospasm, liberal isotonic fluids are used. If needed, volume expansion is added to promote cerebral perfusion. If vasospasm occurs, induced hypertension and hypervolemia are used. With the major goal of increasing cerebral blood flow and cerebral perfusion, the measures used have the potential to precipitate a cardiopulmonary crisis. Simply stated, if the client cannot tolerate an increase in fluid status or an increase in blood pressure, how can the vasospasm be relieved? Table 69-6 is a guide to various clinical interventions. The goal of

---

TABLE 69–6   Example Treatment Protocol for Vasospasm

Interventions	Rationales
1. Glasgow Coma Scale and other neurologic assessments q 1 hr. Compare findings to baseline, and report changes.	1. Hourly observations allow early intervention when change occurs.
2. Maintain patent airway with Po_2 values >85 mm Hg and Pco_2 between 25 and 30 mm Hg.	2. Prevents cerebral hypoxia; hypercapnia increases cerebral blood flow.
3. Continuous hemodynamic monitoring of RAP, PAP, and PAWP. Perform CO/CI assessments as ordered. Titrate medications and fluids to maintain desired ranges. Usual ranges are as follows: ■ RAP: 1-7 mm Hg ■ PAWP (no congestion): 6-12 mm Hg ■ CI: >2.5 L/min ■ Target hematocrit is 33-38%. ■ Hypertensive goals are minimally hypertensive state (10 mm Hg above baseline), with SBP 110-160 mm Hg.	3. Hypervolemic, hemodilution, and hypertensive therapies are used to improve perfusion through cerebral vessels. Fluid balance must be monitored closely to prevent fluid volume overload.
4. Nimodipine (Nimotop) 60 mg q 4 hr for at least 3 weeks.	4. Calcium-channel blocker; promotes relaxation of blood vessels, decreasing vasospasm.
5. Morphine as required.	5. Sedative effect; allows for continuous monitoring.
6. Accurate I&O q 1 hr.	6. Fluid balance is crucial to maintaining CPP.

BP, Blood pressure; *CI,* cardiac index; *CO,* cardiac output; *CPP,* cerebral perfusion pressure; *I&O,* (fluid) input and output; *MAP,* mean arterial pressure; *PAP,* pulmonary artery pressure; *PAWP,* pulmonary artery wedge pressure; *RAP,* right atrial pressure; *SBP,* systolic blood pressure.

such therapies is to increase cerebral blood flow and cerebral perfusion pressure (CPP) without producing cerebral infarction or cardiopulmonary compromise. Angioplasty may be employed if medical measures fail; however, its success is limited.

Maintain Cerebral Perfusion Pressure

Medical and nursing management focuses on maintaining blood pressure to facilitate CPP. Once the aneurysm is secured, the blood pressure must be maintained to keep the systemic pressure at a level high enough to provide adequate CPP. Various medications and infusions are used to maintain the blood pressure approximately 10% above the client's normal pressure. In addition to medications supporting the blood pressure, blood products and albumin are used when indicated.

Surgical Management

Successful treatment of the aneurysm requires either a surgical procedure or an endovascular intervention (Figure 69-7). If surgery is the chosen treatment, several different procedures may be used; however, the one most commonly used is clipping of the intracranial aneurysm. Aneurysms not anatomically suited to clipping can be wrapped in a surgical gauze material and coated with an acrylic material.[49,67]

Aneurysm Clipping

Surgical obliteration of the aneurysm with a metal clip eliminates the risk of rebleeding. A craniotomy incision is used; the surgeon dissects down to the aneurysm and places a metal clip over the neck of the aneurysm. The craniotomy is then closed. Surgical obliteration of an aneurysm is usually performed within 24 hours of rupture. Medical instability, delay in transfer from one hospital to another, and client or family reluctance to seek medical care or consent to surgery may also delay prompt intervention.

Postoperatively, the client's neurologic status is carefully monitored. The usual postoperative care is given, including cardiac monitoring. As with any neurologic disorder, the physician must be promptly notified about any neurologic changes.

Endovascular Therapy and Embolization

An embolization procedure involves obliteration of the aneurysm by means of platinum coils. An interventional radiologist performs the procedure in an angiography suite. A cerebral angiogram is first performed to visualize the aneurysm. A small platinum coil is guided carefully into the aneurysm and then detached using a small current of electricity, leaving the coil to remain in the aneurysm. The process is repeated with as many coils as

■ **FIGURE 69–7** Common locations of cerebral aneurysms are around the circle of Willis. Surgical resection of aneurysms includes clipping the neck of the aneurysm or inserting a coil into the sac to obliterate the aneurysm.

needed to block blood flow into the aneurysm but not through the adjacent vessel. As the aneurysm is embolized, it thromboses and closes off.

After embolization, the client is admitted to the ICU. The client may receive heparin for 12 to 24 hours after the procedure. The catheter sheath (from the angiogram site) remains in the femoral/groin area with a saline infusion to maintain patency of the artery. Care of the femoral/groin site includes assessing the puncture site for bleeding and hematoma formation, as well as frequent checking of peripheral pulses of the legs. The client remains flat in bed to avoid bending the leg at the groin. Nursing measures to maintain comfort are provided. Ongoing and frequent assessment of neurologic status is required.

Complications can result from the embolization procedure. If the aneurysm has not bled, there is a risk of rupture at the time of embolization. Ischemic stroke can occur if the coil does not stay in the aneurysm or if the parent vessel thromboses. Other problems may be related to the cerebral angiogram (see Chapter 67). Regardless of the treatment, the most important factor is the extent of SAH. Further details may be found in Chapter 70.

ARTERIOVENOUS MALFORMATIONS

Etiology and Pathophysiology

AVMs are vascular lesions in which there is a congenital lack of capillaries; a tangled array of arteries and veins form. Because of the lack of a capillary bed, the blood is shunted directly from the artery to the vein. At the core or center of the AVM is the major artery, referred to as the *nidus*. From the nidus are multiple feeding vessels. Blood flowing from the higher pressure arterial system after shunting to the lower pressure venous system can contribute to hemorrhage. AVMs range in size from small to those encompassing an entire hemisphere.

AVMs may be found in the brain or spinal cord. The majority of AVMs are found in the cerebral hemispheres. In the spinal cord, AVMs predominantly occur on the posterior aspect of the thoracic cord. Depending on the size of the malformation, the number of feeders, and the magnitude of circulatory steal, the AVM can bleed or undergo thrombosis, resulting in transient to permanent brain or spinal cord damage.

Clinical Manifestations

The onset of clinical manifestations may be seen at any age; however, increased incidence is noted in clients younger than 40 years of age. Manifestations are related to the anatomy of the malformation and the vessels involved, and occur as the result of the weakening of the vessels and of the shunting of blood in the tortuous mass. Manifestations may also be due to increasing size of the AVM. As the AVM expands, the anomalous vessels dilate and require more blood. The process of acquiring more blood flow is referred to as circulatory "steal." In this phenomenon, blood is diverted (stolen) from normal areas to maintain flow through the anomalous vessels. Consequently, localized hypoperfusion and hypoxia occur in the tissue adjacent to the AVM.

When the AVM bleeds, the client may present with any of the following: complaints of headache, seizures, or focal deficits. Bleeding may occur into the subarachnoid spaces or the brain tissue itself (intracerebral hemorrhage). Once an AVM has bled, there is a 25% chance of rebleeding.

OUTCOME MANAGEMENT

The management of an AVM is similar to that of an intracranial aneurysm. Nursing goals are comparable to those for aneurysm management, with limitation of activity, seizure control, and blood pressure management. The goals of AVM treatment are complete and permanent obliteration of the lesion. This goal may be accomplished with surgery, endovascular embolizations, radiosurgery, or a combination of these methods. The client's condition and the characteristics of the AVM determine the course of treatment. For example, in a client who has had a large SAH, vasospasm may develop. In this case, treatment is delayed until the vasospasm is decreased or resolved. With an improvement in the clinical status of the client, a treatment plan can then be developed.[49,67]

Clients commonly require a combination of treatments. Surgical resection may be the preferred treatment. Depending on the size and location of the aneurysm, the client may undergo serial embolizations, and surgery is the final form of treatment. For the serial embolizations, a thrombosing agent, Histoacryl glue, may be used. The goal of the embolization is to place the glue as close to the nidus of the AVM as possible.

Another treatment option for cerebral AVMs is radiosurgery. This approach may constitute the main treatment or may be used in combination with other therapies. Radiosurgery consists of direction of a focused beam of radiation toward the nidus of the AVM. The dose delivered is determined by the size of the AVM. The use of radiotherapy is recommended with small AVMs.

The treatment and management of hemorrhagic cerebral disorders is an area of active research. For example, "liquid coils" (coils that take the shape within the vascular lesion), stent-assisted coils, and new coatings on currently used coils are being studied.

INFECTIONS

The brain and spinal cord are remarkably resistant to infection, but when they become infected, the consequences are usually very serious. Infections may be caused by bacteria, viruses, fungi, and occasionally protozoa or parasites. The most common types of brain infections are discussed here; others are presented in Table 69-7.

BACTERIAL MENINGITIS

Meningitis is characterized by inflammation of the meninges, the membranes lining the brain and spinal cord. Bacterial, viral, fungal, and parasitic organisms can all cause meningitis, but bacterial meningitis is by far the most common and this discussion will focus on bacterial meningitis.

Almost any bacteria entering the body can cause meningitis. The most common are meningococci (*Neisseria meningitidis*), pneumococci (*Streptococcus pneumoniae*), and *Haemophilus influenzae*. These organisms are often present in the nasopharynx. *S. pneumoniae*

TABLE 69-7   Central Nervous System Infections

Type of Infection	Organism	Clinical Manifestations	Management
Viral Infections			
Viral meningitis Aseptic meningitis	Mumps virus Picornaviruses Enteroviruses (coxsackievirus, echovirus)	Drowsiness, headache, weakness, photophobia Nuchal rigidity (Brudzinski's sign) Spine stiffness with flexion (Kernig's sign) Blood in CSF Clinical manifestations usually resolve in 2 weeks Seizures may be present	Symptomatic management to reduce headache, control fever, and increase general comfort Anticonvulsants for seizure Isolation
	Arthropod-borne virus (arbovirus)	Unpredictable course of illness Acute fever, malaise, sore throat, vomiting, listlessness, photophobia Later, mental deterioration, personality changes, hemiparesis May develop coma or seizures Arbovirus encephalitis often leads to severe residual disabilities including mental retardation, seizures, blindness, deafness, speech disorders, and hemiplegia	Symptomatic management with close assessment for neurologic deterioration If antiviral medications, close monitoring of vital signs, lungs, airway, fluid balance, and serum electrolytes
	Herpes simplex 1	Similar to above, plus headache, fever, vomiting, and seizures Permanent neurologic and mental disabilities are common If not aggressively treated, will lead to brain herniation, coma, and brain death	Infectious agent confirmed with biopsy Symptomatic management with close assessment for neurologic deterioration Acyclovir given early in course
Fungal Infections			
Granulomatous meningitis	*Cryptococcus*	Concurrent diseases that reduce immune response Drowsiness, headache, weakness, photophobia, fever Nuchal rigidity Spine stiffness with flexion Cryptococci in CSF	IV antifungal medications, such as amphotericin B, flucytosine, and fluconazole
Parasitic Infections			
Neurocysticercosis	Cysticercosis	Consumption of raw or undercooked pork by history May be asymptomatic unless near a vital portion of brain, which leads to local manifestations CT or MRI shows cysts	Praziquantel Surgical excision of cyst if medication is ineffective
Toxoplasmosis	*Toxoplasma gondii*	Most common opportunistic infection in clients with AIDS Confusion, headache, lethargy, low-grade fever Focal manifestations of weakness, ataxia, speech problems, apraxia, seizures, and sensory changes (depending on location of mass) Multiple brain abscesses	Pyrimethamine, sulfadiazine, leucovorin, or clindamycin Symptomatic treatments

AIDS, Acquired immunodeficiency syndrome; *CSF*, cerebrospinal fluid; *CT*, computed tomography; *IV*, intravenous; *MRI*, magnetic resonance imaging.

and *N. meningitidis* are found most often in adults. Factors predisposing to bacterial meningitis include any circumstance where the dura has been compromised, such as open brain injury or brain surgery, systemic infection, anatomic defects of the skull, immunocompromise, and other systemic illnesses. Close quarters, poor hygiene, and malnutrition also place people at risk.

Pathophysiology
The route of entry into the intact CNS is uncertain. Invasion may occur through the choroid plexus (across the blood-brain barrier) or directly through an opening in the dura. Organisms colonize in the CSF, leading to inflammation of the meninges that contain it. Exudate forms, and

the meninges become thickened, and adhesions form, leading to hydrocephalus. The arteries supplying the subarachnoid space may also become inflamed, leading to rupture or thrombosis of these vessels. If severe enough, underlying brain can become inflamed, leading to cerebral edema and increased ICP, as well as vasculitis and cerebral infarction. The CSF and meninges have no effective immune defense, so infections in this region can spread very quickly.

Clinical Manifestations
The classic manifestations of meningitis are nuchal rigidity (rigidity of the neck), Brudzinski's sign and Kernig's sign, and photophobia. To assess for *Kernig's sign,* begin

A   Kernig's Sign   B   Brudzinski's Sign

■ **FIGURE 69-8**   Assessment of meningeal irritation. Stretching the inflamed meninges by flexing the neck or legs causes pain. **A,** Kernig's sign. **B,** Brudzinski's sign.

with the client recumbent and the thigh flexed at a right angle to the abdomen, and with the knee flexed at a 90-degree angle to the thigh. Then extend the client's lower leg. In meningeal irritation, extending the leg upward causes pain, spasm of the hamstring muscles, and resistance to further leg extension at the knee (Figure 69-8, *A*). To assess for *Brudzinski's sign,* with the client supine lift the head rapidly up from the bed. If meningeal irritation is present, forward neck flexion produces flexion of both thighs at the hips and flexure movements of the ankles and knees (see Figure 69-8, *B*).

Other general manifestations related to infection may also be present, such as headache, fever, tachycardia, prostration, chills, fever, nausea, and vomiting. The client may be irritable at first, but, as the infection progresses, the client appears acutely ill and confused, stuporous, or comatose. Seizures may occur. A petechial or hemorrhagic rash may develop. Diagnosis is made by lumbar puncture. The CSF is cloudy. Gram stain of the CSF reveals organisms in 70% to 80% of cases. When the organism cannot be identified, bacterial antigens can be determined. *H. influenzae* is frequently detected with this technique. Clients with bacterial meningitis demonstrate the following:

- Moderately elevated CSF pressures
- Elevated CSF protein level (normal, 15 to 45 mg/dl)
- Decreased CSF glucose level (normal, 60 to 80 mg/dl, or two thirds of the serum glucose value)
- Elevated white blood cell count, usually increased (100 to 10,000/cm^3), with predominantly polymorphonuclear leukocytes

OUTCOME MANAGEMENT

Bacterial meningitis constitutes a medical emergency. Prognosis varies according to the causative organism. The use of antibiotics has reduced the death rate to less than 5% for all types of bacterial meningitis. If untreated, it can be fatal within hours to days. Deaths most often occur in newborn infants and in older adults. Complications are rare

but may include septic shock, vasomotor collapse, seizures, and increased ICP attributable to hydrocephalus, brain swelling, and fluid overload. Residual neurologic deficits are rare in adults.

Medical diagnosis is made by assessment of clinical manifestations and is confirmed by isolating the causative organism from the CSF. Empirical therapy in bacterial meningitis includes cephalosporins, rifampin, and vancomycin. The empirical use of penicillin or ampicillin in the treatment of CNS infections is avoided because of the beta-lactamase–producing *H. influenzae* and *N. meningitidis.* It is believed that the cephalosporins are more potent against the beta-lactamase organisms. Chloramphenicol and trimethoprim-sulfamethoxazole are recommended for clients allergic to penicillin. Once the organism is known, antibiotics with greater sensitivity may be used. High doses of the appropriate antibiotic are usually prescribed for at least 10 days. Factors contributing to development of meningitis also need to be addressed.

A unique problem in treating CNS infection is that an intact blood-brain barrier prevents complete penetration of the antibiotic. However, inflammation inhibits the blood-brain barrier, so for a short time antibiotics penetrate the CNS. Antibiotics are given intravenously; the blood-brain barrier recovers as inflammation subsides, and high doses are required to reach the CSF.

If meningococcal meningitis is suspected, place the client in respiratory isolation and ensure that all personnel who had contact with the patient receive prophylaxis.   SAFETY ALERT

Adequate fluid and electrolyte balance must be maintained. Frequent assessment of the neurologic status is indicated to detect early manifestations of increasing ICP and seizures. Anticonvulsants may be prescribed for seizure prevention.

Outbreaks of meningitis can be a major health problem in the community, especially when they occur in schools. A vaccine is now available and is recommended for those living in tight quarters, such as dormitories or barracks.

ENCEPHALITIS

Encephalitis is an infection of the brain tissue that may be caused by a virus, bacterium, fungus, or parasite. Viral encephalitis is the most common and many different viruses can cause encephalitis. The disease course is extremely variable. Some viruses have a particular affinity for the nervous system, and the nervous system has a limited ability to mount a host response. Immunocompromised clients are at greatest risk for developing encephalitis, but the very young and very old are also at risk. Organisms can enter the body through oral or respiratory routes, or through animal or insect bites. Post-vaccine transmission can also occur.

Once the organisms invade the neuron, they replicate, and destroy the cell. The infection can be acute or the organism may remain latent and cause a more chronic type of infection years later. In acute encephalitis, the brain becomes inflamed, with a pathophysiology similar to that seen in brain involvement with bacterial meningitis. The exact pathophysiology varies and depends on the organism.

Clinical manifestations vary with the type of organism and the area of brain involved. Common manifestations include mild headache, low-grade fever, and mental status changes such as confusion. Hemiparesis, seizures, aphasia, and cranial nerve deficits may be seen. Diagnosis may be difficult. A comprehensive history must be obtained to include recent illnesses and immunizations, travel, and exposure to animals, birds, or insects. A lumbar puncture will show slight elevation in CSF protein with normal glucose level; lymphocytosis may be present. Enzyme-linked immunosorbent assay (ELISA) or other serologic assays may show elevated immunoglobulin M (IgM) (early) or IgG (late). Polymerase chain reaction (PCR) testing may be positive for specific antigens. It may take many days to weeks to get ELISA and PCR test results, so empirical care may be provided in the interim. Rarely, brain tissue biopsy is necessary to identify the organism.

OUTCOME MANAGEMENT

There is no specific treatment for encephalitis. Vaccines are available against eastern and western equine encephalitis. Prevention is an important factor; remaining indoors at dawn and dusk or, if outdoors, wearing long-sleeved clothing and using diethyltoluamide (DEET)-based insect repellants minimize the risk for insect and tick bites. Anti-inflammatory medications may be used for symptomatic relief while progressive cases of viral encephalitis may be treated with antiviral medications such as acyclovir. Complete supportive care is necessary during the time of acute illness; rehabilitation may be necessary for those with pre-existing neurologic deficits.

BRAIN ABSCESS

A brain abscess is a collection of pus within brain tissue arising from a primary focus elsewhere (e.g., ear, mastoid sinuses, nasal sinuses, heart, distal bones, lungs, or primary bacteremia). A brain abscess may occur after penetrating traumatic brain injuries or intracranial surgery. The frontal lobe is the most common site of a brain abscess. They vary in size; a large abscess may involve most of one cerebral hemisphere. Multiple abscesses are microscopic. Brain abscesses are relatively rare; when they do occur, they are most common in people younger than age 30. Morbidity and mortality increase greatly with multiple brain abscesses.

Staphylococci are the most common organisms in trauma-related cases; however, many organisms may be implicated. *Toxoplasma* is the usual agent found in clients with human immunodeficiency virus (HIV) infection.

In its early stages, the abscess produces inflammation, necrotic tissue, and surrounding edema. Within several days, the center of the abscess is purulent, and a wall of granulation tissue forms, encapsulating the abscess. Infection may spread through thin places in the wall of the capsule, resulting in development of additional abscesses.

Clinical manifestations of a brain abscess are essentially the same as those seen with any space-occupying brain lesion. Headache and lethargy are the most common manifestations. Manifestations of infection (e.g., fever, chills) are present about half the time. The client may experience drowsiness, confusion, and a depressed mental status as a result of the cerebral edema; increasing ICP; and intracranial effects of the brain abscess. Transient focal neurologic disorders (e.g., weakness on one side, loss of speech) occur when the abscess is located in a specific area such as the motor or speech area. Early manifestations may subside, and then within a few days or weeks, indications of increasing ICP may develop (e.g., recurrent headaches, changes in level of consciousness, focal or generalized seizures).

Medical diagnosis of a brain abscess is made by CT or MRI. However, the appearance is similar to a brain tumor and misdiagnosis is possible.

OUTCOME MANAGEMENT

Pyogenic brain abscess may be treated either with 6 to 12 weeks of antibiotic therapy or with antibiotics combined with surgical aspiration or craniotomy for excision. Needle aspiration may be performed stereotactically (guided by CT imaging) with the use of local anesthesia. Corticosteroids may also be given to reduce cerebral edema. Penicillin is the antibiotic of choice for this type of infection. When antibiotics are used to treat the abscess, follow-up CT or MRI scans are used to monitor progress.

HEADACHE

Headache, the most common of pains, may occur either in the absence of organic disease or as a manifestation of serious disease. Most headaches are transient and of only moderate or slight severity. However, a few types are chronic, intense, and recurrent over a period of months or years. Headache is a manifestation of an underlying disorder, rather than a disease itself. The cause of headache must be identified so that appropriate treatment can be given.

Clients often self-treat headaches with over-the-counter medications. Most headaches do not indicate serious disease. However, some headaches and headache patterns require more complete assessment, as shown in the Critical Monitoring feature below. Serious disorders that typically produce headache include intracranial tumors and hemorrhage, CNS infections, acute systemic infections, severe hypertension, and acute or chronic diseases of the eye, ear, or nose.

Assessment of headaches may include detailed history, psychosocial assessment, and physical examination. Neurologic assessment is particularly important. Possible neurologic diagnostic tests include CT, MRI, EEG, and lumbar puncture with CSF examination.

History should determine (1) location of the pain, intensity, and paths of radiation; (2) character of the headache (e.g., sharp, dull, throbbing); (3) mode of headache onset, duration, and frequency; (4) methods used to treat the headache; (5) presence of localized tenderness; (6) associated phenomena or precipitating factors; and (7) familial incidence.

Classification and Etiology

Tension Headaches

Tension headaches result from muscle contraction (Figure 69-9, *A*). This type of headache is described as a tight band-like discomfort that is unrelenting, with few headache-free intervals. The pain typically builds slowly, fluctuates in severity, and may persist more or less continuously for many days. Triggers include fatigue and stress. The diagnosis of tension headache is confirmed when the headaches occur more often than 15 days a month. Clients may report that the head feels as if it is in a vise or that the posterior neck muscles are tight. In some clients, anxiety or depression coexists with tension headache.

Cluster Headaches

Cluster headaches are classified as a form of migraine (see Figure 69-9, *B*). These headaches have a cyclical pattern of one to three short-lived attacks of periorbital pain lasting from 4 to 8 weeks, with an increased incidence in spring and fall. These headaches also have quiescent periods lasting months to years. Cluster headaches occur more often in men.

The headache lasts between 15 minutes and 3 hours. It may occur from every other day to eight times each day and may awaken the client from sleep. The pain is described as deep, boring, intense pain of such severity

---

Headache

Headaches are the most common form of pain and most headaches are due to primary causes, such as migraines or tension. However, headache requires further evaluation when any of the following exists:

- There is a significant change in the progression or pattern of the pain.
- The pain recurs in one particular area, such as over the eye or in the temple.
- The pain is described as "the worst headache" the client has ever had.
- The pain is severe and begins abruptly, waking the client from sleep.
- The client also has neck stiffness or fever.
- The client had a recent injury to the head.
- The client has neurologic changes lasting more than 1 hour, or loss of consciousness.
- There is a change in vision, such as light waves in the line of vision.
- The headache is present in clients with cancer, immunosuppression, or pregnancy.
- The headache is triggered by physical exertion, sexual activity, or the Valsalva maneuver.

FIGURE 69–9 Types of headaches. The red areas show the regions of greatest pain. **A,** Muscle contraction headache. **B,** Cluster headache. **C,** Migraine headache.

that the client has difficulty remaining still. The client may also develop Horner syndrome with constricted pupils, injected conjunctiva, unilateral lacrimation, and rhinorrhea during the headaches. Cluster headaches are triggered by consumption of alcohol.

The most satisfactory treatment is the administration of drugs to prevent cluster attacks until the bout is over. Effective prophylactic drugs are prednisone, lithium, methysergide, ergotamine, and verapamil. Lithium appears to be particularly useful for the chronic form of the disorder. A 10-day course of prednisone, followed by a rapid taper, may interrupt the pain bout for many clients.

For the attacks themselves, oxygen inhalation (9 L/min via a loose mask) is the most effective modality; inhalation of 100% oxygen for 15 minutes is often necessary. The self-administration of intranasal lidocaine, either 4% topical or 2% viscous, to the most caudal aspect of the inferior nasal turbinate can produce a ganglionic block that is usually remarkably effective in terminating an attack.

Migraine Headaches

Migraine headache is often considered to be a "vascular" headache, with vasospasm and ischemia of intracranial vessels being the cause of the pain (see Figure 69-9, *C*). These headaches usually begin in puberty and are more common in women, often associated with hormonal changes following the menstrual cycle. About 66% of cases of migraine are familial.

Migraine headaches last between 4 and 72 hours, with headache-free intervals between attacks. The headache is most often unilateral, but pain may occur on alternate sides with different attacks. Pain is described as throbbing and pulsatile. Photophobia, phonophobia, anorexia, nausea, vomiting, and focal neurologic manifestations are often present. Some clients have a visual aura that precedes the headache by 10 to 60 minutes (usually 20 minutes). The client sees a jagged edge of light in the visual fields. Other premonitory manifestations occur 12 to 24 hours before an attack and may include euphoria, fatigue, yawning, and craving for sweets. Migraine headache can be triggered by relief of intense stress, missing meals, or tyramine-rich foods. The Client Education Guide above, right lists additional triggers and stress-management interventions.

Typically, the client finds pain reduction in a quiet, dark environment. When aspirin and acetaminophen alone fail, the addition of butalbital, caffeine, ibuprofen (600 to 800 mg), and naproxen (375 to 750 mg) is often useful. Isometheptene compound, one to two capsules, is effective for mild to moderate "common migraine." When these measures fail, more aggressive therapy should be considered. Drug absorption is impaired during migrainous attacks because of reduced gastrointestinal motility. Delayed absorption occurs in the absence of nausea and is related to the severity of the attack and not

CLIENT EDUCATION GUIDE

Migraine Headache

- Many things can trigger a migraine headache. Find out what triggers your headaches and avoid those triggers. If this is not possible, consult your physician about adjusting the dosage of your medication.
- If menstruation and ovulation are triggers, consult your physician for adjustments to your medication dosage.
- Alcohol temporarily increases the diameter of your blood vessels (a process called vasodilation), which may trigger migraines.
- Some foods, such as chocolate, cheese, citrus fruits, coffee, pork, and dairy products, contain substances that may trigger migraines.
- Low food intake may lead to a low blood glucose (sugar) level (hypoglycemia), which can trigger migraines. Eat small, frequent meals to decrease this risk.
- Stress management is essential. Adjust your lifestyle to reduce fatigue and exposure to bright sunlight, heat, or humidity. Get enough sleep. If you are having trouble managing the stresses in your life, seek expert guidance.

its duration. Therefore when oral agents fail to cure, alternative therapies, including rectal ergotamine, subcutaneous or intranasal sumatriptan, sublingual zolmitriptan, parenteral dihydroergotamine, and IV chlorpromazine and prochlorperazine, should be tried. Narcotics should be avoided if possible. The Complementary and Alternative Therapy feature on p. 1840 presents one alternative therapy that is effective and inexpensive, with minimal side effects.

A number of drugs have the capacity to stabilize migraine. They must be taken daily. The decision to use daily medication as a prophylactic measure depends on the frequency of attacks and on how well acute treatment is working. The occurrence of at least two or three attacks per month may be an indication for this approach. There is usually a lag of 2 weeks before an effect is seen. The major drugs are propranolol, amitriptyline, valproate, verapamil, phenelzine, and methysergide.

Lumbar Puncture Headaches

Loss of CSF volume with lumbar puncture decreases the brain's supportive cushion. Headache after lumbar puncture usually begins within 48 hours but may be delayed for up to 12 days. Head pain is dramatically positional; it begins when the client sits or stands upright, and reduction is obtained upon reclining or with abdominal compression. The longer the client is upright, the longer the latency before head pain subsides. It is worsened by head shaking and jugular vein compression. The pain is usually a dull ache but may be throbbing; its location is occipitofrontal. Nausea and stiff neck often accompany

High-Dose Vitamin B₂ (Riboflavin) for Headaches

Because of the high cost and side effects of current migraine drug treatments, there is ongoing interest in alternative and cheaper options. For example, in a controlled trial, 55 clients were randomized to 3 months of vitamin B_2 (riboflavin) 400 mg once a day or placebo for 3 months. Clients were included who experienced 2 to 8 migraines a month. Responders were defined as those having a 50% reduction in manifestations. The two groups were similar in terms of age, co-morbidities, and severity of migraine at baseline. After 3 months of treatment, the number of migraines per month for clients taking riboflavin was reduced from 3.83 to less than 2 ($P = .0001$), with parallel reductions in the number of days ($P = .0001$) and the duration of migraines ($P = .018$). There were no changes in the placebo group. These changes were moderate but were also significant. Headache severity and medication use during headache did not change. Side effects were minimal; only one riboflavin recipient left the study, complaining of diarrhea after 2 weeks. Health professionals should keep in mind that riboflavin may work more slowly than other agents (taking 2 to 3 months to reach full effect). High doses of other B vitamins such as B_6 (pyridoxine) may cause peripheral neuropathy. Clients should be warned about the potential of this vitamin to create fluorescent yellow urine, as well as not attempting to obtain the 400 mg of B_2 with a multivitamin, which contains other toxic vitamins in excess. Thus clients should take B_2 as a separate individual supplement.

REFERENCE

Schoenen, J., Jacquy, J., & Lenaerts, M. (1998). Effectiveness of high-dose riboflavin in migraine prophylaxis: A randomized controlled trial. *Neurology, 50*, 466-470.

headache, and occasionally blurred vision, photophobia, tinnitus, and vertigo are reported. The pain usually resolves over a few days but may sometimes persist for weeks to months.

Treatment with IV caffeine sodium benzoate promptly terminates headache in most clients. An epidural blood patch accomplished by injection of 15 ml of autologous whole blood rarely fails for those who do not respond to caffeine. The mechanism for these treatment effects is not certain. The blood patch has an immediate effect, making it unlikely that sealing off a dural hole with a blood clot is its mechanism of action.

Postconcussion Headaches and Syndrome

After seemingly trivial head injuries and particularly after rear-end motor vehicle collisions, many clients report varying combinations of headache, dizziness, vertigo, and impaired memory. Anxiety, irritability, and difficulty with concentration are other hallmarks of *postconcussion syndrome*. Manifestations may remit after several weeks or persist for months and even years after the injury.

Postconcussion headaches may occur whether or not a client was rendered unconscious by head trauma. Typically, findings on neurologic examination are normal, with the exception of the behavioral abnormalities. Chronic subdural hematoma may on occasion mimic this disorder. Although the cause of postconcussive headache disorder is not known, it should not in general be viewed as a primary psychological disturbance. It often persists long after the settlement of pending lawsuits.

Treatment is symptomatic support. Repeated encouragement that the syndrome eventually remits is important.

Other Causes of Headache

Head pain may also develop from disorders of the eyes, ears, teeth, and paranasal structures. Headaches may result from errors of refraction, glaucoma (with increased intraocular pressure), inflammation, and ocular muscle disturbances (see Chapter 65). Pain associated with sinus infection is usually caused by irritation and inflammation of sinus openings. Sinus walls are less sensitive. The pain of a sinus headache may be reduced or eliminated by decongestants and analgesics. Sometimes antibiotics are needed. Surgery to drain the sinuses may also be required (see Chapter 60).

CONCLUSIONS

Because of the complexity of brain disorders and the emotional reactions of the client and family members to these problems, neurologic nursing is one of the most challenging areas of nursing practice. Common nursing problems center on cerebral perfusion and cognition as well as on those related to functional rehabilitation. Prevention and early intervention are key to optimal client outcome.

THINKING CRITICALLY

1. A client suffered a temporal lobe contusion from a motor vehicle accident 3 days ago. He is disoriented to time and place and has short-term memory deficits. During your assessment of the client, he stops answering questions and begins tonic movements of his extremities.

Factors to Consider. What are the highest priorities for this client? What are the interventions related to these priorities? What interventions come next? What significance does the site of injury have?

2. A client with a history of headaches, dizziness, and vertigo experienced a first-time seizure at age 27 years. Immediately after this episode, he noted the onset of blurred vision. Subsequent studies revealed the presence of a brain tumor, and cranial surgery was

scheduled. Two days after surgery, the client is transferred to the regular unit. What are your responsibilities regarding monitoring for an increase in intracranial pressure? What are the general interventions for the client after craniotomy?

Factors to Consider. What is the major complication following intracranial surgery? How do the general interventions prevent complications associated with this type of surgery?

3. You are caring for a client who had a malignant brain tumor resected 72 hours ago. During previous assessments, she was alert and oriented; her pupils were equal, round, reactive to light, and accommodative (PERRLA); her eyes opened spontaneously; and she was moving all four extremities equally and on command. Her Glasgow Coma Scale score was 15. Now, however, she is slow to respond although still oriented to person, place, and time. Her right pupil is equal in size to the left but exhibits a sluggish reaction to direct light. Her left pupil responds normally. She still responds to verbal commands appropriately, has equal motor strength, and opens her eyes spontaneously. Thus her score on the Glasgow Coma Scale is still 15. You decide to notify the physician. Why?

Factors to Consider. How sensitive is the Glasgow Coma Scale? What abnormality may be indicated by the decreased response time and the change in pupil reaction?

4. A 33-year-old woman, Miss Brown, arrives in the emergency department with a severe headache. She has vomited twice. She states, "This is the worst headache I have ever had." The headache has lasted for about 6 hours, and two doses of acetaminophen have given no relief. Miss Brown cannot lift her head off of the pillow or position herself for comfort. Her pupils are equal, and there is no diaphoresis. What further nursing history and assessments should be done? How soon can medication to alleviate the headache be administered?

Factors to Consider. How crucial is a thorough pain assessment? How can a migraine headache mimic manifestations of a cerebral disorder? Would it be advisable to delay giving an analgesic? Why? Why not?

Discussions for these questions can be found on the website.

BIBLIOGRAPHY

Citations appearing in red refer to primary research.

Citations appearing in blue refer to evidence-based practice guidelines and protocols.

1. American Brain Tumor Association. (2000). *A primer of brain tumors* (7th ed.). Chicago: Author.
2. Anderson, S.I., et al. (1999). Mood disorders in patients after treatment for primary intracranial tumors. *British Journal of Neurosurgery, 13*(5), 480-485.
3. Angelle, D. (2002). Brain attack. *Leading Medicine, 1*(Spring), 8-12.
4. Bader, M.K., & Littlejohns, L.R. (2004). *AANN core curriculum for neuroscience nursing* (4th ed.). Philadelphia: Elsevier.
5. Breslau, N., et al. (2000). Headache and major depression. *Neurology, 54*(2), 308-313.
6. Broderick, S., Connolly, E., Feldmann, D., et al. (2007). Guidelines for the management of spontaneous intracerebral hemorrhage in adults: 2007 update: A guideline from the American Heart Association/American Stroke Association Stroke Council, High Blood Pressure Research Council, and the Quality of Care and Outcomes in Research Interdisciplinary Working Group. *Stroke, 38*(6), 2001-2023.
7. Buffalo Neurosurgery Group. (2003). *Endoscopic endonasal removal of pituitary tumors.* Accessed July 2007 from www.buffaloneuro.com/cranial/brain%20tumors.htm.
8. Central Brain Tumor Registry for the United States (CBTRUS), Accessed December 2007 from www.cbtrus.org
9. Clinical Guideline 20. (2004). *The epilepsies: The diagnosis and management of the epilepsies in adults and children in primary and secondary care.* Accessed July 2007 from www.nice.org.uk/CG020NICEguideline.
10. Columbia-Presbyterian Department of Neurological Surgery. (2003). *Endoscopic neurosurgery.* Accessed July 2007 from www.cumc.columbia.edu/dept/nsg/NSGCPMC/specialties/endoscopy.html.
11. Dunleavy, K., Finck, A., Overstreet, W., et al. (2005). Doing it better: Putting research into practice. Improving care of patients with subarachnoid hemorrhage. *Nursing, 35*(11), 26-27.
12. Engle, J., & Pedley, T.A. (Eds.) (2007). *Epilepsy—A comprehensive textbook* (Vol. I, II, and III). Philadelphia: Lippincott, Williams and Wilkins.
13. Faylor, C.R. (1999). Using transcranial Doppler to augment the neurological examination after aneurysmal subarachnoid hemorrhage. *Journal of Neuroscience Nursing, 31*(5), 285-293.
14. Gahart, B., & Nazareno, A. (2008). *Intravenous medications* (24th ed., pp. 362-365). St. Louis: Mosby.
15. Gibson, P.A. (2005). Beyond pharmacologic therapy: Quality of life issues and counseling needs of the newly diagnosed patient. *Advanced Nursing Studies, 3*(3), 79-84, 91–93.
16. Gusa, D. (2004). Clinical updates. Aneurysmal subarachnoid hemorrhage. *Journal of Continuing Education in Nursing, 35*(4), 150-151.
17. Kaniecki, R. (2003). Headache assessment and management. *Journal of the American Medical Association, 289*(11), 1430-1433.
18. Krapohl, B.D., Keutinger, M., & Komurcu, F. (2007). Research for practice. Vagal nerve stimulation: Treatment modality for epilepsy. *MEDSURG Nursing, 16*(10), 39-44.
19. Laino, C. (2003). Changes in brain function associated with recovery identifiable two weeks after stroke. *Neurology Today,* September, 45-46.
20. Lawal, M. (2005). Epilepsy management. Management and treatment options for epilepsy. *British Journal of Nursing, 14*(16), 854-858.
21. Lech, J., Dungay, J., & Dowson, A. (2006). Headache management in primary care. *Primary Health Care, 16*(9), 25-31.
22. Longatti, P., Fiorindi, A., DiPaola, F., et al. (2006). Coiling and neuroendoscopy: A new perspective in the treatment of intraventricular hemorrhages due to bleeding aneurysms. *Journal of Neurology, Neurosurgery, and Psychiatry, 77*(12), 1354-1358.
23. Mayo Clinic. (2003). *Treatment options for brain tumors.* Accessed July 2007 from www.mayoclinic.org/braintumors.
24. McLendon, R.E., Bigner, D.D., & Rosenblum, M.K. (Eds.) (2006). *Russell and Rubinstein's pathology of tumors of the nervous system* (7th ed.). London: Hodder Arnold.
25. Minton, M. (1999). Primer of neuroanatomy and neurophysiology. *Nursing Clinics of North America, 34*(3), 555-572.
26. Moloney, M.F., et al. (2000). Caring for the woman with migraine headaches. *Nurse Practitioner, 25*(2), 17-41.
27. Morrison, S.R. (1997). Guglielmi detachable coils: An alternative therapy for surgically high-risk aneurysms. *Journal of Neuroscience Nursing, 29*(4), 232-237.
28. Mower-Wade, D., Cavanaugh, M.C., & Bush, D. (2001). Protecting the patient with a ruptured cerebral aneurysm. *Nursing, 31*(2), 52-58.
29. Myers, F. (2000). Meningitis: The fears, the facts. *RN, 63*(11), 52-58.
30. Rogers, G. (2003). Emerging guidance for epilepsy. *Primary Health Care, 13*(6), 39-41.
31. Rowan, J.A., & Tuchman, L. (2003). Management of seizures in the elderly. *Profiles in Seizure Management, 2*(4), 4-9.

32. Schiller, Y., et al. (2000). Discontinuation of antiepileptic drugs after successful epilepsy surgery. *Neurology, 54*(2), 346-349.

33. Schmidek, H.H., & Roberts, D.W. (2005). *Schmidek's and Sweet's operative neurosurgical techniques* (5th ed., Vol. I and II). Philadelphia: Saunders.

34. Shafer, P.O. (1999). Epilepsy and seizures—Advances in seizure assessment, treatment and self-management. *Nursing Clinics of North America, 34*(3), 743-759.

35. Shafer, P.O. (2005). Improving quality of life in adults with new-onset epilepsy. *Advanced Studies in Nursing, 3*(4), 120-125, 139-141.

36. Shah, S.M., & Kelly, K.M. (2007). *Emergency, neurology—Principles and practice.* Cambridge: Cambridge University Press.

37. Shuttleworth, A. (2004). Implementing new clinical guidelines on epilepsy management. *Nursing Times, 100*(45), 28-29.

38. Spencer, D.C., et al. (2000). The role of intracarotid amobarbital procedure in evaluation of patients for epilepsy. *Surgery, 42*(3), 302-325.

39. Snively, C., et al. (1998). Vagal nerve stimulator as a treatment for intractable epilepsy. *Journal of Neuroscience Nursing, 30*(5), 286-289.

40. Stewart-Amidei, C. (2005). Managing symptoms and side effects during brain tumor illness. *Expert Reviews in Neurotherapeutics, 5*, S71-S76.

41. Vitners, H.V. (1998). *Diagnostic neuropathology.* New York: Marcel Dekker.

42. Winn, H.R. (2004). *Youmans' neurological surgery: A comprehensive reference guide to the diagnosis and management of neurosurgical problems.* Philadelphia: Elsevier.

43. Wisniewski, A. (2203). Combating infection. Closing in on clues to encephalitis. *Nursing, 33*(4), 70-71.

evolve *Did you remember to check out the bonus material on the Evolve website and the CD-ROM, including NCLEX®-Examination Style Review Questions, Open-Book Quizzes, and Chapter Review Audio Podcasts?*

http://evolve.elsevier.com/Black/medsurg

CHAPTER 70

Management of Clients with Stroke

LISA BOWMAN

STROKE

Stroke is a term used to describe neurologic changes caused by an interruption in the blood supply to a part of the brain. The two major types of stroke are *ischemic* and *hemorrhagic*. Ischemic stroke is caused by a thrombotic or embolic blockage of blood flow to the brain. Bleeding into the brain tissue or the subarachnoid space causes a hemorrhagic stroke. Ischemic strokes account for about 83% of all strokes. The remaining 17% of strokes are hemorrhagic.

Cerebrovascular disorders are the third leading cause of death in the United States and account for about 150,000 mortalities annually. An estimated 550,000 people experience a stroke each year. When second strokes are considered in the estimates, the incidence increases to 700,000 per year in the United States alone. Stroke is a leading cause of adult disability and a leading primary diagnosis in long-term care. More than 4 million stroke survivors are living with varying degrees of disability in the United States. Along with a high death rate, strokes produce significant morbidity in people who survive them. Of stroke survivors, 31% require assistance with self-care, 20% require assistance with ambulation, 71% have some impairment in vocational ability up to 7 years following the stroke, and 16% are institutionalized.

Before 1995 health care professionals could offer only supportive measures and rehabilitation to stroke survivors. Thrombolytic therapies can prevent or limit the extent of damage to brain tissue caused by acute ischemic stroke. Thrombolytic therapy must be administered as soon as possible after onset of the stroke; a treatment window of 3 hours from the onset of manifestations has been established. To convey this sense of urgency regarding the evaluation and treatment of stroke, health care professionals now refer to stroke as a *brain attack*. Public education is focused on prevention, recognition of manifestations, and early treatment.

Etiology and Risk Factors

Blood flow to the brain can be decreased in several ways. Ischemia occurs when the blood supply to a part of the brain is interrupted or totally occluded. Ultimate survival of ischemic brain tissue depends on the length of time it is deprived plus the degree of altered brain metabolism. Ischemia is commonly due to thrombosis or embolism (Figure 70-1). Thrombotic strokes are more common than embolic strokes.

Strokes can also be "large vessel" and "small vessel." Large vessel strokes are caused by blockage of a major cerebral artery, such as the internal carotid, anterior cerebral, middle cerebral, posterior cerebral, vertebral, and basilar arteries. Small vessel strokes affect smaller vessels that branch off the larger vessels to penetrate deep into the brain.

Thrombosis

A thrombus starts with damage to the endothelial lining of the vessel. Atherosclerosis is the primary culprit. Atherosclerosis causes fatty material to deposit and form plaques on vessel walls. These plaques continue to enlarge and cause stenosis of the artery. Stenosis alters the usual smooth flow of blood through the artery. Blood swirls around the irregular surface of the plaques, causing platelets to adhere to the plaque. Eventually the

---

evolve Web Enhancements

Case Management Stroke

Case Study Meningioma, Fractured Hip, and Possible Stroke

Client Education Guide Transfer from Bed to Wheelchair by a Hemiplegic Client (Spanish Translation)

Clinical Pathway Stroke

Be sure to check out the bonus material on the Evolve website and the CD-ROM, including free self-assessment exercises. **http://evolve.elsevier. com/Black/medsurg**

■ **FIGURE 70–1 A,** Events causing stroke. **B,** Hemorrhagic stroke caused by blood leaking into brain tissue and ischemic stroke caused by clot blocking the blood supply to area in brain.

Thrombotic stroke. Cerebral thrombosis is a narrowing of the artery by fatty deposits called *plaque.* Plaque can cause a clot to form, which blocks the passage of blood through the artery.

A   B

vessel lumen becomes obstructed. Rarely occlusion is due to inflammation of the arteries, called *arteritis* or *vasculitis.*

A thrombus can develop anywhere along a carotid artery or its branches. A common site is at the bifurcation of the common carotid into the internal and external carotid arteries. Thrombotic stroke is the most common type of stroke in people with diabetes.

Lacunar strokes are small vessel strokes. The endothelium of smaller vessels is affected primarily by hypertension, which causes a thickening of the vessel wall and stenosis. Lacunar infarctions are also common in people with diabetes mellitus.

Embolism

The occlusion of a cerebral artery by an embolus causes an embolic stroke. An embolus forms outside the brain, detaches, and travels through the cerebral circulation until it lodges in and occludes a cerebral artery. A common embolus is plaque. A thrombus can detach from the internal carotid artery at the site of an ulcerated plaque and travel into the cerebral circulation. Chronic atrial fibrillation is associated with a high incidence of embolic stroke. Blood pools in the poorly emptying atria. Tiny clots form in the left atrium and move through the heart and into the cerebral circulation. Mechanical prosthetic heart valves have a rougher surface than the normal endocardium and can also cause an increased risk of clots. Both bacterial and nonbacterial endocarditis can be sources of emboli. Other sources of emboli include tumor, fat, bacteria, and air. Any cerebrovascular territory may be affected. The incidence of cerebral embolism increases with age.

Hemorrhage

Most intracerebral hemorrhages are caused by the rupture of arteriosclerotic and hypertensive vessels, which causes bleeding into brain tissue. Intracerebral hemorrhage is most often secondary to hypertension and is most common after age 50 years. Aneurysms are another cause of hemorrhage. Aneurysms are weakened outpouchings in a vessel wall. Although cerebral aneurysms are usually small (2 to 6 mm in diameter), they can rupture. An estimated 6% of all strokes are caused by aneurysm rupture.

Stroke secondary to bleeding often produces spasm of cerebral vessels and cerebral ischemia because the blood outside of the vessels acts as an irritant to the tissues. Hemorrhagic stroke usually produces extensive residual functional loss and has the slowest recovery of all types of stroke. The overall mortality of intracerebral hemorrhage varies between 25% and 60%. The volume of the hemorrhage is the single most important predictor of client outcome. Therefore it is not surprising that hemorrhage into the brain causes the most fatalities of all strokes.

Other Causes

Cerebral arterial spasm, caused by irritation, reduces blood flow to the area of the brain supplied by the constricted vessel. Spasm of short duration does not necessarily cause permanent brain damage.

Hypercoagulable states, including protein C and protein S deficiencies and disorders of the clotting cascade, can cause thrombosis and ischemic stroke. Compression of cerebral vessels may result from a tumor, large blood clot, swollen brain tissue, brain abscess, or other disorders. These causes are fairly rare.

Risk Factors

The incidence of stroke and stroke mortalities has gradually declined in many industrialized countries in recent years as a result of increased recognition and treatment of risk factors. Modifiable risk factors can be reduced or eliminated through lifestyle changes. Hypertension is the most important modifiable risk factor for both ischemic and hemorrhagic stroke. Adequate blood pressure control is associated with a 38% reduction in stroke incidence.

Cardiovascular disease and atrial fibrillation are also associated with an increased risk of stroke. The Complementary and Alternative Therapy feature below discusses elevated homocysteine levels. Diabetes mellitus increases the risk of stroke and morbidity and mortality after stroke. The mechanism is related to macrovascular changes in people with diabetes mellitus. Prior stroke, carotid stenosis, and a history of transient ischemic attacks (TIAs) are considered modifiable risk factors for stroke. Reduction in the risk factors for initial stroke may prevent stroke recurrence. Early recognition and treatment of carotid stenosis and treatment of TIAs with antiplatelet agents reduce the risk of stroke.

Other modifiable risk factors for stroke include hyperlipidemia, cigarette smoking, heavy alcohol consumption, cocaine use, and obesity. Current research suggests that although heavy alcohol consumption increases one's risk of a stroke, light or moderate alcohol consumption may protect against ischemic stroke. Stroke is uncommon in women of childbearing age; however, high-dose estrogen oral contraceptives combined with hypertension, cigarette smoking, migraine headaches, and increasing age increase the risk of stroke in women. The Complementary and Alternative Therapy feature below examines whether vitamin E has any value in preventing stroke.

Client education is aimed at stroke prevention. *Primary* prevention of stroke includes the following:

- Maintaining an ideal body weight
- Maintaining safe cholesterol levels
- Smoking cessation
- Using low-dose estrogen contraceptives only in the absence of other risk factors
- Reducing heavy alcohol consumption
- Eliminating illicit drug use

Secondary prevention includes the following:

- Adequate blood pressure control
- Care of diabetes mellitus
- Treatment of cardiovascular disease, TIA, and atrial fibrillation

Nonmodifiable risk factors cannot be prevented or treated. Advancing age is one of the most significant risk factors for stroke. The incidence of stroke in men is

---

COMPLEMENTARY AND ALTERNATIVE THERAPY

Elevated Homocysteine Levels and Stroke

A recent meta-analysis of studies from 1966 to 1999 was conducted to evaluate the ability of homocysteine levels to predict heart disease or stroke. A total of 30 studies were found (12 prospective and 18 retrospective) that met the inclusion criteria. Researchers found that lower plasma homocysteine levels were associated with a modest reduction in cardiovascular disease (CVD) risk, but a true causal association cannot be concluded. None of the studies that were reviewed adjusted for the presence of renal impairment, a condition known to increase both plasma homocysteine levels and risk for CVD. Also, genetic studies and large intervention trials are required to establish causation. Interestingly, plasma homocysteine levels can be lowered in most clients using 1 mg/day oral folic acid, with or without vitamins B_{12} and B_6. Some researchers suggest that until ongoing primary and secondary prevention trials of homocysteine reduction and CVD are completed, the measurement of homocysteine levels should be done only in those with unexplained premature CVD.

REFERENCE

The Homocysteine Studies Collaboration. (2002). Homocysteine and risk of ischemic heart disease and stroke: A meta-analysis. *Journal of the American Medical Association, 288,* 2015-2022.

COMPLEMENTARY AND ALTERNATIVE THERAPY

Vitamin E and Stroke

In a randomized, controlled clinical trial of 29,133 Finnish male smokers, the overall net stroke morbidity and mortality with alpha-tocopherol (vitamin E) and beta-carotene was not significantly different from that of the placebo group. However, a trend toward higher rates of subarachnoid hemorrhages was found (relative risk [RR] = 1.5, number needed to harm = 833), but the cerebral infarction rate was decreased (RR = 0.86, number needed to treat = 239).[2] The Italian GISSI* study of 11,324 clients with a recent myocardial infarction showed no effect of vitamin E on the combined outcomes of death, myocardial infarction, and stroke.[1] Therefore recommending vitamin E supplements for cardiovascular disease reduction cannot be advocated at this time.

REFERENCES

1. GISSI Investigators. (1999). Dietary supplementation with n-3 polyunsaturated fatty acids and vitamin E after myocardial infarction: Results of the GISSI Prevenzione Trial. *Lancet, 354,* 447-455.
2. Leppala, J., et al. (2000). Controlled trial of alpha-tocopherol and beta-carotene supplements on stroke incidence and mortality in male smokers. *Arteriosclerosis, Thrombosis, and Vascular Biology, 20,* 230-235.

*Gruppo Italiano per lo Studio della Streptochinasi Nell'Infarto Miocardico (Italian Group for the Study of Streptokinase in Myocardial Infarction).

slightly higher than that in women. Stroke is also more prevalent in African Americans than in whites or Hispanics. This difference is probably related to the increased incidence of hypertension and diabetes mellitus in this group. Family history of stroke increases one's risk for stroke.

Pathophysiology

The brain is very sensitive to a loss of blood supply. Hypoxia can cause cerebral ischemia because unlike other body tissues, such as muscle, the brain cannot use anaerobic metabolism in the absence of oxygen and glucose. The brain is perfused at the expense of other less vital organs to preserve cerebral metabolism. Short-term ischemia leads to temporary neurologic deficits or a TIA. If blood flow is not restored, brain tissue sustains irreversible damage or infarction within minutes. The extent of infarction depends on the location and size of the occluded artery and the adequacy of collateral circulation to the area it supplies.

Ischemia quickly alters cerebral metabolism. Cell death and permanent changes can occur within 3 to 10 minutes. The client's baseline oxygen level and ability to compensate determine how quickly irreversible changes occur. Blood flow can be altered by localized perfusion problems, such as stroke, or by generalized perfusion problems, such as hypotension or cardiac arrest. Cerebral perfusion pressure must fall to two thirds of normal (a mean arterial pressure of 50 mm Hg or below assuming a normal baseline) before the brain does not receive adequate blood flow. A client who has lost compensatory autoregulation experiences manifestations of neurologic deficit sooner.

Decreased cerebral perfusion is usually caused by occlusion of a cerebral artery or intracerebral hemorrhage. Occlusion produces ischemia in the brain tissue supplied by the affected artery and edema in the surrounding tissue. Cells in the center of the stroke area, or the core, die almost immediately after stroke onset; this is referred to as *primary neuronal injury*. A zone of hypoperfusion also exists around the infarcted core; this zone is called the *penumbra*. The size of this zone depends on the amount of collateral circulation present. Collateral circulation describes the vessels that augment the major circulatory vessels of the brain. Differences in the size and number of collateral vessels help to explain variations in the severity of manifestations experienced by clients with strokes in the same anatomic area.

A cascade of biochemical processes occurs within minutes of cerebral ischemia. Neurotoxins, including oxygen free radicals, nitric oxide, and glutamate, are released. Local acidosis develops. Membrane depolarization occurs. This results in an influx of calcium and sodium. Cytotoxic edema and cell death are a result; this is secondary neuronal injury. Penumbral neurons are highly susceptible to the effects of the ischemic cascade. The area of edema after ischemia may lead to temporary neurologic deficits. Edema may subside in a few hours or sometimes in several days, and the client may regain some function.

Clinical Manifestations
Early Warnings

Some strokes have early warning signs, called transient ischemic attacks (TIAs, see later discussion also). Manifestations of impending ischemic stroke include *transient* hemiparesis, loss of speech, and hemisensory loss. Manifestations of a thrombotic stroke develop over minutes to hours to days. The slow onset is because the thrombus is still increasing in size. First there is partial, and then complete, occlusion of the affected vessel. In contrast, manifestations of embolic strokes occur suddenly and without warning.

Hemorrhagic stroke also occurs rapidly, with manifestations developing over minutes to hours. Common manifestations include severe occipital or nuchal headaches, vertigo or syncope, paresthesias, transient paralysis, epistaxis, and retinal hemorrhages.

Manifestations of deficit must persist longer than 24 hours to be diagnostic of stroke. TIAs are focal neurologic deficits lasting less than 24 hours.

Generalized Findings

Most clients are hypertensive when arriving in the emergency department. General findings of stroke unrelated to specific vessel sites include headache, vomiting, seizures, changes in mental status, fever, and changes on the electrocardiogram (ECG). ECG changes may include atrial fibrillation, which can help indicate the cause of the stroke. Recent myocardial infarction can be seen with T-wave changes, shortened PR interval, prolonged QT interval, premature ventricular contractions, sinus bradycardia, and ventricular and supraventricular tachycardias. Subarachnoid hemorrhage (SAH) can lead to ST-segment and T-wave abnormalities also. Fever can indicate hypothalamic injury.

Specific Deficits After Stroke

Stroke manifestations can be correlated with the cause (Table 70-1) and with the area of the brain in which perfusion is impaired (Table 70-2). The middle cerebral artery is the most common site of ischemic stroke. The client's deficit also varies according to whether the dominant or the nondominant side of the brain is affected. The degree of deficit can also vary from little impairment to serious functional loss.

Hemiparesis and Hemiplegia. *Hemiparesis* (weakness) or *hemiplegia* (paralysis) of one side of the body may

TABLE 70–1   Clinical Manifestations of the Various Causes of Stroke

Cause	Clinical Manifestations
Thrombosis	Tends to develop during sleep or within 1 hour of arising
	Ischemia is produced gradually; therefore clinical manifestations develop more slowly than those caused by hemorrhage or emboli
	Relative preservation of consciousness
	Hypertension
Embolism	No discernible time pattern, unrelated to activity
	Clinical manifestations occur rapidly, within 10-30 seconds, and often without warning
	May have rapid improvement
	Relative preservation of consciousness
	Normotension
Hemorrhage	Typically occurs during active, waking hours
	Severe headache and nuchal rigidity occur (if client is able to report manifestations)
	Rapid onset of complete hemiplegia, occurs over minutes to 1 hour
	Usually results in extensive, permanent loss of function with slower, less complete recovery
	Rapid progression into coma

occur after a stroke. These deficits are usually caused by a stroke in the anterior or middle cerebral artery, leading to an infarction in the motor strip of the frontal cortex. Complete hemiplegia involves half of the face and tongue as well as the arm and leg of the ipsilateral side of the body. Infarction in the right side of the brain causes left-sided hemiplegia and vice versa because nerve fibers cross over in the pyramidal tract as they pass from the brain to the spinal cord. Strokes causing hemiparesis or hemiplegia usually affect other cortical areas in addition to the motor strip. As a result, hemiparesis and hemiplegia are often accompanied by other manifestations of stroke, including hemisensory loss, hemianopia, apraxia, agnosia, and aphasia. Muscles of the thorax and abdomen are usually not affected because they are innervated from both cerebral hemispheres.

Over time, when voluntary muscle control is lost, strong flexor muscles overbalance the extensors. This imbalance can cause serious contractures. For example, a hemiplegic client's affected arm tends to rotate internally and to adduct because adductor muscles are stronger than abductors. The elbow, wrist, and fingers also tend to flex. The affected leg tends to rotate externally at the hip joint, flex at the knee and plantar flex, and supinate at the ankle joint (Figure 70-2).

Aphasia. *Aphasia* is a deficit in the ability to communicate. Aphasia may involve any or all aspects of communication, including speaking, reading, writing, and understanding spoken language. The primary language center is usually located in the left cerebral hemisphere

and is affected by stroke in the left middle cerebral artery. Several different types of aphasia exist; the most common are described here.

Wernicke's (sensory or *receptive) aphasia* affects speech comprehension as a result of an infarction in the temporal lobe of the brain. *Broca's (expressive* or *motor) aphasia* affects speech production as a result of an infarction in the frontal lobe of the brain. Branches of the middle cerebral artery supply both areas. *Global aphasia* affects both speech comprehension and speech production.

Other methods of classifying aphasia are by fluency or by the degree of difficulty in articulation. Clients with fluent aphasia (Wernicke's) have speech that is well articulated and grammatically correct but lacks content. Clients with nonfluent aphasia (Broca's) have varying degrees of difficulty in producing speech, and what words are spoken are uttered slowly, with great effort and poor articulation. Clients with global aphasia typically repeat the same sounds they hear and have poor comprehension.

Sensory or fluent aphasias involve loss of the ability to comprehend written, printed, or spoken words. A client with acoustic aphasia can hear the sounds of speech, but the parts of the brain that give meaning to these sounds are damaged. Clients have difficulty understanding what is being said. They hear sound but cannot make sense of it because they cannot understand the symbolic communication associated with the sound. Visual aphasia is similar. Affected clients cannot read words but can see them. They cannot understand the symbolic content of printed or written symbols.

Motor or nonfluent aphasias include aphasias in which the ability to write, make signs, or speak is lost. For example, with motor aphasia, words may be recalled but the client cannot combine speech sounds into words and syllables. Pure motor or pure sensory aphasias are rare. Most aphasias are mixed, affecting both expressive and receptive elements.

Most aphasias are partial rather than complete. The severity of aphasia varies with the area involved and the extent of cerebral damage. Severe damage may deprive the client of any meaningful relationship with the environment and family. Global aphasia can be so extensive that neither expressive nor receptive language abilities are retained. Early determination of the client's yes-no reliability facilitates communication. Verbal skills are often the best. Reading and writing are usually more impaired. The use of gestures can aid in communication.

Aphasia is frequently associated with hemiplegia involving the dominant hemisphere. The speech center for a right-handed client is usually located in the left cerebral hemisphere; the speech center for a left-handed client may be in the brain's right or left side. Thus a right-handed client with right-sided hemiplegia usually has

TABLE 70–2 Clinical Manifestations of Stroke Associated with Area of Brain Affected

Location	Middle Cerebral Artery	Anterior Cerebral Artery	Posterior Cerebral Artery
Motor changes	Contralateral hemiparesis or hemiplegia, face and arm deficits greater than leg	Contralateral hemiparesis, foot and leg deficits greater than arm, footdrop, gait disturbances	Mild contralateral hemiparesis (with thalamic or subthalamic involvement) Intention tremor
Sensory changes	Contralateral hemisensory alterations Neglect of involved extremities	Contralateral hemisensory alterations	Diffuse sensory loss (thalamic)
Visual or ocular changes	Homonymous hemianopia Inability to turn eyes toward affected side	Deviation of eyes toward affected side	Pupillary dysfunction (brain stem) Loss of conjugate gaze, nystagmus Loss of depth perception Cortical blindness Homonymous hemianopia
Speech changes	Dyslexia, dysgraphia, aphasia	Expressive aphasia	Perseveration Dyslexia
Mental changes	Memory deficits	Confusion, amnesia Flat affect, apathy Shortened attention span Loss of mental acuity	Memory deficits
Other changes	Vomiting may occur	Apraxia (inability to carry out purposeful movements in unaffected areas) Incontinence	Visual hallucinations
Contralateral hemiparesis with facial asymmetry	Alternating motor weaknesses Ataxic gait, dysmetria (uncoordinated actions)	Ipsilateral ataxia Facial paralysis	Ataxia Paralysis of larynx and soft palate
Contralateral sensory alterations	Contralateral hemisensory impairments	Ipsilateral loss of sensation in face, sensation changes on trunk and limbs	Ipsilateral loss of sensation in face, contralateral on body
Homonymous hemianopia	Double vision Homonymous hemianopia	Nystagmus	Nystagmus
Ipsilateral periods of blindness (amaurosis fugax)	Nystagmus, conjugate gaze paralysis		
Aphasia if dominant hemisphere is involved	Dysarthria Memory loss Disorientation		Dysarthria
Mild Horner syndrome	Drop attacks	Horner syndrome	Horner syndrome
Carotid bruits	Tinnitus, hearing loss Vertigo Dysphagia Coma or locked-in syndrome	Tinnitus, hearing loss	Hiccups and coughing Vertigo Nausea, vomiting

"Frozen" shoulder
Subluxation of the shoulder
Painful shoulder-hand dystrophy
Adduction of arm with internal rotation; flexion of elbow, wrist, and fingers

External rotation of leg at hip joint; flexion at knee; and plantar flexion and supination at ankle

Shortened heel cord

■ **FIGURE 70–2** Hemiplegic contractures. The elbow is bent, the wrist is flexed, and the fingers are curled into palmar flexion; the knee is bent and the heel cord is shortened.

aphasia because the speech center is in the damaged left hemisphere. Most people have left-sided speech dominance.

Dysarthria. *Dysarthria* is imperfect articulation that causes difficulty in speaking. It is important to differentiate between dysarthria and aphasia. With dysarthria the client understands language but has difficulty pronouncing words and may slur them, enunciating poorly. No disturbance is evident in grammar or in sentence construction. A dysarthric client can understand verbal speech and can read and write (unless the dominant hand is paralyzed, absent, or injured).

Dysarthria is caused by cranial nerve (CN) dysfunction from a stroke in the vertebrobasilar artery or its branches. It may result from weakness or paralysis of the muscles of the lips, tongue, and larynx or from a loss of sensation. In addition to speaking problems, clients with dysarthria often have difficulty chewing and swallowing because of poor muscle control.

Dysphagia. Swallowing is a complex process that requires the function of several cranial nerves. The mouth must open (CN V), the lips must close (CN VII), and the tongue must move (CN XII). The mouth must sense the quantity and quality of the food bolus (CN V and VII) and must send messages to the swallowing center (CN V and IX). During swallowing, the tongue moves the food bolus toward the oropharynx. The pharynx elevates and the glottis closes. Contraction of the pharyngeal muscles transports food from the pharynx to the esophagus. Peristalsis moves food to the stomach. A stroke in the territory of the vertebrobasilar system causes dysphagia.

Apraxia. *Apraxia* is a condition that affects complex motor integration and therefore can result from a stroke in several areas in the brain. Clients who have apraxia cannot carry out a skilled act such as dressing even when they are not paralyzed. A client with apraxia may be able to conceive or conceptualize the content of messages to send to muscles. The motor patterns or schema necessary to convey the impulse message cannot be reconstructed, however. Thus accurate "instructions" do not reach the limb from the brain, and the desired action or movement does not happen. Apraxia ranges from relatively simple to highly complex disorders. For example, a client may have less difficulty writing than speaking or vice versa.

Visual Changes. Vision is a complex process controlled by several areas in the brain. Parietal and temporal lobe strokes may interrupt visual fibers of the optic tract en route to the occipital cortex and impair visual acuity. Depth perception and visual perception of horizontal and vertical planes may also be impaired. In clients with hemiplegia, this causes motor performance problems in gait and posture (Figure 70-3). Clients may or may not be aware of a perceptual difficulty, but it may cause them to be accident prone, and their behavior may appear bizarre. Visual disorders can interfere with a client's ability to relearn motor skills. Infarcts affecting the function of CN III, IV, and VI may produce CN palsies and result in diplopia.

Homonymous Hemianopia. *Homonymous hemianopia* (Figure 70-4) is a visual loss in the same half of the visual field of each eye, so the client has only half of normal vision. For example, the client may see clearly on one side of the midline but see nothing on the other side. Clients with homonymous hemianopia cannot see past the midline without turning the head toward that side.

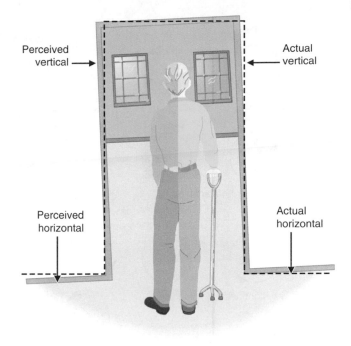

■ **FIGURE 70–3** Perceptual disturbances in left-sided hemiplegia. Such disturbances can be both unpleasant and unsafe.

Horner Syndrome. *Horner syndrome* is paralysis of the sympathetic nerves to the eye, causing sinking of the eyeball, ptosis of the upper eyelid, slight elevation of the lower lid, constriction of the pupil, and lack of tearing in the eye.

Agnosia. *Agnosia* is a disturbance in the ability to recognize familiar objects through the senses. The most common types are visual and auditory. Agnosia may result from an occlusion of the middle or posterior cerebral arteries supplying the temporal or occipital lobes.

A client with visual agnosia sees objects but is unable to recognize or attach meaning to them. Disorientation occurs because of an inability to recognize environmental cues, familiar faces, or symbols. Such a client may examine objects curiously but might be unable to determine their function. This can cause considerable self-care deficit when common, necessary objects, such as silverware, clothing, or toilet articles, are unfamiliar. Visual agnosia greatly increases the risk for injury because the client cannot recognize danger or symbols that warn of danger. Extensive visual agnosia can produce such extreme behavioral effects that the client's condition may be inaccurately diagnosed as diffuse dementia.

A client with auditory agnosia cannot attach meaning to sounds in the absence of hearing loss or decreased level of consciousness. Some degree of aphasia is almost always present. Often these people are initially considered hysterical or psychotic.

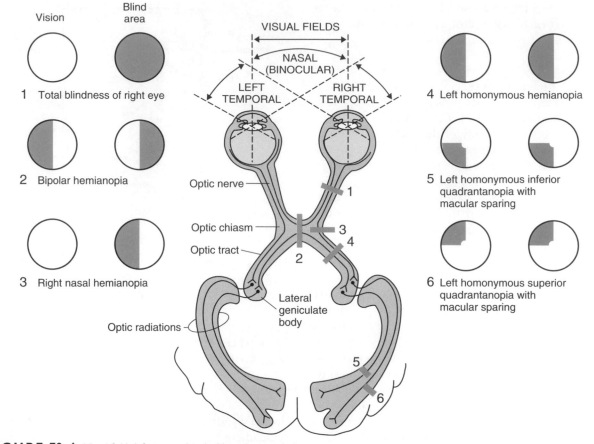

■ **FIGURE 70–4** Visual-field defects associated with optic nerve lesions.

Unilateral Neglect. *Unilateral neglect* is the inability of a person to respond to a stimulus on the contralateral side of a cerebral infarction. Clients with injury to the temporo-parietal lobe, inferior parietal lobe, lateral frontal lobe, cingulate gyrus, thalamus, and striatum as a result of a middle cerebral artery occlusion most commonly develop neglect. Because of the dominance of the right hemisphere in directing attention, neglect is most commonly seen in clients with right hemisphere damage.

Clinical manifestations of unilateral neglect include failure to (1) attend to one side of the body, (2) report or respond to stimuli on one side of the body, (3) use one extremity, and (4) orient the head and eyes to one side. Unilateral neglect may be accompanied by inaccurate beliefs about the position of a limb in space or its existence or ownership. For example, a man with unilateral neglect may not believe that his arm is part of his body, he may be unaware of his arm's position, or he may deny that a limb is paralyzed when it is.

Sensory Deficits. Several types of sensory changes can result from a stroke in the sensory strip of the parietal lobe supplied by the anterior or middle cerebral artery. The deficit is on the contralateral side of the body and is frequently accompanied by hemiplegia or hemiparesis. *Hemisensory loss* (a loss of sensation on one side of the body) is generally incomplete and may not be noticed by the client. The superficial sensations of pain, touch, pressure, and temperature are affected in varying degrees. *Paresthesia* is described as persistent, burning pain; feelings of heaviness, numbness, tingling, or prickling; or heightened sensitivity. *Proprioception* (the ability to perceive the relationship of body parts to the external environment) and postural sense disturbances may occur with loss of muscle-joint sense. This may seriously interfere with the client's ability to ambulate because of a lack of balance control and inappropriate movements. The risk of falling is high because of the tendency to malposition the feet when walking.

Behavioral Changes. Various portions of the brain assist with control of behavior and emotions. The cerebral cortex interprets stimuli. The temporal and limbic areas modulate emotional responses to stimuli. The hypothalamus and pituitary glands coordinate the motor cortex and language areas. The brain can be seen as a modulator of emotions, and when the brain is not fully functional, emotional reactions and responses lack this modulation.

Behavioral changes after a stroke are common. People with stroke in the left cerebral, or dominant, hemisphere are frequently slow, cautious, and disorganized.

People with stroke in the right cerebral, or nondominant, hemisphere are frequently impulsive, overestimate their abilities, and have a decreased attention span, which increases their risk of injury. Frontal lobe infarcts from a stroke in the anterior or middle cerebral arteries can lead to disturbances in memory, judgment, abstract thinking, insight, inhibition, and emotion. The client may exhibit a flat affect, a lack of spontaneity, distractibility, and forgetfulness. The client may have emotional lability and burst into tears or, less commonly, laughter without provocation. There is little or no relationship between the emotion and what is occurring in the person's environment. Significant clinical depression occurs in 25% to 60% of clients with strokes. Because depression can interfere with rehabilitation and functional recovery, it is important to identify it and initiate treatment.

Incontinence. Stroke may cause bowel and bladder dysfunction. One type of neurogenic bladder, an uninhibited bladder, sometimes occurs after stroke. Nerves send the message of bladder filling to the brain, but the brain does not correctly interpret the message and does not transmit the message not to urinate to the bladder. This results in frequency, urgency, and incontinence. Sometimes clients with a type of neurogenic bowel seem fixated on having a bowel movement. Other causes of incontinence may be memory lapses, inattention, emotional factors, inability to communicate, impaired physical mobility, and infection. The duration and severity of the dysfunction depend on the extent and location of the infarct.

Diagnostic Findings

With the advent of thrombolytic therapy in the treatment of acute ischemic stroke, accurate brain imaging plays an important role in the diagnosis and treatment of stroke. A noncontrast computed tomography (CT) scan of the head is performed to rule out hemorrhagic stroke as a cause of acute neurologic deficits. Cellular changes that are diagnostic of stroke do not appear on the head CT scan acutely. Standard magnetic resonance imaging (MRI) has limited value in diagnosing acute ischemic stroke because the infarct is usually not apparent until 8 to 12 hours after the onset of symptoms. New MRI techniques—diffusion-weighted imaging (DWI) and perfusion imaging (PI)—may improve the diagnosis and treatment of acute stroke. These techniques have greater sensitivity and anatomic resolution and the potential to allow earlier detection and characterization of acute ischemic stroke.

Further diagnostic studies include ECG to rule out atrial fibrillation and echocardiogram if atrial emboli are suspected. Carotid duplex scanning is used to identify carotid artery stenosis or occlusion.

OUTCOME MANAGEMENT

Medical Management

Medical management of the client with stroke is directed at early diagnosis and early identification of the client who can benefit from thrombolytic treatment. Preserving cerebral oxygenation, preventing complications and stroke recurrence, and rehabilitating the client are other goals.

Identify Stroke Early

A critical factor in the early intervention and treatment of stroke is the proper identification of stroke manifestations and establishing the onset of the manifestations. Because manifestations vary by the location and size of the infarct, standardized assessment tools, including the Acute Stroke Quick Screen and the National Institutes of Health Stroke Scale (NIHSS) (Table 70-3), can be used to identify rapidly which clients might benefit from thrombolytic therapy. The assessment must be complete and accurate to provide a baseline for ongoing assessments. A score of less than 5 on the 42-point scale indicates a minor stroke.

The initial assessment of the client who is thought to have had a stroke includes the level of consciousness, pupillary response to light, visual fields, movement of extremities, speech, sensation, reflexes, ataxia, and vital signs. These data are often recorded and scored in addition to the information assessed on the Glasgow Coma Scale (GCS). In addition, if intracranial pressure monitors are in place, baseline pressure values and waveforms should be noted.

A complete history of the presenting problem as well as past medical and social history can provide data about the cause of the stroke. This information also guides stroke treatment. The time of onset of manifestations must be determined because thrombolytic therapy must be administered within 3 hours of the onset of manifestations. A history of hypertension or cardiac valve disorders is commonly associated with stroke.

Maintain Cerebral Oxygenation

Emergency care of the client with stroke includes maintaining a patent airway. The unconscious client should be turned on the affected side to promote drainage of saliva from the airway. The collar of the shirt should be loosened to facilitate venous return. The head should be elevated, but the neck should not be flexed. The client should be kept quiet, and emergency help should be contacted.

Once the client is in the emergency department (ED), a patent airway is maintained and oxygen is supplied. If the client demonstrates poor ventilatory effort,

TABLE 70–3 National Institutes of Health (NIH) Stroke Scale

Administer stroke scale items in the order listed. Scores should reflect what the client does, not what the clinician thinks the client can do. Except where indicated, the client should not be coached (i.e., repeated requests to client to make a special effort). For the total score, 0 = normal examination, >4 often represents acute stroke, and >20 often represents profound neurologic deficit.

Instruction	Scale Definition
1a. Level of Consciousness The investigator must choose a response, even if a full evaluation is prevented by such obstacles as an endotracheal tube, language barrier, or orotracheal trauma or bandages. A 3 is scored only if the client makes no movement (other than reflexive posturing) in response to noxious stimulation.	0 = Alert, keenly responsive 1 = Not alert, but arousable by minor stimulation to obey, answer, or respond 2 = Not alert, requires repeated stimulation or painful stimulation to make movements (not stereotyped) 3 = Responds only with reflex motor or autonomic effects, or totally unresponsive, flaccid, areflexic
1b. LOC Questions The client is asked the month and his or her age. The answer must be correct—there is no partial credit for being close. Aphasic and stuporous clients who do not comprehend the questions will score 2. Clients unable to speak because of endotracheal intubation, orotracheal trauma, severe dysarthria from any cause, language barrier, or any other problem not secondary to aphasia are given a 1. It is important that only the initial answer be graded and that the examiner not "help" the client with verbal or nonverbal cues.	0 = Answers both questions correctly 1 = Answers one question correctly 2 = Answers neither question correctly
1c. LOC Commands The client is asked to open and close the eyes and then to grip and release the nonparetic hand. Substitute another one-step command if the hands cannot be used. Credit is given if an unequivocal attempt is made but not completed because of weakness. If clients do not respond to command, the task should be demonstrated to them (pantomime) and score the result (i.e., follows none, one, or two commands). Clients with trauma, amputation, or other physical impediments should be given suitable one-step commands. Only the first attempt is scored.	0 = Performs both tasks correctly 1 = Performs one task correctly 2 = Performs neither task correctly
2. Best Gaze Only horizontal eye movements will be tested. Voluntary or reflexive (oculocephalic) eye movements will be scored, but caloric testing is not done. If the client has a conjugate deviation of the eyes that can be overcome by voluntary or reflexive activity, the score will be 1. If a client has an isolated peripheral nerve paresis (CN III, IV, or VI), score a 1. Gaze is testable in all aphasic clients. Clients with ocular trauma, bandages, pre-existing blindness, or other disorder of visual acuity or fields should be tested with reflexive movements, and a choice made by the investigator. Establishing eye contact and then moving about the client from side to side will occasionally clarify the presence of a gaze palsy.	0 = Normal 1 = Partial gaze palsy; this score is given when gaze is abnormal in one or both eyes, but where forced deviation or total gaze paresis is not present 2 = Forced deviation or total gaze paresis not overcome by the oculocephalic maneuver
3. Visual Visual fields (upper and lower quadrants) are tested by confrontation, using finger counting or visual threat as appropriate. Client must be encouraged, but if he or she looks at the side of the moving fingers appropriately, this can be scored as normal. If there is unilateral blindness or enucleation, visual fields in the remaining eye are scored. Score 1 only if a clear-cut asymmetry, including quadrantanopia, is found. If client is blind from any cause, score 3. Double simultaneous stimulation is performed at this point. If there is extinction, client receives a 1 and the results are used to answer question 11.	0 = No visual loss 1 = Partial hemianopia 2 = Complete hemianopia 3 = Bilateral hemianopia (blind, including cortical blindness)
4. Facial Palsy Ask or use pantomime to encourage the client to show teeth or smile and close eyes. Score symmetry of grimace in response to noxious stimuli in the poorly responsive or noncomprehending client. If facial trauma or bandages, orotracheal tube, tape, or other physical barrier obscures the face, these should be removed to the extent possible.	0 = Normal symmetrical movement 1 = Minor paralysis (flattened nasolabial fold, asymmetry on smiling) 2 = Partial paralysis (total or near total paralysis of lower face) 3 = Complete paralysis (absence of facial movement in the upper and lower face)

TABLE 70–3   National Institutes of Health (NIH) Stroke Scale—Cont'd

Instruction	Scale Definition
5 and 6. Motor Arm and Leg The limb is placed in the appropriate position: extend the arms 90 degrees (if sitting) or 45 degrees (if supine) and the leg 30 degrees (always tested supine). Drift is scored if the arm falls before 10 seconds or the leg before 5 seconds. The aphasic client is encouraged using urgency in the voice and pantomime but not noxious stimulation. Each limb is tested in turn, beginning with the nonparetic arm. Only in the case of amputation or joint fusion at the shoulder or hip may the score be 9, and the examiner must clearly write the explanation for scoring as a 9.	0 = No drift; limb holds 90 degrees (or 45 degrees) for full 10 seconds 1 = Drift; limb holds 90 degrees (or 45 degrees) but drifts down before full 10 seconds; does not hit bed or other support 2 = Some effort against gravity; limb cannot get to or maintain (if cued) 90 degrees (or 45 degrees); drifts down to bed but has some effort against gravity 3 = No effort against gravity; limb falls 4 = No movement 9 = Amputation, joint fusion; explain: 5a = Left arm 5b = Right arm 0 = No drift; leg holds 30 degrees for full 5 seconds 1 = Drift; leg falls by the end of the 5-second period but does not hit bed 2 = Some effort against gravity; leg falls to bed by 5 seconds but has some effort against gravity 3 = No effort against gravity; leg falls to bed immediately 4 = No movement 9 = Amputation, joint fusion; explain: 6a = Left leg 6b = Right leg

7. Limb Ataxia
This item is aimed at finding evidence of a unilateral cerebellar lesion. Test with eyes open. In case of visual defect, ensure testing is done in intact visual field. The finger-nose-finger and heel-shin tests are performed on both sides, and ataxia is scored only if present out of proportion to weakness. Ataxia is absent in the client who cannot understand or is hemiplegic; only in the case of amputation or joint fusion may the item be scored 9, and the examiner must clearly write the explanation for not scoring. In case of blindness, test by touching nose from extended arm position.
	0 = Absent
	1 = Present in one limb
	2 = Present in two limbs
	If present, is ataxia in
	  Right arm: 1 = Yes 2 = No
	9 = Amputation or joint fusion; explain:
	  Left arm: 1 = Yes 2 = No
	9 = Amputation or joint fusion; explain:
	  Right leg: 1 = Yes 2 = No
	9 = Amputation or joint fusion; explain:
	  Left leg: 1 = Yes 2 = No
	9 = Amputation or joint fusion; explain:

8. Sensory Sensation or grimace to pinprick when tested or withdrawal from noxious stimulus in the obtunded or aphasic client. Only sensory loss attributed to stroke is scored as abnormal, and the examiner should test as many body areas (arms [not hands], legs, trunk, face) as needed to accurately check for hemisensory loss. A score of 2, "severe or total," should only be given when a severe or total loss of sensation can be clearly demonstrated. Stuporous and aphasic clients will therefore probably score 1 or 0. The client with brain stem stroke who has bilateral loss of sensation is scored 2. If the client does not respond and is quadriplegic, score 2. Clients in coma (question 1a = 3) are arbitrarily given a 2 on this item.	0 = Normal; no sensory loss 1 = Mild to moderate sensory loss; client feels pinprick is less sharp or is dull on the affected side, or there is a loss of superficial pain with pinprick but client is aware of being touched 2 = Severe to total sensory loss; client is not aware of being touched
9. Best Language A great deal of information about comprehension will be obtained during the preceding sections of the examination. The client is asked to describe what is happening in the attached picture, to name the items on the attached naming sheet, and to read from the attached list of sentences. Comprehension is judged from responses here as well as to all of the commands in the preceding general neurologic examination. If visual loss interferes with the tests, ask the client to identify objects placed in the hand, repeat, and produce speech. The intubated client should be asked to write a sentence. The client in coma (question 1a = 3) will arbitrarily score 3 on this item. The examiner must choose a score in the client with stupor or limited cooperation, but a score of 3 should be used only if the client is mute and follows no one-step commands.	0 = No aphasia; normal 1 = Mild to moderate aphasia; some obvious loss of fluency or facility of comprehension, without significant limitation on ideas expressed or form of expression. Reduction of speech and/or comprehension, however, makes conversation about provided material difficult or impossible. For example, in conversation about provided materials, examiner can identify picture or naming card from client's response. 2 = Severe aphasia; all communication is through fragmentary expression; great need for inference, questioning, and guessing by the listener. Range of information that can be exchanged is limited; listener carries burden of communication. Examiner cannot identify materials provided from client response. 3 = Mute, global aphasia; no usable speech or auditory comprehension

(Continued)

TABLE 70-3 National Institutes of Health (NIH) Stroke Scale—Cont'd

Instruction	Scale Definition
10. Dysarthria If the client is thought to be normal, an adequate sample of speech must be obtained by asking client to read or repeat words from the attached list. If the client has severe aphasia, the clarity of articulation of spontaneous speech can be rated. Only if the client is intubated or has other physical barriers to producing speech may the item be scored 9, and the examiner must clearly write an explanation for not scoring. Do not tell the client why he or she is being tested.	0 = Normal 1 = Mild to moderate; client slurs at least some words and, at worst, can be understood with some difficulty 2 = Severe; client's speech is so slurred as to be unintelligible in the absence of or out of proportion to any dysphasia, or is mute/anarthric 9 = Intubated or other physical barrier; explain:
11. Extinction and Inattention (formerly Neglect) Sufficient information to identify neglect may be obtained during the prior testing. If the client has severe visual loss preventing visual double simultaneous stimulation, and the cutaneous stimuli are normal, the score is normal. If the client has aphasia but does appear to attend to both sides, the score is normal. The presence of visual spatial neglect or anosognosia may also be taken as evidence of neglect. Because neglect is scored only if present, the item is never untestable. *Additional item, not part of the NIH Stroke Scale score.*	0 = No abnormality 1 = Visual, tactile, auditory, spatial, or personal inattention or extinction to bilateral simultaneous stimulation in one of the sensory modalities 2 = Profound hemi-inattention or hemi-inattention to more than one modality; does not recognize own hand or orients to only one side of space
12. Distal Motor Function The client's hand is held up at the forearm by the examiner, and client is asked to extend his or her fingers as much as possible. If the client cannot or does not extend the fingers, the examiner places the fingers in full extension and observes for any flexion movement for 5 seconds. The client's first attempts only are scored. Repetition of the instructions or of the testing is prohibited.	0 = Normal (no flexion after 5 seconds) 1 = At least some extension after 5 seconds but not fully extended; any movement of the fingers that is not a command is not scored 2 = No voluntary extension after 5 seconds; movement of the fingers at another time is not scored a. Left arm b. Right arm

CN, Cranial nerve; *LOC,* level of consciousness.
Modified from National Institutes of Health, Bethesda, Md.

intubation and mechanical ventilation may be required to prevent hypoxia and increased cerebral ischemia. An ECG is performed to assess for cardiac disorders, such as atrial fibrillation, that increase the risk for embolic stroke. Blood pressure is also evaluated, and hypertension may be reduced with vasodilators. Caution is exercised when treating blood pressure because lowering the blood pressure too far may lower cerebral perfusion pressure and increase cerebral ischemia. Laboratory tests for hematology, chemistry, and coagulation are obtained to rule out stroke-mimicking conditions and to detect bleeding disorders that would increase the risk of bleeding during thrombolytic therapy.

Restore Cerebral Blood Flow

The client is evaluated as a candidate for thrombolytic therapy once an intracerebral hemorrhage is ruled out. The goal of thrombolytic therapy is recanalization of the occluded vessel and reperfusion of ischemic brain tissue. Thrombolytic agents are exogenous plasminogen activators, which dissolve the thrombus or embolus blocking the cerebral blood flow. Clients who receive recombinant tissue plasminogen activator (rt-PA) within 3 hours of the onset of stroke are 30% more likely to have minimal or no disability from acute ischemic stroke without an increase in mortality. Several contraindications to thrombolytic therapy are shown in Box 70-1.

> **BOX 70-1 Inclusion Criteria for Intravenous rt-PA Therapy for Acute Ischemic Stroke**
>
> - Diagnosis of ischemic stroke with a measurable neurologic deficit
> - Neurologic signs are not clearing spontaneously
> - Neurologic signs should not be minor and isolated
> - Caution should be used in treating clients with major deficits
> - Symptoms should not be suggestive of subarachnoid hemorrhage
> - Onset of manifestations <3 hours before the start of probable infusion
> - No head trauma or prior stroke in past 3 months
> - No myocardial infarction in prior 3 months
> - No GI/GU hemorrhage in past 21 days
> - No arterial puncture in a noncompressible site during prior 7 days
> - No major surgery in prior 14 days
> - No history of prior intracranial bleed
> - Systolic BP <185, diastolic BP <110
> - No evidence of acute trauma or bleeding
> - Not taking an oral anticoagulant, or if so INR <1.7
> - If taking heparin within 48 hours must have a normal aPTT
> - Platelet count >100,000
> - Blood glucose level >50 mg/dl (2.7 mmol)
> - No seizure with residual postictal impairments
> - CT does not show evidence of multilobar infarction
>
> *aPTT,* Activated partial thromboplastin time; *CT,* computed tomography; *INR,* International Normalized Ratio.

Treatment should begin immediately after the client is deemed to be a candidate for rt-PA. The dose of rt-PA for acute ischemic stroke is 0.9 mg/kg administered intravenously over 1 hour. Ten percent of the total dose is given as a bolus over 1 minute before initiation of the intravenous dose. The pharmacologic half-life of rt-PA is approximately 5 to 7 minutes. After thrombolytic therapy, the client is sent to the intensive care unit (ICU) for careful monitoring of blood pressure, neurologic status, and bleeding.

The risk-benefit ratio for the use of thrombolytic therapy must be considered in certain client populations. The choice of whether to pursue aggressive treatment focuses on several factors, such as the client's age, the client's preference (if known), the presence and severity of other disorders, the severity of the stroke, and how much time has elapsed since the infarction. The risk of intracerebral hemorrhage after rt-PA is greater in clients with early signs of a major infarct on CT scan. Clients who have severe neurologic deficits at presentation (NIHSS >22) are at increased risk for intracerebral hemorrhage and poor outcome.

At present the treatment for most clients with large areas of infarction or large intracerebral hemorrhage is supportive care. It is hoped that future research can improve the treatment outcomes for these clients.

Prevent Complications

Bleeding. After administration of rt-PA, the client is monitored for potential complications of rt-PA, which may include intracranial hemorrhage and systemic bleeding. In the initial studies of rt-PA in acute ischemic stroke, symptomatic intracranial hemorrhage occurred in 6.4% of clients within the first 36 hours after treatment. Intracranial hemorrhage carries a death rate greater than 50%. All fatal intracranial hemorrhages occurred within the first 24 hours of treatment. The expanding clot of an intracranial hemorrhage destroys brain tissue. The pressure of the clot also disrupts blood flow and causes additional ischemia. Increased intracranial pressure (ICP) results from the space-occupying clot and surrounding edema of ischemic tissue and can lead to midline shift of intracranial contents, possible brain stem herniation, and death. To decrease the risk of intracranial or systemic bleeding, administration of anticoagulants and antiplatelet medications is not recommended until 24 hours after administration of rt-PA.

Stringent blood pressure management is the single most important measure to prevent intracranial hemorrhage after thrombolysis. Frequent vital signs and neurologic checks are necessary to prevent hypertension and detect manifestations of intracranial hemorrhage. Hypertension frequently accompanies acute ischemic stroke. Therefore blood pressure is usually not treated unless it increases to 185 mm Hg systolic or 105 mm Hg diastolic. In addition, the mean arterial pressure should be lowered by no more than 10% and in gradual increments. This is less likely to lead to hypoperfusion and worsening cerebral ischemia.

An intracranial hemorrhage should be suspected if the client has new complaints of headache, nausea, and vomiting, or a sudden change in level of consciousness. An intracranial hemorrhage should be assumed with any acute worsening of neurologic function until it can be ruled out by CT scan. If the rt-PA is still infusing, the infusion should be stopped. A complete blood count, coagulation studies, and type and crossmatch are done. If a head CT scan reveals intracranial hemorrhage, fresh frozen plasma with fibrinogen or cryoprecipitate is administered to correct coagulopathies.

Systemic bleeding may also occur as a complication of rt-PA. Clinical manifestations include change in level of consciousness (LOC), tachycardia, hypotension, and cool, clammy, and pale skin. Thrombolytic therapy may be stopped depending on the site and severity of the bleeding.

Cerebral Edema. Increased ICP is a potential complication of large ischemic strokes. Increased ICP is also a potential complication of intracerebral hemorrhage, either primary or secondary to thrombolytic therapy. Manifestations of increased ICP include change in LOC, reflex hypertension, and worsening neurologic status. Invasive monitoring of ICP is done for clients with decreased LOC who are at high risk for increased ICP. All clients are placed on bed rest with the head of the bed elevated to 30 degrees to decrease ICP and to facilitate venous drainage. Ideally the degree of head elevation is based on the response of the client's ICP for those clients on ICP monitoring.

External *ventriculostomy* drainage is sometimes used to reduce pressure from cerebrospinal fluid (CSF) accumulation. A burr hole is placed through the skull, and a catheter is passed into the lateral ventricle to allow for controlled drainage of CSF. Blood pressure is closely monitored. The goal is to maintain blood pressure low enough to prevent another stroke or hemorrhage without decreasing cerebral perfusion. The client may require continuous mechanical ventilation and hyperventilation to decrease ICP. Mannitol, an osmotic diuretic, helps in lowering increased ICP. Surgical evacuation of the intracerebral hematoma may be performed. Increasing ICP, central herniation, and brain stem hemorrhage can lead to death from depression of the vital centers in the medulla, that is, brain stem failure.

Blood Glucose Control. Severe hyperglycemia can lead to poor outcomes and reduced perfusion of the brain during thrombolysis. Even nondiabetic clients should not be given excessive glucose via intravenous fluids.

Stroke Recurrence. The incidence of stroke recurrence in the first 4 weeks after acute ischemic stroke ranges from 0.6% to 2.2% per week. The risks of anticoagulation include intracranial hemorrhage, systemic bleeding, and death. Therefore the general use of heparin in all clients with acute ischemic stroke is no longer recommended. Heparin is indicated to prevent stroke recurrence in clients at risk for cardiogenic emboli. Initially unfractionated heparin, dose based on body weight, is administered intravenously, and then warfarin is administered orally.

> **SAFETY** ⚠ **ALERT**
>
> **Intravenous heparin is delivered with an infusion pump for accurate and safe delivery. Monitoring of clotting times is important to detect over-anticoagulation, which increases the risk of bleeding. Activated partial thromboplastin time (aPTT) should be at 1.5 to 2.5 times control for anticoagulation to be effective.**

After a therapeutic anticoagulant level has been achieved with heparin therapy, warfarin administration is begun. Because warfarin has a long half-life, the physician initiates the warfarin therapy while the client is still receiving intravenous heparin. Once the client has a therapeutic response to heparin, in about 24 to 48 hours, the physician discontinues the heparin and continues the warfarin therapy. The therapeutic International Normalized Ratio (INR) for prophylaxis against cardiogenic embolization is 2.0 to 3.0. Clients receiving anticoagulation therapy should be assessed for bruising, hematuria, blood in feces, bleeding from mucous membranes, and new-onset or worsening headaches.

The long-term risk for stroke recurrence is 4% to 14% per year. Antiplatelet agents, including aspirin, ticlopidine, extended-release dipyridamole plus aspirin, and clopidogrel, decrease the risk for secondary stroke. Antiplatelet agents inhibit platelet function to decrease the risk of thrombus formation. The selection of the specific antiplatelet agent is individualized according to the client's medical history.

Aspiration. Clients with stroke are at high risk for aspiration pneumonia, which is the direct cause of death in 6% of clients following stroke. Aspiration is most common in the early period and is related to loss of pharyngeal sensation, loss of oropharyngeal motor control, and decreased LOC. Oral food and fluids are generally withheld for 24 to 48 hours.

> **SAFETY** ⚠ **ALERT**
>
> **Feeding by mouth must proceed cautiously; check gag reflex to determine if the client can swallow fluids. Hold feeding if there is any sign of aspiration.**

If the client cannot eat or drink after 48 hours, alternate feeding routes are used, such as tube-feeding or hyperalimentation. When the swallowing mechanism has returned, the client can be fed orally. Progressive feeding programs for dysphagia are based on the degree of swallowing ability.

Other Potential Complications. Other complications of stroke depend primarily on the location of the lesion or infarcted tissue. If the brain stem is affected, blood pressure fluctuations, altered respiratory patterns, and cardiac dysrhythmias are all possible. Physical injury related to the client's inability to realize his or her limitations can occur. Complications of immobility can also occur.

Coma can follow strokes of various causes. The blood supply to the brain stem or reticular activating system, which controls consciousness, may have been directly occluded. Similarly, the deep structures of the thalamus that relay information to the cerebral cortex may be involved. Vascular occlusion of the internal carotid artery or one of its major branches may also decrease LOC. Sometimes the cerebral edema that follows stroke may produce midline shifts, resulting in coma.

Hyperthermia is treated immediately with antipyretics. Temperature elevations lead to increased cerebral metabolic needs, which in turn cause cerebral edema and increased risk for cerebral ischemia. Antipyretics are given and, if needed, a hypothermia blanket or ice packs to reduce body temperature. Causing the client to shiver should be avoided, however, because shivering increases oxygen consumption and ICP. If seizures develop, phenytoin (Dilantin) may be used.

Strokes caused by occlusive disease (e.g., thrombus, embolus) rarely cause sudden death. When stroke is fatal, death may occur within 3 to 12 hours, but it occurs more often between 1 and 14 days after the original episode. Typically, with any type of fatal stroke, a rise in temperature, heart rate, and respiratory rate occurs along with deepening coma several hours or days before death. These manifestations result from damage to the vasomotor and heat-regulating centers. The Case Study on p. 1857, which is continued on the website, presents 🔵*evolve* a scenario of a client at risk for stroke.

Rehabilitation After Stroke

From the onset of stroke, interventions are aimed at maximizing the client's physical and cognitive recovery. Early pre-mobilization efforts are aimed at preventing the complications of neurologic deficit and immobility. After the first few days of the acute event, cerebral edema has usually subsided and the residual deficits of stroke can be identified. Clients with stroke and their families face difficult adjustments as the acute stages pass and residual disabilities become obvious.

Previously it was thought that damage to the central nervous system (CNS) was irreversible. Now it has been shown that even in adults with significant brain injury, relearning can take place. It is extremely important that relearning take place as soon as possible after the injury. Early rehabilitation makes this relearning possible. The severity of a client's stroke will impact the length of time it may take to recover function.

Meningioma, Fractured Hip, and Possible Stroke

Mrs. Olsen is a 72-year-old white woman who resides at Shady Oaks Care Center. She fell today and could not get up again because of the pain. An x-ray examination obtained at the nursing home showed a proximal femoral fracture near the right hip joint. She has been transferred to your hospital for a preoperative medical evaluation in preparation for possible surgical repair of her right hip fracture later today ...

Case Study continued on the website and the CD-ROM with discussions, multiple-choice questions, and a nursing care plan.

An interdisciplinary rehabilitation team is necessary to assist and support clients and their families during this time. Assessing the functional abilities of the client and setting realistic goals are part of this approach. Because stroke is a common health care problem, many facilities have developed clinical pathways to guide care. (See the CareMap of the Clinical Pathway feature on Stroke on the website.)

INTERDISCIPLINARY MANAGEMENT

Several disciplines facilitate recovery of the client following a stroke. It is the coordinated effort of the entire team that best serves the client and family.

The recommended plan of care includes using interdisciplinary services to do the following:

- Document the client's condition and course fully, including deficits, status of other diseases, complications, changes in status, and functional status before stroke.
- Begin physical activity as soon as the client's medical condition is stable; use caution with early mobilization in clients with progressing neurologic deficit, subarachnoid or intracerebral hemorrhage, severe orthostatic hypotension, acute myocardial infarction, or acute deep vein thrombosis.
- Assist in managing general health functions throughout all stages of treatment, such as managing dysphagia, nutrition, hydration, bladder and bowel function, sleep and rest, co-morbid conditions, and acute illnesses.
- Prevent complications, including deep vein thrombosis and pulmonary embolism, aspiration, skin breakdown, urinary tract infections, falls, spasticity and contractures, shoulder injury, and seizures.

- Prevent recurrent strokes through control of modifiable risk factors, oral anticoagulation, antiplatelet therapy, or surgical intervention.
- Assess throughout acute and rehabilitation stages.
- Use reliable standardized instruments for evaluation.
- Evaluate for formal rehabilitation during the acute stage.
- Choose an individual or interdisciplinary program based on the client's and family's needs; success of the program requires full support and active participation of the client and family; families must be involved at the outset.
- Choose the local rehabilitation program that best meets the client's and family's needs.

Physical Therapy

Physical therapists work with the client to build strength and preserve range of motion (ROM) and tone in noninvolved muscles. Physical therapy also builds ROM and tone and retrains muscles affected by the stroke. The client also works on balance and proprioception skills. This may enable the client, with continued improvement, to sit on the edge of the bed and eventually to ambulate. Exercise and bed mobility skills are taught at the client's bedside, as are wheelchair mobility and transfers. Clients who would benefit from the use of an orthosis are identified and instructed on how to apply and remove it. A hemiplegic client is usually able to ambulate using a quad cane following gait training.

Occupational Therapy

Occupational therapists work with the client to relearn activities of daily living (ADL) and to use assistive devices that promote independence. For example, a client with hemiplegia may be able to dress if the clothing can be closed with self-fastening tape (Velcro) fasteners rather than buttons.

Many clients experience severe pain in the affected shoulder and hand after a stroke. This pain can be so severe that it results in lack of balance and loss of ROM, which further restricts mobility and self-care. Overstretching from turns and transfers can aggravate the problem. Some clients have experienced partial dislocation or subluxation of the shoulder both from having the shoulder pulled on and from the weight of the arm pulling it. Chronic subluxation results in shoulder-hand syndrome, characterized by a painful or frozen shoulder and hand edema. Occupational therapists assist in treating this problem and in instructing the client and caregivers in proper transfer and positioning techniques to prevent further injury.

Speech Therapy

Speech pathologists work with the client to foster the maximum amount of speech recovery possible through relearning, accentuation of speech sounds, or use of alternative communication devices. The speech pathologist also assesses the client's swallowing mechanism and makes recommendations for initiation and progression of foods and fluids to decrease the risk of aspiration.

Case Management

Case managers are often assigned to clients following stroke. Their role is to facilitate all care providers and to advocate for the client and family. (See Case Management feature on Stroke on the website.)

Nursing Management of the Medical Client

Assessment. Ongoing assessments of all body systems are needed. The use of a standardized neurologic assessment tool such as the GCS assists the nurse in documenting changes in the client's status and in monitoring progress. The NIH stroke scale (Table 70-3) is also commonly assessed. In addition to the neurologic assessment, the client's blood pressure, heart sounds, heart rate and rhythm, respiratory rate and rhythm, temperature, levels of nutrition, ability to swallow, bladder and bowel elimination, and communication need to be assessed. The client's and family's psychosocial and learning needs should be assessed daily.

Diagnosis, Outcomes, Interventions

Diagnosis: Ineffective Tissue Perfusion. Cerebral perfusion of the cerebrum is critical for survival and long-term outcome. Therefore it should be the first priority in the care of clients with acute stroke. Decreased cerebral blood flow may be secondary to thrombus, embolus, hemorrhage, edema, or spasm. Ongoing assessment and intervention are required beyond the critical stage. Data indicating that the risk for altered perfusion has become an actual problem are shown in the Critical Monitoring box above, right.

Outcomes. The client will have improved cerebral tissue perfusion as evidenced by ICP less than 15 mm Hg, cerebral perfusion pressure (CPP) greater than 65 mm Hg, no type A waves (when using intracranial monitors), no reports of headache, no decreases in LOC, and stable or improving GCS score.

Interventions. Serial assessments of these data may be required as often as every 15 minutes for unstable clients to every 2 to 4 hours for stable clients. Analyze data for trends, and if the client is deteriorating neurologically, notify the physician. Manifestations of progressive deterioration include decreasing LOC, changes in motor or sensory function, pupillary changes, respiratory difficulty, and development of visual or perceptual defects or aphasia.

CRITICAL MONITORING

Manifestations Indicating an Acute Change in Cerebral Perfusion

- Intracranial pressure greater than 15 mm Hg sustained for 15 to 30 seconds or longer
- Cerebral perfusion pressure less than 70 mm Hg
- Decrease in Glasgow Coma Scale score of 2 or more points from baseline
- Decreasing levels of consciousness
- Mean arterial pressure of less than 80 mm Hg or systolic blood pressure less than 100 mm Hg
- Bradycardia
- Altered pattern of breathing
- Loss of response to painful stimuli
- Change in pupil size or response to light
- Headache
- Vomiting
- Abnormal flexion or extension posturing

Maintain the client's blood pressure within the range prescribed by the physician to maintain perfusion without promoting cerebral edema. Maintain normothermia to reduce cerebral glucose and oxygen consumption. Cluster nursing interventions to reduce unneeded movement and stimulation. Elevate the head of the bed 30 degrees to reduce cerebral edema. Maintain the client's head in a neutral position to improve venous drainage.

Administer medications to improve cerebral tissue perfusion as prescribed. Anticoagulants or antiplatelet agents will be used to decrease risk of further thrombus formation. Nimodipine, a calcium-channel blocker, is used to treat vasospasm secondary to subarachnoid hemorrhage.

Delirium and restlessness should be controlled, with sedatives if necessary. Be certain, however, that restlessness is not the result of treatable causes, such as hypoxia, full bladder, bowel impaction, or pain. Restraints should be avoided because they often increase agitation and ICP.

Straining at stool or with excessive coughing, vomiting, lifting, or use of the arms to change position should be avoided, because the Valsalva maneuver increases ICP. Mild laxatives and stool softeners are often prescribed.

Collaborative Problem: Hemorrhage. Because of the increased risk for systemic bleeding secondary to the use of thrombolytic therapy or anticoagulation, monitoring for bleeding is an important collaborative problem. Write the collaborative problem as *Risk for Prolonged Bleeding Times related to use of thrombolytic agents or anticoagulation.*

Outcomes. The nurse will monitor for hemorrhage and, if present, will control bleeding and notify the physician.

Interventions

SAFETY

⚠

ALERT

For the client who is receiving thrombolytic therapy, certain interventions can prevent systemic bleeding, including the following: do not perform arterial punctures or insertions of nasogastric tubes, rectal thermometers, or rectal medications for 24 hours after the infusion; monitor all puncture sites and body fluids for manifestations of bleeding for 24 hours; and maintain bed rest for 24 hours after completion of the infusion.

Gingival bleeding and oozing from intravenous sites have been associated with intracranial hemorrhage. Pressure may be applied to any compressible bleeding sites.

For the client who is receiving anticoagulation, monitor the aPTT and INR and adjust the client's dosage based on the physician's orders. Report any manifestations of bleeding to the physician immediately.

Diagnosis: Risk for Aspiration. The nursing diagnosis *Increased Risk for Aspiration* is listed here because of its importance in maintaining airway and oxygenation. Not all clients are at risk for aspiration after stroke, and the risk depends on the time since injury and the area of infarction. When considering this nursing diagnosis, use the following causes of aspiration to guide your analysis: impaired swallowing, depressed cough and gag reflexes, and decreased LOC.

Outcomes. The client will have a reduced risk of aspiration as evidenced by easily managing saliva, no choking or coughing while eating, no fever, and no crackles or rhonchi.

Interventions. Assess the client for clinical manifestations of aspiration, such as fever, dyspnea, crackles and rhonchi, confusion, and decreased Pao_2 in arterial blood gases. Use caution in feeding the client, either orally or enterally. If the client is receiving enteral feedings, add food coloring to the tube feeding to assist with identifying aspiration via suctioned aspirate. Monitor chest x-ray results, and report findings of pulmonary infiltrate.

Diagnosis: Impaired Physical Mobility. Almost all clients have some degree of immobility after a stroke. In the early phases of stroke recovery, the client may be completely immobile and need assistance just to turn over in bed. Later in recovery, mobility may be hampered in one extremity only. Various causes can be used to individualize this diagnosis. These include (1) loss of muscle tone secondary to flaccid paralysis or spasticity and (2) reluctance to move because of the fear of self-injury or prolonged disuse.

Outcomes. The client will achieve maximal physical mobility within the limitations imposed by the stroke as evidenced by more normal movement of the affected extremity, improved muscle strength, and effective use of adaptive devices. This outcome may require a long time frame; shorter outcomes may be indicated for acute care.

Interventions. Assess the client's degree of muscle strength to use as a baseline value and for determining and evaluating outcomes. A comprehensive assessment by a physical therapist helps to determine appropriate activity levels.

Encourage Bed Exercises. Encouraging clients with hemiplegia to exercise while on bed rest not only prepares them for later activities but also offers hope and a sense of optimism about recovery. A hemiplegic client can learn to move the weak leg by sliding the unaffected leg under it to lift and move the weak leg. The client can also use the unaffected arm to move the affected arm and hand. Keep in mind that clients may have difficulty crossing the midline.

Frequent gluteal and quadriceps muscle setting exercises during the day help to prepare the client for later ambulation. Begin with 5 repetitions, and increase gradually to 20 repetitions each time. Instruct the client as follows:

- *Gluteal setting:* "Pinch" or contract the buttocks together and count to five. Then relax and count to five. Repeat.
- *Quadriceps setting:* Contract the quadriceps muscles on the anterior portion of the thigh while raising the heel and trying to squash a rolled towel placed under the popliteal fossa against the mattress. While keeping the muscle contracted, count to five. Then relax and count to five. Repeat. Perform on both legs if possible. Start quadriceps setting exercise as soon as the client is conscious. The quadriceps muscle is the most important in giving knee joint stability in walking.

Help the Client Sit Up

Help the client out of bed as soon as the client's condition is medically stable. Remember, however, that hemiplegia can severely affect balance. Assistance is needed to provide security and safety. Raise the head of the bed slowly to reduce orthostatic hypotension.
    Assist the client to sit up the first time and closely monitor for balance and safety awareness.

SAFETY

⚠

ALERT

When the client first sits up, support the affected side, especially the back and the head. Gradually the client will learn to sit alone with the head of the bed elevated and then to sit on the edge of the bed with the feet on a firm surface. Help the client maintain balance by extending the affected arm and placing the palm flat on the bed. Be patient and encouraging as the client regains balance. When the client is sitting in a chair, support the weak side with pillows.

Eventually the client will learn to raise the weak leg with the unaffected leg and to swing both legs laterally over the side of the bed onto the floor. It is safest to have the client pivot on the unaffected leg. Therefore position the chair at a right angle to the unaffected side.

Teach the Client How to Use a Wheelchair. A hemiplegic client needs to learn safe transfers from the bed to the chair, commode, or wheelchair. The Client Education Guide below shows one method of moving safely from the bed to a wheelchair. The client with hemiplegia can propel a wheelchair with the unaffected arm and leg; one-arm-drive wheelchairs also are available. Once in a wheelchair, the client's level of independence increases greatly. Deficits in spatial relations, decreased awareness, and unilateral neglect can result in problems such as falling and running into doors. Clients must not be allowed to perform wheelchair self-transfers until they have demonstrated competence.

Promote Walking. A tilt table may be used in physical therapy to help the client assume a standing position if difficulty with balance is a problem. The client can begin standing as soon as the quadriceps muscles on the unaffected side have normal strength. Have the client seated on the edge of the bed. Encourage the client to rise by using the muscle power of the unaffected leg. The client may tend to swing around toward the affected side. Gradually the client will learn to take increasing amounts of weight onto the weaker side.

Despite weakness in the affected limb, a hemiplegic client often develops an extensor reflex, which facilitates

standing. Position yourself on the weaker side when helping the client to stand. To avoid pulling on the affected arm and increasing the risk for shoulder injury, provide support with ambulation by using a gait belt. A quad cane should be used on the unaffected side to allow walking with a three-point gait.

Most hemiplegic clients can be taught to walk. Remind them to keep the body weight forward over the feet. Practice is important for learning to walk correctly. Incorrect habits, once developed, may be difficult to overcome later. Supervise clients carefully until they can safely walk alone without fear of falling. When walking, the client should not show circumduction or toe scraping or stoop forward. Heel-toe walking with a reciprocal gait pattern is the goal of ambulation.

Teach Bracing. If bracing is used, teach the client and family how to apply and remove the brace, to observe skin for breakdown, to give proper skin care, and to care for the brace itself.

Diagnosis: Risk for Hyperthermia. Bleeding or edema of the hypothalamus can lead to ischemia of the thermoregulatory center of the brain.

Outcomes. The client will have a reduced risk of hyperthermia or will have a normal temperature.

Interventions. Treat fever with antipyretics. A hypothermia blanket may be used to bring down a high temperature quickly. When hypothermia blankets are used, assess the skin frequently for pressure points and cold injury. Shivering must be avoided because the muscle activity increases body temperature. Keeping the feet warm with blankets may decrease shivering. Phenothiazine agents may be used to help stabilize neuronal membranes if fever is related to damaged brain structures.

Diagnosis: Risk for Impaired Skin Integrity. The loss of protective sensation and decreased ability to move increase the risk for injury to the skin. In addition, skin damage may develop from friction and shearing or increased skin fragility from inadequate nutritional status or edema.

Outcomes. The client's skin will remain intact as evidenced by an absence of stage I pressure ulcer development and an absence of manifestations of redness from friction or shearing.

Interventions. Assess the skin every 2 hours. Turn the client with hemiplegia or decreased LOC every 2 hours. Develop a written turning schedule for other health care providers and family members to follow. When positioning the client on the affected side, make sure that body weight does not harm affected limbs. Support the affected arm and leg when turning and positioning

---

CLIENT EDUCATION GUIDE

Transfer from Bed to Wheelchair by a Hemiplegic Client

- Lock the wheelchair for safety, and keep it beside the bed on your unaffected side.
- Use your unaffected arm and leg to move your affected arm and leg.
- As your legs drop over the edge of the bed, swing your torso up to a sitting position.
- Push yourself up to a standing position by using your unaffected arm and leg.
- Reach across the wheelchair to grasp the far arm of the chair, and turn to seat yourself.
- Shading on the right side of the client indicates the affected side.

a hemiplegic client. Complete shoulder and hip dislocation can occur if the flaccid extremity is not supported properly. Place a pillow between the client's legs to provide support. The client may be able to tolerate lying only for 30 minutes on the affected side because of the impaired circulation or pain.

Collaborative Problem: Risk for Contracture. Normally the brain inhibits spastic muscle contraction. Early in stroke recovery, flaccidity is usually present because of a loss of cerebral connections for afferent sensory and efferent motor nerves. During recovery affected muscles may be spastic because the injured brain cannot inhibit spastic muscle contraction. Therefore the collaborative problem *Risk for Contracture* is due to flaccid paralysis or spasticity.

Outcomes. The nurse will monitor for the development of contractures as evidenced by no muscle shortening and by maintaining normal ROM.

Interventions. Assess the client's ROM in both the involved and noninvolved joints. These findings can be used as a baseline and as an expected outcome.

Perform passive ROM exercises two times daily after the first 24 hours following a stroke unless otherwise prescribed. Motor impulses usually begin to return between 2 and 14 days after a stroke. The affected part (initially flaccid) becomes spastic as the spinal cord motor systems establish their autonomy, and the potential for contractures increases. Passive ROM exercises are more difficult to perform once affected muscles begin to tighten.

Do not force extremities beyond the point of initiating pain or continuous spasm. Always support the joint you are exercising, and move the extremity smoothly, without jerking movements. Frequent passive ROM exercises (1) prevent joint immobility, tendon contractures, and muscle atrophy; (2) stimulate circulation; and (3) help reestablish neuromuscular pathways. Performing these exercises before dressing and undressing the client may facilitate self-care.

Teach the client to use the unaffected hand to lift the weak arm and to put it through ROM exercises. Exercise each finger separately. While in bed, teach the client (1) to exercise the affected arm by grasping it at the wrist with the unaffected hand and raising it above the head and (2) to stretch and rub the fingers of the affected hand several times each day. Active ROM to the unaffected extremities assists in maintaining or increasing muscle strength.

Once some voluntary movement returns, encourage the client with assisted movements. As motor strength increases, resisted movements may strengthen weakened muscles and help restore muscle bulk. Shoulder slings are not recommended because they may increase the risk of contractures.

Several interventions are used to reduce the risk for joint contracture:

- Allow the client to sit upright for short periods only; sitting can contribute to hip and knee flexion deformities.
- When the client is on one side, do not flex the hip acutely.
- Do not place a pillow under the affected knee when the client is supine; this encourages flexion deformity and impedes circulation.
- If the client's knees tend to hyperextend, place a folded towel under the knee for short periods while the client is lying supine.

If the client can tolerate the prone position, place the client in this position for 15 to 30 minutes several times a day, with a small pillow placed under the pelvis (from the umbilicus to the upper third of the thigh) to hyperextend the hip joints.

Prevent footdrop, heel cord shortening, and plantiflexion by (1) avoiding pressure on the feet, (2) performing frequent passive ROM exercises, and (3) having the client sit in a chair as soon as possible with the feet flat on the floor. While the client is in bed, keep the foot flexed at 90 degrees by using high-top tennis shoes or orthotics.

A trochanter roll, extending from the crest of the ilium to mid thigh, prevents external hip rotation by wedging under the projection of the greater trochanter and stopping the femur from rolling. Because trochanter rolls increase the risk of skin impairment, assess the skin beneath the roll often.

When the client is in bed, prevent adduction of the affected shoulder by placing a pillow in the axilla, between the upper arm and the chest wall, to keep the arm abducted about 60 degrees. Keep the arm slightly flexed in a neutral position. Place the forearm on another pillow with the elbow above the shoulder and the wrist above the elbow. This position stretches the shoulder's internal rotators. Elevating the arm also helps to prevent edema and resultant fibrosis.

Place the affected hand in a position of function (i.e., slightly supinated with fingers slightly flexed and the thumb in opposition). Frequent passive ROM exercises are important. The use of splints to prevent flexion contractures is more effective if the splints are designed individually by occupational therapists and scheduled for on-and-off periods to allow for skin assessment and ROM. Squeezing a rubber ball is not recommended because it promotes flexion when extension is desired.

The weight of an immobile arm may cause pain and movement limitation (frozen shoulder) or subluxation of the shoulder joint. Prevent these manifestations by supporting a completely flaccid arm with a pillow when the client is in bed or seated in a chair.

Diagnosis: Self-Care Deficit. Self-care deficits may range from not being able to reach with a weak arm to full dependence on others. This diagnosis is applicable if an achievable outcome can be obtained. Clients with complete paralysis and cognitive deficits may not be able to perform self-care. Other nursing diagnoses may be more applicable, such as *Impaired Physical Mobility* and *Impaired Skin Integrity.* Several nursing diagnoses can be used to describe *Self-Care Deficit,* including *Impaired Physical Mobility, Disturbed Sensory Perception (Visual), Unilateral Neglect,* or *Disturbed Thought Processes.*

Outcomes. The client will perform as many ADL as possible within limitations as evidenced by use of adaptive devices and techniques.

Interventions. Initially a client who has had a stroke may need considerable help with all self-care activities, including washing, eating, and grooming. Encourage clients to perform as many self-care activities as possible and to use the affected arm to avoid the tendency to do everything with the unaffected arm. This activity helps to preserve independent self-care, prevents complications of immobility, and enhances self-esteem.

Remember that stroke clients are easily frustrated and may need a lot of encouragement. Self-care activities provide an excellent opportunity for family teaching. Family members find it difficult to watch a loved one struggle with a task, and they often perform the task for the client. Explain how it benefits the client to be as independent as possible.

In clients with diplopia, an eye patch over one eye removes the second image and promotes better vision. Alternating the patch daily helps to maintain the function and strength of the extraocular muscles in both eyes. Provide mouth care at least three or four times a day, giving special attention to the affected side of the tongue and mouth. Focus rehabilitation plans on self-care deficits and ADL.

Diagnosis: Risk for Injury. The *Risk for Injury* and trauma continues throughout recovery from stroke. It may also extend into the home environment, where clients attempt to perform former activities, such as cooking or driving. Factors that increase the risk for injury include decreased LOC, weakness, flaccidity, spasticity, impulsive behavior, altered thought processes, and motor, visual, and spatial-perceptual impairments.

Outcomes. The client will remain free from injury as evidenced by an absence of abrasions, burns, or falls. The client will also seek needed help to perform tasks that are beyond his or her capabilities.

Interventions. Keep the side rails of the bed raised for clients with recent hemiplegia to protect them from rolling out of bed. As recovery proceeds, the client may pull against side rails when sitting up or turning. Once the client can get out of bed unassisted, half side rails may be more useful. Full side rails hinder ambulation.

A client with impaired sensation is especially prone to injury. Frequent skin inspections for manifestations of injury are essential. Visual disturbances may also increase a hemiplegic client's potential for injury. Weakness on one side makes clients susceptible to falls.

Remind clients to walk slowly, rest adequately between intervals of walking, use effective lighting, and look where they are going. Be especially alert during toileting. Make sure that support staff and family members know not to leave these clients alone in the bathroom. SAFETY ⚠ ALERT

Diagnosis: Imbalanced Nutrition: Less Than Body Requirements. Use the nursing diagnosis *Imbalanced Nutrition: Less Than Body Requirements* if your client has an inability to swallow secondary to stroke. Support the diagnosis with data on intake and output, ability to swallow, caloric intake and weight change over the past 3 days, and levels of hemoglobin, hematocrit, albumin, prealbumin, and lymphocyte count over the past 3 days.

Outcomes. The client will demonstrate manifestations of adequate nutrition as evidenced by (1) maintenance of stable weight; (2) consumption of adequate calories for age, height, and weight; (3) intake equaling output; (4) hemoglobin and hematocrit levels within normal limits for age and gender; (5) lymphocyte count, prealbumin levels, and albumin levels within normal limits; and (6) healing of incisions and wounds within 12 to 14 days, as applicable.

Interventions. Carefully assess the client's diet to ensure adequate nutrition. Assess total intake. Feeding clients with partial paralysis of the tongue, mouth, and throat requires patience and care for prevention of choking and aspiration. Clients often fear choking and are embarrassed and frustrated by eating difficulties. Consequently, they may avoid eating and may not obtain adequate nutrition. Give supplemental meals as necessary. If the client cannot swallow at all, tube-feeding may be used. With help and encouragement, hemiplegic clients can usually learn to feed themselves. Many helpful orthotic devices are available through consultation with an occupational therapist. These might include utensils with built-up handles or scoop plates. Make mealtimes pleasant and unhurried. Serve food attractively and at an appropriate temperature.

Feeding can be very frustrating for a dysphagic client, especially if the caregiver is not familiar with the client's specific disabilities. Support personnel and family members need to be taught basic feeding techniques and also to be informed of each client's individual needs and limitations. To facilitate feeding, assess the following and intervene as necessary. The speech pathologist can recommend additional feeding techniques based on the client's specific deficits and needs.

Promote Head Control. If the client has limited or no voluntary head control, placing a hand on the forehead may help. The caregiver approaches the client from the midline rather than from the side so that the client does not have to turn the head to be fed. Remind the client not to throw the head back to propel food because this can lead to aspiration. The head should be midline and flexed slightly forward.

Assist in Positioning. Have the client in an upright position, as close to 90 degrees as possible, either in bed or in a chair. Support the client's head to counteract hyperextension.

Promote Mouth Opening. If the client does not open the mouth, lightly touch both lips with the tip of a spoon. If this does not work, apply light pressure with a finger to the chin just below the lower lip. Ask the client to open at the same time. Stroking the muscle under the chin (digastric muscle), without crossing the midline, also stimulates mouth opening.

Stimulate Mouth Closing. If a client does not close the lips, swallowing is more difficult. Stimulate lip closure by stroking the lips with a finger or ice or by applying gentle pressure just above the upper lip with your thumb or forefinger.

Help the Client with Swallowing. A dysphagic client must concentrate on swallowing. A quiet environment, free from distractions, is helpful. Feed the client slowly and offer small amounts. Begin feeding the client with foods that require no chewing and are easy to swallow (Table 70-4). Gradually progress to foods that require more chewing and swallowing effort as tolerated. Alternate liquids with solids whenever possible to prevent food from being left in the mouth. Avoid unthickened liquids. Place food in the unaffected side of the mouth. Encourage the client to chew each bite thoroughly. After clients have swallowed, teach them to check for food on the paralyzed side by turning the head to the unaffected side and sweeping the mouth with the tongue.

Diagnosis: Impaired Verbal Communication. The inability to speak is frustrating for clients. Early recognition of this problem decreases some of the frustration in meeting everyday needs. Loss of verbal communication is usually caused by ischemia of the dominant cerebral hemisphere, leading to loss of the function of muscles that produce speech.

Outcomes. The client will be able to communicate effectively, the client's needs will be understood and met, and the client will indicate understanding of the communication of others.

Interventions. Communication involves the dual processes of sending and receiving language. Although either can be affected, the expressive deficit is usually greater than the receptive deficit after initial recovery. Clients may understand more than they can respond to clearly.

Most aphasic clients regain some speech through spontaneous recovery or speech therapy. Speech therapy should be started early. Occasionally residual brain function is not adequate for an aphasic client to relearn the complicated processes of communication. A picture board may be helpful.

TABLE 70–4 Progressive Feeding Program for Clients with Dysphagia

	Stage I	Stage II	Stage III	Stage IV
Description	Severe swallowing difficulty	Chewing and swallowing difficulty with various textures	Less difficulty swallowing, beginning to control foods better in mouth, able to tolerate various food textures and consistencies	Able to swallow most foods very well
Meats	Puréed meat with gravy, baby food, egg yolks	Junior baby food meats with gravy; scrambled, soft, or poached eggs; cottage cheese	Ground meat with gravy, soft meats (tuna) in casseroles, macaroni and cheese, fish without bones, chopped meats	Soft diet
Starch	Mashed potatoes with gravy	Muffins (no seeds), pancakes, French toast, cooked cereal (thick)	Toast (no seeds), rice, soft baked potato	Soft foods
Vegetables	Puréed	Junior vegetables	Peas, squash, cooked carrots; avoid stringy foods (celery, spinach)	Soft foods
Fruits	Puréed	Cooked fruit, ripe banana, soft canned fruit	Grapefruit and orange sections; peeled ripe peaches, pears, and nectarines	Soft foods
Dessert	Custard, pudding	Cakes (no seeds, nuts)	Pies, cakes, sherbet, ice cream	Soft foods
Liquids	None	None	Thick liquids, nectars, strained cream soups, eggnog, liquid caloric supplements, milk shakes	May be able to have thickened liquids

Assessment of dysarthria usually includes examination of the peripheral muscles of speech, tests for specific speech skills, and assessment of the client's functional ability based on the clarity of speech in conversation. Speech therapy is beneficial for many dysarthric clients.

Reinforce the lessons that a speech therapist has initiated. Remember, the client may have a short attention span. Use every encounter to encourage and support communication, and yet be careful not to cause frustration and fatigue. In general, when working with an aphasic client, speak at a slower rate and give the client time to respond. Listen and watch carefully when an aphasic client attempts to communicate. Try hard to understand. This reduces the client's frustration. Anticipate an aphasic client's needs to reduce feelings of communication helplessness.

When a client *cannot identify objects by name,* give the client practice in receiving word images. For example, point to an object and clearly state its name. Then ask the client to repeat the word.

When a client *cannot understand spoken words or has receptive difficulty,* repeat simple directions until they are understood. Do not shout; the client can hear. Speak slowly and clearly. Talk without pressing for a response. Use nonverbal methods of communication to reinforce your words. Stand within 6 feet, and face the client directly. Gradually shift topics of conversation, and tell the client when you are going to change the topic.

When a client has *difficulty with verbal expression,* give the client practice in repeating words after you. Begin with simple words and then progress to simple sentences.

Help the family to communicate with the aphasic client. Act as a role model for such communication by being calm, patient, and gentle. Explain how damaging it can be to the client's self-image if others appear to be embarrassed or amused by the client's attempts to communicate. Likewise, the family should not do all of the speaking for the client.

Always try to put aphasic clients at ease. Reduce the feelings of panic that may occur when they first realize that they cannot communicate as before. The fact that others understand the problem is helpful. Offer calm reassurance. Demonstrate the use of the call light and allow the client to practice. Use gestures and one-step commands.

Collaborative Problem: Risk for Corneal Abrasion. Following stroke, clients may lose their ability to blink. Without a blink reflex, the cornea will dry and become abraded. The collaborative problem is *Risk for Corneal Abrasion.*

Outcomes. Monitor the client for risk factors for the development of corneal abrasion, including the absence of eye closure or blinking and lack of eye moisture.

Interventions. Protect the eye with an eye patch if no blinking is noted. Instill prescribed artificial tears or consult the physician for a prescription if none exists.

Diagnosis: Disturbed Thought Processes. Sometimes it is difficult to make a nursing diagnosis of *Disturbed Thought Processes* unless you spend time with the client. Asking simple or common questions may get fixed, yet correct, answers. Often, after spending a morning with a client, you may note difficulty with thought processing that was not evident on first assessment. Changes in behavior may be caused by alterations in body image, sensation, vision, mobility, and perception. Cerebral edema may also increase confusion.

Outcomes. The client will have improved thought processing as evidenced by recall of information, improved Mini-Mental State Examination scores, decreased agitation, cooperation with interventions, and appropriate responses to questions about recent and past events.

Interventions. Try to prevent disorientation by reorienting the client as LOC improves. Continually reorient a confused client. Glasses and hearing aids assist the client in maintaining awareness of the environment and thus improve thought processes. Activity such as sitting up in a chair for meals or at scheduled times throughout the day also improves LOC and orientation. Position a calendar and a clock where the client can see them. Stroke contributes to altered behavioral patterns, including confusion, memory loss, and emotional lability. To decrease agitation, explain all nursing activities before initiating them. Avoid sensory overload.

Diagnosis: Disturbed Sensory Perception: Visual. Ischemia of visual pathways can lead to altered vision. The client may not notice you when you approach from one side or may not eat food from one side of the food tray. A thorough assessment of visual fields is usually needed for this diagnosis.

Outcomes. The client will successfully compensate for altered visual perceptions as evidenced by safely performing ADL and safely compensating for visual deficit through scanning or other techniques.

Interventions. Approach the client from the side that is not visually impaired. Position the call light and telephone on that side. If possible, position the bed so that the client's side that is not visually impaired is toward the center of the room. Teach clients to position the head to increase the visual field. Warn hemiplegic clients to be careful when crossing streets because they may not see traffic approaching from the affected side. An eye patch over one eye in clients with diplopia removes the second image and assists vision.

A client with perceptual deficits benefits from simplicity. A busy or noisy environment is difficult to interpret and may increase confusion. Reduce complexity and the need for decision-making. The following are examples:

- Obtain clothing that is simply designed and easy to put on.
- Give brief, simple directions.
- Prepare food trays with a minimum number of utensils, dishes, and foods.

Diagnosis: Unilateral Neglect. *Unilateral Neglect* is a pattern of lack of awareness of one side of the body. The client behaves as if that part is simply not there. He or she does not look for the paralyzed limb when moving about. It is caused by damage to portions of the non-dominant cerebral hemisphere. Unilateral neglect creates an increased risk of injury. It is possible to relearn to look for and to move the limb.

Outcomes. The client will be able to compensate for unilateral neglect as evidenced by being free from injury and demonstrating an increased awareness of the neglected body side.

Interventions. Initially adapt the environment to the deficit by focusing on the client's unaffected side. Greet the client as you enter the room, especially if the entrance is toward the neglected side. Keep personal care items and a bedside chair and commode on the unaffected side. Set up the client's food tray toward the unaffected side. Position the client's extremities in correct alignment. Gradually begin to focus the client's attention to the affected side. Move the personal items, bedside chair, and commode to the affected side. Assist the client from the affected side. Have the client groom the affected side first. Cue the client to scan the entire environment and remind the client to keep track of the affected extremities.

Diagnosis: Ineffective Coping. Coping strategies are quite varied among people. Any major illness or change in the body challenges a client's or family's coping skills. This process is particularly true after a stroke because of the physiologic changes and frustrations associated with the resulting deficits. The term *coping* refers to the use of all forms of coping strategies: emotional, cognitive, support systems, and risk appraisal.

Outcomes. The client will develop effective coping strategies as evidenced by appropriate lifestyle modifications, use of the assistance of others, and appropriate social interactions.

Interventions. After a stroke, the client may experience grief over lost mobility, inability to communicate, alterations in sensation and vision, and loss of roles within society. Stroke clients express feelings of profound suffering related to the sudden, devastating changes that accompany stroke. Be understanding and kind. Supportive statements are often helpful, such as "I am sure it's hard for you not to be able to dress alone." The client needs to feel listened to and cared about.

Loss of independence is of particular concern for the stroke client. Care for clients in a way that encourages their independence. Arrange the environment and anticipate needs to reduce frustration. Praise all successes, however small. Break a long-term goal into several short-term goals so that the client can experience successes along the way. For example, a long-term goal may be to walk independently, but short-term goals such as sitting on the side of the bed and ambulating with a quad cane will allow the client to have successes and the long-term goal will seem more attainable. Inappropriate behavior may occur. When necessary, point out the behavior in a matter-of-fact manner and ask the client to stop. Significant others often need help to understand that these behaviors may be caused by damage to the inhibitory centers in the brain or they may be a part of the normal grief response. Provide support by helping the client and family understand this.

Aphasic clients often express their emotional state by irritability and "moodiness." These frustrated clients are often anxious, bewildered, and depressed. Emotional lability may also be present. Accept such behavior in a matter-of-fact but kind manner, without embarrassment. Help families by encouraging short visits by one or two people. If children are allowed to visit, ensure that they are adequately supervised.

Psychosocial Nursing Diagnoses. Various psychosocial nursing diagnoses may be appropriate for clients experiencing stroke, depending on the client and the circumstances. These include *Interrupted Family Processes, Deficient Diversional Activity, Anxiety, Fear, Powerlessness, Situational Low Self-Esteem,* and *Social Isolation.* Shift in spousal roles often occurs. The ways a couple copes will determine how satisfying their lives are after a stroke. Include significant others in the plan of care; let them help care for the client if they wish. Provide them with the information they need to understand the client's condition. Many clients with strokes are in ICUs during the acute phase. The complexity of equipment and activity within an ICU may be frightening to the client and to significant others. Explain carefully what is happening, and provide opportunities for questions and discussion. Give frequent reassurance and support.

Evaluation. Evaluate the degree of outcome attainment on an ongoing basis. After a stroke, some outcomes, such as cerebral perfusion, are achieved early; others, such as self-care deficit, may require long-term rehabilitation. Monitor progress toward outcomes, working with both the client and the family.

Surgical Management

Several criteria are used to identify candidates for rapid evacuation of the hematoma in hemorrhagic stroke. The clients most likely to benefit from surgery are those who are younger than 70 years of age, can open their eyes and follow commands, have elevated ICP (>30 mm Hg), or are rapidly deteriorating neurologically. Clients who have large blood clots removed often can recover a substantial portion of speech. Surgery is usually not performed in clients with bleeding in deep cerebral structures such as the basal ganglia or thalamus.

Most therapies are aimed at reducing increased ICP. Surgery is also performed on some intracranial aneurysms and on the carotid arteries to reduce the risk for stroke.

Modifications for Older Clients

Because stroke affects older people more than it affects others, the nursing care discussed here does not have to be significantly altered for older clients. Older people often have multiple medical problems that must be monitored and treated simultaneously.

Self-Care

Clients who have experienced a stroke often are transferred to a rehabilitation unit after they are medically stable. The client is evaluated for rehabilitation potential, and plans are made for ongoing therapy. The plan of care established during acute care can continue. The major nursing diagnoses and collaborative problems include *Impaired Physical Mobility, Self-Care Deficit, Impaired Verbal Communication, Risk for Contracture, Imbalanced Nutrition: Less Than Body Requirements,* and *Ineffective Coping.*

The following are adjuncts to discharge from rehabilitation settings to home:

- Self-medication
- Use of therapeutic passes
- Rehabilitation home visits

Self-medication means that clients can manage their own medications. Goals are to help the client learn about the medications, including dosage, action, and side effects. Provide a supervised trial to evaluate the client's knowledge and compliance and to enable clients to develop increased responsibility for their own care. A clear and accurate medication chart is helpful.

Therapeutic passes allow the client to return to home or family for short stays. They facilitate discharge planning and improve the transition into the community. Passes help the stroke survivor adjust to the home environment and to practice self-care activities at home, and help the family adjust to living with the stroke survivor and to any alterations in physical, cognitive, and emotional functioning. Clients and family members can practice problem solving and can perform some physical care skills needed after discharge from the facility. Much effort goes into planning for the passes and preparing the client and family. Passes are usually for 8 hours at first and then are increased to a weekend. When the client returns to the facility, the client and family discuss any difficulties they had during the pass interval. Team members intervene with information, retraining, or procurement of needed supplies.

For the *rehabilitation home visit,* team members, including the nurse, social worker, and physical and occupational therapists, visit the client's home.

SAFETY ALERT

The purpose is to evaluate the accessibility of the home and the safety of the home environment based on the client's level of functioning, specifically the client's ability (1) to get in and out of the house; (2) to perform specific tasks in each room; (3) to transfer onto and off of the toilet, bed, and chair; and (4) to move about from room to room. The client's ability to use the telephone and various appliances safely is also evaluated. On the basis of findings from the visit, the team recommends home modifications, further teaching, or adaptive equipment.

The family needs a clear understanding of the client's residual deficits. If spatial or perceptual deficits or unilateral neglect is present, emphasize the need for assistance with ADL and the need for adherence to safety precautions to prevent injury.

Writing lists of tasks or activities may help clients with impaired memory. Reinforce measures to improve mobility and the ability to perform ADL. The client should have a plan for exercises. Equally important, the family and client need to have realistic expectations about the client's abilities so that they can encourage independence when and where the client is able.

Provide written documentation of any anticoagulant schedule as well as a list of warning signs of bleeding. Reinforce the need for caution when the client is using sharp instruments and tools. If appropriate, contact sports must be curtailed while the client is receiving anticoagulants. The INR is closely monitored, and medications are adjusted as needed. The client should be taught to carry Medic-Alert identification.

Provide information about community resources that can assist the client and family with home management and adjustments to residual deficits. These resources include Meals-on-Wheels, the American Stroke Association (a division of the American Heart Association), the National Stroke Association, stroke support groups, social services, local service groups to assist with the purchase of equipment, and individual and family counselors.

At times the stroke client may not be able to tolerate the intensive therapy of a rehabilitation setting, and placement in an extended care facility may be necessary. This is usually very stressful for the client and family, particularly an older spouse. In some cases, care by nurses and allied health professionals in the home may prevent placement in an extended care facility. If both partners are older or in poor health, placement in an extended care facility may be the only option, which can create feelings of guilt and abandonment. Emotional support must be provided to both the client and family members. Education in how to choose a facility and how to monitor care can be helpful.

TRANSIENT ISCHEMIC ATTACKS

Transient ischemic attacks (TIAs) are sudden, brief episodes of neurologic dysfunction caused by temporary, focal cerebral ischemia. Recovery is complete. By definition, a TIA lasts less than 24 hours, and most TIAs last only 5 to 20 minutes. TIAs that last longer than 1 hour are often caused by small infarcts. TIAs often serve as warning signs of an impending stroke, especially in the first few days.

Etiology and Risk Factors

During a TIA, a transient decrease in blood supply to a focal area of the cerebrum or brain stem occurs. Many factors can cause this ischemia. Thromboembolism from ulcerated plaque on the carotid arteries is the most common cause of TIAs, accounting for 80% of cases. Thromboemboli may originate in the vertebrobasilar system. Other sources of emboli include blood clots forming on diseased or prosthetic heart valves, atrial fibrillation, or breakdown of plaque.

Pathophysiology

The pathophysiology of a TIA is similar to that of a stroke. The major differences are the short duration of ischemia and the lack of permanent deficits associated with TIAs.

Clinical Manifestations

Manifestations of TIAs vary, depending on which area of the brain is affected. Common manifestations of a TIA in the carotid artery circulation include a rapid onset of weakness or numbness in an arm or leg, aphasia, and visual-field cuts. Manifestations of a TIA in the vertebrobasilar circulation include two or more of the following: vertigo, diplopia, dysphagia, dysarthria, and ataxia.

Transient ischemic attacks are often recurrent; however, some clients have only one or two episodes before having a complete stroke. TIAs may occur for 1 to 6 years before cerebral infarction, or clusters of TIAs may first appear only a few hours or days before a cerebral infarction. Between episodes, neurologic assessment findings are normal.

The diagnosis of TIA is confirmed by the client's reported clinical manifestations. The causes of the TIA and the potential risk for stroke are diagnosed by the following examinations:

- Auscultation for a carotid bruit
- CT to rule out stroke or other causes of neurologic deficit
- Doppler, computed tomographic angiography (CTA), or magnetic resonance angiography (MRA) studies of the carotid arteries
- Cerebral angiogram
- ECG to assess for atrial fibrillation
- Transthoracic or transesophageal echocardiography (TTE and TEE, respectively) to rule out mural thrombosis and valvular disorders

The results of the noninvasive carotid artery studies, which include the Doppler, CTA, and MRA, determine whether the more invasive cerebral angiogram is performed. The TTE is often performed before the TEE because it is less invasive; however, the TEE may better visualize prosthetic valves and the left atrium.

Conditions that mimic a TIA include intracranial hemorrhage, seizures, hypoglycemia, migraine, and inner ear disorders.

OUTCOME MANAGEMENT

Medical Management

Preventing the progression of a TIA to a stroke is the goal of medical management. Every effort is made to determine the cause of the TIAs. If the TIA is not from the heart or from embolism, the client is placed on antiplatelet therapy. Common agents include aspirin and sustained-release dipyridamole. For clients with persistent or paroxysmal atrial fibrillation, anticoagulation is recommended to maintain an INR of 2.5. Another important medical intervention is to identify and decrease the client's modifiable risk factors for stroke. All smokers should be encouraged to stop smoking. Physical activity of at least 10 minutes of exercise daily should be encouraged. Lowering blood pressure and serum lipid levels is also advised. Diabetic clients should keep fasting blood glucose levels below 126 mg/dl.

Teach the client and family about the manifestations of stroke, risk factors for stroke, and emergency care if a stroke occurs at home. If the client is hospitalized, assess neurologic status frequently for progressive ischemia.

Clients experiencing TIAs are often afraid that they are having a stroke. They need emotional support and education during this stressful time. The diagnostic work-up as well as the manifestations themselves can produce anxiety. Thorough, simple explanations of upcoming events can help. Stress the importance of completing the work-up. Baseline neurologic status must be recorded for postoperative comparison.

Surgical Management

Clients who are considered for surgery are those who have a low risk for postoperative morbidity and mortality and one of the following: (1) asymptomatic carotid artery disease with 50% or greater stenosis or (2) symptomatic carotid artery disease with 70% or greater stenosis. In these clients, the incidence of stroke with surgical management is significantly reduced compared with those with medical management. Clients considered at increased risk for postoperative morbidity and mortality include those with coronary artery disease, pulmonary disease, and moderate to severe stroke on the ipsilateral side. Surgery is usually performed only on stenotic arteries, not on those that are totally occluded. A client may require bilateral endarterectomy. The interval between surgeries is determined by the client's tolerance of the procedure and the likelihood of symptom progression from the remaining stenotic vessel.

Cerebral angiography may be performed before carotid artery surgery to establish the degree of carotid stenosis. The risk for stroke from cerebral angiography is 1% to 3%. Because of the vast improvements in the technology of noninvasive carotid artery studies (carotid ultrasound, carotid duplex, and MRA), these studies may also be used to evaluate stenosis and guide the planning for surgery. Preoperative aspirin is often administered to decrease the formation of embolism at the carotid suture line. If the client is receiving heparin, it is usually stopped on arrival to the operating room.

Carotid Endarterectomy

Carotid endarterectomy is useful in preventing stroke. Carotid endarterectomy is the opening of the carotid artery to remove obstructing and embolizing plaque (Figure 70-5). An incision is made on the anterior border of the sternocleidomastoid muscle. The vessel is clamped, and the plaque or atheroma is removed. Some surgeons use intraoperative electroencephalogram (EEG) and transcranial Doppler monitoring to detect decreased cerebral perfusion while the carotid artery is clamped. In addition, some surgeons shunt blood from below the targeted carotid artery incision to above it to provide a temporary blood supply to the brain. Neurologic status is closely monitored following surgery and the client is usually discharged the following day.

Prognosis. Follow-up Doppler studies are performed at 3 months postoperatively to assess for artery patency

■ **FIGURE 70–5** Carotid endarterectomy. **A,** The common carotid artery is clamped, and an incision is made along the carotid bifurcation. **B,** Plaque is removed. Sometimes portions of the artery are also removed and reconstructed with vein grafts or polyester, such as Dacron. **C,** The artery is sutured closed, and the clamps are removed.

and again at 6 months to 1 year to detect restenosis on the operated side and disease on the nonoperated side. Restenosis may occur in about 1% to 37% of clients after carotid endarterectomy.

Complications. Neurologic complications of carotid endarterectomy include the following:

- Embolization during surgery, causing cerebral vessel occlusion and ischemia
- Thrombosis of the artery at the endarterectomy site, causing cerebral ischemia
- Inadequate cerebral perfusion from intolerance of the temporary artery clamping during surgery

Other Techniques

Recent advances in microcatheter and microballoon technology have led to the investigational use of interventional neurovascular procedures to treat and prevent cerebrovascular disorders. Results of studies of the use of carotid angioplasty and stenting have been promising. The less invasive procedures would treat severe carotid stenosis in a less invasive way than traditional surgery.

Cerebral angioplasty is similar to coronary angioplasty. A balloon catheter is threaded through the arterial system via the femoral artery to the area of carotid stenosis. A small balloon is inflated to dilate the lesion. A stent catheter can also be used to further open the area of stenosis. The U.S. Food and Drug

Administration (FDA) considers both these procedures to be experimental. The complications and complication rate are comparable to those of carotid endarterectomy.

Nursing Management of the Surgical Client

Postoperative care after carotid endarterectomy includes neurologic assessments every 1 to 2 hours. Immediately report indications of deterioration of neurologic status. In addition, several cranial nerves (CNs) are close to the operative site. The function of the following CNs is assessed: facial (VII), vagus (X), spinal accessory (XI), and hypoglossal (XII). CN dysfunction is usually temporary but may last for months. The most common CN damage causes vocal cord paralysis, difficulty managing saliva, or tongue deviation.

Keep the client's head aligned in a straight position to help maintain airway patency and to minimize stress on the operative site. Antiplatelet agents are often administered. The client can lie supine or on the side, as long as the neck is not flexed. Elevate the head of the bed when vital signs are stable. Local applications of cold to the operative site may be prescribed.

Frequently assess the client's breathing pattern, pulse, and blood pressure. Maintain the client's blood pressure within 20 mm Hg of the preoperative normal values. Hypertension or hypotension may lead to hemorrhage, ischemia, or occlusion of the anastomosis. Labile blood pressure is a common postsurgical problem. Baroreceptors located in the lining of the carotid sinus are one of the primary mechanisms of maintaining normotension. Manipulation of the baroreceptors during surgery causes a short-term disruption in blood pressure regulation.

Observe the operative site. Airway obstruction can occur from excessive swelling of the neck or hematoma formation. Bleeding and hemorrhage are a concern because anticoagulation from intraoperative heparin is not yet reversed. Risk factor modification is essential to the long-term success of the surgery and the general health of the client.

🪔 CLIENT AND PUBLIC EDUCATION

The general public has limited knowledge of the manifestations of stroke. In one study, only slightly more than half of the respondents could name at least one stroke manifestation. In addition, only 68% could name a risk factor for stroke. A public education campaign is under way to promote awareness of the manifestations of a stroke. In this campaign, stroke is referred to as a "brain attack" to indicate the need for emergency care with the same intensity as a heart attack. Prompt recognition allows for early treatment of a stroke, which may

---

CLIENT EDUCATION GUIDE

I Am a Stroke

Warning signs are clues your body sends that your brain is not receiving enough oxygen. If you observe one or more of these signs of a stroke or "brain attack," do not wait; call a doctor or 911 right away!

- Sudden numbness or weakness of face, arm, or leg, especially on one side of the body
- Sudden confusion, trouble speaking, or understanding
- Sudden trouble seeing in one or both eyes
- Sudden trouble walking, dizziness, loss of balance or coordination
- Sudden severe headache with no known cause

Other danger signs that may occur include double vision, drowsiness, and nausea or vomiting. Sometimes the warning signs may last only a few moments and then disappear. These brief episodes, known as transient ischemic attacks or TIAs, are sometimes called "mini-strokes." Although brief, they identify an underlying serious condition that is not going away without medical help. Unfortunately, since they clear up, many people ignore them. Do not ignore them! Heeding them can save your life.

Retrieved June 2007 from www.brain attack.org.

---

lessen residual deficits and decrease disability. Recognition and modification of risk factors for stroke, shown in the Client Education Guide above, is the most effective prevention available.

CONCLUSIONS

Stroke is being managed today as a treatable problem if recognized early; however, because of the limited knowledge of the public about early warning signs, many clients still suffer the consequences of stroke. Treatment of the client with stroke is aimed at maximizing function and preventing disability.

THINKING CRITICALLY

1. A 70-year-old man had a left-side stroke 2 days ago. While obtaining his assessment, you note that his blood pressure is elevated at 200 mm Hg systolic; his usual systolic blood pressure is 140 to 160 mm Hg. He is receiving oxygen at 5 L, but his oxygen saturation has dropped from 95% to 88% in the last hour. The client was oriented to person, place, and time an hour ago but has become increasingly restless and slightly confused. The confusion has led him to pull out the nasogastric tube that had been placed for nutritional maintenance. What other neurologic assessments should you do? What is the first priority? Is the suddenness of this change significant?

Factors to Consider. How has the client's assessment changed from baseline values? Is there any relationship between the increased blood pressure and the hypoxia? Is the removal of the nasogastric tube an immediate problem?

2. A 78-year-old woman with a history of hypertension has a stroke. Her family reports that she has felt good and has refused to take her antihypertensive medication. She now has hemiparesis and is able to respond verbally. She does not recognize people or objects in her line of vision on the left side. Three days after her stroke, she is able to move her fingers and wiggle her toes on the affected side, and she is transferred to the rehabilitation unit. What are the most likely rehabilitation goals for this client? How should you proceed with teaching about the complications, motivation to comply with the prescribed therapies, and the importance of antihypertensive medications?

Factors to Consider. What types of rehabilitation will she require? How soon can teaching begin? How will you teach the client and family to provide her care after discharge?

3. A client is seen in the emergency department at 9 AM on Monday morning. His chief complaint is a severe headache. He states, "I am having the worst headache of my life. The pain awakened me around 5 AM and has gotten worse and worse." On examination, the client scores 15 on the Glasgow Coma Scale, complains of nausea, and has a stiff neck. The left-hand grip is slightly weaker than the right-hand grip, and there is a slight pronator drift of the left arm. In addition, there is flattening of the left nasolabial fold. A computed tomography scan of the brain reveals moderate hemorrhage on the right side with increased blood present in the right sylvian fissure. What tests would you expect to be ordered? What complications are important to assess for in this client?

Factors to Consider. What problem is probably in progress? Is the client a surgical candidate, either at the present time or in the future?

evolve   *Discussions for these questions can be found on the website.*

BIBLIOGRAPHY

🔴 Citations appearing in red refer to primary research.

🔵 Citations appearing in blue refer to evidence-based practice guidelines and protocols.

1. Adams, H.P., del Zoppa, G., Alberts, M.J., et al. (2007). Guidelines for the early management of adults with ischemic stroke. *Stroke*, *38*(5), 1655-1711.
2. Ailawadi, G., et al. (2002). Carotid stenosis: Medical and surgical aspects. *Cardiology Clinics*, *20*(4), 599-609.
3. American Heart Association. (2002). *Heart disease and stroke statistics—2003 update*. Dallas, Tex: American Heart Association.
4. Barch, C., et al., and the NINDS rt-PA Stroke Study Group. (1997). Nursing management of acute complications following rt-PA in acute ischemic stroke. *Journal of Neuroscience Nursing*, *29*(6), 367-372.
5. Biller, J., & Love, B.B. (2000). Ischemic cerebrovascular disease. In W.G. Bradley (Ed.), *Neurology in clinical practice: Principles of diagnosis and management* (3rd ed.). Boston: Butterworth-Heinemann.
6. Biller, J., et al. (1998). Guidelines for carotid endarterectomy, a statement for healthcare professionals from a special writing group of the Stroke Council, American Heart Association. *Circulation*, *97*, 501-509.
7. Broderick, J., et al. (1998). The greater Cincinnati/northern Kentucky stroke study: Preliminary first-ever and total incidence rates of stroke among blacks. *Stroke*, *29*(2), 415-421.
8. Caplan, L.R. (1998). 10 most commonly asked questions about stroke. *The Neurologist*, *4*(4), 227-231.
9. Cates, C. (2000). 10 most commonly asked questions about carotid angioplasty and stenting. *The Neurologist*, *6*(1), 58-62.
10. Coombs, U.E. (2007). Spousal caregiving for stroke survivors. *Journal of Neuroscience Nursing*, *39*(2), 112-119.
11. Kase, C.S. (2000). Intracerebral hemorrhage. In W.G. Bradley (Ed.), *Neurology in clinical practice: Principles of diagnosis and management* (3rd ed.). Boston: Butterworth-Heinemann.
12. Kasner, S.E. (2000). Stroke treatment-specific considerations. *Neurologic Clinics*, *8*(2), 399-417.
13. King, R.B., Hartke, R.J., & Denby, F. (2007). Problem-solving early intervention: A pilot study of stroke caregivers. *Rehabilitation Nursing*, *32*(2), 68-76, 84.
14. Hershey, L. (1999). 10 most commonly asked questions about stroke in women. *The Neurologist*, *5*(3), 166-168.
15. Hinkle, J.L. (1998). Biological and behavioral correlates of stroke and depression. *Journal of Neuroscience Nursing*, *30*(1), 25-31.
16. Johnson, S.C., Nguyen-Huynh, M.N., Schwarz, M.E., et al. (2007). *National Stroke Association Guidelines for the Management of TIA*. Accessed June 2007 from Stroke.org.
17. Lee, J., Soeken, K., & Picot, S.J. (2007). A meta-analysis of interventions for informal stroke caregivers. *Western Journal of Nursing Research*, *29*(3), 344-356.
18. Manno, E.M., et al. (1999). The effects of mannitol on cerebral edema after large hemispheric cerebral infarct. *Neurology*, *52*, 583-587.
19. Mayo, N.E., et al. (2000). There's no place like home: An evaluation of early supported discharge for stroke. *Stroke*, *31*(5), 1016-1023.
20. Michael, K.M., & Shaughnessy, M. (2006). Stroke prevention and management in older adults. *Journal of Cardiovascular Nursing*, *21*(5 Suppl), S21-26.
21. National Center for Health Statistics, Centers for Disease Control and Prevention. (2007). *Fast stats A to Z, stroke*. Retrieved June 2007 from www.cdc.gov/nchs/fastats/stroke.htm.
22. National Institute of Neurological Disorders and Stroke rt-PA Stroke Study Group. (1995). Tissue plasminogen activator for acute ischemic stroke. *New England Journal of Medicine*, *333*(24), 1581-1587.
23. Pancioli, A., et al. (1998). Public perception of stroke warning signs and knowledge of potential risk factors. *Journal of the American Medical Association*, *279*(16), 1288-1292.
24. Pilkington, F.B. (1999). A qualitative study of life after stroke. *Journal of Neuroscience Nursing*, *31*(6), 336-347.
25. Post-stroke Rehabilitation Guideline Panel. (1995). *Post-stroke rehabilitation: Assessment, referral and patient management. Quick reference guide for clinicians (Pub No. 95-0663)*. Rockville, Md: U.S. Department of Health and Human Services, Agency for Health Care Policy and Research.
26. Rapp, K., et al., and the NINDS rt-PA Stroke Study Group. (1997). Code stroke: Rapid transport, triage and treatment using rt-PA therapy. *Journal of Neuroscience Nursing*, *29*(6), 361-366.
27. Reynolds, K., et al. (2003). Alcohol consumption and risk of stroke. A meta-analysis. *Journal of the American Medical Association*, *289*(5), 579-588.
28. Siroky, M.B. (2003). Neurological disorders, cerebrovascular disease and parkinsonism. *Urologic Clinics of North America*, *30*(1), 27-47.
29. Smith, G.R., & Mahoney, C. (1995). Coping and marital equilibrium after stroke. *Journal of Neuroscience Nursing*, *27*(2), 83-89.
30. Suarez, J.L., et al. (1999). Predictors of clinical improvement, angiographic recanalization, and intracranial hemorrhage after intra-arterial thrombolysis for acute ischemic stroke. *Stroke*, *30*, 2094-2100.

31. Swanson, R.A. (1999). Intravenous heparin for acute stroke: What can we learn from the megatrials? *Neurology, 52*, 1746-1750.

32. Tanne, D., et al. (2002). Markers of increased risk of intracerebral hemorrhage after intravenous recombinant tissue plasminogen activator therapy for acute ischemic stroke in clinical practice, The Multicenter rt-PA Acute Stroke Survey. *Circulation, 105*, 1679-1685.

33. Testani-Dufour, L., & Marano Morrison, C.A. (1997). Brain attack: Correlative anatomy. *Journal of Neuroscience Nursing, 29*(4), 213-222.

34. Wardlaw, J.M., Zoppo, G., Yamaguchi, T. & Berge, E. (2003). Thrombolysis for acute ischemic stroke. *Cochrane Data Base Systematic Review* (2), CD000213.

35. Williams, L.S., et al. (2002). Effects of admission hyperglycemia on mortality and costs in acute ischemic stroke. *Neurology, 59*, 67-71.

evolve *Did you remember to check out the bonus material on the Evolve website and the CD-ROM, including NCLEX®-Examination Style Review Questions, Open-Book Quizzes, and Chapter Review Audio Podcasts?*

http://evolve.elsevier.com/Black/medsurg

CHAPTER 71

Management of Clients with Peripheral Nervous System Disorders

SHARON R. REDDING

The peripheral nervous system is that portion of the nervous system that exists outside of the brain and spinal cord itself. The peripheral nervous system is made up of three types of nerves:

- Motor nerves (responsible for voluntary movement)
- Sensory nerves (responsible for sensing temperature, pain, touch, and limb positioning)
- Autonomic nerves (responsible for involuntary functions, e.g., breathing, blood pressure, sexual function, digestion)

This chapter addresses problems with the spine and cranial nerves.

LOWER BACK PAIN

Lower back pain is the second most common reason for visits to health care providers (the most common reason being respiratory problems) and because of treatment and lost work hours it results in more health care costs than any other medical condition. The problem of lower back pain is a source of fascination, frustration, and often confusion by clinicians and scientists who attempt to study and treat this problem. The spine is the only organ that consists of bones, joints, ligaments, fatty tissue, multiple layers of muscles, peripheral nerves, sensory ganglia, autonomic ganglia, and the spinal cord. These structures are in turn fed by an intricate system of arteries and veins. Furthermore, the movement of the spine is complex and injury to the spine and other structures leads to unique patterns of pain.

Etiology

The spine is a mechanical organ that has been described as a crane with the ability to support weight, maintain balance, and counter numerous daily strains during normal work and recreational activities. Although it has tremendous ability to withstand most mechanical stresses, it can be stressed beyond its limits. Forces that exceed the capacity of the tissues to stretch can lead to injury and pain.

The origin of back pain is not well-known and has never been fully described. Many groups have given up trying to describe the cause of lower back pain and instead have listed several *red flag* conditions that are associated with the problem. Four groups of problems lead to back pain:

1. *Biomechanical and destructive* origins include compression of the disks, herniation of the disks, torsion injury, and vibration. These problems are seen when clients have occupations that require strenuous or repetitive lifting in a stooped position or jobs that require operating vibrating machinery.
2. *Destructive origins* include infection, tumors, and rheumatoid disorders. These conditions can place pressure on the spinal roots or cord, or alter the structure of the vertebrae.
3. *Degenerative* problems include osteoporosis and spinal stenosis. Osteoporosis can cause collapse of the vertebrae and lead to compression of the nerve roots. The spinal canal can narrow and compress the nerves, a condition called *spinal stenosis*,

evolve **Web Enhancements**

Client Education Guide Lower Back Care (English Version and Spanish Translation)

Home Care After Cervical Laminectomy or Fusion (English Version and Spanish Translation)

Home Care After Carpal Tunnel Release (English Version and Spanish Translation)

Be sure to check out the bonus material on the Evolve website and the CD-ROM, including free self-assessment exercises. **http://evolve.elsevier. com/Black/medsurg**

usually occurring in older people. The severity ranges from entrapment of one nerve root to compression of the entire cord.

4. *Other disorders* include those that have no clear physiologic cause, yet lead to loss of income and pain. There is a growing body of data that show strong psychological influences on the response of clients to lower back pain. The primary determining factors for disability from lower back pain appear to be based on whether the client is depressed, is unhappy in a work setting, or involved in litigation. These psychosocial issues do not negate the presence of real pain. The manner in which the brain processes pain may be implicated. The psychosocial aspects may suppress the serotonergic pathways and limit the secretion of endorphins.

Specific Injuries to the Back

There are many causes of back pain (Figure 71-1). It is important to differentiate those conditions that are non-emergent from those that require surgery.

Back Strain

Back strain is an acute injury leading to lower back pain. Back strain occurs when the client flexes the back without bending the knees or makes rotating movements, creating significant stress on the intervertebral disks and muscles of the lower back.

Disk Herniation

Strenuous activity or degeneration of the disk or vertebrae can permit movement of the disk from its normal location. With aging, changes in disk cartilage and elasticity of the disk may cause the disk to prolapse. Displacement of intervertebral disk material may be referred to as *prolapse, herniation, rupture,* or *extrusion.* Ruptured intervertebral disks may occur at any level of the spine. Lumbar disks are more likely to rupture than cervical disks, because of the force of gravity, continual movement in this region, and improper movements of the spine as with lifting or turning. Thoracic disk disorders are the least common. More than half of people with clinical manifestations of a herniated disk give a history of a previous back injury. Heavy physical labor, strenuous exercise, and weak abdominal and back muscles all increase the risk of herniated disk. Repeated stress progressively weakens the disk, resulting in bulging and herniation.

Spinal Stenosis

Spinal stenosis is narrowing of the spinal canal, nerve root canals or foramen. It is due to excess bone growth from chronic stress on the bone. The excess bone produces pressure on the entire spinal cord. If compression remains untreated, weakness or paralysis of the innervated muscle groups may result.

Lordosis

Lordosis is an excessive backward concavity in the lumbar spine. It is commonly associated with sagging shoulders, medial rotation of the legs, and an exaggerated pelvic angle. Excessive lordosis may result in swayback and kyphosis. Back pain is common.

Spondylolisthesis

Spondylolisthesis is the forward slipping of one vertebra. It commonly occurs at L4–5, where the upper vertebra slips forward out of alignment. Spondylolisthesis is graded from 1 to 4. Grades 1 and 2 are managed conservatively. Grades 3 and 4 usually require surgery for stabilization (Figure 71-2).

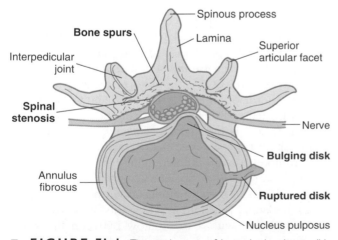

■ **FIGURE 71-1** The usual causes of lower back pain are disk herniation and spinal stenosis.

■ **FIGURE 71-2** Preoperative radiograph of spondylolisthesis. Note the slippage of the vertebrae. *(Courtesy James Manz, MD, Mayo Clinic, Eau Claire, Wis.)*

Spondylolysis

Spondylolysis is structural defect in which repeated microtrauma causes the vertebral arch to slip forward, resulting in stress fractures. The fifth lumbar vertebrae is most commonly involved.

Pathophysiology

Compressive loads have different effects on the intervertebral disk, body of the vertebrae, facets, and spinal ligaments. Under compressive loads, the annular fibers of the disks are stretched. The vertebrae are also compressed and may fracture at the end-plates. Spinal ligaments tend to buckle easily and the facet joints offer little resistance to compression.

The result is that the disk can herniate. When the disk only bulges, the annulus remains intact. With herniation, the annulus is usually torn, allowing extrusion of the nucleus pulposus (Figure 71-3). Compression of spinal nerve roots may result from herniation of the disk. The disks that separate and pad the vertebrae are innervated with fine nerve endings. When the disk impinges on the sciatic nerve, the condition and resulting pain is called *sciatica*. Sciatica is a severe, usually constant pain in the leg that occurs along the course of the sciatic nerve and its branches.

Clinical Manifestations

Rupture or herniation of a lumbar disk leads to lower back pain that radiates down the sciatic nerve into the posterior thigh as a result of compression of the spinal nerve roots. Typically, the pain of sciatica begins in the buttocks and extends down the back of the thigh and leg to the ankle. Disk herniation can result in groin pain. The client frequently has muscle spasms and hyperesthesia (numbness and tingling) in the area of distribution of affected nerve roots. The pain is aggravated by straining (coughing, sneezing, defecation, bending, lifting, and straight-leg raising) or prolonged sitting and is reduced by assuming the side-lying position with the knees flexed. Any movement of the lower extremities that stretches the nerve causes pain and involuntary resistance. Straight-leg raising on the affected side is

■ **FIGURE 71-3** Magnetic resonance imaging of the lumbar spine showing herniation of the disk between L5 and S1.

limited. Complete extension of the leg is not possible when the thigh is flexed on the abdomen (Lasègue's sign). There may be depression of deep tendon reflexes.

Manifestations of spinal stenosis usually begin slowly and are due to pressure placed on nerve roots as they exit the vertebrae. The most common manifestations are aching pain with standing and walking, paresthesias, and heaviness in the legs that progressively worsens with walking. There is rapid improvement in manifestations with trunk flexion, stooping, or sitting. The manifestations of spinal stenosis must be differentiated from claudication.

Diagnostic Findings

Computerized tomography (CT) and magnetic resonance imaging (MRI) scans provide precise images of the spine, disk, spinal cord, and paraspinal tissues (see Figure 71-3). Myelography and diskography are seldom used for initial evaluation.

OUTCOME MANAGEMENT

Medical Management

Goals of medical care include reducing pain and spasms, improving mobility, and repairing any structural problems in the spine or disks. Initial assessment of the client with lower back pain helps pinpoint the cause. The client's medical history is obtained to help determine whether a serious underlying condition is responsible for the pain, such as a fracture, tumor, or infection. The client's psychological and socioeconomic history is obtained, because these problems can complicate both assessment and management. The client is also asked to rate the pain. Physical examination determines whether lumbar nerve roots are involved by testing for reflexes, muscle strength, and the presence of neurologic deficits (Figure 71-4).

Control Pain and Spasms

Initial care of acute lower back pain is directed at managing the client's pain and directing activities. Pain is usually managed with nonsteroidal anti-inflammatory drugs (NSAIDs), COX-2 inhibitors, muscle relaxants, and short-term opioids. Ice has been shown to reduce pain with acute disk herniation for the first 48 hours. After that, heat is usually a better analgesic. A semi-sitting position (in a recliner chair) is usually comfortable and promotes forward lumbar spine flexion, thus reducing back strain. Other positions of comfort include (1) the supine position with pillows under the knees or legs or (2) the lateral position, in which the client lies on the unaffected side with a thin pillow between the knees and with the painful leg flexed to reduce tension on the sciatic nerve. Lying in a prone position and sleeping

Nerve root	L4	L5	S1
Pain			
Numbness			
Motor weakness	Extension of quadriceps	Dorsiflexion of great toe and foot	Plantar flexion of great toe and foot
Screening Exam	Squat and rise	Heel walking	Walking on toes
Reflexes	Knee jerk diminished	None reliable	Ankle jerk diminished

■ **FIGURE 71–4** Assessment of lumbar nerve root compromise includes testing for motor weakness and reflexes, and eliciting pain (screening examination). *(Redrawn from Agency for Health Care Policy and Research. [1994]. Acute low back problems in adults: Assessment and treatment. Quick reference guide for clinicians (No. 14). Rockville, Md: Author.)*

with thick pillows under the head should be avoided. Physical therapists may be able to reduce pain and spasm with stretching exercises, massage, ultrasonic heat treatments, or transcutaneous electrical nerve stimulation (TENS). Work space or environmental modifications may also be necessary. Acupuncture and yoga exercises may be of therapeutic benefit.

For the client with nonspecific lower back pain, manipulation may be used by a physical therapist or chiropractor. *Spinal manipulation* is the use of the hands on the spine to stretch, mobilize, or manipulate the spine and paravertebral tissues. It is usually performed for clients with manifestations of back pain for more than 1 month's duration. There is no evidence that spinal traction with weights is effective in reducing lower back pain. Although unproven, deep ultrasonic heat treatment and moist local heat applications may

help reduce pain. Progressive muscle relaxation exercises, muscle stretching, and other stress reduction techniques can be helpful.

For severe lumbar disk problems with leg pain, conservative intervention involves 2 to 4 days of bed rest on a firm mattress. Bed rest reduces back pain by relieving the back muscles and vertebrae of the stresses. The forces of gravity (e.g., weight of the head with cervical problems) and motion can increase back pain during activity.

Improve Mobility

Activity modifications are prescribed to reduce back irritation and prevent debilitation from inactivity. Most clients do not require bed rest; in fact, more than 4 days of bed rest can be debilitating and slow recovery. The client is taught to minimize the stress of lifting by using good body mechanics, keeping objects close to the body, and to avoid twisting when lifting. Sitting may aggravate leg pain and clients who sit at work should change positions often. Aerobic activities should be prescribed to help avoid debilitation.

Walking, stationary bicycling, and even light jogging can be performed. Exercise should begin within the first 2 weeks after injury and each activity should be performed for 20 to 30 minutes, two or three times a week, for best aerobic conditioning.

Work activities need to be individualized for each client based on his or her job requirements. See the Client Education Guide feature on Lower Back Care on the website.

A back brace or corset is often prescribed for a client with a ruptured lumbar disk. Back supports are usually not recommended once clinical manifestations are relieved, because restricted back motion progressively weakens muscles and causes further degeneration of spinal structures. Strengthening the back and abdominal muscles helps prevent further problems when the exercises are done daily throughout life.

Nursing Care of the Medical Client

Nursing care focuses on assisting the client to adjust his or her lifestyle to reduce the risk of further back injuries. Many clients are frustrated with the lack of cure of their back pain. Clients have become accustomed to having a well-defined cause of a health problem and a well-researched approach for management. Many clients with lower back pain have pain for years without relief. This level of chronic pain can lead to depression and personality changes or relationship difficulties. Nurses should remain sensitive to the exasperation felt by the clients as well as the health care team. Clients reported higher satisfaction with treatment programs for low back pain when they received effective communication regarding treatment plans and care that was given.

Surgical Management

Surgery is indicated for spinal disk problems when (1) sciatica is severe and disabling, (2) manifestations of sciatica persist without improvement or worsen, and (3) physiologic evidence of specific nerve root dysfunction is present. Surgery is also used to stabilize spinal fractures and correct scoliosis and kyphoscoliosis. Some surgeons use other criteria.

Microdiskectomy

Microdiskectomy is the use of microsurgical instruments to remove the herniated fragment of disk. Use of this technique results in less trauma to the surgical site than standard diskectomy and more tissue integrity is preserved. Advantages of microsurgery include (1) minimal nerve root retraction, (2) preservation of an intact joint capsule (no bone is removed), (3) improved hemostasis, and (4) minimal stripping of the muscle and fascia from the spine.

Decompressive Laminectomy

The term *laminectomy* is confusing and is used loosely. The term *laminectomy* means complete removal of the bone between the spinous process and the facet. This much surgical removal is seldom necessary. The more correct term for what is done is *laminotomy,* which is the creation of a hole in the lamina. However, since the term is so common, it is used here.

Decompressive laminectomy is surgical removal of the posterior arch of a vertebra, exposing the spinal cord (Figure 71-5). This gives access to the spinal canal for (1) removing a spinal cord tumor, (2) removing portions of the facets, or (3) decompressing bony infringement on the spinal cord. Sometimes foraminotomy is performed to enlarge the intervertebral foramen if it is narrowed and osteophytic processes (overgrowth of bone) entrap the nerve root and impinge on neural structures.

Artificial Disk Replacement

Recent advances in research have developed replacement disks to provide spinal motion rather than fusion.

Postoperative care is similar to other spinal surgery except that clients are ambulated sooner. Outcomes of ambulation and recreation are positive.

Spinal Fusion/Arthrodesis

Spinal fusion is the placement of bone grafts (bone chips) between vertebrae (Figure 71-6). The new bone that grows fuses the two vertebrae and immobilizes them to reduce the pain. Usually no more than five vertebrae are fused; fusing more than five vertebrae causes considerable loss of movement in the spine. Bone grafts may be obtained from a bone bank or the anterosuperior iliac crest. During healing, the graft gradually grows onto the vertebrae and forms a bony union. This union causes permanent stiffness in the area. After a while, the stiffness is hardly noticed in the lumbar area but is noticeable in the cervical area. The client cannot be guaranteed that back pain will be relieved permanently or that further surgery will not be required.

Spinal Fusion with Instrumentation

Metal rods may be used to straighten and fuse the spine in disorders such as scoliosis or multiple vertebral

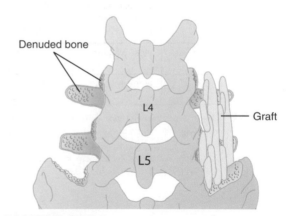

■ **FIGURE 71-6** Lumbar interbody spinal fusion. Bone grafts are taken from the iliac crest and inserted between the vertebrae. In this illustration, the "bed" of raw bone is shown on the left, and the graft material is shown in place on the right.

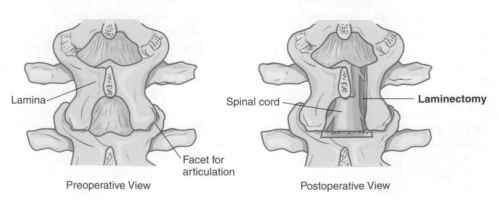

Preoperative View   Postoperative View

■ **FIGURE 71-5** Laminectomy for the interlaminal removal of a herniated disk.

fractures. Orthotic devices and braces can also be used to provide additional support while the bones heal in a fused manner (see Figure 27-4).

Complications

General potential complications following spinal disk surgery at any level include infection and inflammation, injury to nerve roots, dural tears, cauda equina syndrome, and hematoma. Non-union of the surgical area is also a risk and is associated with smoking. Some surgeons assess serum or salivary nicotine levels before surgery to reduce the risk of non-union and validate statements of smoking cessation.

Prognosis

The Agency for Healthcare Research and Quality (AHRQ) reviewed outcomes of surgery for lower back problems.[29] In general, lumbar diskectomy often relieved manifestations of pain in clients with severe and disabling leg pain faster than continued medical management. However, in individuals with no leg pain, there appeared to be little difference in outcome between diskectomy and conservative care. Most clients who had chymopapain injections required eventual diskectomy for permanent pain relief. More research is needed to determine who is best served by the various techniques; client preference also plays a big role in the technique chosen.

Nursing Management of the Surgical Client

The nursing care of clients having spinal surgery is shown in the Care Plan. (See Care Plan titled Management of the Client Undergoing Spinal Surgery, pp. 1878-1880.) Before surgery, encourage the client to become actively involved in their own care

Assessment. Following spinal surgery, assessment is similar to that performed for other surgical clients beginning with a head-to-toe assessment and evaluation of current pain level including response to analgesia. Assess neurologic function by asking the client to move his or her legs and comparing the results with those of the baseline evaluation. Question the client about the presence of numbness or tingling and changes in sensation or pain. New paresthesias may be a consequence of the edema from the surgery and the surgeon should be notified of them. If progressive weakness or paralysis of the lower extremities, loss of sphincter control, anal numbness, or urinary retention (called the *cauda equina syndrome*) occurs, notify the surgeon immediately. Emergency surgical decompression may be required.

Assess the wound for bulging or clear drainage, which may indicate cerebrospinal fluid (CSF) leakage. If the client had an anterior approach for surgery, usual care following abdominal surgery is required (e.g., assessment for atelectasis and ileus). Dressings and drains are checked, including those at the donor site. Blood salvage during surgery is common and the client may return to the nursing unit with blood salvage equipment connected to incisional drains. Follow agency protocol and equipment guidelines to collect, filter, and reinfuse the client's salvaged blood.

Immediately following lumbar diskectomy, the client typically is not turned for an hour or so but remains flat to aid hemostasis. Begin side-to-side logrolling and repeat every 2 hours. If a dural tear was repaired, the surgeon may order the client to remain flat longer to minimize the risk of spinal headache, CSF leak, or a tear in the dural sutures.

After lumbar fusion, the bed is generally kept flat. The client logrolls from side to side, usually beginning about 4 hours after surgery and then every 2 to 4 hours thereafter; initially, extra assistance may be necessary (Figure 71-7, A-C on p. 1881). Spinal bone grafts are delicate and heal slowly. Eventually, turning is permitted without help, while keeping the spine rigid. Keep the bed linens loose at the foot of the bed to promote independent movement. If the client requires assistance to turn, or when turning to place a bedpan, turn the client in the logrolling manner. A fracture bedpan is used to reduce back arching and strain. Use of a trapeze over the bed is contraindicated because it promotes twisting. Usually the client is assisted to a chair the morning following surgery. Be sure to follow the physician's activity prescriptions.

Clients who have had fusions are on bed rest longer and thus are at greater risk for deep vein thrombosis (DVT). Compression devices on the legs may be used to improve venous return. Continuous compression stockings may be used, and the client is encouraged to move his or her legs and feet while on bed rest to promote venous return. If a client is supine following spinal surgery (e.g., using a bedpan), the lower back muscles may be relaxed somewhat if pillows are placed under the entire length of the legs. This may also prevent thrombophlebitis in the femoral vessels. Do not flex the client's knees by placing anything under the popliteal space, because the flexion increases the risk of DVT. Observe for and report any manifestations of DVT: redness or swelling in the one leg, Homans' sign (not a very specific sign, however), or sudden chest pain, dyspnea, and anxiety, which may indicate a pulmonary embolism.

After spinal surgery, a brace or corset may be required temporarily to support the spine. Clients who have lumbar or thoracic spinal fusions wear a fiberglass brace, which resembles a shell. Initially, back braces or corsets may be worn constantly, whether the client is in or out of bed. As the client's muscles strengthen, the use of braces or corsets is usually decreased. Again, follow the physician's activity prescriptions. Casts may be used for a while following any thoracic spinal surgery for clients with unstable thoracic spines (e.g., thoracic spinal cord trauma).

Management of the Client Undergoing Spinal Surgery

Nursing Diagnosis: Deficient knowledge related to client and family understanding of the preoperative, operative, and postoperative phases of spinal surgery.

Outcomes: Client and family will be able to explain the surgical procedure, preoperative preparations, and the postoperative precautions and needs. The client will demonstrate safe mobility, including logrolling, and transfer to and from the bed.

NOC OUTCOMES   Knowledge: Treatment Regimen

Interventions	NIC INTERVENTIONS	Rationales

1. Obtain baseline neurologic assessment:
  a. Motor and sensory function
  b. Psychological readiness
	Neurologic Monitoring	1. Establishes baseline motor and sensory function for later comparisons
		Determines level of ability and knowledge.

2. Explain logrolling.	Teaching: Preoperative	2. Protects back and enhances mobility.
3. Discuss activity limitations and avoidance of straining.	Teaching: Preoperative	3. Prevents damage (flexion, extension, twisting) to surgical site.
4. Explain need to seek assistance with ADL.	Teaching: Preoperative	4. Avoid stretching when reaching.
5. Explain use of stool softeners.	Teaching: Preoperative	5. Minimize straining with bowel movements.
6. Explain reason for non-ambulation.	Teaching: Preoperative	6. Clients with recent injury may exacerbate condition.
7. Encourage clients who smoke to stop smoking.	Teaching: Preoperative	7. Increases cardiovascular complications, risk of poor wound healing, and non-union if fusion is performed.
8. Evaluate for autologous blood donation.	Surgical Precautions	8. Two or three units should be donated at least 1 week before surgery. Older adults may require more time.
9. Review care of bone autograft donor site and pain management.	Teaching: Preoperative	9. Prepares client for additional pain.

10. Discuss changes in home environment:
  a. Bathroom facilities
  b. Shower/toilet use
  c. Ambulation devices
  d. Seat rises/grab bars
	Teaching: Preoperative	10. Anticipate home care needs.

Evaluation: Client and family will be knowledgeable of upcoming surgical procedure, understand postoperative nursing care, and have fears and concerns allayed. If questions arise about the operation, ask the surgeon to answer them. Do not attempt to provide information outside of your area of expertise.

Nursing Diagnosis: Fear and anxiety related to postoperative problems such as paralysis and chronic pain.

Outcomes: Client and family will express low level of fear or anxiety related to upcoming surgery and will use positive coping strategies to decrease fear or anxiety.

NOC OUTCOMES   Fear Level, Anxiety Level

Interventions	NIC INTERVENTIONS	Rationales
1. Encourage client and family to express fears and concerns.	Emotional Support	1. Allays concerns and fears.

Evaluation: Client and family will express fears and concerns, thus reducing anxiety level and improving compliance with surgical treatment regimen. For example, clients need to be aware that some edema is expected at the surgical site and therefore some of the preoperative deficit may still exist after surgery, but the client's condition should improve as the edema lessens.

Nursing Diagnosis: Acute Pain related to tissue trauma secondary to back (and/or abdominal) incision.

Outcomes: The client will express comfort, for example, a low level of tolerable pain, such as a 3 on a pain scale of 0 to 10.

NOC OUTCOMES   Pain Level

Interventions	NIC INTERVENTIONS	Rationales

1. Monitor pain:
  a. Incisional
  b. In extremity
	Pain Management	1. Incisional pain is expected, and leg pain is often significantly less after herniated disk surgery.

2. Administer pain medications:
  a. Basal (continuous) dose of opioid via IV pump and/or patient-controlled analgesia (PCA)
  b. PO
	Pain Management	2. Provide for client comfort. Provide PCA assistance. Avoid breakthrough pain. Combination strategy may be more effective.

Interventions	NIC INTERVENTIONS	Rationales
3. Teach client to ask for PO pain med before pain is too great.	Pain Management	3. Provide for client comfort.
4. Monitor epidural catheter for basal dose of analgesic.	Pain Management	4. Catheter to be maintained in position.
5. Avoid low-molecular-weight heparin injections.	Medication Safety	5. LMWH injections are associated with epidural hematoma when epidural catheters are in place.
6. Apply ice bag to incision using abdominal wrap to lumbar area and to bone graft donor site.	Pain Management: Cold Application	6. Provide for client comfort.

Evaluation: The client may have immediate relief from pain as many surgeons inject long-acting local anesthetics into disk spaces during surgery. This promotes a positive attitude toward the outcome of surgery. Often the pain recurs on the second postoperative day. This is due to both the increase in swelling and the fact that the local anesthetic is wearing off.

Nursing Diagnosis: Impaired Physical Mobility related to pain, leg weakness, prolonged immobility, or fear of pain and spasms. Choose the etiology that best fits your client.

Outcomes: The client will resume a maximal level of progressive activity, starting with logrolling on the day of surgery, progressing to independent movement from the bed to a standing position, followed by independent ambulation before discharge.

NOC OUTCOMES   Immobility Consequences: Physiologic, Mobility

Interventions	NIC INTERVENTIONS	Rationales
1. Use transfer device and ample people to assist with initial transfer to bed from surgery.	Body Mechanics Promotion	1. Support spine and maintain alignment. Transfer is smooth and gentle. Ensure safety.
2. Begin side-to-side logrolling every 2-4 hours; use extra help in turning.	Body Mechanics Promotion	2. Support spine and maintain alignment. Avoid twisting spine and hips. Ensure safety.
3. Administer analgesics before moving.	Pain Management	3. Lessens discomfort caused by spasms and pain with movement.
4. Tilt client back onto pillows; flex upper leg and place pillow between legs; place pillow to support upper arm; splint abdominal incision.	Body Mechanics Promotion Pain Management	4. Reduces pressure on donor site (iliac crest); keeps spine straight; prevents upper shoulder from sagging; reduces incisional pain.
5. Elevate head of bed as ordered.	Body Mechanics Promotion	5. Provides for client comfort and facilitates breathing and digestion.
6. Use pressure-redistribution mattress.	Pressure Management	6. Reduces risk of pressure ulcers.
7. Keep call light and PCA control so client can access them.	Body Mechanics Promotion	7. Avoid straining and twisting.
8. Instruct client about contraindicated positions and activities.	Body Mechanics Promotion	8. Avoid straining and twisting.
9. Assist client into chair; keep bed flat; have client roll onto side (see Fig. 71-7); have client then push torso from bed with arms to rise from the bed.	Body Mechanics Promotion	9. Lessen strain on spine. Client may already be familiar with technique.
10. Anticipate spasms with turning and rising from the bed. Teach client to relax, deep breathe through spasm. Consider antispasmodics if prolonged or impaired movement.	Body Mechanics Promotion	10. Spasms are common with movement. Most spasms are transient. Prolonged or intense spasm will impair mobility.

Evaluation: Clients who have spinal surgery will have varying degrees of mobility limitations. Return to activity may depend upon the client's ability to manage pain, the extent of proper bone healing, muscle strength, and the use of proper body mechanics. Spasm control following surgery may be needed for some clients.

Nursing Diagnosis: Impaired Urinary Elimination related to pain and spasms with movement, inability to void in a supine position, and side effects from opioids.

Outcomes: The client will resume normal bladder emptying by the time the client is ambulating.

NOC OUTCOMES   Urinary Continence

Interventions	NIC INTERVENTIONS	Rationales
1. Assess for bladder distention and pain 8 hours after surgery.	Urinary Elimination Management	1. Urine is manufactured continuously by functional kidneys, even though the client has been NPO.
2. Try noninvasive methods to assist client to void	Urinary Elimination Management	2. Urinary catheterization increases the risk of urinary tract infection. Noninvasive measures do not carry this risk.

(Continued)

C A R E   P L A N   *evolve*

Management of the Client Undergoing Spinal Surgery—Cont'd

3. Straight catheterization is usually done twice.	Urinary Elimination Management	3. Straight catheterization empties the bladder, allowing time for resumption of normal voiding sensations.
4. Indwelling catheter is inserted if client still cannot void.	Urinary Elimination Management	4. Bladder or prostate problems may be present, preventing the client from voiding normally.
5. Maintain indwelling catheter until client is ambulating and using less pain medication.	Urinary Elimination Management	5. Pain and decreased activity hinder bladder function.
6. Assist client to urinate when standing or sitting.	Urinary Elimination Management	6. Lying supine can hinder sphincter function.
7. Straight catheterization is done to check for residual urine, if ordered.	Urinary Elimination Management	7. Promotes return of normal bladder function and prevents urinary tract infection.

Evaluation: Urinary retention occurs when the cauda equina is affected. Normal bladder function is dependent upon adequate pain management and resumption of ambulation and ADL.

Collaborative Problem: Risk for Paralytic Ileus is a common bowel problem after laminectomy and spinal fusion. Loss of bowel sounds and abdominal distention is due to lack of peristalsis from a sudden loss of parasympathetic function innervating the bowels and manipulation of the intestines in anterior approaches to spinal surgery.

Outcomes: The nurse will assess the client for return of normal bowel function, including normal bowel sound patterns, and evacuation without straining, by the time he or she is ambulating. This problem is expressed as a collaborative problem; therefore the outcome is written in terms of the nurse's actions. The nurse's actions cannot independently alter the outcome, as occurs with nursing diagnoses.

NOC OUTCOMES	Bowel Continence

Interventions	NIC INTERVENTIONS	Rationales
1. Assess abdominal status every 4 hours.	Bowel Management	1. Common findings include anorexia, nausea, vomiting, hard and possibly distended or tympanic abdomen, absence of bowel sounds.
2. Insert and maintain nasogastric tube to low intermittent suction.	Bowel Management	2. Reduce gastric distention and/or prevent paralytic ileus.
3. Maintain NPO status.	Bowel Management	3. Reduce gastric secretions.
4. Provide oral hygiene every 2 hours.	Oral Health Maintenance	4. Oral mucosa dries quickly when the client is NPO.
5. Resume clear liquid diet; advance diet as tolerated, when ordered.	Bowel Management	5. Hunger, bowel movement, or passing flatus indicates return of bowel function.
6. Encourage client to sit to defecate.	Bowel Management	6. Clients find it difficult or impossible to defecate when flat.

Evaluation: Expect bowel function to return within 12 to 24 hours after surgery; however, it may be longer if the client requires potent opioids. Return of hunger and reduced anorexia and nausea are the earliest signs that peristalsis has resumed. Ambulation is helpful in resuming peristalsis. The client should be able to eat before discharge.

Ileus is common for several days postoperatively. Inactivity and the use of opioid analgesia slow peristalsis. Fluids are forced as ordered; a regular time for bowel movements and bowel care is encouraged; fiber is provided in the diet (when allowed), and prescribed medications (e.g., stool softeners, mild bulk laxatives, or a suppository) and enemas are administered. Instruct the client not to strain for a bowel movement, because this increases pain and CSF pressure. Bowel movements are documented.

Disk problems often create fears and concerns related to pain, treatments, sexual activity, possible length of illness, and possible lifestyle changes. Provide psychosocial support to the client and family. Impaired mobility and altered urinary or bowel elimination are also common problems experienced after disk surgery. Smoking cessation is imperative because smoking delays the healing of bone. Considerations about employment and finances should be referred to a social worker.

Self-Care

Approximately 80% of the population experience lower back pain at some point in their lives. It is estimated that 10% of those who seek medical attention for back pain have herniated disks. Because of the frequency of herniated disk problems, health promotion is an essential activity for health care providers. See the Client Education Guide feature Lower Back Care on the website.   *evolve*

■ **FIGURE 71–7** Helping the client stand after lumbar fusion. **A,** Logroll the client to the edge of the bed using a turning sheet if needed. Leave the bed in that position. **B,** The client pushes off the bed with the hand and the other elbow to sit up without twisting. The client drops his or her legs off the side of the bed at the same time. **C,** With the client seated on the edge of the bed, the nurse assesses for orthostatic hypotension. The client stands from the bed without flexing the back.

CERVICAL DISK DISORDERS

Disks may become entrapped in the cervical spine. The process is much like that with herniated lumbar disks. Manifestations include arm pain, neck pain and spasms, and loss of function (grip strength) and changes in sensation in the hands.

OUTCOME MANAGEMENT

Initial treatment is with NSAIDs, muscle stretching, and teaching proper body mechanics. Opinions differ concerning the advisability of performing head and neck range-of-motion exercises in the presence of significant cervical disease. Tell the client to avoid activities that increase cervical disk pain. To prevent neck extension when in bed, only one flat pillow (to prevent neck flexion) is recommended. The neck should not be hyperextended. Intermittent traction may be applied for cervical disk herniation (5- to 8-lb weight) to reduce pain. The head of the bed may be slightly elevated with cervical traction. Otherwise, it is best kept flat when cervical pain is present.

A review of posture at work is important for clients who work at computer terminals. Keyboards, screens, and written materials should be kept at a height that reduces strain on the neck and shoulders. Stretching routinely also allows muscles to relax.

A soft cervical collar may be prescribed for mild to moderate cervical disk problems to keep the head slightly flexed. After fracture of a cervical vertebra, cervical disk rupture, or whiplash injury, the client may wear a neck brace (fitted so the chin rests on a cup and the neck is kept hyperextended), a hard collar (which extends up under the chin and prevents flexion of the neck), or a soft collar. Neck braces tend to limit vision, because people wearing them cannot look down at their feet.

> **Implement safety precautions when clients wear neck braces. Vision is impaired because they cannot turn the head or look down. Teach the client to climb stairs using a handrail.**

SAFETY
⚠
ALERT

Surgical Management

Sometimes conservative treatment does not work and clients require surgery. Surgery to stabilize bone fragments is necessary when a neck injury involves a bone fracture. Cervical fusion is most commonly performed through an anterior approach, so the incision will be on the front of the neck. Immediately after a posterior cervical diskectomy, a cervical collar is worn (Figure 71-8). A hard cervical collar is usually prescribed following fusion.

Treat any reports of nausea after cervical fusion. Vomiting can lead to aspiration because of difficulty in clearing the airway and not being able to turn the head or flex the neck.

Complications after posterior cervical surgery include soft tissue hematoma, air embolism, and subcutaneous wound dehiscence. Complications following anterior cervical surgeries include laryngeal nerve damage and injury to neck structures such as the carotid arteries, trachea, esophagus, and soft tissue.

After microdiskectomy, the client may have the head of the bed elevated to whatever position is comfortable. Following cervical spine fusion, the surgeon indicates

■ **FIGURE 71–8**   A cervical collar with a chin piece. This orthosis provides additional support for the head and some restriction of cervical spine motion. (Courtesy Zimmer, Inc., Dover, Ohio.)

the degree of head elevation for comfort and to reduce edema. Make sure the spine is in anatomic alignment by keeping the head placed in neutral alignment. The client's head may be elevated and a folded small towel, bath blanket, or small pillow is placed under the head to maintain spinal alignment while the client lies supine or on the side.

Assess and document the client's neurologic status frequently.

SAFETY

⚠

ALERT

The development or worsening of a neurologic deficit must be promptly reported to the surgeon. During the first 24 hours after an anterior cervical diskectomy, assess the client's ability to breathe, check the operative site for excessive swelling, and changes in the client's voice. Laryngeal nerve damage during surgery may cause permanent vocal impairment, such as hoarseness. Watch for indications of respiratory paralysis resulting from spinal cord edema. Emergency tracheostomy equipment is kept at hand. If a spinal fusion was performed with the anterior cervical diskectomy, the surgeon is notified if upper extremity pain suddenly recurs. This could mean that the bone graft has moved out of place and surgery needs to be repeated.

Also assess the client for indications of postoperative improvement such as absence of paresthesias.

Tell the client that it is not unusual for preoperative manifestations to persist for a few days secondary to edema at the operative site, although these manifestations are usually less uncomfortable. Difficulty

swallowing and throat discomfort are usually present for several days and are commonly a result of local irritation from the endotracheal tube. A soft diet, throat lozenges, humidified air, minimal talking, and other comfort measures lessen the discomfort.

A wound drain may be present and is usually removed by the surgeon on the second postoperative day, after drainage has decreased. Bladder and bowel management are the same as for clients after lumbar surgery. Cervical surgery may affect the parasympathetic chain, causing urinary retention.

Self-Care

With shorter postoperative hospital stays, most clients are discharged before suture or staple removal. Instruction for care of the incision includes keeping the sutures or staples clean and dry and noting any increased redness or drainage from the wound. Clients need clear instructions on walking, lifting, driving, and returning to work. Most clients can resume regular activity 6 weeks after surgery. Specific physician instructions need to be followed.

Prolonged sitting or standing in one position strains the healing back. Contraindicated activities vary. The client is instructed to ask the surgeon when it will be safe to perform activities that could damage the back (climbing stairs, lifting a weight greater than 5 lb, prolonged travel, sexual activity, sports, exercise, and driving a car). Clients must not smoke. Smoking reduces blood supply to the tissues and delays healing. See the Client Education Guide feature on Home Care After Cervical Laminectomy or Fusion on the website.

POST-POLIO SYNDROME

Poliomyelitis is an acute form of paralysis characterized by destruction of motor cells in the spinal cord and brain stem. The disease has been controlled since the 1950s when mass immunization was used. However, post-polio syndrome can develop in polio survivors 30 years after the original disease. No form of prevention of post-polio syndrome has been identified.

Post-polio syndrome is a new onset of progressive weakness, fatigue, decreased temperature tolerance, emotional distress, dysphagia, pain in the joints and muscles, and respiratory problems. The onset is insidious, and weakness occasionally extends to muscles that were not involved during the initial illness. The prognosis is generally good; progression to further weakness is usually slow, with plateau periods that range from 1 to 10 years. The syndrome is thought to be due to progressive dysfunction and loss of motor neurons that compensated for the neurons lost during the original infection and not to persistent or reactivated poliovirus infection.

Management of post-polio syndrome has three components: energy conservation and lifestyle modification, medications, and measures to promote quality of life. Energy conservation includes pacing of activities, making the environment more ergonomic, sitting rather than standing, and use of electric mobility. Assistive devices to correct and minimize postural and gait abnormalities (e.g., canes, crutches, walkers) and braces designed to provide support to weakened muscles and joints can reduce pain, improve safety, and enhance energy conservation; they also help clients reduce fatigue, avoid overuse, and recover faster after activity. Occupational therapists can help clients assess their lifestyles and design appropriate changes. Despite the benefits of assistive devices, many polio survivors are reluctant to use them. They remember the intense rehabilitation efforts during their childhood and how they were encouraged to become independent and "like everyone else" again. It is important for a knowledgeable orthotist to fully explain the advantages of assistive devices and discuss the newer designs and materials.

Polio survivors may have also been instructed not to exercise, in order to avoid activity-induced muscle pain and "save" what muscle strength they have. This advice results in declining strength as a result of muscle deconditioning and increased long-term risk of cardiac deconditioning. Currently, several studies have demonstrated both the safety and the efficacy of nonfatiguing exercise for polio survivors. Progressive resistive strength training with reduced repetitive motion (e.g., 3 sets of 4 to 10 repetitions) done every other day demonstrated significant increases in static and dynamic strength without manifestations of injury or worsening manifestations.

Medications are used to reduce fatigue. Pyridostigmine (Mestinon) is commonly prescribed, but side effects of increased muscle twitching, nausea, diarrhea, and frequency are common. The weakness is treated with strengthening exercises, steroids to reduce inflammation, and electrical stimulation. Other manifestations are also treated symptomatically.

Symptomatic treatment of pain is important for optimizing both functional ability and quality of life. Polio survivors with pain can benefit from a multidisciplinary approach to pain management, which may include medication. The cause of the pain determines the choice of drug used to treat it. Primary post-polio muscle pain may have features of neuropathic pain. Additionally, primary neuropathic pain from nerve compression may be present. Neuropathic pain responds to NSAIDs, topical capsaicin, lidocaine (Xylocaine) preparations, and membrane-stabilizing agents. Biomechanical pain can be treated with steroids (oral or injectable), NSAIDs, or muscle relaxants, as well as with rehabilitation techniques, topical cold or heat, TENS, and relaxation/biofeedback. Overuse pain and cramps should not be

casually medicated, because they are signs that changes in lifestyle and body mechanics are overdue.

Quality of life can be affected when post-polio syndrome develops in clients who have successfully adapted to their disease and disability. Respiratory distress may bring back memories of the initial infection and treatment in an iron lung (a very early form of a respirator in which the client's entire body was placed in a large metal cylinder).

Perceived barriers to health that furthered disablement in polio survivors have included fatigue, lack of money and time, lack of convenient resources, and lack of supportive health care providers. Additional restrictions are difficult to accept. Emotional support is vital. Teach the client to balance rest and activity.

SPINAL CORD DISORDERS

SPINAL TUMORS

Spinal tumors are similar in nature and origin to intracranial tumors but occur much less often. They are most common in young or middle-age adults and most often involve the thoracic region. Spinal tumors may occur outside of the spinal cord, such as in the meninges, nerve roots, or vertebrae (extramedullary), or within the substance of the spinal cord (intramedullary). Neurofibromas and meningiomas are the most common spinal cord tumors. Both are benign and operable and may not produce permanent damage if removed early.

Clinical manifestations of spinal tumors vary according to their location. Extramedullary tumors cause manifestations by compressing the spinal cord or some of its nerve roots or by occluding blood vessels supplying the cord. Early characteristics of spinal cord compression include pain, sensory loss, muscle weakness, and muscle wasting. Progressive cord compression is manifested by spastic weakness below the level of the lesion, decreased sensation, and increased reflexes. Severe cord compression at the cervical level destroys cord function and produces quadriplegia; compression at the thoracic or lumbar level results in paraplegia.

Intramedullary tumors produce more variable clinical manifestations. High cervical cord involvement causes spastic quadriplegia and sensory changes. Tumors in descending areas of the spinal cord produce motor and sensory changes appropriate to functions at that level.

Medical diagnosis is made after a complete general neurologic examination. Diagnostic testing includes CT scan or MRI scan.

Intervention for spinal tumors is usually surgery, radiation therapy, or both. Immediate surgery is indicated if compression of the cord or nerve roots is evident. Often, surgery results in marked improvement or even complete restoration of function, especially when the tumor is benign and encapsulated (e.g., meningioma or lipoma). However, functional improvement is less common when cord necrosis has developed. Complete surgical removal of an intramedullary tumor is rare. However, partial resection followed by radiation may improve the client's condition. Usually the course of the condition is gradually progressive.

SYRINGOMYELIA

Syringomyelia is often associated with Arnold-Chiari malformation (an abnormal protrusion of the medulla into the spinal canal) or spina bifida. Syringomyelia consists of abnormal cavities filled with dense, glue-like tissue in the spinal cord substance, especially the cervical cord. Scar tissue surrounds the cysts. Syringomyelia is characterized by (1) muscular weakness and wasting, (2) sensory defects, and (3) indications of injury to the long tracts of the spinal cord, such as hyperreflexia.

Early manifestations of cervical syringomyelia often include the following:

- Atrophy, weakness, and fibrillations of the small muscles of the hands
- Loss of pain sensation in the fingers or forearms
- Weakness and atrophy of the shoulder girdle muscles
- Horner syndrome, which is characterized by ptosis (droop) of the upper eyelid, constriction of the pupil, anhidrosis (absence of sweating), and flushing of the affected side of the face
- Nystagmus
- Vasomotor and trophic disturbances of the upper extremities

Although there is segmental loss or impairment of pain and temperature sensation, sensation for light touch remains. Segments of sensory loss may be separated by zones of normal sensation. Spasticity, ataxia, or paralysis of the lower extremities may occur, as may disturbed bladder control, if the lumbosacral region of the spinal cord is involved.

Cranial nerve involvement may produce additional problems such as impairment of facial pain and temperature sensation, loss of the corneal reflex (necessitating protection of the eye), dysphagia, dysarthria, laryngeal stridor (possibly necessitating tracheostomy), nystagmus, and atrophy and fibrillation of the tongue muscles.

Syringomyelia may progress rapidly at first and then become quiescent for many years. Some clients live 40 years after onset. Others become incapacitated (from paralysis or sensory defects) or die within a few years.

Treatment includes relieving increased pressure on the cord from the fluid content of the cavities within the spinal canal. The fluid buildup can be removed and CSF outflow restored by direct surgical drainage or by shunt placement.

NEUROSYPHILIS

Neurosyphilis is a chronic or late stage of syphilis involving infection of the brain or spinal cord. The oculomotor nerves may be affected, leading to an inability of the pupil to react to light, called an Argyll Robertson pupil. The posterior columns and nerve roots of the spinal cord may be affected, which is called *tabes dorsalis*. Because these are sensory nerves, the most common manifestation is pain. The pain can occur almost anywhere in the body, although abdominal pain is most common. The pain is severe enough to be confused with gastric ulcers and gallbladder disease. In addition to pain, areas of paresthesias may be noted. A common finding in tabes dorsalis is the loss of position sense in the feet and legs. As a result, clients walk with a slapping step. They are at increased risk of falls when walking in the dark because they must rely on visual cues for placement of their feet with each step. In addition, because the gait is abnormal, bone alignment with walking is altered. Eventually the foot is abnormally shaped (called *Charcot's joint*). This alteration in foot structure can lead to foot ulcerations, because the client bears the body weight on abnormal areas. The brain can also be involved in later stages of syphilis. A general deterioration of mental status can develop.

With improved case finding and the use of penicillin to treat syphilis in its early stages, the management of syphilis is improving. However, with development of resistant strains of organisms and a recent increase in the incidence of sexually transmitted diseases, problems may recur in the future.

UPPER/LOWER MOTOR NEURON LESIONS

Any lesion that destroys the UMNs initially results in contralateral paralysis, such as is seen with stroke. Initially, the involved area is flaccid and hyporeflexic. The flaccidity gradually recedes, and the reflex arc becomes hyperactive because of the lack of inhibition by the UMNs. Muscle tone is hypertonic and the extremity becomes spastic. Despite the spasms, the muscle becomes atrophied from disuse. The atrophy seen with UMN lesions occurs later than that seen with lower motor neuron (LMN) problems. The Babinski reflex is present.

When a lesion develops in lower motor neurons, the client develops flaccid muscle weakness or paralysis, loss of reflexes, loss of muscle tone, and atrophy of the involved muscles. The degree to which these clinical manifestations develop depends on the extent of the lesion. Each anterior horn cell innervates several separate muscle fibers, and because several anterior horn cells exist at each spinal level, a lesion confined to one spinal segment may not damage all of the anterior horn cells innervating an entire muscle. This type of lesion would cause muscle weakness rather than paralysis. Paralysis occurs when a lesion involves the column or anterior horn cells in several spinal segments. When all the peripheral motor nerves are involved, the entire muscle becomes flaccid. The muscles atrophy early from lack of innervation. LMN lesions are often associated with spinal cord injury or tumors and surgery on the aorta, which alters blood flow to the spinal cord.

DISORDERS OF THE CRANIAL NERVES

Cranial nerves can be affected in many ways by various nervous system disorders. For example, they may be secondarily affected by compression resulting from increased intracranial pressure or they may be directly damaged as a result of head injuries. In this section, only the two most common disorders specific to the cranial nerves, not those associated with other disorders, are discussed. Other cranial nerve disorders do exist. Regeneration of the cranial nerves can occur except for the first (olfactory) or second (optic) cranial nerve, because these nerves are actually part of the central nervous system (CNS).

TRIGEMINAL NEURALGIA

Chronic irritation of the fifth cranial nerve results in trigeminal neuralgia, also called *tic douloureux*. Although most commonly occurring in 50- to 70-year-old people, trigeminal neuralgia can occur in adults of any age. Approximately 60% of clients are women. The trigeminal nerve has three divisions: the ophthalmic, maxillary, and mandibular (Figure 71-9). Trigeminal neuralgia may occur in any one or more of these divisions.

Causes of trigeminal neuralgia can be divided into intrinsic and extrinsic lesions within the nerve itself, such as gross abnormalities of the axon or myelin, as may occur with multiple sclerosis. Extrinsic lesions are outside the trigeminal root and include mechanical compression by tumors, vascular anomalies, dental abscesses, or jaw malformation.

Trigeminal neuralgia is characterized by intermittent episodes of a sudden onset of intense pain. The pain is rarely relieved by analgesics. Tactile stimulation, such as touch and facial hygiene, and even talking, may trigger an attack. Trigeminal neuralgia is more prevalent in the maxillary and mandibular distributions and on the right side of the face. Bilateral trigeminal neuralgia is rare but does occur. The pain from trigeminal neuralgia can become so intense that the client ponders suicide.

None of the current diagnostic studies identify trigeminal neuralgia. Angiography, CT scan, and MRI can identify a causative lesion. The actual diagnosis is made on the

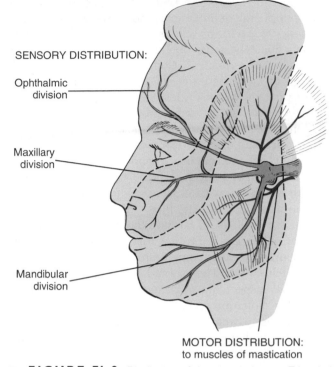

SENSORY DISTRIBUTION:

Ophthalmic division

Maxillary division

Mandibular division

MOTOR DISTRIBUTION: to muscles of mastication

■ **FIGURE 71–9**   Distribution of the trigeminal nerve. Trigeminal neuralgia develops along the course of this nerve.

basis of an in-depth history with attention paid to triggering stimuli and the nature and site of the pain. A careful history is obtained from the client regarding stimuli that trigger an attack. This information is used to plan care so as to minimize triggering events. The client's dental hygiene and nutritional intake are evaluated. These clients often do not eat enough to meet their daily nutritional needs and neglect their teeth because of the pain.

OUTCOME MANAGEMENT

Anticonvulsants such as carbamazepine (Tegretol) and gabapentin (Neurontin) are often prescribed as the initial treatment of trigeminal neuralgia. These drugs may dampen the reactivity of the neurons within the trigeminal nerve. For some clients, these medications are all the treatment that is ever needed. Liver impairment may result from administration of both carbamazepine and phenytoin. Liver enzymes must be monitored before and during therapy. If the client cannot tolerate the dose needed for pain control, phenytoin can be used. These medications should be used cautiously in clients with a history of alcohol abuse. Baclofen (Lioresal) is an antispasmodic that may be used alone or in conjunction with anticonvulsants. Opioids are not particularly effective in relieving trigeminal neuralgia pain. Help clients use and improve any pain control strategies they have developed. Clients with trigeminal neuralgia need emotional support to help them deal with pain that has often been present for a long time.

Surgery includes nerve blocks with alcohol and glycerol, peripheral neurectomy, and percutaneous radiofrequency wave forms that create lesions that alter pain transmission. The relief obtained with these procedures is not always permanent. Complications include development of facial paresthesias and muscular weakness. These procedures, being less invasive, are often better tolerated by older or debilitated clients.

More invasive techniques include major surgical procedures. Microvascular decompression involves removing the vessel from the posterior trigeminal root. A rhizotomy is the resection of the root of the nerve. These procedures require a craniotomy to allow access to the nerve.

Complications include those of any surgical procedure, as well as facial weakness and paresthesias. If facial numbness is present following surgery, clients must learn to test the temperature of food before putting it into their mouth. They should chew on the unaffected side and inspect mucous membranes for irritation. Assess for aspiration and advance the diet slowly. Teach clients to use a water jet device instead of a toothbrush for dental hygiene and advise them to visit their dentist as soon as possible after surgery.

If the corneal reflex has been impaired, the client should be taught eye care. During the acute postoperative period, apply eye drops and a protective shield. The client assumes these tasks with supervision and then independently.

BELL'S PALSY

Bell's palsy affects the motor aspects of the facial nerve, the seventh cranial nerve (Figure 71-10). Bell's palsy is the most common type of peripheral facial paralysis. It affects both women and men in all age groups. However, it occurs most commonly between ages 20 and 40 years.

Bell's palsy results in a unilateral paralysis of the facial muscles of expression. There is no obvious pathologic cause although there is accumulating evidence that reactivation of herpesvirus (simplex type 1 or zoster) and Lyme disease may be implicated. Facial paralysis may be central or peripheral in origin. Central facial palsy is an upper motor neuron paralysis or paresis. Sometimes it produces dissociation of motor function. In this situation, the client cannot voluntarily show his or her teeth on the paralyzed side, but can show them with emotional stimulation such as that causing smiles or laughter. This phenomenon is called *voluntary emotional dissociation*.

Typical clinical manifestations include (1) upward movement of the eyeball on closing the eye (Bell's phenomenon), (2) drooping of the mouth, (3) flattening of the nasolabial fold, (4) widening of the palpebral fissure, and (5) a slight lag in closing the eye. Eating may be difficult.

There is no known cure for Bell's palsy. Care is palliative and includes analgesics if discomfort occurs from herpetic lesions, corticosteroids to decrease nerve tissue edema and often in combination with antiviral agents such as Acyclovir, physical therapy with moist heat, gentle massage, and stimulation of the facial nerve with faradic current. The cornea is protected with artificial tears, sunglasses, an eye patch at night, and periodic gentle closure of the eye.

Clients experiencing Bell's palsy often think they have had a stroke. Reassure the client that this is not the case. Most clients recover from Bell's palsy within a few weeks without residual manifestations. If permanent complete facial paralysis occurs, surgery may be necessary. Anastomosis of the peripheral end of the facial nerve with the spinal accessory or hypoglossal nerve allows closure of the eye during sleep and restores tone to the facial musculature.

DISORDERS OF THE PERIPHERAL NERVES

Peripheral neuropathy is a general term referring to disorders of peripheral nerves. Peripheral neuropathy can be associated with poor nutrition, a large number of diseases, and pressure or trauma. Many people suffer from the disorder without ever identifying the cause.

Peripheral neuropathy also can be classified by where it occurs in the body. Nerve damage that occurs in one area of the body is called *mononeuropathy;* that which occurs in many areas is called *polyneuropathy.* Radiculopathy is the term for neuropathy that affects nerve roots.

Neuropathy also can be categorized by cause, such as diabetic neuropathy and nutritional neuropathy. When a cause cannot be identified, the condition is called *idiopathic neuropathy.*

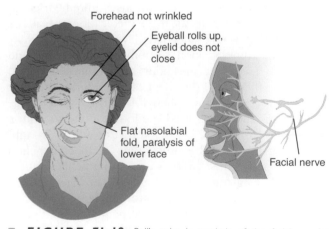

Forehead not wrinkled

Eyeball rolls up, eyelid does not close

Flat nasolabial fold, paralysis of lower face

Facial nerve

■ **FIGURE 71–10** Bell's palsy is paralysis of the facial muscles innervated by the seventh cranial nerve.

Peripheral neuropathy can be caused by disease; nerve compression, entrapment, or laceration; exposure to toxins; or inflammation. In many cases, especially in clients older than age 60 years, no cause can be determined. Several conditions are associated with neuropathy, including alcoholism, amyloidosis (metabolic disorder), autoimmune disorders (e.g., Guillain-Barré syndrome), Bell's palsy, cancer, carpal tunnel syndrome, renal failure, connective tissue diseases (rheumatoid arthritis), diabetes, Lyme disease, and vitamin deficiencies.

Clinical manifestations depend on the type of nerve affected (motor, sensory, autonomic) and where the nerve is located in the body. One or more types of nerve may be damaged.

Muscle weakness, cramps, and spasms are associated with motor nerve damage. In some cases, there may be loss of balance and coordination.

Sensory nerve damage can produce tingling, numbness, and pain. Pain associated with sensory nerve damage is variably described in the following manner:

- Sensation of wearing an invisible "glove" or "sock"
- Burning, freezing, or electric-like
- Extreme sensitivity to touch

If the autonomic nerves are damaged, involuntary functions may be affected. Orthostatic hypotension, bradycardia, reduced ability to perspire, constipation, bladder dysfunction, and sexual dysfunction may occur.

Because analgesics (e.g., aspirin, ibuprofen) are usually ineffective against pain caused by neuropathy, treatment often involves medications that target nerve cells. Anticonvulsants and antidepressants such as gabapentin (Neurontin) and amitriptyline (Elavil) are usually the first medications prescribed. Topical treatment with capsaicin cream (Zostrix) may be prescribed for focal neuropathy. The area surrounding the affected nerves may also be injected with lidocaine (Xylocaine) to temporarily reduce pain. Vitamin supplements may be used to treat nutritional neuropathy. Physical therapy (e.g., exercise, massage, heat) and acupuncture may be used to reduce manifestations.

CUMULATIVE TRAUMA DISORDERS

Cumulative trauma disorders (CTDs) include a group of overuse syndromes that predominantly affect the wrist and hand. They are also called *repetitive strain injuries* because some repetitive work activities seem to cause or exacerbate the manifestations. There are several forms (see Table 71-1). The client often describes fatigue in the extremity, and aching and tiredness during the activity. Rest generally relieves the manifestations in the first clinical stage. As the disorder progresses, manifestations persist despite rest. Finally, chronic aching, fatigue in the extremity, and weakness develop despite rest. To minimize the incidence and effects of CTDs, health specialists in business and industry have modified work tasks, workstations, work environment, tools, and equipment. Prevention focuses on exercises to reduce muscle strain and tension of the hands and wrist.

CARPAL TUNNEL SYNDROME

Carpal tunnel syndrome (CTS) is an entrapment neuropathy that occurs when the median nerve is compressed as it passes through the wrist along a pathway to the hand. The tunnel, called the *carpal tunnel,* is bordered by the flexor retinaculum, which is a band of fibrous tissue that prevents the wrist tendons from bowing when the wrist is flexed. Compression causes sensory and motor changes in the thumb, the index and middle fingers, and the radial aspect of the ring finger. CTS also leads to atrophy of the radial half of the thenar eminence.

CTS may develop spontaneously without a known cause or may result from disease or injury. The most commonly reported cause of CTS is repetitive motion of the wrist, with the wrist in constant flexion. A higher incidence of CTS is reported among homemakers, factory workers, bricklayers, cashiers, musicians, secretaries, and computer operators. Pregnancy, hypothyroidism, gout, and rheumatoid arthritis are other conditions associated with CTS.

Initially, the client may be awakened at night by pain and paresthesia. Although these initial manifestations are temporary and relieved by shaking the hand, later stages may be accompanied by motor loss (e.g., progressive weakness, inability to perform fine motor activities, and burning or numbness in the thumb, index finger, or middle finger) and daytime pain.

Assessment of the client begins with a thorough history, including occupational tasks. Diagnostic assessment for CTS includes assessing for Tinel's and Phalen's signs (Figure 71-11, *A* and *B*). Tinel's sign is the development of tingling in the hands and fingers when the wrist is tapped. Phalen's test is assessing for the development of numbness and tingling following forceful flexion of the wrists for 20 to 30 seconds (see Figure 71-11, *B*). Finally, the wrist compression test is done. The wrist compression test is manual application of 30 seconds of pressure over the flexor retinaculum (see Figure 71-11, *C*). If paresthesias develop after compression, the result is positive. The wrist compression test has been demonstrated to be 87% accurate in diagnosing CTS. Electromyography may also be used in differential diagnosis to rule out other possible causes.

OUTCOME MANAGEMENT

Initially the wrist is splinted in a neutral position to prevent mechanical irritation of the nerve. Injection of steroids into the flexor tendons is done less frequently than in the past because of reported problems with scarring, median nerve damage, and infection. In

TABLE 71-1 Repetitive Motion Injuries

Condition	Manifestations	People/Occupations at Risk	Usual Treatment
Neck			
Tension neck syndrome	Stiff, aching neck; headache	Typists, keypunch operators, cashiers, and others who must maintain a restricted posture	Prevention is key: (1) pause frequently when typing or keying to stretch about 30 sec every 30 min; (2) place screen directly in front of typist, avoid twisting; (3) place material to be typed at eye level if possible; avoid having materials to be typed consistently on one side of typist; conservative*
Cervical syndrome	Pain on flexion or extension of the neck with radiation down the arm	Common in people who assume awkward positions for a long time, such as painters, dentists	Conservative,* cervical collar, surgery
Shoulder			
Thoracic outlet syndrome	Numbness, pain, ischemia, and weakened pulse in upper extremity with hyperextension of shoulder	Overhead assembly workers, automobile repair mechanics, letter carriers	Conservative,* transcutaneous nerve stimulation, surgery
Supraspinatus tendinitis	Pain on elevating arm above 70 degrees at shoulder	People who must maintain abduction with elbow extended: painters, construction workers	Conservative,* physical therapy, steroid injections
Bicipital tendinitis	Pain over bicipital tendon in bicipital groove	Window washers, construction workers, shipping clerks	Conservative,* physical therapy, steroid injections
Elbow, Hand, and Wrist			
Lateral or medial epicondylitis (tennis elbow)	Local pain and pain on resisted hand motion	Repeated and forceful rotation of forearm with wrist bent; can be seen in bowlers, tennis players, and pitchers	Conservative,* steroid injections, surgery
de Quervain's tenosynovitis (inflammation of the extensor pollicis brevis tendons)	Gradual onset of pain, and sometimes swelling of radial styloid; popping sensation on extension of thumb	Middle-age women and those subject to repetitive stress of thumb	Conservative,* steroid injections, surgery
Carpal tunnel syndrome	Pain and paresthesias on percussion over median nerve at wrist (Tinel's sign) or with flexed wrists pressed together (positive Phalen's maneuver); night pain after 3-4 hr of sleep, morning stiffness, daytime numbness	Repetitive forced hand movements, keypunch operators, cashiers, typists, people with degenerative joint disease	Prevention is key: (1) while typing pause frequently, at least 30 sec every 30 min; (2) adjust keyboard so elbows are at 90-degree angle and wrists are straight; (3) do not rest wrists on a hard surface or restpad; wrists should "float" above keyboard; (4) use a light touch when striking keys; conservative,* steroid injections, surgery
Ulnar nerve entrapment	Pain and paresthesias on percussion of ulnar nerve over epicondyle (Tinel's sign); local swelling and tissue hypertrophy around elbow	Rheumatoid arthritis clients, occupational stress on elbow	Conservative,* surgery

*Conservative treatment consists of restriction of the harmful motion, splinting (if appropriate and only for short periods of time or at night), application of ice or heat, use of mild analgesics and nonsteroidal anti-inflammatory drugs, and performing gentle stretching exercises.

addition to rest, pyridoxine hydrochloride (vitamin B_6) has been reported to be helpful. For some clients, pain can be relieved by gently squeezing the distal metacarpal heads together with the affected hand palm up; in some instances, stretch of digits III and IV is also required. This maneuver may also help in the clinical diagnosis of CTS.

Surgery is indicated with (1) severe manifestations of long duration, (2) muscle atrophy, or (3) progressive sensory loss in the fingers and hand. Carpal tunnel release can be performed by opening the wrist or through an endoscope. General or regional anesthesia can be used. During the surgery, the transverse carpal ligament is divided to relieve pressure.

After surgery, blood flow is assessed hourly by checking the color, capillary refill, and warmth of the fingertips. When the anesthetic has worn off, assess the fingers for sensation.

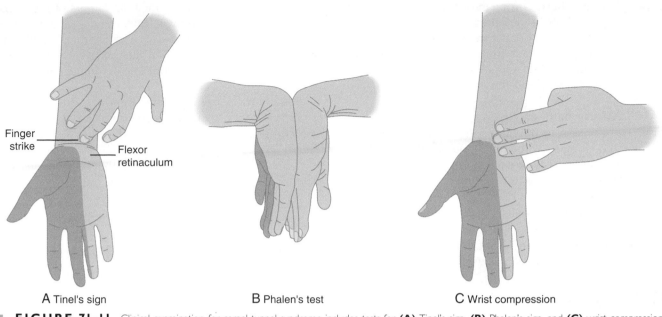

Finger strike

Flexor retinaculum

A Tinel's sign   B Phalen's test   C Wrist compression

■ **FIGURE 71–11** Clinical examination for carpal tunnel syndrome includes tests for **(A)** Tinel's sign, **(B)** Phalen's sign, and **(C)** wrist compression. Each of these maneuvers elicits numbness and pain in the thumb, the index and middle fingers, and the radial aspect of the ring finger when carpal tunnel syndrome is present.

Initially, postoperative care centers on wrist immobilization using bulky dressings and a wrist splint. The arm is elevated on pillows to reduce edema. Encourage the client to try to move the fingers, even though they are splinted. Heavy gripping and pinching should be avoided for up to 6 weeks. These actions need to be avoided to keep the tendons from pushing out against the healing transverse ligament. After 6 weeks, the client should be safe to resume gripping and pinching without irritating the wrist. The client often returns to the same type of work, so recovery of strength and flexibility are imperative. Work site analysis should also be completed to avoid reinjury.

The client and family are the care providers beyond the immediate postoperative period. Because this surgery is usually performed on an outpatient basis, provide detailed instructions on home care. See the Client Education Guide feature on Home Care After Carpal Tunnel Release on the website.

CUBITAL TUNNEL SYNDROME

Cubital tunnel syndrome results from a combination of local pressure and stretching of the ulnar nerve at the elbow as it passes behind the medial epicondyle. The problem may arise following local trauma, but most often is spontaneous, with elbow position during sleep being the largest contributing factor. Problems include pain, numbness, altered sensation, and weakness, and may be permanent if nerve damage has occurred. Electrical nerve testing may be helpful in assessing nerve damage, but may be normal even in clients with symptomatic nerve compression. Nerve irritation at the neck may produce similar manifestations and may coexist with

this problem. Most mild cases can be treated with a splint or elbow pad and avoidance of flexion and direct pressure on the nerve. More advanced cases require surgery to decompress and transpose the nerve out of the cubital tunnel.

TARSAL TUNNEL SYNDROME

Tarsal tunnel syndrome is the counterpart of the CTS in the lower extremity. In this syndrome, the posterior tibial nerve is trapped beneath the flexor retinaculum and deep fascia along the foot's medial border. Entrapment compresses the nerve, causing pain, burning, and tingling on the sole of the foot; it usually worsens as the day progresses. This pain can usually be reduced by rest, elevation, or massage.

Conservative treatment, such as arch supports and wider shoes, may successfully relieve the discomfort of tarsal tunnel syndrome. If inflammation of the nerve is causing the compression, NSAIDs may be prescribed. Steroid injections may also be effective. If the problem is caused by flat feet, custom orthotics can help restore the foot's natural arch.

Surgery to release the laciniate ligament may be required to provide room for expansion of the nerve. If a cyst is impinging on the nerve, it can be removed.

DUPUYTREN'S CONTRACTURE

Dupuytren's contracture is permanent flexor contracture of the fourth and fifth fingers. Dupuytren's contracture is inherited as an autosomal dominant trait and is common in people of Northern European descent. It is also more common in alcoholic and diabetic clients.

In severe forms of contracture, a longitudinal fibrous cord forms, which extends from the fingers to the palm and pulls the fingers into a locked position. Milder forms have less contracture and fewer nodules in the palmar fascia.

Ten years or more may pass before surgery is necessary. The decision to operate is usually made when the client can no longer lay the hand outstretched on a table. The operation consists of excision of part of the palmar fascia. After surgery, the hand is dressed in a large compression dressing. Range of motion is encouraged. Frequent assessments of capillary refill and finger color are needed. Splints are often used at night to promote extension. Many months of physical therapy may be needed, and even then, full function may not be achievable.

GANGLION CYST

A ganglion can be described simply as a fluid-filled sac arising from an adjacent joint capsule or tendon sheath. A ganglion can form from almost any joint or tendon sheath in the wrist and hand. Trauma or degenerative changes in the fibrous joint capsule are thought to contribute to development of ganglia.

Ganglions may limit motion in the adjacent joints, or produce discomfort from compression or distention of local soft tissues. Large ganglions can be cosmetically unpleasant. Ganglion cysts of the distal interphalangeal (DIP) joint may produce deformities of the fingernail. Ganglion cysts arising from the flexor tendon sheath at the base of the finger may produce pain when grasping. On rare occasions, ganglion cysts (particularly those associated with the wrist) may cause changes in the bone. Ganglion cysts can frequently be diagnosed simply by their location and shape. They are usually not adherent to the overlying skin and are firmly attached to the underlying joint or tendon sheath. Large ganglions may permit the passage of light through their substance (transillumination). X-ray studies are sometimes helpful in diagnosing ganglion cysts, particularly around the DIP joint where associated degenerative arthritis is often found.

To relieve pain or numbness, the ganglion may be aspirated or surgically excised. The area may then be injected with a corticosteroid before a pressure dressing and splint are applied. NSAIDs are commonly used for pain. Wrist ganglions may recur in up to 30% of clients.

PERIPHERAL NERVE TUMORS

Although solitary tumors (generally neurofibromas) may develop on any peripheral nerve, multiple tumors most often occur and are part of a syndrome known as *neurofibromatosis* (von Recklinghausen's disease). This hereditary disorder is characterized by multiple tumors of the spinal and cranial nerves along with involvement of many other systems. The disease is usually not life-threatening, and lesions are excised only when they interfere with normal activity. Intracranial and intraspinal tumors are usually removed.

Surgery for peripheral nerve tumors is often done on an outpatient basis. In the recovery room, the dressings are checked for drainage; circulation, motion, and sensation in the extremity are also assessed. Clients are encouraged to perform range-of-motion exercises. Clients and family members are taught the manifestations of circulatory compromise and infection, medication management, and care of the dressing and incision.

PERIPHERAL NERVE INJURIES

The peripheral nerves most commonly subjected to external pressure are the median, radial, ulnar, sciatic, common peroneal, tibial, and long thoracic nerves. The common peroneal nerve (a terminal branch of the sciatic) is injured more frequently than any other nerve. Because of its course and distribution, the sciatic nerve is exposed to internal and external trauma and inflammation more than any other nerve. The sciatic nerve may also be injured directly during medication injections. The median nerve is most often injured by constriction from fascial bands. The axillary nerve may be injured as the result of an allergic reaction to serum injections or secondary to improper crutch walking. Any peripheral nerve can be injured by bone fractures or perforating wounds. Nerves can also be injured in common household accidents (cut on glass) or in motor-vehicle accidents.

Assessment includes a full examination of the injured area. Assessment findings with nerve damage depend on the type of nerve injured and the extent of damage. Damaged motor nerves cause clinical manifestations such as flaccid paralysis, and reflex loss in the muscle innervated by the injured nerve. Damaged mixed nerves or sensory nerves cause vasomotor and trophic disturbances following either partial or complete interruption of the nerve. Following partial injury or incomplete division of a nerve, the person may experience stabbing pains, paresthesias ("pins and needles" sensation), and, occasionally, the burning pains of causalgia. Damaged sensory nerves cause loss of sensation in the nerves' area of anatomic distribution. If the hand is injured, document the client's occupation and the dominant hand.

Conservative management may include splinting, ice, elevation of the limb, administration of anti-inflammatory and analgesic agents, or a combination of these modalities. If a peripheral nerve is traumatically severed, the ends should be surgically anastomosed to enable healing. The nearer the site of injury occurs to the CNS, the less chance of regeneration. When nerves are only slightly damaged, mild edema occurs at the injury site. This may cause temporary manifestations that recede in a few days or possibly weeks.

Postoperative care of clients having nerve repair or grafting includes elevation of the extremity. Elevation is critical to reduce edema and improve venous return. The procedure is usually performed with local anesthesia, so assessment of neurovascular status is not conclusive until the anesthesia has worn off. Color, warmth, movement, sensation, capillary refill, and strength are assessed. Some of these assessments can be hampered by dressings, but as many as possible should be performed. Monitor the fingertips for blood flow with Doppler laser or standard Doppler ultrasonography and temperature probes. The temperature of the hand is usually less than the core temperature and the surgeon indicates acceptable ranges of temperature. Physical therapy begins within a few days to promote movement after severe injuries.

If the injury is severe, the client may have recurring dreams about the accident and his or her injury. These dreams are generally normal, but if they are bothersome to the client, a psychiatric consultant may be helpful.

CONCLUSIONS

The physical and psychological impairments vary with the degree of damage as well as the client's response and ability to cope with the body changes. The coping response is not always related to the degree of physiologic damage. A client can have facial paralysis or trigeminal neuralgia and be more compromised psychologically than a client with spinal cord injury who has strong coping skills. It is imperative that nurses comprehend the severity of the client's dysfunction as it relates to quality of life, as well as the impact it has on family dynamics.

THINKING CRITICALLY

1. The client, a 34-year-old woman, had a lumbar laminectomy done earlier today. A prior assessment showed that movement and sensation of both lower extremities were intact. During the current postoperative assessment, she states that her right toes feel numb, and the dorsiflexion and plantiflexion of the right foot are weaker than earlier. She has requested an analgesic because she is starting to get a headache. What are the priorities for her care? What assessments and interventions might be used?

Factors to Consider. What assessment methods can be used to determine the extent of vascular insufficiency? What type of neurologic checks should be done?

A discussion for this question can be found on the website.

BIBLIOGRAPHY

Citations appearing in red refer to primary research.

Citations appearing in blue refer to evidence-based practice guidelines and protocols.

1. Ashkenazi, A., & Levin, M. (2004). Three common neuralgias. *Postgraduate Medicine, 116*(3), 16-32.
2. ASPAN pain and comfort clinical guideline. (2003). *Journal of Peri-Anesthesia Nursing, 18*(4), 232-236.
3. *Bell's palsy fact sheet.* National Institute of Neurological Disorders and Stroke website. Accessed 07/16/06 at www.ninds.nih.gov/disorders/bells/detail_bells.htm.
4. Boswell, M.V., Shah, R.V., Everett, C.R., et al. (2005). Interventional techniques in the management of chronic spinal pain: Evidence-based practice guidelines. *Pain Physician, 8*(1), 1-47.
5. Bridwell, K.H., Anderson, P.A., Boden, S.D., et al. (2005). What's new in spine surgery? *Journal of Bone and Joint Surgery, 87*(8), 1892-1901.
6. Brigham and Women's Hospital. (2003). *Upper extremity musculoskeletal disorders. A guide to prevention, diagnosis and treatment.* Boston, Mass: Brigham and Women's Hospital.
7. Cain, J.E. (2006). Gentle yoga effective for chronic low-back pain. *American Journal of Nursing, 106*(3), 22.
8. Canter, P. (2006). How effective is spinal manipulation? *General Practitioner, April 14*, 30-31.
9. Carlson, D. (2005). When your patient has acute facial paralysis. *Nursing, 35*(4), 54-55.
10. Childs, S.G. (2005). Dupuytren's disease. *Orthopaedic Nursing, 24* (2), 160-165.
11. Chronic pain relief. (2006). *British Journal of Community Nursing, 11*(4), 175.
12. D'Arcy, Y. (2006). Treatment strategies for low back pain relief. *Nurse Practitioner, 31*(4), 16-27.
13. Exercises for aching hands. (2005). *Harvard Women's Health Watch, 13*(3), 2-3.
14. Implant eases low back pain. (2006). *Nursing, 36*(2), 34-35.
15. Institute for Clinical Systems Improvement (ICSI). (2005). *Adult low back pain.* Bloomington, Minn: ICSI.
16. Institute for Clinical Systems Improvement (ICSI). (2005). *Assessment and management of chronic pain.* Bloomington, Minn: ICSI.
17. Kramasz, V.C., & Roman, L.M. (2005). Polio patients take a second. *RN, 68*(11), 33-37.
18. Kwon, B. (2006). A review of the 2001 Volvo Award winner in clinical studies: Lumbar fusion versus nonsurgical treatment for chronic low back pain: A multicenter randomized controlled trial from the Swedish Lumbar Spine Study Group. *Spine, 31*(2), 245-249.
19. Lively, M.W. (2005). Acute lumbar disk injuries in active patients: Making optimal management decisions. *Physician and Sportsmedicine, 33*(4), 21-27.
20. Low level heat wrap therapy helps low back pain. (2006). *Journal of Pain & Palliative Care Pharmacotherapy, 20*(1), 78-79.
21. Meadows, G.R. (2005). Microendoscopic lumbar diskectomy. *Operative Techniques in Sports Medicine, 13*(2), 122-124.
22. Mueller, D.M., & Oro, J.J. (2004). Prospective analysis of presenting symptoms among 265 patients with radiographic evidence of Chiari malformation type I with or without syringomyelia. *Journal of the American Academy of Nurse Practitioners, 16*(3), 134-138.
23. New concepts in Bell's palsy improve treatment options. (2005). *American Family Physician, 72*(1), 169-170.
24. National Institute of Dental and Craniofacial Research website. Accessed 10/12/05 at www.nidcr.nih.gov/.
25. Posture and back health. (2005). *Harvard Women's Health Watch, 12*(12), 6-7.
26. Shaw, W.S., Zaia, A., Pransky, G., et al. (2005). Perceptions of provider communication and patient satisfaction for treatment of acute low back pain. *Journal of Occupational and Environmental Medicine, 47*(10), 1036-1043.
27. Stevenson, K., Lewis, M., & Hay, E. (2006). Does physiotherapy management of low back pain change as a result of an evidence-based educational programme? *Journal of Evaluation in Clinical Practice, 12*(3), 365-375.

28. University of Michigan Health System. (2004). *Acute low back pain.* Ann Arbor, Mich: University of Michigan Health System.

29. U.S. Preventive Services Task Force (USPSTF). (2004). *Primary care interventions to prevent low back pain in adults: Recommendation statement.* Rockville, Md: Agency for Healthcare Research and Quality (AHRQ).

30. Schoen, D.C. (2005). Injuries of the wrist. *Orthopaedic Nursing, 24* (4), 304-307.

31. Washington State Department of Labor and Industries. (2005). *Antiepileptic drugs guideline for chronic pain.* Provider Bulletin (PB 05-10), 1-3.

32. Watkins, J. (2005). Independent nurse: Clinical—Diagnosis and care of Bell's palsy. *General Practitioner, June 6,* 119-120.

33. Work Loss Data Institute. (2006). *Carpal tunnel syndrome (acute & chronic).* Corpus Christi, Tex: Work Loss Data Institute.

34. Work Loss Data Institute. (2006). *Forearm, wrist & hand.* Corpus Christi, Tex: Work Loss Data Institute.

35. Work Loss Data Institute. (2006). *Low back—Lumbar & thoracic (acute & chronic).* Corpus Christi, Tex: Work Loss Data Institute.

36. Work Loss Data Institute. (2006). *Neck and upper back (acute & chronic).* Corpus Christi, Tex: Work Loss Data Institute.

evolve *Did you remember to check out the bonus material on the Evolve website and the CD-ROM, including NCLEX®-Examination Style Review Questions, Open-Book Quizzes, and Chapter Review Audio Podcasts?*

http://evolve.elsevier.com/Black/medsurg

CHAPTER 72

Management of Clients with Degenerative Neurologic Disorders

PATRICIA E. GRAHAM

Degenerative neurologic disorders pose a great challenge to the client, the family, and the caregiver, whether it is a nurse, a family member, or a significant other. By their very nature, these disorders cause progressive decline in neurologic function. Some progress relatively quickly (over months to 1 or 2 years), whereas others progress more gradually, sometimes over decades. Common nursing diagnoses for clients with these disorders are *Altered Thought Processes, Memory Deficit, Visual-Perceptual Alteration, Impaired Physical Mobility, Incontinence, Self-Care Deficit,* and *Impaired Individual and Family Coping.* A major goal of intervention is to help the client achieve an optimal level of functioning in light of chronic neurologic deficits. The family should also be taught what to expect, such as the usual areas of decline, how to provide care and support to the client, and how to manage stress and cope with the progressive nature of the disorder.

The diagnosis of degenerative neurologic disease is most often made in an outpatient setting; however, hospital admission may be necessary when acute relapses or life-threatening events occur. Many clients return to their homes and have regular follow-up in outpatient clinics; however, some may require rehabilitation, in either inpatient or outpatient settings, for newly acquired deficits. Other clients may require transfer to long-term care facilities because of a significant decline in their ability to provide self-care. Still other clients may not survive their acute illness.

ALZHEIMER'S DISEASE AND RELATED DEMENTIAS

The term *dementia* refers to the loss of memory, reasoning, judgment, and language to such an extent that it interferes with everyday life. The changes may occur gradually or quickly, and how they come about is key to determining whether the condition causing dementia is temporary.

Cognition is the act or process of thinking, perceiving, and learning. Cognitive activities that become impaired in dementia include decision-making, judgment, memory, spatial orientation, thinking, reasoning, calculation, personality, and verbal communication. A client with dementia may undergo behavioral and personality changes as well, depending on the area(s) of the brain affected. There are many causes of dementia. Because the brain is quickly injured from hypoxia, reduced blood flow, or drugs, the causes are numerous (Box 72-1).

Types of Dementia

Alzheimer's disease (AD) is the most common form of dementia among people over age 65. AD constitutes at least half of all dementias. Alzheimer's disease affects about 4 million Americans. Slightly more than half of these people receive care at home, and the remainder receive institutional nursing care. The prevalence of AD doubles every 5 years after the age of 65. In fact, some estimates indicate that nearly half of all people older than 85 have AD.

---

evolve Web Enhancements

Bridge to Home Health Care   Respite Care for Caregivers of People with Alzheimer's Disease

Client Education Guide   Caring for Family Members with Alzheimer's Disease (English Version and Spanish Translation)

Parkinson's Disease (Spanish Translation)

Complementary and Alternative Therapy   Use It or Lose It: Reducing the Risk of Dementia

Ethical Issues in Nursing   In Revealing Information About Huntington's Disease, Which Should Take Precedence: Client Confidentiality or Beneficence?

Be sure to check out the bonus material on the Evolve website and the CD-ROM, including free self-assessment exercises. **http://evolve.elsevier.com/Black/medsurg**

BOX 72-1 Causes of Dementia

- Alzheimer's disease
- Multi-infarct dementia (arteriosclerotic dementia)
- Parkinson's disease
- Lewy body disease
- Alcoholic dementia
- Binswanger's disease
- Creutzfeldt-Jakob disease
- Huntington's chorea
- AIDS-related dementia
- Normal pressure hydrocephalus
- Genetic or metabolic disease (e.g., thyroid)
- Toxic or traumatic injury
- Malignant disease: primary, metastatic, or iatrogenic from the treatment

---

Multi-infarct (multiple stroke) disease is the second most common cause of irreversible dementia. Blood clots block small blood vessels in the brain and destroy brain tissue. Typically multiple infarct dementias occur in men more than 50 years old. The effect of multiple infarcts (strokes) over time leads to the progressive decline in cognition.

Lewy body dementia is similar to Alzheimer's disease but may progress more rapidly. Abnormal brain cells called cortical Lewy bodies occur throughout the brain and produce manifestations. Lewy bodies are also associated with Parkinson's and Alzheimer's diseases, but it is not clear whether dementia with Lewy bodies is a distinct clinical entity or perhaps a variant of Alzheimer's or Parkinson's disease.

Pick's disease also is a form of dementia but differs from AD in several ways. First, the two diseases produce different abnormalities in the cells of the brain. Pick's disease is marked by "Pick bodies," rounded, microscopic structures found within affected cells. Neurons swell, taking on a "ballooned" appearance. Neither of these changes appears in Alzheimer's disease, and the pathology of Alzheimer's disease (plaques and tangles) is not found in Pick's disease. Second, Pick's disease is usually sharply confined to the front parts of the brain, particularly the frontal and anterior temporal lobes. This contrasts with Alzheimer's disease, which is more widely distributed.

Etiology and Risk Factors

The cause of AD has not been found, although several risk factors have been identified. Increasing age is a risk factor. Genetic factors are also linked to AD. At least five chromosomes (1, 12, 14, 19, and 21) are involved in some forms of familial AD. Four genetic loci have also been identified as contributing to AD, including the amyloid precursor gene, the presenilin 1 gene, the presenilin 2 gene, and the apolipoprotein E gene on chromosome 19. Research has also shown that the age of AD development is also

genetic. The Genetic Links feature on p. 1895 describes other genetic disorders in addition to AD.

Clinical situations associated with AD development include elevated homocysteine levels (also a risk factor for heart disease), inflammation, stroke, and oxidative damage from free radicals. (The Complementary and Alternative Therapy feature on p. 1896 summarizes promising research findings in using omega-3 fatty acids to lower the risk of Alzheimer's disease.) Research is active in these areas to find the pathophysiologic connections and prevent them.

Pathophysiology

Alzheimer's disease disrupts the three neuronal processes that keep neurons healthy: communication, metabolism, and repair. Alois Alzheimer first described presenile dementia in 1907. He used a new staining technique of human brain tissue to demonstrate the pathologic changes. The changes he noted are now termed *beta-amyloid plaques* and *neurofibrillary tangles* (Figure 72-1). *Plaque* is a cluster of beta-amyloid, a protein fragment snipped from a larger protein, called *amyloid precursor protein*. Plaques have been described as dense, mostly insoluble deposits of protein and cellular material outside and around the neuron. Plaques develop in the hippocampus, an area of the brain that helps encode memories. Degenerating nerve terminals, both dendritic and axonal, contain amyloid protein. Healthy neurons have an internal support structure, called *microtubules*. These tubules serve as tracts to guide nutrients to the end of the axon and back. The tubule is stable because of a protein called tau. In AD, the tau is changed chemically and becomes tangled. Once tangled, the tubules degenerate and so do the cells they support. The destruction leads to memory failure, personality changes, and problems carrying out activities of daily living (ADL).

Gross brain changes evident in clients with AD include thickening of the leptomeninges, shrunken gyri, widened sulci, enlarged ventricles, hippocampal shrinkage, and generalized atrophy (Figure 72-2). In addition to structural changes, neurotransmitter changes, for example acetylcholine, are evident in the brain of clients with AD. Acetylcholine decreases because there is a decline in cholinergic neurons in the basal nucleus that leads to loss of choline acetyltransferase in the neocortex and hippocampus.

Clinical Manifestations

Clinically, AD is characterized by a relentless impairment of decision-making that generally begins insidiously and can progress for a decade or so. Manifestations can vary depending on the portion of the brain involved and on genetic predisposition. The onset of AD typically occurs in late middle age (age 65 years and older), although some familial cases occur in a person's 40s and 50s.

GENETIC LINKS

Examples of Neurodegenerative Genetic Disorders

Disorder	Features	Inheritance	Gene Defect	Genetic Testing Available?
Huntington's disease (HD)	Progressive disorder of motor, cognitive, and psychiatric disturbance; onset 35-44 yr; median survival 15-18 yr after onset	AD	*HD*	Yes
Early-onset familial Alzheimer's disease (EOFAD)	Early onset of progressive impairment of memory, judgment, decision making, and language; mean onset under age 65 yr; comprise <2% of all AD cases	AD	*PSEN1* *APP* *PSEN2*	Yes No Yes
Late-onset Alzheimer's disease (AD2)	Multiple affected family members, with onset of dementia after age 60-65 yr; estimated to account for ≈25% of Alzheimer's disease	Complex trait; one or more susceptibility genes	*APOE*	Yes*
Parkinson's disease (familial PD)	Progressive disorder characterized by resting tremor, akinesia, and rigidity; rare occurrence	AD	*PARK1* *PARK2* *PARK3* *PARK4* *UCH-L1* *PARK6* *PARK7* *PARK8*	Yes No No No No No No No
Spinocerebellar ataxias, 21 types	Poor coordination of movement and wide-based uncoordinated, unsteady gait; poor coordination of limbs and speech often present; onset, frequency, and features vary and overlap	AD AR XL	*SCA1* *SCA2* *SCA3* *SCA6* *SCA7* *SCA8* *SCA10* *SCA12* *SCA17*	Yes Yes Yes Yes Yes Yes Yes Yes Yes
Friedreich's ataxia	Slowly progressive ataxia; onset age <25 yr; depressed tendon reflexes	AR	*FRDA*	Yes
Early-onset primary dystonia (DYT1)	Onset age <21 yr; involuntary sustained muscle contractions that cause posturing of limbs	AD	*DYT1*	Yes

AR, Autosomal recessive; *AD*, autosomal dominant; *XL*, X-linked.
*Presymptomatic testing is not routinely performed.

Preclinical Alzheimer's Disease

Alzheimer's disease begins near the hippocampus, a structure essential to the formation of both short- and long-term memories. Affected regions begin to shrink and in time (10 to 20 years perhaps) lead to memory loss.

Mild Alzheimer's Disease

As the cerebral cortex begins to shrink, other cognitive losses become apparent. *Memory disturbance* is usually noticed by family members or co-workers before the client does. The client may demonstrate poor judgment and problem-solving skills and become careless in work habits and household chores. Clients may become confused about where they are and they begin to get lost

easily. Routine activities such as bill paying and other daily tasks take longer. The client may do well in familiar surroundings and may be able to follow well-established routines but lacks the ability to adapt to new challenges. The person may become irritable, suspicious, or indifferent. Agitation, apathy, dysphoria, and aberrant motor behavior are associated with cognitive impairments.

Moderate Alzheimer's Disease

The client may demonstrate *language disturbance*, characterized by impaired word-finding and *circumlocution* (talking around a subject rather than about it directly). Later, spontaneous speech becomes increasingly empty, and *paraphasias* (words used in the wrong context)

COMPLEMENTARY AND ALTERNATIVE THERAPY

Omega-3 Fatty Acids from Fish and a Lower Risk of Alzheimer's Disease

A prospective study conducted from 1993 to 2000 followed 815 individuals (ages 65 to 94 years) in a community in the United States for an average of 3.9 years. These individuals completed a dietary questionnaire on average 2.3 years before clinical evaluation. A total of 131 individuals developed Alzheimer's disease in this study. Individuals who consumed fish once per week or more had 60% less risk of developing Alzheimer's disease compared with those who rarely or never ate fish.

REFERENCE

Morris, M., et al. (2003). Consumption of fish and omega-3 fatty acids and risk of incident Alzheimer disease. *Archives of Neurology, 60,* 940-946.

BRAIN CROSS-SECTIONS

Normal   Alzheimer's

■ **FIGURE 72–2** Alzheimer's disease affects many portions of the brain, especially those required for memory and speech.

---

are used. Clients may repeat words and phrases just spoken by themselves *(palilalia)* or by others *(echolalia)*. Motor disturbance *(apraxia)* is characterized by difficulty in using everyday objects such as a toothbrush, comb, razor, and utensils. Apraxia combined with forgetfulness can create serious safety problems. The person may leave a stove burner on in the kitchen or forget to extinguish a cigarette. Indifference worsens, and restlessness with frequent pacing appears. *Hyperorality* (the desire to take everything into the mouth to suck, chew, or taste) may develop. Swallowing may become difficult.

Depression and irritability may worsen, and delusions and psychosis may appear. The person fears personal harm, theft of property, or infidelity of the spouse. Clients may see bugs crawling on the bed or throughout the house. Wandering at night is common. Occasional incontinence may occur.

■ **FIGURE 72–1** Neurofibrillary tangles. In clients with Alzheimer's disease and some other neurologic disorders, these tangles replace the normal neuronal cytoplasm. The tangles are often seen with senile plaques and appear throughout the cortex, hippocampus, and amygdala. The number of plaques and tangles correlates roughly with the severity of the dementia.

Severe Alzheimer's Disease

In the final stage, plaques and tangles are widespread throughout the brain. Clients cannot recognize family or friends and do not communicate in any way. Voluntary movement is minimal, and the limbs become rigid with flexor posturing. Urinary and fecal incontinence is frequent. Aspiration and aspiration pneumonia are frequent.

Diagnostic Findings

A diagnosis is best made by a multidisciplinary group that can assist the client and family to understand what is happening and what interventions or assistance will be needed. Because there is no definitive test for AD, the diagnosis is made by exclusion of known causes of dementia (e.g., toxic or metabolic alterations, drug side effects, cerebrovascular disease, cancer, infection). The diagnosis is confirmed with (1) the presence of dementia involving two or more areas of cognition, (2) insidious onset and steady progression, and (3) loss of normal alertness.

Computed tomography (CT) scan can be used to identify ventricular dilation and sulcal enlargement and cerebral atrophy of the portions of the brain most affected. Magnetic resonance imaging (MRI), single-positron emission computed tomography (SPECT), and positron emission tomography (PET) are also used to detect changes in brain function.

Finally, laboratory studies are performed to rule out metabolic and drug-related causes of dementia. These studies include urinalysis, complete blood count (CBC), erythrocyte sedimentation rate (ESR), electrolytes, blood urea nitrogen (BUN) and creatinine values, thyroid and liver function tests, calcium, serum B_{12} levels, syphilis serology, and human immunodeficiency virus (HIV) testing.

Manifestations of Other Dementias

Manifestations of multi-infarct dementia (MID) often develop in a stepwise manner and include confusion, problems with recent memory, wandering or getting lost in familiar places, incontinence, emotional lability such as laughing or crying inappropriately, difficulty following instructions, and problems handling money. Usually the damage is so slight that the change is noticeable only as a series of small steps. Over time, however, as more small vessels are blocked, gradual mental decline occurs. MID, which typically begins between the ages of 60 and 75, affects men more often than women.

Manifestations of Lewy body dementia can range from traditional parkinsonian effects, such as loss of spontaneous movement *(bradykinesia),* rigidity (muscles feel stiff and resist movement), tremor, and shuffling gait, to effects similar to those of AD, such as acute confusion, loss of memory, and loss of or fluctuating cognition. Visual hallucinations may be one of the first manifestations noted, and clients may suffer from other psychiatric disturbances such as delusions and depression.

OUTCOME MANAGEMENT

No cure has been found for AD. Management of the client centers on helping maintain mental function and slowing the process of deterioration.

Medical Management

Maintain Mental Function

Several medications are used to retain ACh in the neuro-junctions. Tacrine (Cognex), donepezil (Aricept), galanthamine (Reminyl), and rivastigmine (Exelon) are used to maintain memory. These drugs can have small but noticeable effects, depending on the stage of disease, differences in the way the drugs act in different clients, and other factors. At least temporarily, many clients taking these drugs experience improvements in their thinking abilities and are less likely to demonstrate common manifestations of advanced AD, such as wandering, agitation, and socially inappropriate behaviors. None of these drugs prevents AD from worsening over time.

In an effort to combat the effect of oxygen free radicals, alpha-tocopherol (vitamin E) and selegiline have been studied. Both agents have been reported to delay the development of the later stages of AD and show some improvement in levels of independent and behavioral manifestations. The Complementary and Alternative Therapy features here and on p. 1898 summarize research findings in the use of vitamin E supplements for Alzheimer's disease and in the use of ginkgo biloba to improve memory in healthy people. An extract of ginkgo biloba may improve cognitive function for 6 to 12 months. Propentofylline has been effective in the management of AD. See the Complementary and Alternative Therapy

---

COMPLEMENTARY AND ALTERNATIVE THERAPY

Vitamin E Supplements for Clients with Alzheimer's Disease

The only agent that has been shown to slow the progression of Alzheimer's disease in a prospective study (in clients diagnosed with this condition) is vitamin E supplements. A multi-institutional, double-blind, placebo-controlled prospective study included 341 moderately impaired clients (Clinical Dementia Rating score of 2). Clients were randomly assigned to receive 2000 international units of vitamin E; 10 mg of selegiline; vitamin E and selegiline; or placebo for 2 years. The primary end-point was the time to progression to any of the following end-points: institutionalization, loss of any two of three basic activities of daily living (eating, dressing, and toileting), a rating of 3 on the Clinical Dementia Rating Scale, or death. Using an intention-to-treat analysis and after adjusting for differences among the groups in the baseline Mini-Mental State Examination score, the researchers observed a significant delay in the primary outcome among the treatment groups. There was an increase in median survival of 230 days for clients taking vitamin E alone, 215 days for clients taking selegiline, and 145 days for clients taking vitamin E and selegiline compared with clients receiving placebo.[2] The interpretation of this trial was somewhat controversial because of the need to include the baseline Mini-Mental State Examination score as a covariant in order to reveal a statistically significant difference between the treatment and placebo groups. Regardless, the American Academy of Neurology now recommends 2000 international units of vitamin E daily (1000 international units twice daily) as a standard care for the treatment of clients with Alzheimer's disease.[1]

REFERENCES

1. Doody, R., et al. (2001). Practice parameter: Management of dementia (an evidence-based review). Report of the Quality Standards Subcommittee of the American Academy of Neurology. *Neurology, 56,* 1154-1166.
2. Sano, M., et al. (1997). A controlled trial of selegiline, alpha-tocopherol, or both as treatment for Alzheimer's disease. The Alzheimer's Disease Cooperative Study. *New England Journal of Medicine, 336,* 1216-1222.

---

feature Use It or Lose It: Reducing the Risk of Dementia on the website.

Over the short term, other medicines can somewhat relieve anxiety, agitation, depression, and psychotic or inappropriate behavior: anxiolytics for anxiety and agitation, neuroleptics for unusual or troublesome behavior, and antidepressants or mood stabilizers for mood disorders and specific problems such as spells of anger or rage. No specific drugs or dosages address the wide range of problems that clients with AD experience. Medications such as risperidone (Risperdal), olanzapine (Zyprexa), quetiapine (Seroquel), sertraline (Zoloft), or citalopram (Celexa) should be used as seldom as possible and at the lowest effective doses. This will help minimize side effects in frail

COMPLEMENTARY AND ALTERNATIVE THERAPY

Ginkgo Biloba in Healthy Individuals for Memory Enhancement

Extracts or compounds from ginkgo have shown some initial promise in enhancing memory in demented older individuals.[1] However, researchers wanted to test the potential claims of some manufacturers that ginkgo could, in general, enhance mental focus and improve memory and concentration. Community-dwelling, functionally independent individuals older than 60 years volunteered for this study of memory.[2] Participants were excluded if they scored less than 27 out of a possible 30 points on the Mini-Mental State Examination at baseline. Highly educated or intelligent participants with mild dementia may have been included in this study. Participants in this randomized controlled trial received 40 mg of ginkgo biloba three times daily (dose recommended by many manufacturers) or placebo for 6 weeks. This duration was 2 weeks longer than the manufacturer's suggested onset of action. A total of 230 participants were included. No statistically significant differences were observed between ginkgo and placebo on any of the scales measured. No significant changes from baseline to post-treatment and no adverse effects were noted in the groups. In other words, ginkgo, in standard doses for 6 weeks, was ineffective in improving memory, intelligence, and concentration in older clients without dementia.

REFERENCES

1. Le Bars, P., et al. (2002). Influence of the severity of cognitive impairment on the effect of the ginkgo biloba extract Egb 761 in Alzheimer's disease. *Neuropsychobiology, 45,* 19-26.
2. Solomon, P., et al. (2002). Ginkgo for memory enhancement: A randomized controlled trial. *Journal of the American Medical Association, 288,* 835-840.

older clients. The use of these medications to "control behavior problems" is avoided; rather, the behavior should be considered an attempt to communicate a specific need.

Nursing Management of Alzheimer's Disease

Assessment. When AD is suspected, a complete history should be taken to assess for other causes of dementia. Data should be obtained from the client, family, and co-workers (if possible). Secondary sources are used because the client is often unaware of a problem with thought processing and minimizes it. Ask specific questions about difficulties with ADL, increasing forgetfulness, and changes in personality. Assess past medical history for previous head injury or surgery, recent falls, headache, and a family history of AD. A Mini-Mental State examination may provide objective data for ongoing evaluation of the client (see Chapter 67). AD has a profound impact on psychosocial behaviors. Ask about the client's reactions to changes in routine or in the environment. It is not uncommon for a client with AD to become very agitated over small

changes, and apathy, social isolation, and irritability may be noted. As the brain continues to atrophy and the limbic system becomes dysfunctional, the client may become paranoid, use abusive language, and become suspicious of others.

Alzheimer's disease has a profound impact on the family. Assess the family for strengths and weaknesses, their ability to provide care for the client, and their financial concerns. In large centers, assessment of the client and family is performed through a team approach. The Client Education Guide website feature titled Caring for Family *evolve* Members with Alzheimer's Disease provides instructions and resources for caregivers of people with AD.

The home environment should be evaluated for safety before the client is sent home from the hospital: SAFETY

- Is the home on a busy street?   ALERT
- Can doors be secured so that the client cannot leave without supervision?
- Are potentially dangerous appliances out of reach?

Diagnosis, Outcomes, Interventions

Diagnosis: Impaired Verbal Communication. Use the nursing diagnosis of *Impaired Verbal Communication related to loss of cognitive function* to describe the client with AD.

Outcomes. The client's needs will be communicated effectively, as evidenced by making her or his needs known and by interacting meaningfully with others. This outcome is only possible in the early stages. In later stages, a more appropriate outcome might be expressed as the client's needs are interpreted appropriately.

Interventions. In the initial stage of AD, the client's receptive and expressive language skills are relatively intact. The nurse must be prepared to adapt to the communication level of the client. If the client speaks only single words or short phrases, the nurse should do likewise. It is best to speak slowly and simply, with a firm volume and low pitch. The tone of voice should always be calm and reassuring and project control of the situation. When language becomes impaired in the second stage of the illness, be prepared to apply new techniques for communicating with the client.

Nonverbal behavior can provide clues about specific needs. Clients with AD often avert their eyes, look down, back away, and increase hand gesturing when they do not understand. If they are frustrated, angry, or hostile, they may increase motor activity by pacing, rattling doorknobs, waving their arms or shaking their fists, frowning, raising their voice volume and pitch, or tightening their facial muscles. These behaviors should signal staff to increase their alertness, search for the cause of the distress, and prepare to intervene.

The identification of pain or discomfort in clients with advanced AD is also difficult. Behavioral indicators of discomfort include noisy breathing, negative vocalization (constant muttering, making sounds with a negative quality), a sad or frightened facial expression, frowning, tense body language, and fidgeting.

Diagnosis: Impaired Memory. *Impaired Memory* is an ideal diagnosis for clients with AD. State this diagnosis as *Impaired Memory related to loss of short-term memory, inability to execute complex mental processes, or inability to concentrate or focus on specific tasks.*

Outcomes. The client will retain information to maximal capacity, maintain maximal orientation, and share meaningful life experiences.

Interventions. Because memory deficit occurs in all stages of AD, continually apply interventions to enhance memory. Reorient the client as necessary by placing a calendar and clock in obvious places. Because the client's long-term memory is retained longer than short-term memory, allow clients to reminisce. Become aware of a client's past experiences so that they can be shared meaningfully. Repetition is useful for ensuring maximal retention of information.

The client's memory loss can be an advantage in distracting him or her from the stressful situation. If removed from the situation and provided with calm, nonthreatening environment, clients may forget why they are upset. Elicit listening behavior by reaching out and touching, holding a hand, putting an arm around the waist, or in some way maintaining physical contact with the client. Dementia sufferers can perceive nonverbal behavior of others and can become agitated or upset if they sense negative nonverbal behavior from them. Having activities or interests, exercise periods, and opportunities to wander in a safe environment can do much to reduce anxiety and stress. The Management and Delegation feature at right discusses Communicating with Agitated Clients.

Diagnosis: Risk for Injury. Altered thought processes lead to impairments in judgment and forgetfulness. These changes increase risk for injury. State this common nursing diagnosis as *Risk for Injury related to impaired judgment, forgetfulness, and/or motor impairments.*

Outcomes. The client will be at reduced risk of injury by having the staff maintain a safe physical environment and the client having no physical injuries, near-falls, or falls.

Interventions

SAFETY
⚠
ALERT

In the inpatient setting, ensure that clients cannot leave the premises without being noticed, that they wear an identification badge in case they become lost, and that doors and windows are secured. In the home, electrical devices, toxic substances, loose rugs, hot tap water, inadequate lighting, and unlocked doors can be sources of injury. Teach family members how to eliminate these safety hazards. Dangerous objects should be kept out of

reach, and potentially dangerous activities, such as cooking, should be supervised. The client's driving skill should be evaluated at regular intervals. The Bridge to Home Health Care feature on p. 1900 addresses additional safety considerations for clients with AD.

Diagnosis: Self-Care Deficit. Clients in the middle stage of AD require assistance to put clothes on properly, bathe, and toilet. State this diagnosis as *Self-Care Deficit related to loss of memory and motor impairments.*

Outcomes. Clients will maintain self-care ability as evidenced by completing the tasks they are capable of performing and receiving assistance with ADL that they are incapable of performing.

Interventions. Encourage the client with AD to do as much as possible, as long as it is safe and appropriate. Carefully balance helping the client with maintaining his or her autonomy; this can boost the client's confidence and self-respect, which can be very fragile during

---

MANAGEMENT AND DELEGATION

Communicating with Agitated Clients

Many aspects of client care are performed by unlicensed assistive personnel. Almost all of these activities, from taking vital signs to giving a bath, require communicating with the client. When clients are demented, they often cannot understand spoken directions and respond with aggressive or frightened behavior.

Communication with clients who have dementia is difficult. They do not always understand what you are saying and may respond differently each time you attempt to work with them. For clients who need help to put on clothes, bathe, and get to the bathroom, spoken words can usually be understood if the words are simplified and the caregiver is patient. Identify yourself and call the client by name. Be certain that the client is wearing a hearing aid and glasses, if necessary. Do not startle the client or speak to the client in a derogatory manner. Use simple, direct statements, speaking slowly and calmly. Look at the face of the client and have light shining on your face. For example, do not stand with your back toward the window; you will be in a shadow from the client's view.

If the client makes no attempts to speak, nonverbal forms of communication become more important. Avoid approaching the client from the side or from behind. Keep your facial expression positive, your body language open. You should continue to speak using a calm tone of voice. A person with dementia who feels threatened or confused by your communication may react in negative ways, such as striking out or crying. Try to use the same caregiver each day. Use nonverbal cues, such as moving your arms and hands, to indicate "Please come with me" or "Please take this pill." Do not give more than one instruction at a time.

BRIDGE TO HOME HEALTH CARE

Safety Solutions for People with Alzheimer's Disease

To live with damaged thinking and judgment is to live at risk. People with Alzheimer's disease cannot take responsibility for their own safety. They are unable to evaluate the potential consequences of their actions and they forget quickly. Verbal reminders and written notes have little value, but there are many other ways to promote safety.

Many older people love to live surrounded by their treasures. Although a neat home is always safer than a cluttered one, anticipate that only small changes can be made. Suggest moving knickknacks so that the edges of surfaces can be used for balance. Retain the existing furniture arrangements but consider removing or altering furniture with sharp corners, rocking chairs that tip easily, coffee tables, and fragile antiques. Block off unsafe areas by placing a sturdy chair in front of them. Eliminate hazards such as trailing wires, extension cords, or telephone cords. Caution caregivers to watch for paper or wooden objects that are tossed into gas fireplaces.

Most accidents happen in the kitchen and the bathroom. Therefore it is important to thoroughly assess how the person with Alzheimer's disease uses those areas. Disable stoves by removing knobs, installing a special switch behind the stove, removing a fuse, or turning the stove off at the breaker. Because people with AD may retain overlearned food preparation skills, they may be able to use sharp utensils and hot surfaces safely, but do need to be supervised. Encourage them to participate in meal preparation by doing single steps of a task, such as tearing lettuce for a salad or putting plates on the table.

Remove rugs and runners that tend to slide, especially those in the bathroom. Install grab bars to help prevent falls during transfers into or out of the tub or shower. Bars should be attached to structural supports rather than drywall or plaster. Consider using a raised toilet seat if rising is difficult and a bedside commode at night if urgency is a problem. Bath benches with nonskid feet are best, and hand-held showers minimize the need for the person to move about. Lower the temperature on the water heater to 120° F so that the water cannot become hot enough to scald anyone. If hot pipes are exposed, cover them with insulation.

While walking is good exercise and can reduce stress, wandering can become a safety issue. If the environment is secured with a fence, camouflaged doors, or locks, people with dementia may move freely within a relatively safe area, reducing the stress of caregivers who are afraid to let them out of sight. It is important to balance freedom, safety, and client rights. If wandering away from home is a potential hazard, the Alzheimer's Association has an excellent program called "safe return." More information about this low-cost program is available by calling 1-800-272-3900; website www.alz.org.

SAFETY

ALERT

---

the early and middle stages of the disease. Give directions one at a time and plenty of time to complete a task.

Diagnosis: Urge Urinary and Fecal Incontinence. Clients in the middle stage of AD develop both urinary and bowel incontinence in the absence of pathology. State this nursing diagnosis as *Urge Urinary Incontinence or Self-Care Deficit: Toileting related to neuronal degeneration and forgetfulness.*

Outcomes. The client will have optimal bowel and bladder continence as evidenced by having dry, clean clothing and bedding as much as possible, having intact skin, and voiding appropriately in the bathroom.

Interventions. Anticipation of elimination needs and scheduled voiding and defecation times can help in the initial stages. The client may show nonverbal signs of needing to void or defecate, such as restlessness, grasping the genital area, or picking at clothing. Sometimes the client forgets where the bathroom is located. Having clear, bright signs indicating where the bathroom is and frequently taking the client there may help control incontinence. Fluid intake after the dinner meal can be restricted to help maintain continence during the night.

Try to arrange a bowel program to coincide with the client's usual pattern. In the later stages of AD, clients may need to wear incontinence briefs during the day and external urinary drainage devices at night. Indwelling catheters should be avoided because of the risk of infection and injury. Several varieties of disposable and extra-absorbent washable underwear, bed pads, and mattress covers are available. If the client is male, choose undergarments that allow him to urinate through an opened fly.

Diagnosis: Caregiver Role Strain. Family members and especially caregivers (usually the spouse or adult children) of the client with AD face a great deal of emotional and physical burden. (See Translating Evidence into Practice feature on p. 1901.) State this nursing diagnosis as *Caregiver Role Strain related to grieving the loss of a family member to AD, a change in social role, and intense demands for time commitment and provision of care.*

TRANSLATING EVIDENCE INTO PRACTICE

Caregivers and Caregiver Role Strain

The annual direct and indirect cost of caring for the 4.5 million people with Alzheimer's disease in the United States is estimated to be at least $100 billion. By 2030, when the entire Baby Boomer generation is age 65 and older, the increased number of people with Alzheimer's disease could exceed the ability to absorb the added cost. Historically, most of the long-term care for functionally impaired older adults has been provided by informal caregivers. Family caregivers provide 80% of chronic illness home care services to clients age 50 and older by providing day to day services. It is noted that as AD progresses, caregivers spend as many as 70 hours per week primarily monitoring and managing the cognitive decline of AD clients.[1] In 1997 the National Family Caregiver Survey found that nearly 1 in 4 (23% or 22.4 million) U.S. households was involved in helping care for an individual 50 years old or older, at some point during the previous 12 months. In telephone interviews of 1002 households, the results showed only 20% of the informal caregivers received any assistance in providing care from the formal health care system. Further, 60% of the caregivers reported they had had no formal training in the care they were providing.[2]

The burden of providing care for clients with dementia is particularly troublesome. The degree of cognitive impairment, amount of help required with activities of daily living, personality changes, and presence of psychiatric symptoms and behavioral disturbances cause the greatest concern.[2,3] The relationship between the client and the caregiver can become strained and isolation from friends and activities creates additional social isolation. Caregivers often experience clinically significant changes in physical and mental health, particularly depression.[1,4]

In a series of interviews, family members reported that they coped in two styles. One style, emotion-focused, was seen as grieving, worrying, and self-accusation. They were also the only ones using wishful thinking and stoicism as strategies. Problem-based copers confronted the problem and sought information and social support. The problem-based copers also used the emotion-focused strategy of acceptance in combination with seeking information and social support.[2] Spirituality was identified as an important coping mechanism among wife caregivers of people with dementia. It was shown that caregivers of persons with AD relied on prayer and religious coping to help them through the caregiving experience. To mix approaches like these seems to be an effective choice of strategy.[5]

Interventions on the communication techniques, behavioral strategies, and environmental modifications improved the quality of life of primary caregivers while reducing the anxiety and depression levels.[6,7] Family caregivers can provide practical training to enable health care professionals to provide better care for their family member. In addition, family caregivers need information and support in self-care activities that promote their health and well-being. A community-based interventional study investigated the effectiveness of a comprehensive educational program exploring problems most likely to be experienced by caregivers of Alzheimer's clients. Results of this study indicate that problems among caregivers of Alzheimer's clients, especially in an environment with limited respite care options, were improved by participating in the comprehensive educational intervention program.[8]

REFERENCES

1. Burns, A. (2000). The burden of Alzheimer's disease. *International Journal of Neuropsychopharmacology, 3*(7), 31-38.
2. Navaie-Waliser, M., Feldman, P.H., Gould, D.A., et al. (2001). Long-term care provision: Striking a balance between informal and formal caregiving. *Abstracts from the Academy of Health Service Research and Health Policy Meeting, 18,* 97.
3. Almberg, B., Grafstrom, M., & Winblad, B. (1997). Major strain and coping strategies as reported by family members who care for aged demented relatives. *Journal of Advanced Nursing, 26*(4), 683-691.
4. Takano, M., & Arai, H. (2005). Gender difference and caregivers' burden in early-onset Alzheimer's disease. *Psychogeriatrics, 5*(3), 73-77.
5. Spurlock, W.R. (2005). Spiritual well-being and caregiver burden in Alzheimer's caregivers. *Geriatric Nursing, 26*(30), 154-161.
6. Yahas, N., McGowan, B., et al. (2006). Psychosocial interventions for disruptive symptoms of dementia. *Journal of Psychosocial Nursing and Mental Health Services, 44*(11), 34-42.
7. Perry, J. (2002). Wives giving care to husband's with Alzheimer's disease: A process of interpretive caring. *Research in Nursing and Health, 25*(4), 307-316.
8. Kuzu, N., Beser, N., Zencir, M., et al. (2005). Effects of a comprehensive educational program on quality of life and emotional issues of dementia patient caregivers. *Geriatric Nursing, 26*(6), 378-385.

Outcomes. The family will demonstrate reduced role strain as evidenced by voicing their emotional concern, seeking appropriate assistance, and providing adequate care for the client.

Interventions. AD is called a "long goodbye" because the client with AD remains alive for many months to years during which time the client cannot interact with the family. Family members grieve the loss of the person they used to know. Each decline in cognitive function becomes another source of grief. Two stages of grief in the family have been described. The process of grief begins during the caregiving stage and continues after the client's death. Normal family routines are lost, and the relationship between the family member and the dementia sufferer changes. Factors that have the most profound effect on the emotional well-being of caregivers include incontinence, overly demanding behavior, and the need for constant supervision.

Wives tend to experience a higher degree of emotional burden as caregivers than husbands do. Paradoxically, the closer the emotional bond between caregiver and dementia sufferer, the less the strain for the caregiver. Conversely, a low past level of intimacy is associated with an increased level of both perceived strain and depression in the spouse caregiver. According to the literature, caregivers tend to be women.

Support for Caregivers. Interview family members to determine their understanding of the diagnosis and prognosis of AD and to allow them to discuss their concerns about caring for the client:

- Do they know about community resources?
- Do they have someone to call when they can no longer cope with caregiving?

The Alzheimer's Disease and Related Disorders Association has local chapters that offer support groups in many major cities in the United States (Phone: 1-800-272-3900).

A variety of options are available to caregivers. Chore service workers can help with household chores and relieve the caregiver of these duties. Other paid help can provide in-home respite care by observing the dementia sufferer while the caregiver tends to business outside the home, seeks social interaction, or meets recreational needs.

Adult day care provides time away from home for the dementia sufferer. Day care usually offers a lunchtime meal as well as several hours of scheduled activities that are tailored to the client's abilities. These activities may include games, crafts, music, and exercise.

Respite care involves admission of the client to an extended care facility for a few days to a few weeks to allow the caregiver time to recover from the demands of providing 24-hour care (see the Bridge to Home Health Care website feature on Respite Care for Caregivers of People with Alzheimer's Disease). Assisted living facilities with dementia units can also be used. These settings are home-like and can provide needed supervision as long as the client is ambulatory.

Nursing home care is usually the final and most difficult and trying option for a caregiver. This decision creates guilt, self-doubt, and anxiety; however, it may be the only option when the caregiver suffers burnout and becomes unable to provide adequate care. Table 72-1 lists nursing guidelines for meeting family needs.

Diagnosis: Decisional Conflict. State this diagnosis as *Decision Conflict related to the need to make crucial decisions about life and death for a loved one.*

Outcomes. The family will experience comfort that the decisions that they have made meet the needs and wishes of the client with AD and will be acceptable to themselves and other family members.

Interventions. When the person with AD reaches the terminal stage of illness, the family needs to plan for the inevitable end-of-life issues. Questions about CPR and use of feeding tubes and antibiotics for the treatment of pneumonia and other infections will need answers. Ideally, decisions about these questions are raised and discussed with the client and family members before the person loses the capacity to make decisions.

Two forms of *advance directives* (means of expressing one's wishes about life-sustaining treatment after losing the mental capacity to make informed decisions) are available. One is the *living will,* a written document signed by the individual (while he or she is still mentally capable of making informed decisions) in the presence of a witness. The living will lists conditions under which the person wishes life-sustaining treatments to be withheld or withdrawn. The other advance directive is a *durable power of attorney for health care.* This is a legal document in which the person (while still mentally capable) assigns someone to act on his or her behalf in matters of health care decisions if the person loses decisional capacity (e.g., becomes demented). The family needs to be advised early to seek legal assistance to set up trusts, power of attorney documents for finances and for health care, and a living will.

The nurses' role during this time is to listen and facilitate discussion and comprehension of decisions. For example, if the family decides not to tube-feed the client, they may later ask "is she hungry?" for which the answer is "no, she has no sensation of hunger." The nurse may also have to guide the family through grieving over the finality of the decisions they made. Consultation with clergy is often beneficial.

PARKINSON'S DISEASE

Parkinson's disease (PD) is a chronic, progressive, neurologic disorder that results from the loss of the neurotransmitter dopamine in a group of brain structures that control movements. Its major manifestations are variable but can include hand tremor, slowness of movements, limb stiffness, and difficulties with gait and balance. For the vast majority of individuals, PD is not thought to be an inherited disease. Even when a second person within a family is diagnosed with PD, this is thought to be more of a coincidence than an emerging genetic pattern because PD is a fairly common disorder among the older population. Parkinson's disease develops most often in people in their 60s, although it can strike much younger people as well. It occurs worldwide. About 1% of people older than age 50 have PD.

Parkinsonian manifestations may also develop from other problems, such as long-term use of phenothiazines; poisoning from carbon monoxide, mercury, or manganese; or traumatic injury to the midbrain.

When PD occurs, degenerative changes are found in an area of the brain known as the *substantia nigra,* which produces *dopamine,* a chemical substance that enables people to move normally and smoothly. Once

TABLE 72–1   Nursing Guidelines for Meeting the Needs of the Family of the Client with Dementia of the Alzheimer's Type

Goals	Selected Interventions
Physical	
Monitor chronic health problems or physical limitations of family caregiver.	Obtain health history of family caregiver to identify past and new health problems.
	Support family in following through with routine health examinations.
	Refer family members to physician when health problems are observed.
Identify development of new health problems.	Assess family's understanding of medical management of own health problems.
	Teach family members to preserve own health in order to continue caring for client with Alzheimer's disease.
Identify cues for stress.	Emphasize family's need for adequate nutrition, hydration, exercise, and rest.
Examine somatic health problems.	Help family members to be alert to signs of caregiver stress.
Psychosocial	
Assist family in coping positively with stress.	Instruct family to get respite regularly for rest and relaxation.
	Teach stress management techniques (e.g., relaxation, supportive relationships, goal setting, time management, diversion).
Identify destructive methods of coping (e.g., alcohol, drugs, tobacco, overeating or under-eating, physical abuse of client).	Refer family to physician, therapist when stress remains unmanageable even with social or psychological resources.
Assess family dynamics.	Refer signs of physical abuse to adult protective services.
Assist family members in dealing with role change and conflict.	Recognize the family's role, discuss capacity to provide care, and give reinforcement for care provided.
	Counsel family in dealing with role conflicts, unmet expectations, or interpersonal conflicts.
	Teach family the need to maintain roles and social activities outside caregiving experience.
	Administer burden interview.
	Reinforce family's attempt to cope.
	Acknowledge family fears of being unable to continue with caregiving.
If need for support identified, direct family members to sources (e.g., in-home respite care or senior day services, nursing home).	Refer family to a support group to share with others in similar situations.
	Refer family to nearest office on aging or Alzheimer's Disease and Related Disorders Association, Inc. (ADRDA), to identify benefits in community available to Alzheimer's disease clients.
Identify family's mixed emotions (e.g., depression, anger, resentment, pity, embarrassment, guilt).	Listen to family and facilitate sharing of emotions and feelings in supportive, empathic environment.
Identify alternative plans for care if family members or social support systems become unable to provide care or are ineffective.	Counsel and support family if client placed in care of others; allay feelings of guilt.
	Facilitate family meeting to identify time for socialization.
Identify financial limitations.	Encourage family to be specific about financial limitations.
	Offer family referrals (legal, financial, or social service) for information on eligibility for private, county, state, or federal financial support for home services; advise and counsel regarding power of attorney or guardianship, trust or estate planning.
Assess family's ability to make funeral plans.	Help family anticipate and cope with grief process.
	Assist family in making prefuneral arrangements.
	Address family's fear regarding the possible role of heredity in development of Alzheimer's disease, and assist in making decision regarding autopsy.
Environmental	
Identify compatibility of environment with family and client.	Conduct a family meeting to discuss relationship of family, client, and environment.
Assess learning needs regarding client care tasks.	Teach management of concurrent physical health problems of the client with Alzheimer's disease.
	Include family in development of client care plan.
	Teach family to encourage the client to continue daily habits to extent possible.
	Complete behavior problems' checklist.
	Anticipate likely problems and teach how to manage them.
	Teach environmental modification (consistent, simple, calm routines) to maximize family endurance and enhance safety.
	Teach family to relate to client with creative connectedness (touch, humor, flexibility, reminiscence, music, planned activities).
Assess family's need and desire for information about Alzheimer's disease and how it affects the client's behavior.	Assist family in understanding symptoms related to memory loss, nature of the illness, symptoms, stages of disease progression, and behavior manifestations.
	Provide written material to reinforce education and understanding (e.g., *The 36-Hour Day, Coping and Caring: Living with Alzheimer's Disease;* literature from local, state, or national ADRDA chapters).
	Supply ADRDA 24-hour hotline number: 1-800-272-3900; website: www.alz.org.

Modified from Stevenson, J.P. (1990). Family stress to home care of Alzheimer's disease patients and implications for support. *Journal of Neuroscience Nursing,* 22(3), 185.

cell loss in the substantia nigra reaches 80%, manifestations appear. The cause of nigral cell degeneration is not known. PD is characterized by a severe shortage of dopamine in relation to ACh in the basal ganglia, which leads to the clinical characteristics of PD.

Clinical Manifestations

The diagnosis of Parkinson's disease (PD) can be difficult. It is recommended that all people suspected of having PD be referred to a neurologist for diagnosis and initial planning of care. The manifestations do not appear until about 60% of the normal amount of dopamine is lost. The disease has six cardinal features: (1) tremor at rest on one side, the first manifestation in 70% of clients; (2) rigidity, increased tone, and stiffness in the muscles at rest; (3) bradykinesia (slow movement), fine movements become clumsy; (4) flexed posture of the neck, trunk, and limbs; (5) loss of postural reflexes; and (6) freezing movement.

Early in the disease, the client may notice a slight slowing in the ability to perform ADL *(bradykinesia)*. A general feeling of stiffness *(rigidity)* may be noticed, along with mild, diffuse muscular pain. *Tremor* is a common early manifestation that usually occurs in one of the upper limbs. It occurs at rest and involves a coarse "pill-rolling" movement of the thumb against the fingers that can vary in intensity and distribution. Voluntary movement stops or reduces the tremor in some people; however, others may have tremor during voluntary movement *(intention tremor)* as well.

Bradykinesia makes voluntary movements difficult to execute. When manifestations are severe, total lack of movement *(akinesia)* may occur and the client is literally frozen in one spot. Bradykinesia also affects gait. Initially there may be a slight stiffness of one leg while walking, and the ipsilateral arm may be held flexed at the elbow and abducted at the shoulder. The person may catch or drag one foot. Later, when both sides of the body are involved, the typical shuffling gait with short steps may develop. There is lack of associated swinging of the arms while walking. In advanced PD, the client stands with head, shoulders, and spine flexed forward, giving the appearance of a stooped posture (Figure 72-3).

The face of someone with advanced PD appears stiff, mask-like, and without expression. Speech is low in volume, monotonous in tone, and slow. Words are poorly articulated *(dysarthria)*. Saliva may flow involuntarily from the mouth because of the lack of spontaneous swallowing. PD clients may also exhibit *micrographia*—small, cramped handwriting.

Usually PD does not affect intellectual ability; however, a dementia similar to that of AD develops in 15% to 20% of clients with PD. Fatigue is a common occurrence; everyday tasks take longer and require more concentration. PD symptoms can disturb sleep. Immobility

■ **FIGURE 72–3** Gait changes seen in Parkinson's disease. Some of the clinical manifestations of Parkinson's disease are stooped posture, bradykinesia, and a festinant gait.

slows gastric motility, and drug therapy contributes to constipation. Mood disturbance can occur, and emotional stress may intensify clinical manifestations. As many as 50% of PD clients have an episode of depression during this illness.

The course of the disease is slowly progressive. The person becomes more rigid and more disabled, eventually requiring full assistance with ADL.

OUTCOME MANAGEMENT

The goal of management of PD is to control the manifestations with the lowest possible dose of medication in order to avoid side effects. Medication selection and dosage are tailored to the client; factors considered are the severity of manifestations, the age of the client, and the presence of other medical conditions. Every client responds differently to a medication or dosage level, so this process involves experimentation, persistence, and patience.

Because clients with PD lack dopamine, it follows that a pharmacologic replacement of dopamine would be used. Dopamine does not cross the blood-brain barrier, but its precursor, L-dopa does. L-dopa is combined with carbidopa to prevent the breakdown of L-dopa so that smaller doses can be used. In general, most clients are treated with selegiline, a monoamine oxidase inhibitor, to block one pathway in the breakdown of dopamine. When manifestations become more pronounced, L-dopa/carbidopa (Sinemet) or a dopamine receptor agonist (pergolide) is used. Anticholinergics and antivirals are also used. These medications are gradually increased until the optimal therapeutic response is achieved. This process may take several months. When the daily dose of L-dopa approaches the desired level, the client often has involuntary *dyskinesias* (jerky, writhing movements), especially of the face, mouth, and tongue. Some clients prefer this stage to being severely bradykinetic because at least they can be mobile and perform voluntary movements more easily. Anticholinergics are used to reduce the tremor. The Complementary and Alternative Therapy feature below describes the possible benefits of coenzyme Q_{10} therapy.

Medical Management

Manage the Parkinsonian Crisis

Occasionally clients with PD experience a parkinsonian crisis as a result of emotional trauma or sudden or inadvertent withdrawal of anti-parkinsonian medication. Severe exacerbation of tremor, rigidity, and bradykinesia, accompanied by acute anxiety, sweating, tachycardia, and hyperpnea, occur. Intervention for parkinsonian crisis includes respiratory and cardiac support. The client should be placed in a quiet room with subdued lighting. Barbiturates may be prescribed in addition to anti-parkinsonian drugs.

Manage the On/Off Response

An *on/off response* (rapid fluctuation of clinical manifestations) may occur in clients with PD; the client may be mobile and active ("on") one moment and akinetic and rigid ("off") the next. This transition may happen quickly, within 1 to 2 minutes. Initially the off periods tend to occur 3 to 4 hours after a dose of anti-parkinsonian medication. Later the transition may happen any time and may be unrelated to medication ingestion. Apparently, off periods are due to dopamine deficit, but this factor is not clear. A person experiencing on/off response may be temporarily helped by shortening the interval between medication doses or by gradually increasing the total dosage.

Medications such as ropinirole may be given in addition to other PD medications to help stabilize the fluctuations.

COMPLEMENTARY AND ALTERNATIVE THERAPY

Coenzyme Q_{10} Supplements and Parkinson's Disease

Parkinson's disease is a neurologic disorder that currently has no treatment that has demonstrated a reduction in the progression of this disease. Researchers conducted a multicenter, randomized, parallel-group, placebo-controlled, double-blind, dosing-ranging trial. The participants in this trial were 80 individuals with early Parkinson's disease that did not require treatment for their condition. Clients were randomly assigned to placebo or coenzyme Q_{10} at dosages of 300, 600, or 1200 mg/day. Clients were followed for 16 months or until disability requiring treatment with levodopa had developed. Researchers found that coenzyme Q_{10} supplements were safe and well tolerated at dosages of up to 1200 mg/day. Less overall disability developed in clients assigned to coenzyme Q_{10} than in those assigned to placebo, and the benefit was greatest in the clients consuming the highest dose. Coenzyme Q_{10} seemed to slow the progressive deterioration of function in Parkinson's disease. Clients taking the highest dosage (1200 mg/day) had deterioration slowed by 44%. The greatest benefit was observed for daily activities such as feeding, dressing, bathing, and walking. By the eighth month, clients taking the highest dose scored significantly better than the placebo group.

REFERENCE

Shults, C., et al. (2002). Effects of coenzyme Q10 in early Parkinson disease: Evidence of slowing of the functional decline. *Archives of Neurology, 59,* 1541-1550.

Nursing Management of Parkinson's Disease

Nursing care of the PD client includes health assessment, medication instruction and monitoring, liaison with other members of the health care team, and client and family education. Case managers are often used to guide transitions from one facility to the next.

Advise the client to maintain fluid intake of 2 L every 24 hours and to increase the intake of dietary fiber. Stool softeners and mild laxatives can be used. A regular time for bowel movements should be established, usually ½ hour after the morning or evening meal.

Teach the client various techniques to enhance voluntary physical movement. Clients often need to try different strategies on their own to find what helps most. Some clients grasp coins in their pocket to reduce embarrassing hand tremor. Others grip the arms of a chair. Mental thoughts, such as walking over imaginary lines, can aid ambulation. One client may find that tossing small scraps of paper in front of him aids his walking, and another may find that rocking back and forth helps initiate movement. Encourage daily range-of-motion exercises to avoid rigidity and contractures. Remind the client to maintain good posture and to avoid flexion of the neck and shoulders. The client should sleep on a firm mattress. When resting, the client should avoid using a pillow to prevent flexion of the spine. Periodically lying prone also helps.

The benefits of regular daytime rest should be encouraged. The PD client should be encouraged to rest in bed laying flat for 30 minutes to 1 hour at the same time every day. By resting during the day, the PD client will experience renewed energy for the rest of the day.

Because self-care activities are performed more slowly by the client with PD, extra time should be allowed for completion of tasks such as dressing, bathing, and eating. Warming trays can keep food hot. Recommend rest periods during meals to avoid aspiration. Activities of daily living (ADL) or exercise should be performed when drugs are working well to avoid injury to the client and caregiver.

As PD progresses, clients become rigid and unresponsive to verbal stimuli. During these stages, continue to treat clients with dignity, speaking to the clients rather than ignoring them.

Teach the client about home safety. Loose carpeting should be removed. Grab bars should be placed in the bathroom. An elevated toilet seat should be installed. Clients with severe tremor should avoid carrying hot liquids. Walking aids such as a cane or walker can provide added stability. The Client Education Guide below suggests additional interventions for clients with Parkinson's disease.

SAFETY
ALERT

CLIENT EDUCATION GUIDE

Parkinson's Disease

Make sure that you understand how to take your medications on schedule and to not forget a dose. Know the importance of following the correct diet, and what side effects you can expect from your medications.

To avoid rigidity and the development of contractures:

■ Exercise and stretch regularly.
■ Perform the exercises recommended in your self-help booklets.
■ Exercise first thing in the morning, when your energy levels are highest.
■ Exercise in bed if getting to the floor is difficult.
■ Get out of a chair by bending over slowly so that your head is over your toes; avoid soft, deep chairs.

If your health care provider has told you that you have bradykinesia (slow movements):

■ Rock back and forth to get going.
■ Imagine that you are stepping over an imaginary line when you walk.
■ Throw small objects (e.g., small scraps of paper) in front of you to practice fine motor movements.
■ Count to yourself while walking.
■ Visualize your intended movement.
■ Maintain a wide-based gait.
■ Maintain upright posture and look up, not down, especially when walking.

If you have a tremor:

■ Hold change in your pocket or squeeze a small rubber ball.
■ Use both hands to accomplish tasks.
■ Lie face down on the floor and relax your entire body.
■ Sleep on the side that has the tremor.

If you have trouble getting dressed:

■ Dress and undress in front of a mirror.
■ Use adaptive devices such as long-handled shoehorns and button fasteners.
■ Buy clothes with self-fasteners (e.g., Velcro) and slide-locking buckles.

To ensure safety:

■ Wear good, sturdy shoes.
■ Use a cane or walker.
■ Concentrate on standing upright.
■ Consciously pick up your feet to take steps.
■ Remove all throw rugs, electrical cords, and clutter from the floor.
■ Make sure that you have adequate lighting.
■ Arrange essential items so that they are within easy reach.
■ Use a bath chair and a hand-held shower nozzle.
■ Have grab bars installed in the bathroom.
■ Have a raised toilet seat installed.

To ensure good communication:

■ Pause between every few words.
■ Exaggerate the pronunciation of words.
■ Finish saying the final consonant of a word before starting to say the next word.
■ Express ideas in short, concise phrases.
■ Plan what to say.
■ Face the listener.

To ensure adequate swallowing and prevent aspiration:

■ Think through the steps of swallowing:
  ■ Keep your lips closed.
  ■ Keep your teeth together.
  ■ Put food on your tongue.
  ■ Lift your tongue up and back.
  ■ Swallow.
■ Eat slowly, taking small bites.
■ Chew hard and move food around with your tongue.
■ Finish one bite before taking another.
■ Eat in an upright chair.
■ Consume a high-fiber diet to prevent constipation.
■ Avoid caffeine; caffeine increases PD symptoms.

To keep saliva from building up in your mouth:

■ Make a conscious effort to swallow saliva often.
■ Keep your head in an upright position so saliva will collect in the back of your throat and *stimulate automatic swallowing*.
■ Swallow excess saliva before attempting to speak.

The client and family need emotional support. Support groups are available in most major cities. Refer the client and family to the American Parkinson Disease Association (1-800-223-APDA) or the website www.apdaparkinson.com.

Surgical Management

Surgical interventions are used for PD. Intractable tremor *(dyskinetic movement)* may be ameliorated by pallidotomy. Fetal tissue transplantation and genetically engineered cells that produce dopamine are in experimental stages. Deep brain stimulation is also used to treat uncontrollable movement. Deep brain stimulation involves electrodes implanted in the thalamus or globus pallidus. The device uses electrical currents to "jam" abnormal brain signals.

CREUTZFELDT-JAKOB DISEASE

Creutzfeldt-Jakob disease (CJD) is a rare, fatal brain disease that produces progressive dementia, myoclonus, and distinctive electroencephalographic (EEG) changes. CJD is a unique disease that apparently can arise from two separate mechanisms: genetic and infectious. People with the genetic form have a mutated gene. The infectious form does not develop from a known virus or other pathogen; therefore words such as *virion, slow virus,* and *prion* are sometimes used to describe the etiologic agent. Several reports document human-to-human spread of CJD from transplanted tissue from a person with CJD. Incubation periods have ranged from 4 to 21 years, which indicates the enormous difficulty of tracing the infection. In 1996 CJD was associated with ingestion of infected beef. This led to the popular term *mad cow disease.*

Clinical Manifestations

Manifestations include vague psychiatric or behavior changes suggesting a personality change. About one third of clients report weight loss, anorexia, insomnia, malaise, and dizziness for a period of weeks to months. In the early stages, there is progressive memory loss, visual impairment, and dysphagia. Within a few weeks or months, a relentlessly progressive dementia develops and marked deterioration is noted from week to week. *Myoclonus* (twitching) is usually present. Deterioration is rapid, with 90% of clients dying within 1 year.

A definitive diagnosis attempts to differentiate CJD from AD, which has a more protracted course and no myoclonus or EEG changes. Lithium toxicity can mimic the manifestations, but they clear within about 2 weeks after discontinuation of the drug. Brain biopsy during hospitalization or on autopsy is the usual method of establishing a definitive diagnosis. According to the World Health Organization, diagnostic criteria for CJD include progressive dementia and the presence of at least two of the following: myoclonus, extraocular or cerebellar disturbance, pyramidal/extrapyramidal dysfunction, and akinetic mutism. In addition there should be at least one of the following findings: electroencephalogram (EEG) typical for CJD regardless of the clinical duration of the disease; a positive 14-3-3 assay for cerebrospinal fluid. Laboratory values have been more helpful than EEGs in diagnosing CJD.

OUTCOME MANAGEMENT

No effective treatment is available, and CJD appears to be uniformly fatal. Nursing care is directed at supportive care—preventing skin breakdown, supplying nutrition, and providing emotional support to the client and family. Families require much support, care, and concern as they try to cope with the sudden onset of this debilitating disease and with managing the day-to-day care of the client.

Although CJD can be transmitted, the risk to health care workers and others having contact with the client is no more than that to the general population. Isolation of clients is not indicated, but personnel should wear gloves when handling tissues, blood, and spinal fluid. Accidental skin contact with possibly infected material should be followed by washing in 10% normal sodium hydroxide or a solution of 5% household chlorine bleach. The agent can be inactivated on surfaces by using a 10% bleach solution for 1 hour. Surgical and pathologic instruments should be steam-autoclaved for 1 hour at 132° C. No organs, tissue, or tissue products from clients with CJD or any other ill-defined neurologic disorders should be used for transplantation or replacement therapy.

HUNTINGTON'S DISEASE

Huntington's disease (HD), also known as *Huntington's chorea,* is an autosomal-dominant degenerative neurologic disease. It is characterized by abnormal movements *(chorea* has the same word root as *choreography),* intellectual decline, and emotional disturbance. Clinical manifestations usually begin in the 30s and 40s, although occasionally they begin in young adulthood or even in children. Women and men are equally affected. The disease is relentlessly progressive, leading to disability and death within 15 to 20 years. Death usually results from respiratory tract complications caused by aspiration. According to 1 report in the United States alone, about 30,000 people have HD and its prevalence is estimated to be about 1 in every 10,000 people. It is estimated that at least 150,000 others have a 50% risk of developing the disease and thousands more of their relatives live with the possibility that they may develop HD.

The disease is autosomal dominant; offspring of an affected person have a 50% chance of inheriting the disease. Because HD does not skip generations, offspring who have not inherited the disease will not pass it on to their offspring. The abnormal gene has been isolated on chromosome 4.

Pathophysiology

The pathologic changes of HD involve degeneration of the striatum (caudate and putamen) in the basal ganglia. Other subtle changes occur in the cortex and cerebellum, namely, loss of neurons and an increased number of glial cells (gliosis). The degeneration of the caudate nucleus leads to a reduction in several neurotransmitters, including gamma-aminobutyric acid, ACh, substance P, and metenkephalin, and their synthetic enzymes. This change leaves relatively higher concentrations of the other neurotransmitters—dopamine, and norepinephrine. The relative excess of dopamine in HD, a disorder of excessive movement, can be contrasted to the lack of dopamine in Parkinson's disease (PD), a disorder of lack of movement.

Clinical Manifestations

Emotional disturbances and mental deterioration may precede the abnormal movements. The person may become negative, suspicious, and irritable. This condition may progress to depression and psychosis. Temper outbursts and sexual promiscuity may also occur. Severe mood swings are common. Cognitive decline progresses, and eventually the person becomes demented, incontinent, and completely unable to provide self-care.

The abnormal movements in HD are subtle at first. The person may appear restless or fidgety. The person may be aware of these movements and try to mask them by making them seem to be parts of intentional movements, such as head scratching or leg crossing. As the disease progresses, the rapid, jerky choreiform movements become more pronounced and involve all muscles. The person is constantly in motion. Stress, emotional situations, and attempts to perform voluntary movement can aggravate the abnormal movements. During sleep the movements diminish or disappear.

The diagnosis of HD is made on the basis of clinical manifestations and family history because there is no specific diagnostic test for the disease itself. CT or MRI imaging of the brain may show atrophy of the head of the caudate, but this factor alone is not diagnostic of HD.

OUTCOME MANAGEMENT

Medical Management

There is no pharmacologic treatment for HD. Haloperidol, a dopamine blocker, can control the abnormal movements and some behavioral manifestations. Diazepam can be used to lower anxiety, thereby aiding in control of movements. Antidepressants can help depression.

The duration of HD ranges from 10 to 30 years. The most common causes of death are infection (most commonly pneumonia) and injuries related to a fall or other complications.

Nursing Management of Huntington's Disease

One of the most common and dangerous problems in the middle to late stages is dysphagia. Several interventions should be tried. Medications need to be evaluated for their anticholinergic and sedative effects, which may impair swallowing. Mealtimes should be free of stress and clutter and have an unhurried atmosphere. Use of adaptive eating utensils can encourage and extend independence in eating. The diet should include foods that are easy to swallow and form a bolus in the mouth (e.g., canned peaches, chopped meat in gravy and mashed potatoes, custards). Many clients with HD may require an intake of 5,000 calories a day without gaining weight because of their excessive movements. They should try eating frequent, small meals containing high-calorie foods. Vitamins or other nutritional supplements may be added to their diet. Clients should sit upright when eating. While swallowing, they should keep the chin down toward the chest. They can be trained to hold their breath before swallowing and cough after each mouthful is swallowed to clear the throat of any residual food. Clients with HD are at risk for dehydration and may require large quantities of fluids, especially during hot weather. In some cases water may be thickened with commercial additives to give it the consistency of syrup.

If the client continues to have difficulty eating and loses weight despite dietary and environmental modifications, a feeding tube may become necessary; however, artificial feeding methods often frighten families, and they pose ethical dilemmas about prolonging life. Nurses can help clients and their families make these difficult decisions by clarifying the issues and providing information on the types, risks, benefits, and long-term effects of artificial feeding methods.

Poor control of oral and respiratory muscles can make communication difficult. The nurse can assist the family in developing signals such as raising a hand or keeping the eyes open or closed for yes and no responses. If physical signals are not an option, cards with printed words may be helpful. Keep communication simple and unstrained. Repeat words that are understood to let the client know that communication has been successful.

Excessive movements and falls may cause physical injury and can restrict independence. Pads on wheelchairs and beds, shin guards, and walking belts can prevent injury. Aids for ambulation (e.g., walking behind a wheelchair) can extend independence. Clothing should be light and simple to put on and take off. SAFETY ⚠ ALERT

Huntington's disease has a major impact on the family, not only because of the burden of caregiving but also because of the risk to offspring of inheriting the disease. Many ethical dilemmas surrounding the issue of privacy can surface in cases of HD. Whether test results are positive or negative, the results are of interest to the spouse, other family members, employers, and insurers; however, principles of confidentiality forbid disclosure of medical information to anyone without the client's consent. Be sensitive to the client's desire for confidentiality, but use this opportunity to teach the client about the effect the disease may have on other family members. Because a blood test is now available to check for the presence of the abnormal gene, family members face difficult choices about whether to find out if they have the Huntington gene. Information is available for clients and families living with HD from the Huntington's Disease Society of America (telephone: 1-800-345-HDSA, website: www.hdsa.org).

MULTIPLE SCLEROSIS

Multiple sclerosis (MS) is a chronic demyelinating disease that affects the myelin sheath of neurons in the central nervous system (CNS). The myelin sheath is essential for normal conduction of nerve impulses. Patches of myelin deteriorate at irregular intervals along the nerve axon, causing slowing of nerve conduction. Axonal destruction also occurs in MS.

The onset of MS usually occurs between 20 and 40 years of age, and it affects women twice as often as men. Whites are affected more often than Hispanics, blacks, or Asians. The disease is most prevalent in the colder climates of North America and Europe. If someone is born in an area of high risk for MS and moves to an area of low risk after age 15, the person carries the risk of the area of origin.

Etiology and Risk Factors

The exact cause of MS is unknown. Most theories suggest that MS is an immunogenetic-viral disease, that is, an immune-mediated demyelination triggered by a viral infection, probably with the Epstein-Barr virus. A genetic susceptibility apparently alters the body's immune response to viral infection. Multiple genes are probably involved; however, the only consistently identified disease locus is on the human leukocyte antigen (HLA) gene complex on chromosome 6.

A variety of precipitating factors can precede the onset or an exacerbation of MS, such as infection, physical injury, emotional stress, pregnancy, and fatigue. Most pregnancy-related exacerbations occur 3 months postpartum and may relate more to the stress of labor and fatigue during the puerperium than to the pregnancy itself.

Pathophysiology

Myelin is a highly conductive fatty material that surrounds the axon and speeds conduction of nerve impulses along the axon. Myelin is made by oligodendrocytes. Both autoimmune processes and infectious agents have been implicated in the pathogenesis of multiple sclerosis. Activated T cells, which recognize self-antigens expressed in the CNS, and macrophages enter the brain from the peripheral circulation and initiate the inflammation. Through the production of inflammatory cytokines and reactive oxygen species, activated T lymphocytes and microglia/macrophages cause the demyelination and destruction of oligodendrocytes. Plaques form along the myelin sheath, eventually causing scarring and destruction (Figure 72-4). When edema and inflammation subside, some remyelination occurs but is often incomplete. Although plaques may occur anywhere in the white matter of the CNS, the areas most commonly involved are the optic nerves, cerebrum, and cervical spinal cord.

Clinical Manifestations

The wide variety of manifestations possible with MS and the unpredictable nature of the disease pose many challenges to the client and family. The course of illness varies from person to person. Four clinical patterns have been identified (Figure 72-5). The most common initial pattern is *relapsing-remitting* MS. Clients experience manifestations that eventually remit with little or no progression of disability.

■ **FIGURE 72–4** Changes in the nerve sheath, as seen in multiple sclerosis. Myelin is made by oligodendrocytes and coats peripheral nerves, facilitating the nerve impulse. In clients with multiple sclerosis, the myelin degenerates in patches, causing nerve transmission to become erratic.

Disease Category	Pattern	Definition
Relapsing-remitting		Episodes of acute worsening with recovery and a stable course between relapses
Secondary progressive		Gradual neurologic deterioration with or without superimposed acute relapses in a client who previously had relapsing-remitting multiple sclerosis
Primary progressive		Gradual, nearly continuous neurologic deterioration from the onset of manifestations
Progressive relapsing		Gradual neurologic deterioration from the onset of manifestations but with subsequent superimposed relapses

■ **FIGURE 72–5** Clinical patterns of multiple sclerosis. *(Modified from Lublin, F.D., & Reingold, S.C. [1996]. Defining the clinical course of multiple sclerosis: Results of an international survey. Neurology, 46, 907-911.)*

The random distribution of MS plaques leads to several clinical manifestations:

- Weakness or tingling sensations (paresthesias) of one or more extremities caused by involvement of the cerebrum or spinal cord
- Vision loss from optic neuritis
- Incoordination that is due to cerebellar involvement
- Bowel and bladder dysfunction as a result of spinal cord involvement

Bladder dysfunction can take several forms, depending on which neural pathways are affected. Dysfunction may involve hesitancy, frequency, loss of sensation, incontinence, and retention. Increased or decreased detrusor muscle, bladder neck, or external sphincter tone, or a combination of these problems, may occur. The ultimate bladder dysfunction, however, is usually hyperreflexia in association with sphincter dyssynergia (sphincter contraction during detrusor contraction).[3] Proper diagnosis of the type of bladder dysfunction requires a thorough history, laboratory assessment of kidney function, and identification of possible infection. If bladder emptying is defective, further investigation with urography, cystoscopy, and urodynamic studies should be performed.

Constipation is commonly experienced by clients with MS. Dysfunction can result from one or more of the following factors: spinal cord lesion, immobility, dehydration, medications, and nutritional deficiencies. Fecal incontinence, although rarer, is also possible. Sexual dysfunction can also occur as a result of lesions in the ascending or descending autonomic and sensory fibers in the spinal cord.

Fatigue is a common manifestation of MS and usually one of the most disabling. Spasticity can reduce energy, inhibit motor control, and interfere with self-care, sexuality, vocational responsibilities, and recreation. Physical fatigue can be easily induced in MS by a short walk or other physical activity. For some reason, also not fully

understood, the efficiency of demyelinated nerves deteriorates very rapidly with use. Almost everyone whose physical functioning has been disturbed through MS finds that their ability to perform an activity is reduced each time it is attempted.

Because MS strikes young adults during their years of establishing a family and an occupation, the impact of the disease can be devastating. Depression often occurs in clients, but it is not clear whether depression is a reaction to disability or a function of the disease itself. Others may experience euphoria, emotional instability, or apathy.

Because there is no definitive test for MS, clinicians rely on a detailed history, clinical findings, and a variety of diagnostic tests. The history often reveals several episodes of neurologic dysfunction, separated by time and by different locations in the CNS. Current research looking at clients who experience only one manifestation, such as optic neuritis, is changing the way clinicians diagnose MS.

Diagnostic tests include the following:

- Cerebrospinal fluid (CSF) evaluation for the presence of oligoclonal banding
- Evoked potentials of the optic pathways and auditory system to assess the presence of slowed nerve conduction
- MRI of the brain and spinal cord to determine the presence of MS plaques

OUTCOME MANAGEMENT

Medical Management of Multiple Sclerosis

The most important therapeutic aim of any disease-modifying treatment of MS is to prevent or postpone long-term disability. Long-term disability in MS often evolves slowly over many years. Treatment generally falls into one of three categories: (1) treatment of acute relapses, (2) treatment aimed at disease management, and (3) symptomatic treatment.

Treat Acute Relapses

Treatment of acute relapses usually involves the use of intravenous (IV) or oral corticosteroids, which have both anti-inflammatory and immunosuppressive properties. They are often used to enhance recovery from an exacerbation. Methylprednisolone is standard therapy for acute exacerbations sometimes followed by an oral prednisone taper. Azathioprine (Imuran) and cyclophosphamide (Cytoxan), other immunosuppressive agents, may be used for more severe exacerbations or progressive MS.

Treat Exacerbations

Interferon-β_{1b} (Betaseron) is used for ambulatory clients with relapsing-remitting MS. Interferon-β_{1b} is a genetically engineered complex protein with both antiviral and immunoregulatory properties that can reduce the number of MS exacerbations. The drug is injected subcutaneously every other day. Interferon-β_{1a} (Avonex) is also available for the treatment of relapsing forms of MS. In addition to reducing the number and severity of relapses, interferon-β_{1a} has provided a delay in disability in placebo-controlled studies.

The third disease-modifying agent available for use in the United States is glatiramer acetate (Copaxone), a synthetic polypeptide approved for use in relapsing-remitting MS. It is not an interferon but is believed to work by mimicking myelin basic protein and interrupting the inflammatory cascade to prevent damage to myelin.

Side effects of the interferons include fever, fatigue, and flu-like manifestations. Clients taking interferon-β_{1a} have also reported increased depression and injection site reactions. Copaxone does not produce the interferon-type side effects of fever and flu-like manifestations, but rare episodes of face flushing, chest tightness, and shortness of breath lasting less than 15 minutes have been reported. Numerous other therapeutic agents are undergoing clinical trials.

Symptomatic Treatment

Several strategies are available for symptomatic management in MS. Pharmacologic interventions can be used for bladder dysfunction (oxybutynin, propantheline), constipation (psyllium hydrophilic mucilloid, bisacodyl pills or suppositories), fatigue (amantadine, modafinil), spasticity (baclofen, diazepam, dantrolene), tremor (propranolol, phenobarbital, clonazepam), and dysesthesias and trigeminal neuralgia (carbamazepine, phenytoin, amitriptyline).

Transcutaneous electrical nerve stimulation (TENS) is also helpful for dysesthesias. Areas of numbness should be inspected regularly to prevent injury and development of pressure ulcers. Skin should be kept dry and free of urine and feces. A seat cushion that distributes pressure should be used for wheelchair-bound clients with insensate buttock skin. Blindness or severely impaired vision may occur. In this case, refer the client to Services for the Blind for rehabilitation. Cognitive and perceptual impairment necessitates psychometric and functional testing for accurate assessment and rehabilitation services.

Nursing Management of Multiple Sclerosis

Assessment. If the client is being assessed for possible MS, you should assess the client for clinical manifestations of the disorder. Ocular manifestations are very common. As a result of the fluctuations of clinical manifestations, the client may report a past history of similar findings that disappeared. The Care Plan on pp. 1912-1913 includes applicable nursing diagnoses and interventions for a client with multiple sclerosis.

If the client is being hospitalized for an exacerbation of MS, focus on the client's ability to perform ADL as well as other areas that require fine motor movements. Gross motor activities, such as walking, may also be impaired and may lead to problems with bowel and bladder continence.

Depression is commonly seen in clients with MS. It may be caused by the situation or stress. The potential for MS to progress to permanent disability can instigate depression. Likewise, MS may destroy the insulating myelin that surrounds nerves that transmit signals affecting mood, thus causing depression. Depression is also a side effect of some drugs used to treat MS, such as steroids or interferon.

Fatigue is common in clients with MS. Sleep disturbance is cited as one possible explanation; clients with MS are three times as likely to have disturbed sleep as the rest of the population. A number of factors contribute to this, including a reduction in sleep efficiency (demonstrated by polysomnographic studies), periodic involuntary leg movements, and urinary urgency.

The client with MS needs to have a clear understanding of the unpredictability of this disorder. The client may be free of manifestations for many weeks to months, even years, and then experience them. If the client can identify stressors that exacerbate the clinical manifestations, sometimes these stressors can be avoided. The National Multiple Sclerosis Society can be an excellent resource for education and support. For clients receiving one of the three disease-modifying pharmacologic agents, each pharmaceutical company has a support program to offer education, financial information, and support for clients with MS and their families.

Evaluate the client's social support system, which contributes to a sense of well-being. Grieving the loss

C A R E   P L A N   *evolve*

Client with Multiple Sclerosis

Nursing Diagnosis: Impaired Urinary Elimination. Demyelination of the nerves supplying the bladder may result in altered bladder function (neurogenic bladder). This nursing diagnosis is stated as *Impaired Urinary Elimination related to bladder dysfunction.*

Outcomes: The client will maintain urinary continence and normal bladder filling as evidenced by residual volumes of less than 100 ml, application of appropriate bladder elimination procedures, and verbalization of personal satisfaction with urinary elimination status.

NOC OUTCOMES   Urinary Elimination

Interventions	NIC INTERVENTIONS	Rationales
1. Assess skin for incontinence-associated dermatitis with each voiding.	Urinary Incontinence Care	1. Urine in contact with skin causes injury to the skin and denudement.

2. Maintain fluid intake of 2000 ml/24 hr:
  a. 400-500 ml with each meal
  b. 200 ml tid between meals
  c. Limited fluid intake after 6 PM
	Fluid Management	2. Adequate fluid intake promotes adequate urine production and improves urine volume at each voiding. Limited fluids after the evening meal reduces nighttime voiding/incontinence.

3. Toilet every 3 hr while awake.	Urinary Elimination Management	3. Bladder training with routine voiding reduces the risk of incontinence.
4. Scan bladder to confirm postvoid residual (PVR) volume.	Urinary Elimination Management	4. Urinary retention is determined by measuring the postvoid residual (PVR) urine volume 10-20 min after the person has voided.
5. If PVR is >100 ml, catheterize the bladder using sterile technique in the hospital.	Urinary Catheterization: Intermittent	5. A PVR volume >100 ml indicates incomplete bladder emptying. In older adult clients, a PVR of 150-200 ml or greater (measured on 2 separate occasions) indicates incomplete bladder emptying.
6. Instruct client on self-catheterization with a clean catheter.	Urinary Catheterization: Intermittent	6. Sterile equipment is not required for ongoing catheterization at home. A clean red rubber catheter can be reused for up to 1 week so long as it is washed thoroughly with soap and water and placed in a clean, tightly sealed plastic bag after every catheterization.

Nursing Diagnosis: Constipation. Immobility and demyelination lead to constipation. State this common nursing diagnosis as *Constipation related to immobility and demyelination.*

Outcomes: The client will have bowel movements of normal consistency and frequency.

NOC OUTCOMES   Bowel Elimination, Bowel Continence

Interventions	NIC INTERVENTIONS	Rationales
1. Assess normal bowel movement pattern.	Bowel Training Intervention	1. Daily BM is not everyone's pattern.
2. Develop a bowel program with suppositories or digital stimulation 45 min after breakfast.	Bowel Management Intervention	2. The gastrocolic reflex is most intense after breakfast.
3. Avoid routine use of enemas and laxatives.	Bowel Management Intervention	3. Routine use of laxatives and enemas leads to dependence for BMs.
4. Perform manual disimpaction if other methods do not work.	Bowel Management Intervention	4. Manual disimpaction is the last step of any bowel program.
5. Teach client to consume a high-fiber diet and 2000 ml of fluid.	Bowel Training Intervention	5. Fiber is not digested, so it adds to the bulk of BM, making it easier to pass. Fluid is absorbed from the large colon; so maintaining fluid intake softens stool.

Nursing Diagnosis: Fatigue. State this common nursing diagnosis as *Fatigue related to fatigue and muscle weakness.*

Outcomes: The client will demonstrate reduced fatigue as evidenced by (1) maintaining a balance between work, rest, and exercise and recreation; (2) performing ADL without excessive fatigue; (3) using energy-saving devices and techniques; (4) avoiding elevations in environmental and body temperatures; and (5) consuming a diet adequate in calories and protein for body size, frame, and age.

| NOC OUTCOMES | Activity Tolerance, Endurance, Energy Conservation |

Interventions	NIC INTERVENTIONS	Rationales
1. Keep the environment cool.	Energy Management	1. Mental fatigue can vary between mild and severely disabling and is usually exacerbated by exercise or increased body or ambient temperature.
2. Teach client to plan activities during peak energy periods.	Energy Management	2. Promotes optimal synchrony between the client's circadian rhythms and physical demands.
3. Plan for rest periods during the day.	Energy Management	3. Prevents some fatigue.
4. Facilitate sleep by reducing nighttime interruptions, noise, and light.	Energy Management	4. Sleep disturbance may lead to fatigue.

Nursing Diagnosis: Impaired Physical Mobility. Several aspects of MS lead to difficulties with mobility. State this common nursing diagnosis as *Impaired Physical Mobility related to weakness, contractures, spasticity, and ataxia.*

Outcomes: The client will demonstrate improved mobility as evidenced by performing ADL without excessive fatigue.

| NOC OUTCOMES | Ambulation: Walking, Joint Movement: Active, Mobility Level |

Interventions	NIC INTERVENTIONS	Rationales
1. Assess degree of muscle spasticity.	Exercise Therapy: Joint Mobility	1. Muscle spasticity can be painful and limit mobility. Some clients rely on muscle spasms to stabilize limbs for ambulation.
2. Stretch muscles and perform ROM on joints bid.	Exercise Promotion: Stretching	2. Muscle flexibility and joint mobility can be preserved with ROM exercises.
3. Administer antispasmodics as ordered.	Exercise Therapy: Muscle Control	3. Antispasmodics are often prescribed to control muscle spasm.
4. Position in neutral alignment.	Exercise Therapy: Joint Mobility	4. Maintaining body alignment prevents contractures.
5. Consult with physical therapists for mobility aids.	Exercise Therapy: Ambulation	5. Canes, walkers, and wheelchairs are used to promote mobility; they must be fit to the client and the client taught how to use them.
6. Consult with occupational therapists for utensils and splints.	Exercise Therapy: Joint Mobility	6. Splints help to maintain joint position and reduce contractures.
7. Avoid intense aerobic exercise.	Exercise Therapy: Joint Mobility	7. Exercise can exacerbate muscle fatigue in involved muscles because demyelinated nerve fatigues easily.

Nursing Diagnosis: Situational Self-Esteem. Because of the client's age, loss of independence and fear of disability or need for institutionalization can be devastating. State this diagnosis as *Situational Self-Esteem related to loss of independence and fear of disability.*

Outcomes: The client will achieve improved self-esteem as evidenced by verbalizing awareness that personal goals and body image will need to be adjusted, willingness to maintain appropriate independence, and positive thoughts and statements about self.

| NOC OUTCOMES | Self-Esteem |

Interventions	NIC INTERVENTIONS	Rationales
1. Assess for the presence of depression and any previous treatment for depression.	Coping Enhancement	1. Depression may be due to MS or caused by MS or the medications used for treatment.
2. Assess the client's problem-solving strategies.	Coping Enhancement	2. Identifies coping behavior strengths and defense mechanisms such as denial, avoidance, or intellectualization used to mask depression.
3. Evaluate the client's support systems.	Socialization Enhancement	3. The family and other people can be great assistance to the client, both physically and emotionally.
4. Provide experiences that increase the client's autotomy.	Self-Esteem Enhancement	4. Doing activities for oneself promotes a positive self-esteem.
5. Assist client to accept dependence on others.	Self-Esteem Enhancement	5. Accepting limitations resulting from disease and accepting help are crucial steps in being realistic about the disease and its impact.

Evaluation: The degree of expected outcome attainment for all of the above diagnoses should be evaluated on an ongoing basis. Most outcomes are long-term and may require weeks to months to attain.

of function in MS can lead to a reactive depression and require provision of support group therapy for both the client and the family. Some clients may not benefit from this type of therapy, however, because they may see people whose condition is much worse than their own and fear developing that level of disability. Online computer services for MS clients can provide a means of social support.

PARALYTIC DISEASES

Paralysis, the lost of both motor and sensory function, can occur from virus-like poliomyelitis or Guillain-Barré syndrome. Unfortunately, it can also develop from botulism. The Terrorism Alert feature below describes manifestations of and interventions for this rare paralytic condition.

GUILLAIN-BARRÉ SYNDROME

Guillain-Barré syndrome (GBS) is an inflammatory disease of unknown origin that involves degeneration of the myelin sheath of peripheral nerves. GBS is seen worldwide and affects people of all ages and races. Since the virtual elimination of poliomyelitis, GBS has become the most common cause of acute generalized paralysis, which affects between 1 and 4 per 100,000 of the population annually throughout the world. In one half to two thirds of cases, an upper respiratory or gastrointestinal tract infection precedes the onset of the syndrome by 1 to 4 weeks.

Although many organisms have been suspected, including cytomegalovirus and Epstein-Barr virus, *Campylobacter jejuni* is the organism most often implicated. This gram-negative rod is found in poultry, pets, raw milk, and contaminated water. *C. jejuni* targets the myelin

---

TERRORISM ALERT

Botulism

Botulism is a serious paralytic illness caused by a nerve toxin that is produced by the bacterium *Clostridium botulinum*. Botulinum is the most poisonous substance known. Two types of botulinum toxin are of concern in bioterrorism: food-borne and inhalational forms. Food-borne botulism can be especially dangerous because many people can be poisoned by eating a contaminated food. Food-borne botulism can occur from contaminated low-acid foods such as asparagus, green beans, beets, and corn. Outbreaks of botulism have been reported from chopped garlic in oil, chili peppers, tomatoes, improperly handled baked potatoes wrapped in aluminum foil, and home-canned or fermented fish. Inhalational botulism has been released intentionally via weapons.

The classic clinical manifestations of botulinum toxin exposure depend on the amount of toxin absorbed into the circulation. Manifestations include double vision, blurred vision, drooping eyelids, slurred speech, difficulty swallowing, dry mouth, and muscle weakness. All manifestations are due to muscle paralysis caused by the bacterial toxin. If untreated, these manifestations may progress to cause paralysis of the arms, legs, trunk, and respiratory muscles. In food-borne botulism, symptoms generally begin 18 to 36 hours after eating a contaminated food, but they can occur as early as 6 hours or as late as 10 days. Accordingly, food suspected of being contaminated should be refrigerated until it is retrieved by the public health department staff. The most direct way to confirm the diagnosis is to detect the botulinum toxin in the serum or stool.

Therapy for botulism is considered supportive with passive immunization with equine antitoxin. According to current reports, optimal use of botulism antitoxin requires early suspicion of botulism. Apparently, timely administration of

passive neutralizing antibody will help minimize nerve damage and the severity of the disease, but will not reverse existent paralysis. Supportive care may include enteral or parenteral nutrition, intensive care, and mechanical ventilation. The respiratory failure and paralysis that occur with severe botulism may require mechanical ventilation for weeks. After several weeks, the paralysis slowly improves. Because of the risk of respiratory failure and aspiration, the client should be frequently assessed for the gag and cough reflexes and control of oropharyngeal secretions and oxygen saturation.

If diagnosed early, food-borne and wound botulism can be treated with an antitoxin that blocks the action of the toxin. Contaminated food still in the gut can be partially removed by inducing vomiting or by using enemas. A careful travel and dietary history should be taken on any client suspected of botulism. Wounds should be treated, usually surgically, to remove the source of the toxin-producing bacteria. After exposure to suspected botulism, clothing and skin should be washed with soap and water. Contaminated surfaces should be cleaned with 0.1% hypochlorite solution.

Botulism is a rare disease. Intentional exposure should be considered if a large number of clients are seen with flaccid paralysis, if unusual types are found that are not seen in food poisoning, or if outbreaks are occurring in unusual settings (e.g., airports). Suspected outbreaks of botulism are quickly investigated. If they involve a commercial product, the appropriate control measures are coordinated among public health and regulatory agencies. Physicians should report suspected cases of botulism to the hospital epidemiologist or infection control practitioner and the state health department.

REFERENCE

Arnon, S., et al. (2002). *Bioterrorism: Guidelines for medical and public health management* (pp. 141-165). Chicago, Ill: American Medical Association.

sheath. Macrophages penetrate the basal lamina surrounding the axon, displace the Schwann cell from the myelin sheath, and phagocytose the myelin lamellae. An association between HIV and GBS has also been reported, and clients with GBS should be tested for HIV.

Clinical Manifestations

A characteristic feature is ascending weakness, usually beginning in the lower extremities and spreading, sometimes rapidly, to the trunk, upper extremities, and even the face. The weakness evolves over hours to days, with maximal deficit by 4 weeks in 90% of cases. Deep tendon reflexes are lost. Paresthesias (tingling sensation) in the limbs may occur early in the course of the illness.

This *initial phase* is usually followed by a *plateau phase* during which the disease no longer seems to progress, but the client does not recover functions initially lost. Deep, aching muscle pain in the shoulder girdle and thighs is common. The two most dangerous features of the disease are respiratory muscle weakness and autonomic neuropathy involving both the sympathetic and parasympathetic systems. The latter feature can involve orthostatic hypotension, hypertension, pupillary disturbances, sweating dysfunction, cardiac dysrhythmias, paralytic ileus, and urinary retention.

The third phase of the disease is the *recovery phase.* Improvement and recovery occur with remyelination. If nerve axons are damaged, however, some residual deficits may remain. Remyelination occurs in a descending pattern; the functions lost last are thus the first to be regained. Recovery is usually maximal at 6 months, although severe cases may take up to 2 years for maximal recovery. Fortunately, 85% to 90% of clients with GBS recover completely.

Diagnosis of GBS is based on history and physical examination, CSF examination, and electrophysiologic studies. The CSF contains increased protein, with few or no white blood cells. Nerve-conduction velocity is slowed, although it may be normal in the early stage of the illness. *Conduction block,* a diminution in amplitude or an absence of elicited muscle action potentials from stimulation of a peripheral nerve, also occurs.

OUTCOME MANAGEMENT

The focus of therapy is supportive care. Monitor respiratory or cardiovascular status carefully: vital signs, serial measurement of vital capacity, peripheral oxygen saturation, and electrocardiography. When vital capacity falls to 15 ml/kg of body weight, intubation and artificial ventilation are usually necessary.

Medical Management

Current practice guidelines for GBS include treatment with plasma exchange (PE) or IV immunoglobulin (IVIg), which hastens recovery from GBS. In addition, corticosteroids are not recommended for the treatment of GBS. Early treatment with (PE) may accelerate recovery, although the exact mechanism for this effect is not known. Hypotheses include the removal of circulating antibodies or other humoral myelinotoxic or immunopathogenic factors. IV immunoglobulin G (IVIG) therapy may prove to be the treatment of choice because it can be administered easily and can be given with other drugs simultaneously (PE removes co-medication jointly with adverse disease factors).

Nursing Management

During the first several days after hospital admission, it is crucial to assess the client's respiratory, swallowing, and autonomic function. The Critical Monitoring feature below summarizes nursing assessments for clients with Guillain-Barré syndrome who are in respiratory distress. Assess the following at least every 4 hours: vital signs, forced vital capacity, swallowing, strength in the extremities, and intake and output balance. If ascending weakness is noted, increase the frequency of assessment to every 2 hours or even more often. Cardiac monitoring and supplemental oxygen are often needed. Common complications include bladder infection, deep vein thrombosis, pulmonary emboli, pneumonia, and syndrome of inappropriate antidiuretic hormone (SIADH).

CRITICAL MONITORING

Respiratory Distress with Guillain-Barré Syndrome

Monitor the client for the following:
- Complaints of headache
- Myoclonic jerks
- Drowsiness
- Confusion
- Restlessness
- Reduced cough
- Decreased ability to move pulmonary secretions

Assess pulmonary function studies for the following:
- Decreased forced vital capacity (<15 ml/kg)
- Decreased tidal volume (<3-4 ml/kg)
- Decreased maximum inspiratory pressure (<10-20 cm H_2O)
- Decreased maximum expiratory pressure (<40 cm H_2O)

Assess arterial blood gases for the following:
- Decreased Pao_2 (<80 mm Hg on 50% Fio_2 with normal Pco_2)
- Alveolar-arterial gradient >300 on 50% Fio_2
- $Paco_2$ >50 mm Hg
- V_D/V_T >0.6

Fio$_2$, Fraction of inspired oxygen; *Paco$_2$,* partial pressure of arterial carbon dioxide; *Pao$_2$,* partial pressure of arterial oxygen; V_D/V_T, ratio of dead space volume to tidal volume.

Interventions to control infection and prevent complications of immobility are vital. Proper body alignment should be maintained to prevent deformities and injury to paralyzed limbs. Once the client's condition is stabilized, rehabilitative interventions can be implemented.

Assist the client in coping with the progressive nature of GBS. During the early stages, clients are frightened because their paralysis can ascend rapidly. They are often admitted to an acute care agency with progressive weakness and within days are completely paralyzed. Clients fear they will never recover. Help clients in verbalizing their fears, and offer support and encouragement that although the disorder is progressive, most clients gain full recovery. Encouragement is not hollow, however. The client is not taught to expect immediate resolution but is assisted to realize the usual time frames for recovery.

MYASTHENIA GRAVIS

Myasthenia gravis (MG) is an autoimmune disease that presents as muscular weakness and fatigue that worsens with exercise and improves with rest. The manifestations result from a loss of ACh receptors in the postsynaptic neurons of the neuromuscular junction. The cause of MG is unknown, but 80% of people with the generalized form of the disease have elevated titers of antibodies to the ACh receptor in their serum. MG may appear at any age, although there are two peaks of onset. In early-onset MG, at age 20 to 30 years, women are more often affected than men. In late-onset MG, after age 50, men are more often affected.

Clinical Manifestations

The primary feature of MG is increasing weakness with sustained muscle contraction. For instance, if the person is asked to hold the arms up, the power of muscle contraction diminishes and the arms gradually drift downward. After a period of rest, the muscles regain their strength. Muscle weakness is greatest after exertion or at the end of the day.

Ocular manifestations are most common, with *ptosis* (drooping of the upper eyelid) or *diplopia* (double vision) occurring in many clients. Ptosis is due to weakness of the levator palpebrae muscles of the eye. If not present at the examination, ptosis can be elicited by prolonged upward gaze, which creates fatigue of the muscle.

Diplopia is a result of weakness or fatigue of the extraocular muscles. Other manifestations are weakness of the orbicularis oculi muscles (which help close the eye), the facial muscles, the muscles of chewing and swallowing, and the limb muscles. Weakness of the facial and levator palpebrae muscles produces an expressionless face, with droopy eyelids, smoothed features, and a tendency for the mouth to hang open.

An attempt to smile often turns into a snarl because of the weakness. A person may hold a hand under the jaw to keep it closed. Dysphagia and a nasal quality to speech occur when the muscles of chewing and swallowing are involved. In severe cases, respiratory muscle weakness may occur, which may necessitate intubation and mechanical ventilation (see The Critical Monitoring Box on p. 1917).

The course of MG varies, and remissions and exacerbations may occur. Clinical manifestations may progress quickly or slowly and may fluctuate from day to day. The severity of the disease varies greatly from person to person.

Diagnostic Findings

The diagnosis of MG is based on the clinical presentation and can be confirmed by testing the client's response to anticholinesterase drugs. These drugs inhibit cholinesterase, an enzyme that breaks down ACh in the neuromuscular junction, thereby allowing more ACh to bind to the remaining ACh receptors. Edrophonium (Tensilon) is a short-acting drug that is given intravenously *(Tensilon test)*. A test dose of 2 mg (for adults) is injected first. If no untoward reaction occurs (such as increased weakness, change in heart rate or rhythm, nausea, or abdominal cramps), the remaining 8 mg is injected. The client is then observed for objective manifestations of improvement in muscle strength. The effect is transitory, wearing off after 3 to 5 minutes. Another drug, neostigmine methylsulfate (Prostigmin), may be used because of its longer duration of effect on muscle strength (1 to 2 hours), which allows better analysis of its effect.

When either drug is used, IV atropine sulfate should be available to inject as an antidote. This medication counteracts any severe cholinergic reactions (cardiac dysrhythmias or abdominal cramping). Electromyography (EMG) helps confirm the diagnosis. Repetitive stimulation of the nerve with recording from the involved muscle shows a characteristic decrementing response of the muscle action potential. Generally, after the initial diagnostic testing is performed by the practitioner, referral to a neurologist and/or pulmonologist may be necessary for long-term management.

OUTCOME MANAGEMENT

No cure for MG exists as yet. Pharmacologic intervention consists of two groups of medications: (1) short-acting anticholinesterase compounds and (2) corticosteroids. The most effective anticholinesterase drugs are pyridostigmine (Mestinon) and neostigmine (Prostigmin). Dosages are highly individualized, based on physiologic response to the medication. The goal is to achieve the maximum benefit (muscle strength and endurance) with the fewest side effects (excessive salivation, sweating, nausea, diarrhea, abdominal cramps, or tachycardia). Corticosteroids (usually prednisone) are directed toward reducing the levels of serum ACh receptor antibodies. Corticosteroids may temporarily worsen manifestations; however, this is followed by gradual improvement in muscle strength.

After a peak of improvement is reached and maintained for several weeks, the dosage of both prednisone and anticholinesterase medication may be gradually decreased. A low maintenance dose of alternate-day prednisone may be effective for many months or years. Precautions with any steroid therapy are important, including potassium supplements if indicated and liberal use of antacids.

Potential complications of steroid use are cataracts, hypertension, diabetes, fluid retention, delayed wound healing, insomnia, and osteoporosis. Other treatments include azathioprine (Imuran) and cyclosporine (Sandimmune), which reduce the level of circulating ACh receptor antibodies, and plasmapheresis and IVIG.

Plasmapheresis

Plasmapheresis is an adjunctive therapy for clients with refractory MG. It is a process by which plasma is separated from formed elements of blood. The plasma is discarded and the packed red blood cells are joined with albumin, normal saline, and electrolytes and returned to the client. The purpose is to remove plasma proteins containing antibodies that are believed to cause MG. Plasmapheresis may produce transient improvement in clients who have actual or pending respiratory failure.

Usually, three to five treatments given once daily over 5 to 7 days are required. Potential complications include myasthenic or cholinergic crisis and, rarely, hypovolemia. Muscle strength should be assessed before and after the procedure, with particular attention paid to vital capacity, swallowing ability, diplopia, and ptosis to evaluate the effectiveness of the treatment.

Complications

Two major complications of MG may occur: *myasthenic crisis* and *cholinergic crisis*. The Critical Monitoring feature at right highlights clinical manifestations of these medical emergencies and outlines appropriate nursing interventions.

Myasthenic Crisis

Clients with moderate or severe generalized MG, especially those who have difficulty swallowing or breathing, may experience a sudden worsening of their condition. This is usually precipitated by an intercurrent infection or sudden withdrawal of anticholinesterase drugs, but it may occur spontaneously. If an increase in the dosage of the anticholinesterase drug does not improve the weakness, endotracheal intubation and mechanical ventilation may be required. In many instances, drug responsiveness returns in 24 to 48 hours, and weaning from the respirator can proceed.

CRITICAL MONITORING

Myasthenic and Cholinergic Crises in Clients with Myasthenia Gravis

MYASTHENIC CRISIS IS CAUSED BY UNDERMEDICATION

Clinical Manifestations
- Sudden marked rise in blood pressure because of hypoxia
- Increased heart rate
- Severe respiratory distress and cyanosis
- Absent cough and swallow reflexes
- Increased secretions, increased diaphoresis, and increased lacrimation
- Restlessness, dysarthria
- Bowel and bladder incontinence

Intervention
- Increased doses of cholinergic drugs as long as the client responds positively to edrophonium treatment
- Possible mechanical ventilation if respiratory muscle paralysis is acute

CHOLINERGIC CRISIS IS CAUSED BY DEPOLARIZATION BLOCK RESULTING FROM EXCESSIVE MEDICATIONS

Clinical Manifestations
- Weakness with difficulty swallowing, chewing, speaking, and breathing
- Apprehension, nausea, and vomiting
- Abdominal cramps and diarrhea
- Increased secretions and saliva
- Sweating, lacrimation, fasciculations, and blurred vision

Intervention
- Discontinue all cholinergic drugs until cholinergic effects decrease
- Provide adequate ventilatory support
- 1 mg intravenous atropine may be necessary to counteract severe cholinergic reactions

Cholinergic Crisis

Cholinergic crisis occurs as a result of overmedication. The muscarinic effect of a toxic level of anticholinesterase medication causes abdominal cramps, diarrhea, and excessive pulmonary secretions. The nicotinic effect paradoxically worsens weakness and can cause bronchial spasm. If respiratory status is compromised, the client may need intubation and mechanical ventilation.

Nursing Management of Myasthenia Gravis (MG)

Because MG may involve the muscles of respiration, the client may experience dyspnea and ineffective cough and swallow mechanisms, which may lead to aspiration and pneumonia. Encourage deep breathing and coughing. Have suction equipment available at the bedside, and instruct the client on how to use it. Instruct the client to sit upright when eating, to swallow only when the chin is tipped downward toward the chest, and never to speak while food is in the mouth. Oxygen and, in severe cases, mechanical ventilation may be required.

In MG, weakness is usually greatest following exertion and at the end of the day. Activities should be carefully planned to include rest periods so that energy is conserved and the muscles have a chance to regain their strength. Rearrangement of the home environment may help prevent unnecessary energy expenditure. Vocational retraining may be indicated for those who can no longer meet the physical demands of their jobs. Clients with severe disease or an acute exacerbation will be totally dependent on nursing care for ADL. This level of care requires that complications of immobility be avoided.

Provide the client and family with information about MG and its treatment. They should be aware of adverse reactions of both anticholinesterase drugs and steroids. Explain how to recognize myasthenic and cholinergic crises and how to have a plan to seek medical intervention, if necessary.

Surgical Management

Thymectomy can be used for treatment. The thymus gland, located in the superior mediastinum, is important during fetal growth for development of the immune system. It is usually atrophied and nonfunctioning in adulthood. The effect of thymectomy is not fully understood. It may alter some immunologic control mechanism that affects the production of antibodies to the ACh receptor, or it may eliminate a trigger to antibody production. Thymectomy is indicated for clients with thymoma, selected clients with generalized MG without thymoma, and selected clients with disabling ocular MG.[14] The procedure is recommended early in the course of the disease. Nursing management is similar to care following thoracic surgery.

AMYOTROPHIC LATERAL SCLEROSIS

Amyotrophic lateral sclerosis (ALS) is the most common of the motor neuron diseases. It is an age-dependent, fatal paralytic disorder also known as *Charcot's disease* and *Lou Gehrig's disease.* Onset is usually in middle age. Men are affected more often than women.

Amyotrophic lateral sclerosis involves degeneration of both the anterior horn cells and the corticospinal tracts. Consequently, both upper and lower motor neuron clinical manifestations are seen. Lower motor neuron clinical manifestations include weakness, atrophy, cramps, and fasciculations (irregular twitchings of muscle fibers or bundles). Upper motor neuron manifestations include spasticity and hyperreflexia. Involvement of the corticobulbar tracts causes dysphagia (difficulty swallowing)

and dysarthria (slurred speech). These clients are at risk for suboptimal caloric and fluid intake and a worsening of muscle atrophy, weakness, and fatigue. The sensory system is not involved, and cognition is not affected. The client remains alert and mentally intact throughout the course of the disease. The course of the disease is relentlessly progressive. Death usually results from pneumonia caused by respiratory compromise within 2 to 5 years.

Weakness typically begins in the upper extremities and progressively involves the upper arms and shoulders and then the muscles of the neck and throat. The trunk and lower extremities are usually not affected until late in the disease. When the intercostal muscles and diaphragm become involved, respirations are shallow and coughing is ineffective. Cognition, as well as bowel and bladder sphincters, remains intact, even when the client is totally debilitated. In some cases, weakness begins in the brain stem, causing problems with speech and swallowing. This is called *bulbar ALS.*

Diagnosis of ALS is made by the clinical presentation and EMG. The EMG criteria for the diagnosis of ALS include the presence of widespread anterior horn cell dysfunction with fibrillations, positive waves, fasciculations, and chronic neurogenic motor unit potential changes in multiple nerve root distribution in at least three limbs and the paraspinal muscles in the presence of normal sensory responses.

OUTCOME MANAGEMENT

Supportive therapy was the only intervention for ALS until riluzole (Rilutek) was approved in 1996. Its mechanism of action is unknown, but it is thought to have a neuroprotective effect. The drug extends the life of ALS clients by a few months. Clients with ALS are usually admitted to health care facilities only twice in their illness, first for diagnosis and later in the final stage of debilitation.

The antibiotic minocycline is being studied for ALS. Laboratory studies have linked inducible nitric oxide and caspase enzyme activation to motor nerve cell death in ALS. Minocycline is in the tetracycline group of antibiotics that penetrates barriers around the CNS when taken orally and helps to inhibit caspase enzymes, which are involved in cell death pathways. Genetic treatments are also being researched.

Supportive nursing care is an important aspect of managing the ALS client. In the outpatient arena, the nurse can provide ongoing assessment of daily living needs and make suggestions for modifications in activity level, clothing, and diet. Often just allowing the client or family to talk about problems reduces anxiety and helps them find solutions to problems.[19] Interventions should be aimed at conserving energy. Activities should be spaced during the day. Muscle stress, strenuous activity, and extremes of hot and cold should be avoided. Leg braces, canes, and walkers can prolong independence in ambulation. Hand braces, special utensils, and adaptive devices such as buttonhooks can help with dressing and self-feeding. Pressure ulcers are not usually a problem because the sensory system remains intact and the client can feel when pressure on a body part is too great.

In the acute care setting, gather information from the client and family about communication needs and which positions are best for respiration, handling secretions, eating, and turning routines.

Encourage fluid intake regularly, when the client is not fatigued. Proper positioning is imperative. Providing a cup with a spout may prevent liquid from running out of the corners of the mouth. Give liquids by using a large syringe with short tubing on the tip. The tube is placed on the anterior portion of the tongue, and gentle force is used to deliver small amounts of liquid.

Encourage small, frequent, high-nutrient feedings. Tell the client to sit upright, with the head slightly flexed forward while eating. Papase tablets placed under the tongue 10 minutes before meals can make thick saliva less sticky. Plenty of time should be allowed for eating, and the client should not attempt to speak while food is in the mouth. Have suction equipment available during meals to reduce the risk of aspiration of food and secretions that become lodged in the mouth and pharynx. The head may need to be stabilized with a soft cervical collar. Consult the dietitian for special diet recommendations. As dysphagia progresses, percutaneous endoscopic gastrostomy (PEG) should be considered as an alternative or supplemental route for oral nutrition.

Although speech remains intelligible, the client can be trained to slow the rate of speech and exaggerate articulation. As manifestations progress, the client may need to repeat words or have an interpreter (usually the spouse). At this stage, it is important to eliminate extraneous noise, face the client when he or she is talking, and maintain eye contact. When the client's speech contains only one-word phrases or is no longer possible, writing can be an effective means of communicating and should be encouraged. When writing is no longer possible, a speech pathologist can provide communication devices such as alphabet boards and portable memo writers.[9]

If the client is a smoker, encourage him or her to stop. Exposure to people with respiratory tract infections should be avoided. Remind the client to use good posture. Pulmonary function tests should be performed regularly to assess ventilatory status. Clients generally experience respiratory fatigue when vital capacity is less than 1.5 L. Some clients can be taught to use their abdominal muscles to enhance respirations when the intercostal muscles and diaphragm become weak. A manifestation of pending respiratory insufficiency is shortness of breath while eating.

Encourage the client and family to talk about the losses they are experiencing and the feelings associated with them. Family members should be encouraged to take time for rest and activities away from the client. Refer the client and family to an ALS support group.

Eventually clients face the difficult choice of deciding whether they will accept artificial ventilation. Encourage them to discuss this with family and friends and to seek input from ALS support groups. Encourage clients to complete advance directives to indicate whether they desire life-sustaining treatments such as cardiopulmonary resuscitation, but this should be reassessed at regular intervals. Clients may change their minds on the basis of their experience with their illness, changes in their subjective appreciation of their quality of life, or changes in their evaluation of the benefits and burdens of life-sustaining measures as they come to terms with the imminence of death.[21]

CONCLUSIONS

Degenerative neurologic disorders have many causes, including viruses, autoimmune responses, and heredity. Some have no known cause. In general, they are relentlessly progressive, slowly taking away both physical and mental ability. Nurses should focus care on the management of clinical manifestations and prevention of complications. Family support throughout the process of care is essential.

THINKING CRITICALLY

1. A 52-year-old man with multiple sclerosis is wheelchair-bound and has a neurogenic bladder. He complains of a sudden onset of generalized weakness, fever, and chills and is admitted to the hospital. What priorities should be set for his care?

Factors to Consider. What do generalized weakness, fever, and chills suggest in *any* client? If your client has not been following good bladder management, how can you intervene?

2. A 70-year-old man with Parkinson's disease is admitted to the hospital after experiencing severe nightmares and periods of confusion. During lucid periods, he is very disturbed by these manifestations. At other times, he believes that his wife is participating in a conspiracy to harm him. What assessments and interventions should you consider?

Factors to Consider. Are hallucinations and paranoia typical manifestations of Parkinson's disease? Might the client's manifestations be related to treatment or to some cause other than Parkinson's disease?

3. A 41-year-old woman with myasthenia gravis is taking pyridostigmine and prednisone. She is complaining of increased fatigue and weakness and has difficulty breathing. What concerns should you have?

Factors to Consider. Might the client's difficulty breathing be related to her fatigue and weakness? Could these manifestations be related to myasthenia gravis or its treatment?

evolve *Discussions for these questions can be found on the website.*

BIBLIOGRAPHY

Citations appearing in red refer to primary research.

Citations appearing in blue refer to evidence-based practice guidelines and protocols.

1. American Academy of Neurology Guideline Summary for Clinicians. (2006). *Manage ALS from the beginning: Care makes a difference* (pp. 1-2). St. Paul, Mn: American Academy of Neurology.

2. Andrews, K.L., & Husmann, D.A. (1997). Bladder dysfunction and management in multiple sclerosis. *Mayo Clinic Proceedings, 74*, 1176-1183.

3. Armstrong Mortenson, S., & Schumann, L. (2003). Myasthenia gravis: Diagnosis and treatment. *Clinical Practice, 15*(2), 72-78.

4. Brown, P. (1997). The risk of bovine spongiform encephalopathy ('mad cow disease') to human health. *Journal of the American Medical Association, 278*(12), 1008-1011.

5. Calne, S. (2005). Late-stage Parkinson's disease for the rehabilitation specialist: A nursing perspective. *Topics in Geriatric Rehabilitation, 21*(3), 233-246.

6. Friedlander, R. (2003). Apoptosis and caspases in neurodegenerative diseases. *New England Journal of Medicine, 348*(14), 1365-1375.

7. Goodwin, D.S., Frohman, E.M., & Garmany, G. (2002). Disease modifying therapies in multiple sclerosis. *Neurology, 58*(2), 169-178.

8. Gwyther, L.P. (2000). Family issues in dementia: Finding a new normal. *Neurology Clinics, 18*(4), 993-1010.

9. Haberman, B., & Davis, L.L. (2005). Caring for family with Alzheimer's disease and Parkinson's disease: Needs, challenges, and satisfaction. *Journal of Gerontological Nursing, 31*(6), 49-54.

10. Halper, J., et al. (2003). Rethinking cognitive function in multiple sclerosis: A nursing perspective. *Journal of Neuroscience Nursing, 35*(2), 70-81.

11. Handley, J. (2005). Using drugs to treat Parkinson's disease: A nurse's perspective. *Practice Nurse, July* 8, *30*(1).

12. Hecht, M.J., et al. (2003). Burden of care in amyotrophic lateral sclerosis. *Palliative Medicine, 17*(4), 327-333.

13. Hogancamp, W.E., Rodriguez, M., & Weinshenker, B.G. (1997). The epidemiology of multiple sclerosis. *Mayo Clinic Proceedings, 74*, 871-878.

14. Hughes, R.A.C., Wijdicks, E.F.M., & Barohn, R. (2003). Practice parameters: Immunotherapy for Guillain-Barré syndrome. *Neurology, 61*, 736-740.

15. Jones, P.S., & Martinson, I.M. (1992). The experience of bereavement in care givers of family members with Alzheimer's disease. *Image—The Journal of Nursing Scholarship, 24*(3), 174-176.

16. Knopman, D.S., Boeve, B.F., & Petersen, R.C. (2003). Essentials of the proper diagnosis of mild cognitive impairment, dementia and major subtypes of dementia. *Mayo Clinic Proceedings, 78*, 1290-1308.

17. Lang, A.E., & Lozano, A.M. (1998). Parkinson's disease. *New England Journal of Medicine, 339*(16), 1130-1143.

18. Le Bars, P.L., et al. (1997). A placebo-controlled, double-blind, randomized trial of an extract of ginkgo biloba for dementia. *Journal of the American Medical Association, 278*(16), 1327-1332.

19. Levin, L.I., Munger, K., Ruberton, M., et al. (2003). Multiple sclerosis and Epstein Barr virus. *Journal of the American Medical Association, 289*(12), 1533-1536.

20. Lucchinetti, C.F., & Rodriguez, M. (1997). The controversy surrounding pathogenesis of the multiple sclerosis lesion. *Mayo Clinic Proceedings, 74*, 665-678.

21. Mayo Foundation for Medical Education and Research. (1996, Oct). Alzheimer's disease: Living with a 'long goodbye.' *Mayo Clinic Health Letter* (Suppl), 1-8.

22. McGonigal-Kenney, M.L., & Schultte, D.L. (2004). *Non-pharmacologic management of agitated behaviors in persons with Alzheimer's disease and other chronic dementing illnesses.* University of Iowa Gerontological Nursing Interventions Research Center, Research Dissemination Core.

23. Mezey, M., et al. (1996). Life-sustaining treatment decisions by spouses of patients with Alzheimer's disease. *Journal of the American Geriatrics Society, 44*(2), 144-150.

24. Miller, R.G., Rosenberg, J.A., Gelinas, D.F., and the ALS Practice Parameters Task Force. (2003). Practice Parameters: The care of the patient with amyotrophic lateral sclerosis (an evidence based review). *Report of the Quality Standards of Subcommittees of the American Academy of Neurology, 52*(7), 1311-1323.

25. National Institute of Neurological Disorders and Stroke Publication. (2006). *Huntington Disease: Hope through research* (NIH Pub No. 98-49). Bethesda, Md: NIH.

26. Nowotny, M.L. (1998). My journey with amyotrophic lateral sclerosis. *Journal of Neuroscience Nursing, 30*(1), 68-70.

27. Palmieri, R. (2005). Is it myasthenia gravis or Guillain-Barré syndrome? *Nursing, 35*(12), 1-4.

28. Perry, J. (2002). Wives giving care to husbands with Alzheimer's disease: A process of interpretive caring. *Research in Nursing and Health, 25*(4), 307-316.

29. Post, S.G., et al. (1997). The clinical introduction of genetic testing for Alzheimer disease: An ethical perspective. *Journal of the American Medical Association, 277*(10), 832-836.

30. Prusiner, S. (2001). Neurodegenerative diseases and prions. *New England Journal of Medicine, 344*(20), 1516-1524.

31. Robinson, L. (2003). The importance of touch for the patient with dementia. *Home HealthCare Nurse, 21*(1), 16-19.

32. Robinson, B.E. (1997). Guideline for initial evaluation of the patient with memory loss. *Geriatrics, 52*(12), 30-39.

33. Rodriguez, M. (1997). Multiple sclerosis: Insights into molecular pathogenesis and therapy. *Mayo Clinic Proceedings, 74*, 663-664.

34. Rudick, R.A., et al. (1997). Management of multiple sclerosis. *New England Journal of Medicine, 337*(22), 1604-1611.

35. Schechter, R., Inglesby, T.V., & Henderson, D.A. (2002). *Botulinum toxin as a biological weapon: Medical and public health management. (2) Botulinum toxin as a biological weapon. (Addendum)* (pp. 141-165). Chicago, Ill: American Medical Association.

36. Spurlock, W.R. (2005). Spiritual well-being and caregiver burden in Alzheimer's caregivers. *Geriatric Nursing, 26*(30), 154-161.

37. Vrabec, N.J. (1997). Literature review of social support and caregiver burden, 1980 to 1995. *Image—The Journal of Nursing Scholarship, 29*(4), 383-388.

evolve **Did you remember to check out the bonus material on the Evolve website and the CD-ROM, including NCLEX®-Examination Style Review Questions, Open-Book Quizzes, and Chapter Review Audio Podcasts?**

http://evolve.elsevier.com/Black/medsurg

CHAPTER 73

Management of Clients with Neurologic Trauma

Norma D. McNair and Judi L. Kuric

The complexity of the central nervous system (CNS) allows the human organism to evaluate information about the outside world. Failure of the brain or the spinal cord to process information correctly prevents the affected person from accurately performing tasks and may impair interactions with others as well as self-appraisal.

Admission of a client with CNS trauma to the emergency department requires rapid mobilization of a trauma team. The team provides initial assessment and resuscitation of the trauma victim and performs triage to the appropriate radiologic studies and surgical service. Ultimately the management of a client with a head injury, spinal cord injury, or a combination of neurologic injuries is directed by the neurosurgical service. This chapter examines the needs of clients with CNS trauma, including head and spinal cord injuries.

The discussion will begin with crucial information in caring for any client with neurologic disease or trauma. Discussions about specific diseases will follow.

INCREASED INTRACRANIAL PRESSURE

The skull is a hard, bony vault filled with brain tissue, blood, and cerebrospinal fluid (CSF). A balance between these three components maintains the pressure within the cranium. The modified *Munro-Kellie hypothesis,* a theory for understanding intracranial pressure (ICP), states that because the bony skull cannot expand, when one of the three components expands, the other two must compensate by decreasing in volume for the total brain volume and pressure to remain constant.

Intracranial pressure is the pressure exerted in the cranium by its contents: the brain, blood, and CSF (Figure 73-1). ICP is measured with a monitor in the ventricle, the brain parenchyma, or the subarachnoid space. The normal ICP is 5 to 15 mm Hg. Pressures greater than 20 mm Hg are considered to represent *increased ICP,* which seriously impairs cerebral perfusion. Recognition of increased ICP is one of the most important assessments made by nurses caring for clients with neurologic disorders.

Cerebral perfusion pressure (CPP) is the amount of blood flow from the systemic circulation required to provide adequate oxygen and glucose for brain metabolism. *Mean arterial pressure* (MAP) represents the average pressure during the cardiac cycle. It is calculated by adding the systolic pressure to twice the diastolic pressure and dividing by 3. (Diastole is twice as long as systole.) The formula for calculating CPP is as follows:

$$CPP = MAP - ICP$$

When MAP and ICP are equal, there is no CPP and brain perfusion ceases. Therefore it is crucial to maintain control of both ICP and MAP.

Etiology and Risk Factors

Increased ICP is most often associated with a space-occupying lesion (such as a tumor, edema, or bleeding). However, a cerebral infarction, an obstruction to the outflow of CSF, an abscess, an ingested or accumulated toxin,

evolve Web Enhancements

Case Study Spinal Cord Injury

Client Education Guide Monitoring Family Members After Head Injury (English Version and Spanish Translation)

Use of a Halo Vest (English Version and Spanish Translation)

Ethical Issues in Nursing What is the Government's Obligation to Put Care for Its Citizens Above Care for Noncitizens, Given Scarce Resources?

Figure A Neurologic Observation Chart

Be sure to check out the bonus material on the Evolve website and the CD-ROM, including free self-assessment exercises. **http://evolve.elsevier.com/Black/medsurg**

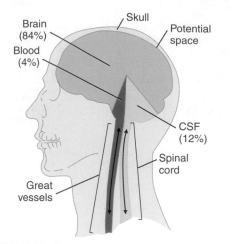

■ **FIGURE 73–1** Components of the intracranial vault. A balance between these three compartments maintains normal intracranial pressure.

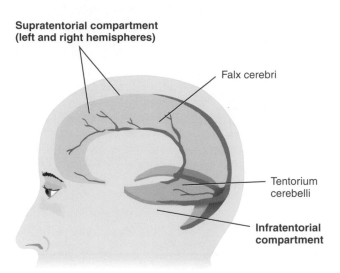

■ **FIGURE 73–2** The intracranial compartments are divided by inelastic fibers to provide support.

impaired blood flow to or from the brain, vasodilation from increased carbon dioxide ($PaCO_2$) or decreased partial pressure of oxygen (PaO_2), systemic hypertension, or increased intrathoracic pressure can also increase the pressure. Risk factors include head injury, brain tumors, cerebral bleeding, hydrocephalus, and edema from surgery or injury.

Pathophysiology

As an intracranial mass enlarges, initial compensation occurs through *displacement of CSF* into the spinal canal. The ability of the brain to adapt to increasing pressure without increasing ICP is called *compliance*. The movement of CSF out of the cranium is the first and major compensatory mechanism, but the cranial vault can accommodate increasing intracranial volume only to a point. When the compliance of the brain is exceeded, the ICP rises, clinical manifestations develop, and other compensatory efforts to reduce pressure begin.

The second form of compensation is *reduction of blood volume* in the brain. *Autoregulation* is the occurrence of compensatory changes in the diameter of intracranial blood vessels designed to maintain a constant blood flow during changes in CPP. Autoregulation is lost with increasing ICP. Small increases in brain volume can then cause dramatic increases in ICP, with a longer time required to return to baseline level. When ICP approaches systemic blood pressure, cerebral perfusion decreases and the brain suffers severe hypoxia and acidosis.

When blood flow is reduced by 40%, cerebral tissue becomes acidotic. When 60% of blood flow is lost, the electroencephalogram (EEG) begins to change. This stage of compensation alters cerebral metabolism, eventually leading to brain tissue hypoxia and areas of brain tissue ischemia.

The last stage of compensation and the most lethal is *displacement of brain tissue* across the dividing structures of the brain. The brain is supported within various intracranial compartments (Figure 73-2). The supratentorial compartment contains all the brain tissue from the top of the midbrain upward. This section is divided into right and left chambers by the tough, inelastic fibers of the falx cerebri. The supratentorial compartment is separated from the infratentorial compartment (containing the brain stem and cerebellum) by the tentorium cerebelli. The brain is capable of some movement within these compartments. Pressure increases in one compartment affect surrounding areas of lower pressure.

When swollen, the brain can bulge into the tentorium, under the falx cerebri, or through the foramen magnum into the spinal canal. This process is called *herniation* and often results in death from brain stem compression.

Cerebral Edema

The terms *cerebral edema, brain swelling,* and *increased ICP* are sometimes used interchangeably, but they are not the same. Cerebral edema and brain swelling are causes of increased ICP. An increase in brain bulk caused by an increase in cerebral blood volume is called *brain swelling*. *Brain edema,* in contrast, is an increase in the fluid surrounding the tissues of the brain, such as in the extracellular spaces or the white matter, or within the cells themselves. The distinction between these two conditions is important because the interventions differ.

After head injury, edema develops because of a disruption of the blood-brain barrier. This type of edema is similar to other forms of edema, such as that seen in a sprained ankle. The fluid contains electrolytes, proteins, and blood. Edema reaches its maximum within 48 to 72 hours after brain surgery or injury. The fluid returns to the systemic circulation via the CSF or the venous system. This form of edema is usually treated with osmotic diuretics.

Brain swelling is caused by increased blood volume resulting from dilated cerebral blood vessels. Brain swelling, in conjunction with cerebral edema, appears to be a major mechanism responsible for increasing ICP and for decreasing the size of the ventricles when compensation occurs. This form of swelling may be treated with therapeutic hyperventilation using mechanical ventilation to cause vasoconstriction.

Clinical Manifestations

Manifestations of increased ICP are caused by traction on the cerebral blood vessels from swelling tissues and by pressure on the pain-sensitive dura mater and various structures within the brain. The pathologic process of increased ICP actually comprises several entities that occur at the same time. No single set of clinical manifestations occurs in all clients. Indications of increased ICP relate to the location and cause of the raised pressure and to the speed and extent of its development.

Initial manifestations of increased ICP are subtle, and diligent observation for changes in the client's condition is necessary. Clinical manifestations include *any* alteration in level of consciousness (e.g., restlessness, irritability, confusion) and may include a decrease in the Glasgow Coma Scale (GCS) score. In addition, the client may have changes in speech, pupillary reactivity, motor or sensory ability, or cardiac rate and rhythm. Headache, nausea, vomiting, or blurred or double vision (diplopia) may be reported. The optic nerve is an extension of the brain, and increased tension in the skull is transmitted to the optic nerve to cause papilledema. *Papilledema* is swelling and hyperemia of the optic disc and can be observed only through an ophthalmoscope. Early detection of increased ICP (i.e., before clinical manifestations develop) by means of ICP monitoring in the critical care unit can greatly improve a client's outcome.

Cushing's triad—increased systolic blood pressure with widened pulse pressure and bradycardia—is a late response and indicates severe increased ICP with failure of autoregulation. Respiratory patterns progress from Cheyne-Stokes respiration to central neurogenic hyperventilation to apneustic breathing and ataxic breathing as ICP increases (see Chapter 68). These respiratory patterns will not be noticed in the client receiving mechanical ventilation, however. Hyperthermia is typically present when the hypothalamus is first affected by the increase in pressure, followed by hypothermia as ICP increases (Figure 73-3).

Common diagnostic studies performed to determine the source of increased ICP include skull radiography, computed tomography (CT) scanning, and magnetic resonance imaging (MRI). A lumbar puncture is not usually performed because of the risk of causing herniation of

■ **FIGURE 73–3** A late response to increased intracranial pressure is Cushing's triad (also called Cushing's response): bradycardia, systolic hypertension, and a wide pulse pressure, which result from pressure on the medulla. These manifestations can occur with intracranial hypertension or herniation. Alterations in the respiratory pattern also accompany Cushing's triad.

the brain stem when the pressure of the CSF in the spinal cord is lower than that in the cranium. In addition, the CSF pressure at the lumbar level is not always an accurate reflection of the intracranial CSF pressure.

Herniation Syndromes

Herniation syndromes have been classified into five types (Figure 73-4). These conditions occur late in the course of increased ICP and represent the body's last attempt to restore normal brain volume and pressure through displacement of blood, brain tissue, or CSF.

Herniation, regardless of the type, always constitutes an emergency. Notify the physician immediately of any manifestations that indicate a worsening of the client's condition as a result of increasing ICP.

Supratentorial Herniation Syndromes

Transcalvarial Herniation. Transcalvarial herniation occurs with open head injuries when brain tissue is extruded through an unstable skull fracture. Clinical manifestations vary greatly, depending on the location and extent of the open skull fracture.

Central Transtentorial Herniation. Central transtentorial herniation is the downward displacement of the diencephalon through the tentorial notch. It is caused by injuries or masses located in the cerebral tissue or on the outward perimeter of the cerebrum. An early indication of central transtentorial herniation is a rapid change in the level of consciousness. As the pressure increases,

■ **FIGURE 73–4** Types of intracranial herniation. In *transcalvarial* herniation, edematous brain tissue is extruded through the skull. In *central transtentorial* herniation, the lesion is located centrally or superiorly in the cranium, and compression of central and midbrain structures may result. In *lateral* (or *uncal*) herniation, the lesion is located laterally within the cranium and can cause pressure on the midbrain. *Cingulate* herniation occurs between the two frontal lobes; the brain is pressed under the falx cerebri. In *tonsillar* herniation, the cerebellar tonsils are driven between the posterior arch of the atlas and the medulla and may be compressed.

changes in respiratory patterns are seen: first, Cheyne-Stokes respirations and then central neurogenic hyperventilation; later, apneustic breathing and also ataxic breathing (Biot's respiration); and, finally, apnea (see Chapter 68). Pupils become small but at first remain reactive, with progression to a dilated and fixed state. Pathologic reflexes begin with Babinski's sign (see Chapter 67) and then progress from abnormal flexion to abnormal extensor posturing. Doll's eye reflex and a positive response to caloric testing are noted when brain stem function is still intact but are absent if the brain stem dies (see Chapter 68). The Critical Monitoring feature on p. 1925 lists the specific areas of brain involvement that are correlated with pathologic manifestation.

Lateral Transtentorial Herniation. Lateral transtentorial herniation occurs from displacement by masses in or along the temporal lobe. It is also called *uncal herniation* because as the temporal lobe is compressed, the *uncus* (the anteromedial portion of the hippocampus) or the hippocampal gyrus shifts from the middle fossa through the tentorial notch into the posterior fossa. As the herniation progresses, the pupils first become sluggish in response to light and then become unresponsive; lack of response is seen first in the ipsilateral pupil and then in the contralateral pupil, as a result of third cranial nerve compression at the midbrain level. Other progressive clinical manifestations include a decreasing level of consciousness (stupor to coma), Cheyne-Stokes respirations

followed by central neurogenic hyperventilation, and abnormal flexor posturing that progresses to abnormal extensor posturing.

Cingulate Herniation. Cingulate herniation occurs when the frontal lobes of the cerebrum are compressed, resulting in compression of the cingulate gyrus (an arch-shaped convolution situated just above the corpus callosum) under the falx cerebri. Manifestations are related to cerebral artery compression resulting in ischemia and congestion, edema, and increasing ICP.

Infratentorial (Tonsillar) Herniation Syndrome

Tonsillar herniation, also known as *cerebellar herniation,* occurs when the cerebellar tonsil shifts through the foramen magnum, compressing the medulla and upper portion of the spinal cord. Increasing pressure in the posterior fossa, often secondary to cerebellar bleeding, is the usual underlying problem. Manifestations often progress rapidly and include erratic changes in blood pressure, pulse rate, and breathing; decreased level of consciousness; an arched, stiff neck; and quadriparesis.

OUTCOME MANAGEMENT OF HERNIATION SYNDROMES

Hyperventilation has been the standard treatment for herniation for many years. Based on the reduction in cerebral blood flow by vasoconstriction from "blowing off carbon dioxide," CPP is reduced in the brain. The tradeoff, however, is a serious reduction in arterial blood flow to the brain; therefore the routine practice of hyperventilation is questioned because the lack of arterial blood flow causes secondary brain injury. Today hyperventilation is used as a temporary measure for clients who exhibit manifestations of herniation.

Management of clients with head injury and increased intracranial pressure begins at the scene of injury and continues until the client reaches maximal function. This discussion begins in the emergent settings.

Medical Management

The goals of medical management are to maintain cerebral oxygenation, to decrease ICP, to maintain optimal neurologic function, and to ready the client for rehabilitation.

Maintain Cerebral Oxygenation

The swollen or bruised brain has an increased need for oxygen and glucose because of an increased metabolic rate. The Pa_{O_2} must be kept between 90 and 100 mm Hg. Hypoxemia (apnea, cyanosis, oxygen saturation below 90%) is corrected immediately by opening the airway or intubating the client (cervical spine injury must be considered). Routine prophylactic hyperventilation

Manifestations of Changes in Neurologic Status

"Change" is the key word. Notify the physician whenever there is a change in the client's neurologic status. The following manifestations are listed in the order that indicates a *worsening* in the client's condition. Remember, a client may display a "transient" deterioration in neurologic responses that does not warrant calling a physician. For example, after you have just performed suctioning of the client's airway or have turned the client, you would anticipate a possible change in neurologic status. If you hyperoxygenate the client and ensure proper positioning for venous return from the jugular veins and airway maintenance, however, any manifestations of increased deficit should last only a few seconds or no more than 4 or 5 minutes. Worsening deficit that lasts longer than this increases the risk for irreversible brain injury and requires immediate attention.

NORMAL

- Alert, oriented to person, place, time
- Responds appropriately to verbal commands
- Eyes open spontaneously with any stimulus, unless in a deep sleep

ABNORMAL; CHANGES RESULTING FROM ALTERED PERFUSION OF THE CEREBRAL CORTEX

- Altered level of consciousness
- Altered perception of time, then place, and lastly person
- Motor deficits (e.g., hemiparesis, hemiplegia)
- Speech deficits (e.g., expressive or receptive speech or both)
- Memory deficits (e.g., recent, intermediate, remote)
- Hyperreflexia
- Babinski's sign
- Seizures
- Decorticate rigidity
- Emotional lability
- Altered sensory interpretation
- Cheyne-Stokes respiration
- Headache, nausea, vomiting, papilledema

ABNORMAL; CHANGES RESULTING FROM ALTERED PERFUSION JUST INFERIOR TO THE CORTEX

- Pupillary changes: asymmetry of size, shape, or time-responsiveness
- Loss of reaction to direct light
- Visual field changes (e.g., homonymous hemianopsia; see Chapter 70)

CN, Cranial nerve.

ABNORMAL; CHANGES RESULTING FROM ALTERED PERFUSION OF THE DIENCEPHALON

- Altered temperature; first high fevers, then hypothermia
- Cheyne-Stokes respiration

ABNORMAL; CHANGES RESULTING FROM ALTERED PERFUSION OF THE POSTERIOR PITUITARY GLAND

- Diabetes insipidus (decreased antidiuretic hormone)

ABNORMAL; CHANGES RESULTING FROM ALTERED PERFUSION OF THE MIDBRAIN

- Dysfunction of CN III (loss of reaction to indirect or consensual light, disconjugate eye movement)
- Dysfunction of CN IV (disconjugate eye movement)
- Central neurogenic hyperventilation

ABNORMAL; CHANGES RESULTING FROM ALTERED PERFUSION OF THE UPPER PONS

- Dysfunction of CN V (altered sensory function to cornea, nasal membranes, face, oral cavity, tongue, teeth, or altered mastication)
- Dysfunction of CN VI (altered lateral eye movement)
- Dysfunction of CN VII (altered facial expression, taste, and salivation)
- Central neurogenic hyperventilation
- Abnormal extension posture
- Pinpoint pupils

ABNORMAL; CHANGES RESULTING FROM ALTERED PERFUSION OF THE LOWER PONS

- Apneustic breathing
- Flaccidity

ABNORMAL; CHANGES RESULTING FROM ALTERED PERFUSION OF THE MEDULLA

- Dysfunction of CN VIII (altered equilibrium and hearing)
- Dysfunction of CN IX (altered taste, pharyngeal sensations, and cough and swallowing)
- Dysfunction of CN X (altered sensations in pharynx, larynx, external ear, and altered cough and swallowing; altered parasympathetic nervous system functions in thoracic and abdominal viscera)
- Dysfunction of CN XI (altered neck and shoulder movement)
- Dysfunction of CN XII (altered tongue movement)
- Projectile vomiting
- Cushing's triad (increased systolic blood pressure, wide pulse pressure, bradycardia)
- Ataxic (Biot's respiration)

is avoided unless the client shows evidence of cerebral herniation (see later discussion).

Steroids have been prescribed for decades to control cerebral edema, and their use was shown to improve outcomes over 30 years ago. Recent studies, however, have not shown improved client outcomes with steroids, and so their use is no longer recommended.

Decrease Intracranial Pressure

Emergency care of the client at high risk for development of increased ICP focuses on maintaining the airway, improving breathing, and promoting circulation. Hypoxemia and hypotension are often associated with poor outcomes in head injuries. Immediate interventions may include intubation followed by hyperventilation, administration of osmotic diuretics, and elevation of the head to promote venous drainage.

Cerebral Perfusion

Intravenous (IV) fluids are administered to avoid or limit hypotension and to prevent secondary brain injury. Vasoactive medication, given either to raise or to lower blood pressure, may be required to maintain CPP at a normal level. CPP is a result of the relationship between blood pressure and ICP. If the physician has not left orders to treat blood pressure changes, notification must occur if the blood pressure range is below 100 or above 150 mm Hg systolic. Several clinical studies suggest that a CPP of 70 to 80 mm Hg is the critical threshold, although some recommend maintaining CPP over 60 mm Hg. Often physician orders specify titration of medication to maintain the CPP at greater than 60 mm Hg. General reduction measures include elevating the head of the bed, preventing obstruction of the jugular veins, controlling body temperature, preventing seizures, and providing sedation and analgesia. Nurses often titrate several medications simultaneously to achieve ideal CPP.

Hyperventilation

Hyperventilation had been recommended as the primary treatment of head-injured clients because elevated carbon dioxide levels cause cerebral blood vessels to dilate. By manually hyperventilating or increasing the ventilator settings to cause hyperventilation, a hypocarbic (low carbon dioxide) blood level is created. A partial pressure of CO_2 ($Paco_2$) level between 30 and 35 mm Hg results in vasoconstriction of the cerebral blood vessels, leading to decreased blood flow and thus decreased ICP. In traumatic brain injury, however, cerebral blood flow is reduced by as much as two thirds of normal and hyperventilation can seriously compromise cerebral perfusion. Therefore routine hyperventilation is no longer recommended unless the client is manifesting herniation. If the client has extensor posturing or pupillary asymmetry or nonreactivity, the client should be hyperventilated at a rate of 20 breaths/min until blood gas analyses can provide guidelines for ventilation rates.[9]

Osmotic Diuresis

Mannitol, a hyperosmotic agent, is used to immediately expand the volume of plasma and increases cerebral blood flow and oxygen delivery. Mannitol has a delayed effect of creating an osmotic gradient that pulls fluid out of the cells, resulting in diuresis over the following hours. Mannitol may accumulate in the brain over time; so to reduce this risk, it is usually given in bolus doses rather than by continuous infusion. Renal function, levels of electrolytes, and serum osmolality need to be monitored when the client is receiving mannitol. Diuresis is

expected, and the client may become hypotensive and dehydrated with the excessive use of mannitol. Monitoring for dehydration is crucial; it is manifested by increased serum sodium and osmolality values.

Hypertonic Saline. Hypertonic saline is any saline solution that is at a concentration higher than 0.9%. Common concentrations are 3%, 5%, 7%, and 23% sodium chloride. Hypertonic saline causes osmotic diuresis because its concentration is higher than that of tissue. Administration of hypertonic saline leads to an increase in plasma osmolarity and establishes an osmotic gradient that moves excess water from the cerebral tissue into the vasculature. By decreasing the water content of brain tissue, hypertonic saline can decrease mass effect and decrease ICP.

Prevent Complications

Many complications are associated with head injury (Box 73-1). Antibiotics may be prescribed, especially with an open head injury, the placement of an ICP monitor, or an infection in another body system. Infections increase metabolism and thus raise ICP.

Antiseizure medications (e.g., phenytoin, carbamazepine) may be given prophylactically to reduce the risk of seizures. Seizures significantly increase metabolic requirements and cerebral blood flow and volume and thus increase ICP. Chapter 69 describes the care of the client with seizures.

Intravenous fluids are given by IV infusion pump to help monitor the amount of fluids given. The client is maintained in a state of euvolemia. Hypotonic IV solutions are avoided because of the risk of promoting cerebral edema.

Temperature reduction decreases metabolism and cerebral blood flow and thus ICP. Antipyretics should be the first intervention to reset the hypothalamic thermostat. Other cooling measures include hypothermic blankets, bathing with tepid water, or placement of ice packs. Muscle relaxants are given to prevent shivering.

BOX 73-1 Complications of Head Injury

- Cerebral edema
- Stress ulcers
- Seizures
- Infections
- Acute hydrocephalus
- Diabetes insipidus
- Syndrome of inappropriate secretion of antidiuretic hormone
- Cardiac dysrhythmias
- Neurogenic pulmonary edema
- Subarachnoid hemorrhage/aneurysms
- Altered behavior
- Post-trauma response

Malnutrition, with wasting of lean muscle mass, can develop quickly because of the metabolic response to severe head injury. Hypoglycemia must be avoided; glucose is the primary fuel for the brain. Hypoglycemia should be avoided by close monitoring. Furthermore, severe hypoglycemia can also result in seizures and coma. Nutritional support is provided with jejunal feeding to reduce the risk of gastric regurgitation and aspiration. Recommended calorie intake is 140% of resting metabolic expenditures in nonparalyzed clients and 100% of resting metabolic expenditures in paralyzed clients with 15% of caloric intake as protein. Nutritional support should begin no later than the seventh day after injury.

Monitor Intracranial Pressure

Continuous ICP monitoring is used for clients experiencing conditions associated with potentially elevated ICP (e.g., head trauma with GCS scores of 8 and lower), preoperative and postoperative aneurysms, tumors, and posterior fossa lesions. ICP monitoring aids in earlier detection of intracranial mass lesions; it can limit the use of indiscriminate therapies to control ICP, which themselves can be harmful; it can reduce ICP by draining CSF and thus improve cerebral perfusion; it helps to determine prognosis; and it may improve outcomes.

Several methods of ICP monitoring are available. The most common types measure CSF pressure in the ventricles, brain parenchyma, or subarachnoid space. Intraventricular catheters provide the most accurate results. All monitoring devices are invasive and carry a risk of infection/colonization, hemorrhage, and obstruction, especially when the device is left in place for over 5 days.[9] Most surgeons prescribe antibiotics, limit the length of time for which the ICP monitor remains in place, and monitor CSF samples on a regular basis. The Bridge to Critical Care feature on Intracranial Pressure Monitoring below describes the nurse's role in caring for clients with these devices.

Monitoring ICP also allows the measurement of intracranial compliance. Introducing a known volume of fluid

---

BRIDGE TO CRITICAL CARE

Intracranial Pressure Monitoring

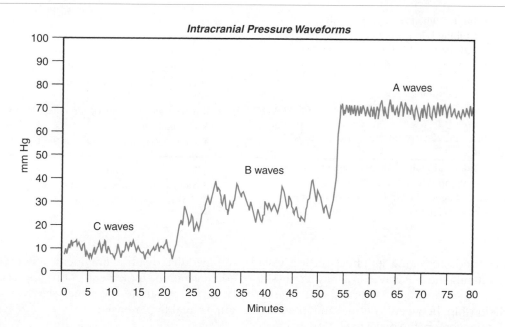

The shape of the waves is influenced by cardiac pulsations and respirations as well as by intracranial pressure (ICP).

C waves occur 4 to 8 times per minute and reflect fluctuations in arterial pressure. C waves are not considered significant.

B waves occur at intervals of 30 seconds to 2 minutes and represent increases in ICP to 50 mm Hg. They may be precursors to A waves and may indicate a decrease in compliance.

A waves are most pronounced when the amount of cranial contents is increased. Also called *plateau waves,* A waves represent recurrent ICP elevations to 100 mm Hg. An A wave may be caused by coughing or straining but, if recurrent or sustained, may indicate a reduced ability of the brain to compensate. The client may also show other manifestations of increasing ICP.

(Continued)

BRIDGE TO CRITICAL CARE

Intracranial Pressure Monitoring—Cont'd

To monitor

Ventricular catheter (ventriculostomy)

To monitor

Subarachnoid screw (bolt) (ventriculostomy)

GENERAL INTERVENTIONS FOR MONITORING INTRACRANIAL PRESSURE AND VENTRICULOSTOMY DEVICES

- Use sterile technique when setting up the device.
- Ensure that the tubing is long enough to allow the client to be moved in bed but that it is no longer than 14 feet. Use of tubing longer than 14 feet may cause inaccurate readings.
- Prevent kinks in the tubing.
- Level the transducer at the tragus of the ear (level with foramen of Monroe).
- Zero or calibrate the device per the manufacturer's recommendations.
- Do baseline and serial neurologic assessments.
- Analyze ICP/PCP and CSF drainage trends.
- Medicate client as needed to reduce risk of dislodgement.
- Monitor response to stimuli.

- If head of bed is lowered, turn drainage device off to avoid draining the ventricles.
- Monitor insertion site for bleeding, drainage, CSF leakage.
- Monitor CSF for manifestations of infection (cloudy, increased volume).
- Notify the physician if the readings show damping (lessening of amplitude) of the waves. The catheter may need to be flushed by the physician or advanced practice nurse.
- If inaccurate readings occur, check for the following:
  - Leaks in the system
  - Differences in the height of the transducer and the device
  - Kinks in the tubing
  - Valsalva maneuver in client
  - Obstruction in the system

into the ventricle and measuring its effect on ICP tests compliance. Examining the ICP waveform may also assist in determining brain compliance. Detecting a change in the critical relationship between volume and pressure allows early treatment before the onset of clinical manifestations or sustained elevated ICP. Measurements of CPP can be made with ICP monitors. Ideally, CPP should be maintained at greater than 60 mm Hg.

Prevent Intracranial Hypertension

Intracranial hypertension is defined as an ICP greater than 20 to 25 mm Hg and can lead to a fatal herniation of the brain. When the herniation occurs at the level of

the medulla, death is imminent. CSF drainage, mannitol administration, hyperventilation, and sedation/chemical paralysis constitute the usual steps in management of intracranial hypertension.

Sedation/Paralysis. Some clients have refractory intracranial pressures and require very advanced methods to reduce cerebral metabolism. Methods can include sedation and paralysis.

Barbiturates. High-dose barbiturates (pentobarbital or thiopental) induce coma, lower ICP, and decrease mortality in clients with uncontrollable ICP that is refractory to all other medical and surgical treatments. These agents, however, can lead to hypotension, and their use is limited to clients with severe traumatic brain injury. Prophylactic use of barbiturates is not warranted. Barbiturate therapy requires sophisticated monitoring and special training. The client is intubated and placed on ventilatory support, and a pulmonary artery catheter is inserted. Additional monitoring modalities include jugular venous oxygenation ($Sjvo_2$) and brain tissue oxygenation (tbO_2).

Monitor serum drug levels daily; the dose should be reduced if serum levels exceed 5 mg/dl or if the burst suppression pattern on the EEG lasts longer than 10 seconds. Monitor temperature because barbiturates reduce metabolism, thereby cooling the body. If the temperature falls below 36° C, active warming is indicated. Propofol has been used instead of barbiturates to provide similar management of increased ICP but may not be as beneficial as barbiturates. The advantage of propofol is that it is short-acting, allowing for daily assessment of neurologic status. Similar monitoring of the EEG occurs as does care of the client.

Continue pupillary assessment. Even when a client is in a coma, the pupils dilate if the brain stem becomes compressed. Notify the physician of this change. Barbiturate therapy eliminates the client's normal protective functions. The client is completely dependent on nursing care for all basic needs (see Chapter 68). Wean clients slowly from barbiturate therapy/propofol to prevent rebound intracranial hypertension.

Neuromuscular Blocking Agents. Nondepolarizing neuromuscular blocking agents are sometimes used to induce skeletal muscle relaxation and to promote synchronous breathing during mechanical ventilation. Decreasing muscle activity may be necessary to control ICP. Nurses use a peripheral nerve stimulator to monitor for adequacy of drug dosage as well as for the risk of overdose (see Chapter 63). Pentobarbital and neuromuscular blocking agents usually are not given concomitantly. If the client is receiving a neuromuscular blocking agent, sedation and analgesia must be given because the neuromuscular blocking agents do not provide it. Other complications may result and are described in Box 73-1.

Nursing Management

Assessment. The Glasgow Coma Scale (GCS) is the most commonly used neurologic assessment tool in clinical care (Box 73-2). This scale provides objective measurement of three essential components of the neurologic examination: spontaneity of eye opening, best verbal response, and best motor response. The total score can range from 3 to 15. The client who is unresponsive to painful stimuli, does not open the eyes, and has complete muscular flaccidity has a score of 3. The client who is oriented, opens the eyes spontaneously, and follows commands scores 15. A score of 8 or less indicates coma. Because the scoring of the GCS is based on the client's ability to respond and to communicate, the following criteria may render the GCS invalid:

- The client is intubated and cannot speak.
- Eyes are swollen closed.
- The client is unable to communicate in English.
- The client has a hearing loss.
- The client is blind.
- The client is aphasic.
- The client is paralyzed or hemiplegic.

The first GCS score recorded for the client becomes the baseline score. Subsequent scores allow assessment of trends or changes in neurologic status and provide a significant and reliable indicator of the severity of head injury. A single measurement cannot predict outcome; however, a decrease of 2 points in the GCS with a score of 9 or lower indicates serious injury. The use of consistent criteria for client assessment is more important than the specific tool used. Specific behaviors dictating a given score should be indicated. If variations occur in scoring criteria, the value of the scale is lost, and serious changes in the client's condition can be overlooked or treated unnecessarily (see the neurologic observation chart on the website). While the Glasgow Coma Scale is quick and easily repeated, more detailed neurologic assessments are conducted to identify specific trends in responses.

Level of Consciousness

The first change in a client who presents with altered cerebral tissue perfusion is a change in the level of consciousness (LOC). When decreased LOC is noted, serial and detailed assessments are required until the client has achieved maximum recovery. To eliminate the subjectivity associated with use of terms such as *lethargy, obtundation, semi-coma,* or *coma,* the GCS both objectifies the client's LOC and assists in identifying very subtle changes (see Box 73-2).

SAFETY

ALERT

Pupil Response. A pupil check includes assessing pupil appearance and physiologic response. The affected pupil is usually on the same *(ipsilateral)* side as the brain lesion, whereas the motor and sensory deficits are usually on the opposite *(contralateral)* side. Be careful not to mistake a prosthetic eye for a fixed pupil.

Pupil Equality. Document pupil equality, noting the relative size of each pupil.

BOX 73-2   Assessment of Clients Using the Glasgow Coma Scale

The Glasgow Coma Scale (GCS) is a numeric expression of cognition, behavior, and neurologic function. It is the most commonly used scale and was designed to measure level of consciousness and severity of injury through eye opening, verbal responsiveness, and motor response. The total of the three scores ranges from 3 to 15, with 3 being the most severe and 15 being normal. Assessments of abstract thought and problem solving should be combined with the GCS to give a more complete picture of neurologic status.

Documentation should contain specific descriptive terms. For example, instead of just indicating that the client is "stuporous," record the evidence of stupor that you observe: "no response to verbal commands, responded only to tracheal suctioning with abnormal flexor posturing." Words such as "lethargic," "stuporous," or "comatose" are open to individual interpretation, and a clear description of behavior is less likely to be misunderstood.

SCALE COMPONENTS

Eye Opening

Observe eye opening without speaking to the client. Does the client open the eyes and look around? If the eyes are closed, call the client's name. If no response is noted, raise your voice. If there is still no response, use a mildly painful stimulus, given in the central part of the body, such as squeezing the trapezius muscle or rubbing the sternum.

Avoid supraorbital pressure, as it can cause damage to the eyes. Pinching of the body can cause severe bruising and is unnecessary in a neurologic examination.

Motor Response

Asking the client to follow specific commands such as "Raise your right arm" or "Wiggle your toes" assesses motor responses. Do not ask the client to squeeze your hand, because grasp is a reflexive response that can occur with head injury. If agency protocol lists grasp as a neurologic assessment component, ask the client to "let go" after grasping to measure cognitive ability to control movement.

In a client who is unable to follow commands, observe the response to a painful stimulus. Responses may include (1) localizing (trying to remove the stimulus), (2) withdrawing, and (3) posturing. In addition, a response may not be elicited and the client may remain motionless.

Compare the right and left sides and the upper and lower extremities. Record the best response while also recording any abnormality that indicates decreased movement in a particular extremity.

Motor Activity

Motor activity assessment is the measure of strength of voluntary movement of the arms and legs. If a client cannot cooperate with testing, paralysis may be difficult to detect. Observe the client carefully. If a client is restless, paralysis may become obvious because the paralyzed part does not move as

other body parts move. Additional information may be obtained in the following ways:

1. Comparing the tone of one side of the body with that of the other
2. Lifting the arms or legs on both sides, releasing them, and watching them drop to the bed
3. Observing the position of the limbs at rest

If a client can cooperate, assessing "drift" may demonstrate subtle tone and strength alterations. For this assessment, have the client hold both arms up in front of the body with the palms upward and the eyes closed. This position should be maintained for 10 seconds. Muscles are weak if one arm "drifts" (gradually moves) downward or if the hand pronates (turns over). This maneuver is often referred to as the *pronator drift test*. Drift can also be assessed in the lower extremities by having the patient raise one leg off the bed and hold it for five seconds with eyes closed. If the leg cannot be held up, it is weak and therefore has a drift.

Posturing

Review posturing in Chapter 68. As the client's intracranial pressure increases at the cortical level, abnormal flexor posturing occurs. As pressure reaches the pons level, abnormal extensor posturing occurs. When the pressure reaches further to the medullary level, flaccidity is noted, or a response is totally lacking—the gravest of all signs.

Verbal Response

Verbal responses assess the client's orientation to self, environment, and time. Ask appropriate questions such as the following: "What is your name? Where are you? What is the month, year, season, nearest holiday?" Avoid asking questions about the date or day of the week.

Being hospitalized can alter the accuracy of that response even in a person with normal cognitive function. Structure the conversation to elicit information that can be verified by family members, such as home address or employer's name. In many cases, a slight degree of confusion is not noticeable until some time is spent with the client. An apparently oriented client may ask the same question a few minutes after it was originally asked and answered, or the client may have "learned" the answers to common questions such as "What is your name?" and "What hospital are you in?" Therefore it is helpful to reassess the client regularly to check memory or to challenge cognitive integrity with various questions. If addition, observing the patient during the course of a normal conversation may provide evidence of confusion or disorientation.

SCORING

After obtaining the data for all three parts of the GCS, total the points for each part and compare the score obtained with the client's baseline score. If a decrease in the score of even 1 point occurs, complete a detailed neurologic assessment, including pupillary responses, cranial nerves, and motor/sensory examinations and notify the physician.

Pupil Size. Estimate the size of each pupil in millimeters (mm) before and after light stimulation. A penlight provides more accurate data than obtainable with a flashlight because of the smaller size of the light and the ability to focus the beam directly at the pupil.

Pupil Position. Note whether the pupil is positioned in the midline or deviated from midline.

Pupil Reaction to Light. Bring the penlight from the lateral aspect of the client's head toward the eye. Observe for constriction in that eye as well as in the opposite eye. Then test the opposite eye in the same way. The detection of subtle change may require four approaches with the penlight. Brisk and equal constriction of the pupils to direct and indirect light is a normal response. Sluggish or unequal direct or indirect *(consensual)* response is abnormal. *Anisocoria,* or unequal pupils, occurs normally in about 17% of the population, with one pupil being about 1 mm larger. It is important to ascertain information about pupil inequality from the client or family members so that an unnecessary procedure is not performed.

Pupil Shape. Normally, pupils are round. Describe abnormal shapes with a drawing. Pupils may be oddly shaped as a result of previous eye surgery. A pupil that looks oval may be early evidence of increasing ICP.

Pupil Accommodation. Normally, the size of the pupil and the lens (which is not visible to the naked eye) accommodates (adjusts) to varying focal lengths. Having the conscious client focus on a distant object and then quickly focus on a close object tests accommodation. Pupils should become smaller as the object is brought nearer the eye and should dilate when the object is moved away from the eye. Accommodation is often not tested in the acute care setting because of the client's inability to cooperate.

The acronym PERRLA is often used in practice and indicates that the *p*upils are *e*qual, *r*ound, and *r*eactive to *l*ight and *a*ccommodation. Notify the physician immediately if any change occurs in the pupillary response.

Eye Movement. Document any changes in eye movement. Observe the position of the eyes when assessing the pupils. The eyes should move together. If *disconjugate* (not together) movement is noted, the physician should be notified.

Vital Signs. Initially vital signs should be assessed continuously and recorded every 15 minutes until they are stable. Body temperature should be monitored every 2 hours. If hypothermia or hyperthermia occurs,

temperature should be monitored continuously; axillary thermometers or thermometers within urinary catheters are commonly used. Trends in vital signs and respiratory patterns should be analyzed. As ICP increases and herniation occurs at the level of the medulla, Cushing's response occurs (see Figure 73-3).

Vital sign changes are *late* changes. See the following discussion of altered cerebral tissue perfusion for care of a client with increasing ICP. Once the vital signs begin to deteriorate, many other changes have already occurred, such as a decrease in LOC. Ongoing monitoring for such changes is imperative; do not wait for vital signs to change because the delay may prove fatal for the client. Any changes in neurologic status may be significant and must be reported to the physician, no matter how minor they may seem.

Other assessments can also be made of the cranial nerves. Extraocular movements are tested on clients who are awake enough to follow directions. Ask the clients to follow your fingers with their eyes without moving the head. Move your fingers in a figure H, and observe both eyes as they move across, up, and down. Conjugate eye movements occur when both eyes move in a parallel motion. Disconjugate eye movements occur when the eyes do not move in a lateral direction together (one eye may move laterally while the other is fixed or moves in another direction). Tracking occurs when the client is consciously following someone's or something's movement around the room.

The *blink reflex* can be tested by lightly stroking the eyelashes. When the eyelids are closed, they will flutter slightly if the reflex is present. Observe for blinking in the conscious and alert client. The *gag reflex* is tested by asking the alert client to cough or swallow. If the client is unable or unconscious, stroke the back of the client's throat with a long cotton-tipped swab. The gag reflex should be swift; do not continue to test gagging once it is present because it will provoke vomiting.

Note the symmetry of the facial muscles. Note the ability of the eyelids to open spontaneously and equally. Ask the client to close the eyes as tightly as possible. Ask the client to smile, and note the corners of the mouth to identify symmetrical patterns. Ask the client to frown/wrinkle the forehead. Finally, note whether speech is clear, slurred, rambling, or aphasic.

Diagnosis, Outcomes, Interventions

Diagnosis: Ineffective Cerebral Tissue Perfusion. If the client is in a coma because of increased ICP, use this diagnosis to reflect the risk to cerebral tissue perfusion. Write the diagnosis as *Ineffective Tissue Perfusion: Cerebral related to increased ICP.* The term *patient* is used to refer to a person in a coma. The *client* in this case is the patient's family, who serves as his or her advocate.

Outcomes. The patient will maintain normal cerebral perfusion as evidenced by (1) stable or improving levels of consciousness; (2) stable or improving GCS score; (3) ICP of 15 mm Hg or less; (4) no restlessness, irritability, or headache; and (5) no pupillary changes, no seizures, no widening pulse pressure, no respiratory irregularity, and no hypertension or bradycardia.

Interventions. Administer the medications ordered to reduce cerebral edema (e.g., osmotic diuretics) and to decrease the risk of seizure (e.g., anticonvulsants), and monitor the patient's response to these medications. If the patient's baseline manifestations of increased ICP are not improving, if the patient's status deteriorates, or if seizures develop, notify the physician. Also, consult the physician for medication to promote bowel evacuation without straining because straining increases ICP. Disimpaction is not advised because of the vasovagal response that occurs.

Position the Patient. Place the patient supine with the head elevated 30 degrees unless contraindicated (e.g., with some spinal injuries, some aneurysms). Keep the patient's head in a neutral position to facilitate venous drainage from the brain. Avoid extreme rotation and flexion of the neck because these positions compress the jugular veins and increase ICP. Also avoid extreme hip flexion because this position increases intra-abdominal and intrathoracic pressures, which increase ICP. As the coma lightens, the patient may become disoriented and combative, making it difficult to maintain proper positioning. If restraints must be used, remember that they often increase agitation, which increases ICP.

If the patient's condition indicates that it will be considerable time before the neurologic condition will improve, consider placing the patient on a pressure-redistribution surface if turning from side to side cannot occur.

Maintain a Patent Airway. Patients need to maintain a patent airway even in the presence of increased ICP. Suctioning prevents the buildup of secretions, which results in elevations of CO_2 levels that lead to an increase of ICP. Adequately oxygenate intubated patients before initiating suctioning, between suctioning efforts, and after suctioning. Try to limit suctioning to three passes, and limit each pass to 10 seconds. Nasal drainage may indicate a dural tear; therefore suctioning of the nares is contraindicated because of the risk of injury to the dura and meningitis.

Balance Fluid Levels. In the past, only small amounts of fluids were administered to clients with head injury, in an effort to decrease cerebral edema. Current data indicate that fluid restriction may actually reduce blood volume and decrease cerebral circulation. The lack of volume causes the blood to be thick and sluggish and may decrease the mobilization of nutrition and toxins into and out of the circulation. Patients should be maintained in a euvolemic state rather than a fluid-restricted state. Fluid restriction may be appropriate for certain conditions (such as syndrome of inappropriate secretion of antidiuretic hormone [SIADH]) but otherwise is contraindicated. Strict intake and output measurement every 1 to 4 hours is necessary to assess fluid balance.

Control Body Temperature. Hyperthermia increases ICP because it increases metabolic demand. Therefore notify the physician immediately if hyperthermia occurs. If a patient's temperature is being managed with a hypothermia blanket, notify the physician if the patient's response is not within the prescribed parameters. Administer any ordered antipyretics. Observe for shivering because this phenomenon also increases metabolism and ICP. Assess for skin breakdown if cooling blankets are used for extended periods, especially in patients who are thin.

Monitor Intracranial Pressure. The ICP reading should be less than 15 mm Hg, the MAP reading 80 mm Hg or higher, and the CPP reading greater than 60 mm Hg.

Plateau waves (A waves) are noted when ICP is greater than 50 mm Hg and can be sustained for longer than 5 minutes. Whenever these sustained pressures are present, assess for contributing factors and intervene appropriately. For example, neck flexion, excessive hip flexion, airway secretions, excess water in the ventilator tubing, taping the endotracheal tube tightly over the jugular veins, and discussing the patient's condition at the bedside have all been known to increase ICP. Plan and space nursing interventions (e.g., turning the patient) for when the patient's ICP is not elevated to help prevent plateau waves. Plateau waves may not be obvious on the ICP monitor screen; a printout generated at a slow rate may be required for accurate observation of these waves. Whenever ICP is greater than 20 mm Hg, interventions to decrease ICP should begin. Use caution when adjusting the patient's position when intracranial monitoring systems are in use. If the system is open to the patient, changing position will quickly alter ventricular fluid levels.

Always close the stopcock on intracranial monitors before moving the patient or lowering the head of the bed. SAFETY ⚠ ALERT

Assessing the ICP monitor site for infection and leakage, using sterile technique for dressing and drainage bag changes, and maintaining a closed system are helpful in preventing infection or in promoting early intervention if infection occurs. If CSF drainage is required, most systems have a stopcock for attaching the tubing and drainage bag that maintains the closed system, decreasing the likelihood of infection. The system is opened only to change the drainage bag. The drainage bag is changed using strict sterile technique.

Evaluation. Evaluate the client's response to treatment as often as every 15 minutes, progressing to hourly, then every 2 to 4 hours, and every 8 hours as the client improves. Once the physician has determined that the client's clinical condition has been optimized, the frequency and extent of evaluation can diminish even further. In the immediate and acute stages, anticipate ongoing modification in the care plan to help the client reach maximum recovery.

Surgical Management

Various surgical techniques are used to treat increased ICP. Optimally, the cause of increased ICP is located and removed. Decompressive surgery removes some brain tissue (e.g., part of the temporal lobe) or a large portion of the skull to give the remaining structures room to expand. If brain compliance is low during surgery, the bone flap removed to gain access to the brain is not replaced, or the dura may not be closed. Subsequent surgery is then required to repair the defect. Postoperative care is the same as that required after craniotomy (see Chapter 69). If the bone flap remains unattached, special care is required to keep the patient off the side of the defect and a helmet may be required until the bone flap is replaced. Surgical placement of a ventriculoperitoneal shunt to allow drainage if CSF circulation is blocked can be done for chronic problems (Figure 73-5).

TRAUMATIC BRAIN INJURY

Traumatic brain injury is an insult to the brain that is capable of producing physical, intellectual, emotional, social, and vocational changes. In the United States, a head injury is experienced approximately every 15 seconds. Head injuries occur in about 7 million Americans every year. Among these head-injured people, more than 500,000 are hospitalized, 100,000 experience chronic disability, and about 2000 are left in a persistent vegetative state.

In more than 30% of cases, because of the seriousness of the injury, head injuries are fatal before the injured person arrives at the hospital. An additional 20% die later because of secondary brain injury. Secondary brain events include ischemia from hypoxia and hypotension, secondary hemorrhage, and cerebral edema.

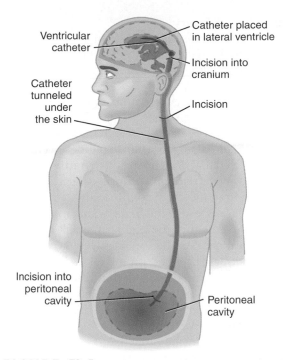

■ **FIGURE 73–5** Ventriculoperitoneal shunt placed for chronic hydrocephalus.

Clients with traumatic head injuries often have other major injuries, including injury to the facial structures, lungs, heart, cervical spine, abdomen, and bones. Facial fractures and lung injuries may contribute to respiratory insufficiency. Airway obstruction and decreased ability to breathe (e.g., from pulmonary contusion, flail chest, pneumothorax) contribute to respiratory insufficiency and poor oxygenation of the brain and other tissues. Ischemia of brain tissue may result.

Hemorrhagic shock in clients with multiple trauma is rarely caused by head injury alone. Frequently shock is due to ruptured abdominal organs or musculoskeletal injuries (e.g., fractured femur and pelvis). Circulation may be further compromised by cardiac contusion and associated dysrhythmias.

Etiology and Risk Factors

Motor-vehicle accidents are the leading cause of head injuries. Of clients admitted to the emergency department, most are males younger than 30 years and 50% have evidence of ingestion of alcohol or other substances of abuse. Alcohol slows the reflexes and alters cognitive processes and perception. These physiologic changes increase the chances of being involved in an accident or altercation. A second risk factor is driving without seat belts. Peak occurrence is during evenings, nights, and weekends. Other causes are assaults, falls, and sports-related injuries.

Mechanisms of Injury

Head injuries are caused by a sudden impact force to the head or inertial forces within the skull (Figure 73-6). The results are complex. Three mechanisms contribute to head trauma.

Primary injuries occur on impact and are the direct result of the impact resulting in injury to the area of the brain beneath the contact site. Skull fractures commonly occur (see Figure 73-6, *A*). Diffuse injuries occur when a blow is received that does not result in fracture but causes the brain to move enough to shear or tear some of the veins going from the cortex of the brain to the skull (see Figure 73-6, *B*). Because the brain is able to move within the skull, movement of the brain can result in injuries at different locations. As the brain moves, it scrapes over the skull's irregular inner prominences, which bruise and lacerate brain tissue. Disruption of the brain's small surface blood vessels may occur. Changes in capillary integrity lead to fluid shifts and petechial hemorrhages. Cranial nerves, nerve tracts, larger blood vessels, and other structures may be stretched, twisted, or rotated, and their functions disrupted. An example is an automobile accident in which the head hits the steering wheel.

Coup-Contrecoup Injuries. A unique term can be used for this complex head injury: *coup-contrecoup injury*. From the French word *coup,* which means "blow," this diagnosis indicates that the client has sustained a combined injury at the point of impact and an injury on the side of the brain opposite from the movement of the brain within the skull. That is, a contrecoup injury (see Figure 73-6, *C*) from the French for "counterblow." Figure 73-7, *A* depicts a contrecoup injury as shown in an MRI scan.

Penetrating Trauma. *Penetrating injuries* are a form of primary injury and include head wounds made by foreign bodies (e.g., knives or bullets) or those made by bone fragments from a skull fracture. The damage caused by a penetrating injury often relates to the velocity with which a penetrating object pierces the skull and brain. Bone fragments from a skull fracture may cause local brain injury by lacerating brain tissue and damaging other structures (e.g., nerves, blood vessels). If a major blood vessel is severed or ruptured, a large clot *(hematoma)* may form, with resultant damage to adjacent or remote structures (e.g., brain compression as in a herniation syndrome). Thus a hematoma itself can cause extensive brain tissue damage.

High-velocity objects (e.g., bullets) produce shock waves in the skull and brain. The shock waves may significantly damage brain structures beyond those in the object's path. Frequently penetrating wounds create an open communication between the external environment and the cranial cavity, and infection is thus a possible complication.[8]

Scalp Injuries. Scalp injuries can cause lacerations, hematomas, and contusions or abrasions to the skin. These

A   B   C

■ **FIGURE 73–6**   Some mechanisms of head injury. **A,** Penetrating injury may fracture the skull. **B,** Diffuse injuries such as a blow to the skull do not result in fracture; they may cause the brain to move enough to tear some of the veins traversing from the cortical surface to the dura. Subdural hematoma may then develop. Note the areas of cerebral contusion (dark brown). **C,** Rebound of the cranial contents may result in an area of injury opposite the point of impact. Such an injury is called a *contrecoup* injury. In addition to the direct damage sustained in the three injuries depicted, additional brain damage may occur.

■ **FIGURE 73–7** A magnetic resonance imaging scan showing coup (A) contrecoup (B) injury after head injury.

injuries may be unsightly and may bleed profusely. Clients with minor scalp injuries not accompanied by damage to other areas do not require hospitalization. The care of these injuries is discussed in Chapter 82.

Skull Fractures. Skull fractures are often caused by a force sufficient to fracture the skull and cause brain injury. The fractures themselves do not signal that brain injury is also present; however, skull fractures often cause serious brain damage. Depressed skull fractures injure the brain by bruising it (resulting in a contusion) or by driving bone fragments into it (causing lacerations). The site of a fracture and the extent of brain injury may not correlate.

The three types of skull fractures are as follows:

- *Linear skull fractures* appear as thin lines on x-ray and do not require treatment; they are important only if there is significant underlying brain damage.
- *Depressed skull fractures* may be palpated and are seen on x-ray.
- *Basilar skull fractures* occur in bones over the base of the frontal and temporal lobes. These are not observable on plain x-ray but may be manifested as ecchymosis around the eyes or behind the ears or by blood or CSF leakage from the ear.

Brain Injuries

A single classification of brain injuries does not exist; however, the terms *open, closed, contusion,* and *concussion* are often applied to brain injuries. Open head injuries are those that penetrate the skull. Closed injuries are from blunt trauma.

Concussions. A *concussion* is head trauma that may result in loss of consciousness for 5 minutes or less and retrograde amnesia. There is no break in the skull or dura, and no damage is visible on CT or MRI scans.

Contusions. Contusions are associated with more extensive damage than that from concussions. With contusions the brain itself is damaged, often with multiple areas of small hemorrhage and bruised areas in brain tissue. Diffuse axonal injury resulting in anatomic disruption of the white matter may result from serious contusions. Microscopic nerve fiber lesions also occur. Abnormalities may be located primarily in one area of the brain, but other areas may also be injured. This is particularly true of brain stem contusions, which are a very serious type of lesion.

Diffuse Axonal Injury. Diffuse axonal injury is the most severe form of head injury because there is no focal lesion to remove. The injury involves the tissue of the entire brain and occurs at the microscopic level. Diffuse axonal injury is classified as mild, moderate, or severe. With *mild diffuse axonal injury,* loss of consciousness lasting 6 to 24 hours is characteristic, and short-term disability may be associated with it. With *moderate diffuse axonal injury,* coma lasting less than 24 hours is the predominant clinical feature, with incomplete recovery on awakening. *Severe diffuse axonal injury* also involves primary injury to the brain stem. The patient may present with abnormal posturing and in coma, but there may not be evidence of cerebral edema or increased ICP. Diffuse axonal injury begins with immediate loss of consciousness, prolonged coma, abnormal flexion or extensor posturing, hypertension, and fever.

Focal Injuries

Epidural Hematoma. An epidural hematoma, also called an *extradural hematoma,* forms between the skull and the dura mater (Figure 73-8). It occurs in about 10% of severe head injuries and is usually associated with a skull fracture. An epidural hematoma occurs from injury to the cerebral blood vessels, most often the middle meningeal artery. Bleeding is usually continuous, and a large clot forms, which separates the dura from the skull.

Manifestations are usually acute in onset because the bleeding is often arterial. With an epidural hematoma, the following sequence of events may occur:

1. The client is unconscious immediately after head trauma.
2. The client awakens and is quite lucid.
3. Loss of consciousness occurs and pupil dilation response rapidly deteriorates, with onset of eye movement paralysis, on the same side as that of the hematoma.
4. The client lapses into a coma.

Dura

A Subdural hematoma   B Epidural hematoma   C Intracerebral hematoma

■ **FIGURE 73–8** Formation of a hematoma after head injury. Note the shift of the brain structures.

Although these manifestations are often described as "classic" for an epidural hematoma, few clients present with such classic manifestations and astute assessment is necessary to prevent death.

Computed tomography scanning confirms the diagnosis. Rapid diagnosis and prompt intervention are essential with an epidural hematoma. Careful, ongoing assessment of neurologic status is also necessary.

Subdural Hematoma. Subdural hematoma is a collection of blood in the subdural space (i.e., between the dura mater and arachnoid mater). Tearing of the bridging veins over the brain causes most subdural hematomas.

Subdural hematomas may be classified as acute, subacute, or chronic, depending on how rapidly clinical manifestations develop. Another classification system recognizes only acute and chronic, combining the acute and subacute categories.

Acute and Subacute Subdural Hematoma. Acute subdural hematoma usually results from brain or blood vessel laceration. Acute subdural hematomas are a serious complication requiring prompt treatment because they compress and distort an already damaged, edematous brain. Acute subdural hematoma is symptomatic within 24 to 48 hours of injury and is seen in about 24% of clients with severe head injuries.

Clinical manifestations of acute subdural hematoma are similar to those of acute epidural hematoma. The onset and development of the clinical manifestations may be somewhat slower because the bleeding is more often venous rather than arterial. Recognition of clinical manifestations may be difficult because subdural hematoma is often associated with moderate or severe brain injury. A patient who develops an acute subdural hematoma may remain unconscious after injury or may have a variable LOC (depending on the extent of injury). A conscious client usually has a headache. The client may become irritable and confused and lapse into a coma or show a fluctuating LOC. Manifestations of increasing ICP appear. Subtle changes in LOC and development

of lateralizing changes (i.e., on one side) such as hemiparesis, pupillary dilation, or extraocular eye movement paralysis may be the only findings.

Chronic Subdural Hematoma. Chronic subdural hematoma is most common in older and alcoholic clients (Figure 73-9). These clients experience atrophy of the brain, which results in stretching of the bridging veins and an increase in the size of the subdural space. These stretched veins are easily ruptured in a fall, even if the fall does not result in other injuries. It develops several weeks or even months after injury because of a slow accumulation of fluid in a larger-than-normal space. Older or alcoholic clients may not even recall the mechanism of injury. The initial injury may have been relatively minor, and the client may not associate current

■ **FIGURE 73–9** *A,* Magnetic resonance image of a chronic subdural hematoma with an area of acute bleeding. *B,* Severe midline shift results.

clinical manifestations with the past injury. In addition, family members may not recognize the subtle neurologic changes or may not give credence to them because of the client's age or alcohol use.

Gradually the enlarging blood clot creates pressure on the brain. There is an interval during which the client appears to be recovering or seems completely recovered. Later, manifestations of neurologic deterioration develop. The client may become drowsy, inattentive, and incoherent and display personality changes. Headaches are another prominent symptom. These indications of chronic subdural hematoma may be overlooked until focal or lateralizing signs appear (e.g., hemiparesis, pupil signs). Changes in LOC continue, and LOC may fluctuate widely. Clinical assessment with subdural hematoma is similar to that with epidural hematomas. Surgical intervention usually consists of placing several burr holes or performing a craniotomy to remove the hematoma. Treatment results depend on the client's condition before surgery and the degree of primary brain tissue damage.

A client who has undergone evacuation of a chronic subdural hematoma usually has a drain placed in the cavity to prevent reaccumulation of the fluid and blood. These clients are typically kept flat during the immediate postoperative period, which allows the brain to reexpand to fill the cranial cavity.

Intracerebral Hematoma. Intracerebral hematomas occur less often than epidural or subdural hematomas. They are caused by bleeding directly into brain tissue and may occur at the area of injury, some distance away, or deep within the brain. These hematomas cause problems with increased ICP. Surgical resection may cause as much damage as the clot itself and is usually not performed unless the clot is easily accessible. Clinical manifestations are similar to those that occur with epidural or subdural hematomas, although hemiplegia is more common than hemiparesis. Many assessment findings relate to the lesion's mass effect. Various other clinical manifestations may also be present, depending on the location of the intracerebral hematoma. A diagnosis is established as with other types of hematomas. One form of hematoma, called *delayed traumatic intracerebral hematoma,* occurs after a few days. It is most common in people with disseminated intravascular coagulation, hypertension, a history of alcohol abuse, or hypoxia. It carries a poor prognosis.

Pathophysiology

Major head injuries cause direct damage to the parenchyma of the brain. Kinetic energy is transmitted to the brain, and bruising analogous to that seen in soft tissue injuries results. A blow to the surface of the brain results in rapid brain tissue displacement and disruption of blood vessels, leading to bleeding, tissue injury, and

edema. Damage to the brain and skull includes the blow itself *(primary injury)* and continuing injury from edema, inflammation, and hemorrhage within the brain *(secondary injury).* Secondary injury can result in more severe manifestations than those attributable to the impact itself. Inflammation leads to cerebral edema and increased ICP. Hemorrhage may be diffuse if it is due to tearing of several small vessels within the brain. Whenever pressure is increased within the brain, the brain can become hypoxic. The secondary problems occur hours to days after the initial impact.

A concussion usually causes injury to the brain that is reversible. Some biochemical and ultrastructural damage, such as depletion in mitochondrial adenosine triphosphate and changes in vascular permeability, also can occur.

Clients with diffuse axonal damage have microscopic injury to the axons in the cerebrum, the corpus callosum, and the brain stem. Widespread white-matter injury, white-matter degeneration, neuronal dysfunction, and global cerebral edema are characteristic features.

Studies have noted a significantly increased mortality in the client who experiences hypotension, especially early in the postinjury period. When autoregulation is disrupted, as in head injury, cerebral hypoperfusion leads to brain tissue ischemia. Hypoxia has a diminished effect on mortality so long as cerebral perfusion is adequate because the brain can extract extra oxygen for short periods. The combination of arterial hypotension and hypoxemia is significant in the progression of secondary injury. Other causes of secondary brain injury include increased ICP, respiratory problems, electrolyte imbalance, and infection.

Reperfusion injury occurs when ischemia is reversed and blood flow is reestablished; it also leads to secondary injury. Reperfusion injury is also recognized in myocardial infarction and stroke. Reperfusion injury is probably caused by oxygen free radicals, which are normal by-products of aerobic metabolism that usually break down into oxygen and water. In cell injury, breakdown of these radicals is impaired so that they accumulate, causing destruction of nucleic acids, proteins, carbohydrates, and lipids and, eventually, cell membranes in the brain tissue. Currently, research is targeted at developing neuroprotective agents that prevent delayed injury progression.[61]

Clinical Manifestations
Skull Fractures

Other than a history of skull fracture, clients may not have clear manifestations of the injury. Therefore they need careful ongoing assessment. They may develop other clinical signs, including the following:

- CSF or other fluid draining from the ear or nose
- Evidence of various cranial nerve injuries

- Blood behind the tympanic membrane
- Periorbital ecchymoses (bruises around the eyes)
- Later, a bruise over the mastoid process (Battle's sign)

Indications of cranial nerve and inner ear damage may be noted at the time of the initial injury or may not appear until later. They include the following:

- Vision changes from optic nerve damage
- Hearing loss from auditory nerve damage
- Loss of the sense of smell from olfactory nerve damage
- Squint or fixed, dilated pupil and loss of some eye movements from oculomotor nerve damage
- Facial paresis or paralysis (unilateral) from facial nerve damage
- Vertigo caused by damage from otoliths in the inner ear
- Nystagmus from damage to the vestibular system

Basilar skull fractures, depressed fractures, and other open (compound) fractures allow communication between the external environment and the brain. Infection is therefore a possible complication. See Chapter 69 for a discussion of brain abscess and meningitis. Increasing ICP with basilar skull fractures can be difficult to assess because the pressure is not exerted on the motor strip of the frontal lobes, which means that there will be no weakness in the contralateral extremities. Assess for subtle changes in vital signs, especially heart rate and rhythm and breathing patterns. Headache may be present if there is bleeding at the site of injury.

Concussions

After concussion, observers report loss of consciousness for 5 minutes or less. Retrograde amnesia, post-traumatic amnesia, or both may be present. The duration of amnesia may directly correlate with the severity of the concussion. The client usually has a headache and dizziness and may complain of nausea and vomiting. There is no break in the skull or dura, and no visible damage is seen on CT or MRI scans.

Contusions

The clinical manifestations of contusions are varied, partly because any area of the brain can suffer contusion. Contusions are often associated with other serious injuries, including cervical fractures. Secondary effects (e.g., brain swelling and edema) accompany serious contusions. Increased ICP and herniation syndromes may result. Contusions may be divided into cerebral contusions and brain stem contusions.

Cerebral Contusions. Manifestations of cerebral contusions vary, depending on which areas of the cerebral hemispheres are damaged. An agitated, confused head-injured client who remains alert may have a temporal lobe contusion. Hemiparesis in an alert head-injured client may indicate a frontal contusion. An aphasic head-injured client may have a frontotemporal contusion. Other findings indicate contusions in other areas. Although these findings correlate with cerebral contusion, they do not rule out other abnormalities, such as a developing mass lesion. Adverse changes in the client's condition require immediate medical attention. If treated early, these complications may be reversible.

Brain Stem Contusions. Brain stem contusions render a client immediately unresponsive or partially comatose because of significant brain stem disruption. Typically an altered LOC continues for at least several hours and usually days or weeks. The client may regain partial consciousness within hours or remain in a coma.

Damage to the reticular activating system may render the client permanently comatose. Other neurologic abnormalities are present and are usually symmetrical (i.e., evenly distributed on both sides of the body). Some may be lateralized (asymmetrical, or on one side of the body only), indicating development of a secondary event, such as a hematoma.

In addition to the altered LOC that is always present with brain stem contusion, respiratory, pupillary, eye movement, and motor abnormalities may occur.

- Respirations may be normal, periodic, very rapid, or ataxic.
- Pupils are usually small, equal, and reactive. Damage to the upper brain stem (third cranial nerve) may cause pupillary abnormalities.
- Loss of normal eye movements may occur because pathways controlling eye movements traverse the midbrain and pons.
- The client may respond to light or noxious stimuli by purposeful movements, such as pushing the stimulus away, or the client may have no response to stimuli (i.e., may be in a flaccid state). In the presence of profound alteration in LOC, flexor or extensor posturing may be elicited with or without noxious stimuli (see Chapter 68).

Brain stem contusions do not usually injure the brain stem alone. Localized swelling or direct injury to the hypothalamus may produce autonomic nervous system effects. The client may have a high temperature and a rapid pulse rate and respirations and may perspire profusely. These effects may wax and wane but, if sustained, can lead to serious complications.

These clinical manifestations often vary from one observation to another, whereas findings with a developing hematoma are more consistent. Careful documentation of assessment findings to identify patterns or trends in the client's condition is important.

Diagnostic assessments such as CT or MRI scanning may reveal fractures and areas of bleeding or brain shift (see Figure 73-9). Lumbar puncture can also be used to assess for bleeding within the subarachnoid space if any possibility of increased ICP has been ruled out. Currently, CT scans can identify blood in the subarachnoid space, and lumbar punctures are rarely done for this purpose.

OUTCOME MANAGEMENT

Major goals in the care of severely head-injured clients are as follows:

- Prompt recognition and treatment of hypoxia and acid-base disorders that can contribute to cerebral edema
- Control of increasing ICP resulting from factors such as cerebral edema or expanding hematoma
- Stabilization of other conditions.

Medical Management

The medical management of severely head-injured clients focuses on supporting all organ systems while recovery from the injuries takes place. This involves (1) ventilatory support, (2) management of fluid balance and elimination, and (3) management of nutrition and gastrointestinal function. Head trauma affects all systems of the body, and managing its effects requires a holistic perspective. The Translating Evidence into Practice feature on Management of Fever in Clients with Head Injury on p. 1940 describes assessments and interventions related to hyperpyrexia. Clinical manifestations may be the result of the initial head injury or may arise from a complicating process.

Initial Management

The initial management of clients with head injury is the same as for any other injured client: airway, breathing, and circulation. There is a high association of cervical fracture with head injury; therefore the client must be immobilized at the scene of the injury. Lateral cervical spine x-ray films are obtained before the client's head is moved, or the immobilization devices are removed. The client with head injury is protected from possible complications of cord injury by immobilizing the head and neck immediately, using a cervical collar or sandbags until a collar can be obtained.

If intubation is necessary, a jaw thrust maneuver must be used rather than neck flexion to open the airway without possible injury to the spine. A baseline assessment of the client's motor and sensory function is obtained at the scene of the accident. Interventions include achieving oxygenation and lowering the ICP with hyperventilation by mechanical ventilation or by manually hyperventilating the client with a bag-valve-mask device if the client has evidence of herniation.[9]

An IV line is placed and fluids are given to stabilize the blood pressure to systolic pressures over 90 mm Hg. Head injury alone does not cause major loss of blood. If substantial blood loss is suspected, look for other injuries (e.g., fractures, abdominal injury, and severe scalp laceration).

A complete history, including the mechanism of injury, is important. These data allow the physician to determine the probable extent of injury and allow emergency department personnel to prepare for the client's arrival. Open head wounds should be covered and pressure applied to control bleeding unless there appears to be an underlying depressed or compound skull fracture.

Do not attempt to remove foreign objects or any penetrating objects from the wound. Uncomplicated scalp wounds (that do not lie over depressed or compound skull fractures) are anesthetized with a local anesthetic agent, cleansed, and sutured. In the emergency department, primary and secondary surveys of the client's injuries are performed. Resuscitation continues with fluid administration.

Laboratory studies are performed, as are necessary radiologic studies. If any identified injuries require emergency surgery, the client is taken directly to the operating room (OR) before admission to the intensive care unit (ICU). Once the client is stabilized enough for transfer to the ICU, the neurosurgical and trauma teams and the nursing staff maintain ongoing care.

Ongoing Management

Ongoing care to maintain cerebral perfusion and reduce ICP is the focus of critical care. The cerebral metabolic rate is reduced with sedatives, paralytic agents, antipyretics, barbiturates, and hypothermia. Morphine is a commonly used opioid for the head-injured client. It reduces pain and can be given intravenously. Respiratory depression is controlled in the client who is intubated and ventilated. Paralytic agents may be used to promote adequate ventilation and should be administered in conjunction with a sedative and an analgesic because paralytic agents have no sedative or analgesic effect.

Prognosis

Few clients die instantly from head injury; however, many head-injured clients die within the first few minutes after injury from shock or impaired respiration. Early death may also result from brain stem damage. According to the results of several studies, coma duration is the best predictor of damage severity because it correlates highly with the probability of death, intellectual deficit, and social skill impairment. These studies classified a *mild* head injury as loss of consciousness

TRANSLATING EVIDENCE INTO PRACTICE

Management of Fever in Clients with Head Injury

Fever is defined as a core temperature greater than 38° C or 100.4° F. Other definitions of fever include two or more consecutive elevations greater than 38.3° C or 101° F.[5,6] Fever (hyperpyrexia) implies that the thermoregulatory response is intact but that the body temperature is maintained at a higher level. In the presence of fever, compensatory cooling responses occur. Hyperthermia is the loss of thermoregulatory ability, which can occur with injury to the hypothalamus or in malignant hyperthermia. Hyperthermia requires aggressive treatment to prevent cellular damage as the temperature approaches 40° C.

The management of fever in the head-injured patient can be complex because the etiology of fever is not always clear. Assessment of the fever is the first step in management. The nurse needs to evaluate the diagnosis of the patient, the disease processes that might be occurring in conjunction with the fever, and the pattern of the fever that the patient is experiencing. In addition, the presence of intravenous lines or other invasive devices (e.g., ICP monitor or indwelling bladder catheter) needs to be evaluated as causes of the fever.

Infectious causes of fever include ventilator-acquired or nosocomial pneumonia, bacteremia from central lines, and drug fever from antimicrobials, diuretics, or other medications. Noninfectious fever can occur as a result of neurologic events (stroke, head injury, seizure, or hemorrhage), malignancies, or acute myocardial infarction.

Whereas the literature suggests that fever can enhance the host defense by activating the body's physiologic adaptive response, in certain vulnerable populations (neurologic, cardiac, immune compromised, and older clients), evidence shows that fever is maladaptive and needs aggressive management.[2,4,6]

When fever is present, the physician is notified, and appropriate cultures are obtained. Antipyretics should be given as the first line of therapy for temperatures greater than 38.5° C. Acetaminophen, aspirin, or nonsteroidal anti-inflammatory drugs are given to "re-set" the hypothalamic thermoregulatory mechanism or "thermostat."[5,6]

Which cooling measures to use and when to use them have not been answered in the literature in scientifically rigorous studies. Cooling measures should be directed toward increasing heat loss. Examples of this include placing ice packs at the groin or axilla or sponging with alcohol and tepid water. It is important to prevent shivering, however, because shivering increases metabolic activity and the potential to increase rather than decrease the fever. Cooling measures that allow evaporation may be more effective than the use of cooling blankets.[1,4]

The use of cooling blankets should be reserved for clients whose core temperatures rise to 39° to 40° C (>103.5° F). The cooling blanket should be set at 23.9° C to prevent shivering episodes and clients should not be cooled at greater than 0.5° C every 30 minutes. The cooling blanket should be turned off once the patient temperature reaches a desirable level (<38° C).[1] Skin integrity should be assessed while on the cooling blanket because areas of "frost bite" can develop, especially if the skin is damp.

REFERENCES

1. Caruso, C.C., et al. (1992). Cooling effects and comfort of four cooling blanket temperatures in humans with fever. *Nursing Research, 41*(2), 68-72.
2. Henker, R. (1999). Evidence-based practice: Fever-related interventions. *American Journal of Critical Care, 8*(1), 481-489.
3. Kluger, M.J. (1986). Is fever beneficial? *Yale Journal of Biological Medicine, 58*, 89-95.
4. McIlvoy, L.H. (2005). The effect of hypothermia and hyperthermia on acute brain injury. *AACN Clinical Issues, 16*(4), 488-500.
5. O'Donnell, J., et al. (1997). Use and effectiveness of hypothermia blankets for febrile patients in the intensive care unit. *Clinical Infectious Diseases, 24*, 1208-1213.
6. Vaughn, L.K., Veale, W.L., & Cooper, K.E. (1980). Antipyresis: Its effect on mortality rate of bacterially infected rabbits. *Brain Research Bulletin, 5*, 69-73.
7. Wright, J.E. (2005). Therapeutic hypothermia in traumatic brain injury. *Critical Care Nursing Quarterly, 28*(2), 150-161.

for 20 minutes or less, a *moderate* head injury as 21 to 59 minutes of unconsciousness, and *severe* head injury as coma for 1 hour or longer.

Nursing Management

Assessment. A description of the mechanism of injury is helpful in understanding the nature of a head injury. Whenever there are witnesses to the accident, information obtained can be valuable in determining the extent of the injury. Information about the client's activity and LOC before and after the injury is also helpful. Also important is whether the client was conscious at all or unconscious after injury.

As soon as possible after head injury, assess and document the client's vital signs and neurologic status. This initial assessment and the data obtained from witnesses at the accident scene establish a baseline for later observations. Carefully document all assessment findings. Assessment data collection is described earlier in this chapter.

The physician should be notified promptly of any findings that indicate the possible development of complications. It is particularly difficult to accurately assess the condition of a head-injured client who has ingested large amounts of alcohol or other drugs before injury because the effects of these substances may obscure significant clinical abnormalities.

Diagnosis, Outcomes, Interventions. Many nursing and collaborative problems are present in the client with a head injury, such as risk for *Ineffective Airway Clearance, Ineffective Tissue Perfusion,* seizures, paralysis, infection, diabetes insipidus, and *Post-trauma Syndrome.* Other problems that a client with a head injury may experience include the following:

- Risk for contractures
- Impaired skin integrity
- Impaired oral mucous membranes
- Imbalanced nutrition
- Risk for imbalanced fluid volume
- Risk for falls
- Risk for increased ICP
- Disturbed thought processes
- Interrupted family processes

Nursing diagnoses for these problems are discussed in Chapters 68 and 69. Investigation of the underlying causes of these problems and the interventions for them must be individualized according to the client's needs. A sample care plan for managing clients with traumatic injury appears on pp. 1942 to 1947.

Diagnosis: Risk for Ineffective Airway Clearance. The client with traumatic brain injury may have an altered state of consciousness and may not be able to expectorate secretions. The client is also at increased risk for aspiration.

Outcomes. The client will have effective airway clearance. The upper airway should be free of secretions. Respirations should be of a regular rate (16 to 22 breaths/min), rhythm, and depth. Breath sounds should be clear in both lungs, and the chest should have symmetrical movement. The trachea should be in a midline position, and no dyspnea or accessory muscle use should be noted. Aspiration should be prevented. The Pao_2 should be maintained greater than 90 mm Hg and the $Paco_2$ between 30 and 35 mm Hg initially. The chest film should be clear.

Interventions. Nursing actions aimed at maintaining adequate airway clearance include clearing the mouth and oral pharynx of foreign bodies (e.g., broken teeth) and suctioning the oropharynx and trachea every 1 or 2 hours and as needed. Avoid suctioning the nasopharynx until after a basilar fracture or meningeal tear is ruled out. A semiprone lateral position may facilitate drainage of secretions and prevent aspiration but is contraindicated with increased ICP or a cervical fracture. Humidified oxygen, endotracheal intubation, mechanical ventilation, or a tracheostomy may be required to maintain the client's Pao_2 and $Paco_2$ within set parameters.

Diagnosis: Ineffective Cerebral Tissue Perfusion. In clients who suffer from traumatic brain injuries, another appropriate nursing diagnosis is *Risk for Ineffective Cerebral Tissue Perfusion secondary to hypotension, hypertension, intracranial hemorrhage, hematoma, or other injuries.*

Outcomes. The client will have adequate cerebral tissue perfusion. The client will have a stable or improving LOC with a stable GCS score and an ICP of less than

15 mm Hg. Temperature will be maintained at less than 38.5° C. The client's blood pressure will be maintained within established parameters. Urine output will be a minimum of 0.5 ml/kg/hour and not greater than 200 ml/hour. Laboratory values will remain within normal limits.

Interventions. Although anticipatory, prudent monitoring is key to early detection of ineffective cerebral tissue perfusion, nursing interventions can actually prevent, delay, or minimize ineffective cerebral perfusion. These interventions are discussed earlier in this chapter. Briefly they include maintaining all physiologic parameters within normal limits, positioning the client for optimal venous return, and monitoring extracerebral systems for complications. Communicating a client's neurologic status accurately and completely through verbal reporting and documentation is essential to early identification of change and early intervention. ICP monitoring may be required (see earlier discussion).

Surgical Management

Conditions that may require surgery include subdural and epidural hematomas, depressed skull fractures, and penetrating foreign bodies. An epidural clot may be surgically evacuated through burr holes (Figure 73-10) or a craniotomy. During surgery the wound may be drained and bleeding vessels ligated. After surgery nursing care is the same as that for any client recovering from a craniotomy. Simple skull depressions are treated electively by surgically elevating the depressed bone tissue, removing fragments, and repairing lacerated dura. Compound depressed skull fractures are immediately treated surgically. The scalp, skull, and devitalized brain are debrided, and the wound is cleaned thoroughly. Unless all foreign material is removed, a brain abscess or seizures may develop. Debridement of a penetrating wound or depressed skull fracture frequently leaves a cranial

■ **FIGURE 73-10** Placement of burr holes in the skull.

C A R E   P L A N   *evolve*

Management of the Client with Traumatic Brain Injury

Nursing Diagnosis: Airway Clearance, Ineffective (NANDA) related to decreased level of consciousness, loss of protection of airway and inability to maintain positioning.
Outcomes: Client will be free of respiratory distress or aspiration pneumonia.

NOC OUTCOMES   Aspiration Prevention; Respiratory Status: Airway Patency; Respiratory Status: Ventilation

Interventions	NIC INTERVENTIONS	Rationales
1. Maintain patent airway using suctioning or coughing.	Airway Suctioning	1. A clear airway allows for adequate oxygenation and ventilation.
2. Position patient with HOB elevated 30 degrees.	Cough Management Aspiration Precautions: Positioning	2. Reduces risk of secretions from entering the lungs.
3. Assess client's ability to maintain own airway (cough, gag reflexes present).	Airway Management	3. Clients who are comatose may have lost reflexes needed to maintain airway.
4. Assess patency of artificial airway (ETT or tracheostomy).	Airway Management	4. Artificial airways can become plugged with mucus or from biting. Maintaining airway patency allows for effective oxygenation and ventilation.
5. Monitor oxygenation using pulse oximetry.	Respiratory Monitoring	5. Pulse oximetry provides information about oxygen status and should be >90%.
6. Provide oxygen support as needed.	Ventilation Assistance	6. Supplemental oxygen may be necessary to support the injured brain.

Evaluation: With interventions, client will be able to maintain/protect airway and oxygenate and ventilate without difficulty.

Nursing Diagnosis: Tissue Perfusion: Cerebral, Ineffective (NANDA) related to edema from traumatic brain injury.
Outcomes: The client will maintain cerebral perfusion.

NOC OUTCOMES   Circulation Status; Cognition; Neurologic Status; Neurologic Status: Consciousness; Tissue Perfusion: Cerebral

Interventions	NIC INTERVENTIONS	Rationales
1. Maintain blood pressure within ordered range. Assess hemodynamic status to ensure appropriate cardiac output.	Cerebral Perfusion Promotion	1. Cerebral perfusion should be maintained to ensure oxygenation and nutrient delivery to brain tissue.
2. Monitor neurologic examination as per unit standard.	Neurologic Monitoring	2. Neurologic status is the most important indicator of the client's condition.
3. Maintain ICP <20 mm Hg. Treat ICP >25 mm Hg with diuresis, CSF drainage, mild hyperventilation.	Intracranial Pressure Monitoring	3. ICP monitoring provides an early warning system of possible changes within the cranial vault that could lead to a change in neurologic status.

Evaluation: The client will maintain a stable neurologic examination with ICP <20 mm Hg and CPP >60 mm Hg.

Nursing Diagnosis: Intracranial Adaptive Capacity, Decreased (NANDA) related to traumatic brain injury, increased ICP, and cerebral edema.
Outcomes: The client will return to a functional neurologic status and will be seizure-free.

NOC OUTCOMES   Neurologic Status; Neurologic Status: Consciousness; Seizure Control; Tissue Perfusion: Cerebral

Interventions	NIC INTERVENTIONS	Rationales
1. Assess neurologic status per unit standard and client condition, including mental status and motor, sensory, and cranial nerves.	Cerebral Edema Management Cerebral Perfusion Promotion	1. Changes in neurologic status are the first indicators of problems developing within the cranial vault.
2. Monitor ICP and CPP to ensure oxygen and nutrients are delivered to the brain.	Intracranial Pressure Monitoring Neurologic Monitoring	2. ICP and CPP provide additional information about the status of the brain.
3. Monitor for seizures. Administer antiseizure medications as ordered.	Seizure Precautions Seizure Management	3. Seizures increase metabolic rate in the brain and lead to poor outcomes after TBI.

Evaluation: The client will maintain a stable neurologic examination.

Nursing Diagnosis: Confusion, Acute (NANDA) related to traumatic brain injury, hospitalization in an unfamiliar environment, effect of medications provided.

Outcomes: Client will be alert, oriented to person, place, and situation.

NOC OUTCOMES   Cognitive Orientation; Neurologic Status: Consciousness

Interventions	NIC INTERVENTIONS	Rationales
1. Evaluate the possible causes of delirium or delusion such as medications, environment, or lack of sleep.	Delirium Management Delusion Management	1. Determining the causes of changes in orientation will provide direction for management.
2. Attempt to modify those causes that can be modified.	Reality Orientation	2. When possible, a quiet environment with minimal stimulation will assist in calming and reorienting the client.
3. Orient the patient as much as is possible.		3. Reorienting the client may not be possible. It is important not to argue with the patient's current reality.
4. Provide medication that will decrease the delirium or delusion.		4. Use of sedative medications is a last resort, but should be used when the client indicates potential for self-harm or harm to others.
5. Ensure that a total assessment is completed by the medical team.		5. Ensuring that the change in orientation is not related to a structural change in the brain is a priority.
6. Determine the need for a psychiatric consultation.		6. Psychiatric consultation can assist with medication management for delirium/delusion.
7. Monitor neurologic status as required for area of care.	Neurologic Monitoring	7. Provides early identification of changes in level of consciousness.
8. Maintain ICP <20 mm Hg and CPP >60 mm Hg.	Cerebral Perfusion Promotion	8. Prevents secondary brain injury from edema or poor blood flow.

Evaluation: With interventions, client will show no evidence of delirium or delusion and will be aware of current situation. ICP and CPP will be maintained within normal limits.

Nursing Diagnosis: Fluid Volume Deficit or Excess (NANDA) related to need for fluid resuscitation after traumatic brain injury or need for diuresis.

Outcomes: Client will maintain fluids and electrolytes within normal limits and will maintain a regular diet.

NOC OUTCOMES   Electrolyte and Acid-Base Balance; Fluid Balance; Hydration; Nutritional Status: Food and Fluid Intake

Interventions	NIC INTERVENTIONS	Rationales
1. Monitor acid-base balance, fluid intake and output, and electrolyte results.	Acid-Base Management Fluid/Electrolyte Management	1. Values outside of normal range can cause changes in mentation and ability to participate in rehabilitation activities.
2. Assess fluid volume status.	Fluid Management Fluid Monitoring Hypovolemia Management Hypervolemia Management	2. Management of fluid volume will avoid hypovolemia and hypervolemia.
3. Provide fluid and electrolytes via IV access until client able to take liquids by mouth.	Intravenous Therapy	3. IV therapy provides hydration and electrolytes until the client can eat or be fed through a nasogastric tube.

Evaluation: The client will have stable fluid volume and electrolyte status.

Nursing Diagnosis: Hyperthermia (NANDA) related to traumatic brain injury or infection.

Outcomes: The client will be maintained without a fever.

NOC OUTCOMES   Thermoregulation; Vital Signs

Interventions	NIC INTERVENTIONS	Rationales
1. Monitor temperature per unit standard.	Temperature Regulation	1. Fever can occur from infection or from inability of the hypothalamus to regulate properly.
2. Initiate treatment of fever once >38.5° C.	Fever Treatment	2. Treatment of fever will reset the thermostat to decrease the event of further fever.

Evaluation: The client will maintain a temperature <38.5° C.

(Continued)

CARE PLAN ⬛evolve⬛

Management of the Client with Traumatic Brain Injury—Cont'd

Nursing Diagnosis: Pain, Acute or Chronic (NANDA) due to injuries sustained at the time of the traumatic brain injury.
Outcomes: The client will have pain control and will not become depressed as a result of pain.

NOC OUTCOMES Comfort Level; Pain Control; Pain Level; Depression Level

Interventions	NIC INTERVENTIONS	Rationales
1. Educate client regarding medications, dosage, side effects.	Medication Management	1. Understanding of all medications allows for more appropriate choices.
2. Provide information about appropriate pain management and weaning from pain medication.	Pain Management	2. Excessive use of pain medication can lead to tolerance and may require additional support for weaning.
3. Assess the client's level of pain and if the client is not able to verbally express pain, use other pain assessment tools.	Pain Assessment Analgesic Administration	3. Pain management begins with assessment of level of pain.
4. Educate the client about analgesics and appropriate management of pain using various types of analgesia.	Sedation Management	4. Understanding all analgesia options helps the client in decision making for pain relief.
5. Provide information about the sedative effects of certain analgesics so that the client will not drive.		5. Sedation caused by medication can impair the ability to drive or perform complex tasks.

Evaluation: The client will have comfort at a tolerable level and will develop a self-management plan for pain control if needed.

Nursing Diagnosis: Skin Integrity, Impaired (NANDA) related to prolonged bed rest.
Outcomes: The client will have no evidence of skin breakdown or poor wound healing.

NOC OUTCOMES Tissue Integrity: Skin and Mucous Membranes; Wound Healing: Primary/Secondary Intention

Interventions	NIC INTERVENTIONS	Rationales
1. Assess skin every shift to identify potential pressure areas and begin treatment if necessary.	Pressure Management	1. Clients who are on bed rest have increased risk of skin breakdown from pressure.
2. Turn the client q 2 hours.	Pressure Ulcer Care Skin Surveillance	2. Turning relieves pressure and decreases risk of skin breakdown.
3. Assess incision line to ensure that it remains clean, dry, and intact.	Incision Site Care	3. Incision line infection causes a delay in wound healing.
4. Provide appropriate care to incisions or pressure ulcers to promote healing.	Wound Care Pressure Ulcer Care Wound Care	4. Delay in wound healing leads to delays in mobility and rehabilitation.

Evaluation: The client's skin will remain intact and incisions will heal in a timely manner without evidence of infection.

Nursing Diagnosis: Nutrition: Imbalanced: Less Than or More Than Body Requirements (NANDA) related to inability to consume food or from eating too much food as a result of traumatic brain injury.
Outcomes: The client will maintain a normal weight and will consume a balanced diet.

NOC OUTCOMES Appetite; Nutritional Status: Food, Fluid and Nutrient Intake; Weight Control

Interventions	NIC INTERVENTIONS	Rationales
1. Assess caloric consumption.	Nutrition Therapy Nutritional Monitoring	1. Too many calories or too few calories can inhibit healing and mobility.
2. Provide information about appropriate dietary intake.	Nutrition Management Weight Gain/Loss Assistance	2. Many clients need education about proper dietary intake, which will prevent future health care problems.
3. Educate regarding weight loss or gain as appropriate.		3. Weight gain or loss may affect strength and ability to regain independence.

Evaluation: The client will maintain an appropriate intake without excessive weight gain or loss.

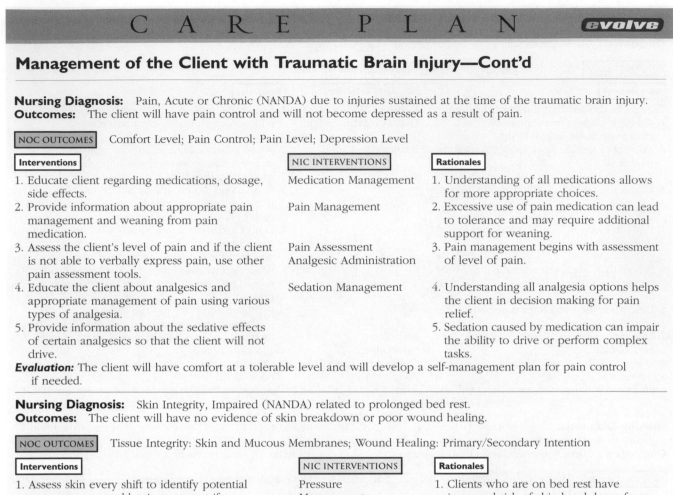

Nursing Diagnosis: Self-Care Deficit: Bathing/Hygiene, Dressing/Grooming, Feeding, Oral Hygiene, Toileting (NANDA)

Outcomes: The client will have a satisfactory level of self-care as evidenced by independently performing as many activities of daily living as possible. The client will direct a caregiver to provide any needs not independently met.

| NOC OUTCOMES | Self-Care Activities of Daily Living; Nutritional Status; Swallowing Status |

Interventions	NIC INTERVENTIONS	Rationales
1. Assist the client in activities of daily living.	Self-Care Assistance: Bathing/Hygiene	1. Allowing the client to do as much as possible leads to increased independence.
2. Provide education regarding feeding and swallowing.	Oral Health Maintenance Self-Care Assistance: Dressing/Grooming	2. Careful monitoring of food intake and appropriate feeding/swallowing techniques will minimize aspiration.
3. Provide education about bowel management.	Self-Care Assistance: Feeding Swallowing Therapy Self-Care Assistance: Toileting Bowel Management	3. A regular bowel regimen will promote bowel continence and decrease constipation.

Evaluation: The client will become as independent as possible in all activities of daily living.

Nursing Diagnosis: Urinary Retention (NANDA) due to traumatic brain injury affecting neuronal control of the bladder.

Outcomes: The client will be continent and without bladder distention.

| NOC OUTCOMES | Urinary Continence; Urinary Elimination |

Interventions	NIC INTERVENTIONS	Rationales
1. Assess for bladder distention, particularly after urinary catheter is removed; use bladder scan if available.	Urinary Retention Care Urinary Catheterization	1. Bladder distention is a common problem after neurologic injury and can contribute to urinary tract infections.
2. Insert urinary catheter if client is unable to void, has history of urinary retention or prostatic hypertrophy, or has a post-void residual of >250 ml.		2. Catheterization removes excess urine and decreases the likelihood of infection from retention of urine. Good catheter care decreases the risk of infection from the catheter.
3. Assess for volume, color, odor of urine; frequency of urination; difficulty with urination; and overflow urination.	Urinary Elimination Management Urinary Retention Care	3. Voiding high volumes of urine could be related to diuresis or to diabetes insipidus. Clients with urinary retention may void frequently and in small amounts.

Evaluation: The client will be able to void or be able to notify caregivers of need to void.

Nursing Diagnosis: Sleep Deprivation (NANDA) due to traumatic brain injury, lack of sleep in the hospital, and changes in diurnal patterns from hospitalization.

Outcomes: The client will report a normal sleep pattern.

| NOC OUTCOMES | Mood Equilibrium; Rest; Sleep; Symptom Severity |

Interventions	NIC INTERVENTIONS	Rationales
1. Assess the client's mood and ability to tolerate stressful situations. Provide opportunities for sleep.	Mood Management Sleep Enhancement	1. Inability to sleep leads to intolerance of stressful situations, delays healing and recovery, and slows the rehabilitation process.
2. Assess medications provided to temper mood and promote sleep.	Medication Management	2. Medications may be necessary for the short-term to assist with stabilizing the sleep pattern.
3. Encourage increased activity during the day.	Energy Management	3. Increasing activity will promote sleep.
4. Avoid long naps during the day.	Sleep Enhancement	4. Naps during the day will prevent long periods of sleep at night.

Evaluation: After interventions, the client will return to a normal sleep schedule and will be able to tolerate stress and daily activities.

(Continued)

C A R E   P L A N   *evolve*

Management of the Client with Traumatic Brain Injury—Cont'd

Nursing Diagnosis: Communication, Impaired Verbal (NANDA) related to the results of traumatic brain injury.
Outcomes: Client will be able to communicate within limitations.

NOC OUTCOMES Communication: Expressive and Receptive; Information Processing

Interventions	NIC INTERVENTIONS	Rationales
1. Assess the client's ability to understand verbal and visual input and follow instructions, utilizing occupational therapists and speech/language pathologists.	Active Listening Communication Enhancement: Speech Deficit Communication Enhancement: Visual Deficit	1. Understanding communication deficits will assist in identifying alternate strategies for communication. The therapists will be able to provide opportunities for learning for the client and caregivers.
2. Identify anxiety that may be present in the client related to inability to communicate or remember.	Anxiety Reduction Memory Training	2. Providing strategies for dealing with communication and memory deficits will decrease the client's anxiety about functioning in society.

Evaluation: Client will develop strategies to enhance memory and communication.

Nursing Diagnosis: Mobility, Physical: Impaired (NANDA) related to prolonged bed rest, traumatic brain injury, and physical injuries from the cause of the brain injury.
Outcomes: The client will be able to ambulate and transfer to achieve independence.

NOC OUTCOMES Ambulation; Balance; Coordinated Movement; Mobility; Transfer Performance

Interventions	NIC INTERVENTIONS	Rationales
1. Provide early ambulation and out of bed activities.	Exercise Promotion: Strength Training Exercise Therapy: Ambulation	1. Increasing activity will lead to increased strength. Being able to ambulate out of the room improves the client's overall outlook.
2. Assist with balance activity when the client is out of bed.	Exercise Promotion: Strength Training Exercise Therapy: Balance	2. Reinforcing information taught by therapists will assist the client in improving balance.
3. Teach client and caregiver range-of-motion and isometric exercises that can be conducted in bed.	Exercise Therapy: Joint Mobility Exercise Therapy: Muscle Control	3. Exercises conducted in bed will improve client's strength and increase independence.
4. Provide opportunities for the client to transfer from bed to chair and back.	Self-Care Assistance: Transfer	4. Self-transfer allows the client to become more independent.

Evaluation: The client will increase strength and mobility within bed or be able to be placed in a wheelchair with tolerance for sitting and ability to propel self.

Nursing Diagnosis: Activity Intolerance (NANDA) related to prolonged bed rest, fluid and electrolyte imbalance, poor nutrition and physical deficits.
Outcomes: Client will feel rested with fewer complaints of fatigue and increasing tolerance for activities.

NOC OUTCOMES Activity Tolerance, Endurance; Self-Care: Activities of Daily Living (ADL)

Interventions	NIC INTERVENTIONS	Rationales
1. Alternate rest and activity.	Energy Management Activity Therapy	1. Conserves energy and reduces demands on musculoskeletal system. Increases activity tolerance and endurance.
2. Assist with activities.	Self-Care Assistance	2. Being assisted as needed with activity of daily living (ADL) conserves energy and reduces demands on musculoskeletal system.
3. Monitor fluids and electrolytes. Assist with treatment of abnormal results.	Fluid/Electrolyte Management	3. Allows detection and treatment of abnormal laboratory results.

Evaluation: Upon discharge from the intensive care unit (ICU), if interventions are successful, the client will have an increased tolerance to activity, perform more ADL, and experience fewer fluid/electrolyte changes. Fluid/electrolyte replacement will improve tolerance to activity. Activity therapy will result in an increase in activity endurance.

Nursing Diagnosis: Adjustment, Impaired (NANDA) related to body and cognitive changes due to traumatic brain injury.

Outcomes: Client will be able to adjust to changes in health status, cognitive and physical disabilities.

| NOC OUTCOMES | Acceptance: Health Status, Adaptation to Physical Disability, Coping, Motivation, Psychosocial Adjustment: Life Change |

Interventions	NIC INTERVENTIONS	Rationales
1. Assist with identifying strategies for adjusting to body and cognitive changes.	Anticipatory Guidance	1. Helps client begin to realistically accept changes that might be permanent.
2. Provide opportunities for client to express concerns	Coping Enhancement Emotional Support Counseling	2. Respects the client's concerns about changes in body and loss of cognitive function.
3. Provide resources and opportunities for venting of feelings, particularly social services or psychiatric consultation service.	Crisis Intervention	3. Assists the client during the early emotional period of adjustment after injury.

Evaluation: With interventions, the client will begin to accept changes that have occurred from the traumatic brain injury and will identify resources to assist with emotional recovery.

Nursing Diagnosis: Self-Esteem Disturbed (NANDA) related to changes in physical abilities, mental abilities, and appearance as a result of traumatic brain injury.

Outcomes: Client will be able to acknowledge changes in physical and cognitive abilities resulting from the brain injury. Client will cope with body image disturbance, avoid isolation, and initiate or reestablish support systems.

| NOC OUTCOMES | Adaptation to Physical Disability; Psychosocial Adjustment: Life Change; Self-Esteem |

Interventions	NIC INTERVENTIONS	Rationales
1. Assess the client's response to body changes.	Body Image Enhancement	1. Determines the extent of body image disturbance
2. Promote accepting and nonjudgmental attitude.	Active Listening Emotional Support Self-Esteem Enhancement	2. Respects the client's sensitivity to body image changes.
3. Listen and encourage ventilation of feelings.	Active Listening Emotional Support	3. Helps the client feel valued.
4. Provide information regarding adaptive equipment and/or techniques.	Anticipatory Guidance Coping Enhancement	4. Helps provide the client some control over the situation.

Evaluation: Some degree of change in body functioning may persist and the client will learn to accept the altered body image. In addition, it is expected that the client will maintain or establish new interpersonal relationships and activities.

Nursing Diagnosis: Caregiver Role Strain (NANDA) related to efforts to care for client, other family members and running of a household.

Outcomes: Caregiver will maintain an emotionally and physically stable relationship with the client by assuring that the caregiver achieves respite from care.

| NOC OUTCOMES | Caregiver Emotional Health; Caregiver Lifestyle Disruption; Caregiver-Patient Relationship; Caregiver Physical Health; Caregiver Well-Being |

Interventions	NIC INTERVENTIONS	Rationales
1. Assist primary caregiver in identifying resources to relieve the burden of caring for a brain-injured client.	Caregiver Support Coping Enhancement Respite Care	1. Helping the caregiver adjust to role changes enables caregiver to identify additional resources for support. Care of a client with TBI is demanding and draining and the caregiver will need breaks.
2. Allow the caregiver to express concerns about the role changes that the TBI has presented.	Coping Enhancement Presence Role Enhancement	2. When the caregiver can express concerns and begin to identify role changes, the caregiver is more prepared to care for the client.
3. Provide education to the caregiver regarding the need for rest, healthy eating, and exercise.	Energy Management Nutrition Management	3. Ensuring that the caregiver is rested and healthy will enable the caregiver to provide care without becoming ill.
4. Provide education to the caregiver regarding how to manage the day to day needs of the client.	Caregiver Support Respite Care Teaching: Individual	4. Providing the caregiver with information early in the recovery period will assist in identifying needs for learning.

Evaluation: Caregiver will recognize the additional demands of caring for a brain-injured individual and will develop strategies to minimize strain, provide respite, and maintain own activities and interests.

defect that is cosmetically unsightly. The defect may be surgically corrected by cranioplasty later.

Before surgery ICP is reduced as much as possible. Baseline neurologic data are documented. Informed consent needs to be obtained from the family if the patient is unconscious or confused. After surgery, provide nursing care for the client following the guidelines for craniotomy (see Chapter 69).

Self-Care

Clients with possible head injury or mild head injury were previously hospitalized for observation for a minimum of 6 hours (ideally for 48 hours) because of the risk of extradural hemorrhage. If the client is sent home, give clear instructions to help the client's caregiver assess for complications (see the Client Education Guide website feature on Monitoring Family Members After Head Injury).

Rehabilitation

Most clients hospitalized for more than 48 hours because of a head injury ultimately require some rehabilitation. Clients with mild head injury may be overlooked in the population of people who need follow-up care. Mild head injuries can cause headache, memory difficulties, difficulty performing simple tasks, and irritability. These clinical manifestations may persist for a month or longer.

Rehabilitation may take place in an inpatient or outpatient setting, depending on the client's condition. Rehabilitation may include physical, occupational, speech and cognitive therapy and is essential in returning the client to maximal function. Nurses play a major role in the rehabilitation of the head-injured client and in the education of significant others.

More severely injured clients may be sent to rehabilitation facilities with feeding tubes or tracheostomy tubes in place. Clients and families need assistance in choosing a new health care facility that can deliver the level of care needed. If recovery is unlikely, the client may need to be transferred to an extended-care facility. Because many head-injured clients are young, previously healthy people, placement in a nursing home may be a very difficult reality for family members to accept. Teaching and support can greatly improve coping. Involvement of disciplines such as social services, pastoral care, or discharge planning can increase the family members' understanding of the next phase of care.

The rehabilitation of clients with brain injuries is challenging. In some cases, community reintegration is unsuccessful. Studies have reported improvement in the client's ability to lead a productive life with the use of interdisciplinary techniques that include rehabilitation in cognition, compensatory techniques, social skills, emotional adjustment, leisure skills, physical fitness, and health maintenance. Most clients require at least 6 months in an ongoing program of rehabilitation both in-patient and out-patient. The ability of a client in a persistent vegetative state to respond to stimuli is constantly being reviewed. Hopefully, with continued research families will be given accurate and compassionate answers to their questions and concerns about the patient's ability to respond.

Modifications for Older Clients

Although most head injuries caused by motor-vehicle accidents do not occur in the older population, injury caused by falls is common. Diagnosis of a head injury is often more difficult in older adults because of an atypical presentation. These clients also experience more complications. An older client may be less able to tolerate respiratory problems or cardiac dysrhythmias. The presence of chronic diseases such as chronic obstructive pulmonary disease or heart failure can make managing ventilation and fluid balance more difficult. If any type of mental impairment was present before the injury, recovery to full independence is less likely. Poor stamina and medical complications may impede rehabilitation.

SPINAL CORD INJURY

Injury to the spinal cord can range in severity from mild flexion-extension "whiplash" injuries to complete transection of the cord with permanent quadriplegia. Trauma to the cord can occur at any level but most commonly occurs in the cervical and lower thoracic-upper lumbar vertebrae. These common cord injuries are due in part to the support given by the ribs to the thoracic spine and the flexibility of the cervical and lumbar spinal segments.

Although this discussion focuses on nursing management of *acute* spinal cord injury (SCI), it should be appreciated that about 200,000 people with spinal cord injury are living in the United States.

Etiology and Risk Factors
Trauma is the most common cause of SCI. Each year about 10,000 people sustain such injury. Most victims are males between the ages of 16 and 30 years; only 9% of injuries occur in people over the age of 60. Traumatic SCI is most often caused by automobile or motorcycle accidents, gunshot or knife wounds, falls, and sports mishaps. More than half of all SCIs involve the cervical spine, and the rest occur in the thoracic, lumbar, and sacral spinal segments.

The feeling of immortality often experienced by adolescents and young adults contributes strongly to their risk of SCI. Young people may believe they can engage in dangerous behavior without being injured. The use of alcohol and illicit drugs can reinforce this belief in immortality. A young person who has experienced the devastation of SCI may best deliver the message of primary prevention. In several nationwide programs, head-injured and spinal cord–injured people are available to speak at school-sponsored educational programs.

Nontraumatic disorders may also result in SCI. These problems include the following:

- Cervical spondylosis with myelopathy (spinal canal narrowing with progressive injury to the cord and roots)
- Myelitis (infective or noninfective)
- Osteoporosis causing vertebral compression fractures
- Syringomyelia (central cavitation of the cord)
- Tumors, both infiltrative and compressive
- Vascular diseases, usually infarction or hemorrhage

Whatever the cause, SCI produces distinctive and debilitating damage. Nowhere else in the body can a local insult produce such devastation in proportion to the extent of tissue involved.

Flexion-Rotation, Dislocation, and Fracture-Dislocation Injuries

By far the most common SCI is flexion injury. When the head strikes the steering wheel or windshield, the spine is forced into acute hyperflexion (Figure 73-11, *A*). Rupture of the posterior ligaments results in forward dislocation of the vertebrae. Nutrient blood vessels may be damaged, leading to ischemia of the spinal cord. The cervical spine, usually at the C5-6 level, is most commonly affected by a flexion injury. In the thoracic-lumbar spine, this type of injury is most frequently seen at the T12-L1 level.

Hyperextension Injuries

Hyperextension injuries result after a fall in which the chin hits an object and the head is thrown back (see Figure 73-11, *B*). The anterior ligament is ruptured, with fracture of the posterior elements of the vertebral body. Hyperextension of the spinal cord against the ligamentum flavum can lead to dorsal column contusion and posterior dislocation of the vertebrae. Complete transection of the cord can follow a hyperextension injury, although transection of the cord is rare. Clients who have complete lesions of the spinal cord do not necessarily have transection of the cord. Complete lesions of the cord result in loss of all voluntary movement and sensation below the lesion and loss of reflex function in isolated segments of the cord.

Compression Injuries

Compression injuries are often caused by falls or jumps in which the person lands directly on the head, sacrum, or feet (see Figure 73-11, *C*). The force of impact

fractures the vertebrae and the fragments compress the cord. Disk and bone fragments may be propelled into the spinal cord on impact. The lumbar and the lower thoracic vertebrae are the most commonly injured regions after a compression impact when the person lands on the feet. If the person lands on the head (as in diving into shallow water), the injury is to the cervical spine. About 50% of these injuries result in incomplete lesions. Incomplete lesions occur when some of the spinal tracts remain intact.

Unique Cervical Injuries

Three types of fractures are unique to the cervical spine (Figure 73-12):

1. *Fractures of the odontoid process* (the superior projection on C2) may be intact, with no detectable movement, or may be displaced, with movement and entrapment of the spinal cord.
2. A *hangman's fracture* is a bilateral fracture through the pedicles of C2, separating the posterior elements from the body of the vertebra.
3. The *Jefferson fracture* involves bursting of the ring of C1. The spinal canal usually widens.

These injuries are usually associated with other spinal injuries. Clients with these cervical fractures either die of the injury immediately or are stable and may walk into the emergency department reporting only neck pain.

Pathophysiology

Most often SCIs occur as a result of injury to the vertebrae. The most common sites of injury are at the C1-2, C4-6, and T11-L2 vertebrae. These segments of the spine are the most mobile and therefore the most easily injured.

The cord is injured as the result of acceleration, deceleration, or another force (e.g., impact) applied to the spine. The forces injure the spinal cord by compressing, pulling, or tearing the tissues. Microscopic bleeding occurs immediately after injury, primarily in the gray matter of the cord. Within the first hour, edema develops and often spreads along segments of the spinal cord. Arachidonic acid and its metabolites (prostaglandins, thromboxanes, and leukotrienes) cause edema. Cord edema peaks within 2 to 3 days and subsides within the first 7 days after injury. Although the site of the initial injury has the most edema and bleeding, some edema and bleeding extend at least for two cord segments on either side of the injury. The edema of the cord leads to temporary loss of sensation and function. Spinal cord tissue injury is related to the initial insult, biochemical changes, and hemodynamic instability. Therefore immediately after injury, it is not easy to determine the ultimate degree of permanent impairment.

Further changes include fragmentation of the axonal covering and loss of myelin. Phagocytic cells can injure

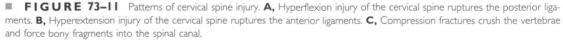

■ **FIGURE 73–11** Patterns of cervical spine injury. **A,** Hyperflexion injury of the cervical spine ruptures the posterior ligaments. **B,** Hyperextension injury of the cervical spine ruptures the anterior ligaments. **C,** Compression fractures crush the vertebrae and force bony fragments into the spinal canal.

surviving axons as they scavenge cellular debris. Chemotactic and inflammatory mediators further extend tissue necrosis. Macrophages engulf the spinal cord tissue and may cause a central cavity (called *post-traumatic syringomyelia*) to develop as early as 9 days after injury.

In addition, the oligodendroglial cells that support the cord are lost. Injury to the cord leads to rapid loss of axonal conduction from ion changes, such as very rapid increases in extracellular potassium and influx of calcium into the cell. Finally, free radicals are produced.

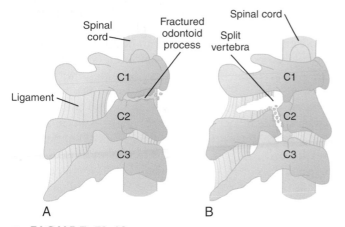

■ **FIGURE 73-12** Fractures of the cervical spine. **A,** Odontoid fractures are fractures of the superior projection of C2 that normally projects into C1. **B,** Hangman's fractures are of the pedicle of C2. The vertebra is split in half.

Free radicals are normally found in the body but are quickly controlled by antioxidant enzyme systems. When the antioxidant systems are overwhelmed, the free radicals damage tissues.

The physiologic response to SCI extends beyond changes within the spinal cord. For example, the sympathetic nervous system stress response results in reduced perfusion of the gastrointestinal tract and reduced production of gastric mucus to protect the lining. Ulceration and bleeding may develop.

Spasticity is the increased tone or contraction of muscles, producing stiff movements. Various CNS injuries or diseases such as SCI, strokes, and cerebral palsy may result in spasticity. After SCI, the brain can no longer influence reflex movements through the spinal cord. Eventually the lower part of the cord, using spinal reflex arcs, begins to work automatically. Spinal reflex activities include the flexor withdrawal reflex and reflex emptying of the bladder and bowel. These primitive spinal mechanisms, normally kept inactive by higher centers, are "released" when the normal inhibitions of the higher centers are destroyed. As recovery progresses, flexor responses are interspersed with extensor spasms. These movements ultimately develop into predominantly extensor activity. The client's limbs spasm into extension with movement. Spasticity may remain indefinitely or gradually decrease over time.

Clinical Manifestations
Level of Injury
The initial clinical manifestations of acute SCI depend on the level and extent of injury to the cord. Below the level of injury or lesion, the following functions are lost:

■ Voluntary movement
■ Sensation of pain, temperature, pressure, and *proprioception* (the ability to know where the body is in space)
■ Bowel and bladder function
■ Spinal and autonomic reflexes

The level of injury may be described in terms of (1) skeletal injury and (2) neurologic level of injury. Skeletal injury refers to the vertebral damage demonstrated by x-ray study. The criterion of the American Spinal Injury Association (ASIA) is useful in describing the level of spinal cord involvement: *The neurologic level of injury is the lowest segment of the spinal cord with bilateral intact sensory and motor function.* Sensory function is assessed according to dermatomes to identify the areas of skin with normal sensation. Motor function is measured by testing myotomes to identify muscles with active movement and full range of motion (ROM) against gravity. The ASIA Impairment Scale is as follows:

■ Normal with sensory and motor function preserved
■ Incomplete with the majority of motor function preserved
■ Incomplete with nonfunctional motor function preserved
■ Incomplete with only sensation preserved
■ Complete with loss of sensation and motor function

Injury to the cervical cord produces quadriplegia. Injuries above the C4 level may be fatal because of loss of innervation to the diaphragm and intercostal muscles. Without immediate rescue breathing after the accident, the injured person will die of asphyxiation. Today, with the general public's knowledge of cardiopulmonary resuscitation, many people survive this injury to the cervical spine. Injuries to the remainder of the cervical spine create specific patterns of motor loss. Note that a person with a C7 injury is able to lift the shoulders, elbows, and wrists and has some hand function, but below C7 no motor function or sensation remains.

Injuries to the thoracic or lumbar spinal segment produce paraplegia. People with such injuries have function in their upper extremities and can be mobile in a wheelchair or with crutches and braces. People with L5 injury can extend the great toe and dorsiflex the ankle. They have no sensation in the perianal area, calf, heel, or small toe.

Changes in Reflexes
Reflexes, which normally cross the spinal cord and return to the stimulated limb, are absent in early SCI because of spinal shock. Blood pressure and temperature in denervated (without nervous function or innervation) areas fall markedly and respond poorly to reflex stimuli.

After spinal shock subsides, some body functions may return by reflex (e.g., control of the urinary bladder), but they lack integration with other visceral activities. Visceral activities may be initiated by atypical stimuli. For example, scratching the skin may cause vasodilation, sweating, and urination. Nervous system lesions may produce a type of defective urinary bladder function known as *neurogenic bladder*. For example, stimulation of the skin on the lower abdomen or thighs may cause reflex urination. This form of cord bladder is called a *reflex bladder*. Such stimulation may also cause reflex ejaculation and priapism (persistent abnormal penile erection without sexual desire) in paralyzed men.

Muscle Spasms

Intense and painful muscular spasms of the lower extremities occur following a traumatic complete transverse spinal cord lesion. In assisting the client and the family members to understand these movements, it should be explained that these muscle spasms are involuntary and do not mean that voluntary movement is returning. This information, although disappointing, is essential.

Muscle spasms range in intensity from mild muscular twitching to vigorous mass reflexogenic states. Extreme, involuntary muscle spasms can actually throw a client out of bed or wheelchair. Bed side rails are kept up and restraining straps are comfortably secured over the client lying on a stretcher. Muscle spasms, often aggravated by cold weather, prolonged periods of sitting, infections, or emotionally upsetting events, may become intolerable. Reflex spasms may be triggered by extrinsic or visceral stimuli, such as a distended bladder.

Emotion (e.g., anxiety, crying, anger, laughing) or cutaneous stimulation (e.g., tickling, stroking, pinching) may initiate spastic movements. By learning to recognize events that trigger such reflex spasms, the client may use these potentially annoying movements to achieve functional activities such as urination.

Autonomic Dysreflexia

Autonomic dysreflexia, also known as *autonomic hyperreflexia,* is a life-threatening syndrome. It is a cluster of clinical manifestations that results when multiple spinal cord autonomic responses discharge simultaneously. This syndrome, observed in as many as 85% of clients with cord injury above the T6 level, can occur anytime after spinal shock has resolved. Dysreflexia often lessens as time after injury passes, but it may recur. The manifestations of autonomic dysreflexia result from an exaggerated sympathetic response to a noxious stimulus below the level of the cord lesion. Common stimuli are bladder and bowel distention but may also include pressure ulcers, spasms, pain, pressure on the penis, excessive rectal stimulation, bladder stones, ingrown toenails, abdominal abnormalities, or uterine contractions.

Exaggerated sympathetic responses cause the blood vessels below the level of injury to constrict. As a result, the client develops hypertension (readings of 20 mm Hg above baseline are considered hypertensive), a

pounding headache, flushing above the level of the lesion, nasal stuffiness, diaphoresis, piloerection ("gooseflesh"), dilated pupils with blurred vision, bradycardia (30 to 40 beats/min), restlessness, and nausea. The manifestations are a result of compensatory efforts to overcome the severe hypertension. Initially baroreceptors sense the hypertensive stimuli and stimulate the parasympathetic nervous system, which results in vasodilation above the level of cord injury (headache, flushing) and bradycardia. The problem is that the visceral and peripheral vessels do not dilate because the efferent impulses cannot pass through the damaged cord. Thus the overall effect is one of extreme hypertension (with pressures possibly as high as 300 mm Hg). Seizures and cerebral hemorrhage occur in about 10% to 15% of cases. See the later discussion on Risk for Autonomic Dysreflexia for interventions.

Clinical Syndromes Causing Partial Paralysis

Five spinal cord syndromes cause partial paralysis (Figure 73-13): central cord syndrome, anterior cord syndrome, Brown-Séquard syndrome, conus medullaris syndrome, and cauda equina syndrome. Each has distinctive neurologic features.

Central Cord Syndrome. Central cord syndrome (most common with hyperextension-hyperflexion injuries) produces more weakness in the upper extremities than in the lower extremities. This type of injury occurs most often in the older adult who has a pre-existing spinal stenosis. This injury may also occur in a person who lands on the head such as when diving into shallow water and hitting the bottom. The common mechanism of injury is a fall forward. The weakness is caused by edema and hemorrhage in the central area of the cord, which is predominantly occupied by nerve tracts to the hands and arms.

Anterior Cord Syndrome. A lesion in the anterior spinal cord causes anterior cord syndrome, with complete motor function loss and decreased pain sensation. Deep pressure, position sense, and two-point discrimination sensations remain intact. Often the anterior spinal artery is affected, causing an infarction of spinal cord tissue. Cervical cord concussion may produce various degrees of motor and sensory deficit, which completely resolve within hours. Occasionally cervical cord trauma produces only root injuries, which may paralyze isolated muscles or muscle groups in the arms and shoulders. These deficits are usually permanent.

Brown-Séquard Syndrome. Brown-Séquard syndrome is caused by lateral hemisection of the cord (i.e., when half the cord is cut or otherwise damaged, as in a bullet or knife wound). This injury results in ipsilateral (same

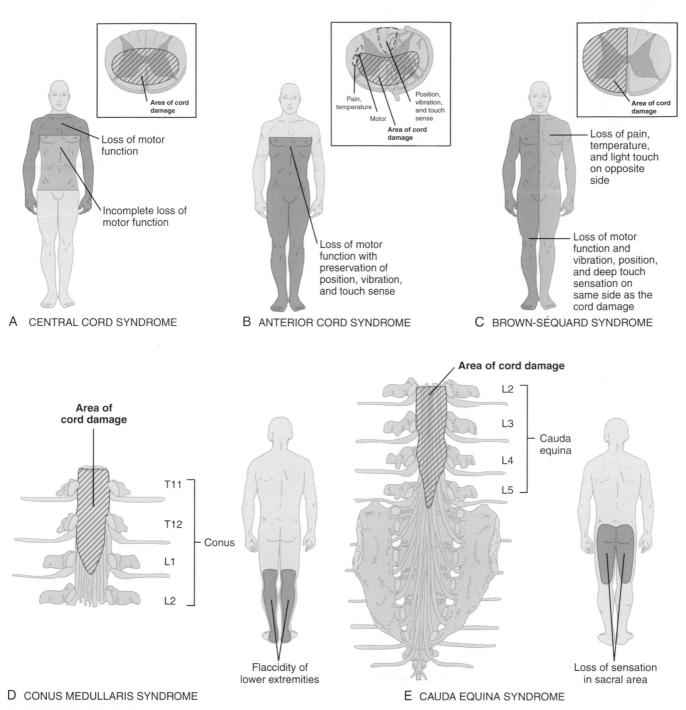

A CENTRAL CORD SYNDROME

Area of cord damage

Loss of motor function

Incomplete loss of motor function

B ANTERIOR CORD SYNDROME

Pain, temperature

Motor

Position, vibration, and touch sense

Area of cord damage

Loss of motor function with preservation of position, vibration, and touch sense

C BROWN-SÉQUARD SYNDROME

Area of cord damage

Loss of pain, temperature, and light touch on opposite side

Loss of motor function and vibration, position, and deep touch sensation on same side as the cord damage

D CONUS MEDULLARIS SYNDROME

Area of cord damage

T11
T12
L1
L2

Conus

Flaccidity of lower extremities

E CAUDA EQUINA SYNDROME

Area of cord damage

L2
L3
L4
L5

Cauda equina

Loss of sensation in sacral area

■ **FIGURE 73–13** Patterns of injury leading to partial paralysis. **A,** Central cord syndrome. **B,** Anterior cord syndrome. **C,** Brown-Séquard syndrome. **D,** Conus medullaris syndrome. **E,** Cauda equina syndrome.

side) motor paralysis, loss of vibratory and position sense, and contralateral (opposite side) loss of pain and temperature sensation.

Conus Medullaris Syndrome. *Conus medullaris syndrome* follows damage to the lumbar nerve roots and the conus medullaris in the spinal cord. The client usually has bowel and bladder areflexia and flaccid lower

extremities. The bulbocavernosus penile (erection) and micturition reflexes may be preserved when damage is limited to the upper sacral segments of the spinal cord.

Cauda Equina Syndrome. Injury to the lumbosacral nerve roots below the conus medullaris results in the cauda equina syndrome. The client experiences areflexia of the bowel, bladder, and lower extremities.

Spinal Shock

The immediate response to cord transection is called *spinal shock*. The client with SCI experiences a complete loss of skeletal muscle function, bowel and bladder tone, sexual function, and autonomic reflexes. Loss of venous return and hypotension also occur. The hypothalamus cannot control temperature by vasoconstriction and increased metabolism; therefore the client's body assumes the environmental temperature. Spinal shock is most severe in clients with higher levels of SCI. Clients with thoracic or lumbar injuries are often unaffected because the sympathetic nervous system is spared with these levels of injury.

Spinal shock may last for 1 to 6 weeks. Indications that spinal shock is resolving include return of reflexes, development of hyperreflexia rather than flaccidity, and return of reflex emptying of the bladder. The earliest reflexes recovered are the flexor reflexes evoked by noxious cutaneous stimulation. The return of the bulbocavernosus reflex (anal sphincter contraction in response to squeezing the glans penis or tugging on the urinary catheter) in male patients is also an early indicator of recovery from spinal shock. Babinski's reflex (dorsiflexion of the great toe with fanning of the other toes when the sole of the foot is stroked) is an early returning reflex.

Diagnostic Findings

Lateral cervical spine x-rays may show dislocation of the vertebrae. Normally, the vertebrae are aligned. Dislocation of the vertebrae appears as one or more segments being offset. If present, there is likely also damage to the ligaments that connect one vertebra to another. CT scans are used to see in great detail how the vertebrae are aligned and whether other structures are injured. MRI can detect damage to the spinal cord, ligaments, and disks. MRI can also detect edema or bleeding in the spinal cord.

OUTCOME MANAGEMENT

Both initial (especially during the first hour after injury) and long-term interventions provided for a client who has sustained an SCI significantly influence the following:

- The extent of the injury and associated deficits
- How well the person survives the acute phase of injury
- The success of recovery and rehabilitation

People with SCI can lead productive and, in many cases, independent lives. As with head injury, information obtained from witnesses to the accident can assist in diagnosis and treatment. Information from witnesses or the client should include the mechanism of injury, the presence and duration of loss of consciousness, and impairment of motor function. It is also important to diagnose SCI correctly. Delays in diagnosis can be attributed to alcohol intoxication, concomitant head injury, or other multiple injuries.

Initial Care

At the scene of the accident, the injured person should be moved only when adequate numbers of people are present to accomplish while keeping the spinal immobile. The neck should be stabilized in a neutral position without flexion or extension until a fixed immobilizing device can be applied. Cervical traction should not be applied. Without x-ray films to guide movements, the spinal cord can be injured. The simplest method of immobilizing the spine is to place the affected person on a spine board and to secure the spine with a hard collar around the neck and self-fastening ties across the torso and legs. Transparent stiff collars have become popular because they allow visualization of the carotid arteries and trachea. Excellent on-the-scene care has increased the number of people who are neurologically intact despite vertebral column fractures. Accurate reporting of the person's baseline deficits is essential to help the physician plan the aggressiveness of treatment interventions.

Spinal trauma is often associated with other injuries, such as head injury, chest trauma, extremity fractures, and abdominal injury. Anyone who has sustained multiple trauma should be handled as though spinal injuries are present until assessment proves otherwise. In handling a client in whom cervical spine injury is present, the spine is kept in neutral alignment and flexion is prevented.

When turning is required, a *logrolling* maneuver is used. The client is placed in a supine position on a firm surface. The head is supported in alignment with the body and is immobilized with a firm, padded cervical collar. Some physicians use halter traction immediately to keep the cervical spine aligned and prevent movement. Clothing is cut off rather than removed. The client is transported on a flat, firm stretcher with the neck immobilized. SCI-trained personnel should remain with the client while x-ray studies are taken to ensure that the cervical spine is not moved.

Cervical spine injury may produce respiratory distress. When breathing difficulty is noted, immediate action is taken to maintain a patent airway and to provide adequate oxygenation. It is important that the client's neck not be hyperextended during intubation; therefore the jaw thrust technique is used. Suctioning is performed as necessary to maintain a patent airway. Mechanically assisted ventilation is required when definite loss or impairment of respiratory muscle function occurs. Respiratory parameters can be used to guide the decision of whether to ventilate the client mechanically. Serial decreases in vital capacity (less than 15 ml/kg), along with an increase in the partial pressure of arterial carbon dioxide ($Paco_2$), constitute a good predictor of impending pulmonary failure.

In the emergency department, a client who has sustained a severe cervical injury should be placed immediately in skeletal traction to immobilize the cervical spine and reduce the fracture and dislocation. Gardner-Wells tongs are inserted through the outer table of the skull (Figure 73-14). Traction is applied to the tongs via rope, pulleys, and weights. Traction weight is begun with 10 to 20 pounds (4.5 to 9.1 kg) and is gradually increased to accomplish bone reduction. When proper alignment is obtained and verified by x-ray examination, the traction weight may be lessened to maintain the reduction. Traction is not used to stabilize and immobilize thoracic or lumbar spinal fractures or fracture-dislocations because there is no effective way to provide it. Therefore the spine is kept in alignment, and logrolling is used as needed, until surgical stabilization can be performed.

A cross-table lateral x-ray film of the cervical spine is obtained before transport of the injured person. Lateral and anteroposterior x-ray studies are not usually sufficient. To visualize lower cervical fractures, it is necessary either to apply downward traction to the arms or have the arms in the swimmer's position during x-ray examination. If a high-level cervical lesion is suspected, a view of the odontoid bone through the open mouth may be required. CT and MRI are often used to establish the extent of the injury. A brief but thorough neurologic examination is made to assess the extent of injury and to establish a baseline of function and involvement for later comparison.

Common emergency interventions include insertion of an IV line and infusion of normal saline, insertion of an indwelling catheter, administration of high-dose steroids, administration of vasoactive medications to maintain systolic blood pressure, insertion of a nasogastric tube, and provision of oxygen if oxygen saturation is low.

Once orthopedic and medical stabilization of the fracture has been achieved, the client is transferred to an ICU or to an SCI center. It is important that the client be appropriately immobilized before transport.

Medical Management

Maintaining Vital Functions

Respiratory compromise may occur, and if the client develops diaphragmatic fatigue mechanical ventilation may be needed. Arterial blood gases are monitored closely. The client may be transferred to a kinetic treatment bed to reduce the risk of pressure ulcer development, improve pulmonary function, and minimize complications of immobility. These beds are shown in Figure 68-2 on p. 1801.

Vasoactive agents are commonly used to support blood pressure immediately after injury. Short-term high-dose methylprednisolone therapy is started in people with SCI less than 8 hours old. A bolus dose of 30 mg/kg infused over 1 hour followed by 5.4 mg/kg infused over 23 hours is usual. Other therapies may include the use of neuropeptides and thyrotropin-releasing hormone, which may induce some reversal of lesions by decreasing post-traumatic ischemia. Histamine-2 (H_2) receptor-blocking agents are often given to reduce the risk of gastric and intestinal bleeding. Long-term pharmacologic management may include urinary antiseptics, anticoagulants, laxatives, and antispasmodics.

Respiratory impairment, position, emotional status, or gastrointestinal function may compromise nutritional intake. Intubation eliminates the possibility of oral intake, whereas a tracheostomy does not. Clients with a tracheostomy require time to adjust to swallowing with the tube in place and must be carefully monitored to prevent aspiration.

Aspiration is also a risk for clients who must remain flat while in tongs and traction. Although these clients may be capable of swallowing, it is unlikely that they

■ **FIGURE 73–14** Gardner-Wells tongs are used to provide skeletal traction on the cervical spine before operative stabilization.

will be able to consume safely enough food to meet their metabolic needs. Clients wearing a halo jacket (Figure 73-15) often experience difficulty eating because the halo jacket immobilizes the head. They should be encouraged to take small bites, eat slowly, and concentrate on swallowing.

Assessment of Other Injuries

Once the client's spine and emergency medical conditions have been stabilized, a complete neurologic assessment is performed. Several associated injuries are commonly seen with SCI. These include orthopedic injury to the spine, head injury, chest injury, abdominal injury, and genitourinary injury. Some of these injuries may not be immediately evident in the emergency department, and ongoing assessments are made until the problem is ruled out.

Monitoring for Complications

Potential complications include spinal shock, atelectasis, pneumonia, bradycardia, hypotension, deep vein thrombosis (DVT), gastrointestinal bleeding, pressure ulcers, joint contractures, and psychological dysfunction such as denial and depression. Depression is a common reaction to SCI and may be associated with inhibition of the appetite. Choosing when and what to eat may be one of the few areas of control left to the person with SCI.

■ **FIGURE 73–15** Halo traction. This form of traction immobilizes the cervical spine so that the client can move without risk of further injury. *(Courtesy DePuy Spine, a Johnson & Johnson Company, Raynham, Mass.)*

As much free choice of dietary intake as is feasible should be encouraged. Any of these conditions can severely limit a spinal injury client's oral intake at a time when a high-calorie, high-protein diet is needed. Enteral feeding or total parenteral hyperalimentation is often prescribed until oral intake is sufficient to meet the body's needs.

Initial Nursing Management of the Client with Spinal Cord Injury

Assessment. A holistic assessment approach is essential in planning for nursing care of clients with SCI. Every system of the body is affected with these injuries. A complete baseline assessment is obtained initially. The results of subsequent assessments are then compared with the baseline results. Specific components in the assessment of the client with an SCI depend on the client's phase of treatment. Therefore assessment is addressed within the following sections.

Careful monitoring of hemodynamic parameters is essential. Heart rate, blood pressure, temperature, respirations, fluid balance, and peripheral oxygen saturation (by pulse oximetry) should be monitored continuously.

If the client is conscious, ask whether there is any pain. Sensation of touch and pinprick is assessed in the feet, legs, trunk, hands, and arms. Levels of sensation are documented according to dermatomes. To assess motor function, ask the client to wiggle toes, move ankles, flex knees, and move hands and arms. The location, symmetry, and strength of muscle movement are documented (Table 73-1). The major reflexes—that is, the Achilles, patellar, biceps, and triceps tendon reflexes—are briefly tested. Assessment for intact sensation in areas such as the perineum is also necessary. If the patient is

TABLE 73–1	Motor Assessment After Spinal Cord Injury
Spinal Nerve(s)	**Assessment Technique**
C4-5	Shoulders are shrugged against downward pressure of examiner's hands
C5-6	Arm is pulled up from resting position against resistance
C7	From flexed position, arm is straightened out against resistance
C7	Index finger is held firmly to thumb against resistance to pull it away
C8	Hand grasp strength is evaluated
L2-4	Leg is lifted from bed against resistance
L2-4	From flexed position, knee is extended against resistance
L5-S1	Knee is flexed against resistance
L5	Foot is pulled up toward nose against resistance
S1	Foot is pushed down (as in stepping on automobile gas pedal) against resistance

unresponsive, assessment is more limited. Assess respiratory status by observing for spontaneous movement and thorax expansion. Sensation and movement of extremities are assessed by watching the client for a few moments or by applying a painful stimulus (nail bed pressure) and observing for withdrawal.

Usually the client is awake and may be concerned about obtaining pain relief, the chances of survival, and the safety of any other people in the accident. Once these issues are addressed, the client may begin to appraise the severity of his or her own injury.

Rehabilitation begins when the client is admitted to the acute health care facility. During the acute stage, nursing and medical attention is appropriately focused on immediate needs. It is also imperative to remember that the client probably will have severe residual disabilities and must make major lifestyle changes. Care provided in the acute period can significantly affect the client's later life. Prevention of complications such as infection, pressure sores, and contractures facilitates rehabilitation and reduces suffering, disability, and expense. Challenges in caring for clients with SCI are presented in the Case Study below.

Diagnosis, Outcomes, Interventions

Collaborative Problem: Risk for Hypotension. Clients suffering from SCI are at risk for the development of hypotension. The collaborative problem of *Risk for Hypotension* is related to vasodilation and the inability to vasoconstrict attributable to loss of reflexes rather than to volume depletion.

Outcomes. The nurse will monitor for hypotension and pulmonary fluid overload as evidenced by systolic blood pressure greater than 90 mm Hg, heart rate more than 60 beats/min, and the client alert and oriented with an adequate urine output.

Interventions. Hypotension associated with spinal shock is initially treated with IV fluid. It is important to remember that fluid depletion is seldom the cause of hypotension; rather, lack of reflexes is the likely cause. Therefore fluid resuscitation should be carefully monitored to avoid fluid

---

CASE STUDY *evolve*

Spinal Cord Injury

Ben Brown is a 21-year-old college junior who was admitted to the intensive care unit (ICU) via the emergency department for evaluation and treatment of a spinal cord injury (SCI) sustained in a diving accident. Consider the type of fracture most typical from this type of accident. He is accompanied by his fiancée and his parents. . . .

Case Study continued on the website and the CD-ROM with discussions, multiple-choice questions, and a nursing care plan.

---

overload, which can lead to pulmonary edema. Vasopressor agents are often given in the acute phase of SCI to maintain blood pressure. Elevating the feet can aid venous return in acute situations.

Diagnosis: Impaired Spontaneous Ventilation, Ineffective Airway Clearance, Impaired Gas Exchange. Cervical-level SCI carries a high risk of respiratory compromise. Any or all three of these nursing diagnoses may be appropriate.

Outcomes. The client will show no manifestations of respiratory compromise as evidenced by clear lung sounds; Pao_2, Pco_2, pH, and oxygen saturation values within normal limits; unlabored respirations; and normal vital capacity.

Interventions. Chest physical therapy can help mobilize secretions and prevent pneumonia, as can suctioning and assisted coughing. When spinal cord edema has temporarily impaired respiratory function, mechanical ventilation is used to support respiration. Intubation and ventilation can be frightening to a person who has been able to breathe independently. Sedation is administered as needed after intubation. Provide reassurance that mechanical ventilation will probably not be permanent. Clients may also be placed on a kinetic bed to maximize pulmonary function.

For extended airway management, a tracheostomy may be required to allow for long-term controlled ventilation, to facilitate the removal of tracheobronchial secretions, and to seal off the esophagus from the trachea for the prevention of aspiration. An abdominal binder is often used to provide abdominal support, to facilitate diaphragmatic breathing, and to increase venous return.

Diagnosis: Risk for Aspiration. Clients without a tracheostomy or with ineffective airway clearance or in whom the gag reflex is absent are at higher risk for aspiration. Aspiration is a common cause of morbidity in SCI clients.

Outcomes. The client will exhibit no manifestations of aspiration as evidenced by clear lung sounds; absence of stridor and fever; minimal amounts of clear mucus upon suctioning; and Pao_2, $Paco_2$, pH, and oxygen saturation values within normal limits.

Interventions. Suctioning equipment should be kept available and breath sounds assessed every 1 or 2 hours in acutely ill clients. The results of arterial blood gas analysis and pulse oximetry are monitored to determine the degree of oxygenation provided with mechanical ventilation or supplemental oxygen administration. Tracheobronchial suctioning is performed frequently to prevent or reduce the accumulation of secretions from immobility, lack of a cough reflex, or pneumonia. Monitor the electrocardiogram for dysrhythmias (e.g., premature ventricular contractions) resulting from hypoxia during suctioning.

Diagnosis: Ineffective Thermoregulation. Thermoregulation may be altered because of loss of hypothalamic control of the sympathetic nervous system in clients with SCI above the T6 level.

Outcomes. The client will maintain normothermic status.

Interventions. Rectal or core temperature is monitored every 4 hours during the first 72 hours after injury. Skin surfaces are palpated for areas of warmth, coolness, and moisture. Control the environmental temperature by using bed linens as needed to warm the client, eliminating drafts in the room, and using hypothermia blankets cautiously.

Evaluation. The problems identified in the early period of SCI care may resolve within 72 hours, especially if no other serious injuries or medical problems are present. If the client remains in an ICU for a prolonged time, implement other aspects of SCI care as discussed later.

■ **FIGURE 73–16** Fractures of the spine are often stabilized with internal fixation devices.

Surgical Management

The goal of surgical intervention is to stabilize the spine. Decompressive laminectomy, in which the laminae of the vertebrae are removed to minimize pressure on the spinal cord, can be used for complete SCIs. Stabilization by surgical fusion can be done by insertion of metal plates and screws or the use of bone grafts alone or in combination.

Cervical fractures can also be allowed to heal with stabilization of bone fragments achieved by immobilization in a brace or halo jacket (see Figure 73-15). The halo jacket has a ring that is fixed to the skull with pins. This ring is then attached to the jacket by rods. This system provides the traction required to maintain cervical alignment. A halo jacket allows early mobilization and rehabilitation.

SAFETY

⚠

ALERT

The wrench that comes with the brace should always be taped to the front of the jacket to allow quick removal in case of emergency. If the client has some mobility remaining, always assist during the client's first attempt at any activity. The halo jacket changes the client's center of gravity, making falls a constant risk. Never grasp the rods to help reposition the client. Perform pin site care around the pin insertion sites daily. See your agency's policy manual for guidelines.

Burst fractures of the thoracic and lumbar spinal segments can be treated with body casts, Harrington rods, or other devices for spine stabilization. Spine stabilization devices are commonly inserted through a posterior incision (Figure 73-16). After the operation, perform the usual postoperative assessments, including an assessment of the neurovascular status of the legs. Chest tubes and nasogastric tubes are inserted during surgery. The client is logrolled to facilitate maintenance of respiration and skin perfusion. Pain is managed with continuous-infusion or injected opioids. The client usually is fitted for a body brace, and mobilization begins on the fourth day.

Complications of surgery include infection and poor wound healing as well as those related to anesthesia. Both infection and impaired wound healing are more likely to occur in a malnourished client.

Spinal Cord Injury Rehabilitation

Clients with all levels of injury and of all ages benefit from rehabilitation. The client and family are involved in all phases. In all phases of rehabilitation, it is imperative that a motivated client be given the opportunity to perform any skill, even if the nurse or the physician can accomplish it more quickly. Allowing the client to attempt a complex skill demonstrates support of the client's self-care abilities. The key to rehabilitation is a multidisciplinary team of physicians, nurses, and allied health care providers (physical therapists, occupational therapists, speech and language pathologists) to reduce morbidity, maximize functional recovery, and promote independence.

Establish Functional Goals

Prediction of functional ability after SCI can generally be guided by the degree of residual muscle function (Table 73-2). It is intended to be a guide and might not represent ability in all clients with various levels of injury.

Promote Mobility

Wheelchairs provide mobility, and having the proper wheelchair is crucial. The wheelchair design must provide the client with the ability to propel the chair and prevent development of spinal deformities and pressure

TABLE 73–2 Functional Goals in Rehabilitation After Spinal Cord Injury

Spinal Cord Level	Muscle Function/Sensory Impairment	Functional Goals
C1-2	No phrenic nerve function; no sensation below neck	Respirations managed with phrenic pacemaker
C3-4	Neck control; scapular elevators; diaphragm function may be weak or absent	Manipulate electric wheelchair with breath control, chin control, or voice activation
C5	Fair to good shoulder control; functional deltoids/biceps; elbow flexion	Dress upper trunk; turn self in bed with or without arm slings
	No sensation below clavicles	Propel wheelchair with hand splints or after tenodesis
		Assist in getting into and out of bed; may learn to write or type
C6	Ability to lift shoulders, elbows, and wrists (partial)	Dress upper trunk; sometimes dress lower trunk
	Sensation as in C5 but more in arms and thumbs	Propel wheelchair with hand rim projections
		Self-feeding with hand splints
		Transfer from wheelchair to bed with or without minimal assistance (e.g., sliding board)
		Assist in getting to and from bedside commode; self-catheterization
C7	Ability to lift shoulders, elbows, wrists, and hands (partial)	Independent in transfer to bed, car, and toilet
	Sensation as in C6 level, with more in arms and middle fingers	Total dressing independence
		Propel wheelchair with standard hand rims
		Self-feeding with no assistive devices
C8	Ability to lift shoulders, elbows, wrists, and hands (partial)	Independent in transfer to bed, car, and toilet
	Sensation as in C7 level, with more in arms and little fingers	Total dressing independence
		Propel wheelchair with standard hand rims
		Self-feeding with no assistive devices
T1-4	Ability to use arms and hands normally	Independent in transfer to bed, car, and toilet
	No sensation below nipple line	Total dressing independence
	No trunk control	Propel wheelchair with standard hand rims
		Self-feeding with no assistive devices
		Transfer from wheelchair to floor and return
		Propel wheelchair up and down curb
		Transfer from wheelchair to tub and return
T5-L2	Partial to good trunk stability	Total wheelchair independence
	Able to use intercostal muscles	Limited ambulation with bilateral long leg braces and crutches (injury at T12 or below)
	No sensation below level of injury	
L3-4	All trunk-pelvic stabilizers intact; hip flexors, adductors, quadriceps	Ambulation with short leg braces with or without crutches depending on level of injury
L5-S3	Hip extensors, abductors; knee flexors; ankle control	No equipment needed if plantar flexion is strong enough for push-off at end of stance
	No sensation below midanterior thigh or in perianal area	

■ **FIGURE 73–17** A wheelchair with power hand controls for clients with C1-3 cervical spine injury. A respirator can be attached to the wheelchair. *(Courtesy Graham-Field Health Products, Atlanta, Ga.)*

ulcers. A high back and head support are needed for clients without arm function (Figure 73-17). For clients who can use their arms, the back of the wheelchair should be at the level of the scapula and the wheelchair should be lower than normal to facilitate transfers. Cushions help reduce pressure and the risk of pressure ulcers. Cushions, however, do not prevent pressure ulcers, and weight shifts are still needed every 10 to 15 minutes of time spent in the wheelchair. Physical therapists work with the client to teach how to transfer from bed to a wheelchair, from a wheelchair into and out of a car, and from the wheelchair onto a toilet.

Current emphasis is on strengthening muscles rather than using braces; however, back braces may be prescribed after lumbar spinal injury or for intervertebral disk problems. More frequently, a thoracolumbosacral orthosis is used. This device is a custom-made plastic brace with front and back pieces that attach together with self-fastening straps. This brace provides stability for the healing spine. The nurse is responsible for supervising the unlicensed professional whenever he or she is assisting with positioning transfers for a client with a spinal abnormality.

Reduce Spasticity

Spasticity often interferes with positioning and functional activities. However, spasticity also maintains muscle bulk, facilitates venous return, prevents DVT, and can aid in transfers. Treatment includes ROM exercises. Oral antispasmodic medications such as baclofen, dantrolene sodium, and clonidine are used only when the spasms cause discomfort or safety concerns. An implanted pump designed to deliver baclofen through a catheter into the intrathecal space can be used to increase the efficacy of the baclofen and decreasing dosages.

Improve Bladder and Bowel Control

The term *neurogenic bladder* is used to describe bladder control changes that occur with both upper and lower motor neuron disorders. Upper motor neuron disorders produce a spastic or reflex bladder. Lower motor neuron disorders produce a flaccid bladder. The bladder can be managed in many ways, and treatment options must be tailored to fit the client's preferences and lifestyle as well as the client's functional abilities.

Intermittent urinary catheterization is begun when the urine output drops to less than 600 ml in 4 to 6 hours. Intermittent catheterization reduces the risk of infection and bladder stone formation caused by indwelling catheters. Clients with injuries at the C6 level and lower can perform self-catheterization, if they have adequate hand function and can manage lower extremity clothing. External catheters are used for men who void between catheterizations or for those who leak urine during bladder spasms. Clients with arm function are taught to facilitate the emptying of their bladder using the Credé maneuver over the bladder to relax the sphincter and express urine (see Promote Bladder Retraining in the later nursing management section).

Urinary complications occur because of incomplete emptying of the bladder, necessitating catheterization. Catheterization may predispose the client to infection and vesicoureteral reflux, which may lead to kidney complications. Renal calculi, pyelonephritis, and hydronephrosis are major causes of considerable disability and even death in paralyzed clients.

Compared to indwelling catheters, suprapubic catheters seem to offer the advantages of less infection and urethral injury. Indwelling catheters are not ideal from a medical standpoint but are preferred by many clients because of the ease of management. Complications from catheters include infection, bladder stones, urethral damage, and a reported increased incidence of bladder cancer. A neurogenic bladder may also be managed pharmacologically with medications such as bethanechol (Urecholine) to stimulate bladder contraction or oxybutynin (Ditropan) to reduce bladder contraction. Urine-acidifying agents may also be prescribed to reduce the risk of infection.

A neurogenic bowel is similar to a neurogenic bladder in that the client cannot control defecation. The goal is to develop a bowel elimination method that is convenient, effective, and least expensive for the client. Sufficient fluid and fiber intake is essential. Consistent timing and position are important to a successful program. When fiber is added to or increased in the diet, it must be done slowly to avoid cramping and diarrhea. Stool softeners and bulk laxatives may also be used.

Bowel movements of clients with upper motor neuron damage are generally regulated with suppositories or digital stimulation every day or every other day to reduce the risk of autonomic dysreflexia. A lower motor neuron neurogenic bowel is more difficult to regulate, and often the client requires manual removal of impacted fecal material.

Prevent Pressure Ulcers

Numb skin is associated with an increased frequency of pressure ulcers. During the acute care period, the risk of pressure ulcer development is related to the level of injury, completeness of the injury, and duration of immobilization. Once the client is seated in a wheelchair, pressure ulcers can develop on the ischia as a result of prolonged sitting. Clients should be turned every 2 hours when in bed. If the client can reposition or turn without assistance in bed, an overlay mattress should be used and an alarm clock set to ring every two hours as a reminder during sleep.

A client with spinal fractures may be placed on a rotating bed (see Figure 68-2). It is equipped with supportive packs and straps that keep the body in neutral alignment while the bed continuously oscillates from side to side. If rotation is greater than 40 degrees, the continuous motion helps to prevent skin breakdown, reduce urinary stasis, and promote lung aeration. Skin inspection must be performed closely on the sacrum for signs of shearing. Unfortunately, the constant movement may also stimulate peristalsis, resulting in severe diarrhea. Some clients also experience disorientation from the constant movement and have reported fear of falling. Staff members should remain with the client initially to provide emotional support and reassurance. Also, it is important to pull window curtains at night because a client in a rotating bed who can see himself or herself "floating" in the window reflection can become disoriented or frightened.

Reduce Respiratory Dysfunction

Respiratory dysfunction is a significant cause of morbidity and mortality after SCI. Clients with injury to C3 have paralyzed diaphragms and will need phrenic pacing once they are weaned from a ventilator. In injuries lower than C3, the diaphragm may be the only functional muscle that is active in respiration because the intercostal and abdominal muscles are often paralyzed. Vital capacity and inspiratory reserve volume are markedly diminished. The client should be taught to use incentive spirometry and diaphragmatic breathing to enhance vital capacity. Glossopharyngeal breathing uses the tongue and muscles of the pharynx to force air into the lungs. This technique enhances vital capacity and promotes chest expansion.

Promote Expression of Sexuality

Sexual function in spinal cord–injured men depends on the location of the lesion (Box 73-3). Reflex erection is possible in some clients with upper motor neuron lesions and also with some lower motor neuron lesions. Ejaculation is possible with lower motor neuron lesions and if the lesion is more caudal. Fertility after SCI remains low but has been improved by electroejaculation, artificial insemination, and in vitro fertilization. Sexual dysfunction is approached from two avenues: psychological counseling and education about technological advances in the facilitation of sexual activity. Erection can be restored with external aids, an implantable penile prosthesis, or medications.

Female clients retain fertility after SCI. Problems with sexual function generally relate to positioning and the lack of vaginal lubrication. These problems can usually be addressed through client education.

Control Pain

Long-term pain occurs frequently in spinal cord–injured clients with intact sensation. Dysesthetic pain, which is distal to the site of injury, is extremely disabling. It is similar to the phantom sensation experienced after amputation. It is described as cutting, burning, piercing, radiating, or tightening. The usual treatment is with nonopioid analgesics and transcutaneous nerve stimulators. An "as-needed" approach to pain management is not recommended for chronic pain; however, routine analgesics may need to be supplemented with other

---

BOX 73-3   Sexual Function in Clients with Spinal Cord Injury

FEMALES

Lesions at C1-3: Reflex lubrication is probable; erogenous areas may develop above injury; libido is intact

Lesions at C4-6: Psychogenic lubrication is unlikely; nongenital orgasm may be experienced

Lesions at C7: Able to use hands for holding and caressing

Lesions at T12-L5: Psychogenic stimulation of the clitoris, lubrication, labial swelling, and skin flush are possible but unlikely

MALES

Lesions at C1-3: Reflex erection is caused by genital stimulation; psychogenic erection is not possible; erogenous zones above injury site may develop; libido is intact

Lesions at C4-6: Reflex erection is possible; nongenital orgasm may be experienced; no ejaculation; oral sex is possible; libido is intact

Lesions at C7: Able to use hands for holding

Lesions at T12-L6: Psychogenic stimulation and erection are possible; no reflex erection

Lesions at S2-4: Reflex erection is possible; ejaculation is possible but may be retrograde pain-relieving medications given as needed during a client's pain peaks. Gabapentin (Neurontin) has been used successfully for patients with neuropathic pain.

Reduce Abnormal Bone Growth

Heterotopic ossification is the formation of bone in abnormal locations, occurring most often around the hips and knees after SCI. The client may develop swelling in the joint or loss of ROM. Heterotopic ossification is diagnosed by x-ray study or bone scan. Treatment includes the use of etidronate disodium (Didronel) and ROM exercises of the affected joints. Sometimes the bone is removed surgically.

Promote Psychological Adjustment

Psychological counseling is ongoing. Commonly, spinal cord–injured clients participate in peer group counseling sessions in which experiences and solutions are shared to help newly injured clients to cope better with their losses. Vocational rehabilitation may help clients reach their maximum rehabilitation potential.

Ongoing Nursing Management of the Client with Spinal Cord Injury

Assessment. The client usually is transferred to a rehabilitation setting when the acute illness is stable. Clients with high cervical injuries may remain on ventilators. The care of the ventilator-dependent client is discussed in Chapter 63. Some of the nursing diagnoses that applied in the acute care setting may still apply after transfer. The client remains at risk for skin impairment and may still have difficulty swallowing, with attendant risk for aspiration. A baseline assessment should be completed at transfer.

Diagnosis, Outcomes, Interventions

Diagnosis: Impaired Physical Mobility. Spinal cord injury that causes permanent impaired physical mobility produces problems with ambulation and potential complications arising from immobility. The relevant nursing diagnosis is *Impaired Physical Mobility related to inability to move upper and/or lower extremities secondary to paralysis.*

Outcomes. The client will have maximal physical mobility as evidenced by absence of tendon contractures, joint ankylosis, and muscle shortening and will demonstrate effective use of adaptive devices.

Interventions. Throughout the acute and rehabilitative phases of nursing care, make every effort to maximize functional abilities and independence by encouraging the client to perform independently any activities of daily living (ADL) for which capability remains.

Provide Positioning and Adaptive Equipment. Improper positioning of the client in the bed or chair and lack of joint movements (e.g., related to spasticity or immobility) lead to tendon contractures, joint ankylosis, and muscle shortening. Interventions to prevent such problems include the following:

- Frequent position changes
- Proper positioning of joints
- Use of splints and removable casts
- Intermittent turning to a prone position
- Positioning of upper extremities away from the body
- Draping of bed linen over frames to keep pressure off the feet
- Keeping knee joints flexed 15 degrees when the client is supine
- Use of active and passive conditioning exercises (see Risk for Contractures)

Wristdrop and footdrop are inevitable sequelae in paralyzed extremities unless specific preventive measures are used. Footdrop may be prevented by keeping the client's feet firmly supported in dorsiflexion at right angles to the hips to counteract the force of gravity on weakened muscles. Many devices are available to prevent footdrop; they are designed to stretch the Achilles tendons. Wearing shoes also helps prevent footdrop when the client lies down. Support a paralyzed arm in a sling when the client is out of bed and in a cock-up splint when the client is in bed. Usually the hand end of the splint is elevated 2 inches to support the wrist, and the fingers are maintained in a position of function. Posterior molded casts may be used instead of splints to support a paralyzed wrist while the client is in bed. For some clients, pillows and a hand roll are adequate. Skin must be frequently assessed under any braces or splints.

Assist with Transfers and Ambulation. Rehabilitative programs often require strength and endurance. To prepare a client for ambulation, the unaffected parts of the body must be strengthened and suitable exercises started early. Tolerance for activity gradually increases. Take care not to fatigue the client. Periods of planned rest and recreation are important.

Braces or corsets should be applied before the client is assisted to get out of bed. A thin, knitted undershirt is worn under the brace or corset to protect the skin and to keep the appliance clean. To apply the brace or corset, turn the client to one side, place the appliance against the back, and then roll the client back into it. The brace or corset is secured while the client lies supine. As recovery and rehabilitation progress, many clients learn to apply their own brace or corset while in bed. Others continue to need help. The degree of arm and hand function determines the client's ability to apply a brace.

■ **FIGURE 73–18** Bed-to-wheelchair lateral transfer using a sliding board.

Physical therapy is essential for all clients with SCI. Paraplegic clients need to learn various transfers to become self-sufficient. One transfer method is illustrated in Figure 73-18. Learning to sit up precedes learning to transfer. Take care in helping clients to stand or sit in a chair for the first time. Because of the loss of venous return from reflexes with movement, these clients are prone to orthostatic hypotension. Always check blood pressure before and after transfers. Syncope during a wheelchair transfer may be avoided in the quadriplegic client by using an abdominal binder, thigh-high support hose, and slowly elevating the head of the bed to 90 degrees. Using a recliner or a wheelchair with an adjustable back will help achieve gradual elevations.

Weight-bearing begins as early as possible after SCI. Weight-bearing stimulates osteoblastic (bone formation) activity and thus decreases demineralization of bone (*osteoporosis*) that develops with prolonged immobilization. Use of a standing board or tilt table assists the client to tolerate gradually a standing position. Having the client stand periodically each day also helps prevent contractures (e.g., hip contractures resulting from long periods of sitting).

Clients easily lose balance when wearing braces, particularly the halo brace, and must be careful to avoid falling. (See the Client Education Guide website feature on Use of a Halo Vest.) A brace feels surprisingly

heavy at first, especially if the client is weak. For safety, shoes (rather than slippers or just stockings or socks) should be worn during ambulation. Shoes should tie or have self-fastening straps for firm support and have a low heel. High-top athletic shoes give added support. Slick soles, high or narrow heels, and stocking feet are hazardous.

SAFETY

⚠

ALERT

The fit, comfort, and appearance of braces, corsets, and shoes are important to the client. Try to accommodate the preferences of clients who want to be as stylish as possible as well as benefit from therapeutic garments. Disabled clients are helped by being encouraged to express their feelings concerning their self-image and by having their desires taken into consideration when being fitted for therapeutic garments. Some garments can be painful when first worn. The pain worsens if the garments do not fit properly.

Diagnosis: Ineffective Airway Clearance. Airway clearance may be impaired because of paralysis of the abdominal and intercostal muscles. The relevant nursing diagnosis is *Ineffective Airway Clearance related to inability to cough*.

Outcomes. The client has adequate airway clearance as evidenced by participating in "quad-assisted" coughing, remaining afebrile, and having normal blood gas or pulse oximetry values and clear sputum.

Interventions. Use the "quad-assisted" cough maneuver to promote airway clearance. Quad-assisted coughing is accomplished by placing a fist or heel of the hand between the umbilicus and the xiphoid process. Press inward and upward during the client's cough (Figure 73-19). Other interventions, such as turning, hydration, and chest physical therapy, may also be used.

Collaborative Problem: Risk for Thrombophlebitis. Muscular activity is a major factor in venous circulation. A paralyzed client experiences slowed venous return and pooling of blood in dependent limbs. These phenomena constitute the basis for the collaborative problem *Risk for Thrombophlebitis*.

Outcomes. The nurse will monitor for thrombophlebitis as evidenced by unilateral leg edema, erythema, and warmth.

Interventions. In the acute phase of SCI, anti-embolism stockings, sequential compression devices, and subcutaneous heparin may be used prophylactically.

Education is vital to preventing vascular complications and minimizing their impact. Teach the client the importance of all preventive activities. During assessment of the legs for manifestations of clot formation (i.e., redness and unilateral swelling and warmth), explain the components of assessment and emphasize the importance of incorporating this activity into daily

Sternum

Outline of lungs

■ **FIGURE 73-19** Cough assistance. In this technique, which can be performed with the client sitting in a wheelchair, the hands are placed on the midline of the upper abdomen. After the client inhales, pressure is directed inward and upward as the client attempts to cough. *(From AACN, & Carlson, K. [Eds.] [2008]. AACN advanced critical care nursing, St. Louis: Saunders.)*

routines. Measuring calf diameter on both legs daily to detect any changes is a more objective way of assessing swelling. Clients also learn not to cross their legs while sitting in a wheelchair.

Collaborative Problem: Risk for Contractures. Active ROM is severely limited or nonexistent in the upper extremities and nonexistent in the lower extremities in a client with cervical cord damage; it is also nonexistent in the lower extremities in a client with thoracic or lumbar cord damage. This deficit increases the risk for contractures. The collaborative problem is *Risk for Contractures related to inability to move purposefully secondary to spinal injury.*

Outcomes. The client will have reduced risk of contractures as evidenced by maintaining ROM present before the injury.

Interventions. Monitor the degree of ROM in all involved joints. Passive exercises prevent contractures and painful reflex dystrophies of the hand and shoulder. Such exercises may be prescribed as soon as 48 to 72 hours after injury. Active exercises, massage, and electrical stimulation may also be prescribed. Begin shoulder and arm exercises early. Strength in these areas and in the chest and back is essential for effective self-transfers and

ambulation. Clients may find that the prone position is helpful to prevent hip flexure contracture.

Diagnosis: Self-Care Deficit. The client who has suffered an SCI is often unable to perform many self-care activities.

Outcomes. The client will have a satisfactory level of self-care as evidenced by independently performing as many ADL tasks as possible. If unable to perform an activity independently, the client will be able to direct a caregiver's performance. These goals will be evaluated by observing successful performance of ADL by the client or under the client's direction.

Interventions. Self-care deficit can lead to a feeling of powerlessness. Assisting the client to maximize independence can lessen this feeling. The client is assisted with muscle-strengthening exercises and the use of adaptive devices. Clients with high cervical injuries are able to perform few activities independently. Allow them adequate time to accomplish whatever tasks they can. If help with ADL is needed, adapt nursing care to the client's routine. In collaborating to maintain intact oral mucous membranes, a schedule is established for brushing the teeth at least twice daily and cleaning the tongue, roof of the mouth, and gums with agents that do not contain lemon or alcohol.

Diagnosis: Risk for Imbalanced Nutrition: Less Than Body Requirements. After traumatic injury metabolic demand increases because of the response to stress and the body's requirements for healing. The relevant nursing diagnosis is written *Risk for Imbalanced Nutrition: Less Than Body Requirements related to increased metabolic demand and inability to access nutrients.* Anorexia related to depression may be another etiologic factor.

Outcomes. The client will have balanced nutrition as evidenced by maintaining a reasonable weight for height.

Interventions. The client should be weighed on admission to obtain a baseline measurement. Compare current weight to ideal body weight. Whereas weight loss is not encouraged during the healing phase of injury, once the client is stable, excess weight should be shed to promote activity and transferring. For clients below ideal body weight, nutrient supplementation should begin by 72 hours after injury if the client is not eating. Enteral feeding can be used if the client has bowel sounds. If the client still has paralytic ileus, hyperalimentation is commonly used. Weigh the client at least once a week to monitor progress. Laboratory values for albumin and prealbumin should also be monitored.

Diagnosis: Total Urinary Incontinence. Urinary bladder *atony* (absence of tone) may last several weeks or months after SCI. In clients with upper motor neuron lesions, when spinal shock subsides and the reflexes return, a reflex contraction may empty the bladder.

Observe the client carefully for indications of problems with bladder control and infection, including incontinence, retention, urgency, dribbling, frequency, enuresis, and precipitate micturition. Document such observations and inform the physician. The relevant nursing diagnosis is written *Total Urinary Incontinence related to paralysis.*

Outcomes. The client will have improved bladder control as evidenced by absence of infection and by emptying of the bladder every 4 to 6 hours.

Interventions. Nursing intervention is planned to prevent urinary tract infection, to preserve existing bladder capacity and muscle tone, and to establish and maintain a routine pattern of elimination requiring minimal artificial assistance.

It is important to check a postvoid residual or to use an ultrasound to measure bladder volume to ensure near-complete bladder emptying. During the period of atony, a retention catheter may be inserted to prevent bladder distention and keep the client dry and comfortable.

SAFETY

⚠

ALERT

Bladder overdistention causes stretching and fissure formation—a predisposing factor for infection—and may result in bladder rupture. When sensory pathways are damaged, the client does not feel the discomfort of bladder distention; however, prolonged catheter use also predisposes to infection. Therefore catheterization every 4 to 6 hours to keep urine volumes less than 600 ml is preferred over a retention catheter.

Urinary complications may be avoided by periodically examining the client for bladder distention, accurately documenting fluid intake and output, using aseptic technique when handling urinary catheters, and observing for manifestations of bladder infection. Encourage the client to drink water to keep the urine diluted, which lessens the possibility of infection.

Urine acidifiers may be prescribed. To prevent development of renal calculi, encourage the client to drink about 3000 ml of fluid per day, unless contraindicated by other medical conditions. This is sufficient to maintain a minimal urine output of 2000 ml/day. Drinking this much fluid may increase incontinence but is necessary to prevent renal calculi.

Self bladder care is discussed later, under Therapeutic Regimen Management.

Diagnosis: Bowel Incontinence or Constipation. Bowel dysfunction is a common but manageable problem in a client with SCI. This common nursing diagnosis is written as *Constipation related to paralysis.*

Outcomes. The client will have reduced risk of bowel incontinence or constipation as evidenced by a bowel movement every 1 to 2 days, no manifestations of fecal impaction, no incontinence, and no manifestations of hyperreflexia.

Interventions. Nursing intervention is planned to prevent constipation, distention, and impaction; to detect and treat these conditions if they occur; and to reestablish habitual, controlled bowel movements by conditioned reflex activity. Paralytic ileus is common after SCI. By frequently assessing bowel sounds and documenting the passage of stool, return of peristalsis can be determined and the client can resume oral intake. The client is observed carefully for indications of constipation, diarrhea, or *tenesmus* (straining at stool). If the bowel becomes impacted, a cleansing enema may be prescribed to initially empty the lower bowel. Enemas should be avoided for long-term bowel management, however. A paraplegic or quadriplegic client cannot retain an enema solution, nor can the degree of intestinal distention be felt. Therefore enemas must be administered carefully to avoid overdistending the intestine with excessive fluid; 500 ml or less is usually given.

Document the client's intake of fluid and food and elimination patterns. A bowel program should be established early. The program should occur at the same time every day (or every other day), after a meal or large snack with the patient as upright as possible. The use of water-based suppositories or digital stimulation provides a signal to the body for reflex evacuation.

A daily fluid intake of 3000 ml/day is important for proper bowel function as well as bladder function. Also, the diet must be high in bulk and roughage, such as bran, whole grains, fresh and dried fruits, and leafy green and raw vegetables. A stool softener such as docusate sodium (Colace) may be taken daily, but laxatives should be carefully administered. Bulk-forming medications (e.g., psyllium hydrophilic mucilloid [Metamucil]) are effective for spinal cord–injured clients so long as adequate hydration is maintained. Self bowel care is discussed later, under Therapeutic Regimen Management.

Diagnosis: Risk for Impaired Skin Integrity. Clients with SCI are at higher risk of impairment of skin integrity because of immobility and loss of protective functions.

Outcomes. The client will have intact skin as evidenced by no reddened areas over bony prominences and no areas or manifestations of skin irritation or dryness.

Interventions. The spinal cord–injured client cannot respond to the sensory cues to local tissue hypoxia resulting from being in one position for an extended period. Therefore, the development of pressure ulcers is frequent. Spinal cord–injured clients should be placed on pressure-redistributing beds or mattresses. Use of these special beds does not, however, eliminate the need to assess the skin every shift, turn the client every 2 hours, or eliminate the risk of pressure ulcers. In addition, the client's nutritional needs must be met to reduce the risk of pressure ulcers.

Wheelchairs need to be fitted with pressure reduction seating cushions that allow movement for transfers as well as pressure reduction. Because ischial pressure ulcers can develop quickly, clients should be taught to inspect their own skin with a long handled mirror or have their caregiver do so daily. The cushion also needs to be assessed; air columns should be full, foam should not be compressed, and gel cushions should not show wear. Seating evaluation for pressure areas is helpful to choose a chair cushion that provides pressure redistribution. Once an ulcer forms, complete bed rest may be needed to heal the ulcer; so prevention and early detection are crucial.

Once the client is seated, he or she should be taught to perform a daily systematic skin inspection. For example, at bedtime the client can use a long-handled mirror to see the buttocks before transferring to bed. Clothing should be worn that does not have seams, pockets, or rivets because these items cause unusual pressure points. Prevention of pressure ulcers should include use of pressure-relieving devices in both chair and bed. Wheelchairs should be fitted with gel cushions for those clients who transfer and with air column cushions for those who do not transfer. Pressure relief in wheelchairs is usually accomplished by pushing off the arms of the wheelchair or leaning forward every 15 to 30 minutes.

Diagnosis: Chronic Pain. Clients with SCI may experience pain at the level of the injury and radiating along spinal nerves originating in the area. Phantom sensation may also be experienced. The onset of pain is usually later than that for muscle spasms. Some paraplegic and quadriplegic clients experience both pain and spasm. Pain most often occurs in the lower extremities.

Outcomes. The client will experience adequate pain relief as evidenced by verbalization of improvement in comfort, ability to rest without interruption by pain, and ability to participate in therapies without hindrance by pain.

Interventions. Analgesics such as aspirin and nonsteroidal anti-inflammatory drugs (NSAIDs) may be prescribed. Opioids are seldom used after the initial injury and are contraindicated in clients with high cervical-level injuries because of the risk of respiratory depression.

Clients with thoracic pulmonary injuries tend to breathe more shallowly to avoid pain. Inadequate depth of respirations can lead to complications. Give prescribed pain medication and encourage deep breathing and coughing to aerate the lungs and remove secretions from the respiratory tract.

Antispasmodics, NSAIDs, and non-opioid analgesics are prescribed for pain associated with spasticity. Surgery (e.g., neurectomy, chordotomy) is sometimes required for pain relief.

Collaborative Problem: Risk for Autonomic Dysreflexia. Autonomic dysreflexia/hyperreflexia is a serious complication of SCI when injury is above the T6 level. This collaborative problem is documented as *Risk for Autonomic Dysreflexia related to spinal cord injury.*

Outcomes. The nurse will monitor for clinical manifestations of autonomic dysreflexia and respond to them quickly.

Interventions. Assess the client for sudden onset of severe hypertension, severe throbbing headache, profuse diaphoresis, flushing of the skin above the level of the lesion, nasal stuffiness, pilomotor spasm, blurred vision, nausea, and bradycardia. The Critical Monitoring feature below lists additional assessment findings related to this serious complication.

Educate the client about early warning signs and symptoms of autonomic dysreflexia and the importance of calling for a nurse immediately if any occur. Adaptive call lights are available to facilitate calling for assistance. If autonomic dysreflexia does occur, institute the following measures:

1. Elevate the head of the bed to a sitting position immediately.
2. Check blood pressure.
3. Check for possible sources of irritation (e.g., kinked or clogged catheter or distended bladder or lower bowel).
4. Remove the stimulus if it can be done quickly. Once the source of irritation is removed, manifestations of autonomic dysreflexia usually subside.
5. If blood pressure remains elevated, antihypertensive medication (nitrates, hydralazine, guanethidine, or diazoxide) may be administered according to prescription or procedural policy (intravenously, intranasally, or sublingually).
6. If there is no order or policy or if these measures do not correct the problem, notify the physician.

CRITICAL MONITORING

Features of Autonomic Dysreflexia

- Severe hypertension (up to 300 mm Hg)
- Pounding headache
- Flushing (above the level of the lesion)
- Piloerection
- Diaphoresis
- Dilated pupils, blurred vision
- Nasal stuffiness
- Bradycardia (pulse rate <60 beats/min)
- Restlessness
- Nausea

Once manifestations have subsided, observe the client's vital signs and neurologic status closely for 3 to 4 hours. If an antihypertensive medication has been given, the client may become hypotensive after the stimulus is removed. Autonomic dysreflexia may recur if the stimulus is not completely removed. If the identified source is bladder distention, use caution when emptying the bladder. Remove 500 ml every 5 to 15 minutes. If the identified source of irritation is bowel distention, be careful when removing the impacted material from the bowel. An anesthetic lubricant is used, and another nurse must monitor the client's blood pressure every few minutes. The stimulation of trying to remove the impacted material can increase the severity of the autonomic response.

SAFETY

⚠️

ALERT

When a quadriplegic client complains of a headache, *do not automatically give analgesics without first checking the blood pressure.*

Diagnosis: Risk for Injury. In clients with SCI, another appropriate nursing diagnosis is *Risk for Injury related to abnormal reflexes, spasms, and corneal drying.* Corneal abrasions may result unless proper interventions are instituted.

Outcomes. The client will sustain no injuries from spasms as evidenced by no abrasions or bruising. Corneal abrasions will not occur.

Interventions. Injections should be avoided whenever possible. Medications should be given orally or intravenously if needed. When injections must be given, inject them above the level of the cord lesion whenever possible. Absorption may be compromised in denervated areas of the body with impaired capillary and precapillary circulation. Moisten the cornea with natural tears every 4 hours for a client with altered blinking reflexes.

Clients can also be injured from involuntary spasms. Avoid unnecessary stimulation of areas that elicit reflex spinal automatisms. When such reactions do occur, an unembarrassed, accepting response helps relieve the client's anxiety and embarrassment. Gentle, slow hyperextension of a limb in spasm can often override the trigger points and interrupt the spasm. Abnormal spinal reflexes make clients respond to stimuli in ways that may be puzzling to both the client and others unless the origin of such responses is explained. For example, stimulation of the limbs (perhaps toe flexion while the person's foot is being dried) may cause mass flexion of the upper and lower extremities. Mass flexion reactions may be accompanied by massive contractions of the abdominal wall, evacuation of the urinary bladder and bowel, and automatic response such as sweating, flushing, penile erection, or pilomotor reactions below the level of the lesion.

Diagnosis: Ineffective Coping. When the reality of the injury and the permanent deficits are understood, coping skills may need to be taught. The nursing diagnosis can be written as *Ineffective Coping related to awareness of the permanent paralysis and its effect on life goals.*

Outcomes. The client will use adaptive coping strategies and resources appropriately.

Interventions. Clients need to find appropriate methods for coping with new approaches to performing ADL and managing bodily functions. The learning needs of spinal cord–injured clients and their family members are complex and ongoing. In the acute phase, education about spinal anatomy and physiology is needed. This teaching begins in the acute phase of hospitalization and should be incorporated into all aspects of care. Successful learning in this stage affects the client's entire life. Over time many SCI clients develop unique and resourceful adaptations to their living and work environments to facilitate independence.

Diagnosis: Anticipatory Grieving. Clients with SCI experience many changes (e.g., functional ability, role definition, body image, financial security). Grief is a normal response to these losses. Write the nursing diagnosis as *Anticipatory Grieving related to multiple losses.*

Outcomes. The client will progress through the grieving process and develop adaptive coping strategies as evidenced by verbalizing his or her feelings about the injury and the future, participating in community activities, and expressing positive thoughts about the future.

Interventions. Adjusting to paralysis is difficult physically and psychosocially for the client and family. Family members may experience the same reactions as those experienced by the disabled client and may need the same type of help. Sudden paralysis in a previously healthy, active person can be devastating. Typically the sudden lifestyle changes brought about by serious SCI produce a grief reaction. The reaction may involve initial shock and denial, leading to depression and anger. Crying and talking about the injury may be helpful. Social services or pastoral care may also be of assistance during this time of grief.

It takes time to adjust to disability and to develop ways of coping. Psychological adjustment occurs when the client can function appropriately in the real world. A client may use psychological defense mechanisms in adjusting to paralysis. When caring for such a client, assess the possible reasons for observed behavior. Hostility, depression, anger, or withdrawal may be upsetting to staff and family. These emotions and behaviors represent coping mechanisms and should not be taken personally.

Paralysis may cause complex changes in self-concept and body image. In the acute phase, immobilization can contribute to sensory deprivation and its consequences (e.g., hallucinations). Providing visual, auditory, and tactile stimulation as desired by the client may minimize the experience of deprivation.

Paralyzed clients are often helped initially by being with others who are experiencing similar problems. Clients should be allowed to wear their own clothing as soon as possible and encouraged to be out of bed and out of the hospital room. Planned social activities may reduce feelings of social isolation and may help clients regain self-confidence. Peer counseling, in which newly disabled clients are provided opportunities to talk with others who have adjusted to similar disabilities, may be helpful. Young clients may find enjoyment in sports designed for people in wheelchairs (Figure 73-20).

A sense of security is particularly important for a newly paralyzed client adjusting to enforced dependency. A paralyzed client should always have a means of summoning help and yet needs to learn that it is safe to be alone at times. Blow lights, minimal-pressure call lights, pads, and voice-activated call lights are now available in many settings.

Gradually the client develops trust in his or her abilities and resources and relinquishes some reliance on others. These feelings and attitudes develop slowly as the client experiences genuinely trustworthy relationships.

To avoid unnecessary frustrations, try to keep the client's environment comfortable, with necessary items conveniently placed. It is difficult and depressing for the client to have to ask for help repeatedly. Although recent advances have been made in the rehabilitation prognosis of paraplegic and quadriplegic clients, it is important to be realistic as well as optimistic. Nurses need to understand the tremendous lifestyle changes disabled clients must make. Some clients can be rehabilitated to a level of near-independence: walking (perhaps with braces or other appliances), driving a car, and coping with full-time employment outside the home. Quadriplegic clients usually rely on a wheelchair and other devices and appliances.

Most paralyzed clients can become productive and happy. After his devastating SCI, actor Christopher Reeve served as a positive role model regarding *abilities* that remain after SCI. Even if some clients are unable to be "productive," all disabled clients have a right to a satisfying, happy life. Although many paralyzed clients achieve complete rehabilitation, others lead lives that are difficult, frustrating, and psychophysiologically complex. At times, severe mental depression develops. Depression is assessed, and professional counseling is offered as indicated. Unfortunately, ideations of suicide are frequent.

Diagnosis: Disabled Family Coping. A family is a unit. A trauma as devastating as SCI to one of the members of the family unit affects the entire family. The relevant nursing diagnosis can be written *Disabled Family Coping: related to multiple changes in the family roles.*

Outcomes. The client and family members will use adaptive coping by identifying areas of significant or potential loss and changes in family roles, working together to overcome obstacles, seeking appropriate support services, and being able to restore a supportive family structure.

Interventions. The injury affects not only physical functioning but also the psychological, vocational, educational, and social aspects of life. An organized team approach is vital to helping the injured client and family cope with lifestyle changes. Nurses are often the first health care professionals to assess client and family coping. An open, empathetic manner can allow the people involved to express their grief and uncertainty and to ask questions. Educate the family about the normal grief response. Carefully probe into persistent denial of grief or lack of progression through grieving. Encouraging as much optimism as possible while remaining truthful and realistic may help SCI survivors to face the future.

Assess the previous roles of the client and other family members and how they have handled stressful situations or losses. Identify the family's sources of strength. Assess patterns of interaction between family members; their spiritual, social, and economic status; and their lifestyle. Cultural or ethnic influences should also be noted. These variables often influence how the family responds to grief. Sometimes the nurse can play a valuable role simply by giving family members permission to have a day off from visiting.

■ **FIGURE 73-20** The Paralympics offer young athletes opportunities to play sports.

Diagnosis: Ineffective Therapeutic Regimen Management. Clients with SCI have bladder and bowel function changes. Bladder emptying has to be learned using a different approach, and bowel retraining is often necessary. A common nursing diagnosis in this circumstance is *Ineffective Therapeutic Regimen Management.*

Outcomes. The client will be able to manage his or her bowel and bladder or instruct others how to do so.

Interventions. One of the most common stimuli for autonomic dysreflexia, a life-threatening complication in people with SCI, is bladder distention. Therefore intervention leading to bladder management is crucial.

Promote Bladder Retraining. When the initial indwelling catheter is removed, a program of intermittent catheterization is commonly prescribed to empty the bladder regularly every 4 to 6 hours for several weeks. During this time, the client may be taught methods of emptying the bladder without catheterization. Such methods promote urination by increasing intra-abdominal pressure on the bladder. For some clients with SCI, urinary flow can be initiated by using the Credé maneuver, the Valsalva maneuver, or the rectal stretch.

The *Credé maneuver* involves placing the fist or fingers directly over the bladder and pressing down toward the pubic bone with a kneading motion. This motion is continued until the bladder is empty.

The *Valsalva maneuver* involves inhaling deeply, holding the breath, and bearing down as hard as possible, as if for a bowel movement.

The *rectal stretch* involves inserting a lubricated, gloved finger into the rectum. When the anal sphincter is relaxed, the client maintains the relaxation by gently pulling on the sphincter. This relaxes the perineal floor. The Valsalva maneuver is performed at the same time.

Urination may also be prompted by reflex stimulation. The following stimuli may be successful: tapping the suprapubic area; stroking the glans penis, thigh, or vulva; tugging pubic hairs; or flexing the toes. The client or caregiver may apply the stimulation. As training continues, less stimulation is needed to initiate urination.

Catheterization may be required at home. Teach the client and caregiver clean, rather than sterile, technique. This technique has the same infection rate as for sterile insertion methods used for home catheterization. Suprapubic catheters may be inserted for long-term bladder management.

Occasionally a surgical procedure such as sphincterotomy is necessary. The bladder then empties continuously. An external, condom-type catheter connected to a closed drainage bag may be used to collect urine in men. External appliances for females are not consistently effective. The Mitrofanoff procedure is a surgical option that creates an opening from the bladder to the umbilicus. It allows for catheterization of the stoma and bladder emptying with less hand function and disrobing needed.

Teach Bowel Retraining. Bowel retraining is possible for most paraplegic and quadriplegic clients. It involves developing controlled bowel movements by conditioned reflex activity. Begin bowel retraining as soon as feasible. Ensure privacy during the daily bowel routine, and if possible, have the client sitting upright. When possible, include appropriate family members in the bowel retraining program because they may be involved in this aspect of long-term management. Always assess the family members' willingness to participate in such care. If the sexual partner is also responsible for hygiene and personal care, problems in role separation and intimacy may result. These issues should be openly discussed between partners.

With an effective bowel program, a client has a bowel movement once a day or every other day and is not incontinent at other times. Attaining continence may influence a paralyzed client's vocational future and positively affect ability to have satisfying social relationships. It can also give the client the confidence to cope with other problems.

Diagnosis: Sexual Dysfunction. Spinal cord–injured clients are often concerned about sexuality and their ability to achieve sexual fulfillment. They often worry about such concerns long before they express them to others. Nurses are often asked about sexuality issues before other professionals are approached, perhaps because nurses provide intimate care. Such care can promote a high degree of trust.

Outcomes. The client will develop personally satisfying and socially acceptable means of expressing sexuality as evidenced by interacting appropriately in social situations, verbalizing the effects of the injury on sexual function, discussing sexual issues with a health care team member, verbalizing methods of sexual expression, and verbalizing understanding of contraceptive implications.

Interventions. To be helpful, nurses need to be able to talk about sexuality without embarrassment. They also need accurate information about "normal" sexuality and how physiologic changes that occur because of the injury affect sexual function. Some clients discuss their own sexual potential directly. Others refer to it subtly or appear crude in the way they introduce the topic, such as making inappropriate sexual comments or gestures. Such behaviors are attempts to acknowledge sexuality. Try to look beyond the behavior to the underlying emotional concerns. Acknowledge the client's concerns and offer to open a discussion, by saying, for example, "You seem concerned about your sexuality, James. This is a common concern that others with spinal cord injury have had. Sometimes talking about it helps. If you like, we can talk about how this has affected you, and when you are ready, I can share with you interventions that have helped others who have had similar problems."

The client can be referred to another person or an agency if appropriate. Referral should not be made too hastily, however. If a client talks with a nurse about this subject, it is probably because the client feels most comfortable speaking with that nurse at that time. Allow the client to lead the conversation, which may be difficult. Professionals must be aware that they do not always know what a client needs and wants and should listen carefully to the client's voiced concerns.

In general, a physiologic sexual response requires an intact nervous system. For example, psychogenic erection requires an intact spinal cord with preservation of S2-4 nerve roots and spinal reflexes; ejaculation is a function of skeletal muscle controlled by the somatic center in the pudendal nerve originating in the S2-4 roots; and orgasm involves contraction of both smooth and skeletal muscle. It should be remembered, however, that there is more involved in sexual expression than physiologic response.

To some extent, sexual function can be predicted by the level of the spinal cord lesion (see Box 73-3). For example, psychogenic erection is often difficult or impossible after SCI. Although physical limitations certainly exist, every person is different. Many men do have reflex erections after SCI. Many disabled people enjoy *paraorgasm* (phantom orgasm) by developing alternative erogenous zones. The genitals are not the only body areas where sexual stimulation is possible, and intercourse is not the only means of sexual expression.

Some people find it disappointing, perhaps devastating, that they can no longer function sexually as they did before the injury; however, they can be helped to learn new ways of giving and receiving sexual pleasure. Sexual and relationship counseling is sometimes helpful. Some form of sexual expression is possible for anyone, regardless of disability. Before making specific suggestions for alternative expressions of sexuality, discussion with the client should occur to identify past sexual behavior and cultural taboos. Some clients may find some methods of giving and receiving sexual pleasure unacceptable. Lack of a sexual partner may be a deterrent but should not preclude discussion of sexuality. Society as a whole is becoming progressively more open about sexuality.

Increasingly, the parenting potential of disabled people is receiving societal attention. Physical assessment is needed to determine a client's ability to reproduce. Male infertility is a frequent complication of SCI because of testicular atrophy, decreased sperm formation, and infrequent ejaculation. Most men are unable to ejaculate after SCI. Women usually remain fertile and can conceive and deliver a child. Adoption is a viable option, and conception by artificial insemination is possible.

Disabled people may have contraception concerns. Little is known about the effects of various kinds of contraceptives on disabled people. Oral contraceptives may be contraindicated. Paralyzed women often have slowed circulation, increasing the potential circulatory complications of oral contraceptives. To use an intrauterine device, a woman must have feeling in her pelvis to be able to recognize early manifestations of pelvic inflammatory disease. Many paralyzed women do not have such sensation. Barrier devices, such as a diaphragm, a condom, or foam, may be used if at least one partner has enough manual dexterity to insert the diaphragm or foam or put on the condom.

Diagnosis: Risk for Injury. Sensory loss poses serious problems for paralyzed clients because they cannot feel the pain or pressure that normally warns of tissue damage.

Outcomes. The client will be free of injury as evidenced by absence of abrasions, reddened areas, ulcerations, or burns.

Interventions. Spinal cord–injured clients should not wear tight, restrictive clothing or ill-fitting shoes or braces. They need to develop the habit of preventive thinking to avoid potential danger.

> **Dangerous situations include getting too close to heaters, radiators, and fireplaces; using heating pads or hot-water bottles; and rubbing against shoes or parts of the wheelchair. Burns can be a serious problem because impaired circulation delays healing. External heat should not be applied if there is a loss of sensation, and the bath water should not be too hot.**
>
> SAFETY ⚠ ALERT

Regular foot and nail care is required to prevent overgrown nails from rubbing or cutting the skin and to prevent ingrown nails. Instruct the client not to cut corns or calluses; cutting too deep is easy to do and may lead to a foot infection. Cocoa butter or oils without alcohol may be used to soften calluses and reduce cracking.

Diagnosis: Ineffective Health Maintenance. Spinal cord injuries result in many alterations in physiologic functioning that place the client at risk for maintaining normal health status. A possible nursing diagnosis is *Ineffective Health Maintenance.*

Outcomes. The client and family members will be able to meet the client's needs as evidenced by intact skin, bowel and bladder continence, ability to transfer into and out of a wheelchair, absence of infection, maintenance of appropriate weight, and satisfaction with personal relationships.

Interventions. Teaching should be conducted in short sessions, using easily understood terms. For example, teach the caregiver the importance of providing good skin care on the hands and skin folds to prevent

Candida overgrowth. Complex tasks should be taught in steps, with return demonstrations provided by the client or caregiver.

Most spinal cord–injured people are transferred from an acute care hospital to a rehabilitation facility. After functional capabilities have been maximized, the person is then discharged from the rehabilitation facility. The Bridge to Home Health Care feature on Managing the Immobile Client in Chapter 27 on p. 534 provides suggestions for helping caregivers support the client with SCI who lives at home.

Evaluation. Spinal cord–injured clients are hospitalized for a long time. Therefore certain functions important to expected outcomes need to be evaluated frequently, such as respiratory and cardiac function. Other expected outcomes will not be achieved for months, such as independence in performing ADL. The plan of care must reflect these individual needs of the client.

Modifications for Older Clients

For older adults with SCI, the most important modification of the nursing care plan is increased vigilance. Older people are more prone to the complications of immobility. A person with heart failure may have difficulty breathing when lying flat. Before initiation of halo traction in this age group, some neurosurgeons perform a temporary prophylactic tracheostomy because the older client has difficulty swallowing oral secretions and eating. Older people are also more susceptible to sensory deprivation. The nurse must make sure the client has his or her eyeglasses and hearing aid. If a window or clock is not within the range of vision, the client should be reoriented as needed. Discharge plans for older clients may be complicated if the caregiver is also an older adult. The spouse of an older spinal cord–injured person may not have the physical strength to provide the needed care. Learning to provide home care may also be problematic.

Self-Care

The skills learned in a rehabilitation setting must be adapted to the home environment and community setting before hospital discharge. This process can be accomplished by the use of therapeutic weekend passes and participation in community activities as a part of the rehabilitation process. The client needs to learn how to delegate needed skills to another caregiver so that care can be provided at home.

Paraplegic clients can usually live independently. Most quadriplegic clients need assistance with ADL. Depending on the amount of assistance needed and the specific situation, this care may be provided by family members or by a part-time or full-time paid attendant. By using a wheelchair, clients may become completely independent in ADL, with minimal help of social services personnel, a home health aide, or family members. Many clients drive and hold outside jobs.

Ventilator-dependent people who cannot obtain in-home care and others who do not have the personal or financial resources for in-home care may have no option except institutional living. The problem of limited government resources for all clients requiring rehabilitative care remains an important ethical issue in nursing. Group-living situations, especially for young adults, are becoming more available, however.

CONCLUSIONS

Brain and spinal cord injuries are some of the most complex injuries the human can endure. Nurses who work with the neurologically impaired must develop and maintain astute assessment skills to detect the subtle signs of neurologic deterioration quickly. The physical and psychological impairments vary with the degree of damage as well as the client's response to and ability to cope with the body changes. The coping response is not always related to the degree of physiologic damage. It is imperative that nurses comprehend the severity of the client's dysfunction as it relates to quality of life as well as the impact it has on family dynamics.

THINKING CRITICALLY

1. A 23-year-old man was admitted from the emergency department (ED) following a car accident in which he sustained a concussion and thoracic injuries with thoracic spinal cord involvement. The client's baseline data included loss of consciousness for 15 minutes, headache, nausea, and an inability to move or feel any sensation from his thorax down. One hour after this man arrived in the intensive care unit (ICU), additional assessment changes included an inability to move his fingers and hands and to flex or extend his arms. Shoulder movement was still intact. He was fully conscious, and his vital signs were stable. What critical interventions initiated in the ED need to be continued in the ICU? What do these changes in data indicate? What nursing interventions are appropriate both initially and as precautions?

   Factors to Consider. What are the implications when a high thoracic injury occurs? What changes indicate ascending cord dysfunction?

2. A 22-year-old man was admitted 4 hours after sustaining a C6 spinal cord compression injury. No neurologic deficits were found, but his blood alcohol level was very high on admission. Initially, he kept falling asleep after you completed your assessments. Gardner-Wells tongs with 10 pounds of traction were placed. Now that the client is more awake, he has begun thrashing his arms and attempting to roll over in bed. What are the priorities for his care? What nursing interventions should be used?

Factors to Consider. What is the purpose of the Gardner-Wells tongs? How would edema and microscopic bleeding compromise recovery in this client?

evolve   *Discussions for these questions can be found on the website.*

BIBLIOGRAPHY

🔴 Citations appearing in red refer to primary research.

🔵 Citations appearing in blue refer to evidence-based practice guidelines and protocols.

1. Aito, S., Cariaggi, B., & Perazza, S. (2002). The use of high-dose methylprednisolone in acute spinal cord injuries: NASCIS review. National Acute Spinal Cord Injury Study. *Europa Medicophysica, 38*(2), 89-95.
2. American Association of Neuroscience Nurses. (2005). *AANN Reference Series for Clinical Practice: Guide to the care of the patient with intracranial pressure monitoring.* Chicago: Author.
3. American Spinal Injury Association (ASIA). (2002). *International standards for neurological classification of SCI.* Chicago: Author.
4. Anson, K., & Ponsford, J. (2006). Coping and emotional adjustment following traumatic brain injury. *Journal of Head Trauma Rehabilitation, 21*(5), 248-259.
5. Bader, M.K., Arbour, R., & Palmer, S. (2005). Refractory increased intracranial pressure in severe traumatic brain injury: Barbiturate coma and bispectral index monitoring. *AACN Clinical Issues, 16*(4), 526-541.
6. Bauman, W.A., & Spungen, A.M. (2000). Metabolic changes in persons after spinal cord injury. *Physical Medicine and Rehabilitation Clinics of North America, 11*(1), 109-140.
7. Bell, G.B. (1999). Spinal cord injury, pressure ulcers, support surfaces. *Ostomy and Wound Management, 45*(6), 48-50, 52–53.
8. Blank-Reid, C., & Reid, P.C. (2000). Penetrating trauma to the head. *Critical Care Nursing Clinics of North America, 12*(4), 477-487.
9. Bond, A.E., Draeger, C.R.L., Mandleco, B., Donnelly, M. (2003). Needs of family members of patients with severe traumatic brain injury: Implications for evidence-based practice. *Critical Care Nurse, 23*(4), 63-72.
10. Brain Trauma Foundation. (2000). *Management and prognosis of severe traumatic brain injury.* New York: Author.
11. Brewer, T., & Therrien, B. (2000). Minor brain injury: New insights for early nursing care. *Journal of Neuroscience Nursing, 32*(6), 311-317.
12. Bryce, T.N., & Ragnarsson, K.T. (2000). Pain after spinal cord injury. *Physical Medicine and Rehabilitation Clinics of North America, 11*(1), 157-168.
13. Chamberlain, D.J. (2006). The experience of surviving traumatic brain injury. *Journal of Advanced Nursing, 54*(4), 407-417.
14. Chaviano, A.H., et al. (2000). Mitrofanoff continent catheterizable stoma for pediatric patients with spinal cord injury. *Topics in Spinal Cord Injury Rehabilitation, Summer Suppl* (6), 30-35.
15. Chen, D., & Nussbaum, S.B. (2000). The gastrointestinal system and bowel management following spinal cord injury. *Physical Medicine and Rehabilitation Clinics of North America, 11*(1), 45-56, viii.
16. Christensen, M.A., Janson, S., & Seago, J.A. (2001). Alcohol, head injury and pulmonary complications. *Journal of Neuroscience Nursing, 33*(4), 184-189.
17. Clear, D., & Chadwick, D.W. (2000). Seizures provoked by blows to the head. *Epilepsia, 41*(2), 243-244.
18. Consortium for Spinal Cord Medicine. (2001). *Autonomic dysreflexia in individuals with spinal cord injury presenting to health care facilities* (2nd ed). Washington, DC: Paralyzed Veterans of America.
19. Consortium for Spinal Cord Medicine. (1999). *Neurogenic bowel management in adults with spinal cord injury.* Washington, DC: Paralyzed Veterans of America.
20. Consortium for Spinal Cord Medicine. (1999). *Outcomes following traumatic spinal cord injury.* Washington, DC: Paralyzed Veterans of America.
21. Consortium for Spinal Cord Medicine. (2000). *Pressure ulcer prevention and treatment following spinal cord injury.* Washington, DC: Paralyzed Veterans of America.
22. Consortium for Spinal Cord Medicine. (1999). *Prevention of thromboembolism in spinal cord injury.* Washington, DC: Paralyzed Veterans of America.
23. Davis, A.E. (2000). Mechanisms of traumatic brain injury: Biomechanical, structural and cellular considerations. *Critical Care Nursing Quarterly, 23*(3), 1-13.
24. Davis, A.E. (2000). Cognitive impairments following traumatic brain injury. *Critical Care Nursing Clinics of North America, 12*(4), 447-456.
25. Domeier, R.M., et al. (2002). Multicenter prospective validation of prehospital clinical spinal clearance criteria. *Journal of Trauma: Injury, Infection, and Critical Care, 53*(4), 744-750.
26. Dubendorf, P. (1999). Spinal cord injury pathophysiology. *Critical Care Nursing Quarterly, 22*(2), 31-35.
27. Ellenbogen, P.S., Meade, M.A., Jackson, M.N., et al. (2006). The impact of spinal cord injury on the employment of family caregivers. *Journal of Vocational Rehabilitation, 25*(1), 35-44.
28. Fan, J. (2004). Effect of backrest position on intracranial pressure and cerebral perfusion in individuals with brain injury: A systematic review. *Journal of Neuroscience Nursing, 36*(5), 278-288.
29. Flanagan, S.R., Hibbard, M.R., Riordan, B., et al. (2006). Traumatic brain injury in the elderly: Diagnostic and treatment challenges. *Clinics in Geriatric Medicine, 22*(2), 449-468.
30. Franzen, M.D. (2000). Neuropsychological assessment in traumatic brain injury. *Critical Care Nursing Quarterly, 23*(3), 58-64.
31. Goldstein, B. (2000). Musculoskeletal conditions after spinal cord injury. *Physical Medicine and Rehabilitation Clinics of North America, 11*(1), 91-108, viii-ix.
32. Hauber, R.P., & Testani-Dufour, L. (2000). Living in limbo: The low-level brain-injured patient and the patient's family. *Journal of Neuroscience Nursing, 32*(1), 22-26.
33. Henker, R. (2000). Use of blood cultures in the critically ill. *Critical Care Nurse, 20*(1), 45-50.
34. Henker, R. (1999). Evidence-based practice: Fever-related interventions. *American Journal of Critical Care, 8*(1), 481-489.
35. Hickey, J.V. (2003). Craniocerebral trauma. In J.V. Hickey (Ed.), *The clinical practice of neurological and neurosurgical nursing* (5th ed., pp. 373-406). Philadelphia: J.B. Lippincott.
36. Hickey, J.V. (2003). Vertebral and spinal cord injuries. In J.V. Hickey (Ed.), *The clinical practice of neurological and neurosurgical nursing* (5th ed., pp. 407-450). Philadelphia: J.B. Lippincott.
37. Hickey, J.V. (2003). Intracranial hypertension: Theory and management of increased intracranial pressure. In J.V. Hickey (Ed.), *The clinical practice of neurological and neurosurgical nursing* (5th ed., pp. 285-318). Philadelphia: J.B. Lippincott.
38. Iacono, L.A. (2000). Exploring the guidelines for the management of severe head injury. *Journal of Neuroscience Nursing, 32*(1), 54-60.
39. Iacono, L.A., & Lyons, K.A. (2005). Making GCS as easy as 1, 2, 3, 4, 5, 6. *Journal of Trauma Nursing, 12*(3), 77-81.
40. Johnson, M., Bulechek, G., Butcher, H., et al. (2006). *NANDA, NOC and NIC linkages* (2nd ed). St. Louis: Mosby.
41. Jumisko, E., Lexell, J., & Soderberg, S. (2005). The meaning of living with traumatic brain injury in people with moderate or severe traumatic brain injury. *Journal of Neuroscience Nursing, 37*(1), 42-50.
42. Karlet, M.C. (2001). Acute management of the patient with spinal cord injury. *International Journal of Trauma Nursing, 7*(2), 43-48.
43. Kavchak-Keyes, M.A. (2000). Autonomic hyperreflexia. *Rehabilitation Nursing, 25*(1), 31-35.
44. Kemp, B., & Thompson, L. (2002). Aging and spinal cord injury: Medical, functional, and psychosocial changes. *SCI Nursing, 19*(2), 51-60.
45. Kinder, R.A. (2005). Psychological hardiness in women with paraplegia. *Rehabilitation Nursing, 30*(2), 1-27.
46. Kirkness, C.J. (2005). Cerebral blood flow monitoring in clinical practice. *AACN Clinical Issues, 16*(4), 476-487.
47. Kirshblum, S.C., & O'Connor, K.C. (2000). Levels of spinal cord injury and predictors for neurologic recovery. *Physical Medicine and Rehabilitation Clinics of North America, 11*(1), 1-27, vii.

48. LeJeune, G., & Howard-Fain, T. (2002). Nursing assessment and management of patients with head injuries. *Dimensions of Critical Care Nursing, 27*(6), 226-229.

49. Lohne, V. (2001). Hope in patients with spinal cord injury: A literature review related to nursing. *Journal of Neuroscience Nursing, 82*(2), 173-187.

50. March, K. (2000). Intracranial pressure monitoring and assessing intracranial compliance in brain injury. *Critical Care Nursing Clinics of North America, 12*(4), 429-435.

51. Marion, D.W. (2004). Controlled normothermia in neurologic intensive care. *Critical Care Medicine, 32*(2, Suppl), S43-S45.

52. Marion, D.W., & Speigel, T.P. (2000). Changes in the management of severe traumatic brain injury: 1991-1997. *Critical Care Medicine, 28*(1), 16-18.

53. McIlvoy, L.H. (2005). The effect of hypothermia and hyperthermia on acute brain injury. *AACN Clinical Issues, 16*(4), 488-500.

54. McIlvoy, L., et al. (2001). Successful incorporation of the severe head injury guidelines into a phased-outcome clinical pathway. *Journal of Neuroscience Nursing, 33*(2), 72-78.

55. Mitchell, P.H., Ozuna, J., & Lipe, H. (1981). Moving the patient in bed: Effects on intracranial pressure. *Nursing Research, 30*(4), 212-218.

56. Moore, K.N., Burt, J., & Voaklander, D.C. (2006). Intermittent catheterization in the rehabilitation setting: A comparison of clean and sterile technique. *Clinical Rehabilitation, 20*(6), 461-468.

57. Mortimer, D.S., & Jancik, J. (2006). Administering hypertonic saline to patients with severe traumatic brain injury. *Journal of Neuroscience Nursing, 38*(3), 142-146.

58. Oertel, M., Kelly, D.F., Lee, J.H., et al. (2002). Metabolic suppression therapy as a treatment for intracranial hypertension: Why it works and when it fails. *Acta Neurochirurgica, 81*(Suppl), 69-70.

59. Olson, D.M., & Graffagnino, C. (2005). Consciousness, coma, and caring for the brain-injured patient. *AACN Clinical Issues, 16*(4), 441-455.

60. Pagni, C.A., & Zenga, F. (2005). Posttraumatic epilepsy with special emphasis on prophylaxis and prevention. *Acta Neurochirurgica, 93*(Suppl), 27-34.

61. Pryor, J. (2004). What environmental factors irritate people with acquired brain injury? *Disability and Rehabilitation, 26*(16), 974-980.

62. Pryor, J. (2006). What do nurses do in response to their predictions of aggression? *Journal of Neuroscience Nursing, 38*(3), 177-182.

63. Quint, D.J. (2000). Indications for emergent MRI of the central nervous system. *Journal of the American Medical Association, 283*(7), 853-855.

64. Ronne-Engstrom, E., & Winkler, T. (2006). Continuous EEG monitoring in patients with traumatic brain injury reveals a high incidence of epileptiform activity. *Acta Neurologica Scandinavica, 114*(1), 47-53.

65. Roth, P., & Farls, K. (2000). Pathophysiology of traumatic brain injury. *Critical Care Nursing Quarterly, 23*(3), 14-25.

66. Rovlias, A., & Kotson, S. (2000). The influence of hyperglycemia on neurologic outcome in patients with severe head injury. *Neurosurgery, 46*(2), 335-342.

67. Stempien, L., & Tsai, T. (2000). Intrathecal baclofen pump use for spasticity: A clinical survey. *American Journal of Physical Medicine & Rehabilitation, 79*(6), 536-541, 547-550, 564.

68. Sullivan, J. (2000). Positioning of patients with severe traumatic brain injury: Research based practice. *Journal of Neuroscience Nursing, 32*(4), 204-209.

69. Verhaeghe, S., Defloor, T., & Grypdonck, M. (2005). Stress and coping among families of patients with traumatic brain injury: A review of the literature. *Journal of Clinical Nursing, 14*(8), 1004-1012.

70. Wells, R., Dywan, J., & Dumas, J. (2005). Life satisfaction and distress in family caregivers as related to specific behavioural changes after traumatic brain injury. *Brain Injury, 19*(13), 1105-1115.

71. Wilensky, E.M., Bloom, S., Leichter, D., et al. (2005). Brain tissue oxygen practice guidelines using the LICOX CMP monitoring system. *Journal of Neuroscience Nursing, 37*(5), 278-288.

72. Winemuller, M.K., et al. (1999). Prevention of venous thromboembolism in patients with spinal cord injury: Effects of sequential pneumatic compression and heparin. *Journal of Spinal Cord Medicine, 23*(3), 182-191.

73. Winkelman, C. (2000). Effect of backrest position on intracranial and cerebral perfusion pressures in traumatically brain-injured adults. *American Journal of Critical Care, 9*(6), 373-380.

74. Winter, C.D., Adamides, A.A., & Rosenfeld, J.V. (2005). The role of decompressive craniectomy in the management of traumatic brain injury: A critical review. *Journal of Clinical Neuroscience, 12*(6), 619-623.

75. Wood, R.L.L., & Rutterford, N.A. (2006). Demographic and cognitive predictors of long-term psychological outcome following traumatic brain injury. *Journal of the International Neuropsychological Society, 12*(3), 350-358.

76. Wong, F.W.H. (2000). Prevention of secondary brain injury. *Critical Care Nurse, 20*(5), 18-27.

77. Wright, J.E. (2005). Therapeutic hypothermia in traumatic brain injury. *Critical Care Nursing Quarterly, 28*(2), 150-161.

78. Zuccarelli, L.A. (2000). Altered cellular anatomy of acute brain injury and spinal cord injury. *Critical Care Nursing Clinics of North America, 12*(4), 403-411.

evolve   *Did you remember to check out the bonus material on the Evolve website and the CD-ROM, including NCLEX®-Examination Style Review Questions, Open-Book Quizzes, and Chapter Review Audio Podcasts?*

http://evolve.elsevier.com/Black/medsurg

U N I T 17

PROTECTIVE DISORDERS

ANATOMY AND PHYSIOLOGY REVIEW:

The Hematopoietic System

Robert G. Carroll

Survival depends on maintaining a barrier separating the inside of the body from pathogens outside of the body and on employing effective defense mechanisms against those pathogens that break that barrier. The epithelium of the skin and of the gastrointestinal (GI), respiratory, urinary, and reproductive tracts provides the barrier. The body defends itself against attack by viruses, bacteria, and other parasites using two sets of separate but interrelated functions: (1) innate immunity and (2) adaptive immunity. Both of these systems must be present and operating properly in order to block establishment of infectious agents, to minimize damage caused by disease in progress, and to expel, destroy, or isolate infectious agents that gain access to inner tissues.

Together, the body is protected using both *surveillance* ("inside" threats) and *defense* ("outside" threats) functions. The importance of these mechanisms to our health and well-being becomes apparent when the defenses of a healthy body are compromised by infection or suppressed by medication or chemotherapy. Parts of the defense system in a healthy body may function inappropriately to reject organ and tissue transplants and may produce autoimmune disease or hypersensitivity states that cause pathologic changes and sometimes death.

RESISTANCE: A FORM OF NONSPECIFIC DEFENSE

The first line of defense in the body is the aspect of resistance that stops a threatening agent or condition. Defenses provide a form of resistance against disease by combating anything not recognized as *self*. Resistance components are usually the first to encounter infectious agents or parasites. Many of these functions operate independently of the immune system but, as shown later, some of the components and features participate in or amplify acquired immune responses.

SURFACE DEFENSES

Intact skin and mucous membranes, combined with surface-clearing mechanisms, are sufficient to provide barriers that prevent penetration to underlying tissues by many pathogens. Lysozyme in tears and bile in the gut inhibit gram-positive bacteria; hydrochloric acid in the stomach is lethal to many pathogens; and fatty acids help protect the skin from infectious agents.

The *reticuloendothelial system* (RES) includes mononuclear phagocytic cells (macrophages). Fixed (attached) macrophages in the sinusoids of the liver, spleen, and bone marrow monitor the circulating blood and remove all foreign particulates and any moribund self cells. Resident mobile macrophages in lymph nodes remove foreign particulate matter. Macrophages in the alveolar spaces are the most active of the RES cells and help remove inspired particulates that reach the lower recesses of the lung.

ORGANS OF THE IMMUNE AND HEMATOLOGIC SYSTEMS

The organs of the immune and hematologic systems are shown in Figure A&P17-1. There are both (1) peripheral sites for the production of the molecules and cells that serve as effector units of the immune response and (2) central organs that prepare antigens for recognition.

Lymph Nodes

Lymph nodes are mostly small organs (many are less than 5 mm in diameter) that are present throughout the body and interconnected by means of lymph vessels. Their structure is fairly complex and provides both RES and immune functions. The lymph node receives fluids, particulates, and solutes that are taken up by lymphatic capillaries from distal tissue sites. Resident macrophages within the node monitor the lymph fluid passing through the node for the presence of foreign particulates and remove them by phagocytic action. Antigenic substances, either particulates or solutes, are taken up by the macrophages or dendritic cells serving as antigen-presenting cells (APCs). Immunocompetent cells in the lymph node can initiate either a humoral immune response or a cell-mediated immune response.

Lymph nodes are found in large numbers in the thoracic and abdominal cavities. Those lying close to the body surface are called *superficial nodes*. Cervical nodes lie alongside the neck, axillary nodes in the armpit, and inguinal nodes in the crease between the upper thigh and the trunk. When inflamed, these nodes become swollen and may be palpated, serving as diagnostic signs.

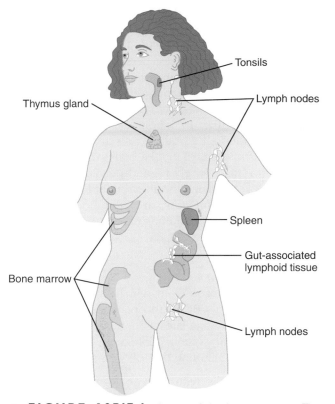

■ **FIGURE A&PI7–I** Organs of the immune system. The bone marrow, spleen, lymph nodes, tonsils, and gut-associated lymphoid tissue (GALT) function in both specific and nonspecific immunity, whereas the thymus functions primarily in specific immunity.

Lymph Nodules

The structure of the lymph nodules is much less organized than that of the lymph nodes. The nodules occur in the mucosal epithelium lining the respiratory, GI, and urogenital tracts. Antigenic materials are translocated across the epithelium through a special cell (M cell). The translocated material is deposited directly into the nodule structure where it is taken up by APCs. Immunocompetent B cells in lymph nodules produce either immunoglobulin E (IgE) or immunoglobulin A (IgA). These immunoglobulins provide for the development either of an allergic response of the immediate hypersensitivity type or, for IgA, of a mucosal immune response.

Spleen

The spleen is the largest lymphoid organ in the body. Its defensive functions include the blood-clearing process via fixed macrophages in sinusoids as well as serving as a major site of humoral immune responses to blood-borne antigens. The splenic pulp is divided into red zones and white zones. The white zones are accumulations of lymphocytes and APCs. Loss of the spleen or diminished function resulting from injury or infection greatly increases the risk of infection with extracellular bacteria.

Other functions of the spleen include (1) assisting in recycling iron by capturing hemoglobin released from destroyed red blood cells (RBCs) and (2) performing pitting (removal of particles from RBCs without destroying the cell itself).

Thymus

The thymus is located in the mediastinum, and reaches peak development during childhood. After puberty, it begins to atrophy but remnants persist into old age. The thymus is an endocrine organ that secretes hormones that contribute to the maintenance and function of peripheral T-cell populations.

A fundamental paradigm in immunology is the rearrangement of germ line genes during differentiation of lymphocytes in the central lymphoid tissues, leading to the production of molecules for the recognition of antigen. In both cell types, the antigen recognition unit is inserted into the membrane with the antigen-reactive ends extending out into the extracellular environment. The T cell uses the T-cell antigen receptor, and the B cell has a tetrapeptide monomer called *surface immunoglobulin* (SIg). The individual cells each have a unique receptor capable of reacting only with a single antigenic determinant (Figure A&P17-2). Each specifically reacting cell is called a *clonotype;* when properly stimulated by an antigen, the clonotype produces effector units (either antibody molecules or specially reactive cells) and a memory cell clone, both of which have the identical specificity of the original clonotype.

The positive and negative selection processes acting on cells in the thymus make it possible for the mechanism to discriminate between *self* and *non-self* in

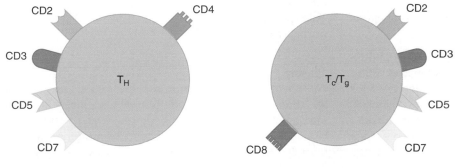

■ **FIGURE A&PI7–2** T cells can be distinguished by distinctive molecules located on their cell surfaces. They are called cluster designations (CDs). All mature T cells carry markers known as T2 (or CD2), T3 (or CD3), T5 (or CD5), and T7 (or CD7). T helper (T_H) cells carry a T4 (CD4) marker, and suppressor and cytotoxic T (T_c/T_g) cells carry a T8 (CD8) marker.

immune function. This distinction is accomplished by making antigen recognition absolutely dependent on the variable but individually unique composition of the transcription products of gene loci located in the major histocompatibility region of the genome.

The major histocompatibility complex (MHC) consists of integral cell membrane glycoproteins. Class I MHC molecules are found on nearly all nucleated cells in the body and represent a major antigenic distinction between individuals of a given species with different genotypes. This molecule is necessary for antigen recognition by cytotoxic T cells with CD8 surface markers. Class II MHC molecules are found on some APCs, on all B cells, and on antigen-activated T cells. This molecule is necessary for antigen recognition by helper T cells with CD4 surface markers. MHC antigens in humans were initially discovered on leukocyte membranes and are thus called *human leukocyte antigens* (HLAs). It is this recognition system that forms the basis for the rejection of foreign or transplanted tissue. The cells in the recipient's immune system recognize the surface HLA proteins of the donor's tissue as being non-self.

Bone Marrow

Bone marrow constitutes one of the largest organs in the body, with an aggregate weight in adults of about 3000 g (comparable in mass to the liver). Based on visual appearance, the marrow mass was originally described as being either red or yellow. *Red marrow* consists of a mass of supporting cells surrounding aggregates of hematopoietic cells and interspaced with sinusoidal capillaries. *Yellow marrow* is less active in hematopoiesis, with the light color resulting from adipose cells.

Function of Bone Marrow

Bone marrow provides for the following:

- Maintenance of a self-renewing pluripotent stem cell population from which all blood cells are derived
- An environment for the differentiation and maturation of blood cells
- A storage site for large numbers of neutrophils and erythrocytes
- Transformation of undifferentiated lymphocytes into mature B cells
- A site of antibody production in a secondary immune response to thymic-dependent antigens administered intravenously

Sinusoids bearing fixed macrophages serve an RES function in blood clearing. This is a defensive action based on the phagocytic activity of the macrophages attached to the luminal side of the marrow sinuses. These phagocytes, part of the RES or mononuclear phagocytic system, monitor the blood for the presence of foreign particulate matter, remove it, and destroy it.

Formation of Blood Cells

Hematopoiesis, the process of formation and development of blood cells, begins early in the development of the human embryo and must persist unabated throughout one's lifetime. The demands made on this function are enormous. Cells in the peripheral blood have a finite life span and must be continuously renewed at a rate probably greater than 10 billion cells per day.

During childhood, all blood cells are essentially produced in marrow sites of the flat bones of the skull, clavicle, sternum, ribs, vertebrae, and pelvis. After puberty, hematopoiesis becomes localized within the flat bones of the sternum, ilium, ribs, and vertebrae, sometimes occurring in the proximal ends of long bones (humerus and femur).

Blood

Blood is a complex fluid in which a variety of RBCs, white blood cells (WBCs), and platelets are suspended in plasma. Blood circulates continuously through the heart and vascular system. Circulating blood performs many functions, including the following:

- Supplying cells with oxygen from the lungs and absorbed nutrients from the GI tract
- Removing waste products from tissues to the kidney, skin, and lungs for excretion
- Transporting hormones from their origin in the endocrine glands to their targets in other parts of the body
- Protecting the body from dangerous microorganisms
- Promoting *hemostasis* (the arrest of bleeding)
- Regulating body temperature by heat transfer

Composition

About 8% of our total body weight is blood; for example, a healthy young female has 4 to 5 L and a male has about 5 to 6 L. Blood volume also varies by age and body composition. The less body fat, the more blood per kilogram of body weight is present.

Arterial blood is bright red because of the oxygen bound to the hemoglobin within RBCs. Venous blood is dark red because of the lower amount of oxygenated hemoglobin. Pulse oximetry uses this change in color to estimate the oxygen saturation in tissues. Blood is three to four times more viscous (thick) than water. The specific gravity of blood is 1.048 to 1.066. Blood normally has a pH of 7.35 to 7.45.

Plasma

Plasma, the liquid portion of the blood, is one of the three major body fluids (along with interstitial and intracellular fluids). A straw-colored, watery substance, plasma is composed of 92% water, 7% proteins, and less than 1% nutrients, metabolic wastes, respiratory gases, enzymes, hormones, clotting factors, and inorganic salts. Serum albumin and gamma-globulin contribute to colloidal osmotic pressure (see the Anatomy and Physiology Review for Unit 12). Gamma-globulin also contains the antibody immunoglobulins IgM, IgG, IgA, IgD, and IgE, which are essential in the body's defense against microorganisms.

Plasma makes up about 55% of the blood, and solid suspended particles (blood cells and platelets) compose the other 45%. If a tube of blood is allowed to stand or is spun in a centrifuge, the cells separate. The term *packed cell volume* or *hematocrit* is used to express the volume or percent of the RBCs in the sample. Normal hematocrit levels are 35% to 45%. Hematocrit can be increased from loss of plasma (e.g., dehydration) or increased production of RBCs (polycythemia). Low hematocrit levels are seen in overhydration, during enhanced RBC loss, or during diminished RBC synthesis (Figure A&P17-3). The WBCs and platelets make up less than 1% of the blood volume. These cells form a buffy coat or white layer and are seen at the interface of the RBCs and plasma.

Hematopoiesis

Stem cells are poorly characterized, undifferentiated cells that exist within the red marrow. These totipotent, or pluripotent, stem cells are self-replicating and maintain a small population throughout the lifetime of the individual. Following stimulation by one or more signal

■ **FIGURE A&P17-3** Tubes showing hematocrit levels of normal blood, anemia, and polycythemia. Note the buffy coat located between the packed red blood cells (RBCs) and the plasma. **A,** A normal percentage of RBCs (45%). **B,** Anemia (a low percentage of RBCs, 30%). **C,** Polycythemia (a high percentage of RBCs, 60%). *WBCs,* White blood cells. *(Modified from Thibodeau, G., & Patton, K. [2007]. Anatomy and physiology [6th ed.]. St. Louis: Mosby.)*

molecules called *poietins,* the stem cells can undergo differentiation into erythrocytes (RBCs), megakaryocytes, and leukocytes. The steps of hematopoiesis and the divisions of each cell, once it takes a committed path, are shown in Figure A&P17-4.

Control of Hematopoiesis. Growth factors *(cytokines)* control blood cell growth, proliferation, and differentiation. Growth factors are usually identified by using acronyms that are a legacy from original studies of colony-forming cells. The suffix "-CSF" (colony-stimulating factor) describes the growth factor that stimulates or regulates the development of the corresponding cell type identified by the prefix "CFU-." For example, G-CSF is the growth factor for CFU-G (colony-forming unit–granulocytic series), and M-CSF is the growth factor regulating the development of monocytes (CFU-M). Other growth factors—interleukins (ILs)—are given numbers to distinguish between different molecules.

Red Blood Cells

RBCs (erythrocytes) carry oxygen to the cells and help transport carbon dioxide back to the lungs. RBCs also assist with acid-base balance. They contain carbonic anhydrase, an enzyme that joins carbon dioxide to water to form carbonic acid. The acid dissociates to form bicarbonate and hydrogen ions, which diffuse out of the RBC.

The mature RBC has no nucleus and is only 7.5 mm in diameter. Each RBC has a depression on the flat surface that provides a thin center and thicker edges. The unique structure of the RBC supplies a large surface area relative to its volume (to facilitate exchange by diffusion) and allows the cell to change shape passively as it flows through capillaries that are smaller than 7.5 mm in diameter. The average RBC count is 5,500,000 cells/mm^3 of blood.

Packed within each RBC are about 200 to 300 million molecules of hemoglobin. Each hemoglobin molecule is composed of four protein chains (globin). The globin is bound to a heme group that contains one iron atom. In healthy men, 100 ml of blood contains 14 to 16 g of hemoglobin. Women have slightly less, about 12 to 14 g. Anemia is present when hemoglobin levels decrease to less than 10 g per 100 ml of blood.

Erythrocyte Production. The production of erythrocytes is termed *erythropoiesis.* Normally, more than 100 million RBCs, or about 1% of the body's total, are formed to replace an equal number of destroyed cells. Erythropoietin increases the rate of RBC production when oxygen levels decrease or during pregnancy. Healthy bone marrow has the capacity to increase its production of erythrocytes six to eight times over the normal rate and is thus able to keep pace with increased destruction or

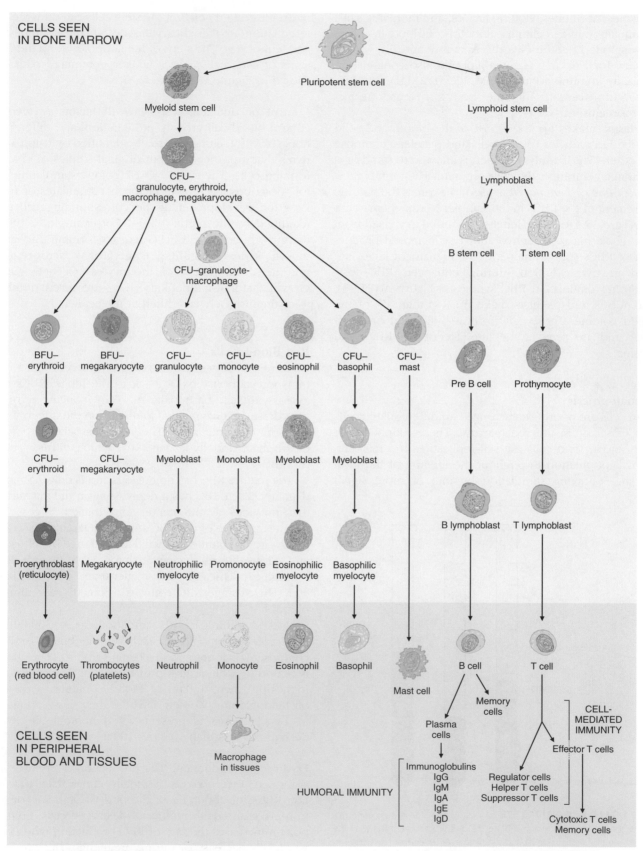

CELLS SEEN
IN BONE MARROW

Pluripotent stem cell

Myeloid stem cell

Lymphoid stem cell

CFU–
granulocyte, erythroid,
macrophage, megakaryocyte

Lymphoblast

CFU–granulocyte-
macrophage

B stem cell

T stem cell

BFU–
erythroid

BFU–
megakaryocyte

CFU–
granulocyte

CFU–
monocyte

CFU–
eosinophil

CFU–
basophil

CFU–
mast

Pre B cell

Prothymocyte

CFU–
erythroid

CFU–
megakaryocyte

Myeloblast

Monoblast

Myeloblast

Myeloblast

B lymphoblast

T lymphoblast

Proerythroblast
(reticulocyte)

Megakaryocyte

Neutrophilic
myelocyte

Promonocyte

Eosinophilic
myelocyte

Basophilic
myelocyte

Erythrocyte
(red blood cell)

Thrombocytes
(platelets)

Neutrophil

Monocyte

Eosinophil

Basophil

Mast cell

B cell

T cell

Memory
cells

CELLS SEEN
IN PERIPHERAL
BLOOD AND TISSUES

Macrophage
in tissues

Plasma
cells

CELL-
MEDIATED
IMMUNITY

Effector T cells

Immunoglobulins
IgG
IgM
IgA
IgE
IgD

HUMORAL IMMUNITY

Regulator cells
Helper T cells
Suppressor T cells

Cytotoxic T cells
Memory cells

■ **FIGURE A&P17–4** Hematopoietic cascade. The pluripotent stem cell is the origin of all cells. Once a pathway is chosen, the cell is committed to the final cell type.

loss of RBCs. This response mechanism leads to a remarkably constant number of erythrocytes.

Erythrocytes are produced in the red bone marrow. Required for this process are (1) precursor cells, (2) a proper microenvironment, and (3) adequate supplies of iron, vitamin B_{12}, folic acid, protein, pyridoxine, and traces of copper. If any of these factors is missing, the resultant erythrocytes are fragile, misshapen, abnormally large or small, deficient in hemoglobin, or too few in number. Erythrocytes arise from nucleated cells called *hematopoietic stem cells*. *Stem cells* can maintain a constant population of newly differentiating cells. Differentiation takes about 7 days and involves about six stages (see Figure A&P17-4).

Immature erythrocytes leave the bone marrow via veins in the marrow and enter the general circulation as nucleated reticulocytes. After their release from the marrow sites, the reticulocytes travel to the spleen, where they undergo conditioning and evolve into mature erythrocytes before being released into the general circulation.

The life span of RBCs is about 105 to 120 days. As erythrocytes age, they become increasingly fragile and eventually rupture. The released hemoglobin and the empty membranes ("ghost cells") are taken up by macrophages within the liver, spleen, lymph nodes, and bone marrow. The hemoglobin is broken down into heme (iron and porphyrin) and globin (polypeptide chain) fractions. The iron of the heme fraction is returned to the liver, spleen, and bone marrow to be reused in making hemoglobin. The liver converts the porphyrin of the heme fraction into bilirubin, an orange pigment, and secretes it into the bile to be excreted from the body in the feces and urine (Figure A&P17-5). During periods of increased RBC destruction (e.g., in hemolytic anemia),

excessive amounts of bilirubin are formed and may accumulate in the body's tissues.

Nutritional Influences on Red Blood Cell Production. Vitamin B_{12} and folic acid are essential for normal RBC maturation and nervous system function. Because it is not synthesized in the body, vitamin B_{12} must be a component of the daily diet. Animal products such as meat and dairy products are primary sources of this vitamin. When released from food during digestion, vitamin B_{12} binds with *intrinsic factor,* and the complex is absorbed in the distal ileum. Folic acid, a B-group vitamin synthesized by many plants and bacteria, is also necessary for RBC formation and maturation.

Iron is essential to hemoglobin production. The adult human body contains about 50 mg of iron per 100 ml of blood. Total body iron ranges between 2 and 6 g, depending on the size of the person and the amount of hemoglobin sequestered within the cellular compartment. Hemoglobin accounts for about two thirds of the total iron (called *essential iron*). The other one third resides in the bone marrow, spleen, liver, and muscle. When an iron deficiency develops, the latter iron stores are depleted first, followed by a gradual loss of the iron contained in hemoglobin.

Megakaryocytes and Platelets

Platelets *(thrombocytes)* have two essential roles in hemostasis: (1) occlusion of small openings in blood vessels (a hemostatic function) and (2) provision of chemical components in the molecular cascade leading to coagulation (a thromboplastic function).

Individual platelets are produced by a fragmentation process from giant multinucleated cells in the red bone marrow called *megakaryocytes* (see Figure A&P17-4). The time required for the formation of human platelets is about 5 days. Cytoplasmic extensions from megakaryoblasts are extruded into sinusoids, and platelets are formed by fragmentation at the terminal ends of the filaments. Normal human marrow may have up to 6 million megakaryocytes per kilogram of body weight, with each megakaryocyte being able to produce 1000 or more individual platelets. Platelet production in a normal person appears to be under tight control by the hepatic hormone *thrombopoietin* and is remarkably consistent, with the numbers in a healthy person often remaining constant for years.

Hemostasis. Normal hemostasis is a process that repairs vascular breaks to reduce blood loss from blood vessels while maintaining the flow of blood through the vascular system. Hemostasis occurs in three stages: (1) *vasoconstriction* of the blood vessels, (2) formation of a platelet plug, and (3) coagulation or formation of a fibrin clot. Once the fibrin clot has served its purpose, further

■ **FIGURE A&P17–5** Destruction of red blood cells. *(From Thibodeau, G., & Patton, K. [2007]. Anatomy and physiology [6th ed.]. St. Louis: Mosby.)*

clot formation is balanced by anticoagulation and by *fibrinolysis* (clot dissolution).

Whenever bleeding results from injury or disease, the blood vessels that supply the damaged site constrict. Vasoconstriction slows the flow of blood to the injured area, decreasing blood loss. Vasoconstriction results from muscular tissue and reflex nervous system reactions. *Thromboxane A₂*, a potent local vasoconstrictor, is secreted by platelets and promotes constriction of small blood vessels following injury.

Adequate numbers of platelets (150,000 to 400,000/mm³) are required in the peripheral blood for hemostasis. When platelets come into contact with an alteration of the endothelial cell lining of a blood vessel, they become sticky and adhere to one another, thus sealing the surface of the vessel lining. These platelet constituents can activate additional platelets that aggregate to form a *thrombus*.

Platelets control hemostasis unless large blood vessels have been damaged. If bleeding is severe, coagulation factors must join with platelets to form a permanent clot. The coagulation system consists of a series of interactions that result in the formation of a fibrin clot. The system consists of clotting proteins, most of which circulate in the plasma in an inactive state.

The formation of a fibrin clot can result from activation of one of two pathways: *intrinsic* or *extrinsic* (Figure A&P17-6). Various factors are needed by these two pathways for completion of a final common pathway that results in a fibrin clot. The *extrinsic pathway* is initiated when tissue injury occurs outside the vessels, such as a burn. The *intrinsic pathway* involves the blood itself (i.e., antigen-antibody reactions and endotoxins) or damage to the blood vessels. Blood in normal vessels that is stagnant for a long time can form clots.

Activated factor X is responsible for the conversion of prothrombin to thrombin and of soluble fibrinogen to an insoluble fibrin clot. The protein fibrin forms dense interlacing threads that entrap erythrocytes and platelets. The platelets then release a contractile protein, which causes shrinkage and retraction of the clot into a firm, insoluble fibrin mass. The process of retraction squeezes out the clear yellow serum. Serum differs from plasma in that it does not contain clotting factors.

In some cases, formation of a fibrin clot is unnecessary because hemostasis occurs at an early stage. Temporary clots are sometimes insufficient. For example, bleeding from a small pinprick can normally be ended by a platelet plug, whereas more serious cuts require the interaction of the various coagulation factors.

Fibrinolysis and Anticoagulants. The coagulation system is controlled by several mechanisms to maintain a flow of blood through the vascular space. The blood carries natural anticoagulants (e.g., heparin, antithrombin, antithromboplastin) that act continuously to inhibit

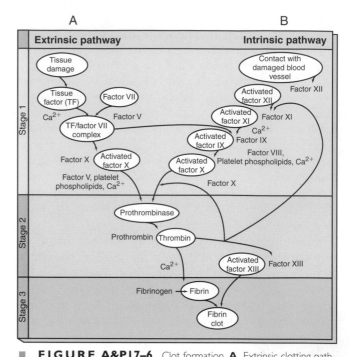

■ **FIGURE A&P17–6** Clot formation. **A,** Extrinsic clotting pathway. *Stage 1:* Damaged tissue releases tissue factor (TF), which with factor VII and calcium ions activate factor X. Activated factor X, factor V, phospholipids, and calcium ions form prothrombinase. *Stage 2:* Prothrombin is converted to thrombin by prothrombinase. *Stage 3:* Fibrinogen is converted to fibrin by thrombin. Fibrin forms a clot. **B,** Intrinsic clotting pathway. *Stage 1:* Damaged vessels cause activation of factor XII. Activated factor XII activates factor XI, which activates factor IX. Factor IX, along with factor VIII and platelet phospholipids, activates factor X. Activated factor X, factor V, phospholipids, and calcium ions form prothrombinase. *Stages 2* and *3* take the same course as in the extrinsic clotting pathway. *(From Thibodeau, G., & Patton, K. [2007]. Anatomy and physiology [6th ed.]. St. Louis: Mosby.)*

coagulation. The liver and RES also aid in controlling coagulation by removing activated clotting factors and fibrin.

In fibrinolysis, the fibrin clot is dissolved. The fibrinolytic mechanism activates in less than a day after clot formation. Formation of plasmin by *tissue plasminogen activator* is the major mechanism for dissolving a clot. Plasmin, a proteolytic enzyme, can dissolve such protein material as fibrin, fibrinogen, and factors V and VIII. Plasminogen, a serum globulin, is the inactive precursor of plasmin. Lysis of the clot produces formation of fibrin split products (or fibrin degradation products), which also act as anticoagulants.

Blood vessels break and are repaired continuously in the body. The multiple and complex interactions between clot formation, clot lysis, and anticoagulation allow normal vessel repair without precipitating a massive clot throughout the vascular system. Clots formed in the venous system often break free (embolus) and are transported to the lung capillaries, which have enhanced clot lysis properties. In contrast, emboli formed on the arterial system travel progressively through the arteriolar tree until they occlude an arteriole and block blood flow to areas distal to the occlusion. Clots lodging in the coronary circulation can cause a myocardial infarction, and clots lodging in the cerebral circulation can cause a stroke.

Roles of the Liver and Spleen

The spleen and liver both have important roles in the hematopoietic system. The spleen, lung, and liver sequester some of the peripheral blood erythrocytes, providing a ready reserve supply whenever the RBC count decreases significantly. The liver is also important in the blood-clearing process. Fixed macrophages *(Kupffer cells)* remove inanimate particulates and bacterial cells that appear in the peripheral blood. The roles of the liver in hematopoiesis are mostly indirect, related to the synthesis of plasma proteins and clotting factors, the decomposition of hemoglobin into bilirubin, and the storage of iron in the form of *ferritin.*

White Blood Cells (Leukocytes)

There are five types of WBCs, or *leukocytes,* classified according to the presence or absence of granules and the staining characteristics of their cytoplasm. As a group, the leukocytes appear brightly colored when stained. *Granulocytes* are derived from a myeloid stem cell that differentiates (see Figure A&P17-4). Granulocytes include three types of WBCs that have large granules in their cytoplasm. Their names are derived from the staining properties: (1) *neutrophils,* (2) *eosinophils,* and (3) *basophils.* There are two types of agranulocytes (WBCs without cytoplasmic granules): (1) *monocytes* and (2) *lymphocytes.*

Granulocytes

Neutrophils. Neutrophils stain very light pink-purple with neutral dyes. The granules in their cytoplasm make them appear "coarse," and they have nuclei with many lobes. Because of the appearance of their nuclei, they are also called polymorphonuclear leukocytes ("polys").

The neutrophil is the primary cell to respond during an acute inflammatory response (see Figure A&P17-4). About 90% of mature neutrophils remain in the bone marrow, a storage arrangement that enables the body to quickly release large numbers of these cells when inflammation occurs. The remaining 10% of neutrophils in the peripheral blood are subdivided, about half and half, into a circulating cell group and a cell group that adheres to endothelial linings in small blood vessels.

Thus a complete blood count (CBC) for a healthy person accounts for only about 5% of the total number of mature neutrophils actually present in the body at that time. The increases seen in peripheral WBC counts during episodes of inflammation are the result of large numbers of neutrophils being released from the bone

marrow reserve. If the inflamed state is prolonged, the supply of mature cells with lobed nuclei becomes exhausted, and immature neutrophils with a banded nucleus appear in the circulating blood. The life span of the neutrophil is hours to 3 days.

Eosinophils. Eosinophils contain numerous large granules that stain orange. Under normal circumstances, mature eosinophils do not remain long in the marrow; they are present only in small numbers in the peripheral blood (less than 3% of the total WBC count in a healthy person). These cells exit the peripheral blood compartment and accumulate in extravascular sites near epithelial surfaces. From there, they can be recruited to protect against parasitic infections and to modulate IgE-mediated allergic responses. Their life span is hours to 3 days.

Basophils. The basophil stains purple and has large granules. Details of its normal role in body homeostasis are lacking. The intracytoplasmic granules (storage vesicles) include heparin, histamine, and a chemotactic factor for eosinophils. There is disagreement as to whether this cell is a precursor to a similar cell found in solid tissues: the mast cell. Vesicular contents in the mast cell are similar to those found in the basophil, and the human mast cell is known to bind IgE and to be a primary participant in the induction of IgE-mediated allergic cascades.

Agranulocytes

Monocytes. The monocyte is derived from a precursor cell that is indistinguishable from a myeloblast. Subsequent differentiation, however, leads to a cell structure that is markedly different from that of the granulocyte. The monocyte released from the bone marrow into the circulation is a hypoactive phagocytic cell. After becoming attached to sinusoidal endothelium in the spleen, bone marrow, and liver, or after emigrating from the blood into lung, connective, or lymphoid tissue, this cell becomes transformed into a *macrophage* with full phagocytic function. These cells constitute the RES and are responsible for removing all foreign particulate material that enters the body.

The macrophage is attracted secondarily to acute inflamed sites and is the characteristic cell in chronic and in many secretory T-cell–orchestrated inflammatory lesions. Some macrophages also have immune functions by serving as antigen-processing cells and APCs.

Lymphocytes. In their mature form, lymphocytes are assigned to one of three groups according to the presence of characteristic surface markers and cell function (see Figure A&P17-2): (1) Some lymphocytes are programmed in the thymus to become *T cells;* (2) others are programmed in the bone marrow to become *B cells;*

(3) some lymphocytes, not identifiable as either T cells or B cells, are *natural killer (NK) cells*. *B cells* function in antibody-mediated immune responses, helping to defend the body against invasive types of bacteria, bacterial toxins, and some viruses. *T cells* are the basis of cell-mediated immune functions that defend against facultative and obligate intracellular pathogens, fungi, and viruses. *NK cells* make up about 5% to 10% of the circulating lymphocytes. They are involved in killing some tumor cells and some virally infected cells. Their cytotoxicity can be enhanced by exposure to cytokines, which convert a naive NK cell into a lymphokine-activated cell. After binding to a target cell, the NK cell secretes *perforins*, which cause holes to form in the target cell membrane in a manner analogous to the membrane attack complex (MAC) of complement. Interestingly, people who have normal T-cell and B-cell populations but who are deficient in NK cells experience repetitive life-threatening infections by viruses such as varicella and cytomegalovirus.

Inflammation

Inflammation is a complex response to sublethal injury to a tissue, having both local and systemic consequences. The process can be initiated by products released from damaged cells, by components from microbial cells, and by the interaction of effector units and antigen. Within the injured tissue site, the first indication is a transient constriction followed by a sustained dilation of small blood vessels. Swelling at the site is caused by increased capillary permeability and the escape of plasma (with its solutes: complement, fibrinogen, immunoglobulins). At about the same time that the vessels are responding, WBCs begin to stick to the vascular endothelium, a process called *margination*. Neutrophils are the first to escape from the vessels *(diapedesis)* and, in response to a chemotactic gradient, accumulate at the site of injury.

After a few hours, monocytes from the local circulation and macrophages present in local connective tissues begin to infiltrate the site of injury. In a limited type of injury, the healing and resolution begin shortly afterward. Some cytokines produced by stimulated macrophages act locally to stimulate vascular changes and to activate fibroblasts and other cells. The same or other cytokines are distributed systemically and help to initiate the *acute phase response*. This systemic response accompanies a strong local inflammatory response. Many aspects of the acute phase response are initiated by the action of cytokines produced by stimulated macrophages. These stimulatory molecules include interleukin-1 (IL-1), tumor necrosis factor (TNF), and IL-6. The systemic responses of the host include (1) elevation of serum cortisol level, (2) induction of fever, (3) leukocytosis, (4) the de novo appearance of C-reactive protein, an opsonizing protein

that aids in phagocytosis, (5) increased production of complement components, and (6) increased production of siderophores (iron-binding proteins).

IMMUNITY

We can become immunized following *direct* (active) exposure to an antigen and generation of our own effector units or following *indirect* (passive) receipt of effector units produced by an animal, by another human, or by gene-engineering procedures. Indirect natural immunity occurs in utero via colostrum (topologic protection in humans) and across the placenta (systemic protection in humans). Artificial indirect immunity is produced through pooled gamma (immune)-globulin, $RH_o(D)$ immunoglobulin (RhoGAM), and genetically engineered human antibody.

ACQUIRED IMMUNITY

Four types (or compartments) of active immunity are identified based on the type and body location of the effector units:

1. *Humoral immunity*. The effector units are immunoglobulins (IgM, IgG, and IgA) present in the peripheral blood.
2. *Mucosal immunity*. The effector unit is an immunoglobulin (secretory IgA) present in mucous secretions of the respiratory tract, GI tract, and urogenital tract.
3. *Cell-mediated immunity*. The effector units are cytotoxic T cells that circulate in peripheral blood and are present in peripheral lymphoid tissues.
4. *Atopic hypersensitivity (type I hypersensitivity)*. The effector unit is IgE, which is attached to surface receptors on mast cells found in connective tissues and subsurface tissues of the respiratory and GI tracts.

THE PRIMARY IMMUNE RESPONSE AND THE IMMUNE CASCADE

A primary immune response arguably occurs only once (Figure A&P17-7). The quality and quantity of the primary immune response depend on many factors, some of which are host-related whereas others depend on the composition of the antigen and how it is presented to the recipient. The primary immune response can be divided into three stages (the immune cascade).

Phase 1: Afferent Phase
Application or Exposure to the Antigen
Topical (skin) exposure is successful only with certain materials called *proantigens*. Examples of these substances include plant secretions (poison oak, poison ivy),

Antibody concentration in serum

1st injection of antigen

2nd injection of antigen

Primary response

Secondary response

IgG

IgM

0   10   20   30   60   70   80   90

Days

■ **FIGURE A&P17–7** Primary and secondary antibody response. The second exposure of an antigen to the host causes a more rapid, stronger, and longer-acting response than the first exposure, owing to the presence of memory cells. Immunoglobulin M (IgM) is most often produced in the primary response, whereas IgG is more likely to be produced predominantly in the secondary response.

salts of nickel and chromium, and formaldehyde. Mucosal exposure, through epithelia in the respiratory, GI, or urogenital tract, is triggered by foods (strawberries, peanuts), drugs (aspirin), pollens, or house dust. Parenteral (subcutaneous, intradermal, intravenous) exposure is via vaccines or allergens for testing.

Transport of Antigen

Lymph nodules lie immediately under modified mucosal epithelium (M cells in the gut). No transport of antigen is required. Antigen deposited into solid tissues gains access to draining lymphatics and is then carried to the nearest regional lymph node. Antigen introduced intravenously localizes in the white pulp of the spleen. Proantigens applied to the skin are absorbed and, in conjunction with Langerhans cells in the subepithelial tissues, are coupled with an autogenous protein. The resultant complex is transported to a regional lymph node.

Arrival of Antigen

Arrival of antigen in peripheral lymphoid tissue is followed by its uptake by APCs. Any exogenous molecule or any cell that does not have the self-markers of the recipient can serve as an antigen. Antigens may be natural, artificial, or synthetic.

1. *Natural* antigens include unmodified bacteria, fungi, viruses, parasites, foreign tissue cells, and large individual molecules such as proteins.
2. *Artificial* antigens are natural antigens that have been altered, usually to produce a vaccine (e.g., killed or attenuated bacteria, inactivated viruses, and toxoids).
3. *Synthetic* antigens are not found in nature but are produced in the laboratory (e.g., molecules genetically engineered to improve current or proposed immunization protocols).

The reactive sites of antigens are called determinant sites (or *epitopes*) and consist of three to five monosaccharide or amino acid residues that act together as a unit. The determinant sites are complementary to the reactive sites of the T-cell antigen receptor (on T cells) and the serum immunoglobulin (on B cells). Each natural antigen has many different epitopes, each of which is capable of stimulating a specific B-cell or T-cell clonotype (Figure A&P17-8).

Phase 2: Central Phase

In phase 2, the central phase, antigen is taken up by or becomes affiliated with processing and presenting cells. Protein antigens are processed intracellularly by the APCs into peptide fragments. The fragments, in association with the major histocompatibility molecules, are placed on the surface of the APCs for presentation to T cells. B cells can react to antigen in solute form, or the antigen can be adsorbed to the surfaces of follicular dendritic cells. T and B lymphocytes become activated and produce effector units and memory clonotypes.

Phase 3: Efferent Phase

Effector units and memory clonotypes are exported to all body sites. If residual antigen remains in the tissues, effector units may combine with it, causing manifestations until the antigen is neutralized or removed. Residual antigen is most often seen with obligate or facultative intracellular parasites or pathogens. This condition is not likely to occur with an extracellular pathogen.

THE SECONDARY IMMUNE RESPONSE

The secondary immune response occurs when a person who has been previously immunized with an antigen is rechallenged later with the same substance. In this second (and any subsequent) response, effector units are generally produced in greater quantity for a longer

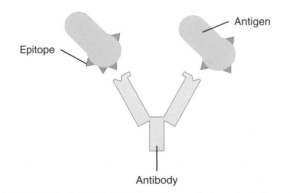

Antigen

Epitope

Antibody

■ **FIGURE A&P17–8** Epitopes protrude from the surface of an antigen and combine with the appropriate receptor of an antibody, much as a key fits into a lock.

period, and antibody molecules may exhibit a higher affinity for antigen (see Figure A&P17-7).

Antigen Processing and Presentation

T-cell recognition of antigen is limited to peptide fragments presented by an APC in conjunction with an MHC molecule. The recognition process is assisted by CD4 or CD8 molecules on the T-cell surface. Class I MHC molecules are used to present peptides to CD8 cells, and class II molecules present peptides to CD4 cells. This recognition process is said to be self-MHC–restricted; that is, the APC and the T cell both must have the same MHC molecules (each must recognize the other as self). The cells that can function as APCs in peripheral lymphoid tissue sites are B cells, dendritic cells, and some macrophages. Other locations include endothelial cells in peripheral vasculature (in humans) and Langerhans cells in the skin.

B Cells and the Antibody Response

B cells recognize antigen in one of two forms:

1. When free, unprocessed antigen (characteristically carbohydrate) is encountered, the response is limited; only IgM is produced, and there are no memory B clonotypes developed.

2. When proteins or protein conjugates are used as antigens, the APCs must first process the molecules to produce peptide fragments, which are combined with MHC molecules and then presented to T helper cells (Figure A&P17-9).

The activated T cells secrete cytokines, which assist the B cell in responding to its own set of determinant sites present on the protein antigen. The cytokines stimulate growth and maturation in B cells, induce isotype switching, and make possible the development of memory clonotypes in both T and B cell lines.

After being activated by antigen and stimulated by cytokines, the B cell is transformed morphologically and physiologically into a distinct cell type: the *plasma cell*. Plasma cells are highly differentiated and specialized cells that are capable of producing large quantities of secreted immunoglobulin.

Immunoglobulins

Antibodies, or immunoglobulins (Ig), are a family of glycoprotein molecules that are present in the body as solutes in body fluids (plasma and mucous secretions) and attached to a group of cells in solid tissues. Once attached, they inactivate and bind to antigens to facilitate phagocytosis and initiate inflammation by activating the complement cascade (Figure A&P17-10). The terminal amino acid residues react with receptors on the surface of macrophages, neutrophils, B cells, and mast cells. There are five types (Table A&P17-1).

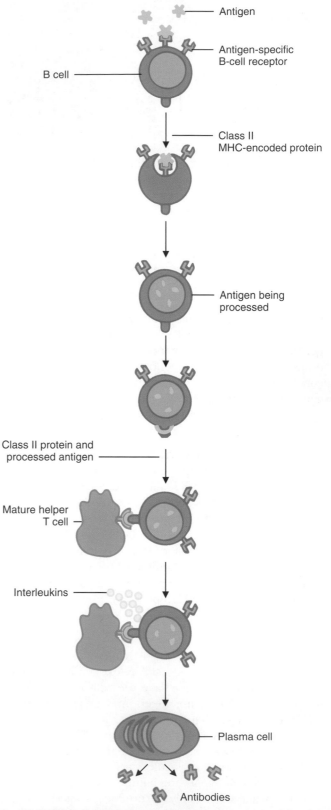

■ **FIGURE A&P17–9** Activation of B cells to make antibody. The B cell uses its receptor to bind matching antigen, which it engulfs and processes. The B cell then presents a piece of antigen, bound to class II protein, on its surface. The complex binds to the mature T helper cell, which releases interleukins that transform the B cell into an antibody-secreting plasma cell. *(Redrawn from Schindler, L.W. [1991]. Understanding the immune system. Washington, DC: National Institutes of Health.)*

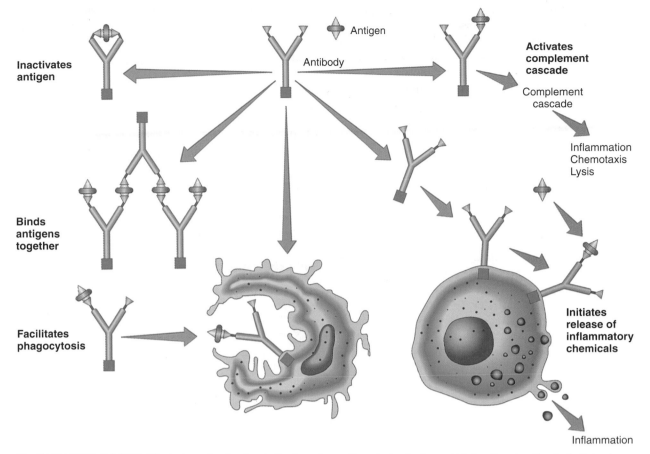

■ **FIGURE A&P17–10** Actions of antibodies. Antibodies act on antigens by inactivating and binding them together to facilitate phagocytosis and by initiating inflammation and activating the complement cascade. *(From Thibodeau, G., & Patton, K. [2007]. Anatomy and physiology [6th ed.]. St. Louis: Mosby.)*

TABLE A&P17–1		Classes and Characteristics of Immunoglobulins (Ig)
Class	**% of Total**	**Characteristics**
IgG	75	Present in circulation and tissue spaces Opsonizes antigen Activates complement Transferred transplacentally First Ig synthesized in secondary immune response
IgA	15	Present in circulation and seromucous secretions Prevents adherence of microorganisms to mucosal surface
IgM	10	Present primarily in circulation Powerful agglutinating antibody First Ig of primary immune response Activates complement
IgE	<1.0	Mediates hypersensitivity reactions Binds to mast cells and triggers mediator release
IgD	<1.0	Lymphocyte differentiation Full function unknown

IgG

IgG is available to react either by opsonizing antigens for accelerated uptake by RES cells or by activating complement via the classic pathway. When inflammation occurs in extravascular tissues, IgG is carried out of the vascular compartment to the septic site. There are four subclasses of IgG based on variation in amino acid composition in the heavy chain.

IgA

IgA is the predominant immunoglobulin in saliva, tears, colostrum, breast milk, and intestinal and bronchial secretions. The secretory (or mucosal) form of IgA prevents the adherence of microorganisms to mucosal epithelium and thus supplements resistance mechanisms against local infections in the respiratory, GI, and urogenital tracts.

IgM

IgM is normally present as a pentamer stabilized by a peptide J chain. It is the largest of the immunoglobulin molecules and is the class identified by the designation "natural." It is produced in response to challenge by bacteria in the normal gut flora and not only acts against these and similar bacteria that may infect tissue sites but also is the main immunoglobulin composing the iso-agglutinins reacting with blood group antigens.

IgM is more effective than IgG in activating complement, because only a single pentameric molecule bound to a cell is sufficient to initiate the cascade sequence (IgG requires the presence of two adjacent molecules bound to the cell surface). IgM is the early antibody seen in response to a thymic-dependent antigen and is the sole antibody produced against a thymic-independent antigen.

IgE

In most people, IgE is normally present only in trace amounts within the blood. Exceptions occur in people who have active atopic allergies or who are infected with parasitic worms. In humans, IgE is normally bound to a surface receptor on mast cells, where, following antigen binding, it triggers the release of chemical mediators such as histamine, which helps initiate the cascade of events leading to the expression of atopic allergy.

IgD

The physiologic function of IgD is unknown. It is present in large numbers on the cell membrane of naive B lymphocytes, and its only role is thought to be for antigen recognition.

MONOCLONAL ANTIBODIES

Monoclonal antibodies are immunoglobulins that can be synthesized by fusing a normal plasma cell (for antibody) with a myeloma cell (for longevity). The products of such a hybrid cell are immunoglobulins with an identical specificity. Current technology enables large quantities of immunoglobulins with almost any specificity to be produced at reasonable cost. Because they have a single specificity, they are widely used in research and for diagnostic and therapeutic regimens. Some of the applications include leukocyte identification, parasite and pathogen identification, quantitative estimation of peptide hormones, antitumor therapy, immunosuppression, and fertility control.

COMPLEMENT AND AMPLIFICATION OF ANTIBODY FUNCTION

Complement refers to a group of dissolved plasma proteins. When activated, the various components react in a cascade fashion. Complement activated by antibodies forms holes in the plasma membrane of the bacterium.

Sodium and water diffuse into the cell and cause it to swell and burst (Figure A&P17-11). Plasma complement can be activated by either of two methods: (1) a classic pathway requiring the participation of antibody and (2) an alternative pathway that is independent of antibody.

Activation of complement by the classic pathway must be preceded by the interaction of antigen with antibody (either IgG or IgM). The advantage of this pathway is that complement can be recruited to assist in the removal of any solute or of any cell against which antibody can be produced. The alternative pathway helps defend against pathogens. Surface molecules of many bacterial species can initiate the complement cascade, leading to the destruction of the bacterial cell either indirectly by opsonization or directly by cell lysis.

T LYMPHOCYTES AND CELL-MEDIATED IMMUNITY

Cell-mediated immunity (CMI) includes immune responses in which antibodies are not involved. CMI is vital in protecting the body against infection by viruses, slow-growing bacteria, and fungal infections. It also has a major role in immunosurveillance, reacting to abnormal clones of self cells, some of which are malignant. Such altered self cells can be destroyed in early stages by cytotoxic T cells or by NK cells, preventing them from becoming established tumors. Other CMI functions include primary rejection of allografts and development of delayed hypersensitivity reactions such as contact dermatitis (poison oak) and hypersensitivity to products of the tubercle bacillus. Many of the biologic actions of T lymphocytes are mediated through the secretion of factors called *lymphokines* (cytokines). Although humoral and

■ **FIGURE A&P17-11** Complement fixation. **A,** Complement molecules activated by antibodies form doughnut-shaped complexes in a bacterium's plasma membrane. **B,** Holes in the complement complex allow sodium (Na⁺) and then water (H₂O) to diffuse into the bacterium. **C,** After enough water has entered, the swollen bacterium bursts. *(From Thibodeau, G., & Patton, K. [2007]. Anatomy and physiology [6th ed.]. St. Louis: Mosby.)*

cell-mediated responses are often discussed separately, these two arms of the immune system work together (Figure A&P17-12), sometimes inseparably, and failure or malfunction in one part of the system frequently alters the effectiveness of the other.

The T lymphocytes that play a predominant role in CMI belong to a variety of T-cell subsets. Some have a regulatory function and are designated as *T helper cells* or *T suppressor cells;* others act as effector cells. Cytokines from antigen-activated T helper cells assist B cells to mature and produce antibody and also modulate the maturation and function of cytotoxic T cells (see Figure A&P17-12). The importance of T helper cell function is reflected by the severe consequences seen when it is suppressed by physical or chemical means or depleted during infection with human immunodeficiency virus (HIV); the T helper cell is a primary target of HIV. The decline of T helper cells in infected people is almost inevitably followed by recurrent episodes of opportunistic infections and the development of malignancy in people with acquired immunodeficiency syndrome (AIDS).

The homeostatic reduction or suppression of B- and T-cell responses to antigen is no longer considered to be restricted to a single suppressor cell population (once thought to be a subset of T cells bearing the CD8 marker). It is currently hypothesized that this type of negative regulation may be a function of essentially all T cells. Whether a given cell will act to produce a positive immune response (produce effector units) or will mediate a negative response (tolerance) may be a function of the mechanism by which an individual T cell is activated by antigen.

The cytotoxic T lymphocyte reacts individually with target cells to establish a contact boundary that is required for target cell destruction. The intimate contact between the target cell and the cytotoxic T lymphocyte is mediated by an antigen-specific process and allows the cytotoxic T lymphocyte to release lytic molecules *(porins)* directly into the membrane of the target cell. Cytokines produced and released by the cytotoxic T lymphocyte during the cell contact phase enhance the action of porins. The cytotoxic T-lymphocyte function

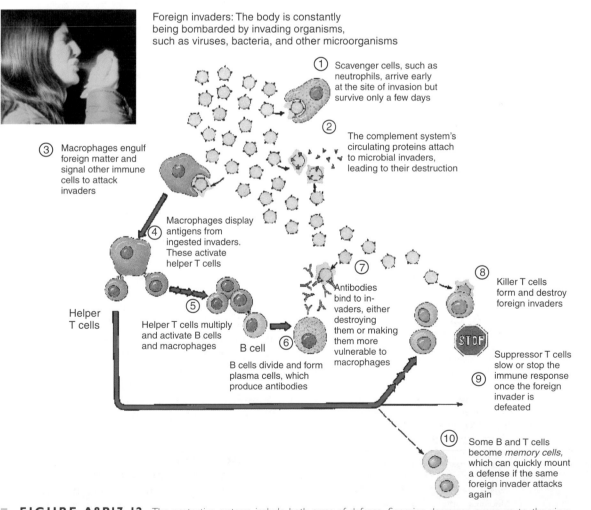

Foreign invaders: The body is constantly being bombarded by invading organisms, such as viruses, bacteria, and other microorganisms

① Scavenger cells, such as neutrophils, arrive early at the site of invasion but survive only a few days

② The complement system's circulating proteins attach to microbial invaders, leading to their destruction

③ Macrophages engulf foreign matter and signal other immune cells to attack invaders

④ Macrophages display antigens from ingested invaders. These activate helper T cells

Helper T cells

⑤ Helper T cells multiply and activate B cells and macrophages

B cell

⑥ B cells divide and form plasma cells, which produce antibodies

⑦ Antibodies bind to invaders, either destroying them or making them more vulnerable to macrophages

⑧ Killer T cells form and destroy foreign invaders

STOP

⑨ Suppressor T cells slow or stop the immune response once the foreign invader is defeated

⑩ Some B and T cells become *memory cells,* which can quickly mount a defense if the same foreign invader attacks again

■ **FIGURE A&P17–12** The protective systems include both arms of defense. Sneezing decreases exposure to the virus. Humoral immunity is shown in steps *1* and *2,* cell-mediated immunity in steps *3* and *10. (From Thibodeau, G., & Patton, K. [2007]. Anatomy and physiology [6th ed.]. St. Louis: Mosby.)*

is to kill viral-infected host cells, malignant cells, and cells in allograft transplants.

CYTOKINES

The *cytokine* is a general term for cell-derived factors that mediate interactions between cells. Cytokines produced by lymphocytes are called *lymphokines;* those produced by monocyte-macrophage cells are called *monokines.* Some of these factors are called interleukins, indicating service as regulatory signals between various leukocytes (Table A&P17-2).

Cytokines are a diverse group of proteins with four areas of function:
1. Enhancement of mononuclear phagocytes
2. Regulation of lymphocyte growth, differentiation, maturation, and secretory activities
3. Inflammation
4. Systemic effects such as fever induction and induction of hemopoietic activity in the bone marrow

One of the best known cytokines is *IL-1,* originally described in the early 1960s. Produced by macrophages, IL-1 plays a role in induction of fever, acts as a coactivator of T cells, assists in activation of B cells and NK cells, and initiates the acute-phase response.

IL-2 is also well-known from its first identification as a T-cell growth factor. The growth-enhancing function was crucial in the original studies of some of the retroviruses. Current research efforts are directed toward finding an application for IL-2 for treatment of malignant conditions.

IL-3 and *IL-4* are necessary for inducing antigen-stimulated B cells to undergo isotype switching to

change from synthesis and secretion of IgM to IgG (or IgA or IgE). IL-3 also stimulates bone marrow stem cells to differentiate into monocytic and granulocytic precursors.

Interferons (IFNs) are another group of molecules that serve as intercellular messengers. There are three major types: IFN-α, produced by many cells; IFN-β, produced by fibroblasts; and IFN-γ, produced by T lymphocytes. All interferons have antiviral activity and have a downregulating effect on proliferation of both normal and malignant cells.

Tumor necrosis factor acts as a growth factor for fibroblasts and has a necrotizing effect on tumor cells. TNF participates in inducing the acute-phase response and is apparently one of the major factors in inducing endotoxic shock (sometimes seen in infections with gram-negative bacteria). This cytokine is thought to be a major cause of infection-related cachexia.

BLOOD GROUPS AND BLOOD TYPING

Human RBCs display antigens that are either glycoproteins or glycolipids on the surface of the membrane. Together the various blood group systems contribute more than 400 characterized antigens. Antigens are inherited from the parents. Fewer than a dozen of these blood group antigens attract frequent clinical notice, and of these only the ABO and rhesus (Rh) systems are major determinants of compatibility testing.

The ABO Blood Group System

The ABO blood type is inherited as an autosomal trait. The four major blood types of clinical importance in this genetic system are A, B, AB, and O. Blood is typed according to the antigens found on the RBC and the antibodies found in the serum.

The two major antigens within the blood group system are antigens A and B. For the antibodies to be formed, usually there must be exposure to foreign or homologous RBC antigens through pregnancy or transfusion. The major exceptions are the A and B antigens, for which there are structurally similar proteins in the environment, resulting in antibody formation against the missing A or B, or both antigens by the age of 3 months. Table A&P17-3 shows the antigen and antibody combinations for the different blood groups.

The Rh System

The Rh blood groups are nearly equal in clinical importance to the ABO groups. Although Rh serology involves more than 20 different antigens, the D antigen has the most clinical significance because of the high risk of formation of an anti-D in an Rh-negative recipient. The

TABLE A&P17–2	Major Cytokines
Cytokine	**Principal Effects**
Interleukin-1 (IL-1)	Lymphocyte activation
	Macrophage and neutrophil stimulation
	Stimulation of acute-phase proteins
	Fever and sleep
	Pituitary hormone regulation
Interleukin-2 (IL-2)	Enhances T-cell growth and function
Interleukin-3 (IL-3)	Stimulates differentiation of hematopoietic cells (colony-stimulating factor)
Interleukin-4 (IL-4)	B-cell growth factor
Interleukin-5 (IL-5)	B-cell growth and differentiation
Interleukin-6 (IL-6)	B-cell growth and differentiation
	Stimulates acute-phase response
Colony-stimulating factor	Stimulates division and differentiation of bone marrow stem cells
Interferon	Antiviral factor
Tumor necrosis factor	Activates macrophages, granulocytes, and cytotoxic cells
	Cachexia
	Mediates septic shock
	Increases leukocyte adhesion
	Enhances antigen presentation

TABLE A&P17–3   The ABO Blood Group System

Blood Type	Agglutinogens on RBCs	Agglutinins in Plasma	Frequency in United States
A	A	Anti-B	41%
B	B	Anti-A	10%
AB	A and B	None	4%
O	None	Anti-A and anti-B	45%

RBCs, Red blood cells.

term *Rh-positive* means that the client has the D antigen; the *Rh-negative* client has no D antigen.

The most striking difference between the ABO and Rh systems is that, in the ABO system, there is spontaneous development of antibodies directed against A and B antigens not present on the RBC. In the Rh system, antibody formation is never spontaneous. Instead, a client must first be exposed to the Rh antigen, for example, through a blood transfusion or pregnancy. Thus clients with Rh-negative blood, transfused for the first time with Rh-positive blood, do not experience a reaction because their blood does not yet contain anti-Rh antibodies (anti-D). About 50% of people, however, develop sensitivity and form antibodies against the D antigen as a result of exposure to it from transfusion or pregnancy. If a sensitized client receives a second transfusion or has a second pregnancy with exposure to the D antigen, some degree of RBC destruction will occur. However, it is usually possible to prevent sensitization from occurring the first time by administering a single dose of anti-Rh antibodies in the form of $Rh_o(D)$ immune globulin (RhoGAM) immediately following exposure to the D antigen.

THE HLA SYSTEM

HLAs are also called *histocompatibility antigens* because the antigens (glycoproteins) are found on the surface of most cells in the body except RBCs (including circulating and tissue cells). The HLA system is a series of closely linked genes located on the short arm of chromosome 6. The major function of the HLA antigen is regulation of the immune response, distinguishing self from non-self. This plays a major role in the rejection of transplanted tissues when donor and recipient HLA antigens do not match. There also is an association between HLA antigens and some diseases. For example, in ankylosing spondylitis, the association with HLA factor is so strong that HLA typing can be used diagnostically.

CONCLUSIONS

The immune system is extremely complex. It has evolved through the years to become a pervasive and highly structured group of complex functions that defend the body against pathogens and parasites from the outside and that are able to detect and attack altered self cells that pose threats to an individual's homeostasis.

BIBLIOGRAPHY

1. Goldsby, R.A., et al. (2000). *Kuby immunology* (4th ed.). Philadelphia: W.H. Freeman.
2. Thibodeau, G., & Patton, K. (2007). *Anatomy and physiology* (6th ed.). St. Louis: Mosby.
3. Travers, P., Walport, M., & Shlomchik, M. (2001). *Immunobiology* (5th ed.). New York: Garland.
4. Actor, J.K., DeBord, C. (2007). *Elsevier's integrated immunology and microbiology*. St. Louis: Mosby.

CHAPTER 74

Assessment of the Hematopoietic System

Linda H. Yoder

HISTORY

The nature of the presenting problem determines the focus of the health history for the hematopoietic and immune system. Clients may present with manifestations that suggest a hematologic or immunologic problem.

Biographical and Demographic Data

The immune response is diminished in both very young and older people. Some hematologic and immunologic disorders occur more frequently at certain ages, in women or men, and in those of a particular race or ethnic background. Collect family health history data because several hematologic and immunologic disorders are inherited. In addition, the normal values of some hematologic tests have age-specific and gender-specific norms. For example, hemoglobin and hematocrit levels are lower in women, particularly during the menstrual years, than in men. Hemoglobin values in African Americans are about 0.5 g/dl lower than those in whites.[14]

Current Health

Disorders of the protective system often affect all organs and tissues of the body, resulting in widespread pathophysiologic manifestations. Manifestations may be vague and nonspecific, such as fatigue, malaise, fever, anorexia, weight loss, and chronic diarrhea.

The body's defense against infectious or malignant disease occurs through the immune system. Two main functions of the immune system are to recognize substances that are foreign (non-self) and to eliminate these foreign substances with return to homeostasis. Factors that may affect immune responses are stress, aging, gonadal hormones (specifically estrogen, progesterone, and testosterone), nutrition, alcohol and other central nervous system acting drugs, physical exercise, and sleep.

Chief Complaint

It is important to note the timing; quality and quantity; severity and location; and precipitating, aggravating, and relieving factors associated with hemapoietic system manifestations. The chief complaint of the client may be fever, fatigue, or bleeding. Figure 74-1 provides an overview of the assessment of clinical manifestations related to the hematopoietic system.

Clinical Manifestations

In general, anemias often manifest with fatigue, paleness, and weakness; bleeding disorders with bruising, petechiae, epistaxis, and bleeding gums; and immunodeficiencies with recurrent infections and fever. Allergic manifestations may present as simple skin rashes, nasal stuffiness, and cough, or they may be more severe, such as wheezing and respiratory distress. Assess if different allergens trigger different responses and if the client ever experienced an anaphylactic reaction. Allergic manifestations range from mild to severe and can be systemic or organ specific, such as integumentary, respiratory, gastrointestinal, or cardiovascular reactions.

Fever. Clients with severe neutropenia or immunosuppression may be unable to mount the inflammatory

---

evolve Web Enhancements

Assessment Terms English and Spanish

Appendix B A Health History Format that Integrates the Assessment of Functional Health Patterns

Web Tables Sequence and Palpation Technique for Lymph Nodes

Lymphocyte Immunophenotyping

Immunoglobulin (Ig) Isotopes

Be sure to check out the bonus material on the Evolve website and the CD-ROM, including free self-assessment exercises. **http://evolve.elsevier.com/Black/medsurg**

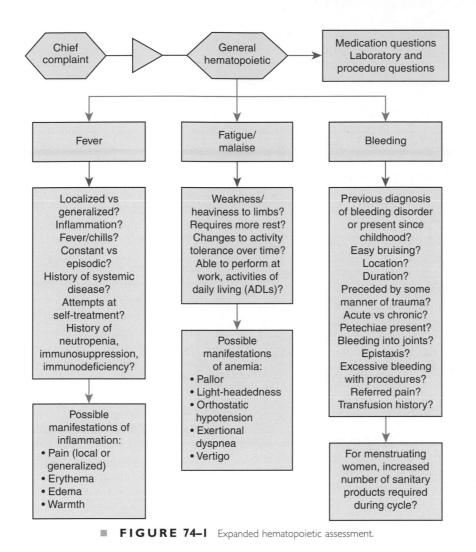

■ **FIGURE 74–1** Expanded hematopoietic assessment.

response of fever, redness, and pus formation. Assess for local inflammation (redness, heat, swelling, pain). Immunodeficiencies may be present at birth or may develop later in life, and they may be *iatrogenic* (a result of treatment with cytotoxic agents, corticosteroids or other immunosuppressants, or radiation). Immunodeficiencies also may result from protein-deficiency malnutrition, protein-losing enteropathy, nephrotic syndrome, or hypercatabolic states (major trauma, severe thermal injury). Immunodeficiencies may be related to loss of anatomic integrity from instrumentation (catheters), impaired dermatologic barrier function (burns, psoriasis, atopic dermatitis), mucosal inflammation (atopic diseases, irritants such as cigarette smoke), or mucociliary elevator dysfunction (cystic fibrosis or immotile cilia syndrome). Any episode of fever should be detailed as completely as possible, including any associated manifestations such as chills or night sweats.

Fatigue/Malaise. Anemia is characterized by pallor, weakness, and lightheadedness; severe anemia manifests with chronic severe fatigue, exertional dyspnea, headache, or vertigo. Does the client have sufficient energy to perform normal activities and occupational tasks? Do fatigue, dyspnea, or other manifestations interfere with a productive lifestyle? Has the client missed time from work or school, resulting in financial loss or other economic concerns, such as health or life insurance eligibility? Does the client feel rested after sleeping? The fatigue from anemia will not improve with increased amounts of sleep. The client should be questioned about a feeling of weakness or heaviness in the limbs.

Bleeding. Assess for bleeding disorders. Ask whether the disorder might be related to genetic factors, exposure to toxins, or liver disease. Cirrhosis, hepatitis, and other liver diseases can result in reduced production of clotting factors as well as reduced clearance of factors that inhibit clotting or promote fibrinolysis. Clients with hemophilia and other congenital coagulation disorders have a history of lifelong bleeding tendencies, such as excessive or prolonged bleeding after circumcision or dental extraction, repeated episodes of spontaneous bleeding into joints (hemarthrosis), and life-threatening hemorrhages (retroperitoneal, intracranial, or paratracheal).

When assessing the client for a suspected bleeding disorder, ask the following: How long has there been a bleeding problem? Was it present in childhood, or did it appear recently? Do any family members have a history of bleeding disorders? Is the bleeding linked to any specific event or procedure? Clients with bleeding disorders may manifest petechiae, purpura, and ecchymoses (bruises); spontaneous bleeding from the nose, gingiva, vagina, and rectum; oozing of blood from cuts and venipuncture sites; jaundice; conjunctival or retinal hemorrhage; hemoptysis, hematemesis, hematuria, and back and flank pain.

Ask about illnesses and hospitalizations. Have there been retroperitoneal, intracranial, or paratracheal hemorrhages? Has the client received a blood or blood product transfusion, and for what reason? Were there problems or reactions to the blood or blood products? Does the client know his or her blood type, including Rh factor? This information is important for the pregnant client who is Rh negative.

Review of Systems

The review of systems in Figure 74-2 demonstrates a systematic history relative to the hematopoietic system. Specific manifestations can vary if the disorder is related to allergy, anemia, bleeding, or immunodeficiency.

Past Medical History

Assess for hematologic disorders by asking whether there is a history of anemia, concurrent disorders (such as renal, liver, or autoimmune disease), cancer, or organ transplantation.

Clients with immunodeficiencies have a history of recurrent infections, especially of mucous membranes (such as the oral cavity, anorectal area, genitourinary tract, or respiratory tract). There may be a history of poor wound healing, diarrhea, or manifestations of systemic activation of the inflammatory response (fever, malaise, fatigue, anorexia, unexplained weight loss, headache, and irritability). There may be a history of unusually frequent bacterial infections, unusually severe viral infections, or development of an infection with an unusual microorganism (fungus or protozoa). When assessing lymphatic problems, inquire about trauma or other injury, especially to an extremity. Has the client had a recent infection or cancer?

Did the client experience an unusually severe course of measles, mumps, or other infectious diseases of childhood? Were there severe reactions to vaccinations, especially immunizations with live virus vaccines such as measles and mumps? Are vaccinations current? Has the client recently donated blood or blood components?

Donating whole blood, erythrocytes, leukocytes, platelets, or plasma can affect laboratory values for days or weeks.

Ask the client about the occurrence of any major illnesses, including cancer, lymphoproliferative diseases (lymphoma, leukemia, multiple myeloma), infection (especially HIV-1, HIV-2, rubella, cytomegalovirus, influenza, varicella zoster), systemic inflammatory diseases (rheumatoid arthritis, systemic lupus erythematosus, sarcoidosis, vasculitis), diabetes mellitus, renal or liver disease, and sickle cell anemia or disease. Is there a history of diseases involving the terminal ileum, Crohn's disease, tropical sprue, ulcers, or severe atrophic gastritis?

Surgical History

Surgical procedures can influence the development of hematologic disorders or immunodeficiency. For example, cardiac valve replacement may cause erythrocyte hemolysis and subsequent anemia. Anemia may also occur following partial or total gastrectomy or removal of the terminal portion of the ileum because of the consequent reduction in absorption of vitamin B_{12}. Surgical removal of duodenal tissue can decrease iron absorption and thus produce iron deficiency anemia. Splenectomy increases the risk of overwhelming infections with encapsulated bacteria such as *Streptococcus pneumoniae*. Surgical instrumentation and loss of anatomic integrity increase the risk of infection.

Allergies

If the client has a history of transfusions with blood or blood products, ask about complications. Reactions to blood products include fever, chills, back or flank pain, wheezing, headache, vomiting, urticaria (hives), and shock. Inquire about food and drug allergies or sensitivities. Has the client ever had an anaphylactic reaction or been hospitalized for an allergic reaction?

Clients with allergies may have rhinitis, sinusitis, urticaria, and pruritus. Ask whether allergic manifestations have been present since childhood. Can the client identify triggers? Is there a seasonal pattern associated with the manifestations? Has hospitalization or emergency treatment been necessary for a severe allergic reaction? Was desensitization therapy (allergy shots) undertaken, and if so was it effective?

Medications

Note the client's past and current use of both prescription and over-the-counter (OTC) drugs as well as herbal or complementary remedies and alcohol intake. Many medications can prolong bleeding; cause hemolysis of red blood cells; or, through selective or general bone marrow suppression, produce anemia, thrombocytopenia, or leukopenia. Medications also can inhibit folic acid

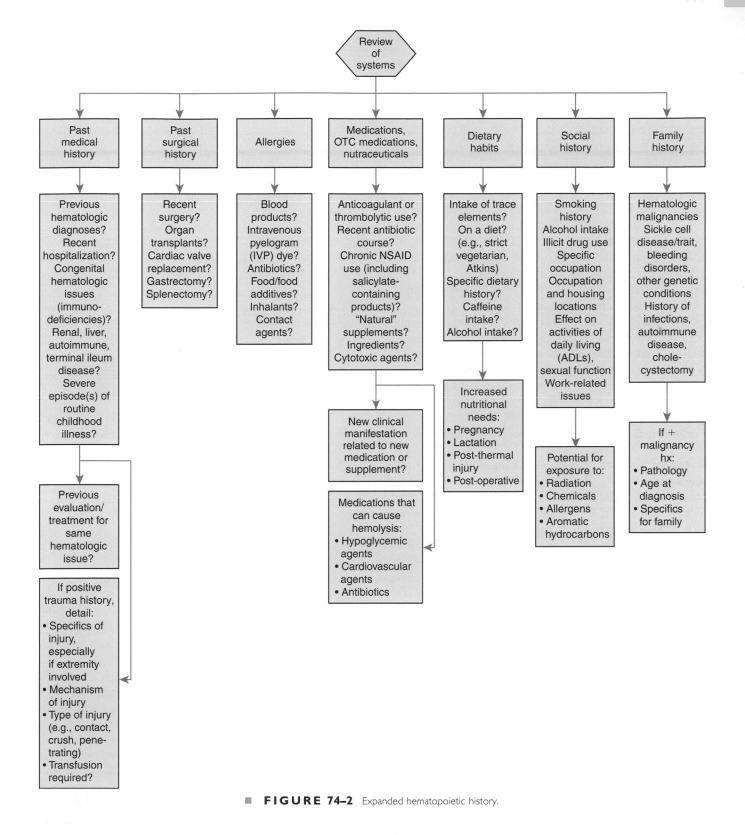

■ **FIGURE 74–2** Expanded hematopoietic history.

absorption from the intestine, leading to folic acid deficiency and anemia.

Ask about current or recent anticoagulant therapy or thrombolytic treatment. The anticoagulants heparin and warfarin prolong bleeding, and heparin may also cause immune-mediated thrombocytopenia. The thrombolytic agents streptokinase, tissue plasminogen activator (t-PA), and urokinase also prolong bleeding.

Has the client taken corticosteroids, cytotoxic agents (cyclophosphamide, chlorambucil, cisplatin, etoposide), other immunosuppressants (gold salts, nonsteroidal anti-inflammatory drugs [NSAIDs]), or therapies (irradiation) for the treatment of cancer or autoimmune diseases? These agents may suppress bone marrow production of blood cells or the immune response. Effects may continue long after the medications have been stopped. Treatment with cytotoxic agents or high doses of corticosteroids can mask fever and other manifestations until an infection is serious and widespread.

Has the client received other medications for which myelosuppression is an adverse effect? These include chloramphenicol, cephalosporins, clindamycin, penicillin, tetracycline, sulfonamides, D-penicillamine, amphotericin B, antimalarials, captopril, phenothiazines, antithyroid drugs, zidovudine, and ganciclovir. Determine whether the client has received intravenous immune globulin (IVIG) or intramuscular immune globulin (IMIG) to treat an immunoglobulin deficiency or other conditions.

Ask the client about herbal preparations and nutritional supplements including comfrey (*Symphytum officinale*), echinacea (*Echinacea angustifolia, E. pallida, E. purpura*), evening primrose (*Oenothera biennis*), ginseng (*Panax ginseng, P. quinquefolius, Eleutherococcus senticosus*), goldenseal (*Hydrastis canadensis*), licorice (*Glycyrrhiza glabra, G. uralensis*), maitake (*Grifola frondosa*), St. John's wort (*Hypericum perforatum*), and stinging nettle (*Urtica dioica*).

Assess the client for potential interactions of herbal preparations with prescription medications. Ephedra (*Ma-huang, Ephedra sinica*), a sympathomimetic, might reduce the effect of prednisone. St. John's wort can reduce warfarin levels.[26] There is some limited anecdotal evidence that gingko, garlic, fish oil, and the Chinese herbs danshen and dong quai may exert an anticoagulant effect.[26] The use of these products may need to be avoided in people with bleeding disorders or receiving anticoagulant therapy.

Dietary Habits

The hematopoietic and immune systems depend on the adequate intake of protein, calories, vitamins (A, B_{12}, folic acid), minerals, and trace elements such as iron and zinc. Inadequate intake of any of these substances can lead to anemia or immunodeficiency. Assess for conditions that increase nutritional needs, such as pregnancy, lactation, and hypercatabolic states that occur with thermal injuries. When assessing anemia, obtain a dietary history focusing on the intake of foods such as meat, fish, eggs, dairy products, whole grains, dark green vegetables, legumes, and nuts. Strict vegetarians who do not eat foods of animal origin may be at higher risk for a deficiency anemia, especially related to inadequate intake of vitamin B_{12} (see Chapter 28).

Social History

Encourage the client to discuss current levels of stress and whether they seem to relate to the appearance of allergic manifestations. Some clients may report breaking out in hives when under emotional stress. Their appearance triggers more emotional distress and can lead to further outbreaks; a cycle may develop that is difficult to interrupt.

Ask about occupational exposure to agents that might predispose the client to the development of hematopoietic disorders: radiation, aromatic hydrocarbons (kerosene, gasoline), benzene (used in the manufacture of pharmaceuticals, rubber, leather, and explosives), inorganic arsenics, trinitrotoluene, insecticides, weed killers, lead, and phenylbutazone. Exposure to toxic chemicals and ionizing radiation may occur in several industries (chemicals, plastics, ceramics, steel, metal refinery); in the manufacturing of rubber tires, shoes, incandescent lamps, vacuum tubes, glue, and varnish; in nuclear reactors, uranium mines, research laboratories, hospital radiology, or sterile supplies; and in farming and horticulture. Exposure to allergens at work may trigger reactions. Ask about the heating and cooling systems if airborne allergens are suspected.

Geographical location may be associated with exposure to possible health hazards. Living at altitudes above 10,000 feet may result in increased hemoglobin levels and other physiologic adaptations. Immunologic disorders may be more prevalent in certain geographical areas. High levels of air pollution can increase the incidence of allergy-related respiratory problems. Ask about home and work environments. Are pets, houseplants, or fresh-cut flowers present? What type of vegetation is in the immediate vicinity?

Does the client have sufficient energy to perform normal activities and occupational tasks? Do fatigue, dyspnea, or other manifestations interfere with a productive lifestyle? Has the client missed time from work or school, resulting in financial loss or other economic concerns, such as health or life insurance eligibility? Assess the client's current and past use of tobacco (including exposure to second-hand smoke that can aggravate allergies), alcohol, and illicit drugs. Excessive use of alcohol in particular often results in poor nutrition, folic acid deficiency, and decreased immunity as well as acute or chronic loss of blood from gastritis and esophageal varices. Many substances, most notably alcohol, damage the structure and function of liver cells, decreasing the production of clotting factors and reducing the clearance of factors that promote clot dissolution; the result is a bleeding tendency.

Family Health History

Explore the family history for common hematopoietic conditions, such as anemia, thrombocytopenia, bleeding disorders such as hemophilia or von Willebrand's disease, and congenital blood disorders such as sickle cell anemia. Inquire about a family history of jaundice; infections that were unusually frequent, unusually severe, or caused by an unusual organism; or a history of delayed healing. There may also be a history of cancer or autoimmune disease. A family history of neonatal jaundice or early cholecystectomy (gallbladder removal) may indicate a genetic hematologic disorder. Ask the client to identify allergies and sensitivities in family members, particularly atopic reactions. Hay fever tends to occur among family members.

PHYSICAL EXAMINATION

The physical examination of the hematopoietic system can entail both a complete head-to-toe examination and examinations of specific systems, depending on the nature of the client's problem. For example, anemia or fever can cause tachycardia and systolic ejection murmur; immunodeficiency manifested by repeated episodes of pulmonary infections may result in adventitious breath sounds. See Chapters 54 and 59, respectively, for discussions of cardiac and respiratory assessment. The Physical Assessment Findings in the Healthy Adult feature below outlines expected normal findings for the hematopoietic system.

The portions of the lymphatic system accessible for a physical examination are the superficial lymph nodes, liver, and spleen. Note the presence of a surgical splenectomy scar. For more specific information about physical assessment see the physical assessment texts provided in the references for this chapter. Table 74-1

describes possible abnormal physical findings related to the hematopoietic system and possible causes.

Inspection

Inspect surfaces overlying the lymph nodes for masses, scars, swelling, and redness. Note extremity swelling or edema. Look for symmetry and compare with the contralateral side.

Palpation

Use a methodical approach to examine the lymph nodes; do not overlook single nodes or chains of nodes. Palpate nodes for location, size, shape, consistency, symmetry, discreteness, mobility, tenderness, temperature, overlying edema, or red streaks.

Lymph nodes are generally nonpalpable; however, small (1 cm in diameter), single, round, soft, mobile, nontender nodes are common, particularly in the head, neck, and inguinal areas, and are usually not significant. Nodes that are inflamed, tender, large (>1 cm in diameter), hard, matted together, or fixed to underlying structures are abnormal. Describe their characteristics thoroughly. If you see a mass, palpate the area and compare with the contralateral side. The supraclavicular area is a frequent site of metastatic disease; investigate palpable nodes in this site.

The nodes of the head and neck and the clavicular and epitrochlear areas are most easily palpated while the client is sitting. Palpate the inguinal and popliteal nodes when the client is lying down. Axillary nodes may be palpated with the client sitting or lying. Specific guidelines for palpating the lymph nodes are presented in the website table Sequence and Palpation Technique `evolve` for Lymph Nodes.

DIAGNOSTIC TESTING

Diagnosis of hematologic, bleeding, or immunologic disorders depends primarily on laboratory analysis. No particular preprocedure or postprocedure care is associated with the simple blood tests involved in most hematopoietic assessments.

Although dozens of specific tests are used to diagnose individual disorders, all cases generally call for (1) a complete blood count (CBC) to determine the number of leukocytes, erythrocytes, and platelets; (2) a white blood cell (WBC) differential count to indicate the relative percentages of the different leukocytes; (3) coagulation studies such as prothrombin time (PT), partial thromboplastin time (PTT), and bleeding time; and (4) a peripheral blood smear for red blood cell (RBC) morphology to differentiate various anemias and blood dyscrasias.

Physical Assessment Findings in the Healthy Adult

The Hematopoietic System

INSPECTION

Alert and oriented; afebrile. Skin color even, without pallor, flushing, jaundice, bruises, or petechiae. Lumps or masses absent; no draining lesions. Sclerae white. Lingual papillae visible; oral lesions absent. Eupneic. Joints not swollen; full range of motion.

PALPATION

Lumps, masses absent. Lymph nodes, liver, and spleen nonpalpable and nontender. Joints nontender. Several round, small (0.5 cm), discrete, soft, mobile nodes palpable in submandibular area.

AUSCULTATION

Heart sounds regular, without murmurs or palpitations.

TABLE 74–I **Abnormal Assessment Findings**

Anatomic Area	Manifestation	Possible Cause
Eyes	Visual disturbances	Anemia, polycythemia
	Blindness	Retinal hemorrhage related to
	Scleral jaundice	thrombocytopenia or bleeding disorder
	Conjunctivitis, tearing, eye rubbing, styes, dark circles or "allergic shiners," "raccoon eyes"	Hemolytic anemia
		Allergies
Ears	Vertigo or tinnitus	Severe anemia
	Blood in external auditory canal or bluish tympanic membrane, suggesting blood in middle ear	Bleeding disorders
	Chronic otitis media, mastoiditis	Immunodeficiencies or chronic infections and treatment with ototoxic drugs
	Hearing impairment related to eardrum rupture, scarring, perforated tympanic membrane	
Nose	Epistaxis	Thrombocytopenia and bleeding disorders
	Crusting around nares, sinopulmonary drainage, and indications of chronic sinusitis	Immunodeficiency
		Allergies
	Sneezing, sniffling, rhinitis, nasal polyps, nasal voice quality	
Mouth	Smooth, glossy, bright red, and sore tongue	Pernicious anemia, iron deficiency anemia
	Gingival bleeding	Thrombocytopenia, bleeding disorders
	Oral ulcers, candidiasis, gingivitis, periodontitis, dental caries, and tooth loss	Immunodeficiencies
		Allergies
	Tonsils may be enlarged, inflamed, or pustular; lip and tongue swelling, frequent throat clearing from postnasal drip, sore throat, itching of palate, throat, or neck, and hoarseness	
Respiratory tract	Dyspnea and orthopnea	Anemia, sickle cell crisis
	Wheezing, frequent cough, ineffective cough, and respiratory arrest	Allergies
Cardiovascular system	Tachycardia, palpitations, murmurs, particularly systolic and angina	Anemia
Gastrointestinal tract	Dysphagia	Mucous membrane atrophy related to iron deficiency anemia
	Abdominal pain	
	Hepatomegaly, splenomegaly	Sickle cell disease, retroperitoneal bleeding, acute hemolysis
	Hematemesis and melena	
	Vomiting, cramping, and diarrhea	Hemolytic anemia resulting in increased need for removal of erythrocytes
		Thrombocytopenia and bleeding disorders
		Allergies
Genitourinary tract	Hematuria	Hemolysis and bleeding disorders
	Amenorrhea and menorrhagia	Iron deficiency and bleeding disorders
	Decreased fertility	Severe anemia
Musculoskeletal system	Back pain	Hemolysis
	Sternal tenderness and excruciating bone pain, joint pain	Sickle cell crises
		Hemarthroses or bleeding into joints, often related to hemophilia
Nervous system	Headache and confusion	Anemia, polycythemia
	Brain hemorrhage	Thrombocytopenia or bleeding disorder
	Peripheral neuropathy, paresthesias, loss of balance	Pernicious anemia

The diagnosis of deficiency anemias may require measuring serum levels of iron, total iron-binding capacity (TIBC), transferrin saturation, ferritin, folic acid, and vitamin B_{12} (Table 74-2). Bone marrow aspiration and biopsy are performed to determine both the cellularity of the bone marrow and the morphology of the cells present. The diagnosis of particular hematologic disorders requires specialized blood tests, such as the Schilling test, hemoglobin electrophoresis, and measurement of levels of specific clotting factors. These specialized tests are discussed in Chapter 75. Table 74-3 and the website tables Lymphocyte Immunophenotyping and Immunoglobulin (Ig) Isotopes provide additional information concerning

TABLE 74–2 **Laboratory Tests Used in the Diagnosis of Anemia**

Test	Normal Value
Iron	50-150 mcg/dl
Total iron-binding capacity (TIBC)	250-350 mcg/dl
Transferrin	250-430 mg/dl
Transferrin saturation	20-55%
Ferritin	Men: 15-200 mcg/ml
	Women: 11-200 mcg/ml
Folate	7-20 mcg/ml
Vitamin B_{12}	200-800 pg/ml
Schilling test (vitamin B_{12} absorption)	8.5-28% excretion in 24-48 hr

dl, Deciliter; *mcg,* microgram; *ml,* milliliter; *pg,* picogram.

TABLE 74–3   Diagnostic Tests of the Hematopoietic System

Test Description	Purpose	Findings
Bone Marrow Aspiration and Biopsy		
Most commonly taken from posterior iliac crests; alternative site is sternum	Used to assess and identify most blood dyscrasias such as aplastic anemia, leukemias, pernicious anemia, thrombocytopenia	Reveals number, size, and shape of RBCs, WBCs, and platelet precursors
Lymphocyte Immunophenotyping		
Lymphocyte subpopulation analysis by flow cytometry	Measures total numbers and percentages of B lymphocytes, T lymphocytes, and T lymphocyte subsets (CD4, CD8) in a peripheral blood sample	See table on Lymphocyte Immunophenotyping on website *evolve* Lists normal levels of T and B lymphocytes and conditions in which abnormal levels of T cells and B cells occur
Immunoglobulin isotypes	Measures serum level of various immunoglobulins: IgG, IgA, IgM, IgD, and IgE; subclasses of IgG may also be measured (IgG1, IgG2, IgG3, IgG4)	See table on Immunoglobulin (Ig) Isotypes on website *evolve*
Radiography		
Chest x-ray	Assesses upper chest and lower part of the neck	Detects congenital absence of thymic tissue or tumor of thymus gland
Computed tomography (CT)	Assesses integrity of sinuses	See diagnostic testing textbook
Lymphangiography	Allows visualization of lymphatic system to assess malignancy, metastases, or obstruction	See diagnostic testing textbook
Skin Tests		
Skin tests confirm sensitivity to a specific allergen; antigens are applied by one of three methods:	A known antigen is placed on or directly beneath skin to detect presence of antibodies	
1. Patch tests		See Chapters 48 and 76
2. Scratch tests (tine tests or prick tests)		See Chapter 76
3. Delayed-type hypersensitivity skin testing		See Chapter 76

diagnostic tests that may be used with clients who have hemapoietic disorders.

Hematologic Tests
Complete Blood Cell Count (CBC)
The CBC includes the RBC count, hemoglobin, hematocrit, RBC indices, WBC count with or without differential, and platelet count. Table 74-4 presents the purpose for the various indices within a CBC and Table 74-5 presents reference values for the CBC. Table 74-6 reviews the effects of diseases, disorders, and conditions on the CBC and the RBC indices.

Peripheral Blood Smear
A peripheral blood smear is obtained to determine variations and abnormalities in erythrocytes, leukocytes, and platelets. Cells of normal size and shape are termed *normocytes;* cells of normal color are *normochromic.* Abnormalities of erythrocyte size, shape, and color usually indicate some form of anemia.

Antiglobulin Tests
The *direct* antiglobulin test (Coombs' test) is used to detect certain antigen-antibody reactions between serum antibodies and RBC antigens, differentiate between various forms of hemolytic anemia, determine unusual blood types, and identify hemolytic disease in newborns. This test examines erythrocytes for the presence of antibodies (agglutinins) that damage erythrocytes without causing clumping or hemolysis. It is used to crossmatch blood for blood transfusions, test umbilical cord blood for erythroblastosis fetalis, and diagnose acquired hemolytic anemia.

The *indirect* antiglobulin test identifies antibodies to erythrocyte antigens in the serum of clients who have a greater than normal chance of developing transfusion reactions. Both the direct and the indirect tests are agglutination procedures that use a suspension of RBCs.

Coagulation Screening Tests
Laboratory studies are the most crucial for pinpointing the type and cause of bleeding disorders. Initially, four basic laboratory tests are performed to discern whether the bleeding problem is related to a platelet, coagulation, or vascular defect: platelet count, PT, PTT, and bleeding time. Most bleeding disorders are diagnosed by the PT and PTT (Table 74-7).

Because the normal and therapeutic ranges for PT vary according to the type of reagent used in the assay, the PT is standardized by conversion to the International Normalized Ratio (INR). For most clinical

TABLE 74–4   Purpose of Complete Blood Cell Count Indices

Test Component	Purpose
Red blood cell count	Measures number of RBCs per cubic millimeter (mm^3) of blood. Normal values vary with age and gender.
Hemoglobin level	Used to evaluate hemoglobin content (iron and oxygen-carrying capacity) of erythrocytes by measuring number of grams of hemoglobin per 100 ml of blood (dl).
Hematocrit level	Measure of volume of RBCs in whole blood expressed as a percentage. Normal values vary with age and gender.
Red blood cell indices	
Mean corpuscular volume (MCV)	Measures erythrocyte size and hemoglobin content.
	Normal value: 76-100 μm^3.
	MCV <76 μm means abnormally small *(microcytic)* RBCs.
	MCV >100 μm means abnormally large *(macrocytic)* RBCs.
Mean corpuscular hemoglobin (MCH)	Measures hemoglobin content within one RBC of average size.
	Normal value: 27-33 pg.
	MCH <27 pg indicates hemoglobin deficiency, hypochromic RBCs.
	MCH >33 pg indicates macrocytic cells with abnormally large volume of hemoglobin.
Mean corpuscular hemoglobin concentration (MCHC)	Measures average hemoglobin concentration within 100 ml (1 dl) of packed RBCs.
	Normal value: 32-36 g/dl of packed RBCs.
	MCHC <32 g/dl indicates hemoglobin deficiency.
	MCHC remains normal when MCH >32 g/dl because cells are oversized (fewer cells can be packed together within 1 dl).
Platelet count	Platelets have a key role in blood clotting.
	Number of platelets (thrombocytes) per cubic millimeter (mm^3) of blood.
White blood cell count	Number of WBCs in a cubic millimeter of blood.
White blood cell differential	Determines proportion of each of the 5 types of WBCs in a sample of 100 WBCs.
Reticulocyte count	A reflection of RBC production, reticulocyte count measures responsiveness of bone marrow to a decreased number of circulating erythrocytes. Specifically, this test measures number of reticulocytes released from bone marrow into blood.

dl, Deciliter; *pg*, picogram; *μm^3*, cubic micrometer.

TABLE 74–5   Normal Values for Complete Blood Cell Counts in Adults

Measure	Value*
Erythrocytes	
RBC count (number of cells/mm^3 of blood)	Women: 4.2-5.4 million/mm^3
	Men: 4.7-6.1 million/mm^3
Hemoglobin (oxygen-carrying pigment of RBC)	Women: 12-16.0 g/dl
	Men: 13.5-18.0 g/dl
Hematocrit (% volume of RBCs in whole blood)	Women: 37%-47% (pregnancy >33%)
	Men: 42%-52%
Reticulocytes	0.5%-2% of total erythrocytes
Leukocytes	
WBC count (number of cells/mm^3 of blood)	4000-9000/mm^3
WBC differential	
Granulocytes	
Neutrophils	55%-70%
Eosinophils	1%-4%
Basophils	0.5%-1.0%
Agranulocytes	
Lymphocytes	20%-40%
Monocytes	2%-8%
Platelets	
Platelet (thrombocyte) count (number of cells/mm^3 of blood)	150,000-450,000/mm^3

g/dl, Grams per deciliter; *mm^3*, cubic millimeter; *RBC*, red blood cell; *WBC*, white blood cell.
* Normal values may differ significantly among laboratories.

conditions that necessitate anticoagulation, the recommended INR is 2 to 3.0. Clients with mechanical prosthetic valves or recurrent systemic embolism may need higher INR levels.

Immunologic Status Tests

Most immunodeficiencies can be identified through three blood tests: (1) WBC and differential, (2) immunoglobulin levels, and (3) total serum complement.

TABLE 74-6 Diseases, Disorders, and Conditions Affecting the Complete Blood Cell Count and Red Blood Cell Indices

CBC, RBC Index	Increased by	Decreased by
RBC count	Polycythemia vera, cardiac and pulmonary disorders characterized by cyanosis, dehydration, acute poisoning	Anemia, fluid overload, recent hemorrhage, leukemia
Reticulocyte count	Hemolytic anemia, hemorrhage, following effective treatment for pernicious anemia	Bone marrow failure, pernicious anemia
Hemoglobin	Hemoconcentration from polycythemia or dehydration	Hemodilution (fluid overload), anemia, recent hemorrhage
Hematocrit	Hemoconcentration from loss of fluid, dehydration, polycythemia	Hemodilution, anemia, acute massive blood loss
Mean corpuscular volume	Pernicious anemia, macrocytic anemia, folic acid, or vitamin B_{12} deficiency anemias	Microcytic anemia, iron deficiency anemia, hypochromic anemia, thalassemia, lead poisoning
Mean corpuscular hemoglobin	Macrocytic anemia	Microcytic anemia
Mean corpuscular hemoglobin concentration	Spherocytosis	Microcytic anemia, hypochromic anemia, thalassemia, iron deficiency anemia
WBC count	Infection, leukemia, tissue necrosis	Bone marrow depression
Neutrophils	Inflammatory disease or response, tissue necrosis (burns, myocardial infarction), granulocytic leukemia and other malignancies, acute stress response, bacterial infection	Bone marrow depression, viral diseases, drugs (chemotherapy, some antibiotics, psychotropics)
Eosinophils	Allergic reactions, parasitic infections, skin diseases, cancers, pernicious anemia	Stress response, Cushing's syndrome
Basophils	Leukemia, some hemolytic anemias, polycythemia vera	Corticosteroids, allergic reactions, acute infections (*Note:* decline is unlikely to be detected because normal count is 0%-2%)
Lymphocytes	Infectious mononucleosis, chronic bacterial infections, tuberculosis, pertussis, lymphocytic leukemia	AIDS, corticosteroids, immunosuppressive drugs
Monocytes	Infections (tuberculosis, malaria, Rocky Mountain spotted fever), collagen-vascular diseases, monocytic leukemia	Drug therapy, prednisone
Platelet count	Malignancies, polycythemia vera, splenectomy (rebound thrombocytosis)	Idiopathic thrombocytopenia purpura, aplastic anemia, hemolytic disorders, chemotherapeutic drugs or radiation, hypersplenism or splenomegaly, infiltrative bone marrow disease, disseminated intravascular coagulation, viral infections, AIDS

AIDS, Acquired immunodeficiency syndrome; *RBC,* red blood cell; *WBC,* white blood cell.

TABLE 74-7 Laboratory Tests Used in the Diagnosis of Hemorrhagic Disorders

Name of Test	Purpose	Normal Values	Interpretation of Findings
Platelet count	Measures number of circulating platelets in venous or arterial blood	150,000-450,000/mm³	Low count results in prolonged bleeding time and impaired clot retraction; diagnostic of thrombocytopenia
Prothrombin time (PT)	Determines activity and interaction of factors V, VII, and X, prothrombin, and fibrinogen; determines dosages of oral anticoagulant drugs	11-15 sec (one-stage) INR: 2-3	Prolonged PT is seen in clients receiving anticoagulant therapy; with low levels or deficiencies of fibrinogen, clotting factors II, V, VII, and X; impaired prothrombin activity; in presence of circulating anticoagulants as seen in SLE
Partial thromboplastin time (PTT, aPTT)	Complex method for testing normalcy of intrinsic coagulation process; used to identify deficiencies of coagulation factors, prothrombin, and fibrinogen; used to monitor heparin therapy	25-38 sec	Prolongation of time indicates coagulation disorder that is related to deficiency of a coagulation factor; not diagnostic for platelet disorders
Thrombin time	Measures functional fibrinogen available, as shown by time needed to form fibrin clot after thrombin is added	10-15 sec	Prolonged time indicates DIC or hypofibrinogenemia; presence in blood of excess heparin or other anticoagulants
Thromboplastin generation test (TGT)	Measures generation of thromboplastin; if result abnormal, second stage is done to identify missing coagulation factor	<12 sec (100%)	Abnormal values found in hemophilia
Fibrinogen level	Measures level of fibrinogen	200-400 mg/dl	Abnormally low values may indicate DIC, liver disease, congenital or acquired afibrinogenemia
Fibrin split products (FSPs), fibrin degradation products (FDPs) test	Measures products that result from breakdown of fibrin	Less than 10 mcg/ml	Abnormally high levels are seen in DIC; helpful in monitoring fibrinolytic therapy
D-dimer	Measures a specific product resulting from breakdown of fibrin	Less than 0.5 mcg/ml	Abnormally high levels confirm diagnosis of DIC; screen for abruptio placentae (placental abruption)
Activated clotting time	Crude measure of coagulation process in venous blood; used to control heparin therapy; commonly used during cardiovascular surgery and in ICU	7-120 sec (depends on type of activator used)	Prolonged time occurs in severe coagulation problems and therapeutic administration of heparin
Bleeding time	Measures ability to stop bleeding after a small puncture wound	3-8 min in adults (varies with test method)	Prolonged bleeding time occurs in vascular maladies and after aspirin ingestion
Capillary fragility test (tourniquet test, Rumpel-Leede test)	Crude test of vascular resistance and platelet number and function; BP cuff is placed on arm and inflated to pressure midway between systolic and diastolic BP for 5 min; petechiae in area are counted	No petechiae	Petechiae (five or more) are seen in thrombocytopenia and vascular purpura
Clot retraction	Indicates function and number of platelets; measures time needed for contraction of an undisturbed clot	50%-100% in 24 hr	Clot retraction is retarded in thrombocytopenia; clot is small and soft with thrombasthenia (functional disturbance of platelets)

BP, Blood pressure; DIC, disseminated intravascular coagulation; ICU, intensive care unit; INR, International Normalized Ratio; SLE, systemic lupus erythematosus.

Additional immunodeficiencies can be determined through more complex tests, including lymphocyte immunophenotyping, measures of immunoglobulin subclasses, complement assays, and the presence of specific antibodies (after immunizations or exposure to antigens as with communicable diseases).

CONCLUSIONS

The hematopoietic and immune systems are extremely complex. Understanding the structure, function, and assessment of the protective system will help you care for clients with any of the wide variety of disorders that affect this highly complex system.

BIBLIOGRAPHY

Citations appearing in red refer to primary research.

Citations appearing in blue refer to evidence-based practice guidelines and protocols.

1. Abbott, M.B., & Levin, R.H. (2001). Anaphylactoid reactions to radiocontrast agents. *Pediatric Revue, 22*(10), 356.
2. Ahya, S., et al. (Eds.) (2001). *The Washington manual of medical therapeutics* (30th ed.). Philadelphia: Lippincott Williams & Wilkins.
3. Anderson, K.N. (Ed.) (2002). *Mosby's medical, nursing, & allied health dictionary* (6th ed.). St. Louis: Mosby.
4. Bickley, L.S., & Szilagyi, P.G. (2005). *Bates' guide to physical examination & history taking* (9th ed.). Philadelphia: Lippincott Williams & Wilkins.
5. Cavanaugh, B.M. (2003). *Nurse's manual of laboratory and diagnostic tests* (4th ed.). Philadelphia: F.A. Davis.
6. Chernecky, C.C., & Berger, B.J. (Eds.) (2003). *Laboratory tests and diagnostic procedures* (4th ed.). Philadelphia: Saunders.
7. Corbett, J.V. (2003). *Laboratory tests and diagnostic procedures with nursing diagnoses* (6th ed.). Upper Saddle River, NJ: Prentice Hall.
8. Doenges, M.E., et al. (2006). *Nurse's pocket guide: Diagnosis, prioritized interventions and rationales* (10th ed.). Philadelphia: F.A. Davis.
9. Etkin, S., et al. (Eds.) (2005). *Professional guide to diseases* (8th ed.). Philadelphia: Lippincott Williams & Wilkins.
10. Ferri, F.F. (2006). *Ferri's clinical advisor: Instant diagnosis and treatment*. Philadelphia: Saunders.
11. Fishbach, F.T. (2003). *A manual of laboratory and diagnostic tests* (7th ed.). Philadelphia: Lippincott Williams & Wilkins.
12. Goldman, L., & Ausiello, D.A. (Eds.) (2003). *Cecil's textbook of medicine* (22nd ed.). Philadelphia: Saunders.
13. Guyton, A.C., & Hall, J.E. (2005). *Textbook of medical physiology* (11th ed.). Philadelphia: Saunders.
14. Harmening, D. (Ed.) (2001). *Clinical hematology and fundamentals of hemostasis* (4th ed.). Philadelphia: F.A. Davis.
15. Healey, P.M., & Jacobson, E. (2006). *Common medical diagnoses: An algorithmic approach*. Philadelphia: Saunders.
16. Kasper, D.L., et al. (Eds.) (2004). *Harrison's principles of internal medicine* (16th ed.). New York: McGraw-Hill.
17. McPherson, R.A., & Pincus, M.R. (Eds.) (2006). *Henry's clinical diagnosis and management by laboratory methods* (21st ed.). Philadelphia: Saunders.
18. Jacobs, D.S., et al. (Eds.) (2001). *Jacobs & DeMott laboratory test handbook* (5th ed.). Cleveland: Lexi-Comp.
19. Jarvis, C. (2003). *Physical examination and health assessment* (4th ed.). Philadelphia: Saunders.
20. Kee, J.L. (2004). *Laboratory and diagnostic tests with nursing implications* (7th ed.). Upper Saddle River, NJ: Prentice Hall.
21. Mandell, G.L., et al. (Eds.) (2000). *Mandell, Douglas, and Bennett's principles & practice of infectious diseases* (5th ed.). Philadelphia: Churchill Livingstone.
22. Miller-Keane, B.F., & O'Toole, M.T. (Ed.) (2005). *Encyclopedia & dictionary of medicine, nursing, & allied health* (7th ed.). Philadelphia: Saunders.
23. Pagana, K.D., & Pagana, T.J. (2004). *Mosby's diagnostic and laboratory test reference* (7th ed.). St. Louis: Mosby.
24. Seidel, H.M., et al. (Eds.) (2006). *Mosby's guide to physical examination* (6th ed.). St. Louis: Mosby.
25. Shils, M.E., et al. (Eds.) (2006). *Modern nutrition in health & disease* (10th ed.). Philadelphia: Lippincott Williams & Wilkins.
26. Skidmore-Roth, L. (2005). *Mosby's handbook of herbs & natural supplements* (3rd ed.). St. Louis: Mosby.
27. Tierney, L.M., et al. (Eds.) (2006). *Current medical diagnosis and treatment* (45th ed.). New York: McGraw-Hill.
28. Turgeon, M.L. (2004). *Clinical hematology: Theory and procedures* (4th ed.). Philadelphia: Lippincott Williams & Wilkins.

evolve   **Did you remember to check out the bonus material on the Evolve website and the CD-ROM, including NCLEX®-Examination Style Review Questions, Open-Book Quizzes, and Chapter Review Audio Podcasts?**

http://evolve.elsevier.com/Black/medsurg

CHAPTER 75

Management of Clients with Hematologic Disorders

Linda H. Yoder

This chapter provides information about disorders that affect red blood cells (erythrocytes), white blood cells (leukocytes), the spleen, platelets, and clotting factors. Priorities of nursing care center on the lack of oxygenated blood flow and risk of hemorrhage. Leukemia and lymphoma are discussed in Chapter 79.

DISORDERS AFFECTING RED BLOOD CELLS

THE ANEMIAS

Anemia is a clinical condition that results from an insufficient supply of healthy red blood cells (RBCs), the volume of packed RBCs, and/or the quantity of hemoglobin. Hypoxia results because the body's tissues are not adequately oxygenated. Not a disease in itself, anemia reflects a number of underlying pathologic processes leading to an abnormality in RBC number, structure, or function. When anemia is identified, further testing must be done to determine its cause.

Risk Factors, Etiology, and Classification

Anemia can arise from primary hematologic problems or can occur as a secondary consequence of defects in other body systems. Those at risk for developing anemia differ with the various etiologies. Because the prevalence of anemia increases with age, adults 65 and older are at particular risk; the estimated prevalence in this age-group is 20%. Aging cannot be assumed to be the cause of anemia, however, without excluding other reversible causes. Hereditary anemias have several cultural and ethnic considerations. The prevalence of sickle cell disease and thalassemia is high in African Americans. Thalassemia is also high in people of Mediterranean

origin. Pernicious anemia rates are high in Scandinavians and African Americans.

The anemias are classified by either the etiology or the morphology of the specific anemia. Anemia is caused in one of three ways: (1) decreased production of healthy RBCs, (2) increased RBC destruction (hemolysis), or (3) loss of blood. A number of underlying problems lead to these conditions. Etiologic categories are listed in Box 75-1.

Morphologic classification is based on erythrocyte size, shape, and color. Normal RBCs are shown in Figure 75-1, A. Morphologic categories include normocytic/normochromic (normal size and color), macrocytic/normochromic (large size, normal color), and microcytic/hypochromic (small size, pale color). Some anemias are named for the abnormal shape of the RBCs. For instance, normal RBCs have a biconcave shape, and sickle cell anemia has sickle-shaped RBCs (Figure 75-1, B); spherocytosis, a hereditary disorder leading to hemolytic anemia, has spherical-shaped RBCs.

Table 75-1 gives a general overview of blood components, including composition, compatibility, special considerations, and outcomes. (See Table 74-6 on p. 2001 for other abnormalities of erythrocytes and their associated conditions.)

---

evolve Web Enhancements

Concept Map Understanding DIC and Its Treatment

Ethical Issues in Nursing Should Parents Who Are Jehovah's Witnesses Have the Right to Refuse a Life-Saving Transfusion for Their Child?

Be sure to check out the bonus material on the Evolve website and the CD-ROM, including free self-assessment exercises. **http://evolve.elsevier.com/Black/medsurg**

BOX 75-1   Etiologic Categories of Anemia

DECREASED RBC PRODUCTION

Defective DNA Synthesis
- Cobalamin/vitamin B_{12} deficiency
- Folic acid deficiency

Decreased Hemoglobin Synthesis
- Iron deficiency
- Thalassemia (decreased globin synthesis)
- Sideroblastic anemia (failure to completely form heme)

Decreased Number of Erythrocyte Precursors
- Aplastic anemia
- Anemia of leukemia and myelodysplasia
- Chronic diseases

INCREASED RBC DESTRUCTION (HEMOLYSIS)

Intrinsic
- Abnormal hemoglobin (sickle cell anemia)
- Enzyme deficiency
- Membrane abnormalities

Extrinsic
- Physical trauma
- Antibodies (autoimmune and isoimmune)
- Infectious agents
- Toxins (snake venom; chemotherapy)

BLOOD LOSS

Acute
- Trauma
- Blood vessel rupture

Chronic
- Gastritis
- Hemorrhoids
- Menstruation

Pathophysiology

Transport of oxygen is impaired with anemia. Hemoglobin is lacking or the number of RBCs is too low to carry adequate oxygen to tissues and hypoxia develops. The body attempts to compensate for tissue hypoxia by increasing the rate of RBC production, increasing cardiac output by increasing stroke volume or heart rate, redistributing blood from tissues of low oxygen needs to tissues with high oxygen needs, and shifting the oxygen-hemoglobin dissociation curve to the right to facilitate the removal of more oxygen by the tissues at the same partial pressure of oxygen.

Clinical Manifestations

Manifestations accompanying anemia are due primarily to the body's response to hypoxia. The manifestations differ depending on the severity and speed of blood loss, the chronicity of the anemia, the client's age, and the presence of other disorders. Hemoglobin (Hb) levels are used to determine the severity of anemia. Clients with mild anemia (Hb levels of 10 to 14 g/dl) are usually asymptomatic. If manifestations do occur, they typically follow strenuous exertion. Clients with moderate anemia (Hb levels of 6 to 10 g/dl) may suffer from *dyspnea* (shortness of breath), palpitations, *diaphoresis* (profuse perspiration) with exertion, and chronic fatigue. Some clients with severe anemia (Hb levels <6 g/dl), such as those with chronic renal failure, may be asymptomatic because their anemia develops gradually; others may have significant clinical manifestations involving multiple body systems. Additional manifestations are due to the underlying etiology; a careful work-up can provide clues to the etiology. Table 75-2 on p. 2009 lists typical manifestations of severe anemia by body system. The Translating Evidence into Practice feature on p. 2011 provides additional information on how anemia can cause fatigue and compromise quality of life.

The RBC count, hemoglobin level, and hematocrit value confirm the presence of anemia. A bone marrow specimen may be required to confirm the type of anemia. A peripheral blood smear (RBC indices) is needed to determine the size of the RBC. Table 75-3 on p. 2010 identifies laboratory study findings in various anemias.

■ **FIGURE 75-1   A,** Normal red blood cells. **B,** Sickle cell anemia. (Magnification ×875.) Note the elongated and sickle-shaped cells. (*From Rodak, B. [2002]. Hematology: Clinical principles and applications [2nd ed.]. Philadelphia: Saunders.)*

TABLE 75–1 Blood Components

	Whole Blood	Red Blood Cells	Platelet Concentrates	Fresh Frozen Plasma	Cryoprecipitate	Granulocyte Concentrates	Plasma Derivatives	Coagulation Factor Concentrates
Composition	RBC, plasma, plasma proteins (globulins, antibodies), 63 ml of anticoagulant-preservative	RBC with CPDA-1 solution (anticoagulant-preservative only), final hematocrit no higher than 80% (80% RBC, 20% plasma) RBC with 100 ml of additive solution, final hematocrit about 55%-60%	Single-unit platelets contain minimum of 5.5×10^{10} (1 unit) platelets in 50-70 ml of plasma obtained by separating platelet-rich plasma from 1 unit of fresh whole blood; 6-10 units may be pooled for 1 transfusion Single-donor platelets contain minimum of 3.0×10^{11} platelets (6 units) obtained from single donor by use of automated cell separator during apheresis; recipient exposed to fewer donors, which decreases complications	91% water, 7% protein (globulin, antibodies, clotting factors), and 2% carbohydrates Freezing within 8 hr of collection preserves all clotting factors	Each unit contains 50% of antihemophilic factor VIII (80-120 units) and 20-30% of factor XIII originally present in a unit of whole blood, as well as vWF and 250 mg of fibrinogen suspended in 10-20 ml of plasma	Unit obtained by granulocytaphresis contains minimum of 1×10^{10} granulocytes, variable amounts of lymphocytes (usually <10%), 30-50 ml of RBC and 100-400 ml of plasma, and 6-10 units of platelets; platelets can be separated from the unit if granulocyte recipient is not thrombocytopenic	*Albumin:* 96% albumin, 4% globulin and other proteins extracted from plasma; available as a 5% solution, oncotically equivalent to plasma, and also concentrated 25% solution *Plasma protein fraction:* 83% albumin and 17% globulins extracted from plasma; less pure than albumin and has higher degree of contamination with other plasma proteins; in 5% solution only	*Factor VIII:* Lyophilized concentrate containing large quantities of factor VIII; prepared from large pools of donor plasma, but heat treatment during fractionation process significantly reduces risk of transmitting viral disease *Factor IX:* Lyophilized concentrate containing large quantities of factor IX; also contains factors II, VII, and X; product prepared from large pools of donor plasma, but heat treatment during fractionation process significantly reduces risk of transmitting viral disease
Volume	500 ml/unit	250-350 ml/unit 350-400 ml/unit	50-70 ml/unit 200-400 ml/unit	200-250 ml	5-10 ml/unit	200-400 ml with platelets 100-200 ml without platelets	Albumin: 250 and 500 ml (5%); 50 and 100 ml (25%)	Multiple-dose vial

ABO/Rh Compatibility							
ABO type of donor should be identical with recipient's Rh− blood can be given to an Rh− or Rh+ recipient	A can match with A or O; B can match with B or O; O can match only with O; AB can match with A, B, or O Rh− blood can be given to either Rh+ or Rh− recipient	Whereas platelets have no ABO or Rh antigens, they are suspended in 200-400 ml of plasma containing donor antibodies and a small number of RBC ABO and Rh compatibility is recommended	A can match with A or AB; B can match with B or AB; AB can match only with AB; O can match with A, B, AB, or O Rh− and Rh+ blood can be given to either Rh+ or Rh− recipient	Cryoprecipitate contains no RBC and a small volume of plasma ABO crossmatching not needed, and plasma compatibility preferred but not required	Granulocytes contain a significant number of RBC and plasma; therefore ABO of donor should be identical with recipient's Rh− components may be transfused to Rh+ recipient	Antibodies destroyed during processing; therefore compatibility not a factor	Antibodies destroyed during processing, so compatibility not a factor
Special Considerations							
Whole blood transfusion is rarely indicated Treatment with specific blood components is usually recommended	RBC may be viscous; thus 0.9% saline may be added to achieve optimal flow rates For some clients, leukocyte depletion filter may be used to prevent complications	Because platelet concentrates contain few RBC, crossmatch testing is not required Plasma ABO and Rh compatibility is recommended, especially when total volume of transfusion exceeds 150-200 ml Only filters specially designed for platelet transfusion should be used	Plasma carries same risk of disease transmission as does whole blood If only volume expansion is required, products of choice are crystalloid or colloid solutions, such as saline or albumin Plasma contains no RBC, and Rh compatibility and crossmatching are not required ABO compatibility must be confirmed before administration	Single units of cryoprecipitate may be pooled into 1 container by blood collection center If individual bags are issued, 0.9% saline may need to be added to rinse residual cryoprecipitate from bags and tubing	Granulocytes have short survival (<24 hr); infuse as soon as possible Granulocyte concentrates contain significant number of RBC; pretransfusion testing recommended Increased incidence of febrile, nonhemolytic reactions with granulocyte transfusions; infuse slowly, observe client closely; premedication with antihistamine, acetaminophen, steroids advised	PPF and albumin cannot transmit hepatitis or HIV infection; pasteurization process used to prepare products destroys such viruses Hypotension has been associated with rapid infusion of PPF; 25% albumin can cause significantly increased blood pressure because of its ability to draw fluid into intravascular space	Factor VIII and factor IX assays should be performed at appropriate intervals to assess response Factor VIII concentration lacks vWF and should not be used in treatment of von Willebrand's disease

(Continued)

TABLE 75-I Blood Components—Cont'd

	Whole Blood	Red Blood Cells	Platelet Concentrates	Fresh Frozen Plasma	Cryoprecipitate	Granulocyte Concentrates	Plasma Derivatives	Coagulation Factor Concentrates
						Do *not* administer amphotericin B within 4 hr of granulocyte transfusion to avoid pulmonary insufficiency		Client will develop hemostasis because of increased levels of factor VIII and factor IX activity
Outcomes	Prevention or resolution of hypovolemic shock and anemia. In a nonbleeding adult, 1 unit of whole blood should increase hematocrit by 3% and hemoglobin by 1 g/dl	Resolution of manifestations of anemia. In a nonbleeding adult, 1 unit of RBC should increase hematocrit by 3% and hemoglobin by 1 g/dl	Prevention or resolution of bleeding caused by thrombocytopenia or platelet dysfunction. 1 unit should raise peripheral platelet count 5000-10,000/mm³ if underlying cause is resolved or controlled. Efficacy of platelet transfusion can be determined by obtaining platelet counts at 1 hr and 18-24 hr after infusion	Treatment effectiveness is assessed by monitoring coagulation function (specifically PT and PTT) or by specific factor assays	Correction of factor VIII, vWF, factor XIII, and fibrinogen deficiency; cessation of bleeding in uremic clients. Laboratory values required to assess effectiveness of treatment	Improvement in or resolution of infection. Increase in peripheral WBC count not usually seen after granulocyte transfusion in adults, although increase may be seen in children. An improvement in clinical condition because of resolving infection is only measure of treatment effectiveness	Client will acquire and maintain adequate blood pressure and volume support	

CPDA-I, Citrate-phosphate-dextrose-adenine; *FFP,* fresh frozen plasma; *HIV,* human immunodeficiency virus; *IV,* intravenous; *PPF,* plasma protein fraction; *PT,* prothrombin time; *PTT,* partial thromboplastin time; *RBC,* red blood cells; *vWF,* von Willebrand's factor; *WBC,* white blood cells.

TABLE 75–2 Clinical Manifestations of Severe Anemia (Hb <6 g/dl)

Area	Clinical Manifestations
General	Pallor, severe fatigue, malaise, weakness, lightheadedness, fever, exertional dyspnea, headache, vertigo, sensitivity to cold, weight loss
Skin (integumentary)	Pallor (anemia); jaundice (HA); dry skin, brittle nails, spoon-shaped concave nails with longitudinal ridges (IDA)
Eyes	Blurred vision (anemia, PV); sclera jaundice and retinal hemorrhage (HA)
Ears	Vertigo, tinnitus
Mouth	Smooth, glossy, bright red, and sore tongue (PA, IDA)
Lungs	Dyspnea, orthopnea (anemia, HbS crisis)
Cardiovascular	Tachycardia, palpitations, murmurs (particularly systolic), angina, hypertension, cardiomegaly, intermittent claudication, heart failure, MI
Gastrointestinal	Anorexia; dysphagia (IDA); abdominal pain (HbS, HA); hematemesis (vomiting blood), tarry stools (HA); hepatomegaly, splenomegaly
Genitourinary	Amenorrhea and menorrhagia (IDA); decreased fertility (anemia); hematuria (HA)
Musculoskeletal	Back pain (HA); sternal tenderness and severe bone and joint pain (HbS)
Nervous system	Headache, confusion (anemia); peripheral neuropathy, paresthesias, and loss of balance (PA); mental depression, anxiety, coping difficulties (especially life-threatening conditions)

AP, Aplastic anemia; *HA*, hemolytic anemia; *HbS*, sickle cell anemia; *IDA*, iron deficiency anemia; *MI*, myocardial infarction; *PA*, pernicious anemia; *PV*, polycythemia vera.

OUTCOME MANAGEMENT

Medical Management

The goals of care for clients with anemia include (1) alleviating or controlling the causes, (2) relieving the manifestations, and (3) preventing complications. Treatment varies in intensity and duration because some anemias resolve after blood transfusion, others resolve within a few weeks or months, and still other forms require lifelong intervention.

Alleviate and Control the Causes

Depending on the etiology of the anemia, interventions may include (1) supplemental iron therapy, (2) nutritional therapy, (3) surgery to repair sites of hemorrhage, (4) splenectomy, (5) removal of toxic agents that cause aplasia, (6) stem cell or bone marrow transplantation, (7) corticosteroid therapy, and (8) immunosuppressive therapy.

Relieve Manifestations

Oxygen Therapy. Oxygen therapy may be prescribed for clients with severe anemia because their blood has a reduced capacity for oxygen. Oxygen helps to prevent tissue hypoxia and lessens the workload of the heart as it struggles to compensate for the lower Hb levels.

Erythropoietin. Subcutaneous injections of erythropoietin can be given to treat anemias of chronic disease because this drug increases the production of RBCs. For this drug to be effective, the client must have bone marrow capable of producing RBCs and sufficient nutrients for the production of RBCs.

Iron Replacement. Iron can be given to augment oral intake in cases where the need for iron is immediate or the demands are beyond dietary measures (e.g., pregnancy). The oral form of iron should be used because it is inexpensive and convenient. It is usually given for mild forms of anemia. The medications of choice are ferrous sulfate (Feosol) or ferrous gluconate (Fergon), 200 to 325 mg orally in three or four doses a day, with or after meals. Taking iron with vitamin C or orange juice aids in the absorption of iron. Clients usually receive iron supplements for at least 6 months for repletion of the body stores. Side effects may include nausea, vomiting, constipation or diarrhea, and blackened stools. The consequences of iron replacement therapy are outlined in the Integrating Pharmacology feature on p. 2012.

Blood Component Therapy

Traditionally the term *blood transfusion* has meant the administration of whole blood. The term now has a broader meaning because of the ability to administer specific blood components such as platelets or plasma. Blood component therapy is used to manage hematologic diseases and some surgical/therapeutic procedures depend on blood product support. Blood products obtained from another person are called homologous. Those reinfused from the client's own blood are called autologous.

Risks Associated with Homologous Blood Transfusions. Blood transfusions should not be used as a substitute for a specific therapy to treat the underlying cause of the anemia.

TABLE 75–3 Laboratory Study Findings in Erythrocytic Disorders

	Iron Deficiency	Thalassemia Major	Cobalamin B$_{12}$	Folic Acid Deficiency	Aplastic Anemia	Hemolytic Anemia	Sickle Cell Anemia	Polycythemia Vera	Hemachromatosis
RBC count	–	N to –	–	–	–	–	–	+	+
Hb/HcT	–	– (beta trait +)	–	–	–	–	–	+	+
RBC	Mic/H	Mic/H	Mac/N	Mac/N	N/N	N/N			
Morphology		Target cells	Hypersegmented Polymorphonuclear Leukocytes	Hypersegmented polymorphonuclear leukocytes		Fragmented Bizarre shape	Sickle cell Target cell	Few cells N/N	
Reticulocyte	N or –	–	–	–	–	+	+		
Platelets	N or –	–	+	+	N		+	+	
MCV	–	–	– to N	– to N	N			+	
MCH	–	–	+	+	N		+	+	
MCHC	–	–	+	+	N	+ with spherocytosis >36			
Serum iron	–	+	– with malabsorption			+	N or +	–	+
TIBC	+	+	–			–	N or –	–	+
Serum ferritin	–	–							+
Bilirubin	N or –	+				N or + – Indirect bilirubinemia	+		
Marrow aspirate	Absence of hemosiderin		Megaloblasts	Megaloblasts	– Aplastic: remaining cells normal Myelodysplastic: remaining cells abnormal			Hyperplastic	
Other	– Transferrin saturation	Hb electrophoresis Amniocentesis	– Serum vitamin B$_{12}$ + Schilling	– Serum folate	– WBC	– Folate	+ HbS on Hb electrophoresis – Haptoglobin + Fibrinogen + Urobilinogen + Stercobilinogen Amniocentesis	– Serum erythropoietin + Serum B$_{12}$ + Fibrinogen + WBC (neutrophils)	+ Transferrin saturation Liver biopsy: +iron stores Genetic test to detect *HFE* gene mutation

+, Increase or positive; –, decrease or negative; *Hb*, hemoglobin; *Hb/HcT*, hemoglobin/hematocrit; *HbS*, sickle hemoglobin; *HFE*, hemachromatosis gene symbol; *Mac/N*, macrocytic/normochromic; *MCH*, mean corpuscular hemoglobin; *MCHC*, mean corpuscular hemoglobin concentration; *MCV*, mean corpuscular volume; *Mic/H*, microcytic/hypochromic; *N*, normal; *N/N*, normocytic/normochromic; *RBC*, red blood cell; *TIBC*, total iron-binding capacity; *WBC*, white blood cell.

TRANSLATING EVIDENCE INTO PRACTICE

Fatigue and Quality of Life

One of the most debilitating manifestations of anemia is profound fatigue that significantly affects the client's quality of life. A growing body of literature documents that fatigue not only is often overlooked and undertreated but also is considered an inevitable sequela of disease and treatment to be endured. Most of the research into fatigue and its management has occurred in the cancer model; however, manifestations accompanying fatigue in the ill client are endemic to all client populations. For example, clients with anemia experience classic clinical manifestations of profound fatigue, dyspnea, shortness of breath, pallor, weakness, and below normal Hb serum blood levels.[1,2]

Only recently have researchers found that fatigue is so far reaching that it is known to decrease the quality of life in the four domains of living: physical, psychological, social, and spiritual well-being. The correlation between fatigue and physical well-being is well-known but not always well understood. Clients most often report they cannot keep pace with their normal activities of functioning as a parent, work at their jobs, exercise, or have energy for pleasurable activities such as going to the movies or visiting friends.[1-4]

Psychological well-being is affected by emotional distress, fears of the unknown, the inability to concentrate, forgetfulness, and the notion that their disease is worsening. Cognitive dysfunction secondary to cancer treatment is only beginning to be explored.[4,5] Studies suggest that women with cancer who have been treated with adjuvant therapy show cognitive dysfunction 2 years after treatment.[6] The cognitive functions that appear to be affected by chemotherapy include verbal and short-term memory, verbal fluency, and concentration.[6] A randomized study about the effect of the use of epoetin alfa on cognitive function, fatigue, and quality of life in women with breast cancer who had received adjuvant or neoadjuvant chemotherapy found that less fatigue and better quality of life were seen in the epoetin alfa arm than in the placebo arm during chemotherapy.[7] However, in a longitudinal study of breast cancer clients, the strongest predictor for fatigue was poor mental health.[8]

Social well-being affected by fatigue is manifested in the client's reluctance to attend support groups or attend community activities because of the profound fatigue. Clients find themselves becoming isolated and often depressed because they must conserve their energy for the basic tasks of daily living.[1]

Finally, the spiritual well-being domain encompasses the client's concern for his or her mortality and often causes a shift in life priorities from the need to accumulate tangible goals (e.g., promotions at work, gaining more financial security) to focus on the small but joyous events of even one day (e.g., the change of seasons, gardening, or return to a religion that might have been abandoned for some years).

More research is required to understand fully the manifestations of fatigue and its enormous consequences for the client and the client's family. Although the impact of fatigue is well documented in its physical consequences, psychological, social, and spiritual consequences are only beginning to be researched. Similar to shifts in understanding and treating the manifestations of pain in a humanistic and nonjudgmental fashion, fatigue is emerging as an important manifestation to be managed by health care clinicians.[9]

Nursing research is emerging to document that all the domains of fatigue can be diminished by teaching clients and their families to practice certain behaviors.[10-12]

1. Treating anemia with erythropoietin colony-stimulating factors or RBC transfusion when appropriate
2. Promoting sleep and rest
   a. Take short naps instead of long ones.
3. Providing optimal nutritional support
   a. Eat low-fat, high-fiber meals.
4. Alternative therapies
   a. Use relaxation techniques, biofeedback, or massage therapy.
5. Energy conservation and body mechanics
   a. Wash hair in the shower, not in the tub or over a sink.
   b. Use a terry-cloth robe instead of a towel to dry off.
   c. Use a hand-held shower while sitting in the tub.
   d. Install a handrail.
6. Exercise
   a. Exercise moderately.
   b. Take walks.
7. Cognitive dysfunction
   a. Do crossword puzzles.
   b. Do jigsaw puzzles.

REFERENCES

1. Nail, L.M. (2004). Fatigue. In C.H. Yarbro, M.H. Frogge, & M. Goodman (Eds.), *Cancer symptom management* (3rd ed., pp. 47-60). Boston, Mass: Jones & Bartlett.
2. Fletchner, H., & Bottomley, A. (2003). Fatigue and quality of life: Lessons from the real world. *The Oncologist, 8*(Suppl 1), 5-9.
3. Ferrell, B.R., et al. (1996). "Bone tired": The experience of fatigue and impact on quality of life. *Oncology Nursing Forum, 23,* 1539-1547.
4. Fu, M.R., McDaniel, R.W., & Rhodes, V.A. (2005). Fatigue. In C.H. Yarbro, M.H. Frogge, & M. Goodman (Eds.), *Cancer nursing: Principles & practice* (6th ed., pp. 741-760). Boston, Mass: Jones & Bartlett.
5. Holzner, B., et al. (2002). The impact of hemoglobin levels on fatigue and quality of life in cancer patients. *Annals of Oncology, 13,* 965-973.
6. Schagen, S.B., et al. (1998). Impairment of cognitive function in women receiving adjuvant treatment for high-risk breast cancer; high dose versus standard-dose chemotherapy. *Journal of the National Cancer Institute, 90,* 210-218.
7. O'Shaughnessy, J., et al. (2002). *Impact of epoetin alfa on cognitive function, asthenia, and quality of life in women with breast cancer receiving adjuvant or neoadjuvant chemotherapy: Analysis of a 6-month follow-up data.* Presented at the 25th Annual San Antonio Breast Cancer Symposium, Dec 11-14, San Antonio, Tex.
8. Nieboer, P., et al. (2005). Fatigue and relating factors in high-risk breast cancer patients treated with adjuvant standard or high-dose chemotherapy: A longitudinal study. *Journal of Clinical Oncology, 23*(33), 8296-8304.
9. National Cancer Institute (NCI). Fatigue. Retrieved 04/18/07 from www.cancer.gov/cancertopics/pdq/supportivecare/fatigue/HealthProfessional/.
10. Crimpton, B. (1995). Symptom management: Loss of concentration. *Seminars in Oncology Nursing, 11,* 279-288.
11. Swartz, A. (1998). Patterns of exercise and fatigue in physically active cancer survivors. *Oncology Nursing Forum, 25*(3), 1-12.
12. Young-McCaughan, S. (2006). Exercise in the rehabilitation from cancer. *MEDSURG Nursing: The Journal of Adult Health, 15*(6), 384-388.

INTEGRATING PHARMACOLOGY

Oral and Parenteral Iron Replacement Therapy

Iron deficiency anemia is often treated with oral ferrous sulfate and, more recently, with parenteral iron administration. Although oral iron is an over-the-counter medication, its frequent side effects often cause the client to discontinue the medication. Nurses can teach clients the nature of the side effects and how to manage them. You may teach your client to drink ginger tea or suck on ginger candy to avoid or minimize nausea and vomiting. Stool softeners to avoid constipation are also important. Conversely, IV iron replacements, long discouraged because of the danger of anaphylactic shock, are being replaced by newer preparations with fewer adverse effects. Because of the history of adverse events, fear of administering the IV iron agent warrants discussion of this new preparation.

Functional iron deficiency may develop in clients with normal ferritin levels but low transferrin saturation (<20%) because of the inability of the client to mobilize iron stores rapidly enough to support increased erythropoiesis. Some factors that influence the absorption of iron include the dose, iron stores, the degree of erythropoiesis, diet, and the route of administration. In iron deficient clients, the amount of iron absorbed can be 10% to 30% and as high as 60%. In healthy clients, about 5% to 10% of dietary iron is absorbed. In clients with iron deficiencies such as iron deficiency anemia, oral or IV iron replacement may be needed.

Oral iron supplementation therapy is preferred, provided the client can adequately absorb iron and can tolerate oral therapy. If no blood is lost, the usual adult daily dose of elemental iron is in the range of 180 to 200 mg in divided doses preferably taken on an empty stomach. Oral iron supplementation is available as ferrous sulfate, ferrous gluconate, or ferrous fumarate. These iron salts are absorbed equally; however, they differ in the amount of elemental iron they contain. Ferrous gluconate, ferrous sulfate, and ferrous fumarate provide about 11%, 20%, and 33% of elemental iron, respectively. All three iron salts are known to be associated with GI side effects such as nausea and vomiting, constipation, diarrhea, or dark coloration of feces.

Some clients may inadequately respond to oral iron supplementation because of poor absorption, noncompliance, or intolerance of therapy.

Parenteral iron therapy does not induce GI side effects, thereby reducing client noncompliance, and it is convenient to take; however, parenteral iron preparations are also known to be associated with hypersensitivity reactions, including anaphylactic reactions and local adverse reactions. Three different IV iron preparations are currently available for iron deficiency anemia: (1) iron dextran, (2) sodium ferric gluconate, and (3) iron sucrose. All iron dextran products are indicated for use as a second-line therapy only after clients fail oral iron therapy.

SAFETY

⚠

ALERT

A homologous transfusion can have significant risks for the client. These risks include hemolytic transfusion reactions and the possibility of contracting infectious diseases such as human immunodeficiency virus (HIV)/acquired immunodeficiency syndrome (AIDS), hepatitis B or C, graft-versus-host disease (GVHD), cytomegalovirus (CMV), Epstein-Barr virus (EBV), and West Nile virus. 🪔 Transfusions should be avoided in clients who might be candidates for bone marrow transplantation (BMT) (e.g., those with aplastic disorders or sickle cell disease) because transfusion decreases the probability of cure. In addition, clients who may have multiple antibodies against RBCs and those with autoimmune antibodies are at a higher risk for complications because of the complexities of obtaining crossmatched donor blood. Considering the potential risks, alternative interventions should be taken when possible to reduce the need for transfusion. The Joint Commission (TJC) requires that all blood transfusions be evaluated to confirm that clear medical indications for the transfusion exist and that the client responds as expected.

Because of the risks associated with blood transfusion, a client's informed consent is required. Blood is administered only after informed consent is obtained. Consent includes an explanation to the client or family member, if necessary, of medical indications for homologous transfusion and its benefits, risks, and alternatives. Documentation of informed consent may consist of a form in the medical record stating that this information was presented in a manner understandable to the client or family member (e.g., the risks of and alternatives to blood transfusion were explained, and the client consented). If no family member is available or time does not allow, place a note to this effect in the chart.

Transfusion Reactions Associated with Homologous Blood Transfusions. A blood transfusion reaction is an adverse reaction to blood component therapy that can range from mild symptoms to a life-threatening condition. Complications can be acute or delayed, occurring days to years after a transfusion. Acute reactions may be immunogenic or nonimmunogenic. Immunogenic reactions include allergic, acute hemolytic, and anaphylactic reactions as well as fever; nonimmunogenic reactions include circulatory overload and septicemia. Table 75-4 details acute transfusion reactions.

Delayed reactions may include a delayed hemolytic reaction, hepatitis B, hepatitis C, HIV, GVHD, iron overload, and other infections and agents such as CMV, EBV, human T-cell leukemia virus type 1 (HTLV-1, the organism

TABLE 75–4   **Acute Transfusion Reactions**

Reaction	Cause	Clinical Manifestations	Management	Prevention
Immunogenic				
Allergic Incidence: 1%	Sensitivity to foreign proteins in plasma	Urticaria, flushing, itching (no fever)	Administer antihistamines as directed If manifestations mild and transient, transfusion may resume	Treat prophylactically with antihistamines
Febrile, nonhemolytic Incidence: 0.5-1%	Sensitization to donor white blood cells, platelets, or plasma proteins	Fever and/or pulmonary symptoms Sudden chills and fever (rise in temperature >1° C [1.8° F]), headache, flushing, anxiety, muscle pain	If fever and/or pulmonary manifestations occur, *do not* resume transfusion Give antipyretics as prescribed; avoid aspirin thrombocytopenic clients	Consider leukocyte-poor blood products (filtered, washed, or frozen) if fever occurs more than once
Acute hemolytic Incidence: 1:25,000 Fatal: 2:1 × 10^6	Infusion of ABO-incompatible RBCs	Chills, fever, low back pain, flushing, tachycardia, tachypnea, hemoglobinuria, hemoglobinemia, hypotension, vascular collapse, bleeding, acute renal failure, shock, cardiac arrest, death	Treat shock Send blood samples for serologic testing, and send urine samples to lab Maintain blood pressure Give diuretics as prescribed to maintain urine flow Insert indwelling catheter or measure hourly output Dialysis may be needed	Meticulously verify recipient from sample collection to transfusion
Anaphylactic Incidence: 1:150,000	Infusion of IgA proteins to IgA-deficient recipient who has developed anti-IgA antibodies	Anxiety, urticaria, wheezing progressing to cyanosis, shock, and possible cardiac arrest	Do not transfuse additional RBCs Initiate CPR if indicated Have epinephrine ready for injection (0.4 ml of a 1:1000 solution subcutaneously)	Give blood components from IgA-deficient donors or remove *all* plasma by washing
Nonimmunogenic				
Circulatory overload Estimated incidence: 1:10,000 (not usually reported to blood bank)	Infusion of blood at a rate too rapid for size, cardiac status, or clinical condition of recipient	Cough, dyspnea, pulmonary congestion (rales), headache, hypertension, tachycardia, distended neck veins	Place client in upright position with feet in dependent position Administer diuretics, oxygen, and morphine as prescribed Phlebotomy may be required	Adjust transfusion volume and flow rate on basis of client size and clinical status If slow transfusion will exceed 4 hr, request that unit be aliquoted into smaller volumes
Septicemia Incidence: very rare	Transfusion of component contaminated with microorganism	Rapid onset of chills, high fever, vomiting, diarrhea, marked hypotension, and shock	Treat manifestations and administer antibiotics, IV fluids, vasopressors, and steroids as directed Obtain culture of client and blood containers	Collect, process, store, and transfuse blood according to industry standards Infuse within 4 hr of starting time

CPR, Cardiopulmonary resuscitation; *Ig,* immunoglobulin; *IV,* intravenous; *RBC,* red blood cells.

that causes malaria), and West Nile virus. Table 75-5 provides details on delayed transfusion reactions.

Autologous Blood Transfusion. *Autologous* blood transfusion is the alternative to *homologous* (random) transfusion and should be considered. Clients who do not have leukemia or bacteremia should be offered the option of donating their own blood before a scheduled surgical procedure when there is a reasonable expectation that blood will be required. Although the risk-benefit ratio should be evaluated, experience to date indicates that even clients with heart disease and other high-risk conditions tolerate donating blood well. The elimination of disease transmission, alloimmunization, and other potential transfusion complications makes this a reasonable option for many surgical clients.

Autologous donations can be made every 3 days if the donor's Hb level remains at or above 11 g/dl. For the blood to be maintained in a liquid state, donations should begin within 5 weeks of the transfusion date. Donations should cease at least 3 days before the date of transfusion.

Transfusion Procedures

Confirm Physician's Order. The physician's order for transfusion should specify blood component, volume, and rate of infusion.

Obtain Venous Access. The gauge of the needle used for transfusion varies with the product being infused.

When packed RBCs weighing less than 300 g are infused, a 19-gauge or larger needle is needed to achieve the maximal flow rate. If a smaller-gauge needle must be used, the RBCs can be diluted with 0.9% saline. To prevent hemolysis, add no solution other than normal saline to blood components.

SAFETY

⚠

ALERT

TABLE 75–5   Delayed Transfusion Reactions

Reaction	Clinical Manifestations
Delayed hemolytic	Fever, mild jaundice, decreased hemoglobin and hematocrit
	Occurs as early as 3 days or as late as several months but usually 7 to 14 days posttransfusion as result of destruction of transfused RBCs by alloantibodies not detected during crossmatch
	Generally, no acute treatment is required, but hemolysis may be severe enough to warrant further transfusions
	Although uncommon, severe complications such as renal failure and DIC have been reported
Hepatitis B*	Elevated liver enzymes (AST and ALT), anorexia, malaise, nausea and vomiting, fever, dark urine, jaundice
	Incubation period is about 8-12 wk, although it may extend to 6 mo or longer
	Usually resolves spontaneously within 4-6 wk; chronic carrier state can develop and can result in permanent liver damage
	Treat symptomatically
Hepatitis C*	Similar to hepatitis B, but manifestations are usually less severe
	Approximately 20% of acute infections resolve
	Chronic liver disease and cirrhosis may develop
	Before introduction of anti-HCV test, accounted for 90%-95% of all posttransfusion hepatitis
	Treat symptomatically
Human immunodeficiency virus (HIV)	Can be asymptomatic for up to several years or may develop flu-like manifestations within 2-4 wk
	Later manifestations include weight loss, diarrhea, fever, lymphadenopathy, thrush, *Pneumocystis* pneumonia
Iron overload	Heart failure, dysrhythmias, impaired thyroid and gonadal function, diabetes mellitus, arthritis, cirrhosis
	Excess iron is deposited in heart, liver, pancreas, and joints, causing dysfunction
	Commonly occurs in clients receiving >100 units for chronic anemia over a period of time
	Prevented by iron chelation therapy [deferoxamine (Desferal)], which chelates and removes accumulated iron via kidneys, may be administered IV or subcutaneously
	Treat clinical manifestations
Graft-versus-host disease	Fever, rash, diarrhea, nausea, jaundice, hepatitis
	Result of replication of donor lymphocytes (graft) in transfusion recipient (host)
	Onset 3-30 days posttransfusion
	No effective therapy available
	To prevent, irradiate blood products before transfusion in at-risk recipient
	Some believe that irradiated blood products are indicated for first-degree family members' donations also
Other	Other infectious diseases and agents may be transmitted via transfusion, including cytomegalovirus, HTLV-1, and those causing malaria

ALT, Alanine aminotransferase; *AST*, aspartate aminotransferase; *HTLV-1*, human T-cell leukemia virus, type 1; *IV*, intravenous; *RBCs*, red blood cells.
*New cases of transfusion-related hepatitis B and C are not common.
From Blaney, K.D., & Howard, P.R. (2000). *Basic and applied concepts of immunohematology.* St. Louis: Mosby; and Hillyer, C.D., et al. (2003). *Blood banking and transfusion medicine: Basic principles and practice.* Philadelphia: Churchill Livingstone.

Components that contain a significant volume of plasma or other diluent can be safely infused at a rapid rate through smaller-gauge needles or catheters.

SAFETY ALERT

A central venous catheter is an acceptable access option for blood transfusion; however, a large volume of refrigerated blood infused rapidly into the ventricle of the heart may cause cardiac dysrhythmias. Warming the blood can reduce the risk of this complication.

Another issue of concern is the use of multilumen catheters, which may allow blood to mix with incompatible solutions and medications as they exit the catheter tips. Experience indicates that the circulation achieved through a blood vessel that is suitable for central line placement results in rapid mixing of fluids. As a result no harmful effects have been reported.

Preparation for the Infusion. Blood-bank regulations state that refrigerated components may not be returned to inventory if they have been warmed to more than 10° C (50° F). To meet this requirement, most transfusion medicine services consider 30 minutes to be the maximal allowable time out of monitored storage. To avoid wasting a scarce commodity, certain procedures should be performed before blood is requested: (1) An intravenous (IV) catheter appropriate for transfusing the requested component should be functional, flushed with normal saline, and maintained at a keep-vein-open (KVO) rate. (2) Vital signs should then be taken and recorded. (3) The existence of a fever may be a reason for delaying the transfusion. In addition to masking a possible manifestation of an acute transfusion reaction, fever can also compromise the efficacy of platelet transfusions. (4) Premedication may be required if the client has a history of adverse reactions. In many cases, febrile reactions can be prevented by administering acetaminophen. A history of allergic reactions may warrant prophylactic administration of antihistamines (e.g., diphenhydramine HCl). To ensure effectiveness, administer oral medication 30 minutes before the transfusion is started. IV medication may be given immediately before the transfusion is initiated.

Confirm Blood Acceptability

SAFETY ALERT

The most crucial phase of transfusion is confirming product compatibility and verifying the client's identity. The name and identification number of the recipient must be provided, and a permanent record of this information must be maintained in the blood bank. To avoid delivery to the wrong client, blood should be transported to only one client at a time.

An estimated 90% of transfusion reactions are due to improper product-to-client identification. Before going to the client's bedside, verify ABO and Rh compatibility, usually by comparing the bag label with the medical record and forms issued from the blood bank. Also check the bag label to ensure that the correct component has been issued, and check for the expiration date.

Inspect the unit for leaks, abnormal color, clots, excessive air, and bubbles. Check carefully for important labels (e.g., "autologous" or "directed") or instructions (e.g., "use a leukocyte-depleting filter"). Cellular components (whole blood, RBCs, and platelets) for an immunosuppressed client should be clearly marked "irradiated."

At the bedside compare the name and number on the identification bracelet with the tag on the blood bag. If applicable, check the secondary identification system. The American Association of Blood Banks recommends that two qualified people perform this critical step.

Infuse Blood. Most blood products should be infused through administration sets designed specifically for this use. The set usually contains a 170-micrometer filter designed to trap fibrin clots and other debris that accumulates during blood storage. Most standard filters can filter 4 units of blood. Tubing is available in two basic configurations: straight or Y-type. The use of Y-type tubing simplifies the process of adding normal saline to RBCs and provides ready access to a saline flush if the transfusion must be interrupted. Straight tubing usually has a medication injection site a few inches from the needle. If an adverse reaction develops, a KVO saline drip initiated at this site maintains patency of the IV line but avoids exposure to the 30 to 50 ml of blood remaining in the tubing and filter.

SAFETY ALERT

To reduce the risk of septicemia, change the administration set every 4 to 6 hours or according to institution policy.

Blood warmers may be used to prevent hypothermia, which can be induced by rapid infusion of large volumes of refrigerated blood.

Monitor During the Transfusion

SAFETY ALERT

The first 10 to 15 minutes of any transfusion are the most critical. If a major ABO incompatibility exists or a severe allergic reaction such as anaphylaxis occurs, it is usually evident within the first 50 ml of the transfusion. Therefore it is recommended that the transfusion begin slowly and that the client be closely monitored. If no evidence of a reaction is noted within the first 15 minutes, flow can be increased to the prescribed rate.

Before leaving the client unattended, instruct the client to report anything unusual immediately. Take and record vital signs before the transfusion begins, after the first 15 minutes, and every hour until 1 hour after the transfusion has been discontinued. Check vital signs immediately if the client displays any untoward manifestations.

The recommended rate of infusion varies with the blood component being transfused. Components such as platelets, plasma, and cryoprecipitate may be infused rapidly, but you must take care to avoid circulatory overload, especially with geriatric clients and clients with cardiac disease. To avoid the risk of septicemia, infusions should not exceed 4 hours. If the client's size or medical condition does not allow infusion within 4 hours, the unit may be split into smaller aliquots in the blood bank. Regulatory agencies require complete documentation of the transfusion, including identification of personnel starting and ending the transfusion, unique product number, and outcome (e.g., "no reaction noted").

SAFETY

⚠️

ALERT

Watch for Transfusion Reaction

Exposure to foreign blood elements may mediate immunologic and nonimmunologic reactions affecting all major body systems. Consider any unusual manifestation that occurs during or immediately after a transfusion a potential reaction. Monitor unconscious clients closely because manifestations of a reaction may be inhibited in the unconscious state. The acute reactions most frequently seen are described in Table 75-4.

Although treatment may vary depending on the manifestations, certain standard procedures must be followed when a reaction is suspected. It is important to know your institutional policies regarding management of transfusion reactions; however, the following steps are indicated:

1. Stop the transfusion.
2. Keep the IV line open with normal saline.
3. Contact the client's physician and the blood bank.
4. Recheck identifying tags and numbers on the blood and the client.
5. Monitor vital signs and urine output.
6. Treat symptoms per physician's orders.
7. Save blood bag and tubing and send it to the blood bank for examination with transfusion reaction report.
8. Complete transfusion reaction report.
9. Obtain blood and urine samples, in accordance with institutional policy.
10. Document client's condition and all actions taken in the client's record and transfusion reaction forms per hospital policy.

Nursing Management of the Medical Client

Assessment. The general nursing care of clients with anemia includes adequate assessment by the nurse to help identify the cause of the anemia and client education deficits relating to the underlying illness causing the anemia. You can help in the diagnosis by taking a complete health history focusing on the elements outlined in Chapter 74. Client and family teaching is extremely important in treating the anemias because most of the care takes place in an outpatient clinic or in the client's home. Help the client and family to become knowledgeable about self-care in both preventing and treating anemia.

Diagnosis, Outcomes, Interventions

Diagnosis: Activity Intolerance and/or Fatigue. Write the nursing diagnosis as *Activity Intolerance and/or fatigue related to decreased blood supply or low hemoglobin levels as evidenced by complaints of fatigue and lack of energy, dyspnea, pallor, tachycardia, and cognitive dysfunction.*

Outcomes. The client will tolerate activity as evidenced by being able to sit up without fatigue, dyspnea, pallor, or tachycardia; walking increasing distances; and participating in activities of daily living such as bathing, dressing, grooming, and feeding, to the greatest extent possible.

Interventions. Teach the client about the condition, self-care activities, lifestyle changes, nutritional needs, and medication information. Inform the client that iron salts are gastric irritants and should always be taken with or after meals. Liquid iron preparations should be well diluted and taken through a straw (undiluted liquid iron stains teeth). The client can avoid constipation, commonly seen during iron therapy, by eating a high-fiber diet and using stool softeners or laxatives as required. 🪔 Avoid consumption of coffee and tea with iron; absorption is hampered by the tannates. See the discussion of transfusion therapy procedures earlier in the chapter if a blood transfusion is required.

Evaluation. Resolution of anemia requires time. When packed RBCs are used, anemia will be corrected immediately. When oral iron preparations are used, it takes weeks for anemia to resolve; the client will thus need assessments at intervals to monitor the progress of therapy. Ultimate prognosis depends on how well the underlying disease is resolved or controlled; progress in this regard should also be monitored.

Modifications for Older Clients

Older adults have an especially high prevalence of anemia, primarily attributable to poor nutrition with decreased intestinal absorption of iron, often resulting from debilitation or depression or both. Anemia in older clients is often asymptomatic or mistakenly diagnosed as normal aging changes. Such manifestations include fatigue, confusion, angina, ataxia, and heart failure. 🪔 Special care should be taken to provide a thorough work-up of these clients to determine whether an etiology exists that might be reversible and thus treatable.

ANEMIA CAUSED BY DECREASED ERYTHROCYTE PRODUCTION

Normally the production and destruction of erythrocytes are in equilibrium in the body. In situations where the production of erythrocytes is decreased, anemia results. Decreased production may be due to (1) decreased synthesis of normal hemoglobin, as seen in iron deficiency anemia, thalassemia, and sideroblastic anemia; (2) defective DNA synthesis, as seen in megaloblastic anemia resulting from cobalamin (vitamin B_{12}) and folate deficiency; or (3) reduced availability of erythrocyte precursors, as seen in aplastic anemia and anemia of chronic disease.

IRON DEFICIENCY ANEMIA

Iron deficiency anemia (IDA) is a chronic, hypochromic, microcytic anemia resulting from an insufficient supply of iron in the body. Without iron, hemoglobin concentration in the RBCs is reduced and the cells are unable to oxygenate the body's tissues adequately, resulting in anemia.

Etiology and Risk Factors

The National Academy of Sciences recommends an iron intake of 15 mg daily for women and 10 mg daily for men. An average diet supplies the body with about 12 to 15 mg/day of iron, of which only 5% to 10% (0.6 to 1.5 mg) is absorbed. IDA is associated with either inadequate absorption or excessive loss of iron. Major risk factors for IDA include (1) insufficient dietary intake of iron, (2) blood loss, (3) impaired absorption of iron, and (4) excessive demands for RBC production as a result of hemolysis. It is important to know the population groups that have a higher association with these risk factors.

Populations in poor countries and people whose diets lack meat are at particular risk for iron deficiency anemia from insufficient dietary intake of iron, the most prevalent hematologic disorder worldwide. About 30% of the world's population has this anemia. It is an important international economic concern for two reasons: (1) the diminished capacity of individuals to perform physical labor and (2) the impact on the growth, development, and learning of infants and children. Alcoholics are also at increased risk because of poor diets.

Other populations may have increased requirements for iron intake at particular times in their lives. The amount of iron normally absorbed daily is sufficient for meeting the needs of healthy men and women past childbearing age, but it does not meet the additional needs of menstruating and pregnant women, infants, children, adolescent females, older adults (>65 years),

regular blood donors, and those on strict vegetarian diets. These groups are at a sufficiently high risk to warrant consideration of prophylactic iron therapy. In the United States women have twice the prevalence of IDA as men (8% versus 4%) because of the excess needs of women of childbearing age. An estimated 4% to 8% of premenopausal women are iron deficient. The most common etiologies of IDA for women are menstruation and pregnancy. Normal iron excretion is less than 1 mg daily. Iron is excreted in urine, sweat, bile, and feces and from the skin in desquamated cells. The average woman loses another 15 mg monthly during menses. About 500 mg of iron is lost during a normal pregnancy.

Older adults are a population at risk for IDA. An estimated 20% of adults more than 65 years of age suffer from this condition. Economic constraints, poor dentition, lack of interest in food preparation, malnutrition, and increased rates of chronic disease and cancers, particularly of the gastrointestinal (GI) tract, contribute to a higher prevalence rate in older adults.

Blood loss is the most common etiologic factor in men, and the GI tract is the most common site. Hemorrhage may result from peptic ulcers, hiatal hernia, gastritis, gastroesophageal reflux disease (GERD), cancer, hemorrhoids, diverticula, Crohn's disease, ulcerative colitis, or salicylate poisoning. It may also be related to gastritis from the use of aspirin, steroids, or nonsteroidal anti-inflammatory drugs (NSAIDs). Bleeding from the GI tract is usually chronic and occult (too small to be seen). A chronic blood loss of as little as 2 to 4 ml daily can result in iron deficiency anemia because every 2 ml of blood contains 1 mg of iron. The body can compensate for such losses to some degree by excreting less than 0.5 mg of iron daily rather than the normal 1 mg.

Malabsorption of iron may result from alterations in the mucosa of the duodenum and proximal jejunum (as in chronic diarrhea, malabsorption syndromes such as sprue and celiac disease, gastrectomy, and removal of the proximal small bowel), resulting in IDA. Tannates (in tea and coffee), carbonates, the chelating agent ethylenediaminetetraacetic acid (EDTA), and the medicinal antacid magnesium trisilicate all hinder nonheme iron absorption. Eating starch and clay, which occurs in some cultures, also leads to malabsorption.

Pathophysiology

Iron is present in all RBCs as heme in Hb; heme accounts for two thirds of the body's iron. Iron is also vital for the metabolic processes of DNA synthesis and electron transport. Iron concentration in the body is regulated by the absorptive cells in the proximal small intestine; these cells alter iron absorption to match body losses of iron intake. Errors in this balance also lead to anemia. Fortunately the GI tract can increase its absorption of iron from 10% daily to about 20% to 30% daily. In this way, the body often compensates for diminishing iron stores resulting from inadequate iron intake or excessive iron loss. The other one third of the body's iron (non-heme) is stored in the form of ferritin, an iron-phosphorus-protein complex that contains about 23% iron.

Clinical Manifestations

In mild cases of iron deficiency anemia, the client is asymptomatic; in more severe cases, assessment reveals the general manifestations of anemia, including fatigue; headache; dyspnea; palpitations; pallor in the face, palm of the hand, nail bed, and mucous membranes of the mouth and conjunctiva; *angular stomatitis* (inflammation of the mucosa of the mouth), *glossitis* (inflammation of the tongue), and *cheilitis* (inflammation of the lips); and brittle nails. Laboratory results characteristic of iron deficiency anemia are presented in Table 75-3. Once a diagnosis of iron deficiency anemia is confirmed, studies are conducted to find the cause. Radiographic studies (GI tract series), stool examination for occult blood, esophagoscopy, gastroscopy, and sigmoidoscopy are commonly done to identify the site of blood loss. Correction of the underlying problem (malnutrition, alcoholism, hemorrhage) must follow so that the deficiency does not recur.

OUTCOME MANAGEMENT

Management of IDA focuses on (1) diagnosis of and correction of the underlying cause and (2) treatment through diet and supplemental iron preparations. Supplemental iron is administered to increase iron available in the blood. Monitoring the client to ensure compliance is important. An increase in reticulocytes 5 to 10 days after initiation of iron therapy can document a positive response. Clients with increased daily needs should be given supplemental iron prophylactically (during pregnancy) (see the Integrating Pharmacology feature on Oral and Parenteral Iron Replacement Therapy, p. 2012).

Diets high in iron should be planned with the client and family members. The nurse plays a key role in this intervention. Clients and families may need to be taught the elements of high-iron diets, both in terms of the food to be consumed (Box 75-2) and with respect to how it should be prepared to increase (cooking in iron skillets) or prevent the loss of dietary iron.

THALASSEMIA

Thalassemia is an autosomal-recessive genetic disorder that results in inadequate normal Hb production. Whereas IDA affects heme synthesis, thalassemia disrupts the synthesis of globin.

Etiology and Risk Factors

Thalassemia is frequently found in people of Mediterranean, African, and Southeast Asian origin. Individuals

---

BOX 75-2 Foods High in Iron, Vitamin B₁₂, and Folic Acid

EXCELLENT SOURCE OF IRON

Almonds, asparagus, bran, beans, Boston brown bread, carrots, cauliflower, celery, chard, dandelions, egg yolk, graham bread, kale, kidney, lettuce, liver, oatmeal, oysters, soybeans, spinach, and whole wheat. (Cook foods in iron pans.)

GOOD SOURCE OF IRON

Apricots, beef, beets, cabbage, cornmeal, cucumbers, currants, dates, duck, goose, greens, lamb, molasses, mushrooms, oranges, parsnips, peanuts, peas, peppers, potatoes, prunes, radishes, raisins, rhubarb, pineapple, tomatoes, and turnips.

VITAMIN B₁₂

Red meats, especially liver, dairy products, and eggs.

FOLIC ACID

Asparagus, broccoli, spinach, lettuce, lemons, bananas, melons, green leafy vegetables, fish, legumes, whole grains, liver, organ meats, mushrooms, strawberries, milk, eggs, yeast, wheat germ, kidney beans, beef, potatoes, dried peas and beans, and nuts. (Foods should not be cooked with excessive heat or large amounts of water.)

---

who inherit an alpha-gene(s) have alpha-thalassemia, the most common of the thalassemias; the alpha-trait (*heterozygous* state) is asymptomatic in about 30% of African Americans. Those who inherit just one beta-gene (*heterozygotes*) have thalassemia minor, also called *thalassemia trait,* the carrier state of thalassemia major. Those who inherit both beta-genes (*homozygotes*) have thalassemia major, which results in a profound and life-threatening anemia.

Pathophysiology

In alpha-thalassemia, there is a mutation in the alpha-globin gene(s). In thalassemia minor, one beta-globin gene is mutated, leading to minor disruptions in beta-globin synthesis. In thalassemia major, a mutation exists in both beta-genes, resulting in significant impairment of beta-globin synthesis, marked reduction in hemoglobin production, and profound anemia. Hemolysis results from an imbalance in the alpha- and beta-globin chains, which are normally paired. The excess unpaired alpha- or beta-globin chains aggregate and form a precipitate that damages RBC membranes, leading to intravascular hemolysis.

Clinical Manifestations

Individuals with alpha-thalassemia may have very mild anemia and are typically asymptomatic. Those with thalassemia minor have clinical manifestations of mild to moderate anemia. These disorders may be undiagnosed for several years.

Individuals with thalassemia major are diagnosed early in life because the lack of Hb becomes quickly apparent. Affected children appear normal at birth because fetal Hb contains no beta-globin; however, in the first few months of life, as Hb synthesis switches from fetal to adult form, manifestations of severe anemia begin to appear. The children also have pain, failure to thrive, frequent infections, diarrhea, splenomegaly, hepatomegaly, jaundice from RBC hemolysis, and bone marrow hyperplasia.

Fetal diagnosis for a specific type of thalassemia can be made through amniocentesis. Molecular diagnostic tests can determine whether a mutation is present after 8 weeks of gestation.

OUTCOME MANAGEMENT

Thalassemia minor usually does not require treatment. For thalassemia major, the treatment goals are to provide adequate normal Hb for erythropoiesis and to alleviate the effects of iron overload. Chronic transfusions are administered to correct the anemia with the targeted Hb level at 9 to 10 g/dl. Iron chelation with deferoxamine is necessary to prevent iron overload. Iron supplementation should not be used. Because RBCs may be sequestered in the spleen, a splenectomy may be necessary to decrease transfusion requirements. Genetic counseling and testing for families should be encouraged.

MEGALOBLASTIC ANEMIAS

Megaloblastic anemias are a group of disorders caused by impaired DNA synthesis resulting in defective, large RBCs (megaloblasts). They are caused by deficiencies of vitamin B_{12} (cobalamin) and folic acid.

Cobalamin/B_{12} Deficiency (Pernicious Anemia)

Pernicious anemia is an autoimmune disorder characterized by the absence of intrinsic factor (IF) in gastric secretions, leading to malabsorption of cobalamin (vitamin B_{12}). Pernicious anemia has been incorrectly used to describe any cobalamin deficiency, but it is actually only one cause of inadequate cobalamin.

Etiology and Risk Factors

Pernicious anemia (PA) is the most prevalent form of vitamin B_{12} deficiency in the United States and Canada (Box 75-3). It is associated with gastric atrophy and loss of IF as well as a rare genetic autosomal-recessive disorder (congenital pernicious anemia) in which IF is lacking without gastric atrophy. Ninety percent of people with PA have antibodies that react specifically against the parietal gastric cells where IF is produced; 60% have anti-IF antibodies. It occurs more often in families of PA clients and is associated with human leukocyte

---

BOX 75-3 Causes of Cobalamin and Folate Deficiencies

- Insufficient dietary intake: Rare with cobalamin (Cbl) but common with folate
- Drugs that impede absorption in the stomach: Purine analogs (azathioprine), pyrimidine analogs (5-fluorouracil [5-FU]), ribonucleotide reductase inhibitors (hydroxyurea), anticonvulsants (phenytoin), and oral contraceptives
- Drugs that impair uptake in the ileum: Nitrous oxide, cholestyramine, *p*-aminosalicylic acid, neomycin, metformin, phenformin, and colchicine
- Genetic disorders causing defects in the ileal receptors of intrinsic factor (IF): Imerslund-Graesbeck syndrome, hereditary transcobalamin II (TCII) deficiency
- Impaired absorption resulting from medications, cancers, gastrointestinal (GI) diseases, or surgical resection of the terminal ileum
- GI disorders: Gastric atrophy, gastrectomy, gastric stapling, bypass for pancreatic insufficiency of protease, which releases Cbl from R-protein binders so that Cbl can bind with IF
- Zollinger-Ellison syndrome

---

antigen (HLA) types A2, A3, and B7 and in type A blood groups. PA typically arises in people between 40 and 70 years of age with peak incidence around 70 years of age. It is more prevalent in people of Celtic and Scandinavian ancestry.

Pathophysiology

Cobalamin (B_{12}) and folate deficiency is believed to lead to attenuated production of DNA. In normal metabolism cobalamin (extrinsic factor) is released from its ingested protein-bound state by gastric acid. It is bound to IF, a glycoprotein produced by parietal cells of the gastric lining, and absorbed in the terminal ileum. It is then bound to the protein transcobalamin II (TCII) and transported to storage sites in the liver. Problems with any of these steps can lead to deficiency. Without cobalamin, DNA synthesis and cell replication are impaired. RBC precursors (erythrocytes/reticulocytes) do not divide normally, and large, poorly functioning RBCs are created. Production of myelin on nerves is greatly affected, also resulting in neurologic deterioration.

Clinical Manifestations

The major manifestations of PA are low Hb, hematocrit (HcT), and RBC levels. The diagnosis is based on the presence of anemia, GI manifestations (weight loss, appetite loss, nausea, vomiting, abdominal distention, diarrhea, constipation, steatorrhea), and neurologic disorders (paresthesias of feet and hands, poor gate, memory loss, cognitive problems, depression). Laboratory studies include a complete blood count (CBC), peripheral smear, reticulocyte count, Hb and HcT levels, serum iron level, total iron-binding capacity, and serum ferritin levels (see Table 75-3). In addition the Schilling test is the definitive test for PA and is used to diagnose and determine the cobalamin deficiency. The Schilling test measures the absorption of orally administered radioactive vitamin B_{12} (tagged with cobalt 60) before and after parenteral administration of IF. Gastric secretion analysis to check for the presence of free HCl is another important test. Most clients with pernicious anemia have low-volume gastric secretions with high pH and free hydrochloric (HCl) acid levels. These findings do not change, even after the administration of histamine, which normally stimulates gastric secretion.

OUTCOME MANAGEMENT

Medical Management

Cobalamin/Vitamin B_{12} Therapy

Clients with PA need both immediate treatment and lifelong therapy with maintenance vitamin B_{12}. The standard treatment is parenteral administration of cobalamin (cyanocobalamin or hydroxocobalamin) at 1000 mcg daily for 2 weeks and then weekly until the HcT returns to normal. Once the HcT is normal, monthly injections for life are required. An intranasal form of cyanocobalamin (Nascobal) is available as a nasal gel that is self-applied weekly. The response to the injections is usually quick and dramatic, often occurring within 24 to 48 hours. Within 72 hours, reticulocytes begin to increase; by the end of the first week, the total RBC count rises significantly. Cardiovascular involvement usually lessens with improved erythropoiesis. Peripheral nerve function may improve, but long-term neuromuscular complications are rarely reversed with treatment.

Iron Supplements

Additionally the client may need oral or IV iron supplements if the Hb level fails to rise in proportion to an increased RBC count. Iron deficiency may be an etiologic factor in pernicious anemia and must be corrected if it is present. Iron deficiency anemia can also develop during treatment of pernicious anemia. Injections of vitamin B_{12} may cause a rapid regeneration of RBCs that depletes iron. As a result the Hb level remains low, although the total RBC count rises. Once the acute stage of the illness is past, the client with pernicious anemia must undertake a lifelong program of maintenance therapy. Monthly injections of vitamin B_{12} are needed to avoid relapse. Encourage the client to eat a diet high in folic acid and iron to supplement the medication used to treat the anemia (see Box 75-2).

If the cause involves altered absorption of vitamin B_{12}, nutritional supplements are useless. If the disease is related to decreased intake of the vitamin, a diet high in vitamin B_{12} is encouraged.

Digestants

Digestants may be given to enhance the metabolism of vitamins; for example, HCl acid may be diluted in water and given with meals during the first few weeks of vitamin B_{12} therapy.

Treat Neurologic Complications

Multidrug combinations of high doses of folate, cobalamin, and pyridoxine have been proposed to help prevent neurologic complications.

Nursing Management of the Medical Client

Because clients with PA must receive weekly or monthly treatment for life, the nurse plays an important role in monitoring client progress. Response to treatment should be carefully monitored with blood counts and clinical blood chemistry tests. The client must be educated about the importance of adherence to the treatment regimen on a lifelong basis if the anemia is to be controlled and about the life-threatening consequences of not doing so. The progress of neurologic complications should be continually assessed. Clients with existing neurologic problems should be monitored for and educated about the possibility of injuries attributable to diminished sensitivity to heat and pain from nerve damage. Because gastric carcinoma is commonly associated with PA, clients should be evaluated frequently for the presence of this cancer.

Folic Acid Deficiency Anemia

Etiology and Risk Factors

Anemia associated with folic acid deficiency is common. There are many causes, most of which are the same as those of vitamin B_{12} deficiency. Usually folic acid deficiency results from a diet lacking in such foods as green leafy vegetables, liver, citrus fruits, nuts, grains, and yeast. Clients with chronic alcoholism or eating disorders, such as anorexia, because of their typically inadequate diets, are particularly at risk. High levels of alcohol in the blood also partially block the response of the bone marrow to folic acid, which thereby interferes with RBC production. Hemodialysis clients have to be carefully watched for folic acid deficiency because folic acid is lost during dialysis.

Folic acid deficiency, like vitamin B_{12} deficiency, can develop with malabsorption syndromes (e.g., sprue, celiac disease, steatorrhea). Certain medications can also impede folic acid absorption and utilization.

For example, a serious anemia may develop under the following conditions:

- Long-term use of anticonvulsant medications (e.g., primidone, phenytoin, phenobarbital)
- Administration of antimetabolites (e.g., folic acid antagonists, purine, pyrimidine analogs) to clients with cancer and leukemia
- Use of certain oral contraceptives

Finally, folic acid deficiency may occur with increased demands for folate, such as during pregnancy and the growth spurts of childhood and adolescence.

Clinical Manifestations

Folic acid, like vitamin B_{12}, is necessary for DNA synthesis; unlike PA, however, folic acid deficiency does not cause neurologic manifestations. The presence of neurologic problems generally rules out folic acid deficiency as the etiology. Anemia resulting from folic acid deficiency has a slow and insidious onset. The client, often thin and emaciated, usually appears quite ill. The client's malnourished and debilitated state frequently leads to other deficiencies, for example, of iron, protein, minerals, and other vitamins. Some clients may also have an electrolyte imbalance, and neurologic manifestations may develop as a result of thiamine, calcium, or magnesium deficiency (commonly linked with alcoholism).

The megaloblastic anemia caused by folic acid deficiency is the same as that seen in pernicious anemia (see Table 75-3). The diagnosis is confirmed by blood smear and bone marrow examinations. With folic acid deficiency, the serum folate level is less than 4 ng/ml (normal: 7 to 20 ng/ml); the Schilling test finding is normal. HCl is probably present in the gastric juice. Neurologic manifestations are absent; and the client responds favorably to a therapeutic trial of 50 to 100 mg of folic acid administered intramuscularly (IM) daily for 10 days.

OUTCOME MANAGEMENT

For correction of anemia caused by folate deficiency, the client receives oral doses of folic acid 0.1 to 5 mg daily until the blood profile improves or the cause of intestinal malabsorption is corrected. Clients with malabsorption syndromes may need parenteral folic acid initially, followed by maintenance therapy with oral doses. Folic acid is administered IM in the form of folinic acid (leucovorin calcium injection). In addition, vitamin C is sometimes prescribed because it increases the role of folic acid in promoting erythropoiesis. Diets with foods rich in folic acid (see Box 75-2) and food preparation methods that ensure that folate is not destroyed are important. Lifelong monthly doses of folate may be necessary for clients with partial or total gastrectomies.

Multivitamins with folate are often prescribed for older clients. Nursing interventions are similar to those discussed for the client with PA.

ANEMIAS CAUSED BY INCREASED ERYTHROCYTE DESTRUCTION
HEMOLYTIC ANEMIA

Hemolytic anemia is an end result of conditions that lead to hemolysis. Hemolysis, the premature destruction of erythrocytes, can result from physical damage, intrinsic membrane defects, abnormal Hb, erythrocytic enzymatic defects, immune destruction of RBCs by macrophages, or hypersplenism. Anemia occurs when the bone marrow fails to replace RBCs at the rate they are destroyed.

Etiology and Risk Factors

Hemolytic anemias constitute about 5% of all anemias. Hemolysis can result from hereditary disorders or acquired hemolytic conditions. Hemolysis can happen because of problems intrinsic or extrinsic to the RBCs. Extrinsic hemolytic anemias are the most common type and are acquired. In this type of hemolytic anemia, the RBCs are normal, but damage is caused by external factors such as toxins, mechanical injury (prosthetic heart valves), or trapping of cells within the sinuses of the liver or spleen. Intrinsic hemolytic anemias are caused by defects in the RBCs themselves resulting from abnormal Hb (e.g., sickle cell disease), enzyme deficiencies that alter glycolysis (glucose-6-phosphate dehydrogenase deficiency [G-6-PD]), or RBC membrane abnormalities.

The two sites of hemolysis are either intravascular or extravascular. Intravascular destruction takes place in the circulation whereas extravascular hemolysis takes place in the liver, spleen, and bone marrow.

Clinical Manifestations

The clinical manifestations of hemolytic anemia are numerous and diverse and are due primarily to anemia, the extent of compensation, previous treatment, and the underlying cause. The client with hemolytic anemia may suffer from all the general manifestations of anemia discussed previously (weakness, fatigue). Manifestations of specific disorders may be present, such as *hemochromatosis* (bronze skin tone and diabetes), or *hemoglobinuria* (dark urine) caused by intravascular hemolysis. Renal failure may be caused by an increased load of RBC breakdown products. Jaundice is often present because of the increased destruction of RBCs, causing an elevation in bilirubin levels. The spleen and liver may enlarge because of hyperactivity.

Because of the large number of causes for hemolytic anemia, numerous laboratory tests are conducted to determine or rule out known etiologies. These include a CBC, peripheral smear and morphologic examination, RBC indices, increased red blood cell distribution width (RDW), reticulocyte count, lactic acid dehydrogenase level, serum haptoglobin level, indirect bilirubin level, and other studies suggested by the history or physical examination (see Table 75-3). Increased RBC fragility, shortened erythrocyte life span, increased fecal and urinary urobilinogen levels, and hemoglobinemia in cases of massive intravascular hemolysis are typically seen.

OUTCOME MANAGEMENT

Interventions are undertaken to counter the complications of the hemolysis and to treat the underlying disorder. Removal of the offending agent, if it is known, is key. Transfusion therapy may be necessary (packed RBCs should be administered slowly to avoid cardiac arrest). Adequate fluids are given to flush the kidneys. In addition, sodium bicarbonate or sodium lactate is administered to alkalize the urine, which decreases the likelihood of precipitation in the renal tubules. Folate acid may be given to offset the consumption of folate that results from active hemolysis. Corticosteroids (prednisone) may be indicated and iron replacement therapy may be needed for those with severe intravascular hemolysis to counter persistent hemoglobinuria. Erythropoietin is given for anemia that has resulted from renal failure. Finally, clients should be educated to recognize the manifestations of hemolysis and to seek immediate medical attention if they occur.

SICKLE CELL DISEASE

Sickle cell disease (SCD) is a group of inherited disorders of mutant hemoglobin (hemoglobin S [HbS]) that causes the characteristic sickling of RBCs. Sickling occurs only under conditions of low oxygenation. The abnormally shaped RBCs become trapped in capillaries, causing organ damage from infarcts and tissue hypoxia, or are damaged in transit, leading to severe anemia. The most common variant, *sickle cell anemia,* is an autosomal-recessive disorder in which the person is homozygous for HbS. The heterozygous form, known as *sickle cell trait,* is a much milder form of the disease and the carrier state of HbS. SCD is a lifelong condition that manifests in the first year of life and persists throughout one's life span.

Etiology and Risk Factors

Sickle cell disease is found in races of people from areas of the world where malaria is endemic, including Africa, the Mediterranean, the Middle East, and India. It is the most common form of anemia worldwide; there are more than 200 million carriers of sickle cell trait worldwide. In the United States, about 1 in 375 African Americans are affected, and 8% of African Americans carry the gene and have the sickle cell trait. It is also found, although rarely, in people of Mediterranean, Middle East, or East Indian descent. The prevalence rate is less than the incidence rate because of high early mortality. Whether an individual will have sickle cell anemia or sickle cell trait or will be free of the disorder depends on the Hb genes inherited from each parent. Figure 75-2 shows the distribution of the sickle cell gene and the inheritance pattern for the gene. Life expectancy is currently 42 years for males and 48 years for females. The leading cause of death is *acute chest syndrome.*

Pathophysiology

The genetics, molecular biology, and pathophysiology of SCD are well understood. The defective hemoglobin (HbS), when exposed to a decrease in oxygen, becomes viscous, has decreased solubility, and forms a gel-like substance containing hemoglobin crystals within the affected RBCs. These crystals clump together into long chains that form a parallel array of filaments, which disrupt the membrane, and the cell assumes a crescent or classic sickle shape (see Figure 75-1, *B*). The sickled cells become rigid, sticky, and fragile. These cells agglutinate and impede circulation in the capillaries, causing microinfarcts, tissue hypoxia, and further sickling. These responses to HbS

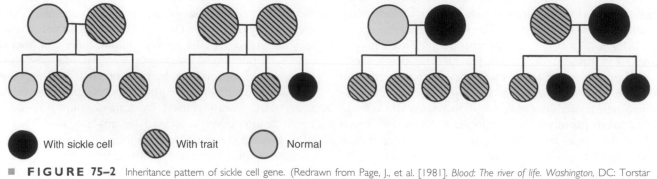

With sickle cell   With trait   Normal

■ **FIGURE 75–2** Inheritance pattern of sickle cell gene. (Redrawn from Page, J., et al. [1981]. *Blood: The river of life.* Washington, DC: Torstar Books.)

lead to the profound clinical manifestations of sickling disorders: hemolytic anemia, painful sickle cell crisis, and multiple organ system damage.

Sickle cell crisis is an acute, episodic exacerbation of the disorder instigated by reduced oxygen levels and associated crises. Exposure to low oxygen levels (low oxygen tension) triggers the process of sickling, such as living in high altitudes, flying in planes that are not pressurized, exercising strenuously (including military boot camp), acquiring respiratory tract infections, or undergoing anesthesia without receiving adequate oxygenation. A sickle cell crisis is most typically the result of vaso-occlusion in tissues and organs *(vaso-occlusive crisis)*. This crisis is the most common reason for seeking medical care. It may be induced by stress, exposure to cold water or temperature, hypoxia, or infection; most crises occur with no obvious cause.

Organ-damage syndromes are also a hallmark of SCD. Organ damage is due to increased fibrinogen levels and plasma-clotting factors (products of hemolysis) that contribute to the formation of microthrombi and the resultant microinfarcts and tissue necrosis of vital organs. The organs most vulnerable to infarction and necrosis are the brain, heart, lung, and kidneys because of their constant demand for oxygen and the bone marrow and spleen because of increased demands on these organs to replace damaged erythrocytes.

Clinical Manifestations

The typical clinical picture of SCD is associated with profound manifestations of chronic hemolytic anemia, painful sickle cell crisis, and manifestations of the various associated organ-damage syndromes. Many people with SCD are in good health and asymptomatic, except for the occasional but painful periods of vaso-occlusive crisis, the most common manifestation of SCD in adulthood.

Chronic hemolytic anemia is universally present but usually well tolerated. Clients often present with the classic manifestations of chronic anemia such as pallor of the mucosa, fatigue, and low tolerance for exercise. Jaundice is a common side effect of chronic hemolysis. Folate deficiency with resulting megaloblastic changes is also common because of increased demands for folate required for the replacement of destroyed cells.

Sickle cell crisis is predominantly a *vaso-occlusive crisis* (sometimes referred to as *pain crisis*), a serious manifestation that requires immediate medical attention. It has a sudden onset and results in severe pain in the long bones, joints, the chest, the back, and the abdomen (resembling an acute condition of the abdomen); the face may also be involved. The painful bone infarction of the *hand-foot syndrome* is often the first symptom of SCD. Fever, malaise, and leukocytosis may be present. The duration of crises is extremely variable from client to client and may range from six or more per year, to relatively few over a lifetime, to none. Individual clients

appear to have established frequency patterns. About 50% of individuals with homozygous HbS have vaso-occlusive crises.

Aplastic, hemolytic, and sequestration crises are seen much less frequently but also require immediate medical attention. *Aplastic crisis* is a serious complication caused by infection with the parvovirus B19. This virus infects red cell progenitors in the bone marrow, leading to cessation of erythropoiesis. Hb levels drop precipitously; however, this condition is self-limiting because bone marrow usually recovers in 7 to 10 days. Pain may be a presenting manifestation of this condition. *Hemolytic crisis,* resulting from the abnormal destruction of RBCs, also may be seen. This condition presents with manifestations of severe hemolytic anemia. The client is usually febrile. *Sequestration crisis* occurs when there is a sudden and massive trapping of destroyed RBC components by visceral organs; splenic sequestration is a common and painful complication.

Acute chest syndrome is the current most common cause of SCD-related mortality followed by cerebrovascular, cardiac, and pulmonary infarcts. This syndrome presents with chest pain, fever, cough, tachypnea, leukocytosis, and pulmonary infiltrates. Fat emboli resulting from bone marrow infarction are thought to be the major cause of this syndrome. It is a medical emergency and, if not treated immediately, can result in acute respiratory distress and death.

The involvement of multiple organ systems, caused primarily by microinfarcts and resulting tissue necrosis, is the basis for the complications most commonly seen in SCD. Nearly every major organ system is affected (Table 75-6). Cerebrovascular, myocardial, and pulmonary infarctions are serious complications. The most severe manifestation is stroke, typically of thrombotic origin. It is a life-threatening condition and often leads to brain-related deficits (e.g., sensory, motor, cognitive, affective) and paralysis. Heart involvement, caused by ischemia from chronic anemia and microinfarcts, usually includes hemosiderin deposits in the myocardium, systolic murmur, and dilation of the ventricles and left atrium, leading to heart failure. Pulmonary infarcts lead to pulmonary hypertension, heart failure, and eventually cor pulmonale.

Splenomegaly is evident by the latter part of the person's first year of life and may present as a sudden and painful splenic sequestration crisis. Impaired function follows, and eventually the spleen shrinks *(autosplenectomy)*. As a result immune deficiency develops, and infections are commonly seen, particularly with encapsulated microorganisms such as *Streptococcus pneumoniae*. Hepatomegaly- and infarction-related hepatopathy is often present, as are bile stones, as a result of chronic hemolysis with hyperbilirubinemia. Renal medullary ischemia may be present, resulting in a diminished capacity to concentrate urine; nephritic syndrome, although uncommon, may occur.

TABLE 75–6 Organ System Manifestations in Sickle Cell Anemia

Organ Systems	Clinical Manifestations
Central nervous system	Thrombosis- or hemorrhage-related paralysis, cerebral deficits, or death
Cardiac	Systolic murmur, cardiomegaly, heart failure
Pulmonary	Acute chest syndrome, hypertension, infiltrates, pneumonia, heart failure
Renal	Hematuria, renal failure
Spleen	Splenomegaly, splenic atrophy (autosplenectomy)
Hepatic	Hepatomegaly, gallstones
Skeletal	Hand-foot syndrome, osteonecrotic skeletal deformities, osteomyelitis, osteoporosis
Genital	Penile priapism
Optic	Hemorrhage, retinal detachment, retinopathy, blindness
Dermis	Stasis ulcers of extremities

Hyperactivity of the bone marrow can lead to spindly legs, a short trunk, and a tower-shaped skull. Skeletal manifestations of aseptic necrosis, especially on the heads of weight-bearing long bones, are due to repeated infarction of the bone, joints, and growth plates, and may lead to osteomyelitis, osteoporosis, and osteosclerosis. Related pain in the joints and long bones is common and usually severe; necrotic bone marrow with associated development of infection is often present. Skeletal and joint involvements are associated with chronic pain and disability and may require changes in lifestyle and employment. This is the single most important economic effect of the disease.

Impaired circulation leads to edema of the hands and feet and often results in leg and foot ulcers because of delayed healing and opportunistic infections. Leg ulcers are a chronic painful problem and are found in about 75% of older children and adults with the disease. Ophthalmologic manifestations may include ptosis from periorbital infarction, retinal vascular changes, and proliferative retinitis, which may result in a loss of vision. Diagnosis of HbS disease is suggested by findings of chronic hemolytic anemia and vaso-occlusive crisis and is confirmed by the existence of homozygous HbS. Typical laboratory study findings are shown in Table 75-3.

Four specific laboratory procedures demonstrate the presence of HbS in either homozygous or heterozygous clients. A stained blood smear is examined for the presence of sickle cells. A sickle slide preparation is used to detect the sickling phenomenon after deoxygenation of the blood. This test is accurate but time-consuming. The sickle-turbidity tube test is an excellent mass screening test to detect HbS. After a finger prick, blood is mixed with Sickledex solution in a test tube. Five minutes later, the specimen is observed for cloudiness, which indicates the presence of HbS. Solutions mixed with normal Hb will remain clear. If the test demonstrates HbS, it does not however differentiate SCD from sickle cell trait and other variants. The final study, Hb electrophoresis, is the diagnostic test for HbS and also differentiates SCD from sickle cell trait.

Imaging studies are also frequently used. Skeletal x-rays may show deformities and flattening of the bones and joints and areas of infarction. Magnetic resonance imaging (MRI) can demonstrate areas of avascular necrosis and distinguish between osteomyelitis and bony infarction. An abdominal sonogram can document spleen size and the presence of bile stones. Transcranial Doppler ultrasonography can identify clients at risk for stroke.

Many African Americans are unaware that they carry the sickle cell trait and that they can transmit this trait to their future children. Consequently, researchers are perfecting mass screening tests for the detection of HbS among the African-American population. Clients who have only the sickle cell trait may never be detected unless they are exposed to extremely low oxygen tension, strenuous work or exercise, or pregnancy. When exposed to extreme stressors, the client with the trait may experience manifestations of SCD.

OUTCOME MANAGEMENT

Medical Management

No safe, effective treatment is currently available. Treatment strategies are aimed at control of manifestations and management of disease complications and include management of the following: (1) vaso-occlusive crisis; (2) acute and chronic pain; (3) chronic hemolytic anemia; (4) acute chest syndrome and organ-damage syndromes; and (5) infections. Vaso-occlusive crisis is typically treated with hydration and analgesics. Intravenous fluids (normal saline or 5% dextrose in saline) are administered to correct dehydration and to replace continuing loss.

Reduce Pain

Acute pain control is best accomplished by the administration of opioids, with morphine sulfate being the drug of choice. The drug is given IV, hourly at first, until an effective dose is established; then the dose is tapered off once pain control is achieved, usually in 24 to 48 hours. Often patient-controlled analgesia (PCA) pumps are used to provide the best pain control. When the client is discharged, sustained-release morphine is given with the dose gradually reduced over several days. Morphine elixir is most commonly used for breakthrough pain. Chronic pain control is achieved with acetaminophen and NSAIDs. The NSAIDs are best for treating deep bone pain, although the use of opioids may be required. If so, codeine and hydrocodone should be tried first; morphine should be used only for more severe cases. Tricyclic antidepressants may reduce the dose of opioids because of their ability to interfere with pain perception. Many clients are depressed, and lifting depression may have a positive effect on the pain. Non-pharmacologic measures, such as physical therapy, heat and cold applications, transcutaneous nerve stimulation (TENS), hypnosis, and acupuncture, may also be used.

Pharmacologic Agents

Hydroxyurea is the only drug currently approved by the Food and Drug Administrative (FDA) for the treatment of SCD. Hydroxyurea increases the production of HbF, which retards sickling, the Hb level increases, and vaso-occlusive crises become less frequent and less severe or totally eliminated. A decrease in chronic pain and a lowering of reticulocyte levels also occur; however, hydroxyurea has been identified as a potential leukemogenic and carcinogenic agent. Data on long-term use are currently not available. Candidates for this therapy should include only those who have frequent, painful crises (>6 per year), uncontrolled pain using conservative treatment, acute chest syndrome, or a history of or high risk for stroke. For clients receiving hydroxyurea, frequent blood tests to monitor for leukopenia or thrombocytopenia are necessary.

Sodium cromoglycate has shown promising results in significantly reducing the percentage of sickle cells in venous blood. This effect appears to be retained when the blood is deoxygenated. The drug is given by inhalation or the nasal route.

Folic acid supplementation is required because all clients have a folate deficiency. Iron supplementation may also be required for menstruating women.

Blood Transfusion

Blood transfusion is indicated only for special situations such as acute chest syndrome, stroke, aplastic crisis, pregnancy, and general anesthesia. The goal of the transfusion is to reduce the concentration of HbS to 30% or less. Those receiving repeated transfusions should be given iron-chelating agents.

Acute chest syndrome is treated with analgesics, oxygen, antibiotics, and transfusion. The goal of treatment is to reduce the level of HbS to 30% or less. If the HcT is 30% or higher, an exchange transfusion is required. This entails removing 1 unit of blood, transfusing 1 unit, and repeating the process or using a continuous-flow phoresis machine.

Prevent Infection

Prevention of infection greatly improves survival. In the past, infection was the leading cause of mortality. Penicillin prophylaxis, beginning in infancy, and pneumococcal vaccination at 2 years with a booster at 5 years, controls infections of pneumoniae origin. All infections must be treated promptly with broad-spectrum antibiotics until the causative organism is identified and appropriate antibiotic therapy instituted.

Nursing Management of the Medical Client

Assessment. Assess the client for the patterns that may indicate sickle cell crisis. Assess for the ability of the family and client to cope with the disorder and their understanding of the disease and triggers of crisis.

Diagnosis, Outcomes, Interventions
Diagnosis: Acute Pain. Because of the long bone pain, joint swelling, and abdominal pain secondary to sickling crisis, one nursing diagnosis is *Acute Pain related to sickle cell crisis.*

Outcomes. The client will experience diminished pain as evidenced by verbalization of pain reduction and reliance on fewer opiates for control of pain.

Interventions. Assess for the earliest manifestations of vaso-occlusive crisis and initiate analgesics as needed and ordered. Monitor for the effectiveness of analgesia. Apply heat to joints as ordered. Provide rest periods. Administer fluids to prevent dehydration and recurrence of pain crisis. Increase oral fluid intake, and monitor intake and output.

Diagnosis: Readiness for Enhanced Self-Care. Another nursing diagnosis is *Readiness for Enhanced Self-Care related to disease, treatment, and prevention of crises.*

Outcomes. The client and family will understand the disease, treatment, and prevention of crises as evidenced by the client's and the family's statements and the absence or lessened frequency of crises.

Interventions. When educating clients about sickle cell anemia or sickle cell trait, remember the following:
1. Explain the nature of the disease and answer any related questions the client or family may have.
2. Explain that because SCD is a lifelong condition, adherence to therapy and follow-up visits is critical for effective control of the disease.
3. Encourage African-American parents to have themselves and their children tested for the presence of HbS. Advise parents-to-be that sickle cell screening procedures for the fetus and newborn are available, as is genetic counseling.
4. Advise the client and family to have routine medical examinations that include an RBC count.
5. Encourage young adults who carry HbS to ask their physician for genetic counseling before marrying or having children.
6. Alert young women with sickle cell anemia that pregnancy carries a high risk for them.

7. Explain that multiple organ system complications, particularly pulmonary, cerebrovascular, cardiovascular or renal complications, may develop. The client and family should be taught the manifestations of these complications and be advised to seek prompt medical attention if any arise.

8. Explain how to prevent crises, such as (a) avoiding lower oxygen tension and (b) taking caution against becoming dehydrated. Instruct the client and family to call a physician if vomiting, diarrhea, high fever, or any other cause of water loss develops.

The nurse plays an important role in the lifelong management of this disease. The nurse should be aware that the risk for failure to maintain the treatment regimen might be high. Many clients may be of lower socioeconomic and education levels and without adequate health insurance coverage. These factors often lead to noncompliance with treatment regimens.

Evaluation. An appropriate outcome for the client with SCD is that the disease will remain in remission as long as possible. It is impossible to prevent every crisis; however, with education and an effort by the client and family, the number of attacks can be reduced and the severity lessened.

POLYCYTHEMIA VERA

Polycythemia vera (PV), the excessive production of erythrocytes, leukocytes, and platelets, is caused by excessive activation of pluripotent stem cells in the bone marrow. It is a chronic, life-shortening, pan-hyperplastic, malignant, neoplastic marrow disorder. The inordinate mass production of these three cell lines results in (1) an increase in blood viscosity; (2) an increase in the total blood volume, which may be twice or even three times greater than normal; and (3) severe blood congestion of all tissues and organs.

Etiology and Risk Factors

In the United States, PV is relatively rare; its prevalence is 0.6 to 1.6 per million population. Although it occurs in people of every age group, its peak incidence is in the group 50 to 70 years of age. All ethnic groups are affected, and predilection of people of Jewish descent may exist. No cure is currently available. With the advent of new therapeutic regimens for management of PV, survival is now between 10 and 20 years. The most common causes of mortality are thrombosis, particularly pulmonary emboli (up to 40%), and hemorrhagic complications, especially for those with myelofibrosis or pancytopenia (up to 30%).

Pathophysiology

Polycythemia vera is due to the excessive production of a single line of clonal stem cells present in the bone marrow. These cells interfere with or stimulate normal stem cell growth and maturation. Unregulated neoplastic proliferation is thought to be the etiology. The origin of the abnormal clonal cells is currently unknown; however, these cells have an increased sensitivity to growth factors for maturation, indicating the presence of a defect in the signal pathway common to different growth factors.

Clinical Manifestations

In its early stages polycythemia usually remains asymptomatic (an increased HcT level may be an incidental finding). Presenting manifestations are usually related to hypoxia from impairment of the microcirculation caused by blood hyperviscosity secondary to hypervolemia. Manifestations include dizziness, headache, vertigo, tinnitus, visual disturbances, and angina pectoris. Other manifestations can appear depending on the body system that is affected. The client may also have a ruddy complexion and dusky, red mucosa; cardiovascular hypertension and heart failure (shortness of breath, orthopnea); increased clotting leading to stroke, myocardial infarction, or peripheral gangrene; bleeding (hemorrhage in capillaries, venules, and arterioles), which causes rupture of vessels, GI peptic ulcers, and enlargement of liver and spleen; and skeletal gout (painful swollen joints, usually the big toe) characterized by an increased uric acid level.

Diagnostic findings (see Table 75-3) include (1) an RBC count as high as 8 to 12 million/mm^3; (2) Hb level of 18 to 25 g/dl; (3) HcT greater than 54% in men and 49% in women; (4) platelet count usually increased; (5) normal arterial blood gas (ABG) values; (6) hyperplastic bone marrow; and (7) a serum uric acid level three to four times normal.

OUTCOME MANAGEMENT

A permanent cure for PV is currently unavailable, but remission of many years can be achieved. The goals of care in PV are 2-fold: reduction of (1) blood volume and viscosity and (2) myeloproliferative activity. These decreases are accomplished through phlebotomy, administration of myelosuppressive agents, and radiation therapy. Emergency phlebotomy can be used to normalize red cell mass as quickly as possible (removal of 500 to 2000 ml of blood until the HcT reaches 45%). Clients with hematocrits of less than 70% may be bled twice a week. Clients who are older or who have cardiovascular compromise or cerebrovascular complications should receive volume replacement with saline solution to avoid postural hypotension. If platelet counts are elevated, a myelosuppressive agent should be used in combination with aspirin (300 mg three times a day) to avoid thrombotic or hemorrhagic complications. Women of childbearing age should be treated only with phlebotomy. Once normal HcT levels are reached, subsequent phlebotomies should be carried out as frequently (monthly) as necessary to maintain the HcT at about 45%. Iron deficiency will likely result, but as it supervenes, RBC production will be retarded so that clients managed by phlebotomy alone may require as few as two or three phlebotomies a year.

The myelosuppressive agent hydroxyurea is commonly used in clients older than 50 years of age. ✎ Radioactive phosphorus, chlorambucil, busulfan (Myleran), and melphalan (Alkeran) have also been tried but are not indicated for long-term use because of the increased incidence of acute leukemia (17%) after 15 years. Radioactive phosphorus, however, may be used for clients older than 80 years or for those with co-morbid conditions in which life expectancy is shorter than 5 to 10 years. Anagrelide may be used in younger clients (50 to 70 years) if hydroxyurea is contraindicated. In young males, myelosuppressive therapy can lead to aspermia; use of this treatment should be carefully evaluated for these clients.

Hyperuricemia is treated with allopurinol until remission is attained; acute gouty attacks are treated with colchicine or other anti-inflammatory agents.

HEMOCHROMATOSIS

Hemochromatosis (HH), also called *iron overload disease,* is the most common genetic disorder in the United States. It is an inherited metabolic disorder that causes increased absorption of iron that is deposited in the body tissues and organs, particularly the liver, heart, and pancreas. As iron levels increase, toxicity results and leads to damage of vital organs.

Etiology and Risk Factors

Hemochromatosis is associated with a defect in a gene (*HFE)* that helps regulate the amount of iron absorbed from food. The body's normal iron concentration is 2 to 6 g. Individuals with HH accumulate between 0.5 and 10 g/year and eventually may have in excess of 50 g. Individuals who inherit a defective gene from each parent (*homozygous)* may develop the disease. Those with only one defective gene from each parent (*heterozygous)* are carriers and rarely develop the disease. HH is present at birth, but manifestations seldom manifest before adulthood.

Hemochromatosis is the most common genetic disorder among Caucasians, with an incidence of 1 in 100 to 500 Caucasians of European heritage. About 0.5% (5 in 1000) of the American Caucasian population is homozygous for the disorder. About 1 person in 10 is a carrier. Men and women are equally at risk for HH, but men are five times more likely to be diagnosed than women and to have manifestations at a much younger age. Women seldom have manifestations before menopause.

Clinical Manifestations

Joint pain is the most common manifestation of HH. Other manifestations include fatigue, lack of energy, irritability, depression, loss of body hair, abdominal pain, loss of sex drive, and heart problems. Early diagnosis and treatment are critical to a positive outcome in HH. If the disease is not detected early and treated before the accumulation of iron in the body tissues, serious disorders such as arthritis, liver disease, pancreatic disease, heart complications, impotence, bronzing of the skin, and other problems can arise.

Hemochromatosis is one of the most underdiagnosed disorders. Certain blood tests can determine whether iron stores in the body are higher than normal. The transferring saturation test (TS) can calculate how much iron is bound to the protein that carries iron in the blood. The serum ferritin test shows the level of iron in the liver. ✎ If HH is suspected, a special blood test to detect the *HFE* mutation can be ordered as a definitive diagnosis. A liver biopsy is sometimes undertaken to determine how much damage the liver has sustained (see Table 75-3).

OUTCOME MANAGEMENT

Treatment is simple, inexpensive, and safe. The major goal of treatment is to rid the body of excess iron, which is accomplished with phlebotomy. Depending on the severity of iron overload, 500 ml of blood can be drawn each week for up to 2 or 3 years until iron levels return to normal limits. Then maintenance phlebotomy, usually once every 2 to 4 months for life, is initiated. Clients with HH should not take iron supplements, and dietary intake of iron may be limited. Those with liver damage should avoid alcoholic beverages. If tissue damage has occurred, specialists in the organ system involved usually treat the resulting organ system complications.

DISORDERS AFFECTING WHITE BLOOD CELLS

White blood cells (WBCs), also called *leukocytes,* are divided into two groups:

- *Granulocytes* (polymorphonuclear leukocytes)
- *Agranulocytes* (mononuclear cells)

Granulocytes, in turn, are divided into three groups: (1) neutrophils, (2) basophils, and (3) eosinophils. The names denote affinity for the dyes used in staining. Agranulocytes include lymphocytes (B and T) and monocytes.

Plasmacytes (plasma cells) are derived from B lymphocytes. Plasmacytes are formed within the bone marrow and lymph nodes and are active in producing immunoglobulins (antibodies). Leukemia and lymphoma are discussed in Chapter 79.

AGRANULOCYTOSIS

Agranulocytosis (granulocytopenia, malignant neutropenia) is an acute, potentially fatal blood dyscrasia characterized by profound *neutropenia* (a reduced number of circulating neutrophils). Because neutrophils make up roughly 93% of all granulocytes, the terms *neutropenia* and *agranulocytosis* are often used interchangeably.

Etiology and Risk Factors

Agranulocytosis is a fairly rare condition. For unknown reasons, females are much more susceptible to this condition than males, although even among females, agranulocytosis is relatively rare.

Agranulocytosis results from either inadequate neutrophil production or excessive destruction of neutrophils. The most common cause of agranulocytosis is drug or chemical toxicity or hypersensitivity. Any drug or chemical that leads to aplasia can also cause agranulocytosis. More than 75 drugs have been associated with development of agranulocytosis. Agents that also produce neutropenia, when given in sufficiently large does over time, include many cancer chemotherapeutic agents, ionizing radiation, and benzene. Agents that frequently produce neutropenia (usually only in clients sensitive to the drug) include tranquilizers (phenothiazine, chlorpromazine), antithyroid agents (thiouracil, propylthiouracil), anticonvulsants (phenytoin), antibiotics (chloramphenicol, sulfonamides), and analgesics (aminopyrine, phenylbutazone). Some of these agents (including valproic acid, carbamazepine, and beta-lactam antibiotics) inhibit myelopoiesis, whereas others induce the formation of antibodies that destroy granulocytes (antithyroid drugs, gold compounds, aminopyrine).

Additional causes include (1) anemias related to diminished erythropoiesis (aplastic and megaloblastic anemias); (2) certain diseases such as uremia, tuberculosis, typhoid fever, malaria, yellow fever, EBV, hepatitis B, CMV, and influenza; (3) ionizing radiation exposure; (4) autoimmune diseases such as systemic lupus erythematosus and rheumatoid arthritis; and (5) genetic aberrations, which may be suspected if a family history of recurrent infections beginning in childhood exists.

Pathophysiology

The exact mechanisms of neutropenia are not clearly understood. Bone marrow and the peripheral blood are the organ systems most affected in neutropenia. Neutrophils are the first blood cells to respond to an injury and constitute a swift and powerful defense against invading microorganisms through normal surveillance and phagocytosis. Failure to produce adequate numbers of neutrophils leads to a greater susceptibility to bacterial invasion, especially when the absolute neutrophil count (ANC) drops below 500/mm^3. In profound neutropenia (<100/mm^3), infection occurs in nearly 100% of cases.

Clinical Manifestations

The manifestations of agranulocytosis are a result of neutropenia. Typically the onset of this acute disease is rapid. For the first 2 or 3 days, severe fatigue and weakness occur, followed by a sore throat, ulcerations of the pharyngeal and buccal mucosa, dysphagia, high fever, weak and rapid pulse, and severe chills. The mucous membranes of the throat and mouth are particularly vulnerable. Without prompt antibiotic treatment, the disorder usually causes septicemia and death within a week.

OUTCOME MANAGEMENT

Treatment of clients with agranulocytosis involves eliminating potentially toxic agents that may be responsible for marrow suppression. Agranulocytosis caused by toxic substances is usually reversed within 2 to 3 weeks after their elimination. An allogenic bone marrow transplant (BMT) may be required for survival if agranulocytosis is not reversed when the cause is removed.

Surveillance cultures of blood, throat, sputum, urine, and stool should be taken at frequent intervals to monitor the status of infections. Broad-spectrum antibiotics are usually administered until the offending organism is identified and appropriate antibiotic therapy, along with rehydration, is initiated to treat the infection. Control of oral and gingival pain is performed with meticulous mouth care, saline rinses, and local anesthetic gels and gargles. Diet needs include soft or liquid foods until mouth and gum sores are diminished.

Treatment of agranulocytosis includes various *colony-stimulating factors*, such as granulocyte colony-stimulating factor (G-CSF), granulocyte macrophage colony-stimulating factor (GM-CSF), recombinant neutrophil cytokine filgrastim (Neupogen), and erythropoietin (EPO). These factors are given after the offending agent has been eliminated. If given before a serious infection is established, the duration of the infection is shortened and recovery hastened.

MULTIPLE MYELOMA

Multiple myeloma is a malignancy of the plasma B cell characterized by infiltration of the cells into the bone marrow, which leads to destruction of other marrow cells, destruction of the bone cortex, and the secretion by the cells of the monoclonal paraprotein (Bence-Jones).

Etiology and Risk Factors

The etiology of multiple myeloma is a neoplastic proliferation of the plasma B cells. Risk factors include an increased incidence in some families, ionizing radiation, and occupational chemical exposures. The incidence rate is 4 per 100,000 people. Men are affected twice as often as women and African Americans twice as often as Caucasians. It usually develops after the age of 40 and peaks in the sixth decade. It accounts for 1% of all malignancies and 10% of hematologic malignancies.

Pathophysiology

Multiple myeloma is characterized by an abnormal proliferation of plasma B cells. These cells infiltrate the bone marrow and produce abnormal and excessive amounts of immunoglobulin *(myeloma protein)*. Accumulation of these cells in the marrow disrupts RBC, leukocyte, and platelet production, which leads to anemia, increased vulnerability to infection, and bleeding tendencies, respectively. In addition, abnormal and excessive amounts of cytokine are produced, which plays an important role in bone destruction (lytic lesions and osteoporosis). Cell destruction leads to hypercalcemia, which can cause renal problems and failure (polyuria, hyperuricemia), GI problems (nausea, anorexia), and neurologic manifestations (confusion). Further complications include hematopoietic suppression, immunosuppression, chronic infections, proteinuria, and soft tissue masses.

Clinical Manifestations

Once manifestations appear, they typically involve the skeletal system, particularly the pelvis, spine, and ribs. The most common presenting complaint is bone pain (70%). The most common cause of the pain is pathologic fractures and bone lesions, which occur in 93% of clients over the course of the illness. Diffuse osteoporosis is common and manifests as multiple osteolytic lesions of the skull, sternum, rib cage, and spine (10% to 20% have spinal cord compression). Thirty percent of clients present with manifestations of hypercalcemia (confusion, somnolence, bone pain, constipation, nausea, and thirst); renal stones may be seen with this condition. Hyperuricemia is usually present and manifests as renal impairment/renal failure attributable to renal tubule obstruction and interstitial nephritis. Infections resulting from the high volume of monoclonal proteins, bleeding attributable to thrombocytopenia, and carpal tunnel syndrome may also be present.

A diagnosis of multiple myeloma is made with radiographic studies, bone marrow biopsy, and blood and urine examinations. Radiographic studies may reveal diffuse lesions in the bone, widespread demineralization, and osteoporosis. The CBC shows anemia, leukopenia, and thrombocytopenia. The bone marrow contains large numbers of immature plasma cells, which usually constitute 5% of the bone marrow cell population. Because of the abnormal number of plasma cells producing immunoglobulins, peripheral blood samples sent for plasma electrophoresis reveal a large amount of abnormal immunoglobulins. Another diagnostic manifestation of multiple myeloma is the appearance of Bence Jones paraprotein in a 24-hour urine test. A beta$_2$-microglobulin test is an important test because it is an overall marker of the total body tumor burden and (along with the level of renal damage) is a strong indicator of outcome. Median survival is 3 years.

OUTCOME MANAGEMENT

Currently no cure for multiple myeloma exists. Management is aimed at early recognition and treatment of complications of the disease. Clients may require hospitalization for pain management and treatment of bone-related complications. Not all clients with multiple myeloma should be treated initially. Clients who are asymptomatic are often carefully monitored until the disease progresses and then are treated with chemotherapy.

Medical Management

Suppress the Bone Marrow

If overt manifestations are present, chemotherapy is the preferred initial treatment. Some controversy exists over which chemotherapy regimen is most effective. The most commonly used regimen is melphalan and prednisone given orally for 4 to 7 days and repeated at 4- to 6-week intervals. It is well tolerated and has a 50% to 60% response rate. Other combinations of alkylating agents can also be effective. The VAD regimen of vincristine (Oncovin), doxorubicin (Adriamycin), and dexamethasone (Decadron) is used for clients who do not respond to alkylating agents and is well tolerated. Thalidomide has recently been shown to have positive results, with a 30% response rate. Leukocyte and platelet counts are monitored regularly and doses are adjusted until modest cytopenia occurs. Chemotherapy may continue for 1 to 2 years, but almost all cases recur when chemotherapy is discontinued. Interferon-alfa appears to be beneficial in prolonging the duration of remission.

Autologous bone marrow and peripheral blood stem cell transplantation in combination with high-dose chemotherapy has had a significantly higher response rate (80% versus 57%) and better 5-year event-free survival (28% versus 10%) than those treated with chemotherapy alone.

Reduce Serum Calcium Levels

Corticosteroids and hydration are used to reduce serum calcium levels. A new group of corticosteroid agents now exists for treating hypercalcemia. The most effective agent to date is pamidronate sodium (Aredia); etidronate disodium (Didronel) and gallium nitrate (Ganite) are also effective agents. Medications such as furosemide (Lasix), steroids, etidronate, gallium, or pamidronate are used to increase calcium excretion and to decrease calcium loss from bone. If the client is able, encourage activity that places stress on the long bones to increase calcium absorption.

Administer IV fluids in amounts adequate to maintain an output of 1.5 to 2 L daily. Clients with multiple myeloma usually require about 3 to 4 L of fluid per day. The client needs sufficient fluid not only to dilute the calcium overload, but also to prevent protein from precipitating in the renal tubules.

Treat Complications

Nursing care is focused primarily on management of the various complications caused by dissemination of the disease. Bone pain management can be obtained with palliative radiotherapy of localized myeloma lesions and with NSAIDs, acetaminophen, or an acetaminophen-opioid combination.

Antiemetics may be required for relief of nausea and vomiting. Small, frequent feedings may be better tolerated, and stool softeners may be routinely required. Closely monitor intake, output, and blood studies to determine the effectiveness of treatment. Weigh the client daily so that any significant loss can be noted and corrected. Measure the client's calcium level at regular intervals for assessment of the development of hypercalcemia.

Because of skeletal complications, care should be taken when moving the client because there is a high potential for pathologic fractures. Closely monitor the client's mental status. If disorientation or confusion occurs, remove sharp objects and other potentially hazardous items from the environment. The side rails should be raised, and light restraints may be required.

Teach the client and family about the manifestations of hypercalcemia and instruct them to report any manifestations immediately to the physician.

SAFETY

⚠️

ALERT

Instruct family members or significant others on how to institute safety measures to prevent falls and injuries. The client may need some assistive devices at home, such as a toilet riser and handhold bars in the bathroom.

Counseling may be needed for the client and family to deal with the eventual fatal outcome of multiple myeloma.

INFECTIOUS MONONUCLEOSIS

Infectious mononucleosis is an acute disorder that is self-limiting and usually is benign.

Etiology and Risk Factors

The cause of 85% of infectious mononucleosis-like cases is the EBV, a herpesvirus. Infectious mononucleosis should be suspected in clients 10 to 30 years of age and is most common in populations with many young adults such as college students and military personnel. The mode of transmission is primarily through saliva during close contact and the incubation period is 4 to 6 weeks.

Clinical Manifestations

The epithelial cells of the oropharynx, nasopharynx, and salivary glands are infected first before spreading to the lymphoid tissue via infected B lymphocytes. The infection is characterized by painful enlargement of the lymph nodes, numerous large lymphoblasts, lymphocytosis, sore throat, and fever. The onset of infectious mononucleosis follows an incubation period of 4 to 8 weeks. Before frank clinical manifestations occur, the person may experience fatigue, headaches, malaise, and myalgias.

Clients present with sore throat; palatal petechiae; posterior, cervical, or auricular adenopathy; or marked diffuse adenopathy and significant fatigue. Subsequently, assessment may reveal temperatures up to 39° C (102.2° F), pharyngitis, and lymphadenopathy that is more pronounced in the cervical regions. Splenic enlargement causes left upper quadrant pain. In rare cases, liver involvement may develop into a hepatitis-like syndrome. When infectious mononucleosis is severe, two complications may develop: (1) splenic rupture resulting from the infiltration of the spleen by massive numbers of lymphocytes and (2) streptococcal pharyngitis secondary to bacterial invasion of the throat.

The diagnosis of infectious mononucleosis is based on three criteria: (1) physical assessment, (2) laboratory tests (WBC with differential), and (3) tests specific for EBV antibodies (*Monospot;* heterophile antibody test). The WBC count usually ranges from 12,000 to 20,000/mm³, of which >50% are lymphocytes and 10% are atypical lymphoblasts.

OUTCOME MANAGEMENT

No specific intervention either mitigates or shortens the disease process. Because infectious mononucleosis must simply run its course, treatments are directed at control of manifestations. Symptomatic treatment is the focus of care, which includes adequate hydration, analgesics, antipyretics, and adequate rest. Bed rest should not be enforced; the client's energy level should guide appropriate activity. Aspirin is avoided in children because of the risk of Reye's syndrome; therefore nonsteroidal anti-inflammatory drugs (NSAIDs) are used to treat fever, headache, sore throat, and myalgias. Amoxicillin and ampicillin should be avoided because they may cause a morbilliform rash in clients with infectious mononucleosis. Cool sponge baths and a large fluid intake help control fever. Warm saline or 2% lidocaine solution throat gargles may relieve sore throat. Contact sports must be avoided for at least 4 weeks after the onset of clinical manifestations to reduce the risk of splenic rupture. Corticosteroids are recommended only in clients with significant pharyngeal edema that causes or threatens respiratory compromise.

Although complications sometimes develop, the prognosis for clients with infectious mononucleosis is generally excellent. During the long convalescence, the client slowly regains strength and energy although between 9% and 22% of clients report persistent fatigue or hypersomnia 6 months after infectious mononucleosis.

SPLENIC RUPTURE AND HYPERSPLENISM

Rupture of the spleen, complicated by severe hemorrhage, is the most frequent indication for splenectomy. Hypersplenism is the second most important indication for splenectomy.

Etiology and Risk Factors

Causes of splenic rupture include the following:

- Trauma (e.g., automobile accidents, bullet or knife wounds, severe blows to the spleen)
- Accidental tearing of the splenic capsule during surgery on neighboring organs
- Disease of the spleen that causes softening or damage (e.g., infectious mononucleosis and malaria)

In hypersplenism the spleen destroys, in excessive numbers, one of the blood cell types (i.e., erythrocytes, leukocytes, or platelets). Primary hypersplenism occurs in idiopathic thrombocytopenic purpura and congenital spherocytosis. Some etiologic factors associated with secondary hypersplenism include lymphomas (including Hodgkin's disease), leukemia, polycythemia vera, acute infections (including infectious mononucleosis), chronic infections, malaria, syphilis, hemoglobinopathy, and cirrhosis of the liver.

Clinical Manifestations

Manifestations of hypersplenism include moderate to massive splenomegaly, anemia, leukopenia, or thrombocytopenia and a compensatory increase in the production of the affected blood cell line by the bone marrow. Overactivity of the spleen develops either as a primary condition of unknown origin or as a condition secondary to another disease.

OUTCOME MANAGEMENT

Primary hypersplenism can be alleviated by splenectomy. Splenectomy is palliative only for clients with secondary hypersplenism because the surgery has little or no effect on the course of the primary illness. When the diagnosis is confirmed, it is important to teach the client to prevent complications associated with the specific cytopenia.

The spleen has an important role in the phagocytosis of circulating opsonized organisms. Clients are at increased risk for infection, especially during the first 3 years after surgery. The splenectomized client should be advised to seek medical treatment at the earliest manifestations of infection.

The unique functions performed by the spleen are eventually assumed by other organs; however, loss of the spleen because of the cessation of function or splenectomy does require the client to be monitored for potentially serious complications. Nursing care of the client undergoing splenectomy is generally the same as that discussed in Chapter 14 for any client undergoing surgery.

DISORDERS OF PLATELETS AND CLOTTING FACTORS

Disorders of hemostasis that affect platelets and clotting factors include (1) purpura and (2) coagulation disorders (Box 75-4). They are classified with the hemorrhagic disorders. The Terrorism Alert feature on p. 2032 discusses viruses that can cause hemorrhage.

HEMORRHAGIC DISORDERS

Normal clot formation and lysis depend on (1) intact blood vessels, (2) an adequate number of functioning platelets, (3) sufficient amounts of the 12 clotting factors (I to XIII; VI is no longer used), and (4) a well-controlled fibrinolytic system. Consequently, the four basic problems underlying hemorrhagic (bleeding) disorders are as follows:

- Weak, damaged vessels that rupture easily or spontaneously
- Platelet deficiency (*thrombocytopenia*) resulting from hypoproliferation, excessive pooling of platelets in the spleen, or excessive platelet destruction
- Deficiency or total lack of one of the clotting factors
- Excessive or insufficient fibrinolysis

The diagnosis of a hemorrhagic disorder is based on a complete health and family history, physical examination, and laboratory tests for platelet and clotting defects. The

---

BOX 75-4 Classification of Disorders of Hemostasis

PURPURA

Vascular Defect Purpura
- Familial hemorrhagic telangiectasia
- Anaphylactoid purpura (allergic purpura)
- Toxic purpura

Platelet Disorder Purpura
- Idiopathic thrombocytopenic purpura
- Secondary thrombocytopenias

COAGULATION DISORDERS
- Hemophilia
- Hypoprothrombinemia
- Disseminated intravascular coagulation (DIC)

TERRORISM ALERT

Hemorrhagic Fever Viruses

HEMORRHAGIC FEVER VIRUSES

Historically, hemorrhagic fever viruses (HFVs) refer to a clinical illness associated with fever and a bleeding disorder caused by a virus belonging to one of four distinct families: Filoviridae, Arenaviridae, Bunyaviridae, and Flaviviridae. Ebola and Marburg are in the Filoviridae family; Lassa and New World Arenaviridae are in the Arenaviridae family; Rift Valley fever is in the Bunyaviridae family; and Dengue, Omsk hemorrhagic fever, Kyasanur Forest disease, and yellow fever are in the Flaviviridae family.

The HFVs are transmitted to humans via contact with infected animal reservoirs or arthropod vectors, although the reservoirs and vectors for Marburg and Ebola viruses are unknown. The Working Group on Civilian Biodefense previously established nine features that characterize biologic agents that pose serious risks if used as biologic weapons against civilian populations. Several HFVs exhibit a number of these features and pose serious risk as biologic weapons, including Ebola and Marburg viruses, Lassa fever and New World arenaviruses, Rift Valley fever, yellow fever, Omsk hemorrhage fever, and Kyasanur Forest disease. These viruses can be spread through unannounced aerosol attacks. The overall incubation period is 2 to 21 days.

A variety of clinical manifestations follow infection with HFVs, including fever, headache, hypotension, abdominal pain, diarrhea, myalgias, skin rash, encephalitis, and eventually manifestations of progressive hemorrhaging such as conjunctival hemorrhage, petechiae, hematuria, hematemesis, and melena. DIC and circulatory shock may ensue. Therefore in the event of a bioterrorist attack with one of these agents, infected clients may have a variety of clinical presentations, complicating early detection and management.

The mainstay of treatment of HFV is supportive, with careful maintenance of fluid and electrolyte balance, circulatory volume, and blood pressure. Vasopressor support is with hemodynamic monitoring as well as mechanical ventilation and renal dialysis. IM injections, aspirin, NSAIDs, and anticoagulant therapies are contraindicated. Steroids are not indicated. No antiviral drugs have been approved by the U.S. FDA for treatment of HFVs. Ribavirin (used for treatment of chronic hepatitis C) has some in vitro and in vivo activity against Arenaviridae and Bunyaviridae but no utility against Filoviridae or Flaviviridae.

Protective measures against nosocomial transmission of HFVs include double gloves, impermeable gowns, strict hand hygiene, N-95 masks or powered air-purifying respirators, a negative isolation room with 6 to 12 air changes per hour, leg and shoe coverings, face shields, goggles for eye protection, restricted access of nonessential staff and visitors, environmental disinfection with 1:100 dilution of household bleach, and placing all clients with HFVs in the same part of the hospital to minimize exposures to other clients and health care workers.

Data from Borio, L, et al. (2002). Hemorrhagic fever viruses as biological weapons: Medical and public health management. *Journal of the American Medical Association, 287*(18), 2391-2405.

history usually offers numerous clues to the type of bleeding problem and its cause. *Petechiae* (tiny hemorrhagic spots caused by intradermal or submucosal bleeding) are usually present in vascular and thrombocytopenic purpuras. The presence of *ecchymoses* (large, blotchy subcutaneous hemorrhagic areas), *hematomas* (subdermal hemorrhage), and *hemarthrosis* (blood within the joints) points to *hemophilia;* however, ecchymoses may develop in any hemorrhagic disorder. Clients who hemorrhage severely from several areas during childbirth or a major surgical procedure may have a fibrinogen deficiency. In addition to any evidence of bleeding, search for manifestations of hepatic cirrhosis (e.g., hepatomegaly, jaundice) and splenomegaly. Laboratory studies provide the most crucial evidence for pinpointing the type and cause of a bleeding disorder.

Clients with hemorrhagic disorders need to understand (1) why they are at risk for bleeding, (2) the manifestations of bleeding, and (3) preventive measures to avoid bleeding. Those who can be managed by home health care should be referred to appropriate health care agencies. Clients with bleeding disorders should carry an identification card at all times that indicates their diagnosis, name of their physician or health care agency, and blood type.

IMMUNE THROMBOCYTOPENIC PURPURA

Immune thrombocytopenic purpura (ITP) is the most common thrombocytopenic disorder. It was previously called idiopathic thrombocytopenic purpura because its cause was unknown, but it is now clearly considered to be a hemorrhagic autoimmune disease that results in the destruction of platelets.

Etiology and Risk Factors

ITP is an acquired disorder in which circulating platelets are destroyed because of autoantibodies that bind with antigens on the platelet membrane. Although the platelets perform normally in the bloodstream, they are recognized as foreign and are destroyed by the macrophages when they reach the spleen and liver. The decrease in the number of platelets results in bruising and spontaneous bleeding into the skin and mucous membranes (purpura). Platelets normally survive 8 to 10 days within the circulation; with ITP, however, platelet survival is as brief as 1 to 3 days or less. ITP may be acute or chronic; in most cases, the course is one of remissions and exacerbations that, if untreated, may continue for years. Chronic ITP occurs most commonly in women between 20 and 40 years of age.

Clinical Manifestations

Clinical manifestations include petechiae, ecchymosis, epistaxis, bleeding from the gums, and easy bruising. Women may have extremely heavy menses or bleeding between periods.

Diagnostic findings that confirm the presence of ITP include the following:

- A platelet count below 100,000/mm^3
- Prolonged bleeding time with normal coagulation time (all coagulation factors are present and normal)
- Increased capillary fragility as demonstrated by the tourniquet test
- Positive platelet antibody screening
- Bone marrow aspirate containing normal or increased numbers of megakaryocytes

Complications of ITP include (1) spontaneous cerebral hemorrhage, which proves fatal in 1% to 5% of clients with ITP; (2) severe hemorrhages from the nose, GI tract, and urinary system; (3) bleeding into the diaphragm, which can result in pulmonary complications; and (4) nerve pain, extremity anesthesia, or paralysis resulting from the pressure of hematomas on nerves or brain tissues.

OUTCOME MANAGEMENT

Idiopathic thrombocytopenic purpura is treated with high-dose corticosteroids to inhibit the macrophage ingestion of the antibody-coated platelets. Plasmapheresis is sometimes used as short-term therapy until the steroid therapy takes effect. If the client is actively bleeding or requires surgery, IV gamma-globulin can be used to increase the platelet count.

If the client does not have a sustained remission, splenectomy may be needed. In 60% to 80% of cases, removal of the spleen results in complete and permanent remission. Danazol (Danocrine) has been used with success in some clients. Immunosuppressive therapy used in refractory cases includes vincristine, vinblastine (Velban), azathioprine (Imuran), and cyclophosphamide.

Nursing care of clients at high risk for bleeding is discussed in Chapter 79.

COAGULATION DISORDERS

Coagulation disorders stem from a defect in the clotting mechanisms. One or more of the clotting factors (I-XIII) is depleted or absent. The important coagulation disorders discussed here are (1) disseminated intravascular coagulation (DIC) and (2) the hemophilias. See Figure A&P17-6 on p. 1982 for an explanation of the coagulation cascade.

DISSEMINATED INTRAVASCULAR COAGULATION

Disseminated intravascular coagulation is a complex syndrome of activated coagulation that results in bleeding and thrombosis. It is basically a loss of balance between the clotting and lysing systems in the body caused by the simultaneous presence of thrombin and plasmin. Too much thrombin tips the balance toward the prothrombic state, resulting in thrombosis; too much plasmin triggers excessive clot lysis *(fibrinolysis),* in which clotting factors are consumed to such an extent that generalized bleeding occurs. This concept is referred to as *consumptive coagulopathy.* In DIC these seemingly contradictory states of excessive thrombosis and excessive lysis occur simultaneously.

Etiology and Risk Factors

The causes of DIC are many. Four categories of causative factors are (1) infection, (2) tissue coagulation factors traveling into the circulation, (3) damage to the vascular endothelium, and (4) stagnant blood flow. Infection is the leading cause (e.g., gram-negative septicemia, typhoid fever, Rocky Mountain spotted fever, viremia, parasites). Conditions that may lead to DIC are listed in Box 75-5. The key to managing DIC is treatment of the underlying cause/disease.

Pathophysiology

Excessive clotting can be precipitated through extrinsic or intrinsic coagulation pathways (see Figure A&P17-6). The extrinsic pathway is a response to massive tissue damage (e.g., burns or trauma); the intrinsic pathway is a response to damaged blood vessels (endothelium). Both release substances that activate thrombin, which in turn activates fibrinogen. This results in deposition of fibrin throughout the microcirculation. The formation of fibrin is triggered by increased production of thrombin, the suppression of anticoagulation mechanisms, and delayed removal of fibrin because of impaired fibrinolysis.

Platelet aggregation or adhesiveness is increased, enabling fibrin clots and microthrombi to form in the brain, kidneys, heart, and other organs; microinfarcts and tissue necrosis ensue. RBCs become trapped in the fibrin strands and are destroyed (hemolysis). The resultant sluggish circulation of blood reduces the flow of nutrients and oxygen to the cells. Platelets, prothrombin, and other clotting factors are consumed in the process, which compromises coagulation and predisposes to bleeding.

Excessive clotting activates the fibrinolytic mechanism, which causes the production of fibrin degradation products. Fibrin degradation products act to inhibit platelet clotting functions, which causes further bleeding. Ultimately, with lysis of clots and depletion of clotting factors,

BOX 75-5 Conditions That May Precipitate Disseminated Intravascular Coagulation

- Shock
- Cirrhosis
- Purpura fulminans
- Glomerulonephritis
- Acute fulminant hepatitis
- Acute bacterial and viral infections (septicemia)

CONDITIONS THAT MAY CAUSE THE RELEASE OF PLATELET FACTOR III

- Fat emboli
- Snakebites

Hemolytic processes caused by

- Infection
- Transfusion reactions
- Immunologic disorders

Tissue damage caused by

- Trauma
- Heatstroke
- Extensive burns
- Transplant rejections
- Surgery—particularly if extracorporeal circulation was used
- Glomerulonephritis
- Acute anoxia
- Prosthetic devices

CONDITIONS THAT MAY CAUSE THE RELEASE OF THROMBOPLASTIN FROM TISSUES

- Neoplastic growths
- Adenocarcinomas
- Acute leukemias
- Prostatic cancer
- Bronchogenic cancer
- Giant cavernous hemangioma
- Obstetric conditions
- Abruptio placentae (placental abruption)
- Retained dead fetus
- Amniotic fluid embolism
- Septic abortion
- Eclampsia

the blood loses its ability to clot (Concept Map feature on Understanding DIC and Its Treatment, p. 2035).

Clinical Manifestations

Clinically, DIC is termed acute, subacute, or chronic. *Acute* DIC usually presents as a hemorrhagic condition associated with excess plasmin formation. The onset is usually within days to hours after an initial assault to the body system. *Subacute* DIC may not be apparent initially but may become fulminant as the clinical course progresses. *Chronic* cases of DIC are typically seen in clients with cancer or in women carrying a dead fetus.

Subacute and chronic cases usually present as thrombosis attributable to excessive formation of thrombin.

Manifestations of acute DIC (hemorrhagic) include (1) purpura, petechiae, and ecchymoses on the skin, mucous membranes, heart lining, and lungs; (2) prolonged bleeding from venipuncture; (3) severe, uncontrolled hemorrhage during surgery or childbirth; (4) excessive bleeding from gums and the nose; (5) intracerebral and GI bleeding; (6) renal hematuria; (7) tachycardia and hypotension; and (8) dyspnea, hemoptysis, and respiratory congestion. Manifestations of microvascular thrombosis include oliguria and acute renal failure; pulmonary emboli and acute respiratory distress; delirium, convulsions, and coma; hemorrhagic necrosis; and ischemia of the peripheral tissue (acral cyanosis) with the risk of gangrene.

The prognosis for clients with DIC varies. Associated mortality is quite high, primarily because of the underlying illness. Hemorrhage, organ damage (especially acute respiratory distress syndrome [ARDS]), or even death may occur within a matter of hours if associated with gram-negative sepsis. In severe cases the mortality reaches 80%.

Diagnostic tests include screening assays and confirmatory assays. Findings of the screening assays show prolonged prothrombin time (PT) and activated partial thromboplastin time (PTT), a very low (and falling) platelet count ($<100,000/mm^3$), reduced fibrinogen level, and prolonged clotting times. Confirmatory tests such as fibrinogen degradation product (FDP), D-dimer, and factor assays identify the presence of products of DIC pathology. Table 75-7 provides the laboratory tests used in the diagnosis of DIC.

OUTCOME MANAGEMENT

Medical Management

The treatment of DIC is controversial, and efforts are under way to determine the most suitable regimen for managing this syndrome. Goals of treatment include (1) identification and correction of the precipitating cause or problem (e.g., infection, delivery of a fetus, surgery, or irradiation for cancer); (2) reestablishing hemostasis by replacing missing blood components; and (3) supportive therapy to control manifestations of hemorrhage and thrombosis.

Appropriate treatment is determined when (and if) the underlying cause is identified; for instance, antibiotic therapy to control infections or surgery to control severe obstetric complications. In the meantime, manifestations of hemorrhage and thrombosis must be addressed. Replacement of missing blood components is an important first step, particularly if bleeding is present. Washed packed RBCs can be administered to replace blood volume lost through hemorrhage without introducing anticoagulant substances. The specific blood product to be transfused is determined by the deficiency. Platelets

CONCEPT MAP

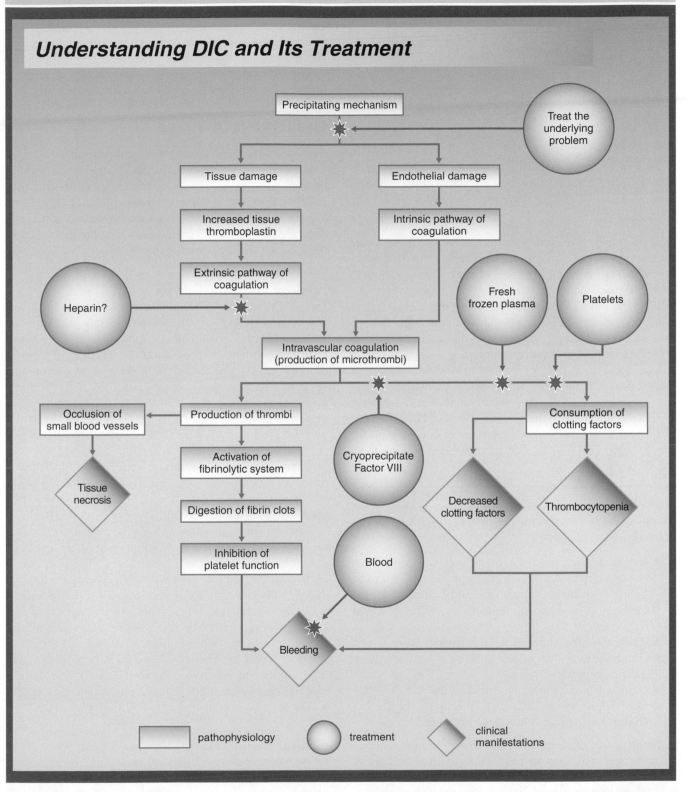

Understanding DIC and Its Treatment

are given for thrombocytopenia. If fibrinogen levels are below 100 mg/dl, transfusions of cryoprecipitate are given until fibrinogen levels can be maintained at 100 to 150 mg/dl. Fresh frozen plasma is transfused if coagulation factors are decreased. Concerns that this may reaccelerate coagulation are unfounded because the plasma protease inhibitors in the plasma are sufficient to control such a reaction. The protease

TABLE 75–7 Laboratory Tests Used in Diagnosis of Disseminated Intravascular Coagulation

Test	Results
Prothrombin time	Prolonged (75%)
Partial thromboplastin time	Usually prolonged
Thrombin time	Usually prolonged
Fibrinogen level	Usually depressed
Platelet count	Usually depressed
Fibrin degradation products	Elevated (75%-100%)
D-Dimer (cross-linked fibrin fragments)	Positive*
Protamine sulfate test	Strongly positive
Antithrombin III	Reduced (90%)
Factor assays II, V, VII, VIII, X, XIII	Reduced

*Important diagnostic test. Identifies presence of both thrombin and plasmin. More reliable than fibrin split products (FSP).

inhibitors gabexate and aprotinin (Trasylol) have been used in studies to control bleeding with some success. The most controversial of the current treatments is the use of IV heparin to control thrombosis. Heparin inhibits the production of thrombin and other coagulation enzymes, but it can also accelerate bleeding. If heparin induces bleeding, ε-aminocaproic acid (Amicar) is given; cardiac, renal, and electrolyte studies should be followed closely during its use because Amicar enhances thrombosis. Antithrombin III (Desirudin), a natural coagulation inhibitor, may also be given and appears to shorten the course and reduce the complications of DIC. Hirudin, a thrombotic inhibitor and neutralizer is currently under study. Chronic DIC can be controlled by long-term use of heparin.

Nursing Management of the Medical Client

Assess all body systems for the effects of DIC, including the following:

- Integumentary bleeding or oozing of blood from venipuncture sites or mucosal surfaces and wounds, pallor, petechiae, ecchymoses, and hematomas
- Respiratory tachypnea, hemoptysis, orthopnea, and basilar rales
- Cardiovascular tachycardia and hypotension
- GI abdominal distention, guaiac-positive stools or gastric contents
- Genitourinary hematuria and oliguria
- Neurologic vision changes, dizziness, headache, changes in mental status, and irritability

Nursing care of clients with DIC is complex and requires extreme vigilance because the client must be treated simultaneously for the primary causative problem as well as the related manifestations of DIC. Generally the goal is to monitor and quantify blood loss and provide supportive therapy with blood components to resolve manifestations of hemorrhage and control further bleeding. Monitor appropriate laboratory values to determine treatment

effectiveness and observe for manifestations of thrombosis or transfusion reactions. To prevent further injury, avoid injections when possible, apply pressure to bleeding sites, and turn and reposition the client frequently and gently. Overt bleeding from body orifices and other clinical manifestations can be frightening to clients and their significant others, who all will require intense emotional support, especially if the client does not survive.

HEMOPHILIA

Hemophilia is an X-linked genetic disorder that results in a deficiency of coagulation factors. Two major forms are hemophilia A (HA), the classic form, which is due to a deficiency of factor VIII; and hemophilia B (HB), also known as Christmas disease, which is due to a deficiency of factor IX. Inherited clotting disorders are discussed in the Genetic Links feature on p. 2037.

Etiology and Risk Factors

Factor VIII and factor IX deficiencies result in an insufficient production of thrombin through the intrinsic pathway of the coagulation cascade, which creates a profound tendency for spontaneous bleeding. Both conditions are usually found only in males. Factor VIII (FVIII) deficiency also may be caused by a congenitally acquired molecular defect in the FVIII binding domain of von Willebrand factor (vWF). FVIII circulates in the blood bound to vWF. This disorder, von Willebrand disease, is the most common congenital bleeding disorder and may affect both genders. A comparison of the three forms of hemophilia appears in Table 75-8. Because HA makes up 80% of all hemophilia, the discussion of manifestations and treatment refers only to this form.

Hemophilia is classified as severe (<1% of normal factor level), moderate (1% to 5% of normal factor level), or mild (5% to 40% of normal factor level). The prevalence of HA in the United States is 20.6 cases per 100,000 males, with 60% having severe disease; the HB rate is 5.3 cases per 100,000 males, with 40% having severe disease. Female carriers of the disease will transmit the genetic defect to 50% of their sons and 50% of their daughters will be carriers. Men with hemophilia will not transmit the defect to their sons, but all their daughters will be carriers. Rare female hemophilia can occur if a man with hemophilia mates with a female carrier.

Clinical Manifestations

All manifestations are related to bleeding. Severe hemophilia often presents at circumcision or at the beginning of ambulation or primary dentition. The hallmark of this disorder is *hemarthrosis* (bleeding into the joints) in the knees, ankles, elbows, wrists, fingers, hips, and shoulders. Hemarthrosis is painful and leads to deterioration of the joints, which may become deformed and permanently

GENETIC LINKS

Examples of Inherited Clotting Disorders

Disorder	Features	Inheritance	Metabolic/Gene Defect	Genetic Testing vailable?
von Willebrand disease	Mucocutaneous bleeding; prolonged bleeding time	AD	Mutation in von Willebrand factor (VWF) gene on chromosome 12	Yes
Hemophilia A (factor VIII deficiency; classic hemophilia)	Easy bruising and hemorrhage into joints and muscles because of deficient clotting ability	XR	Mutation in factor VIII (FVIII) gene on chromosome 10	Yes
Hemophilia B (factor IX deficiency; Christmas disease)	Similar to hemophilia A	XR	Mutation in factor IX (FIX) gene on chromosome 10	Yes
Hemophilia C (factor XI deficiency)	Mild to moderate bleeding; mucocutaneous bleeding	AR	Mutation in factor XI (FXI) gene on chromosome 4; deficiency of plasma thromboplastin antecedent (PTA)	Yes

AD, Autosomal dominant; *AR,* autosomal recessive; *XR,* X-linked recessive.

crippled. Synovial hypertrophy, hemosiderin deposition, fibrosis, damage to the cartilage, and subchondral cyst formation are seen with this condition.

HA typically manifests in the following ways:

- Slow, persistent bleeding from cuts, scratches, and other minor traumas
- Delayed hemorrhage that follows minor injuries; bleeding may not start from a site until hours or even days after the traumatic event
- Severe hemorrhaging from the gums after dental extraction or even brushing the teeth with a hard toothbrush
- Severe, sometimes fatal, epistaxis after injury to the nose
- Overwhelming gastric hemorrhage, which may be linked to gastric disorders such as ulcers and gastritis
- Recurrent hematoma formation in the deep subcutaneous tissue in the intramuscular tissues (muscular atrophy sometimes results) and around the peripheral nerves, causing compression that can result in severe pain, anesthesia of the innervated part, nerve damage, and paralysis
- Hematuria from genitourinary trauma
- Splenic rupture from falls or abdominal trauma
- Intracranial bleeding, which is the leading cause of hemorrhagic death

Life expectancy dramatically increased with the advent in the 1960s of antihemophilic factor (AHF) replacement therapy and prophylactic therapy with lyophilized concentrates that eliminate bleeding. Before this time, the life expectancy for clients with severe HA was 5 to 11 years; today it is 50 to 60 years. Intracranial hemorrhages currently account for about one third of HA-related deaths.

Platelet function, platelet count, bleeding time, and prothrombin time are normal. The activated partial thromboplastin time (aPTT) is prolonged. Quantitative assays for factor VIII determine the severity of the disease.

TABLE 75–8   Comparison of the Three Forms of Hemophilia

Form of Hemophilia	Etiology	Transmission	Major Laboratory Findings
Hemophilia A (classic hemophilia)	Inherited factor VIII (antihemophilic globulin) deficiency	Transmitted as sex-linked *recessive* trait; transmitted by females; occurs in males and, rarely, homozygous females	Coagulation time prolonged but bleeding time normal; factor VIII missing from plasma
Hemophilia B (Christmas disease)	Inherited factor IX (plasma thromboplastin component) deficiency	Transmitted as sex-linked *recessive* trait; transmitted by females; occurs in males and, rarely, homozygous females	Laboratory findings and symptoms same as in hemophilia A; factor IX missing
von Willebrand's disease	Inherited factor VIII deficiency and defective platelet dysfunction	Transmitted as autosomal *dominant* trait to both sexes; occurs in both males and females	Both coagulation time and bleeding time prolonged; low factor VIII levels; platelet adhesiveness decreased

OUTCOME MANAGEMENT

The goals of care for clients with hemophilia are as follows:

- Stop topical bleeding as quickly as possible.
- Supply the missing factor causing hemorrhage.
- Prevent complications leading to and caused by bleeding.

The nurse can control topical bleeding quickly by applying pressure or ice to the injured site, packing the area with fibrin foam, and applying topical hemostatic agents such as thrombin.

Primary factor replacement therapy should be initiated as ordered. This typically is the immediate transfusion of factor VIII (or IX) concentrate supplied as a lyophilized powder. One unit per kilogram of concentrate increases the plasma level of FVIII by 2%, with a reaction half-time of 8 to 12 hours. Because the procoagulant activity of AHF disappears rapidly, clients need transfusions every 12 hours until bleeding stops. For mild hemorrhage, an FVIII level of 30% should be maintained; for major hemorrhage, the level should be maintained at 50%; life-threatening bleeds require a level of 80% to 90%. Plasma levels must be maintained at higher than 50% for a minimum of 7 to 10 days. Prophylactic administration of FVIII to a level 50% above normal is recommended in cases of minor injury, surgery, and dental extractions. Transfusion of packed RBCs or WBCs is used only to replace blood volume when there has been severe loss.

With repeated transfusions and AHF therapy, some clients become sensitized to AHF and develop alloantibody inhibitors that can neutralize FVIII and complicate replacement therapy. These antibodies are seen in about 30% of clients with severe cases by the age of 10. In case of major and life-threatening hemorrhages, these clients are treated with massive doses of factor VIII from animal sources (bovine and porcine), inactivated prothrombin complex concentrates (Konyne 80, Proplex T), or activated prothrombin complex concentrates (Feiba VH Immuno, Autoplex T). Recent treatment with FVIIa for hemarthrosis has been effective for these clients. Clinicians are using various experimental treatments such as immunosuppressive therapy to combat this problem.

Hemarthrosis may be controlled if the client receives AHF in the early stages of bleeding. Joint immobilization and local chilling (such as packing ice around the joint) may bring relief. If pain is severe, it may be necessary to aspirate blood from the joint. Once bleeding stops and swelling subsides, the client should perform active range-of-motion exercises without weight-bearing to prevent further complications such as deformity and muscle atrophy.

Prophylactic home infusion of AHF can greatly reduce bleeding episodes and related complications. Training programs with strict guidelines for this regimen have been developed. As a result, clients with hemophilia lose less time from work or school and need fewer visits to the emergency department.

Analgesics and corticosteroids often reduce joint pain and swelling and the pain of chronic arthritis. Avoid all aspirin products. In mild hemophilia, the use of IV desmopressin may eliminate the need for AHF. Desmopressin acts by causing an increase in plasma factor VIII activity.

Although most clients with hemophilia are successfully maintained with home health care, they may be seen in the hospital during acute bleeding episodes or for unrelated treatments. If even a minor invasive procedure is planned, it is crucial to assess the factor VIII level and to administer a sufficient quantity of factor concentrate before the procedure. During routine medical examinations, these clients should be assessed for the frequency of bleeding episodes and the effectiveness of home therapy. Examine joints for manifestations of bleeding and related atrophy.

Teach the client and family to recognize early manifestations of bleeding and why it is critical to intervene with treatment immediately. Effective and prompt administration of factors to reduce the incidence of bleeding episodes and resultant complications is a priority. The client and family will need to learn IV infusion administration techniques to control the bleeding. Discuss situations that require medical consultation. Discuss the need to curtail physical activities such as contact sports, minor invasive procedures, falls, and cuts that may precipitate a bleeding episode. If a client has HIV seroconversion, arrange for a referral for appropriate care.

CONCLUSIONS

Hematologic diseases are complex disorders that require the nurse to understand the hematopoietic system. The nurse is often involved in the administration of blood and blood products for treatment of these various disorders. Many of the blood disorders are life-threatening; others are easily controlled with proper nutrition or regular medication.

Because blood and blood product transfusions are widely used in the treatment of hematologic disorders, it is vital that you understand these procedures, the implications of these procedures, and the proper techniques of administration so the client will receive safe and effective care.

THINKING CRITICALLY

1. A 62-year-old client underwent a gastric resection for peptic ulcer disease 3 months ago at a hospital in another state. She comes to the nursing clinic complaining of shortness of breath and fatigue

with minimal physical exertion. She currently takes ranitidine (Zantac). What assessments should you make now?

Factors to Consider. What is the significance of the history of gastric resection? How might this contribute to the client's lethargy? What might be causing the shortness of breath and fatigue? What laboratory results would be appropriate to evaluate? What teaching should you consider with this client?

2. A 40-year-old client has recently been told that she has multiple myeloma. She has been admitted to the oncology inpatient unit for initial evaluation and treatment. On her fourth day after admission, she becomes confused and difficult to arouse. Bowel sounds are diminished, and she begins to vomit. What priority assessment should you make now?

Factors to Consider. What might predispose the client to this change in her level of consciousness? What additional assessments would you need to make? What interventions should you anticipate at this time?

Discussions for these questions can be found on the website.

BIBLIOGRAPHY

Citations appearing in red refer to primary research.

Citations appearing in blue refer to evidence-based practice guidelines and protocols.

1. Agaliotis, D. (2006). Hemophilia overview. *EMedicine*. Available: www.eMedicine.com/med/topic3528.htm.
2. Ahmed, S., Shahid, R.K., & Russo, L. (2005). Unusual causes of abdominal pain: Sickle cell anemia. *Best Practice & Research Clinical Gastroenterology, 19*(2), 297-310.
3. Auwaeter, P.G. (2004). Infectious mononucleosis: Return to play. *Clinics in Sports Medicine, 23*, 485-497.
4. Besa, E., & Woermann, U. (2003). Polycythemia vera. *eMedicine*. Available: www.emedicine.com/med/topic1864.htm.
5. Bryan, S. (2002). Hemolytic transfusion reaction: Safeguards for practice. *Journal of PeriAnesthesia Nursing, 17*(6), 399-403.
6. Busch, M., Kleinman, S., & Nemo, G. (2003). Current and emerging infectious risks of blood transfusions. *Journal of the American Medical Association, 289*(8), 959-961.
7. Conrad, M. (2006). Anemia. *EMedicine*. Available: www.emedicine.com/med/topic132.htm.
8. Conrad, M. (2006). Iron deficiency anemia. *EMedicine*. Available at www.emedicine.com/med/topic1188.htm.
9. Conrad, M. (2006). Pernicious anemia. *EMedicine*. Available at www.emedicine.com/med/topic132.htm.
10. De Franceschi, L., & Corrocher, R. (2004). Established and experimental treatments for sickle cell disease. *Haematologica, 89*(3), 348-356.
11. Distenfeld, A., & Woermann, U. (2005). Sickle cell anemia. *EMedicine*. Available at www.emedicine.com/med/topic12126.htm.
12. Distenfeld, A. (2006). Agranulocytosis. *EMedicine*. Available at www.emedicine.com/med/topic82.htm.
13. Doenges, M.E., et al. (2006). *Nurse's pocket guide:Diagnosis, prioritized interventions and rationales* (10th ed). Philadelphia, Pa: F.A. Davis.
14. Ebell, M.H. (2004). Epstein-Barr virus infectious mononucleosis. *American Family Physician, 70*(7), 1279-1287, 1289-1290.
15. Edwards, C.L., Scales, M.T., Loughlin, C., et al. (2005). A brief review of the pathophysiology, associated pain, and psychosocial issues in sickle cell disease. *International Journal of Behavioral Medicine, 12*(3), 171-179.
16. Epstein-Barr virus and infectious mononucleosis. Accessed 02/22/07 at www.cdc.gov/ncidod/diseases/ebv.htm.
17. Ferri, F.F. (2006). *Ferri's clinical advisor: Instant diagnosis and treatment*. Philadelphia: Saunders.
18. Gaines, K. (2003). Aminocaproic acid (Amicar): Potent antifibrolytic agent for treating hematuria. *Urologic Nursing, 23*(2), 156-158.
19. Gando, S., Iba, T., Eguchi, Y., et al. (2006). A multicenter, prospective validation of disseminated intravascular diagnostic criteria for critically ill patients: Comparing current criteria. *Critical Care Medicine, 34*(3), 625-631.
20. Grethlein, S. (2006). Multiple myeloma. *EMedicine*. Available at www.emedicine.com/med/topic1521.htm.
21. Hebert, P., et al. (2003). Clinical outcomes following institution of the Canadian universal leukoreduction program for red blood cell transfusions. *Journal of the American Medical Association, 289*(15), 1941-1949.
22. Hess, J.R., & Lawson, J.H. (2006). The coagulopathy of trauma versus disseminated intravascular coagulation. *Journal of Trauma, 60*, S12-S19.
23. Mehta, S.R., Afenyi-Annan, A., Byrns, P., et al. (2006). Opportunities to improve outcomes in sickle cell disease. *American Family Physician, 74*, 303-310, 313-314.
24. National Institute of Diabetes, Digestive, and Kidney Diseases. (2003). *Hemochromatosis*. National digestive diseases information clearinghouse. Available at www.niddk.nih.gov/health/digest/pubs/hemochrom/hemochromatosis.htm.
25. Rajkumar, S., et al. (2002). Current therapy for multiple myeloma. *Mayo Clinic Proceedings, 77*, 813-822.
26. Raphael, R.L., & Vichinsky, E.P. (2005). Pathophysiology and treatment of sickle cell disease. *Clinical Advances in Hematology & Oncology, 3*(6), 492-505.
27. Reed, W., & Vichinsky, E. (1999). Transfusion practice for patients with sickle cell disease. *Current Opinions in Hematology, 6*(6), 432-436.
28. Rosenfeld, S., et al. (2003). Antithymocyte globulin and cyclosporine for severe aplastic anemia: Association between hematologic response and long-term outcome. *Journal of the American Medical Association, 289*(9), 1130-1135.
29. Schick, P. (2005). Hemolytic anemia. *EMedicine*. Available at www.emedicine.com/med/topic979.htm.
30. Schick, P. (2005). Megaloblastic anemia. *EMedicine*. Available at www.emedicine.com/med/topic1420.htm.
31. Levi, M., & Schmaier, A. (2006). Disseminated intravascular coagulation. *EMedicine*. Available at www.emedicine.com/med/topic557.htm.
32. Siddiqui, A.K., & Ahmed, S. (2003). Pulmonary manifestations of sickle cell disease. *Postgraduate Medicine Journal, 79*, 384-390.
33. Steinberg, M. (2006). Pathophysiologically based drug treatment of sickle cell disease. *Trends in Pharmacological Sciences, 27*(4), 204-210.
34. Steinberg, M., et al. (2003). Effect of hydroxyurea on mortality and morbidity in adult sickle cell anemia: Risks and benefits up to 9 years of treatment. *Journal of the American Medical Association, 289*(13), 1645-1651.
35. Takeshita, K. (2006). Thalassemia beta. *EMedicine*. Available at www.emedicine.com/med/topic2260.htm.
35a. The Joint Commission. (2008). National Patient Safety Goals Hospital Program. Available at www.JointCommission.org/PatientSafety/NationalPatientSafetyGoals/08_hap_npsgs.htm.
36. Weiner, D., & Brugnara, C. (2003). Hydroxyurea and sickle cell disease: A chance for every patient. *Journal of the American Medical Association, 289*(13), 1692-1695.

evolve *Did you remember to check out the bonus material on the Evolve website and the CD-ROM, including NCLEX®-Examination Style Review Questions, Open-Book Quizzes, and Chapter Review Audio Podcasts?*

http://evolve.elsevier.com/Black/medsurg

CHAPTER 76

Management of Clients with Immune Disorders

Linda M. Scott

The immune system constitutes the body's defense system against invading foreign substances. A functioning immune system must protect the body from potential pathogens. An immune system that is malfunctioning predisposes an individual to the development of a wide variety of diseases ranging from severe infection to autoimmune disease and the resultant tissue injury. The Unit 17 Anatomy and Physiology Review describes the normally functioning immune system; this chapter looks at alterations in the immune system and examines how these changes affect the human organism.

HYPERSENSITIVITY DISORDERS

As health care providers, nurses deal with allergic conditions far more often than might be suspected. Allergic rhinitis, asthma, and dermatitis are a few examples of these immunologic diseases.

The tendency to develop allergies for which there is a genetic predisposition and that involve immunoglobulin E (IgE) antibody formation is known as *atopy*. The terms *atopic, allergic,* and *hypersensitive* are frequently used interchangeably. *Allergy* (or, more appropriately, hypersensitivity) describes the increased immune response to the presence of an allergen, also known as an *antigen*. Between 20% and 30% of the population have allergies. We cannot predict who will have allergies; however, there is a higher incidence of allergies among children of allergic parents.

People must progress through a two-step process to become allergic. Step 1 starts with *sensitization*. Sensitization occurs when one develops IgE antibodies against a substance that is inhaled, ingested, or injected. Newly formed IgE antibodies stick to basophils and mast cells, which are found in the skin's mucosal surfaces and in the respiratory and gastrointestinal (GI) tracts. Hypersensitivity can be claimed only after IgE antibodies against a certain foreign substance have formed and are bound to the surface of tissue mast cells and circulating basophils.

Hypersensitivity does not produce any of the manifestations typically associated with allergic disease. It is not until step 2, *reexposure to the allergen,* that allergic manifestations such as sneezing, asthma, and anaphylaxis occur. Although the cellular events for all immediate allergic reactions tend to be similar, differences are found in the clinical sequelae that occur, based on the state of the individual's host defenses, the nature of the allergen, the concentration of the allergen, the route by which the allergen enters, the amount of allergen exposure received, and which organ is affected.

Etiology and Risk Factors
Host Defenses
Some people are more susceptible to hypersensitivity than others for reasons that are unclear (see the Complementary and Alternative Therapy feature on p. 2041). The increasing prevalence of allergic disease suggests that environmental factors acting either before or after birth contribute to the regulation of the development of Th$_2$ cells or their function. Th$_2$ cells play a triggering role in the activation and recruitment of IgE antibody–producing B cells, mast cells, and eosinophils—the cellular triad involved in allergy. The decrease in the number of reported childhood infectious

evolve Web Enhancements

Bridge to Home Health Care Managing Immunosuppression and Nutrition

Be sure to check out the bonus material on the Evolve website and the CD-ROM, including free self-assessment exercises. **http://evolve.elsevier. com/Black/medsurg**

Allergies

Several studies have found a number of environmental factors that may be associated with a lower incidence of allergic disease. For example, taking oral supplements of a probiotic supplement such as *Lactobacillus ruminus*,[3] having a dog or other pet in the home,[5] attending a day care center or having siblings in the home,[1] and farm exposure[4] have all been found to decrease the incidence of allergic disease. However, exposure to tobacco smoke increased the production of allergen-specific IgE and exacerbated allergic responses in clients with allergies,[2] which suggests that clients with allergies should avoid tobacco smoke.

REFERENCES

1. Celedon, J., et al. (2002). Day care attendance, respiratory tract illnesses, wheezing, asthma, and total serum IgE level in early childhood. *Archives of Pediatric Adolescent Medicine, 156,* 241-245.
2. Diaz-Sanchez, D., et al. (2006). Challenge with environmental tobacco smoke exacerbates allergic airway disease in human beings. *The Journal of Allergy and Clinical Immunology, 118*(2), 441-446.
3. Kalliomaki, M., et al. (2001). Probiotics in primary prevention of atopic disease: A randomised placebo-controlled trial. *Lancet, 357,* 1076-1079.
4. Leynaert, B., et al. (2006). Association between farm exposure and atopy, according to the CD14 C-159T polymorphism. *The Journal of Allergy and Clinical Immunology, 118*(3), 658-665.
5. Reijonen, T., et al. (2000). Predictors of asthma three years after hospitalization admission for wheezing in infancy. *Pediatrics, 106,* 1406-1412.

diseases that has resulted from vast vaccination programs, antimicrobial therapy, and changing lifestyles are important influences on an individual's outcome in the Th response to an allergen. Specific IgE formation can be influenced by viral infections, especially those caused by cytomegalovirus (CMV) and mononucleosis. Factors such as air pollution, gender, age, and exposure to second-hand smoke can influence the manifestations of allergies.

Nature of the Allergen

Allergens are antigens that produce a clinical allergic reaction. In atopic diseases, allergens are capable of inducing IgE antibody, thus triggering an allergic response. Molecules that combine with proteins to produce antibodies are called *haptens*. Haptens, along with other environmental allergens, are carried on vectors that may become airborne (e.g., pollen, molds, dust particles, animal dander). Contact with these allergens causes sensitization and atopy and evokes the acute manifestations of allergy. Some haptens (e.g., penicillin) are highly antigenic.

Concentration of the Allergen

Higher concentrations usually result in hypersensitivity responses of greater intensity. Lower concentrations of the allergen may then cause severe manifestations when reexposure occurs.

Route of Entrance into the Body

Routes by which allergens enter the body include inhalation, injection, ingestion, and direct contact. Most allergens are inhaled.

Exposure to the Allergen

Sensitization to allergens is necessary for hypersensitivity to occur. A few factors that influence the likelihood of development of allergy are a person's age at the time of exposure (exposure early in life), the type of allergen (house dust mite, cockroach, various medications, and pollen), the allergen load (lower levels are capable of inducing specific IgE production), and the month of a person's birth (a greater affinity for allergies is seen in those born in the spring and fall).

Pathophysiology

The key intermediate in allergic disease is the IgE antibody. The production of IgE in response to an allergen renders an individual allergic. The two general categories of hypersensitivity reactions are (1) *immediate* (humoral or antigen-antibody) and (2) *delayed* (cell-mediated).

Immediate Reaction

The immediate (antigen-antibody) reaction occurs within minutes after exposure to the allergen. The resultant IgE production mediates the immediate response by activating mast cells and basophils, causing them to degranulate and release mediators such as histamine, leukotrienes from basophils and prostaglandins, and platelet-activating factor from eosinophils.

The mediators, whether preformed or newly formed after activation, are able to increase vascular permeability, dilate vessels, cause bronchospasm, contract smooth muscle, and ignite other inflammatory cells. Table 76-1 describes chemical mediators of the allergic reaction, their action, and the associated manifestations.

Manifestations of mediator release vary, depending on the organ where the mediators' receptors are found. For example, histamine is a preformed mast cell mediator that has receptors in various organs, including skin, oral and nasal mucosa, lungs, and the smooth muscle in the GI tract. Once histamine binds to its receptor, it can cause many reactions. Vasodilation causes edema; smooth muscle contraction results in dangerous airway narrowing; and glandular stimulation leads to increased mucus secretion in the nose, lungs, and GI tract.

TABLE 76–1   Chemical Mediators of the Allergic Reaction

Mediator	Action	Manifestations
Histamine	Dilates blood vessels and increases vascular permeability	Erythema, tissue swelling, and shock
	Constricts smooth muscles in bronchial airways	
	Stimulates nerve endings	Shortness of breath and wheezing
	Increases mucus production in airways and GI tract	Itching and painful skin
		Congestion, gastric reflux, and heartburn
Platelet-activating factor	Dilates blood vessels and constricts bronchial airways	Same as for histamine
	Aids in secretion and aggregation of platelets	Same as for histamine
Eosinophil chemotactic factor of anaphylaxis (ECF-A)	Increases eosinophil migration	Inflamed airways
Neutrophil chemotactic factor	Increases neutrophil migration	Inflamed airways
Heparin	Anticoagulation	Increased bleeding and bruising
Bradykinin	Slows smooth muscle contraction	Mucus plugging
	Increases vascular permeability	Swelling
	Increases mucus production	Congestion
Lipid Mediators or SRS-A		
Leukotrienes	Increase vascular permeability	Same as for histamine
	Increase smooth muscle contraction	
Prostaglandin D	Constricts bronchial airways	Wheezing, shortness of breath, and cough
	Vasodilation	Flushing and swelling
Cytokines (IL-4, IL-5, TNF-α)	Allow cells to influence activity and development of other unrelated cells	Inflammation, edema, and fibrosis
	Aid in eosinophil production	
	Increase vascular permeability	

GI, Gastrointestinal; *IL*, interleukin; *SRS*, slow-reacting substance of anaphylaxis; *TNF*, tumor necrosis factor.

Newly formed mediators, including lipid mediators and cytokines, are made after the mast cell has been activated and have similar actions to those of histamine, but their effects tend to last much longer. Once released into the blood and after binding to their receptors, these mediators cause more bronchial smooth muscle contraction, vasodilation in the skin, nasal congestion, and edema.

Delayed Reaction

The delayed (cell-mediated or late-phase) reaction is seen when there is a prolonged response to the initial allergen. T cells govern the delayed inflammatory response that occurs about 2 to 8 hours after mast cells have been activated by the initial allergen exposure.

Hypersensitivity reactions are divided into four main types (Table 76-2):

- Type 1, immediate or anaphylactic
- Type 2, cytolytic or cytotoxic
- Type 3, immune complex
- Type 4, cell-mediated or delayed

Type 1 (Anaphylactic) Hypersensitivity. The anaphylactic response (described previously) is a rapidly

TABLE 76–2   Types of Hypersensitivity Reactions

	Type	Causative Component	Pathologic Process	Reaction
1	Immediate/ anaphylactic	IgE	Mast cell degranulation ↓	Anaphylaxis
				Atopic diseases
			Histamine and leukotriene release	Skin reactions
2	Cytolytic/cytotoxic	IgG	Complement fixation	ABO incompatibility
		IgM	↓	Drug-induced hemolytic anemia
		Complement	Cell lysis	
3	Immune complex	Antigen-antibody complexes	Deposition in vessels and tissue walls ↓	Arthus reaction
				Serum sickness
			Inflammation	Systemic lupus erythematosus
				Acute glomerulonephritis
4	Cell-mediated/delayed	Sensitized T cells	Lymphokine release	Tuberculosis
				Contact dermatitis
				Transplant rejection

Ig, Immunoglobulin.

occurring reaction that is mediated by IgE antibodies. The allergen binds to IgE antibodies, which are attracted to the surface of mast cells and basophils, causing the release of mediators (see Table 76-1). Examples of type 1 hypersensitivity reactions include anaphylaxis, allergic rhinitis, asthma, and acute allergic drug reactions.

Type 2 (Cytolytic or Cytotoxic) Hypersensitivity. Cytolytic or cytotoxic reactions are complement dependent and thus involve IgG or IgM antibodies. The antigen-antibody binding results in activation of the complement system and destroys the cell on which the antigen is bound, usually a circulating blood cell, thus causing tissue injury. Examples of tissue injury caused by type 2 hypersensitivity include hemolytic anemia, Rh hemolytic disease in newborns, autoimmune hyperthyroidism, myasthenia gravis, and blood transfusion reactions.

During a blood transfusion, blood group incompatibility causes cell lysis, which results in a transfusion reaction. The antigen responsible for initiating the reaction is a part of the donor red blood cell membrane. Manifestations of a transfusion reaction result from intravascular hemolysis of red blood cells and include headache and back pain (flank), chest pain similar to angina, nausea and vomiting, tachycardia and hypotension, hematuria, and urticaria.

Transfusions of more than 100 ml of incompatible blood can result in severe, permanent renal damage, circulatory shock, and death. Therefore if manifestations develop, stop the transfusion at once, maintain an open intravenous (IV) line, check the client's vital signs, and notify the physician immediately. For detailed nursing interventions related to transfusion reactions, see Chapter 75.

Type 3 (Immune Complex) Hypersensitivity. Immune complex reactions result when antigens bind to antibodies, leading to tissue injury. The molecular size of the antigen-antibody complexes is an important feature in eliciting immune complex reactions. Larger complexes are rapidly cleared by phagocytic cells. The smaller complexes formed in antigen excess persist longer in the circulation because they are not so easily captured by phagocytic cells in the spleen and liver. Inflammation results and leads to acute or chronic disease of the organ system in which the immune complexes were deposited.

Immune complex–mediated inflammation is produced by IgG or IgM antibodies, antigen, and complement. The mediators of inflammatory injury include the complement cleavage peptides, which can activate mast cells, neutrophils, monocytes, and other cells. The release of lysosomal granules from white blood cells and macrophages causes further tissue injury.

The antigen may be tissue-fixed or released locally, as in Goodpasture's syndrome, in which circulating antibodies react with autologous antigens in the glomerular basement membranes of the kidneys, causing inflammation of the glomerulus.

Antigen-antibody complexes are formed in the bloodstream and get trapped in capillaries or deposited in vessel walls, causing urticaria, arthritis, arteritis, or glomerulonephritis. Alternatively, antigen-antibody complexes may form in the joint space, with resultant synovitis, as in rheumatoid arthritis and systemic lupus erythematous. The Arthus reaction is a localized area of tissue necrosis that results from immune complex hypersensitivity.

The antigen may also be circulating, as in serum sickness. Serum sickness develops 6 to 14 days after injection with a foreign serum. Deposition of complexes on vessel walls causes complement activation, with resultant edema, fever, inflammation of blood vessels and joints, and urticaria. Classic serum sickness is rare because large doses of heterologous sera (e.g., horse antisera to human lymphocytes) are seldom used.

A serum sickness–like reaction may occur, however, after administration of such medications as penicillin, sulfonamides, streptomycin, thiouracils, and hydantoin compounds. Rather than being dominated by cutaneous vasculitis, these reactions more often manifest with fever, arthralgias, lymphadenopathy, and urticaria. The illness is usually benign and self-limiting, and it resolves after discontinuation of the offending medication.

Nursing care of the client with serum sickness depends on the severity of the reaction. For a mild reaction, care includes control of fever and pain with aspirin and antihistamines. For a severe reaction, care may require steroids.

Serum sickness can be prevented by avoiding allergen exposure. Obtain an allergy history and information about any previous reactions to drugs or vaccines. Document findings in the client's chart, care plan, and medication record so that the risk of subsequent exposure is minimized.

Type 4 (Cell-Mediated, Late-Phase, or Delayed) Hypersensitivity. In cell-mediated hypersensitivity, sensitized T cells respond to antigens by releasing lymphokines, some of which direct phagocytic cell activity. This reaction occurs 24 to 72 hours after exposure to an allergen. Delayed hypersensitivity is induced by chronic infection (e.g., tuberculosis) or by contact sensitivities, as in contact dermatitis.

Type 4 reactions occur after the intradermal injection of tuberculosis antigen or purified protein derivative (PPD). If the client has been sensitized to tuberculosis, sensitized T cells react with the antigen at the injection site. The reaction leads to edema and fibrin deposits, which result in the induration characteristic of a positive tuberculosis reaction.

Graft-versus-host disease (GVHD) and transplant rejection are also type 4 reactions. In GVHD, immunocompetent donor bone marrow cells (the graft) react against various antigens in the bone marrow recipient (the host). Various clinical manifestations result, including skin, GI, and hepatic lesions. Transplant rejection is discussed in Chapter 80, and GVHD is discussed in Chapter 79.

Contact dermatitis is another type 4 reaction that occurs after sensitization to an allergen, commonly a cosmetic, adhesive, topical medication, drug additive (such as lanolin added to lotions), or plant toxin (such as poison ivy). With the first exposure, no reaction occurs, but antigens are formed. On subsequent exposures, hypersensitivity reactions are triggered, which lead to itching, erythema, and vesicular lesions.

Clinical Manifestations

During an allergic response, mast cell activation and the release of chemical mediators result in increased vascular permeability, edema, dilation of blood vessels, smooth muscle contraction, bronchospasm, and increased mucus secretion in the nose, lungs, and GI tract.

The diagnosis of an allergic disease is based on the client's history, manifestations experienced during or after allergen exposure, and the results from commonly used allergy tests. Common allergy tests include (1) skin testing; (2) radioallergosorbent test (RAST) or fluoroenzyme immunoassay test (ImmunoCAP FEIA), which are used to measure IgE levels to certain allergens in vitro; (3) pulmonary function tests (PFTs) to diagnose asthma; and (4) blood assays for IgE levels.

Skin Testing

Skin tests are the diagnostic test of choice for allergic diseases. In prick skin testing, the clinician introduces a small quantity of allergen into the skin by quickly pricking, scratching, or puncturing it. A wheal and flare reaction peaks in 15 to 20 minutes if the client is allergic. Skin testing is generally considered safe and is more specific, though less sensitive, than intradermal testing, but it always carries a risk of causing a systemic reaction such as anaphylaxis.

Intradermal testing is used if the prick skin test is negative. The allergen is injected directly below the skin by holding the skin taught and inserting the 26-gauge needle parallel to its surface, just far enough to cover the beveled portion and produce a bleb. There is a higher incidence of severe allergic reactions with this kind of testing. Therefore it should be used with extreme caution and under close supervision. A patch test can be used to evaluate contact allergies; the allergen is applied directly to the skin and then covered with a gauze dressing.

Nurses often administer skin tests and interpret test results. An *immediate* reaction (i.e., appearing within 10 to 20 minutes after the injection), marked by erythema and wheal formation greater than 3 mm of the positive control (usually histamine), denotes a positive reaction. *Positive* reactions indicate antibody response to previous exposure to this antigen and suggest that the client is allergic to the particular substance that causes the reaction. *Negative* reactions may be inconclusive, requiring further assessment. Negative results may indicate the following: (1) antibodies have not formed to this antigen, (2) the antigen was deposited too deeply into the skin (e.g., subcutaneously), (3) the client is immunosuppressed from disease or therapies (e.g., steroids, chemotherapy, radiation therapy), or (4) the client has taken antihistamines within the past 72 hours.

Problems that arise from skin testing range from minor itching to anaphylaxis. Itching and discomfort at the injection site are common and can be relieved by the application of cool compresses or topical steroid or antihistamine creams, and by the administration of oral antihistamines such as diphenhydramine (Benadryl). Ulceration of the injection site is best treated by keeping the area clean and dry. Anaphylactic shock is a rare but potentially lethal complication of skin testing. A client with a history of an anaphylactic reaction to a substance should never undergo skin testing for an allergy to that substance. This is especially true of allergens such as penicillin, which can produce lethal anaphylaxis in susceptible clients.

Radioallergosorbent Test

The RAST uses the principle of immunoabsorption and reveals elevated levels of allergen-specific IgE antibodies in the client's blood. The allergen of interest is first bound to some solid surface, usually a paper disk. The client's blood is then incubated with the disk. If the client has antibodies specific to the allergen being tested, they bind to that allergen. The unbound antibodies are washed away, and the level of antigen-specific IgE can be measured. This test is somewhat less sensitive than skin testing and is more time-consuming and costly. However, this may be indicated if the client is unable to omit certain medications, like antihistamines, before testing, has suffered from anaphylaxis to a known allergen, or has dermographism or a widespread skin disease.

ImmunoCAP FEIA (Fluoroenzyme Immunoassay Test)

This method uses as the solid phase a flexible, hydrophobic cellulosic disk to which an allergen has been linked. The advantage of this system compared to RAST testing is that it has a very high antigen-binding capacity and has minimal nonspecific binding with high total IgE output. This test is more readily used worldwide based on its increased sensitivity and equal specificity.

Pulmonary Function Test

The PFTs are done to confirm the diagnosis or to evaluate respiratory status in asthmatic disease, to assess the severity of lung obstruction, and to guide the medical treatment of asthma. The principal abnormality associated with asthma is reversible airway obstruction, reflected by a reduction in the forced expiratory volume measured in 1 second (FEV_1). Reversibility is noted if an increase of more than 15% in the FEV_1 is observed after giving a bronchodilator such as albuterol (Ventolin).

Blood Assays

Immunometric blood assays measure the total amount of IgE normally present in the circulation. Most studies have shown that blood concentrations of IgE are increased in the presence of allergic disease; however, a normal or even decreased level may occur in IgE-mediated sensitivities. Elevated serum eosinophil levels also may suggest hypersensitivities.

OUTCOME MANAGEMENT

Medical Management

Allergies are among the most common disorders seen in the medical community. The client often requires a combination of treatments, ranging from avoidance of known allergens to environmental control, immunotherapy, and follow-up.

Identify Allergen

It is imperative to obtain a detailed history that identifies any previous allergic problems in the client and also the presence of allergy in close family members, to perform a thorough assessment and examination, and to ensure that appropriate diagnostic tests are performed. The clinician must know the times of the year during which manifestations occur to determine a correct diagnosis on the basis of the offending allergen. If year-round manifestations are present, find out whether they are worse at any time. A careful search for environmental factors should be undertaken. The client should be questioned in detail regarding the home environment: location, type of heating, insulation, humidity, nature of the bedding, presence of carpeting, method of house cleaning, and so on.

Avoid Allergen

Avoidance of the allergen is often the easiest, cheapest, and safest way of dealing with allergies; however, identification of the specific allergen is sometimes difficult, especially if the client refuses, cannot afford, or cannot locate allergen-testing services. Even if the allergen can be identified, complete avoidance may not be possible, as with pollens and food additives.

Control Environment

Environmental control sometimes helps to eliminate airborne allergens. Figure 76-1 illustrates ways to desensitize a room. These environmental controls, combined with air filters that remove small particles from the air, can help to eliminate many allergens.

Administer Medications

Atopic clients benefit greatly from selected prescriptions and over-the-counter medications. Usually, clients self-administer these agents, although in some settings the nurse or a family member administers them. For more information on allergy medications, see the Integrating Pharmacology feature on p. 2047.

Promote Desensitization

Immunotherapy ("desensitization therapy") is designed for the treatment of type 1, IgE-mediated hypersensitivity reactions. Precise doses of allergens are injected at intervals over a prolonged period with the goal of altering the immune system's response to an allergen, thus reducing manifestations of rhinitis, sneezing, and generalized pruritus triggered by subsequent exposures. The doses are increased gradually over time, or injections may be given several times a day in increasing doses in "rush" protocols. Immunotherapy increases IgG antibody levels and may increase suppressor T-cell function. Specific IgG interferes with IgE binding to allergens and thus mitigates the hypersensitivity response. Immunotherapy is widely used in the treatment of allergic rhinitis (hay fever), for which its greatest success has been achieved because immunotherapy blunts the seasonal rise in specific IgE antibody levels. It also is used for Hymenoptera sensitivity (bee, yellow jacket, wasp, and hornet stings) with reportable success. There is some controversy regarding the efficacy of this treatment in the management of asthma.

Nurses often administer these injections and assess and treat side effects. Clients are asked to wait at least 30 to 40 minutes after receiving the injections so that immediate reactions can be treated. Side effects are similar to those seen in skin testing.

Nursing Management of the Medical Client

Assessment. As a nurse, you play a crucial role in obtaining a detailed medical history of the client and ensuring that appropriate diagnostic tests are performed. The most important part of evaluating the allergic client is the history. The history should elicit all the client's current manifestations. It is important for clinicians to know

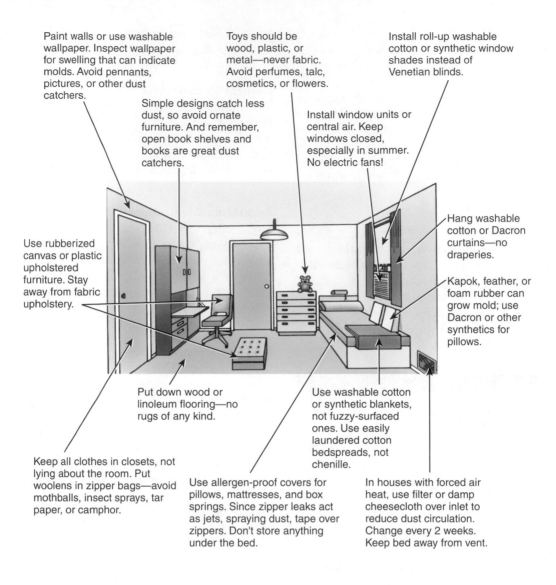

Paint walls or use washable wallpaper. Inspect wallpaper for swelling that can indicate molds. Avoid pennants, pictures, or other dust catchers.

Toys should be wood, plastic, or metal—never fabric. Avoid perfumes, talc, cosmetics, or flowers.

Install roll-up washable cotton or synthetic window shades instead of Venetian blinds.

Simple designs catch less dust, so avoid ornate furniture. And remember, open book shelves and books are great dust catchers.

Install window units or central air. Keep windows closed, especially in summer. No electric fans!

Use rubberized canvas or plastic upholstered furniture. Stay away from fabric upholstery.

Hang washable cotton or Dacron curtains—no draperies.

Kapok, feather, or foam rubber can grow mold; use Dacron or other synthetics for pillows.

Put down wood or linoleum flooring—no rugs of any kind.

Use washable cotton or synthetic blankets, not fuzzy-surfaced ones. Use easily laundered cotton bedspreads, not chenille.

Keep all clothes in closets, not lying about the room. Put woolens in zipper bags—avoid mothballs, insect sprays, tar paper, or camphor.

Use allergen-proof covers for pillows, mattresses, and box springs. Since zipper leaks act as jets, spraying dust, tape over zippers. Don't store anything under the bed.

In houses with forced air heat, use filter or damp cheesecloth over inlet to reduce dust circulation. Change every 2 weeks. Keep bed away from vent.

■ **FIGURE 76–1** Controlling the environment of a room. Dacron is a trade name for polyester. *(Courtesy A.H. Robins Co., Richmond, Va.)*

whether the manifestations are always present or what times of the year they worsen.

Indoor allergens are causing increasing amounts of distress. House dust mites and cockroach and animal allergens are problematic and are present year-round in many homes. Assess whether animals are present in the home and, if so, how many. Is the house filled with plants that could harbor mold spores? Is the client exposed to moist rooms, such as a basement, that is constantly damp?

Environmental factors such as smoke can exacerbate manifestations. Determining where these manifestations present is very important. Many occupations involve exposure to certain allergens such as smoke, latex, chemicals, and animals. Manifestations may be reported as worse during the workweek compared with the weekend. Inquiries such as these help to narrow down possible causes of manifestations.

Diagnosis, Outcomes, Interventions

Diagnosis: Health-Seeking Behaviors and Readiness for Enhanced Self-Care. The key nursing diagnoses for the client with hypersensitivity disorders is *Health-Seeking Behaviors* and *Readiness for Enhanced Self-Care related to the desire to learn about the disease process, treatment regimen, and risk control methods.*

Outcomes. The client will follow a mutually agreed on health maintenance plan that includes stated understanding of the disease process, treatment regimen, and control of risk factors.

Interventions

Provide Teaching. Although clients usually self-administer medications, as described under the medical management section, you are responsible for instructing clients and their significant others about these medications.

INTEGRATING PHARMACOLOGY

Medications for Allergies

In addition to avoiding the allergen, several medications are available to minimize manifestations and decrease the inflammatory process.

Antihistamines are the major group of prescription and over-the-counter drugs used to alleviate the early phase allergic manifestations. These medications relieve sneezing, rhinitis, itching, and other manifestations of allergic rhinitis. They bind to the H_1 receptor. Traditional antihistamines such as diphenhydramine (Benadryl) pass the blood-brain barrier and can produce significant drowsiness. Because newer agents (cetirizine [Zyrtec], fexofenadine [Allegra], and loratadine [Claritin]) do not cross the blood-brain barrier (or do so poorly), they do not cause the drowsiness that limits the use of traditional medications.

Decongestants (oral sympathomimetics) such as pseudoephedrine and phenylephrine help relieve nasal congestion by stimulating the alpha-adrenergic receptors that control the capillary sphincters at the entrance to the venous plexuses of the turbinates. Nasal decongestants such as oxymetazoline hydrochloride and phenylephedrine sprays act primarily on turbinate swelling and are more effective and rapid in onset when used topically rather than orally. Because the prolonged use of topical nasal sprays can cause rhinitis medicamentosa (recurrence of congestion), however, it is advisable to limit their use to no more than 3 to 5 days. Practitioners are cautioned against the use of oral agents by clients with heart disease, hypertension, thyroid disease, diabetes, and urinary difficulties resulting from prostatic hypertrophy. These drugs can be combined with antihistamines to treat the multiple manifestations of allergy.

Corticosteroids, anti-inflammatory agents, and immunosuppressants can be used to treat allergic manifestations. Corticosteroids are the most effective drug for the treatment of rhinitis. Oral steroids are in general more effective and rapid in onset than topical forms, but their systemic effects can produce a myriad of complications. Topical steroid creams can be used to treat dermatitis. Beclomethasone dipropionate (Beconase), triamcinolone (Nasacort), flunisolide (Nasarel), budesonide (Rhinocort), and fluticasone (Flonase) are nasal sprays useful in treating allergic rhinitis, and they evoke few systemic side effects.

Cromolyn sodium is a topical or aerosol medication used to treat allergic rhinitis (Nasalcrom) and asthma (Intal). Its mechanism of action is not completely understood, but it helps prevent the release of chemical mediators (e.g., histamine and leukotrienes) by stabilizing mast cells during both immediate and late-phase reactions. Cromolyn sodium should be administered before allergen exposure. It should be started a week before allergy season to be most effective in the treatment of seasonal allergic rhinitis. It must be used on a regular basis and, unfortunately, dosing is required four to six times a day. Nasal steroids such as Flonase and Rhinocort are the mainstay of therapy for allergic rhinitis.

Inhaled steroids are fundamental to the treatment of asthma. New inhaled steroids with a greater topical potency ratio and fewer systemic effects allow greater control in asthma management. Fluticasone (Flovent), fluticasone and Serevent (Advair), triamcinolone (Azmacort), and beclomethasone (Vanceril) are examples of inhaled steroids.

Anticholinergics are used primarily to treat allergic rhinitis and rhinorrhea caused by the common cold. Ipratropium (Atrovent) was a major advance in the therapeutic regimen for asthma. It does not cross the blood-brain barrier and is relatively free of side effects. Anticholinergics inhibit the effects of acetylcholine by blocking its binding to receptors at neurotransmitter sites on glandular tissue, thereby decreasing the amount of watery discharge in clients with rhinitis. Anticholinergics are also available in oral forms in combination with antihistamines and decongestant preparations (Dura-Vent DA, Extendryl SR).

$Beta_2$ agonists are commonly used to control bronchospasm in asthma. Albuterol (Ventolin) and other short-acting bronchodilators have proved to be well tolerated. The drawback of the older bronchodilators is their short duration of action (only 4 to 6 hours), which limits their use for manifestations experienced at night. This problem has been addressed with the new generation of long-acting $beta_2$ agonists such as salmeterol (Serevent).

Anti-leukotrienes are used to treat manifestations of asthma and anaphylaxis. They block the synthesis or action of leukotriene mediators, which are known to contribute to airway edema, smooth muscle contraction, and the process of inflammation. These drugs include zafirlukast (Accolate), zileuton (Zyflo), and montelukast (Singulair).

The client needs to learn what the medication is, why it is being prescribed, how to take it, when to take it, and what the possible side effects might be. In addition, the client needs to know what to do during an anaphylactic reaction (see Anaphylaxis, Insect Sting Allergy, and Latex Allergy).

If an inhaler is prescribed, the client must be taught how to use it correctly (see Chapter 61). A spacer (an attachment added to the inhaler that holds the medication in the additional chamber or space until the client inhales) may be recommended to help the client obtain the maximal effect. Some clients are taught to perform desensitization injections themselves. In this case, teach clients the proper injection technique and the manifestations of any untoward reactions to the medications, such as shortness of breath, hoarseness, urticaria, and generalized flushing.

Clients may need to carry medications for anaphylaxis with them at all times. In such instances, clients should also wear a medical alert bracelet. Other nursing interventions are described in the following sections under specific disorders.

Evaluation. It is expected that the client will obtain relief from allergic manifestations when the treatment regimen is followed. The client will be able to avoid or control risk factors for allergic manifestations. Ideally, the client will be able to avoid anaphylactic events and obtain treatment before serious problems develop.

ALLERGIC DISORDERS

FOOD ALLERGY

Adverse food reactions can be classified in one of two ways: (1) *food allergies,* which occur by a specific IgE-mediated response to the offending food, such as food-induced anaphylaxis from peanuts; and (2) *food intolerances,* which do not result from an IgE-mediated response but cause manifestations such as diarrhea and vomiting. The prevalence of food intolerances is much higher than that of food allergies. Although food allergies can occur at any age, the condition is more common among infants and very young children, affecting about 8% of those under age 3.

A thorough history is the most important factor in the diagnosis of food allergy or intolerance. Eight foods account for nearly 90% of all food allergies: milk, eggs, peanuts, tree nuts, fish, shellfish, soybeans, and wheat. Fortunately, most food allergies are outgrown; however, allergies to peanuts, tree nuts, and shellfish are lifelong. Food allergies can be determined through skin testing. Food diaries (a record of events, including dietary intake for subsequent episodes) are used to provide insight for the correct diagnosis.

The standard of diagnosis in food allergy is the double-blind, placebo-controlled food challenge. The suspected food is eliminated from the diet for 10 to 14 days. Antihistamines are not to be taken for at least 24 hours before the challenge, and a fasting state should be maintained for 12 to 18 hours before testing. The challenge starts with the introduction of a very low dose of the suspected food, and the dose is gradually increased every 20 to 30 minutes until a reaction is noted or the amount of food present in a normal feeding is reached. *Elimination diets* are also used and consist of removing one food at a time until the adverse manifestations are relieved.

Measuring serum blood tryptase levels can also prove helpful because elevations in tryptase occur and are detectable in the blood for up to 2 hours after a severe systemic reaction. Negative results do not, however, rule out a positive reaction.

See the Bridge to Home Health Care website feature *evolve* on Managing Immunosuppression and Nutrition.

ATOPIC DERMATITIS

Atopic dermatitis occurs in about 10% of the population. Clients typically have a history of or complaints about itchy skin, in addition to a history of rashes in the area of skin creases. Other common complaints are of generally dry skin initially experienced in children younger than 2 years of age, accompanied by manifestations of asthma, hay fever, or dermatitis. Lesions of atopic dermatitis are red and pruritic, contain exudates, and are maculopapular in younger clients, becoming drier and thicker as clients age (Figure 76-2). The lesions are typically found on the cheeks, scalp, and forehead; in later years, they may occur on the trunk and extremities.

Medical Management

Treatment is aimed at controlling and reducing the manifestations because there is no true cure. Antihistamines are used with good results to help alleviate the itch-scratch cycle that is common to atopic dermatitis. The mainstay of therapy is topical corticosteroids, which control the inflammation in the skin lesions. Gels

■ **FIGURE 76–2** Contact dermatitis.

penetrate more effectively but are drying. Ointments should be used in more severe cases because they promote hydration; however, some clients prefer not to use them because they are oily and become messy in the heat. Creams and lotions are the least penetrating but are preferred by most clients. They are absorbed quickly and promote comfort. Antibiotics may be needed to treat superficial skin infections caused by intense pruritus and scratching.

Nursing Management of the Medical Client

Teach clients the importance of environmental control. A key strategy is to minimize allergen exposure and physical stimuli that provoke pruritus. Explain that the client can reduce itching by avoiding severe changes in temperature, wearing loose cotton clothing, using gentle detergents, and rinsing clothing completely. Advise clients to avoid chemical irritants, emotional stress, aeroallergens such as dust and animal dander, and dietary allergens. Teach the client general skin care measures, such as how to perform the following:

1. Maintain good skin hydration by bathing in lukewarm water.
2. Use gentle soaps (e.g., Basis, Dove).
3. Apply a lubricant such as Alpha Keri, petroleum jelly, Eucerin, or Aquaphor to the skin immediately after bathing.
4. Avoid scratching.
5. Keep fingernails trimmed to avoid infection.

URTICARIA

Urticaria (or hives) is a cutaneous reaction associated with several different causes (Figure 76-3). It occurs in as many as 25% of all people at some time. Hives that are present daily or intermittently over a period of less than 6 weeks are termed *acute* urticaria. Hives present for more than 6 weeks are referred to as *chronic* urticaria.

■ **FIGURE 76–3** Allergic urticaria.

Lesions of urticaria tend to be papules or plaques that fade within 24 hours. They do not leave areas of hyperpigmentation. Hives are round or oval and range in size from a few millimeters to several centimeters. Numerous agents can trigger the onset of urticaria: cold, heat, the sun, vibrations, rubbing, or pressure. Urticaria can also be caused by medications, foods, and infections.

Mast cells and their mediators may play a key role in urticaria, causing intense pruritus and vascular changes. A lesional skin biopsy to identify which types of inflammatory cells are present in the lesion is useful in structuring treatment. Some known provoking stimuli of urticaria are medications, foreign substances, foods and food additives, infections, insect bites and stings, contact irritants, inhalants, heat, cold, light, and pressure.

Medical Management

Although management focuses on identifying and eliminating any known causative factors, in about 80% of chronic cases no cause of urticaria is found. All clients with urticaria should be cautioned about aspirin and nonsteroidal anti-inflammatory drugs (NSAIDs), which may exacerbate existing hives. Opiates should be used cautiously as well because they are typically mast cell degranulators.

Antihistamines are the mainstay of therapy for urticaria. Nonsedating antihistamines are recommended during the day; more sedating antihistamines may be preferred at night. Doxepin (Sinequan), a tricyclic antidepressant, is sometimes used for treatment because of its actions on both H_1 and H_2 receptors. Corticosteroids should not be used except for short-term therapy.

Nursing Management of the Medical Client

Urticaria tends to evoke anxiety and frustration in both clients and clinicians. The most effective treatment is to eliminate any triggers. Help the client identify factors that may be suspect, and suggest elimination diets and challenges if foods or food additives are thought to provoke manifestations. Encourage clients to avoid initiating physical factors, such as pressure from tight clothing, heat, vibration, sunlight, and rubbing of the skin. Good skin hydration is mandatory; counsel the client to avoid harsh soaps and irritants and to apply moisturizing lotions after bathing while the skin is still damp.

ANAPHYLAXIS, INSECT STING ALLERGY, AND LATEX ALLERGY

The most common causes of anaphylaxis are drugs, foods, latex exposure, and insect bites and stings. Common food offenders in adults are peanuts, tree nuts, and shellfish (Box 76-1). Insect stings cause many deaths

---

BOX 76-1 Common Agents Causing Anaphylaxis

DRUGS
- Penicillins (most common)
- Cephalosporins
- Tetracyclines
- Streptomycin
- Kanamycin
- Neomycin
- Heparin
- Protamine
- Vancomycin
- Amphotericin B
- Polymyxin
- Bacitracin
- Aspirin, other anti-inflammatory agents
- Colchicine
- Tranquilizers

FOODS
- Peanuts
- Seafood
- Eggs
- Nuts
- Milk
- Citrus fruits
- Strawberries
- Legumes

INSECT VENOMS
- Hymenoptera (honeybees, wasps, yellow jackets, hornets, fire ants)

BIOLOGICALS
- Heterologous antisera (especially equine)
- Enzymes
- Hormones
- Vaccines (especially egg-cultured types)

BLOOD PRODUCTS
- Plasma
- Cryoprecipitate
- Whole blood
- Gamma-globulin

ALLERGEN EXTRACTS
- Skin-testing agents
- Desensitization

DIAGNOSTIC AGENTS
- Sulfobromophthalein
- Iodinated contrast media

---

tract obstruction, which can occur immediately and without other manifestations, are the primary cause of death from anaphylaxis. Although manifestations usually begin 5 to 30 minutes after the offending trigger has been encountered, there can be a delay of an hour or more. The more rapid the onset, the more severe the episode.

The incidence of anaphylaxis related to insect stings ranges from 0.3% to 3% in the general population. The sting insects are members of the order Hymenoptera. People may be allergic to one or all of the stinging insects, but the sting of the yellow jacket is the most common cause of allergy. Common reactions to an insect sting include pain, swelling, and redness that may be localized or may extend over a large area. The swelling usually peaks in 24 to 48 hours and may last for 7 to 10 days. There are no factors that identify those at potential risk for anaphylaxis from an insect sting other than a prior history. Those who have had severe anaphylaxis have an 80% chance of another reaction.

Health care workers are at particular risk for latex allergy. About 700,000 health care workers are affected. Workers with allergies to latex also have a high incidence of reactions to certain foods, such as chestnuts, bananas, kiwi, avocado, apricot, and papaya. Manifestations range from simple dermatitis to generalized itching, urticaria, sneezing, coughing, wheezing, hypotension, and shock on exposure. The diagnosis of type 1 hypersensitivity to latex is confirmed by in vivo skin testing with raw latex extracts or in vitro blood assays that measure specific IgE responses to latex.

Medical Management

Anaphylaxis is treated by (1) administering epinephrine, (2) removing or discontinuing the causative agent, (3) administering emergency oxygen, (4) maintaining an open airway, (5) placing the client in the Trendelenburg position, and (6) giving supportive IV fluids, such as 0.9% normal saline or lactated Ringer's solution as necessary.

SAFETY
ALERT

Nursing Management of the Medical Client

The nursing diagnoses *Risk for Latex Allergy Response* and *Latex Allergy Response* are more specific nursing diagnoses for latex allergy reactions. Most of the interventions for these diagnoses have been described under the nursing diagnoses *Health-Seeking Behaviors* and *Readiness for Enhanced Self-Care*. In addition, the incidence and severity of anaphylactic reactions are decreased by both general and specific measures.

Take a thorough history for drug, food, insect, pollen, and animal allergies from every client. Counsel all clients with a history of anaphylaxis or anaphylactic-like reactions to carry epinephrine with them at all

SAFETY
ALERT

---

in the United States every year. The incidence of anaphylaxis related to latex exposure, especially in health care workers, has dramatically increased since the 1990s with the increased use of latex gloves.

Anaphylactic events commonly present with hives and angioedema and often with dyspnea, wheezing, syncope, hypotension, nausea, vomiting, diarrhea, abdominal pain, flushing, headache, rhinitis, substernal pain, and itching. Cardiovascular collapse, shock, and respiratory

times in the form of an EpiPen or Ana-Kit for self-injection. Recommend that they carry a medical alert bracelet or necklace and an identification card in their wallet or purse and that they register with the proper authorities.

ALLERGIC RHINITIS

Manifestations of allergic rhinitis are persistent and show seasonal variation. Nasal manifestations are often accompanied by eye irritation, which causes pruritus, erythema, and excessive tearing. Numerous allergens may cause these manifestations, such as tree pollens (most common in the spring), grasses (summer), ragweed (fall), or dust mites and animal dander (year-round).

When the nasal mucosa is exposed to an allergen, a series of events is set in motion. Allergen exposure increases the production of IgE, which binds to the receptors on mast cells and basophils and eventually causes a release of mediators. The mediator release leads to increased swelling and congestion, watery discharge, sneezing, and nasal itching that persists for a period of at least 1 hour per day.

Medical Management

Avoidance therapy, symptomatic therapy, and immunotherapy are the three types of management for allergic rhinitis. Nasal glucocorticoid sprays are used with good results for the treatment of allergic rhinitis. The newer, nonsedating antihistamines are beneficial in maintaining control over allergic rhinitis and are a crucial component of therapy. Sympathomimetic agents such as pseudoephedrine help to vasoconstrict the nasal mucous membranes but should be used for short-term therapy only.

Nursing Management of the Medical Client

Educating the client is the most important component of therapy. Teach clients to avoid allergens and to use air filters and air conditioning. Emphasize that compliance with medication is essential. Explain the reasoning behind daily medication use as well as how to adjust the medication to control minor flare-ups and to prevent progression of the disease.

ASTHMA

Because the diagnosis and treatment of asthma account for a substantial number of outpatient visits in allergy clinics, a heightened awareness and thorough understanding of the disease are warranted. See Chapter 61 for a thorough discussion of asthma management.

CONCLUSIONS

The immune system is a complex, interrelated system that affects the whole body. As a nurse, you must understand immune responses to provide clients with complete and individualized care. Because the care of these clients requires multifaceted interventions, you must be able to develop and implement complex care plans to meet their needs.

THINKING CRITICALLY

1. L.S. is a 41-year-old woman admitted for surgery. After surgery, she was to receive prophylactic IV cephalosporin but received a dose of penicillin by mistake. She has a known allergy to penicillin. With a history of allergy to penicillin, what type of hypersensitivity reaction is L.S. most likely to experience? Using the concepts of hypersensitivity, explain this process.

Factors to Consider. What reactions might the nurse expect? What should be the nurse's first actions? What medications might the nurse expect the physician to prescribe to treat this reaction? How can such a reaction be prevented from occurring in the future?

2. A.W. is a 21-year-old college student admitted with an asthmatic attack that has not responded to his usual treatments. He is admitted for a course of IV medications and respiratory treatments. When you enter the room to start the IV line, his wheezing is audible. He is also anxious and gasping for air. What actions should you implement? What problems might you experience when you start the IV line?

Factors to Consider. After the acute phase is over, what might the nurse assess to determine the cause of the asthma attack and why the typical interventions were unsuccessful? What additional teaching might be required?

3. R.H. is a newly graduated registered nurse on an oncology unit. She has been wearing gloves more than ever during the past 2 weeks following orientation. A rash develops on her hands, and she complains of itching all over her body. What type of allergic reaction might be occurring? What actions to assess the allergy should be taken?

Factors to Consider. Can R.H. expect to continue in her new job? Does the organization have a responsibility to keep her employed?

Discussions for these questions can be found on the website. evolve

BIBLIOGRAPHY

Citations appearing in red refer to primary research.

Citations appearing in blue refer to evidence-based practice guidelines and protocols.

1. Brown, S. (2006). Anaphylaxis: Clinical concepts and research priorities. *Emergency Medicine Australasia, 18*(2), 155-169.

2. Casale, T., et al. (2001). Effect of omalizumab on symptoms of seasonal allergic rhinitis: A randomized controlled trial. *Journal of the American Medical Association, 286*(23), 2956-2968.

3. Craig, T.J. (2002). Allergic rhinitis remains an important disease. *Journal of the American Osteopathic Association, 102*(6 Suppl 2), S1-S2.

4. DiLorenzo, G. (2006). Is there a role for antileukotrienes in urticaria? *Clinical and Experimental Dermatology, 31*(Issue 3), 327-334.

5. Mohrenschlager, M. (2006). Atopic eczema: What's new? *Journal of the European Academy of Dermatology and Venereology, 20*(5), 503-513.

6. Price, D. (2006). International primary care respiratory group (IPCRG) guidelines: Management of allergic rhinitis. *Primary Care Respiratory Journal, 15*(1), 58-70.

7. Rote, N. (2006). Alterations in immunity and inflammation. In K. McCance & S. Huether (Eds.), *Pathophysiology: The biologic basis for disease in adults and children* (5th ed., pp. 249-291). St. Louis: Mosby.

8. Rote, N., & Trask, B. (2006). Adaptive immunity. In K. McCance & S. Huether (Eds.), *Pathophysiology: The biologic basis for disease in adults and children* (5th ed., pp. 211-248). St. Louis: Mosby.

9. Ryan, D. (2005). Management of allergic problems in primary care: Time for a rethink? *Primary Care Respiratory Journal, 14*(4), 195-203.

10. Solomon, W. (2003). Atopic dermatitis and urticaria. In S. Price & L. Wilson (Eds.), *Pathophysiology: Clinical concepts of disease processes* (6th ed., pp. 149-153). St. Louis: Mosby.

11. Solomon, W. (2003). Bronchial asthma: Allergic and otherwise. In S. Price & L. Wilson (Eds.), *Pathophysiology: Clinical concepts of disease processes* (6th ed., pp. 139-148). St. Louis: Mosby.

12. Solomon, W. (2003). Familiar (IgE-mediated) allergic disorders: Anaphylaxis and the atopic diseases. In S. Price & L. Wilson (Eds.), *Pathophysiology: Clinical concepts of disease processes* (6th ed., pp. 129-138). St. Louis: Mosby.

13. Sommers, M. (2003). Alterations in immunocompetence. In V. Carrieri-Kohlman, A. Lindsay, & C. West (Eds.), *Pathophysiological phenomena in nursing: Human responses to illness* (3rd ed., pp. 297-317). Philadelphia: Saunders.

14. Walker, S. (2005). Management of urticaria. *Primary Care Respiratory Journal, 14*(3), 166-168.

15. Willsie, S.K. (2002). Improved strategies and new treatment options for allergic rhinitis. *Journal of the American Osteopathic Association, 102*(6 Suppl 2), S7-S14.

evolve *Did you remember to check out the bonus material on the Evolve website and the CD-ROM, including NCLEX®-Examination Style Review Questions, Open-Book Quizzes, and Chapter Review Audio Podcasts?*

http://evolve.elsevier.com/Black/medsurg

CHAPTER 77

Management of Clients with Rheumatic Disorders

PATRICIA A. MACDONALD

Rheumatic disorders comprise autoimmune and inflammatory disorders, which have been called "the primary crippling diseases" of the developed world. The term arthritis literally means "inflammation of a joint" but arthritis is actually a collection of more than 100 related, but distinct, conditions. Approximately 49% of all Americans older than 65 feel that they have arthritis; this is 1 in every 7 Americans and 1 in every 3 families. The Centers for Disease Control and Prevention (CDC) reports that 70 million Americans currently suffer from arthritis and that by 2035 more than 20% of the U.S. population will be 65 years of age or older. Arthritis is the primary reason for work-related disability and is the leading cause of disability among people ages 65 or older.

Given the high prevalence and significant impact of rheumatic disorders in terms of economic, functional, social, and psychological consequences, these disorders should receive considerable attention from us all. The United Nations, the World Health Organization, and 37 countries have proclaimed the years 2000 to 2010 as the Bone and Joint Decade. This global initiative is intended to improve the lives of people with musculoskeletal disorders, such as arthritis, and to advance understanding and treatment of musculoskeletal disorders through prevention, education, and research. A consortium of national organizations produced the *National Arthritis Action Plan: A Public Health Strategy,* a comprehensive and ambitious plan for addressing the management of arthritis. In addition, autoimmunity was named a major priority women's health issue by the Office of Research on Women's Health, a unit of the National Institutes of Health, as these disorders target women 75% of the time. As the incidence of autoimmune and inflammatory disorders continues to rise, research efforts focus on the role of overuse, injury, obesity, gene defects, infection, immunosuppression, amino acids, interleukin, and environmental agents in both the development and the treatment of these life-altering diseases. The ultimate goals in managing rheumatic disorders are to relieve pain and clinical manifestations, assuage psychological distress, improve physical function, and generally aid in the well-being of the client. Equally important, however, are interventions to prevent and ameliorate socioeconomic problems. A majority of the costs, both economic and social, are due to lost function rather than direct medical costs. Until a cure for the many types of rheumatic disorders is found or far more effective therapies to prevent joint damage and physical disability are developed, people will continue to suffer severe, premature economic and social dislocations that will seriously affect their lives. As the population ages, society can expect that these impacts will mushroom.

Rheumatic disorders are characterized by chronic pain and progressive physical impairment of joints and soft tissues. They encompass more than 100 diseases and conditions including osteoarthritis (OA) (discussed in Chapter 26), rheumatoid arthritis (RA), psoriatic arthritis (PsA), systemic lupus erythematosus (SLE), fibromyalgia syndrome (FMS), systemic sclerosis (SSc), ankylosing spondylitis (AS), reactive arthritis, polymyositis (PM), dermatomyositis (DM), vasculitis, bursitis, polymyalgia rheumatica, and Lyme disease.

Because RA is the classic autoimmune and inflammatory disease, it is helpful to refer to the discussion of RA while studying the other disorders, which are outlined in

---

evolve Web Enhancements

Bridge to Home Health Care Increasing Independent Living with Rheumatoid Arthritis

Web Tables Extra-Articular Manifestations of Rheumatoid Arthritis

Common Diagnostic Studies Used in Rheumatic Disorders

Principles of Joint Protection and Associated Work Simplification Strategies

Be sure to check out the bonus material on the Evolve website and the CD-ROM, including free self-assessment exercises. **http://evolve.elsevier. com/Black/medsurg**

Chapter 26. Although the conditions have different clinical patterns, pain and impaired mobility are common problems among clients with these disorders.

Clinical trials and their results are used to support evidence-based practice (EBP). The American College of Rheumatology has set the standard for what is an acceptable indicator of disease improvement. The difficulty in evaluating the results of clinical trials is due to differences in designs (single agent vs. combination) and differences in client populations (early vs. late disease, rheumatoid factor positive vs. negative). Standardizing clinical trial designs ensures that the efficacy and safety of the treatments for rheumatic disorders is clearly demonstrated, subjectively as well as objectively, leading to the practice of evidence-based medicine. The treatment of RA is explored in the Translating Evidence into Practice feature on p. 2055.

AUTOIMMUNITY

Relationships between altered immune function and rheumatic disease are better understood as a result of continued research efforts. Autoimmune diseases are defined as conditions in which immunologic self-tolerance has been disrupted, with resultant damage to body tissues or cells normally recognized as self. Autoimmune disorders with muscle and joint involvement include SLE, RA, dermatomyositis (DM), scleroderma (SSc), Sjögren's syndrome, and mixed connective tissue disease.

To understand systemic, arthritic autoimmune diseases, it is important to briefly review key components of the immune system. Please see the anatomy and physiology review of the hematopoietic system at the beginning of Unit 17.

The ability of the immune system to distinguish self from non-self depends in large part on cell-surface antigens. These antigens (which are unique to every person) are encoded by a large cluster of genes called the *major histocompatibility complex* (MHC) located on the short end of chromosome 6. Histocompatibility antigens are also more typically referred to as *human leukocyte antigens* (HLAs) because they were first discovered on leukocytes. Seven closely related gene loci have been identified: HLA-A, HLA-B, HLA-C, HLA-D, HLA-DR, HLA-DQ, and HLA-DP. Each of these gene loci is occupied by multiple alleles (alternate genes) that code the development of each surface antigen. At least 23 gene products are associated with the HLA-A group, and 47 are associated with the HLA-B group.

HLAs have been categorized into two groups. Found on the surface of nucleated cells, class I antigens include HLA-A, HLA-B, and HLA-C. Class II antigens (D, DR, DQ, and DP) are found on macrophage and B cells, among others.

As a result of aberrations in HLA activity genetic coding, the body may lose some of its ability to recognize and differentiate self from non-self, resulting in autoimmune disorders. In other words, the body has decreased self-tolerance. Abnormalities of the HLA system, however, are but one key to the development of autoimmunity. Other factors involve abnormal T-cell or B-cell reactivity, resulting in altered recognition of foreign antigens and self by the immune system. For example, altered T-cell function has been implicated in the pathogenesis of arthritic diseases, such as RA. Research has begun to identify the specific roles of various T cells in these disease processes. For example, $CD4^+$ T cells have been shown to have a crucial role in the pathogenesis of arthritis, and $CD8^+$ T cells may play an immunoregulatory role. In addition, research suggests that B cells in the synovial membrane of joints expand as a result of local antigen stimulation. It is also likely that the immune system can be altered by interactions with chemical, environmental, viral, and bacterial agents.

Another important aspect of autoimmune disease is familial aggregation (or clustering), which suggests that there is a genetic predisposition to the development of specific disorders. This possibility is not surprising because an individual's HLA type is inherited. Indeed, some HLA types appear more frequently in certain disease conditions. For example, in Caucasians HLA-B27 appears in 80% to 90% of people with ankylosing spondylitis but in only 7% to 10% of the general population.

RHEUMATOID ARTHRITIS

Rheumatoid arthritis (RA) is a chronic, systemic autoimmune disorder whose major distinctive feature is chronic, symmetrical, and erosive inflammation of the synovial tissue of joints. The severity of the joint disease may fluctuate over time, but progressive development of various degrees of joint destruction, deformity, and disability is the most common outcome of established disease. Associated nonarticular manifestations may include subcutaneous nodules, vasculitis, pulmonary nodules or interstitial fibrosis, and pericarditis.

Rheumatoid arthritis occurs worldwide and affects all racial and ethnic groups. It can occur at any time of life, but its incidence tends to increase with age, peaking between the fourth and sixth decades. Women are affected two to three times more often than men. Clients with RA have a substantially reduced life expectancy, and mortality can be predicted, in most instances, by more severe clinical status.

The incidence of RA is estimated to range from 0.5% to 1.5% of the population. After age 55, the incidence rates for men and women are estimated to be 2% and 5%, respectively. Incidence rates for African Americans are similar to those for Caucasian Americans. RA appears to be a relatively "recent" disease. It was first described

TRANSLATING EVIDENCE INTO PRACTICE

Rheumatoid Arthritis Treatment

Have new pharmacologic treatments made a difference in treatment outcomes for rheumatoid arthritis (RA)? RA is a chronic, systemic autoimmune disorder whose major distinctive feature is exhibited primarily by chronic, symmetrical, and erosive inflammation of the synovial tissue of joints. Pharmacologic treatment of this disorder is one of the most thoroughly researched areas in the treatment of rheumatic disorders. However, this has not always been true. Many of the early treatments were based on anecdotal reports written by health care providers about clients treated within their own practice.

Careful review of the literature relating to new therapies as well as new evidence about older treatment standards is necessary. Recent studies that address the use of biologic response modifiers (BRMs) in addition to the more traditional disease-modifying antirheumatic drugs (DMARDs) have been reviewed. As a result of these studies, much more is known about RA, its progression, and the damage that occurs to joints without overt clinical manifestations.

All 10 of the studies used double-blind, controlled methods to evaluate the medications studied. Many measured ACR20 and Sharp Scores as recommended by the American College of Rheumatology.[2,3,5-7,9] Others used quality of life measurement instruments or radiographic findings.[1,4,5,7,8-10]

Methotrexate (MTX) and placebo were found to be less effective than methotrexate and infliximab combined[1] or MTX and abatacept combined.[4,10] Findings also found that combination therapy of MTX with adalimumab was superior to either MTX alone or adalimumab alone;[2] in addition, MTX with etanercept was superior to either MTX alone or etanercept alone.[8] Etanercept was also found to decrease fatigue for nearly 4 years in clients who received it.[7] Adalimumab was more effective than placebo at inhibiting the progression of structural joint damage, reducing the clinical manifestations of RA, and improving physical function in clients with active RA who had demonstrated an incomplete response to MTX.[6] Similarly, clients with an incomplete response to DMARDs showed improved responses when etanercept or infliximab was added to the treatment regimen.[3]

Dosages of 5 mg/day of prednisolone[9] or infliximab[3,5,9] in combination with DMARD therapy substantially decreased radiographic progression in early RA clients.[3,5,9] The use of more than one drug provided better outcomes than did single use of a drug.[1-5,8,9]

However, one study reported increased rates of serious adverse advents when abatacept was combined with DMARDs.[10]

Greater joint damage at baseline was associated with poorer physical function at baseline and less improvement in physical function after treatment, underlining the importance of early intervention to slow the progression of joint destruction.[1]

IMPLICATIONS

The most common finding was the improvement in clients who received more than one DMARD for the treatment of RA. Additional research is needed to determine whether continued long-term use of multiple agents will result in less progression of RA over time while also limiting adverse side effects. As more pharmacologic agents are introduced for treatment of RA, the nurse will need to monitor results of studies according to ACR20, Sharp, and other scores that measure client outcomes associated with treatment of rheumatoid arthritis. All of these agents have potential toxic side effects that need to be monitored closely by the nurse and the client.

REFERENCES

1. Breedveld, F., Han, C., et al. (2005). Association between baseline radiographic damage and improvement in physical function after treatment of patients with rheumatoid arthritis. *Annals of the Rheumatic Diseases, 64*(1), 52-55.
2. Breedveld, F., Weisman, M., et al. (2006). The PREMIER study: A multicenter, randomized, double-blind clinical trial of combination therapy with adalimumab plus methotrexate versus methotrexate alone or adalimumab alone in patients with early, aggressive rheumatoid arthritis who had not had previous methotrexate treatment. *Arthritis and Rheumatism, 54*(1), 26-27.
3. De Filippis, L., et al. (2006). Improving outcomes in tumor necrosis factor α treatment: Comparison of the efficacy of the tumor necrosis factor vs blocking agents etanercept and infliximab in patients with active rheumatoid arthritis. *PAN Minerva Medica, 48*(2), 129-135.
4. Emery, P., et al. (2006). Treatment of rheumatoid arthritis patients with abatacept and methotrexate significantly improved health-related quality of life. *The Journal of Rheumatology, 33*(4), 681-689.
5. Goekoop-Ruiterman, Y., et al. (2005). Clinical and radiographic outcomes of four different treatment strategies in patients with early rheumatoid arthritis (the BeSt study): A randomized, controlled trial. *Arthritis and Rheumatism, 52*(11), 3381-3390.
6. Keystone, E., et al. (2004). Radiographic, clinical, and functional outcomes of treatment with adalimumab (a human anti-tumor necrosis factor monoclonal antibody) in patients with active rheumatoid arthritis, receiving concomitant methotrexate therapy: A randomized, placebo-controlled, 52-week trial. *Arthritis and Rheumatism, 50*(5), 1400-1411.
7. Moreland, L., et al. (2006). Effect of etanercept on fatigue in patients with recent or established rheumatoid arthritis. *Arthritis and Rheumatism, 55*(2), 287-293.
8. Van der Heijde, D. (2006). Patient reported outcomes in a trial of combination therapy with etanercept and methotrexate for rheumatoid arthritis: The TEMPO trial. *Annals of the Rheumatic Diseases, 65*(3), 328-334.
9. Wassenberg, S., et al. (2005). Very low-dose prednisolone in early rheumatoid arthritis retards radiograph progression over two years: A multicenter, double-blind, placebo-controlled trial. *Arthritis and Rheumatism, 52*(11), 3371-3380.
10. Weinblatt, M., et al. (2006). Safety of the selective costimulation modulator abatacept in rheumatoid arthritis patients receiving background biologic and non biologic disease-modifying antirheumatic drugs: A one-year randomized, placebo-controlled study. *Arthritis and Rheumatism, 54*(9), 2807-2816.

in the mid-18th century and has not been found in skeletal remains from ancient European or Asian civilizations. However, erosive polyarthritis has been documented in the skeletons of prehistoric (3000 to 5000 years ago) Native Americans, which might indicate an infectious agent confined to a small geographic area before the 18th century.

Etiology and Risk Factors

RA is characterized by the presence of rheumatoid factor (RF), an autoantibody directed against immunoglobulin G (IgG), in more than 80% of those with the disease. In addition to RF, antibodies against collagen, Epstein-Barr virus, encoded nuclear antigen, and certain other antigens have been identified. The role of autoantibodies in RA is still unclear, but research has focused attention on pre-illness immunologic status. Antikeratin antibody (AKA) and anti-perinuclear factor (APF) appear to be markers that predict the development of RA in RF-positive clients. However, RA develops in only a proportion of cases. Other immunogenetic markers may aid in the identification of clients with early RA and those with more severe disease.

Genetic factors are important in the epidemiology of the disease. A genetic predisposition for RA is seen with a higher concordance rate of 32% in identical twins rather than the 9% rate observed in fraternal twins. Research suggests that the consistent reports by female RA clients that joint pain and swelling disappear during pregnancy, may be due to the genetic differences between mother and fetus. This is an exciting area for continuing research. The strongest genetic evidence, however, is seen in the association of RA with HLA-DR4, a genetically determined allele of the MHC on the short arm of chromosome 6.

Pathophysiology

The histologic changes in RA are not disease specific but largely depend on the organ involved. The primary joint lesion involves the synovium. Rheumatoid factor (RF) antibodies develop there against the immunoglobulin IgG, the largest of the five classes of immunoglobulins, to form immune complexes. Ironically, immunoglobulins (IgG) are natural human antibodies. It is not clear, however, why the body produces an antibody (RF) against its own antibody (IgG) and, in effect, transforms IgG to an antigen or foreign protein that must be destroyed. The products of macrophages and lymphocytes are thought to have critical roles in the pathogenesis of RA, as part of the immune response to an unidentified antigen. Moreover, it is the formation of these antibody-antigen immune complexes that leads to the activation of the complement system and the release of lysosomal enzymes from leukocytes. Both of these reactions cause inflammation. Initial

research has demonstrated that interleukin-8, known as neutrophil-activating peptide 1 (NAP-1), has a definite role in the inflammatory process of RA and that circulating autoantibodies may provide a clinically useful marker for RA severity. With the initial formation of immune complexes, synovitis develops as the synovial membrane becomes swollen, irritated, and inflamed.

As the immune complexes are deposited onto the synovial membrane or the superficial layers of the articular cartilage, they are phagocytized by polymorphonuclear (PMN) leukocytes, monocytes, and lymphocytes. Unfortunately, phagocytosis deactivates the immune complexes and simultaneously produces additional enzymes (oxygen radicals, arachidonic acid) that lead to hyperemia, edema, swelling, and thickening of the synovial lining. The hypertrophied synovium literally invades the surrounding tissue, including cartilage, ligaments, joint capsule, and tendons. Eventually, granulation tissue forms to cover the entire articular cartilage, leading to the formation of *pannus,* a highly vascularized fibrous scar tissue composed of lymphocytes, macrophages, histiocytes, fibroblasts, and mast cells. Undoubtedly the most destructive element in RA, pannus can erode and destroy articular cartilage, eventually resulting in subchondral bone erosions, bone cysts, fissures, and development of bone spurs and osteophytes. Research has concluded that tumor necrosis factor (TNF) is produced by cells at the cartilage-pannus junction and may lead to cartilage destruction. Pannus can also scar and shorten tendons and ligaments, leading in turn to ligamentous laxity, subluxation, and contractures. The Concept Map on p. 2057 explores the pathophysiology and treatment of rheumatoid arthritis.

Clinical Manifestations

Rheumatoid arthritis may be mild and relapsing, involving a few joints for a brief period, or markedly progressive, with the development of deformities and severe systemic disease. Overall, RA is characterized by cycles of exacerbation and remission, the duration of which adds to the feelings of powerlessness and uncertainty that clients often experience, A small percentage of clients have severely progressive disease that does not respond to aggressive therapy.

Table 77-1 illustrates the seven criteria for the 1987 revised American College of Rheumatology (ACR) classification of RA. The 1987 criteria for the classification of RA serve as a framework for the clinical diagnosis. The classification system, however, is not intended to explicitly define diagnosis. It is important to remember that RA is a clinical diagnosis. Other findings, including the results of laboratory tests, radiologic examination, and synovial fluid analysis, help to confirm the diagnosis. The criteria highlight the symmetrical involvement of inflamed joints of the wrist, the metacarpophalangeal (MCP) joints, and the proximal interphalangeal (PIP)

CONCEPT MAP

Understanding Rheumatoid Arthritis and Its Treatment

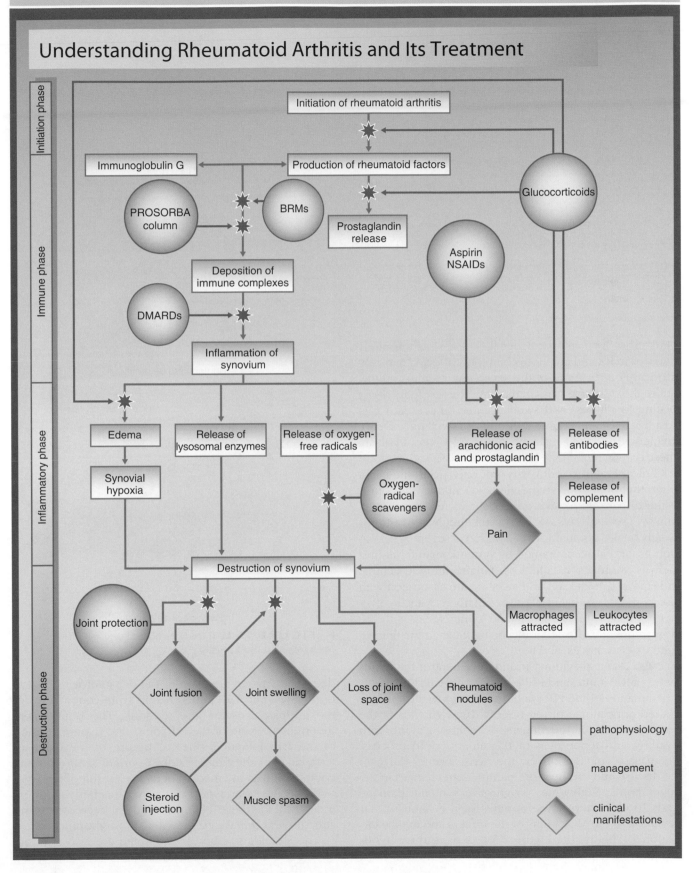

TABLE 77-1 1987 Revised Criteria of the American Rheumatism Association for the Classification of Rheumatoid Arthritis*

Criterion	Description
1	Morning stiffness in and around joints lasting at least 1 hr before maximal improvement
2	Soft tissue swelling (arthritis) of three or more joint areas (including right and left PIP,[†] MCP, wrist, elbow, knee, ankle, and MTP joints)
3	Swelling of at least one wrist, MCP, or PIP joint
4	Simultaneous symmetrical swelling in joints listed in criterion 2
5	Subcutaneous rheumatoid nodules
6	Presence of rheumatoid factor
7	Radiographic erosions or periarticular osteopenia in hand or wrist joints

* *Note:* Rheumatoid arthritis is defined by the presence of four or more criteria. Criteria 1 through 4 must have been present for at least 6 weeks. The American Rheumatism Association 1987 revised criteria for the classification of rheumatoid arthritis.
†*MCP,* Metacarpophalangeal; *MTP,* metatarsophalangeal; *PIP,* proximal interphalangeal.
Data from Arnett, F.C., et al. (1988). The American Rheumatism Association 1987 revised criteria for the classification of rheumatoid arthritis. *Arthritis and Rheumatism, 31,* 315-324.

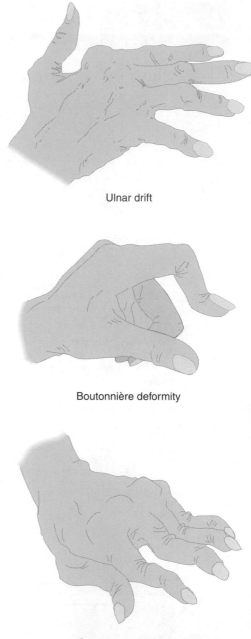

Ulnar drift

Boutonnière deformity

Swan-neck deformity

■ **FIGURE 77–1** Three types of hand deformity characteristic of clients with rheumatoid arthritis.

joints. The distal interphalangeal (DIP) joints are rarely involved in RA and are more commonly affected in osteoarthritis. Four or more of the seven criteria must be met before the disease is classified as RA. The first four criteria relating to stiffness and swelling must be present for at least 6 weeks, and criteria 2 through 5 (swelling and subcutaneous nodules) must be observed by a physician. These criteria remain the hallmark for classification of RA.

Clinical features of RA vary not only from one client to another but also in an individual client over the course of the disease. Explosive acute polyarticular onset evolving over several days also can occur. Rheumatoid arthritis usually begins gradually, over a period of several weeks to months, and is accompanied by systemic manifestations, such as anorexia, weight loss, fatigue, muscle aching, and stiffness. Joint pain and swelling are associated with morning stiffness that can last several hours. Joint involvement is usually polyarticular and symmetrical, with the most frequently affected joints being those in the fingers, hands, wrists, knees, and feet.

Bilateral symmetrical involvement of the hands (wrists, MCP joints, and PIP joints) is characteristic of RA. Inflammation of the PIP joints contributes to the spindle-shaped appearance of the fingers. Tenosynovitis of the flexor tendons of the fingers is common, along with swelling and tenderness of the ulnar styloid process. Decreased dorsiflexion of the wrist occurs early in the disease and can be more painful than changes in the finger joints. With time, progressive synovial damage leads to characteristic deformities of the hands: ulnar deviation of the MCP joints of the fingers and medial deviation of the wrist. Figure 77-1 depicts three types of hand deformities characteristic of RA. A swan-neck deformity (hyperextension of the PIP joint with flexion of the MCP and DIP joints) results from contractures of the intrinsic muscles and tendons. The boutonnière deformity (flexion of the PIP joints and hyperextension of the DIP joints) is due to rupture of the extensor tendons over the fingers. Carpal tunnel syndrome, the compression of the median nerve as a result of tenosynovitis on the volar aspect of the wrist, is fairly common in RA. All of these changes lead to decreased hand strength and the ability to maintain a tight pinch.

The shoulders, elbows, and spine are also affected. Shoulder arthritis is seen with late disease, whereas the elbows can become flexed and contracted with early disease. Spinal involvement is usually limited to the cervical area. Atlantoaxial subluxation can lead to tenderness, muscle spasm, persistent head tilt, and occipital headache.

In the lower extremities, RA frequently affects the feet and knees. Cock-up toes result from plantar subluxation of the metatarsal heads. Walking can be difficult because of limited flexion and extension of the ankle. Active synovitis is often seen in swelling over the medial and lateral aspects of the patella. Popliteal cysts (Baker cysts) can develop behind the knee joint.

As a systemic disease, RA can affect almost every body system. Extra-articular manifestations of RA are summarized in the Extra-Articular Manifestations of Rheumatoid Arthritis table on the website. Three of these manifestations, however, are the most frequently seen in RA. These include rheumatoid nodules (Figure 77-2), Sjögren's syndrome, and Felty's syndrome. Rheumatoid nodules, granuloma-type lesions that develop around small blood vessels, can develop in up to 50% of clients with RA. Usually, those affected have high titers of RF. Generally firm, mobile, and painless, rheumatoid nodules appear over the extensor surfaces of joints, such as elbows and fingers, but may be found elsewhere in the body, including in the lungs. These nodules can easily break down or become infected.

Secondary Sjögren's syndrome, keratoconjunctivitis sicca, is seen in approximately 10% to 15% of clients. It may occur by itself or with other diseases, such as SLE or polymyositis. Clients with Sjögren's syndrome have diminished lacrimal and salivary gland secretion. They may complain of gritty, burning, or sandy eyes, with decreased tearing, itching, and photosensitivity.

Felty's syndrome was originally described as the combination of RA, splenomegaly, leukopenia, and leg ulcers. Subsequent observations have shown an association with lymphadenopathy, thrombocytopenia, and the HLA-DR4 haplotype. Felty's syndrome occurs most commonly in clients with severe, nodule-forming RA. Other extra-articular problems seen in RA include inflammatory eye disorders, infection, pulmonary disease, vasculitis, and cardiac abnormalities.

Diagnostic Testing

Laboratory Testing. The laboratory evaluation of clients with rheumatic disease is often informative but rarely definitive. Serum and urine chemistries are usually normal in RA. Anti-CCP (cyclic citrullinated protein antibodies) is a diagnostic marker and is predictive of the future development of rheumatoid arthritis. It is as sensitive as rheumatoid factor, but is more specific. Elevated erythrocyte sedimentation rates (ESRs) and C-reactive protein (CRP) levels are typical of active disease, with the CRP level being a more definitive indicator of inflammation. Hematologic studies often indicate a mild normocytic, hypochromic anemia along with thrombocytosis. An underlying iron deficiency anemia is usually present if the hemoglobin level is less than 10 g/ml and ferritin levels are low. Low eosinophil counts occur with increased disease activity, and granulocytopenia may indicate Felty's syndrome. Occasionally, proteinuria and microscopic hematuria are seen as a result of amyloid deposits in the kidney.

Serologic tests used to confirm the diagnosis of RA include antinuclear antibodies (ANAs) and RF. Antinuclear antibody titers are seen in 15% to 20% of clients, over half of who have Felty's syndrome. Rheumatoid factor, an autoantibody directed against the immunoglobulin IgM, is positive in only 80% of clients. Higher titers are seen in active disease. The presence of IgM RF, however, is not specific for RA. Increased levels can be seen in older adults or after infections or immunizations. Rheumatoid factor titers are also present in other rheumatic disorders, including SLE, dermatomyositis, and SSc, and in liver and pulmonary disease. The absence of a positive RF test does not exclude the diagnosis of RA in a client with typical clinical characteristics. Clients can convert from negative to positive with an exacerbation in their clinical manifestations. Clients with seronegative RA, however, have better outcomes and rarely have extra-articular involvement. Recent evidence points to recognition that seronegative and seropositive polyarthritis are separate entities. See the Common Diagnostic Studies Used in Rheumatic Disorders table on the website.

Radiologic Studies. Radiologic findings help to confirm disease activity and monitor treatment results. In the early stages, soft tissue swelling is indicated by increased shadowing on the x-ray around the affected joint (Figure 77-3). Massive tissue swelling of the entire joint often precedes further destructive changes, such as periarticular osteoporosis. Subchondral cysts may develop from the invasion of granulation tissue. As the disease progresses, subchondral bone erosions develop, ultimately causing a narrowing of the joint space. In mild disease, erosions may not develop for 6 to 12 months. Initially

■ **FIGURE 77–2** Rheumatoid nodules.

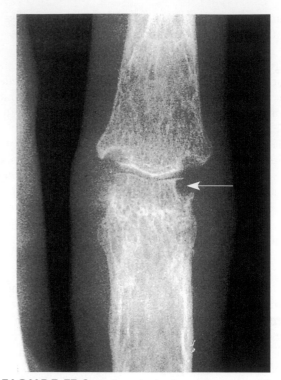

■ **FIGURE 77–3** Radiograph of an interphalangeal joint affected by rheumatoid arthritis. Pocket erosion is shown with the arrow. Pocket erosions can spread into trabecular bone and weaken the bone surface. There is also joint space narrowing and soft tissue swelling. *(From Resnick, D., Berthiaume, M.J., & Sartoris, D. [1993]. Imaging. In W.N. Kelley, et al. [Eds.], Textbook of rheumatology [4th ed., p. 600]. Philadelphia: Saunders.)*

occurring at the joint margins where the capsule is attached, erosions are first seen in the small joints of the hands and feet, where the bone is less dense. Subluxation and malalignment of the joints can be seen on x-ray, reflecting the destructive changes seen on physical examination. With advanced disease, subchondral bone destruction and diffuse osteoporosis appear.

Other Procedures. Synovial fluid analysis indicates a change from the normal transparent color to a milky, cloudy, or dark yellow fluid. Arthroscopic examinations typically show pale, thick, edematous synovial villi, cartilage destruction, and fibrous scar formation (pannus). Bone and joint scans can be used to detect early joint changes and more readily confirm the diagnosis.

OUTCOME MANAGEMENT

There has been considerable effort devoted to the development of outcome measures in RA. A proposed set of core RA measures includes pain measurement, disability, physician and client global assessment, number of tender and swollen joints, and acute-phase reactants. In addition, the American College of Rheumatology (ACR) developed a statistically powerful definition of improvement in

RA: 20% improvement in tender and swollen joint counts and 20% improvement in three of the five remaining ACR core set measures of client and physician global assessments, pain, disability, and an acute-phase reactant. These research advances continue to clarify effective and appropriate management strategies for RA clients. At the very least, the plan of care for clients with manifestations suggestive of RA should (1) establish a diagnosis of RA as early as possible, (2) determine the stage of disease (joint destruction) and disease activity (inflammation), (3) define relevant factors that will affect prognosis, (4) establish a plan for treatment as early as possible, (5) monitor disease activity and response to treatment, and (6) modify the treatment when client response is absent or inadequate.

Medical Management

Effective management of RA involves a combination of medications, rest, exercise, and methods of joint protection. The primary goals of RA treatment strategies are to provide pain relief, to decrease joint inflammation, to maintain or restore joint function, and to prevent bone and cartilage destruction. Proven treatments for arthritis must show in repeated, controlled scientific clinical trials that they are safe and provide benefit in one or more of the following areas:

- Pain reduction
- Reduction of inflammation
- Safe joint mobility
- Avoidance of stress damage to joints

The treatment and management of RA requires successful collaboration between the client and the entire health care team—health care provider (physician, physician's assistant, and nurse practitioner), nurse, and physical and/or occupational therapist. Other team members—orthopedic surgeon, nutritionist, social worker, and orthotist—may be required, as the client's needs change. The totally dependent RA client is uncommon today, in large part because of advances in joint replacement surgery and the advent of new therapies.

Education is critical in the successful treatment of RA. Clients and their families must be educated about the disease process and its impact on the entire unit. Families must be helped to become partners with the client to effectively manage the disease and enable the client to function at the highest level of his or her abilities.

Collaboration between health care providers is necessary for teaching and reinforcing the unpredictable nature of the disease. Clients need to understand that the disease is chronic, characterized by remission and exacerbation, and is therefore somewhat unpredictable. This unpredictability can affect, on a daily basis, the client's ability to do simple tasks, and the lack of certainty with which the client and family can plan ahead for outings and special activities can be frustrating for all involved. Individual and family stress can escalate to the point where family counseling is required. Reinforcing positive coping strategies and recommending stress-management techniques, however, can help to avoid feelings of powerlessness and helplessness.

Reduce Pain and Inflammation

Reduction of pain and inflammation is most often achieved with pharmacologic management, which usually combines a nonsteroidal anti-inflammatory drug (NSAID), a disease-modifying antirheumatic drug/biologic response modifier (DMARD/BRM), and short intermittent courses of oral glucocorticoids. Medications are changed in response to lack of efficacy or if the initial improvement fades. The use of single-drug therapy has been shown to be of limited benefit in the treatment of RA. The majority of clients who are prescribed a single agent are no longer on that agent 3 years later. Combination therapy is most effective if introduced within the first 2 years after diagnosis of RA. Methotrexate (MTX), in combination with the BRMs, has shown a synergistic effect, as well as with the immunodmodulator leflunomide. As explained in the Integrating Pharmacology feature on pp. 2062-2063, these medications reduce pain and inflammation as well as control systemic involvement. Also, see the Translating Evidence into Practice feature on p. 2055 for information related to pharmacologic management of RA.

PROSORBA Column

PROSORBA column, a medical device used in conjunction with apheresis, employs approximately 200 mg of protein A covalently bound to an inert silica matrix that is contained within a 300-ml polycarbonate housing. Each column contains 123 ± 2 g of this matrix. Protein A is a component of certain strains of the *Staphylococcus* bacterium, and it has the propensity to bind immunoglobulin G (IgG) and IgG bound to an antigen, i.e., circulating immune complex. The PROSORBA column is indicated for use in the therapeutic reduction of the clinical manifestations of severe RA in adult clients with long-standing disease who have failed to respond to or are intolerant of DMARDs. The procedure requires 12 weekly apheresis procedures. A plasma volume of 1250 ± 250 ml is passed through the column. Clients must have good intravenous access. The therapeutic effect is usually not noticed until completion of the 12 weeks.

Protect Articular Surfaces

One important interrelated area of medical management involves the principles of joint protection and work simplification. In a multidisciplinary setting, principles of joint protection and work simplification can be taught by the occupational therapist and reinforced by the nurse. Education in these areas can have a positive effect on increased energy levels and decreased fatigue, thereby improving the client's coping abilities and sense of control.

Specific suggestions or anticipatory guidance about self-care can be beneficial. For example, clients should select easy-to-grip combs and brushes with large handles. These devices are readily available at almost all stores. Using a long-handled bath brush to reach the feet and back during bathing is much less stressful on the joints. Selecting attractive, adaptable clothing is easier now that many stores and mail-order catalogs have included a home care section. Jogging suits with pull-on pants and large, easily zippered tops are comfortable and attractive. Adaptive equipment for dressing includes long-handled shoehorns, zipper pulls, and buttoners. Involvement of the feet, the metatarsalphalangeals (MTPs), can seriously affect the ability to ambulate and enjoy life. Referral to an orthotist for proper supportive shoes and/or orthotics is essential to reduce pain and prevent further joint damage. See the Principles of Joint Protection and Associated Work Simplification Strategies table on the website.

Maintain Function

Therapeutic exercise is another important modality in the initial and ongoing treatment of RA. Three types of exercises are typically used: range-of-motion (ROM), strengthening, and endurance. The purpose of ROM exercises is to improve joint motion. ROM exercises can be passive, assisted, or active. Carried out by the therapist, without any client effort, passive exercises are most often done when the client is totally unable to move the joint because of the lack of strength or voluntary control. The purpose of passive ROM is to ensure joint movement when there is a risk of developing contractures. Research has identified a safe role for progressive resistance exercise training in selected clients, leading to significant improvements in strength, pain, and fatigue without exacerbating disease activity or joint pain. Whatever form of exercise is prescribed, the client should not perform these exercises if joint inflammation or a flare-up exists. Although clients may be able to enjoy other therapeutic and recreational exercises, they need to understand that engaging in other activities or activities of daily living (ADL) is not a substitute for a ROM program.

Strengthening exercises are done to preserve or improve the muscle's ability to perform work. Two types of strengthening exercises are commonly used: isometric and isotonic. With isometric exercises, the muscle is contracted for 5 to 6 seconds, but the joint is not permitted to move. Common isometric techniques include gluteal folds and quadriceps-setting exercises. Isotonic exercises are used carefully in clients with RA because

INTEGRATING P H A R M A C O L O G Y

Medications Used in the Treatment of Rheumatoid Arthritis

Pharmacologic treatment of rheumatoid arthritis (RA) is directed at (1) relieving manifestations of pain, inflammation, and stiffness; (2) maintaining joint function and range of motion; (3) minimizing systemic involvement; and (4) delaying disease progression.

ANALGESICS

Acetaminophen (Tylenol) is given only for pain relief because it has analgesic and antipyretic properties equivalent to those of aspirin. However, acetaminophen does not have any anti-inflammatory or antirheumatic actions and is not helpful in reducing the inflammation and swelling of rheumatic arthritis.

NSAIDs

Nonselective nonsteroidal anti-inflammatory drugs (NSAIDs) such as aspirin, ibuprofen (Motrin, Advil), meloxicam (Mobic), nabumetone (Relafen), and diclofenac (Voltaren) are used to treat inflammation and swelling. They suppress inflammation by inhibiting the synthesis of prostaglandins, which play a major role in the process of inflammation. The most common side effects of NSAID therapy include nausea, GI irritation, and gastric and duodenal ulcers. NSAIDs do not alter the course of RA because they do not prevent joint damage or slow disease progression.

Cyclooxygenase is the key enzyme involved in the production of prostaglandins that is inhibited by NSAIDs. There are two forms of this enzyme—cyclooxygenase-1 (COX-1) and cyclooxygenase-2 (COX-2). COX-1 is present in all cells at all times and its purpose is to produce prostaglandins that regulate normal cellular processes; drugs that inhibit this enzyme are called nonselective NSAIDs. COX-2 is expressed almost completely in response to inflammation. COX-2 produces prostaglandins in the joints and synovium; drugs in this class are called selective NSAIDs. Celecoxib (Celebrex) is currently the only available COX-2 NSAID, and it is less likely to cause stomach ulcers and GI irritation than traditional NSAIDs.

The COX-2 NSAIDs and traditional NSAIDs have been shown to equally relieve arthritis pain and to share many of the same side effects, including the potential to cause fluid retention, high blood pressure, heart failure, and liver and kidney problems in some clients. As with all medications, clients are urged to use the lowest effect dose.

An additional important side effect of some of the COX-2 NSAIDs is an increase in the risk of heart attacks and strokes, especially when they are used at higher doses. Although all NSAIDs have the potential to cause high blood pressure and worsen congestive heart failure, present studies have not clearly shown traditional NSAIDs to cause an increase in heart attacks and strokes as was seen with some of the COX-2 NSAIDs pulled from the market (valdecoxib [Bextra] and rofecoxib [Vioxx]). More research is needed to understand if some or all of the traditional NSAIDs also increase the risk of these events.

DMARDs AND BRMs

Disease-modifying antirheumatic drugs (DMARDs) reduce joint destruction and retard disease progression, but they are more toxic than NSAIDs and require close monitoring. DMARDs are considered when the client does not show a decrease in pain, swelling, and stiffness or if x-rays show evidence of bony erosions within the first 30 to 60 days of onset. First-choice DMARDs include methotrexate (MTX), sulfasalazine (Azulfidine), and the antimalarial agent hydroxychloroquine (HCQ, Plaquenil). MTX is considered the first-choice drug among the DMARDs because of its efficacy, relative safety, low cost, and extensive use in RA. Other DMARDs include gold salts, penicillamine (Depen), azathioprine (Imuran), and cyclosporine (Sandimmune). Since 1998, seven new DMARDs, classified as biologic response modifiers (BRMs) and tumor necrosis factor (TNF) blockers, have been released in the United States: etanercept (Enbrel), infliximab (Remicade), anakinra (Kineret), adalimumab (Humira), rituximab (Rituxan), abatacept (Orencia), and leflunomide (Arava).

> **All of the DMARDs, including TNF blockers and BRMs, are toxic to multiple body organs including the liver, kidneys, GI tract, lungs, bone marrow, and eyes (HCQ), and must be monitored closely. These drugs suppress the bone marrow and place clients at risk for infection, anemia, and bleeding.**

SAFETY
⚠
ALERT

Many of the DMARDs may take days, weeks or months to begin controlling the manifestations of RA, which is why clients continue to receive, glucosteroids and/or NSAIDs while the DMARDs are initiated. MTX may result in a therapeutic effect in 3 to 6 weeks, but HCQ may require 3 to 6 months.

GLUCOCORTICOIDS

Glucocorticoids produce an immediate and profound anti-inflammatory response in clients with RA. At low doses, glucocorticoids demonstrate characteristics that are primarily anti-inflammatory rather than immunosuppressive. At higher doses, these agents are immunosuppressive by appearing to exert the greatest suppressive effect on T helper cells. Higher doses are reserved for rapid relief of acute manifestations seen with exacerbation of RA. Low-dose prednisone is used as a bridge, to carry clients from unsuccessful NSAID therapy until they experience the benefits of the slow-acting, disease-modifying agents. The bridge time has shortened considerably with the advent of the BMRs and TNFs. Long-term prednisone use is correlated with the development of several adverse effects, specifically serious infections, fractures and osteoporosis, increased urinary calcium excretion that can cause urolithiasis, and GI bleeding. Treatment guidelines have been published for treatment of steroid-induced osteoporosis. The defect in calcium absorption is treated with daily doses of 1500-mg calcium supplements and 800 units of vitamin D. Bisphosphonates (alendronate sodium and risedronate) are most frequently used for the treatment of osteoporosis.

INTEGRATING PHARMACOLOGY

Medications Used in the Treatment of Rheumatoid Arthritis—Cont'd

SAFETY

⚠️

ALERT

Determining if a surgical client is glucocorticoid dependent has important implications for those undergoing surgery. Taking a drug history of the client with RA requires exploration of the use of glucocorticoids: when they were initiated, dosage history, and date they were discontinued. Steroid-dependent clients are those currently taking glucocorticoids as well as those weaned from chronic glucocorticoid therapy within the last year. Other clients at risk of steroid dependency include those who received regular intra-articular injections of steroids, psoriasis clients who routinely used topical steroids on large areas of the skin, and clients with inflammatory bowel disease who routinely used steroid enemas. Steroid-dependent clients who undergo

general anesthesia must receive stress doses of glucocorticoids to prevent intraoperative shock. Three doses of intravenous hydrocortisone (100 mg each) are usually given before, during, and immediately after the surgical procedures.

COMBINATION THERAPIES

A combination of one or two medications may be used to provide relief of pain, swelling, and stiffness and to slow degeneration of a joint. The benefit of giving more than one medication is to maximize the therapeutic effect and minimize the side effects with smaller dosages of all medications prescribed. Common combinations include MTX + HCQ, MTX + Enbrel, or MTX + Arava.

INVESTIGATIONAL AGENTS

Rheumatoid arthritis research continues to focus on the pathogenesis of disease, halting disease progression and treating earlier in the course of the disease. For more information regarding clinical trials being conducting in RA and other rheumatic diseases, see the website www.clinicaltrials.gov.

---

they require repetitive joint motion. After joint pain and inflammation have been controlled, however, and the client has achieved increased isometric strength, dynamic, low-resistance exercises are appropriate. Appropriate low-resistance exercises for the client with RA include bike riding, swimming, golf, Ping-Pong, and dancing.

Other physical therapy modalities are also useful. 🪔 For severely inflamed joints, splints appear to help resolve inflammation more quickly than does leaving the joint unsplinted. Heat therapy and cold therapy are important adjuncts to an exercise and rehabilitation program.

Superficial heat therapy can be given with hot packs, hydrotherapy, or paraffin baths. Deep heat is achieved through the use of diathermy or ultrasound. Superficial heat appears to cool joints by increasing the local blood flow, but deep heat actually raises the intra-articular joint temperature. As a result, superficial heat is generally preferred to deep heat. Heat seems to be more beneficial in the treatment of chronic conditions characterized by minimal swelling and inflammation. It also permits more effective stretching exercises.

Many clients find cold therapy provides relief of pain and stiffness. Cold packs, however, should not be used in clients with Raynaud's phenomenon, cold sensitivity, or cryoglobulinemia, or in anyone who finds it uncomfortable. The Arthritis Foundation has developed a wide selection of literature about RA. Support groups, self-help classes, and water-based or land-based exercises are available. To obtain this information from The Arthritis Foundation, call 1-800-283-7800. Requests for information can also be mailed to The Arthritis Foundation,

1414 Spring Street, NW, Atlanta, GA 30309, or visit their website at www.arthritis.org.

Nursing Management of the Medical Client

The goal of nursing care for clients with RA is to promote a healthy, positive life course adaptation. To achieve this goal, the nurse focuses on four domains of human response: comfort, self-care, control, and coping.

Adapting to a chronic illness is a demanding, complex process physically, emotionally, and socially. The energy required to achieve this adaptation can be easily exhausted, especially in the early stages of RA. Achieving normalcy, regulation, or adjustment can become a lifelong process, consuming increasing amounts of energy, unless clients learn to participate actively in modulating their responses to the illness. By working together, the nurse helps the client master adaptive strategies in each of the four domains so physical, psychological, and social energy is renewed.

The nurse's role is to assess, educate, and coordinate treatments, facilitate adaptations in the home, reevaluate periodically, and serve as client advocate. Providing information to help the client deal with chronic pain, comply with treatment, and cope with a chronic disease are some of the challenges faced in managing clients with RA. The nurse provides information and encourages the client's self-management by allowing choices about when to exercise, which adaptive equipment to use, and what other self-care techniques to use. Clients with RA appreciate caring and empathy by nurses. See the Bridge to Home Health Care feature on Increasing *evolve*

Independent Living with Rheumatoid Arthritis on the website.

Assessment. Nursing assessment begins by identifying the client's concerns and needs. The history should include information about the duration of clinical manifestations and ways the client has been managing those manifestations, particularly pain. The client's current understanding of RA and the coping strategies used for dealing with pain and fatigue are important. Determine the methods that the client is now using to reduce pain and the amount of pain the client considers tolerable. Find out what methods the client is using for joint protection.

Evaluate the amount of swelling and pain in each joint and the number of affected joints to obtain a "joint count." Determine physiologic measures of function such as a timed walk, measures of grip strength, and results of self-reported instruments that evaluate flexion and extension. Assess for clinical manifestations in the client's eyes, heart, lungs, and peripheral nerves. It is important to note new manifestations and marked changes in previous clinical manifestations.

Also evaluate the client's perception of his or her quality of life, usual role in the family, and social involvement. Physical changes in the body can lead to lower self-esteem. Clients may find it psychologically difficult to be seen in public and manage stares instigated by a hand deformity and other changes. Be sensitive to these issues and bring them into the discussion if the client or family hints at suicidal thoughts.

Diagnosis, Outcomes, Interventions

Diagnosis: Chronic Pain/Impaired Physical Mobility. The primary diagnosis of clients with RA is *Chronic Pain related to inflammation and swelling from pressure on surrounding tissues, joint deformity, and joint destruction.* Another common and related nursing diagnosis is *Impaired Physical Mobility related to pain, stiffness, and joint deformity.* The amount of pain these clients experience permeates all aspects of their lives including physical mobility.

Outcomes. The client's pain will be controlled at a level that permits the client to perform ADL. The client will maintain mobility at the highest level possible to carry out desired activities.

Interventions. Achieving a reasonable degree of comfort is a continuous challenge. Pain can be so pervasive and encompassing that it becomes a veil over daily activities, only to lift at unpredictable moments. Clients frequently use military terms, such as "struggle," "battle," "siege," "in the trenches," "attack," "fight," and "surrender," to describe their experiences with pain and discomfort. The importance of covering up the pain and keeping up with activities as a means of rejecting or disengaging from the disease has been emphasized. In fact, achieving some degree of comfort is the primary predictor of psychological well-being as well as maintaining mobility.

Teach About Medications. Numerous strategies can be used to help clients achieve pain relief and maintain mobility. Obviously, teaching clients about their medications and monitoring their response are important nursing responsibilities. Clients should receive information about the purpose, dose, frequency, and anticipated side effects of each medication. See the Integrating Pharmacology feature on Medications Used in the Treatment of Rheumatoid Arthritis, pp. 2062-2063. Clients need to understand clearly when they are to report adverse manifestations to the health care team and what to do if they miss a dose. Some of the new therapies include self-injectable medications, requiring that clients and their families be taught injection and preparation techniques. Preprinted or written instructions are essential to help clients recall the information. Appropriate educational materials on a variety of pharmacologic agents are available from The Arthritis Foundation and the pharmaceutical manufacturer.

Nurses play an important role in teaching clients to participate in their care by keeping a medication history. Clients can use a notebook or flow sheet to record essential medication information useful to themselves and other health care providers, such as dentists, other medical specialists, or emergency personnel. Initially, many clients find it helpful, as does the health care provider, to list the medications, date started, dosage, date discontinued, and reason for discontinuing the drug. This list should be reviewed and updated at each visit.

Promote Comfort with Nonpharmacologic Measures. Modulating the client's response to the experience of joint pain is another key principle of pain management. The uncertainty and unpredictability of the disease, with its concomitant impact on comfort, have been well documented. The following four interventions are used to help clients with the pain of RA: (1) making them comfortable, according to what has worked for them in the past; (2) listening to and learning from clients; (3) reducing anxiety; and (4) enlisting family and community support. Not all clients with RA have the same pain or the same experience with pain, so it is critical to understand the phenomenon from the individual client's perspective.

Other nonpharmacologic pain management strategies can be very useful. They not only can help to relieve pain but also can decrease anxiety and, thus, enhance overall comfort and a sense of control.

Positioning the client, ensuring that the limbs are correctly supported, and reinforcing the use of heat and cold are all important measures for promoting comfort. Some clients find that flannel nightwear, sleeping blankets, and thermal underwear are helpful means of retaining warmth while reducing pain and stiffness. A variety of relaxation techniques, including imagery, self-hypnosis, and controlled, rhythmic breathing, have been suggested. Progressive muscle relaxation techniques should be used with caution in clients with RA, however, because there is a danger that muscles could be tensed too tightly, thus exacerbating joint and muscle pain.

Manage Stiffness. Other comfort-promoting activities include the management of stiffness and the promotion of adequate sleep. If these areas are addressed through the nurse-client partnership, fatigue can also be significantly reduced. Clients need to be taught to distinguish between pain and stiffness and to understand why the nurse is interested in differentiating between the two manifestations. As one of the most important diagnostic criteria of RA (as well as several other arthritic diseases), *morning stiffness* can vary in duration or quality depending on disease activity. Typically, clients with morning stiffness wake up feeling comfortable until they begin to move. If the morning stiffness lasts longer than 1 hour or does not show evidence of decreasing, they may require additional rest and sleep plus changes in their medical regimen. Exercise can also decrease morning stiffness, pain, and fatigue. Clients may use pain medication before exercise to permit increased freedom of movement.

Occasionally, if stiffness is severe, family members may need to provide early morning assistance so the client is prepared for the day ahead. Another option is for clients to begin (or organize) as many tasks as possible the night before so they have enough time to complete ADL without rushing or undue anxiety. Clients might also be able to rearrange schedules so chores normally performed in the morning, when stiffness is most pronounced, are deferred until later in the day. Daytime stiffness can occur, but frequent position changes and pacing or alternating the types of activities usually alleviates it.

One unusual aspect of stiffness is that it is a disabling phenomenon that is not readily understood by other family members. Initially, family and co-workers may wonder if the client is feigning his or her inability to move rapidly or perform optimally in the morning. Helping the client and family understand the need for additional time to complete activities is an important measure in decreasing the family's frustration and the client's anxiety about moving slowly.

Promote Sleep and Rest. Disturbed sleep can significantly affect the client's level of comfort, especially when the client has a chronic illness. With RA, sleep is often interrupted because of joint pain, excessive fatigue, stiffness, or generalized musculoskeletal aching. Other important causes are anxiety and poor sleep hygiene. Before specific interventions are suggested, the nurse needs to determine how the sleep has been disturbed—for example, difficulty falling asleep, frequent periods of waking up during the night, or early morning awakening. Often the nurse's first interventions are to reinforce good sleep habits, such as maintaining a regular sleep schedule, avoiding caffeine or alcohol before bed, or engaging in soothing activities before retiring.

Other strategies address specific causes of impaired sleep in clients with RA. For example, warming the bed or taking a bath before bedtime can ease painful joints. Taking the prescribed NSAID (with a light snack of milk and crackers) half an hour before retiring can also promote sleep by relieving joint pain. If clients are awakened during the night because of pain or stiffness, they may need to use a smaller pillow, bed boards, or even lighter weight blankets. Those clients who have difficulty falling asleep because of worries or diffuse anxiety may benefit from using relaxation-imagery exercises. Avoidance of alcohol and caffeine before bed or engaging in soothing activities such as reading are also helpful.

Whole body rest can decrease joint inflammation and pain. Alternating rest and activity throughout the day may help with maintenance of mobility and management of pain. An afternoon nap also helps reduce fatigue.

Diagnosis: Readiness for Enhanced Self-Care. The nursing diagnosis is *Readiness for Enhanced Self-Care related to complex medication schedules, high risk of side effects of medications, health maintenance, and self-care.* Self-care includes taking medications as ordered, maintaining mobility with exercise and rest, and ensuring good nutrition. Self-care also includes all practices that clients undertake to promote their health and well-being despite having a chronic illness. Other modalities besides medications, such as heat, exercise, rest, positioning, or joint protection, are examples of these practices. Self-care practices must be taught and reinforced so the client does not develop self-care deficits.

Outcomes. The client will make informed decisions about the management of RA that will lead to a satisfactory quality of life despite the disease and will demonstrate ability to cope with the chronic illness.

Interventions. In general, clients with RA have a difficult time learning to live in partnership with the disease. RA clients may experience the fears of becoming crippled, being perceived as being old and nonproductive, and not being understood by loved ones. As with any chronic illness, clients need to maintain some degree of physical and psychological control over the disabling effects of their clinical manifestations. For some clients, however, the need to exercise control is so great that they can experience extreme powerlessness and helplessness during exacerbations of the illness. Clients who can view their relationship with RA as an evolving partnership have better outcomes, both physically and psychosocially, than clients who perceive the disease to be the "enemy." This sense of partnership helps the client let go (i.e., rest and take care of himself or herself) during exacerbations of the disease yet respond actively by agreeing to engage in health-promoting, self-care practices. It can also help clients not to waste precious energy with anxiety, anger, and unresolved grief or guilt.

Promote Balanced Nutrition. Nutrition is an important aspect of self-care that is often misunderstood by the client with RA. This misunderstanding can occur because the popular press has promoted nutrition and unique diet therapies as instant cures for arthritis. Clients with RA may become overweight (because of decreased activity or mobility) or underweight (because of the anorexia of a chronic illness, the side effects of medications, or alterations in oral mucous membranes). In addition, diets may not provide sufficient iron to restore the deficit that results from the anemia of a chronic illness.

Clients need to understand that it is just as important to consume nutritionally sound diets as it is to achieve a reasonable body weight. Strategies to promote nutrition in anorectic clients include good oral hygiene before and after meals; small, frequent feedings; and high-calorie snacks. Clients with a dry mouth (xerostomia) benefit from moister foods and extra fluids with meals. Eliminating spicy or acidic foods, sitting upright to eat, and taking all medications with food and a full glass of water can ameliorate gastrointestinal distress. Clients with stiffness or hand deformities need assistive devices to feed themselves or require help to open cartons or packages.

Promote Decision Making. Exercising healthy control over the disease may include formulating causes of the illness. Clients who reported causes for their arthritis (such as fate, personal habits, heredity, or the environment) were less anxious, depressed, and hostile than were those who did not report any cause. Most likely, clients who continue to ask "Why me?" and are unable to identify a specific cause of the illness have a more difficult time feeling in control.

Powerlessness can have physically and mentally detrimental effects on the client and can lead to anxiety, depression, and hopelessness. The key intervention for powerlessness is to increase the client's active participation in decision making by allowing the client as many choices as possible, for example, when to take medications or how to perform required ADL. Helping clients

to reframe their relationship with the disease to one of active partnership, as was previously mentioned, can also increase the sense of control.

Client education and hope are important to the client's perception of control. Arthritis education provides information that clients can use to make informed decisions about their care. Knowledge about the disease, its course, the appropriate treatment, and what clients can do to promote their well-being increases their mastery of the unknown. Client education in the safe environment of a support group can also decrease the uncertainties of the disease and thus enhance control.

Promote Hope. Having a sense of hopefulness about the future is a powerful ally against powerlessness. Everything clients do can be based on some level of hope. Nursing interventions to promote hope include avoiding false reassurance, helping clients to set realistic goals, praising them for all accomplishments (no matter how small), and active listening. Being sensitive to changes in mood and affect is important, particularly for clients receiving glucocorticoid therapy. When clients are taking steroids, views about the future often change from hopeful and positive to depressed, despairing expressions about their lives. If medication changes are not possible or if dosage adjustments do not relieve the depression, the nurse should consult the physician about the need for a psychiatric evaluation.

Promote Coping. Successful coping strategies help the client with RA to integrate the disease into the demands of daily living. Coping strategies can be viewed as either approach (positive or healthy) or avoidance strategies. Healthy approach strategies include seeking out information and assistance, finding strength through spiritual support, verbalizing feelings and concerns, setting goals, expressing positive thoughts, and maintaining realistic independence. The less adaptive, avoidance strategies include denial, excessive sleeping, other passive behaviors, and depression. Depression is often associated with increased levels of pain and functional impairment and increased use of health care services. As with clients who have other chronic illnesses, treatment with antidepressants may improve coping and pain control. In addition, the relationship between depression and pain may be influenced by the use of adaptive or maladaptive coping strategies and by clients' beliefs about their abilities to control their pain. Therefore the nurse's goal is clearly to help the client realize the benefits of the healthier approach strategies. Healthy coping strategies and the reframing of negative behaviors can be discussed, modeled, and safely tested in nurse-led client support groups.

For some clients, coping may be impaired because of changes in their body image and self-esteem. As the disease progresses, disfiguring joint changes or systemic alterations, such as rheumatoid nodules, may contribute to clients' sensitivity about their appearance and attractiveness. If changes occur in the performance of occupational, family, or social roles, self-esteem can be significantly affected. When clients with RA maintain employment with high levels of functional disability and exposure to stressful work, men and women, are at equal risk of experiencing emotional distress.

Evaluation. Rheumatoid arthritis is progressive and improvement can be slow. It may take several weeks to months for the expected outcomes to be achieved. Nevertheless, despite the many problems that people with RA face daily, many of these people courageously overcome these problems to maintain active, productive lives. There are multiple websites for arthritis that clients or health care providers can access, with the most comprehensive being The Arthritis Foundation at www. arthritis.org.

Surgical Management

Surgical procedures may be helpful for clients with arthritis. Surgery may be used to relieve pain, improve function, and correct deformities. When joints are already severely damaged and pain is uncontrollable, joint replacement may become an option. Previously, surgery was considered only late in the course of arthritis, often after severe joint destruction or deformity had developed. Now, however, early surgery is used to prevent deformities during the early phases or active stages of the disease.

Tendon Transfer and Osteotomy

Tendon transfers can prevent progressive deformity. During these procedures, nodules or benign bony tumors (exostoses) may be surgically removed and flexion contractures surgically relieved. Osteotomies (excising or cutting through bone) may improve the function of deformed joints or limbs. For example, a femoral head osteotomy may give symptomatic relief by changing the position of the head of the femur when it is being subjected to the stress of impact against the acetabulum. Postoperative care varies, depending on the joint treated. Postoperative physical therapy is critical.

Synovectomy

Synovectomy (surgical removal of synovia, as in the elbows, wrists, fingers, or knees) may be used in clients with RA to help maintain joint function. With RA, joint destruction begins in the synovial tissue and then proceeds to involve bone, cartilage, and other structures.

Short-term immobilization and physical therapy are needed after surgery.

Arthrodesis

Arthrodesis is an operation to produce bony fusion of a joint and is used for clients with bone loss after joint infection, tumors, musculoskeletal trauma, and paralysis. Arthrodesis may also help certain clients with RA or degenerative arthritis to regain some mobility. Although arthrodesis immobilizes the joint, the procedure may eliminate some of the discomfort of the arthritic process and improve functional mobility. The ankle is the joint most commonly treated with arthrodesis, usually to relieve post-traumatic arthritis. Arthrodesis often results in stiffness in adjacent joints and increases the energy required for ambulation. After surgery, the limb is casted. Nursing care is the same as for clients with casts (Chapter 27).

Joint Replacement

Arthroplasty (joint replacement) is the surgical replacement of diseased joints or joint components with artificial joints or joint components. The operation restores motion to a joint and function to the muscles, ligaments, and other soft tissue structures that control a joint. The selection of a prosthesis will require collaboration between the client and health care provider and will be dependent on the joint involved as well as the age and sex of the client. Joint prostheses can be a combination of a metal surface articulating with a polyethylene surface. The metal surfaces are made of strong, light-weight alloys such as cobalt-chromium and titanium-aluminum-vanadium. In some instances both surfaces of an arthritic joint may be replaced. Arthroplasties of the shoulder and hand are discussed next; hip and knee replacement is described in Chapter 26 following discussion of osteoarthritis.

Shoulder Arthroplasty. Disorders of the shoulder that require arthroplasty are much less common than those problems in weight-bearing joints. The shoulder relies on soft tissue and ligaments for stability, particularly the rotator cuff muscle-tendon unit. Shoulder arthroplasty is the replacement of the humeral head and glenoid articulating surface with a metal and polyethylene prosthesis (Figure 77-4). The primary indication for total shoulder replacement is pain and, secondarily, improvement in function and ROM.

Contraindications include infection and inability to comply with rehabilitation, such as clients with physiologic (e.g., neuropathy) or psychological problems. Complications include brachial nerve palsy, prosthetic loosening, joint dislocation or subluxation, and impingement syndrome.

■ **FIGURE 77–4** Total shoulder arthroplasty.

Postoperative Care

SAFETY

⚠

ALERT

Nursing assessment includes neurovascular examination of the operative arm at least every 4 hours. As shown in the Critical Monitoring feature at right, a possible complication is development of impingement syndrome because of the proximity of the brachial plexus.

Hemovac drainage should be less than 100 ml during the first 12 hours. Elevate the head of the bed 30 degrees to reduce swelling and improve comfort. Aggressive pain management is needed; shoulder arthroplasty usually causes more pain during the first 24 hours than the other joint replacements.

Patient-controlled analgesia (PCA) works well when supplemented with non-opioid anti-inflammatory agents. Ice is applied to the shoulder and the shoulder is positioned for comfort. Shoulder rehabilitation begins quickly after surgery and continues for about 6 weeks. For no other joint is rehabilitation as important as for the shoulder. The shoulder is placed through progressive external and internal ROM, hyperextension, and finally exercises with resistance once the rotator cuff has healed (approximately 6 weeks). Usually, the client can be taught how to use the nonoperative arm to move the operative arm through ROM.

Hand Arthroplasty. Various hand deformities develop from synovitis. Synovitis stretches the central portion of the extensor tendon, causing it to shift. Eventually, the tendons become shortened and fixed. Ulnar drift occurs when the imbalance of damaged extensor tendons and intact flexor tendons causes subluxation of the MCP joint. Other hand deformities develop from synovitis of the PIP joint: boutonnière deformity and swan-neck deformity.

CRITICAL MONITORING

Postoperative Brachial Plexus Compromise

■ To assess median nerve status, have the client grasp your hand. Note the strength of the first and second fingers. A weak grip may indicate compromise of the median nerve.

■ To assess radial nerve status, note the movement of the client's thumb toward the palm and then back to neutral. Problems with this motion may indicate compromise of the radial nerve.

■ To assess ulnar nerve status, have the client spread all the fingers wide and resist pressure. Weakness against pressure may indicate compromise of the ulnar nerve.

■ To assess cutaneous nerve status, assess for flexion of the biceps by having the client raise the forearm. Poor biceps flexion may indicate compromise of the cutaneous nerve.

■ To assess axillary nerve status, have the client push the elbow outward against pressure. Hold the arm still while you palpate the deltoid for contraction. Weak contraction may indicate compromise of the axillary nerve.

A boutonnière deformity is flexion of the PIP joint and hyperextension of the DIP joint. There is no loss of MCP joint mobility. In the swan-neck deformity, the DIP joint is flexed and the PIP joint is hyperextended. Surgery includes tendon transfers to improve pinch grasp and arthrodesis for strength and position of the thumb for opposition. Hinge implants are placed to restore function to the fingers.

Postoperative Care. After surgery, neurovascular assessments are performed every hour for several hours. If the client has regional block anesthesia, the hand may be numb. The hand is elevated off the bed to prevent ulnar pressure. The hand is usually placed in a stockinette and suspended from the bed. An opening is made to assess the fingers. Encourage the client to exercise the fingers 10 times every hour, attempting full extension and flexion. Finger exercises reduce edema and pain. Place the client's personal items within easy reach of the nonoperative arm. If the opposite hand is equally deformed from RA, the client is often quite helpless and will require assistance with most components of ADL.

Encourage the client to use the nonoperative arm as much as possible. Some clients may express great concern about being dependent. Promote independence, and praise actions that foster self-care. Rehabilitation is a long process. Most clients are fitted with outrigger splints with rubber bands that allow exercise with resistance after 1 week. Therapy continues for several weeks to assist the client to regain strength and control.

Modifications for Older Clients

Older clients may have adapted to RA very well but often find any further dependency needed after surgery difficult to handle. They tend to be slower in their recovery from total joint replacement surgery. They may require prolonged hospitalization in an extended-care facility or subacute care setting until they regain adequate mobility to function independently or with some assistance and safety.

CONNECTIVE TISSUE DISORDERS

SYSTEMIC LUPUS ERYTHEMATOSUS

The term *lupus*, Latin for wolf, to describe various disfiguring cutaneous disorders, dates to the medieval period. The first clinical description of rashes that continue to be recognized as lupus was by Biett, in 1833. Credit is usually given to Kaposi for describing the systemic nature of the disease, including fever, weight loss, lymphadenopathy, and mental disturbances. Insights into the pathogenesis of systemic lupus erythematosus (SLE) were enhanced by the discovery of the lupus erythematosus (LE) cell phenomenon and the antinuclear factor.

SLE is a multisystem, inflammatory disorder associated with abnormalities of the immune system. It is a chronic condition characterized by various degrees of increased disease activity that are generally followed by a less active, remitting course. So many classic immunologic abnormalities can be present in SLE that it is considered the prototype of an autoimmune disease. Typically, multiple body organs and systems are affected at different times, thus producing widespread damage to connective tissues, blood vessels, and serous and mucous membranes.

SLE is primarily a disease of young women. Peak incidence occurs between the ages of 15 and 40 during the childbearing years, with a female to male ratio of 5:1. However, the onset can range from infancy to advanced age. In both pediatric and older-onset clients, the female to male ratio approximates 2:1. The 1982 revised criteria for the classification of SLE are listed in Table 77-2. The diagnosis of SLE is confirmed if a client has any 4 of the 11 criteria present, either serially or simultaneously, during any observation period.

Etiology and Risk Factors

In the general population, SLE affects approximately 1 in 2000 individuals. Incidence rates have increased over the past 40 years, most likely because of an increased availability of serologic tests and increased awareness of the disease. The disease has a predilection for women in

TABLE 77-2 1982 Revised Criteria for the Classification of Systemic Lupus Erythematosus

Criterion	Definition
Malar rash	Fixed erythema, flat or raised, over the malar eminences, tending to spare nasolabial folds
Discoid rash	Erythematous raised patches with adherent keratotic scaling and follicular plugging; atrophic scarring may occur in older lesions
Photosensitivity	Skin rash as a result of unusual reaction to sunlight, by client history or physician observation
Oral ulcers	Oral or nasopharyngeal ulceration, usually painless, observed by physician
Arthritis	Nonerosive arthritis involving two or more peripheral joints, characterized by tenderness, swelling, or effusion
Serositis	Pleuritis—convincing history of pleuritic pain or rub heard by a physician or evidence of pleural effusion *or* Pericarditis—documented by electrocardiogram or rub or evidence of pericardial effusion
Renal disorder	Persistent proteinuria greater than 0.5 g/day or greater than 3 g if quantification not performed *or* Cellular casts—may be red cell, hemoglobin, granular, tubular, or mixed
Neurologic disorder	Seizures—in the absence of offending drugs or known metabolic derangements, e.g., uremia, ketoacidosis, or electrolyte imbalance *or* Psychosis—in absence of offending drugs or known metabolic derangements, e.g., uremia, ketoacidosis, or electrolyte imbalance
Hematologic disorder	Hemolytic anemia—with reticulocytosis *or* Leukopenia—less than 4000/mm³ total on two or more occasions *or* Lymphopenia—less than 1500/mm³ on two or more occasions *or* Thrombocytopenia—less than 100,000/mm³ in absence of offending drugs
Immunologic disorder	Positive lupus erythematosus cell preparation *or* Anti-DNA—antibody to native DNA in abnormal titer *or* Anti-Sm—presence of antibody to Sm nuclear antigen *or* False-positive serologic test for syphilis known to be positive for at least 6 months and confirmed by *Treponema pallidum* immobilization or fluorescent treponemal antibody absorption test
Antinuclear antibody	Abnormal titer of antinuclear antibody by immunofluorescence or an equivalent assay at any point in time and in absence of drugs known to be associated with "drug-induced lupus" syndrome

Data from Tan, E., et al. (1982). The 1982 revised criteria for the classification of systemic lupus erythematosus (SLE). *Arthritis and Rheumatism, 25,* 1271-1277.

their childbearing years, with young African-American women the majority group affected. The prevalence of SLE varies with race, ethnicity, and socioeconomic status. The Lupus Foundation of America (www.lupus.org) estimates that 1,500,000 Americans have either systemic or limited forms of lupus. The female to male prevalence ratio is 10:1 for women in the childbearing years. However, men and African-American females have a worse renal outcome than women.

Once considered a fatal disease in young women, SLE now has improved outcomes. Over 85% of people with the disorder live longer than 15 years after diagnosis. Increased mortality, however, has been noted in African Americans, Asians, Puerto Ricans, and people of Hispanic descent living in the southwest United States. Poor survival has been associated with high serum creatinine levels, low hematocrit levels, proteinuria, and the source of medical care funding. The most common causes of death in SLE are active lupus nephritis, vascular events, and infections.

An underlying hormonal change may explain why the disease affects so many more women. Genetic factors may also be involved. Familial aggregation occurs in 10% of people having a first-degree relative with SLE, including its occurrence in identical twins.

Pathophysiology

The pathologic findings of SLE occur throughout the body and are manifested by inflammation, blood vessel abnormalities that encompass both bland vasculopathy and vasculitis, and immune complex deposition. SLE results from an abnormal reaction of the body against its own tissues, cells, and serum proteins. In other words, as an autoimmune disease, SLE is characterized by a decreased self-tolerance. In the North American Caucasian population, there is a positive association between SLE and two HLA antigens (DR2 and DR3) that are coded by the MHC. People with SLE have increased numbers of both self and non-self antigens, suggesting hyperactivity of the B cells. Interleukin-6 may have a role in B-cell hyperactivity. Another antibody, anti-DNA of the IgG type, may be responsible for the development of the engulfed LE bodies in the LE cells. The relationship between the serum LE factor and the pathologic changes that occur with SLE is not clear. The absence of the LE factor, however, is a strong indication that the disease is not present. Increased levels of anti–double-stranded DNA (anti-dsDNA) antibodies are associated with increased disease activity in clients with SLE.

Clinical Manifestations

SLE can be differentiated by the presence or development of glomerulonephritis, photosensitivity, characteristic skin rashes, central nervous system disease, and various cytopenias such as the Coombs' test positive hemolytic anemia, leukopenia, and thrombocytopenia. The clinical manifestations vary considerably, from general complaints of fever, fatigue, and malaise; to painful, swollen joints; to the psychological distress of a variety of skin lesions. The latter can include the classic butterfly rash over the bridge of the nose and cheeks, erythematous discoid lesions (which can result in permanent scars on the scalp, ears, face or neck), the temporary loss of hair on the scalp, painless mouth ulcers, and cutaneous vascular lesions. Sunlight may trigger a local dermatitis. Systemic manifestations (renal, cardiac, or pulmonary) as well as a variety of serum, immunologic, and antibody abnormalities may be present. Table 77-3 summarizes the changes in organ systems that occur in SLE.

The *most specific tests* for SLE are antibodies to double-stranded DNA and antibodies to Sm and ribosomal P proteins, which are seen exclusively in SLE. Measuring C-reactive protein levels can sometimes be a useful test for distinguishing between a lupus flare-up and infection. It usually remains normal in a flare-up but is elevated in infection.

The *most sensitive test* for SLE is the relatively nonspecific fluorescent anti-nuclear antibody (ANA) assay. Almost all clients with SLE have ANAs, but they also occur in many other situations, such as infections, advanced age, and RA, and with certain drug therapy regimens. Complements C3, C4, and CD 50 are useful measures of disease activity.

TABLE 77–3 System Changes with the Pathogenesis of Systemic Lupus Erythematosus

System	Pathogenesis with Systemic Lupus Erythematosus
Integumentary	Immune complex deposition, inflammation of dermal-epidermal junctions, vasculitis
Gastrointestinal	Collagen degeneration and vasculitis leading to mucous membrane ulcers; vasculitis leading to organ infarction and necrosis
Musculoskeletal	Increased fibrin deposits at synovial surfaces; inflammation of arterioles, venules, and tendon sheaths; eventual necrosis, degeneration, and fibrosis of muscle tissue
Pulmonary	Pleural inflammation, pneumonitis, pulmonary hypertension
Cardiovascular	Diffuse vasculitis; inflammation and scarring of atrioventricular and sinoatrial nodes; inflammation of pericardial sac
Renal	Deposition of immune complexes in glomerular basement membranes
Neurologic	Immune complex deposition; antineuronal antibody activity leading to cerebritis, seizures, organic brain syndrome, and peripheral neuropathies

OUTCOME MANAGEMENT

Medical Management

In general, the clinical pattern and prognosis of SLE are variable. The illness may develop rapidly with an acute fulminant course. More commonly, it develops insidiously and becomes chronic, with remissions and exacerbations. The course of the disorder is more severe when onset occurs at a young age. The survival rate has improved dramatically in recent years, although the disease is still potentially fatal. Improvements in early diagnosis and treatment allow clients the opportunity to live longer.

The primary management of SLE involves the use of drugs that suppress end-organ inflammation or interfere with immune function. Very few drug therapies have been subjected to randomized clinical trials. Treatment of acute SLE is based on the use of steroids, immunosuppressive agents, and experimental therapies. It is critical in the management of these clients to be aware of and to aggressively treat the co-morbid conditions that commonly occur in SLE—hypertension, infections, seizures, hyperlipidemia, and osteoporosis.

Reduce Inflammation and Minimize Complications

Only three drugs have been approved for the treatment of lupus, with the last approved more than 40 years ago. They are aspirin, glucocorticoids, and hydroxychloroquine. Off-label use includes NSAIDs, cyclophosphamide, and azathioprine. Medications used to treat lupus are reviewed in the Integrating Pharmacology feature on p. 2072.

Dialysis or Kidney Transplantation

Clients with end-stage lupus nephropathy are managed with dialysis or kidney transplantation. There is a tendency for decreased clinical and serologic lupus activity following the onset of end-stage renal disease. Survival rates of lupus clients and other end-stage renal clients are comparable. Most studies note an increased incidence of infections among SLE clients on dialysis. Kidney transplantation during an acute exacerbation of SLE is controversial and may increase the risk of poor outcome. Recurrence of lupus nephritis in transplanted allografts, often with the same histopathology as in the native kidney, develops in 2% to 4% of transplanted kidneys.

Promote Rest and Coping

Although drug therapy and the use of experimental treatments play a significant part in the management of SLE, perhaps the more important aspects of treatment are the supportive therapies of physical and emotional rest, diet and nutrition, and skin protection. Nurses have

an important role in teaching clients how to manage the daily stress of coping with a chronic illness.

Nursing Management of the Medical Client

Obtain Nursing History

The nursing history of people with confirmed or suspected SLE must be sufficiently thorough to capture the range of possible manifestations that accompany an autoimmune disease. Clients need to be asked about general problems, such as fever, weight loss, and fatigue, and about changes in energy levels. A detailed medication history is essential in identifying the need for additional client teaching as well as in determining that the condition has not been drug induced. Clients should be asked about the names of their current medications, dosage, purpose, side effects, and length of time that they have been taking these drugs. Approximately 25 drugs have been implicated as causing a lupus-like syndrome, but only a few (hydralazine, procainamide, isoniazid) cause the disorder with any great frequency.

Questions about changes in skin should be elicited. The presence, location, and nature of rashes need to be explored as well as if the rashes are associated with exposure to sunlight or even fluorescent lighting. Clients should be asked about changes in their nails and nail beds, loss of hair on the scalp, and mouth or nasal sores.

Because SLE is occasionally characterized by generalized cerebritis, careful attention should be paid to the neuropsychiatric system. If seizure activity occurs, it is usually the generalized tonic-clonic type. The client should be asked about visual disturbances, vertigo, facial weakness, and presence of headaches. Changes in emotional status, including anxiety, insomnia, disorientation, and mood swings, are fairly common as a result of the disease and/or steroid therapy. The client may also complain of impaired cognition, such as mental dullness or a slow reaction time.

Complete Physical Assessment

The nursing assessment should begin with an examination of the integumentary and musculoskeletal systems because clients with SLE have a high percentage of physical changes involving the skin, muscles, and joints. Inspect the entire body carefully, noting the location, nature, and size of cutaneous and vascular lesions. Transient rashes can appear in any location, particularly after exposure to sunlight. Interestingly, the classic butterfly rash over the bridge of the nose and cheeks affects fewer than half of those with SLE. Discoid lesions, characterized by annular erythematous plaques, can appear as atrophied, scaling areas on the face, neck, and arms. Severe scarring is also possible. Fingers can be affected by erythema under the nail beds or by digital gangrene.

INTEGRATING PHARMACOLOGY

Medications Used to Treat Systemic Lupus Erythematosus

Systemic lupus erythematosus (SLE) is a chronic disease similar in many ways to rheumatoid arthritis (RA). However, with SLE, inflammation is not limited to joints; rather, it occurs throughout the body. Clinical manifestations include pleuritis, pericarditis, and nephritis and a severe episode can be fatal. Fortunately, the manifestations of SLE can usually be controlled with prompt and aggressive glucocorticoid therapy.

NSAIDs

Nonsteroidal antiinflammatory drugs (NSAIDs) are used to reduce musculoskeletal manifestations, mild serositis, and fever.

SAFETY ALERT

Care must be taken when using NSAIDs in clients with SLE. NSAIDs inhibit prostaglandin synthesis within the kidney and impair renal blood flow. Clients with lupus nephritis are particularly susceptible because of a heightened dependency on prostaglandins to maintain renal function compromised by glomerular inflammation. Clients should be questioned about their nonprescription use of NSAIDs. Renal abnormalities produced by NSAIDs, particularly impaired renal function, are generally promptly reversible.

GLUCOCORTICOIDS

Glucocorticoids are required to control serious complications, such as thrombocytopenic purpura, hemolytic anemia, myocarditis, pericarditis, seizures, and nephritis. Prednisone is usually given orally in low doses (up to 15 mg/day), moderate doses (16 to 40 mg/day), or high doses (up to 120 mg/day). Divided doses are generally administered to ensure more sustained anti-inflammatory action and greater lupus-suppressing activity than the same amount of drug given as a single morning dose.

SAFETY ALERT

Once the disease is under control, however, gradual reduction (tapering) is essential. Clients on a multiple daily dose regimen must first be converted to a single morning dose before attempting to reduce the actual drug dose. The length of time the client has been on the drug directly affects the length of drug taper. Many methods have been used with the most common being to decrease the dose by 10 mg in weekly increments.

See the discussion of surgery clients receiving glucocorticoid therapy in the Integrating Pharmacology feature on Medications Used in the Treatment of Rheumatoid Arthritis.

An alternative to the use of high-dose oral glucocorticoids is bolus intravenous steroid pulse therapy. Usually 1 to 1.5 g of methylprednisolone is given daily for 3 days to clients with severe disease, such as active nephritis, fulminating central nervous system disease, and hematologic crises. Generally, oral glucocorticoids (up to 60 mg/day of prednisone) are also given following this treatment period. Dysrhythmias and seizures have been associated with sudden death after administration of pulse therapy.

OTHER IMMUNOSUPPRESSANTS

The use of immunosuppressive agents has gradually become an accepted therapy for SLE. Methotrexate in low doses (7.5 to 15 mg/week) appears to be useful in managing arthritis, skin rashes, serositis, and other clinical manifestations. Treatment regimens, including azathioprine (Imuran) or cyclophosphamide (Cytoxan), have been able to halt the progression of glomerulonephritis or result in significantly less renal deterioration. Azathioprine, intravenous cyclophosphamide, and HCQ can also be given. See the Integrating Pharmacology feature on Medications used in the Treatment of Rheumatoid Arthritis for more information.

OTHER AGENTS

The attenuated androgen danazol has been shown to be useful in managing SLE thrombocytopenia. The mechanism of action has not been defined, but it is thought to involve endocrine influences such as the suppression of pituitary follicle-stimulating hormone and luteinizing hormone on immune or reticuloendothelial functions.

Intravenous immunoglobulin has been shown to be useful in managing severe SLE thrombocytopenia. The platelet count rises rapidly within hours of administration, occasionally peaking with extraordinarily high counts in which thrombotic events become a clinical concern. The rate of relapse following treatment is high. The primary role is to control acute bleeding associated with lupus thrombocytopenia or to rapidly increase the platelet count to allow for splenectomy or other surgery.

Dapsone, an antimicrobial agent used to treat leprosy (Hansen's disease), has been used to manage cutaneous manifestation of lupus, including discoid, subacute cutaneous lupus, bullous, and lupus profundus lesions. Hematologic side effects are common and require close monitoring.

There are several drugs in clinical trials for the treatment of lupus nephritis, including the use of mycophenolate mofetil (CellCept) and tolerogens that arrest the production of dsDNA antibodies. A placebo-controlled trial of dehydroepiandrosterone (DHEA) has reported benefits in clients with mild to moderate lupus activity. Stem cell transplant is also being aggressively explored.

Mild to moderate loss of scalp hair can occur when the disease is active. Vascular lesions can include petechiae, purpuric lesions, and Raynaud's phenomenon.

Joint manifestations, with or without active synovitis, occur in over 90% of those affected. Along with Raynaud's phenomenon, these findings are often the earliest features of the disease. Therefore the musculoskeletal examination should focus on a full assessment of the ROM of all joints, noting the location and presence of synovitis, diffuse swelling, joint and muscle pain, and stiffness. Joint involvement is symmetrical in SLE, but deformities are usually the result of soft tissue stresses rather than erosive changes. One of the more common deformities is Jaccoud's arthropathy, a rheumatoid-like deformity of the hands present in about 10% of clients with SLE. In this condition, the MCP joints are subluxed, ulnar deviation develops, and hyperextension of the PIP joints can be observed.

Manage Exacerbations

During exacerbations, clients may become acutely and seriously ill. Infectious complications can develop in about one half of clients with SLE, especially bacterial infections of the skin, respiratory tract, and urinary tract. Nursing care during this time is directed toward the assessment and management of acute confusional states, the prevention of seizures, the maintenance of skin integrity, the prevention of additional infection, the assessment of renal function, and the management of impaired gas exchange associated with lung disease and infection.

During this acute phase, increased fatigue, joint pain, and stiffness are often present as a result of inflammation and increased disease activity. Nursing activities to manage these acute flare-ups are similar to those used during exacerbations of RA. Self-care deficits are often exacerbated because of the increased disease activity. It is important to help clients maintain as much independence as possible during periods of acute flare-ups so both self-esteem and physical functions are enhanced. Clients may require considerably more time to complete even one task, so nursing interventions may need to help the client focus on conserving energy and prioritizing self-care actions.

Promote Orientation and Decision Making

Caring for a client with acutely impaired thought processes can be perplexing. Several factors can contribute to the cause of this nursing diagnosis, including increased inflammation of the central nervous system and psychosis from high doses of steroids. Clients typically have severe throbbing headaches that are sometimes accompanied by generalized tonic-clonic seizures. They may display impaired judgment, inappropriate speech and behavior, difficulty concentrating or comprehending simple instructions, or short-term memory deficits. As the disease progresses, they may have personality changes, with a decreased ability to carry out purposeful activity. Clients with impaired thought processes should be cared for in a quiet environment, particularly when headaches are severe. Clocks and calendars should be provided to help with orientation. Communication must be caring but clear and concise to decrease ambiguity and anxiety.

Provide Seizure Precautions

If clients are prone to seizures, they should be observed carefully for auras or specific activities that might trigger the seizure. During the seizure, the client should be protected from injury by removing dangerous objects, providing padding and blankets, and by turning the client to the side after muscle activity has stopped to prevent aspiration. Restraints should never be applied during the seizure because the intense muscular activity beneath the restraint could lead to fractures.

SAFETY ALERT

Monitor Fluid Status

Another focus of nursing care during exacerbations of the disease is the management of excess fluid volume typically seen in peripheral edema. The goal is to maintain optimal renal function by assessing urinary output and urine specific gravity every 2 to 4 hours, monitoring fluid intake and electrolyte levels, and assessing changes in the level of consciousness.

Maintain Skin Integrity

The skin of a steroid-dependent client with SLE is characteristically tissue thin and fragile, so clients with peripheral edema must be moved and handled gently. The excess osmotic pressure beneath the skin surface can stress it easily so that minimal shearing forces can quickly denude the dermal layers.

SAFETY ALERT

Promote Coping and Self-Esteem

During the chronic phase of the illness, clients can experience intense frustration because they often do not appear ill. The extreme weakness and fatigue they encounter during exacerbations of the disease, however, can lead to feelings of powerlessness and helplessness, ineffective coping, and a disturbance in self-concept. Helping clients with SLE develop a traditional support group is difficult. Lupus clients are often homebound because of extreme fatigue, impaired mobility, and commitment to their roles of spouse and parent. In these situations, the use of telephone support networks or Internet support networks for clients with SLE can be a powerful nursing strategy. At the same time that these networks provide social support and counseling for the homebound, they also encourage personal growth and development among other clients with SLE who have developed positive coping skills. Nurses can play an important role in helping to establish this type of network through the education and support of peer counselors.

Discuss Reproductive Issues

During remissions, clients often wonder about whether they can safely have children. This is a natural concern because most clients are women of childbearing age. Because fertility in clients with SLE is comparable to that of the general population, initiating and responding to clients' requests for health information are important functions of the nurse. Relapses of SLE can occur at any time during pregnancy but have not shown to result in an increase in the risk of fetal loss. The incidence of relapses during pregnancy has been reported to vary from 22% to 58%. However, most disease exacerbations can be reasonably well controlled with increasing doses of prednisone. Oral contraceptives containing low doses of estrogen are safe with mild lupus but should be used with caution by clients with severe lupus, as they can cause a flare-up. In addition, most studies report good neonatal outcomes in infants born to women with SLE, although a high incidence of prematurity has been observed.

SYSTEMIC SCLEROSIS

Systemic sclerosis (SSc), literally "hard" (scleros) "skin" (derma), encompasses both a disease restricted to the skin (localized scleroderma) and a disease with internal organ involvement (diffuse scleroderma or systemic sclerosis). One of the earliest definite descriptions of scleroderma was published by W.D. Chowne (1842, London), pertaining to a child, and in an adult by James Startin (1846, London). Maurice Raynaud (1862, Paris) described the vasospastic phenomenon that bears his name.

SSc is one of the least well understood of the rheumatic disorders. It occurs as a multisystem inflammatory disease characterized by skin thickening (scleroderma) and deposition of excessive quantities of connective tissue (particularly collagen), which eventually results in severe fibrosis. The skin, blood vessels, synovium, and skeletal muscles are affected along with the microvasculature of internal organs, such as the heart, lung, kidney, and gastrointestinal tract. Widespread vascular involvement, perhaps the earliest and most significant pathologic change, is also a prominent feature of SSc.

SSc is seen worldwide. The incidence for women is more than three times greater than that for men, especially for those between the ages of 14 and 40 years. The incidence has been calculated to be 10 per 100,000 people, with a total estimate of 250,000 to 300,000 cases in the United States.

SSc is considered one of the eight types of scleroderma, the classification of which depends on the degree and extent of skin thickening. The term "scleroderma" was first introduced in the mid-19th century to describe skin induration. Later, others used the term "progressive systemic sclerosis" to reflect its often-generalized multisystem course. Currently, the term "systemic sclerosis" is preferred because many clients have limited skin and organ involvement.

Etiology and Risk Factors

Several risk factors have been associated with SSc. Overproduction of collagen and fibrous skin thickening have been associated with environmental factors (working with plastics, coal, or silica dust) and a high alcohol intake. Scleroderma-like conditions can also be present as a result of genetic factors (phenylketonuria), metabolic disorders (Hashimoto's thyroiditis), malignancies, postinfectious disorders, and neurologic conditions.

Pathophysiology

SSc is the result of an excessive production of collagen by fibroblasts. It seems likely that lymphocytes accumulate in the lower dermis. These cells, almost entirely T lymphocytes, generate lymphokines, which in turn stimulate fibroblasts to produce excessive amounts of procollagen. After the procollagen is secreted from the cell, it undergoes cross-linking in the extracellular environment to produce mature, relatively insoluble collagen. The skin undergoes fibrotic changes, leading to loss of elasticity and movement.

Vascular changes are also important in the development of SSc. When the vascular endothelium is injured, damaged blood vessels release vasoactive substances, which are stimulated to overproduce collagen and mucopolysaccharides. Proliferation of the subintimal connective tissue results, along with fibrous thickening and narrowing of the lumina, thus leading to tissue ischemia. A small number of clients with CREST (see Clinical Manifestations) develop pulmonary hypertension and intestinal malabsorption, which are the leading causes of death for these clients.

Clinical Manifestations

The two major types of SSc are classified according to the degree of their skin and systemic involvement. The first type, characterized by diffuse, cutaneous scleroderma, begins with symmetrical widespread thickening of the skin on the extremities, the face, and the trunk. In the early stages of the disease, bilateral symmetrical swelling of the fingers, face, and feet can be seen, and the skin has a tense, wrinkle-free appearance (Figure 77-5). As

■ **FIGURE 77–5 A,** Long-term scleroderma. Note wrinkle-free appearance and shininess of the skin. **B,** Appearance of the hands in a client with scleroderma. Note thickening of the skin and swelling of the fingers.

the disease progresses, the skin becomes more thickened, hidebound, and shiny. Changes in pigmentation (both hypopigmentation and hyperpigmentation) are associated with the loss of normal skin folds. Distal thickening is always more severe than proximal thickening, so the extremities may show more changes than the face. Eventually, the face can become mask-like. The mouth is rigid, and the overall expression is blunted or immobile. Clients with this diffuse type have a tendency to develop early problems in the gastrointestinal tract, heart, lungs, and kidneys. The esophagus is particularly affected. Because of the early development of visceral changes, the pace, progression, and complications can be rapid.

The second type, limited cutaneous scleroderma, is characterized by skin changes that are usually confined to the fingers and distal portions of the extremities and face. In general, skin changes progress much more slowly than they do in the diffuse type of SSc. Truncal scleroderma is absent. Visceral changes (e.g., severe pulmonary arterial hypertension and biliary cirrhosis), if they do appear, are rare and are seen late in the course of the disease. Clients with limited scleroderma often develop "CREST":

- **C**alcinosis: Calcium deposits in the tissues
- **R**aynaud's phenomenon: Intermittent vasospasm of the finger tips
- **E**sophageal hardening: Sclerosis of the esophagus
- **S**clerodactyly: Scleroderma of the digits
- **T**elangiectasias: Capillary dilations that form vascular lesions on the face, lips, and fingers

The presence of the CREST manifestations is a poor prognostic indicator. The 10-year survival rate after diagnosis is approximately 65%.

Raynaud's phenomenon, a generally bilateral vasospastic condition, can be an especially important predictor of SSc. Tricolor changes affecting the fingers in Raynaud's disease consist of pallor (white) accompanying vasoconstriction, followed by cyanosis (blue) as capillary blood is desaturated of oxygen, followed by hyperemia (redness) secondary to vasodilation. Clients with the CREST syndrome often develop painful ulcers on the finger tips or in the areas of calcinosis because of chronic vascular insufficiency. Although not listed in the acronym CREST, there is evidence of pulmonary involvement in the majority of clients. An occasional client with limited cutaneous scleroderma will develop pulmonary artery hypertension.

Laboratory findings are relatively normal in clients with scleroderma. Mild hemolytic anemia is often present because of mechanical damage to red cells from diseased small vessels. Mild hypergammaglobulinemia (IgG) and rheumatoid factor are found in 30% of those affected. Slight elevation of the ESR is also common. Proteinuria is common with renal involvement. Most clients have positive titers for ANA. Anticentromere and anticentriole antibodies seem to be relatively specific for scleroderma. Clients with the serum anticentromere antibody have a more favorable prognosis. SCL-70, an antibody to topoisomerase, is found in about 35% of clients with diffuse SSc but is rarely seen in clients with limited cutaneous involvement and the CREST syndrome. The anticentromere ANA is seen in 80% of those with limited cutaneous involvement and in only 5% of those with diffuse cutaneous involvement.

A definite diagnosis of SSc requires the presence of one major or two minor criteria. The major criteria for proximal scleroderma are skin thickening and tightening of areas proximal to the MCP joints. These changes can affect the entire extremity, face, neck, thorax, and abdomen. The three minor criteria are (1) sclerodactyly (in which the skin changes are limited to the fingers); (2) digital pitting scars, with depressed areas at the tips of the fingers or loss of fingerpad tissue; and (3) bibasilar pulmonary fibrosis.

OUTCOME MANAGEMENT

Medical Management

The treatment of SSc involves the shared management of a chronic illness and pharmacologic support. Members of the health care team should educate the client about the nature, course, and treatment of SSc, the importance of avoiding cold, stress management techniques as a means to control Raynaud's phenomenon, the prevention of hand contractures and facial rigidity, the nutritional management of constipation and diarrhea and ideal body weight, and the prevention of injury. Protecting digits by using gloves or wearing warm socks, avoiding cold temperatures, and not smoking are important self-care measures that may require behavior modification to help the client have some control over the illness.

Reduce Inflammation, Sclerosis, and Vasospasm

Many medications are used in systemic sclerosis, but no single agent has been proved convincingly effective. Treatment and prevention of complications are the current goals of therapy. Three types of therapeutic agents have been used to treat SSc: (1) vasoactive agents, (2) anti-inflammatory medications, and (3) immunosuppressive drugs.

In Raynaud's disease, calcium-channel blockers have become widely prescribed. Nifedipine, 10 to 20 mg three times a day, was effective for Raynaud's disease in a controlled, double-blind trial. Digital ulcers and digital infarcts have been somewhat successfully treated with digital sympathectomies.

Glucocorticoids are the major anti-inflammatory agents used in SSc when clients have significant joint and muscle involvement or extensive skin disease. Low-dose steroid therapy (prednisone, 10 mg/day or every other day) is preferred. Overall, immunosuppressive agents (azathioprine, cyclophosphamide, cyclosporine, and methotrexate) have not consistently been proved effective in the

treatment of SSc. Cyclophosphamide is often used in clients with progressive lung fibrosis.

Penicillamine, an immunomodulating agent that also interferes with the cross-linking of collagen, is a widely used drug in treating scleroderma. A large retrospective study showed significant improvement in skin thickening after 2 years of therapy and improved 5-year survival compared with untreated clients Not all clinicians, however, accept penicillamine as established therapy for SSc. Initial doses should be low (125 mg/day) and the dose should increase gradually. Reduction of skin thickness requires long-term therapy, so clients need considerable support and monitoring while they are taking penicillamine. In addition, numerous toxic side effects can occur, including lupus-like syndrome, myasthenia gravis, glomerulonephritis, pemphigus, excessive skin wrinkling, and blood and liver dyscrasias. Clients taking penicillamine must be carefully instructed to report skin rashes, burning, bleeding, sore throats, or fevers that might indicate serious side effects. The nurse and physician must explain the importance of periodic laboratory follow-up of liver, kidney, and renal function to the client.

Various other agents are used to treat specific system problems. Minocycline has been effective in the treatment of diarrhea associated with malabsorption syndrome. This drug may reduce inflammation by blocking metalloproteases. A proton pump inhibitor should be administered to reduce the acidity of gastric reflux. Etanercept, a biologic response modifier (BMR), in an initial small (10 client), open-label pilot study was encouraging, as was the long-term extension, but further research is necessary to determine its effectiveness in SSc management.

Reduce Renal Complications

Renal crisis and associated hypertension was the most feared complication of systemic sclerosis. The introduction of angiotensin-converting enzyme (ACE) inhibitors, which are capable of reversing underlying hyperreninemia and controlling hypertension, has improved the outcome of renal crisis. Clients now have an 80% 1-year survival and a 60% 5-year survival, in contrast to a 15% 1-year survival without the use of ACE inhibitors.

Treat Pulmonary Arterial Hypertension

Pulmonary arterial hypertension (PAH) is a leading cause of mortality in SSc. Two-year survival of clients with PAH has been 40% to 55%. Pulmonary vascular disease can occur in isolation or in the setting of the later stages of interstitial lung disease, complicating both diffuse and limited scleroderma. Initial endothelial cell injury results in abnormal vascular reactivity, related to factors such as local release of the vasoconstrictive mediator endothelin and loss of the endothelial-derived vasodilators prostacyclin and nitric oxide (NO). Functional lesions progress to structural lesions of arteriolar fibrosis.

The newly approved pharmacologic treatments, epoprostenol (Flolan), bosentan (Tracleer), and terprostinil (Remodulin), are well matched to current understanding of the underlying pathophysiology. All three agents have been demonstrated in controlled clinical trials to have beneficial effects on exercise capacity and pulmonary hemodynamics. Factors affecting the use of these agents include the short half-life of the prostacyclin analogs (epoprostenol, 2 to 5 minutes; trepostinil, 3 hours), necessitating continuous infusion; the need for a central line for administration of epoprostenol; the potential teratogenicity (risk for congenital defects) of bosentan; and availability issues (e.g., bosentan is distributed only through centralized pharmacies).

Nursing Management of the Medical Client

Complete Nursing History

Clients should be interviewed with great sensitivity because of their possible fears about the disease and the changes in body image. The first manifestation of SSc is often puffiness of the fingers and toes and in limited scleroderma, Raynaud's phenomenon. Question clients carefully about their experiences. Ask them if they have had the sequence of blanching, cyanosis, and erythema that is associated with periodic vasospasm of the peripheral blood vessels. Ask which parts of the body have been affected. Although Raynaud's phenomenon is commonly seen in the hands and toes, it can affect the earlobes, nose, and tongue. It is also important to ask clients under what circumstances (i.e., cold or stress) they have experienced Raynaud's phenomenon.

Clients should be asked about changes in the texture, color, consistency, and moisture of their skin. Because skin changes can be widespread, it is usually helpful to tell clients you would like to review changes according to body location. Clients should be asked about subcutaneous nodules that they may have noticed under their finger tips.

Other systemic changes to be explored include those associated with the gastrointestinal tract. Clients should be asked about the ease with which they swallow food and the types of food they have had difficulty swallowing. The presence of diarrhea (related to bacterial overgrowth) or a malabsorption syndrome can occur; constipation (related to colonic hypomotility), nausea, vomiting, and abdominal distention should be explored within the framework of onset, severity, duration, aggravating factors, and relieving factors. The respiratory system can be affected, secondary to interstitial pulmonary fibrosis. Therefore ask clients if they have had any cough, shortness of breath, or dyspnea with activity.

Clients should be asked questions about their musculoskeletal health. The presence of bilateral symmetrical joint pain and swelling should be elicited. Changes in endurance and muscle strength, as indicated by the ability to perform ADL, should be explored.

Complete Physical Assessment

A careful assessment is required of the entire integumentary system, including the skin on the feet, trunk, and abdomen. The face and lips (as well as fingers, palms, and fingernails) may have telangiectasias, which are macular dilations of superficial blood vessels that collapse after firm palpation. The hands are inspected and palpated for edema, thickened or hardened skin, loss of skin folds, or wrinkles (see Figure 77-5, B). Fingers are also inspected and palpated for subcutaneous calcific nodules and dilated capillary loops or venules or ulcers on the tips of the fingernails. Nail beds are inspected for pitting, changes in contour, and the appearance of suppurative cuticles.

Changes in the skin over the forearms, face, legs, and trunk can occur in diffuse cutaneous scleroderma. Therefore each area should be carefully assessed for edema, thickening, or tightening. The face should be inspected for mobility of expression and ability to open the mouth. Clients with SSc are often unable to open the mouth fully as the disease progresses. Skin thickening is often accompanied by areas of hypopigmentation and hyperpigmentation, so these changes are most commonly observed on the extremities and chest.

The musculoskeletal assessment includes a thorough evaluation of ROM because reduced joint mobility and polyarthritis characterize SSc. Flexor and extensor tendons should be palpated for the presence of friction rubs. Often, coarse crepitus caused by fibrin deposits can be heard with tendon motion—a sign that is often considered specific for SSc. Eliciting Tinel's sign (see Figure 71-11, A, p. 1889) to rule out or confirm carpal tunnel syndrome is useful. Muscle strength should be assessed and graded because SSc may have a polymyositis-type myopathy affecting the proximal muscles.

Other body systems should be assessed to provide baseline data or to determine possible organ involvement. The respiratory system should be assessed for the ease and extent of thoracic excursion, presence of dyspnea, and presence of adventitious lung sounds. The heart is examined for changes in rhythm or signs of heart failure. Blood pressure must be monitored closely because sudden malignant hypertension associated with renal disease can occur in SSc.

Facilitate Muscle and Joint Movement

Most clients with SSc have significant muscle and joint involvement, including arthralgias, myalgia, and fibrosis of the tendons. When contractures develop, they are often due to the fibrotic changes in the skin. These muscle and joint changes lead to problems often encountered in clients with RA—joint pain, stiffness, fatigue, self-care deficits, and impaired physical mobility.

From the client's perspective, coping with an altered body image that accompanies extensive skin changes can be an overwhelming task. Nurses can help clients understand that successful coping often means assuming responsibility for self-care and the prevention of complications. Nursing interventions, therefore, are targeted at maintaining a full ROM of the mouth and hands as well as suggesting creative use of clothing and makeup to enhance the appearance.

Maintain Skin Integrity

Changes in skin integrity require meticulous nursing care. For the acutely ill client, all digits and extremities must be handled carefully and gently. If possible, the client should try to move or reposition himself or herself so minimal discomfort occurs. Debilitated or steroid-dependent clients or those undergoing orthopedic surgery should be placed on pressure-reducing beds or air mattresses to prevent the development of skin breakdown over bony prominences. Dressings must be removed carefully so that additional trauma does not occur. Although moist dressings are applied to injured areas, they should be dampened with sterile saline if they do not come off easily. Tape should be used only when absolutely essential, for example, to stabilize an intravenous catheter needle. Otherwise, all dressings should be secured with stretchable gauze.

Whenever possible, the administration of injections and intravenous therapy should be in sites free of fibrosis and sclerosis. Areas of tough, thickened skin and sclerotic veins cannot be easily punctured. It is possible, also, to cause additional damage (and a portal for infection) if needle punctures are not made successfully.

Provide Education

Client education is the cornerstone to effective nursing care of the client with Raynaud's phenomenon. Clients must be assisted to modify their dress and health practices so all controllable sources of vasospasm are eliminated. Newly diagnosed clients may need anticipatory guidance about how to dress protectively in cold weather and in air conditioning. They may readily recognize the need for gloves but not realize the importance of protecting the head, ears, nose, lips, and feet. Keeping a pair of gloves in a tote bag or pocket is helpful when in air-conditioned stores or when taking frozen items out of the grocery freezer. Clients must maintain their core temperature, always dressing warmly. Clients must often be helped to change their health practices so they eliminate the use of vasoconstrictive substances, such as alcohol and caffeine. Learning biofeedback or other stress

management skills is indicated when clients identify stress as a cause of altered tissue perfusion.

Promote Adequate Nutrition

Clients with SSc often have difficulty maintaining their weight because of esophageal changes leading to dysphagia, esophagitis, and decreased intestinal motility. Consultation with the dietitian can help the nurse provide appropriate, easy-to-swallow, high-calorie snacks. The dietitian can plan meals to avoid foods contributing to esophagitis and gastric reflux. Remaining upright for 1 to 2 hours after eating also helps to prevent esophageal reflux. Avoiding heavy snacks close to retiring, using a large wedge pillow to elevate the head and shoulders, or elevating the head of the bed on shock blocks can prevent bedtime reflux. The client's ability to chew and swallow dry, compact foods, such as meat and bread, should be carefully evaluated. Often, these foods cause severe choking spells. Moistening them with gravies, sauces, or jellies helps them to be more easily tolerated. The achievement of nutritional goals is often affected by dental hygiene practices. Because of sclerotic skin changes, clients may have a difficult time completely opening the mouth. Mucous membranes may become inflamed or ulcerated because of lack of moisture or inadequate brushing and rinsing. Using a small angled toothbrush or Waterpik can help prevent these problems. Reinforcing the need to perform facial exercises to prevent rigidity of the face and mouth is a priority nursing intervention.

Promote Bowel Elimination

Chronic constipation and diarrhea are two other problems that are usually amenable to nursing intervention. Chronic constipation is associated with the decreased motility of the gastrointestinal tract that accompanies SSc. Nursing interventions include eating easy-to-swallow, high-fiber foods along with drinking more fluids and participating in exercise. The use of bulk stool softeners and suppositories may be needed as part of the bowel program. Diarrhea is associated with the malabsorption syndrome. Foods known to precipitate diarrhea should be eliminated from the diet, and natural antidiarrheal agents can be added to meals. When infectious organisms are present, antibiotic agents are prescribed, often tetracycline.

Monitor for Complications

Nursing care is also directed toward the monitoring and detecting of potential problems. The potential for impaired gas exchange exists when interstitial fibrosis of the lungs occurs. The presence of dyspnea, changes in activity tolerance, and an increased rate and depth of respirations may be noted. Auscultation of lung sounds may indicate fine crackles. Oxygen is usually administered as supportive therapy, and clients are educated about factors (pollen, smoking, humidity) that exacerbate the pulmonary condition.

SPONDYLOARTHROPATHIES

The *spondyloarthropathies* are a group of interrelated disorders that include psoriatic arthritis (PsA), reactive arthritis, arthritis-associated inflammatory bowel disease, and ankylosing spondylitis (AS). Spondyloarthropathies are distinguished from RA by the following three characteristics: (1) a negative test for RF, (2) the absence of rheumatoid nodules, and (3) an inflammatory peripheral arthritis that is typically asymmetrical. Three other features of the spondyloarthropathies have been noted. First, inflammation occurs where the ligament inserts into the bone (enthesis) rather than at the synovium. Extraskeletal changes can occur in the eye, skin, lung parenchyma, or aortic valve. Second, there is considerable overlap between the various spondyloarthropathies. For example, a person with PsA can develop the classic sacroiliitis seen in AS. Finally, there is a tendency toward familial aggregation in the development of the disease, with genes other than *B27* probably playing a role.

■ **FIGURE 77–6** Ankylosing spondylitis.

ANKYLOSING SPONDYLITIS

Literally, ankylosing spondylitis (AS) refers to fusion (ankylosis) of inflamed vertebrae (spondylitis) (Figure 77-6). The disease typically begins in the spine of young men in their late teens or early twenties. The majority of clients have bilateral sacroiliitis that causes pain and some degree of restricted motion in the lumbar spine. Peripheral arthritis of the large joints, usually the hips and shoulders and more rarely the knees, occurs in 20% to 30% of people with AS. Small joint involvement is not usually seen. Chest expansion can also be decreased because of an associated costovertebral arthritis. By the time the client is 50 or 60, the fusion of the lumbar spine has proceeded to the cervical region. If AS is not treated, the disease tends to progress with remissions and exacerbations to a final stage of rigid lumbar and thoracic kyphosis that leaves the neck in a flexed position. Ankylosing spondylitis is associated with a shortening of the life span.

Etiology and Risk Factors

The average annual age-adjusted incidence rate of AS has been reported to be 6.6 per 100,000 population, with men affected three times as frequently as women. Although the usual age of onset has been established as between 15 and 35 years, the age group with the highest incidence rate is the 25- to 34-year-old group.

The overall incidence rate is estimated to be 129 per 100,000 population. Thus the overall incidence rate for the entire population has been estimated to fall between 1 and 2 per 1000 population.

Risk factors associated with AS include gender (with a 3:1 to 4:1 predominance of males over females), the young adult years of adolescence through adulthood (15 to 35 years old), and a genetic predisposition. A strong tendency toward familial aggregation has been seen and a sex-linked hormone may be important. The presence of HLA-B27 may also be a risk factor, as it appears frequently in the high-risk Indian population but is almost nonexistent in the low-risk U.S. African-American population. Although the disease is generally seen in men in the third decade of life, the condition may go undetected in women because of its milder course and the usual caution in performing pelvic x-rays in women of childbearing age.

Clinical Manifestations

Initially, morning backache and stiffness begin during young adulthood. The back pain and stiffness subside with movement but often return with inactivity. Back pain throughout the spinal column, difficulty sleeping, and neurologic changes such as bowel and bladder incontinence, paresthesia, and numbness may also occur.

Several other systemic manifestations of AS can be seen, such as uveitis, pulmonary fibrosis, inflammatory bowel disease, and aortic insufficiency. Uveitis occurs in up to 25% of all clients with AS, especially in HLA-B27-positive clients with peripheral joint disease, but its incidence seems to be unrelated to the severity of the spondylitis. Upper lobe pulmonary fibrosis is rare, but it has been reported. Intestinal inflammation is frequent in clients with spondylarthropathy, and one fourth of clients have early features of Crohn's disease. Aortic insufficiency, accompanied by a typical diastolic murmur, occurs in 5% of those with AS, and this problem frequently leads to the need for an aortic valve replacement. Cardiac problems, however, do not usually appear for several years.

The diagnosis of AS is based on the results of the history and physical examination and on radiologic findings. Positive physical examination findings include the presence of sacroiliitis, spinal muscle spasms, and decreased hip mobility. Decreased chest expansion is seen later in the disease. Along with symptomatic sacroiliitis, radiologic confirmation of sacroiliac joint changes is probably the most important finding early in the disease. Although radiographs taken early in the disease may show no abnormalities, later the typical changes of sacroiliitis develop, with patchy sclerosis at the joint margins. Early changes in AS include a squaring off of the anterior lumbar vertebral surfaces. This squaring is caused by erosion of the upper and lower margins of the vertebrae at the site of insertion of the annulus fibrosus. The intervertebral ligaments involved in the inflammatory process heal by ossification, leading to the formation of syndesmophytes in the outer layers of the annulus fibrosus. Eventually, the disk space becomes bridged by these bony syndesmophytes. In the end stage of the disease, complete spinal fusion (bamboo spine) and fusion of the sacroiliac joints occur along with ossification of all of the ligamentous structures.

Generally, laboratory studies are not helpful in diagnosing AS. Although the HLA-B27 antigen is seen in 90% of clients with AS, it is found in up to 10% of those without the disease, thus limiting its specificity in diagnosis. An elevated ESR is seen in most clients, but it may be normal in those with severe disease. Other findings may include elevated creatine kinase (CK) and alkaline phosphatase levels, but these are not confirming diagnostic tests.

OUTCOME MANAGEMENT

Medical Management

The treatment goals for AS are to maintain mobility, decrease inflammation, and control pain. As with other chronic conditions, treatment is more successful when clients are engaged in and assume responsibility for health promotion and other self-care activities.

Maintain Mobility

Instructing the client to perform appropriate exercises and engage in ADL is critical if the client is to maintain mobility with minimal spinal curvature. Good posture must be encouraged through exercises that promote stretching and extension of the spine. Swimming is an excellent general conditioner as well as an activity that promotes spinal extension without increased pain. The nurse may need to help the client solve problems about awkward furniture or equipment that reinforces spinal flexion. For example, the client who has a desk job may need to invest in a tilting artist's table so the neck and head are not forced into flexion with constant activity. Selecting ergonomic chairs or ensuring the correct placement of a computer workstation can also be beneficial for the client's comfort. Appropriate sleep posture must be reinforced, particularly in those with mild cervical flexion who are accustomed to sleeping with two pillows. Spinal extension is maximized during sleep if clients lie on a firm mattress, preferably with bed boards underneath, in a supine position, without a pillow. If the client insists on using a pillow, it should be as flat as possible.

Reduce Pain and Inflammation

As with many other chronic arthritic conditions, successful pain management depends on reducing inflammation and stiffness. NSAIDs are used to reduce inflammation, and the application of heat (or a warm shower or bath) helps to relieve morning pain and stiffness. Sulfasalazine and methotrexate have shown beneficial effects but their use is being supplanted by the approval of the "Tumor-Necrosis-Factor alpha (TNF-α) blockers," which have been shown to slow or even halt the progression of AS and to be highly effective in treating spinal arthritis. Etanercept and infliximab have been approved by the FDA for the treatment of AS.

Nursing Management of the Medical Client

Obtain Nursing History

Questions should focus on the typical clinical manifestations of pain, stiffness, and fatigue and their effects on performing ADL, as well as screening for extra-articular involvement. Question clients about the nature, onset, location, duration, and quality of their pain. Ask what self-care measures (e.g., use of heat or cold, showers or baths) they have used to cope with the pain-stiffness-fatigue cycle and which measures have been effective.

Determine whether the pain is in the lower back, thorax, or cervical area and if other large peripheral joints, such as the knees, hips, or shoulders, cause discomfort. During the early phase of AS, clients complain of lumbosacral pain that radiates to the buttocks and thighs. Sleep for clients with AS is different from normal sleep.

Therefore an assessment of sleep patterns should be completed. Ask clients if the pain is worse on rising, if it is associated with morning stiffness, and if it decreases with activity. Also determine the length of time that the client has been affected with back pain. These points are important because the following five features strongly suggest inflammatory spinal disease: (1) insidious onset of discomfort, (2) being younger than 40 years, (3) persistence of discomfort for more than 3 months, (4) association with morning stiffness, and (5) improvement with exercise.

Clients should also be questioned about fatigue, weight loss, and the presence of a low-grade fever. With advanced disease, cord compression can occur as a result of spinal fractures, so it is important to elicit information about neurologic changes, such as decreased motor activity, paresthesias, numbness, and bowel and bladder incontinence. Because of the possibility of extra-articular disease, it is important to ask clients about their eyes, respiratory status, and heart. The following are suggested screening parameters for each system:

Eyes: Presence of blurred vision, decreased vision, pain, excessive tearing, photophobia

Respiratory status: Presence and quality of cough, sputum production, dyspnea, shortness of breath, smoking history

Cardiovascular status: History of murmurs, tachycardia, and extra heart sounds

Complete Physical Assessment

The spinal assessment is often normal early in the disease, or there can be tenderness with deep palpation of the sacroiliac joint. As the disease progresses into the upper spinal segments, loss of the normal lumbar lordosis occurs, followed by decreased flexion, extension, and lateral movement. Asking the client to flex at the waist and observing the flattening of the lumbar spine can assess loss of lumbar lordosis. Tenderness along vertebral structures and marked paravertebral spasm can also be present with decreased lumbar lordosis.

A useful measure of lumbar flexion is the Schober's test. With the client standing erect, the nurse makes a mark at the L5-S1 area and another 10 cm above it. When the client bends forward in maximal flexion, the distance between the two marks normally should increase to 15 cm. In AS, however, this measurement does not significantly increase. The Schober's test is most useful in evaluating young clients because spinal flexion generally decreases with age. Alternatively, when screening for AS, measure the distance from fingers to floor when clients attempt to touch their toes. Clients with decreased flexion have a greater distance between their fingers and the floor. The tendency to develop a kyphotic posture in AS is reflected in diminished thoracic expansion. To assess chest expansion, place the tape measure at the nipples and then note the chest measurement with full lung expansion. A distance of less than 3 cm, along with other physical signs, is highly suggestive of AS.

As the disease progresses, loss of ROM in the neck leads to a fixed kyphosis that can seriously impair visual function. The serial tracking of measurements of the distance from the client's head to the wall can be used to detect the progression of cervical kyphosis. Positioning the client with the heels against the wall and instructing the client to extend the neck fully can obtain consistent results.

Clients with AS should also be assessed for two other musculoskeletal changes. The first change is the development of an inflammatory peripheral joint involvement, particularly of the hips, knees, and shoulders. Assess these joints bilaterally for changes in ROM, pain, tenderness, and synovitis. Also observe for signs of enthesitis, a problem commonly seen in juvenile AS and occasionally present in adults. Enthesitis can involve the plantar aspect of the foot (plantar fasciitis), the heel (Achilles tendinitis), and the knee. Other sites include the greater trochanters, superior anterior iliac crests, and ischial tuberosities. Attachment sites may or may not be swollen, but typically they are extremely painful to palpation. Because of the potential for developing extraskeletal problems with the eyes, lungs, and heart, these systems should be carefully assessed during the baseline screening.

Provide Education

The nurse plays a key role in educating the client about health promotion activities, exercise, and the management of pain. One of the most critical areas for skillful nursing intervention involves being attentive and providing positive, unconditional regard for those clients with changing appearances. If the disease progresses rapidly or if the client has not sought help until skeletal changes are noticeable, the client may be quite self-conscious and even depressed about the appearance. Businessmen may have found it increasingly more difficult to find clothing that fits. Some men have been known to avoid buying suits because of their embarrassment about being seen by salespersons or tailors. The client may be so concerned about appearance that he or she avoids social interaction outside of the job. Helping clients who have an altered body image or who are socially isolated is a significant challenge and an opportunity to establish a meaningful, therapeutic relationship. Although specific nursing interventions can be implemented that encourage group participation and interaction, it is often the nurse's positive, unconditional regard that helps the client work toward reintegration of self. Approximately one third of clients experience depression and women report more depression than men.

Promote Effective Breathing

Another important area for nursing intervention, especially as the disease progresses, is the maintenance of effective breathing patterns and adequate oxygenation. Ongoing assessment of chest wall expansion, instructions in deep-breathing exercises, and the avoidance of smoking and respiratory depressants can help the client to maintain optimal breathing. If dyspnea becomes a problem, instruct the client in pursed-lip breathing and the pacing of activities. For those clients with cervical involvement who become acutely ill or require surgery, notify the anesthesia department. Ankylosing spondylitis in the cervical area frequently causes problems with intubation.

REACTIVE ARTHRITIS

Reactive arthritis and Reiter's syndrome are both designations for a form of peripheral arthritis, often accompanied by one or more extra-articular manifestations, which appear shortly after certain infections of the genitourinary or gastrointestinal tracts. The majority of affected individuals, usually young men, have inherited the human leukocyte antigen HLA-B27. Reiter's syndrome originally referred to the clinical triad of nongonoccocal urethritis, conjunctivitis, and arthritis. Because of many overlapping clinical, epidemiologic, and genetic features, reactive arthritis is classified as a seronegative spondylarthropathy. Approximately 80% of clients experience chronic problems marked by periods of remission and exacerbation.

Etiology and Risk Factors

Reactive arthritis occurs following exposure to a bacterial gastrointestinal or genitourinary infection. Although the exact mechanism remains unclear, certain infective agents and a specific genetic background (presence of HLA-B27) are associated with reactive arthritis. Epidemic reactive arthritis has occurred in association with dysentery. Endemic or postvenereal reactive arthritis is the more common type found in the United States.

Endemic reactive arthritis occurs more frequently in young men (9:1) and is linked to the greater prevalence of HLA-B27 antigen in this population. Cases following food-borne enteric infections affect both genders equally. Caucasians are affected more commonly than African Americans or other racial groups who have a lower frequency of HLA-B27. Reactive arthritis is difficult to diagnose and probably occurs more frequently than reported.

Clinical Manifestations

Reactive arthritis demonstrates features in almost every system of the body. The most common features are polyarthritis, urethritis or cervicitis, and conjunctivitis. There is a link between the genitourinary system and reactive arthritis. Urethritis can occur symptomatically (discharge, slight burning on urination) or can be asymptomatic, which is a component in the difficulty in establishing a diagnosis. Reactive arthritis has been reported frequently in clients with human immunodeficiency virus (HIV) infection. There is a high incidence of prostatitis and acquired immunodeficiency syndrome (AIDS). The role of AIDS in the pathogenesis of reactive arthritis is still being investigated. Urethral infection is commonly accompanied by stomatitis, balanitis, and keratoderma blennorrhagicum. The keratodermal lesions are similar to psoriatic lesions and can appear on the soles of the feet, glans penis, and toes.

Conjunctivitis, considered a classic manifestation, is typically a transient, mild phenomenon. If a sterile discharge is present, it subsides within a few days. Uveitis can become a more significant clinical problem in this disorder.

Reactive arthritis is characteristically additive, asymmetrical, and oligoarticular, affecting an average of four joints. The arthritic process generally affects weight-bearing joints, especially of the knees and ankles. Large effusions can accompany it.

Diagnostic work-up includes radiography and laboratory examinations. Early in the disease, there are no radiographic changes. With disease progression, joint space narrowing and erosive changes can be seen. In advanced disease, the individual may develop sacroiliitis, as found in AS.

Laboratory findings may show an elevated erythrocyte sedimentation rate (ESR), but the ESR may be normal despite active joint involvement. Mild hypochromic or normochromic anemia may be present. Routine typing for HLA-B27 is considered unnecessary.

OUTCOME MANAGEMENT

Medical Management

Reactive arthritis usually runs a self-limited course of from 3 to 12 months in the majority of clients; however, some studies suggest that many clients continue to be plagued by minor musculoskeletal manifestations. Management of the client targets client education and management of clinical manifestations. There is a general recognition that reactive arthritis has a greater propensity for chronicity than previously appreciated, which should temper an overly optimistic prognosis. One study reported that at 1 year after diagnosis 40% of clients with post-genitourinary-acquired reactive arthritis and 20% of post-gastrointestinal-acquired reactive arthritis still had active disease, but almost all had recovered at 2-year follow-up.

Administer Medications

Pharmacologic management is similar to that used for AS. The attacks tend to be self-limiting, lasting 2 to 4 months, with a recurrence rate of 15% per year. The use of antibiotic therapy in the prevention or management of reactive arthritis remains controversial. For clients with ocular manifestations, steroid eye drops or subconjunctival preparations may be needed. Severe uveitis is relatively common and is a difficult clinical management problem.

Provide Physical Therapy

Joint pain and dysfunction are managed with a regimen of physical therapy. Splinting for joint protection along with a managed exercise and activity program are indicated.

Nursing Management of the Medical Client

Obtain Nursing History and Complete Physical Examination

The history should examine the pattern of orthopedic pain. Joint pain, back pain, heel pain, and a tendinitis-type pain can manifest in reactive arthritis. Clients with a nonspecific arthritis should be questioned about the presence of genitourinary and ocular manifestations. Ask the client if he or she has noted any atypical urethral discharge or slight pain or burning on urination for even a few days. An examination of past history of sexually transmitted diseases is important, as is the sexual history in relation to number and frequency of sexual partners. Question the client specifically about eye disease. Has the client experienced recent eye irritation and perhaps attributed it to smog or other chemical irritants? The client may have noted dermatologic lesions. Ask the client about any lesions for which he or she may have used a glucocorticosteroid cream. Has the client noticed any other vesicle-type lesions?

Physical examination targets the involved joints and inspects for dermatologic lesions and the presence of localized infections.

Provide Education

As with any chronic disease, client education plays a crucial role in helping the individual understand and manage the disease. Similar to RA (see prior discussion), clients and their families need information about the disease process and management. Because of the link to genitourinary pathology, education must target safe sexual practices. There is some evidence that use of a condom protects the client from postvenereal exacerbation of reactive arthritis. Clients are advised to avoid multiple sexual partners.

PSORIATIC ARTHRITIS

Psoriasis is a common skin disorder characterized by stippled nails, pruritus, and silvery scales on bright red plaques, usually on the elbows, knees, and scalp. It is a genetically determined disease associated with several histocompatibility antigens, including HLA-B14, HLA-Bw17, and HLA-Cw6. About 5% to 10% of those with psoriasis develop a distinctive inflammatory arthritis—psoriatic arthritis (PsA).

Three to five types of PsA have been proposed. In asymmetrical oligoarthropathy, there is asymmetrical involvement of both large and small joints, and sausage-shaped joints are common. With this type of arthritis, the asymmetrical pattern involves the interphalangeal and metatarsophalangeal joints of the feet and the DIP joints of the fingers. The second type, symmetrical polyarthropathy, closely resembles RA. Arthritis mutilans, a severe form of destructive arthritis, is characterized by telescoping digits also known as the "opera-glass hand." Psoriatic spondylitis is characterized by the sacroiliitis of AS. Clients with this last type, characterized by DIP involvement, often have nail changes, such as pitting, transverse depressions, and subungual hyperkeratosis, along with DIP joint disease.

The overall incidence of PsA is approximately 0.1% in the United States. Arthritis occurs in approximately 5% to 7% of clients with psoriasis but it may affect 40% of hospitalized clients with extensive skin involvement. Two percent of Caucasian North Americans and Europeans are believed to be affected with psoriasis but it is relatively uncommon in Asians. The male to female ratio is equal but varies in subsets of this disease. In contrast to psoriasis, where the peak age is between 5 and 15 years, the peak age of PsA is between 30 and 55 years, which is similar to RA.

Etiology and Risk Factors

The cause of PsA appears to be a complex combination of immunologic, genetic, and environmental factors. Immunologic changes seen in some clients include elevated titers of IgG and IgA and the presence of immune complexes. There is an increased prevalence of the disease among family members who have psoriatic arthritis. Possible environmental factors include group A streptococci and trauma.

Clinical Manifestations

The diagnosis of PsA is usually confirmed after a positive history of psoriasis and specific x-ray findings. It is important to realize that in some clients, particularly children, joint changes precede skin changes. Nevertheless, most rheumatologists agree that the diagnosis cannot be made without evidence of psoriatic skin or nail changes.

Some changes that appear on x-ray are suggestive of PsA. In early cases, soft tissue swelling can be seen in clients with psoriasis similar to that observed in RA. Periarticular demineralization of the bone, however, is less common in psoriatic arthritis. Radiologic findings indicative of the disease include erosions of the DIP joints (both hands and feet), which can lead to a whittled, "pencil-in-cup" appearance. Clients with spinal involvement have radiologic evidence of sacroiliitis, but the distribution of the joint changes is less predictable than it is in AS.

Laboratory tests often reveal a slightly elevated sedimentation rate and hypochromic anemia. Many clients have mild hyperuricemia, which is a confusing finding that could initially lead to the diagnosis of gout. Tests for RF are negative in 75% of clients; among the 25% with positive tests, many have coexisting psoriasis and RA.

OUTCOME MANAGEMENT

Medical Management

Although clients with PsA can have an explosive onset of polyarticular or monoarticular joint pain, erythema, and swelling, treatment goals are directed to the management of a chronic illness. Clients can be confused or discouraged when they first realize their diagnosis. They may perceive themselves as having not just one but two chronic diseases and thus feel increasingly powerless or helpless about their illness. Nurses and physicians, therefore, must work collaboratively to educate clients about the cause of the disease and the expected course of treatment. As with all other arthritic diseases, engaging the client's interest and partnership in actively managing the disease is essential for the best outcomes.

Nurses work with physicians to educate clients about key treatment strategies, many of which are similar to those implemented in RA and AS. During exacerbations of the disease, clients must avoid stressing inflamed joints, participate in active assistive ROM exercises to prevent joint contractures, and alternate periods of rest with activity. Those with foot and toenail involvement must be instructed to select appropriate footwear to protect swollen digits and keratotic nail beds.

Reduce Inflammation
The initial treatment for stable plaque psoriasis is topical. However, topical therapy may be impractical for clients with extensive psoriasis (more than 20% involvement) and systemic therapy may be indicated at the outset. Topical treatment includes emollients and keratolytic agents alone or in combination with anthralin, glucocorticoids, and vitamin D derivatives. Stress and certain drugs (beta-adrenergic blockers, angiotensin-converting enzyme inhibitors, lithium, and antimalarial drugs) may exacerbate psoriasis and should be used with caution.

Unlike rheumatoid arthritis, which usually requires constant treatment, psoriatic arthritis may only require therapy when manifestations arise. When they subside, therapy can be stopped until further problems develop. Initial treatment usually consists of NSAIDs. If the arthritis does not respond, DMARDs may be used. These include sulfasalazine, methotrexate, and cyclosporine and the more recently available "anti-TNF agents" such as etanercept, infliximab, and adalimumab. The antimalarial drug hydroxychloroquine may be effective, but some people taking this will experience a flare-up of their psoriasis, so it is usually avoided. Azathioprine may benefit those with severe forms of PsA.

For severely swollen joints, glucocorticosteroid injections can be useful for controlling the inflammation. Surgery can be helpful to repair or replace badly damaged joints. Simultaneous joint and skin disease activity has been observed in up to one third of clients, particularly those with non–spondylitis disease.

For clients with intractable pain or loss of joint function, surgery may be indicated. Although several reports have raised concerns about a higher risk of infections, recurrent contracture or stiffness, or excessive bone formation after surgery, most of these fears seem ill founded and surgery should not be withheld.

Nursing Management of the Medical Client

Obtain Nursing History
The focus of the nursing history for clients with psoriatic arthritis is similar to that for clients with RA. Asymmetrical pauciarticular arthritis, however, often occurs in psoriatic arthritis, so clients should be questioned about the nature, onset, and location of any acutely occurring painful, swollen joints. Questions about back pain and stiffness can help to identify psoriatic spondylitis. In addition, clients should be asked about their psoriasis-associated skin changes—location, size, color, and degree of scaling of the plaques—as well as changes in the nail beds of the fingers and the toes. Because the disease seems to be caused by several other factors, ask clients if there is a family history of arthritis, psoriatic arthritis, or psoriasis. Determine whether the client has a history of severe infection before or after developing clinical manifestations of the disease or any episodes of local trauma to the hands, feet, or spine.

Complete Physical Assessment
Assessment of the client with psoriatic arthritis begins with a thorough assessment of the skin for evidence of psoriatic plaques or nail bed changes. Such completeness is essential because the disease cannot be confirmed, even with characteristic radiologic changes,

unless there is evidence of psoriasis. Usually located on extensor surfaces, psoriatic skin lesions are either macular or papular round scales that tend to bleed when they are removed. If clients deny that they have any skin involvement, examine all areas carefully, particularly the scalp, axillae, and umbilicus. Look carefully for pitting nails, which often precede skin rashes and are highly suggestive of psoriasis.

Defer the assessment of the musculoskeletal system until the examination of the integument is complete, so that subtle changes in either system are not overlooked. Because the range of joint involvement in psoriatic arthritis is extensive (e.g., asymmetrical or symmetrical, small or large, pauciarticular or monoarticular), each joint must be assessed for swelling, bogginess, and erythema. Pay particular attention to the small joints of the hands and feet, watching for swollen, sausage-shaped digits, which result from tenosynovitis of the flexor tendon sheath. Note whether any of the digits have assumed a spindle or telescopic shape.

Maintain Skin Integrity

Nursing interventions are especially important for the client with PsA experiencing impaired skin integrity. Clients with PsA may need basic instruction about how to care for their skin. If skin changes are severe, the client should be referred to a dermatologist, or the nurse (and physician) should collaborate with the dermatologist if the client has previously sought care from this specialist. The nurse should review skin care principles, such as the purpose and application techniques of emollients to keep the skin soft, patting the skin dry after bathing instead of vigorous towel drying, and the correct application of topical ointments with a thin layer, sparingly applied. If the client is hospitalized, it is important that he or she assume responsibility for skin care as soon as it is feasible.

Enhance Body Image

Because of the changes in both the skin and the joints, it is likely that the client has experienced a significant body image disturbance. Being sensitive to clients' expressions can help to assess the degree of integrity they perceive they have. It is not unusual for people to be so affected by their appearance that they wear long-sleeved shirts on the hottest days and buy only clothes with pockets to hide their altered fingers. The communication of positive unconditional regard by the nurse—and all members of the health care team—can be a powerful tool to help clients begin to feel comfortable exploring their feelings.

FIBROMYALGIA SYNDROME

Not all people complaining of musculoskeletal pain have arthritis. Fibromyalgia syndrome is an increasingly recognized chronic musculoskeletal pain disorder of unknown cause. It occurs in about 2% to 5% of the general population, predominantly in girls and young women. Active research is being conducted to find the cause. Clinical manifestations include fatigue, morning stiffness, non-refreshing sleep because of lack of stage 4 sleep, and postexertional muscle pain. About one third of clients have associated problems such as irritable bowel syndrome, tension headaches, premenstrual syndrome, numbness and tingling, and Raynaud's phenomenon. Fatigue is the most common clinical manifestation, and the most common cause of the fatigue is chronic depression.

OUTCOME MANAGEMENT

Management is symptomatic and includes L-tryptophan to increase sleep, tricyclic antidepressants to inhibit serotonin uptake, benzodiazepines for the treatment of anxiety associated with depression, and glucocorticoids and NSAIDs for pain control. Low-intensity exercise is also important and helps to decrease pain. Biofeedback, acupuncture, and hypnotherapy have also been used to help manage nonmuscular problems such as functional diarrhea, tension headache, and fatigue. The efficacy of these treatments is yet to be fully ascertained.

Many clients with fibromyalgia perceive themselves to be significantly disabled and have a reduced quality of life that rivals conditions such as RA and terminal emphysema. Clients with fibromyalgia have difficulty coping with "daily hassles" and this, in turn, increases the psychological stress. Cognitive behavioral therapy is often effective in providing these clients a sense of control over their lives.

IDIOPATHIC INFLAMMATORY MYOPATHY (POLYMYOSITIS AND DERMATOMYOSITIS)

Inflammatory diseases of muscle are a heterogeneous group of disorders characterized by proximal muscle weakness and nonsuppurative inflammation of skeletal muscle. Traditionally, the terms polymyositis and dermatomyositis have been used to represent these diseases. Today it is more appropriate to use the term *idiopathic inflammatory myopathy* to describe the entire group and reserve the terms polymyositis (PM) and dermatomyositis (DM) for more specific conditions or subsets.

The idiopathic myopathies are relatively rare diseases. Accurate estimates of their prevalence are difficult to obtain because the diseases are uncommon and lack universally accepted specific diagnostic criteria. Estimates of incidence range from 0.5 to 8.4 cases per million. The incidence appears to be increasing, although this may simply reflect increased awareness and more accurate diagnosis. Although polymyositis and dermatomyositis affect all age groups, there is a bimodal distribution of the age of onset with peaks at ages 10 and 15 years in children and between 45 and 60 years in adults. As with other rheumatic diseases, there is a 2:1 female to male predominance in PM-DM with the exception of inclusion body myositis, which affects men twice as often. Racial differences are apparent. In adults the lowest rates are reported in the Japanese and the highest in African Americans. Although no direct relationships have been established between an inflammatory myopathy and a specific genetic marker, several associations have been recognized. The strongest associations are for HLA-B8, HLA-DR3, and HLA-DRW52 phenotypes with polymyositis and dermatomyositis in all age groups.

Etiology and Risk Factors

The idiopathic myopathies are believed to be immune-mediated processes that are triggered by environmental factors in genetically susceptible individuals. This is supported by the following two observations: (1) there is a recognized association with other autoimmune and connective tissue diseases and (2) there is a high prevalence of circulating autoantibodies. The autoantibodies associated with PM-DM include the myositis-specific autoantibodies (MSAs) found almost exclusively in these diseases.

The triggering event of PM-DM is unknown, but viruses have been strongly implicated. The seasonal variation in the onset of disease is direct evidence that infectious agents play a role as well as the evidence found in animal models. Genetic factors play an important role. Individuals with HLA-DR3 are at increased risk for developing inflammatory muscle disease including polymyositis and juvenile dermatomyositis. All clients with the anti-Jo-1 antibodies have the HLA antigen DR52, and Caucasian clients also have a high prevalence of HLA-B8, HLA-DR3, and HLA-DR6. Inclusion body myositis is more likely associated with HLA-DR1, HLA-DR6, and HLA-DQ1.

A subset of clients with inflammatory myopathies develops muscle weakness with an underlying malignancy. Malignancy may precede or follow the onset of muscle weakness. The association is rare in children, but has occurred in clients of all ages in all subsets of disease, although associated malignancy may be more common with dermatomyositis. Subsequent studies seem to indicate that the types of tumors found roughly paralleled those found in the general population with the exception of ovarian cancer, which is over-represented in women with dermatomyositis.

Pathophysiology

The results of muscle biopsies, usually of the deltoid or quadriceps muscles, have provided useful information about the pathology of the disease. Several changes have been noted, including focal or extensive degeneration of muscle fibers caused by inflammatory infiltrates of lymphocytes and macrophages. In some cases, necrosis of parts or entire groups of muscle fibers can occur. Fibers, however, can also show evidence of regeneration.

Clinical Manifestations

The most frequently occurring idiopathic myopathies in adults, polymyositis and dermatomyositis are diffuse, systemic, inflammatory connective tissue diseases. Although these disorders can have an acute onset and progress rapidly, more typically there is a slower progression. Clients gradually develop significant weight loss, fatigue, and weakness over a period of months, sometimes not even being aware of when the changes began. Both diseases cause symmetrical progressive weakness of the proximal or limb-girdle muscles and occasionally atrophy of the muscles of the limbs, neck, and pharynx. Decreased muscle strength occurs in the pelvic girdle first, followed by weakness of the legs and shoulders and arms. Weakness of the flexor muscles of the neck occurs in about half of those affected with PM-DM. In acute disease, muscles can be tender or swollen and doughy. When classic skin changes are associated with polymyositis, the disease is classified as *dermatomyositis*. The classification of idiopathic inflammatory myopathies, to which polymyositis and dermatomyositis belong, includes the following seven groups: (1) polymyositis, (2) dermatomyositis, (3) amyopathic dermatomyositis, (4) juvenile dermatomyositis, (5) myositis associated with neoplasia, (6) myositis associated with collagen vascular disease, and (7) inclusion body myositis.

The criteria developed in 1975 for the diagnosis of PM and DM continue to be used: (1) proximal, symmetrical muscle weakness, with or without dysphagia or respiratory muscle weakness; (2) elevation of serum muscle enzyme levels; (3) characteristic electromyographic changes; (4) muscle biopsy evidence of myositis; and (5) the typical skin rash of DM. In addition, the diagnosis is confirmed after excluding other neuromuscular diseases, such as myasthenia gravis, amyotrophic lateral sclerosis, polymyalgia rheumatica, and Guillain-Barré syndrome. Research continues to refine the diagnostic criteria for PM-DM, and four additional criteria may become standard in the future.

The most important laboratory test is the measurement of the muscle enzyme creatine kinase (CK) (formerly creatine phosphokinase). An elevated CK level indicates muscle injury, but it is not specific to PM-DM. Elevated CK levels can be seen after intramuscular injections, muscle biopsies, or exercise, for example. The level of CK changes according to the activity of the disease. Other muscle enzymes are also elevated in most cases, including aldolase, ALT, AST, and LDH. The sedimentation rate is normal in 50% of clients.

Electromyographic (EMG) results often show bizarre, high-frequency discharges with spontaneous fibrillations and positive spikes at rest. Muscle biopsies are done if there is doubt about the diagnosis. The muscle chosen should be affected by the disease but not atrophied. The site should not be one where a previous EMG needle has been introduced. When biopsies are performed using general anesthesia, a permanent scar usually forms, and the area is sore for several weeks. For these reasons, physicians may prefer not to perform the biopsy unless it is essential to making the diagnosis. Muscle biopsy results, as was previously mentioned, show changes associated with necrosis and degeneration as well as evidence of regeneration. Fibrosis may be seen.

OUTCOME MANAGEMENT

Medical Management

The treatment of PM-DM usually begins with the daily administration of high doses of oral glucocorticosteroids. Prednisone (1 to 2 mg/kg/day) is given until elevated levels of muscle enzymes begin to decrease toward normal and clients show improvement in their ability to perform ADL. In severe cases, the daily dose can be divided or intravenous methylprednisolone may be used. Reduction in steroid dosages to alternate-day therapy may not be possible for several months. Some clients require long-term treatment with maintenance doses of steroids because the disease can recur when the steroids are withdrawn. Clients who do not respond to steroids or who cannot tolerate the high steroid doses usually require the addition of an immunosuppressive agent, such as daily azathioprine (50 to 150 mg/day) or weekly methotrexate therapy (7.5 mg/week PO or 0.5 to 0.8 mg/kg/week IV). Other immunosuppressive agents have been used in steroid-resistant clients. Cyclophosphamide, 6-mercaptopurine, chlorambucil, total-body (or total-nodal) irradiation, and intravenous immunoglobulins have also been used. Hydroxychloroquine can be used to treat the cutaneous lesions of dermatomyositis, although it has no recognized effect on the myositis.

Nursing Management of the Medical Client

Obtain Nursing History

Eliciting the history of a person with PM-DM begins with the client's perspective. The client seeks health care because of the nonspecific changes, usually occurring over several months, of increasing fatigue, weight loss, and malaise. When questioned about the nature of the fatigue and how it affects the ability to carry out activities of daily living, clients usually describe difficulty in performing tasks because of muscle weakness. Good screening questions include queries about the changes in ability to perform ADL that require the use of large muscle groups. Questions about the onset, duration, location, and quality of muscle pain should be asked. Muscle pain or tenderness may or may not be present in the early phases of the disease. Ask the client if he or she has had difficulty brushing the hair, reaching over the head for objects on a shelf or putting on clothes, or performing repetitive chores, such as mowing the lawn, hanging up laundry, or putting away groceries.

For a history of pelvic limb weakness, determine if the client has had difficulty rising from an armless chair, getting out of a car, climbing steps, or riding a bike. Ask if the client has had difficulties in raising the neck off the bed or pillow. Question the client about associated joint pains because arthritis and arthralgia occur in many clients who are in the overlap group V (i.e., they have both polymyositis and dermatomyositis and evidence of another collagen vascular disease, such as RA or SSc). Some clients may report a tendency to fall that is unrelated to balance, so explore changes in gait patterns with them. Because muscle weakness in the face and larynx is seen in PM-DM, determine if there has been any difficulty in chewing or swallowing, facial swelling, or hoarseness.

Because PM-DM is a systemic disease, questions must also be included about the integumentary, pulmonary, and cardiovascular systems. Determine whether the client has experienced any skin or nail changes—rash, reddened areas, scaling—typical of those seen in dermatomyositis. Common respiratory complications of PM-DM include aspiration pneumonia (because of a weakened cough, slow protective movements with vomiting, and pharyngeal muscle weakness) and interstitial lung disease. Questions about whether the clients had previous respiratory diseases, particularly pneumonia and influenza-like illnesses, and about how they recovered provide important information to surgical nurses for preoperative and postoperative pulmonary care. The client's cardiac history should be assessed via questions about dysrhythmias and the existence of a prolapsed mitral valve.

Complete Physical Assessment

The examination of the client with PM-DM requires a meticulous assessment of the skin and nail beds for the presence of erythema, macular-papular rashes, plaques, scaling, and nodules. Skin changes can help to direct this examination. To confirm the presence of a heliotrope rash on the client's face, hold the neck and head securely while it is lowered off the examination table or the side of the bed. This maneuver elicits increased suffusion to cause the distinctive color of the bluish red hue of the rash.

Initially test for muscle weakness by asking the client to walk, get up from a chair without arms, raise the neck off the bed or table, or lift a heavy book. Loss of hand strength is less noticeable, but it can be detected by a test of grip strength. Asking the client to shrug the shoulders upward against the nurse's hands can test proximal weakness of the shoulder girdle. Weakness of the masseter muscles (which can be seen in clients who have difficulty chewing) is assessed by palpating their strength when the client clenches the teeth. All muscle groups should be palpated for symmetry, atrophy, pain or tenderness, and the presence of contractures. Atrophy generally appears late in the disease, but contractures develop early if muscle weakness has been severe. As muscles are being assessed, large and small joints should be inspected for erythema, pain, presence of synovitis, and limitations in ROM.

Although the focus of the examination is on the integumentary and musculoskeletal systems, thorough assessment of the cardiopulmonary system is required because of the systemic nature of the disease. The bilateral assessment of chest expansion (diaphragmatic excursion) helps the nurse to know how compliant the muscles of respiration are. The quality of the breathing, the presence of dyspnea with simple activities, and the presence of a cough can indicate an acute or chronic respiratory problem with muscle disease. The quality of the lung sounds should be carefully assessed for fine rales (crackles) because aspiration pneumonia is a frequent complication of advanced PM-DM.

Provide Medication Teaching

The education of clients receiving high-dose steroid therapy focuses on teaching them about the potential side effects of long-term prednisone. Clients should be aware that they have an increased risk of infection, so they should monitor and report any manifestations, such as low-grade fevers, chills, or joint pain, to their primary caregivers. Other long-term effects include facial edema, increased appetite, and the development of diabetes mellitus, osteoporosis, and avascular necrosis.

SAFETY ⚠ ALERT

Clients should also be instructed to wear a medical alert identification tag as long as they are receiving prednisone therapy. Clients must clearly understand that they should never change a dose of prednisone. Steroids must be tapered slowly after high-dose or long-term use because the body cannot respond quickly to changes in cortisol levels. During the period in which high doses of steroids have been administered, the hypothalamus-pituitary-adrenocortical axis has been suppressed, thus leading to negative feedback for the natural production of cortisol. Steroid-dependent clients who abruptly discontinue their therapy can experience an addisonian crisis (characterized by circulatory collapse, vomiting, and severe weakness) with minimal stress.

Prevent Aspiration

SAFETY ⚠ ALERT

Clients with involvement of the pharyngeal and respiratory muscles must be carefully monitored for the prevention of aspiration pneumonia. Helping clients maintain or regain effective swallowing can significantly reduce aspiration. Resting before meals, eating easily swallowed foods (such as those of a smooth, slippery consistency), and sitting upright during meals are measures that can enhance the client's ability to swallow.

Prevent Falls

SAFETY ⚠ ALERT

Clients with PM-DM are also at risk of falling because of muscle weakness, gait changes, and the possibility of osteoporosis from high-dose prednisone therapy. Balancing a muscle-strengthening program with the use of assistive devices and instructions about safe ambulation helps to keep the client injury free.

BURSITIS

Bursitis is a painful inflammation of the bursae, those closed, minimally fluid-filled sacs that are lined with a synovium similar to the lining of joint spaces. The purpose of bursae is to reduce friction between adjacent tissues—tendon and bones or tendons and ligaments—by lubricating these enclosed structures with synovial fluid from the bursal sac. There are approximately 150 bursae in the body. They typically cover bony prominences, such as the olecranon, trochanter, or patella, and provide protection between the skin and other structures. They are usually quite thin, but with repeated stress, they can become thickened and fluid-filled secondary to inflammation. Bursitis can be either an acute or a chronic condition.

Approximately 3% of the adult population has been estimated to have painful, symptomatic bursitis. The problem peaks between the ages of 40 and 50, presumably as active adults first experience the beginning of degenerative changes in the joints. The shoulder joint is the most commonly affected, followed by the elbow, knee, and hip. When bursitis involves the upper extremities, the dominant arm is usually affected.

Risk factors associated with the development of bursitis include acute or chronic trauma, typically through participation in mechanical, highly repetitive activities. Other causes include such arthritic conditions as RA, gout, tumors, and degenerative changes associated with increasing age. Bursitis is considered a true inflammatory condition with the classic signs of inflammation, local redness, warmth, and swelling.

Typically, the client with acute bursitis complains of exquisite localized pain in the target area. Clients may experience point tenderness and can point specifically to the spot of greatest discomfort. They may also have diffuse soreness radiating to the tendons at the site. Depending on the location of the bursitis, clients may complain of interrupted sleep (e.g., with subacromial bursitis, calcaneal bursitis), difficulty walking (trochanteric bursitis, calcaneal bursitis), or difficulty performing ADL (subacromial or olecranon bursitis).

Occupational or avocational activities can also provide insight into the nature of the pain, for example, a woodcarver who has developed acute subacromial bursitis or a businesswoman who walks long distances in medium to high heels.

The diagnosis of bursitis is generally based on the results of the history and physical examination. Radiographs of the affected joint are usually normal in acute bursitis, whereas in chronic conditions calcium deposits may be present. Results of laboratory tests and synovial fluid analysis are normal unless the bursa has become infected.

OUTCOME MANAGEMENT

Acute bursitis is treated with rest and immobilization of the affected joint, non-opioid analgesics, and ROM exercises. In general, the pain of acute bursitis is controlled with NSAIDs. Client education focuses on the causes of bursitis, the prevention of additional attacks (by avoiding activities that cause constant friction or pressure), the correct application of moist heat, and medication and exercise instruction.

Relieve Pain

Helping clients obtain pain relief is the primary focus of nursing interventions. Without pain relief, joint mobility is impaired through frozen, protective measures. Nurses must instruct clients about the purpose of anti-inflammatory medications as well as the appropriate dose and untoward side effects.

Pain relief is also achieved by resting or immobilizing the joint or by elevating or compressing the involved area to control edema. Teaching clients about the correct application of ice and heat is important so they receive maximum pain relief. If clients receive intra-articular injections of cortisone, they should be informed about the possibility of a post-injection flare-up. They should also be reassured that the pain responds quickly to the application of ice packs.

Promote Self-Care

Self-care deficits are usually temporary in acute bursitis. If the condition becomes chronic, clients may experience more difficulties, particularly if the shoulder or elbow is involved. Dressing is easier if oversized garments are worn, especially those with long sleeves or wide pant legs. Shirts and tops that button in the front are also helpful. Clients can be taught to minimize shoulder or elbow pain by putting clothing on the affected arm first and by taking it off the affected arm last.

VASCULITIS

Vasculitis comprises a group of disorders leading to inflammation and necrosis of blood vessel walls. Soluble immune complexes are deposited in blood vessel walls in areas where capillaries have increased permeability. After deposition, the immune system is activated and the complex is destroyed along with the blood vessel wall. These disorders include polyarteritis nodosa, systemic necrotizing vasculitis, and allergic granulomatous angiitis. Inflammation and damage to large and small vessels result in end-stage organ damage.

Specific manifestations vary, depending on the organs affected. Steroids are the treatment of choice for these disorders.

POLYMYALGIA RHEUMATICA

Polymyalgia rheumatica is a clinical syndrome occurring more commonly in women than in men. It is a disease of aging, rarely occurring before age 60 years. It is characterized by pain and stiffness in the neck, shoulder, back, and pelvic girdle, especially in the morning. Headaches or painful areas on the head may be present. The client also may have a low-grade fever or temporal arteritis. Laboratory findings include an elevated ESR, mild anemia, and possible elevation of immunoglobulins. Steroids usually produce symptomatic relief within days.

GIANT CELL ARTERITIS

Giant cell arteritis, also known as temporal or cranial arteritis, is also a disease of older people. The client often has manifestations of polymyalgia rheumatica for months, and then suddenly experiences the severe headaches associated with temporal arteritis. The onset of this disorder is usually sudden, with severe pain often appearing in the temporal area. The pain also may be felt in the occipital area, face, jaw, or side of the neck. It is usually associated with hyperesthesia, which makes any touch exquisitely painful. The client may experience visual changes, including sudden onset of blindness in one or both eyes.

It is very important to diagnose and treat this disorder before blindness occurs. Because older women are often affected, their complaints of decreased vision and headaches are sometimes ignored as normal aging. Treatment is with glucocorticoids, which are highly effective in controlling this disorder.

MIXED CONNECTIVE TISSUE DISEASE

Mixed connective tissue disease is a combination of several connective tissue diseases. Clients have manifestations that are not typical of any one disorder. Frequent combinations are SLE and SSc and RA. Mixed connective tissue diseases are managed according to their manifestations.

LYME DISEASE

Lyme disease is one form of rheumatic joint disease with a known cause. It is included as a connective tissue disorder because the skin, joints, nervous system, and heart are involved. This complex multisystem disease is caused by the tick-borne spirochete *Borrelia burgdorferi*. Clinical manifestations found from 3 to 32 days after the bite may include a red, flat rash that clears in the center, severe headache, stiff neck, fever, chills, myalgias, joint pain, severe malaise, and fatigue.

The disease can be treated with a course of antibiotic therapy. Doxycycline is the most common antibiotic used. Neurologic abnormalities may occur if treatment is ineffective. Intra-articular steroids and NSAIDs may be used to relieve joint inflammation and pain. Long-term effects include fatigue and arthralgia for many years after the initial infection.

CONCLUSIONS

Nursing clients with rheumatic disorders can prove to be challenging. Clients can experience acute exacerbations or crises with almost all of these diseases. Systemic manifestations can be as devastating as the musculoskeletal manifestations. Whether in remission or exacerbation these diseases are always present. This results in considerable uncertainty, which can lead to a cycle of ineffective coping, disturbed self-esteem, helplessness, and powerlessness. In many respects, the psychological and social problems that are associated with these chronic illnesses can be as disabling as the physical complaints.

Physiologically, clients with rheumatic disorders (autoimmune, spondylarthropathies, or inflammatory arthritis) experience many common problems. The triad of pain, fatigue, and stiffness must be controlled so that function is enhanced or maintained. Difficulty with self-care is usually accompanied by sleep disturbances, altered nutrition, and impaired mobility. These can adversely affect the individual's self-concept and self-esteem and lead to social isolation.

Because of the chronicity of these disorders, clients need skilled, knowledgeable nursing care that draws on the disciplines of rehabilitation, counseling, and self-care. The unique role of the nurse for these clients is one that assumes accountability and responsibility for guiding and directing the client through the health care maze. Clients with chronic, usually systemic illnesses require multiple therapies and follow-up appointments for pharmacologic management, nutritional counseling, lifestyle assessment, physical and occupational therapy, and psychological support. The personal and financial cost can exhaust the client's enthusiasm, job security, support systems, and sense of purpose in life. The nurse can provide a sense of consistency, hope, and reassurance that the client can learn to cope with, and positively adapt to, the demands of a chronic illness. Clients with arthritis need the nurse's expertise to teach them how to explore new self-care strategies so successful adaptation to the disease is a reality. Nurses help clients learn to become partners with the entire health care team as well as with themselves. When clients assume the role of partner, they exhibit greater control, greater accountability, and increased self-esteem as they learn self-management skills. This is nowhere more evident than clients giving themselves their bi-weekly or daily injections of some of the newer treatments.

THINKING CRITICALLY

1. You are working in an outpatient clinic and receive a call from a 66-year-old woman who is experiencing a flare-up of rheumatoid arthritis. She was seen 2 days ago in the clinic and was given a high dose of prednisone. Now she reports epigastric abdominal pain. She reports that her pain has a burning quality, is worse between meals, is relieved by food, and is aggravated by coffee. She has taken some over-the-counter ibuprofen for the pain but states, "It didn't help." What other information do you need to collect? What interventions would you advise?

Factors to Consider. Consider the side effects of glucocorticoids and NSAIDs.

2. A 55-year-old woman with a history of joint pain is scheduled for shoulder arthroplasty. She has experienced increasing pain while working as a waitress and handling orders that must be carried to tables of restaurant guests. She hopes to be able to work pain-free so she can resume her job as a waitress. What nursing assessments are pertinent to this type of condition and proposed surgery? How realistic is the client's desire to return to work as a waitress?

Factors to Consider. How will assessments help in the prevention of postoperative complications? Are clients able to return to an improved level of functioning after joint replacement surgery?

Discussions for these questions can be found on the website. **evolve**

BIBLIOGRAPHY

Citations appearing in red refer to primary research.

Citations appearing in blue refer to evidence-based practice guidelines and protocols.

1. Acorn, J., Joachim, G., & Wachs, J. (2003). Scleroderma: Living with unpredictability. *AAOHN Journal, 51*(8), 358-359.

2. American College of Rheumatology and Association of Rheumatology Health Professionals. (2007). *Rheumatoid arthritis.* Accessed 03/04/07 from www.rheumatology.org.

3. American College of Rheumatology, Subcommittee on Rheumatoid Arthritis Guidelines. (2002). Guidelines for the management of rheumatoid arthritis, 2002 update. *Arthritis and Rheumatism, 46*(2), 238-346. (Also available at www.rheumatology.org/research/guidelines.)

4. Arnett, F., et al. (1988). The American Rheumatism Association 1987 revised criteria for the classification of rheumatoid arthritis. *Arthritis and Rheumatism, 31*, 315-324.

5. Cooper, G., & Stroehla, B. (2003). The epidemiology of autoimmune diseases. *Autoimmune Review, 2*(3), 119-125.

6. Crowther, C., & McCance, K. (2006). Alterations of musculoskeletal function. In K. McCance & S. Huether (Eds.), *Pathophysiology: The biological basis for disease in adults and children* (5th ed., pp. 1497-1545). St. Louis: Mosby.

7. Egan, M., et al. (2006). Splints and orthosis for treating rheumatoid arthritis. *The Cochrane Library, 1*, CD004018.

8. Graham, D., et al. (2002). Ulcer prevention in long-term users of nonsteroidal anti-inflammatory drugs. *Archives of Internal Medicine, 162*, 169-175.

9. Hansen, A., Lipsky, P., & Dorner, T. (2003). New concepts in the pathogenesis of Sjögren's syndrome: Many questions, fewer answers. *Current Opinion in Rheumatology, 15*(5), 563-570.

10. Harris, E., et al. (2005). *Kelley's textbook of rheumatology* (7th ed.). Philadelphia: Saunders.

11. Koopman, E., & Moreland, L. (2005). *Arthritis and allied conditions: A textbook of rheumatology* (15th ed.). Philadelphia: Lippincott Williams & Wilkins.

12. Marchesoni, A., et al. (2003). Radiographic progression in early rheumatoid arthritis: A 12-month randomized controlled study comparing the combination of cyclosporine and methotrexate with methotrexate alone. *Rheumatology, 42*, 1-5.

13. Mayes, M., et al. (2003). Prevalence, incidence, survival, and disease characteristics of systemic sclerosis in a large U.S. population. *Arthritis and Rheumatology, 48*(8), 2246-2255.

14. Meenan, R., Callahan, L., & Helmich, C. (1999). The Arthritis Action Plan: A public health strategy for a looming epidemic. *Arthritis Care and Research, 12*, 79-81.

15. National Center for Chronic Disease Prevention and Health Promotion. (1999). *National Arthritis Action Plan: A public health strategy.* Atlanta: Centers for Disease Control and Prevention.

16. Neumann, L., & Buskila, D. (2003). Epidemiology of fibromyalgia. *Current Pain and Headache Reports, 7*(5), 362-368.

17. Robinson, V., et al.. (2006). Thermotherapy for treating rheumatoid arthritis. *The Cochrane Library, 1*, CD002826.

18. Roth, S. (2004). Effects of Prosorba Column apheresis in patients with chronic refractory rheumatoid arthritis. *Journal of Rheumatology, 31*(11), 2131-2135.

19. Schneider, J., Matthews, J., & Graham, B. (2003). Reiter's syndrome. *Cutis, 71*(3), 198-200.

20. Tan, E., et al. (1982). The 1982 revised criteria for the Classification of Systemic Lupus Erythematosus (SLE). *Arthritis and Rheumatism, 25*, 1271-1277.

21. Turesson, C., O'Fallon, W., & Crowson, C. (2003). Extra-articular disease manifestations in rheumatoid arthritis: Incidence trends and risk factors over 46 years. *Annals of Rheumatic Diseases, 62*(8), 722-727.

22. Wolfe, F., et al. (2003). Predicting mortality in patients with rheumatoid arthritis. *Arthritis and Rheumatology, 48*(6), 1530-1542.

23. Wolfe, F., et al. (1990). The American College of Rheumatology 1990 Criteria for the classification of fibromyalgia: Report of the multicenter criteria committee. *Arthritis and Rheumatism, 33*(2), 160-172.

INTERNET RESOURCES

Arthritis Foundation: www.arthritis.org

Clinical Trial Information: www.Clinicaltrials.gov

Lupus Foundation of American: www.lfa.org

National Sjögren's Syndrome Association: www.sjogrens.org

Rheumatology Resources: www.rheumatology.org/resources.htm

Scleroderma Foundation: www.scleroderma.org

Sjögren's Syndrome and Anesthesia: www.sjogrens.org/ane.htm

Fibromyalgia: www.fibromyalgia.org

evolve *Did you remember to check out the bonus material on the Evolve website and the CD-ROM, including NCLEX®-Examination Style Review Questions, Open-Book Quizzes, and Chapter Review Audio Podcasts?*

http://evolve.elsevier.com/Black/medsurg

CHAPTER 78

Management of Clients with Acquired Immunodeficiency Syndrome

Meg Blair

HIV/AIDS

The year 2006 marked the 25th anniversary of the onset of HIV/AIDS. In June 1981 the first cases of what would come to be called HIV/AIDS were reported to the Centers for Disease Control (CDC). Currently, HIV/AIDS is one of the world's greatest public health crises. Globally, in 2006 more than 65 million people were living with HIV/AIDS. In 2005 there were 4.9 million people newly infected, and there were more than 3.1 million AIDS-related deaths. HIV kills more people than any other infectious disease and ranks fourth among the leading causes of death worldwide. In the United States, more than 944,000 cases have been recorded to date. The number of diagnosed cases continues to rise, with minority populations being among the hardest hit. African Americans comprise half of current HIV/AIDS cases, and AIDS was the leading cause of death for black women ages 25 to 44 years in 2002. Other groups heavily affected in the United States include men who have sex with other men, injecting drug users, women, older adults, and adolescents.

Infection with the human immunodeficiency virus (HIV) results in destruction of the body's host defenses and immune system. For many years, because of a lack of understanding and effective treatment, HIV was considered a rapidly progressing fatal disease. Today HIV infection is viewed more optimistically as a chronic disease that can be controlled with appropriate health care. The cost of such health care (which may top $28,000 per year, per person), however, limits its accessibility to developed, industrialized nations such as the United States. Because many parts of the world, such as Africa and Asia, lack adequate economic resources to treat this disease, HIV infection continues to be a rapidly progressing fatal illness in these areas.

From both a medical and a nursing perspective, clinical management parallels the HIV illness trajectory. Once infected with HIV, a person who receives appropriate treatment can live for many years and continue to function without major problems. In the latter stages of disease, for a variety of reasons to be discussed, the illness progresses, wearing out the immune system. The person is then given the diagnosis acquired immunodeficiency syndrome (AIDS). Because of this dual clinical picture, the material presented in this chapter is divided into (1) caring for the person with HIV disease and (2) caring for the person with AIDS.

Etiology and Risk Factors
Etiology

The etiologic agent associated with AIDS was first isolated by French scientists in 1983 and named the lymphadenopathy-associated virus. One year later, an American scientist claimed the discovery of the etiologic agent and named it the human T-cell lymphotropic virus type III. This led to much confusion, since both scientists actually identified the same virus. In 1986 the International Society on the Taxonomy of Viruses renamed the virus, calling it the human immunodeficiency virus (HIV). In that same year, a second and distinctly different strain of the

evolve **Web Enhancements**

Bridge to Home Health Care Living with HIV/AIDS

Case Study Human Immunodeficiency Virus

Diversity in Health Care HIV and AIDS in Minority Populations

Ethical Issues in Nursing Should a Client's Sexual Lifestyle Influence Nursing Care?

Boxes HIV and AIDS Classification System for Adolescents and Adults

Common Nursing Diagnoses for Clients with HIV and AIDS

Be sure to check out the bonus material on the Evolve website and the CD-ROM, including free self-assessment exercises. **http://evolve.elsevier. com/Black/medsurg**

virus was discovered in Africa. Therefore since 1986 the scientific names use to distinguish the two viruses are HIV-1 and HIV-2.

This was a major—and alarming—discovery because it was the first clue that HIV could change its appearance, or mutate, rapidly. This capability is called genetic promiscuity, and it has become the hallmark of the virus, creating a monumental challenge for scientists and researchers alike. HIV-1 is distributed worldwide, but it is most prevalent in Europe and the United States. HIV-2 predominates in West African nations but has been isolated in other parts of the world. By 1996 scientists discovered that HIV-1 had also mutated several times. It has two major subtypes: (1) HIV-1 major (group M) viruses and (2) HIV-1 outlier (group O) viruses.

HIV-1 Group M

Group M viruses are assigned to 10 genetic subtypes, designated HIV-1, group M, subtypes A, B, C, D, E, F, G, H, I, and J, according to the phylogenetic analysis of their genes. The distribution of subtypes varies worldwide.

HIV-1 Group O

The designation O was deliberate because this mutation was an outlier and differed from the others. Group O was identified primarily in west and central Africa, with a few isolated cases found through special tests in France and the United States.

It is important to mention these complexities to illustrate the rapidly changing nature of HIV. The virus poses a considerable challenge to researchers investigating new drugs to treat the disease or developing vaccines because their work is usually limited to one specific subtype of HIV-1. Indeed, vaccine trials have shown that a vaccine for one subtype may not work for other subtypes.

Risk Factors

Modes of transmission have remained constant throughout the course of the HIV pandemic. The virus is spread through certain sexual practices, through exposure to blood and body fluids, and through perinatal (vertical) transmission. The patterns in the spread of HIV changed considerably during the first 19 years of the epidemic in the United States. Although most Americans infected with HIV continue to be men who have sex with men, significant increases have been noted in intravenous (IV) drug users, women, and heterosexuals. This decline, however, has been limited to white men; the number of new HIV infections among racial and ethnic minority men who have sex with men continues to increase, as outlined in the Diversity in Health Care website feature on HIV and AIDS in Minority Populations. In

young adults (ages 19 to 29), the number of new infections has been increasing, especially in the South and Midwest. Increased numbers of cases are also seen in rural areas and in smaller cities. HIV infection and AIDS are the second leading causes of death among adults ages 25 to 44.

Perhaps the most overlooked population in the HIV epidemic is adults ages 50 and older. Cumulatively they represent 12% of all known cases, but in 2004 they represented 16% of new infections. People in this age group may not be tested promptly for HIV because neither they nor their health care providers perceive them to be at risk for this disease. Women older than 50 acquire HIV infection primarily through heterosexual contact.

The principal mode of transmission of HIV throughout the world has been through sexual exposure. Except in Australia, Europe, and the United States, most HIV transmission has been through heterosexual activity. One important lesson health care professionals have learned from this epidemic is that sexual practices, not sexual preferences, place people at risk for sexually transmitted infections (STIs), including HIV/AIDS. Homosexual men who do not engage in unprotected sex or expose themselves to another person's body fluids are no more at risk for acquiring HIV infection than anyone else; similarly, heterosexual or homosexual couples in long-term, monogamous relationships are at low risk. Unsafe sexual encounters outside of these relationships do, however, pose a risk.

Sexual practices that are completely safe include (1) autosexual activities (such as masturbation), (2) mutually monogamous relationships between noninfected partners, and (3) abstinence. Very safe sexual practices include noninsertive activity. Insertive practices with a condom are considered probably safe so long as the condom is used correctly, does not break, and no contact with body fluids occurs. Everything else is considered risky. Other cofactors, such as engaging in sexual activities while under the influence of drugs or alcohol, having multiple sex partners, and the presence of sores in the genital area, increase the risk of acquiring HIV. Although the number of reported cases is small, oral sexual practices, whether performed on a man or a woman, have been implicated in transmission.

Transmission by exposure to blood is a broad category encompassing numerous possible routes, the most obvious being through transfusion of infected blood products and through transplantation of infected donated tissue or organs. Prevention of HIV infection by any of these means is possible by donor exclusion (excluding people from high-risk groups), routine serologic testing of donated tissues or fluids for HIV antibodies, and heat inactivation of certain blood products, such as factor VIII concentrate. Other means of preventing HIV infection related to blood products are adhering to autologous (self-donated) blood programs and limiting the administration of any blood product to situations in which it is absolutely necessary.

Use of injected drugs accounts for the largest number of HIV infections through exposure to contaminated blood. The only absolutely safe injecting drug use behavior is not to inject. Very safe practice is to use sterilized injection paraphernalia and never share needles and syringes. A probably safe practice is to clean injection paraphernalia with full-strength bleach before injecting, although disposable needles and syringes are difficult to clean. Anything else is considered risky. Other cofactors that increase the chances of acquiring HIV by drug injection include the seroprevalence of HIV in the geographical area of the drug user, the social setting of the drug use (e.g., "shooting galleries," where injection paraphernalia is shared), and the frequency of injection.

Needle exchange programs provide sterile injection equipment, latex condoms, counseling, and access to social and health programs, including drug treatment. Numerous studies have shown that needle exchange programs decrease the spread of HIV and hepatitis B and C and do not increase or promote injection drug use. Despite the proven success of this approach to disease prevention, state and federal legislators have been reluctant to appropriate funds to support this model of care. In the United States, needle exchange programs may operate as legal, illegal but tolerated, or illegal underground programs. In Europe, where this approach has more support, government studies have found that needle exchange programs not only reduce the incidence of HIV but also reduce health care spending for other diseases associated with IV drug injection.

HIV transmission to health care workers by clients is an ongoing concern for workers, employers, and public health officials. In the United States, the total number of health care workers with documented, occupationally acquired HIV or AIDS in 2002 was 57. The number with possible transmission was 139. Although most occupationally-related HIV infections are due to percutaneous exposure, other modes of transmission included mucocutaneous exposure and direct exposure to HIV in the laboratory setting. The actual average risk to a health care worker for exposure to HIV is extremely low (0.4% after a needle-stick or sharp instrument injury and 0.09% after a mucous membrane exposure). The risk is increased in situations in which a deep injury occurs, when there is visible blood on the device causing the injury, when the device involved was previously placed in a client's artery or vein, and when AIDS was diagnosed in the source client who died within 60 days after the health care worker's exposure.

SAFETY

⚠️

ALERT

Accidental needle-stick exposure poses the greatest hazard to health care workers. Nurses must learn and follow standard precautions when handling blood and body fluids and when performing procedures that could lead to exposure to blood and body fluids. One of The Joint Commission's National Patient Safety Goals recommends following standard precautions and complying with the CDC guidelines. When any incident reflects potential exposure to blood-borne pathogens, seek medical treatment immediately. The CDC has guidelines for evaluating and possibly treating exposures to HIV.

In the United States, only one case of HIV transmission from a health care worker to clients has been documented. It was reported in 1990 and involved a Florida dentist. Six clients reportedly became infected with HIV after receiving dental care. The circumstances of this case implied inadequate disinfection and sterilization of instruments in the dental office. Since this incident, retrospective studies of possible HIV transmission from infected health care workers to clients have not identified any other cases in the United States. There have been two reported incidents of clients infected with HIV in France, one documented and one suspected.

Occupational exposure to blood and body fluids is a potential problem not only for health care workers but also for members of other occupations, such as police and corrections officers.

Perinatal HIV exposure can occur during pregnancy, during vaginal delivery, and post-partum through breast-feeding. In 2001 there were fewer than 200 neonatal cases of HIV in the United States; however, there were more than 700,000 new cases in sub-Saharan Africa alone. This is mostly because women in this resource-poor area do not have access to testing and treatment. Administration of zidovudine to pregnant women has been shown to reduce the rate of vertical HIV transmission from 23% to 8%. The CDC has published guidelines for the use of zidovudine and other antiretroviral therapies for pregnant women and their newborn infants.

The only absolute method of preventing perinatal exposure is to avoid pregnancy. Health care workers should discuss HIV infection as part of routine prenatal care with all clients because many mothers may be unaware that they are infected with HIV. Infected women who carry to term should be advised against breast-feeding because this is a mode of HIV transmission. However, a woman living where a reliable supply of clean, safe drinking water does not exist may expose her infant to more danger from other infectious illnesses with bottle feeding.

Primary prevention of HIV infection for exposed individuals is an emerging concept being applied not only to health care workers but also to the treatment of other accidental exposures. Post-exposure prophylaxis is being used as a health maintenance strategy by some clinicians for people who engage in some high-risk activities. Considerable controversy surrounds the use of post-exposure prophylaxis except in cases of rape, and the ethical aspects of providing such treatment continue to be discussed.

Vaccine research has been ongoing since 1987. However, the mainstay of disease prevention continues to be education and reduction of risky behaviors.

Pathophysiology

HIV-1 is a member of the lentivirus subfamily of human retroviruses. Diseases caused by lentiviruses are characterized by an insidious onset and progressive involvement of the central nervous system (CNS), and may result in disorders of the immune system. HIV-1 is one of five viruses in the lentivirus family (Figure 78-1). The others are HIV-2 and human T-lymphotropic virus (HTLV) types I, II, and IV.

A retrovirus belongs to the family Retroviridae and possesses ribonucleic acid (RNA)-dependent deoxyribonucleic acid (DNA) polymerase (reverse transcriptase). HIV infects T helper cells (T4 lymphocytes), macrophages, and B cells. HIV does not directly affect the CNS or peripheral neurons, astrocytes, or oligodendrocytes. HIV infection in the CNS is indirectly caused by neurotoxins produced by infected macrophages or chemical substances produced by the dysregulation of cytokines and chemokines.

T helper cells are infected more readily than other cells. The depletion of T helper cells occurs in the following steps:

1. Once inside the host, HIV attaches to the target cell membrane by way of its receptor molecule, CD4.
2. The virus is uncoated, and the RNA enters the cell.
3. The enzyme known as reverse transcriptase is released, and viral RNA is transcribed into DNA.
4. This newly created DNA moves into the nucleus and the DNA of the cell.
5. A provirus is created when the viral DNA integrates itself into the cellular DNA or genome of the cell.
6. Once the provirus is in place, its genetic material is no longer pure host DNA but is part viral DNA.
7. The cell may function abnormally.
8. The host cell dies, and viral budding occurs (Figure 78-2). The new virus now infects other cells.

The main target for HIV is the T4 helper cell; however, the "glue" to which HIV is attracted is the CD4 molecule, which acts as the receptor for HIV on the T4 helper cell. Even though the CD4 molecule is also found on other cells, such as macrophages and monocytes, clinicians usually refer to T4 helper cells as CD4$^+$ cells. Therefore in articles, research papers, or laboratory reports about HIV, the labels T4, T4 helper, CF4$^+$, and CD4$^+$ T helper cell are used synonymously. Another substance, chemokine, acts as a messenger to facilitate

■ **FIGURE 78–1** Schematic diagram of the human immunodeficiency virus-1 (HIV-1) virion. *RNA,* Ribonucleic acid. *(Redrawn from Sande, M., & Volberding, P. [1999]. The medical management of AIDS [6th ed.]. Philadelphia: Saunders.)*

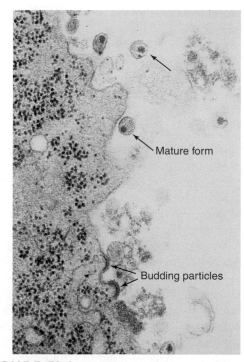

■ **FIGURE 78–2** Human immunodeficiency virus. Electron micrograph of the virus budding from a T lymphocyte. *(From Friedman-Kien, A., & Cockerell, C. [1996]. Color atlas of AIDS [2nd ed., p. 11]. Philadelphia: Saunders.)*

HIV entry into cells. In 1996 scientists discovered that certain people have a genetic defect in a gene related to chemokines and, despite repeated exposure to HIV, never become infected.

The $CD4^+$ T helper cells are regulating cells in the immune system. They interact with monocytes, macrophages, cytotoxic T cells, natural killer cells, and B cells. In the analogy of an orchestra and a conductor, the T cells are the "conductor" of the immune system, directing all the activity ("music") produced by the other immune cells ("orchestra"). Therefore the loss of the $CD4^+$ T helper cells results in significant decreases in coordinated immune activity. The body loses its ability to maintain a consistent state of health. With significant losses of these regulatory cells, the HIV-infected person becomes highly susceptible to acquired infection. Pathogens that previously caused disease may reactivate and also cause infection. An example is the varicella zoster virus, which may have caused chickenpox when an HIV-infected person was a child and may reappear as shingles when the $CD4^+$ T-cell count drops to low levels.

The average laboratory range for the $CD4^+$ T-cell count is $500/mm^3$ to $1600/mm^3$. A gradual physiologic decline occurs in these cells over an individual's lifespan. In fact, $CD4^+$ T-cell counts in newborns are almost double those of an adult. In the adult, $CD4^+$ cell counts below $200/mm^3$ are considered dangerously low and infection is likely to develop. Other laboratory changes that indicate immune dysfunction include the following:

- An overall decline in the total numbers of white blood cells
- Decreases in both the total number and the percentage of lymphocytes
- Significant changes in the $CD4^+/CD8^+$ ratio
- Decreased $CD4^+$ T-cell test findings
- Absent or decreased skin test reactivity (anergy)
- Increased immunoglobulin levels

The cause of this immune system damage is the extensive amount of HIV activity taking place in an infected person from the time of infection. HIV replicates at a rapid rate. In fact, it may produce 10 million new virions (viral particles) daily. Although a person with HIV may be asymptomatic with a normal $CD4^+$ cell count, insidious destruction of the immune system is taking place. Antiretroviral drugs interrupt the disease process by inhibiting the ability of the virus to replicate or to enter the cell, thus reducing the amount of circulating virus in the body and halting its destructive activity. Once this happens, the immune system begins to heal and restore itself, as noted by rising $CD4^+$ cell counts.

Sustaining the beneficial effects of antiretroviral therapy is challenging. The greatest problem is HIV's ability to mutate and become resistant to antiretroviral drugs. When this drug failure occurs, plasma viral load rises and the $CD4^+$ cell count decreases. The treatment regimen must then be changed. Because two to three drugs are usually used at the same time and the list of available approved drugs is still small, the number of combinations that can be prescribed is limited. Additionally, although the drugs can contain the disease in plasma, the virus

can hide in many other cells in the body. Finally, because most antiretroviral agents do not cross the blood-brain barrier in the CNS, treatment of CNS problems caused by HIV infection can be very difficult.

The course of HIV illness varies from person to person. Several cofactors may accelerate immunodeficiency, including malnutrition, continued substance abuse, allergic conditions, genetics, age, pregnancy, gender, and presence of other infections. Factors that have been linked to increased mortality and morbidity include being of lower socioeconomic status, lacking access to adequate care, receiving care in a hospital with limited AIDS experience, and being treated by a physician with little experience in AIDS care.

Overall, survival among clients with AIDS has improved dramatically since the advent of highly active antiretroviral therapy (HAART) in 1996, which uses varying combinations of drugs from four different classes of antiretroviral medications. Since 2006, HAART has been called antiretroviral therapy (ART). Combined with prophylactic treatment for commonly occurring opportunistic infections, ART has led to HIV disease changing from a rapidly fatal disease to a chronic, mostly manageable condition (Figure 78-3).

To illustrate further the differences observed in HIV-infected people, scientists have reported that about 5% are perfectly healthy after many years and show no manifestations of disease progression. These long-term nonprogressors have the following:

- Documented evidence of HIV infection for more than 10 years
- Lack of manifestations
- Normal, stable immune profiles
- Never required any treatment for HIV disease

Long-term nonprogressors (LTNPs) appear to produce vigorous amounts of serum antibodies that keep HIV activity at extremely low levels, thus preventing damage to the immune system. LTNPs may have one part of a two-part genetic defect. People with both alleles on two genes cannot be infected with HIV. Do not confuse a long-term nonprogressor with a long-term survivor, defined as someone who has lived for more than 8 years after an AIDS diagnosis, who shows all clinical and laboratory manifestations of disease, and who continuously requires treatment.

Although the main target of HIV is the immune system, considerable damage occurs to other parts of the body as a result of HIV in body tissues. Examples of clinical conditions that can be directly attributed to HIV include cranial and peripheral neuropathies, uveitis, cardiomyopathy, pneumonitis, malabsorption in the small intestine, nephritis, cervicitis, arthritis, psoriasis, gonad dysfunction, and adrenalitis. Additionally, damage to the hematologic system—caused in part by impaired blood cell production—commonly results in anemia, granulocytopenia, and thrombocytopenia.

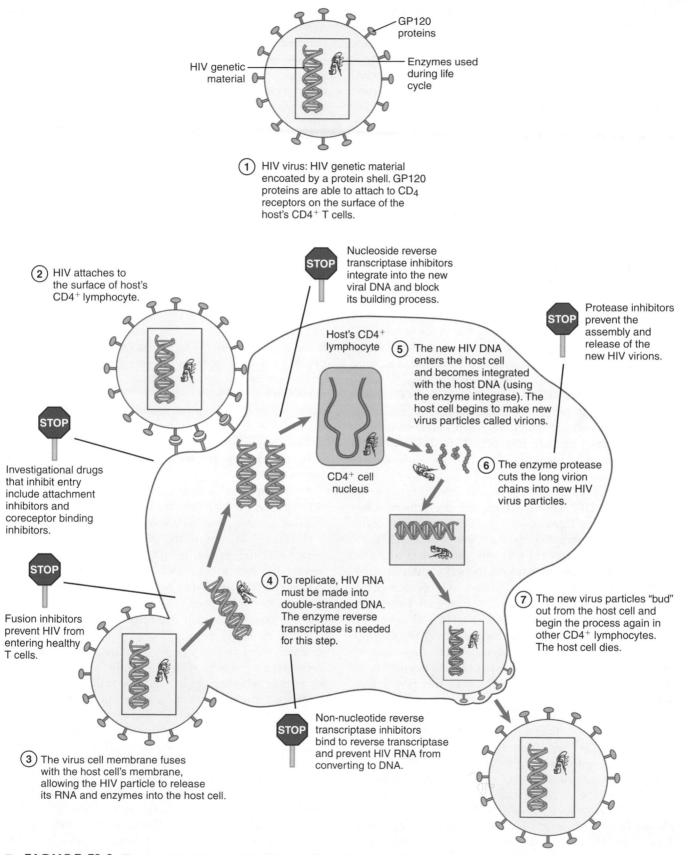

GP120 proteins

HIV genetic material

Enzymes used during life cycle

(1) HIV virus: HIV genetic material encoated by a protein shell. GP120 proteins are able to attach to CD$_4$ receptors on the surface of the host's CD4$^+$ T cells.

(2) HIV attaches to the surface of host's CD4$^+$ lymphocyte.

STOP Nucleoside reverse transcriptase inhibitors integrate into the new viral DNA and block its building process.

STOP Protease inhibitors prevent the assembly and release of the new HIV virions.

Host's CD4$^+$ lymphocyte

(5) The new HIV DNA enters the host cell and becomes integrated with the host DNA (using the enzyme integrase). The host cell begins to make new virus particles called virions.

STOP Investigational drugs that inhibit entry include attachment inhibitors and coreceptor binding inhibitors.

CD4$^+$ cell nucleus

(6) The enzyme protease cuts the long virion chains into new HIV virus particles.

STOP Fusion inhibitors prevent HIV from entering healthy T cells.

(4) To replicate, HIV RNA must be made into double-stranded DNA. The enzyme reverse transcriptase is needed for this step.

(7) The new virus particles "bud" out from the host cell and begin the process again in other CD4$^+$ lymphocytes. The host cell dies.

(3) The virus cell membrane fuses with the host cell's membrane, allowing the HIV particle to release its RNA and enzymes into the host cell.

STOP Non-nucleotide reverse transcriptase inhibitors bind to reverse transcriptase and prevent HIV RNA from converting to DNA.

■ **FIGURE 78–3** The steps in the life cycle of the HIV virus with correlation to medications.

In addition to managing HIV disease, clinicians are challenged with addressing illnesses that existed before the person acquired HIV infection. These not only require continuing treatment and attention but also may complicate the course of illness. Frequently encountered pre-existing and co-morbid conditions seen in HIV-infected clients include, but are not limited to, alcoholism, drug dependence, liver disease, kidney disease, psychiatric illness, and a history of STIs. As therapy improves and people with HIV disease live longer, they will also require treatment for such illnesses as cancer, coronary artery disease, chronic obstructive lung disease, hypertension, and diabetes, all of which may occur in the aging population not infected with HIV.

Clinical Manifestations

As knowledge has evolved regarding the HIV disease process, the CDC has developed and revised numerous classification systems (see the box on HIV and AIDS Classification System for Adolescents and Adults on the website). The most recent classification system for HIV disease in adults and adolescents is based on two monitoring parameters used to follow a client: (1) laboratory data ($CD4^+$ cell counts) and (2) clinical presentation (the person's clinical manifestations of diseases). The period in which a person becomes infected is referred to as primary infection. If HIV is detected at the time of initial infection, the client is considered to be in category A.

Primary infection is the initial period after a person has acquired HIV. The length of time the primary infection lasts varies from several weeks to a few months. During primary infection, 50% to 70% of people become sick. Many clinicians are unaware of this fact and tend to think that primary infection is silent. In addition to systemic manifestations (fever, fatigue, lymphadenopathy, nausea, vomiting), the infected person may experience headache; truncal (torso and arms) rash; ulcers of the mouth, genitals, or both; thrush; pharyngitis; diarrhea; hepatomegaly; myalgia; arthralgia; anemia; thrombocytopenia; and leukopenia. In some people, the manifestations are mild and similar to mononucleosis. Other people have severe manifestations requiring hospitalization.

During primary infection, a sudden and intense burst of HIV activity results in a high viral load and a dramatic drop in the $CD4^+$ cell count. In fact, during this time, the $CD4^+$ cell count may drop to below $100/mm^3$, with the concomitant development of an AIDS-defining illness. This is also the period in which most newly infected people develop antibodies to HIV, which can then be detected through enzyme immunoassay testing. There is a "window" period for seroconversion (the time it takes for a newly infected person to develop antibodies to HIV that can be detected in a laboratory specimen). On average, antibodies can be detected in 4 to 12 weeks.

Unfortunately, in most instances the diagnosis is not confirmed at the time of primary infection, either because the person does not seek medical care or because the clinician does not take an adequate history that raises the suspicion of HIV infection. This is quite a serious situation because preliminary studies have shown that starting antiretroviral therapy at the time of initial infection may prevent damage to the immune system and to other body systems.

Previously, the decision to seek an HIV test was left up to the individual, except in certain instances, such as when seeking a federal job or when donating blood or solid organs. However, in 2006, the CDC began recommending routine HIV screening for all adolescent, adult, and pregnant clients in all health care settings. Clients will be notified that testing will be done with other routine screening unless the client defers. This is a change from past practice in which clients had to be asked specifically and had to give consent. Testing also involves pre- and post-test counseling. Testing may be performed either anonymously or confidentially. If testing is performed too early in the initial infection period, a false-negative result may occur. False-positive results are extremely rare but may occur in clients with autoimmune disorders such as lupus erythematosus, or in clients who have taken part in HIV vaccine studies. Other methods for detecting HIV infection include home test kits, salivary tests, and urine tests. HIV/AIDS is reportable in all 50 states and in the territories.

In general, test results are reported as (1) positive, (2) negative, or (3) indeterminate. If the enzyme immunoassay result is positive, a second test, the Western blot, is performed to confirm the diagnosis. A positive result means that the person is HIV-infected, but it does not predict the future course of disease. A negative result means that HIV antibodies were not detected. Indeterminate results usually mean that the enzyme immunoassay test was positive, but the Western blot test did not confirm the findings. Repeated testing later is commonly recommended as a means of validating initial test results. Repeated annual screening is recommended by the CDC for people who engage in high-risk activities.

The person usually remains asymptomatic for many years during the period following primary infection; therefore clients with HIV disease are commonly categorized in group A for extended periods. Although the clients have no obvious major manifestations, they may start to notice recurrent infections of the sinuses or respiratory tract or may feel increasing fatigue. Although no significant disease is apparent, viral destruction takes place throughout the body. The majority of this destruction occurs in lymph tissue, resulting in a slowly declining $CD4^+$ cell count. The damage to lymphatic structures also has a negative effect on the quality of $CD4^+$ cells that continue to be produced. After a while, although the numbers may be adequate, $CD4^+$ cells lose their ability to contain the destructive nature of HIV.

Since the beginning of the HIV epidemic, clinical monitoring has focused on evaluating the quantity of $CD4^+$ cells. In essence, $CD4^+$ cell counts are an indirect measurement of the clinical course of HIV disease, showing the end result of HIV activity. In 1996 viral load testing became available to directly measure viral activity in a person with HIV. Viral load tests measure the amount of HIV RNA in plasma, quantify HIV activity, determine prognosis, indicate the need for treatment, evaluate the biologic response to treatment, and detect treatment failure. $CD4^+$ cell counts should not be a substitute for viral load testing because the correlation between the two is weak. High viral loads may not always correlate with clinical manifestations and a low $CD4^+$ cell count and vice versa. Viral load results may be reported in copies per milliliter (e.g., 10,000 copies/ml). The actual numbers may be reported as follows:

- Decimal numbers, as in 10,000 copies
- Exponents, as in 10^4, where the exponent 4 indicates the number of zeros after the 1
- A logarithm, in this case 4, which indicates 10^4 or 10,000

Thus a report that sets viral activity at 5 logs would be interpreted as 10^5 or 100,000 copies/ml.

As the disease progresses, manifestations such as thrush or vulvovaginal candidiasis usually appear, which are distinct manifestations of an underlying immunodeficiency. This development is what commonly causes people to seek HIV testing. Those who have symptomatic illness are then classified into group B (see the box on HIV and AIDS Classification System for Adolescents and Adults on the website). Eventually a client with HIV infection develops one or more AIDS-defining diseases and is finally classified into group C. Once again, this may be the first time that HIV infection is discovered.

OUTCOME MANAGEMENT FOR HIV INFECTION

The outcomes for medical and nursing management of the client infected with HIV are to maintain the person's health, initiate and maintain an effective antiretroviral regimen, and prevent infectious complications. This requires follow-up at specified intervals and an understanding that to achieve these outcomes the client has to make lifestyle changes.

Medical Management of the Client with HIV Infection

Maintain Health

Initiating a plan of care for any client infected with HIV requires a detailed laboratory and clinical assessment.

Initial and follow-up laboratory testing provides invaluable information on disease progression, serves as a guide for treatment decisions, and determines the efficacy of treatment. A complete blood count is needed to identify anemia, thrombocytopenia, leukopenia, and developing infections. Multichannel chemistry panels and urinalysis disclose renal, liver, metabolic, or nutritional disease. Both tests are repeated at 6- to 12-month intervals to detect any abnormalities from disease progression or treatment complications. These results are also needed to modify dosages of antiretroviral drugs for clients with impaired kidney or liver function.

An annual tuberculin skin test detects mycobacterial disease, and a chest x-ray identifies pulmonary problems. For women, a pregnancy test and Papanicolaou (Pap) smear are usually performed. Pap smears are performed twice during the first year after a diagnosis of HIV infection and then at least annually. Screening for STIs includes testing for syphilis, gonorrhea, and *Chlamydia*. These are repeated annually if the client is sexually active. Hepatitis antibody testing is performed to identify acute or prior infection and to determine the need for immunization. There is a high incidence of hepatitis C in people infected with HIV.

Testing for pathogens known to cause opportunistic infections in people infected with HIV includes serologic tests intended to detect previous exposure to toxoplasmosis, histoplasmosis, cryptococcosis, and cytomegalovirus. For seronegative clients, repeated testing may reveal a primary exposure. For seropositive clients, rising titers of antibodies to these pathogens indicate the need for prophylactic therapy.

Finally, $CD4^+$ cell counts, ratios, and percentages are performed to determine the degree of immunodeficiency, and viral load testing is ordered to calculate the amount of viral activity. Viral load test result interpretations are as follows:

- 10,000 copies/ml: poses a low risk for AIDS
- 10,000 to 100,000 copies/ml: doubles risk for AIDS
- >100,000 copies/ml: poses a high risk for AIDS

The initial test, without any treatment, may reveal viral loads of 80,000 to 1 million copies per milliliter or even higher. These same tests are repeated at intervals determined by the presence or absence of manifestations or disease in the client through the course of illness. Because several viral load tests have been approved for use, clinicians are advised to use the same viral load test when performing serial measurements to control variations in test results. Diseases such as influenza, herpes, or pneumonia, as well as testing immediately after the influenza vaccine is administered, can cause a temporary increase in test results. Therefore testing may be deferred in any of these situations.

Initiate and Maintain Antiretroviral Therapy

The decision to treat HIV disease should involve both the primary care provider and the client. Many clients, because of personal experience or preference, may refuse recommended antiretroviral therapy. Clinicians should, in a noncoercive manner, provide as much objective information as possible so that the person with HIV can make an informed choice about taking these drugs. Most clinicians recommend starting an antiretroviral combination therapy regimen early in the course of disease; however, this has become somewhat controversial. This debate is outlined in the Translating Evidence into Practice feature on p. 2101.

Current guidelines from the U.S. Department of Health and Human Services are as follows:

- Symptomatic clients: Treat
- Asymptomatic clients with a CD4 count <200/mm^3: Treat
- Asymptomatic clients with CD4 counts 200-350/mm^3: Therapy should generally be offered
- Asymptomatic clients with CD4 counts >350/mm^3: Defer or consider therapy if viral load is high

The following classes of antiretroviral agents are most commonly used:

- Nucleoside/nucleotide reverse transcriptase inhibitors (NRTIs)
- Protease inhibitors (PIs)
- Non-nucleoside reverse transcriptase inhibitors (NNRTIs)
- Fusion inhibitors

Also called nucleoside/nucleotide analogs, NRTIs block HIV replication of HIV in newly infected cells. PIs attack infected cells and prevent the virus from maturing appropriately. NNRTIs work in a manner similar to that of NRTIs. Fusion inhibitors, the newest class of drugs for treatment of HIV, prevent HIV from entering healthy T cells in the body (see Figure 78-3 and the Integrating Pharmacology feature on p. 2102). The only approved entry inhibitor is enfuvirtide (Fuzeon). Enfuvirtide blocks HIV fusion with the cell membrane, thus preventing entry of the virus into the cell. Enfuvirtide is given by twice daily subcutaneous injection. Use of entry inhibitors is reserved for HIV-positive clients who have become resistant to PIs, NRTIs, and NNRTIs.

Combination pills are available that greatly decrease the number of pills needed daily and facilitate adherence to treatment (see the Translating Evidence into Practice feature on p. 2101). In ART, a combination of three drugs from two of the first three drug classes (NRTIs, PIs, and NNRTIs) is used. Atripla, a combination of an NNRTI and two NRTI drugs, was approved by the FDA in July 2006. This is the first once-a-day combination antiretroviral pill. Clinicians and clients strive to find combinations that are the least toxic and that produce the largest and most long-lasting viral response (lowest viral load) and the best immune response (highest CD4$^+$ cell counts). The goals of therapy are to inhibit the replication of HIV, reduce the viral load to undetectable levels, and stabilize the disease.

Perhaps the greatest challenge in treating HIV infection has been the genetic promiscuity of this virus. As stated earlier, HIV mutates rapidly. In the presence of an antiretroviral drug, it can develop resistance to the drug and continue to grow in the presence of the drug. Three types of drug resistance are of concern:

- Genotypic resistance, in which the virus mutates
- Phenotypic resistance, in which the virus shows a decrease in sensitivity to the drug
- Cross-resistance, in which the virus, having developed resistance to one drug, becomes resistant to other drugs in that class

Monotherapy (prescription of one antiretroviral agent at a time) is more likely to result in drug resistance than is combination therapy. Subtherapeutic levels of a drug also lead to drug resistance. Subtherapeutic levels can occur when the client does not take the prescribed dosage or does not take doses at specified intervals, or both, and can also occur when other prescribed drugs interact with the antiretroviral drug and cause lower blood levels.

Attempting to prevent drug resistance, clinicians order combination therapy, believing that combinations of drugs "confuse" the virus, thus interfering with its ability to develop resistance. Unfortunately, preliminary data show that even in combinations of three drugs at once, resistance may develop to one or more of the agents being taken over time. Evaluation of antiretroviral therapy is based on the client's clinical manifestations and on laboratory tests of viral load and CD4$^+$ cell counts. The most reliable objective determinant is viral load testing, which is performed 3 to 4 weeks after initiating or changing therapy. If the decrease in viral load is not at least three times the original laboratory reports, or decreased by at least 0.5 log, the therapy is usually changed. Repeated testing is usually performed at 3- to 4-month intervals.

Drug failure, in which the ordered combination is no longer effective, can occur after trying several standard combinations of antiretrovirals. The challenge to the clinician at that point is to try combinations of four to six drugs in an effort to suppress HIV activity once again. This approach to therapeutic intervention is commonly called salvage therapy. In many instances, salvage therapy fails because the HIV-infected person has developed drug resistance to most of the available drugs.

Studies are also being conducted to identify other chemotherapeutic strategies to control HIV infection. Scientists are looking at the use of HIV vaccines

Adherence to Antiretroviral Therapy (ART)

Adherence to prescribed medication is known to be problematic. Clients have difficulty fully complying with therapy, whether it is of short duration for an acute episode (for instance, antibiotics) or of long duration (as in the case of chronic illness). It is well documented that adherence declines as the urgency of treating the disease declines and as the duration of therapy lengthens.

The literature shows that overall medication adherence rates vary from 40% to 80%. Unfortunately, HIV presents a unique challenge. Among individuals taking ART (antiretroviral therapy), only 40% to 60% are 90% adherent. Nonadherence to therapy allows the viral load to increase as immune functioning decreases, and is the major contributing factor to the development of resistant strains of HIV, which can be transmitted to others. Compliance with anti-HIV medication must occur at an incredible 95% to prevent these sequelae.

People living with HIV (PLWH) undergoing treatment face a daunting challenge in remaining adherent to their regimen. ART requires that the person take multiple medications, at precise dosing intervals, and with specific restrictions regarding timing the medications with food and fluid. In addition, there may be particular dietary or storage requirements. PLWH may also be taking several drugs to combat or prevent opportunistic infections, nutritional supplements, drugs to counteract unpleasant side effects, and, as the population of PLWH ages, medications to control other chronic conditions.

Many research studies have attempted to shed light on this topic by investigating factors leading to nonadherence as well as factors promoting adherence to therapy. Nonadherence can be a result of personal factors or systems-level factors. Personal factors include such things as forgetfulness, unwillingness to suffer side effects, lack of knowledge, large pill burden, lack of social support, and unwillingness to make lifestyle changes required by the treatment regimen. Systems-level factors include client-health care provider relationship; having multiple services available at one location; ease of obtaining refills; and simplicity of arranging follow-up care, especially in light of new manifestations or side effects. Ongoing substance abuse and psychiatric conditions also are important considerations. Cultural factors also appear to play a role in adherence.

Medication nonadherence seems to be a multifactorial and unique experience to each client. It is incumbent on the nurse to assess this topic gently at every opportunity, attempting to learn, from the client's point of view, what barriers he or she is facing in remaining adherent to the medical regimen.

IMPLICATIONS

Several strategies to improving medication adherence seem to be beneficial. First and foremost is education. PLWH need detailed information about their medications and knowledge regarding the consequences of nonadherence. They also need ongoing information regarding their viral load and $CD4^+$ counts, which can be correlated with medication use. Motivate the client by including him or her in all decisions regarding drug treatment. Give the client information regarding dosing schedule, food and storage requirements, and side effects; then let the client decide whether that treatment is feasible. Some clinics let the PLWH "practice" the regimen with candy or jelly beans for several weeks before the client is asked to commit to the regimen.

Simplify the regimen as much as possible and use drugs that require the least amount of change in the client's lifestyle. Help the client schedule taking medications along with other daily routines. Anticipate unpleasant side effects and be prepared to deal with them promptly. Several "adherence-promoting devices" are available, including simple pill boxes, beepers and alarms, and computer-generated telephone reminder calls. PLWH may need specific skills-building sessions or assistance with problem-solving barriers to taking medications.

Clients with active substance abuse or untreated and undertreated psychiatric conditions (depression, anxiety) may not be able to adhere until these issues are under control. Likewise, a person must fulfill "survival needs" before managing a complex condition such as HIV. If a client is homeless, finding shelter will be a much higher priority than adhering to medications. For these types of clients, it probably is best to delay the start of therapy until these conditions have been stabilized.

Adherence to an HIV medication regimen is demanding and complex, and requires vigilance on the part of the client in maintaining his or her treatment schedule. It also requires the nurse to be vigilant, sensitive, creative, and a partner with the PLWH to design strategies to improve adherence. Adherence to therapy is the most significant determinant of its success. Nurses must be in the forefront to help their clients combat this disease.

REFERENCES

1. Acri, T., Coco, A., Lin, K., et al. (2005). Knowledge of structured treatment interruption and adherence to antiretroviral therapy. *AIDS Patient Care and STDs, 19,* 167-173.
2. Adamian, M.S., Golin, C.E., Shain, L.A., & DeVellis, B. (2004). Brief motivational interviewing to improve adherence to antiretroviral therapy: Development and qualitative pilot assessment of an intervention. *AIDS Patient Care and STDs, 18,* 229-238.
3. Corless, I.B., Nicholas, P.K., Davis, S.M., et al. (2005). Symptom status, medication adherence, and quality of life in HIV disease. *Journal of Hospice and Palliative Nursing, 7*(3), 129-138.
4. Deloria-Knoll, M., Chmiel, J.S., Moorman, A.C., et al. (2004). Factors related to and consequences of adherence to antiretroviral therapy in an ambulatory HIV-infected patient cohort. *AIDS Patient Care and STDs, 12,* 721-727.
5. Enriquez, M., Lackey, N.R., O'Connor, M.C., & McKensey, D.S. (2004). Successful adherence after multiple HIV treatment failures. *Journal of Advanced Nursing, 45,* 439-446.
6. Garcia, P.R., & Cote, J.K. (2003). Factors affecting adherence to antiretroviral therapy in people living with HIV/AIDS. *Journal of the Association of Nurses in AIDS Care, 14*(4), 37-45.
7. Kalichman, S., Cherry, J., & Cain, D. (2005). Nurse-delivered antiretroviral treatment adherence intervention for people with low literacy skills and living with HIV/AIDS. *Journal of the Association of Nurses in AIDS Care, 16*(5), 3-15.
8. Mills, E., Nachega, J., Buchan, I., et al. (2006). Adherence to antiretroviral therapy in sub-Saharan Africa and North America. *Journal of the American Medical Association, 296*(6), 679-690.
9. Oggins, J. (2003). Notions of HIV and medication among multi-ethnic people living with HIV. *Health and Social Work, 28*(1), 53-62.
10. Piliero, P.J., & Colagreco, J.P. (2003). Simplified regimens for treating HIV infection and AIDS. *Journal of the American Academy of Nurse Practitioners, 15,* 305-312.
11. Russel, J., Krantz, S., & Neville, S. (2004). The patient-provider relationship and adherence to highly active antiretroviral therapy. *Journal of the Association of Nurses in AIDS Care, 15*(5), 40-47.
12. Trzynka, S.L., & Erlen, J.A. (2004). HIV disease susceptibility in women and the barriers adherence. *MEDSURG Nursing, 13*(2), 97-104.
13. Tugenberg, T., Ware, N.C., & Wyatt, M.A. (2006). Paradoxical effects of clinician emphasis on adherence to combination antiretroviral therapy for HIV/AIDS. *AIDS Patient Care and STDs, 20,* 269-274.

INTEGRATING PHARMACOLOGY

Understanding Antiretroviral Therapy (ART)

Compared with the early days of the epidemic, many drugs now exist to treat HIV/AIDS and more are being developed. Treating HIV with monotherapy (using one drug) leads to rapid drug resistance. Combination therapy (ART, or antiretroviral therapy) consists of the simultaneous administration of drugs that have different mechanisms of action and without similar toxicities. ART drug combinations attack the HIV virus at different points necessary for its replication. Utilizing multiple drugs decreases the chance of developing resistance.

Since the advent of ART, dramatic declines in AIDS morbidity and mortality have occurred. Inhibiting viral replication allows for "reconstitution" (rebuilding) of the immune system and reducing clinical progression and the risk of death. Drugs to treat HIV/AIDS fall into categories based on where in the viral replication cycle they are effective.

REVERSE TRANSCRIPTASE INHIBITORS

To replicate, HIV's viral RNA must be converted into double-stranded DNA. The enzyme *reverse transcriptase* is responsible for this activity. The first drugs approved to treat HIV/AIDS were reverse transcriptase inhibitors, which prevent the enzyme from changing viral RNA into DNA.

Non-Nucleoside Reverse Transcriptase Inhibitors

Non-nucleoside reverse transcriptase inhibitors (NNRTIs) bind directly to the enzyme and prevent the conversion of RNA to DNA. Examples include the following:

- Rescriptor (delavirdine, DLV)
- Sustiva (efavirenz, EFV)
- Viramune (nevirapine, NVP)

Nucleoside/Nucleotide Reverse Transcriptase Inhibitors

Nucleoside/nucleotide reverse transcriptase inhibitors (NRTIs) incorporate themselves into viral DNA and cause its construction to be terminated. Examples include the following:

- Combivir (zidovudine/lamivudine, AZT + 3TC)
- Epivir (lamivudine, 3TC)
- Retrovir (zidovudine: ZDV or AZT)
- Zerit (stavudine or d4T)
- Ziagen (abacavir or ABC)
- Videx, Videx EC (didanosine, ddI)
- Viread (tenofovir disoproxil fumarate, DF)
- Trizivir (abacavir/lamivudine/zidovudine, ABC + AZT + 3TC)

PROTEASE INHIBITORS

These drugs work by preventing the successful assembly and release of new virus particles (virions). Problems with this class include intolerance, high "pill burden," and poor adherence to treatment. Examples include the following:

- Agenerase (amprenavir, APV)
- Crixivan (indinavir, IDV)
- Fortovase (saquinavir soft gels, SQV-SGC)
- Invirase (saquinavir capsules, SQV-HGC)
- Kaletra (lopinavir/ritonavir, LPV)
- Norvir (ritonavir, RTV)
- Viracept (nelfinavir, NFV)

The optimal time to start therapy has not been definitively determined by research studies. Most clinicians favor the "hit early and hard" approach; however, recent guidelines from the U.S. Department of Health and Human Services and the International AIDS Society—USA Panel delineate several factors to consider before initiating therapy: CD4$^+$ count, viral load, presence of manifestations or opportunistic infections, and the client's willingness to adhere to the regimen. Client willingness is key: nonadherence to this complex regimen leads to drug resistance (see the Translating Evidence into Practice feature on Adherence to ART on p. 2101). Other considerations include drug toxicity profile, "pill burden," dosing/storage/food requirements, and interactions with other drugs the client is taking.

There is no specific prescription for ART. Recommended combinations include the following:

- 2 NRTIs plus either 1 NNRTI or 1 PI or 2 PIs
- 3 NRTIs

In July 2006 the FDA approved Atripla, the first once-a-day combination antiretroviral pill. It is a combination of an NNRTI and two NRTI drugs.

ENTRY INHIBITORS

Entry inhibitors work by preventing HIV from entering healthy T cells. They work differently from the approved anti-HIV drugs described earlier that are active against HIV after it has infected a T cell. These drugs are recommended after initial regimens but before clients become multi-drug resistant. Entry inhibitors include *fusion inhibitors* such as enfuvirtide (Fuzeon, ENF). Fuzeon binds to the gp41 protein on the HIV's surface so that it cannot bind with T cells, thus preventing the virus from infecting healthy cells. Administration is more difficult because enfuvirtide cannot be taken by mouth and must be given as an injection twice a day every 12 hours. Other entry inhibitors are currently under investigation.

Other drugs that work to inhibit different phases of the HIV life cycle are currently being studied. Supervised drug interruptions are also being investigated as a way to boost the client's immune system and decrease the financial and emotional burden of such complex therapy.

as a therapeutic strategy to stimulate host responses and control viral replication. Research continues on immunomodulators—drugs designed to modulate or reconstitute the immune system, such as interleukin-2.

Other novel approaches to therapy include newer entry inhibitor agents, nonpeptidic protease inhibitors, second-generation NNRTIs, integrase inhibitors, and chemokine antagonists.

🪔 Prevent Infection

By 1986 surveillance data indicated that in more than 80% of people with HIV disease, *Pneumocystis (carinii) jiroveci* pneumonia occurred at least once before death. 🪔 Studies eventually showed that morbidity and mortality rates could be reduced significantly by giving a drug prophylactically for *P. jiroveci* pneumonia. Since 1989 the U.S. Public Health Service has recommended that all HIV-infected clients with a $CD4^+$ cell count below $200/mm^3$ receive prophylaxis for *P. jiroveci* pneumonia. Drugs include trimethoprim-sulfamethoxazole (TMP-SMX); dapsone; dapsone, pyrimethamine, and folinic acid; aerosolized, intravenous, or intramuscular pentamidine; or atovaquone. TMP-SMX and dapsone also provide protection against toxoplasmosis.

Although surveillance data alone do not reflect the true incidence of infection with *Mycobacterium avium-intracellulare* complex, postmortem examinations revealed that more than 60% of HIV-infected people had an active infection. 🪔 Since 1993 the U.S. Public Health Service has recommended that all HIV-infected clients with a $CD4^+$ cell count below $50/mm^3$ receive prophylaxis for *M. avium-intracellulare* complex. Recommended drugs include clarithromycin, azithromycin, and rifabutin. However, these drugs may interact with antiretrovirals.

All HIV-infected clients with a positive result to a tuberculin skin test who have no evidence of active tuberculosis should receive 9 months of preventive therapy with isoniazid. Pyridoxine should be added to reduce the potential for peripheral neuropathy. An alternative regimen is rifabutin and pyrazinamide for 2 months; however, these drugs may interact with antiretrovirals.

Other recommended prophylactic measures include prevention of respiratory tract infections by using pneumococcal vaccine and influenza vaccine and prevention of traveler's diarrhea when traveling to countries where diarrhea is common by using antimicrobials such as ciprofloxacin. Finally, prophylactic medication may be ordered to prevent cytomegalovirus infection, recurrent candidiasis, cryptococcosis, or histoplasmosis.

Nursing Management of the Client with HIV Infection

Assessment. To help a client with health maintenance behaviors, nurses should not restrict assessment to the client's immediate clinical status. Instead, focus on potential problems the client may encounter during the illness. For example, if the client has no health insurance or money to pay for follow-up visits, the nurse should initiate social work consultation. There are alternate sources for health care services, such as the federally funded AIDS Drug Assistance Program. If the client lives alone and has no one willing to assist, he or she may need to be placed in an institution when the illness progresses. As a coordinator of care, have information readily available to identify problems and plan ahead.

Before performing any teaching, evaluate the client's existing level of knowledge about HIV infection. Some clients may know little, whereas others may be knowledgeable. Instead of making any assumptions, try to assess exactly what the client does or does not know about transmission and health-promoting behaviors.

The psychological burden of HIV disease can be overwhelming. Crisis points at which the nurse can anticipate anxiety, fear, or depression include the following:

- Time of the initial HIV-positive diagnosis
- Time of the initial AIDS diagnosis
- Changes in treatment
- Development of new manifestations
- Recurrence of problems or relapse
- Terminal illness

Psychological conflicts that clients commonly experience include fear of transmitting HIV to others, constant worry about developing an infection, guilt about a previous lifestyle, and changes in personal relationships. Social stressors may include disclosure of one's HIV status, stigma related to that status, insecurity about employment and insurance, and loneliness and social isolation.

Diagnosis, Outcomes, Interventions

Diagnosis: Risk for Ineffective Therapeutic Regimen Management. The primary nursing diagnosis encountered with newly diagnosed HIV infection is *Risk for Ineffective Therapeutic Regimen Management related to complexity of health care regimen.* Although some clients may know about HIV disease, it is unlikely that they know all that can be done to improve their health.

Outcomes. The client will learn about HIV disease—how to prevent transmission, how to manage the disease, and how to prevent complications.

Interventions

Provide Education. Health teaching should be ongoing and repeated at frequent intervals. An HIV-infected person can adopt several behaviors that not only improve immune function but also increase a sense of well-being. The content outline for teaching health maintenance includes stress management, exercise, safer sex practices, pregnancy and HIV infection, nutrition (emphasizing a high-protein, high-calorie, low-fat diet), food and water safety, skin care, routine mouth care, proper hand-washing, environmental cleaning and safety, pet care, limiting alcohol consumption, use of injected drugs, travel safety and avoiding exposure to infectious pathogens, importance of health care follow-up, and understanding and interpreting viral load tests and CD4$^+$ cell counts.

The Joint Commission (TJC) National Patient Safety Goals related to reducing the risk of infections and hand hygiene guidelines are an important part of promoting health maintenance and preventing infection in clients who are infected with HIV.

Carefully explain viral load test results because many people misunderstand the results. When successful therapy begins, the viral load drops from high levels, such as 750,000 copies/ml, down to what are called "undetectable" levels; however, most laboratory tests can detect HIV copies down to only 50 copies/ml. Because anything lower cannot be measured, the laboratory report reads "undetectable levels." Although this is great news and indicates the success of the prescribed regimen, it does not mean that the person no longer has HIV infection. Some clients with HIV infection leave their primary care provider thinking that they are disease free and no longer at risk of spreading HIV. This must be clarified whenever you report laboratory results to a client; emphasize that the client must still practice safer sex, avoid sharing needles, and so on.

Encourage clients to tell their health care providers about any self-prescribed therapies they are taking because these therapies might have a positive or negative influence on the outcomes of care. Keep track of over-the-counter medications because they may interact with prescribed therapies. Some clients may also obtain drugs through buyers' clubs or underground pharmacies. This not only may be detrimental to the effectiveness of prescribed treatments but also may have an adverse effect on observations made during a drug trial.

Some clients may opt to try alternative or complementary treatments, including (1) spiritual or psychological interventions (e.g., guided imagery, meditation, faith healing), (2) nutritional alternatives (e.g., a macrobiotic diet), (3) drug and biologic therapies (e.g., homeopathy, oxygen, ozone therapy), and (4) physical forces (e.g., acupuncture, acupressure, massage therapy). In most cases, these choices can have a positive effect on the person's emotional well-being but may also have a negative effect. For example, a macrobiotic diet can lead to vitamin and mineral deficiencies as well as weight loss. Herbal remedies may cause nausea, vomiting, diarrhea, or CNS depression or interact with antiretrovirals. Despite these effects, some clients will continue to use these methods.

Initiate and Maintain Antiretroviral Therapy. One of the most important aspects of providing nursing care to the HIV-infected client is helping with the antiretroviral regimen. Studies suggest that clients with chronic diseases such as hypertension and diabetes mellitus take their prescribed drugs about 50% of the time. However,

to sustain the durability and efficacy of antiretroviral therapy, clients must maintain about a 95% compliance rate. This places high expectations on both the HIV-infected client and the physicians and nurses. Because therapy may last for many years, it is vital that the client understand the potential benefits and drawbacks of any regimen and the potential consequences of not adhering to therapy. Potential benefits of antiretroviral therapy include the following:

- Control of HIV replication and mutation, with reduction in viral load
- Prevention of destruction of the immune system and loss of CD4$^+$ T helper cells
- Delayed progression to AIDS-defining illnesses
- Decreased risk for development of HIV resistance to drugs
- Decreased risk of drug toxicity (drugs are started when the client is healthier)
- Increased survival with HIV disease (the most important benefit)

Potential risks of antiretroviral therapy include the following:

- Reduced quality of life from adverse drug effects and the inconvenience of a complex regimen
- Earlier development of drug resistance
- A limited number of drugs available to respond to drug resistance
- Unknown long-term toxicity of antiretroviral therapy
- Unknown duration of the effectiveness of current antiretroviral therapies

The decision of whether to take antiretrovirals is ultimately up to the client. The regimens ordered may be complex and require the client to take large numbers of pills daily (as many as 15 to 20), often at exactly spaced intervals and with differing requirements as to timing the pills related to food. Liquid preparations often taste horrible, and the client must try various strategies to mask the taste. All the drugs have side effects to which the person must learn to adjust and control, and they also interact with numerous other drugs. These drug-drug interactions are usually not life-threatening, but they may interfere with antiretroviral blood levels, causing subtherapeutic effects, drug resistance, and drug failure. Instruct all clients taking antiretrovirals as follows:

- Take the drug at specified intervals.
- Do not skip a dose.
- Do not increase or decrease the number of pills you take.
- Follow meal and fluid requirements.
- If side effects occur, tell your physician or nurse. If side effects are significant, ask your primary care provider for information or medication to help manage them.

■ Store all drugs as instructed.

■ If you do not want to take the drugs, tell your primary care provider.

■ If you take the drugs only periodically, it would be better not to take them at all. Discuss this with your physician or nurse.

■ Remember, the treatment plan is yours. If you do not agree with it, discuss it with your physician or nurse.

Because of concern over the development of drug resistance and drug failure, several studies have been conducted on methods to help people infected with HIV adhere to their drug regimens. Several strategies have proved very helpful, especially when used together (see the Translating Evidence into Practice feature on Adherence to ART on p. 2101). Primary care providers also need to incorporate cultural and religious beliefs when addressing drug adherence behaviors. Meal planning because of fat content requirements or dietary restrictions or preferences as well as the need to abstain from food and water on certain days because of religious practices may be necessary.

Prevent Infection. Nursing strategies to prevent infection include health teaching and helping the client take drugs properly to prevent opportunistic infections. Health teaching focuses on safer sex practices not only to prevent HIV transmission but also to keep clients from acquiring STIs. Practicing food and water safety can prevent such diseases as salmonellosis, cryptosporidiosis, and toxoplasmosis. Simple hand-washing is an effective technique for minimizing food-borne illnesses. Maintaining skin and mucous membrane integrity with good skin and mouth hygiene can reduce the incidence of candidiasis.

Evaluation. Evaluation includes the client's understanding of the teaching provided and the choices available. If a client chooses not to adopt a recommended behavior, it does not mean that the client is noncompliant. Health care providers can have a difficult time evaluating the outcomes of teaching and weighing them against the client's free choice. Remember that the ultimate decision about following a health care provider's advice belongs to the client. The client's decisions do not reflect failure on the part of the health care professional.

Evaluation of a client's ability to adhere to a prescribed drug regimen includes both subjective and objective techniques. Subjective evaluation is by self-report; clients and their care partner describe the client's ability to take all prescribed medications. Objective analysis of the success of the plan of care is by laboratory evaluation of CD4$^+$ cell counts and viral load.

A totally different situation exists when minimal learning takes place because of cognitive impairment. It is well documented that problems with thinking or memory may exist and go unidentified if they are not obvious. This is more likely to occur in clients with less than a 12th grade education and in clients older than 50 years of age. In such a situation, a care partner should be designated who receives all information when it is provided to the client. Whenever the care partner cannot make a clinic or office visit, provide telephone teaching and document that you accomplished this.

OUTCOME MANAGEMENT FOR AIDS

As both the quantity and the quality of CD4$^+$ cells diminish, "AIDS-indicator" diseases occur. The categories of AIDS-defining illnesses include opportunistic infections, cancers, and other conditions specific to HIV disease. The four main types of opportunistic infections are (1) bacterial, (2) fungal, (3) protozoal, and (4) viral (Table 78-1). Neoplasms associated with AIDS include Kaposi's sarcoma (KS), non-Hodgkin's lymphoma, and invasive cervical cancer. Two other conditions unique to AIDS are (1) HIV wasting syndrome and (2) HIV encephalopathy. Hepatitis C is now considered an AIDS-indicator disease. Since the introduction of ART in 1996, the onset of AIDS-defining illness has been delayed and treating these diseases has become easier.

Medical Management of the Client with AIDS

Prevent and Treat Opportunistic Infections

Most of the pathogens responsible for opportunistic infections are ubiquitous; that is, they are all around us. Most people do not become sick from the organisms that cause opportunistic infections because their immune systems are intact. Once the regulators of the immune system (CD4$^+$ cells) are destroyed by HIV, however, infection can occur. Most opportunistic infections result from secondary reactivation of previously acquired pathogens rather than from a new or primary infection. For example, most people are infected with *P. (carinii) jiroveci* in the early preschool years, when it causes respiratory manifestations and is probably dismissed as a common cold. The child's intact immune system brings the infection under control; however, the organism remains dormant in the person's body. The potential then exists for the organism to reactivate, causing disease again in an immunocompromised person. This concept applies to any person with an immunodeficiency, regardless of the cause. Single opportunistic infections are rare, and clients may have multiple infections. Many of these opportunistic infections are not curable. Because the immune system no longer has the strength to contain the infection, it becomes chronic and requires lifetime suppressive therapy. Helping the client comply with the antibiotic regimen to keep opportunistic infections under control is an essential part of the care planning process. Because the client must take antibiotics for extended periods, drug resistance may develop,

TABLE 78–1 Opportunistic Infections Seen in Clients with AIDS

Infection and Source	Manifestations	Treatment and Comments
Bacterial Infections		
Mycobacterium tuberculosis (airborne, droplets)	"Constitutional": fever, chills, weight loss, night sweats, lymphadenopathy, fatigue "Pulmonary": cough, dyspnea, chest pain, hemoptysis	Combination therapy including isoniazid, rifampin, pyrazinamide, ethambutol, or streptomycin. All clients with HIV-positive status should be tested for TB annually; multi-drug resistance is growing problem.
Mycobacterium avium (soil, water, eggs, unpasteurized diary products)	Fever, night sweats, fatigue, anorexia, weight loss, abdominal pain, diarrhea	Difficult to treat; may defer based on severity. Prophylaxis may be considered. Drugs include azithromycin, clarithromycin, ethambutol, ciprofloxacin, rifabutin, amikacin, ampicillin, chloramphenicol, TMP-SMX, ciprofloxacin, norfloxacin.
Salmonellosis (contaminated food and water, handling contaminated feces, sexual activity involving oral-anal contact; food handlers and pets may be source of exposure)	Fever, night sweats, fatigue, anorexia, weight loss, abdominal pain, diarrhea	Prevent and treat perianal skin breakdown. Antibiotic therapy based on culture and sensitivity.
Pneumonia, especially from *Streptococcus pneumoniae* and *Haemophilus influenzae* (airborne)	Cough, productive cough, fever, chills, chest pain, shortness of breath, fatigue	Especially common in IV drug injecting clients. Pneumococcal vaccination recommended every 5 years.
Fungal Infections		
Candida albicans (found in food, soil, on fomites, and normally found on skin and in mouth, vagina, and large intestine)	Related to site of infection: may include dysphagia with esophagitis, oral lesions with thrush, cutaneous lesions with intertrigo, vulvovaginal irritation and discharge, vaginitis; constitutional symptoms occur with disseminated disease	Various antifungals related to the site of infection. Oral: clotrimazole troches, nystatin suspension, fluconazole. Esophagitis: fluconazole, itraconazole, ketoconazole, amphotericin B. Intertrigo and vaginitis: clotrimazole, miconazole, ketoconazole, fluconazole, itraconazole. Disseminated disease: amphotericin B. Most infections are endogenous; that is, the person's own organism is the source of infection. Eating yogurt made with live cultures helps control recurrence.
Cryptococcus neoformans (found in pigeon droppings, nesting places, soil, fruit, and unpasteurized fruit juice; organism is aerosolized and inhaled)	Low-grade fever, fatigue, headache, nausea, vomiting, altered mental status, cough, dyspnea, pleuritic chest pain, cutaneous and oral lesions possible	Amphotericin B, with or without flucytosine, fluconazole, or itraconazole. Maintenance lifetime suppressive therapy may be required.
Histoplasma capsulatum: histoplasmosis (endemic to certain regions of United States, especially middle, central, southern states, and to Puerto Rico)	Fever; weight loss; enlarged lymph nodes, liver, and spleen; abdominal pain; oral and skin lesions; anemia; leukopenia; and thrombocytopenia	Amphotericin B, itraconazole, fluconazole. Maintenance lifetime suppressive therapy may be required.
Coccidioides immitis: coccidioidomycosis (fungus endemic to Southwestern United States; also called valley fever)	Fever, dyspnea, fatigue, weight loss, cough	Amphotericin B, ketoconazole, itraconazole, fluconazile. Lifetime suppressive therapy may be required.
Protozoal Infections		
Pneumocystis (carinii) jiroveci (airborne)	Presentation may be elusive; with pneumonia, cough may be first symptom Productive cough, fever, dyspnea Extrapulmonary infection can occur	TMP-SMX, pentamidine, atovaquone, TMP-dapsone, clindamycin-primaquine, trimetrexate. Lifetime suppressive therapy may be required.
Toxoplasma gondii: toxoplasmosis (contaminated meat, vegetables, eggs, unpasteurized dairy products, in utero transmission, contaminated cat feces)	Headache, impaired cognition, hemiparesis, aphasia, ataxia, vision loss, cranial nerve palsies, motor problems, seizures; infection can occur in other body systems	Pyrimethamine plus sulfadiazine, leukovorin, clindamycin plus pyrimethamine, clarithromycin, azithromycin. Lifetime suppressive therapy may be required. Fewer than 1% of domestic cats are infected and veterinarians can perform a simple blood test to determine if cat is infected.

TABLE 78–1	Opportunistic Infections Seen in Clients with AIDS—Cont'd	
Infection and Source	**Manifestations**	**Treatment and Comments**
Cryptosporidium (mammals, birds, reptiles, fish; water and food-borne; contaminated swimming pools, anal-oral sexual contact)	Malabsorption, dehydration, malnutrition, profuse diarrhea (up to 25 L/day), steatorrhea, flatulence, abdominal cramping and pain, anorexia, nausea, vomiting, fever, fatigue, profound weight loss, myalgia, electrolyte imbalance	Chronic disease, may be fatal. No effective treatment exists; however, drugs that may be tried include paromomycin, azithromycin, clarithromycin, nitazoxanide, thalidomide, and symptomatic therapy to decrease peristalsis and control pain. Monitor for and treat perianal skin breakdown.
Isospora belli: isosporiasis (infected animals, human-to-human, contaminated water)	Diarrhea, anorexia, nausea, vomiting, weight loss, abdominal pain, fever	TMP-SMX, pyrimethamine plus folinic acid.
Viral Infections		
Cytomegalovirus (CMV) (blood and body fluids, including saliva; feces)	May be asymptomatic May cause chorioretinitis, pneumonitis, encephalitis, adrenalitis, colitis, esophagitis, hepatitis, or cholangitis	Ganciclovir, foscarnet, cidofovir plus probenecid. Lifetime suppression may be required. Most healthy people eventually become infected with CMV.
Herpes simplex (direct contact with infectious lesions/secretions)	Painful vesicular lesions on the oral, genital, or perianal regions May also cause encephalitis, esophagitis, bronchitis, keratitis, pericarditis, and hand infections	Acyclovir, foscarnet, famciclovir; topical acyclovir for skin lesions. Chronic disease requires lifetime suppressive therapy.
Progressive multifocal leukoencephalopathy; JC virus (common in nature; most healthy people infected)	Limb weakness, ataxia, cognitive impairment, vision loss, speech impairment, headache May progress to dementia, blindness, paralysis, and death	No effective therapy, but may try acyclovir, foscarnet, adenine arabinoside, cytosine arabinoside, interferon alfa.
Hepatitis		The leading cause of death in AIDS clients remains liver failure, with hepatitis being the most common etiology. See Chapter 47 for a discussion of hepatitis.

and both physicians and nurses must constantly observe the client for recurrence of the infection.

Bacterial Infections. There are several important opportunistic infections caused by bacteria, including *Mycobacterium tuberculosis* (causing TB), *Mycobacterium-avium* complex, and *Salmonella*. Bacterial pneumonia is common and is usually caused by *Streptococcus pneumoniae* and *Haemophilus influenzae*. The risk of bacterial infection rises with low CD4$^+$ counts and often clients will take prophylactic antibiotics to prevent these diseases (see Table 78-1).

Fungal Infections. Fungal infections are a common source of illness in the client with AIDS. *Candida albicans* is a frequent culprit. *Cryptococcus neoformans, Histoplasma capsulatum,* and *Coccidioides immitis* are other fungi found in nature that cause disease when the immune system is severely compromised (see Table 78-1).

Protozoal Infections. *Pneumocystosis (carinii) jiroveci* causes a pneumonia that was once a leading cause of death in the AIDS client. Successful treatment and prophylaxis has greatly reduced the death rate from this

protozoal infection. *Toxoplasma gondii, Cryptosporidium,* and *Isospora belli* are also ubiquitous in nature and cause problems in an immunocompromised state (see Table 78-1).

Viral Infections. Viral infections in the AIDS client are difficult to treat. Cytomegalovirus disease (CMV), herpes, progressive multifocal leukoencephalopathy, caused by the JC virus (initials of the first client in whom it was first discovered), and hepatitis are the most common viral illnesses seen in the AIDS client (see Table 78-1).

Treat Neoplasms
Kaposi's Sarcoma. Four types of KS may be encountered in clinical practice: (1) classic KS, which tends to occur in older men who are black, of Mediterranean descent, or from certain Jewish populations; (2) African KS, seen in Africa; (3) transplant KS, seen in people who receive organ transplants; and (4) HIV-related KS, which differs from the others in that it runs a fulminant course, is disseminated throughout the body, and results in shorter survival.

The only form associated with HIV disease is HIV-related KS. It has been diagnosed predominantly in men who have sex with men and is thought to be associated with a sexually transmitted pathogen that then predisposes the person to development. Researchers think it is caused by either human herpesvirus type 8 (HHV-8) or KS-associated herpesvirus (KSHV). KS differs from most AIDS-defining diseases in that it is unrelated to low CD4$^+$ cell counts and can occur early in HIV infection.

Clinical presentation typically starts with an initial "patch" that is flat and pink, looks like a bruise, and is symmetrical on both sides of the body. Later, it turns into dark violet or black plaques. Clinical presentation of the lesions can include the mouth, skin, mucous membranes, head, neck, torso, limbs (soles of feet), genitals, lung, brain, intestines, testes, liver, spleen, pancreas, adrenal gland, and lymph nodes. They can be painful.

Treatment depends on the extent of tumors (tumor burden), CD4$^+$ cell count, associated manifestations and diseases, and the client's functional ability. Local therapy includes radiation, localized chemotherapy, and cryotherapy. Systemic therapy includes doxorubicin, alpha interferon, bleomycin, paclitaxel, and daunorubicin. Experimental therapies under investigation include possible treatment of the underlying viral cause of KS with foscarnet or ganciclovir. Initially several therapies may be tried, which may be effective in suppressing the course of KS; eventually, however, the clinical decline in the client's condition makes continued treatment impossible.

Non-Hodgkin's Lymphoma. Non-Hodgkin's lymphoma tends to occur late in the course of HIV disease and is related to low CD4$^+$ cell counts. The primary sites of occurrence are the brain, gastrointestinal tract, bone marrow, and liver. The initial clinical presentation may be nonspecific and include fever, night sweats, and weight loss, all of which are associated with *M. avium* complex infection, TB, and CMV infection.

Treatment includes methotrexate, bleomycin, doxorubicin, cyclophosphamide, and vincristine. Despite aggressive treatment, the prognosis is poor except in clients on combination antiretroviral therapy, who tend to survive longer.

Invasive Cervical Cancer. Cervical intraepithelial neoplasia (CIN), the precursor to cervical cancer, occurs at a high rate in women infected with HIV and is related to low CD4$^+$ cell counts. In early stages of disease, the client is asymptomatic; however, it progresses rapidly. Cervical dysplasia is usually detected by Pap smear. Early clinical manifestations include postcoital bleeding, metrorrhagia, and a blood-tinged vaginal discharge. Manifestations of more extensive disease include back, pelvic, and leg pain; weight loss; vaginal bleeding; anemia; lymphadenopathy; and edema of the legs.

Treatment of CIN can include conization, laser therapy, cryosurgery, electrocautery, or hysterectomy. For invasive cancer, treatment may involve surgery, radiation, and chemotherapy with cisplatin, vincristine, bleomycin, or mitomycin. Follow-up care focuses on recurrent disease and control of manifestations and metastasis.

Treat Conditions Specific to AIDS

AIDS Dementia. HIV encephalopathy, also referred to as *AIDS dementia complex,* appears to affect the very young and older HIV-infected clients and clients with anemia and weight loss. In addition, HIV-infected people with less than a 12th grade education may be more likely to show clinical manifestations. Manifestations include cognitive dysfunction, motor problems, and behavioral changes. Cognitive manifestations include an inability to concentrate, decreased memory, impaired judgment, and slowed thinking. Motor impairment may be manifested as leg weakness, ataxia, and clumsiness. Behavioral changes can range from apathy, reduced spontaneity, and social withdrawal to irritability, hyperactivity, anxiety, mania, and delirium.

The staging system for AIDS dementia complex is as follows:

- Stage 1: Minimal manifestations, mild neurologic manifestations, no impairment of work or ability to perform activities of daily living (ADL)
- Stage 2: Obvious intellectual or motor impairment, still able to do all but the most demanding ADL
- Stage 3: Cannot work or perform demanding ADL, still capable of basic self-care, ambulatory but may need a single assistive device
- Stage 4: Major intellectual disability, cannot walk without assistance
- Stage 5: Nearly vegetative, paraplegic or quadriplegic, only rudimentary cognition remains

Some studies have shown a favorable response to combination antiretroviral therapy. Psychotropic drugs may be tried in small doses, but benzodiazepines, drugs with strong anticholinergic properties, and amitriptyline should be used with caution. Follow-up monitoring focuses on detecting the progression of AIDS dementia complex and on evaluating the client's ability to safely maintain independent living and comply with prescribed therapies.

HIV Wasting Syndrome. Weight loss occurs at some point in more than 90% of people with HIV infection. *HIV wasting* is defined as profound involuntary weight loss (>10% of total body baseline weight) with either chronic diarrhea or chronic weakness and fever. The primary causes of HIV wasting syndrome are reduced food intake, malabsorption of nutrients, and altered metabolism of nutrients. The evaluation of a client with HIV wasting syndrome includes determining and treating the cause. Reversing wasting syndrome is very difficult.

The goal of drug therapy in wasting syndrome is to stimulate appetite, produce weight gain, and increase lean muscle mass. Often weight gain is from water and body fat, which is not beneficial. Identified conditions that contribute to wasting should be treated first. Drugs used to treat HIV wasting syndrome include megestrol acetate, anabolic steroids, and dronabinol (the major psychoactive component of marijuana). The drug used most successfully to treat wasting syndrome is human growth hormone. Follow-up therapy includes constant assessment for factors that may interfere with the plan of care.

Nursing Management of the Client with AIDS

The goal of nursing care is to diagnose and treat human responses to actual or potential health problems related to the development of clinical manifestations and the diagnosis of AIDS. All efforts are directed at controlling manifestations. Actual or potential problems seen in people with AIDS include fever, fatigue, weight loss, nausea, diarrhea, dry and painful mouth, dry skin, skin lesions, pain, dyspnea, cough, impaired cognition, impaired vision, insomnia, and sexual dysfunction. Common nursing diagnoses associated with the diagnosis of AIDS are presented in the website box Common Nursing Diagnoses for Clients with HIV and AIDS. Four problems that affect most AIDS clients are described here, in the Case Study feature below, and in the Bridge to Home Health Care website feature on Living with HIV/AIDS.

Assessment. Assessment of clinical manifestations should include both subjective and objective data. All clinical manifestations should be quantified. The easiest way to measure the severity of a clinical manifestation is by asking the client to rate it on a scale from 0 to 10, with 0 being no problem at all and 10 being the worst

CASE STUDY · evolve

Human Immunodeficiency Virus

Edith Jones is a white woman, age 50 years, who presents to an outpatient clinic with complaints of fever, fatigue, "swollen glands," and a sore throat. She is an elementary school teacher and states that she believes she has been exposed to some virus in her classroom. She is concerned because the manifestations have not resolved as quickly as they usually do when she catches a "classroom bug" .... *Case Study continued on the website and the CD-ROM with discussions, multiple-choice questions, and a nursing care plan.*

possible. This method works well for most manifestations, such as fatigue and pain. Fever assessment can be made easy if the client is willing to keep a fever diary (i.e., recording the temperature whenever it is measured). For clients who have no scale at home, the nurse will have to rely on client self-report to detect trends in weight.

Pain is a subjective experience. The single most reliable indicator of the existence and intensity of acute pain and any related discomfort or distress is the client's self-report. Neither behavior nor vital signs can substitute for self-report. A client may be in excruciating pain even while smiling or laughing in an attempt to cope with it.

Diagnosis, Outcomes, Interventions
Diagnosis: Hyperthermia. An important nursing diagnosis and collaborative problem for a client with AIDS is *Hyperthermia related to hypermetabolic state (secondary to chronic HIV infection), opportunistic infections, dehydration, side effects of medication, malnutrition, and sites for potential organism invasion, such as IV lines or Foley catheters.*

Outcomes. After discussing the assessment findings and the nursing diagnosis, select interventions in concert with the client, care partner, or both to control fever and replace fluid loss.

> **Involving the client in planning care and reducing the risk of infections are two of TJC's National Patient Safety Goals.**

SAFETY

ALERT

Interventions. Because of the underlying immunodeficiency and impaired inflammatory response, clinical manifestations of infection, including fever, may be greatly muted. Nonpharmacologic interventions include keeping the client in a warm room to avoid shivering and applying a sheet and a loosely woven blanket. Avoid fanning the bed covers, exposing skin, or rapidly removing clothing that might cause chilling.

Avoid tepid water sponge bathing, which causes defensive vasoconstriction and has not been shown to be an effective coolant in fever. Sponge baths can cause shivering and can be distressing. Avoid alcohol sponging as well, which also causes vasoconstriction, shivering, and toxic fumes. The alcohol also can be absorbed cutaneously, causing hypoglycemia.

Increase caloric and fluid intake by providing a plan for six feedings distributed over 24 hours and high-protein, high-calorie nutritional supplements, especially if the client has anorexia. Provide 2 to 2.5 L of fluid to drink daily.

Maintain comfort and safety by providing dry clothes and bed linens made out of cotton rather than synthetics. Use emollient creams for dry skin. Monitor mental status frequently, especially when the client has a fever. Evaluate the client's need for assistance with all ADL. Teach the client how to manage chronic recurrent night fever and night sweats by doing the following:

- Take the antipyretic agent of choice before going to sleep.
- Have a change of bedclothes nearby in case a change is necessary.
- Keep a plastic cover on the pillow.
- Place a towel over the pillow in case of profuse diaphoresis.
- Keep liquids at the bedside to drink.

Pharmacologic treatment can include aspirin, nonsteroidal anti-inflammatory drugs (NSAIDs), or acetaminophen. Follow-up should include comparing patterns of use of these agents with laboratory evaluation of hepatic and hematologic abnormalities as well as interactions with other agents.

Diagnosis: Fatigue. Another common nursing diagnosis is *Fatigue related to hypermetabolic state secondary to viral infection, muscular weakness/wasting secondary to AIDS, anemia, dehydration, and psychological and situational factors.* Fatigue is the most common complaint both of clients with AIDS and of their caregivers.

Outcomes. After discussing and validating the findings of assessment and nursing diagnosis, select interventions in concert with the client, care partner, or both to increase self-awareness of fatigue, associated clinical manifestations, environmental factors affecting fatigue, and activity tolerance. Identify interventions to highlight the importance of resting when needed and accepting assistance when needed. Develop a plan for a lifestyle that keeps the client independent, socially active, and involved in activities of daily living.

Interventions. Promote self-care and self-awareness by having the client keep a daily fatigue diary for at least 1 week to identify sources of fatigue, appropriate interventions, and patterns of peak fitness. Advise the client to avoid coffee, tobacco, and alcohol, which may increase fatigue. Promote adequate sleep by increasing the amount of sleep each day. Reduce the amount of sleep-cycle interruptions by preparing for sleep and keeping needed items at the bedside.

Promote rest and activity by developing a written 24-hour schedule of daily activities that alternates short activities with rest periods. Identify activity priorities, such as eating breakfast and then resting before bathing in the morning, as opposed to the reverse. Evaluate the client's needs and point out ways to conserve energy, such as sitting down while dressing, shaving, or preparing food; sitting on a shower chair while bathing; or using disposable items for eating so that no cleanup is needed. Help the client write a plan for rest and activities. Encourage the client to always plan activities ahead of time.

Prepare an exercise schedule (immobilization may lead to decreased endurance and increased fatigue) and plan exercises at peak energy times (after a rest period). Follow the exercises with rest. Aerobic exercise, which increases endurance, can reduce fatigue. Additional natural techniques that may be of benefit include progressive muscle relaxation, acupressure, massage, reflexology, imagery and visualization, autogenic relaxation, reframing and positive affirmations, therapeutic touch, and social support and support groups.

Diagnosis: Imbalanced Nutrition: Less Than Body Requirements. A frequently encountered nursing diagnosis is *Imbalanced Nutrition: Less Than Body Requirements related to increased nutrient requirements and decreased food intake secondary to side effects of medications and infection, such as anorexia, nausea, vomiting, altered taste, impaired swallowing or chewing, diarrhea, fatigue, depression, or impaired cognition.*

Outcomes. After discussing and validating the findings of assessment and the nursing diagnosis, select interventions in concert with the client, care partner, or both to increase food intake, preserve lean body mass, and provide adequate levels of all nutrients.

Interventions

Minimize Anorexia. Minimize factors contributing to anorexia. For *hyperosmia* (increased sense of smell), avoid cooking odors by keeping windows open and the home well aerated. Encourage meals that include cold foods. For *hyposmia* (decreased sense of smell), use spices such as basil, oregano, rosemary, thyme, cloves, mint, cinnamon, or lemon juice to enhance the aroma. For alterations in sense of taste (especially related to distaste for red meat), marinate meat in a commercial marinade, wine, or vinegar before cooking it, and use substitutes for red meat, such as eggs, peanut butter, tofu, cheeses, poultry, and fish.

Prevent Weight Loss. Weight loss can be a significant problem for clients who live alone or who have fatigue or depression. Interventions include the following:

- Eating small meals frequently throughout the day
- Eating high-calorie snacks or commercially prepared supplements (liquids or bars)
- Indulging in favorite foods
- Consuming more nutrient-dense foods and beverages rather than filling up on low-calorie items
- Drinking liquids 30 minutes before eating instead of with meals
- Preparing meals (such as soups or casseroles) ahead of time so they can be divided into individual servings and frozen until ready to use
- Keeping easy-to-prepare foods on hand, such as frozen dinners, canned foods, and eggs

- Encouraging the client to dine with friends or family
- Getting family members and friends involved in meal preparation; the pleasant atmosphere they can provide may stimulate the client's appetite

Many communities have home food delivery service for people with AIDS as well.

Improve Food Intake. Minimize factors related to difficulty in chewing, dysphagia (difficulty in swallowing), or odynophagia (painful swallowing) by advising clients to avoid rough foods, such as (1) raw fruits and vegetables; spicy, acidic, or salty foods; (2) alcohol or tobacco; (3) excessively hot or cold foods; (4) sticky foods, such as peanut butter; and (5) slippery foods, such as gelatin, bologna, and elbow macaroni. Encourage the client to do the following:

- Eat foods at room temperature.
- Choose mild foods and drinks, such as apple juice rather than orange juice.
- Eat dry grain foods (such as breads, crackers, and cookies) after softening them in milk, tea, or another mild beverage.
- Eat nonabrasive foods that are easy to swallow, such as ice cream, pudding, well-cooked eggs, noodle dishes, baked fish, and soft cheese.
- Eat Popsicles (frozen dessert) to numb pain.
- Use a straw when drinking.
- Tilt the head forward or back to make swallowing easier.

Increase the Availability of Food. Minimize factors related to the client's inability to obtain food by evaluating the client's financial resources and the need for referral for Medicaid, food stamps, or other services. Evaluate the client's home and ability to prepare and obtain food. Look for problems such as an absence of cooking facilities and the need for alternative housing arrangements. Explore community resources that provide free meals.

Teach Nutritional Requirements. If the client has no metabolic condition that requires a special diet, the prescribed diet for people with HIV disease should include high-protein, high-calorie, low-fat foods. Help the client plan a 24-hour menu, and review the essential elements of a low-microbe diet and food safety and preparation. Nutritional teaching should follow the client's usual pattern of food intake as much as possible, rather than expecting the client to follow a totally new, unfamiliar prescription for meal planning.

Diagnosis: Acute Pain or Chronic Pain. A common nursing diagnosis is *Acute Pain or Chronic Pain related to arthralgia, myalgia, or neuropathy associated with HIV disease, mass lesions associated with opportunistic infection(s) or cancer, side effects of medications, co-morbid disease such as diabetic neuropathy, or interventions such as surgery.*

Outcomes. After discussing and validating the findings of assessment, select interventions in concert with the client, care partner, or both to reduce the incidence and severity of pain, communicate effectively about pain experiences, and enhance comfort and satisfaction.

Interventions

Provide Comfort Measures. Help the client and/or care partner identify activities that increase pain. Provide comfort measures such as using a pressure-relieving mattress, positioning and supporting limbs comfortably when in bed or a chair, and using a "pull sheet" to move clients or help them change positions. For institutionalized clients, encourage family members or significant others to bring in familiar objects that will provide physical and/or emotional comfort. Encourage the client to groom as usual, including using make-up or after-shave lotion, to help maintain a sense of normalcy and dignity during illness.

Provide Physical Therapy. Physical therapy can be very helpful in managing pain. The physical therapist can provide the following:

- Exercise to maintain or increase physical activity levels and endurance
- Ultrasound and physical treatments, such as application of heat or cold, to reduce musculoskeletal pain
- Therapeutic massage
- Instruction and supervision in using a transcutaneous electrical nerve stimulation (TENS) device, commonly called a TENS unit

Administer Pain Medications. Pharmacologic treatments usually include (1) *non-opioid analgesics,* such as aspirin or acetaminophen for mild pain; (2) *weak opioids,* such as codeine and oxycodone for moderate pain; and (3) *strong opioids,* such as morphine for severe pain. For neuropathic pain (such as HIV-associated polyneuropathy, acute and postherpetic neuralgia, and nucleoside toxicity with some antiretroviral medications), adjuvants such as ibuprofen may be used as well as amitriptyline, desipramine, nortriptyline, doxepin, carbamazepine, divalproex, phenytoin, gabapentin, or mexiletine. Primary care providers should anticipate several changes in prescriptions for analgesics when starting the client on a pain-control regimen. A major error in initial pain management occurs when a clinician prescribes a 2-week supply of an analgesic, assumes that the prescription works, and has no further contact until the client returns 2 weeks later for follow-up. On the contrary, during the initial phase of pain control, the clinician should have daily contact with the client, even if by telephone, and should anticipate schedule changes. Dosage frequency should be adjusted to prevent pain from recurring once the duration of analgesic action is determined. Similarly, it is a waste of money to prescribe large amounts of an analgesic, such as a 30-day supply, knowing that the orders will change. Orders for opioid analgesics should include "rescue" doses for breakthrough pain when regularly scheduled doses are insufficient.

Orders for analgesics as needed result in delays in administration and intervals of inadequate pain control. Tell clients and their care partners that the client may sleep for extended periods and may appear very drowsy during the first few days of a pain control regimen. Although this may result in part from the initial effects of the drug, it probably also reflects exhaustion and the need for rest as a result of sleep deprivation caused by pain. This situation usually reverses itself within a few days after a scheduled pain management regimen is begun.

Clients may refuse an analgesic if they are not in pain or may forgo it when they are asleep. Explain that this decision may lower blood analgesia levels and cause a resurgence of pain and failure of the pain control plan. Although the anti-inflammatory effects of aspirin are highly effective as an analgesic adjuvant, because aspirin inhibits platelet function, it may be contraindicated if the client has a low platelet count.

Injecting drug users will experience pain as any other client would. Do not deny this client pain medication. Helpful guidelines for managing pain in these clients include (1) having a single practitioner prescribe medications, (2) refusing to refill lost prescriptions, (3) carefully rationing opioid prescriptions, and (4) limiting rescue doses of opioid analgesics on a monthly basis. Clients who are being treated with methadone maintenance for drug addiction probably will require higher and more frequent doses of analgesia than an opioid-naive client would. Some antiretroviral drugs, such as nevirapine and ritonavir, interfere with the half-life of methadone and may decrease its blood levels. The client will experience mild withdrawal manifestations. Increasing the daily dose of methadone usually resolves the problem.

Because diarrhea is common in clients with HIV disease, especially when protease inhibitors are prescribed, the constipating effects of analgesics may actually be beneficial. Evaluate each client's response to therapy instead of automatically using stool softeners when initiating the pain control plan.

Encourage Complementary Therapies. Complementary therapies that may be used include cognitive-behavioral interventions, such as education and instruction in pain control, relaxation exercises, imagery, music distraction, biofeedback, and therapeutic touch.

Evaluation. It is expected that the client will maintain or increase weight. It is expected that the client, care partner, or both will (1) identify factors related to anorexia, difficulty in chewing, dysphagia, or odynophagia; (2) identify sufficient resources to obtain and prepare food or make use of social work interventions employed to obtain food stamps or public assistance; (3) identify ways to increase protein and calorie intake; (4) identify key concepts in planning a low-microbial diet; and (5) select a balanced 24-hour menu. The client's weight will fluctuate during the course of HIV disease related to new disease processes and the side effects of prescribed medications.

It is expected that the client, care partner, or both will be able to (1) identify appropriate measures to take for a fever, (2) initiate and maintain adequate hydration and nutrition, and (3) demonstrate the ability to take and record the client's temperature accurately. Although infection-related fever can be controlled with appropriate antibiotic therapy, this problem can be expected to recur throughout the illness.

It is expected that the client, care partner, or both will be able to (1) identify causative factors that increase fatigue, (2) plan a schedule of paced activity for a 24-hour period, (3) demonstrate the ability to participate in a program of exercise, and (4) verbalize a decrease in the client's fatigue for a 24-hour period. Fatigue is a manifestation that can be expected to recur throughout HIV disease, especially because it is a side effect of some antiretroviral medications.

It is expected that the client, care partner, or both will (1) identify aggravating factors or precipitating factors related to the pain experienced, (2) identify measures to control pain, and (3) verbalize a decrease in the amount and type of pain experienced over 24 hours. Pain may be either chronic or acute, depending on the cause. In most instances, it can be managed effectively, as with any client with another diagnosis.

CONCLUSIONS

Human immunodeficiency virus is a major threat to human health worldwide. The nature of care is very complex, and the client's clinical needs are numerous. At one time or another, almost all nurses will care for a person with HIV infection or AIDS. To provide adequate care for a person with HIV infection, understanding the illness trajectory and the therapeutic interventions needed to maintain health will result in the ability to provide high-level care.

THINKING CRITICALLY

1. A 30-year-old woman presents with fever, fatigue, lymphadenopathy, thrush, diarrhea, and pain in her muscles and joints. She has

a rash on her torso and arms. What questions would you ask to determine her possible exposure to HIV? How will the client be evaluated and treated?

Factors to Consider. What tests confirm the diagnosis of AIDS? How is the CD4$^+$ cell count used? What is the purpose of the viral load test? What treatment should be used?

2. You are working in a homeless shelter and are scheduled to present a 20-minute program on AIDS prevention. A small class of four men and three women has gathered. They are all known to you, and you suspect that one couple may be infected with HIV. What should you plan to teach?

Factors to Consider. What main areas of HIV education should be addressed? What is an effective method of communicating this information?

3. Your HIV-infected female client leaves the physician's office and comes over to you and says, "I don't have HIV anymore. The doctor just told me that my viral load was undetectable." How would you respond?

Factors to Consider. What does an undetectable viral load test result mean? What would you tell this client about safer sex practices and becoming pregnant?

4. Your 40-year-old male client with AIDS and *P. carinii* pneumonia is about to be discharged from the hospital. His CD4$^+$ cell count is 35/mm^3. He asks you what he should do now. What teaching would you provide?

Factors to Consider. When does a person with HIV infection get an AIDS diagnosis? Does this client need any medication for his pneumonia? Given the fact that the CD4$^+$ cell count is 35/mm^3, does he need any medication to prevent any other opportunistic infections?

evolve *Discussions for these questions can be found on the website.*

BIBLIOGRAPHY

Citations appearing in red refer to primary research.

Citations appearing in blue refer to evidence-based practice guidelines and protocols.

1. CNN.com. (2006). *CDC wants HIV test for everyone*. Available at www. cnn.com/2006/HEALTH/conditions/05/09/hiv.testing.ap/index. html
2. Barroso, J. (2002). HIV-related fatigue. *American Journal of Nursing, 102*(5), 83-86.
3. Centers for Disease Control and Prevention (CDC). (2006). A glance at the HIV/AIDS epidemic. Washington, DC: Author.
4. CDC. (2006). Revised recommendations for HIV testing of adults, adolescents, and pregnant women in health care settings. *Morbidity and Mortality Weekly Report, 55*(RR14), 1-17.
5. CDC. (2006). Rapid HIV test distribution—United States—2003-2005. *Morbidity and Mortality Weekly Report, 55*(24), 673-676.
6. CDC. (2006). *Twenty five years of HIV/AIDS—United States, 1981-2006*. Washington, DC: Author.
7. CDC. (2003). *Surveillance of healthcare personnel with HIV/AIDS as of December 2002*. Available at www.cdc.gov/ncidod/dhqp/bp_hiv_hp_with.html.
8. CDC. (1992). 1993 Revised classification system for HIV infection and expanded surveillance case definition for AIDS among adolescents and adults. *Morbidity and Mortality Weekly Report, 41* (RR-17), 1-19.
9. Charland, M.B. (2003). Management of adverse effects associated with the use of Interleukin-2 in patients with HIV infection. *Journal of the Association of Nurses in AIDS Care, 14*(6), 89-95.
10. Cibulka, N. (2006). Mother-to-child transmission of HIV in the United States. *American Journal of Nursing, 106*(7), 56-64.
11. Conrad, A. (2003). Interleukin-2: Where are we going? *Journal of the Association of Nurses in AIDS Care, 14*(6), 83-88.
12. Coyne-Meyers, K., & Trombley, L.E. (2004). A review of nutrition in human immunodeficiency virus infection in the era of highly active antiretroviral therapy. *Nutrition in Clinical Practice, 19* (8), 340-355.
13. Covington, L.W. (2005). Update on antiviral agents for HIV and AIDS. *Nursing Clinics of North America, 40*(1), 149-165.
14. Demmer, C. (2001). Dealing with AIDS-related loss and grief in a time of treatment advances. *American Journal of Hospice & Palliative Care, 18*(1), 35-41.
15. Foy, K., Bradley-Springer, L., Kempner, T., et al. (2005). Enfuvirtide nursing guidelines: A report from the Association of Nurses in AIDS Care Expert Panel on enfuvirtide. *Journal of the Association of Nurses in AIDS Care, 16*(2), 2-12.
16. Foy, K., & Juethner, S.N. (2004). Enfuvirtide (T-20): Potentials and challenges. *Journal of the Association of Nurses in AIDS Care, 15* (6), 65-71.
17. Garcia, P.R., & Cote, J.K. (2003). Factors affecting adherence to antiretroviral therapy in people living with HIV/AIDS. *Journal of the Association of Nurses in AIDS Care, 14*(4), 37-45.
18. Glutzer, E., & Lalezari, J.P. (2005). Enfuvirtide for nurses: Answering patient questions on activity, safety, and lifestyle impact. *Journal of the Association of Nurses in AIDS Care, 16*(5), 26-34.
19. Gostin, L.O. (2000). A proposed national policy on health care workers living with HIV/AIDS and other blood-borne pathogens. *Journal of the American Medical Association, 284*, 1965-1969.
20. Jaspan, H.B., & Garry, R.F. (2003). Preventing neonatal HIV: A review. *Current HIV Research, 1*, 321-327.
21. Kaiser Family Foundation. (2006). *HIV/AIDS policy fact sheet*. Washington, DC: Author.
22. Kaiser Family Foundation. (2006). *Survey of Americans on HIV/AIDS*. Washington, DC: Author.
23. Kenny, P.E. (2004). The changing face of AIDS. *Nursing 2004, 34* (8), 56-63.
24. Kirton, C.A., Talotta, D., & Zwolski, K. (2001). *Handbook of HIV/AIDS nursing*. St. Louis: Mosby.
25. Kotler, D.P. (2004). The biology of human immunodeficiency virus infection. *Nutrition in Clinical Practice, 19*, 324-329.
26. Manen, L.V., Laschinger, S.J., Stevenson, T., et al. (2005). The nature of multidisciplinary care in the ambulatory setting: A synthesis of the literature. *Journal of the Association of Nurses in AIDS Care, 16*(5), 49-57.
27. Matthews, W.C., Mar-Tang, M., Ballard, C., et al. (2002). Prevalence, predictors, and outcomes of early adherence after starting or changing antiretroviral therapy. *AIDS Patient Care and STDs, 16*(4), 157-172.
27a. McLean, J., Murray, C., Schreibman, F., & Rigsby, M. (2007). *Pneumocystis (carinii) jiroveci pneumonia*. Available at www.emedicine. com/med/topic1850.htm.
28. Moyle, G. (2002). Overcoming obstacles to the success of protease inhibitors in highly active antiretroviral therapy regimens. *AIDS Patient Care and STDs, 16*, 585-597.
29. Murphy, D.A., Lu, M.C., Martin, D., et al. (2002). Results of a pilot intervention trial to improve antiretroviral adherence among HIV-positive patients. *Journal of the Association of Nurses in AIDS Care, 13*(6), 57-69.
30. Nolan, M.L., Greenberg, A.E., & Fowler, M.G. (2002). A review of clinical trials to prevent mother-to-child HIV-1 transmission in Africa and inform rational intervention strategies. *AIDS, 16*, 1991-1999.
31. Peiperl, L. (2002). What are the causes of severe illness and death in individuals being treated for HIV? *HIV InSite*. Available at http://hivinsite.ucsf.edu/InSite?page=cf9croi02&ss=xsl/doc.

32. Piliero, P.J., & Colagreco, J.P. (2003). Simplified regimens for treating HIV infection and AIDS. *Journal of the American Academy of Nurse Practitioners, 15,* 305-312.

33. Powderly, W.G. (2002). Long-term exposure to lifelong therapies. *Journal of Acquired Immune Deficiency and Human Retrovirology, 29*(Suppl 1), S28-S40.

34. Raines, C., Radcliffe, O., & Treisman, G.J. (2005). Neurologic and psychiatric complications of antiretroviral agents. *Journal of the Association of Nurses in AIDS Care, 16*(5), 35-48.

35. Russel, J., Krantz, S., & Neville, S. (2004). The patient-provider relationship and adherence to highly active antiretroviral therapy. *Journal of the Association of Nurses in AIDS Care, 15*(5), 40-47.

36. Scarlotti, G. (2004). Mother-to-child transmission of HIV-1: Advances and controversies of the twentieth century. *AIDS Reviews, 6,* 67-78.

37. Sepkowitz, K.A., & Eisenberg, L. (2005). Occupational deaths among healthcare workers. *Emerging Infectious Diseases, 11,* 1003-1008.

38. Sobieszcyyk, M.E., Jones, J., Wilkin, T. & Hammer, S.M. (2006). Advances in antiretroviral therapy. *Topics in HIV Medicine, 14*(1), 1-42.

38a. The Joint Commission. (2008). *2008 National Patient Safety Goals Hospital Program.* Available at www.jointcommission.org/Patient Safety/NationalPatientSafetyGoals.

39. Young, T.P. (2003). Immune mechanisms in HIV infection. *Journal of the Association of Nurses in AIDS Care, 14*(6), 71-75.

40. UNIADS. (2006). *Report on the global AIDS epidemic: Executive summary.* Geneva, Switzerland: Author.

41. Verheggen, R. (2003). Immune restoration in patients with HIV infection: HAART and beyond. *Journal of the Association of Nurses in AIDS Care, 14*(6), 76-82.

42. Villarreal, H., & Fogg, C. (2006). Syringe-exchange programs and HIV prevention. *American Journal of Nursing, 106*(5), 58-64.

43. Wolf, S.A. (2004, Oct). State of AIDS care 2004: One world, multiple standards. *IAPAC Monthly,* 374-388.

44. World Health Organization. (2002). *AIDS epidemic update.* Available at www.unaids.org/worldaidsday/2002/press/update/epiupdate2002_en.doc.

45. Yenni, P.G., Hammer, S.M., Hirsch, M.S., et al. (2004). Treatment for adult HIV infection: 2004 recommendations of the International AIDS Society—USA Panel. *Journal of the American Medical Association, 292,* 251-265.

evolve *Did you remember to check out the bonus material on the Evolve website and the CD-ROM, including NCLEX®-Examination Style Review Questions, Open-Book Quizzes, and Chapter Review Audio Podcasts?*

http://evolve.elsevier.com/Black/medsurg

CHAPTER 79

Management of Clients with Leukemia and Lymphoma

Susan Newton

Cancers of the hematopoietic system are disorders that result from the proliferation of malignant cells originating in the bone marrow, thymus, and lymphatic tissue. Blood cells that originate in bone marrow are called *hematopoietic cells;* cells that originate in the lymph are called *lymphoid cells. Leukemia* is cancer of the bone marrow, and *lymphoma* is cancer of the lymphoid tissue.

LEUKEMIA

Leukemia is a malignant disease of the blood-forming organs. The American Cancer Society estimated that in 2007 about 44,240 new cases of leukemia would be diagnosed, and about 21,790 deaths would be attributed to the disease.[2] Leukemia is the most common malignancy in children and young adults. Half of all leukemias are classified as *acute,* with rapid onset and progression of disease resulting in 100% mortality within days to months without appropriate therapy. The remaining leukemias, classified as *chronic,* have a more indolent course. In children 80% of leukemias are lymphocytic and 20% are nonlymphocytic. In adults the percentages are reversed, with 80% nonlymphocytic.

Etiology and Risk Factors

Although the cause of leukemia is unknown, several risk factors are associated with leukemia, including (1) genetic factors, (2) exposure to ionizing radiation and chemicals, (3) congenital abnormalities (e.g., Down syndrome), and (4) the presence of primary immunodeficiency and infection with the human T-cell leukemia virus type 1 (HTLV-1). Genetic factors increase the risk of leukemia. A high incidence of acute leukemias and *chronic lymphocytic leukemia* (CLL) is reported in certain families. Hereditary abnormalities associated with an increased incidence of leukemia are Down syndrome, Fanconi's aplastic anemia, Bloom syndrome, ataxia telangiectasia, trisomy 13

(Patau's syndrome), Wiskott-Aldrich syndrome, and congenital X-linked agammaglobulinemia. Identical twins, fraternal twins, and siblings of children with leukemia are also at increased risk. In *chronic myelogenous leukemia* (CML), more than 90% of clients have the Philadelphia chromosome, an abnormal chromosome (see Chronic Leukemia later in this chapter).

Overexposure to ionizing radiation is a major risk factor for development of leukemia, with the disease developing years after the initial exposure. Alkylating agents used to treat other cancers, especially in combination with radiation therapy, increase a person's risk of leukemia. Workers exposed to chemical agents, such as benzene (an aromatic hydrocarbon), are at a much higher risk.

Causal risk factors acting together with a genetic predisposition can alter nuclear deoxyribonucleic acid (DNA). The leukemic cell is then unable to mature and respond to normal regulatory mechanisms. Abnormal chromosomes are reported in 40% to 50% of clients with acute leukemia, and certain chromosomes are repeatedly more involved than others. A mutation in a single cell appears to give rise to some leukemias.

Pathophysiology

In normal bone marrow, efficient regulation ensures that cell proliferation and maturation are adequate to meet a person's needs. Pluripotent stem cells commit to differentiate along the myeloid, erythroid, or lymphoid pathway in the presence of growth factors. In leukemia, control is missing or abnormal. Leukemia is an uncontrolled proliferation of leukocytes. This lack of control

Be sure to check out the bonus material on the Evolve website and the CD-ROM, including free self-assessment exercises. **http://evolve.elsevier. com/Black/medsurg**

A Acute nonlymphocytic leukemia (ANLL)

Myeloblasts

B Acute lymphocytic leukemia (ALL)

Lymphocytes

Lymphoblasts

Platelets

Myelocyte

Neutrophil PMN
(young form)

Neutrophil PMN
(band form)

Neutrophil PMN
(mature form)

Lymphocytes

Immature
lymphocytes

C Chronic myelogenous leukemia (CML)

D Chronic lymphocytic leukemia (CLL)

■ **FIGURE 79–1** Comparison of types of leukemia.

causes normal bone marrow to be replaced by immature and undifferentiated leukocytes, or *blast cells* (Figure 79-1). Abnormal, immature leukocytes then circulate in the blood and infiltrate the blood-forming organs (liver, spleen, lymph nodes) and other sites throughout the body.

The French-American-British (FAB) Cooperative Group developed a classification system that is universally accepted. Under this system, acute leukemias are classified on the basis of morphologic characteristics and histochemical staining of blast cells, which indicates the percentage of immature cells in the bone marrow (Table 79-1).

Acute Leukemia

Acute leukemia is caused by a block in the differentiation of cells in the hematopoietic cell line. The result is a massive accumulation of immature, nonfunctional cells or blasts in the bone marrow or in other organs. *Acute lymphoblastic leukemia* (ALL) is most common in children (median age, 10 years). *Acute nonlymphocytic leukemia* (ANLL), also referred to as *acute myeloid leukemia* (AML), is more common in adults (median age, 65 years). Leukemias are considered clonal disorders in that a single cell undergoes transformation, and leukemic cells then proliferate. An interesting paradox is that leukemic cells apparently

TABLE 79–1 French-American-British (FAB) Classification of Acute Leukemia
Acute Lymphocytic Leukemia
L1 Common childhood leukemia
L2 Adult acute lymphocytic leukemia
L3 Rare subtype, blasts resembling those in Burkitt's lymphoma
Acute Myeloblastic Leukemia
Granulocytic
M1 Myeloblastic leukemia without maturation
M2 Myeloblastic leukemia with maturation
M3 Hypergranular promyelocytic leukemia
Monocytic
M4 Myelomonocytic leukemia
M5 Monocytic
Erythroid
M6 Erythroleukemia

divide more slowly and take longer to synthesize DNA than do other blood precursors. Acute leukemia is not caused by rapid cellular proliferation but instead is caused by the blocking of blood cell precursors. Leukemic cells accumulate relentlessly in most affected individuals, and they compete with normal cellular proliferation. Acute leukemia has also been termed an *accumulation disorder* and *proliferation disorder.*

The development of leukemia occurs in the most primitive blood precursors, pluripotent stem cells, which give rise to all other blood cells (see the Unit 17 Anatomy and Physiology Review). The leukemia blasts, or precursor cells, literally "crowd out" the marrow and cause cellular proliferation of the other cell lines to cease. Normal granulocytic, monocytic, lymphocytic, erythrocytic, and megakaryocytic stem cells cease to function, causing *pancytopenia* (a reduction in all cellular components of the blood). Transformation also may occur, most often in the granulocyte-monocyte series, but transformation could also occur in the erythrocyte series.

Chronic Leukemia

Chronic leukemias are caused by unregulated proliferation of hematopoietic cells or disordered cell death *(apoptosis).* Chronic leukemia is classified as CML or CLL. CML originates in the pluripotent stem cell. Initially the marrow is hypercellular with most cells normal. Typically the peripheral blood smear reveals leukocytosis and thrombocytosis with an increased production of granulocytes. In 90% of cases examination of the bone marrow cells during metaphase shows a translocation of the long arms of chromosomes 9 and 22, called the *Philadelphia chromosome.* After a relatively slow course for a median period of 3 to 4 years, the client with CML invariably enters a *blast crisis* that resembles acute leukemia.

Blast crisis results in the death of more than 70% of clients with CML. During this phase increasing numbers of *blasts* (immature myeloid precursor cells, especially *myeloblasts,* the most primitive granulocyte precursors) proliferate in the blood and bone marrow. In blast crisis the blasts and *promyelocytes* (another myeloid cell precursor type) exceed 20% in the blood and 30% in the marrow. Increased fibrotic tissue in the marrow is another manifestation of blast crisis. Leukopenia, thrombocytopenia, and anemia also are evident. Without treatment death usually occurs within 6 months of onset of the blast crisis.

Chronic lymphocytic leukemia, which is characterized by the proliferation of early B lymphocytes, is an indolent leukemia that is seen most often in men older than 50 years of age. It is usually discovered when the complete blood count (CBC) is performed as part of a routine physical examination. A peripheral blood smear reveals increased numbers of mature and slightly immature lymphocytes. As the disease progresses, lymphocytes infiltrate the lymph nodes, liver, spleen, and ultimately the bone marrow. A staging system is based on the extent of lymphocyte infiltration. Progression of the disease may take up to 15 years, during which the client may not require therapy.

Clinical Manifestations

The manifestations of all types of leukemia are similar. The clinical history usually reveals anemia, thrombocytopenia, and leukopenia.

Clinical manifestations of bone marrow depression include fatigue caused by anemia, bleeding resulting from thrombocytopenia (reduced numbers of circulating platelets), fever caused by infection, anorexia, headaches, and papilledema. Bleeding can occur in the skin, gums, mucous membranes, and gastrointestinal (GI) and genitourinary tracts. Bleeding also is the underlying cause of petechiae and *ecchymosis* (discoloration visible through the skin).

Anorexia is associated with weight loss, diminished sensitivity to sour and sweet tastes, wasting away of muscle, and difficulty swallowing. Liver, spleen, and lymph node enlargement are more common in ALL than in ANLL. Splenomegaly and hepatomegaly usually occur together. The client with leukemia commonly experiences abdominal pain with tenderness and breast tenderness.

Headache, vomiting, and papilledema are associated with central nervous system (CNS) involvement. Facial nerve involvement causes facial palsy. Blurred vision, auditory disturbances, and meningeal irritation can occur if leukemic cells infiltrate the cerebral or spinal meninges. Intracranial hemorrhage and compression also can occur (Figure 79-2).

Complete Blood Cell Count

Complete blood cell count values vary greatly. The total white blood cell (WBC) count may be normal, abnormally low ($<1000/mm^3$), or extremely high ($>200,000/mm^3$). The differential may reveal that one type of leukocyte is overwhelmingly predominant. Abnormal leukocytes, including immature blast forms, may be noted on the peripheral smear. The platelet count and hemoglobin level usually are low.

Bone Marrow Aspiration

Bone marrow aspiration or biopsy is a key diagnostic tool for confirming the diagnosis and identifying the malignant cell type. Typical findings in the bone marrow aspirate and biopsy are an overall increase in the number of marrow cells and an increase in the proportion of earlier forms, suggesting immature cells.

Other Findings

Lumbar puncture determines the presence of blast cells in the CNS; 5% of clients have this abnormality at diagnosis. Lumbar puncture is rarely if ever performed during the acute phase of leukemia secondary to an increased risk of iatrogenic introduction of blast cells into the CNS. It is usually performed post-induction, especially in clients with ALL. Radiography of the chest

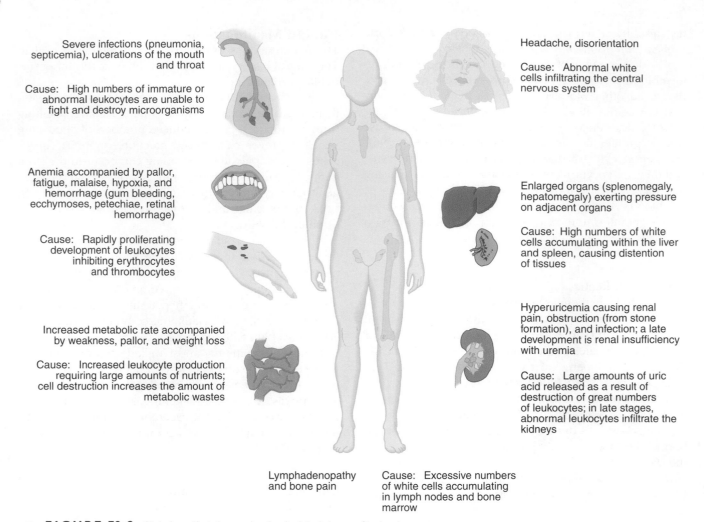

Severe infections (pneumonia, septicemia), ulcerations of the mouth and throat

Cause: High numbers of immature or abnormal leukocytes are unable to fight and destroy microorganisms

Anemia accompanied by pallor, fatigue, malaise, hypoxia, and hemorrhage (gum bleeding, ecchymoses, petechiae, retinal hemorrhage)

Cause: Rapidly proliferating development of leukocytes inhibiting erythrocytes and thrombocytes

Increased metabolic rate accompanied by weakness, pallor, and weight loss

Cause: Increased leukocyte production requiring large amounts of nutrients; cell destruction increases the amount of metabolic wastes

Headache, disorientation

Cause: Abnormal white cells infiltrating the central nervous system

Enlarged organs (splenomegaly, hepatomegaly) exerting pressure on adjacent organs

Cause: High numbers of white cells accumulating within the liver and spleen, causing distention of tissues

Hyperuricemia causing renal pain, obstruction (from stone formation), and infection; a late development is renal insufficiency with uremia

Cause: Large amounts of uric acid released as a result of destruction of great numbers of leukocytes; in late stages, abnormal leukocytes infiltrate the kidneys

Lymphadenopathy and bone pain

Cause: Excessive numbers of white cells accumulating in lymph nodes and bone marrow

■ **FIGURE 79–2** Clinical manifestations and pathophysiologic bases of leukemia.

and skeleton and magnetic resonance imaging (MRI) and computed tomography (CT) scans of the head and body detect lesions and sites of infection. Lymphangiography or lymph node biopsy may be performed to locate malignant lesions and classify the disease accurately.

OUTCOME MANAGEMENT

The treatment goals of all classifications of leukemia are targeted at destroying neoplastic cells and maintaining a sustained remission. During each phase of therapy, the medical treatment may vary, but the basic nursing principles are the same.

Medical Management

Acute Leukemia

The treatment plan for acute leukemia is determined by disease classification, the presence or absence of prognostic factors, and disease progression. The goal of treatment is complete remission with restoration of normal bone marrow function; this means a level of blast cells in the marrow less than 5%. About 70% to 80% of adults with ALL achieve complete remission, with 35% to 45% surviving 2 years. The cure rate remains low without bone marrow transplantation (BMT); however, of adults with ANLL, 60% to 70% achieve complete remission, and about 25% survive 5 years or longer.

Destruction of Neoplastic Cells

Chemotherapy. Chemotherapy is given to destroy the malignant cells of the bone marrow. The treatment protocol for acute leukemia may involve up to three phases: the induction phase, consolidation phase, and maintenance phase. The maintenance phase is usually only used in adult ALL. The three phases of the treatment protocol are as follows:

1. *Induction phase.* The client receives an intensive course of chemotherapy designed to induce complete remission. The usual criteria for complete

remission are blast cells less than 5% of the bone marrow cells and normal peripheral blood counts. Both conditions must be sustained for at least 1 month. Once remission is achieved, the consolidation phase begins.

2. *Consolidation phase.* Modified courses of intensive chemotherapy are given to eradicate any remaining disease. Usually a higher dose of one or more chemotherapeutic agents is administered.

3. *Maintenance phase.* Small doses of different combinations of chemotherapeutic agents are given every 3 to 4 weeks. This phase may continue for a year or longer and is structured to allow the client to live as normal a life as possible. This phase is used more commonly with ALL.

Radiation Therapy. Radiation therapy may be administered as an adjunct to chemotherapy when leukemic cells infiltrate the CNS, skin, rectum, and testes or when a large mediastinal mass is noted at diagnosis (as may occur in ALL).

Targeted Therapy. When AML relapses, treatment options are limited because of the associated toxicities and the health status of the client. Targeted therapies affect only the tumor cells and spare normal cells, hence decreasing the associated toxicities. Gemtuzumab ozogamicin (Mylotarg) is an anti-CD33 monoclonal antibody linked to calicheamicin, which is a potent cytotoxic agent. CD33 antigens are found on the surface of leukemic blast cells and myeloid precursors. This agent is approved for the treatment of CD33-positive AML in clients with first relapse who are 60 or older and who are not candidates for cytotoxic chemotherapy.

Treat or Prevent Tumor Lysis Syndrome. A potentially fatal complication resulting from the treatment of acute leukemia, *tumor lysis syndrome* is a group of metabolic complications associated with the rapid destruction of a large number of WBCs. If the WBC count is high when chemotherapy is initiated, rapid cell lysis can lead to (1) increased serum uric acid, phosphate, and potassium levels and (2) decreased serum calcium levels. Manifestations include confusion, weakness, bradycardia, electrocardiographic (ECG) changes, and dysrhythmias (hyperkalemia); numbness, tingling, muscle cramps, seizures, tetany, and ECG changes (hypocalcemia); and uric acid crystalluria, renal obstruction, and acute renal failure (hyperuricemia). Acute tumor lysis syndrome can be prevented by increasing intravenous (IV) hydration, alkalizing the urine, and administering allopurinol (Zyloprim). Rasburicase (Elitek) is a drug administered once a day for 5 days intravenously in pediatric clients with cancer to lower plasma uric acid

concentrations and manage tumor lysis syndrome (TLS). This drug is also frequently given as a single larger dose in adult clients.[8] Often hemodialysis is necessary to decrease creatinine levels or leukapheresis is necessary to reduce the WBC count.

Replace Cells and Control Infection. Current treatment modalities for acute leukemia destroy normal and aberrant cells. Therapy is aimed at preventing and resolving the complications of acquired and induced pancytopenia: anemia, bleeding, and infection. Transfusions of red blood cells (RBCs) may be required until the marrow produces mature cells. All blood products should be human leukocyte antigen (HLA) matched, cytomegalovirus (CMV) negative, and irradiated. If the client requires IV infusions of RBCs and amphotericin B, an antifungal agent, they should be separated by at least 1 hour so that adverse (e.g., allergic) reactions can be detected.

Chronic Myelogenous Leukemia

Treatment of CML is usually divided into four areas: (1) stem cell transplantation (discussed later in this chapter), (2) interferon alfa therapy with or without chemotherapy, (3) single-agent chemotherapy (hydroxyurea), or (4) the use of specific tyrosine kinase inhibitors.

The goal of therapy in the chronic phase of CML is to control leukocytosis and thrombocytosis. When unwanted cells accumulate, apheresis is a method of blood collection in which blood is withdrawn from the client. The unwanted component is separated, and the remainder of the blood is returned to the client. *Apheresis* is usually performed with use of automated blood cell separators designed to remove selectively the desired blood element. *Leukapheresis* may be performed to lower an extremely high leukocyte count quickly and to prevent acute tumor lysis syndrome (Figure 79-3).

Leukapheresis is rarely performed in CML, however, unless peripheral blast count rises above 300,000/mm^3 and the client is exhibiting abnormal clinical manifestations such as leukostasis. Leukapheresis can lower WBC counts rapidly and safely in clients with WBC counts greater than 300,000/mm^3 and can alleviate acute manifestations of leukostasis, hyperviscosity, and tissue infiltration. This reduction is usually only temporary and often must be combined with chemotherapy and/or targeted therapy for more lasting effects. If painful splenomegaly develops, irradiating or removing the spleen may be recommended; however, splenectomy is considered an avenue of last resort secondary to high surgical mortality in this population.

The most widely used medications used to be interferon alfa administered IV or subcutaneously and hydroxyurea administered orally (PO). Clients with a

■ **FIGURE 79–3** The white blood cell (WBC) level can be temporarily lowered by leukapheresis. Several automated blood cell separators effectively remove large numbers of WBCs and return red blood cells and plasma to the client. The Haemonetics V50 cell separator is commonly used to perform this procedure.

blast crisis (Figure 79-4) require intensive chemotherapy with the same agents as used in acute leukemia. These drugs can destroy leukemic blast cells, transform them into normal granulocytes, or prevent leukemic cells from inhibiting formation of normal granulocytes. Fortunately, the tyrosine kinase inhibitors have transformed the treatment of CML and are the standard of care today.

Targeted Therapy. The class of tyrosine kinase inhibitors have revolutionized the treatment of CML. Imatinib mesylate (Gleevec) inhibits proliferation and induces apoptosis by inhibiting tyrosine kinase activity in cells positive for *bcr-abl*. This agent also targets new leukemic cells in CML that are positive for the Philadelphia chromosome. Data demonstrate 89% overall survival in after five years in patients that received imatinib as initial treatment for CML.

Dasatinib (Sprycel) is a newer drug in the class of tyrosine kinase inhibitors that often works to treat CML in clients when imatinib does not. While still in the class of tyrosine kinase inhibitors, dasatinib has the ability to bind to both the active and inactive conformation of the ABL kinase domain. Dasatinib is indicated for the treatment of adults with chronic, accelerated, or myeloid or lymphoid blast phase CML with resistance or intolerance to prior therapy including imatinib. It is also indicated for the treatment of adults with Ph+ ALL leukemia with resistance or intolerance to prior therapy.

The most recent kinase inhibitor was granted accelerated approval by the FDA in late 2007 is Nilotinib (Tasigna). This oral agent is indicated for use in the treatment of chronic phase (CP) and accelerated phase (AP) Philadelphia chromosome positive chronic myelogenous leukemia (CML) in adult patients resistant or intolerant to prior therapy that included imatinib.

Chronic Lymphocytic Leukemia

The goal of therapy in CLL is palliation or control of undesired manifestations. Local radiation to the spleen may be given as a palliative treatment to reduce complications. Two complications seen during the later stages are hemolytic anemia resulting from autoimmune disorder and hypogammaglobulinemia, which further increases susceptibility to infection. Antibiotics, transfusions of RBCs, and injections of gamma-globulin concentrates may be required for these clients. Leukapheresis is performed when the WBCs are enough to cause vascular thrombosis or embolism, especially in clients who are unresponsive to chemotherapy.

■ **FIGURE 79–4 A,** Microscopic view of a normal bone marrow specimen showing a normal distribution of blood cell types and fatty spaces. Blast cells appear as round, dark gray circles. **B,** During blast crisis the number of blast cells increases and fatty spaces shrink.

A   B

Chemotherapy. Chlorambucil (Leukeran) or cyclophosphamide (Cytoxan) may be given orally to reduce the manifestations of CLL. Chemotherapy generally is given for 2 weeks of every month. When anemia (stage III) and thrombocytopenia (stage IV) develop, daily oral prednisone is given as an adjunct to the alkylating agents. Prednisone has a marked lymphocytolytic effect and may stimulate the production of RBCs and platelets. Fludarabine (Fludara), classified as a nucleoside analog, is another chemotherapeutic agent that is used in treating CLL.

Targeted Therapy. Targeted therapies are now being used in the treatment of CLL. Alemtuzumab (Campath) is a monoclonal antibody approved by the FDA for the treatment of CLL in clients who have been treated with alkylating agents and for whom fludarabine therapy has not been successful. This agent is directed at the CD52 antigen of the lymphocytes, which slows their proliferation. Rituximab (Rituxan), which targets the CD20 antigen, also is effective as a second-line or third-line treatment and is frequently used in combination with IV Cytoxan and Fludarabine in a treatment known as FCR combination therapy.[5]

Nursing Management of the Medical Client

Assessment. Obtain a thorough health history from the client and family members to aid in diagnosis and treatment. The initial history and physical examination provide baseline data to facilitate assessment of complications of ablative chemotherapy and radiation therapy. The severity and longevity of the manifestations of leukemia are important facts to obtain and document.

Ask the client about risk factors and causative factors. Age is important to note because the incidence of leukemia increases with age. The client's occupational history and hobbies may also give hints about environmental exposures. Previous illnesses and medical history may indicate risk factors.

Because leukemia increases the risk of infection resulting from loss of WBC function, ask about the frequency and severity of infections, such as colds, pneumonia, bronchitis, and unexplained fever during the past 6 months. Leukemia reduces the production of RBCs. The client may report activity intolerance, shortness of breath, headache resulting from cerebral hypoxia, increased sleepiness, decreased attention span, anorexia, and weight loss.

The loss of platelet function increases the risk of bleeding. The client may report a tendency to bleed or bruise easily (e.g., nosebleeds), an inability to stop bleeding from small nicks, bleeding gums when brushing teeth, increased menstrual flow, or blood in the stool or urine.

Physical examination findings may include the manifestations shown in Figure 79-2. A complete head-to-toe assessment is performed. Clients with leukemia or blast crisis may have tachycardia, hypotension, tachypnea, murmurs or bruits, and increased capillary fill time resulting from low RBC counts. Skin and mucous membranes may show evidence of bruising and bleeding. *Petechiae* (small, raised red spots) may be present. Lymph node enlargement may be present. If the leukemic cells have infiltrated the spleen or liver, abdominal tenderness may be noted. If the leukemic cells have infiltrated the brain, the client may be confused, have seizures, or become comatose.

The therapeutic relationship initiated during assessment is used to support the psychosocial needs of clients and their families. Leukemia is a life-threatening illness, and working with the client and family as a team is beneficial. Educating the client is an ongoing process to increase understanding of the disease and may help in obtaining compliance with treatment.

The nursing role during the acute phases of leukemia is extremely challenging because the client has many physical and psychosocial needs. Modern therapies offer hope for remission and possibly cure for some clients, but leukemia is still a diagnosis equated with pain, expensive long-term therapy, and potential death.

Diagnosis, Outcomes, Interventions

Diagnosis: Ineffective Protection/Risk for Infection. The nursing diagnosis is written as *Ineffective Protection/Risk for Infection related to neutropenia or leukocytosis secondary to leukemia or treatment.*

Outcomes. Infection will be prevented or will be discovered early and treated effectively as evidenced by a neutrophil count greater than $1000/mm^3$, an absence of fever, and no respiratory difficulty.

Interventions

In compliance with CDC hand hygiene guidelines and The Joint Commission (TJC) National Patient Safety Goals to reduce the risk of health-care–associated infections, it is necessary to institute required hand-washing for everyone coming in contact with the client. The client's risk for infection is estimated by calculating the absolute neutrophil count (ANC). The formula for calculating ANC and an example are given in the Critical Monitoring box on p. 2122. The client should be in protective isolation if the ANC count is below $500/mm^3$. Visitors with possible communicable diseases should be screened for the presence of infection, and visitors or staff with colds or respiratory tract infections should not be allowed near the client. Avoid all live plants and flowers in the client's room.

SAFETY

ALERT

CRITICAL MONITORING

Determining the Absolute Neutrophil Count

A leading complication in oncology clients is infection. To recognize this risk, the absolute neutrophil count (ANC) is calculated daily. The ANC (or granulocyte count) provides a numerical estimate of the client's immune status, risk for bacterial infection, and need for reverse isolation. For example, a client with leukemia may have a high white blood cell (WBC) count or a normal count. On calculating the ANC, however, you may find that the client is at high risk for infection. For example, if a client has a WBC count of 9000/mm³, composed of 10% segmented neutrophils (segs), 60% blast cells, and 30% other WBCs, the client would have an increased risk of infection because the functional neutrophils are only 900.

Three numbers are required:

- Banded neutrophil count
- Segmented neutrophil count
- Total WBC count

Obtain these numbers from the complete blood cell count and differential. The total WBC count is composed of five types of cells; the results from the laboratory show the total count and the percentage of each WBC type. For example, on the differential counts, the value next to monocytes represents the percentage of monocytes among the total number of WBCs.

Then use the following formula to calculate the ANC:

$$(\% \text{ Bands} + \% \text{ Segs}) \times \text{Total WBC count} = \text{ANC}$$

Example:

$$(2\% \text{ Bands} + 55\% \text{ Segs}) \times 1600 = 912$$

When the ANC is less than 1000, the client is at risk for bacterial infection.

When the ANC count is less than 500, the client is at high risk for bacterial infection.

SAFETY ALERT   **The client should be on a low-bacteria diet that excludes raw fruits and vegetables. Assist the client with a daily bath using antimicrobial soap. Encourage the client to perform meticulous oral hygiene several times a day. Female clients should not douche and should avoid the use of tampons. Daily stool softeners are ordered to reduce the risk of anal fissures. Perineal cleansing should occur after every bowel movement. Avoid insertion of rectal suppositories and rectal thermometers.**

SAFETY ALERT   **Oral, axillary, or tympanic temperature should be taken every 4 hours, and the physician should be notified if a temperature is higher than 38° C (100.5° to 101° F) or lower than 36° C (97° to 97.5° F). Fever may be the only manifestation in a neutropenic client.**

Assess the cause of fever before initiation of therapy by obtaining specimens of blood, sputum, urine, central line sites, and other potential sources of infection for culture.

Administer antibiotics as ordered. Therapy usually consists of multiple IV broad-spectrum antibiotics administered on alternating schedules. Administer analgesics as ordered for the relief of discomfort, avoiding aspirin if the client is thrombocytopenic. Aspirin, aspirin-containing products, and acetaminophen should be avoided because they may mask fever.

Invasive procedures should be avoided if possible. Provide meticulous skin decontamination before venipunctures. Maintain sterile occlusion of central venous catheters and perform routine dressing care according to institutional policy. Change IV tubing according to agency policy.

Monitor the client closely for manifestations of fungal or viral infections (i.e., increased respirations, rales, dyspnea, changed oral mucosa). Monitor the respiratory rate and auscultate breath sounds regularly. Viral and fungal pneumonia are common causes of death in the neutropenic client.

Diagnosis: Decreased Cardiac Output. The client eventually becomes thrombocytopenic because of the progression of the disease or because of chemotherapy treatment, leading to the nursing diagnosis of *Decreased Cardiac Output related to thrombocytopenia secondary to either leukemia or treatment*.

Outcomes. Bleeding as a result of injuries, such as falls, punctures, cuts, or other environmental hazards, will be prevented or will be diagnosed and treated successfully as evidenced by absence of bleeding and a platelet count greater than 20,000/mm³.

Interventions

Institute bleeding precautions as follows:

- Provide a soft toothbrush for oral hygiene; avoid flossing, hard toothbrushes, and commercial mouthwashes containing alcohol.
- Instruct the client to avoid blowing or picking the nose, straining at bowel movements, douching or using tampons, or using razors. Men and women should use only electric shavers during the neutropenic phase.
- Do not give any intramuscular (IM) or subcutaneous injections.
- Do not insert rectal suppositories.
- Do not give medications containing aspirin, and instruct the client to avoid aspirin-containing medications.
- Avoid urinary catheters whenever possible. If a catheter must be inserted, use the smallest size possible, lubricate it well, and insert it gently.
- Avoid mucosal trauma during suctioning.

- Remove all potential hazards and sharp objects from the environment. Sharp corners or edges on furniture should be padded.
- Use a pressure-reducing mattress, and turn the client frequently to prevent pressure sores. Use bed cradles to protect extremities.
- Avoid overinflation of the blood pressure cuff, and rotate the cuff to different sites. Avoid prolonged use of tourniquets.
- Use only paper tape, and avoid strong adhesives that may cause skin adhesions.

Teach the client and significant others or family members to institute bleeding precautions during periods of thrombocytopenia. Monitor the client at least every 4 hours for manifestations of bleeding, such as ecchymosis, petechiae, epistaxis, gingival bleeding, hematuria, occult blood in stools, enlarged abdominal girth, disorientation, confusion, and changes in level of consciousness. All urine, stools, and emesis should be tested for blood. Take and record vital signs routinely, noting manifestations of altered tissue perfusion related to anemia (increased respirations and pulse rate, decreased blood pressure).

Check the platelet count, hemoglobin level, and hematocrit daily. Report a hemoglobin level of less than 10 g/dl and a platelet count of less than 20,000/mm³. Administer packed RBCs and platelets as ordered. Keep a current blood sample in the laboratory for crossmatching if needed in an emergency.

Diagnosis: Fatigue. Fatigue is a common complaint by clients. It may be cumulative, a gradually worsening response to treatments for cancer, low hematocrit and hemoglobin levels, altered blood glucose levels, decreased oxygen saturation levels, abnormal electrolyte levels, or unintentional weight loss. Fatigue is the greatest about 2 to 3 days after IV chemotherapy. The nursing diagnosis is written *Fatigue related to side effects of treatments, low hemoglobin levels, pain, lack of sleep, or other causes* as made evident by the client. A scale to rate fatigue numerically may be used, such as the Piper Fatigue Scale (see Evolve website), or, more simply, a 0 to 10 numerical scale (see Chapter 22).

Outcomes. The client will report less fatigue, plan adequate rest periods, and be able to do an increasing amount of usual activities with decreasing assistance from others.

Interventions. Assess for anemia and for the physical, psychological, and treatment-related causes of fatigue. Encourage exercise to maintain strength. Ask a physical therapist to assist with bed and strengthening exercises. An occupational therapist may be able to offer suggestions or devices to conserve energy. If the client has thrombocytopenia or fever or has just received chemotherapy (past 24 hours), exercise is not encouraged, in order to avoid injury. Advocate for adequate pain reduction, minimizing interruptions, and reducing visitors when rest is needed.

Diagnosis: Imbalanced Nutrition: Less Than Body Requirements. The client usually experiences decreased appetite and decreased nutritional intake as a result of the effects of radiation therapy and chemotherapy on the GI tract. Write the nursing diagnosis as *Imbalanced Nutrition: Less Than Body Requirements related to anorexia, pain, or fatigue.*

Outcomes. The client will maintain adequate nutrition and maintain body weight as evidenced by stable weight, adequate caloric intake, and maintenance of fluid and electrolyte balance.

Interventions. Administer antiemetics, as ordered, around the clock as necessary to prevent nausea and vomiting. Premedicate the client with sufficient antiemetics before meals to encourage food and fluid intake. Administer local and IV analgesics, as ordered, to reduce pain caused by mucositis.

Discuss daily dietary requirements with the client and provide high-carbohydrate meals and oral supplements. Allow the client to make food selections. Cold foods, shakes, and sandwiches are tolerated better than hot or spicy foods. Small, frequent feedings may be tolerated better than three large meals a day. Monitor weight daily. If the client cannot tolerate food for an extended period, begin total parenteral nutrition (TPN), as ordered, and monitor intake. The client's own digestive system should be used as long as possible, with TPN used as a last resort. Coordinate and plan rest periods and activities of daily living in increments as needed to minimize fatigue.

Diagnosis: Disturbed Body Image. Most clients experience body image disturbance. The nursing diagnosis is written as *Disturbed Body Image resulting from alopecia, weight loss, and fatigue.*

Outcomes. The client will be able to demonstrate and discuss understanding of the disease condition and the temporary nature of changes in body image and energy.

Interventions. Before treatment, inform the client about the potential for hair loss over the entire body. Encourage the use of scarves, hats, or wigs as desired. Explain the temporary nature of alopecia, although the hair may have a different color or texture when it returns. Alopecia may be permanent with whole-brain radiation therapy (WBXRT).

Encourage the client to balance rest with exercise and activities to maintain muscle tone without developing severe fatigue. Discuss daily dietary requirements with the client, and provide high-carbohydrate meals and oral supplements in an attempt to help clients maintain their body weight and an appearance that is acceptable to them.

Diagnosis: Risk for Sexual Dysfunction. Many clients experience reproductive or sexual dysfunction. The nursing diagnosis is written *Risk for Sexual Dysfunction related to the effects of chemotherapy or radiation therapy on reproductive organs.*

Outcomes. The client will be able to discuss the potential for sterility and decreased libido that may result from therapy.

Interventions. Describe the normal cellular destruction that might lead to temporary or permanent destruction of reproductive function in the client. Inform the client that sexual libido may be altered during and after the acute phase of the illness because of fatigue or other side effects of therapy. Provide the client with emotional support and references to support groups. Provide manuals for alternative sexual positioning and techniques. In appropriate cases, inform the client of reproductive alternatives, such as sperm banking, artificial insemination, and egg harvesting.

Diagnosis: Risk for Ineffective Therapeutic Regimen Management and Risk for Ineffective Family Therapeutic Regimen Management/Readiness for Enhanced Self-Care. Because hospital lengths of stay have become shorter and many oncology clients receive their care in outpatient settings, there is *Risk for Ineffective Therapeutic Regimen Management* and *Risk for Ineffective Family Therapeutic Regimen Management/Readiness for Enhanced Self-Care* related to the chronic nature of the disease process and the risk for complications.

Outcomes. The client and family will manage the therapeutic regimen as evidenced by effective medication administration, an absence of infections and hemorrhage, and the client's ability to remain independent at home.

Interventions. After the induction phase of therapy is completed successfully, the client frequently returns home to recover and to await subsequent courses of therapy that may be given on an outpatient basis if no serious complications arise. It is common for clients to return home with anemia and thrombocytopenia. They also may suffer from the residual effects of chemotherapy or radiation therapy, such as loss of appetite, nausea, and mucositis. Some clients find it difficult to leave the security of the hospital setting because of significantly altered body image, fatigue, and fear.

SAFETY ALERT

Teach the client and the client's significant others how to recognize manifestations of complications as well as appropriate actions to take. Inform them of measures to ensure safety and to reduce risks of bleeding and infection. Provide clients with phone numbers of nursing personnel to call with questions and for suggestions for interventions. The client and **family should be referred to an oncology clinical nurse specialist or case manager as soon as possible after diagnosis. These nurses often educate the client and family about the disease process, the planned treatment, and strategies for successful transition from the hospital to home and outpatient care.**

Evaluation. The desired outcome for the client with leukemia is that the disease will become a chronic condition that the client and family can cope with in a positive manner. If acute leukemia does not respond to therapy, the client's life expectancy is short.

Surgical Management

Bone Marrow Transplantation

To achieve cure with acute leukemia, bone marrow transplantation (BMT) is the most common current recommended treatment. Allogeneic BMT presents a treatment option for clients younger than 60 or 70 years of age, depending on the client's performance status, who have a suitable HLA-matched donor. Transplantation performed during the first remission has a higher success rate than transplantation performed during repeated remissions or in the blast phase of chronic leukemia. BMT is discussed later in this chapter.

Modifications for Older Clients

Older clients are at greater risk for chronic leukemia. The treatment of chronic leukemia in older clients is less vigorous. BMT is an option in older clients if they are otherwise fit and if their organ systems can endure the stress of the procedure. Some older adults with excellent physical and psychological functioning have done quite well with BMT.

LYMPHOMAS

Primary tumors originating from the lymphatic system were identified in 1932. Lymphoma is the most common tumor of the lymphoid system, with about 71,380 new cases diagnosed in 2007 and an estimated 19,730 deaths.[2] About 63,190 new cases of lymphoma will be non-Hodgkin's lymphoma (NHL) and about 8190 Hodgkin's lymphoma (Hodgkin's disease [HD]). *Lymphomas* are tumors of primary lymphoid tissue (thymus and bone marrow) or secondary tissue (lymph nodes, spleen, tonsils, and intestinal lymphoid tissue). Most lymphomas are cancers of secondary lymphoid tissue and involve mostly lymph nodes, the spleen, or both. Malignant lymphoid cells sometimes are found in circulating blood, indicating bone marrow involvement. The major subdivisions of malignant lymphomas are HD and NHL. Bone marrow involvement occurs more often in NHL than in HD.

HODGKIN'S DISEASE

In 1832 Hodgkin reported observations from autopsies showing unusually enlarged lymph nodes and biopsy tissue that showed a distinctive, large cell. Sixty years later Sternberg and Reed described the giant cells, which are called Reed-Sternberg cells of Hodgkin's lymphoma. Today the disease is called *Hodgkin's disease* and is known to be cancer of the lymph, or a lymphoma. Incidence rates differ with respect to age, gender, geographical locations, and socioeconomic class. In 2007 the American Cancer Society estimated the diagnosis of 8190 new cases of HD with 1070 related deaths in the United States.[2]

In economically advantaged countries, the incidence of HD is bimodal, with the first peak occurring in the mid-20s and the second peak occurring after age 50. In economically underdeveloped countries, the overall incidence of HD is lower than that in developed countries but the incidence of HD before age 15 is higher, with only a modest increase into young adulthood. The incidence in people older than age 60 is declining, probably because of improved diagnostic techniques that classify the disease more accurately.

Etiology and Risk Factors

The exact cause of HD is unknown, although indirect evidence indicates a viral cause. The Epstein-Barr virus (EBV) is believed to be a causative agent. EBV-associated lymphomas are well documented in clients who have received organ transplants or who have an immunodeficiency disease. A two-fold to three-fold increase in HD is seen among clients who have a history of mononucleosis, a disease caused by EBV. Researchers have shown that 30% to 50% of HD specimens contained EBV genome fragments in the diagnostic Reed-Sternberg cells.

Some studies indicate a genetic predisposition for HD. The disease occurs more frequently in Jews and among first-degree relatives. Siblings were shown to have a two-fold to five-fold increased risk, and same-sex siblings have a nine-fold increased risk. An increased risk was found among parent-child pairs but not among spouses, suggesting a genetic rather than an infectious cause. Research continues in an attempt to identify the genetic role in the development of HD.

Pathophysiology

Cancerous transformation occurs from a particular site in the lymph node. With continuing growth the entire node becomes replaced, with zones of necrosis obscuring the normal nodular pattern. The mechanism of growth and spread of HD remains unknown. Some have suggested that the disease progresses by extension to adjacent structures. It also may disseminate by the lymphatics because lymphoreticular cells inhabit all tissues of the body except the CNS. Hematologic spread also may occur, possibly by means of direct infiltration of blood vessels.

Clinical Manifestations

Clients often are asymptomatic and may have painless lymphadenopathy. Enlarged lymph nodes most commonly are found in the supraclavicular, cervical, and mediastinal regions (Figure 79-5). Local manifestations produced by lymphadenopathy usually are caused by pressure or obstruction. Involvement of the extremities can be manifested by pain, nerve irritation, and obliteration of the pulse. Clients may experience a nonproductive cough, with the chest radiograph revealing a mediastinal mass, which is present in about 50% of clients.

Pericardial involvement can occur by direct invasion from mediastinal lymph nodes. This involvement can cause pericardial friction rub, pericardial effusion, and engorgement of neck veins. Other manifestations arise when enlarged lymph nodes obstruct or compress an adjacent structure (e.g., edema of the face, neck, and right arm secondary to superior vena cava compression or renal failure secondary to urethral obstruction).

If the tumor infiltrates the spine and presses on the spinal cord, manifestations of spinal cord compression can develop. Manifestations range from early back pain with motor weakness and sensory loss to loss of motor function, urinary retention, constipation, and other manifestations of compression of the cord late in the disease.

Associated clinical manifestations of unexplained weight loss of more than 10% of body weight in 6 months, frequent drenching night sweats, and temperature above 38° C also may be present. Pruritus is a systemic manifestation that can be significant if it is recurrent. These additional manifestations are known as *B symptoms* for staging purposes; they occur in greater frequency in older clients and are negatively related to the prognosis.

The diagnosis is confirmed by lymph node and bone marrow biopsy. A chest radiograph to evaluate complaints of persistent cough or dyspnea may identify mediastinal involvement. The extent of disease is determined by CT scans of the thoracic, abdominal, and pelvic areas as well as gallium scan of mediastinal or hilar lymph nodes and lymphangiography of the lower extremities. If the extent of the disease cannot be determined by these diagnostic tests and confirmation of abdominal disease is necessary for determining treatment choice, a staging laparotomy may be performed.

Staging

Hodgkin's disease is divided into categories, or stages, according to the microscopic appearance of the involved

Severe pruritus is an early sign.

Cause: Unknown

Irregular fever usually present; temperature is elevated for a few days, then drops to normal or subnormal for several days; continuous high fever may indicate impending death

Cause: Apparently related to neoplastic involvement of internal nodes or viscera

Jaundice

Cause: Obstruction of the bile ducts as a result of liver damage causes bilirubin to accumulate in the blood and discolor the skin

Hepatosplenomegaly

Cause: Dissemination of the disorder from the lymph nodes to other organs

Renal failure

Cause: Ureteral obstruction by enlarged lymph nodes

Progressive anemia accompanied by fatigue, malaise, anorexia

Cause: Erythrocyte life span is shortened; erythropoiesis is unable to keep pace with erythrocyte destruction

Edema and cyanosis of the face and neck

Cause: Enlarged lymph nodes place pressure on veins, obstructing drainage of this area

Pulmonary symptoms, including nonproductive cough, stridor, dyspnea, chest pain, cyanosis, and pleural effusion

Cause: Mediastinal lymph node enlargement, involvement of the lung parenchyma, and invasion of the pleura

Alcohol-induced pain in the bones, in involved lymph nodes, or around the mediastinum occurs immediately after drinking alcohol and lasts for 30 to 60 minutes

Cause: Unknown

Bone pain, vertebral compression

Cause: Dissemination of disease from the lymph nodes to the bones

Paraplegia

Cause: Compression of the spinal cord resulting from extradural involvement

Nerve pain

Cause: Compression of the nerve roots of the brachial, lumbar, or sacral plexuses

■ **FIGURE 79–5** Clinical manifestations and pathophysiologic basis of Hodgkin's disease.

lymph nodes, the extent and severity of the disorder, and the prognosis. Accurate staging of HD is important for determining treatment options. Table 79-2 shows the Cotswold staging classification, which modified the Ann Arbor classification system primarily to incorporate the newer diagnostic tests and the evidence that bulky disease is an important prognostic indicator.

OUTCOME MANAGEMENT

Medical Management

Since the advent of combination chemotherapy, adult HD has become one of the most curable malignancies, resulting in a 5-year survival rate of 90% to 95% for stages I and II and 80% to 90% for stages III and IV. The goal of therapy for clients with stage I and II disease is to achieve long-term disease-free survival with minimal acute and long-term complications that affect quality of life. Treatment consists of radiation therapy alone or combined with chemotherapy.

Eradication of Tumor Cells

Radiation. Radiation treatment for HD involves three locations: the mantle, the para-aortic region, and the pelvis (Figure 79-6). The mantle field encompasses the submandibular, cervical, infraclavicular, axillary, mediastinal, subcarinal, and hilar lymph nodes. In clinical stages I and II disease, combined chemotherapy and radiation therapy are recommended for clients with unfavorable prognostic indicators. Most cancer centers classify B manifestations (fever, night sweats, and unexplained weight loss), high erythrocyte sedimentation rate (ESR), or large mediastinal adenopathy as poor prognostic factors. Some centers include large numbers of site involvement and older age as poor prognostic indicators.

TABLE 79–2   Cotswold Staging Classification for Hodgkin's Disease

Stage I	Involvement of a single lymph node region or a lymphoid structure (e.g., spleen, thymus, Waldeyer's ring)
Stage II	Involvement of two or more lymph node regions on same side of diaphragm (e.g., the mediastinum is a single site, hilar lymph nodes are lateralized); number of anatomic sites should be indicated by a subscript (e.g., II$_2$)
Stage III	Involvement of lymph node regions or structures on both sides of diaphragm:
	III$_1$: With or without involvement of splenic, hilar, celiac, or portal nodes
	III$_2$: With involvement of para-aortic, iliac, or mesenteric nodes
Stage IV	Involvement of extranodal site(s) beyond that designated as E

Designation Applicable to Any Disease Stage

A	No manifestations
B	Fever, drenching sweats, weight loss (B symptoms)
X	Bulky disease:
	>⅓ the width of mediastinum
	<10 cm maximal dimension of nodal mass
E	Involvement of a single extranodal site, contiguous or proximal to a known nodal site
CS	Clinical stage
PS	Pathologic stage

Data from Goldman, L., Krevans, J., & Ausiello, D. (2004). *Cecil textbook of medicine* (22nd ed.). Philadelphia: Saunders.

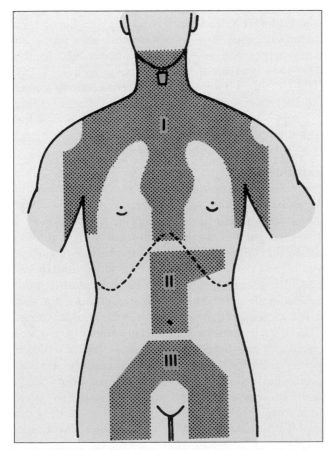

■ **FIGURE 79–6**   Radiation fields in therapy for Hodgkin's disease. *Shaded areas* represent the three treatment fields. The *mantle field* is the uppermost field (I). Lungs and vocal cords are protected by lead blocks; the heart and thyroid gland are within the field. The *para-aortic field,* or middle field (II), extends from the diaphragm to just above the bifurcation of the aorta. When the spleen has not been removed, this field is extended to include the entire spleen and splenic hilum. The *pelvic* or *inverted Y field* is the lowest field (III). It encompasses the pelvic and inguinal nodes and includes a large area of bone marrow.

Chemotherapy. Chemotherapy has become the primary treatment strategy, with or without radiation therapy, in stages I and II disease with poor prognostic indicators and in clients with advanced HD. Numerous chemotherapy regimens are available for HD. For years, MOPP (mechlorethamine, vincristine [Oncovin], procarbazine, prednisone) was the gold standard of therapy; however, ABVD (doxorubicin [Adriamycin], bleomycin, vinblastine, and dacarbazine) has emerged as the best alternative to MOPP. Compared to MOPP, the primary advantages of ABVD are its ease of delivery in full doses, fewer side effects, and less risk of subsequent development of leukemia. With proper treatment, the 20-year disease-free survival rate of HD is 70% to 80%, and the overall survival rate, with salvage chemotherapy for clients who relapse, is 80% to 95%.

Research has shown that clients with advanced disease (stages III and IV) may achieve better treatment results with MOPP plus ABVD than with MOPP alone. Other studies showed that ABVD alone could achieve results similar to MOPP plus ABVD. Many physicians recommend that ABVD alone be given for as many cycles as required to achieve a complete remission plus two consolidation cycles (usually six cycles total). The use of radiation therapy in advanced disease is individualized to the client, especially those with local-regional disease problems.

Clients who relapse after definitive HD therapy generally require some type of systemic therapy, which depends on the type of initial therapy used. Therapies range from chemotherapy and wide-field radiation to high-dose chemotherapy with autologous or allogeneic stem cell transplant. Of clients with stages I to II HD, 20% to 30% relapse within 5 years after radiation therapy. In these cases, the use of combination chemotherapy produces a 57% to 62% disease-free survival at 10 years. At the National Cancer Institute, a 93% second complete remission rate was seen in clients with initial remissions longer than 12 months after chemotherapy. The positive results of several studies investigating the use of stem cell transplant have provided the basis for recommending BMT and stem cell transplantation for all HD clients who relapsed or did not respond to any primary chemotherapy, regardless of the length of the initial remission.

Complications. The complications related to HD are numerous because they are a result of the disease itself or of radiation therapy, chemotherapy, or a combination of several of these factors (Table 79-3).

Nursing Management of the Medical Client

Obtain a thorough health history from the client and family members. The severity and longevity of the manifestations of the disease are important facts to obtain and document. Nurses play an essential role in symptom management associated with therapy. Because of the side effects of chemotherapy, clients may ask for a reduction of the dosage or may want to stop therapy completely. Provide clients with information about the effect of reducing or stopping therapy on long-term survival.

NON-HODGKIN'S LYMPHOMA

Non-Hodgkin's lymphoma comprises a group of malignancies with a common origin in the lymphoid cells. They are heterogeneous in cellular origin, morphologic appearance, and clinical behavior. For 2007 the American Cancer Society estimated that in the United States about 63,190 new cases of NHL were diagnosed, with 18,660 related deaths.[2]

Between 1973 and 1991, the incidence of NHL increased by about 73%. Part of this increase was attributed to acquired immunodeficiency syndrome (AIDS). NHL is about 60 times more common in people with AIDS than in the general population of the United States. NHL is the eighth (male) and seventh (female) most common cause of cancer-related deaths in the United States. Men are affected more often than women, and the incidence is higher in whites than other races. NHL can occur in any age group, but an increase in incidence occurs in the 50s and 60s. Because the average age at diagnosis is in the 50s, the number of years of life lost to these malignancies ranks NHL fourth in economic impact among cancers in the United States.

Etiology and Risk Factors

No hereditary, ethnic, or dietary risk factors have been associated with NHL. An increased risk is associated with immunodeficiency states, autoimmune disorders, and infectious physical and chemical agents. As with HD, a viral or bacterial cause has been implicated (EBV, HTLV-1, human herpes virus 8, *Helicobacter pylori*). A greater than expected incidence of NHL is reported in people with ataxia-telangiectasia, Wiskott-Aldrich syndrome, and Chédiak-Higashi syndrome.

Classifications

Terminology describing NHL is complex, inconsistent, and ambiguous, and several classifications exist. Rappaport's widely used classification, developed in 1956, distinguishes two major histopathologic patterns: nodular and diffuse. These two patterns in NHL illustrate two different pathologic states. The nodular (and diffuse, well-differentiated lymphocytic) pattern involves nodal and extranodal sites. The diffuse pattern does not show the cell aggregates that are evident in the nodular pattern.

Based on expanding knowledge of lymphatic system physiology, six distinct classification systems emerged worldwide in the 1970s. To standardize terminology, the Revised European-American Lymphoma (REAL) classification system was proposed in 1994. This classification includes all lymphoma types as well as the extranodal lymphomas not included in the other classification systems.

Pathophysiology

In clients with NHL, an abnormal proliferation of neoplastic lymphocytes occurs. The cells remain fixed at one phase of development and continue to proliferate. Both T and B lymphocytes mature in the lymph nodes. Clinical manifestations are due to mechanical obstruction of the

TABLE 79–3	Complications of Hodgkin's Disease
Problem	**Cause**
Thyroid dysfunction Thymic hyperplasia	Underlying disease, therapy, or both
Hypothyroidism Thyroid cancer	Direct or indirect radiation exposure
Sexual dysfunction Male impotence Male and female infertility Female dyspareunia	Underlying disease, therapy, or both
Herpes zoster or varicella	Underlying disease, therapy, or both
Pulmonary dysfunction Pneumonitis (acute, chronic, or both)	Direct or indirect radiation exposure, bleomycin, nitrosoureas, radiation recall
Cardiac dysfunction Cardiomyopathy	Mediastinal radiation therapy, pericarditis (acute), doxorubicin, radiation recall
Pericarditis (chronic)	Mediastinal radiation therapy
Dental caries	Salivary changes related to radiation therapy
Myelodysplastic syndrome	Therapy, especially if age >40 yr or lymphocytic leukemia
Non-Hodgkin's lymphoma	Therapy
Solid tumors	Direct or indirect radiation exposure

enlarged lymph nodes. Lymphocytic infiltration of the abdomen or oropharynx also can occur.

Clinical Manifestations

Clients with NHL show localized or generalized lymphadenopathy. The cervical, axillary, inguinal, and femoral chains are the most frequent sites of lymph node enlargement. The swelling is generally painless, and the nodes have enlarged and transformed over months or years. Extranodal sites of involvement are the nasopharynx, GI tract, bone, thyroid, testes, and soft tissue. Some clients have retroperitoneal and abdominal masses with abdominal fullness, back pain, ascites (fluid in the peritoneal cavity), and leg swelling.

Several sites of involvement in NHL are not common in HD, such as Waldeyer's ring (lymphoid tissue that encircles the tonsils), the stomach, the small and large bowels, mesenteric lymph nodes, the thyroid, the skin, the pancreas, the kidneys, and the CNS. With diffuse NHL, clinical manifestations are variable and generally involve more systemic findings. Clients also may experience systemic B symptoms, including night sweats, fever, and weight loss. About one third of clients have hepatomegaly or splenomegaly.

Certain other clinical conditions mimic the malignant lymphomas, including tuberculosis, syphilis, systemic lupus erythematosus, lung cancer, and bone cancer. A thorough diagnostic evaluation is required.

Blood work includes a complete blood cell count (CBC), ESR, and peripheral smear to rule out other causes of lymphadenopathy, such as mononucleosis. Blood cultures and other serologic studies for viral and autoimmune diseases provide important differential information. Elevated lactate dehydrogenase (LDH) levels may be seen in advanced NHL.

A lymph node biopsy is an important diagnostic tool. 🪔 The following are indications for biopsy:

- Adenopathy for longer than 3 weeks, which progresses in size or spreads to other areas
- B symptoms that cannot be attributed to other causes
- Abnormal blood test results indicative of lymphoma
- Radiographs that suggest possible extranodal involvement

Because of the aggressive nature of AIDS-related NHL, any symptomatic client at increased risk or known to be positive for human immunodeficiency virus (HIV) should have a biopsy to rule out high-grade lymphoma.

Just as in HD, once the diagnosis of NHL is made, disease staging should take place. Noninvasive imaging techniques, such as CT and MRI, are useful tools in the initial staging of NHL. Renal and liver function tests are performed to determine the presence of extranodal involvement. Bilateral bone marrow biopsies are important because metastasis to the bone marrow is common, especially in low-grade disease.

Medical Management

Eradication of Tumor Cells

Many classification systems are used to differentiate NHL according to histologic type and cytologic characteristics. Treatment varies based on the histology and stage of the tumor. The treatment of a low-grade lymphoma is different from that for high-grade disease. Low-grade tumors tend to progress slowly and often are asymptomatic for long periods; the natural course of the disease may fluctuate considerably over 5 to 10 years, with or without treatment. Low-grade cells eventually transform into a more aggressive disease process, however, and may quickly cause the death of the client. Because of this process, indolent NHL is believed to be incurable, and many controversies exist concerning treatment standards, especially for clients who have disseminated disease.

Radiation and Chemotherapy. The progression of intermediate-grade and high-grade lymphomas is similar to that of other cancers. Because of their higher growth fraction, however, these tumors tend to be more sensitive to chemotherapy and radiation therapy; the response rate is higher when these tumors are treated. Combination chemotherapy is used to produce tumor shrinkage and remission. Cyclophosphamide and doxorubicin are active against lymphoma. Various combination drug regimens that include these two drugs are used in the treatment of NHL. Controversy regarding first-line standard of care therapy is ongoing. 🪔 Studies comparing various treatment protocols affirmed the practice of using CHOP (cyclophosphamide, hydroxydaunorubicin [doxorubicin], vincristine [Oncovin], and prednisone) as first-line therapy in many academic and community settings.

For clients with low-grade NHL in stage I to II, radiation therapy alone may be curative, although there are reports of recurrence past 10 years. Depending on whether the disease is supradiaphragmatic or subdiaphragmatic, single-mode therapy includes mantle and inverted Y field irradiation (see Figure 79-6).

Clients with stage III to IV intermediate-grade lymphoma require combination chemotherapy as an immediate intervention. Clients who are older than age 60 and have elevated LDH levels, poor performance status, and stage III to IV intermediate disease are at higher risk and should be offered aggressive regimens that provide higher-dose intensities.

The diagnosis of a high-grade NHL warrants immediate and aggressive treatment. Clients may present with rapidly growing disease that has the potential to double in bulk in days or hours. Treatment includes dose-intense chemotherapy, with or without radiation therapy, and prophylactic CNS therapy. It is necessary to provide prophylaxis for the CNS because the blood-brain barrier prevents most chemotherapy drugs from getting into CNS spaces. Without such treatment, lymphoma cells may look for "sanctuary" in the CNS (CNS metastasis). High-grade NHL clients also are excellent candidates for BMT or stem cell transplantation because the tumors respond dramatically to high-dose chemotherapy, which is part of the preparative regimen of transplant.

Monoclonal Antibodies. Rituximab (Rituxan) is an unconjugated chimeric monoclonal antibody that binds to the CD20 antigen found on the surface of most B-cell lymphomas. This surface antigen is present in about 90% of B-cell lymphomas. This intravenous drug is FDA approved as a single agent in the treatment of relapsed low-grade follicular NHL, and also for first-line treatment of diffuse large B-cell, CD20+ NHL in combination with CHOP or other anthracycline-based chemotherapy regimens.

Targeted Therapy. Targeted therapy utilizing radiolabeled monoclonal antibodies is also available for the treatment of NHL. These radiolabeled agents recognize and react with specific antigens to target and kill specific tumor cells. Greater amounts of radiation are delivered to tumor cells than to normal cells, and critical organs that do not express the specific antigen are spared. There are two FDA-approved agents in this class of drugs for the treatment of clients with relapsed or refractory NHL: ibritumomab tiuxetan (Zevalin), which is labeled with yttrium 90, and tositumomab (Bexxar), which uses iodine 131.

Other Therapies. Experimental therapies are emerging in the treatment of NHL. Such therapies include vaccines, high-dose radioimmunotherapy and stem cell transplantation, and antisense anti-angiogenesis agents. These therapies are currently being investigated in clinical trials.

Nursing Management of the Medical Client

Assessment. Although the appearance of an enlarged lymph node in the absence of infection may cause worry, 56% of healthy adults may experience cervical adenopathy; however, any enlargement of lymph nodes warrants further evaluation.

The work-up for NHL begins with a thorough history and physical examination. On examination, lymph nodes involved in infectious processes may be tender or painful, whereas lymphomatous nodes tend to be firm and "rubbery" and are found in generalized patterns. Carcinomatous nodes often are hard and sometimes matted to one another or fixed to underlying structures in contiguous or regional patterns. Other hallmarks of

lymphoma, such as systemic B symptoms (fever, night sweats, unexplained weight loss), are seen in 20% to 30% of clients, but these manifestations also may be seen in other disease states, such as certain infections and connective tissue diseases.

The heterogeneous nature of NHL challenges nurses to meet a variety of physical and psychosocial needs for both clients and their families. The client and family members are confronted with managing a demanding diagnosis and treatment and coping with the effects of the disease on daily routines. Health care professionals often assume that clients with supportive families manage well, but family members share the strain of the illness, are deeply affected (psychologically, financially, and perhaps physically), and need ongoing support. It is crucial that nurses adapt their plans of care for these clients along the disease trajectory, which can wax and wane for many years.

Diagnosis, Outcomes, Interventions. The nursing diagnosis, outcomes, and interventions for HD and NHL are the same as those for the client with leukemia.

Nursing Diagnoses. These clients may have *Ineffective Protection/Risk for Infection* (related to neutropenia or the result of chemotherapy and radiation therapy), *Decreased Cardiac Output* (as a result of thrombocytopenia secondary to treatment), *Fatigue, Risk for Sexual Dysfunction, Imbalanced Nutrition: Less Than Body Requirements, Disturbed Body Image,* and *Risk for Ineffective Therapeutic Regimen Management* (Individuals and Families)/*Readiness for Enhanced Self-Care.*

Outcomes. The desired outcome for the client with lymphoma is that the disease will become a chronic condition that the client and family can cope with in a positive manner. If the disease becomes terminal, the outcome should include a death with dignity, in which comfort measures and psychological support are emphasized.

Interventions. Interventions for these problems were discussed previously for clients with leukemia.

Evaluation. Physiologic problems may resolve quickly with medication. Psychological diagnosis will require prolonged intervention.

BONE MARROW TRANSPLANTATION

Since the 1970s BMT has progressed from a treatment of last resort to a viable therapeutic modality for a variety of hematologic, malignant, and nonmalignant disorders. Peripheral stem cell transplantation and autologous transplants have further revolutionized the field. The status of the disease to be treated by BMT is an important determinant of the outcome for the client.

Transplants for acute leukemias (ALL and AML) in remission at the time of transplant have survival rates of 55% to 68% if the donor is related and 26% to 50% if the donor is unrelated. High-dose chemotherapy and/or radiation therapy followed by bone marrow transplant is also used in the treatment of NHL. BMT has shown long-term survival of approximately 10% to 50% in clients with relapsed or refractory lymphoma.[15]

Indications

Bone marrow transplant may be considered as a treatment for clients with the following conditions:

- Aplastic anemia
- Malignant disorders, specifically myelodysplastic syndromes, leukemia (certain types of acute leukemic, chronic leukemic, and preleukemic states), lymphoma, multiple myeloma, neuroblastoma, and selected solid tumors (breast cancer, ovarian cancer, testicular cancer, poor-risk germ cell tumors)
- Nonmalignant hematologic disorders, such as Fanconi's anemia, thalassemia, and sickle cell anemia
- Immunodeficiency disorders, such as severe combined immunodeficiency disease and Wiskott-Aldrich syndrome

Bone Marrow Harvesting
Sources of Bone Marrow

The three types of bone marrow donors are (1) allogeneic, (2) syngeneic, and (3) autologous.

Allogeneic Bone Marrow. *Allogeneic* bone marrow is obtained from a relative or unrelated donor having a closely matched HLA type. This was the most common type of marrow transplant, but it carried the highest rate of morbidity and mortality because of complications of incompatibility such as graft-versus-host disease (GVHD). The rate of allogeneic transplants has dropped with the decreased birth rate and the increased use of autologous and peripheral stem cell transplants.

Syngeneic Bone Marrow. *Syngeneic* marrow is donated by an identical twin. Although syngeneic marrow is a perfect HLA match, which eliminates the risks of marrow rejection, the incidence of leukemic relapse is higher than when an allogeneic donor is used because GVHD is considered to have an antileukemic effect.

Autologous Bone Marrow. *Autologous* marrow is removed from the intended recipient during the remission phase to allow another course of ablative therapy to be given if a relapse occurs. Although autologous marrow eliminates the risk of adverse immunologic responses, such as GVHD and graft rejection, relapse after autologous BMT is a frequent occurrence. This relapse

may be due to contamination of the harvested bone marrow by malignant cells or the failure of pretransplant chemotherapy to eradicate completely the tumor cells from the body.

Histocompatibility Testing for Allogeneic and Syngeneic Transplantation

Immunologic recognition of the differences in HLA antigens is the first step in host transplant rejection. The HLA system antigens are a complex set of protein structures found on the surface membrane of all human nucleated cells, solid tissues, and circulating blood cells except RBCs. This genetically inherited mixture of antigens is considered representative of the tissue type of each person.

Siblings have a one in four chance of having identical sets of HLA antigens. This situation would provide the optimally matched allogeneic bone marrow donor. Because of the complexity of the HLA system, unrelated clients have less than a 1 in 5000 chance of having identical HLA types. The establishment of the National Bone Marrow Donor Program (NMDP) in 1986 has given hope to many clients who do not have a compatible relative donor. As of April 2007 the NMDP registry contained approximately 5.5 million potential donors and 40,000 cord blood units. This has increased the availability of unrelated donors for allogeneic transplants.

Allogeneic Donor Preparation

An extensive work-up is performed for ensuring compatibility and the mental and physical well-being of the prospective donor. This evaluation includes histocompatibility testing, medical history, physical examination, chest film, ECG, laboratory evaluation (CBC, chemistry profile, viral testing, rapid plasma reagin test [syphilis], ABO and Rh blood typing, coagulation studies), and psychological testing (may include psychiatric consultation).

Before marrow harvest, an informed consent, including potential donor complications (pain, fever, hematoma), must be obtained. In rare instances, the donor may experience serious adverse effects from general anesthesia. Spinal anesthesia is sometimes used instead of general anesthesia during the harvest. Because of the potential for significant blood loss during the harvesting process, syngeneic and allogeneic donors are advised to donate autologous blood for reinfusion before the procedure.

Newborns are currently being considered as potential donors through the use of their cord blood, which is rich in stem cells. Some parents are being encouraged to freeze their newborn's cord blood for potential future use, especially if there is a history of cancer in the family.

Marrow Collection

When collecting marrow, the client or donor is given general or spinal anesthesia in the operating room. The marrow is obtained in 5- to 10-ml aliquots from the marrow spaces of the pelvis or occasionally the anterior iliac crest and sternum. Numerous skin punctures may be required; the aspiration needle is redirected to various marrow spaces without being withdrawn. A total of 500 to 1000 ml of marrow usually is obtained. The blood is placed in heparinized tissue culture media and filtered for removal of fat and bone particles. Marrow can be infused immediately or frozen in a solution containing dimethyl sulfoxide (DMSO), which preserves stem cells in the frozen state.

Peripheral Stem Cell Collection

Peripheral stem (progenitor) cells are harvested by apheresis or leukapheresis, a process that removes blood through a large-bore catheter and runs it through a machine that removes the stem cells before returning the blood to the client. Because stem cell concentration is much lower in peripheral blood compared with bone marrow, a process to increase the concentration in the peripheral blood must be initiated first. To increase the number of circulating stem cells, a stimulus, such as a granulocyte colony-stimulating factor (GCSF), interleukins (ILs), fusion molecules (made from a combination of a CSF and IL-3), or some chemotherapeutic agents, may be given to the donor before the stem cell harvest. As mentioned earlier, the umbilical cord of newborns also is rich in stem cells.

Once the stem cells are harvested, they are preserved in the same manner as bone marrow. The engraftment of stem cells occurs at about the same rate as or slightly faster than with BMT.

Allogeneic Transplant
Recipient Preparation

The physical and psychological evaluation of the recipient is similar to that of the donor. Additional testing may be required to stage existing disease accurately. The recipient must undergo a preparative regimen before transplantation. Such a regimen serves three purposes:

1. Malignant cells are destroyed.
2. The immune system is inactivated, which reduces the risk of GVHD in allogeneic transplant clients.
3. The marrow cavities are emptied to provide space for implantation of the transfused stem cells.

Common protocols combine total body irradiation and high doses of a single chemotherapeutic agent (cyclophosphamide is one of the most common agents used) or fractionated/high doses of multiple agents. A multilumen central venous catheter is inserted to provide suitable access for marrow infusion as well as for antibiotics, blood products, hyperalimentation, and frequent blood sampling.

Bone Marrow Infusion

The infusion of the marrow is commonly anticlimactic after the client has undergone the rigorous preparatory chemotherapy and radiation therapy (often referred to as the *conditioning regimen*). The marrow is usually administered immediately after the conditioning regimen is complete. Before infusion, the client is premedicated with acetaminophen and diphenhydramine to prevent reaction. Marrow is administered from a large blood infusion bag by a multilumen catheter, using an infusion pump, or small volumes may be prefiltered and given by IV push by a physician.

The BMT client remains pancytopenic until the transplanted stem cells make their way to the medullary cavities, where subsequent growth and reconstitution of the marrow are confirmed. Indications of successful engraftment are an increase in platelets and RBCs in the peripheral blood count. This change may occur 14 days after marrow infusion. Each day that recovery is delayed places the client at added risk. Graft rejection is evident if the bone marrow fails to produce peripheral blood cells after several weeks.

Nursing Management

Nursing management of BMT clients follows the plan of care for any completely immunosuppressed client. Clients receiving allogeneic transplants must be observed closely for manifestations of GVHD. Potential immediate adverse reactions are allergic (urticaria, chills, fever), volume overload, and pulmonary complications secondary to fat emboli. Renal damage may occur from too many erythrocytes, or from the dimethyl sulfoxide (DMSO) preservative. The period immediately after transplant is crucial. Multisystem failure related to ablative therapy is common, as are immune reactions caused by the transplanted cells.

GRAFT-VERSUS-HOST DISEASE

The most common and potentially disastrous complication of allogeneic BMT is GVHD, which may occur 7 to 30 days after infusion of viable lymphocytes. The most important factor correlating with incidence and severity of GVHD is HLA disparity. The donor T lymphocytes form an immunologic reaction against the host cells. The clients at highest risk for development of GVHD are those who have had allogeneic BMT. Of those clients, risk is greatest when the donor mismatched two to three antigens and when the client is older than 30 years. With HLA-identical siblings used as bone marrow donors, incidence of moderate-to-severe acute GVHD ranges from less than 10% to 60%, depending on prophylaxis and other risk factors.

ACUTE GRAFT-VERSUS-HOST DISEASE

Acute GVHD is staged according to the organ system affected (Table 79-4). It usually affects the gut, skin, lungs, or liver. *Stage I* GVHD occurs in many allogeneic transplant clients. Skin manifestations may resolve without treatment. Systemic complications may be treated with immunosuppressive drug therapy.

Therapy for GVHD includes high doses of methylprednisolone, antithymocyte globulin, antilymphocyte globulin, cyclosporine, and anti–T-cell immunotoxins. These also leave the client immunosuppressed and vulnerable to infection. The prognosis and treatment depend on the severity of the syndrome. Acute GVHD that does not respond to treatment greatly increases the morbidity and mortality of BMT.

CHRONIC GRAFT-VERSUS-HOST DISEASE

Chronic GVHD, a long-term form of the disease with less acute manifestations, may occur even if the client has not experienced acute GVHD. Chronic GVHD appears about 100 days after transplantation; it may affect the liver, GI system, oral mucosa, and lungs as well as the skin. Chronic GVHD resembles autoimmune collagen-vascular disorders, such as systemic lupus erythematosus. It is characterized by scleroderma-like skin fibrosis and Sjögren's syndrome, in which the mucosa and lacrimal ducts are abnormally dry.

Diagnosis of chronic GVHD is confirmed by skin and oral mucosal biopsy. Although severe GVHD usually is fatal, researchers believe that a complete absence of this immune reaction increases the risk of leukemic relapse.

This situation may be due to a beneficial graft-versus-leukemic reaction that mild GVHD stimulates. In allogeneic BMT recipients with GVHD stages II through IV, the relapse rate is 2.5 times lower than in syngeneic recipients or allogeneic recipients without GVHD.

CONCLUSIONS

Leukemia and lymphoma are complex diseases affecting physiologic and psychological aspects of the client and the family. Nursing care focuses on protection of the client from infection resulting from loss of WBC function, protection from hemorrhage resulting from loss of platelet function, and protection from hypoxia resulting from loss of RBC function.

THINKING CRITICALLY

1. A 68-year-old woman is admitted with acute nonlymphocytic leukemia (ANLL). She is receiving chemotherapy. Her WBC count is 1000/mm³; 3% are banded neutrophils and 54% are segmented neutrophils. What, if any, precautions are needed?

Factors to Consider. How is her risk of sepsis determined? Why does body temperature serve as one marker of infection? What precautions are followed?

2. A 34-year-old man with acute myelogenous leukemia comes to the outpatient oncology facility for his second round of chemotherapy. Three days later the client calls the clinic nurse and is complaining of bleeding gums. What is the priority problem you should address? What instructions should you give the client at this time?

Factors to Consider. What pathologic process underlies the client's manifestations? Are there laboratory results you would want to check? What other precautions should you institute based on the client's other manifestations and the laboratory data? What other data are significant to collect at this time?

Discussions for these questions can be found on the website. **evolve**

BIBLIOGRAPHY

Citations appearing in red refer to primary research.

Citations appearing in blue refer to evidence-based practice guidelines and protocols.

1. Abraham, J., Allegra, C., & Gulley, J. (2005). *Bethesda handbook of clinical oncology.* Philadelphia: Lippincott Williams & Wilkins.
2. American Cancer Society. (2007). *Cancer facts and figures 2007.* Atlanta: American Cancer Society.
3. Burke, J.M. (2006). *Dx/Rx: Leukemia.* Sudbury: Jones and Bartlett.
4. Bush, S. (2002). Monoclonal antibodies conjugated with radioisotopes for the treatment of non-Hodgkin's lymphoma. *Seminars in Oncology Nursing, 18*(1 Suppl 1), 16-21.
5. Cheson, B.D. (2006). Monoclonal antibody therapy for B-cell malignancies. *Seminars in Oncology, 33*(2 Suppl 5), 2-14.
6. Copelan, E.A. (2006). Hematopoietic stem-cell transplantation. *New England Journal of Medicine, 354*(17), 1813-1826.
7. Gleevec Package Insert; accessed at www.gleevec.com on 11/23/3007.

		Liver	Gastrointestinal
Stage	**Skin Manifestations**	**Manifestations**	**Manifestations**
1	Maculopapular rash <25% of body surface area	Bilirubin 2-3 mg/dl	Diarrhea 500-1000 ml/day
2	Maculopapular rash 25%-50% of body surface area	Bilirubin 3-6 mg/dl	Diarrhea 1000-1500 ml/day
3	Generalized erythroderma	Bilirubin 6-15 mg/dl	Diarrhea >1500 ml/day
4	Desquamation and bullae	Bilirubin >15 mg/dl	Abdominal pain or ileus

TABLE 79–4   Stages of Acute Graft-Versus-Host Disease

8. Leukemia and Lymphoma Society. (2007). *Leukemia and lymphoma latest news*. Available at www.leukemia-lymphoma.org.

9. McDonnell, A.M., Lenz, K.L., Frei-Lahr, D.A., et al. (2006). Single-dose rasburicase 6 mg in the management of tumor lysis syndrome in adults. *Pharmacotherapy*, *26*(6), 806-812.

10. NCCN Practice Guidelines in Oncology v.2.2008; Chronic myelogenous leukemia. Available at www.NCCN.org.

11. Oncology Nursing Society. (2007). *Symptom management*. Available at www.ons.org/clinical/SymptomManagement.

12. Seeley, K.M., & DeMeyer, E. (2002). Nursing care of patients receiving Campath. *Clinical Journal of Oncology Nursing*, *6*(3), 138-143.

13. Shannon-Dorcy, K. (2002). Nursing implications of Mylotarg: A novel antibody-targeted chemotherapy for CD33+ acute myeloid leukemia in first relapse. *Oncology Nursing Forum*, *29*(4), 52-59.

14. Sprycel Package Insert; accessed at www.bms.com on 11/24/2007.

15. Steingass, S.K. (2006). Hematopoietic cell transplantation in non-Hodgkin's lymphoma. *Seminars in Oncology Nursing*, 22(2), 107-116.

16. Stolar, K. (1999). A graft versus host disease prevention and management tool: A mechanism for improving continuity of care. *Oncology Nursing Forum*, *26*(6), 977-978.

17. Tasigna Package Insert; accessed at www.tasigna.com on 11/24/2007.

17a. The Joint Commission. (2008). *2008 National Patient Safety Goals Hospital Program*. Available at www.jointcommission.org/PatientSafety/NationalPatientSafetyGoals.

18. Yeager, K.A., et al. (2000). Implementation of an oral care standard for leukemia and transplantation patients. *Cancer Nursing*, *23*(1), 40-47.

evolve *Did you remember to check out the bonus material on the Evolve website and the CD-ROM, including NCLEX®-Examination Style Review Questions, Open-Book Quizzes, and Chapter Review Audio Podcasts?*

http://evolve.elsevier.com/Black/medsurg

UNIT 18

MULTISYSTEM DISORDERS

CHAPTER 80

Management of Clients Requiring Transplantation

CONNIE WHITE-WILLIAMS

The field of organ transplantation has evolved from the early beginnings of experimental kidney transplantation to the current practice of multiple organ transplantation. The advances made have been due largely to the increased knowledge in the areas of immunology and organ preservation, recipient and donor selection, and management of postoperative complications.

Organ transplantation is needed when an organ is irreversibly diseased or injured, leading to end-stage organ failure. Transplantation offers people with end-stage organ failure a chance to live longer and to overcome conditions that were once considered hopeless. Thus nurses have an increasing opportunity to care for clients with end-stage disease who are awaiting transplantation or who have undergone organ transplantation. In addition, nurses may also play a vital role in identification of potential donors and their management during the donor maintenance period.

HISTORICAL PERSPECTIVE

Transplantation had its beginnings in the 17th century with blood transfusions; however, the era of modern transplantation originated with a tooth replacement by John Hunter in the 18th century.[10] In 1912 Alexis Carrel developed the techniques for surgical suturing and vascular anastomosis that opened the pathway to solid organ transplantation.[9] Much of the work during the succeeding years focused on immunology, the importance of ABO and Rh blood group compatibility, and, later, the development of histocompatibility testing, all of which are crucial to organ transplantation today.[9,19] In 1945 Medawar[23] described the immune response of acute rejection, and by 1970 the relationship between donor and recipient histocompatibility in the role of acute rejection was recognized.[10]

Although many attempts at kidney transplantation were made in the early 1900s, it was not until 1954 that Merrell and Murray performed the first successful kidney transplantation between identical twin brothers.[10] Experimental heart transplantation took place in the early 1900s. In 1964 Hardy transplanted a chimpanzee heart (xenograft) into a 68-year-old man. In 1967 Barnard performed the first human-to-human heart transplantation.[5,10,16] The first lung transplantation was performed by Hardy in 1963.[10] Experimental liver transplantation began in the 1950s. The first human liver transplant was performed in 1963 by Starzl.[31] For a summary of the number of transplantation procedures reported by the United Network for Organ Sharing (UNOS), visit www.optn.org/data/annualreport.asp.[34]

With current success and survival statistics, these procedures are no longer deemed experimental. Organ transplantation is clearly an option for clients with end-stage organ disease. Much of the success is due to the availability of new immunosuppressive therapies, advances in organ preservation, improved surgical techniques, and the recognition of risk factors that affect survival after transplantation. Because transplant recipients

evolve **Web Enhancements**

Ethical Issues in Nursing Should Organ Procurement and Donation Be Discussed with the Dying and Their Families?

Do Clients with Transplants Have an Obligation to Comply with Their Post-Transplant Self-Care?

Are Health Care Workers Required to Continue Life- Supporting Interventions Until the Client's Body No Longer Responds?

Figures Transplantation Evaluation Summary Sheet

Tables Religious and Cultural Customs and Beliefs Related to Death and Organ Donation/Transplantation

Appendix A Religious Beliefs and Practices Affecting Health Care

Be sure to check out the bonus material on the Evolve website and the CD-ROM, including free self-assessment exercises. **http://evolve.elsevier.com/Black/medsurg**

now live longer, however, numerous social, economic, ethical, and quality of life (QOL) issues have arisen.

RELATED ISSUES

Cost

Average costs for the surgical procedure plus 5-year post-transplantation expenses are approximately $196,000 for kidney transplantation, $434,000 for heart transplantation, $361,000 for lung transplantation, and $394,000 for liver transplantation.[34] The Social Security Act was amended in 1972 to cover the cost of dialysis and transplantation for end-stage renal disease. Although coverage by private insurance companies, health maintenance organizations (HMOs), preferred provider organizations (PPOs), and Medicare/Medicaid has increased, the high cost remains a factor for clients who wish to undergo transplantation. In 1996 Medicare extended the coverage of immunosuppressive medications to 3 years after transplantation and then in 2001 to lifetime, which was a positive step toward helping clients financially.

Shortage of Organ Donors

The shortage of organ donors is the most significant limitation to transplantation. There are simply not enough organs for the thousands of clients waiting for transplantation. As of November 2007 the numbers of clients with end-stage disease waiting for an organ were as follows: 74,066 for a kidney, 2884 for a heart, 2841 for a lung, 17,471 for a liver, and 1767 for a pancreas.[27,34,35] (Because this information changes hourly, see www.unos.org/data/ for the most current data.[35]) Required request/referral and presumed consent programs are being implemented to increase organ donation. Also, the transplant community is investigating methods to increase donor organ supply. For example, redefining brain death to include cerebral death and anencephaly, use of xenotransplantation (transplanting organs from one species to another), and expanding the donor criteria to include older donors and living extrarenal donors (as in lobar transplantation of lung or liver) are all methods that increase donor organ supply.

Ethical Considerations

Many moral and ethical issues surround transplantation. Religious and cultural customs and beliefs related to death and organ donation and transplantation create challenges for health care professionals (see the website table on Religious and Cultural Customs and Beliefs Related to Death and Organ Donation/Transplantation). As ways to increase the organ donor pool are explored, additional ethical dilemmas may be encountered. The future trends for transplantation include more living-related donation and new experimentation such as cell transplantation. It is important for nurses to be knowledgeable about these issues and to communicate and discuss dilemmas with peers and professionals.

Definition of Death

Debate continues regarding the definition of death. The Uniform Determination of Death Act states that "an individual is considered dead if sustaining either (1) irreversible cessation of circulatory and respiratory function or (2) irreversible cessation of all functions of the entire brain, including the brain stem."[33] Different criteria are recognized for children and infants. In clients in chronic vegetative states or in anencephalic infants, brain stem function is intact but body and mental functions are not. Should death be redefined to include these people as donors? In transplantation, there will always be the dilemma of too few organs available in the face of the need to respect the life of people in a vegetative state who may be potential donors.

Buying and Selling of Organs

The National Organ Transplant Act of 1984 prohibits the sale of human organs and tissues. In addition, the Uniform Anatomical Gift Act of 1968 prohibits the sale or purchase of body parts or organs.[33] The conflict arises with respect to property rights. Supporters of organ sales believe that people own their bodies and have the right to do what they wish with their bodies—including the sale of their organs. The legal sale of blood plasma and sperm, which are body fluids, fuels the debate. The sale of organs in the United States is unlawful. A change in the law would alter the existing practice of free, altruistic donation.[15]

Prisoners as Donors or Recipients

A number of concerns arise in exploring solutions to the organ donor shortage. Once again, payment for organs enters the picture. Should prisoners be allowed to donate a kidney or bone marrow for a reduced sentence? This practice would not comply with current altruistic donation. In the same context, should a convicted criminal be allowed to be a transplant recipient? Some authorities believe that being a convicted criminal should not be an exclusion criterion, whereas others argue that it should be an exclusion criterion because of the prisoner's limited life expectancy outside prison.[15] Criminals may continue a life of crime outside of prison (drugs, guns, robberies), and therefore their chances of early death are greater.

Non–Heart-Beating Donors

Other potential organ donors are people who have experienced a respiratory or circulatory death. The hearts of these potential donors stop beating at the time of organ recovery. Ethical issues here involve the definition of brain death and determining when death occurs after asystole.

Xenotransplantation

Xenotransplantation—the transplantation of organs, tissues, or cells from one species to another (e.g., transplantation of a baboon heart into a human body)—has been proposed as one answer to the organ donor shortage. There are still many medical and ethical issues to consider with this concept. Medical issues include organ rejection, new modes of infection transmission, and incompatible immune system responses. Ethical considerations include informed consent, the use of animals as donors, potential benefits versus risks, and public health issues.[15]

OUTCOME MANAGEMENT

Clients with End-Stage Organ Disease
Referral and Recipient Selection

A primary responsibility of the transplant team is to transplant organs into clients who have the best chance for a long-term successful outcome. It is expected that the transplant recipient will experience an improvement in functional status, maintain long-term graft function, and enjoy improved QOL. This result is accomplished by the selection of an appropriate candidate. The transplant evaluation is a complex, multidisciplinary process that is usually initiated after a referral by the primary physician. The evaluation begins with an initial assessment of medical records and an examination of the client by the transplant team. On the basis of findings from the client's history and physical examination, the transplant team determines whether the client should undergo further evaluation for transplantation. Figure 80-1 shows the referral and evaluation process.

The goals of the evaluation process are to determine the following:

- The medical necessity for transplantation
- The surgical feasibility of the procedure
- Risk factors and the proper timing of transplantation
- Psychosocial suitability
- Immunologic status

The evaluation can be performed on either an inpatient or an outpatient basis and usually takes 3 to 5 days. During this period, extensive testing is completed, client education is provided, and the client and family members meet the members of the transplant team. Tests and procedures performed during the evaluation are listed in Box 80-1. These tests provide the transplant team with information regarding the status of all organ systems, infections, coexisting medical conditions, organ matching, and psychosocial issues that may affect the client and family. Psychosocial factors include

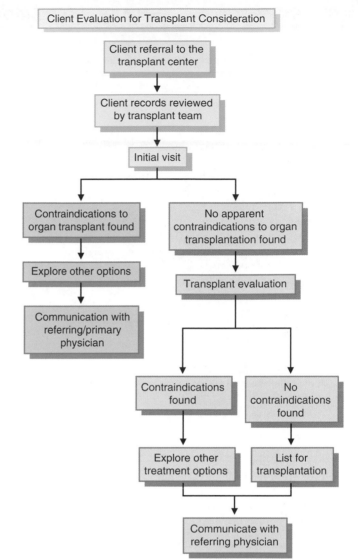

FIGURE 80–1   Client evaluation for transplantation.

neurocognitive status, coping skills, compliance history, availability of support systems, financial status, and extent of resources (Box 80-2). (See the website for an *evolve* example of an evaluation summary sheet to be completed for transplantation candidates.)

The details of the evaluation process may vary between transplant centers and with the organs being evaluated. It is important for you to understand the evaluation process and to know the indications for and contraindications to transplantation. In addition, preoperative education is an important responsibility of the nurse. The goal of education of the potential organ recipient is to provide the client and family with factual information regarding the waiting time for an organ, the surgical procedure, and the post-transplantation regimens, including diet, exercise, medication, routine follow-up, complications, and return to "normal" life expectations (return to work). Many centers provide this

---

BOX 80-1 Evaluation for Organ Transplantation

GENERAL

- Complete medical history and physical examination
- Psychiatric and social evaluation
- Laboratory studies
  - Electrolyte and metabolic profile
  - Liver function tests
  - Hematologic profile
  - Fasting cholesterol/lipid profile
  - Arterial blood gas analysis
  - Urinalysis, urine specific gravity determination
  - Creatinine clearance determination
  - ABO blood typing
  - Antibody screen
  - Human leukocyte antigen (HLA) tissue typing
  - Lymphocyte cytotoxicity screen (assay for preformed reactive antibodies)
- Virologic and microbiologic profile testing for the following:
  - Cytomegalovirus (CMV)
  - Toxoplasmosis
  - Human immunodeficiency virus (HIV)
- Hepatitis B surface antigen (HBsAg)
  - Hepatitis C antibody
  - Epstein-Barr virus (EBV)
  - Syphilis: Venereal Disease Research Laboratory (VDRL) assay
  - Tuberculosis: Purified protein derivative (PPD) testing with controls

KIDNEY

- Laboratory studies
- Glomerular filtration rate determination
- Radiographic and radionuclide scanning studies
  - Renal ultrasound examination
  - Kidney-ureter-bladder radiographic series
  - Renal radionuclide scanning

- Renal angiography
- Magnetic resonance imaging
- Renal biopsy
- Cystourethrography

HEART

- Radiographic and radionuclide scanning studies
  - Posteroanterior (PA) and lateral chest radiographs
  - Sinus and panoramic films
  - Resting radionuclide angiography
  - Pulmonary function tests
  - Ventilation-perfusion lung scan
  - Nuclear magnetic resonance imaging when indicated
  - Computed tomography (CT) studies when indicated
  - Resting and exercise gas exchange studies
- Cardiac catheterization
- Two-dimensional echocardiography
- Electrocardiography

LIVER

- Laboratory studies: additional blood work for diagnosis of specific liver disease may be indicated
- Radiographic and radionuclide scanning studies
  - Ultrasound examination of liver and biliary tree
  - CT scan of head
  - CT scan of abdomen with liver volumes
  - Endoscopic retrograde cholangiopancreatography
  - Percutaneous transhepatic cholangiogram
  - Pulmonary and cardiac evaluation

LUNG

- Radiographic and radionuclide scanning studies
  - CT scan of chest
  - Ventilation-perfusion scan
  - Pulmonary function tests
  - Cardiac evaluation

BOX 80-2 Considerations in the Psychosocial Evaluation for Transplantation

DEMOGRAPHICS

- Age
- Marital status
- Support systems

FINANCIAL

- Insurance
- Savings

SOCIAL HABITS

- Smoking
- Drinking

- Illicit drugs
- Coping skills

HEALTH MAINTENANCE

- Oxygen requirements
- Dialysis
- Compliance with medication regimen
- Compliance with clinical appointments

TRANSPORTATION

- Ability to get to clinic or hospital
- Travel time to transplantation center

HOME ENVIRONMENT

- Telephone
- Running water
- Trailer/home (e.g., financial? Steps? Cleanliness?)
- Heating and air-conditioning

---

education using several teaching skills, such as one-to-one teaching, group classes, and written information. The client uses this information to make an informed decision whether to undergo transplantation.

If contraindications are found during the transplant evaluation (Box 80-3), the transplant team reviews treatment options with the client and family. If no contraindications are found, the client can then be listed on the

---

BOX 80-3 **General Contraindications to Organ Transplantation**

- Presence of active systemic infection (bacteremia, fungemia, viremia)
- HIV/AIDS
- Malignant disease (except skin cancer and some primary tumors of the diseased organ)
- Active peptic ulcer disease
- Active abuse of alcohol or other substances
- Severe damage to organ system(s) other than that to be transplanted (such as severe cardiovascular dysfunction in the potential liver transplant recipient)
- Severe psychiatric disease
- Demonstration of past or current inability to comply with a prescribed medical regimen
- Lack of a functional social support system
- Lack of sufficient financial resources to pay for surgery, hospitalization, medication, and follow-up care

---

national waiting list according to criteria established by UNOS, a nationwide system dedicated to the equitable sharing and distribution of donor organs.

Listing for Transplantation and Waiting for a Donor Organ

The criteria for listing a client for transplantation are governed by UNOS and vary according to the organ to be transplanted. These criteria include urgency, blood type, and recipient weight and height. Liver transplant candidates are assigned a MELD/PELD score, which is indicative of the severity of illness.[34] Likewise, lung transplant clients are assigned a lung allocation score (LAS), which assists in determining the order in which lung offers are made to transplant candidates. This score is a composite of diagnosis, pulmonary function test, and 6-minute walk results.[34]

Stable clients wait at home or near the transplant center. Many clients choose local housing, such as an apartment. A few centers provide hospital-owned housing dedicated to use by pretransplant and post-transplant clients and their families. Cellular telephones or beeper systems must be available to allow the transplant team to contact the client at any time. Usually, a client who lives at a distance from the transplant center requiring more than 2 hours' travel time must relocate or arrange air transportation to arrive at the center within an acceptable time.

Clients whose condition is unstable wait in the hospital, often in an intensive care unit. Some clients, particularly those awaiting heart transplantation, may live outside the hospital with continuous inotropic support. Intermittent hospitalization may be needed throughout the waiting period. Heart transplantation candidates

who become hemodynamically unstable may need an intra-aortic balloon pump or a ventricular-assist device. Clients waiting for renal transplantation may be receiving dialysis, and those waiting for lung transplantation may require ventilator assistance. In liver transplantation candidates, mechanical assistance devices are not used during the wait for the transplant. Cardiac or pulmonary rehabilitation before transplantation is beneficial to optimize the client's strength and aerobic capacity.

Waiting for transplantation is perhaps the most stressful time for clients and families as they cope with terminal illness, altered lifestyles, financial strain, and impending surgery. Both the client and family members may experience feelings of anxiety, depression, and helplessness.[18,28,30] An often forgotten but important component of transplantation nursing is the care of clients with end-stage organ disease who are waiting for transplantation. The transplant nurse may care for clients while they wait in the hospital for a donor organ, in the clinic setting, or in the home. This wait may be days, months, or even years, and it is natural for the nurse to develop strong personal and professional relationships with these clients.

Along with the intense nursing that is involved in keeping the client alive during the waiting period, emotional stress may develop in nurses caring for these clients. It is important for nurses to have periodic meetings to discuss their feelings and difficult cases and to develop plans of care for the clients. More than 20 million people in the United States have chronic renal disease, whereas 400,000 have chronic kidney failure and receive dialysis each year.[25] Approximately 1.1 million Americans are expected to experience new or recurrent heart failure by the year 2010.[1] Cirrhosis is the fourth leading cause of death, accounting for 25,000 deaths yearly.[2] It is important for transplant nurses to understand that, although there may be many happy moments when an organ becomes available for the clients, there will also be tragedies when death occurs before an organ is located. Working with transplant clients can be both emotionally draining and frustrating during the waiting period for organ availability. Nurses can strive to provide excellent care for the client but they have little control over the availability of organs. It is important that emotional support be provided not only for transplant clients and their families but also for health care staff members and their families. Many centers have established support groups vital to the emotional well-being of the people involved.

During the waiting period, the nurse, as part of the transplant team, and the client with end-stage organ disease begin to establish a trusting relationship, participate in the client's education, and work together to grasp the realities of life after transplantation. Many clients and their families unrealistically expect that transplantation will cure all life's problems. The problems of end-stage organ disease may be resolved, but new problems associated with transplantation, including medication side effects, rejection, infections, and financial limitations, are frequently encountered. Help the client understand the post-transplantation regimen, and explain what to expect once the client is discharged from the hospital.

Organ Donation

The gifts of organ and tissue by donation are a vital part of transplantation. Without the gracious decision of the donor or donor family to give the "gift of life" by donation, there would be no post-transplantation miracles.

If the potential donor is a living relative, careful physical and psychosocial assessment is necessary. Potential donors must be psychologically evaluated as to their real desire to donate an organ, usually a kidney, and the ability to make a lifelong adjustment to having one kidney. To avoid conflict of interest, evaluation of the donor is commonly done by a team different from that caring for the recipient. Discussions with the donor should be held in strict confidence; if the potential donor decides not to donate, the medical team frequently cites a physical contraindication in order to allow continued acceptance of that person by the other family members.

Several legislative initiatives have advanced issues of donation and transplantation. In 1968 the Uniform Anatomical Gift Act, aimed at increasing volunteer organ donation, became law. Included in this law were the specifications for notifying legal next of kin of donation wishes, uniform donor cards, and designation of donation preference on the driver's license.[10] The National Transplant Act of 1984 addressed medical, legal, ethical, and social issues of donation such as requiring national scientific registries for assessment by the federal government and declaring it illegal to buy and sell human organs.[33] Also, the Organ Procurement and Transplant Network (OPTN) was established to create a national client registry and to coordinate organ allocation and distribution. UNOS is under contract from the U.S. Department of Health and Human Services to operate OPTN.[10]

The Omnibus Budget Reconciliation Act (OBRA) of 1986 requires hospitals to have written policies and procedures for identification and referral of potential donors. Under the 1987 Organ Donation Request Act, consideration of the donor's religious beliefs is mandated, and guidelines are set forth to guide the health care team's approach to next of kin for donor consent, attainment of consent, and notification of the organ procurement organization (OPO).

OBRA also requires transplant centers and OPOs to be members of OPTN. OPOs are nonprofit organ recovery services in the United States that constitute an integral link in the identification, acceptance, and management of the potential organ donor. In addition to the coordination of organ recovery, transplant procurement coordinators within the OPO provide professional and public education, assist hospitals during donor evaluation, and offer family counseling. Other responsibilities of the procurement coordinators are assisting in donor management, arranging transportation to and from the donor hospital, and assisting surgical personnel in the operating room. The procurement coordinator provides information to the clinical transplantation coordinator and the transplantation surgeon throughout the recovery process.[8,10]

OPOs are either hospital-based or independent. They must meet criteria mandated by the Health Care Finance Administration (HCFA), which includes (1) arranging for appropriate tissue typing, (2) demonstrating a working relationship with 75% of hospitals within the OPO area, (3) discussing accounting procedures, (4) providing a method of transport of donated organs, (5) submitting center-specific data, (6) cooperating with local tissue banks, and (7) having a governing board of directors.

Role of the Nurse in Organ Donation

The nurse plays an important role in organ donation and recovery with early identification of potential donors, making referrals to the OPO, and assisting in the medical management of the organ donor.[8] The nurse may act as a liaison with donor families or may be involved in the clinical management of the donor. This nursing role can be a very emotional experience. A nurse involved in this process must acknowledge the personal loss incurred when faced with the brain death of a donor client. The nurse then begins to focus on managing that client's vital systems until donation is completed.

The nurse's identification of a potential organ donor is a vital link to transplantation. To be a donor, a person must meet certain criteria, including sustaining an injury resulting in brain death.

The nurse may be the first to recognize the manifestations of brain death, including lack of responsiveness; absence of cough, gag, or corneal reflexes; and lack of response to painful stimuli. These findings should be reported to the physician. Refer all clients who meet brain death criteria to the local OPO.[8] It is most often a nurse who notifies the OPO of the potential donor. Notification should occur when brain death is imminent, to allow the procurement coordinator to become familiar with the potential donor's case. Figure 80-2 depicts the organ donor referral and triage procedure.

The first step in the donation process is awareness of potential organ donors. Organ donors are people who have suffered an injury leading to brain death.

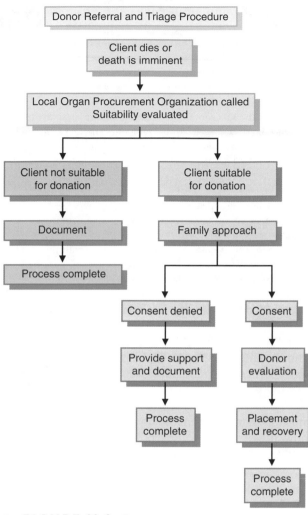

■ FIGURE 80–2 Organ recovery process.

thermoregulation. The ideal organ donor is a person whose fatal injury resulted in brain death but who was otherwise healthy and infection-free. Criteria for organ donation are listed in Box 80-4.

Initiation of the organ donor process should proceed according to hospital policy. Organ recovery occurs in the operating room only after (1) identifying a potential donor, (2) notifying an OPO, (3) diagnosing brain death, (4) obtaining family consent, and (5) managing the donor until organ removal is complete.

Organ Recovery

Multiple organ procurement, or recovery of more than one type of organ from a single donor, is standard practice. As many as four separate surgical teams may be present in the operating room, each focusing on recovery of one organ. Usually, a separate surgical team prepares the recipient for the new organ. After a midline incision is made, dissection of organs occurs. Once cross-clamping of the aorta is done and cardioplegia is begun, the heart is removed. Then lungs, liver, and finally kidneys are procured.

The organs are preserved in a cold storage solution selected by the transplant center. Examples of such solutions are University of Wisconsin solution (UW solution), Euro-Collins solution, Belzer's solution, and other, institution-specific solutions. Organs are preserved in a sterile storage solution, packed in ice, and transported in a cooler to the recipient.

Viability times for donated organs vary. Standard periods after organ recovery are as follows: for kidney, 48 to 72 hours; for heart, 4 to 5 hours; for lung, 4 to 6 hours; for liver, 24 to 30 hours; and for pancreas, 24 hours. For successful transplantation, the timing of organ removal, transport, and preparation of the recipient is essential. Surgical transplantation procedures for specific organs are discussed in their respective chapters.

Preparation of Recipient

While the procurement coordinator manages and coordinates the donor process, the clinical transplant coordinator manages and coordinates the preparation of the potential recipient. The potential recipient (or recipients—in many cases a second client is also told to come to the hospital in case the transplant team encounters a problem with use of the donated organ in the primary potential recipient) is admitted to the hospital and immediately prepared for surgery. Preparation involves obtaining blood work, administering preoperative medications, and performing other standard preoperative interventions such as shaving and skin preparation. Preparation of the recipient may become a race against the clock as the transplant team works within the time constraints of organ viability.

The most common causes of injury are head trauma, strokes, subarachnoid hemorrhage, and primary brain tumors. Once a potential donor is identified, the organ procurement agency should be notified. The next steps are documentation of brain death and family consent of donation.

Next, medical management of the potential donor begins. The goal of donor management is to maintain optimal conditions, ensuring functional and infection-free organs for transplantation. This goal is accomplished by the diligent management of hydration and tissue perfusion, oxygenation, infection control, diuresis, and temperature regulation. ⚗ Guidelines that have been helpful in maintaining organ viability include the "rules of 100's," in which (1) systolic blood pressure is maintained at 100 mm Hg, (2) urine output at 100 ml/hour, (3) heart rate at 100 beats/min, and (4) Pao_2 at 100 mm Hg.[8] Common problems encountered in management of the potential donor are hypotension, shock, electrolyte imbalances, disseminated intravascular coagulation (DIC), and loss of

---

BOX 80-4 Conditions of Participation for Organ Donation

CONDITIONS OF PARTICIPATION

The Department of Health and Human Services (HHS), in an attempt to optimize donor potential and abate the critical shortage of organs for transplantation, issued the Hospital Conditions of Participation (COP) for Medicare and Medicaid on June 22, 1998. This rule took effect on August 21, 1998, and requires all U.S. hospitals to adopt a "routine notification" policy or mandates that hospitals have and implement written protocols to ensure that the organ procurement organization (OPO) is notified of all deaths. According to the COP, the hospital must, "in a timely fashion," notify the OPO of individuals who die or whose death is imminent," thus eliminating the need for hospital staff to identify a potential donor.* All patients who die should be considered a potential organ and/or tissue donor.

Routine notification ensures that an individual who is most familiar with the current criteria on donation, specifically the OPO, evaluates every individual who dies to determine suitability for donation. If the policy were consistently followed, routine notification would make it virtually impossible for the hospital not to refer all potential organ donors. Thus routine notification places the decision making and determination of medical suitability for a person to be a donor in the hands of the procurement and transplant community, not in the hands of hospital staff.

This rule is designed not to exclude hospital professionals from the process but, rather, to ensure that the procurement professionals are included.

Five stipulations are contained in the COP:

- A hospital must have an agreement with an OPO and must contact the OPO in a timely manner about all individuals who die or whose death is imminent. The OPO will then determine medical suitability for donation.
- Every hospital must have an agreement with a designated eye and tissue bank to cooperate in the recovery of eyes and tissues.
- Every hospital must ensure that the family of every potential donor is offered the option to donate organs and/or tissues or not to donate.
- Every hospital must work in collaboration with the OPO and tissue or eye bank in educating their staff, participating in death records to identify potential donors, and maintaining potential donors during the donor management period while necessary testing and the placement of organs and tissues take place.
- Every hospital must provide organ-transplant–related data, as requested by the national Organ Procurement and Transplantation Network and the U.S. Scientific Registry of Transplant Recipients and the OPOs.†

Source: United Network for Organ Sharing.

* Final Rule: *Federal Register,* Vol. 63, No. 119, June 22, 1998. 42 CFR Part 482.4.5. Department of Health and Human Services: Health Care Financing Administration. Medicare and Medicaid Programs; Hospital Conditions of Participation; Identification of Potential Organ, Tissue and Eye Donors and Transplant Hospitals, Provision of Transplant Related Data.

† From Chabalewski, F.L., et al. *Donation and transplantation: Into the new millennium.* Accessed 10/05/2000 at www.medscape.com.

Postoperative Transplant Clients

Management of the post-transplant client involves an intensive collaborative effort of the various members of the transplant team. The transplant team consists of transplant surgeons and other physicians, nurse coordinators, social workers, pharmacists, psychologists, nurse practitioners, nutritionists, members of the clergy, staff nurses, and consultants. Depending on which organ is transplanted, usually the same team members provide care to clients from initial referral throughout the client's lifetime. In many cases, kidney or liver transplant recipients return to their referring physicians for long-term care. Nursing care should be designed to recognize life-threatening clinical problems, to prevent complications, and to promote the client's return to normal activities with improved QOL. These goals are discussed in the Bridge to Critical Care feature on p. 2145.

Basic Immunology Related to Transplantation

To effectively care for the transplant client, you must understand basic immunology concepts related to transplantation (see Chapters 74 and 76). The immune response elicits mechanisms that direct the body to

recognize transplanted organs as foreign (non-self). Although this immune response is normal, it is the goal of immunosuppressive agents to alter this immune response in transplanted clients.

The innate or nonspecific immune responses consist of natural mechanisms for the protection of the client against foreign antigens. These natural defenses are present at birth, lack memory, and do not need prior exposure for antigens to develop. Innate immunity mechanisms include physical barriers, chemical barriers, and leukocyte reactions, all of which play a role in the body's immune response.

Acquired or specific immunity involves mechanisms elicited by the lymphoid system. Lymphoid cells include plasma cells and lymphocytes. Lymphocytes constitute 30% of the white blood cells (WBCs) and are responsible for the recognition of antigens. These lymphocyte defense mechanisms recognize foreign antigens and can elicit rejection of transplanted organs. Two types of lymphocytes can elicit a response: B lymphocytes, which mediate a humoral immune response through the production of antibodies; and T lymphocytes, which are derived from maturing stem cells in the thymus and act to defend the body by interaction with an antigen with

BRIDGE TO CRITICAL CARE

Solid Organ Transplantation

CORE BODY TEMPERATURE CHANGES

The client arrives at the intensive care unit directly from the operating room with the anesthetic agents unreversed. Postoperative hypothermia prolongs clearance of the anesthetic agents and can lead to other complications such as cardiac dysrhythmias, altered platelet function, and decreased oxygen delivery to the tissues. Nursing measures in the early postoperative phase are directed toward supporting and assisting the client while the core body temperature returns to normal. Warming blankets, heat lamps, commercially available rewarming devices, and head covers are important measures to expedite rewarming of the client. Frequent monitoring of arterial blood pressure, cardiac rhythm, central venous pressure, pulmonary artery pressures, and core body temperature is essential during this phase. Arterial blood pressure, systemic vascular resistance, and cardiac output are expected to decrease as core body temperature rises and vasodilation occurs; thus additional support measures often are required during this time of instability.

EARLY GRAFT DYSFUNCTION

The intensive care nurse must be aware of the manifestations of early graft dysfunction. During the first 24 hours, serologic laboratory findings, physical assessments, and objective hemodynamic measurements must be critically evaluated frequently for indications of graft function.

Organ	Indicators of Adequate Early Graft Function
Kidney	High-volume urine output
	Decreasing BUN and creatinine levels
	Normal serum potassium level
	Normal serum glucose level
	Nontender over graft (avoiding incision)
Heart	Normal cardiac output and cardiac index
	Decreasing to normal CVP
	Decreasing to normal PAP and PCWP
	Normal SVR
	Normal sinus rhythm with a ventricular rate of 90-100 beats/min
	Normal LVEF (>55%) by echocardiogram
	Normal S_1, S_2 heart sounds (pericardial rub may be present)
	Decreasing mediastinal drainage (<200 ml/hr in first 4 hr)
Lung	Normal Pa_{O_2}
	Normal CO_2 concentration
	Normal oxygen saturation
	Breath sounds clear and present in all allograft lung fields
	Decreasing pleural drainage
	Chest radiograph clear and well expanded
Liver	Adequate bile output
	Decreasing AST and ALT levels
	Increasing serum protein levels
	Normal to slightly elevated serum glucose level

ALT, Alanine aminotransferase; *AST,* aspartate aminotransferase; *CVP,* central venous pressure; *LVEF,* left ventricular ejection fraction; *PAP,* pulmonary artery pressure; *PCWP,* pulmonary capillary wedge pressure; *SVR,* systemic vascular resistance.

---

a sensitized T lymphocyte.[16,18,26,32,36] There are regulator (T helper and T suppressor) and effector (cytotoxic and memory) T lymphocytes.

In humans, the genetic factor used to determine specific antigen recognition is called the major histocompatibility complex (MHC). The MHC is the human leukocyte antigen (HLA) gene complex, located on chromosome 6. Antigens of the HLA complex are divided into two classes: class I comprises HLA types A, B, and C; class II consists of HLA types DR, DQ, and DP. Histocompatibility testing is used to minimize specific immune responses to the transplanted organ. The type of histocompatibility testing varies according to the organ transplanted and with time limitations.

SAFETY

⚠

ALERT

Before transplantation, the potential recipient undergoes ABO typing, Rh typing, and HLA tissue typing. An assay for preformed reactive antibodies (PRAs) determines the presence of preformed antibodies to HLA antigens. Results range from 0% to 100%. If a potential recipient is found to have antibodies against specific HLA antigens, a donor organ with those antigens is not suitable for transplantation.

Several types of crossmatching procedures can be performed to identify the presence of antibodies in the potential recipient to antigens located on the lymphocytes of the potential donor. A positive result on crossmatching means that antibodies are present, and transplantation is usually inadvisable because of the associated higher risk of rejection. A negative result on crossmatching means that no antibodies are present, with a reduced risk of rejection.

Immunosuppression

The goal of immunosuppressive therapy involves the delicate balance of adequately suppressing the immune response to prevent organ rejection without developing complications from the therapy itself.

SAFETY
⚠
ALERT

This intricate balance of the immunosuppressive medication regimen is individualized for each client and is maintained throughout the client's lifetime. The transplant team aims to keep the dose of each drug within the therapeutic range. Management of the immunosuppressive regimen is crucial to long-term outcomes in post-transplant clients; for example, excessive immunosuppression may lead to increased risk of infection, liver or kidney insufficiency, joint necrosis, cataracts, or malignancies, whereas inadequate immunosuppression may lead to rejection of the transplanted organ. Although in many cases long-term graft acceptance can be maintained with less drug as time passes, most clients require immunosuppression for life to prevent rejection of the transplanted organ.[16]

Immunosuppressive agents are used in the post-transplant population in three categories of use: induction, maintenance, and antirejection. Specific agents and dosages vary according to category of use. Protocols are dependent on the type of organs transplanted, transplant center–specific practices, and the client's history and current health status. See the Integrating Pharmacology feature on Immunosuppressive Agents Used in Transplantation. Most transplant centers use multiple-drug regimens containing agents that act on various functions of the immune system as well as minimize side effects. Many new immunosuppressant medications are being developed and tested in the United States and Europe.

Complications
Rejection

SAFETY
⚠
ALERT

Transplantation of allografts (organs transplanted between genetically different individuals in the same species) elicits an immune response in which the antigens in tissue of the transplanted organ are recognized as foreign; hence a series of events occurs, resulting in rejection of the organ. Rejection is classified into three types: (1) hyperacute, (2) acute, and (3) chronic (Figure 80-3).[16,32]

Hyperacute Rejection. Hyperacute rejection can occur within minutes to hours of implantation of the organ. It is caused by the presence of antibodies. Usually, a destructive humoral or B-cell reaction to antigens on the vascular endothelium results in organ necrosis. Most hyperacute rejection episodes can be prevented by previous panel-reactive antibody (PRA) assay, histocompatibility testing, and crossmatching. If hyperacute rejection occurs, treatment options are limited. Clients who have received kidney or kidney-pancreas transplants may need to return to dialysis. Clients who have received other organ transplants may receive

Immunosuppressive Agents Used in Transplantation

Following transplantation, clients require continuous immunosuppression to prevent rejection of the transplanted organ. These immunosuppressive agents are often given in a combination of two to three agents that may vary from one transplant center to another. There are several classifications of immunosuppressive agents: (1) calcineurin inhibitors (also known as interleukin-2 [IL-2] inhibitors); (2) antiproliferatives; and (3) antibodies.

Calcineurin inhibitors are used to prevent and treat organ rejection and include agents such as cyclosporine (Sandimmune, Neoral, Gengraf), corticosteroids, tacrolimus (Prograf), and sirolimus (Rapamune). These drugs inhibit calcineurin and thereby suppress production of T lymphocytes, suppress T lymphocyte activity, and inhibit production of interleukin-2.

Antiproliferative agents are used to prevent organ rejection and include azathioprine (Imuran), mycophenolate mofetil (CellCept), methotrexate, and cyclophosphamide (Cytoxan). These drugs inhibit proliferation of T and B lymphocytes and interfere with DNA and RNA synthesis.

Antibodies are divided into monoclonal antibodies (muromonab-CD3 [Orthoclone OKT3], daclizumab [Zenapax], basiliximab [Simulect]) or polyclonal antibodies (Thymoglobulin, antithymocyte globulin [ATG]). These drugs inhibit T lymphocyte function, decrease the number of circulating lymphocytes, or block IL-2, which inhibits the activation of lymphocytes. They are used to prevent and treat organ rejection.

Because the client receiving immunosuppressive agents is at increased risk of infection, the client must be taught to recognize the clinical manifestations of infection as well as rejection. Many of the medications may cause serious side effects such as hypertension, fatigue, tremor, diabetes mellitus, renal dysfunction, cataracts, obesity, and various gastrointestinal manifestations such as nausea, vomiting, bleeding, and diarrhea. These problems may also require medical or surgical management.

plasmapheresis, a procedure that removes circulating antibodies from the blood. If this measure fails, retransplantation is indicated.

Acute Rejection. Acute rejection usually occurs in the first 3 months after transplantation; however, it can occur at any time, particularly if the immunosuppression regimen is altered or if an infection develops. Acute rejection can be a purely cellular immune response mediated by T cells or an antibody-mediated response, or a combination of the two.[16,18,26,32] Diagnosis is based on clinical manifestations, laboratory data, or results of tests such

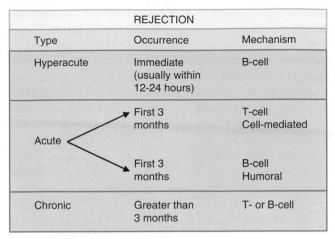

FIGURE 80–3 Transplant rejection.

as organ biopsy. Clinical manifestations of rejection are listed in Box 80-5. Treatment usually consists of high-dose steroids; if recurrent episodes occur, muromonab-CD3 (Orthoclone OKT3) may be administered.

Chronic Rejection. Chronic rejection evolves gradually, usually after the first 3 months after transplantation. It may be the result of frequent episodes of acute rejection, increased ischemic time, or cytomegalovirus (CMV) infection. Chronic rejection results in progressive loss of graft function. The transplanted organ develops a persistent, perivascular inflammation associated with focal myocyte necrosis. Chronic rejection is treated in a similar fashion to test for acute rejection; however, retransplantation may be required as a result of the progressive deterioration of organ function.

Infection

SAFETY ALERT

Infection is the leading cause of morbidity and mortality after transplantation. Many factors contribute to the potential risk of infection, including the client's age, nutritional status, medical condition before transplantation, infection history and exposure, and the immunosuppressive regimen. Infections seen in transplant recipients are usually the result of immunosuppression or altered immune defenses.[18,26,36] During the first month after transplantation, nosocomial infections are common; then, between 1 and 6 months after transplantation, opportunistic infections such as *Pneumocystis (carinii) jiroveci* pneumonia, candidiasis, and CMV infection occur.[26,36] The lungs are the most common site for infection, followed by blood, urine, and the gastrointestinal tract. Common infections seen in transplant recipients are listed in Table 80-1. Infection is the most common indication for hospital readmission after transplantation.[13,36]

Malignancy

SAFETY ALERT

The development of post-transplantation malignancies caused by the immunodeficient state is well documented.[26,36] Types of malignancies seen in the post-transplantation population include basal cell and squamous cell carcinomas of the skin and lip, seen most commonly, followed by the lymphoproliferative disorders and cancers of the vulva, perineum, and lungs. Reduction in the level of immunosuppression, surgical resection, chemotherapy, and radiation therapy are treatment options.

All clients should be screened for development of cancer after transplantation. Routine gynecologic examinations, including mammography and cervical smear in women, annual prostate-specific antigen (PSA) testing in men, and regular physical examination of neck and groin lymph nodes, should be performed to detect any problems. Report any unusual lesions to the transplant team. In addition, monitor clients who are seronegative for Epstein-Barr virus for conversion to seropositivity, which may place them at higher risk for lymphoproliferative disease after transplantation. Clients need to be educated to use sunscreen products with a sun protection factor (SPF) of 15 or greater and to wear protective clothing to help prevent skin malignancies.

Clients Receiving a Specific Organ Transplant
Renal Transplantation

The potential renal transplant recipient has end-stage renal disease, most commonly the result of hypertension, diabetic nephropathy, or a hereditary or congenital disorder.[7,25] In most cases, the renal transplant candidate is anemic and fatigued and has been maintained by chronic hemodialysis (see Chapter 36). Contraindications to renal transplantation include seropositivity for the human immunodeficiency virus (HIV), active infection, severe coronary artery disease with left ventricular dysfunction, malignancy, severe peripheral vascular

TABLE 80-1   Common Infections After Transplantation

Infecting Organism	Site(s) Affected	Therapeutic Agent of Choice
Bacteria		
Gram-negative bacilli		Ticarcillin-clavulanate (Timentin)
Klebsiella	Lung	
Pseudomonas	Blood	
Escherichia coli	CNS	Gentamicin
Legionella	Lung	
Enterobacter		
Gram-positive cocci		Vancomycin
Enterococci		
Staphylococci		
Streptococci		
Viruses		
Cytomegalovirus	Lung	Ganciclovir
	Blood	
	GI tract	
Varicella-zoster virus	Skin	Acyclovir
	Blood	
Protozoa		
Toxoplasma gondii	Transplanted organ	Pyrimethamine Sulfadiazine
	Lung	Folinic acid
	Liver	
Pneumocystis jiroveci	Lung	Trimethoprim-sulfamethoxazole
Fungi		
Aspergillus	Lung	Amphotericin B
	CNS	
Candida	Oral mucosa	Nystatin Fluconazole Amphotericin B

CNS, Central nervous system; *GI,* gastrointestinal.

disease, severe carotid artery disease, and chronic active hepatitis.

Unlike the heart, lung, liver, or pancreas transplant candidate, the kidney transplant candidate has several potential donors: living related, living nonrelated, and cadaver. Eighty-five percent of all renal transplants are from cadaveric donors.

Extensive histocompatibility testing is completed for renal transplantation, because evidence indicates that six antigen matches are necessary for long-term graft survival. Six-antigen-matching means that six antigens recognized on recipient HLA tissue typing match six antigens found on donor HLA tissue typing. A negative result on crossmatching is required for transplantation to occur.

Nursing Care

Nursing care of the renal transplant recipient is focused on the recognition and prevention of complications.

Ongoing assessment of renal function—by determination of blood urea nitrogen (BUN) levels, serum creatinine levels, glomerular filtration rate (GFR), fluid intake and output, weight, and serum electrolyte levels—is routine in these clients. If indicated, a renal scan or ultrasound study may be used to detect complications. Renal biopsy may be performed to make a definitive diagnosis, in that rejection, acute tubular necrosis (ATN), and obstructive complications have similar manifestations.

Goals are to maintain hydration, promote diuresis, avoid fluid overload, and prevent infection. Complications after renal transplantation include fluid and electrolyte imbalances, ATN, obstructive or vascular complications, rejection, and infection. Clinical manifestations of potential complications in the renal transplant client are decreased urine output, graft tenderness or pain, increasing serum creatinine level, fever, and weight gain.

Pancreas and Pancreas-Kidney Transplantation

Pancreas transplantation is indicated for the client with type 1 diabetes mellitus to restore normal glucose metabolism.[11] Pancreas-kidney transplantation is performed in the diabetic client with end-stage renal disease (see Chapter 45).[11] Contraindications are the same as those for renal transplantation.

Nursing Care

Nursing care includes monitoring for fluid and electrolyte imbalances, especially BUN, serum creatinine, bicarbonate, and CO_2 levels. Urine amylase is also monitored to assess pancreatic function. With combined kidney-pancreas transplantation, clinical manifestations of graft thrombosis are a sudden increase in blood glucose concentration, severe graft pain, and increased serum creatinine level.

Heart Transplantation

Potential candidates for heart transplantation are usually New York Heart Association class III or class IV clients who are generally younger than age 65 years and have a life expectancy of less than 12 months. The most common diseases treated by heart transplantation are coronary artery disease and cardiomyopathy.[13,17] Contraindications to heart transplantation include malignancy; active infection; autoimmune disorders; irreversible kidney, lung, or liver disease; and severely elevated pulmonary vascular resistance. Relative contraindications, which vary between transplant centers, are peptic ulcer disease, stroke, peripheral vascular disease, diabetes mellitus, and obesity.[17]

When listed for transplantation, candidates are evaluated periodically, usually every 4 to 6 weeks, to monitor their overall condition. Clients whose condition is stable wait at home or near the hospital, and clients whose condition is hemodynamically unstable wait at the hospital. Clients who become critically ill may need continuous inotropic infusions or ventricular-assist devices.

Cardiac Transplantation Physiology Alterations

Unique to the cardiac transplant recipient is cardiac transplant denervation. Denervation occurs after orthotopic transplantation, in which the vagus nerve is severed. The lack of vagal nerve stimulation results in (1) a higher resting heart rate, (2) a gradual increase in heart rate with exercise and delayed return to baseline, (3) absence of angina, and (4) enhanced response to certain drugs (e.g., adrenaline, adenosine) and decreased response to other drugs (e.g., atropine, digoxin).[6,17] Finally, two P waves may be detected on the electrocardiogram resulting from the presence of both donor and recipient heart sinoatrial (SA) nodes. It is important to note that only the donor heart SA node regulates the electrical conduction of the heart.

Nursing Care

The nursing assessment is a vital component in the care of the cardiac transplant recipient. The physical assessment should include auscultation of heart and breath sounds and assessment of pedal pulses and of the jugular vein for distention. Ongoing assessment of renal and liver function and monitoring of immunosuppressant drug levels and the complete blood cell count (CBC) are important in the overall care of the client. Complications seen after heart transplantation include organ dysfunction, rejection, infection, coronary vasculopathy, and malignancy.[6,17] Chest radiography is used to monitor possible lung infection, whereas echocardiography and endomyocardial biopsy are used to detect rejection. Clinical manifestations of rejection include fever, shortness of breath, fatigue, presence of S_3 or S_4 heart sound, decreased blood pressure, decreased ejection fraction, and jugular vein distention.

Liver Transplantation

Indications for liver transplantation include chronic irreversible liver disease resulting from a number of underlying disorders. In adults, the most common indications are cirrhosis secondary to chronic hepatitis, cryptogenic cirrhosis, primary biliary cirrhosis, and primary sclerosing cholangitis (see Chapter 47).[20,21] Contraindications to liver transplantation are center-specific and may include portal vein thrombosis, active alcoholism, active infection, malignancy outside the hepatobiliary system, and advanced cardiopulmonary disease. The client evaluation takes into account technical feasibility and optimal timing of surgery in addition to the usual physical and psychosocial indications.

Nursing Care

The postoperative care of the liver transplant client is complex. Nursing care focuses on monitoring graft function, managing fluid and electrolyte imbalances, preventing problems with other organ systems, and assessing for manifestations of rejection or infection. Clinical manifestations of rejection include fever, elevation of liver enzymes, and change in color, amount, and consistency of bile drainage through the T tube.

Diagnosis of rejection is confirmed by liver biopsy. In addition, a sudden increase in the International Normalized Ratio (INR) (a system for reporting prothrombin values), serum bilirubin level, or levels of liver enzymes may indicate a complication such as hepatic artery thrombosis or biliary obstruction. If neurologic status is affected, serum ammonia levels may be monitored. Finally, as in all organ transplantation procedures, renal function, immunosuppressant drug levels, and white blood cell (WBC) counts should be closely monitored.

Lung Transplantation

The lung transplantation candidate has end-stage pulmonary disease and (1) is generally younger than 65 years of age for single-lung transplantation, 60 years for two-lung transplantation, or 55 years for heart-lung transplantation and (2) is able to participate in pulmonary rehabilitation (i.e., is not wheelchair-dependent).[3,6,37] The decision whether to perform a single-lung or double-lung procedure varies among transplant centers but is based on the likelihood of achieving the best outcome and most improvement in QOL.

Contraindications to lung transplantation are active malignancy, positive results on hepatitis B antigen assay, hepatitis C infection, autoimmune disorders, and dysfunction of organs other than the lungs. Risk factors that affect eligibility include symptomatic osteoporosis, the need for steroid therapy in doses greater than 20 mg/day, severe musculoskeletal disease, impaired nutritional status (malnutrition or obesity), the need for mechanical ventilation, and colonization with fungi or atypical mycobacteria.

Lung Transplantation Physiology Alterations

Removal of the native lung and lung replacement entail denervation of the transplanted lung. Denervation interferes with autonomic nervous system communication, resulting in dysfunctional ciliary movement, loss of cough reflex, and changes in mucus production, which lead to ineffective clearance of airway secretions. Health maintenance interventions to maintain patent airways are chest vibropercussion, postural drainage, and use of an incentive spirometer.

Nursing Care

The postoperative care of the lung transplant recipient is gratifying. It is a pleasure to watch an oxygen-dependent client who once gasped for breath become an active person requiring no oxygen after transplantation. Immunosuppressant drug levels, electrolyte determinations, liver function tests, CBC, chest radiography, and pulmonary function tests are important monitoring tests in this population.

Complications include surgical side effects, graft dysfunction, rejection, infection, and bronchiolitis obliterans or obliterating bronchiolitis (OB).[3,6,37] OB is the greatest limiting factor to long-term survival after lung transplantation. OB is progressive in nature, resulting in severe shortness of breath, and must be treated aggressively. Usual medical management may include administration of intravenous steroids, cytolytic therapy (with OKT3), administration of Thymoglobulin, photopheresis, and retransplantation. Goals in nursing management are to prevent and recognize complications and to promote return to a functional lifestyle.

Self-Care

Before discharge from the hospital, pertinent information is discussed with the client and family members. Postoperative education after transplantation can be challenging, because many clients are discharged between 1 and 2 weeks after surgery. Many institutions provide client education booklets. Information discussed with the client and family is presented in Box 80-6.

Of special importance are knowledge of the clinical manifestations of rejection and infection and indications for contacting the transplant team. A schedule of return appointments is usually given at discharge. Most clients reside close to the transplant center for 2 to 8 weeks before going home. This proximity allows for frequent medical visits, ongoing education, and familiarization of the client with the postoperative regimen. It also allows the client to become more independent and resume self-care responsibilities. Often it is the nurse who is best able to monitor compliance with the medical regimen and to identify difficulty coping with the post-transplantation regimen. Once the client returns home, it may be necessary for a home health nurse to provide wound care, perform intravenous infusions, or perform other nursing care measures. Findings on home visits are communicated to the transplant coordinator. Box 80-7 lists nursing diagnoses related to care of the post-transplant client.

Meticulous follow-up evaluation (assessing for manifestations of rejection, infection, or other complications)

BOX 80-7 Nursing Diagnoses for the Post-Transplant Client

- *Risk for Imbalanced Nutrition: More Than Body Requirements related to side effects of immunosuppressant agents/Less Than Body Requirements related to increased caloric needs after transplantation*
- *Ineffective Protection and Risk for Infection related to immunosuppression required after organ transplantation*
- *Readiness for Enhanced Self-Care and Deficient Knowledge related to post-transplantation regimen*
- *Pain related to transplantation surgery*
- *Risk for Ineffective Coping after transplantation related to increased stress, anxiety, fear, and lifestyle changes*
- *Risk for Injury: rejection of transplanted organ related to impaired immunocompetence; malignancy/diabetes mellitus/hypertension related to immunosuppression*

BOX 80-6 Client and Family Education After Transplantation

- Members of transplantation team
- When to call the transplant coordinator
- Immunosuppression
  - Administration of medications
  - Side effects of medications
- Rejection
  - Definition, manifestations, diagnosis, treatment
- Infection
  - Definition, manifestations, diagnosis, treatment
- Routine care
  - Temperature
  - Weight
  - Skin care
  - Incision care
  - Fluid intake and output

- Pedal pulses
- Incentive spirometry
- Clinic schedule
- Diet after transplantation
- Activities after transplantation
  - Precautions
  - Exercise
  - Physical therapy
- Self-care
  - Blood pressure
  - Blood glucose levels
  - Medical identification bracelet and card
  - Sun exposure
  - Sexual activity
  - Sending specimens for laboratory monitoring tests

- Vacations
- Over-the-counter medicines to be avoided
- Driving
- Birth control
- Psychosocial issues
  - Physical appearance
  - Family participation and support
  - Writing to the donor family
  - Cost of transplantation
- Health maintenance
  - Dental care
  - Ophthalmologic examinations
  - Gynecologic examinations
  - Yearly evaluations of transplant

is essential to the long-term well-being of the post-transplant client. Long-term care of the transplant recipient requires communication between the client and transplant team. Each client should be assessed for infection, rejection, malignancy, organ dysfunction, and adverse manifestations of immunosuppression such as diabetes mellitus, hypertension, hyperlipidemia, abnormalities on liver function testing, and gastrointestinal distress.

Psychosocial issues that should be investigated are financial status, family dynamics, and ability to return to work. The social worker at the transplant center can assist the client with insurance questions, medication assistance programs, and ways of dealing with the financial stresses of transplantation. 🪔 Coping with QOL may also be an issue for the transplant client, as discussed in the Translating Evidence into Practice feature below.

🪔 Health maintenance areas to evaluate are screening by mammography and Papanicolaou (Pap) smears in women, colon cancer screening, and immunizations such as with the influenza vaccine and pneumococcal vaccine (Pneumovax). Routine dental and ophthalmologic examinations should be scheduled. Communication with the referring physician or the primary health care provider is also important. Constant relaying of information including laboratory findings, clinic visit results, and follow-up plans should occur between the transplant center and the client's primary health care provider.

🪔 TRANSLATING EVIDENCE INTO PRACTICE

Quality of Life After Transplantation

Quality of life (QOL) before and after transplantation, as well as how the client functions, copes, and lives after transplantation, is being investigated by nurses.[2-4,6,8-18,21,23-24] Other health care practitioners have completed similar studies of QOL.[1,5,7,19,20,22] Research studies may evaluate QOL at a specific period either before or after transplantation. Differences in the effects of drug treatment, device intervention, or medical therapy on QOL may be examined also. The diabetic client who is no longer insulin-dependent or the client who had end-stage renal disease who no longer requires dialysis has experienced a major change in lifestyle. Although there are challenges related to immunosuppressive therapy, most clients who undergo successful transplantation report improved QOL. Dew and colleagues reviewed 218 published studies using almost 15,000 total subjects from 1972 through 1996 and evaluated QOL in three areas: physical functioning, mental/cognitive health, and social functioning. Physical functioning was improved in all studies involving pancreas/kidney, pancreas, lung, and heart/lung clients.[1,4,8,22] Mental/cognitive and social improvement were reported in less than 80% of studies reviewed.[4] Of the studies reviewed by Dew and colleagues, few compared QOL ratings by transplant clients to QOL ratings by healthy people.[4]

Hathaway and colleagues and Johnson and colleagues reported improved QOL in renal transplant recipients regardless of race or gender of the client.[10,14] Hathaway and colleagues also completed a longitudinal study of 91 kidney transplant recipients who underwent QOL testing before transplantation and at 6 and 12 months after transplantation. The Sickness Impact Profile, the Adult Self-Image Scale, and the Personal Resource Questionnaire were used for this study. Variables that predicted post-transplantation QOL were employment status, the number of transplantation-related hospitalizations, and available social support.[11] White-Williams and colleagues found that males reported better QOL than females, both before heart transplantation and at 6 months after transplantation.[15,23]

Grady and colleagues reported on compliance at 1 year and at 2 years after heart transplantation in 120 recipients. Compliance was measured with the Heart Transplant Compliance Instrument developed for this study. The heart transplant recipients had no difficulty following medication regimens but did have difficulty with diet, exercise, and taking their vital signs.[8,9] De Geest and associates also examined compliance with taking medications in heart transplant recipients. They found that compliance with immunosuppressive medication was high; however, clients who were considered "moderate noncompliers" had a higher incidence of late acute rejection episodes. The findings in this study suggest that client compliance plays a pivotal role in long-term outcome after transplantation.[3]

Limbos and colleagues studied QOL in women before and after lung transplantation. Overall QOL improved after transplantation; however, the women reported impairments with sexuality and body satisfaction.[16] Manzetti reported that a health maintenance program of education and exercise improved QOL in clients awaiting lung transplantation.[18] Similarly, LoBiondo-Wood and colleagues reported improved QOL over time in 41 liver transplant recipients.[17] Post-transplant anxiety also reduced QOL in transplant recipients.[19,20,22]

IMPLICATIONS

QOL findings may vary from one type of transplant procedure to another, requiring nurses to be familiar with the QOL data for the type of transplant they encounter most frequently. Nurses working with a particular population of transplant clients may also share data about QOL that may be useful for transplant clients and families. It is important to remember that rating one's QOL may be relative because the experience of having a life-threatening illness changes how one thinks about life in general and about one's own particular life. Studies that compare QOL ratings by transplant recipients to QOL ratings by clients who have experienced near-death episodes, life-altering accidents, or medical treatment for severe illness should also be explored. Many studies were short term or asked clients about QOL only once or twice. This suggests that longitudinal studies of QOL are needed to enable nurses to understand and appreciate the impact of chronic illnesses and transplantation on clients and families.

(Continued)

TRANSLATING EVIDENCE INTO PRACTICE

Quality of Life After Transplantation—Cont'd

REFERENCES

1. Almenar-Pertejo, M., et al. (2006). Study on health-related quality of life in patients with advanced heart failure before and after transplantation. *Transplantation Proceedings, 38*(8), 2524-2526.
2. Cicutto, L., et al. (2004). Factors affecting attainment of paid employment after lung transplantation. *Journal of Heart and Lung Transplantation, 23*(4), 481-486.
3. De Geest, S., et al. (1998). Late acute rejection and subclinical noncompliance with cyclosporine therapy in heart transplant recipients. *Journal of Heart and Lung Transplantation, 17,* 854-863.
4. Dew, M., et al. (1997). Does transplantation produce quality of life benefits? A quantitative analysis. *Transplantation, 64,* 1261-1273.
5. Ekberg, H., et al. (2007). Increased prevalence of gastrointestinal symptoms associated with impaired quality of life in renal transplant recipients. *Transplantation, 83*(3), 282-289.
6. Forsberg, A. (2002). Liver transplant recipient's experienced meaning of health and quality of life one year after transplantation. *Theoria Journal of Nursing Theory, 11*(3), 4-14.
7. Girard, F., et al. (2006). Prevalence and impact of pain on the quality of life of lung transplant recipients: A prospective observational study. *Chest, 130*(5), 1535-1540.
8. Grady, K., et al. (1995). Predictors of quality of life in patients with advanced heart failure awaiting transplantation. *Journal of Heart and Lung Transplantation, 14,* 2-10.
9. Grady, K., et al. (1998). Patient compliance at one year and two years after heart transplantation. *Journal of Heart and Lung Transplantation, 17,* 383-394.
10. Hathaway, D., et al. (1996). Racial and gender differences in quality of life prior to and following kidney transplantation. *Proceedings of the Tenth Annual Southern Nursing Research Society Conference,* Feb 29, 2006, Miami, Fla.
11. Hathaway, D., et al. (1998). Post kidney transplantation quality of life prediction models. *Clinical Transplantation, 12,* 168-174.
12. Hilbrands, L., et al. (1995). The effect of immunosuppressive drugs on quality of life after renal transplantation. *Transplantation, 59,* 1263-1270.
13. Houle, N., et al. (2002). Health promoting behaviors, quality of life, and hospital resource utilization of patients receiving kidney transplants. *Nephrology Nursing Journal, 29,* 35-40.
14. Johnson, C., et al. (1998). Racial and gender differences in quality of life following kidney transplantation. *Image: Journal of Nursing Scholarship, 30,* 125-130.
15. Kirklin, J., & White-Williams, C. (2002). Quality of life after heart transplantation. In J. Kirklin, D. McGiffin, & J. Young (Eds.), *Heart transplantation.* New York: Churchill Livingstone.
16. Limbos, M., Chan, C., & Kesten, S. (1997). Quality of life in female lung transplant candidates and recipients. *Chest, 112,* 1165-1174.
17. LoBiondo-Wood, G., et al. (1997). Impact of liver transplantation on quality of life: A longitudinal perspective. *Applied Nursing Research, 10*(1), 27-32.
18. Manzetti, J., et al. (1994). Exercise, education and quality of life in lung transplant candidates. *Journal of Heart and Lung Transplantation, 13,* 297-305.
19. O'Reilly, F., et al. (2006). Baseline quality of life and anxiety in solid organ transplant recipients: A pilot study. *Dermatologic Surgery, 32*(11), 1480-1485.
20. Perez-San-Gregorio, M., et al. (2006). The influence of posttransplant anxiety on the long-term health of patients. *Transplantation Proceedings, 38*(8), 2406-2408.
21. Thomas, D. (1996). Returning to work after liver transplantation: Experiencing the roadblocks. *Journal of Transplantation Coordinators, 6,* 134-138.
22. Vermeulen, K., et al. (2007). Long-term health-related quality of life after lung transplantation: Different predictors for different dimensions. *Journal of Heart and Lung Transplantation, 26*(2), 177-193.
23. White-Williams, C., et al. (1997). Gender differences in quality of life outcomes before and 6 months after heart transplantation. *Journal of Heart and Lung Transplantation, 16,* 100.
24. Zarifian, A. (2006). Symptom occurrence, symptom distress, and quality of life in renal transplant recipients. *Nephrology Nursing Journal, 33*(6), 609-618.

CONCLUSIONS

Nursing care of the transplant client is both challenging and rewarding. With thorough understanding of the end-stage disease process and its manifestations, the organ donation and recovery process, and postoperative management, the nurse has the unique ability to work as a member of the interdisciplinary team caring for this group of clients. The nurse may serve as primary care provider, client advocate, and liaison with other team members. To maximize QOL, caring for the client and family must focus on both the physical and psychosocial aspects of transplantation, including not only medical treatments but also nursing interventions that address the client's specific QOL issues. If psychosocial issues are not fully explored, the client is likely to experience poorer satisfaction with the post-transplantation outcome. Performing meticulous medical care, providing long-term follow-up, and addressing physical and psychosocial QOL issues are all important components of management to improve both survival and QOL in the population of clients who have undergone organ transplantation.

THINKING CRITICALLY

1. A client has been receiving dialysis for several years while awaiting kidney transplantation. She is notified that a kidney donor has been found and that she should proceed to the hospital. What teaching will be completed before she goes to surgery? What psychosocial care should be offered?

Factors to Consider. What teaching and support will the family require? What are the ramifications if the donor kidney is found to be an unsuitable match for the client?

2. A client has recently undergone heart transplantation and is to be discharged from the hospital in 2 days. What client education should be completed? What education should be completed for the family?

Factors to Consider. What living arrangements are required for the client after discharge? What are the long-term concerns related to financial factors, quality of life issues, and long-term immunosuppressive therapy?

3. At a pretransplantation support group, a client makes the following statement: "I think I may need to buy my new organ." How should the nurse react to this statement? What ethical issues are raised by this statement?

Factors to Consider. Of what other ethical considerations regarding organ donation should the transplant nurse be aware?

Discussions for these questions can be found on the website.

BIBLIOGRAPHY

Citations appearing in red refer to primary research.

Citations appearing in blue refer to evidence-based practice guidelines and protocols.

1. American Heart Association. (2007). *Heart transplant: Statistics.* Retrieved 03/01/07 from www.americanheart.org/presenter.jhtml?identifier=4588.
2. American Liver Foundation. (2007). *Liver transplant.* Retrieved 03/01/07 from www.liverfoundation.org/db/articles/1016.
3. American Lung Association. (2007). *Lung transplants fact sheet.* Retrieved 03/01/07 from www.lungusa.org/site/apps/s/content.asp?c=dvLUK9OE&b=34706&ct=3052341.
4. Banner, N., Polak, J., & Yacoub, M. (2003). *Lung transplantation.* Cambridge: Cambridge University Press.
5. Barnard, C.N. (1967). A human cardiac transplant. *South African Medical Journal, 41,* 1271-1274.
6. Baumgartner, W. (2002). *Heart and lung transplantation* (2nd ed.). Philadelphia: Saunders.
7. Danovitch, G. (2005). *Handbook of kidney transplantation* (4th ed.). Philadelphia: Lippincott Williams & Wilkins.
8. Ehrle, R., Shafer, T., & Nelson, K. (1999). Referral, request, and consent for organ donation: Best practice—a blueprint for success. *Critical Care Nurse, 19*(2), 21-33.
9. Guthrie, C (Ed.) (1912). Applications of blood vessel surgery. In *Blood vessel surgery.* New York: Longmans, Green.
10. Hakim, N., & Papalois, V. (2003). *History of organ and cell transplantation.* River Edge, NJ: Imperial College Press.
11. Hakim, N., Stratta, R., & Gray, D. (2002). *Pancreas and islet transplantation.* New York: Oxford University Press.
12. Hornick, P., & Rose, M. (2006). *Transplantation immunology: Methods and protocols.* Totowa, NJ: Humana Press.
13. International Society for Heart and Lung Transplantation. (2003). *Twenty-third annual meeting and scientific sessions,* April 9-12, 2003, Vienna, Austria.
14. Jonsen, A. (2005). *Bioethics beyond the headlines: Who lives? Who dies? Who decides?.* Lanham, Md: Rowman & Littlefield.
15. Kaserman, D., & Barnett, A. (2002). *The U.S. organ procurement system: A prescription for reform.* Washington, DC: AEI Press.
16. Kirklin, J., & George, J. (2002). Immunosuppressive modalities. In J. Kirklin, J. Young, & D. McGiffin (Eds.), *Heart transplantation* (pp. 390-463). New York: Churchill Livingstone.
17. Kirklin, J., Young, J., & McGiffin, D. (2002). *Heart transplantation.* New York: Churchill Livingstone.
18. Kuo, P., Schroeder, R., & Johnson, L. (2001). *Clinical management of the transplant patient.* New York: Arnold.
19. Landsteiner, K. (1928). Cell antigens and individual specificity. *Journal of Immunology, 15,* 589-600.
20. Lucey, M., Neuberger, J., & Shaked, A. (2003). *Liver transplantation.* Georgetown, Tex: Landes Bioscience.
21. Maddrey, W., Schiff, E., & Sorrell, M. (2001). *Transplantation of the liver* (3rd ed.). Philadelphia: Lippincott Williams & Wilkins.
22. Mancuso, D. (2006). *Progress in kidney transplantation.* New York: Nova Science.
23. Medawar, P.B. (1945). A second study of the behavior and fate of skin homografts in rabbits: A report to the War Wounds Committee of the Medical Research Council. *Journal of Anatomy,69,* 157-176.
24. Morris, P. (2001). *Kidney transplantation: Principles and practice* (5th ed.). Philadelphia: Saunders.
25. National Kidney Foundation. *Transplantation.* Retrieved 03/01/07 from www.kidney.org/atoz/atozTopic.cfm?topic=3.
26. Norman, D., & Turka, L. (2001). *Primer on transplantation* (2nd ed.). Mt. Laurel, NJ: American Society of Transplantation.
27. Organ Procurement and Transplantation Network (OPTN). (2007). *Data: Organ datasource: Kidney.* Retrieved 03/01/07 from www.optn.org/organdatasource/about.asp?display=kidney.
28. Palmer, R. (2006). Surgical innovations: Improving the quality of life. *Clinics in Geriatric Medicine, 22*(3), 499-734.
29. Parker, J., & Parker, P. (2004). *Heart transplant: A medical dictionary, bibliography and annotated research guide to internet references.* San Diego: ICON Health Publications.
30. Petty, M. (2003). Lung and heart-lung transplantation: Implications for nursing care when hospitalized outside the transplant center. *MEDSURG Nursing, 12*(4), 250-260.
31. Starzl, T.E., et al. (1963). Homotransplantation of the liver in humans. *Surgery, Gynecology and Obstetrics, 117,* 659-676.
32. Smith, S. (2002). Immunosuppressive therapies in organ transplantation. In S. Smith (Ed.), *Organ transplantation: Concepts, issues, practice, and outcomes.* Available at www.medscape.com.viewarticle/437182.
33. Task Force on Organ Transplantation. (1986). *Organ transplantation: Issues and recommendations* (HRP-0906976). Rockville, Md: Health Resources and Services Administration.
34. United Network of Organ Sharing (UNOS). (2006). *Annual Report of the U.S. Scientific Registry for Transplant Recipients and Organ Procurement and Transplantation Network—Transplant Data.* Richmond, Va: Author. Retrieved 11/20/07 from www.unos.org/data/annualReport.asp.
35. U.S. Department of Health and Human Services. (2006). *Annual Report of the U.S. Organ Procurement Transplantation Network and the Scientific Registry of Transplant Recipients: Transplant Data 1995-2005.* Rockville, Md: Health and Human Services Administration, Healthcare Systems Bureau, Division of Transplantation, United Network of Organ Sharing (UNOS) OPTN and Scientific Registry Data. Retrieved 03/01/07 from www.hrsa.gov/data/.
36. Urden, L., Stacy, K., & Lough, M. (2006). Transplantation. In L. Urden, K Stacey., & M. Lough (Eds.), *Thelan's critical care nursing: Diagnosis and management* (5th ed., pp. 1076-1127). St. Louis: Mosby.
37. White-Williams, C. (2002). Lung transplantation. In S. Smith (Ed.), *Organ transplantation: Concepts, issues, practice, and outcomes.* Available at www.medscape.com/viewpublication704.

evolve Did you remember to check out the bonus material on the Evolve website and the CD-ROM, including NCLEX®-Examination Style Review Questions, Open-Book Quizzes, and Chapter Review Audio Podcasts?

http://evolve.elsevier.com/Black/medsurg

CHAPTER 81

Management of Clients with Shock and Multisystem Disorders

Louise Nelson LaFramboise

SHOCK

Shock is a complex clinical syndrome that may occur at any time and in any place. It is a life-threatening condition often requiring team action by many health care providers, including nurses, physicians, laboratory technicians, pharmacists, and respiratory therapists. Shock causes thousands of deaths and unknown numbers of permanent injuries each year. The economic impact of shock is staggering, with annual health care costs for treatment of shock in the billions of dollars. Because shock is potentially lethal, debilitating, and costly, it is essential that nurses identify clients at risk for shock, recognize the early assessment findings indicating shock, and initiate appropriate interventions before shock ensues.

Shock is defined as failure of the circulatory system to maintain adequate perfusion of vital organs. Disorders leading to inadequate tissue perfusion result in decreased oxygenation at the cellular level. Inadequate oxygenation results in anaerobic cellular metabolism and accumulated waste products in cells. If this condition is untreated, cell death and organ death occur.

Classification

Shock is commonly divided into three major classifications:

- Hypovolemic
- Cardiogenic
- Distributive

Hypovolemic shock is due to inadequate circulating blood volume resulting from hemorrhage with actual blood loss, burns with massive shifts of fluids due to movement of plasma proteins into interstitial spaces, and fluid shifts or dehydration, with or without loss of fluid volume. Hypovolemic shock is the most common type of shock and develops when the intravascular volume decreases to the point where compensatory mechanisms are unable to maintain organ and tissue perfusion.

Cardiogenic shock is due to inadequate pumping action of the heart. The heart muscle can be diseased as a result of primary cardiac muscle dysfunction or mechanical obstruction of blood flow caused by myocardial infarction (MI), valvular insufficiency caused by disease or trauma, cardiac dysrhythmias, or an obstructive condition such as pericardial tamponade or pulmonary embolus. The clinical definition of cardiogenic shock is decreased cardiac output and evidence of tissue hypoxia in the presence of adequate intravascular volume. Hemodynamic criteria for cardiogenic shock are sustained hypotension (systolic blood pressure <90 mm Hg for at least 30 min) and a reduced cardiac index (<2.2 L/min/m^2) in the presence of elevated pulmonary capillary occlusion pressure (>15 mm Hg). Other manifestations of tissue hypoperfusion include oliguria (<30 ml/hour), cool extremities, and altered mentation. Cardiogenic shock occurs in 10% to 15% of all clients after MI and carries an associated death rate of up to 80%. Cardiogenic shock after an MI usually occurs when 40% or more of the myocardium has been damaged.

The term *obstructive shock* is sometimes used to include conditions that lead to a sudden obstruction of blood flow (e.g., cardiac tamponade, tension pneumothorax, pulmonary embolism). Obstructive causes are discussed under the topic of cardiogenic shock because the ability of the heart to pump effectively is the primary problem.

Distributive shock (also called *vasogenic shock*) is due to changes in blood vessel tone that increase the size of the vascular space without an increase in the circulating blood volume. The result is a relative hypovolemia (total fluid volume remains the same but is redistributed). Distributive shock is further divided into three types:

- *Anaphylactic shock* is a severe hypersensitivity reaction resulting in massive systemic vasodilation.
- *Neurogenic shock,* or interference with nervous system control of the blood vessels, can occur with conditions such as spinal cord injury (especially cervical spine injury), spinal anesthesia, or severe vasovagal reactions caused by pain or psychic trauma. Some amount of neurogenic shock is seen with all spinal cord injuries. More dramatic cases of neurogenic shock are seen with cervical spine injuries. The duration of neurogenic shock is usually 1 to 6 weeks as long as there is no irreparable cord injury, but recovery may take as long as 12 months.
- *Septic shock* is caused by a release of vasoactive substances. Current theories suggest there is a cascade of interactions between immune cells that happens rapidly and leads to microcirculatory alterations. Septic shock is the most common cause of mortality in intensive care units. Even with the best treatment, mortality ranges from 15% in clients with sepsis to 40% to 60% in clients with septic shock.

Etiology and Risk Factors

All causes of shock focus on some component of blood distribution throughout the body. There can be an insufficient quantity of blood (hypovolemic shock), an incompetent pump (cardiogenic shock), or an ineffective delivery of blood (distributive shock).

Hypovolemic Shock

The primary event precipitating hypovolemic shock is a large reduction in the circulating blood volume so that the body's metabolic needs cannot be met. Hypovolemic shock may be due to a loss of plasma or blood. Conditions that may cause a reduction in circulating blood volume include hemorrhage, burns, and dehydration.

Health promotion activities to prevent hypovolemic shock include client education to avoid injuries that would put someone at risk for hypovolemic shock. Health maintenance activities are the use of oxygen and maintenance of fluid and electrolyte balance. To restore health, monitor the client with telemetry and hemodynamic monitoring, and give vasoactive medications and blood and fluid replacements as ordered.

Hemorrhage. Hemorrhage is the loss of blood. Clinical manifestations may begin to appear with a blood volume deficit of 15% to 25%, or about 500 to 1500 ml in an adult with a normal circulating volume. Shock fully develops if a previously healthy client loses about one third of the normal circulating blood volume of 5 L. Wounds of the chest, abdomen, and thighs can lead to hemorrhagic shock.

The loss of smaller amounts of blood may cause shock in clients less able to compensate rapidly (e.g., older people with decreased vascular tone and impaired cardiac function). The extent to which shock develops after blood loss also depends on the length of time over which the blood loss occurs. Clients experiencing slow blood loss over a period of days or weeks tolerate their blood loss better than clients whose blood loss occurs rapidly over minutes or hours. Hypovolemic shock following trauma is typically the result of hemorrhage. The classes of hemorrhage and the associated assessment findings are listed in Table 81-1.

Burns. Hypovolemic shock produced by burns occurs most often in people with large partial-thickness or

TABLE 81–1   Assessment Findings and Classifications of Acute Hemorrhage*

Assessment Finding	Class I	Class II	Class III	Class IV
Blood loss (%)	<15	15-30	30-40	>40
Blood loss (ml)	<750	750-1500	1500-2000	>2000
Pulse rate (beats/min)	<100	>100	>120	>140
Respiratory rate (breaths/min)	Normal (14-20)	20-30	30-40	>35
Blood pressure	Normal	Normal	Decreased	Decreased
Pulse pressure	Normal or increased	Decreased	Decreased	Decreased
Central nervous system/mental status	Slightly anxious	Mildly anxious	Anxious, confused	Confused, lethargic
Urine output (ml/hr)	>30	20-30	5-15	Negligible
Intravenous fluid replacement	Crystalloid at 3 ml/1 ml of blood loss	Crystalloid at 3 ml/1 ml of blood loss	Crystalloid plus blood at 3 ml/1 ml of blood loss	Crystalloid plus blood at 3 ml/1 ml of blood loss

*Assumes a normal 70-kg man.
Data from American College of Surgeons Committee on Trauma. (1997). *Advanced trauma life support student manual* (p. 98). Chicago: Author.

full-thickness burns. It is caused primarily by a shift of plasma from the vascular space into the interstitial space. In addition to these fluid losses or shifts, the client may have cardiac dysfunction that is due to the presence of *myocardial depressant factor (MDF),* a polypeptide (see Myocardial Deterioration). MDF affects the contractility of cardiac muscle by depressing myocardial muscle function. The result is impaired cardiac output, even in the presence of a normal circulating volume. Shock related to burns is discussed in Chapter 50.

Other causes of hypovolemic shock that may produce fluid shifts similar to those in burns include nephrotic syndrome, severe crush injuries, starvation, surgery, and conditions causing plasma fluids to accumulate in the abdominal cavity (e.g., cirrhosis of the liver, pancreatitis, bowel obstruction).

Dehydration. Shock may also occur either from reduced oral fluid intake or from significant fluid losses (e.g., rigorous exercise causing fluid loss from sweating and insensible fluid loss through the respiratory tract and in hot environments). Loss of fluid may occur in people with excessive urine output or prolonged vomiting or diarrhea, leading to dehydration-induced hypovolemic shock. Clients with chronic illnesses, especially older people, may be at increased risk because of impaired recognition of thirst, an inability to obtain fluids, inadequate maintenance of chronic conditions (e.g., increased blood glucose levels with diabetes), or inadequate monitoring of therapeutic regimens (e.g., diuretic-induced dehydration). With prolonged fluid deficit, all compartments—intravascular, interstitial, and intracellular—are depleted.

Cardiogenic Shock

Cardiogenic shock results primarily from an inability of heart muscle to function adequately or from mechanical obstructions of blood flow to or from the heart. The major cause of cardiogenic shock is ischemic heart disease of the right and left ventricle. As with other causes of shock, the lack of blood flow decreases tissue and organ perfusion.

Myocardial Infarction. Impaired heart muscle action is most often caused by MI (see Chapter 58). The area of dead or dying tissue that occurs with infarction impairs contractility of the myocardium, and cardiac output decreases. Impaired myocardial contractility may also occur with blunt cardiac trauma, cardiomyopathy, and heart failure.

Prevention of cardiogenic shock related to MI begins with health promotion activities directed at client education to decrease the risk factors associated with coronary artery disease (e.g., increasing exercise and modifying dietary intake). Supportive oxygenation and administration of inotropic agents and vasodilators are health maintenance activities. An intra-aortic balloon pump (IABP) (see Chapter 56) may be needed for health restoration.

Clients in cardiogenic shock may also develop some degree of hypovolemic shock. This is most often due to the therapeutic use of diuretics or to edema in the extremities or other dependent areas (caused by inadequate cardiac pumping activity and venous congestion). Clients in hypovolemic shock are also at risk for cardiogenic shock. The myocardium normally receives its blood supply during diastole. When the heart rate increases to compensate for the decreased blood volume to maintain cardiac output, diastole is shortened, sometimes leading to insufficient time for the coronary arteries to fill with blood. Because these arteries supply blood to the myocardium, the myocardial oxygen supply is impaired. The increased heart rate also increases the need of the myocardium for oxygen, predisposing the myocardium to injury because of the decreased blood flow and resultant decreased oxygen supply. In addition, the decreased venous return associated with hypovolemia results in decreased coronary artery perfusion and inadequate oxygenation of the myocardium.

Obstructive Conditions. Several types of mechanical obstructions of blood flow may cause cardiogenic shock:

1. *Large pulmonary embolism.* An *embolus* is usually the result of a blood clot that breaks loose in a person with deep vein thrombosis (DVT). This embolus travels through the venous system to the right side of the heart and into the pulmonary artery. The size of the embolus determines at what point it lodges in the pulmonary artery. A large embolus can inhibit perfusion of a major portion of the lung, resulting in an increased workload for the right ventricle.
2. *Pericardial tamponade* is an accumulation of blood or fluid in the pericardial space that compresses the myocardium and interferes with the ability of the myocardium to expand.
3. A *tension pneumothorax* is a significant amount of air in the pleural space that compresses the heart and great vessels, thus interfering with venous return to the heart.

Other Causes of Cardiogenic Shock. Most diseases of the heart have the potential to cause cardiogenic shock. They include (1) cardiac valvular insufficiency from trauma or disease, (2) myocardial aneurysms (usually resulting from previous MI or congenital abnormalities), (3) rupture of a valvular papillary muscle, (4) ventricular rupture, (5) aortic stenosis, (6) mitral regurgitation, (7) cardiac dysrhythmias, (8) infectious and inflammatory processes such as myocarditis and endocarditis, (9) pulmonary hypertension, and (10) toxic drugs.

Distributive (Vasogenic) Shock

Distributive shock results from inadequate vascular tone. Blood volume remains normal, but the size of the vascular space increases dramatically because of massive vasodilation. The result is maldistribution of the blood because of decreased blood pressure (BP) and lack of blood returning to the heart; this is why it is often referred to as "relative" hypovolemia. The volume of blood remains constant, but the blood has pooled because of increased capacity of the vascular system. After extensive vasodilation, the BP, return of venous blood to the heart, and cardiac output are decreased. As with other forms of shock, tissue anoxia and cell destruction result. The massive vasodilation present with distributive shock has several major causes.

Acute Allergic Reaction (Anaphylactic Shock). Anaphylactic shock occurs as a result of an acute allergic reaction from exposure to a substance to which the client has been sensitized. Common sensitizing agents are penicillin, penicillin derivatives, bee stings, chemotherapy, latex, chocolate, strawberries, peanuts, snake venom, iodine-based contrast for x-ray studies, seafood, and nonsteroidal anti-inflammatory drugs (NSAIDs).

Re-exposure to the foreign substance results in the offending antigen binding to previously synthesized immunoglobulins (i.e., IgE) on the mast cell. This binding causes the release of histamine (see Chapter 76). Manifestations include massive vasodilation, urticaria (hives), laryngeal edema, and bronchial constriction. Without prompt treatment, a person with anaphylactic shock will die from cardiovascular collapse and respiratory failure.

To help prevent the onset of anaphylactic shock, teach clients to avoid precipitators and to use an epinephrine injection (e.g., EpiPen). Encouraging clients to wear medical alert bracelets and to seek allergy desensitization also decreases their potential for anaphylactic shock.

Spinal Cord Injury (Neurogenic Shock). With injury to the cervical spine, commonly with injuries around the T6 level, the autonomic nervous system is affected. Below the level of injury there is blocking of sympathetic nervous stimulation, and the parasympathetic system acts unopposed. This unopposed stimulation causes vasodilation, decreased venous return, decreased cardiac output, and decreased tissue perfusion. Neurogenic shock is manifested by the triad of hypotension, bradycardia, and hypothermia.

Teaching clients safety measures may help prevent spinal cord injury and neurogenic shock. After injury, protect the client's spine, maintain the airway and breathing, provide circulatory support, and provide for thermoregulation. Health restoration involves rehabilitation when the client is stable.

Infection (Septic Shock). *Sepsis* is the presence of infection and activation of the inflammatory cascade. Systemic inflammatory response syndrome (SIRS) is a term used to define this clinical condition, and it is considered present if abnormalities exist in two of the following four clinical parameters: (1) body temperature, (2) heart rate, (3) respiratory rate, and (4) peripheral leukocyte count. Sepsis is defined as the presence of SIRS in the setting of infection. Severe sepsis is defined as sepsis with evidence of end-organ dysfunction as a result of hypoperfusion. Septic shock is defined as sepsis with persistent hypotension despite fluid resuscitation and resulting tissue hypoperfusion.

Bacteremia is defined as the presence of viable bacteria in blood. Bacteremia may be primary (without an identifiable focus of infection) or, more often, secondary (with a focus of infection). Sepsis is a disease seen most frequently in older adults and in those with co-morbid conditions that predispose them to infection. Clients who are immunocompromised are especially at high risk and include those with cancer who are receiving chemotherapeutic agents, those with end-stage renal or liver disease, those with advanced HIV, or those receiving steroids for chronic conditions. Clients with indwelling vascular catheters and urinary catheters are particularly at high risk. Although sepsis is commonly associated with bacterial infection, bacteremia does not need to be present to activate the massive inflammatory response that results in severe sepsis. In fact, fewer than 50% of cases of sepsis are associated with bacteremia.

Encouraging clients to treat infections immediately and completely may help reduce the incidence of septic shock. Older and immunocompromised clients should be monitored closely for infection, and treatment should begin immediately when infection is diagnosed. Identify high-risk clients and implement measures to prevent shock whenever possible.

Pathophysiology

Shock occurs when there is not adequate circulating volume to maintain aerobic metabolism in the cells. Adequate circulating volume is dependent on three interrelated components of the cardiovascular system: (1) the heart, (2) vascular tone, and (3) blood volume. Blood flows throughout the body because of its driving pressure as it leaves the left ventricle (LV). If there is a reduction in the volume of blood or if the heart muscle cannot pump effectively, cardiac output falls.

Vascular tone refers to the degree of constriction by the smooth muscle in the arteriole. The size of the body's larger blood vessels is regulated by the autonomic nervous system, but this is not true for the microcirculation. Arteriole and capillary sphincters are separate mechanisms governed by different controls. Typically, blood flow through the capillary bed is influenced by the varying needs of the cells located near the vessel. The capillaries open on demand of the cells adjacent to them.

A minor impairment in one component is compensated for by the other two, whereas prolonged or severe impairments lead to shock. Some of the problems with decreased organ and tissue perfusion in shock are due to failure of the normal mechanisms. If one of the three components of circulation fails, other parts of the system initiate compensatory mechanisms. For example, vasoconstriction and increased cardiac output may be used to compensate for decreased volume. As long as two of these factors can maintain a satisfactory compensatory action, adequate blood circulation can be maintained even though the third factor is not functioning normally. If compensatory mechanisms fail or if more than one of the three factors necessary for adequate circulation malfunctions, circulatory failure results and shock develops.

The systemic circulatory bed and the microcirculatory bed apparently do not have sensing devices that would allow a unified, coordinated response throughout the entire circulation. Thus events occurring within one bed do not influence events in the other. The relative autonomy of the microcirculation and the lack of coordination between it and the systemic circulation are important in determining the course of events in shock. Each type of shock progresses uniquely; the following sections discuss of the pathophysiology of each type.

Cardiogenic Shock

Cardiogenic shock is failure of the left ventricle to pump adequate blood volume. When cardiac output falls, the body compensates by releasing catecholamines (epinephrine and norepinephrine) to increase heart rate and systemic vascular resistance to increase venous return. However, these are only temporary measures to restore blood pressure and tissue blood flow to vital organs (heart and brain). The diseased heart cannot maintain its own myocardial tissue oxygenation, which results in a spiral of decreased cardiac output, hypotension, and further myocardial ischemia.

Anaphylactic Shock

Anaphylaxis is a systemic type I hypersensitivity reaction from the sudden release of inflammatory mediators from mast cells and basophils. When a sensitized client comes in contact with an antigen, IgE is stimulated and the mast cells and basophils release large amounts of histamine. Histamine leads to vasodilation, bronchial constriction, bronchorrhea, pruritus, laryngeal edema, and angioedema. Laryngeal edema obstructs the airway.

Septic Shock

Sepsis begins with the unchecked growth of organisms at a tissue site. About 50% of clients with septic shock have

bacteremia, with gram-negative rods and gram-positive organisms being the most common agents. The organisms themselves start the disease. Endotoxins (also called lipopolysaccharides) are produced by gram-negative organisms. Gram-positive cocci also produce exotoxins. Host resistance and organism virulence are both factors that determine the body's response. Initially, there is an overwhelming inflammatory response to the microbes that is regulated by tumor necrosis factor (TNF), interferon, and the interleukins. In addition, complement is activated. These factors promote the systemic inflammatory response. As a result, mediators with vasodilatory and endotoxic properties are released systemically, including prostaglandins, thromboxane A_2, and nitric oxide. This results in vasodilation and endothelial damage, which leads to hypoperfusion and capillary leakage. In addition, cytokines activate the coagulation pathway, resulting in capillary microthrombi and end-organ ischemia.

Stages of Shock

Nonprogressive Stage. During the initial or nonprogressive stage of shock, cardiac output is slightly decreased because of the loss of actual or relative blood volume. During this stage, the body's compensatory mechanisms can maintain BP within a normal to low-normal range and can maintain perfusion to the vital organs. During the compensatory phase, the systemic circulation and microcirculation work together in a hyperdynamic state. This hyperdynamic state leads to an increase in lactic acid levels. Both levels of circulation undergo a major readjustment in which their activities are coordinated to preserve the entire system. Figure 81-1 illustrates these readjustments.

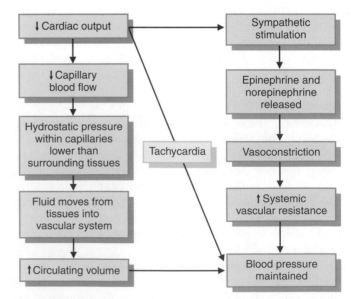

■ **FIGURE 81–1** Nonprogressive stage of shock. Regardless of the cause, decreased cardiac output is generally the stimulus that precipitates the body's response to compensate for the hypovolemia (relative or actual) to maintain blood pressure.

Progressive Stage. If shock and the compensatory vaso-constriction persist, the body begins to decompensate and the systemic circulation and microcirculation no longer work in unison. As vasoconstriction continues, the supply of oxygenated blood to the tissues is reduced. This results in anaerobic metabolism and further lactic acidosis. Acidosis and the increasing $Paco_2$ cause the microcirculation to dilate. This dilation causes decreased venous return and decreased circulation of reoxygenated blood.

Lactic acidosis also causes increased capillary permeability and relaxation of the capillary sphincters. Relaxation of the sphincters allows increased blood in the capillaries and increased capillary pressure. This increased pressure along with the increased capillary permeability allows fluid to move out of the vascular space and back into the tissues. In doing so, the microcirculation reverses its pattern and tries to secure for itself (and the tissue it supplies) more of the limited supply of available blood. Thus the blood supply is progressively retained in the capillary bed, and blood pools in the microcirculation. Because the cells demand greater perfusion time, many or most of the capillaries remain open at any one time, increasing the vascular space in the microcirculation.

Increased vascular capacity, decreased blood volume, or decreased heart action reduces the mean arterial pressure (MAP). In turn, the pressure gradient for the venous return of blood decreases. This also contributes to venous pooling of blood, decreased venous return to the heart, and decreased cardiac output.

Because there are no feedback systems within the body to change this pattern, this cycle of events becomes progressively more severe. Eventually, the circulation is totally disrupted. Once the vascular space enlarges (because of vasodilation of the microcirculation), even normal blood volumes cannot fill all of these vessels. The result is a low central venous pressure (CVP) (except in cardiogenic shock) and inadequate venous return to the right side of the heart, with a further decrease in cardiac output.

This resultant decrease in circulating volume and capillary flow does not allow adequate perfusion and oxygenation of the vital organs. With the prolonged decrease in capillary blood flow, the tissues become hypoxic. This cycle of events is illustrated in Figure 81-2.

Irreversible Stage. The irreversible stage of shock occurs if the cycle of inadequate tissue perfusion is not interrupted. The shock state becomes progressively more severe, even though the initial cause of the shock is not itself becoming more severe. Cellular ischemia and necrosis lead to organ failure and death.

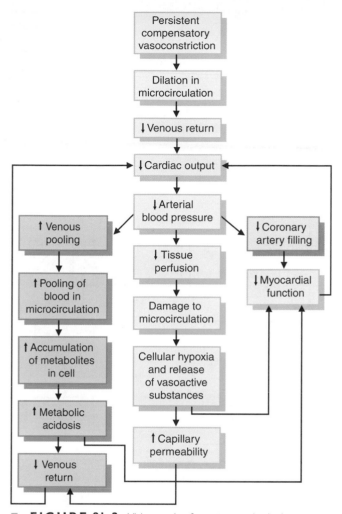

■ FIGURE 81–2   Vicious cycle of events occurring in the progressive stage of shock. The shock syndrome can be initiated anywhere in the cycle depending on the precipitating cause (e.g., impaired myocardial function because of myocardial infarction, blood loss caused by trauma, or the release of vasoactive toxins as a result of sepsis). Hypovolemic shock resulting from blood loss, for example, results in decreased arterial blood pressure, setting in motion a cascade of events that worsen the shock state.

Systemic Effects of Shock

Shock affects every system within the body. Equally important to understanding the cellular level of shock is understanding what happens to the various organs (Figure 81-3).

Respiratory System. Getting oxygen in *(ventilation)* and delivering oxygenated blood to the tissues *(perfusion)* are crucial for survival. Shock produces prolonged circulatory insufficiency that creates variable and inadequate perfusion of certain organs and tissues, particularly at the microcirculation level. Circulatory deprivation results in tissue hypoxia and anoxia. Hypoxia and anoxia can be tolerated for a short time. As the time lengthens, the chances of recovery diminish. A lack of oxygen appears to initiate the irreversible stage of shock. The greater the

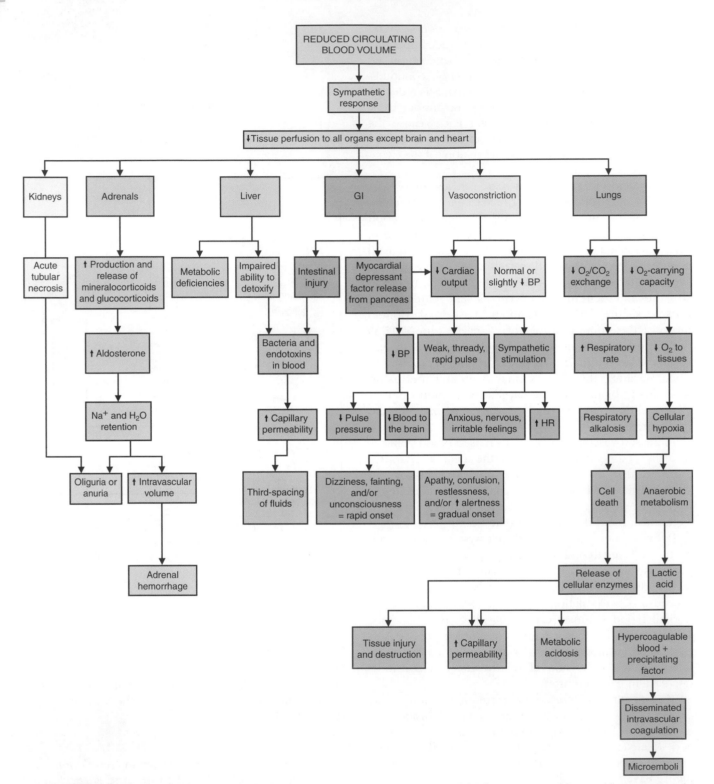

■ **FIGURE 81–3** Systemic effects of shock. The lack of blood flow is compensated by constricting flow to nonessential organs (all organs except the brain and heart).

difference between the amount of oxygen available and the amount needed, the more rapidly irreversible shock develops. If sufficient oxygen is available to the cells to meet the body's needs, irreversible shock is less likely to occur.

Respiratory failure continues to be a major cause of death in shock, despite many advances in shock prevention, early recognition, and management. The magnitude of this problem surfaced during the Vietnam War era when soldiers sustaining massive injuries and profound blood loss were successfully resuscitated, only to die several days later of acute respiratory distress syndrome (ARDS) (see Chapter 63). Although ARDS remains the greatest contributing factor to respiratory failure, other causes of respiratory failure during shock include aspiration and loss of neurologic control of breathing.

Acid-Base Balance. Oxygen and nutrients are essential to life because they synthesize adenosine triphosphate (ATP). ATP is the ultimate source of energy for life processes. When oxygen is not present, ATP is produced through *anaerobic metabolism*. Although production of ATP in this manner is a useful emergency measure, it is inefficient compared with the normal process of *aerobic* (oxidative) *metabolism*. Anaerobic metabolism produces anaerobic metabolites, such as lactic acid (which causes intracellular acidity with consequent cellular damage) and substrates of the adenylic acid system (which depress the heart) (see Figure 81-3).

In response to the chemoreceptors sensing decreased pH, the rate and depth of respirations are increased to "blow off" (exhale) CO_2 to compensate for the metabolic acidosis. This results in respiratory alkalosis. However, the cellular hypoxia is caused not by inadequate ventilation but rather by inadequate tissue perfusion. Therefore the increased respiratory effort does little to correct the problem.

Because lactic acid is not exhaled, it accumulates in tissue fluids, which become increasingly acidic. Metabolic acidosis is eventually produced. During metabolic acidosis, blood pH and bicarbonate levels decrease. Pyruvate, lactate, phosphate, and sulfate levels increase. Unless circulation is restored, the acidotic reaction resulting from metabolic acidosis ultimately kills the cells. The buildup of lactic acid causes such a severe local acidosis that cellular enzymes are inactivated. Cells soon die.

Respiratory alkalosis or *respiratory acidosis* (induced by pulmonary ventilatory or diffusion changes) may be superimposed on the metabolic acidosis. As perfusion and oxygen delivery to the tissues decrease, cellular energy production decreases. To compensate, cells increase anaerobic metabolism, which results in the buildup of lactic acid in the cell. As the pH of the cells decreases, lysosomes within the cell explode, releasing powerful, destructive enzymes. These enzymes destroy the cellular membrane and digest the cell contents. Once this process begins, the cellular changes are irreversible. The final result is cellular death (Figure 81-4).

Lysosomal Enzymes. Lysosomal enzymes are released from dead cells undergoing autolysis. They are also released from injured cells. Lysosomal enzymes become most active in an acid pH range. Thus as long as normal acid-base balance is maintained within the body, these enzymes are repressed within normal cells. During shock, however, the accompanying metabolic acidosis accelerates the activation of these enzymes in hypoxic tissues. The activation of lysosomal hydrolases within the cells and their release into the circulation markedly exacerbate the tissue injury that occurs during shock. The release of active lysosomal proteases and other enzymes from damaged tissue into the bloodstream and their action on extracellular and intracellular structures probably contribute to the progression of injury from cell to cell.

Cardiovascular System

Myocardial Deterioration. As shock progresses, the heart deteriorates. Cardiac deterioration is one of the major causes of death in shock. Although the exact cause of myocardial depression is unclear, much attention has been directed at MDF. MDF, a polypeptide with vasoactive properties, is released in response to ischemia of

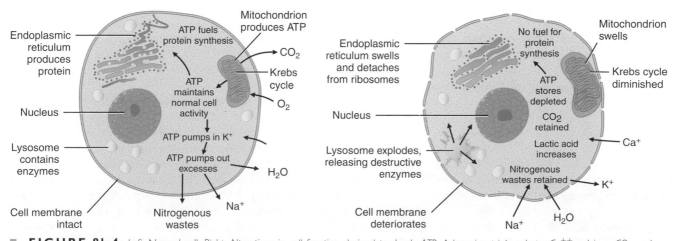

■ **FIGURE 81–4** *Left,* Normal cell. *Right,* Alterations in cell function during late shock. *ATP,* Adenosine triphosphate; *Ca++,* calcium; *CO2,* carbon dioxide; *H2O,* water; *Na+,* sodium; *O2,* oxygen.

the gastrointestinal (GI) tract. It causes a significant reduction in cardiac output, even in the presence of a normal circulating volume of blood. Another factor contributing to cardiac deterioration may be myocardial zonal lesions, which appear in the myocardium after ischemia or infarction. Cells in these areas do not fully repolarize and thus interfere with the usual efficient electrical conduction in the heart, which results in impaired contraction and possibly cardiac failure.

Cardiac depression is often compensated by the large cardiac reserve of a normal person. Because of this reserve, the heart can deteriorate to less than one third (sometimes less than one fifth) of its normal pumping strength without measurable evidence of cardiac failure.

Disseminated Intravascular Coagulation. During shock, tissue hypoxia results from the sluggish movement of blood in the capillaries. Anaerobic metabolism increases the production of lactic acid. The slow-moving acidic blood is hypercoagulable; however, it does not coagulate unless a clot-initiating factor is present. Such factors include bacterial endotoxins and thromboplastin of red blood cells (liberated by hemolysis). Hemolysis (destruction of red blood cells with the liberation of hemoglobin) accompanies trauma, especially when massive crushing injury occurs. When any of these factors is present along with the stagnant, acidic blood of shock, widespread intravascular clotting may occur in the vessels. This disorder is called *disseminated intravascular coagulation* (DIC) (see Chapter 75).

DIC is associated with multiple thrombi or emboli that are deposited in the microvascular circulation, with resultant organ obstruction and increased tissue ischemia. As blood attempts to flow through partially obstructed vessels, widespread hemolysis may occur. When red blood cells are destroyed, hemoglobin is again liberated. Anemia occurs because the liberated hemoglobin is excreted by the kidneys.

Because of the inappropriate clotting that occurs with DIC, the body attempts to reverse the process by breaking down clots. However, clots are destroyed throughout the body, not just the inappropriately formed clots. This results in bleeding in areas previously sealed by clots (e.g., venipuncture sites, vascular leaks in the brain). As DIC progresses, clotting factors are depleted, causing an inability to form normal clots in the presence of bleeding.

Treatment of the precipitating cause, anticoagulant therapy, and replacement of clotting factors must be started as soon as possible for maximal effectiveness. DIC is a serious complication that occurs in almost 40% of clients in septic shock and is often fatal.

Vasoconstriction. Sluggish circulation decreases the removal of CO_2 from the tissues. Increased levels of CO_2 dilate arterioles located in active tissues and constrict those in nonactive tissues. Because of the heart's increased activity, excessive CO_2 is produced in the myocardium. Increased concentration of CO_2 directly dilates the coronary arteries leading to the myocardium, which allows the myocardium to receive more arterial blood. CO_2 is also a powerful stimulant of the vasoconstrictor center in the sympathetic nervous system. With vasoconstriction of nonactive tissues, blood is shunted to the more active tissues, which have a greater immediate need.

Vasoactive Substances. Vasoactive substances (see below) are highly variable in promoting vasoconstriction or vasodilation in a person experiencing shock. The influence they exert may be altered by factors such as pH, the specific tissue (e.g., heart, lung), the presence of drugs or other substances, serum electrolyte levels, and sensitivity of the end organ.

Catecholamines. Catecholamines, such as epinephrine and norepinephrine, are present early in shock and are related to the fight-or-flight response. Their general effects are to increase blood flow to the brain, heart, and striated (skeletal) muscle and to decrease blood flow to the skin, kidneys, and splanchnic bed. Although the initial effect of vasoconstriction in the skin, kidneys, and splanchnic bed (GI tract) increases the intravascular volume, sustained vasoconstriction contributes to stagnant hypoxia and cellular death.

Vasoactive Polypeptides. Among the more important vasoactive polypeptides that appear to play significant roles in shock are the following:

1. *Histamine.* Histamine causes vasodilation, increased capillary permeability, bronchoconstriction, coronary vasodilation, and cutaneous reactions (flares, wheals). The effects of histamine are especially obvious in anaphylactic and septic shock.
2. *Bradykinin.* A kinin peptide, bradykinin produces vasodilation, increased capillary permeability, smooth muscle relaxation, pain, and infiltration of an area with leukocytes. Kinins appear to be most active in late shock. They may be a factor in the development of pulmonary insufficiency associated with shock.
3. *Angiotensin.* Angiotensin results from the action of renal renin on angiotensinogen. This potent substance causes vasoconstriction and increased vascular resistance. Although similar to norepinephrine in effect, angiotensin may produce fewer negative effects. Its role in sodium and water retention (through the stimulation of aldosterone secretion) is discussed under Adrenal Response.
4. *MDF.* MDF is a vasoactive polypeptide that contributes to cardiac failure in clients in shock by depressing cardiac muscle contraction.

Neuroendocrine System

General Adaptation Syndrome Response. Neuroendocrine responses during shock are defensive reactions that occur during the body's stage of resistance in the general adaptation syndrome (GAS). Because the length of the stage of resistance varies among people and is determined by the body's ability to compensate for its deficiencies, one person may be able to combat shock longer than another. For example, a previously healthy person may have a longer stage of resistance against shock compared with a person who is debilitated before shock develops. Various components of the sympathoadrenal (sympathetic part of the autonomic nervous system and adrenal medulla) response to a major stressor are shown in Figure 81-5.

Adrenal Response. Basic features of the neuroendocrine responses include (1) the release of epinephrine and norepinephrine from the adrenal medulla (which results in increased respiratory and heart rates, increased BP, increased blood flow to organs, decreased blood flow to peripheral tissues), and (2) the release of mineralocorticoids (which control fluid and electrolyte balance) and glucocorticoids (which increase blood glucose levels and reduce pain) from the adrenal cortex.

Increased production of adrenocortical mineralocorticoid hormones occurs. The main mineralocorticoids—aldosterone and desoxycorticosterone—help increase intravascular fluid volume by stimulating the kidneys to retain sodium and water. The renal tubular conservation of sodium occurs with any type of fluid loss or blood volume depletion. Aldosterone is essential to the conservation of sodium. Because water is retained in the body along with sodium, urine excretion is diminished during shock. This fluid is retained in the bloodstream to increase blood volume. Increasing the volume of blood in this way is aimed at increasing venous return, cardiac output, and BP.

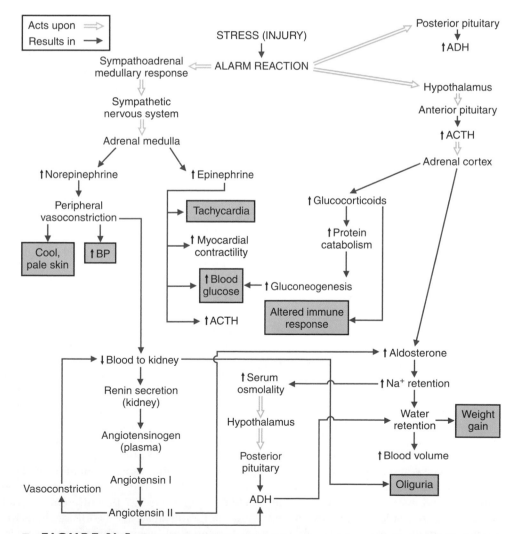

■ **FIGURE 81–5** Components of the neuroendocrine response to a major stressor. Readily observed clinical manifestations as well as laboratory values are indicated by the boxes. *ACTH,* Adrenocorticotropic hormone; *ADH,* antidiuretic hormone; *BP,* blood pressure.

Pituitary Response. Of major importance in regulating water and sodium balance are aldosterone and ADH, also called *vasopressin*. ADH is produced by the posterior pituitary gland. The osmolality (osmotic concentration) of blood increases with dehydration. This stimulates osmoreceptors in the hypothalamus to release ADH from the posterior pituitary gland. ADH is carried via the blood to the kidneys, where it causes the body to retain water.

Metabolic Response. In general, the hormonal response to stress rapidly provides fuel for the body's various tissues, organs, and systems. These fuels (e.g., amino acids, fatty acids, glucose) are produced by the breakdown of food. These substances are then chemically converted into energy, resulting in the formation of ATP. ATP is the main source of energy produced and used inside the body's cells.

The glucocorticoids, particularly hydrocortisone, mobilize energy stores. During the initial phase of shock, the body's small stores of available carbohydrate are rapidly depleted. It then becomes necessary to mobilize protein and fat stores to meet the body's energy requirements. Protein catabolism and negative nitrogen balance occur as part of the metabolic response because of gluconeogenesis (resulting from glucocorticoid action) and starvation.

Neurologic Response. With shock, cerebral blood flow and cerebral metabolism may become insufficient to maintain normal mental functioning and level of consciousness. Because the brain is totally dependent on oxygen and glucose, brain cells are highly sensitive to a shortage of oxygen and glucose and to fluid imbalances. When the brain becomes hypoxic, the cerebral vessels dilate to restore blood flow. Likewise, blood is diverted to the brain from the other, less vital organs.

Immune System. All forms of shock severely depress macrophages, which are located in both the blood and the tissues. The capacity of macrophages to remove bacteria is greatly reduced. Alterations in the blood itself are partially due to tissue hypoxia and impairment of monitoring activities of the macrophage. The stasis, sludging, tendency for venular thrombosis, impaired capillary permeability, and subnormal vascular reactivity that occur during shock can all be traced to macrophage dysfunction.

The impaired ability of macrophages to ward off toxic agents is critical. Reduced blood flow through the intestines during shock extensively impairs the integrity of intestinal tissue. This results in the movement of normal GI flora across the impaired intestinal tissue into the bloodstream, leading to a possible bacteremic state. The person in a state of shock is more susceptible to bacterial products, particularly bacterial endotoxins, because of alterations in macrophage function.

Gastrointestinal System. Under sympathetic stimulation, vagal stimulation to the GI tract slows or stops, resulting in ileus with an absence of peristalsis. A lack of nutrient blood supply to the intestines increases the risk of tissue necrosis and sepsis. GI changes appear to have a more important role in the progression of shock than previously thought. The submucosa of the intestine becomes ischemic early in shock. If ischemia is prolonged, actual tissue necrosis of intestinal mucosa occurs. The intestinal arterioles and venules seem highly susceptible to the extensive vasoconstriction that occurs during shock. The massive amount of tissue destruction within the intestines that results from vasoconstriction and tissue anoxia is sufficient to cause tissue death even if bacteria are not present. Bacteria and their toxins contribute to shock by escaping into the systemic circulation following destruction of the intestinal mucosa barrier.

Shock causes serious changes in the functions of the liver, the major organ of detoxification. The liver suffers from this impaired circulation and appears to be a source of toxic materials. Normally, the liver protectively traps and disposes of toxic materials (released from the bowel contents) that are products of bacterial enzyme actions. During shock, the anoxic liver develops metabolic deficiencies, has an impaired ability to detoxify, and may release vasoactive substances. In addition, enhanced bacterial invasion of the liver from the intestine apparently occurs.

Finally, during shock, pooling of blood occurs in the viscera. Pooling of blood in the liver and portal bed may result when masses of agglutinated (clotted) blood plug numerous small hepatic vessels, sinusoids, and intrahepatic radicles of the portal vein and hepatic artery.

Renal System. The kidneys do not receive adequate blood during shock. As a result, urine production decreases and levels of urea nitrogen and creatinine increase. When blood flow is restored to the brain and heart, blood flow will again be provided to the kidneys. Therefore urine output indicates the status of circulation through the vital organs even if BP is below normal.

Altered Capillary Blood Pressure and Glomerular Filtration. Glomerular filtration within the kidneys depends on the pressure at which the blood is circulating through the glomerular capillaries. The average capillary pressure of blood is usually much higher in the glomeruli than in other capillaries. Under usual circumstances, the kidneys can maintain this heightened capillary pressure in the glomeruli even though there are changes in systemic BP. Afferent arterioles supplying the glomeruli dilate as the BP declines and constrict as it increases. However, this adaptive mechanism cannot protect the kidneys indefinitely against damage from a decreasing systemic BP.

When blood volume and BP decline steadily during shock, glomerular filtration is progressively reduced, which leads to an inability of the kidneys to excrete sodium and water. To compensate, the body excretes some sodium and water through the sweat glands. Damaged kidneys also lose their crucial ability to regulate electrolyte and acid-base balance.

Inadequate perfusion of renal capillaries is believed to be the cause of early prerenal failure in shock. The afferent and efferent arterioles constrict, shunting blood away from the glomeruli. If shock persists, actual renal shutdown occurs from focal tubular necrosis. Vasoconstriction in the kidneys may continue for a prolonged time after the systemic BP is restored to normal levels.

Renal Ischemia. During shock, the kidneys may experience renal ischemia. Because the kidneys have a high rate of metabolism, they are highly susceptible to injury of the tubule cells when the blood supply is deficient. When injury to the kidneys is extensive and renal failure ensues, acute tubular necrosis (ATN) occurs. With appropriate intervention, including careful fluid administration, the kidneys can heal. Normal kidney function usually returns after 10 to 14 days.

Clinical Manifestations
Systemic Manifestations of Shock
Because shock affects every system within the body, there are numerous clinical manifestations. Subjective complaints are usually nonspecific and may not be particularly helpful to the clinician attempting to diagnose shock and treat the client. The client may report feeling sick, weak, cold, hot, nauseated, dizzy, confused, frightened, thirsty, or short of breath. Observable and measurable manifestations are often conflicting (Figure 81-6). BP, cardiac output, and urine output are usually decreased. Respiratory rate is usually increased. Variable indicators of shock include alterations in heart rate, core body temperature, skin temperature, systemic vascular resistance, and skin color. Dyspnea, altered sensorium, and diaphoresis may be present. The manifestations discussed in the sections that follow are usually present in people with shock of any type.

Respiratory System. Rapid, shallow respirations (tachypnea) typically occur during shock because of decreased tissue perfusion. The respiratory rate increases as the oxygen-carrying capacity of the blood decreases. These changes may signal the development of hypoxemia and respiratory alkalosis.

Cardiovascular System
Tachycardia. Increased heart rate is the result of increased sympathetic stimulation. Tachycardia is an attempt to maintain adequate cardiac output and MAP when the blood's circulating volume declines. With increased rate, the pulse becomes typically weak and thready. At the onset of shock, the pulse rate does not

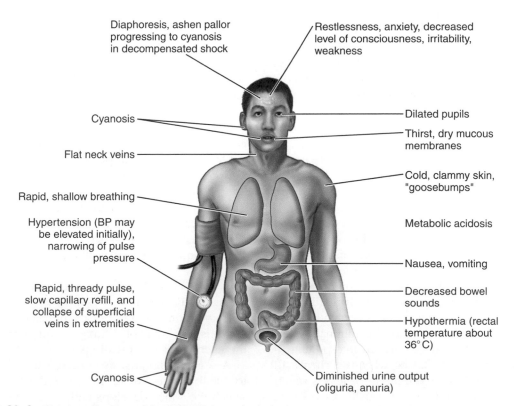

Diaphoresis, ashen pallor progressing to cyanosis in decompensated shock

Restlessness, anxiety, decreased level of consciousness, irritability, weakness

Cyanosis

Dilated pupils

Thirst, dry mucous membranes

Flat neck veins

Rapid, shallow breathing

Cold, clammy skin, "goosebumps"

Hypertension (BP may be elevated initially), narrowing of pulse pressure

Metabolic acidosis

Nausea, vomiting

Rapid, thready pulse, slow capillary refill, and collapse of superficial veins in extremities

Decreased bowel sounds

Hypothermia (rectal temperature about 36° C)

Cyanosis

Diminished urine output (oliguria, anuria)

■ **FIGURE 81-6** Clinical manifestations of the client with hypovolemic shock.

relate as directly to the severity of shock as does BP, because in the early stage of shock, worry, excitement, and fear may influence the heart rate out of proportion to the underlying conditions. However, when emotional factors are no longer significant, serial observations of the pulse rate over a period of time are highly useful to assess the client's condition and the direction of the shock state and to evaluate the effectiveness of intervention.

Older clients (with and without various degrees of heart block) and clients taking beta-blocking medications, however, may show little change in heart rate despite the presence of conditions causing circulatory failure (e.g., hemorrhage). The pulse rate may become extremely slow in the terminal stages of shock and is usually slow in neurogenic shock.

Hypotension. The systolic BP indicates the integrity of the heart, arteries, and arterioles. The diastolic BP indicates the resistance (*systemic vascular resistance* [SVR] or *vasoconstriction)* of blood vessels. For example, an increasing diastolic BP indicates increasing systemic blood vessel resistance. Conversely, a declining diastolic BP indicates decreasing SVR. When the diastolic BP decreases significantly, vasoconstriction is being lost as a compensatory mechanism. When vasoconstriction is replaced by marked vasodilation, there is no resistance to blood flow and an adequate BP is difficult to maintain.

Usually, the BP begins to decrease when total blood volume is decreased by about 15% to 20%, although some clients may lose as much as 25% of the total blood volume without having a decline in BP. This is especially true in young adults; therefore in young adults, declining BP is a *very* late manifestation of shock. Typically, as shock progresses, both the systolic and the diastolic BPs drop, with the systolic pressure dropping more than the diastolic. The pulse pressure narrows because it is equal to the difference between the systolic and diastolic BPs.

During shock, pulse pressure is actually more significant than BP because it tends to parallel cardiac stroke volume. Pulse pressure is affected by stroke volume and by peripheral resistance. If stroke volume is decreased from a reduced circulating blood volume, pulse pressure decreases. In shock, pulse pressure may decrease even in the presence of an acceptable systolic BP. This may provide a clue to worsening shock. In shock, pulse pressure is often less than 20 mm Hg. The Critical Monitoring feature above, right, lists additional manifestations that require immediate intervention.

To maintain coronary circulation, a minimal systolic BP of 60 to 70 mm Hg is necessary. In interpreting BP readings, it is important to know what the client's BP has been. A systolic BP of 100 mm Hg or less is significant for clients whose systolic BP usually ranges from 110 to 140 mm Hg. When a client is supine, a decline

---

CRITICAL MONITORING

Worsening Shock

- Systolic blood pressure decreased more than 20 mm Hg with heart rate increased more than 20 beats/min indicates actual or relative hypovolemia requiring immediate assessment of need for fluid replacement and support of cardiovascular status.
- Decreased oxygen saturation or any manifestations of respiratory distress require immediate intervention. Interventions may range from administration of supplemental oxygen via a nasal cannula to endotracheal intubation with mechanical ventilation. Other interventions to support respiratory status (e.g., decreasing anxiety, positioning to support optimum respiratory functioning) are also important.

---

in BP may be a late finding. Hypotension by itself is not shock. Healthy clients often have BP readings lower than textbook normal values.

Additional problems need to be considered in assessment of BP that makes BP an unreliable criterion for assessing the presence and severity of shock. In the early, nonprogressive stage of shock, BP changes are generally unreliable because the arterial pressure may actually be normal or slightly elevated even though shock is present. In fact, blood volume deficits of 1 L or more may occur even though arterial and venous pressures are normal or elevated. When severe vasoconstriction is present, BP may be normal even though the circulation is actually highly inadequate. Conversely, the blood flow may be adequate even though BP is decreased (e.g., because of mechanisms such as vasodilation).

Valuable information about the level of arterial pressure in clients with vasoconstriction can be gained by assessing the strength of the femoral pulses. Doppler study may also be appropriate to obtain an accurate peripheral BP. Arterial lines are also used to monitor arterial pressures. With displaced or depleted blood volume, it is important to consider adequate venous filling. Hypovolemia, whether actual or relative, causes superficial veins to flatten. This change may hamper attempts to insert intravenous (IV) catheters for fluid replacement.

Neuroendocrine System. Early in shock, hyperactivity of the sympathetic nervous system with increased secretion of epinephrine usually causes the client to feel anxious, nervous, and irritable. Anxiety and worry are seen in the client's facial expressions.

Assessment findings associated with lack of blood flow to the brain are determined by the suddenness with which the shock develops and by its severity. With sudden, severe shock, the body may not have time to initiate its compensatory adjustment mechanisms. Consequently, the brain is deprived of its blood supply. The client may feel dizzy and faint on sitting up from a horizontal position because of postural hypotension. Fainting and unconsciousness may occur. If shock develops gradually over a period of hours, early assessment findings may include apathy and confusion or the opposite—restlessness and unusual alertness.

The systolic BP is important in maintaining blood flow to the brain. A cerebral perfusion pressure (CPP) of at least 50 mm Hg is required to deliver blood to the brain. Cerebral perfusion pressure can be computed by subtracting intracranial pressure from MAP (see Chapter 73 for measurement of intracranial pressure):

$$CPP = MAP - ICP$$

Usually, a decrease in systolic BP is accompanied by a reduced flow of blood to the brain. The vessels of the brain, like those of the heart, however, are not constricted by the vasoconstrictor center in the medulla oblongata. Thus blood from the peripheral vessels can be shifted to the brain as an emergency compensatory measure.

A client's level of consciousness decreases as circulation to brain tissue becomes increasingly impaired. Confusion, agitation, and restlessness may occur. In trauma situations, restlessness can be mistaken for pain. If opioids are given, the client's situation may be worsened or it may be difficult to detect worsening hypoxia. Drowsiness and stupor are more likely in shock related to severe infection than in shock caused by trauma and hemorrhage. As compensatory mechanisms fail, apathy may ensue. Ultimately, coma may develop.

Renal System. A decrease in urinary volume, often the earliest manifestation of developing shock, may occur even while arterial BP and pulse remain stable. Although urine output is one of the most sensitive indices in shock, any form of shock that develops rapidly shows other manifestations before decreased urine output is noticed.

Urine output should be kept greater than 0.5 ml/kg/hour. If the hourly output diminishes significantly, treatment must be instituted to prevent renal failure. Urinary flow of less than 0.5 ml/kg/hour can cause ATN from inadequate renal circulation.

Clinical Manifestations of Specific Types of Shock

Hypovolemic Shock. Initially, urine osmolality and specific gravity increase because of sodium and water reabsorption, which attempts to support circulating volume. As altered tissue perfusion and the hypovolemic shock progress, urine osmolality and specific gravity decrease because of the inability of the kidneys to reabsorb sodium and water. Sympathetic stimulation increases

pulse rate and respirations and decreases tissue perfusion to the skin, causing the skin to feel cool, clammy from diaphoresis, and to appear pale. Clients may sweat profusely, which increases insensible fluid loss, leading to further hypovolemia and temperature instability. Cyanosis may indicate either decreased tissue perfusion or decreased oxygenation, or both. Cyanosis is a late manifestation of decreased oxygenation.

Cardiogenic Shock. Because of the impaired muscle action or mechanical obstruction that caused the cardiogenic shock, blood is inadequately pumped through the heart. This results in a back-up of blood. When the shock is due to right-sided heart failure, this back-up is evidenced as jugular venous distention and increased CVP. (See Chapters 56 and 63 for discussions of cardiac tamponade and tension pneumothorax, respectively.) When the shock is due to left-sided failure, blood backs up into the pulmonary circulation, resulting in pulmonary edema, crackles in the lungs, and increased pulmonary capillary wedge pressure (PCWP). As in hypovolemic shock, there is stimulation of the sympathetic nervous system because of decreased cardiac output and decreased BP and all of the resultant clinical manifestations.

Distributive Shock

Anaphylactic Shock. Initially, the client may complain of a vague feeling of uneasiness or a feeling of impending doom. The massive vasodilation that occurs with anaphylaxis may cause complaints of headache as well. This may be followed by severe anxiety, dizziness, disorientation, and loss of consciousness.

The respiratory system develops many manifestations. The initial complaint may be a feeling of a lump in the throat, which is due to laryngeal edema and is followed by hoarseness, coughing, dyspnea, and stridor. Diffuse wheezes and a prolonged expiratory phase are heard on auscultation. If a pulse oximeter is in use, there may be a rapid decline in oxygen saturation. Additional complaints may include pruritus and urticaria. Direct observation may also demonstrate edema of the eyelids, lips, or tongue (angioedema).

Neurogenic Shock. Neurogenic shock may not present like the other forms of shock. The client often has bradycardia and hypotension (which cannot be corrected because of loss of the inability to vasoconstrict vessels). Below the level of injury, skin temperature takes on the same temperature as the room (poikilothermia). Skin is dry to the touch because of an inability to sweat.

Septic Shock. A person with severe sepsis develops the hypotension, coagulation disorders, and multisystem organ dysfunction of septic shock due, in part, to a dysregulated expression of the body's mediators of inflammation. The relationship between the outcomes of sepsis and the inflammatory response has led to a multitude of research.

Sepsis is diagnosed when two or more of these manifestations are present:

- Temperature greater than 38° C or less than 36° C
- Heart rate greater than 90 beats per minute
- Respiratory rate greater than 20 breaths per minute or a $Paco_2$ in arterial gas less than 32 mm Hg
- WBC count greater than 12,000 cells/ml, less than 4000 cells/ml, or greater than 10% band forms

In the early stages of septic shock, the body experiences massive vasodilation. Warm, dry, flushed skin is apparent during this hyperdynamic stage of septic shock. The compensatory increase in cardiac output and resultant increased perfusion of the skin give this stage the name "warm shock." During later stages, when compensatory mechanisms fail, the release of MDF and decreased venous return result in decreased perfusion and "cold shock," or the hypodynamic stage. At this point, the skin becomes pale, cold, clammy, and mottled. Body temperature decreases to subnormal levels. Auscultation of the lungs reveals crackles and wheezes, which develop secondary to pulmonary congestion as ARDS ensues. In addition to the clinical manifestations seen with shock in general, changes in the level of consciousness may include drowsiness and stupor progressing to coma. The Concept Map on p. 2169 illustrates the pathology, clinical manifestations, and related treatment interventions for the various stages of septic shock.

Diagnostic Assessment

Diagnostic assessments of clients in shock should include oxygenation, organ perfusion, and fluid balance. Assessment of respiratory status can be accomplished to some degree by noninvasive procedures such as spirometry, pulse oxymetry. Other noninvasive assessment and monitoring tools are the cardiac monitor and the 12-lead electrocardiogram (ECG). Laboratory studies include a complete blood cell count, blood chemistry, and blood and body fluid cultures for certain clients.

ABG analysis may also be done to determine whether the metabolic acidosis that occurs with shock is being effectively combated by hyperventilation. A low $Paco_2$, along with low pH and bicarbonate levels (metabolic acidosis), indicates that hyperventilation is trying to compensate. However, an increasing $Paco_2$ in the presence of a persistently low pH indicates that respiratory assistance is needed. It is also important to monitor Pao_2 levels to determine whether the client is being adequately oxygenated (see the Critical Monitoring feature on worsening shock on p. 2166).

CVP measurement is one of the first invasive assessments made in the presence of shock to estimate fluid loss. A pulmonary artery or Swan-Ganz catheter may also be inserted to assist with assessments of fluid status, cardiac function, and tissue oxygen consumption (see Chapter 54).

OUTCOME MANAGEMENT

Treatment should generally be instituted for shock whenever at least two of the following three conditions occur: systolic BP of 80 mm Hg or less, pulse pressure of 20 mm Hg or less, and pulse rate of 120 beats/min or more. Pulse pressure is calculated by subtracting diastolic BP from systolic BP and is normally between 30 and 50 mm Hg.

The therapeutic management of shock has changed markedly over recent years. Lowering the head, raising the feet, and administering potent vasoconstrictor drugs were once the foundation of treatment for a client in shock. Now, emphasis is placed on maintaining adequate circulating volume, using body positions that do not interfere with pulmonary ventilation, and the use of medications having both vasoconstrictor and vasodilator effects.

The following discussion addresses the general interventions for shock. Tables 81-2, 81-3, and 81-4 give specific interventions for hypovolemic, cardiogenic, and distributive shock, respectively.

Medical Management

Correct the Causative Factor

Assessment and an accurate differential medical diagnosis, which establish the specific cause of the shock state, form the basis for treatment. The differential medical diagnosis is usually readily made unless the shock is in an advanced stage, at which point several specific forms of shock may exist at the same time. Some forms of shock more easily recognized are hypovolemic shock that is due to extensive burns or trauma and cardiogenic shock with severe chest pain and acute MI. Septic shock is also treated initially with fluids because of ongoing capillary leakage. Of course, antibiotics are used and if the organisms are not known, antibiotics are prescribed empirically, based on what the suspected organisms might be. Blood cultures are drawn, allowing the antibiotics to be refined for specific bacteria.

Improve Oxygenation

Maintaining the client's airway is vital to the treatment of shock. In all types of shock, supplemental oxygen is administered to protect against hypoxemia. Oxygen can be delivered via a nasal cannula, a mask, a high-flow non-rebreathing mask, an endotracheal tube, or a tracheostomy tube.

Endotracheal intubation, or tracheostomy, may be performed to rest an exhausted client during severe or

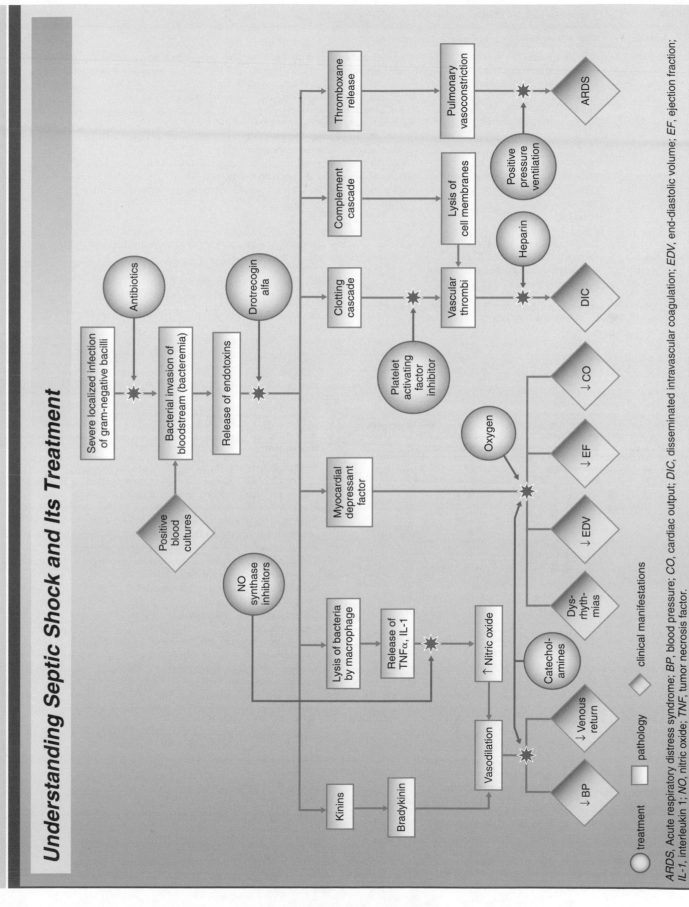

CONCEPT MAP

Understanding Septic Shock and Its Treatment

ARDS, Acute respiratory distress syndrome; BP, blood pressure; CO, cardiac output; DIC, disseminated intravascular coagulation; EDV, end-diastolic volume; EF, ejection fraction; IL-1, interleukin 1; NO, nitric oxide; TNF, tumor necrosis factor.

○ treatment   ▢ pathology   ◇ clinical manifestations

TABLE 81–2 Summary of the Management of Hypovolemic Shock

Etiology	Clinical Situation	Intervention*
Blood loss	Massive trauma	Stop external bleeding with direct pressure, pressure dressing, tourniquet (as last resort)
	Gastrointestinal bleeding	Reduce intra-abdominal or retroperitoneal bleeding or prepare for emergency surgery
	Ruptured aortic aneurysm	
	Surgery	Administer lactated Ringer's solution or normal saline
	Erosion of vessel from lesion, tubes, or other devices	Transfuse with fresh whole blood, packed cells, fresh frozen plasma, platelets, or other clotting factors, if significant improvement does not occur with crystalloid administration
	DIC	Use non-blood plasma expanders (albumin, hetastarch, dextran) until blood is available
		Conduct autotransfusion if appropriate
Plasma loss	Burns	Administer low-dose cardiotonics (dopamine, dobutamine)
	Accumulation of intra-abdominal fluid	Administer lactated Ringer's solution or normal saline
	Malnutrition	Administer albumin, fresh frozen plasma, hetastarch, or dextran if cardiac output is still low
	Severe dermatitis	
	DIC	
Crystalloid loss	Dehydration (e.g., diabetic ketoacidosis, heat exhaustion)	Administer isotonic or hypotonic saline with electrolytes as needed to maintain normal circulating volume and electrolyte balance
	Protracted vomiting, diarrhea	
	Nasogastric suction	

DIC, Disseminated intravascular coagulation; *MAST,* military or medical antishock trousers.
*Assumes that airway management and cardiac monitoring are ongoing.

TABLE 81–3 Summary of the Management of Cardiogenic Shock

Etiology	Clinical Situation	Intervention*
Myocardial disease or injury	Acute myocardial infarction	Fluid-challenge with up to 300 ml of normal saline solution or lactated Ringer's solution to rule out hypovolemia, unless heart failure or pulmonary edema is present
	Myocardial contusion	Insert CVP or pulmonary artery catheter; monitor cardiac output, pulmonary artery pressure, and PCWP; administer IV fluids to maintain left ventricular filling pressure of 15-20 mm Hg
	Cardiomyopathies	Administer inotropics (e.g., dopamine or dobutamine)
		Vasodilators (e.g., sodium nitroprusside, nitroglycerin, calcium-channel blockers, morphine)
		Diuretics (e.g., mannitol or furosemide)
		Cardiotonics (e.g., digitalis)
		Beta-blockers (e.g., propranolol)
		Glucocorticosteroids[†]
		Intra-aortic balloon pump or external counterpulsation device if unresponsive to other therapies
Valvular disease or injury	Ruptured aortic cusp	Same as above: if rapid response does not occur, prepare for prompt cardiac surgery
	Ruptured papillary muscle	
	Ball thrombus	
External pressure on heart interferes with heart filling or emptying	Pericardial tamponade caused by trauma, aneurysm, cardiac surgery, pericarditis	Relieve tamponade with ECG-assisted pericardiocentesis; repair surgically if it recurs
	Massive pulmonary embolus	Thrombolytic (streptokinase) or anticoagulant (heparin) therapy; surgery for removal of clot
	Tension pneumothorax	Relieve air accumulation with needle thoracostomy or chest tube insertion
	Ascites	
	Hemoperitoneum	Relieve fluid accumulation with paracentesis
	Mechanical ventilation	Reduce inspiratory pressure
Cardiac dysrhythmias	Tachydysrhythmias	Treat dysrhythmias; be prepared to initiate CPR, cardiac pacing
	Bradydysrhythmias	
	Pulseless electrical activity	

CPR, Cardiopulmonary resuscitation; *CVP,* central venous pressure; *ECG,* electrocardiogram; *IV,* intravenous; *PCWP,* pulmonary capillary wedge pressure.
*Assumes that airway management and cardiac monitoring are ongoing.
†Controversial.

TABLE 81–4 Summary of the Management of Distributive Shock

Etiology	Clinical Situation	Intervention*
Anaphylactic shock	Allergy to food, medicines, dyes, insect bites, stings, or latex	Prepare for surgical management of airway
		Decrease further absorption of antigen (e.g., stop IV fluid, place tourniquet between injection or sting site and heart if feasible)
		Epinephrine (1:100) 2 inhalations every 3 hr, *or*
		Epinephrine (1:1000) 0.2-0.5 ml every 5-15 min given subcutaneously, *or*
		Epinephrine (1:10,000) 0.5-1.0 ml every 5-15 min given at a rate of 1 mg/min
		IV fluid resuscitation with isotonic solution
		Diphenhydramine HCl or H_1-receptor antagonist IV
		Theophylline IV drip for bronchospasm
		Steroids IV
		Vasopressors (e.g., norepinephrine, metaraminol bitartrate, high-dose dopamine)
		Gastric lavage for ingested antigen
		Ice pack to injection or sting site
		Meat tenderizer paste to sting site
Septic shock	Often gram-negative septicemia but also caused by other organisms in debilitated, immunodeficient, or chronically ill clients	Identify origin of sepsis; culture all suspected sources
		Vigorous IV fluid resuscitation with normal saline
		Empirical antibiotic therapy until sensitivities are reported
		Administer cardiotonic agents (e.g., dopamine or dobutamine, norepinephrine, isoproterenol, digitalis, calcium)
		Naloxone (narcotic antagonist)
		Prostaglandins
		Monoclonal antibodies
		Drotrecogin alfa
		Temperature control (both hypothermia and hyperthermia are noted)
		Heparin, clotting factors, blood products if DIC develops
Neurogenic (spinal) shock	Spinal anesthesia	Normal saline to restore volume
	Spinal cord injury	Treat bradycardia with atropine
		Vasopressors (e.g., norepinephrine, metaraminol bitartrate, high-dose dopamine, and phenylephrine) may be given
		Place client in modified Trendelenburg position
Vasovagal reaction	Severe pain	Place client in a head-down or recumbent position
	Severe emotional stress	Give atropine if bradycardia and profound hypotension; eliminate pain

DIC, Disseminated intravascular coagulation; *IV*, intravenous.
*Assumes airway management and cardiac monitoring are ongoing.

prolonged shock and to correct respiratory failure. By increasing the rate of pulmonary ventilation (through spontaneous or mechanical hyperventilation), it is possible to compensate for minor degrees of metabolic acidosis. This increased "blowing off" of carbon dioxide with hyperventilation begins to compensate for acid-base imbalance. Positive end-expiratory pressure may be added when the client is being mechanically ventilated. This assists in preventing atelectasis and may provide a higher Pao_2 for the client at a lower oxygen concentration setting. The goal of therapy is to maintain a Pao_2 greater than 50 mm Hg and an Sao_2 greater than 90% to avoid anaerobic metabolism. If the chest is congested, chest physical therapy, including vibration, percussion, and postural drainage, may be required.

Sometimes the interventions discussed cannot establish optimal tissue oxygenation. In these instances, hyperbaric oxygenation (HBO) or extracorporeal membrane oxyge-

nation may be used. HBO involves the administration of 100% oxygen under 2 to 3 atmospheres of pressure. This raises tissue oxygen tension to normal or above-normal levels. HBO requires the use of special chambers, which usually are available only in highly specialized institutions.

Extracorporeal membrane oxygenation is most commonly used in adults as a temporary intervention for refractory ARDS. Arterial and venous catheters are inserted, and some of the client's blood is diverted through them into a machine that artificially oxygenates the blood. This is a relatively expensive form of therapy and is usually done only in large medical centers.

Restore and Maintain Adequate Perfusion

The primary aim in treating shock is to maintain an adequate circulating blood volume. Unless this is accomplished early, subsequent therapeutic measures are of no avail, and death can be anticipated. During shock intervention, all of the basic pathophysiologic changes associated with the development of shock must be corrected.

Some problems that must often be treated are (1) the vascular problem of vasoconstriction with the diminished tissue perfusion it causes, (2) the intravascular problem of coagulation and sludging of blood cells, and (3) the extravascular problem of extravasation of fluid into the extravascular space. The Integrating Pharmacology feature below discusses vasoactive medications commonly used to treat shock.

Nitric Oxide. Inducible nitric oxide synthase is a complex found in endothelial and vascular smooth muscle cells. Endothelial cells continually produce low levels of nitric oxide to maintain normal vascular tone. During inflammatory states, nitric oxide production is increased, resulting in hypotension and vasodilation.

Vasoconstrictors. Vasoconstrictors elevate the systemic BP by constricting peripheral arterioles. Vasoconstrictor

---

INTEGRATING PHARMACOLOGY

Vasoactive Medications for Shock Management

It may seem contradictory to use medications that vasoconstrict and medications that vasodilate in caring for individuals in shock. However, both actions are needed at times during shock and many of the medications used have actions that are beneficial during each stage.

In the nonprogressive stage of shock, when the body is experiencing significant vasodilation, vasoconstrictors, such as high-dose dopamine, norepinephrine, and phenylephrine, help maintain blood pressure (BP). Adding medications that increase cardiac contractility, such as amrinone and dobutamine, further support BP by increasing cardiac output. As shock progresses and vasoconstriction ensues, these same drugs, with some changes in dosing, are still effective in supporting the client's hemodynamic stability. Low-dose dopamine causes vasodilation of the renal and mesenteric blood vessels, helping to support perfusion of the kidneys and gut. Amrinone and dobutamine contribute to vasodilation of blood vessels in the heart and skeletal muscle, ensuring adequate oxygenation to those organs and tissues. If significant systemic vasoconstriction continues, relaxation of the vascular smooth muscle may be necessary with drugs such as nitroglycerin and nitroprusside.

Titration and changing of medications are continued until the client's shock is clearly reversed. If the client progresses to the irreversible stage of shock despite the health care team's best efforts, these drugs will have little, if any, effectiveness.

---

agents may be used briefly in shock if compensatory vasoconstriction is unable to maintain blood flow to vital organs. They may also be used to correct hypotension secondary to vasoconstrictor nerve paralysis, as in spinal anesthesia or conditions associated with massive vasodilation. However, vasoconstrictors should not be used exclusively but should be given concomitantly with IV fluids to restore adequate circulation and perfusion.

Perfusion of vital organs with blood is impossible when systolic BP is less than 50 mm Hg. Usually, the goal of using vasoconstrictors is to achieve and maintain a mean BP of 70 to 80 mm Hg, which is sufficient to perfuse tissues. Generally, attempts to increase the BP beyond this level are not advisable because vasoconstrictors increase the oxygen demand of the heart and may cause fatal dysrhythmias. Vasoconstrictors are used with extreme caution in cardiogenic shock. Other major adverse effects of vasoconstrictors include decreased renal and splanchnic blood flow, excessive or sudden increase in arterial BP (which may precipitate heart failure), pulmonary edema or left ventricular (LV) decompensation, and gangrene of the fingers and toes from prolonged vasoconstriction.

Although the use of vasoconstrictors during shock is being critically evaluated, they do favorably increase blood flow to the brain and heart in severely hypotensive clients. Reduced tissue perfusion when systolic pressures are less than 60 to 70 mm Hg may precipitate an MI or a stroke.

Vasodilators. Agents that induce vasodilation or inhibit vasoconstriction may promote recovery from shock in which intensive vasoconstriction is contributing to the problem. These include adrenergic blocking agents, ganglionic blocking agents, and direct-acting peripheral vasodilators.

Adrenergic blockade prevents harmful effects of prolonged vasoconstriction such as increased pressure in capillaries, promoting fluid loss from the vascular to the interstitial compartment, and altered blood flow, especially in the splanchnic area. These agents are also used to keep coronary arteries open. Prolonged vasoconstriction also impairs cellular nutrition and allows accumulation of waste products. Adrenergic blockade prevents these changes in circulation and may also induce opposite beneficial changes.

Vasodilators may be helpful during shock when vasoconstriction is severe and persists even though fluids have been infused in what should be adequate amounts for fluid replacement. Vasodilators may be administered to inhibit vasoconstriction of peripheral blood vessels (the result of norepinephrine from sympathetic stimulation) so that blood can be redistributed to enhance tissue perfusion and increase vascular volume. Vasodilator medications are sometimes given in combination with vasoconstrictor medications to offset the profound effects that may occur with some vasoconstrictors and to provide the benefits both types of drugs have to offer.

When shock is caused by hypovolemia, rapid and adequate fluid replacement is essential before vasodilators are used. Vasodilators are dangerous because they lower arterial BP if they are given while circulating blood volume is deficient. When the circulating blood volume is inadequate, the body depends on vasoconstriction to maintain arterial pressure. However, when the vascular space is full and cardiac venous return is adequate, vasodilation should open arterioles in the lungs and elsewhere. This lets blood circulate, increasing cardiac output and capillary perfusion without lowering systemic BP. In fact, a vasodilator may produce a dramatic, sustained increase in the systemic arterial pressure.

Keep clients who are receiving vasodilators lying relatively flat. Elevation of the head can produce dangerous orthostatic hypotension. Older clients may have sclerotic blood vessels and may not tolerate the hypotension that may accompany administration of vasodilators. In this situation, a cardiotonic drug (such as dobutamine) may be given with the vasodilator to increase cardiac output.

Characteristically, impaired tissue perfusion is correctable during early shock. However, it may be fatal if treatment is not received or is inadequate. In the later stages of shock, impaired tissue perfusion becomes irreversible, leading to death despite treatment. However, treatment for irreversible shock is never abandoned while the client remains alive. Before a client's shock state is viewed as probably irreversible, identification and treatment of occult bleeding and restoration of circulating volume, correction of any factors interfering with cardiopulmonary function, and treatment of overwhelming infection must be attempted.

Assist Circulation

Mechanical devices that assist circulation or decrease the workload of the heart may be used as temporary measures in managing clients in shock.

Intra-Aortic Balloon Pump (IABP). An IABP is used primarily in clients with cardiogenic shock. The ability of the heart to adequately pump blood is augmented by a balloon-tipped catheter placed in the descending thoracic aorta. The catheter is attached to a unit that inflates during diastole and deflates just before systole. This counterpulsation displaces blood back into the aorta and improves coronary artery circulation. In cardiogenic shock, use of the IABP reduces afterload, allowing the heart to more efficiently empty, thereby increasing cardiac output. Details of the IABP are found in the Bridge to Critical Care feature on Intra-Aortic Balloon Pumping in Chapter 56.

Modified Trendelenburg Position. A client in shock is usually placed in a modified Trendelenburg position with the lower extremities elevated 30 to 45 degrees, the knees straight, the trunk horizontal or very slightly raised, and the neck comfortably positioned with the head level with the chest or slightly higher (Figure 81-7). This position promotes increased venous return from the lower extremities without compressing the abdominal organs against the diaphragm. The traditional Trendelenburg position (head down, with legs elevated at least 30 degrees above the head) was once the classic shock position but is no longer used for shock management because it compresses the abdominal contents against the diaphragm, interfering with pulmonary excursion, and promotes congestion of blood in the brain, possibly contributing to cerebral edema.

Elevating the legs mobilizes blood that has pooled in the lower extremities. As a result of gravity, the additional circulating blood increases venous return to the heart, thus improving cardiac output. The position is of temporary value in moderate hypovolemia. However, it does not help in severe hypovolemia, because the extremities have very little blood in them in such a state. Generally, the modified shock position is not used with cardiogenic shock, when there is already circulatory overload.

Replace Fluid Volume

The mainstay of hypovolemic shock therapy is expansion of circulating blood volume by IV administration of blood or other appropriate fluids. Fluid replacement should be administered through large-bore peripheral lines, central venous lines, or both. A sizable amount of fluid (about 4 L in moderately severe shock) leaves the interstitial space. This is in addition to fluid lost from the circulating volume. Thus fluid replacement therapy must replace both blood lost from the circulation and fluid lost from the interstitial space. Fluid replacement therapy must be closely monitored to prevent circulatory overload. Hypervolemia can be lethal; thus aggressive fluid replacement should be tapered off when urine output is at least 0.5 ml/kg/hour, systolic BP is greater than 100 mm Hg, or the heart rate is 60 to 100 beats/min.

■ **FIGURE 81–7** Positioning of the person in shock. This position is a modification of Trendelenburg position and includes elevating the legs, leaving the trunk flat, and elevating the head and shoulders slightly.

In replacing fluids, enough volume must be administered to fill the capillaries and run through into the veins. Such fluid replacement maintains CVP and provides an adequate venous return to the heart. In addition, adequate fluid replacement decreases the sympathetic response and thus produces a vasodilation that promotes capillary flow. Adequate flow of fluids in the capillaries in turn perfuses tissues and prevents sludging and coagulation of blood within the vessels.

Blood. When hemorrhage is the primary cause of shock, the rapid administration of large volumes of packed cells or whole blood may be necessary. Type-specific, crossmatched blood is the most desirable form of blood replacement. However, if the client is hemorrhaging, it may be necessary to administer type-specific, uncrossmatched blood: O-negative blood or O-positive, low antibody titer blood. Women should receive Rh-negative blood.

When shock resulting from hemorrhage is treated, a crystalloid is usually given as an initial emergency treatment to sustain BP. Later, the acute anemia resulting from hemorrhage must be corrected by administration of packed cells for the prevention of hypoxemia.

During fluid replacement, a normal red blood cell mass should be maintained. Fluids given in excess of normal volume should be fluids other than blood so that they can be easily removed from the circulation by the kidneys once the shock is corrected. If the normal red blood cell mass is exceeded, it is difficult for the body to eliminate the excess red blood cells after the vascular volume returns to normal (after adequate perfusion of tissues with blood is achieved). Because dangers also are involved in blood transfusions, blood should not be used if another fluid can satisfactorily maintain an adequate oxygen-carrying capacity and can sufficiently increase blood volume. Blood can become so dilute that there are relatively few blood cells as the result of up to 8 to 12 L of fluid being administered in only a few hours.

Autotransfusion. Autotransfusion involves collecting and retransfusing blood into the same client. Autotransfusion is used to prevent or treat hypovolemic shock caused by hemorrhage. It is common in the treatment of chest injuries.

Crystalloid or Balanced Salt Solutions. Various fluids are given to correct specific problems, such as electrolyte or protein deficiencies or other defects of the blood, including acidosis and hyponatremia. However, in treating hypovolemic shock, the immediate results of therapy seem to depend less on the type of fluid administered for fluid replacement than on the amount of fluid administered. In general, enough fluid is given to exceed the normal blood volume. This "extra" fluid is required to replace intracellular fluid that was mobilized into the circulation as an early response to the hypovolemia. To assist with fluid administration, a three-to-one rule has been developed. For a client's estimated blood loss, three times as much crystalloid solution must be administered for adequate volume resuscitation. Crystalloid solutions that may be administered include normal saline, Ringer's lactate, or half-normal saline.

IV fluids used in shock management may include warmed crystalloids or balanced salt solutions, colloids, and blood. Dextrose and water should not be used to resuscitate a client; once the dextrose is metabolized, only hypotonic water remains, which leads to greater fluid shifts. Electrolyte solutions such as Ringer's lactate help expand extracellular volume, reduce viscosity, and prevent sludging. In a client with impaired liver function, a solution containing lactate could further compound the problem of lactic acidosis. In a normally functioning liver, lactate is converted to bicarbonate and does not accumulate. Because the liver is not an organ of primary perfusion during times of stress for the body and may not be functioning normally, other solutions should be considered before Ringer's lactate.

Abnormalities of electrolyte and acid-base balance are corrected with the specific substance needed rather than with a solution that administers multiple electrolytes and acid-base components. Therapy is gauged by serial ABG and electrolyte determinations.

Colloid Solutions. Colloid solutions contain proteins normally too large to exit at the capillary; thus they remain in the vascular compartment and increase osmotic pressure of the capillaries. This increased osmotic pressure helps pull fluid back into the vascular compartment and maintain circulating volume. These solutions may be used in conjunction with crystalloid solutions in treating hypovolemic shock to maintain an adequate circulating volume. The most commonly used colloid solutions include plasma and its components, plasma substitutes (e.g., dextran), oxygen-carrying solutions other than blood (e.g., perfluorocarbons and ultra-purified, stroma-free hemoglobin solutions), and hetastarch. (See discussions of blood and blood transfusions, Chapter 75.)

Colloid solutions cannot be used in clients with inflammatory conditions such as sepsis and burns. In these clients, capillary leakage is large enough that even the proteins escape.

SAFETY ⚠ ALERT

Fresh frozen plasma (FFP) is the form commonly used to improve serum protein levels. FFP may be administered after massive transfusions to restore some clotting factors deficient in "banked" blood. Because FFP requires 15 to 30 minutes to thaw, it is not used in initial fluid resuscitation with shock.

Albumin may also be used to achieve adequate osmotic pressure. Occasionally, it is administered when sufficient amounts of other fluids fail to restore an adequate circulating volume. Use of albumin is controversial because it may move into the pulmonary interstitial space, drawing water along with it. Thus albumin may contribute to the development of ARDS.

Dextran may be used in both high- and low-molecular-weight forms. The advantage in using dextran is that it contains large molecules that should effectively and rapidly expand the intravascular volume. Dextran can interfere with blood type and crossmatch procedures and with clotting factors. It should therefore be used only after type and crossmatch have been done and until blood is available for transfusion. By initiating therapy with low-molecular-weight dextran and then progressing to high-molecular-weight forms, the incidence of hypersensitivity reactions to dextran can be lowered.

Blood Substitutes. Perfluorocarbons (e.g., Fluosol, Oxygent) are non-blood, oxygen-carrying solutions that remain in the circulation for about 12 to 24 hours. Major limitations associated with the use of perfluorochemicals relate to limited immediate availability (the product must be stored frozen), administration of 80% to 100% O_2 for the solution to be effective, and accumulation of the chemicals in the body. Advantages include the high solubility of perfluorocarbons, making them readily available to the tissues, and their acceptability to clients whose religious beliefs prohibit the use of blood products. Perfluorocarbons have been researched since the 1970s and are still in various stages of experimentation.

Hemoglobin-based oxygen carriers (e.g., stroma-free hemoglobin, PolyHeme, Hemopure, Hemolink) are made from hemoglobin that has been extracted from red blood cells and have been developed from bovine, recombinant, and human sources. Advantages are that no type and crossmatch is required for administration, so oxygen-carrying solutions are more readily available for situations in which major traumas occur or during periods of diminished blood availability. Concerns that still exist relate to the toxicity of the solutions, their short half-life, and their relatively high colloid oncotic pressure.

Hetastarch, a glycogen-like synthetic colloid, has been used to treat hypovolemic shock and may provide alternatives to blood administration. Its effects last between 3 and 24 hours. Pentastarch is also available as a volume expander.

Goal-Directed Therapy for Sepsis

Early goal-directed therapy (EGDT) is used for the treatment of sepsis. EGDT emphasizes early recognition of clients with potential sepsis in the ED and early use of broad-spectrum antibiotics and a rapid crystalloid fluid bolus, followed by goal-directed therapy for those clients who remain hypotensive or severely ill after this initial therapy (Box 81-1). EGDT is a three-step process aimed at optimizing tissue perfusion.

Step 1. Titrate crystalloid fluid administration to CVP, or administer 500-ml boluses of fluid until the CVP measures between 8 and 12 mm Hg. CVP is a surrogate for intravascular volume, as excess circulating blood volume is contained within the venous system. Only after the CVP is greater than 8 mm Hg should vasopressors be considered. A central venous catheter in the internal jugular or subclavian vein is placed to measure central venous pressure (CVP) and an arterial catheter to directly measure arterial blood pressure for those clients who did respond to fluids.

Step 2. If the client has not improved with fluid alone, vasopressors are administered to attain a mean arterial pressure (MAP) greater than 65 mm Hg.

Step 3. Evaluate the central venous oxygen saturation (Svo_2). The sample is obtained from the CV line, the blood from which is a surrogate for peripheral tissue oxygenation and cardiac output. An Svo_2 of less than 70% is considered abnormal and indicative of suboptimal therapy. In this case, the hematocrit is checked and blood transfused until a hematocrit greater than 30% is attained. Once this is attained and the Svo_2 is still low, dobutamine is initiated to increase cardiac output.

BOX 81-1   Sepsis Bundle

To improve quality and outcomes of care, a "sepsis bundle" was developed. For implementation of the bundle of care, a client must meet the following criteria:

1. Two or more of the following four items:
   a. Temperature >38.3° C or <36.0° C
   b. Heart rate >90 beats/min
   c. Respiration >20 breaths/min
   d. White blood cell count >12,000/mm^3 or <4000/mm^3, or >10% bandemia (banded leukocytes)
2. A suspected infection
3. SBP <90 mm Hg after 20 ml/kg fluid bolus or lactate >4 mmol/L

6-HOUR EMERGENCY DEPARTMENT SEVERE SEPSIS BUNDLE

1. Initiate CVP/Svo_2 monitoring within 2 hours of meeting bundle criteria.
2. Give broad-spectrum antibiotics within 4 hours (preferably 1 hour) of meeting bundle criteria.
3. Complete early goal-directed therapy (CVP ≥8 mm Hg, SBP ≥90 mm Hg, or MAP ≥65 mm Hg and Svo_2 ≥70%) at 6 hours of meeting bundle criteria.
4. Give steroid if client is receiving vasopressor or if adrenal insufficiency is suspected.
5. Monitor for lactate clearance.

From Nguyen, H.B., Corbett, S.W., Steele, R., et al. (2007). Implementation of a bundle of quality indicators for the early management of severe sepsis and septic shock is associated with decreased mortality. *Critical Care Medicine, 35* (4), 1105-1112.

Evaluate Fluid Replacement

Often, fluid replacement is the only treatment required for shock. However, it is difficult to evaluate whether fluid replacement is adequate. Internal losses of circulating fluid volume, including whole blood, into areas of traumatized tissue or into third spaces are difficult to estimate. If a vasoconstrictor drug has been administered or if prolonged vasoconstriction occurs, an additional considerable loss of circulating volume may also occur because of vasoconstriction. Large volumes of IV fluid may be administered either until systemic BP, urinary volume, and lactate levels become relatively normal or until central venous or pulmonary artery pressures, or both, stabilize or become elevated.

Infusion of blood or other fluids usually continues only as long as the CVP is low, that is, less than 4 cm H_2O or 2 mm Hg. When the CVP is higher than normal (e.g., greater than 15 cm H_2O or 11 mm Hg), benefit cannot be expected from the continued infusion of fluids or blood beyond maintenance amounts. When the CVP is low and the lungs are clear, with no indications of heart failure, fluids are administered to improve the return of blood to the heart. However, some clients have a normal or low CVP despite faulty LV function. They readily develop heart failure or pulmonary edema. Thus a low or normal CVP does not always mean that fluid administration is advisable.

If there is an adequate systemic response, IV fluid administration should be stopped before extremely high elevations of pulmonary artery pressures occur. An adequate volume of circulating fluid causes an ample venous return to the right side of the heart and increases the right-sided output. Pulmonary artery hypertension may develop if continued pulmonary obstruction is present because of coagulation in the microcirculation or vasoconstriction. This appears as increased pulmonary artery pressure. In the presence of right-sided heart failure, this increased pressure may back up through the right side of the heart, causing an abnormal elevation in CVP. Vasodilators may help open this partially blocked pulmonary microcirculation.

Prevent Complications

Prevent Renal Impairment. To prevent acute renal damage, the urine output is monitored, and diuretics (e.g., furosemide) may be given if fluid volume has been corrected. The normal rate of urinary excretion from the kidneys is 0.5 ml/kg. A client who becomes acutely hypovolemic or is experiencing a redistribution of circulating volume cannot maintain an hourly output of 40 to 60 ml of urine. Decreased urine output (oliguria) typically occurs in shock. Anuria may develop. When anuria is present, the client is said to be in renal shutdown or renal failure. Oliguria does not contraindicate the administration of large volumes of fluid in the treatment of

shock. In fact, restoring renal capillary perfusion along with that of other vital capillaries restores urine volume production as long as tubular necrosis is not already present. If acute tubular necrosis is present, peritoneal dialysis or hemodialysis may be needed until regeneration of functioning renal tubular epithelium occurs (see also Chapter 36).

Correcting metabolic acidosis (see Chapter 13) and using other measures to increase blood volume and improve cardiac output also benefit the kidney. If a large amount of tissue damage (e.g., crush injuries) is present, myoglobin may be released from damaged muscle tissue. Because the myoglobin molecule is large, a type of mechanical renal failure may result from attempts to excrete it. Increased fluids to flush the myoglobin through the kidney are important to decrease damage to the tubules; occasionally osmotic diuretics are used.

Prevent Gastrointestinal Bleeding. An early physiologic response to shock is a decrease in splanchnic circulation. This reduces the nutrient blood supply to the stomach and bowel, causing inadequate GI tissue perfusion and delayed gastric emptying; thus vomiting with aspiration of gastric contents into the lung may occur. For this reason and for diagnostic purposes, nasogastric (NG) suction is often used during treatment of shock. A double-lumen, 16F NG tube is usually used in adults. In addition, because of the ischemia, the gastric mucosa does not produce mucus and may quickly ulcerate. Proton pump inhibitors, sucralfate, or histamine-2 blockers are given prophylactically to reduce the risk of bleeding.

When shock is caused by GI bleeding, other NG tubes may be used. If the suspected cause of bleeding is a gastric ulcer, a 36F Ewald tube may be used. The many large holes in this tube facilitate saline lavage and removal of blood clots. If esophageal varices are suspected or present, a Sengstaken-Blakemore tube may be used. This triple-lumen tube exerts pressure on the lower portion of the esophagus and the upper portion of the stomach, where varices are most prominent. Pressure is created by esophageal and gastric balloons inflated with air. Gentle traction is applied to keep the balloons in proper position (see Chapter 31).

Provide Pharmacologic Management

Antibiotics. Antibiotics are essential for septic shock. Draw blood samples for culture and sensitivity. Cultures of urine, sputum, and fluid from draining wounds, sinuses, and so forth will provide information about the source of the sepsis.

Cultures should be drawn before antibiotics are initiated. However, it is imperative that intravenous antibiotic therapy be started as soon as possible after the recognition of sepsis, ideally within 1 hour.

SAFETY

⚠

ALERT

Effective anti-infective administration within the first hour of documented hypotension is associated with increased survival in septic shock. Selection of the initial antibiotics depends on the probable site and presumed organisms of infection and local susceptibility patterns. Initially, empirical anti-infective therapy should include one or two agents with activity against the most highly suspected pathogens that can penetrate to the presumed site of infection. The potential for resistance of the pathogens should also be considered. For these reasons, vancomycin and/or aminoglycosides (e.g., gentamicin, amikacin) are common first-line choices for antibiotic therapy. Antibiotic therapy should be reevaluated within 48 to 72 hours based on culture and sensitivity results and client response to therapy. If resistant strains are found to be the cause of the infection and resultant sepsis, some of the newer antibiotics with activity against resistant strains (e.g., linezolid, daptomycin, telithromycin, tigecycline) may be initiated. Antibiotics may also be administered along with appropriate surgical management to clients with open or potentially contaminated wounds who are experiencing shock.

Drotrecogin Alfa. Drotrecogin alfa (Xigris) is used for severe sepsis and SIRS. Drotrecogin alfa is a recombinant form of human activated protein C and has the ability to inhibit inflammation, inhibit coagulation, and promote fibrinolysis. The main effect of protein C is to reduce the production of thrombin by inactivating factors Va and VIII. Thrombin is proinflammatory, procoagulant, and antifibrinolytic. In addition, protein C reduces the production of IL-1, IL-6, and TNF-α by monocytes and has profibrinolytic properties. Large clinical trials have shown significant benefit from the use of this medication in septic shock. Bleeding remains a significant side effect.

Heparin. The anticoagulant effect of heparin may help prevent complications or treat DIC. The dosage is usually initiated based on body weight and adjusted according to clotting studies. Heparin is also used because of the prolonged immobility often associated with shock. Immobility predisposes clients to venous thrombosis and pulmonary emboli. The treatment of DIC may include heparin administration to minimize consumption of clotting factors. Heparin also may be appropriate for clients with ARDS if the primary cause of the respiratory insufficiency is suspected to be DIC or massive microembolism.

Steroids. Steroids have several effects that may assist the client in neurogenic shock after spinal cord injury. They are given to reduce edema in the cord and have been shown to improve recovery. They assist in treatment by stabilizing lysosomal membrane and preventing intracellular release of enzymes. Complications from high-dose steroid therapy include acute GI bleeding, aggravation of diabetes, and immunosuppression.

In septic shock, low-dose steroid use for 5 to 7 days with tapering has demonstrated increases in survival rate and shock reversal in clients with vasopressor-dependent septic shock.

Naloxone. Naloxone (Narcan), an opiate antagonist, is commonly used to treat opioid and synthetic opioid overdosages. During stress, opiate-like substances known as *enkephalins* and *endorphins* are released from the brain. Although the mechanisms of action are not clear, endorphins may play a role in capillary bed vasodilation found in all forms of shock. Studies indicate that when naloxone is administered in the absence of shock, no significant cardiovascular effects are noted. However, when administered during shock, naloxone reverses the hypotension and decreases cardiac contractility, resulting in significant hemodynamic improvement and decreased mortality. It is believed that naloxone blocks the effects of endorphins and enkephalins.

Insulin. Recent research studies have indicated a significant reduction in mortality and morbidity in ICU clients when intensive insulin therapy is provided. Average blood glucose levels should be between 80 and 110 mg/dl. Tight regulation of blood glucose level does place clients at risk for hypoglycemic episodes, but studies show that hypoglycemia does not increase the risk of mortality whereas hyperglycemia does.

Epinephrine. Epinephrine is the drug of choice for emergency treatment of allergic reactions (anaphylaxis). Epinephrine inhibits histamine release and antagonizes its effects on end organs, resulting in reversal of the bronchial constriction, increased capillary permeability, and vasodilation that occur with acute anaphylactic reactions. The overall effect is improved respiratory status and cardiovascular stability. Antihistamines, like diphenhydramine (Benadryl), can be used to relieve clinical manifestations associated with anaphylaxis rather than to stop the release of histamine.

Proton Pump Inhibitors, Sucralfate, and Histamine H$_2$-Receptor Antagonists. These agents inhibit gastric acid secretion. Stress ulcers are often lethal complications of severe illness or injury produced by continuous shunting of blood from the GI tract due to extended sympathetic nervous system stimulation.

Opioids. The need for pain reduction may be obvious in clients experiencing different types of shock. However, the use of opioids for pain management may be dangerous. Opioids can lead to vasodilation that interferes with vasoconstriction, the only mechanism by which the client's BP is maintained. However, morphine sulfate may be helpful in cardiogenic shock because it causes pooling of blood in the extremities and contributes to a decrease in anxiety.

Cardiotonic Medications. Medications that improve myocardial contraction are basic in treating those forms of shock that decrease cardiac output (e.g., hypovolemic shock and cardiogenic shock):

- Rate-regulating medications such as beta-blockers and calcium-channel blockers can be used to reduce cardiac oxygen consumption. If digitalis is used, blood levels are monitored to assess for toxicity (e.g., bradydysrhythmias or tachydysrhythmias, ST-segment depression).
- Amiodarone, lidocaine, bretylium, quinidine, and procainamide may treat dysrhythmias that tend to reduce cardiac efficiency. However, these medications reduce myocardial contractility. Amiodarone is considered first-line therapy because of the significantly higher survival rate over lidocaine.
- Atropine may treat bradycardia, which predisposes clients to cardiogenic shock.

Calcium. The value and dosages of calcium in treating shock are not clear. However, calcium may be administered if impaired cardiac function is evident.

SAFETY
⚠
ALERT

Calcium chloride should be given intravenously only and through large veins.

Calcium gluconate requires greater doses for the same outcome but is less toxic to tissues if the IV infiltrates. Although calcium chloride and calcium gluconate are both available as 10% solutions, they are not identical in concentration. Do not substitute one for the other. Indications of hypocalcemia may be subtle. Careful assessment is essential. (See discussions of calcium disorders in Chapter 12.) Calcium may also precipitate toxic effects in a person who has received digitalis and should be given cautiously.

Nursing Management of the Medical Client

Nursing outcomes are similar to medical outcomes in that the overall goals of care are to correct the causative factor if possible, improve oxygenation, restore and maintain adequate tissue perfusion, and prevent complications. However, most of the interventions provided for clients in shock require a physician's order and are not independent nursing actions. The nurse's major responsibilities in shock include assessment of the client's condition and timely and accurate performance of dependent interventions.

Assessment. Because a client's condition can change rapidly in shock, frequent nursing assessment is essential. Documentation of the progress and response to interventions needs to be concise, yet convey the client's status minute by minute. Initiate a flow sheet containing all pertinent data in an easily read format. This flow sheet must contain the assessments essential in treating shock. Blood chemistries, blood gases, oxygen saturations, and electrolytes need to be determined frequently and reported promptly so therapy can be adjusted to the client's rapidly changing physiologic status.

The first step in assessing a person in shock is a general overview, giving attention to airway, breathing, and circulation (ABC).

Oxygenation Monitoring. Several assessments should be performed to determine that no airway or breathing problems exist. To determine airway patency, assess for the presence of noisy respirations and check for obstructions. Listen to lung sounds to determine adequate air movement. Assess the respiratory rate and effort to evaluate the adequacy of breathing. Evaluate chest wall expansion and assess for chest wall bulges or defects. Monitor for tracheal deviation, which could indicate tension pneumothorax.

When caring for clients experiencing shock, carefully differentiate nursing diagnoses concerning pain and impaired gas exchange. Restlessness is an assessment finding common to both and can thus be easily misinterpreted. Too often clients who are restless, especially trauma victims, are given opioids because their behavior is incorrectly interpreted as resulting from pain. However, the restlessness frequently is actually due to hypoxia, and opioids worsen the problem. The decision to administer opioids is often a nursing decision. It is important to assess the need for these medications carefully. Attention to positioning, splinting of injured areas, breathing techniques, and comfort measures may provide safer and more effective pain reduction than opioids. (Pain is discussed in detail in Chapter 20.)

Perfusion Monitoring. To complete the critical assessment of ABCs, circulation must be evaluated. Assess the client's pulse, BP, skin color, temperature, heart sounds, peripheral pulses, state of hydration, and skin perfusion (e.g., capillary refill time less than 3 seconds). Check the condition of the mucous membranes, sclera, and conjunctivae; the presence of pallor or cyanosis; and fullness of the neck veins (jugular venous distention, which may suggest right heart failure and cardiogenic shock).

It is imperative that the adequacy of blood volume be determined before administration of opioids to a client suffering from multiple trauma. Opioid administration causes vasodilation, which results in severe hypotension or shock. If an opioid is administered intramuscularly to a client in shock, it also may not be completely absorbed because of the vasoconstriction that is present. Because the client experiences little or no pain reduction, a second injection may be given. Once fluid resuscitation is complete and the circulating volume is restored, the client may absorb both doses of the opioid.

SAFETY ⚠ ALERT **No one in shock should be given intramuscular medications when rapid onset of action of the drug is needed.**

When opioids are appropriate for a client in shock, they are most effective if administered intravenously in small doses. When caring for trauma victims, especially those with massive injury, the extent of the injury does not necessarily coincide with the amount of pain being experienced. Careful assessment is necessary once opioid administration seems safe (in terms of the client's hemodynamic status). Assess the client's BP more closely after IV administration of opioids to watch for hypotension.

Even though a person in shock may feel cold and may be hypothermic, do not apply heat to the skin. Heat application dilates peripheral blood vessels and draws blood away from the vital organs (where it is life-sustaining) into the vessels of the skin. This interferes with the body's initial compensatory mechanism of peripheral vasoconstriction. Heat also increases the body's metabolism. In turn, this increases the need for oxygen and puts an added strain on the heart.

This approach does not mean that the person is kept in a cold environment. The environment is kept warm because it is important that the person not become chilled. Chilling and shivering expend energy needed to maintain vital functions. Chilling also contributes to sludging of blood in the microcirculation. Hypothermia slows the heart, increases the likelihood of ventricular fibrillation, and inhibits the body's reparative processes.

After potentially life-threatening problems are treated, obtain complete vital signs, with BP taken in both arms to rule out other causes of hypovolemic shock (i.e., thoracic dissection, aneurysm). It is important to take postural vital signs if applicable, and if it is safe to do so. Do not take postural vital signs (1) if the client has multiple traumatic injuries; (2) if there is evidence of vertebral, pelvic, or femoral fracture; or (3) if hypotension already exists. Clients with postural hypotension should not be sent to the x-ray department for upright films until they are adequately volume-resuscitated. If x-ray studies must be obtained, clients require constant attendance by a nurse, who monitors vital signs, administers IV fluids, and provides guidance to x-ray department personnel regarding movement, positioning, and timing of studies.

Measurement of postural vital signs is done when there is a history or presence of significant blood loss, unexplained tachycardia, a history of fluid loss (e.g., diarrhea, vomiting, diuretic therapy, or third-space loss), unexplained syncope, blunt chest or abdominal trauma, or abdominal pain.

Blood Pressure Monitoring. Often when a client is in shock, it is difficult to auscultate BP with a standard stethoscope. Two commonly used techniques to obtain BP measurements are palpation of the radial or brachial pulse during deflation of the BP cuff and use of a Doppler instrument. When palpation is used, the first palpable pulse noted during deflation of the cuff is the systolic BP. Document the BP as such (e.g., 90/palp). A Doppler instrument amplifies arterial and venous pulsations by ultrasonography. Various Doppler probes are available and are used instead of a stethoscope to measure BP. Systolic BP is easily heard by placing the probe over the brachial artery after applying transmission gel. The diastolic BP is not obtainable when the Doppler is used. Direct measurement of arterial BP by use of an arterial line often is done during shock. Discussion of arterial lines is found in Chapter 54.

For clarity and accuracy, document the method by which BP readings are taken (in addition to the readings themselves) and whether palpation or a Doppler monitor is used. This is important because these readings may be higher or lower than those obtained in the standard way with a cuff and stethoscope. Likewise, document whether readings are obtained by automatic BP machines even though readings from these machines may not differ from those taken in the standard way.

Once the airway is patent, air exchange is adequate, a pulse is present, and the cervical spine is immobilized (if it is a trauma situation), perform a rapid, cursory initial head-to-toe physical assessment. The initial assessment goal is to identify major problems and gross abnormalities. Give further detailed attention to specific injuries or problems after shock is stabilized.

Temperature Monitoring. An accurate core temperature measurement is important in assessing a client in shock. Sometimes an indwelling flexible rectal probe connected to a continuous display monitor is more accurate and less traumatic than intermittent rectal temperature measurements with a standard thermometer. Core temperature can also be measured with an indwelling urinary catheter that contains a thermometer. Tympanic temperatures are commonly used in critical care settings and provide core temperature measurements. Core temperature can also be obtained if the client has a thermodilution (Swan-Ganz) catheter in place.

Oral temperature measurement is neither accurate nor safe. During shock, the buccal mucosa is poorly perfused, and the client should be receiving oxygen by mask or nasal prongs. (Because clients in shock are hypoxemic, the procedure of removing the oxygen long enough to obtain an oral temperature is not routinely recommended.)

Cardiac Monitoring. For assessment and evaluation purposes, the electrocardiogram needs to be continuously monitored in all clients in shock, regardless of age. Nurses caring for clients experiencing shock need to be able to initiate cardiac monitoring, recognize cardiac dysrhythmias, and initiate treatment for any potentially lethal dysrhythmias that occur (see Chapter 57).

During the initial resuscitation period, it may be more appropriate to place the ECG monitor electrodes on the client's shoulders than on the chest. This placement does not interfere with chest film findings. It also allows better access to the chest for thoracic procedures such as insertion of chest tubes, pericardiocentesis, and CVP line placement. Once the client's condition is stabilized, the electrodes may be moved to the chest.

Hemodynamic Monitoring. Measurement of CVP is one hemodynamic technique that may be used in initial shock management, especially with hypovolemic shock. However, because CVP only provides information regarding preload, peripheral intra-arterial lines or a pulmonary artery catheter is inserted as soon as possible. Blood volume needs to be expanded as the vascular space enlarges, and CVP measurements are used to determine the amount of fluid needed to fill the enlarging vascular space. The rate of fluid replacement is adjusted to maintain the desired CVP. It is serious if the CVP continues to decrease despite fluid replacement. This means that the rate and volume of fluid replacement are not sufficient to meet the client's physiologic needs.

Peripheral arterial catheters are commonly used in shock to measure arterial BP and MAP and to obtain blood samples for chemical and blood gas analysis. These catheters are usually placed in the radial artery but may also be placed in the femoral or brachial arteries. Pulmonary artery and pulmonary capillary wedge pressure (PCWP) measurements are monitored to assess left-sided heart function and to guide fluid administration. These pressures are measured through a Swan-Ganz catheter. The PCWP reflects the LV end-diastolic pressure. This is the pressure in the LV just before contraction. An increase in this pressure in a client with cardiogenic shock may indicate left-sided heart failure. A low value in a client with hypovolemic shock may indicate that volume replacement is needed. In a client with septic shock, lower values would be expected during the warm phase and higher values during the cold phase.

Depending on the type of Swan-Ganz catheter used, additional measurements may be obtained. Some catheters have a fiberoptic tip that allows measurement of oxygen saturation of hemoglobin in the venous blood (Svo_2). Svo_2 is measured in the pulmonary artery, just before reoxygenation of the blood in the lungs. This reading gives an average of the tissue uptake or use of oxygen in the body. The normal range for Svo_2 is 60% to 80%. When the Svo_2 goes below 60%, it may indicate either decreased arterial oxygenation or increased tissue oxygen demand. If the Svo_2 is greater than 80%, the indication, in relation to shock, is that the oxygen is unable either to reach the tissues or to be extracted by the tissues.

Most Swan-Ganz catheters also have a thermistor bead just proximal to the balloon. This may be used to determine cardiac output by a thermodilution technique. A fourth lumen opens at the level of the right atrium, and CVP measurements (preload) can be obtained through this lumen.

Cardiac Output Monitoring. Cardiac output, measured in liters per minute, is the amount of blood pumped by the LV into the aorta each minute. During shock, cardiac output may be decreased because of myocardial damage resulting from an MI or, in hypovolemic shock, from inadequate volume replacement.

Because of the widespread use of Swan-Ganz catheters and the ease of obtaining measurements, cardiac output monitoring is used in managing all types of shock. These measurements assess overall cardiac function and the function of the LV. Factors that may alter cardiac output include heart rate, SVR, age, body size, exercise, and (in people with cardiac problems) decreased filling or emptying of the LV.

Cardiac index is the cardiac output divided by the body surface area. Cardiac output as a separate reading does not take into account the amount of tissue that needs to be perfused. By figuring body size into the calculation, a more accurate assessment is obtained.

SVR can be computed by dividing the cardiac output by the MAP (SVR = MAP/CO). SVR measures afterload and provides information regarding vasoconstriction or vasodilation. Decreased SVR indicates systemic vasodilation and may indicate the need for administration of vasoconstrictors. Increased SVR indicates systemic vasoconstriction and the potential need for vasodilators. Arterial BP and cardiac function should always be taken into consideration before administering vasoconstrictors or vasodilators.

Prevent Complications. Although it is important to begin assessments and interventions with the ABCs, additional assessments are necessary to evaluate the client's overall condition and prevent complications.

Additional assessments important in preventing complications include evaluation of the following:

- Level of consciousness and orientation × 3 (i.e., person, place, time)
- Ability to move extremities
- Sensation in all extremities
- Hand grasps
- Response to verbal and painful stimuli
- Pupil size and reaction to light
- Presence of abnormal posturing; presence, location, intensity, and duration of pain, and what reduces the pain
- Bowel sounds
- Abdominal distention or rigidity
- Circumference of abdomen or extremities
- Presence of lacerations, contusions, ecchymoses, petechiae, and purpura (also check for bruising over flank area)
- Bone deformities
- Presence of medical alert tags or bracelets

Prevent Renal Impairment. An indwelling urinary catheter is a simple means of monitoring a client during shock. Continuously measuring urinary flow provides important information about peripheral blood flow and kidney function. Because the amount of urine excreted during shock is often small, it is important to have an accurate, calibrated urine collector. In some settings, the catheter may be attached to a urinometer collector or to a more complex electric urinometer.

Urinary volume changes can be highly important as an index of the success or failure of therapy. Minimal (less than 0.5 ml/kg/hour) or absent urine output indicates treatment is not successful. Increasing urine output is a favorable sign. Assess the client's urine output routinely and record it at least every hour.

Prevent Gastric Ulceration. Assess gastric aspirate periodically for blood. Guaiac solution can be used to check for blood; litmus paper checks the pH to determine the acidity of the stomach. Promptly report new findings of blood or increases in the amount of blood.

Diagnosis, Outcomes, Interventions

Diagnosis: Ineffective Tissue Perfusion. The nursing diagnosis *Ineffective Tissue Perfusion* can be used to describe the reduced tissue perfusion and inadequate effective circulating intravascular blood volume. This diagnosis does not describe the oxygen-carrying capacity of the blood, but rather the volume of circulating blood and its ability to reach the tissues. The nursing diagnosis can be written *Ineffective Tissue Perfusion (specify type) related to actual or relative (specify type) hypovolemia secondary to shock (specify type).* Other potential nursing diagnoses for the client in shock are listed in Box 81-2.

BOX 81-2   Potential Nursing Diagnoses for the Client in Shock

- Activity Intolerance
- Acute Pain
- Anticipatory Grieving
- Anxiety
- Bathing/Hygiene, Dressing/Grooming, Toileting Self-Care Deficit
- Compromised Family Coping
- Constipation
- Decreased Cardiac Output
- Deficient Fluid Volume
- Disturbed Body Image
- Disturbed Personal Identity
- Disturbed Sleep Pattern
- Disturbed Sensory Perception: Visual, Auditory, Kinesthetic, Gustatory, Tactile, Olfactory
- Fear
- Imbalanced Nutrition: Less Than Body Requirements
- Impaired Gas Exchange
- Impaired Physical Mobility
- Impaired or Risk for Impaired Skin Integrity
- Impaired Tissue Integrity
- Impaired Verbal Communication
- Ineffective Airway Clearance
- Ineffective Breathing Pattern
- Ineffective Protection
- Ineffective Tissue Perfusion: Cerebral, Cardiopulmonary, Gastrointestinal, Renal, Peripheral
- Interrupted Family Processes
- Spiritual Distress

Outcomes. Nursing care of the client with shock is complex. Specific nursing and medical interventions vary according to individual needs and the setting in which care is delivered (e.g., emergency department versus intensive care unit). However, two major physiologic outcomes of care are desired:

1. Adequate blood flow (tissue perfusion) and cellular oxygenation are achieved to maintain the integrity of the tissue or organ.
2. The metabolic needs of the tissue or organ are reduced or maintained.

Interventions. Provide continuous assessment of the client. Keep equipment and supplies (e.g., suction, emergency drugs) available and in working order. Cardiovascular and respiratory changes can occur rapidly, and interventions must be adjusted promptly. Document observations clearly and concisely.

Help decrease tissue oxygen demand. Because shock states can double the body's O_2 consumption, promote factors that decrease tissue oxygen need. Interventions are aimed at decreasing total body work, pain, anxiety, and temperature to decrease tissue oxygen demand.

Implement appropriate, planned nursing interventions to prevent complications that can develop from enforced immobilization. Provide adequate pain reduction, because pain intensifies shock. Base this intervention on careful assessment.

🪔 Diagnosis: Interrupted Family Processes. Sudden changes in the family's communication and ability to problem-solve without the client and concerns about the cause of illness, or worry about the outcome, create a situational crisis. The appropriate nursing diagnosis is *Interrupted Family Processes.*

Outcomes. The goal is that the usual processes of coping for the family remain intact or that a new process be adopted to facilitate problem solving. Outcomes may include that the family members remain supportive of each other, cope reasonably well with the crisis, and participate in problem solving or decision making with the health care team. Another goal might be that the client and significant others understand the cause of the problem and modify their lifestyle to minimize or eliminate the causative factor.

Interventions. Facilitate expression of concerns and questions by the client and family. For example, try to reduce the client's fears and anxieties about what is happening and about the equipment being used.

A client in shock is extremely ill and may die. In addition, the stress of the situation is compounded by emergency medical treatment, with all the people, equipment, and movement this entails. During shock management, nurses attend to numerous delegated medical care activities. However, there must be sufficient nursing resources to provide psychosocial care (e.g., reassurance, emotional support) to the client and family.

Keep the client's family informed of what is happening. They need information on which to base decisions. Because of the family's anxiety, the nurse may need to calmly repeat information several times. The Client Education Guide at right highlights information to be conveyed to the families of clients with shock. Remember that the client and significant others may be experiencing "psychological shock." They often need, and greatly appreciate, opportunities to discuss with care providers their important concerns.

Help the client (and family) feel physically and emotionally comfortable. Do not keep loved ones away from the client unnecessarily. Because of limited space, there may be times when they must wait in another room for a period of time. However, they should not be kept away long and should be given a reasonable explanation of why it is necessary to leave their loved one.

A client experiencing shock requires emotional support. When caught up in the sudden drama of an emergency or critical care, health professionals sometimes forget that the experience and setting are often new and very frightening for the client. Unfortunately, "dehumanization" of the client may occasionally occur during the rush of emergency treatment. Whether a client appears to be conscious or not, always explain what is happening. Keep the atmosphere as quiet and orderly as possible. Eliminate unnecessary chatter. Commonly, recovered clients remember hearing what was said and were aware of what happened to them even though they appeared to be unconscious.

Provide care to the family. Among a nurse's greatest responsibilities are providing support, comfort, and advocacy to clients receiving care and to their significant others. All of the people involved may be frightened, anxious, confused, and dependent. The Translating Evidence into Practice feature on p. 2183 addresses how to help families best manage the multiple, often overwhelming concerns related to the sudden onset and complex condition of shock. This is very important for nursing clients who are critically ill and are experiencing shock.

Evaluation. It is expected that the client will achieve adequate tissue perfusion and make a full recovery without complications from the type of shock being experienced, be transferred to a medical unit, and eventually be dismissed to home. Recovery from the cause of the shock may be delayed because of the complications created from the shock episode (e.g., wound healing).

CLIENT EDUCATION GUIDE   🔲

Family Support for the Client with Shock

- It is difficult to prevent the occurrence of shock because the causes are often unpredictable. If your family member is in shock, obtain precise, consistent information about his or her current status and prognosis.
- Learn about the monitoring equipment in use.
- Learn how to communicate with the client who is intubated or unconscious.
- Learn how to demonstrate love and caring to someone surrounded by equipment.
- Participate in your family member's care during the hospital stay; this increases your ability to provide care at home.
- Learn how to prevent recurrence if the cause was avoidable.

TRANSLATING EVIDENCE INTO PRACTICE

Helping Family Members Deal with Life-Threatening Illnesses

The etiologies leading to the various types of shock usually have a sudden onset. Families and significant others have little warning or preparation for the life-threatening nature of their loved one's illness, and few have had experience with a family member being critically ill. The illness trajectory is often characterized by periods of stability and instability, and the critically ill client may move back and forth between the two states. All of this leads to a great deal of uncertainty for the families of individuals with shock.

Uncertainty as a concept has been described as having four components: (1) ambiguity concerning the state of the illness, (2) complexity concerning treatment and the system of care, (3) lack of information regarding diagnosis and the severity of illness, and (4) unpredictability of the course of illness and outcome.[2] All four of these components may be experienced by families of an individual shock.

Three studies were reviewed to determine the factors that lead to uncertainty and to identify those interventions most effective in alleviating the uncertainty for families of critically ill clients.

Uncertainty may stem from the tension between the capabilities of modern medicine (i.e., high-tech interventions) to maintain life and the philosophical perspective held by some of death with dignity and the obligation to honor their loved one's wishes related to extraordinary measures to sustain life. Contributors to uncertainty include (1) the client's current health status, (2) treatments necessary to save the loved one's life and the decisions families make about those treatments, (3) lack of information overall, (4) unfamiliarity with the setting, and (5) the need to be with and to be vigilant for their loved one. The experiences families have described resemble a vortex in which there is a downward spiral of prognoses, difficult decisions, feelings of inadequacy, potential for loss despite best efforts, and the possibility that the loved one may remain unconscious and die with no opportunity to say goodbye.

Despite the best efforts of the health care team, sometimes critically ill clients die. However, there are many opportunities during the care of a critically ill client to diminish the family's feelings of uncertainty. Families describe "living it one day at a time" and often need "just in time" information rather than the entire trajectory of information laid out before them. Family members may feel positive about what they have to offer their loved one if they are allowed to participate in the loved one's care.

Families remain vigilant for their loved one. It is unhelpful to provide false hope, but it is equally unhelpful to paint a bleak picture if the outcomes for the client are not yet certain. Families have also described "drawing on God's strength" as something that helps them cope with the uncertainty. Family members may find comfort in talking with someone from pastoral care if that service is available.

Implications for practice include allowing open visitation so that families can spend as much time as they need with their loved one. Families also need to have access to the physicians, nurses, and other health care providers who will listen to their concerns, provide information, and correct any misconceptions they may have. Contact pastoral care or other hospital personnel who can help families find comfort if the family requests it.

Implications for research include exploring the interventions most helpful to families of clients in shock. How much information can families take in at one time? How can the overwhelming nature of the technology be made more manageable for families? Considering the time constraints of health care professionals, how can families' questions and concerns be addressed in a timely manner?

REFERENCES

1. Kirchhoff, K.T., et al (2002). The vortex: Families' experiences with death in the intensive care unit. *American Journal of Critical Care, 11*(3), 200-209.
2. Mishel, M.H. (1981). The measurement of uncertainty. *Nursing Research, 30*, 258-263.
3. Pelletier-Hibbert, M., & Sohi, P. (2001). Sources of uncertainty and coping strategies used by family members of individuals living with end stage renal disease. *Nephrology Nursing Journal, 28*(4), 411-419.
4. Plowfield, L.A. (1999). Living a nightmare: Family experiences of waiting following neurological crisis. *Journal of Neuroscience Nursing, 31*(4), 231-238.

Surgical Management

Although surgical interventions that can help in shock states are limited, they may be very useful. In hypovolemic shock caused by trauma, surgery can be performed to control sources of bleeding. Once bleeding is controlled, interventions aimed at restoring adequate fluid volume are more effective. In septic shock, surgery may help manage the source of infection.

Self-Care

Shock must be fully resolved before a client is transferred or discharged (unless the client is being transported for the treatment of shock). Clients who survive shock find that recovery from the precipitating problem is delayed. They may also experience some feelings of confusion, depression, or grief when they realize that they lived through a very critical illness.

SYSTEMIC INFLAMMATORY RESPONSE SYNDROME (SIRS)

SIRS is an inflammatory clinical response of the whole body without a proven source of infection. SIRS is non-specific and can be caused by ischemia, inflammation, trauma, infection, or a combination of several insults. SIRS with a confirmed source of infection, through blood or tissue cultures, is called *sepsis* (Table 81-5). SIRS is defined as two or more of the following variables:

- Temperature of more than 38° C or less than 36° C
- Heart rate of more than 90 beats per minute
- Respiratory rate of more than 20 breaths per minute or a $Paco_2$ level of less than 32 mm Hg
- Abnormal white blood cell count (>12,000/μl or <4000/μl or >10% bands)

MULTIPLE ORGAN DYSFUNCTION SYNDROME

Single-organ failure (e.g., heart failure, renal failure) has long been recognized as a cause of morbidity and mortality in critically ill clients. *Multiple organ dysfunction syndrome* (MODS) is present when two or more organs fail. MODS is the presence of altered organ function in a client who is acutely ill such that homeostasis cannot be maintained without intervention.

Etiology and Risk Factors

Causes of MODS include dead tissue, injured tissue, infection, perfusion deficits, and persistent sources of inflammation such as pancreatitis or pneumonitis. Acute lung injury is usually present in some form. People known to be at high risk for developing MODS include those with impaired immune responses, such as older adults, clients with chronic illnesses, clients with malnutrition, and clients with cancer. In addition, clients with prolonged or exaggerated inflammatory responses are at risk, including victims of severe trauma and clients with sepsis.

Prevention is a primary direction of current therapy. Source control is a major emphasis. When possible, the potential source of sepsis or inflammation is excised or removed (e.g., infected central line or pressure ulcer).

TABLE 81–5 The Relationship of SIRS to Sepsis

Condition	Definition
SIRS	Inflammatory state of whole body without a proven source of infection
Sepsis	SIRS caused by known infection
Severe Sepsis	Sepsis with evidence of organ hypoperfusion
Septic Shock	Severe sepsis with hypotension despite adequate fluid resuscitation or requirement for vasopressor or inotropics to maintain blood pressure

In many cases, however, the source cannot be removed, such as pneumonia, pancreatitis, soft tissue injury, and hematoma. When the source cannot be removed, empirical antimicrobial agents are used to reduce risk.

It would be helpful to clinicians to be able to predict which clients are at the highest risk, but accurate prediction remains elusive. The most predictive variables appear to be the ratio of arterial oxygen tension (Pao_2) to the fraction of inspired oxygen (Fio_2) on day 1; the plasma lactate concentration on day 2; the serum bilirubin level on day 6; and the serum creatinine level on day 12 after injury. When nurses note these predictors, increased surveillance should begin.

Pathophysiology

In the healthy person, the normal integrated inflammatory response protects tissue from microbial invasion and rids the body of cellular debris and foreign material. This process of responses continues until the insult slows and the client's condition stabilizes. The inflammatory response also normally stops once it is no longer needed. SIRS is a case of unchecked inflammatory responses. MODS is the end result of the prolonged response.

Once the inflammatory response becomes systemic, it is controlled by chemical mediators of inflammation. Mediators include bradykinin, complement, histamine, interleukin-1, prekallikrein, prostaglandins, and tumor necrosis factor. These powerful mediators of inflammation induce a systemic response. Endothelial cells are a common target for some mediators. The endothelium is destroyed, and blood flow is reduced to the tissues. Endothelial damage is produced by endotoxins from bacteria, tumor necrosis factor, interleukin-1, platelet activating factors, and many others. When this inflammatory response is unchecked, it produces damage to organs and tissues by altering perfusion, disturbing oxygen supply or demand, or changing metabolic dysfunctions. Metabolism increases under the direction of mediators such as cortisol and the catecholamines.

Many organs are affected by MODS. The lungs are usually the first to malfunction, because of the large surface area of pulmonary epithelium combined with the presence of bacterial contamination from systemic blood return. The GI tract is generally the second system to malfunction, and it propagates conditions for further deterioration of other organs. Once the GI tract is malfunctioning, bacteria quickly relocate from the GI tract to other organs. Additionally, the hypermetabolic state increases gastric acid production, increasing the risk of ulceration and bleeding. The most serious metabolic problem is hypermetabolism. The hypermetabolic state is continued by cell-to-cell communication, and the sympathetic nervous system responds with its usual "fight-or-flight" response.

Classification

There are two types of MODS. *Primary* MODS results directly from a well-defined insult in which organ dysfunction occurs early and is directly attributed to the insult itself. The direct insult initially causes a localized inflammatory response that may or may not progress to SIRS. An example of primary MODS is a primary pulmonary injury, such as aspiration. Only a small percentage of clients develop primary MODS.

Secondary MODS is a consequence of widespread systemic inflammation, which develops after a variety of insults, and results in dysfunction of organs not involved in the initial insult. The client enters a hypermetabolic state that lasts for 14 to 21 days. During this time, the body catabolizes muscle and fat for energy, which causes profound changes in the body's metabolic processes. Unless the process can be stopped, the outcome for the client is death. Secondary MODS occurs with conditions such as septic shock and ARDS.

Clinical Manifestations

There is usually a precipitating event to MODS, including aspiration, ruptured aneurysm, or septic shock, which is associated with resultant hypotension. The client is resuscitated, the cause is treated, and the client appears to do well for a few days. The following possible sequence of events often develops.

The client experiences SIRS before MODS develops. Within a few days, there is an insidious onset of a low-grade fever, tachycardia, increased numbers of banded and segmented neutrophils on the differential count (called a left shift), and dyspnea with the appearance of diffuse patchy infiltrates on the chest x-ray film. The client often has some deterioration in mental status, with reasonably normal renal and hepatic laboratory results. Dyspnea progresses, and intubation and mechanical ventilation are required. Some evidence of consumptive coagulopathy (DIC) is usually present. The client is usually stable hemodynamically and has relative polyuria, an increased cardiac index (greater than 4.5 L/min), and systemic vascular resistance of less than 600 dynes cm^{-5}. Clients often have increased blood glucose levels in the absence of diabetes. Some physicians use the criteria presented in Box 81-3 to make the diagnosis of MODS.

Between days 7 and 10, the bilirubin level increases and continues to increase, followed by an increase in serum creatinine level. Blood glucose and lactate levels continue to increase because of the hypermetabolic state. Other progressive changes include excretion of urinary nitrogen and protein combined with decreased levels of serum albumin, prealbumin, and retinol binding protein. Bacteremia with enteric organisms is also common. In addition, infections from *Candida* and viruses such as herpes and cytomegalovirus are common. Surgical wounds fail to heal, and pressure ulcers may develop. During this time, the client needs increasing amounts of fluids and inotropic medications to keep blood volume and cardiac preload near normal and to replace fluids lost through polyuria.

BOX 81-3 **Modified Apache II Criteria for Diagnosis of Multiple Organ Dysfunction Syndrome**

CARDIOVASCULAR FAILURE (PRESENCE OF ONE OR MORE OF THE FOLLOWING)
- Heart rate <54 beats/min
- Mean arterial pressure ≤49 mm Hg (systolic pressure ≤60 mm Hg)
- Occurrence of ventricular tachycardia or ventricular fibrillation
- Serum pH ≤7.24 with a $Paco_2$ of ≤40 mm Hg

RESPIRATORY FAILURE (PRESENCE OF ONE OR MORE OF THE FOLLOWING)
- Respiratory rate ≤5 breaths/min or ≥49 breaths/min with a $Paco_2$ ≥50 mm Hg
- Alveolar – arterial oxygen difference ≥350 mm Hg (at sea level calculate as follows: [713 × % oxygen in inspired gas] – $Paco_2$ – Pao_2)
- Dependent on ventilator or CPAP on the second day

RENAL FAILURE (PRESENCE OF ONE OR MORE OF THE FOLLOWING)
- Urine output ≤479 ml/24 hr or ≤159 ml/8 hr
- Serum BUN ≥100 mg/dl (35.7 mmol/L)
- Serum creatinine ≥3.5 mg/dl (309 μmol/L)

HEMATOLOGIC FAILURE (PRESENCE OF ONE OR MORE OF THE FOLLOWING)
- WBC count ≤1000/μl (1 × 10^9/L)
- Platelets ≤20,000/μl (20 × 10^9/L)
- Hematocrit ≤20%

NEUROLOGIC FAILURE
- Glasgow Coma Scale score ≤6 (in absence of sedation)

HEPATIC FAILURE (PRESENCE OF BOTH OF THE FOLLOWING)
- Serum bilirubin ≥6 mg%
- Prothrombin time ≥4 sec over control in the absence of systemic anticoagulation

CPAP, Continuous positive airway pressure; *BUN,* blood urea nitrogen; *WBC,* white blood cell.
From Knaus, W.A., & Wagner, D.P. (1989). Multiple systems organ failure: Epidemiology and prognosis. *Critical Care Clinics, 5*(2), 221.

Between day 14 and day 21, the client is unstable and appears close to death. The client may lose consciousness. Renal failure worsens to the point of considering dialysis. Edema may be present because of low serum protein levels. Mixed venous oxygen levels may increase because of problems with tissue uptake of oxygen caused by mitochondrial dysfunction. Lactic acidosis worsens, liver enzymes continue to increase, and coagulation disorders become impossible to correct.

Prognosis

If the process of MODS is not reversed by day 21, it is usually evident that the client will die. Death usually occurs between days 21 and 28 after the injury or precipitating event. Not all clients with MODS die; however, MODS remains the leading cause of death in the intensive care unit, with mortality rates from 50% to 90%, despite the development of better antibiotics, better resuscitation, and more sophisticated means of organ support. For those clients who survive, the average duration of intensive care unit stay is about 21 days. The rehabilitation, which is directed at recovery of muscle mass and neuromuscular function, lasts about 10 months.

OUTCOME MANAGEMENT

Medical Management

Restrain the Activators

Manifestations of potential infection must be quickly treated to restrain the activators of MODS. If the agent is known, antibiotics to which the organism is sensitive should be administered. If the organism is not known, broad-spectrum empirical antibiotics are given. Early aggressive management of sources of infection should be carried out. For example, the client may need to have a large infected wound incised and drained or necrotic tissue excised.

SAFETY ALERT

Extreme caution must be taken to avoid infecting the client. These clients have many invasive monitors and may have open wounds. Unfortunately, clients in critical care units exist in a paradox. The ICU is the only environment with sophisticated equipment and health care professionals to provide safe care, yet it is an environment where the risk of infection is higher. In addition, there is a high prevalence of multiresistant organisms, such as *vancomycin-resistant enterococci* (VRE) and methicillin-resistant *Staphylococcus aureus* (MRSA).

If the severity of the sepsis is identified early and drotrecogin alfa (Xigris) (see earlier discussion) is administered, progression to MODS may be prevented. However, if there is progression, the lungs are often the first organs to fail and so require special attention. Aggressive pulmonary care is needed in all clients who are at risk of MODS. Interventions may be as simple as coughing and deep breathing or ambulation. The client's oxygen saturation should be monitored as well.

Because malnutrition develops from the hypermetabolism and the GI tract often seeds other areas with bacteria, some clinicians require the client to be fed enterally. They believe that feeding enhances perfusion and decreases the bacterial load and the effects of endotoxins. Nutrient intake is usually 30 to 35 kcal/kg/day of carbohydrates. Fats are restricted to 0.5 to 1 g/kg/day. Proteins are given to the client via modified amino acids. Some practitioners administer protein until an increase in plasma transferrin or prealbumin level is noted. Increases in these values indicate hepatic protein synthesis rather than a breakdown of body stores. Decontamination of the GI tract and pharynx decreases infection but has shown no effect on the death rate from MODS.

Control the Mediators

Controlling the mediators of inflammation is directed at (1) general levels of care and (2) specific treatments targeted at the problem cells. Maintenance of a positive nitrogen balance via nutrition, promotion of sleep and rest, and management of pain are important general care areas. Specific treatments include monoclonal antibodies to control mediators such as interleukin-1, endotoxins, and tumor necrosis factors. These therapies are shown in Table 81-6. Outcomes from research in these treatments are conflicting, and it appears that there is no "magic bullet" to cure the problem.

Protect the Affected Organs

Care is directed toward maintaining the function of organs that fail with MODS. The client is intubated and mechanically ventilated to maintain adequate oxygenation. Oxygen is given to the client until blood levels of lactate decrease toward normal. Elevated serum lactate levels indicate the use of anaerobic metabolism. Nurses must recognize that certain clinical problems further increase the need for oxygen. Problems such as fever, seizures, and shivering increase oxygen demands. These problems should be controlled with medications or environmental changes (e.g., warming).

TABLE 81–6 Summary of Potentially Useful Therapies for Multiple Organ Dysfunction Syndrome

Rationale	Therapy
Treatment of infection	Monoclonal antibodies
	Passive antibody protection
	Gut decontamination regimens
Support of gut function	Mucosal trophic agents (e.g., glutamine, bombesin, ketone bodies)
	Early enteral feeding
	Regulation of gut microbial flora
Improved resuscitation	Hypertonic saline
	In-line sensors
	Tissue-specific sensors
	Noninvasive monitoring
Endothelial cell protection	PAF inhibitors
	WBC adherence inhibition
	Antioxidant therapy
	Eicosanoid modulation
Modulation of macrophage function	n3-Polyunsaturated fatty acids
	Signal transduction modulation
Stimulation of lymphocyte function	Arginine
	ω3-Polyunsaturated fatty acids

PAF, Platelet activating factor; *WBC,* white blood cell.
From Lekander, B.J., & Cerra, F.B. (1990). The syndrome of multiple organ failure. *Critical Care Clinics of North America,* 2(2), 338.

Fluids and inotropic drugs are used to support hemodynamic parameters. The client often becomes more unstable and needs continuous monitoring. Nutritional support is also critical to reduce the catabolism that accompanies hypermetabolism. Dialysis is often used to reduce azotemia from renal failure.

Nursing Management of the Medical Client

Care of the client with MODS is multifaceted, balancing the needs of one system against the needs of another while trying to maintain optimal functioning of each system. Nursing diagnoses appropriate for the client with MODS are determined by the system involved and the clinical manifestations identified.

The number of independent nursing interventions for the client with MODS is limited. The overall goal for nursing is effective client and family coping. This complex disorder taxes the client and family. Nurses must remain sensitive to the needs of the family. Caring for the family of critically ill clients is a challenge in that understanding, predicting, and intervening with families in crisis are less exact than the calculation of oxygen needs. There are no easy formulas to use to provide hope, courage, coping, and caring. Nurses must remain alert to the needs of the family as well as the client during this stressful time.

CONCLUSIONS

This chapter discussed shock under three major classifications: hypovolemic, cardiogenic, and distributive. The pathophysiology, clinical manifestations, and medical and nursing management are presented. Shock is a critical condition with a high death rate. Early diagnosis and intervention are necessary for the best possible outcomes. Multiple organ dysfunction syndrome is a syndrome of multiple organs progressively failing because of prolonged inflammatory responses. Again, early diagnosis and intervention are critical for positive outcomes.

THINKING CRITICALLY

1. The client is a 20-year-old man with a gunshot wound to the right chest and massive hemorrhage. His systolic BP is 60 mm Hg (palpated), heart rate is 130 beats/min, and respiratory rate is 36 breaths/min. The skin is pale, cold, and clammy; capillary refill time is greater than 3 seconds; pulses are weak and thready. What priority assessments should be done? What interventions might be performed?

Factors to Consider. What do his vital signs tell you? What injuries might have occurred with a major chest trauma? How can his need for fluid and blood replacement best be met?

2. A 69-year-old man was brought to the emergency department by a rescue squad. He had undergone a colon resection 2 weeks previously. His wife said that he was having increased difficulty breathing, and he could feel his heart beating in his chest. He also has seemed "slower" to her. He is not moving as fast as usual and gets very dizzy when he stands up. He almost passed out, which is why she called the rescue squad. What priority assessments should be done? What interventions might be performed?

Factors to Consider. What might be happening that could lead to all of the problems with breathing, dizziness, and confusion? What risk might be present as a result of the surgery?

3. A 65-year-old man in the coronary care unit had an acute MI 3 days ago. The monitor alarms and assessments reveal that his BP is 76/50 mm Hg, and his respiratory rate is 20 breaths/min. His pulse is rapid (128 beats/min) and thready. His skin is cool and diaphoretic, with a slight ashen color; the capillary refill time is greater than 3 seconds. The client is restless and confused. What priority assessments should be done? What interventions might be performed?

Factors to Consider. What form of shock can quickly develop in a client after an MI? Does he need fluid resuscitation to increase his blood pressure? Why or why not? What medications are commonly used to support a heart in distress? Are special forms of monitoring needed while these medications are used?

Discussions for the questions can be found on the website. **evolve**

BIBLIOGRAPHY

Citations appearing in red refer to primary research.

Citations appearing in blue refer to evidence-based practice guidelines and protocols.

1. Angstwurm, M.W., Engelmann, L., Zimmermann, T., et al (2007). Selenium in intensive care (SIC): Results of a prospective randomized, placebo-controlled, multiple-center study in patients with severe systemic inflammatory response syndrome, sepsis, and septic shock. *Critical Care Medicine, 35*(1), 118-126.
2. Bassi, G., Radermacher, P., & Calzia, E. (2006). Catecholamines and vasopressin during critical illness. *Endocrinology and Metabolism Clinics of North America, 35*(4), 839-857.
3. Bilbault, P., Lavaux, T., Launoy, A., et al (2007). Influence of drotrecogin alpha (activated) infusion on the variation of Bax/Bcl-2 and Bax/Bcl-xl ratios in circulating mononuclear cells: A cohort study in septic shock patients. *Critical Care Medicine, 35*(1), 69-75.
4. Boeuf, B., Poirier, V., Gauvin, F., et al (2003). Naloxone for shock. *Cochrane Database of Systematic Reviews*, (4), CD004443.
5. Boos, L., Szalai, A.J., & Barnum, S.R. (2005). C3a expressed in the central nervous system protects against LPS-induced shock. *Neuroscience Letters, 387*(2), 68-71.
6. Brasel, K.J., Guse, C., Gentilello, L.M., Nirula, R. Heart rate: Is it truly a vital sign? *Journal of Trauma, 62*(4), 812-817.
7. Brown, E.J. (2004). The molecular basis of streptococcal toxic shock syndrome. *New England Journal of Medicine, 350*, 2093-2094.
8. Bulger, E.M., Cuschieri, J., Warner, K., Maier, R.V. Hypertonic resuscitation modulates the inflammatory response in patients with traumatic hemorrhagic shock. *Annals of Surgery, 245*(4), 635-641.
9. Cohn, S.M., Nathens, A.B., Moore, F.A., et al (2007). Tissue oxygen saturation predicts the development of organ dysfunction during traumatic shock resuscitation. *Journal of Trauma, 62*(1), 44-54, discussion 54-55.
10. Dellinger, R.P., Carlet, J.M., Masur, H., et al (2004). Surviving Sepsis Campaign guidelines for management of severe sepsis and septic shock. *Critical Care Medicine, 32*(3), 858-873.

11. Dewachter, P., Jouan-Hureaux, V., Franck, P., et al (2005). Anaphylactic shock: A form of distributive shock without inhibition of oxygen consumption. *Anesthesiology, 103*(1), 40-49.

12. Fisher, C.G., Noonan, V.K., Smith, D.E., et al (2005). Motor recovery, functional status, and health-related quality of life in patients with complete spinal cord injuries. *Spine, 30*(19), 2200-2207.

13. Geppert, A., Dorninger, A., Delle-Karth, G., et al (2006). Plasma concentrations of interleukin-6, organ failure, vasopressor support, and successful coronary revascularization in predicting 30-day mortality of patients with cardiogenic shock complicating acute myocardial infarction. *Critical Care Medicine, 34*(8), 2035-2042.

14. Gross, P.A. (2006). Hypotension and mortality in septic shock: The "golden hour." *Critical Care Medicine, 34*(6), 1819-1820.

15. Habler, O.P., & Messmer, K.F. (2000). Tissue perfusion and oxygenation with blood substitutes. *Advanced Drug Delivery Reviews, 40*(3), 171-184.

16. Hekmat, K., Kroener, A., Stuetzer, H., et al (2005). Daily assessment of organ dysfunction and survival in intensive care unit cardiac surgical patients. *Annals of Thoracic Surgery, 79*(5), 1555-1562.

17. Hotchkiss, R.S., & Karl, I.E. (2003). The pathophysiology and treatment of sepsis. *New England Journal of Medicine, 348*, 138-150.

18. Huang, S.C., Chen, Y.S., Chi, N.H., et al (2006). Out-of-center extracorporeal membrane oxygenation for adult cardiogenic shock patients. *Artificial Organs, 30*(1), 24-28.

19. Kasperska-Zajac, A., & Rogala, B. (2006). Platelet function in anaphylaxis. *Journal of Investigative Allergology and Clinical Immunology, 16*(1), 1-4.

20. Kohsaka, S., Menon, V., Iwata, K., et al (2007). Microbiological profile of septic complication in patients with cardiogenic shock following acute myocardial infarction (from the SHOCK study). *American Journal of Cardiology, 99*(6), 802-804.

21. Kumar, A., Roberts, D., Wood, K.E., et al (2006). Duration of hypotension before initiation of effective antimicrobial therapy is the critical determinant of survival in human septic shock. *Critical Care Medicine, 34*(6), 1589-1596.

22. Lowenstein, C.J., & Michel, T. (2006). What's in a name? eNOS and anaphylactic shock. *Journal of Clinical Investigation, 116*(8), 2075-2078.

23. Mann, H.J., & Nolan, P.E., Jr. (2006). Update on the management of cardiogenic shock. *Current Opinions in Critical Care, 12*(5), 431-436.

24. Minneci, P.C., Deans, K.J., Banks, S.M., et al (2004). Meta-analysis: The effect of steroids on survival and shock during sepsis depends on the dose. *Annals of Internal Medicine, 141*(1), 47-56.

25. Nguyen, H.B., Corbett, S.W., Steele, R., et al (2007). Implementation of a bundle of quality indicators for the early management of severe sepsis and septic shock is associated with decreased mortality. *Critical Care Medicine, 35*(4), 1105-1112.

26. Nguyen, H.B., Rivers, E.P., Abrahamian, F.M., et al (2006). Severe sepsis and septic shock: Review of the literature and emergency department management guidelines. *Annals of Emergency Medicine, 48*(1), 28-54.

27. Poupko, J.M., Baskin, S.I., & Moore, E. (2007). The pharmacological properties of anisodamine. *Journal of Applied Toxicology, 27*(2), 116-121.

28. Powers, J., & Jacobi, J. (2006). Pharmacologic treatment related to severe sepsis. *AACN Advanced Critical Care, 17*(4), 423-432, quiz 434.

29. Revelly, J.P., Tappy, L., Martinez, A., et al (2005). Lactate and glucose metabolism in severe sepsis and cardiogenic shock. *Critical Care Medicine, 33*(10), 2235-2240.

30. Rudiger, A., Gasser, S., Fischler, M., et al (2006). Comparable increase of B-type natriuretic peptide and amino-terminal pro-B-type natriuretic peptide levels in patients with severe sepsis, septic shock, and acute heart failure. *Critical Care Medicine, 34*(8), 2140-2144.

31. Schmidt, H., Muller-Werdan, U., Hoffmann, T., et al (2005). Autonomic dysfunction predicts mortality in patients with multiple organ dysfunction syndrome of different age groups. *Critical Care Medicine, 33*(9), 1994-2002.

32. Sheikh, A., ten Broek, V., Brown, S.G., Simons, F.E. H1-antihistamines for the treatment of anaphylaxis with and without shock. *Cochrane Database of Systematic Reviews,* (1), CD006160.

33. Stephens, C., & Fawcett, T.N. (2007). Nitric oxide and nursing: A review. *Journal of Clinical Nursing, 16*(1), 67-76.

34. Turgeon, A.F., Hutton, B., Fergusson, D.A., et al (2007). Meta-analysis: Intravenous immunoglobulin in critically ill adult patients with sepsis. *Annals of Internal Medicine, 146*(3), 193-203.

35. Zardi, E.M., Zardi, D.M., Dobrina, A., et al (2007). Prostacyclin in sepsis: A systematic review. *Prostaglandins & Other Lipid Mediators, 83*(1-2), 1-24.

evolve *Did you remember to check out the bonus material on the Evolve website and the CD-ROM, including NCLEX®-Examination Style Review Questions, Open-Book Quizzes, and Chapter Review Audio Podcasts?*

http://evolve.elsevier.com/Black/medsurg

CHAPTER 82

Management of Clients in the Emergency Department

JUDITH S. HALPERN AND PATRICIA A. MANION

During the mid-1960s, the need for specialization of emergency services throughout the United States was identified as a national priority to reduce the associated morbidity and mortality resulting from catastrophic illness or injury. Since then, the specialties of emergency medicine, emergency nursing, and prehospital care services have grown. In the United States, emergency department (ED) visits have increased by 18% (from 93.4 million to 110.2 million) during the years from 1994 to 2004. More than 100 million clients use EDs for health care services each year. The number of EDs throughout the United States has not increased over that same time period, however; in fact, they have decreased by about 12%. This equates to approximately 209 visits to U.S. EDs every minute during 2004. The age groups with the most frequent visits were 50 to 64 year olds (up 17%), 22 to 49 year olds (up 15%), and 65 years and older (up 8%). The scope of services provided in an ED range from treatment of acute conditions that threaten the loss of life, limb, or vision to management of non-urgent, chronic conditions. The types of clinical manifestations that accounted for the most frequent visits were general (e.g., fever, fatigue, pain), musculoskeletal, digestive, and respiratory.

EMERGENCY MEDICAL SERVICES

The emergency medical services (EMS) system encompasses all aspects of emergency care. Federal, state, and county EMS systems are designed to complement each other. The systems are responsible for establishing, regulating, coordinating, and monitoring the components involved in the provision of emergency care. These components include entities such as 911 telephone access systems, Emergency Medical Technician (EMT) and paramedical personnel scopes of practice, ground and air ambulance services, dispatch communication between points of incident and responding personnel, and telecommunications between paramedical personnel and specialty-designated EDs known as *base station hospitals.* EMS systems are also instrumental in the coordination of activities for management of disaster situations.

Two goals of the EMS system are (1) to provide emergency care to a client as quickly as possible and (2) to ensure that the "right client arrives at the right hospital in the least amount of time." Consequently, EMS systems are involved with specialty-designated hospital departments and EDs such as local or state trauma centers, burn centers, and pediatric care centers.

EMERGENCY NURSING

Emergency nursing was officially recognized as a specialty in 1970. The national association representing these nurses is the Emergency Nurses Association (ENA). In 2006 the ENA was comprised of approximately 30,000 nurses who have chosen this area of professional nursing. Emergency nurses throughout the world have realized both their similarities and their differences through use of the World Wide Web and increasing international globalization.

According to the ENA, the definition of emergency nursing involves "the assessment, diagnosis, and treatment of perceived, actual or potential, sudden or urgent,

---

evolve Web Enhancements

Ethical Issues in Nursing   Are Emergency Personnel Obliged to Honor Clients' Advance Directives?

Appendix A   Religious Beliefs and Practices Affecting Health Care

Be sure to check out the bonus material on the Evolve website and the CD-ROM, including free self-assessment exercises. **http://evolve.elsevier. com/Black/medsurg**

physical or psychosocial problems that are primarily episodic or acute." These may require minimal care or life-support measures, education of client and significant others, appropriate referral, and knowledge of legal implications.

The ED of the future is being formulated today. Not only is technology changing, but also the day-to-day processes that support the ED infrastructure are being challenged and redesigned. These include concepts such as incorporating multiple triage stations and bedside or back-end client registration; using computerized protocols, guidelines, and electronic medical records; integrating nontraditional health care modalities; initiating wireless communication technology; and creating "virtual" EDs. In addition to the provision of direct client care, other multifaceted roles exist within emergency nursing. The emergency nurse is involved in the initial triaging of clients according to illness severity, may perform as a mobile intensive care nurse (MICN) by directing prehospital care personnel via telecommunication, and frequently provides client care in the prehospital environment. Community clinics use ED nurses, and many emergency nurses have become active in injury prevention programs at both national and local levels. Advanced practice roles such as clinical nurse specialists and nurse practitioners are integrated into many EDs throughout the United States. Nurses in these advanced practice roles often have a master's degree level of education or higher in addition to specialty certification.

Nurses working in an ED must be prepared to provide care to clients of all age-groups who have a myriad of possible illnesses or injuries. It is often cited that emergency nurses must have an understanding of almost all disease processes specific to any age-group. However, ED nursing is not usually addressed in depth in generic nursing programs. The education of ED nurses frequently occurs through hospital orientation programs, post-employment internship courses, and continuing education programs. ED nurses can obtain national specialty certification through an examination process. A certified ED nurse can use the credential of Certified Emergency Nurse (CEN).

LEGAL ISSUES

Nurses deal with a variety of legal issues in whatever specialty area they practice. The ED is no exception; however, certain issues are of paramount importance in this setting.

Federal Legislation

Past federal legislation has mandated that any client who presents to an ED seeking treatment must be rendered aid regardless of financial ability to pay for services. Since the mid-1980s, additional specific legislation

has been enacted requiring ED personnel to stabilize the condition of any client considered medically unstable before transfer to another health care facility—the Consolidated Omnibus Budget Reconciliation Act (COBRA) of 1986 and the Omnibus Budget Reconciliation Act (OBRA) of 1990. This stabilization must occur regardless of the client's financial ability to pay for services. ED personnel who transfer clients to another institution without first providing this initial stabilization can incur substantial fines and penalties, as can the hospital administration.

Clients have continued to seek health care services in the ED, even with the proliferation of managed health care plans and gate-keeping policies. The financial integrity of the ED has been challenged over the years because of the legal obligations of the ED to provide service. Retrospectively, financial reimbursement for rendered services has been denied to EDs from managed health care plans following a determination that the client's problem did not constitute a true emergency. Additional legislation was enacted (Emergency Medical Treatment and Active Labor Act [EMTALA] in 1988, 1989, 1990, and 1994) requiring that a medical screening examination be performed on all ED clients before solicitation of information about ability to pay. This medical screening examination must be inclusive enough to determine whether the client is experiencing an emergency medical condition requiring treatment or, in the case of a pregnant woman, is experiencing labor contractions. An emergency medical condition includes drug abuse, hemodynamic instability, psychiatric illness, intoxication, severe pain, and labor. If a client has an emergency medical condition, stabilization must be rendered. Stabilization is interpreted to mean that deterioration of the client is unlikely during possible transfer or discharge of the client. Continued interpretations of this act have expanded the facilities that come under EMTALA. These include not only EDs, but also hospital-owned urgent care centers, anywhere unscheduled clients appear for medical care, and off-site locations that are within a 250-yard zone of a main hospital that is covered under the 2001 outpatient prospective payment system. Violations of this legislation can again result in fines and penalties. Each congressional year, new legislation and interpretations of existing law are proposed for providing appropriate emergency medical treatment to the public while continuing to acknowledge cost-containment issues.

In 1996 the Health Insurance Portability and Accountability Act (HIPAA), Public Law 104–191, was passed to provide national standards for electronic health care transactions. Subsequently, the rule was further defined, and in 2002, it was extended to protect privacy of protected health information. The Privacy Rule covers information found in medical records, conversations with health care personnel, insurance records, billing information, and other health information that is collected. The rule restricts who can look at and receive a person's health information and stipulates that personal information cannot be used or shared without authorization.

Consent to Treat

Most adult clients seeking treatment in the ED give voluntary consent to the standard and usual treatment performed in this setting. In some instances, however, a client is deemed unable to give consent for treatment. This inability may be due to the critical nature of the client's illness or injury or to other conditions, such as an altered level of consciousness. In these instances, emergency care may be rendered to the client under the implied emergency doctrine. This doctrine assumes that the client would consent to treatment to prevent death or disability if the client were so able.

Children younger than the age of legal majority must have the consent of their parent or legal guardian for medical care to be rendered. Exceptions include (1) emancipated minors; (2) minors seeking treatment for communicable diseases, including sexually transmitted diseases, injuries from abuse, and alcohol or drug rehabilitation; and (3) minor-age females requesting treatment for pregnancy or pregnancy-related concerns. Some states also allow the adult caregiver with whom the child resides to give treatment authorization even though that caregiver may not be the parent.

The issue of informed consent in the ED is the same as that in any other health care setting. Adult clients must be informed about the necessity of required treatments, expected outcomes, and potential complications. Clients must also be mentally competent and understand the information being explained. As in any other setting, a mentally competent adult client always maintains the right to refuse treatment or withdraw previously given consent.

Restraints

Restraining a client while he or she is in the ED may at times be necessary. The need for restraints usually arises because the client is becoming agitated or potentially violent. Hard leather or chemical restraints are used in the ED if the client is in danger of injuring self or others and when nonphysical methods of controlling the client are not viable.

SAFETY ⚠️ **ALERT**   **According to The Joint Commission (TJC) National Patient Safety Goals, restraints may not be used to control a client solely for convenience or because of staffing issues. When restraints are required, departmental and hospital guidelines that are in compliance with The Joint Commission and the Centers for Medicare & Medicaid Services (formerly the Health Care Financing Administration) must be followed. A physician's order for applying restraints as well as the client's behavior mandating the use of restraints must be documented. The client must be periodically reevaluated both for the continued need for restraints and for the integrity of distal circulation, motor movement, and sensory level of the restrained extremities. The findings must be documented. Offering water to the client and providing opportunities to urinate or relieve other body needs are required, as is documentation of this nursing care. No client may be kept in restraints against his or her will unless the client's behavior indicates the existence of safety issues. Behavior modification techniques used in an attempt to release the client from restraints must also be documented. The ED staff must receive appropriate education pertaining to dealing with clients requiring physical restraint.**

Clients in the ED who have psychological conditions that render them a danger to themselves or to others, or who are unable to provide food or shelter for themselves, can be placed and held on a legal psychiatric restraining order. This order mandates that such clients be placed in a locked psychiatric facility for their protection for a maximum of 72 hours. Within that 72-hour period, the client must be evaluated by a psychiatrist to determine whether the legal hold needs to be extended or whether the client can be released. Clients who may be at risk for suicide must be identified according to TJC's National Patient Safety Goals.

Mandatory Reporting

Every state has mandatory reporting regulations that affect emergency nurses. Incidents and conditions may need to be reported to federal, state, or local authorities or to the Department of Public Health, Department of Motor Vehicles, coroner's offices, or animal control agencies. The types of incidents requiring reporting are suspected child, sexual, domestic, and older adult abuse; assaults; motor vehicle crashes; communicable diseases such as hepatitis, sexually transmitted diseases, chickenpox, measles, mumps, meningitis, tuberculosis, and food poisoning; first-time or recurrent seizure activity; death; and animal bites. Every ED has written policies regarding these mandatory reports.

SAFETY ⚠️ **ALERT**   **According to TJC's National Patient Safety Goals, clients and their families must be told how to report concerns about safety and encouraged to report such incidents.**

Evidence Collection and Preservation

Recognition of unusual circumstances surrounding a client's injury or death is an important aspect of ED nursing because of the associated legal implications.

Not only must the legal authorities be notified, but also, in many instances, the ED nurse may be required to collect and preserve evidence taken from the client. This evidence can include bullets, weapons, clothing, and body fluid specimens. All collected evidence must be identified by the client's name, hospital identification number, date and time of evidence collection, type of evidence and source (e.g., venipuncture, hematoma aspiration, vomitus, swab), and the initials or signature of the person collecting the evidence. Once the evidence has been collected, its preservation and the maintenance of the "chain of custody" are extremely important. Table 82-1 and Boxes 82-1 and 82-2 relate to evidence collection.

Violence

In 2005 the United States Department of Labor, Bureau of Labor Statistics, identified 5702 fatal work injuries, of which 14% were attributed to assaults and violent acts.

Violence directed against ED personnel has become an issue of concern throughout the late 1990s and into the 21st century. The environment inherent in the ED, the emotional circumstances often surrounding the illness or injury that affect both clients and family members, and the increasingly violent trends in the United States all play a role in this phenomenon. Administrative changes have been made in some EDs to enhance both public and health care worker safety. These measures have included the installation of items such as metal detectors, "panic buttons," bullet-proof glass, and lock-down doors at public entrances; increasing the visibility of security guards; using patrol guard dogs; and instituting visitor control policies. Changing the perception of the ED from one of fear and isolation for both clients and family members is also occurring.

BOX 82-1   Tips for Preserving Evidence in the Emergency Department

1. Do not contaminate specimens or person—use gloves.
2. Minimally handle the body of a deceased person.
3. Place paper bags on the hands and feet and possibly over the head of a deceased person to protect trace evidence or residue.
4. Collect and place evidence on clean, white sheet until it can be packaged and labeled.
5. Do not place wet clothing in plastic bags as wet clothes can "sweat," thereby destroying evidence. Allow item to air-dry, and then place inside individual paper bags. If item is soaked and continues to leak fluid, place inside another bag and label to alert crime lab that it contains body fluids.
6. Photograph inflicted wounds or injury before cleansing or repair.
7. Do not insert invasive tubes through pre-existing wounds or holes (e.g., do not place chest tubes through chest wounds or intravenous catheters through needle track marks).
8. Do not cut clothing through evidence holes such as stab wounds or bullet wounds.
9. Collect the client's personal items, such as written notes, drugs or medications, and items from clothing pockets.
10. Do not allow family members, significant others, or friends to be alone with the client.

BOX 82-2   Maintaining "Chain of Custody" of Evidence in the Emergency Department

1. Seal evidence with tape and label with client information data, date and time of collection, signature of person collecting evidence.
2. Document all collected evidence on designated forms.
3. Document all transfers of evidence from one person to another, and include the reason for transfer of evidence.
4. Obtain signatures of the person releasing evidence and of the person receiving evidence.
5. *Never* leave collected evidence unattended. Call police or forensic nurse examiner immediately to retrieve evidence.
6. Air-dry evidence before placing it in a collection container or paper envelope.

TABLE 82–1 Evidence Collection in the Emergency Department	
Evidence	**Collection/Container**
Glass fragments, bullets, broken fingernails, paint chips, loose hair follicles, fibers, or trace evidence such as soil	Place each item in a paper envelope or specimen container.
Head or pubic hair samples	Collected samples from combings and cuttings are each placed in a paper envelope.
Blood (from both venipuncture and possible hematoma evacuation), urine, gastric washings, or vomitus	A 20-30-ml sample is placed in a sealed container.
Swabs from wounds, membranes, or orifices	Air-dry before placing in a collection container or paper envelope.

From Selfridge-Thomas, J. (1995). *Manual of emergency nursing* (p. 382). Philadelphia: Saunders.

Instituting family-centered practices that recognize the importance of family participation and addressing the emotional needs of clients and families is a trend in ED management.

However, education of ED personnel in violence prevention is also of paramount importance in reducing the toll of violence. The following areas are crucial to address:

■ **Recognizing potentially violent clients and situations**

SAFETY ALERT

- **Identifying verbally and physically abusive cues from clients, family members, or friends**
- **Understanding the importance of instinct or "gut reactions"**
- **Using simple communication strategies to defuse potentially problematic situations**
- **Requiring clients to completely undress before physical examination**
- **Minimizing the presence of "potential weapons" in client care areas such as scalpels, needles, excess tubing attached to oxygen flow meters, scissors, stethoscopes worn around the neck, and personal jewelry**
- **Restraining clients, when necessary, using a team approach**
- **Avoiding becoming a hostage in a volatile situation**
- **Having a safety committee track all reported assaults on clients and employees**
- **Ensuring Occupational Safety and Health Administration violence guidelines are followed**
- **Encouraging employees to report both verbal and physical assaults**

Once a violent situation has erupted, the protection of ED personnel and others in the department is of utmost concern. Any means necessary to ensure their safety must be undertaken.

ETHICAL ISSUES

The ethical issues confronting ED nurses usually deal with end-of-life concerns. Initial resuscitation and stabilization of clients in critical condition constitute universal standard practice in the ED. At times, however, the desired outcome of client survivability is not achievable.

Unexpected Death

When death occurs in the ED setting, it is usually sudden and unexpected, even if the client has had a prolonged illness. The unexpected nature of the death, or impending death, can present ethical dilemmas for both the family survivors and the ED personnel. One such issue deals with the length of time to which resuscitation is performed. This is usually a physician's decision; however, family members may at times have input. Allowing family members or significant others to be present during client resuscitation is becoming more common. This practice is not necessarily disruptive to the resuscitation process, and it can be of comfort to the survivors and the involved ED personnel.

When death does occur, the ED nurse and the ED physician have important roles in informing the family:

- Inform the family of the client's death, and refer to the deceased client by name.

- Provide the family with an explanation of the course of events related to the death; use simple explanations.
- Offer the family an opportunity to view the body. If a child has died, allow the parent to hold the child. Providing the parent with a lock of the child's hair may be comforting.
- Help the family to focus on decisions requiring immediate attention such as taking possession of the deceased person's valuables, arranging post-mortem examination if desired or required, identifying possible organ or tissue donation, and selecting a funeral home.
- Inform family members when they can leave the ED setting.
- Provide community agency referral as needed.

Advance Directives

In 1991 Congress enacted the Patient Self-Determination Act (PSDA), which allows a client, or the client's health care proxy, to make determinations related to end-of-life measures. Emergency care personnel are obligated to abide by the client's advance directive decisions, if that information is available and provided in writing. When this written information is not available, ED personnel have a responsibility to stabilize or resuscitate any client according to standard treatment guidelines, regardless of a family member's expressed wishes.

Organ and Tissue Donation

Issues related to potential organ or tissue donation often arise in the ED setting. Once a potential donor is identified, the surviving family members need to be approached. A team approach involving a physician, a nurse, and possibly an organ procurement coordinator is optimal. Utmost dignity and professionalism must be maintained. (Chapter 80 reviews religious and cultural customs and beliefs related to death and organ transplantation. Also see the WebLinks for Chapter 80, *evolve* which include links to various agencies, organizations, and the latest medical information.) Whatever decision the family makes regarding organ or tissue donation, that decision must be supported by health care personnel.

Child Abandonment

States are beginning to pass child abandonment laws in response to the number of newborn infants being abandoned following birth. In general, the law allows mothers to bring their newborn child to the ED and abandon the child in the care of the ED personnel. The mother bears no criminal responsibility. Local Departments of Social Services are then contacted so the child can be placed in their custody.

COMPONENTS OF EMERGENCY CARE

Even though treatment decisions in the ED may at first appear to occur in a chaotic fashion, there is an inherent order in the timing and choice of interventions performed throughout a client's stay. The organizational flow of events involves client triage (prioritizing), in-depth nursing assessment of the client, diagnostic testing, formulation of diagnoses, outcome management, evaluation, disposition, and documentation.

Triage

Whether clients arrive in the ED via ambulance or are ambulatory, they are triaged at some point by either an ED physician or an ED nurse. The purpose of this triage process is to expediently determine the severity of a client's problem or condition in order to deliver emergency care in the most appropriate time frame. In other words, which clients need treatment immediately and which can wait is determined. The acuity level of the presenting problem is rated according to predetermined categories; the most frequently used ratings are *emergent* (must be treated immediately otherwise life/limb/vision is threatened), *urgent* (requires treatment but life/limb/vision is not threatened and care can be provided within 1 to 2 hours), and *non-urgent* (requires evaluation and possible treatment, but time is not a critical factor). However, the American College of Emergency Physicians and the Emergency Nurses Association have a joint position paper supporting the adoption of a reliable, valid five-level triage scale. The five-level rating approach is currently being incorporated into client triage in many emergency departments. The five-level rating systems are one of two types. In one type, the previous *urgent* and *non-urgent* categories may be further subdivided into unstable and stable clients. Another five-level rating system is the Emergency Severity Index (ESI). This system is based on the triage nurse identifying the critical clients and then predetermining the number of department resources most likely required to treat the non-urgent client. Figure 82-1 displays this algometric approach. Once an initial determination is made about the severity of the client's condition, a more in-depth nursing and medical assessment is completed. Appropriate diagnostic testing and specific interventions are performed using a team approach as emergency physicians and nurses work collaboratively to provide appropriate and expeditious management of the client's problem.

Nursing Assessment

The nursing assessment process for any client entering the ED is divided into *primary* and *secondary* assessments (Figure 82-2).

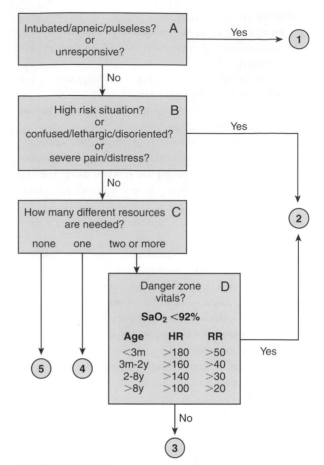

■ **FIGURE 82–1** Emergency Severity Index triage algorithm. *(From Wuerz, R.C., et al [2001]. Implementation and refinement of the Emergency Severity Index. Academic Emergency Medicine, 8, 170-176.)*

The purpose of the *primary assessment* is to immediately identify any client problem that poses a threat, immediate or potential, to life, limb, or vision. Information is gathered primarily through objective data, such as physical examination and vital signs. If any abnormalities are found during the primary assessment, immediate interventions such as Advanced Cardiac Life Support (ACLS) and Advanced Trauma Life Support (ATLS) must be instituted to aid in preserving the client's life, limb, or vision. The primary assessment uses the *ABC* mnemonic:

- *A* Airway patency
- *B* Breathing effectiveness
- *C* Circulation (both peripheral and organ-specific)

For any client arriving in the ED who has been involved in a major traumatic injury, the assessment of the airway also includes evaluation of the adequacy of the C-spine immobilization, and includes *D* for disability. This includes a brief evaluation of level of consciousness and pupil response to light.

Once it is determined that a client's ABC status is satisfactory, the *secondary assessment* is performed to

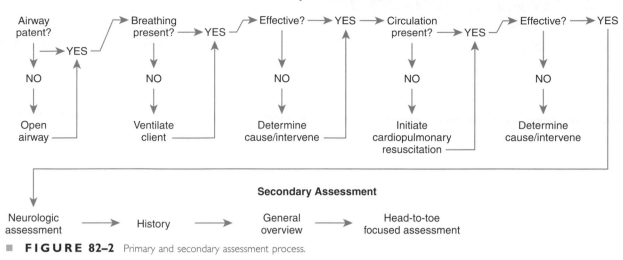

FIGURE 82–2 Primary and secondary assessment process.

identify any other non–life-threatening problems the client may be experiencing. Both subjective information and objective data are obtained. The secondary assessment includes the following elements.

Neurologic Assessment

Determine the client's (1) level of consciousness; (2) orientation to person, place, time, and event; (3) Glasgow Coma Scale (GCS) score (Table 82-2); (4) pupillary size, equality, and reaction to light and accommodation; and (5) motor movement and strength of hand grips and pedal pushes. A brief neurologic assessment can also be determined using the *AVPU* mnemonic:

- *A* Alert (the client is awake and alert and needs no stimulus to respond to the environment)
- *V* Verbal (the client requires a verbal stimulus to elicit a response)
- *P* Pain (the client requires a painful stimulus to evoke a response)
- *U* Unresponsive (the client is unresponsive to any applied stimulus)

History

Elicit the nature of the client's chief complaint, duration of the problem, mechanism of injury from blunt or penetrating forces (Box 82-3), associated manifestations related to the primary problem, past pertinent medical history, current medications and compliance, use of over-the-counter (OTC) medications or herbs, routine use of alcohol or illicit drugs, known medication allergies, and immunization history. Women of childbearing age may need to be questioned about the date of the last normal menstrual period (LNMP) and the number of pregnancies and outcomes. Questions related to potential or actual child, sexual, domestic, or older adult abuse situations also must be addressed.

Pain

The most frequent complaint for which clients seek emergency care is related to both acute and chronic pain. Obtaining specific information regarding pain patterns can be extremely helpful. Asking questions according to the *PQRST* mnemonic often provides useful information:

- *P* Provokes: Are there any specific factors that cause the pain to increase or decrease?
- *Q* Quality: What descriptive terminology identifies the type of pain—dull, sharp, colicky, pressure?
- *R* Region/Radiation: Where is the pain located? Does it move to other areas?
- *S* Severity: Use a rating scale of 1 to 10, visual analogs, or word descriptors to describe pain severity.
- *T* Timing: How long has the pain been present? Are there cycles related to when the pain is present or absent?

TABLE 82–2	Glasgow Coma Scale	
Eye-opening response	Spontaneous	4
	To voice	3
	To pain	2
	None	1
Best verbal response	Oriented	5
	Confused	4
	Inappropriate words	3
	Incomprehensible sounds	2
	None	1
Best motor response	Obeys command	6
	Localizes pain	5
	Withdraws (to painful stimulus)	4
	Flexion (to painful stimulus)	3
	Extension (to painful stimulus)	2
	None	1
Total		3-15

BOX 82-3   History Questions Related to Injury

MOTOR VEHICLE CRASHES

- Do you remember the crash?
- Were you the driver or passenger?
- Were you wearing a seat belt?
- Did the airbag deploy?
- Did you hit the steering wheel or the dashboard? If so, with what part of your body?
- How fast was the vehicle going?
- What did the vehicle hit?
- Where is your pain?

BLUNT INJURY FROM FALLS

- How far did you fall?
- What precipitated the fall?
- What did you land on?
- Where is your pain?
- Self-reported loss of consciousness is not valid information.

GUNSHOT WOUNDS

- How long ago did the incident occur?
- What were you doing when you got shot?
- How many shots did you hear?
- What did the gun look like?
- Where is your pain?

PENETRATING WOUNDS OR STAB WOUNDS

- How long ago did the injury occur?
- How many times were you stabbed?
- What did the knife look like?
- Where is your pain?

Both adult and pediatric clients who rate their pain at a level of 7 or above, or use descriptive words denoting "severe" pain, need to be considered high risk and need to be evaluated by the ED physician as expediently as possible. Clients have a right to have their pain treated appropriately, in a timely manner, and effectively, without exception.

General Overview

Note the client's overall health condition, skin color, gait, posture, unusual skin markings or body odors, and mood and affect. Baseline measurements of blood pressure, heart rate, respiratory rate, pulse oximetry values, and temperature are important. Actual weight in a pediatric client and reported weight in an adult are also important.

Head-to-Toe (Focused) Assessment

Remove the client's clothing and examine the areas where the chief complaint and any other associated complaints are focused. The techniques of inspection, auscultation, percussion, and palpation are used to determine additional normal or abnormal findings.

Diagnosis

Upon completion of the medical and nursing assessment process, diagnostic tests (radiographic, cardiology, laboratory, special studies) may be initiated. Once all pertinent information has been collected, a working diagnosis is formulated. The physician provides a medical diagnosis; in addition, the ED nurse may incorporate a variety of nursing diagnoses. These diagnoses provide a framework on which to build a plan of appropriate client care and against which to measure outcomes.

OUTCOME MANAGEMENT

Client care interventions may be initiated by the ED nurse, the ED physician, or other health care providers. There is frequent collaboration among all health care providers involved, and interventions are assigned priority according to the severity of the client's condition.

Evaluation

The desired goal in client care is to achieve positive client outcomes after medical and nursing management. This is an integral component of ED nursing care. If the client's condition does not improve with initial interventions, the plan of care must be reexamined and additional interventions may be required.

Client Disposition

All clients entering the ED are eventually discharged from the ED. They may be transferred to another health care facility, admitted to the hospital, or released to home or another facility. Most clients are released to home following treatment. Before being discharged from the ED, a client or family members must be given both oral and written instructions concerning follow-up care. These instructions should identify the client's diagnosed problem, explain necessary continued treatments, describe potential complications, and specify time frames for rechecks and the name of the physician to whom the client is being referred. These instructions should be presented in both oral and written form in the client's primary language. At times, a hospital or family interpreter may be required to accomplish this outcome.

Nursing Documentation

Because ED nurses frequently are responsible for an assigned area, zone, or "pod" within the department and because clients enter and exit those areas on a continual basis, nursing documentation is of paramount importance. Documentation must include the recording of all assessment findings, diagnostic tests, interventions and management, responses to treatment, achieved outcomes, and client education. Documentation needs to be complete but concise, providing an ongoing record of the client's condition and responses. The format may be a flow sheet, narrative, computer-generated design, or a combination of these.

EMERGENCY CONDITIONS

INEFFECTIVE AIRWAY CLEARANCE

A compromised or ineffective airway may be due to either complete or partial airway obstruction. Common causes of airway compromise include the presence of a foreign object in the airway, airway edema, airway infection, facial or airway injury, and tongue obstruction.

Clinical Manifestations

The clinical manifestations of airway compromise include absence of breathing, drooling, stridor, intercostal or substernal retractions, alteration in skin color (pallor, gray, cyanotic), and agitation. A decreased level of consciousness may lead to airway compromise as a result of obstruction of the posterior pharynx by the relaxed tongue.

OUTCOME MANAGEMENT

Remove Obstruction

If an obstruction is present, the airway should be opened by a chin-lift or jaw-thrust maneuver (Figures 82-3 and 82-4, respectively). If either of these maneuvers opens the client's airway, patency is maintained via the insertion of a nasopharyngeal or oral airway device. If these maneuvers fail to relieve the obstruction, more aggressive interventions must be instituted, such as

■ **FIGURE 82–3**   Chin-lift maneuver to open the airway.

■ **FIGURE 82–4**   The jaw-thrust maneuver to open the airway is the preferred method for use in clients with head or cervical neck injury.

(1) performing abdominal or chest thrusts if an aspirated foreign object is the suspected cause (Figure 82-5), (2) suctioning the oral cavity to remove secretions or visible foreign objects, (3) intubating via the nasal or oral route, (4) using a laryngeal mask airway (LMA), or (5) assisting with creating a surgical airway via a cricothyroidotomy (Figure 82-6).

Intubate

In some cases, oral or nasal intubation may require the use of *rapid-sequence induction* (RSI). This procedure is used in awake clients who require intubation either to maintain the airway or as a mechanism to provide adequate ventilation. RSI is most frequently used in clients who have sustained a head or spinal injury and in clients who are rapidly tiring from the effort of maintaining effective breathing. RSI involves (1) establishing venous access, (2) hyperventilating the client with 100% oxygen, (3) administering intravenous (IV) lidocaine 1 mg/kg to blunt any transient increase in intracranial pressure from the actual intubation procedure, and (4) administering an IV general barbiturate or anesthetic medication such as thiopental 3 to 5 mg/kg, fentanyl (Sublimaze) 3 to 15 mcg/kg, ketamine (Ketalar) 1 to 2 mg/kg, etomidate (Amidate) 0.3 mg/kg, propofol (Diprivan) 2 mg/kg, or midazolam (Versed) 0.1 mg/kg followed immediately by the administration of an IV muscle-paralyzing agent such as succinylcholine (Anectine) 1.5 to 2 mg/kg, pancuronium (Pavulon) 0.04 to 0.1 mg/kg, or vecuronium (Norcuron) 0.08 to 0.1 mg/kg. Once the client loses consciousness and adequate muscle relaxation and paralysis have been obtained, intubation using equipment such as an intubating laryngeal mask airway, intubating fiberoptic bronchoscope, or nasal/endotracheal tubes is accomplished. The client is then ventilated using 100% oxygen via a bag until a ventilator is attached.

Verify Tube Placement

After an intubation procedure, there is immediate verification of tube placement by auscultation, verification

■ **FIGURE 82–5** Abdominal-thrust maneuver (formerly known as the Heimlich maneuver) used for removal of foreign bodies blocking the upper airway. Vigorous upward chest or abdominal thrusts produce a rush of air that expels the foreign body. The abdominal thrust is the original Heimlich maneuver. The chest thrust is an adaptation that is useful for obese or pregnant victims. Use four quick thrusts in the positions shown. **A,** Hand placement. **B,** Maneuver for conscious victims. **C,** Maneuver for unconscious victims.

A Hand placement for abdominal thrusts

Hand placement for chest thrusts

Position of hands from rescuer's view (conscious victim)

B

Position of hands from rescuer's view (unconscious victim)

C

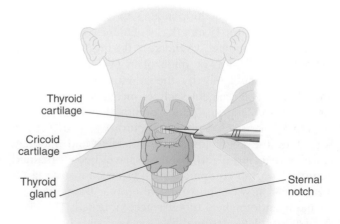

Thyroid cartilage

Cricoid cartilage

Thyroid gland

Sternal notch

■ **FIGURE 82–6** A cricothyroidotomy procedure is performed to create a temporary airway. An opening is made into the trachea and is maintained with a small plastic tube.

of end-tidal CO_2, and then chest x-ray. The ED nurse is immediately responsible for auscultation of the client's epigastric area and then chest during assisted ventilation to confirm the presence of equal bilateral breath sounds. If breath sounds are heard over the epigastric area, the tracheal tube must be removed, the client hyperventilated, and the procedure reattempted. Breath sounds heard more prominently over the upper right chest indicate that the tracheal tube has advanced too far into the right main bronchus. The tube needs to be pulled back and breath sounds reassessed. Once the presence of equal and bilateral breath sounds is confirmed and appropriate end-tidal CO_2 is present, the tube is secured in place and a chest film is obtained to verify correct tube placement.

Securing and maintaining a patent airway constitutes the first priority in any ED client. Other treatments directed at the cause of airway compromise are then instituted. These measures may include administration of IV medications if infection or local edema of the airway is present.

Immobilize the Spine

If the client with an actual or potential airway problem has also sustained a traumatic injury and arrives in the ED without C-spine immobilization, stabilization of the client's cervical, thoracic, and lumbar spine must be instituted and maintained until cleared by the physician. Stabilization is accomplished using a team approach and involves the following steps: (1) manually stabilizing the client's head and cervical spine, (2) applying an appropriate size hard cervical collar around the client's nuchal area, (3) placing the client on an ED stretcher, (4) logrolling as a unit until spine is cleared.

INEFFECTIVE BREATHING PATTERN

Effective breathing is affected if a client is either hyperventilating or hypoventilating. This may occur if the client is breathing too fast or too slowly. The normal respiratory rate for an adult is between 12 and 20 breaths/min; infant respiratory rates are between 30 and 40 breaths/min; and children have respiratory rates between 25 and 30 breaths/min until approximately the age of 10 years.

HYPERVENTILATION

Clinical Manifestations

Respiratory rates faster than normal constitute tachypnea and, in many cases, hyperventilation. Hyperventilation is defined as low arterial carbon dioxide level and may result in respiratory alkalosis. The client may report numbness and tingling sensations in the distal extremities or around the lips, along with carpal or pedal spasms. A sensation of chest pain may also be present. Frequently this condition is caused by client anxiety, but it is important to also investigate other possible causes, such as pain, aspirin toxicity, diabetic ketoacidosis, fluid loss, infection, central nervous system (CNS) lesions, and pulmonary embolism.

OUTCOME MANAGEMENT

The goals of treatment are to return the client's breathing pattern and rate to normal and to restore normal gas exchange. If anxiety is the cause of the hyperventilation, the client needs to be instructed to take slow, deep breaths through the nose and slowly exhale through the mouth. Having clients breathe into a paper bag and rebreathe their own carbon dioxide may be helpful. If another cause is identified as the reason for the client's altered breathing pattern, specific treatments such as administration of oxygen and inhaled, intravenous, or oral medications are initiated to reverse the process.

HYPOVENTILATION

Clinical Manifestations

Hypoventilation occurs when there is a decreased respiratory rate or inadequate exchange of gas at the alveolar level. This may occur when an adult client's respiratory rate falls below 12 breaths/min or, in the case of a child, the respiratory rate is below what is normal for the age group. At these rates, carbon dioxide accumulates in the alveoli, leading to respiratory acidosis. There may also not be enough oxygen available to maintain adequate tissue oxygenation. Clinical manifestations may include a decrease in the client's level of consciousness, pallor, cyanosis, and pulse oximetry readings of less than 96%. Causes of hypoventilation include brain stem lesions, head injury, drug-induced depression of the respiratory center, impaired respiratory muscle innervation from spinal cord injury, and the presence of neuromuscular diseases such as muscular dystrophy or Guillain-Barré syndrome.

OUTCOME MANAGEMENT

Improving ventilation via a bag-valve-mask device and, if necessary, endotracheal intubation is required to reduce carbon dioxide levels to near 38 to 42 mm Hg and to return oxygen levels to between 80 and 100 mm Hg. Recommendations for ventilating infants include using a pediatric size bag-valve-mask instead of an infant bag.

IMPAIRED GAS EXCHANGE

Etiology

Obstructions, infections, and injury within the pulmonary system can lead to the development of gas exchange abnormalities. Common causative disorders include asthma, other reactive airway diseases, chronic obstructive pulmonary disease, pulmonary embolism, pulmonary edema, bronchitis, pneumonia, tuberculosis, pneumothorax, and chest injuries such as a flail chest.

A less common cause of a gas exchange problem is noncardiac pulmonary edema, which results from acute damage to the alveolocapillary membrane. This damage can occur from inhalation injury, near-drowning, sepsis, trauma, and opioid overdose. As the alveolocapillary membrane permeability increases, fluid collects in the interstitial space, surfactant levels decrease, and the alveoli eventually collapse.

Clinical Manifestations

With constriction of the bronchi, accumulation of fluid, or lung consolidation occurs; abnormal lung sounds such as wheezes, rales (fine crackles), or rhonchi (coarse crackles) are often heard throughout the client's lung fields. With pulmonary infections, the client may have concurrent fever. If a pneumothorax is present, breath sounds are diminished or absent on the side of the pneumothorax. Asymmetrical chest wall movement suggests that there is something interfering with air entry or escape from that lung or that the client is splinting that side because of pain. Paradoxical chest wall movement with breathing should raise suspicion of a possible flail chest. In such cases, a chest film or spiral computed tomography (CT) scan provides valuable diagnostic information about the cause of the client's problem.

OUTCOME MANAGEMENT

Administer Oxygen

Oxygen therapy with a flow rate of between 2 and 10 L/min via nasal cannula for lower Fio_2 (fraction of inspired oxygen) or non-rebreather mask for 100% O_2 is the priority intervention for clients with an obstructive or infectious cause of ineffective gas exchange. Biphasic positive airway pressure (BiPAP) or continuous positive airway pressure (CPAP) are noninvasive ventilation masks used when the client requires assistance with ventilation and oxygenation.

Administer Medications to Open Lower Airways

Oxygen administration is frequently followed by administering aerosolized bronchodilator medications such as metaproterenol (Alupent) or albuterol (Ventolin) to open constricted upper or lower bronchi. Subcutaneous epinephrine 1:1000 may be administered to relax constricted bronchi and to reduce the degree of airway or bronchial edema. Administration of steroid medications, either intravenously or orally, is also frequently used as first-line therapy. A client with a pulmonary embolus or deep vein thrombosis may be given heparin or low molecular weight heparin.

Minimize Spread of Infection

Infectious diseases that are the cause of impaired gas exchange are treated with IV or oral antibiotic medications.

SAFETY
⚠
ALERT
 If the client has pneumonia, the IV antibiotic should be administered within 4 hours of arrival in the ED. This is part of The Joint Commission's (TJC) Core Measures.

A client thought to have a highly contagious pulmonary disease such as tuberculosis must be isolated in a reverse or negative airflow room and will need to wear a high-efficiency particulate air (HEPA) filter mask placed over the nose and mouth when not in a reverse pressure room. Anyone entering the reverse pressure TB isolation room will need to wear a HEPA mask or particulate respirator (see Chapter 62).

TRAUMATIC PNEUMOTHORAX

A pneumothorax can be classified as a simple pneumothorax, open pneumothorax, or tension pneumothorax (see Figure 63-9). In a *simple pneumothorax,* air from the bronchus, bronchioles, or alveoli escapes into the pleural space and diminishes lung expansion capacity. With an *open pneumothorax,* a traumatically created opening in the client's chest wall may allow air to move freely into and out of the thoracic cavity during inspiration and exhalation. A tension pneumothorax occurs when air continues to become trapped in the pleural cavity with no mechanism of escape during the exhalation process. This type of pneumothorax is an emergent condition.

Clinical Manifestations

A simple pneumothorax can occur spontaneously but is frequently associated with penetrating injury to the chest or with blunt forces causing a rib fracture. An obvious chest wound is present with an open pneumothorax. If the wound is large enough, a sucking sound is heard as the client breathes. Pain with breathing is present, and diminished or absent breath sounds may be present on the side of the injury. The client may be tachypneic and may have decreased pulse oximetry readings.

A tension pneumothorax produces the clinical manifestations of extreme respiratory distress, distended jugular neck veins, and a mediastinal shift of the heart, trachea, esophagus, and great vessels to the side away from the tension pneumothorax. Hypotension and tachycardia are other findings. Pneumothorax is diagnosed by clinical manifestations, a chest radiograph, or a spiral CT.

OUTCOME MANAGEMENT

Administer Oxygen

Administration of 100% oxygen via a non-rebreather face mask is a priority treatment for a client who has sustained a pneumothorax.

Apply Occlusive Dressing

Any open chest wall wound should be covered with an occlusive gauze dressing, but this intervention may convert an open pneumothorax into the more dangerous tension pneumothorax because the gauze covering blocks the trapped air's escape route. If manifestations of a tension pneumothorax appear, the occlusive dressing must be immediately removed.

Release Trapped Air

If a tension pneumothorax is thought to be the cause of respiratory distress and if it has not been iatrogenically produced by covering an open chest wound, a 14- to 16-gauge catheter needle is immediately inserted into the client's anterior chest wall on the affected side at the second intercostal space, midclavicular line. This life-saving intervention allows the immediate release of trapped air and decompresses the pleural cavity.

Place Chest Tube

The simple, open, and tension varieties of pneumothorax are definitively treated with the insertion of a chest tube that is attached to a suction/collection device. This measure aids in reexpansion of the lung, leading to improvement in the client's gas exchange.

FLAIL CHEST

A flail chest involves serious rib fractures. It occurs when two or more ribs are fractured in two or more places on the same chest wall side or when the sternum is detached from the ribs. The fractured segment has no connection with the remaining rib cage. This segment then moves in a direction opposite that of the rest of the chest wall during the processes of inhalation and exhalation—so-called paradoxical chest wall movement (see Figure 63-8). The client may be tachypneic and in pain, and may complain of dyspnea.

Treatment often involves endotracheal intubation and mechanical ventilation. Pulmonary contusions are commonly present in conjunction with a flail chest, and within 24 to 48 hours, noncardiac pulmonary edema or adult (acute) respiratory distress syndrome (ARDS) may develop.

DEFICIENT FLUID VOLUME

A decrease in circulating blood volume leads to decreased tissue perfusion. Therefore any condition producing a profound volume deficit necessitates immediate intervention. The more common causes of volume loss include actual blood loss from the vascular compartment because of bleeding from solid organ injury, long bone fractures, vascular injuries, or GI bleeding. Illness leading to prolonged vomiting or diarrhea can also produce large fluid losses as can "third-spacing" volume loss or interstitial volume sequestering associated with major burn injury.

As volume loss occurs, various compensatory mechanisms produce vasoconstriction of the vasculature, retain fluid via the renal tubules, and increase cardiac output. These compensatory mechanisms—such as stimulation of the sympathetic nervous system; the release of renin, angiotensin, aldosterone, and antidiuretic hormones; and fluid shifts—continue in an effort to restore tissue perfusion, thus ensuring cell survival. However, these mechanisms are limited in scope, and if the lost volume is not restored, eventually cellular structures incur irreversible damage from the oxygen debt, and death ensues.

Clinical Manifestations

The client or prehospital personnel may provide a history of recent injury or illness with associated volume loss. Clinical manifestations may include agitation or decreasing level of consciousness, pale and diaphoretic skin, delayed capillary refill time of longer than 2 seconds, tachycardia, tachypnea, decreased urine output, and hypotension. Positive orthostatic vital signs (a decrease in systolic blood pressure by 20 mm Hg and an increase in pulse rate by 20 beats/min associated with the client changing from a lying to an upright position) may be present in clients with a mild to moderate volume loss. If blood has accumulated in the thoracic cavity (hemothorax) or abdominal cavity, percussion over the area elicits a dull sound. A collection of blood under the thoracic diaphragm or in the peritoneal cavity can produce Kehr's sign (referred shoulder pain unrelated to injury) or a rigid, hard abdomen with increased rebound tenderness upon palpation.

Diagnostic testing is directed at locating the source of any internal bleeding. Tests may include radiography, ultrasonography, and CT scans of the chest, pelvis, extremities, or abdomen. The laboratory tests of blood typing, complete blood count (CBC), hemoglobin concentration and hematocrit, and electrolyte panel are performed on collected blood samples. A urine specimen should be tested for specific gravity and the presence of blood and leukocytes and, in females, for pregnancy. If gastrointestinal bleeding is suspected, a nasogastric tube is passed and the aspirate tested for the presence of blood. Stool is tested for blood. Diagnostic testing not only helps in identifying the source and severity of volume loss but also aids in determining whether the client requires immediate surgery or hospital admission.

OUTCOME MANAGEMENT

Treatment is directed at preventing further volume loss and replacing fluid volume.

Maintain Blood Flow to Vital Organs

Oxygen (100%) is given via face mask to provide additional oxygen to tissues. The use of Trendelenburg positioning is not recommended.

Stop or Decrease Bleeding

If external bleeding is present, direct pressure should be applied to control further blood loss. The physician may suture or staple actively bleeding lacerations. If the bleeding source is the posterior nasal passages, the client needs to be seated and leaning forward in a high Fowler position. Nasal packing may be required.

Replace Fluids

Venous access must be obtained using a large-bore catheter (14 to 16 gauge). Usually two IV sites are required for fluid replacement. At the time of vein cannulation, blood samples should also be obtained for laboratory testing. If peripheral venous access is not possible, a central line may be inserted or an intraosseous procedure may be performed. This involves inserting an intraosseous needle into the proximal anterior tibia. Fluids, blood, and medications can then be infused into the bone marrow. This is a temporary lifeline and is removed once peripheral venous access can be obtained. The procedure is usually performed by a physician, but it may also be performed by educated personnel such as paramedics and ED nurses. In the past, this procedure was performed only on children younger than age 3 years, but this has recently been expanded so that the procedure can be performed on individuals of any age.

Crystalloids

Crystalloid fluids (normal saline, lactated Ringer's solution) are the replacement fluids of choice. They should be warmed and administered rapidly. If a client with actual loss of blood does not improve after 2 to 3 liters of crystalloid, then blood should be administered. In children, the infusion rate is 20 ml/kg administered as a bolus. This bolus may need to be repeated.

Colloids

Colloid fluids (e.g., blood, hetastarch, albumin) may also be given for fluid resuscitation. If the client has lost blood, then blood is the colloid of choice. These fluids contain proteins and are infused at a 1:1 ratio (1 unit of solution for every 1 unit of blood loss). Blood can be administered as whole blood or as packed red blood cells. It is best if the client's blood has been typed or, optimally, typed and crossmatched with the donor's blood, but universal type O Rh-negative blood can be used if speed is a vital consideration. Blood is usually warmed and can be infused quickly in an adult using a rapid infuser machine. In children, blood is infused at a rate of 40 ml/kg bolus.

Replace Fluids for Burns

Clients who have sustained major partial- or full-thickness burn injuries are at risk for associated fluid loss. Fluid replacement is calculated according to the client's weight in kilograms and the total body surface area (TBSA) involved, as determined by the *rule of 9s* (see Chapter 50). The usual formula is 2 to 4 ml of fluid × body weight in kilograms × TBSA. The calculated amount of fluid is used as the total fluid replacement volume required over the 24-hour period from the time of injury. One half of the total fluid amount is infused in the first 8-hour period, one fourth of the fluid amount in the second 8-hour period, and the remaining one fourth amount in the last 8-hour period.

Institute Other Measures

Once fluid resuscitation is begun, other interventions can be instituted. A nasogastric tube is passed to prevent vomiting and possible aspiration. In clients with gastrointestinal bleeding, gastric lavage is performed, instilling room-temperature normal saline; then, using a large syringe, the fluid is aspirated through the nasogastric tube. This procedure is repeated until there is a clearing of the bloody fluid aspirate. An indwelling urinary catheter is inserted to measure urine output. The client with volume loss is susceptible to the development of mild hypothermia. Keeping the client warm with blankets, warming lights, and infusion of warmed fluids aids in maintaining a normal body temperature. Continual monitoring of cardiac rate and rhythm, blood pressure, pulse oximetry readings, respiratory rate, level of consciousness, and temperature is indicated.

EXCESS FLUID VOLUME

Clients who have an excess of fluid volume can concurrently have pulmonary congestion, leading to respiratory distress. Although clients with renal failure experience fluid volume excess, the disorder most commonly associated with fluid overload in the ED is heart failure. Heart failure results in fluid excess because of the inability of the cardiac muscle to function effectively. Ejection fraction decreases, pressure in the left ventricle increases, and eventually pressure increases affect the left atrium and right ventricle and atrium. The client in heart failure also activates the renin-angiotensin-aldosterone axis and retains fluid.

Clinical Manifestations

The clinical manifestations of heart failure include agitation or restlessness, tachypnea and increased respiratory effort, respiratory rales, distended jugular neck veins, tachycardia, skin pallor, diaphoresis, ascites, and pitting-dependent edema. Pulse oximetry readings are often decreased on room air. The client may also cough up excessive, frothy sputum. Cardiac dysrhythmias, such as atrial fibrillation, may be noted with cardiac monitoring.

Because these clients often have a chronic history of heart failure, their daily medication regimen often includes digoxin, a diuretic, beta-blockers, angiotensin-converting enzyme (ACE) inhibitors, and potassium. Electrolyte imbalances are common, basic metabolic panel (BMP) levels are elevated, and serum levels of digoxin must be assessed via laboratory studies. Chest films provide information about the severity of the heart failure.

OUTCOME MANAGEMENT

Improve Oxygenation

Treatment is directed at improving the client's ability to breathe. Positioning the client in a high Fowler position facilitates the ability to breathe; 100% oxygen should be initiated via a non-rebreather mask although this intervention may be difficult for the client to tolerate. Noninvasive ventilatory assistance via BiPAP may be required. However, if respiratory fatigue develops, the client must be intubated to provide adequate ventilation. The use of RSI before intubation may be indicated.

Administer Medications

Establishing venous access for medication administration is necessary. If pharmacologic interventions with nitrates and diuretics are ineffective, recombinant human B-type natriuretic peptide nesiritide (Natrecor) may be administered to the client. The actions of this medication increase salt and water excretion in addition to producing vasodilation. The client must be monitored for urine output, hypotension, and respiratory improvement. Dobutamine, angiotensin-converting enzyme (ACE) inhibitor, and beta-blocker medications may be administered to reduce afterload. Dobutamine also has a positive inotropic effect.

Monitor Response to Treatment

Continual monitoring of the client's response to treatment is of paramount importance. Assessments should include level of consciousness, cardiac rhythm, blood pressure, respiratory rate and effort, pulse oximetry, and urine output.

DECREASED CARDIAC OUTPUT

Any illness or injury that has a direct effect on the heart can produce a decrease in cardiac output. Such disorders include cardiac dysrhythmias, acute myocardial infarction, cardiac injury, cardiac tamponade, and cardiac infection or myopathy.

When cardiac output decreases, tissue perfusion is adversely affected. Cardiac output (CO) is determined by stroke volume (SV) and heart rate (HR):

$$CO = SV \times HR$$

Therefore any disease process that produces a reduction in stroke volume or an alteration in heart rate has a direct effect on cardiac output. Entities such as cardiac dysrhythmias and acute myocardial infarction have a direct affect on heart rate. Acute myocardial infarction also reduces stroke volume as a result of the death of cardiac muscle. Cardiac tamponade results in compression of the cardiac muscle by the collection of blood or fluid in the pericardial sac. This effect produces a decrease in stroke volume. Infection and cardiac myopathy also affect the cardiac muscle structures, thereby reducing stroke volume.

Clinical Manifestations

Depending on the cause of the reduced cardiac output, clients may present with differing clinical manifestations. Dysrhythmias are self-evident on cardiac monitoring. The most prominent manifestations associated with a decrease in cardiac output include chest pain, skin pallor, diaphoresis, hypotension, nausea, and agitation or a decrease in level of consciousness. External chest wall injury may be evident with blunt cardiac injury. Cardiac tamponade produces the additional findings of distended jugular neck veins and muffled heart sounds. Fever may be present with cardiac infections.

Diagnostic tests include cardiac monitoring, electrocardiography (ECG), chest radiography, ultrasonography, laboratory studies, noninvasive stress testing, two-dimensional echocardiography, myocardial perfusion imaging, CT scans, and invasive coronary angiography. Levels of the cardiac enzymes creatine kinase (CK) and the CK-MB fraction and of the cardiac markers myoglobin and troponin T (cTnT) and troponin I (cTnI) are especially important in diagnosing the occurrences of a myocardial infarction.

OUTCOME MANAGEMENT

Improve Cardiac Output

The goal of treatment is to improve cardiac output. High-flow oxygen should be administered via face mask, and venous access should be secured for the administration of medications. Supraventricular tachycardic dysrhythmias may be treated with IV adenosine (Adenocard), whereas bradycardic rhythms may be treated with IV atropine or with a pacemaker. Ventricular dysrhythmias may be suppressed by treating the cause if possible or by administering amiodarone or lidocaine. Clients who have sustained a blunt cardiac injury from traumatic injury may also develop cardiac dysrhythmias. For further discussion of dysrhythmia treatment, see Chapter 57.

Increase Coronary Artery Blood Flow

An acute myocardial infarction is often caused by an embolus or thrombus that occludes a coronary artery.

According to TJC Core Measures, all clients who arrive to the ED complaining of chest pain must be rapidly evaluated for acute myocardial infarction. An immediate dose of aspirin and a 12-lead ECG within 10 minutes will determine subsequent interventions. If the ECG indicates an ST-elevation MI (STEMI), the client will be transported to the cardiac catheterization laboratory for percutaneous intervention (PCI). If it is not possible to perform PCI within 90 minutes, administration of a fibrinolytic medication is the first-line choice for treatment. Fibrinolytic medication must be given within 30 minutes of arrival. If the ECG is indicative of a non–ST-elevation MI, treatment may then involve the administration of nitroglycerin, IV heparin, or IV enoxaparin

SAFETY

ALERT

glycoprotein (GP) IIb/IIIa inhibitors, while further diagnostic testing occurs. Beta-blocker therapy is also instituted in clients who do not have concurrent heart failure or cardiogenic shock.

Clients who have received fibrinolytic medications must be continuously monitored for the presence of active bleeding. Other monitoring parameters include pain reduction, cardiac rate and rhythm, ST-segment patterns, blood pressure, pulse oximetry readings, and respiratory rate.

Remove Pericardial Fluid

Blunt or penetrating force injury, heart failure, and infections of heart structures can cause cardiac tamponade. If this condition is suspected or diagnosed, treatment involves pericardiocentesis (Figure 82-7). A long spinal needle attached to a 60-ml syringe is inserted beneath the xiphoid process and into the pericardial sac. The accumulated blood is removed, compression of the ventricles is relieved, and cardiac output is restored.

Treat Infectious Causes

Infections of the heart structures, such as pericarditis or endocarditis, may be treated with pain-reducing medications or antibiotics. Pericarditis is frequently caused by a viral organism, whereas endocarditis is of bacterial origin and requires antibiotic therapy.

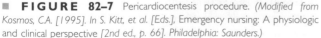

■ **FIGURE 82–7** Pericardiocentesis procedure. *(Modified from Kosmos, C.A. [1995]. In S. Kitt, et al. [Eds.], Emergency nursing: A physiologic and clinical perspective [2nd ed., p. 66]. Philadelphia: Saunders.)*

ACUTE OR CHRONIC PAIN

Pain is one of the most common complaints of clients seeking emergency care. Pain can be caused by almost any entity; therefore identifying the source of pain is of paramount importance. The sensation of pain may be the only complaint, or pain may be associated with other clinical evidence of illness or injury. Pain is assessed as described earlier in the chapter.

OUTCOME MANAGEMENT

Promote Comfort

Pain reduction is the goal of treatment and may be provided by administering oral, intramuscular (IM), or IV analgesic or opioid medications. With isolated orthopedic injuries, such as digit injuries, pain reduction may be obtained by injecting affected nerves with anesthetizing medications. Client comfort measures should also be instituted. Measures may include client positioning to ease stress on painful areas, elevating injured extremities, applying ice or cool compresses to injured areas, and attempting to make the room environment comfortable for the client. Pain is to be assessed before and after each intervention, and the client's response should be documented.

Reduce Procedural Pain

Instituting conscious sedation before painful procedures is a routine practice in many EDs. This procedure involves controlled pharmacologic depression of the level of consciousness that nevertheless allows maintenance of the client's reflexes to protect the airway as well as maintain spontaneous ventilation. Conscious sedation is most commonly induced with medications such as midazolam (Versed), ketamine (Ketalar), or fentanyl (Sublimaze). Dose and route of administration vary with the agent used. It is not uncommon for a narcotic to be given along with a benzodiazepine for painful procedures. The ED nurse's responsibility is to continually monitor the client for airway patency, oxygen saturation levels, cardiac activity, and response to physical or verbal stimulation until recovery from the anesthesia has occurred.

ACUTE CONFUSION

Clients can have an altered level of consciousness from many causes. Underlying disorders such as stroke, metabolic abnormalities, seizure, intoxication, hemorrhage, or injury need to be considered. A helpful guide to use in attempting to determine the cause is the "vowels-TIPS" mnemonic: *A,* alcohol; *E,* epilepsy, encephalopathy, endocrine; *I,* insulin; *O,* overdose; *U,* underdose or uremia; *T,* trauma; *I,* infection; *P,* psychogenic; *S,* stroke or shock.

The normal state of wakefulness and consciousness is controlled by the reticular activating system (RAS) and the brain's cerebral hemispheres. Various factors can produce a decreased state of wakefulness. These include impairment of the central nervous system (CNS) from lesions, infection, or hemorrhage; a decreased supply of oxygen, blood, or glucose to cerebral tissues; and exposure to, ingestion of, or withdrawal from substances toxic to cerebral tissue.

Family members or prehospital personnel may be the only sources for obtaining historical information concerning the client's state of consciousness. It is extremely important to determine any known illnesses of the client, current medications, recent injury, known alcohol or drug use, and duration of the client's altered mental state.

Clinical Manifestations

Clinical manifestations vary according to the cause of the client's illness or injury. The Glasgow Coma Scale (GCS) score is less than 15 or different from baseline. The client may be disoriented or agitated. Pupil size and equality may be altered. Unequal pupil size and reaction may indicate compression of the third cranial nerve caused by increased intracranial pressure. Small, pinpoint pupils may signify opiate overdose, pontine hemorrhage, cholinesterase poisoning, or recent use of miotic eye drops. Cranial nerve abnormalities and unilateral decreased muscle strength may be present with a recent stroke. Tongue lacerations can indicate recent seizure activity. Pale, cool, clammy skin can occur with shock or hypoglycemia. Fresh needle marks on the skin indicate recent IV drug use. A petechial rash on the skin can be an indication of a lethal bacterial meningitis. Bruising of the face, eyes (raccoon eyes), or mastoid process (Battle's sign) or a bluish hue to the tympanic membrane can indicate recent head injury and an associated basilar skull fracture.

Diagnostic testing involves first obtaining a bedside blood glucose level. Other laboratory studies may be indicated, including serum levels of specific medications, serum and urine toxicology screening tests, CBC, blood cultures, electrolyte panel, arterial blood gas analysis, and urinalysis. Urine specimens should also be tested for the presence of myoglobin, because clients who have been comatose for a prolonged time can develop rhabdomyolysis, resulting from ischemia and damage to large muscle groups. Other diagnostic studies include ECG, chest film, and brain CT scan. Occasionally a lumbar puncture may need to be performed.

OUTCOME MANAGEMENT

Establish and Maintain Airway
The first treatment priority in a client with an altered level of consciousness is establishing and maintaining the airway. If the GCS is less than 9, then preparations for intubation should be undertaken. During interventions directed at maintaining airway patency, spinal immobilization should also be considered if there is any suspicion that a traumatic injury may have occurred. Also, 100% oxygen must be administered to provide supplemental oxygen to brain tissue.

Establish Vascular Access for Appropriate Medications
Venous access must be secured for possible IV fluid or medication administration. If a bedside glucose level reading is less than 45 mg/dl, 50% dextrose (D_{50}) is administered IV. If the bedside glucose level reading indicates a high level of glucose, therapy should be instituted for treatment of diabetic ketoacidosis or hyperglycemic hyperosmolar nonketotic coma (see Chapter 45).

Naloxone (Narcan) 2 to 4 mg IV may also be administered. If the cause of the alteration in consciousness is an opiate overdose, naloxone reverses the process.

If a stroke is considered to be the cause of the client's altered level of consciousness, rapid assessment of type of stroke by CT scan is vital to the process of determining the subsequent treatment of the client. Only clients with a nonhemorrhagic stroke, whose onset of clinical manifestations is clearly defined, and who have no contraindications to thrombolytic medication are eligible for thrombolytic therapy. And this is ONLY if the medication is given within 3 hours of the onset of clinical manifestations. If tonic-clonic seizure activity begins, the client is medicated with lorazepam (Ativan) 0.05 to 0.1 mg/kg IV to terminate the seizure. This intervention may need to be followed by IV administration of phenytoin (Dilantin). Phenytoin must be diluted in normal saline solution and infused at a rate of less than 50 mg/min.

IV antibiotic medications are administered in any client with known or suspected bacterial infection within the brain tissue or cerebrospinal fluid. In clients with bacterial meningitis, this can be a life-saving intervention.

Monitor Intoxicated Clients and Treat Toxicity States
Intoxicated clients with an altered level of consciousness must be monitored in the ED. Frequent vital signs and GCS scores must be obtained and documented. If the client sustained any traumatic event, then a brain CT should be obtained to rule out intracranial reasons for altered level of consciousness. Agitation may require RSI in order for CT to be obtained. Treatment involves IV fluid support and nutritional supplementation with thiamine, multivitamins, and occasionally folic acid.

Monitor Clients with Head Trauma and Treat the Injuries
Neurologic trauma can result in minor disturbances such as a concussion. Treatment for concussion varies

according to clinical manifestations. 🪔 A client with a GCS of 13 or higher is considered a mild head injury, a GCS of 9 to 13 is considered a moderate head injury, and a GCS of less than 9 is considered a severe head injury. If asymptomatic, a minor head-injury client is released to home without any definitive treatment. Before leaving the ED, the client or family members must be given instructions on manifestations that indicate worsening of the client's condition.

Other types of neurologic trauma, such as skull fractures, cerebral edema, subdural hematomas, epidural hematomas, and cerebral contusions, may require critical care management or operative intervention. The client must be closely monitored in the ED for any manifestations of increasing intracranial pressure. Mannitol may be administered IV to treat cerebral edema.

Prevent Injury

SAFETY

⚠️

ALERT

Safety is an important issue in a client with an altered level of consciousness. Medication and restraints to avoid dislodging of nasogastric and endotracheal tubes may be indicated. Seizure precautions may be necessary. If in place, spinal immobilization must be maintained and the client should be logrolled. Bed side rails must be up and locked in position at all times. Clients are monitored for changes in level of consciousness along with cardiac rate and rhythm, blood pressure, pulse oximetry, and respiratory rates.

DISTURBED SENSORY PERCEPTION

Sensory perceptions may be disturbed in any of the sensory organs, but an alteration in vision is one of the more common client complaints associated with sensory perceptual changes. Such alterations can be caused by infection, inflammation, or trauma.

Clinical Manifestations

The client may be able to provide information related to the visual changes and the circumstances surrounding the onset of the changes. The affected eye should be assessed for discharge from the eye, excessive tearing, redness of the conjunctiva, presence of a ciliary flush (a ring of inflammation surrounding the corneal-scleral junction), periorbital cellulitis, obvious foreign objects, presence of a cloudy cornea, extruded globe contents, and obvious ecchymosis, laceration, or trauma to the eye and surrounding structures. A baseline visual acuity test must be performed on all clients with a complaint related to the eye.

Changes in vision can be present with non-urgent conditions such as conjunctivitis. This infection of the conjunctival tissue is highly contagious. Foreign objects or chemicals in the eye, corneal abrasions, and deep structure infections or injury are more significant problems, and the client usually presents with a complaint of pain as well as visual changes.

OUTCOME MANAGEMENT 🪔

Anesthetizing ophthalmic drops can be placed in the affected eye to diminish pain and allow for a more thorough examination of the eye. Superficial conjunctival infections are treated with topical ophthalmic antibiotic drops or ointments. Small superficial foreign objects are removed by the ED physician. For exposure to harmful chemicals, the eye must be irrigated with a minimum of 1 L of normal saline. After irrigation, the pH of the eye is checked; if it has not returned to a normal pH of 6 to 7, irrigation may need to be continued. If corneal abrasions are present, the client is given oral pain reduction medications and topical ophthalmic antibiotic medication. Patching of the affected eye is not recommended.

More serious problems associated with the eye necessitate an immediate consultation with, or referral to, an ophthalmologist. These problems include complaints of sudden changes in or loss of vision with or without pain, impaled foreign objects, extensive injury or infection, and globe rupture. Any client who receives treatment from the ED physician for an eye problem should be instructed to be rechecked within 24 hours by his or her primary physician or an ophthalmologist.

RISK FOR INFECTION

Clients frequently present to the ED because of an infectious process. The infection may be caused by either viral or bacterial organisms. The source of the infection may be localized, or the infection may have spread to surrounding tissues or be systemic. It also may be contagious. Hospital employees are frequently treated in the ED for needle-stick injury and prophylactically for hepatitis B and human immunodeficiency virus exposure.

Clinical Manifestations

Clinical manifestations depend on the organism causing the infection, the extent of the infection, and the location of the infection. Bacterial infections usually produce more obvious and severe manifestations than those seen in viral infections. With bacterial infections, the client may have a fever. However, older adults and neonates frequently have subnormal temperatures with an infectious process. The client may complain of pain at the site of the infection, such as in the ear, eye, throat, abdomen, genitourinary tract, or an area of skin. It is important to consider that airway, pharyngeal, and mouth infections can be associated with airway compromise. Meningeal infections can produce headache, vomiting, neck pain, and occasionally petechiae. Pulmonary infections are frequently accompanied by productive cough and sputum. Erythema, edema, lymphadenopathy, and observable discharge or pus may be present with ear, throat, or skin infections. A skin rash or abscess may also be the presenting problem of an underlying infection. Abdominal infections often present with pain and palpable abdominal tenderness. A systemic infectious process can lead to septic shock, in which endotoxins from bacterial organisms are released into the circulation. The client is acutely ill and may have clinical manifestations of fever, tachycardia, hypotension, and decreased urine output. In later stages of sepsis, the client may become hypothermic, the skin may have a mottled appearance, and the level of consciousness becomes diminished. These findings are usually associated with a high death rate.

SAFETY ALERT **A primary decision must be made about whether the infection is considered contagious to other clients in the ED. If the infection is thought to be contagious, the client must be isolated as quickly as possible from other clients. This is in compliance with the TJC National Patient Safety Goal for reducing the risk of health care associated infections.**

It then becomes important to identify the primary source of the infection. The ears, eyes, throat, lungs, skin, and genital and pelvic areas must be assessed for evidence of infection. A chest film is obtained, in addition to possible abdominal and pelvic ultrasound studies. Laboratory studies include a urinalysis, CBC, and culture of discharge and blood specimens. If the source of the infection is not identified, a lumbar puncture may be required.

OUTCOME MANAGEMENT

SAFETY ALERT **When dealing with clients with known or potential infections, it is important that the ED nurse be cognizant of the hospital-wide infection control policies and comply with the TJC National Patient Safety Goal related to reducing the risk of health care associated infections. Appropriate use of standard precautions at all times on all clients is the best protection for the nurse and for all ED clients.**

Administer Medications

Treatment involves administering antibiotic or antiviral medications selected according to the identified or probable source of the infection. These agents may be administered orally, IM, or IV. The antipyretic medications acetaminophen (Tylenol) and ibuprofen can be administered orally or rectally (Tylenol) to reduce temperature. Other treatments to reduce temperature involve undressing the client and allowing heat to dissipate into the environment, but avoid shivering. Abscesses caused by skin infections may need to be incised, drained, and packed.

Hepatitis B prophylaxis treatment for unvaccinated employees exposed to a needle-stick consists of administering HBIG (hepatitis B immunoglobulin) and beginning the series of hepatitis B vaccinations. There is a risk of exposure to hepatitis C from needle-sticks, but to date there is no prophylactic treatment.

Monitor and Treat Sepsis

If sepsis is suspected, it is important to administer 100% oxygen to the client, infuse IV fluids of normal saline, and insert a nasogastric tube and an indwelling urinary catheter. Additional infused medications, after antibiotic administration, may include dopamine and corticosteroids. The client must be closely monitored for changes in blood pressure, heart rate, respiratory rate, oxygen saturation, cardiac rhythm, urine output, level of consciousness changes, and prolonged bleeding times. These clients are at risk for developing disseminated intravascular coagulopathy (DIC).

IMPAIRED PHYSICAL MOBILITY

Any injury to the musculoskeletal system can lead to a decrease in the client's mobility. Other causes of impaired mobility are injuries to the vertebral bodies and possibly the spinal cord. Sprains of ligaments, fractures to bones, dislocated joints, muscle strains, and amputated extremities or digits are the majority of problems for which clients seek emergency care related to mobility deficits.

Spinal cord injury can involve edema of the cord, with transitory or minimal deficits, or other cord injury, or the cord can actually be severed. With marked edema or cord severance, deficits are usually devastating and permanent. Neurogenic shock can develop with loss of the sympathetic component of the autonomic nervous system. With only the parasympathetic nervous system functioning, massive vasodilation occurs, and tissue perfusion is decreased.

Clinical Manifestations

Clinical manifestations in most musculoskeletal injuries include swelling around the injured area, presence of ecchymosis, obvious deformity of the area, palpable tenderness, and limited movement of the area. Amputations are self-evident, and depending upon whether a complete or partial amputation has occurred, active bleeding may be minimal or profuse. With a complete amputation, active bleeding is minimal as a result of constriction of the severed vessels. It is important that the ED nurse assess the effectiveness of circulation, motor movement, and presence and degree of sensation distal to any musculoskeletal injury.

An injury to the spinal cord produces a motor or sensory deficit, or both, below the level of injury. If the injury is in the upper thoracic or cervical area, the diaphragm and thoracic intercostal muscles can be affected, leading to respiratory compromise. A client with neurogenic shock has warm, dry skin caused by the massive vasodilation, hypotension, and bradycardia, with no movement or sensation below the level of injury.

Radiographic films of the injured area are obtained to aid in identifying fractures. Depending on the extent of the injury, additional laboratory tests or other diagnostic studies may be performed.

OUTCOME MANAGEMENT

Treat Sprains, Strains, and Fractures

Treatment of extremity sprains and fractures consists of immediately elevating the extremity above the level of the client's heart, applying ice to the area, and immobilizing the extremity with pillows or cardboard splints. Oral, IM, or IV pain-reducing medication may also need to be administered. More definitive immobilization of the area with the application of splints, molds, or immobilizers is accomplished before the client leaves the ED. Lower extremity injuries may require the client to use crutches. Detailed crutch-walking instructions must be provided, and the client should be able to demonstrate adequate use of the crutches to the ED nurse before his or her discharge from the department.

Pain-reducing medication is also administered to clients with muscle strains. Once clients achieve reduction of pain, they are usually discharged to home with instructions to rest and to apply alternating ice and heat to the injured area for the next 24 hours.

Reduce Dislocations

A joint dislocation requires reduction in the ED. This procedure is performed by the ED physician. Pain-reducing and muscle-relaxant medications may need to be administered before the reduction procedure. Once joint reduction has been achieved, a post-reduction radiographic film must be obtained. After successful reduction, the joint is immobilized with the required orthopedic device.

Treat Amputation

The goal in the management of a client who has sustained an amputation is to attempt to salvage the part so that possible replantation can occur or prevent further loss of tissue. Any profuse bleeding from the stump should be controlled with direct pressure. If the client has sustained significant blood loss, 100% oxygen is administered, venous access is established, and replacement fluids or blood are given.

The stump is then gently cleansed with normal saline. The amputated part is wrapped in sterile gauze moistened with normal saline. It is then placed in a plastic bag or container, and the plastic bag or container is placed on ice. The amputated part should *never* be placed directly on ice, because the resultant freezing of the tissues makes replantation impossible. The client is given pain-reducing medications, antibiotic medications, and possible tetanus prophylaxis with tetanus and diphtheria toxoids (Td) 0.5 ml if more than 5 years have elapsed since the last tetanus immunization. The nurse should be prepared to transfer the client and the amputated part to a facility that performs reimplantations.

Treat Spinal Cord Injury

Clients with a spinal cord injury must be maintained in complete spinal immobilization. At a minimum, a cross-table lateral cervical spine radiograph is required, and this study may be followed by more extensive spinal films or a CT scan. When a high thoracic or cervical injury is present, the client may become fatigued with the effort of maintaining respirations. The need for intubation and assisted ventilation must be considered. IV fluids are necessary to maintain perfusion. Administration of high-dose IV steroids such as methylprednisolone (Solu-Medrol) is controversial. IV administration of a vasopressor to counteract parasympathetic nervous system effects is another treatment consideration. This therapy, however, must be instituted cautiously, because the vasoconstrictive effect of vasopressors may decrease perfusion to the injured cord. A nasogastric tube and indwelling urinary catheter are inserted.

The client must be kept warm with warmed fluids, blankets, and heating lights as necessary, because often the ability to regulate internal body temperature has been lost. Stabilization of cervical fractures may involve applying Gardner-Wells tongs with traction, a halo traction device, or surgical repair. Monitoring of body temperature, cardiac rate and rhythm, blood pressure, respiratory rate and effort, pulse oximetry, urine output, and changes in sensory and motor movement is vital.

IMPAIRED SKIN INTEGRITY

Skin and soft tissue injury is a common problem encountered in ED clients. Injury to the skin and surrounding soft tissue can occur from sharp objects, blunt force injury, scraping mechanisms, or bites resulting in lacerations, contusions, abrasions, avulsions, or puncture wounds.

Clinical Manifestations

Once the skin barrier is interrupted, the potential for infection is increased. Skin flora and other bacteria then have access to the underlying structures. After injury to the skin, natural or secondary healing processes occur, resulting in skin closure and scarring. Primary closure, or suturing, of skin wounds also closes the skin and reduces the amount of scarring. Wounds caused by forces in which bacteria were deeply embedded in the tissues, or that are older than approximately 12 hours, are not routinely managed by primary closure because of the risk for developing infection. Diagnostic tests may involve radiographic films of the wound area. Such studies are important when a foreign object is suspected to be embedded in the wound or when gas in the wound may have developed.

OUTCOME MANAGEMENT

Skin and soft tissue wounds can occur anywhere on the body. Scalp and facial lacerations often bleed profusely because of the high vascularity of these areas. Direct pressure over the wound is usually sufficient to control bleeding.

Cleanse the Wound

Cleansing of wounds is best achieved using high-pressure irrigation and normal saline solution. Directing the stream flow from a 20- to 30-ml syringe directly into the wound adequately cleanses most wounds. A minimum of 100 ml of solution should be used. Shaving an area around a wound to remove hair is controversial. Clipping is the preferred method of removing hair, but any hair removal is controversial. In most instances, shaving is not necessary and should *never* be performed on a wound located in a client's eyebrow.

Open wounds often need to be anesthetized before cleansing and must be anesthetized before primary repair is attempted. A cotton ball can be saturated with a topical solution of tetracaine-adrenaline-cocaine (TAC) or lidocaine-epinephrine-tetracaine (LET) and then applied directly to a face or scalp wound, as long as it is not used near mucous membranes. Other anesthetic agents include lidocaine 1% or 2%, with or without epinephrine, and bupivacaine (Marcaine) 0.25% or 0.5%, with or without epinephrine. Anesthetic agents with epinephrine should never be injected into wounds located on the fingers, toes, ears, nose, or penis because of the vasoconstricting effects of epinephrine. Bupivacaine provides a longer anesthetic effect than that obtained with lidocaine. Sodium bicarbonate at a 1:10 ratio may be added to lidocaine or bupivacaine to reduce pain when the medication is injected into the wound.

Close the Wound

Small, superficial wounds may be closed with adhesive paper strips or Dermabond glue. It is important to evert and bring the wound edges close together and then apply the paper strips or glue.

Larger wounds that are gaping, that involve injury to deeper structures, that occur over joints, or that are

TABLE 82–3	Suture Material
Suture Size	**Indicated Use: Body Area(s)**
2-0, 3-0	Tissue subjected to strong tensile forces (e.g., knees, elbows, over joints)
3-0, 4-0	Epidermal and dermal layers, except for face
5-0, 6-0	Facial area

located in high-tension areas need to be sutured for optimal healing. The type of suture material required varies depending on the size and location of the open wound (Table 82-3).

Abrasion injuries are not sutured. Abrasion injuries need to be thoroughly cleansed in order to remove any particles or debris left in the wound. If particles remain in the wound, a tattooing effect results with the healing process. Human and animal bites are not routinely sutured because of the highly contaminated nature of the wound. The wound is thoroughly irrigated, and prophylactic antibiotic medications are frequently administered. Animal bites should be reported to the local animal control authorities.

Apply a Dressing

Protective dressings must be applied to wounds before the client leaves the ED. Most dressings involve first applying a thin layer of antibacterial ointment or gauze impregnated with petrolatum (Vaseline) or other occlusive substance. Then dry, sterile gauze is applied for padding, followed by a wrap of woven gauze (Kling or Kerlix). Adhesive tape is used to hold the dressing in place.

Administer Tetanus and Rabies Prophylaxis

Clients should be questioned about their tetanus immunization status. Because it is sound public health policy to take advantage of immunizing clients with combined vaccines whenever they are eligible, the CDC has specific recommendations for using vaccines that include protection against diphtheria and pertussis. Table 82-4 presents current recommendations for tetanus prophylaxis that take into consideration the appropriate doses for both children and adults. The vaccines used provide an active (acquired) immunity, but in select situations when immunity is questioned, the wound may be at a high risk for tetanus and the client may also be given passive antibodies in the form of human tetanus immune globulin (TIG) 250 units. If both preparations must be administered, they should be injected in separate sites in different extremities to avoid the globulin from potentially inactivating or inhibiting the immune response from the vaccine. In 2005 the United States licensed the use of a reduced

TABLE 82–4 Tetanus Prophylaxis in Wound Management*

History of Absorbed Tetanus Toxoid? (Doses)	Clean, Minor Wound; Tetanus Toxoid?	Clean, Minor Wound; Tetanus Immune Globulin (TIG)?	All Other Wounds; Tetanus Toxoid?	All Other Wounds; Tetanus Immune Globulin (TIG)?
Unknown or <3	Yes 1. For children <7 years, give DTP (pediatric form) or DT (pediatric form) if pertussis vaccine contraindicated 2. For people >7 years, Td (adult form) preferred 3. For people 11-18 years, give DTaP or Td (DTaP preferred for adolescents who have never received DTaP; Td preferred for adolescents who have received DTaP or if DTaP not available)	Not indicated	Yes 1. For children <7 years, give DTP (pediatric form) or DT (pediatric form) if pertussis vaccine contraindicated 2. For people >7 years, Td (adult form) preferred 3. For people 11-18 years, give DTaP or Td (DTaP preferred for adolescents who have never received DTaP; Td preferred for adolescents who have received DTaP or if DTaP not available)	Yes
+ history of 3 or more doses	If only 3 doses, then give 4th dose of absorbed toxoid Not indicated, unless >10 years since last dose	Not indicated	Yes if >5 years since last dose (more frequent boosters can increase incidence of adverse effects)	Not indicated

* Steps in tetanus prophylaxis include the following: (1) assess client's wound: (a) clean, minor (does not include descriptions listed in b); (b) includes (but is not limited to) wounds contaminated with dirt, feces, soil, saliva; puncture wounds; avulsions, wounds resulting from missiles, crushing injuries, burns, frostbite; (2) assess client's previous immunization history and age: (a) determine if client has received any previous tetanus vaccines (should have a history of receiving 3 doses as a primary series and then boosters as indicated); (b) client's age and wound will determine which vaccine(s) will be indicated.

DTaP, Reduced tetanus and diphtheria toxoid and acellular pertussis vaccine (use in adolescents 11 to 18 years of age); *DTP,* pediatric dose of diphtheria toxoid, tetanus toxoid, and pertussis vaccine (use only in children <7 years of age); *Td,* adult dose of diphtheria toxoid and tetanus toxoid (use only in children >6 years of age); *TIG,* tetanus immune globulin.

diphtheria toxoid and an acellular pertussis vaccine (DTaP) for use with people age 10 to 18 years. The newer vaccines help to reduce the risk of vaccination-related local and systemic reactions.

Rabies prophylaxis should be considered in clients who have been bitten by dogs, cats, skunks, raccoons, bats, squirrels, ferrets, or opossums. Prophylaxis is especially important if the animal cannot be located and placed under quarantine for an observation period.

 Because a bat bite can be relatively minor in comparison to other animal bites, and bats are becoming a significant reservoir for the rabies virus, the Advisory Committee on Immunization Practices (ACIP) recommends that postexposure prophylaxis is appropriate for any bite, scratch, or mucous membrane exposure associated with bats.

 The ACIP recommends two types of vaccine for people potentially exposed to rabies. These include rabies immune globulin (RIG), which provides rapid, passive immunity that persists for approximately 21 days; and rabies vaccine, which produces an active immune response that requires approximately 7 to 10 days to develop. The immunity lasts for approximately 2 years. The dose of human rabies immune globulin (RIG) for passive immunization is 20 units/kg. As much medication as possible should be injected into and around the wound site and the remainder of the dose injected intramuscularly in the buttocks. For active immunization with human diploid cell vaccine (HDCV), the dose is 1 ml

initially and again on days 0 (day 0 is date of exposure), 7, 14, and 28 following the bite incident.

Instruct on Wound Care

Instructions related to the care of the wound are given to the client or family members before they leave the ED. These instructions should identify the manifestations of infection and explain care of the wound. Timing for a follow-up appointment with the appropriate physician for a recheck of the wound and suture removal must also be included in the instructions.

ACCIDENTAL AND INTENTIONAL POISONINGS

Poisonings are either accidental or intentional. Accidental poisonings occur more commonly in the pediatric age group, whereas intentional poisonings are more frequent in the adolescent and adult population. Poisoning can also occur from injected venom, such as snake or insect bites.

Obtaining accurate information about the offending substance, amount, and time of ingestion or exposure can be difficult. Details may be available from family or friends. Other important information to obtain is whether the client has vomited since the exposure, whether the client has been depressed or had any previous episodes of intentional poisoning, if medication containers or drug paraphernalia were found at scene, and any other associated details.

Clinical Manifestations

Assessment must be directed toward the effectiveness of the client's ABCs (airway, breathing, and circulation). There may be few outward clinical manifestations that aid in determining the substance that was ingested, inhaled, or injected.

Diagnostic tests may include electrocardiography and continual cardiac monitoring. Blood and urine specimens need to be obtained for toxicology screening and testing. In many cases, the results of these tests are not rapidly available. Chest films may aid in diagnosing possible aspiration. If envenomation is the source of poisoning, bleeding and coagulation studies must be performed.

OUTCOME MANAGEMENT

Maintain Airway

If the client demonstrates a decrease in level of consciousness, initial interventions include establishing and maintaining a patent airway, possibly with airway adjunct devices. Oxygen should be administered, and venous access should be obtained.

Remove Offending Substance

Treatment is directed at removing or absorbing the offending substance. If the substance was injected, naloxone 2 to 4 mg IV may be administered. If the client's level of consciousness is decreased, a large nasogastric (Ewald) tube is passed either nasally or orally and gastric lavage performed if the ingestion was recent, potentially toxic, or considered significant. This procedure involves instilling approximately 250 to 500 ml of normal saline solution through the tube and then removing the solution either with a syringe or by gravity drainage into a collection bag. This process is repeated until the returned contents are clear of pill fragments. Then liquid-activated charcoal and a cathartic are instilled through the Ewald tube and allowed to remain in the stomach. The charcoal aids in adsorbing any other remaining particles of the toxic substance.

Awake and alert clients are given liquid-activated charcoal to drink. This medication provides the greatest benefit of adsorption if administered within 1 hour of the ingestion. Occasionally, the charcoal slurry may cause the client to vomit, and an additional dose of the charcoal may be required. The purpose of activated charcoal is again to quickly adsorb the ingested toxic substance to minimize its harmful effects. Syrup of ipecac is not routinely administered. It is not effective in removing the toxic substance unless the ingestion occurred within the previous 30 minutes. Its emetic effect prolongs the time until activated charcoal can be administered. Clients who have ingested an alkaline-based substance are not given syrup of ipecac, charcoal, or any substance that can cause emesis.

If a specific toxic substance exposure is known and an antidote is available, the antidote is administered. Table 82-5 provides a list of the more common poisoning substances and antidotes. Dry chemicals that may be present on the client's skin or external surfaces must first be brushed off. Then the contaminated area is copiously irrigated with water or normal saline.

Provide Psychiatric Evaluation as Needed

Any client who is in the ED because of an intentional poisoning must have a psychiatric evaluation before discharge and release from the ED. This is a TJC National Patient Safety Goal.

SAFETY

ALERT

Many communities have psychiatric evaluation teams (PETs) that provide this service.

SNAKE BITE

Snake antivenin is available for clients who have been envenomed by a pit viper (a poisonous snake). The area of the envenomation may be swollen and ecchymotic,

TABLE 82–5	Poisonings and Antidotes
Toxic Substance	**Treatment**
Beta-blocker medications	Treat hypotension initially with fluids; if unsuccessful, administer glucagons 100-150 mcg/kg IV followed by 2-5 mg/hr by infusion
Calcium-channel blocker medications	Calcium chloride 5-10 ml IV, or calcium gluconate 10-20 ml IV
Carbon monoxide	100% oxygen; possibly use of hyperbaric chamber
Iron	Deferoxamine (Desferal) 80 mg/kg IV or IM and repeated q 8 hr
Isoniazid (INH)	Pyridoxine (vitamin B_6) IV in dose equivalent to amount ingested (gram for gram); if ingested amount is unknown, administer 5 g IV over 3-5 min, then repeat q 3-5 min until seizures are controlled
Methanol, ethylene glycol	Fomepizole (Antizol) as an intravenous infusion, initially 15 mg/kg of body weight, followed by 10 mg/kg of body weight every 12 hr for 4 doses, then 15 mg/kg of body weight every 12 hr until ethylene glycol or methanol concentration decreases to less than 20 mg/dl
Phenothiazine medications	Diphenhydramine (Benadryl) 0.5-1 mg/kg IV or benztropine (Cogentin) 1-2 mg IM
Acetaminophen	N-Acetylcysteine (Mucomyst) 140 mg/kg PO, then 70 mg/kg every 4 hr for 17 doses

and pain may be present at the site. Pit viper venom produces both proteolytic and hemotoxic effects. Massive swelling producing a compartment syndrome may develop, and a coagulation disorder such as DIC may result. The wound area should be gently cleansed. Ice should not be applied to reduce swelling. Antivenin is administered intravenously, but skin or conjunctival testing must be performed before administering the antivenin.

HYPERTHERMIA

Hyperthermic emergencies are usually the result of environmental exposure. The pediatric and geriatric populations are at the greatest risk for developing hyperthermia. The types of hyperthermic problems are heat cramps, heat exhaustion, and heat stroke. Heat stroke is the most severe.

Clinical Manifestations

Muscle spasms of the arms and legs are evident with heat cramps. Often there is a depletion of sodium because the client has been perspiring excessively. Excessive sweating can lead to dehydration and heat exhaustion. The client may complain of headache, dizziness, nausea, and weakness. Mild hypotension can be present, and the skin is frequently cool and clammy to the touch.

Heat stroke is an emergent condition. The client is often comatose. Other clinical manifestations include hypotension, tachycardia, hot and flushed-appearing skin, and a core temperature of greater than 105 ° F (40.5 ° C).

OUTCOME MANAGEMENT

Administer Fluids and Electrolytes

For the client with mild heat cramps, administering oral fluids with electrolytes and removal from the hot environment are usually the only necessary treatments. Treatment of a client with heat exhaustion also involves removal from the hot environment and administering either oral or IV fluids to correct the problem.

Resolve Heat Stroke

Heat stroke treatment involves establishing and maintaining a patent airway, administering 100% oxygen, and establishing venous access. IV normal saline is administered to restore fluid volume. Cooling measures must be instituted quickly. These measures include removing all clothing from the client; spraying tepid mist over the client's body and using a fan to increase air flow; placing ice packs on the scalp and neck and in the axillae and groin; and using a cooling blanket. Gastric lavage with cool saline and peritoneal dialysis may be necessary. Cooling measures should continue until the

client's body temperature is 101 ° F (38.4 ° C). As the temperature decreases, administering chlorpromazine (Thorazine) or diazepam (Valium) may be required to reduce shivering. A nasogastric tube and indwelling urinary catheter must be inserted. Continuous cardiac, pulse oximetry, blood pressure, respiratory rate, level of consciousness, and temperature monitoring is performed.

HYPOTHERMIA

Clinical Manifestations

A body temperature less than 94 ° F (34.4 ° C) indicates the condition of hypothermia. The development of hypothermia is usually unintentional and involves accidental and prolonged exposure to cold temperatures.

Hypothermia severity can be divided into stages depending on the client's core temperature. Different clinical manifestations are present with each stage (Table 82-6).

OUTCOME MANAGEMENT

Rewarm the Client

After the establishment and maintenance of a patent airway, heated high-flow oxygen administration, and venous access with warmed fluid replacement, treatment is then directed at rewarming the client. Rewarming must be done slowly, because the hypothermic client is especially susceptible to the development of ventricular fibrillation and cardiovascular collapse if warmed blood is returned too rapidly to a cold heart. Rewarming methods include the following:

1. Passive warming
   a. Removing wet clothing
   b. Covering the client with warm blankets
   c. Placing the client in a warm room
2. Active warming
   a. Immersing the client in a warm bath (104 ° F [40 ° C])
   b. Placing the client on a warming blanket
   c. Placing radiant lamps over the client
3. Active core warming
   a. Infusing warmed IV fluids
   b. Providing heated, humidified supplemental oxygen
   c. Performing warm fluid lavage (peritoneal, gastric, bladder, or colonic lavage)
   d. Performing continuous arteriovenous rewarming (CAVR), hemodialysis, or cardiopulmonary bypass

Insertion of a nasogastric tube and indwelling urinary catheter is an additional component of care. Continuous cardiac, pulse oximetry, blood pressure, respiratory rate, level of consciousness, and temperature monitoring must be instituted.

TABLE 82–6	Stages of Hypothermia
Stage	**Clinical Manifestations**
Mild: 93-95 ° F (34.0-35 ° C)	Person conscious and alert but may have lethargy and confusion
	Shivering
	Bradycardia or tachycardia
Moderate: 86-93 ° F (30-34 ° C)	Decreased level of consciousness or coma
	Hypoventilation
	Bradycardia
	Atrial fibrillation
	Hypovolemia
	Cessation of shivering
	Possible hyperglycemia because of underutilization of glucose
Severe: <86 ° F (<30 ° C)	Coma
	Fixed and dilated pupils
	Bradycardia
	Apnea
	Hypotension
	Ventricular fibrillation
	Asystole

FROSTBITE

Hypothermia to the extremities can lead to frostbite injury. The feet, hands, nose, ears, and cheeks are most commonly affected. Damage to the tissues occurs, and peripheral blood flow is reduced. The area may appear red and swollen or may be pale in color. Formation of blisters containing either clear or purple bloody fluid may be seen. Rewarming of the frostbitten area should begin once the client is removed from the cold environment. The frostbitten part should be immersed in lukewarm water for 20 minutes. The frostbitten area needs to be handled gently so that blood-filled blisters remain intact. Loose, sterile, bulky dressings are then applied and changed daily. The rewarming process is painful; therefore pain-reducing medications must be administered.

INEFFECTIVE COPING

Clients present to the ED not only with medical and traumatically induced problems but also with psychological issues. Psychological disorders can range from mild anxiety to psychosis to deep depression. It is important that clients with psychological problems be taken as seriously as clients seeking treatment for medical problems.

A brief mental status examination needs to be conducted to assess the client's behavior, speech patterns, mood and affect, thought processes, and judgment and insight. Has the client recently experienced a crisis-producing situation? Is the client experiencing auditory or visual hallucinations? A physical examination must be performed to identify any concurrent medical condition or injury that may be compounding the problem.

It is important to communicate with the client in a calm, nonjudgmental, and accepting manner. Focusing the client on reality and explaining expected behaviors constitute part of the therapeutic communication process. In some cases, involuntary psychiatric hospitalization may be required. If the client is discharged from the ED, providing outside agency assistance and referral can be helpful.

DISASTER PLANNING/MASS CASUALTY INCIDENTS

After September 11, 2001 and subsequent national and international events, the U.S. health care system reassessed what constitutes a disaster and how to ensure an effective, unified response. Disasters are also referred to as mass casualty incidents (MCIs) and include such incidents as transportation crashes; forces of nature, such as hurricane, tornado, blizzard, earthquake, tsunami; or intentional events such as terrorist-related. As implied by the term, an MCI can suddenly overwhelm one department or hospital with a surge in clients.

Planning

The ED has typically been involved in both external (i.e., community) and internal (i.e., hospital) disaster planning. During a MCI, the ED serves as a central point for screening and the admission of critically ill or injured clients. They then institute a back-up plan to provide care to others. The entire hospital may be called into action to assist with providing care in the ED or expanding services throughout the institution. To help with emergency preparedness, the Centers for Disease Control and Prevention has developed a core set of competencies that include (1) understanding the necessary roles involved in responding to a disaster, (2) initiating and following the chain of command, and (3) activating the response plan. An ED nurse may help to coordinate responders and transfer clients; provide decontamination; deliver care for critically ill or injured clients admitted to ED; or be reassigned to other clinical areas that need additional nursing assistance.

Effective MCI care begins long before the first incident, and response agencies need a systematic approach to handling large numbers of clients. The United States Department of Homeland Security (USDHS) has worked with public health and acute care providers to develop the National Response Plan (NRP). This plan has several elements, including a standard incident management organizational structure, the National Incident Management System (NIMS), and an Incident Command Structure (ICS), that help individual agencies. In an MCI, an agency can divide their efforts into five functional areas—command, operations, planning, logistics, and finance/administration. The ICS structure can be used for any type of MCI that stresses an ED's ability to provide care, whether the incident is due to a sudden surge of clients from a one-time event or a more wide-spread incident.

All-Hazards Approach

The USDHS also encourages providers to plan for any type and level of MCI and to adopt an "all-hazards approach" to MCI care. The all-hazards approach encourages health care personnel to be aware of the potential for toxic exposure and to protect themselves before initiating care. Agencies involved in an MCI should provide different levels and types of personal protective equipment (PPE) for their staff. Depending on the suspected agents involved, PPE may range from changeable clothing; to protective eyewear and a mask; to full protective gear with self-contained air supply, gloves and boots, and impermeable coverall clothing. In some instances, health care providers may need to be pre-screened or eliminated from initial care if they are pregnant or cannot tolerate wearing PPE for a required time frame. EDs have created specific storage areas for PPE and provide orientation to help staff find what they should use for a given type of incident.

MCI Triage

During an MCI, the ED tends to be the portal through which injured clients are admitted to the hospital. The ED staff will be responsible for triage, decontamination for any suspected noxious substance (e.g., poisons, radiation), and isolation of any suspicious infectious cases. ED personnel may be the first to identify that a terrorist activity has occurred. For example, after a terrorist attack using biochemical weapons, clusters of otherwise healthy individuals may begin appearing at EDs requesting treatment for unknown illnesses (The Terrorism Alert feature above, right discusses staying alert for such patterns of illness.) These illnesses may be caused by the release of substances such as radiation, bacterial agents, toxic agents such as anthrax, nerve gas (see the Terrorism Alert feature on p. 2215 for details on sarin), or viral agents into the atmosphere, food supply, or other medium.

MCI triage is not the same as everyday triage in that clients are evaluated and categorized according to the institution's ability to provide care for the greatest number of victims. Instead of giving the most severely ill or injured person immediate and full attention, some clients receive no care and other lesser ill or injured clients may be sent away or asked to help care for others. The categories of MCI triage can be described as critical with a chance of survival, critical or close to death with minimal chance of survival, clients requiring hospital admission, clients with minor and treatable injuries, and clients with psychological injury. MCI triage allows the ED to rapidly determine which clients are to receive care.

TERRORISM ALERT

Being Alert to Patterns of Illness

All health care providers must remain alert for unusual illness patterns and clinical manifestations that might indicate an unusual infectious disease outbreak associated with intentional release of a biologic agent. The covert release of a biologic agent may not have an immediate impact because of the delay between exposure and illness onset, and outbreaks associated with intentional releases might closely resemble naturally occurring outbreaks. Indications of intentional release of a biologic agent include the following: (1) an unusual temporal or geographic clustering of illness (e.g., people who attended the same public event or gathering or development of a disease at an airport) or clients presenting with clinical manifestations that suggest an infectious disease outbreak (e.g., more than two clients presenting with an unexplained febrile illness associated with sepsis, pneumonia, respiratory failure, or rash or a botulism-like syndrome with flaccid muscle paralysis, especially if occurring in otherwise healthy people); (2) an unusual age distribution for common diseases (e.g., an increase in what appears to be a chickenpox-like illness among adults, but which might be smallpox); and (3) a large number of cases of acute flaccid paralysis with prominent bulbar palsies, suggestive of a release of *botulinum* toxin.

Clinical Manifestations

Each MCI disaster situation is unique in terms of the clients involved and the type of disaster that has occurred. Victims may have traumatic injuries, psychological manifestations, or a constellation of clinical manifestations indicating an exposure to a toxic substance.

Radiation Manifestations

The type and severity of clinical manifestations that clients demonstrate will be a direct result of the exposure to the blast itself and the type and dose of the thermal radiation. The effects may occur within hours of exposure or not appear until up to months afterward. Clinical manifestations of acute radiation exposure include nausea, diarrhea, malaise, development of immunocompromised infections, bleeding, shock, and death.

Chemical Agents

Nerve gas agents, such as sarin (see the Terrorism Alert feature on Sarin), enter the body via inhalation, skin contact, or ingestion. Depending on the route of exposure, clinical manifestations may begin to appear as soon as 20 to 30 minutes after exposure. These include respiratory arrest resulting from muscle paralysis, excessive salivation, diaphoresis, dyspnea, vomiting, incontinence, muscle weakness, and miosis.

TERRORISM ALERT

Sarin

Sarin is one of the dangerous chemical weapons called nerve agents or nerve gases that have dominated chemical warfare since World War II. These gases are the most toxic and rapidly acting of the known chemical warfare agents. Sarin, a colorless and odorless gas, has a lethal dose of 0.5 mg for an adult and is 26 times more deadly than cyanide gas and 20 times more lethal than potassium cyanide. Just 0.01 mg/kg can kill a human. The vapor is slightly heavier than air, so it hovers close to the ground when released. Under cool, wet, and humid weather conditions, sarin degrades swiftly, but as the temperature increases, the lethal duration of the chemical increases despite high levels of humidity. Food and water may also be contaminated with sarin.

Nerve agents (e.g., sarin, tabun, soman, and VX) are potent acetylcholinesterase inhibitors. These agents alter cholinergic synaptic transmission at neuroeffector junctions (muscarinic effects), at skeletal myoneural junctions and autonomic ganglia (nicotinic effects), and in the central nervous system.

EXPOSURE

Following sarin gas release into air, people can be exposed through skin or eye contact or by breathing air that contains sarin. Small containers of sarin gas or liquid can be easily carried and released for an immediate, short-lived attack. Sarin mixes easily with water and can be used to poison water or food. Touching or drinking water that contains sarin or eating food contaminated with sarin may cause clinical manifestations such as those seen with sarin gas exposure.

PROTECTION

Chemical warfare suits that include body (skin and eye) and respiratory (mask) protection are available but are very hot when worn and are rarely available outside military or emergency rescue situations.

If exposure occurs without protection, people should leave the area where sarin was released and get into fresh air immediately, remove clothing, rapidly wash the entire body with soap and water, rinse eyes with plain water, and seek medical attention immediately. Contaminated clothing must be disposed of carefully with placement in plastic bags. Sarin is easily decontaminated with basic solutions.

CLINICAL MANIFESTATIONS

Exposure to large doses of sarin by any route results in loss of consciousness, convulsions, paralysis, and respiratory failure leading to death within seconds and minutes of the exposure if treatment is not initiated immediately. Other clinical manifestations are described below.

Exposure to small doses results in the following clinical manifestations within seconds to hours of exposure:

Muscarinic Effects

- Small, pinpoint pupils
- Blurred vision and eye pain
- Hypersecretion of salivary (drooling), lacrimal (watery eyes), sweat (diaphoresis), and bronchial (coughing) glands
- Runny nose
- Nausea and vomiting
- Diarrhea and abdominal cramps
- Urinary and fecal incontinence
- Slow heart rate

Nicotinic Effects

- Skeletal muscle twitching and weakness
- Convulsions
- Rapid heart rate and high blood pressure (which can mask muscarinic effects)

TREATMENT

Treatment consists of removing sarin from the body as soon as possible and providing supportive medical care. Emergency respondents must be trained and appropriately attired (skin and respiratory protection) before treating clients. Before transport to a hospital, all casualties must be decontaminated (clothing, skin, eyes). A patent airway must be ensured and antidotes, such as 2 mg of atropine IM and 600 mg of pralidoxime chloride (2-PAM Cl) IV, should be administered as soon as possible. These antidotes may be repeated at 5- to 10-minute intervals during transport and upon arrival to an ED. Emesis should not be induced if the client is alert and able to swallow a slurry of activated charcoal. Diazepam may be required to control convulsions. ALS guidelines are followed for clients with cardiac dysrhythmias or hypotension.

Data from CDC Fact Sheet on Chemical Emergencies, Department of Health and Human Services, Centers for Disease Control and Prevention. Retrieved 11/20/07 from www.bt.cdc.gov/agent/sarin/basics/facts.asp.

OUTCOME MANAGEMENT

Depending on the agent used to expose the population, client decontamination may or may not be required. If decontamination is necessary, specialized rooms and equipment must be used to prevent the spread of the agent to other clients or health care workers.

Managing a terrorist incident involves being able to recognize its occurrence and reacting quickly. In the effort to detect the occurrence of possible terrorist activities, emergency nurses must use epidemiologic clues to identify biochemical incidents, such as identifying (1) small or large outbreaks of a disease, (2) an increase in deaths of hospitalized clients within 72 hours of admission, (3) clusters of clients from a single location with the same illness, (4) childhood diseases in adults, (5) healthy people dying of flu, (6) unexplained blood disorders, and (7) unusual increases in complaints of fever, pulmonary, or gastrointestinal manifestations.

CONCLUSIONS

Providing care to clients in the ED setting can be challenging and rewarding. An understanding of the principles of emergency care is the cornerstone of the specialty of emergency nursing. Most clients present to the ED without a working diagnosis but only a cadre of clinical manifestations. Therefore assessing each client using an organized approach is paramount for the ED nurse in order to be able to establish care priorities and institute appropriate interventions. The nursing process from assessment to evaluation is continually used. The scope of ED nursing is constantly changing and expanding beyond the hospital walls into the areas of community practice and community education.

THINKING CRITICALLY

1. A 23-year-old man walks into the emergency department. He tells you that he was in a motor vehicle accident about 4 hours ago. The police were at the scene, but he refused to be transported to the emergency department because he felt fine; he went home. At home, however, the client started to experience worsening shoulder and posterior neck pain. His mother urged him to come to the emergency department. He tells you that he has "numbness" in his fingers and a "tingling" feeling in his right elbow. If you were the triage nurse, what potential problems would you consider that this client might have? Would you classify the client as emergent, urgent, or non-urgent? What measures should you take to ensure the client's safety?

Factors to Consider. What injuries sustained in a motor vehicle accident might account for the client's clinical manifestations?

2. A 35-year-old man is brought into the emergency department by the city police, who were arresting him for drunk and disorderly conduct. He had been involved in a barroom brawl, during which he acquired several small lacerations about the face and arms from broken glass, a hit to the head, and kicks to his ribs. He is conscious, verbally abusive, and threatening to fight his way out of the emergency department because he wants "to go home and be left alone." He has twice threatened you with bodily harm if you persist in preventing him from leaving. How would you proceed with this case?

Factors to Consider. Whom should you call? Would it be appropriate to sedate this client? What should you do if the client actually harms you physically?

3. A 60-year-old man has arrived at the emergency department with a complaint of headache. He states that he never had headaches until about 2 weeks ago, when he began awakening in the mornings with head pain. The headache would go away each day after he had been up and around for a few hours and had taken aspirin. In the last few days, however, neither aspirin nor acetaminophen has helped, and the headache has become nearly continuous. His wife states that his speech and balance have been "off" a little.

He wonders whether there can be any connection between his headaches and a recent fall or a recent elevation in blood pressure. Describe how you would proceed with an evaluation of this client. What further information should you elicit from him? What is your assessment priority? What triage classification would be best for this client? What interventions should you anticipate?

Factors to Consider. What diagnostic assessments should you anticipate? What should you include in your physical examination and nursing history?

4. The client, a 70-year-old man, has been brought to the emergency department by ambulance. His wife states that he has become increasingly confused over the past few months. Within the past few days, he has become worse, is difficult to awaken in the morning, and is "sleepy" all day. This situation progressed until today, when the client's wife could not keep him awake at all; she called an ambulance and had him brought in. The client has a long history of hypertension, coronary artery disease, diabetes mellitus, and depression. Ambulance records show evidence that the client is difficult to arouse, but upon aggressive stimulation, he "wakes up" and can follow basic commands. His vital signs are stable, but his pulse rate is slow and irregular. Blood pressure is lower than his "norm." His wife has brought his medications with her in a large paper bag. What is your priority assessment? What should you include in your physical assessment? What interventions should you anticipate?

Factors to Consider. What body systems should you assess? What diagnostic studies should you anticipate?

Discussions for these questions can be found on the website. **evolve**

BIBLIOGRAPHY

Citations appearing in red refer to primary research.

Citations appearing in blue refer to evidence-based practice guidelines and protocols.

1. Agency for Healthcare Research, National Guideline Clearinghouse. (2003). *Use of physical restraints in the acute care setting.* Retrieved 10/09/06 from www.guideline.gov/summary/summary.aspx?ss=15&doc_id=3515&nbr=2741.
2. Agency for Healthcare Research, National Guideline Clearinghouse. (2006). *Assessment and management of acute pain.* Retrieved 10/09/06 from www.guidelines.gov/summary/summary.aspx?doc_id=9009&nbr=004884&string=pain.
3. Albers, G.W., Amarenco, P., Easton, J.D., et al. (2004). Antithrombotic and thrombolytic therapy for ischemic stroke: The Seventh ACCP Conference on Antithrombotic and Thrombolytic Therapy. *Chest*, 126(3 Suppl), 483S-512S.
4. American Academy of Emergency Medicine. (n.d.). EMTALA. Retrieved 10/09/06 from www.aaem.org/emtala/index.shtml.
5. American Heart Association, ECC Committee, Subcommittees and Task Forces of the American Heart Association. (2005a). 2005 American Heart Association Guidelines for Cardiopulmonary Resuscitation and Emergency Cardiovascular Care. Part 7.1. Adjuncts for airway control and ventilation. *Circulation*, 112(24 Suppl), IV 51-IV 57.
6. American Heart Association, ECC Committee, Subcommittees and Task Forces of the American Heart Association. (2005b). 2005 American Heart Association Guidelines for Cardiopulmonary Resuscitation and Emergency Cardiovascular Care. Part 11: Pediatric Basic Life Support. *Circulation*, 112(Suppl I), IV-156-IV-166.

7. Antman, E.M., Anbe, D.T., Armstrong, P.W., et al. (2004). ACC/AHA guidelines for the management of patients with ST-elevation myocardial infarction—Executive summary: A report of the American College of Cardiology/American Heart Association Task Force on Practice Guidelines (Writing Committee to Revise the 1999 Guidelines for the Management of Patients With Acute Myocardial Infarction). *Circulation, 110*, 588-636.

8. Bracken, M.B. (2006). Steroids for acute spinal cord injury. *The Cochrane Database of Systematic Reviews*, Issue 3. Available from www.cochrane.org/reviews/en/ab001046.html.

9. Bridges, N., & Jarquin-Valdivia, A.A. (2005). Use of the Trendelenburg position as the resuscitation position: To T or not to T? *American Journal of Critical Care, 14*, 364-368.

10. Broder, K.R., Cortese, M.M., Iskander, J.K., et al. (2006). Preventing tetanus, diphtheria, and pertussis among adolescents: Use of tetanus toxoid, reduced diphtheria toxoid, and acellular pertussis vaccines: Recommendations of the Advisory Committee on Immunization Practices (ACIP). *MMWR, 55*(RR03), 1-34.

11. Buller, H.R., Agnelli, G., Hull, R.D., et al. (2004). Antithrombotic therapy for venous thromboembolic disease: The seventh ACCP conference on antithrombotic and thrombolytic therapy. *Chest, 126*(3 Suppl), 401S-428S.

12. Centers for Disease Control and Prevention. (1999). Human Rabies Prevention—United States, 1999. Recommendations of the Advisory Committee on Immunization Practices (ACIP). *MMWR, 48* (RR-1), 1-21.

13. Emergency Nurses Association. (2006a). *ENA history*. Retrieved 10/09/06 from www.ena.org/about/history.

14. Emergency Nurses Association. (2006b). *Violence in the emergency setting* (Position Statement). Retrieved 10/09/06 from www.ena.org/about/position.

15. Epifanio, P. (2000). Ocular emergencies. In K. Jordan (Ed.), *Emergency nursing core curriculum* (5th ed.). Philadelphia: Saunders.

16. Evans, M.M. (2003). Maintaining the chain of custody: Evidence handling in forensic-cases. *AORN Journal, 78*, 563-564, 566-567, 569.

17. Gebbie, K., & Qureshi, K. (2002). Emergency and disaster preparedness: Core competencies for nurses. *American Journal of Nursing, 102*, 46-51.

18. Gilboy, N., Tanabe, P., Travers, D.A., et al.. (2005). *Emergency Severity Index, Version 4: Implementation handbook* (AHRQ Pub No. 05-0046-2). Rockville, Md: Agency for Healthcare Research and Quality. Retrieved 10/09/06 from www.ahrq.gov/research/esi.

19. Heart Failure Society of America. (2006). HFSA 2006 Comprehensive Heart Failure Practice Guideline. *Journal of Cardiac Failure, 12*, e1-2.

20. Intracorp. (2005). Concussion, mild head injury. Retrieved 10/09/06 from www.guideline.gov/summary/summary.aspx?doc_id=7449&nbr=004395&string=concussion.

21. Killian, M. (Ed.) (1999). *Standards for emergency nursing practice* (4th ed.).Park Ridge, Ill: Emergency Nurses Association.

22. McCaig, L.F., & Nawar, E.W. (2006). National hospital ambulatory medical care survey: 2004 emergency department summary. *Advance Data for Vital and Health Statistics*. No. 372. Retrieved 10/09/06 from www.cdc.gov/nchs/data/ad/ad372.pdf.

23. National Heart, Lung, and Blood Institute (NHLBI), NAEPP Expert Panel Report. (2002). *Guidelines for the diagnosis and management of asthma—Update on selected topics 2002*. NIH Pub No. 02-5075.

24. National Institutes of Health. (2002). *Management of Hepatitis C: 2002*. Retrieved 10/09/06 from https://consensus.nih.gov/2002/2002HepatitisC2002116html.htm.

25. Schwartz, B., Weniger, B.G., Iskander, J.K., et al. (2002). General recommendations on immunization. Recommendations of the Advisory Committee on Immunization Practices (ACIP) and the American Academy of Family Physicians (AAFP). *MMWR, 51* (RR02), 1-36.

25a. The Joint Commission. (2008). *2008. National Patient Safety Goals Hospital Program*. Available at www.jointcommission.org/PatientSafety/NationalPatientSafetygoals.

26. The Leapfrog Group. *Quality measures: Pneumonia*. Retrieved 10/09/06 from https://leapfrog.medstat.com/hrp/references/Pneum.htm.

27. Trauma.Org. (2005). *Glasgow Coma Scale*. Retrieved 10/09/06 from www.trauma.org/scores/gcs.html.

28. Trauma.Org. (2005). *Steroids for spinal cord injury*. Retrieved 10/09/06 from www.trauma.org/spine/steroids.html.

29. Tucker, J. (2003). *Toxicity, acetaminophen*. Retrieved 10/09/06 from www.emedicine.com/ped/topic7.htm.

30. United States Department of Health and Human Services (USDHHS), Centers for Disease Control and Prevention. (n.d.), *Public Health Emergency Response Guide for State, Local, and Tribal Public Health Directors*. Retrieved 10/09/06 from www.bt.cdc.gov/planning/responseguide.asp.

31. United States Department of Health and Human Services (USDHHS), Office of Civil Rights. (2006). *Medical privacy—National standards to protect the privacy of personal health information*. Retrieved 10/09/06 from www.hhs.gov/ocr/hipaa/.

32. United States Department of Homeland Security (USDHHS). (2004). *National incident management system*. Available from www.dhs.gov/dhspublic/interapp/press_release/press_release_0367.xml.

33. United States Department of Homeland Security (USDHHS). (2006). *National response plan*. Retrieved 10/09/06 from www.dhs.gov/dhspublic/interapp/editorial/editorial_0566.xml.

34. United States Department of Labor (USDL), Bureau of Labor Statistics. (n.d.). Census of fatal occupational injuries charts, 1992-2005. *Census of Fatal Occupational Injuries (CFOI)—Current and Revised Data*. Retrieved 10/09/06 from www.bls.gov/iif/oshcfoi1.htm#charts.

35. United States General Accounting Office (USGAO). (2001). *Emergency care. EMTALA implementation and enforcement issues*. GAO-01-747.

36. Veenema, T., & Karam, P. (2003). Emergency: Radiation. *American Journal of Nursing, 103*(5), 32-50.

37. Wuerz, R.C., Travers, D., Gilboy, N., et al. (2001). Implementation and refinement of the emergency severity index. *Academic Emergency Medicine, 8*, 170-176.

38. Wyman, C. (n.d.). Conscious sedation a self-study guide. Retrieved 10/09/06 from www.gasnet.org/protocols/sedation/.

evolve   *Did you remember to check out the bonus material on the Evolve website and the CD-ROM, including NCLEX®-Examination Style Review Questions, Open-Book Quizzes, and Chapter Review Audio Podcasts?*

http://evolve.elsevier.com/Black/medsurg

Index

NOTE: Page numbers followed by *f* indicate figures; those followed by *t* indicate tables; and those followed by *b* indicate boxed material.

Institute for Healthcare Improvement
5 Million Lives Campaign

Protecting 5 Million Lives From Harm

Some is Not A Number. Soon is Not A Time.

The 5 Million Lives Campaign challenges American hospitals to adopt 12 changes in care that save lives and reduce patient injuries:

The six interventions from the 100,000 Lives Campaign

- **Deploy Rapid Response Teams** ... at the first sign of patient decline

- **Deliver Reliable, Evidence-Based Care for Acute Myocardial Infarction** ... to prevent deaths from heart attack

- **Prevent Adverse Drug Events (ADEs)** ... by implementing medication reconciliation

- **Prevent Central Line Infections** ... by implementing a series of interdependent, scientifically grounded steps

- **Prevent Surgical Site Infections** ... by reliably delivering the correct perioperative antibiotics at the proper time

- **Prevent Ventilator-Associated Pneumonia** ... by implementing a series of interdependent, scientifically grounded steps

Six new interventions targeted at harm

- **Prevent Harm from High-Alert Medications** ... starting with a focus on anticoagulants, sedatives, narcotics, and insulin

- **Reduce Surgical Complications** ... by reliably implementing all of the changes in care recommended by SCIP, the Surgical Care Improvement Project (www.medqic.org/scip)

- **Prevent Pressure Ulcers** ... by reliably using science-based guidelines for their prevention

- **Reduce Methicillin-Resistant *Staphylococcus aureus* (MRSA) Infection** ... by reliably implementing scientifically proven infection-control practices

- **Deliver Reliable, Evidence-Based Care for Congestive Heart Failure** ... to avoid readmissions

- **Get Boards on Board** ... by defining and spreading the best-known leveraged processes for hospital Boards of Directors, so that they can become far more effective in accelerating organizational progress toward safe care

For more information about the campaign interventions, including how-to guides for each, see the Materials area of IHI.org at www.ihi.org/IHI/Programs/Campaign.

2008 Hospital and Critical Access Hospital National Patient Safety Goals

- Improve the accuracy of patient identification.
  - Use at least two patient identifiers when providing care, treatment, or services.

- Improve the effectiveness of communication among caregivers.
  - For verbal or telephone orders or for telephonic reporting of critical test results, verify the complete order or test result by having the person receiving the information record and "read back" the complete order or test result.
  - Standardize a list of abbreviations, acronyms, symbols, and dose designations that are not to be used throughout the organization (for an example from the Institute for Safe Medication Practices, see the inside front cover of this book).
  - Measure, assess, and take action, if appropriate, to improve the timeliness of reporting and the timeliness with which the responsible licensed caregiver receives critical test results and values.
  - Implement a standardized approach to "hand off" communications, including an opportunity to ask and respond to questions.

- Improve the safety of using medications.
  - Identify and, at a minimum, annually review a list of look-alike/sound-alike drugs used in the organization, and take action to prevent errors involving the interchange of these drugs.
  - Label all medications, medication containers (for example, syringes, medicine cups, basins), or other solutions on and off the sterile field.

- Reduce the likelihood of patient harm associated with the use of anticoagulation therapy.
  - Reduce the risk of health care–associated infections.
  - Comply with current World Health Organization (WHO) Hand Hygiene Guidelines (see the inside back cover of this book) or Centers for Disease Control and Prevention (CDC) Hand Hygiene Guidelines.
  - Manage as sentinel events all identified cases of unanticipated death or major permanent loss of function associated with a health care–associated infection.

- Accurately and completely reconcile medications across the continuum of care.
  - Establish a process for comparing the patient's current medications with those ordered for the patient while under the care of the organization.
  - Communicate a complete list of the patient's medications to the next provider of service when a patient is referred or transferred to another setting, service, practitioner, or level of care within or outside the organization. The complete list of medications is also provided to the patient on discharge from the facility.

- Reduce the risk of patient harm resulting from falls.
  - Implement a fall-reduction program, including an evaluation of the effectiveness of the program.

- Encourage patients' active involvement in their own care as a patient safety strategy.
  - Define and communicate the means for patients and their families to report concerns about safety and encourage them to do so.

- Identify safety risks inherent to the organization's patient population.
  - Identify patients at risk for suicide. (Applicable to psychiatric hospitals and patients being treated for emotional or behavioral disorders in general hospitals.)

- Improve recognition and response to changes in a patient's condition.
  - Select a suitable method that enables health care staff members throughout the organization to directly request additional assistance from a specially trained individual(s) when the patient's condition appears to be worsening.

The full text of the 2008 Goals and Requirements for all accreditation programs is posted on The Joint Commission website, www.jointcommission.org. Compliance with the requirements is a condition of continuing accreditation or certification for Joint Commission–accredited or certified organizations.